a LANGE medical book

CURRENT
Obstetric &
Gynecologic
Diagnosis &
Treatment

9th Edition

Alan H. DeCherney, MD
Professor, Department of Obstetrics & Gynecology,
David Geffen School of Medicine at UCLA,
Los Angeles, California

Lauren Nathan, MD
Associate Professor, Department of Obstetrics
& Gynecology, David Geffen School of Medicine
at UCLA, Los Angeles, California

Lange Medical Books/McGraw-Hill
Medical Publishing Division

New York   Chicago   San Francisco   Lisbon   London   Madrid
Mexico City   Milan   New Delhi   San Juan
Seoul   Singapore   Sydney   Toronto

Current Obstetric & Gynecologic Diagnosis & Treatment, Ninth Edition

1 2 3 4 5 6 7 8 9 0 DOC DOC 0 9 8 7 6 5 4 3 2

ISBN: 0-8385-1401-4

ISSN: 0197-582x

Notice

Medicine is an ever-changing science. As new research and clinical experience broaden our knowledge, changes in treatment and drug therapy are required. The authors and the publisher of this work have checked with sources believed to be reliable in their efforts to provide information that is complete and generally in accord with the standards accepted at the time of publication. However, in view of the possibility of human error or changes in medical sciences, neither the authors nor the publisher nor any other party who has been involved in the preparation or publication of this work warrants that the information contained herein is in every respect accurate or complete, and they disclaim all responsibility for any errors or omissions or for the results obtained from use of the information contained in this work. Readers are encouraged to confirm the information contained herein with other sources. For example and in particular, readers are advised to check the product information sheet included in the package of each drug they plan to administer to be certain that the information contained in this work is accurate and that changes have not been made in the recommended dose or in the contraindications for administration. This recommendation is of particular importance in connection with new or infrequently used drugs.

This book was set in Adobe Garamond by Pine Tree Composition.
The editors were Shelley Reinhardt, Harriet Lebowitz, and Karen G. Edmonson.
The production supervisor was Catherine H. Saggese.
The cover designer was Mary McKeon.
The text was designed by Eve Siegel.
RR Donnelley was printer and binder.

This book is printed on acid-free paper.

INTERNATIONAL EDITION ISBN 0-07-118207-1
Copyright © 2003. Exclusive rights by *The **McGraw-Hill** Companies, Inc.,* for manufacture and export.
This book cannot be re-exported from the country to which it is consigned by McGraw-Hill.
The International Edition is not available in North America.

SECTION III. PREGNANCY AT RISK

Contents

28. **Postpartum Hemorrhage & the Abnormal Puerperium** **531**
   Sarah B.H. Poggi, MD, & Peter S. Kapernick, MD, MPH

29. **Neonatal Resuscitation & Care of the Newborn at Risk** **553**
   Milena Weinstein, MD

SECTION IV. GENERAL GYNECOLOGY

30. **Gynecologic History, Examination, & Diagnostic Procedures** **573**
   Charles Kawada, MD

31. **Pediatric & Adolescent Gynecology** **595**
   Lisbeth Chang, MD, & David Muram, MD

32. **Complications of Menstruation; Abnormal Uterine Bleeding** **623**
   Taaly Silberstein, MD

33. **Contraception & Family Planning** **631**
   Michelle Grewal, MD, & Ronald T. Burkman, MD

34. **Benign Disorders of the Vulva & Vagina** **651**
   Tricia E. Markusen, MD, & David L. Barclay, MD

35. **Benign Disorders of the Uterine Cervix** **677**
   Edward Evantash, MD, Edward C. Hill, MD, & Martin L. Pernoll, MD

36. **Benign Disorders of the Uterine Corpus** **693**
   Sanaz Memarzadeh, MD, Michael S. Broder, MD, MSHS, Alvin S. Wexler, MD,
   & Martin L. Pernoll, MD

37. **Benign Disorders of the Ovaries & Oviducts** **708**
   Karen Purcell, MD, PhD, & James E. Wheeler, MD

38. **Sexually Transmitted Diseases & Pelvic Infections** **716**
   Steven W. Ainbinder, MD, & Susan M. Ramin, MD

39. **Antimicrobial Chemotherapy** **751**
   Ronald S. Gibbs, MD

40. **Endometriosis** **767**
   Sanaz Memarzadeh, MD, Kenneth N. Muse, Jr., MD, & Michael D. Fox, MD

41. **Relaxation of Pelvic Supports** **776**
   Christopher M. Tarnay, MD, & Clyde H. Dorr, II, MD, FACOG

42. **Urogynecology** **798**
   Christopher M. Tarnay, MD, & Narender N. Bhatia, MD

SECTION VII. CONTEMPORARY ISSUES

Authors

Steven W. Ainbinder, MD
Resident, Department of Obstetrics & Gynecology, David Geffen School of Medicine at UCLA, Los Angeles, California
Operative Delivery; Sexually Transmitted Diseases & Pelvic Infections

D. Ellene Andrew, MD
Chief Resident, Department of Obstetrics & Gynecology, Tufts University School of Medicine, & New England Medical Center, Boston, Massachusetts
Hirsutism

Dennis R. Anti, JD
Partner, Morrison, Mahoney & Miller, LLP, Springfield, Massachusetts
danti@mail.mm-m.com
The Borderland Between Law & Medicine

Carol L. Archie, MD
Associate Clinical Professor, Department of Obstetrics & Gynecology, David Geffen School of Medicine at UCLA, Los Angeles, California
carchie@mednet.ucla.edu
The Course & Conduct of Normal Labor & Delivery

Michael P. Aronson, MD, FACOG, FACS
Associate Professor & Director, Benign Gynecologic Services, Department of Obstetrics & Gynecology, University of Massachusetts Medical School, Worcester, Massachusetts
aronsonm@ummhc.org
Perioperative Considerations in Gynecology; Intraoperative & Postoperative Complications of Gynecologic Surgery

Vicki V. Baker, MD
Professor, Department of Obstetrics & Gynecology, Wayne State University School of Medicine, Detroit, Michigan; Karmanos Cancer Center, Detroit, Michigan
Premalignant & Malignant Disorders of the Ovaries and Oviducts

Harrison G. Ball, MD
Professor & Director, Division of Gynecology/Oncology, Department of Obstetrics & Gynecology, University of Massachusetts Medical School & UMASS Memorial Medical Center, Worcester, Massachusetts
ballh@ummhc.org
Radiation Therapy for Gynecologic Cancers

David L. Barclay, MD
Professor & Regional Chair, Department of Obstetrics & Gynecology; Director of Gynecologic Oncology, Texas Tech University Health Sciences Center, Amarillo
barclay@ama.ttuhsc.edu
Benign Disorders of the Vulva & Vagina; Premalignant & Malignant Disorders of the Vulva & Vagina

Joseph D. Bast, PhD
Professor, Department of Anatomy & Cell Biology, University of Kansas Medical Center, Kansas City
jbast@kumc.edu
Embryology of the Urogenital System & Congenital Anomalies of the Female Genital Tract

Narender N. Bhatia, MD
Professor, Department of Obstetrics & Gynecology; Chief, Urogynecology & Section of Gynecology, Harbor/University of California, Los Angeles Medical Center, David Geffen School of Medicine at UCLA, Los Angeles, California
nbhatia@obgyn.humc.edu
Urogynecology

Manoj K. Biswas, MD, FACOG, FRCOG
Associate Professor, Department of Obstetrics & Gynecology, Tulane Medical School, New Orleans, Louisiana
The Course & Conduct of Normal Labor & Delivery; Cardiac, Hematologic, Pulmonary, Renal & Urinary Tract Disorders in Pregnancy

Suzanne Bovone, MD
San Jose Good Samaritan Medical Group, Los Gatos
  Obstetrics & Gynecology Woman's Health Cen-
  ter, Los Gatos, California
Normal Pregnancy & Prenatal Care

Michael S. Broder, MD, MSHS
Assistant Professor, Department of Obstetrics & Gy-
  necology, David Geffen School of Medicine at
  UCLA, Los Angeles, California
mbroder@mednet.ucla.edu
Benign Disorders of the Uterine Corpus

Ronald T. Burkman, MD
Chair, Department of Obstetrics & Gynecology,
  Baystate Medical Center, Springfield, Massachu-
  setts
Contraception & Family Planning

Melissa Bush, MD
Maternal-Fetal Medicine Fellow, Department of
  Obstetrics, Gynecology, & Reproductive Sci-
  ence, Mt. Sinai Medical Center, New York,
  New York
melissa.bush@mssm.edu
Multiple Pregnancy

Mary M. Cadieux, MD
Clinical Professor, Department of Obstetrics & Gy-
  necology, University of Washington School of
  Medicine, Seattle, Washington
mcadieux@u.washington.edu
Approach to the Patient; Infertility

Lisbeth Chang, MD
Private Practice, Northridge Hospital, Northridge
  California
*Complications of Labor & Delivery; Pediatric & Ado-
  lescent Gynecology*

David Chelmow, MD, FACOG
Associate Professor, Department of Obstetrics &
  Gynecology, Tufts University School of Medi-
  cine, Tufts-New England Medical Center,
  Boston, Massachusetts
dchelmow@lifespan.org
*Intraoperative & Postoperative Complications of Gyne-
  cologic Surgery*

C.S. Claydon, MD
Fellow, Department of Obstetrics & Gynecology,
  University of Medicine & Dentistry of New Jer-
  sey, Robert Wood Johnson Medical School,
  Camden, New Jersey
Third-Trimester Vaginal Bleeding

Joseph V. Collea, MD
Professor, Department of Obstetrics & Gynecology;
  Director, Maternal-Fetal Medicine, Georgetown
  University School of Medicine, Washington, DC
Malpresentation & Cord Prolapse

Dipika Dandade, MD
Resident, Department of Obstetrics & Gynecology,
  David Geffen School of Medicine at UCLA, Los
  Angeles, California
*General Medical Disorders During Pregnancy; Thera-
  peutic Gynecologic Procedures*

Alan H. DeCherney, MD
Professor, Department of Obstetrics & Gynecology,
  David Geffen School of Medicine at UCLA, Los
  Angeles, California
adecherney@mednet.ucla.edu
In Vitro Fertilization & Related Techniques

Simie Degefu, MD
Associate Professor, Department of Obstetrics &
  Gynecology, Tulane University School of Medi-
  cine, New Orleans, Louisiana
Chemotherapy for Gynecologic Cancers

Oliver Dorigo, MD
Fellow, Division of Gynecologic Oncology, Depart-
  ment of Obstetrics & Gynecology, David Geffen
  School of Medicine at UCLA, Los Angeles,
  California
*Premalignant & Malignant Disorders of the Uterine
  Corpus; Premalignant & Malignant Disorders of
  the Ovaries & Oviducts; Chemotherapy for Gyneco-
  logic Cancers*

Clyde H. Dorr, II, MD, FACOG
Clinical Professor, Department of Obstetrics & Gyne-
  cology; Associate Chair for Pensacola, University of
  Florida College of Medicine, Gainesville, Florida
cdorr@sacred-heart.org
Relaxation of Pelvic Supports

Adelina M. Emmi, MD
Associate Professor, Department of Obstetrics &
    Gynecology, Reproductive Endocrine Section,
    Medical College of Georgia, Augusta
aemmi@mail.mcg.edu
Hirsutism

Niloofar Eskandari, MD
Staff Physician, Kaiser Permanente Medical Center,
    Baldwin Park, California
nilooesk@yahoo.com
Infertility

Edward Evantash, MD
Assistant Professor, Department of Obstetrics & Gy-
    necology, Tufts University School of Medicine,
    Tufts/New England Medical Center, Boston,
    Massachusetts
eevantash@lifespan.org
Benign Disorders of the Uterine Cervix

Michael D. Fox, MD
Assistant Professor, Department of Obstetrics & Gy-
    necology; Division Director, Reproductive En-
    docrinology, University of Florida College
    of Medicine; Shands Healthcare, Jacksonville,
    Florida
redfoxes@bellsouth.net
Endometriosis

Carol L. Gagliardi, MD
Associate Clinical Director, Department of Obstet-
    rics & Gynecology, Jersey City Medical Center,
    Jersey City, New Jersey
Hirsutism

William F. Ganong, MD
Jack & DeLoris Lange Professor of Physiology Emer-
    itus, University of California, San Francisco
wfganong@aol.com
Physiology of Reproduction in Women

Sara H. Garmel, MD
Staff Perinatologist, Division of Maternal-Fetal
    Medicine, Oakwood Hospital, Dearborn,
    Michigan
garmels@oakwood.org
Early Pregnancy Risks

Brendan P. Garry, MD
Staff Anesthesiologist, Department of Anesthesiol-
    ogy, Beth Israel Deaconess Medical Center,
    Boston, Massachusetts
bgarry@caregroup.harvard.edu
Perioperative Considerations in Gynecology

Ronald S. Gibbs, MD
E. Stewart Taylor Professor & Chair, Department of
    Obstetrics & Gynecology, University of Colorado
    School of Medicine, Denver
ronald.gibbs@uchsc.edu
Antimicrobial Chemotherapy

William L. Gill, MD, FAAP
Head, Section of Neonatology, Tulane Medical
    Center; Medical Director, Level III Regional
    NICU, Tulane Hospital for Children, New Or-
    leans, Louisiana
wgill@tulane.edu
Essentials of Normal Newborn Assessment & Care

Jonathan Gillen-Goldstein, MD
Assistant Clinical Professor, Division of Maternal-
    Fetal Medicine, Department of Obstetrics & Gy-
    necology, New York University School of Medi-
    cine, New York, New York; Director of Prenatal
    Diagnosis & Therapy, Madonna Perinatal Ser-
    vices, Mineola, New York
jggnyu@netscape.net
Methods of Assessment for Pregnancy at Risk

Annekathryn Goodman, MD
Associate Professor of Obstetrics, Gynecology, &
    Reproductive Biology, Harvard Medical School;
    Associate Director, Division of Gynecologic On-
    cology, The Gillette Center for Women's Can-
    cers, Massachusetts General Hospital, Boston,
    Massachusetts
agoodman@partners.org
*Premalignant & Malignant Disorders of the Uterine
    Corpus*

Robert A. Graebe, MD
Director, Division of Reproductive Endocrinol-
    ogy, Department of Obstetrics & Gynecology,
    Monmouth Medical Center, Shrewsbury,
    New Jersey
sherwood81@aol.com
The Role of Imaging Techniques in Gynecology

Jeffrey S. Greenspoon, MD
Associate Professor of Clinical Obstetrics & Gynecology, Department of Obstetrics & Gynecology, David Geffen School of Medicine at UCLA, Los Angeles, California
Diabetes Mellitus & Pregnancy

Michelle Grewal, MD
Private Practice, Greensboro, North Carolina
Cardiac, Hematologic, Pulmonary, Renal & Urinary Tract Disorders in Pregnancy; Contraception & Family Planning

M.K. Guess, MD
Fellow, Division of Urogynecology & Reconstructive Surgery, Albert Einstein College of Medicine, Montefiore Medical Center, Bronx, New York
mguess@montefiore.org
Hirsutism

Alexandra Haessler, MD
Resident Physician, Department of Obstetrics & Gynecology, David Geffen School of Medicine at UCLA, Los Angeles, California
ubergyn@hotmail.com
Psychological Aspects of Obstetrics & Gynecology

Vivian P. Halfin, MD
Associate Clinical Professor of Psychiatry & of Obstetrics & Gynecology, Tufts University School of Medicine; Psychiatric Consultant, Department of Obstetrics & Gynecology, Tufts/New England Medical Center, Boston, Massachusetts
Domestic Violence & Sexual Assault

Kathleen F. Harney, MD
Assistant Professor, Department of Obstetrics & Gynecology, Tufts/New England Medical Center, Boston, Massachusetts; Acting Chief, Department of Obstetrics & Gynecology, Cambridge Hospital, Cambridge, Massachusetts
kharney@challiance.org
The Breast

Eduardo A. Herrera, MD
Vice-Chairman & Associate Professor, Department of Obstetrics & Gynecology, Tulane Medical School, New Orleans, Louisiana
eherrer@tulane.edu
Complications of Labor & Delivery

Darla B. Hess, MD, FACC, FAHA
Lehigh Valley Cardiology Group, Bethlehem, Pennsylvania
darlahess@aol.com
General Medical Disorders During Pregnancy

L. Wayne Hess, MD
Professor of Obstetrics & Gynecology, Pennsylvania State University School of Medicine, Hershey, Pennsylvania; Chairman, Obstetrics & Gynecology, Lehigh Valley Hospital & Health Network, Allentown, Pennsylvania
l_wayne.hess@lvh.com
General Medical Disorders During Pregnancy

Edward C. Hill, MD
Professor Emeritus, Department of Obstetrics, Gynecology, & Reproductive Sciences, University of California, San Francisco
Benign Disorders of the Uterine Cervix

Despina E. Hoffman, BA
Research Assistant, Division of Maternal-Fetal Medicine, Department of Obstetrics & Gynecology, Baystate Medical Center, Springfield, Massachusetts
despina.hoffman@bhs.org
The Borderland Between Law & Medicine

Christine H. Holschneider, MD
Clinical Instructor, Division of Gynecologic Oncology, Department of Obstetrics & Gynecology, David Geffen School of Medicine at UCLA, Los Angeles, California
Surgical Diseases & Disorders in Pregnancy; Premalignant & Malignant Disorders of the Uterine Cervix

Michelle Hugin, MD
Attending Staff Physician, Department of Obstetrics & Gynecology, Santa Clara Valley Medical Center, San Jose, California
hugin.michele@hhs.co.santa-clara.ca.us
Approach to the Patient

Carla Janzen, MD
Clinical Instructor, Department of Obstetrics & Gynecology, David Geffen School of Medicine at UCLA, Los Angeles, California Medical Center
shmonica@yahoo.com
Essentials of Normal Newborn Assessment & Care; Diabetes Mellitus & Pregnancy

Julie Jolin, MD
Resident Physician, Department of Obstetrics & Gynecology, Johns Hopkins University School of Medicine, Baltimore, Maryland
jjolin@ucla.edu
Radiation Therapy for Gynecologic Cancers

Norma L. Jones, MD
Attending Physician, Pomona Valley Hospital Center, Pomona, California, & San Antonio Community Hospital, Upland, California
Menopause & Postmenopause

Theodore B. Jones, MD
Associate Professor of Obstetrics & Gynecology; Associate Chair for Education; Residency Program Director, Wayne State University School of Medicine, Detroit, Michigan
thjones@med.wayne.edu
Methods of Assessment for Pregnancy at Risk

Howard L. Judd, MD
Professor & Chairman, Department of Obstetrics & Gynecology, Olive View/UCLA Medical Center, Sylmar, California
Menopause & Postmenopause

Charles Kawada, MD
Clinical Assistant Professor, Department of Obstetrics & Gynecology, Harvard Medical School, Boston, Massachusetts; Chairman, Department of Obstetrics & Gynecology, Mt. Auburn Hospital, Cambridge, Massachusetts
ckawada@caregroup.harvard.edu
Gynecologic History, Examination, & Diagnostic Procedures

Peter S. Kapernick, MD, MPH
Fort Myers, Florida
pkaper19@earthlink.net
Postpartum Hemorrhage & the Normal Puerperium

Karen Kish, MD
Resident, Department of Obstetrics & Gynecology, David Geffen School of Medicine at UCLA, Los Angeles, California
kkishca@yahoo.com
Malpresentation & Cord Prolapse

Robert A. Knuppel, MD, MPH
Professor & Chair, Department of Obstetrics, Gynecology, & Reproductive Sciences, Robert Wood Johnson Medical School & St. Peter's University Hospital, New Brunswick, New Jersey
knuppero@rwja.umdnj.edu
Maternal-Placental-Fetal Unit; Fetal & Early Neonatal Physiology

Brian J. Koos, MD, DPhil
Professor, Department of Obstetrics & Gynecology, David Geffen School of Medicine at UCLA, Los Angeles, California
bkoos@mednet.ucla.edu
Maternal Physiology During Pregnancy

Kermit E. Krantz, MD, LittD
University Distinguished Professor; Professor of Gynecology & Obstetrics; Professor of Anatomy Emeritus, University of Kansas School of Medicine, Kansas City
Anatomy of the Female Patient

Donelle Laughlin, MD
Private Practice, San Luis Obispo, California
Genetic Disorders & Sex Chromosome Abnormalities; Maternal-Placental-Fetal Unit; Fetal & Early Neonatal Physiology; Amenorrhea

Sondra B. Lee, MD
Resident, Department of Obstetrics & Gynecology, David Geffen School of Medicine at UCLA, Los Angeles, California
Intraoperative & Postoperative Complications of Gynecologic Surgery

Kim Lipscomb, MD
Associate Clinical Professor, Department of Obstetrics & Gynecology, David Geffen School of Medicine at UCLA, Los Angeles, California; Division Chief, Maternal-Fetal Medicine, Department of Obstetrics & Gynecology, Olive View/UCLA Medical Center, Sylmar, California
klipscomb@dhs.co.la.ca.us
The Normal Puerperium

Jessica S. Lu, MPH
Senior Research Associate, Department of Community Health Sciences, School of Public Health, University of California, Los Angeles
Domestic Violence & Sexual Assault

Michael C. Lu, MD, MPH
Assistant Professor, Department of Obstetrics & Gynecology, David Geffen School of Medicine at UCLA, Los Angeles, California; Assistant Professor, Department of Community Health Sciences, School of Public Health, University of California, Los Angeles
mclu@ucla.edu
Domestic Violence & Sexual Assault

William C. Mabie, MD
Professor of Clinical Obstetrics & Gynecology, University of South Carolina School of Medicine, Greenville, South Carolina
bmabie@ghs.org
Hypertensive States of Pregnancy

L. Russell Malinak, MD
Professor Emeritus, Department of Obstetrics & Gynecology, Baylor College of Medicine, Houston, Texas
Therapeutic Gynecologic Procedures

Catherine Marin, MD
Fellow, Division of Reproductive Endocrinology & Infertility, David Geffen School of Medicine at UCLA, Los Angeles, California
cmarin@ucla.edu
Embryology of the Urogenital System & Congenital Anomalies of the Female Genital Tract; In Vitro Fertilization & Related Techniques

Tricia E. Markusen, MD
On-Staff, Community Hospital of the Monterey Peninsula, Department of Obstetrics & Gynecology, Monterey, California
Benign Disorders of the Vulva & Vagina; Gestational Trophoblastic Diseases

John S. McDonald, MD
Professor of Anesthesiology & Obstetrics & Gynecology, David Geffen School of Medicine at UCLA, Los Angeles, California; Chairman, Department of Anesthesiology, Los Angeles County Harbor/ UCLA Medical Center, Torrance, California
jsm5525@aol.com
Obstetric Analgesia & Anesthesia

Sanaz Memarzadeh, MD
Fellow, Division of Gynecologic Oncology, Department of Obstetrics & Gynecology, David Geffen School of Medicine at UCLA, Los Angeles, California
Benign Disorders of the Uterine Corpus; Endometriosis; Premalignant & Malignant Disorders of the Vulva & Vagina

Pamela J. Moore, PhD
Associate Professor Emeritus, Department of Obstetrics & Gynecology, Tulane University School of Medicine, New Orleans, Louisiana
Maternal Physiology During Pregnancy

John C. Morrison, MD
Professor of Obstetrics & Gynecology & Pediatrics, The University Hospital & Clinics, University of Mississippi Medical Center, Jackson
jmorrison@ob-gyn.umsmed.edu
General Medical Disorders During Pregnancy

David Muram, MD
Professor Emeritus, Department of Obstetrics & Gynecology, College of Medicine, University of Tennessee, Memphis, Tennessee; Senior Chemical Research Physician, Eli Lilly & Company, Indianapolis, Indiana
dmuram@lilly.com
Pediatric & Adolescent Gynecology

Kenneth N. Muse, Jr., MD
Associate Professor, Department of Obstetrics & Gynecology, College of Medicine, University of Kentucky, Lexington, Kentucky
ken_muse@hotmail.com
Endometriosis

Mikio Nihira, MD, MPH
Assistant Professor, Department of Obstetrics & Gynecology, Division of Urogynecology & Reconstructive Pelvic Surgery, University of Texas Southwestern Medical Center at Dallas
mikio.nihira@utsouthwestern.edu
Perioperative Considerations in Gynecology

Miles J. Novy, MD
Senior Scientist, Oregon National Primate Research Center/Oregon Health & Sciences University, Beaverton, Oregon; Professor, Department of Obstetrics & Gynecology, School of Medicine, Oregon Health & Sciences University, Portland, Oregon
gibbinsc@ohsu.edu
The Normal Puerperium

John Patrick O'Grady, MD
Professor, Department of Obstetrics & Gynecology, Tufts University School of Medicine; Director, Obstetrical Services, Wesson Women's & Infant Unit, Baystate Medical Center, Springfield, Massachusetts
patrick.ogrady@bhs.org
The Borderland Between Law & Medicine

April Gale O'Quinn, MD
Chairman & Maxwell E. Lapham Professor, Department of Obstetrics & Gynecology, Tulane University School of Medicine, New Orleans, Louisiana
aoquinn@tulane.edu
Gestational Trophoblastic Diseases; Chemotherapy for Gynecologic Cancers

Michael J. Paidas, MD
Assistant Professor, Department of Obstetrics & Gynecology, New York University School of Medicine, New York, New York
mpaidas@aol.com
Methods of Assessment for Pregnancy at Risk

Sue M. Palmer, MD
Private Practice, Maternal-Fetal Medicine, Houston, Texas
spalmer@suempalmer.com
Diabetes Mellitus & Pregnancy

Alan S. Penzias, MD
Assistant Professor of Obstetrics, Gynecology & Reproductive Biology, Harvard Medical School, Boston, Massachusetts; Surgical Director, Boston IVF, Waltham, Massachusetts
alan.Penzias@bostonivf.com
In Vitro Fertilization & Related Techniques

Dorothee Perloff, MD
Clinical Professor Emeritus, Department of Medicine, University of California, San Francisco
Cardiac, Hematologic, Pulmonary, Renal & Urinary Tract Disorders in Pregnancy

Martin L. Pernoll, MD
Formerly: Head, Division of Perinatology, University of Oregon Health & Sciences University School of Medicine, Portland, Oregon; Chair, Department of Obstetrics & Gynecology, Tulane University School of Medicine, New Orleans, Louisiana; Executive Dean, Kansas University School of Medicine, Kansas City, Kansas
mpernoll@att.net
Normal Pregnancy & Prenatal Care; Methods of Assessment for Pregnancy at Risk; Late Pregnancy Complications; Multiple Pregnancy; Third-Trimester Vaginal Bleeding; Complications of Labor & Delivery; Benign Disorders of the Uterine Cervix; Benign Disorders of the Uterine Corpus

Matthew M. Poggi, MD
Clinical Fellow, Radiation Oncology Branch, National Cancer Institute, Bethesda, Maryland
mpoggi@usuhs.mil
The Breast

Sarah B.H. Poggi, MD
Fellow & Lecturer, Division of Maternal-Fetal Medicine, Department of Obstetrics & Gynecology, Georgetown University Hospital, Bethesda, Maryland
Postpartum Hemorrhage & the Normal Puerperium

Ana Polo, MD
Attending Staff, Department of Obstetrics & Gynecology, Vall d'Hebron Hospital, University of Barcelona, Spain
Complications of Labor & Delivery

Karen Purcell, MD, PhD
Resident, Department of Obstetrics & Gynecology, David Geffen School of Medicine at UCLA, Los Angeles, California
Benign Disorders of the Ovaries & Oviducts

Jeannine Rahimian, MD, MBA
Resident, Department of Obstetrics & Gynecology, David Geffen School of Medicine at UCLA, Los Angeles, California
jrahimi@ucla.edu
Disproportionate Fetal Growth

Susan M. Ramin, MD
Associate Professor, Department of Obstetrics, Gynecology, & Reproductive Sciences; Director, Division of Maternal-Fetal Medicine, University of Texas at Houston Medical School, Houston, Texas
susan.m.ramin@uth.tmc.edu
Sexually Transmitted Diseases & Pelvic Infections

Courtney Reynolds, MD
Today's Women's Health Specialists, Chandler, Arizona
carucla@yahoo.com
Hypertensive States of Pregnancy

Ashley S. Roman, MD, MPH
Fellow, Division of Maternal-Fetal Medicine, Department of Obstetrics & Gynecology, New York University, New York, New York
achapinsmith@aol.com
Late Pregnancy Complications

Miriam B. Rosenthal, MD
Associate Professor of Psychiatry & Reproductive Biology, Case Western Reserve University; Chief of Behavioral Medicine, Department of Obstetrics & Gynecology, University MacDonald Women's Hospital, Cleveland, Ohio
miriam.rosenthal@uhhs.com
msr19@juno.com
Psychological Aspects of Obstetrics & Gynecology

Wendy A. Satmary, MD
Assistant Clinical Faculty, Department of Obstetrics & Gynecology, David Geffen School of Medicine at UCLA, Los Angeles, California
Premalignant & Malignant Disorders of the Vulva & Vagina

Baha M. Sibai, MD
Professor & Chairman, Department of Obstetrics & Gynecology, University of Cincinnati College of Medicine, Cincinnati, Ohio
baha.sibai@uc.edu
Hypertensive States of Pregnancy

Taaly Silberstein, MD
Staff Physician, Encino Tarzana Regional Medical Center, Tarzana, California
Complications of Menstruation; Abnormal Uterine Bleeding

Donna M. Smith, MD
Associate Professor, Department of Obstetrics & Gynecology, Division of Gynecologic Oncology, Loyola University Medical Center, Maywood, Illinois
Premalignant & Malignant Disorders of the Vulva & Vagina

Ramada S. Smith, MD
Division of Maternal-Fetal Medicine, Virginia Hospital Center, Arlington, Virginia
Critical Care Obstetrics

Robert J. Sokol, MD
Distinguished Professor of Obstetrics & Gynecology, Wayne State University School of Medicine, Detroit, Michigan; Director, C.S. Mott Center for Human Growth & Development; Former Obstetrician & Gynecologist-in-Chief, The Detroit Medical Center, Detroit, Michigan
rsokol@moose.med.wayne.edu
Methods of Assessment for Pregnancy at Risk

Christopher M. Tarnay, MD
Assistant Clinical Professor, Department of Obstetrics & Gynecology, David Geffen School of Medicine at UCLA, Los Angeles, California; Division of Urogynecology & Reconstructive Pelvic Surgery, Kaiser Permanente Medical Center, Woodland Hills, California
christopher.m.tarnay@kp.org
Relaxation of Pelvic Supports; Urogynecology

Ian H. Thorneycroft, MD, PhD
Professor, Department of Obstetrics & Gynecology, University of South Alabama College of Medicine, Mobile, Alabama
ithorney@aol.com
Amenorrhea; In Vitro Fertilization & Related Techniques

Michael W. Varner, MD
Professor, Department of Obstetrics & Gynecology, Division of Maternal-Fetal Medicine, University of Utah School of Medicine, Salt Lake City, Utah
mvarner@hsc.utah.edu
Disproportionate Fetal Growth

Milena Weinstein, MD
Resident, Department of Obstetrics & Gynecology, David Geffen School of Medicine at UCLA, Los Angeles, California
Neonatal Resuscitation & Care of the Newborn at Risk

Johanna Weiss, MD
Clinical Instructor, Department of Obstetrics & Gynecology, Joan & Sanford I. Weill Medical College, Cornell University, New York, New York
johannaweiss@hotmail.com
Critical Care Obstetrics

Alvin S. Wexler, MD
Associate Professor, Department of Obstetrics & Gynecology, Baylor College of Medicine, Houston, Texas
mpwexler98@aol.com
Benign Disorders of the Uterine Corpus

James E. Wheeler, MD
Professor Emeritus, Department of Pathology & Laboratory Medicine, University of Pennsylvania School of Medicine, Philadelphia, Pennsylvania; Staff Emeritus, Division of Anatomic Pathology, Hospital of the University of Pennsylvania, Philadelphia, Pennsylvania
jewheele@mail.med.upenn.edu
Benign Disorders of the Ovaries & Oviducts

James M. Wheeler, MD, MPH
The Center for Women's Health Care, Houston, Texas
Therapeutic Gynecologic Procedures

Ralph W. Yarnell, MD, FRCPC
Associate Professor, Department of Anesthesiology, Tufts University School of Medicine, Boston, Massachusetts; Director, Obstetric Anesthesia, Tufts-New England Medical Center, Boston, Massachusetts
ryarnell @lifespan.org
Obstetric Analgesia & Anesthesia

Preface

INTRODUCTION

Current Obstetric & Gynecologic Diagnosis & Treatment, 9th edition is a single-source reference for practitioners in both inpatient and outpatient settings. It focuses on the practical aspects of clinical diagnosis and patient management.

OUTSTANDING FEATURES

- Thorough review of all of obstetrics and gynecology
- Medical advances up to time of publication
- More than 1,000 diseases and disorders
- Emphasis on disease prevention and evidence-based medicine
- Covers underlying pathophysiology when relevant to diagnosis and treatment
- Concise format facilitates quick access
- Illustrated with more than 500 anatomic drawings, imaging studies, and diagrams

INTENDED AUDIENCE

Medical students will find *COGDT* to be an authoritative introduction to the specialty and an excellent source for reference and review. House officers will welcome the concise, practical information on commonly encountered health problems. Practicing obstetricians and gynecologists, family physicians, internists, nurse practitioners, nurse midwives, physician's assistants, and other health care providers whose practice includes women's health can use the book to answer questions that arise in the daily practice of obstetrics and gynecology.

SPECIAL TO THIS EDITION

- Extensively revised throughout, with major updates to these chapters:
  "Surgical Diseases & Disorders in Pregnancy"
  "Sexually Transmitted Infections & Pelvic Infections"
  "Benign Disorders of the Uterine Corpus"
  "Premalignant & Malignant Disorders of the Uterine Cervix"
  "Urogynecology"
- The latest on cervical cancer screening guidelines; contraception; prenatal diagnosis and care; domestic violence, and more
- The more than 500 illustrations have been redrawn and enhanced with a second color

Alan H. DeCherney, MD
Lauren Nathan, MD

Los Angeles, California
August 2002

SECTION I
Reproductive Basics

Approach to the Patient

1

Michelle Hugin, MD, & Mary M. Cadieux, MD

An effective relationship between health care provider and patient is based on the knowledge and skill that qualify the provider for effective communication between the individuals, and for the ethical standards that govern the conduct of the participants in the relationship.

THE KNOWLEDGE BASE

The health care of women encompasses all aspects of medical science and therapeutics. Physicians in the practice of obstetrics and gynecology are called upon as consultants, and in addition, they frequently act as primary care providers for their patients. Internists in general practice and family practitioners often find that a major component of their clinical activities involves the special needs of women. These special medical needs and concerns vary with the patient's reproductive status, her reproductive potential, and her desire to reproduce. Certainly the diagnostic possibilities and the choice of diagnostic or therapeutic intervention will be influenced by the possibility of, or desire for, pregnancy, or in some cases by the patient's hormonal profile. In addition, the gynecologic or obstetric assessment must include an evaluation of the patient's general health status and should be placed in the context of the psychologic, social, and emotional status of the patient.

History

To offer each woman optimal care, the information obtained at each visit should be as complete as possible. Whether the contact is a routine visit or is occasioned by a particular problem or complaint, the woman should be encouraged to view the visit as an opportunity to participate in improving her health. The clinical database should include general information about the patient and her goals in seeking care. The history of the present problem, past medical history, family history,

medications used, allergies, and review of systems should be concise but thorough. Portions of the history provided by questionnaire or by other members of the health care team should be reviewed with the patient, in part to verify the information, but also to begin assessing the patient's personality and to determine her attitude toward the health care system. The menstrual history and developmental history may provide a background for presenting complaints in subsequent years. The menstrual history, sexual history, and obstetric history obviously assume central importance for the gynecologic or obstetric visit. In addition, the habit of systematically categorizing the nature of such complaints as pain, abnormal bleeding, or vaginal discharge will usually narrow the differential diagnoses. For example, the categorization of a complaint of pain should include its onset, duration, frequency, and associated behaviors, as well as a description of the nature or type of pain and its location. Such thoroughness will permit assessment of change as well as determination of the appropriate mode of investigation or therapy.

The initial contact with the patient, made while she is fully clothed and comfortable, may be useful in decreasing her anxiety about the physical examination; concerns about the examination may be elicited, and a history of previous unfortunate experiences may alert the examiner to the need for extra attention, time, and gentleness.

Physical Examination

The second component of the patient assessment, the physical examination, should also be directed toward evaluation of the total patient. The patient should again be encouraged to view the examination as a positive opportunity to gain information about her body, and she should be offered feedback regarding the general physical examination and any significant findings. The examination should always include a discussion of any concerns expressed by the patient. The breast examination provides a good opportunity to reinforce the practice of breast self-examination. The pelvic examination is usually an occasion of heightened anxiety for the patient, and every effort should be made to make the experience a positive one. The physician should give the patient as much control over the process as possible, by asking if she is ready, asking for feedback on whether the examination is painful, and seeking her cooperation in relaxation and muscle control. Information about each step of the examination can be provided so the patient is involved and appropriately aware of the value of each maneuver.

Inspection of the external genitalia is followed by the gentle insertion of an appropriately sized, warmed speculum to permit inspection of the vagina and the cervix. For patients with pain or increased anxiety, their cooperation must be continually reinforced by slow, gentle placement of the instrument, maintaining downward pressure against the relaxed perineal body and away from the urethral and anterior vaginal areas. Some women may wish to watch, by the use of a mirror, as the genitalia are inspected and may gain confidence from visualizing the cervix and vagina. The Papanicolaou (Pap) smear may be uncomfortable for some women, and they should be alerted when the test is being done. The bimanual examination should also be explained to the patient. When the uterus is anteflexed, the woman may want to appreciate the size and location of her uterus by feeling it with the guidance of the examiner. The rectovaginal and rectal examinations, if performed while the patient relaxes her anal sphincter, provide additional information and can be another source of reassurance for the normal patient or a means of diagnosis for the patient with disease. If an ultrasound is indicated as part of the gynecologic or obstetric examination, additional participation by the patient in the evaluation can be obtained by explanations of the visualized anatomy.

Implications of Technology

The scientific knowledge base for obstetric and gynecologic care has grown in parallel with general medical advances. In some cases this proliferation of information and technology has profoundly altered the relationship between health care providers and their patients. For example, the change from an intuitive management of labor and delivery to active monitoring and subsequent interpretation of data has provided a more rational basis for decision making. This change of management style has also created a potential for conflict or confusion in the relationship between patient and physician. In seeking to obtain additional information, the physician can

be perceived to be intervening unnecessarily. More than ever before, issues of consumerism and participation in decision making require an understanding of the expectations of each individual woman. Whether a woman perceives herself as a "client" or as a "patient," and the degree to which this perception coincides with the views of her physician, may alter her acceptance of recommendations for care. The fact that several options are available in the management of many obstetric or gynecologic situations may further complicate the relationship. However, this situation provides an opportunity to allow the patient to participate actively in choosing the best therapy for her particular circumstance.

COMMUNICATION

If the first foundation of a strong therapeutic relationship is knowledge, the second is communication. The ability to establish trust, to obtain and deliver complete and accurate information, and to ensure compliance with recommendations depends in large measure on the health care provider's communication skills. In some individuals these skills are innate, but for most the ability to become an effective communicator in a variety of settings requires an active process of learning and a willingness to be evaluated by peers. The information communicated in each encounter, whether by written material, in face-to-face discussion, or by telephone contact, extends beyond the factual content provided to include a demonstration of the provider's willingness to be available to answer questions and to encourage patient involvement in decision making.

One common barrier from the patient's perspective is that medical information is communicated via a foreign language to the layperson. This foreign language is often spoken in a hurried fashion and the listener is not given the opportunity to ask questions for clarification. The patient may also find it difficult to voice her concerns within the traditional doctor-patient relationship. She may be embarrassed to reveal intimate details of her personal life to a provider who does not take the time to show interest in her story. By not allowing the patient to express her fears, concerns, or questions, the provider can miss valuable clues to diagnosis and formulation of a treatment plan.

Solutions to these communication barriers can be found by educating patients and providers. The physician should provide a comfortable environment, encourage the patient to ask questions, listen carefully both to her story and the way she tells it, and explore with her the goals and expectations she has about the treatment. Videotaped interviews are a very effective means of educating providers about these skills. The patient should be asked to repeat instructions, and written material should be provided whenever possible. For her part the patient can be asked to take notes and keep a diary for review at subsequent visits.

Enhanced communication has been shown to dramatically increase compliance. A striking example of lack of compliance occurs with prescription of hormone replacement therapy (HRT). Overall compliance with HRT is approximately 30%. Patients either do not fill or renew their prescriptions because of fear of cancer or due to inadequate or inaccurate information regarding risks and side effects. Long-term continuance rates are highest among patients with the greatest understanding.

For the health care practitioner, the counterbalance of a litigious society that may hold the physician responsible for treatment outcome places a high premium on documentation and scientific justification for each intervention or nonintervention and can place the physician in an adversarial position with respect to the patient's desires. The obligation to inform the patient, to obtain surgical consent, or to advise about choices regarding pregnancy outcome, is becoming in some instances a matter of law rather than established medical practice. These legislative initiatives, while offensive to many, are signals that the public feels it requires protection from manipulation at the hands of those who have the power of knowledge and training not available to the layperson. Regardless of the validity of this perception, it can only be countered by efforts to establish and maintain the trust of each individual with whom the physician has a medical relationship. This trust is rooted in the physician's medical knowledge and is maintained by conscientious structured lifetime learning, the frank assessment and acknowledgment of areas of ignorance, and the willingness to discuss with the patient what is known and what is uncertain.

ETHICS

If the bricks of the foundation of the relationship between physician and patient are knowledge and communication, the mortar that forms the basis for trust is the integrity and ethical behavior of all participants in the relationship. Ethical dilemmas in obstetrics and gynecology are receiving increasing recognition, particularly as they deal with the provocative issues surrounding the beginnings of life, the nature of parenting, and the control of individual patients over their own destiny. Ethical dilemmas only arise when there are conflicting obligations, rights, or claims. Since the delivery of health care involves multiple participants, a consensus of values must often be sought when the patient is cared for by a team, even when significant pluralism of views might be represented. To minimize potential ethical conflicts, to anticipate potential areas of difficulty, and to achieve consistency in behavior, individuals may

avail themselves of a number of resources for ethical decision making. In addition to the growing literature in the field, many hospitals and practice settings have formal consultation services for resolution of ethical dilemmas. Before seeking an external framework, however, the practitioner should be aware of his or her own values and understand the basis of these values. The values of the medical profession and of the institutions in which the physician practices, as formulated by codes and standards, but also as expressed indirectly through past actions, are usually then helpful in providing a decision-making framework. Finally, a familiarity with ethical theories may permit decision making that achieves an acceptable consensus in the face of conflicting values. Discussions based on consideration of the ethical principles of patient autonomy (respect for persons), beneficence (doing good), nonmaleficence (refraining from doing harm), and justice (consideration of resources and fairness of opportunity) will prevent capricious and arbitrary decisions.

The principle of autonomy, or respect for each individual person, may form the underlying basis for resolving many ethical questions and will determine appropriate attitudes toward confidentiality, privacy, right to information, and the ultimate primacy of the patient in making treatment decisions. Since caring for women necessarily involves information regarding sensitive and intimate relationships and activities, as well as access to a woman's thoughts, feelings, and emotions, full disclosure of such information by the patient places a burden of trust on the health care provider to protect the rights and privacy of each patient. The relationship established at an initial gynecologic visit between a young adolescent and the physician may potentially extend throughout her adult life and include such major life events as education about reproductive health, assistance in family planning and childbearing, and preservation of physical fitness and well-being through the postmenopausal years. To successfully establish such an enduring clinical relationship requires a sensitivity to the changing goals and needs of the individual patient. Offering care to some patients or providing some types of services may not be comfortable for all practitioners. For example, establishing a rapport with an adolescent seeking birth control or providing health care for a lesbian woman may require a nonjudgmental approach when one is interviewing the patient and a balanced consideration of lifestyle options. The recognition of these special needs has led to a compartmentalization of health care in some regions, so that specialty practices or clinics directed toward adolescent health care, family planning, fertility, oncology, and menopausal care are frequently available. These resources can best be utilized by referral, with guidance provided by a primary provider, so that appropriate use of such resources can be an integral part of the general health care of each woman.

REFERENCES

Delbarco TL: Enriching the doctor-patient relationship by inviting the patient's perspective. Ann Intern Med 1992;116:414.

Del Mar CB: Communicating well in general practice. Med J Aust 1994;160:367.

DiMatteo MR: The physician-patient relationship, effects on the quality of health care. Clin Obstet Gynecol 1994;37:149.

Eracher SA, Kirscht JP, Becker MH: Understanding and improving patient's compliance. Ann Intern Med 1984;100:258.

Laine C, Davidoff F: Patient centered medicine, a professional evolution. JAMA 1996;275:152.

Quill TE: Recognizing and adjusting to barriers in doctor-patient communication. Ann Intern Med 1989;111:51.

Roberts DK: Prevention: Patient communication. Clin Obstet Gynecol 1988;31:153.

Sarrel PM: Improving adherence to hormone replacement therapy with effective patient-physician communication. Am J Obstet Gynecol 1999;180:S337.

Anatomy of the Female Reproductive System

Kermit E. Krantz, MD, LittD

ABDOMINAL WALL

Topographic Anatomy

The anterior abdominal wall is divided into sections for descriptive purposes and to allow the physician to outline relationships of the viscera in the abdominal cavity. The centerpoint of reference is the sternoxiphoid process, which is in the same plane as the tenth thoracic vertebra. The upper 2 sections are formed by the subcostal angle; the lower extends from the lower ribs to the crest of the ilium and forward to the anterior superior iliac spines. The base is formed by the inguinal ligaments and the symphysis pubica.

The viscera are located by dividing the anterolateral abdominal wall into regions. One line is placed from the level of each ninth costal cartilage to the iliac crests. Two other lines are drawn from the middle of the inguinal ligaments to the cartilage of the eighth rib. The 9 regions formed (Fig 2–1) are the epigastric, umbilical, hypogastric, and right and left hypochondriac, lumbar, and ilioinguinal.

Within the right hypochondriac zone are the right lobe of the liver, the gallbladder at the anterior inferior angle, part of the right kidney deep within the region, and, occasionally, the right colic flexure.

The epigastric zone contains the left lobe of the liver and part of the right lobe, the stomach, the proximal duodenum, the pancreas, the suprarenal glands, and the upper poles of both kidneys (Fig 2–2).

The left hypochondriac region marks the situation of the spleen, the fundus of the stomach, the apex of the liver, and the left colic flexure.

Within the right lumbar region are the ascending colon, coils of intestine, and, frequently, the inferior border of the lateral portion of the right kidney.

The central umbilical region contains the transverse colon, the stomach, the greater omentum, the small intestine, the second and third portions of the duodenum, the head of the pancreas, and parts of the medial aspects of the kidneys.

Located in the left lumbar region are the descending colon, the left kidney, and small intestine. Within the limits of the right ilioinguinal region are the cecum and appendix, part of the ascending colon, small intestine, and, occasionally, the right border of the greater omentum.

The hypogastric region includes the greater omentum, loops of small intestine, the pelvic colon, and often part of the transverse colon.

The left ilioinguinal region encloses the sigmoid colon, part of the descending colon, loops of small intestine, and the left border of the greater omentum.

There is considerable variation in the position and size of individual organs due to differences in body size and conformation. Throughout life, variations in the positions of organs are dependent not only on gravity but also on the movements of the hollow viscera, which induce further changes in shape when filling and emptying. The need to recognize the relationships of the viscera to the abdominal regions becomes most apparent when taking into account the distortion that occurs during pregnancy. For example, the appendix lies in the right ilioinguinal region (right lower quadrant) until the 12th week of gestation. At 16 weeks, it is at the level of the right iliac crest. At 20 weeks, it is at the level of the umbilicus, where it will remain until after delivery. Because of this displacement, the symptoms of appendicitis will be different during the 3 trimesters. Similarly, displacement will also affect problems involving the bowel.

Skin, Subcutaneous Tissue, & Fascia

The abdominal skin is smooth, fine, and very elastic. It is loosely attached to underlying structures except at the umbilicus, where it is firmly adherent. Beneath the skin is the superficial fascia (tela subcutanea) (Fig 2–3). This fatty protective fascia covers the entire abdomen. Below the navel, it consists principally of 2 layers; Camper's fascia, the more superficial layer containing most of the fat; and Scarpa's fascia (deep fascia), the fibroelastic membrane firmly attached to midline aponeuroses and to the fascia lata.

Arteries

The anterior cutaneous branches of the superficial arteries are grouped with the anterior cutaneous nerves (Fig 2–4). The lateral cutaneous branches stem from the lower aortic intercostal arteries and the subcostal ar-

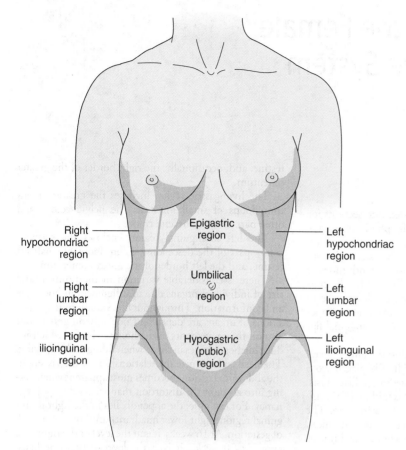

Right hypochondriac region

Epigastric region

Left hypochondriac region

Right lumbar region

Umbilical region

Left lumbar region

Right ilioinguinal region

Hypogastric (pubic) region

Left ilioinguinal region

Figure 2–1. Regions of the abdomen.

teries. The femoral artery supplies both the superficial epigastric and the superficial circumflex iliac arteries. From its origin beneath the fascia lata at approximately 1.2 cm beyond the inguinal ligament, the superficial epigastric artery passes immediately through the fascia lata or through the fossa ovalis. From there, it courses upward, primarily within Camper's fascia, in a slightly medial direction anterior to the external oblique muscle almost as far as the umbilicus, giving off small branches to the inguinal lymph nodes and to the skin and superficial fascia. It ends in numerous small twigs that anastomose with the cutaneous branches from the inferior epigastric and internal mammary arteries. Arising either in common with the superficial epigastric artery or as a separate branch from the femoral artery, the superficial circumflex iliac artery passes laterally over the iliacus. Perforating the fascia lata slightly to the lateral aspect of the fossa ovalis, it then runs parallel to the inguinal ligament almost to the crest of the ilium, where it terminates in branches within Scarpa's fascia that anastomose

with the deep circumflex iliac artery. In its course, branches supply the iliacus and sartorius muscles, the inguinal lymph nodes, and the superficial fascia and skin.

Veins

The superficial veins are more numerous than the arteries and form more extensive networks. Above the umbilicus, blood returns through the anterior cutaneous and the paired thoracoepigastric veins, the superficial epigastric veins, and the superficial circumflex iliac veins in the tela subcutanea. A cruciate anastomosis exists, therefore, between the femoral and axillary veins.

Lymphatics

The lymphatic drainage of the lower abdominal wall (Fig 2–5) is primarily to the superficial inguinal nodes, 10–20 in number, which lie in the area of the inguinal

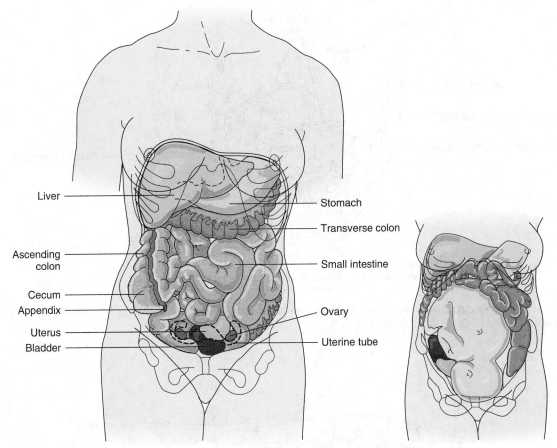

Figure 2–2. Abdominal viscera in situ. Inset shows projection of fetus in situ.

ligament. These nodes may be identified by dividing the area into quadrants by intersecting horizontal and vertical lines that meet at the saphenofemoral junction. The lateral abdominal wall drainage follows the superficial circumflex iliac vein and drains to the lymph nodes in the upper lateral quadrant of the superficial inguinal nodes. The drainage of the medial aspect follows the superficial epigastric vein primarily to the lymph nodes in the upper medial quadrant of the superficial inguinal nodes. Of major clinical importance are the frequent anastomoses between the lymph vessels of the right and left sides of the abdomen.

Abdominal Muscles & Fascia

The muscular wall that supports the abdominal viscera (Fig 2–6) is composed of 4 pairs of muscles and their aponeuroses. The 3 paired lateral muscles are the external oblique, the internal oblique, and the transversus.

Their aponeuroses interdigitate at the midline to connect opposing lateral muscles, forming a thickened band at this juncture, the linea alba, which extends from the xiphoid process to the pubic symphysis. Anteriorly, a pair of muscles—the rectus abdominis, with the paired pyramidalis muscles at its inferior border with its sheath—constitute the abdominal wall.

A. EXTERNAL OBLIQUE MUSCLE

The external oblique muscle consists of 8 pointed digitations attached to the lower 8 ribs. The lowest fibers insert into the anterior half of the iliac crest and the inguinal ligament. At the linea alba, the muscle aponeurosis interdigitates with that of the opposite side and fuses with the underlying internal oblique.

B. INTERNAL OBLIQUE MUSCLE

The internal oblique muscle arises from thoracolumbar fascia, the crest of the ilium, and the inguinal ligament.

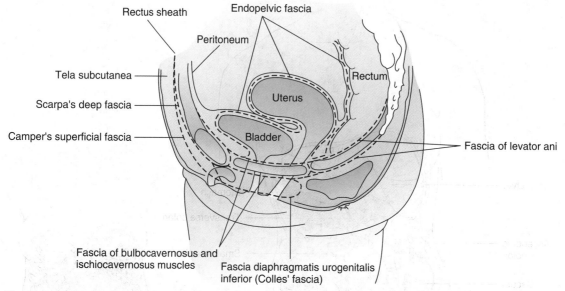

Figure 2–3. **Fascial planes of the pelvis.** (Modified after Netter. Reproduced, with permission, from Benson RC: *Handbook of Obstetrics & Gynecology*, 8th ed. Lange, 1983.)

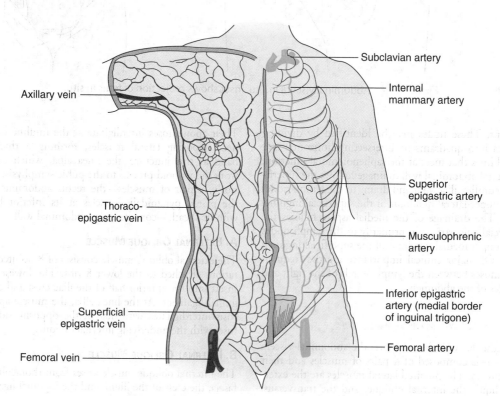

Figure 2–4. **Superficial veins and arteries of abdomen.**

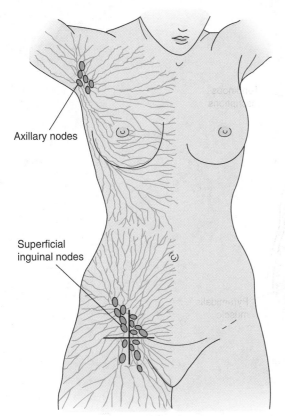

Axillary nodes

Superficial
inguinal nodes

Figure 2–5. Lymphatics of abdominal wall. Only one
side is shown, but contralateral drainage occurs, ie,
crosses midline to the opposite side.

Going in the opposite oblique direction, the muscle inserts into the lower 3 costal cartilages and into the linea
alba on either side of the rectus abdominis. The
aponeurosis helps to form the rectus sheath both anteriorly and posteriorly. The posterior layer extends from
the rectus muscle rib insertions to below the umbilicus.

C. TRANSVERSUS MUSCLE

The transversus muscle, the fibers of which run transversely and arise from the inner surfaces of the lower 6
costal cartilages, the thoracolumbar fascia, the iliac
crest, and the inguinal ligament, lies beneath the internal oblique. By inserting into the linea alba, the
aponeurosis of the transversus fuses to form the posterior layer of the posterior rectus sheath. The termination of this layer is called the arcuate line, and below it
lie transversalis fascia, properitoneal fat, and peritoneum. Inferiorly, the thin aponeurosis of the transversus abdominis becomes part of the anterior rectus
sheath.

D. RECTUS MUSCLES

The rectus muscles are straplike and extend from the thorax to the pubis. They are divided by the linea alba and
outlined laterally by the linea semilunaris. Three tendinous intersections cross the upper part of each rectus
muscle, and a fourth may also be present below the umbilicus. The pyramidalis muscle, a vestigial muscle, is situated anterior to the lowermost part of the rectus muscle.
It arises from and inserts into the pubic periosteum.

Beneath the superficial fascia and overlying the muscles is the thin, semitransparent deep fascia. Its extensions enter and divide the lateral muscles into coarse
bundles.

Abdominal incisions are shown in Fig 2–7. The position of the muscles influences the type of incision to
be made. The aim is to adequately expose the operative
field, avoiding damage to parietal structures, blood vessels, and nerves. The incision should be so placed as to
create minimal tension on the lines of closure.

Abdominal Nerves

The lower 6 thoracic nerves align with the ribs and give
off lateral cutaneous branches (Fig 2–8). The intercostal nerves pass deep to the upturned rib cartilages
and enter the abdominal wall. The main trunks of these
nerves run forward between the internal oblique and
the transversus. The nerves then enter the rectus
sheaths and the rectus muscles, and the terminating
branches emerge as anterior cutaneous nerves. The iliohypogastric nerve springs from the first lumbar nerve
after the latter has been joined by the communicating
branch from the last (12th) thoracic nerve. It pierces
the lateral border of the psoas and crosses anterior to
the quadratus lumborum muscle but posterior to the
kidney and colon. At the lateral border of the quadratus
lumborum, it pierces the aponeurosis of origin of the
transversus abdominis and enters the areolar tissue between the transversus and the internal oblique muscle.
Here, it frequently communicates with the last thoracic
and with the ilioinguinal nerve, which also originates
from the first lumbar and last thoracic nerves. The iliohypogastric divides into 2 branches. The iliac branch
pierces the internal and external oblique muscles,
emerging through the latter above the iliac crest and
supplying the integument of the upper and lateral part
of the thigh. The hypogastric branch, as it passes forward and downward, gives branches to both the transversus abdominis and internal oblique. It communicates with the ilioinguinal nerve and pierces the internal
oblique muscle near the anterior superior spine. The
hypogastric branch proceeds medially beneath the external oblique aponeurosis and pierces it just above the
subcutaneous inguinal ring to supply the skin and symphysis pubica.

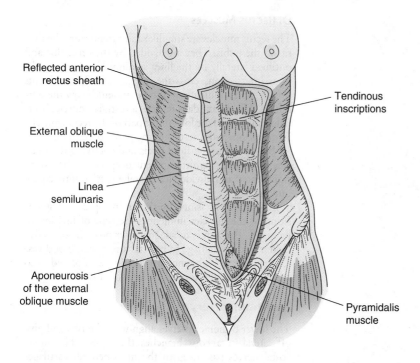

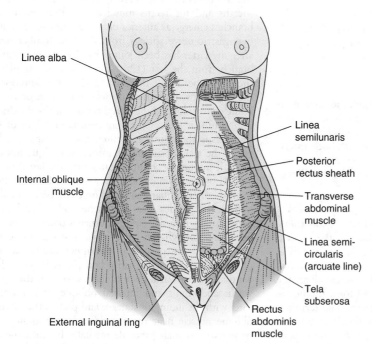

Figure 2–6. Musculature of abdominal wall.

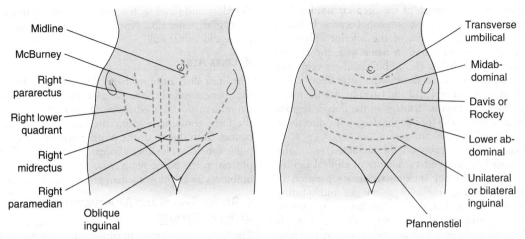

Figure 2–7. Abdominal incisions. Transverse incisions are those in which rectus muscles are cut. A Cherney incision is one in which the rectus is taken off the pubic bone and then sewed back; the pyramidalis muscle is left on pubic tubercles.

Abdominal Arteries

A. ARTERIES OF THE UPPER ABDOMEN

The lower 5 intercostal arteries and the subcostal artery accompany the thoracic nerves. Their finer, terminal branches enter the rectus sheath to anastomose with the superior and inferior epigastric arteries. The superior epigastric artery is the direct downward prolongation of the internal mammary artery. This artery descends between the posterior surface of the rectus muscle and its sheath to form an anastomosis with the inferior epigastric artery upon the muscle. The inferior epigastric artery, a branch of the external iliac artery, usually arises just above the inguinal ligament and passes on the medial side of the round ligament to the abdominal inguinal ring. From there, it ascends in a slightly medial direction, passing above and lateral to the subcutaneous inguinal ring, which lies between the fascia transversalis and the peritoneum. Piercing the fascia transversalis, it passes in front of the linea semicircularis, turns upward between the rectus and its sheath, enters the substance of the rectus muscle, and meets the superior epigastric artery. The superior epigastric supplies the upper central abdominal wall, the inferior supplies the lower central part of the anterior abdominal wall, and the deep circumflex supplies the lower lateral part of the abdominal wall.

B. ARTERIES OF THE LOWER ABDOMEN

The deep circumflex iliac artery is also a branch of the external iliac artery, arising from its side either opposite the epigastric artery or slightly below the origin of that vessel. It courses laterally behind the inguinal ligament lying between the fascia transversalis and the peri-

toneum. The deep circumflex artery perforates the transversus near the anterior superior spine of the ilium and continues between the transversus and internal oblique along and slightly above the crest of the ilium, finally running posteriorly to anastomose with the ili-

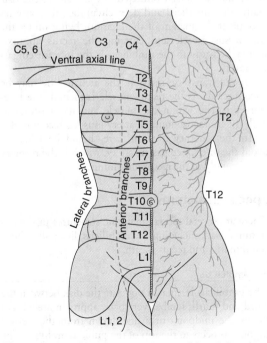

Figure 2–8. Cutaneous innervation of the abdominal wall.

olumbar artery. A branch of the deep circumflex iliac artery is important to the surgeon because it forms anastomoses with branches of the inferior epigastric. The deep veins correspond in name with the arteries they accompany. Below the umbilicus, these veins run caudad and medially to the external iliac vein; above that level, they run cephalad and laterally into the intercostal veins. Lymphatic drainage in the deeper regions of the abdominal wall follows the deep veins directly to the superficial inguinal nodes.

The various incisions on the abdomen encounter some muscle planes and vasculature of clinical significance. The McBurney incision requires separation of the external and internal oblique muscles and splitting of the transversus. The deep circumflex artery may be frequently encountered. The paramedian incision is made in the right or left rectus. Below the arcuate line, the fascia of the external and internal oblique, as well as the transversus muscles when present, go over the rectus abdominis; above the arcuate line, the transversus and part of the internal oblique go under the rectus. The vasculature is primarily perforators and frequently the thoracoabdominal vein. Inferiorly, the superficial epigastric may be encountered. In the Pfannenstiel incision, the fascia of the external and internal oblique go over the rectus muscle as well as the transversus muscle when present. After the fascia over the rectus is incised, the muscles can be separated. The superficial epigastric artery and vein are encountered in Camper's fascia. Laterally, the superficial and deep circumflex iliac arteries may be at the margin of the incision. Lying under the transversus muscle and entering the rectus approximately half-way to the umbilicus is the inferior epigastric artery.

In the transverse incision, the arcuate line may be encountered. As the rectus muscle is incised, the inferior epigastric within the muscle and its anastomosis with the thoracoabdominal artery must be recognized.

In the Cherney incision, care should be taken to avoid the inferior epigastric artery, which is the primary blood supply to the rectus abdominis.

Special Structures

There are several special anatomic structures in the abdominal wall, including the umbilicus, linea alba, linea semilunaris, and rectus sheath.

A. UMBILICUS

The umbilicus is situated opposite the disk between the third and fourth lumbar vertebrae, approximately 2 cm below the midpoint of a line drawn from the sternoxiphoid process to the top of the pubic symphysis. The umbilicus is a dense, wrinkled mass of fibrous tissue en-

closed by and fused with a ring of circular aponeurotic fibers in the linea alba. Normally, it is the strongest part of the abdominal wall.

B. LINEA ALBA

The linea alba, a fibrous band formed by the fusion of the aponeuroses of the muscles of the anterior abdominal wall, marks the medial side of the rectus abdominis; the linea semilunaris forms the lateral border, which courses from the tip of the ninth costal cartilage to the pubic tubercle. The linea alba extends from the xiphoid process to the pubic symphysis, represented above the umbilicus as a shallow median groove on the surface.

C. RECTUS SHEATH AND APONEUROSIS OF THE EXTERNAL OBLIQUE

The rectus sheath serves to support and control the rectus muscles. It contains the rectus and pyramidalis muscles, the terminal branches of the lower 6 thoracic nerves and vessels, and the inferior and superior epigastric vessels. Cranially, where the sheath is widest, its anterior wall extends upward onto the thorax to the level of the fifth costal cartilage and is attached to the sternum. The deeper wall is attached to the xiphoid process and the lower borders of the seventh to ninth costal cartilages and does not extend upward onto the anterior thorax. Caudally, where the sheath narrows considerably, the anterior wall is attached to the crest and the symphysis pubica. Above the costal margin on the anterior chest wall, there is no complete rectus sheath (Fig 2–9). Instead, the rectus muscle is only covered by the aponeurosis of the external oblique. In the region of the abdomen, the upper two-thirds of the internal oblique aponeurosis splits at the lateral border of the rectus muscle into anterior and posterior lamellas. The anterior lamella passes in front of the external oblique and blends with the external oblique aponeurosis. The posterior wall of the sheath is formed by the posterior lamella and the aponeurosis of the transversus muscle. The anterior and posterior sheath join at the midline. The lower third of the internal oblique aponeurosis is undivided. Together with the aponeuroses of the external oblique and transversus muscles, it forms the anterior wall of the sheath. The posterior wall is occupied by transversalis fascia, which is spread over the interior surfaces of both the rectus and the transversus muscles, separating them from peritoneum and extending to the inguinal and lacunar ligaments. The transition from aponeurosis to fascia is usually fairly sharp, marked by a curved line called the arcuate line.

D. FUNCTION OF ABDOMINAL MUSCLES

In general, the functions of the abdominal muscles are 3-fold: (1) support and compression of the abdominal

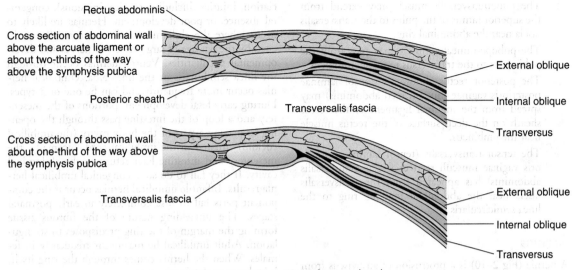

Figure 2–9. Formation of rectus sheath.

viscera by the external oblique, internal oblique, and transversus muscles; (2) depression of the thorax in conjunction with the diaphragm by the rectus abdominis, external oblique, internal oblique, and transversus muscles, as evident in respiration, coughing, vomiting, defecation, and parturition; and (3) assistance in bending movements of the trunk through flexion of the vertebral column by the rectus abdominis, external oblique, and internal oblique muscles. There is partial assistance in rotation of the thorax and upper abdomen to the same side when the pelvis is fixed by the internal oblique and by the external oblique to the opposite side. In addition, the upper external oblique serves as a fixation muscle in abduction of the upper limb of the same side and adduction of the upper limb of the opposite side. The pyramidalis muscle secures the linea alba in the median line.

Variations of Abdominal Muscles

Variations have been noted in all of the abdominal muscles.

A. RECTUS MUSCLE

The rectus abdominis muscle may differ in the number of its tendinous inscriptions and the extent of its thoracic attachment. Aponeurotic slips or slips of muscle on the upper part of the thorax are remnants of a more primitive state in which the muscle extended to the neck. Absence of part or all of the muscle has been noted. The pyramidalis muscle may be missing, only

slightly developed, double, or may extend upward to the umbilicus.

B. EXTERNAL OBLIQUE MUSCLE

The external oblique muscle varies in the extent of its origin from the ribs. Broad fascicles may be separated by loose tissue from the main belly of the muscle, either on its deep or on its superficial surface. The supracostalis anterior is a rare fascicle occasionally found on the upper portion of the thoracic wall. Transverse tendinous inscriptions may also be found.

C. INTERNAL OBLIQUE MUSCLE

The internal oblique deviates at times, both in its attachments and in the extent of development of the fleshy part of the muscle. Occasionally, tendinous inscriptions are present, or the posterior division forms an extra muscle 7–7.5 cm wide and separated from the internal oblique by a branch of the iliohypogastric nerve and a branch of the deep circumflex iliac artery.

D. TRANSVERSUS MUSCLE

The transversus muscle fluctuates widely in the extent of its development but is rarely absent. Rarely, it extends as far inferiorly as the ligamentum teres uteri (round ligament), and infrequently it may be situated superior to the anterior superior spine. However, it generally occupies an intermediate position.

E. OTHER VARIATIONS

Several small muscles may be present.

1. The pubotransversalis muscle may extend from the superior ramus of the pubis to the transversalis fascia near the abdominal ring.

2. The puboperitonealis muscle may pass from the pubic crest to the transversus near the umbilicus.

3. The posterior rectus abdominis (tensor laminae posterioris vaginae musculi recti abdominis) may spread from the inguinal ligament to the rectus sheath on the deep surface of the rectus muscle near the umbilicus.

4. The tensor transversalis (tensor laminae posterioris vaginae musculi recti et fasciae transversalis abdominis) has appeared from the transversalis fascia near the abdominal inguinal ring to the linea semicircularis.

Hernias

A hernia (Fig 2–10) is a protrusion of any viscus from its normal enclosure, which may occur with any of the abdominal viscera, especially the jejunum, ileum, and greater omentum. A hernia may be due to increased pressure, such as that resulting from strenuous exercise, lifting heavy weights, tenesmus, or increased expiratory efforts, or may result from decreased resistance of the abdominal wall (congenital or acquired) such as occurs with debilitating illness or old age, prolonged distention from ascites, tumors, pregnancy, corpulence, ema-

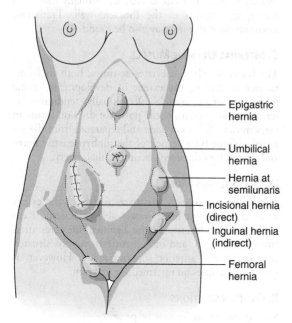

Figure 2–10. Hernia sites.

- Epigastric hernia
- Umbilical hernia
- Hernia at semilunaris
- Incisional hernia (direct)
- Inguinal hernia (indirect)
- Femoral hernia

ciation, injuries (including surgical incisions), congenital absence, or poor development. Hernias are likely to occur where the abdominal wall is structurally weakened by the passage of large vessels or nerves and developmental peculiarities. Ventral hernias occur through the linea semilunaris or the linea alba. Umbilical hernias occur more frequently and can be one of 3 types. During early fetal development, portions of the mesentery and a loop of the intestine pass through the opening to occupy a part of the body cavity (the umbilical coelom) situated in the umbilical cord. Normally, the mesentery and intestine later return to the abdominal cavity. If they fail to do so, a congenital umbilical hernia results. Infantile umbilical hernias occur if the component parts fail to fuse completely in early postnatal stages. The unyielding nature of the fibrous tissue forming the margin of the ring predisposes to strangulation. Adult umbilical hernias occur frequently in females. When the hernia comes through the ring itself, it is always at the upper part.

INGUINAL REGION

The inguinal region of the abdominal wall is bounded by the rectus abdominis muscle medially, the line connecting the anterior superior iliac spines superiorly, and the inguinal ligament inferiorly. The region contains 8 layers of abdominal wall. These layers, from the most superficial inward, are (1) the skin, (2) the tela subcutanea, (3) the aponeurosis of the external oblique muscle, (4) the internal oblique muscle, (5) the transversus abdominis muscle (below the free border, the layer is incomplete), (6) the transversalis fascia, (7) the subperitoneal fat and connective tissue, and (8) the peritoneum. The tela subcutanea consists of the superficial fatty Camper's fascia, which is continuous with the tela subcutanea of the whole body, and the deeper membranous Scarpa's fascia, which covers the lower third of the abdominal wall and the medial side of the groin, both joining below the inguinal ligament to form the fascia lata of the thigh.

Subcutaneous Inguinal Ring

A triangular evagination of the external oblique aponeurosis, the subcutaneous inguinal ring (external abdominal ring), is bounded by an aponeurosis at its edges and by the inguinal ligament inferiorly. The superior or medial crus is smaller and attaches to the symphysis pubica. The inferior or lateral crus is stronger and blends with the inguinal ligament as it passes to the pubic tubercle. The sharp margins of the ring are attributed to a sudden thinning of the aponeurosis. In the female, the ligamentum teres uteri (round ligament) passes through this ring. The subcutaneous inguinal ring is much smaller in the female than in the male, and the abdominal wall is relatively stronger in this region.

Ligaments, Aponeuroses, & Fossae

The inguinal ligament itself forms the inferior thickened border of the external oblique aponeurosis, extending from the anterior superior iliac spine to the pubic tubercle. Along its inferior border, it becomes continuous with the fascia lata of the thigh. From the medial portion of the inguinal ligament, a triangular band of fibers attaches separately to the pecten ossis pubis. This band is known as the lacunar (Gimbernat's) ligament. The reflex inguinal ligament (ligament of Colles or triangular fascia) is represented by a small band of fibers, often poorly developed, and derived from the superior crus of the subcutaneous inguinal ring and the lower part of the linea alba. These fibers cross to the opposite side to attach to the pecten ossis pubis. The falx inguinalis or conjoined tendon is formed by the aponeurosis of the transversus abdominis and internal oblique muscles. These fibers arise from the inguinal ligament and arch downward and forward to insert on the pubic crest and pecten ossis pubis, behind the inguinal and lacunar ligaments. The interfoveolar ligament is composed partly of fibrous bands from the aponeurosis of the transversalis muscle of the same and opposite sides. Curving medial to and below the internal abdominal ring, they attach to the lacunar ligament and pectineal fascia.

Abdominal Inguinal Ring

The abdominal inguinal ring (internal abdominal ring) is the rounded mouth of a funnel-shaped expansion of transversalis fascia that lies approximately 2 cm above the inguinal ligament and midway between the anterior superior iliac spine and the symphysis pubica. Medially, it is bounded by the inferior epigastric vessels; the external iliac artery is situated below. The abdominal inguinal ring represents the area where the round ligament emerges from the abdomen. The triangular area medial to the inferior epigastric artery, bounded by the inguinal ligament below and the lateral border of the rectus sheath, is known as the trigonum inguinale (Hesselbach's triangle), the site of congenital direct hernias.

Inguinal Canal

The inguinal canal in the female is not well demarcated, but it normally gives passage to the round ligament of the uterus, a vein, an artery from the uterus that forms a cruciate anastomosis with the labial arteries, and extraperitoneal fat. The fetal ovary, like the

testis, is an abdominal organ and possesses a gubernaculum that extends from its lower pole downward and forward to a point corresponding to the abdominal inguinal ring, through which it continues into the labia majora. The processus vaginalis is an evagination of peritoneum at the level of the abdominal inguinal ring occurring during the third fetal month. In the male, the processus vaginalis descends with the testis. The processus vaginalis of the female is rudimentary, but occasionally a small diverticulum of peritoneum is found passing partway through the inguinal region; this diverticulum is termed the processus vaginalis peritonei (canal of Nuck). Instead of descending, as does the testis, the ovary moves medially, where it becomes adjacent to the uterus. The intra-abdominal portion of the gubernaculum ovarii becomes attached to the lateral border of the developing uterus, evolving as the ligament of the ovary and the round ligament of the uterus. The extra-abdominal portion of the round ligament of the uterus becomes attenuated in the adult and may appear as a small fibrous band. The inguinal canal is an intermuscular passageway that extends from the abdominal ring downward, medially, and somewhat forward to the subcutaneous inguinal ring (about 3–4 cm). The canal is roughly triangular in shape, and its boundaries are largely artificial. The lacunar and inguinal ligaments form the base of the canal. The anterior or superficial wall is formed by the external oblique aponeurosis, and the lowermost fibers of the internal oblique muscle add additional strength in its lateral part. The posterior or deep wall of the canal is formed by transversalis fascia throughout and is strengthened medially by the falx inguinalis.

Abdominal Fossae

The abdominal fossae in the inguinal region consist of the foveae inguinalis lateralis and medialis. The fovea inguinalis lateralis lies lateral to a slight fold, the plica epigastrica, formed by the inferior epigastric vessels, and just medial to the abdominal inguinal ring, which slants medially and upward toward the rectus muscle. From the lateral margin of the tendinous insertion of the rectus muscle, upward toward the umbilicus, and over the obliterated artery extends a more accentuated fold, the plica umbilicalis lateralis. The fovea inguinalis medialis lies between the plica epigastrica and the plica umbilicalis lateralis, the bottom of the fossa facing the trigonum inguinale (Hesselbach's triangle). This region is strengthened by the interfoveolar ligament at the medial side of the abdominal inguinal ring and the conjoined tendon lateral to the rectus muscle; however, these bands vary in width and are thus supportive.

Ligaments & Spaces

The inguinal ligament forms the roof of a large osseo-ligamentous space leading from the iliac fossa to the thigh. The floor of this space is formed by the superior ramus of the pubis medially and by the body of the ilium laterally. The iliopectineal ligament extends from the inguinal ligament to the iliopectineal eminence, dividing this area into 2 parts. The lateral, larger division is called the muscular lacuna and is almost completely filled by the iliopsoas muscle, along with the femoral nerve medially and the lateral femoral cutaneous nerves laterally. The medial, smaller division is known as the vascular lacuna and is traversed by the external iliac (femoral) artery, vein, and lymphatic vessels, which do not completely fill the space. The anterior border of the vascular lacuna is formed by the inguinal ligament and the transversalis fascia. The posterior boundary is formed by the ligamentum pubicum superius (Cooper's ligament), a thickening of fascia along the public pecten where the pectineal fascia and iliopectineal ligament meet. The transversalis fascia and iliac fascia are extended with the vessels, forming a funnel-shaped fibrous investment, the femoral sheath. The sheath is divided into 3 compartments: (1) the lateral compartment, containing the femoral artery; (2) the intermediate compartment, containing the femoral vein; and (3) the medial compartment or canal, containing a lymph node (nodi lymphatici inguinales profundi [node of Rosenmuller or Cloquet]) and the lymphatic vessels that drain most of the leg, groin, and perineum. The femoral canal also contains areolar tissue, which frequently condenses to form the "femoral septum." Because of the greater spread of the pelvis in the female, the muscular and vascular lacunae are relatively large spaces. The upper or abdominal opening of the femoral canal is known as the femoral ring and is covered by the parietal peritoneum.

Arteries

In front of the femoral ring, the arterial branches of the external iliac artery are the inferior epigastric and the deep circumflex iliac. The inferior epigastric artery arises from the anterior surface of the external iliac, passing forward and upward on the anterior abdominal wall between peritoneum and transversalis fascia. It pierces the fascia just below the arcuate line, entering the rectus abdominis muscle or coursing along its inferior surface to anastomose with the superior epigastric from the internal thoracic. The inferior epigastric artery forms the lateral boundary of the trigonum inguinale (Hesselbach's triangle). At its origin, it frequently gives off a branch to the inguinal canal, as well as a branch to the pubis (pubic artery), which anastomoses with twigs

of the obturator artery. The pubic branch of the inferior epigastric often becomes the obturator artery. The deep circumflex iliac artery arises laterally and traverses the iliopsoas to the anterior superior iliac spine, where it pierces the transversus muscle to course between the transversus and the internal oblique, sending perforators to the surface. It often has anastomoses with penetrating branches of the inferior epigastric via its perforators through the rectus abdominis. The veins follow a similar course.

As the external iliac artery passes through the femoral canal, which underlies the inguinal ligament, it courses medial to the femoral vein and nerve, resting in what is termed the femoral triangle (Scarpa's triangle). The femoral sheath is a downward continuation of the inguinal ligament anterior to the femoral vessel and nerve.

The branches of the femoral artery supplying the groin are (1) the superficial epigastric, (2) the superficial circumflex iliac, (3) the superficial external pudendal, and (4) the deep external pudendal. The superficial epigastric artery passes upward through the femoral sheath over the inguinal ligament, to rest in Camper's fascia on the lower abdomen. The superficial circumflex iliac artery arises adjacent to the superior epigastric, piercing the fascia lata and running parallel to the inguinal ligament as far as the iliac crest. It then divides into branches that supply the integument of the groin, the superficial fascia, and the lymph glands, anastomosing with the deep circumflex iliac, the superior gluteal, and the lateral femoral circumflex arteries. The superficial external pudendal artery arises from the medial side of the femoral artery, close to the preceding vessels. It pierces the femoral sheath and fascia cribrosa, coursing medially across the round ligament to the integument on the lower part of the abdomen and the labium majus, anastomosing with the internal pudendal. The deep external pudendal artery passes medially across the pectineus and adductor longus muscles, supplying the integument of the labium majus and forming, together with the external pudendal artery, a rete with the labial arteries.

PUDENDUM

The vulva consists of the mons pubis, the labia majora, the labia minora, the clitoris, and the glandular structures that open into the vestibulum vaginae (Fig 2–11). The size, shape, and coloration of the various structures, as well as the hair distribution, vary between individuals and racial groups. Normal pubic hair in the female is distributed in an inverted triangle, with the base centered over the mons pubis. Nevertheless, in approximately 25% of normal women, hair may extend upward along the linea alba. The type of hair is depen-

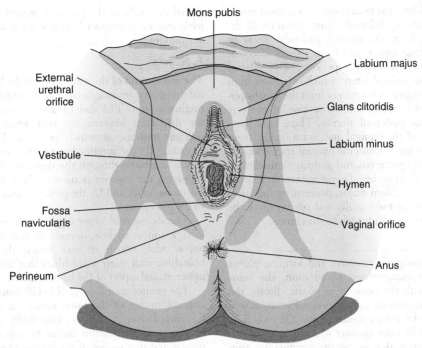

Figure 2–11. External genitalia of adult female (parous).

dent, in part, on the pigmentation of the individual. It varies from heavy, coarse, crinkly hair in blacks to sparse, fairly fine, lanugo type hair in Asian women. The length and size of the various structures of the vulva are influenced by the pelvic architecture, as is also the position of the external genitalia in the perineal area. The external genitalia of the female have their exact counterparts in the male.

Labia Majora

A. SUPERFICIAL ANATOMY

The labia majora are comprised of 2 rounded mounds of tissue, originating in the mons pubis and terminating in the perineum. They form the lateral boundaries of the vulva and are approximately 7–9 cm long and 2–4 cm wide, varying in size with height, weight, race, age, parity, and pelvic architecture. Ontogenetically, these permanent folds of skin are homologous to the scrotum of the male. Hair is distributed over their surfaces, extending superiorly in the area of the mons pubis from one side to the other. The lateral surfaces are adjacent to the medial surface of the thigh, forming a deep groove when the legs are together. The medial surfaces of the labia majora may oppose each other directly or may be separated by protrusion of the labia minora. The cleft that is formed by this opposition anteriorly is

termed the anterior commissure. Posteriorly, the cleft is less clearly defined and termed the posterior commissure. The middle portion of the cleft between the 2 labia is the rima pudendi.

B. DEEP STRUCTURES

Underlying the skin is a thin, poorly developed muscle layer called the tunica dartos labialis, the fibers of which course, for the most part, at right angles to the wrinkles of the surface, forming a crisscross pattern. Deep to the dartos layer is a thin layer of fascia, most readily recognizable in the old or the young because of the large amount of adipose and areolar tissue. Numerous sweat glands are found in the labia majora, the greater number on the medial aspect. In the deeper substance of the labia majora are longitudinal bands of muscle that are continuous with the ligamentum teres uteri (round ligament) as it emerges from the inguinal canal. Occasionally, a persistent processus vaginalis peritonei (canal of Nuck) may be seen in the upper region of the labia. In most women, it has been impossible to differentiate the presence of the cremaster muscle beyond its area of origin.

C. ARTERIES

The arterial supply into the labia majora comes from the internal and external pudendals, with extensive anastomoses. Within the labia majora is a circular arterial pattern originating inferiorly from a branch of the perineal artery, from the external pudendal artery in the anterior lateral aspect, and from a small artery of the ligamentum teres uteri superiorly. The inferior branch from the perineal artery, which originates from the internal pudendal as it emerges from the canalis pudendalis (Alcock's canal), forms the base of the rete with the external pudendal arteries. These arise from the medial side of the femoral and, occasionally, from the deep arteries just beneath the femoral ring, coursing medially over the pectineus and adductor muscles, to which they supply branches. They terminate in a circular rete within the labium majus, penetrating the fascia lata adjacent to the fossa ovalis and passing over the round ligament to send a branch to the clitoris.

D. Veins

The venous drainage is extensive and forms a plexus with numerous anastomoses. In addition, the veins communicate with the dorsal vein of the clitoris, the veins of the labia minora, and the perineal veins, as well as with the inferior hemorrhoidal plexus. On each side, the posterior labial veins connect with the external pudendal vein, terminating in the great saphenous vein (saphena magna) just prior to its entrance (saphenous opening) in the fossa ovalis. This large plexus is frequently manifested by the presence of large varicosities during pregnancy.

E. Lymphatics

The lymphatics of the labia majora are extensive and utilize 2 systems, one lying superficially (under the skin) and the other deeper, within the subcutaneous tissues. From the upper two-thirds of the left and right labia majora, superficial lymphatics pass toward the symphysis and turn laterally to join the medial superficial inguinal nodes. These nodes drain into the superficial inguinal nodes overlying the saphenous fossa. The drainage flows into and through the femoral ring (fossa ovalis) to the nodi lymphatici inguinales profundi (nodes of Rosenmuller or Cloquet; deep subinguinal nodes), connecting with the external iliac chain. The superficial subinguinal nodes, situated over the femoral trigone, also accept superficial drainage from the lower extremity and the gluteal region. This drainage may include afferent lymphatics from the perineum. In the region of the symphysis pubica, the lymphatics anastomose in a plexus between the right and left nodes. Therefore, any lesion involving the labia majora allows direct involvement of the lymphatic structures of the contralateral inguinal area. The lower part of the labium majus has superficial and deep drainage that is shared with the perineal area. The drainage passes, in part, through afferent lymphatics to superficial subinguinal nodes; from the posterior medial aspects of the labia majora, it frequently enters the lymphatic plexus surrounding the rectum.

F. Nerves

The innervation of the external genitalia has been studied by many investigators. The iliohypogastric nerve originates from T12 and L1 and traverses laterally to the iliac crest between the transversus and internal oblique muscles, at which point it divides into 2 branches: (1) the anterior hypogastric nerve, which descends anteriorly through the skin over the symphysis, supplying the superior portion of the labia majora and the mons pubis, and (2) the posterior iliac, which passes to the gluteal area.

The ilioinguinal nerve originates from L1 and follows a course slightly inferior to the iliohypogastric nerve, with which it may frequently anastomose, branching into many small fibers that terminate in the upper medial aspect of the labium majus.

The genitofemoral nerve (L1–L2) emerges from the anterior surface of the psoas muscle to run obliquely downward over its surface, branching in the deeper substance of the labium majus to supply the dartos muscle and that vestige of the cremaster present within the labium majus. Its lumboinguinal branch continues downward onto the upper part of the thigh.

From the sacral plexus, the posterior femoral cutaneous nerve, originating from the posterior divisions of S1 and S2 and the anterior divisions of S2 and S3, divides into several rami that, in part, are called the perineal branches. They supply the medial aspect of the thigh and the labia majora. These branches of the posterior femoral cutaneous nerve are derived from the sacral plexus. The pudendal nerve, composed primarily of S2, S3, and S4, often with a fascicle of S1, sends a small number of fibers to the medial aspect of the labia majora. The pattern of nerve endings is illustrated in Table 2–1.

Labia Minora

A. Superficial Anatomy

The labia minora are 2 folds of skin that lie within the rima pudendi and measure approximately 5 cm in length and 0.5–1 cm in thickness. The width varies according to age and parity, measuring 2–3 cm at its narrowest diameter to 5–6 cm at it widest, with multiple corrugations over the surface. The labia minora begin at the base of the clitoris, where fusion of the labia is continuous with the prepuce, extending posteriorly and medially to the labia majora at the posterior commissure. On their medial aspects superiorly beneath the clitoris, they unite to form the frenulum adjacent to the urethra and vagina, terminating along the hymen on

Table 2–1. Quantitative distribution of nerve endings in selected regions of the female genitalia.

	Touch			Pressure	Pain	Other Types	
	Meissner Corpuscles[1]	Merkel Tactile Disks[1]	Peritrichous Endings	Vater-Pacini Corpuscles[2]	Free Nerve Endings	Ruffini Corpuscles[2]	Dogiel and Krause Corpuscles[3]
Mons pubis	++++	++++	++++	+++	+++	++++	+
Labia majora	+++	++++	++++	+++	+++	+++	+
Clitoris	+	+	0	++++	+++	+++	+++
Labia minora	+	+	0	+	+	+	+++
Hymenal ring	0	+	0	0	+++	0	0
Vagina	0	0	0	0	+ Occasionally	0	0

[1]Also called corpuscula tactus.
[2]Also called corpuscula lamellosa.
[3]Also called corpuscula bulboidea.

the right and left sides of the fossa navicularis and ending posteriorly in the frenulum of the labia pudendi, just superior to the posterior commissure. A deep cleft is formed on the lateral surface between the labium majus and the labium minus. The skin on the labia minora is smooth and pigmented. The color and distention vary, depending on the level of sexual excitement and the pigmentation of the individual. The glands of the labia are homologous to the glandulae preputiales (glands of Littre) of the penile portion of the male urethra.

B. Arteries

The main source of arterial supply (Fig 2–12) occurs through anastomoses from the superficial perineal artery, branching from the dorsal artery of the clitoris, and from the medial aspect of the rete of the labia majora. Similarly, the venous pattern and plexus are extensive.

C. Veins

The venous drainage is to the medial vessels of the perineal and vaginal veins, directly to the veins of the labia majora, to the inferior hemorrhoidals posteriorly, and to the clitoral veins superiorly.

D. Lymphatics

The lymphatics medially may join those of the lower third of the vagina superiorly and the labia majora laterally, passing to the superficial subinguinal nodes and to the deep subinguinal nodes. In the midline, the lymphatic drainage coincides with that of the clitoris, communicating with that of the labia majora to drain to the opposite side.

E. Nerves

The innervation of the labia minora originates, in part, from fibers that supply the labia majora and from branches of the pudendal nerve as it emerges from the canalis pudendalis (Alcock's canal) (Fig 2–12). These branches originate from the perineal nerve. The labia minora and the vestibule area are homologous to the skin of the male urethra and penis. The short membranous portion, approximately 0.5 cm of the male urethra, is homologous to the midportion of the vestibule of the female.

Clitoris

A. Superficial Anatomy

The clitoris is the homologue of the dorsal part of the penis and consists of 2 small erectile cavernous bodies, terminating in a rudimentary glans clitoridis. The erectile body, the corpus clitoridis, consists of the 2 crura clitoridis and the glans clitoridis, with overlying skin and prepuce, a miniature homologue of the glans penis. The crura extend outward bilaterally to their position in the anterior portion of the vulva. The cavernous tissue, homologous to the corpus spongiosum penis of the male, appears in the vascular pattern of the labia minora in the female. At the lower border of the pubic arch, a small triangular fibrous band extends onto the clitoris (suspensory ligament) to separate the 2 crura, which turn inward, downward, and laterally at this point, close to the inferior rami of the pubic symphysis. The crura lie inferior to the ischiocavernosus muscles and bodies. The glans is situated superiorly at the fused termination of the crura. It is composed of erectile tissue and contains an integument, hoodlike in shape,

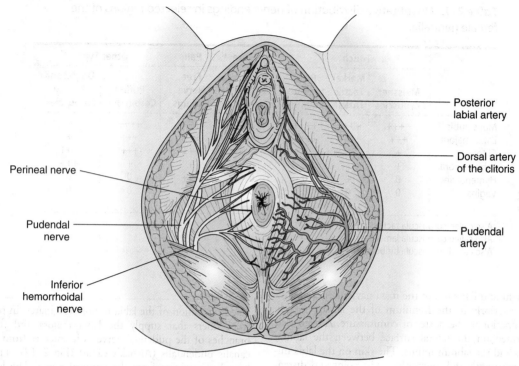

Posterior
labial artery

Dorsal artery
of the clitoris

Perineal nerve

Pudendal artery

Pudendal
nerve

Inferior
hemorrhoidal
nerve

Figure 2–12. Arteries and nerves of perineum.

termed the prepuce. On its ventral surface, there is a frenulum clitoridis, the fused junction of the labia minora.

B. ARTERIES

The blood supply to the clitoris is from its dorsal artery, a terminal branch of the internal pudendal artery, which is the terminal division of the posterior portion of the internal iliac (hypogastric) artery. As it enters the clitoris, it divides into 2 branches, the deep and dorsal arteries. Just before entering the clitoris itself, a small branch passes posteriorly to supply the area of the external urethral meatus.

C. VEINS

The venous drainage of the clitoris begins in a rich plexus around the corona of the glans, running along the anterior surface to join the deep vein and continuing downward to join the pudendal plexus from the labia minora, labia majora, and perineum, forming the pudendal vein.

D. LYMPHATICS

The lymphatic drainage of the clitoris coincides primarily with that of the labia minora, the right and left sides having access to contralateral nodes in the superficial

inguinal chain. In addition, its extensive network provides further access downward and posteriorly to the external urethral meatus toward the anterior portion of the vestibule.

E. NERVES

The innervation of the clitoris is through the terminal branch of the pudendal nerve, which originates from the sacral plexus as previously discussed. It lies on the lateral side of the dorsal artery and terminates in branches within the glans, corona, and prepuce. The nerve endings in the clitoris vary from a total absence within the glans to a rich supply primarily located within the prepuce (Table 2–1). A total absence of endings within the clitoris itself takes on clinical significance when one considers the emphasis placed on the clitoris in discussing problems of sexual gratification in women.

Vestibule

A. SUPERFICIAL ANATOMY

The area of the vestibule is bordered by the labia minora laterally, by the frenulum labiorum pudendi (or posterior commissure) posteriorly, and by the urethra and clitoris anteriorly. Inferiorly, it is bordered by the hymenal ring. The opening of the vagina or junction of the vagina with the vestibule is limited by a membrane stretching from the posterior and lateral sides to the inferior surface of the external urethral orifice. This membrane is termed the hymen. Its shape and openings vary and depend on age, parity, and sexual experience. The form of the opening may be infantile, annular, semilunar, cribriform, septate, or vertical; the hymen may even be imperforate. In parous women and in the postcoital state, the tags of the hymenal integument are termed carunculae myrtiformes. The external urethral orifice, which is approximately 2–3 cm posterior to the clitoris, on a slightly elevated and irregular surface with depressed areas on the sides, may appear to be stellate or crescentic in shape. It is characterized by many small mucosal folds around its opening. Bilaterally and on the surface are the orifices of the para- and periurethral glands (ductus paraurethrales [ducts of Skene and Astruc]). At approximately the 5 and 7 o'clock positions, just external to the hymenal rings, are 2 small papular elevations that represent the orifices of the ducts of the glandulae vestibulares majores, or larger vestibular glands (Bartholin) of the female (bulbourethral gland of the male). The fossa navicularis lies between the frenulum labiorum pudendi and the hymenal ring. The skin surrounding the vestibule is stratified squamous in type, with a paucity of rete pegs and papillae.

B. Arteries

The blood supply to the vestibule is an extensive capillary plexus that has anastomoses with the superficial transverse perineal artery. A branch comes directly from the pudendal anastomosis with the inferior hemorrhoidal artery in the region of the fossa navicularis; the blood supply of the urethra anteriorly, a branch of the dorsal artery of the clitoris and the azygos artery of the anterior vaginal wall, also contributes.

C. Veins

Venous drainage is extensive, involving the same areas described for the arterial network.

D. Lymphatics

The lymphatic drainage has a distinct pattern. The anterior portion, including that of the external urethral meatus, drains upward and outward with that of the labia minora and the clitoris. The portion next to the urethral meatus may join that of the anterior urethra, which empties into the vestibular plexus to terminate in the superficial inguinal nodes, the superficial subinguinal nodes, the deep subinguinal nodes, and the external iliac chain. The lymphatics of the fossa navicularis and the hymen may join those of the posterior vaginal wall, intertwining with the intercalated lymph nodes along the rectum, which follow the inferior hemorrhoidal arteries. This pattern becomes significant with cancer. Drainage occurs through the pudendal and the hemorrhoidal chain and through the vestibular plexus onto the inguinal region.

E. Nerves

The innervation of the vestibular area is primarily from the sacral plexus through the perineal nerve. The absence of the usual modalities of touch is noteworthy. The vestibular portion of the hymenal ring contains an abundance of free nerve endings (pain).

Vestibular Glands

The glandulae vestibulares majores (larger vestibular glands or Bartholin glands) have a duct measuring approximately 5 mm in diameter. The gland itself lies just inferior and lateral to the bulbocavernosus muscle. The gland is tubular and alveolar in character, with a thin capsule and connective tissue septa dividing it into lobules in which occasional smooth muscle fibers are found. The epithelium is cuboid to columnar and pale in color, with the cytoplasm containing mucigen droplets and colloid spherules with acidophilic inclusions. The epithelium of the duct is simple in type, and its orifice is stratified squamous like the vestibule. The secretion is a clear, viscid, and stringy mucoid substance with an alkaline pH. Secretion is active during sexual activity. Nonetheless, after about age 30, the glands undergo involution and become atrophic and shrunken.

The arterial supply to the greater vestibular gland comes from a small branch of the artery on the bulbocavernosus muscle, penetrating deep into its substance. Venous drainage coincides with the drainage of the bulbocavernosus body. The lymphatics drain directly into the lymphatics of the vestibular plexus, having access to the posterior vaginal wall along the inferior hemorrhoidal channels. They also drain via the perineum into the inguinal area. Most of this minor drainage is along the pudendal vessels in the canalis pudendalis and explains, in part, the difficulty in dealing with cancer involving the gland.

The greater vestibular gland is homologous to the bulbourethral gland (also known as Cowper's glands, Duverney's glands, Tiedemann's glands, or the Bartholin glands of the male). The innervation of the greater vestibular gland is from a small branch of the perineal nerve, which penetrates directly into its substance.

Muscles of External Genitalia

The muscles (Fig 2–13) of the external genitalia and cavernous bodies in the female are homologous to those of the male, although they are less well developed.

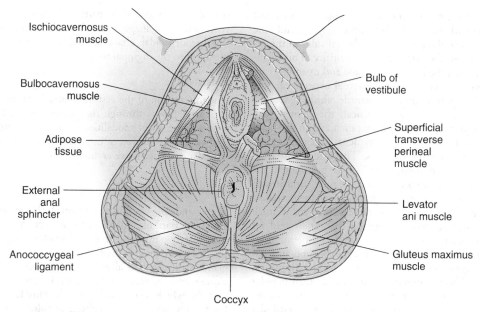

Ischiocavernosus muscle

Bulbocavernosus muscle

Adipose tissue

External anal sphincter

Anococcygeal ligament

Bulb of vestibule

Superficial transverse perineal muscle

Levator ani muscle

Gluteus maximus muscle

Coccyx

Figure 2–13. Pelvic musculature (inferior view).

A. BULBOCAVERNOSUS MUSCLE

The bulbocavernosus muscle and deeper bulbus vestibuli or cavernous tissue arise in the midline from the posterior part of the central tendon of the perineum, where each opposes the fibers from the opposite side. Each ascends around the vagina, enveloping the bulbus vestibuli (the corpus cavernosum bodies of the male) to terminate in 3 heads: (1) the fibrous tissue dorsal to the clitoris, (2) the tunica fibrosa of the corpus cavernosa overlying the crura of the clitoris, and (3) decussating fibers that join those of the ischiocavernosus to form the striated sphincter of the urethra at the junction of its middle and lower thirds. The blood supply is derived from the perineal branch of the internal pudendal artery as it arises in the anterior part of the ischiorectal fossa. Deep to the fascia diaphragmatis urogenitalis inferior (Colles' fascia) and crossing between the ischiocavernosus and bulbocavernosus muscles, the pudendal artery sends 1–2 branches directly into the bulbocavernosus muscle and vestibular body, continuing anteriorly to terminate in the dorsal artery of the clitoris. The venous drainage accompanies the pudendal plexus. In addition, it passes posteriorly with the inferior hemorrhoidal veins and laterally with the perineal vein, a branch of the internal pudendal vein. The lymphatics run primarily with those of the vestibular plexus, with drainage inferiorly toward the intercalated nodes of the rectum and anteriorly and laterally with the labia minora and majora to the superficial inguinal

nodes. Contralateral drainage in the upper portion of the muscle and body is evident.

B. ISCHIOCAVERNOSUS MUSCLE

The ischiocavernosus muscle and its attendant cavernous tissue arise from the ischial tuberosity and inferior ramus to the ischium. It envelops the crus of its cavernous tissue in a thin layer of muscle ascending toward and over the medial and inferior surfaces of the symphysis pubica to terminate in the anterior surface of the symphysis at the base of the clitoris. It then sends decussating fibers to the region of the upper and middle thirds of the urethra, forming the greater part of the organ's voluntary sphincter. The blood supply is through perforating branches from the perineal artery as it ascends between the bulbocavernosus and ischiocavernosus muscles to terminate as the dorsal artery of the clitoris. The innervation stems from an ischiocavernosus branch of the perineal division of the pudendal nerve.

C. TRANSVERSUS MUSCLE

The transversus perinei superficialis muscle arises from the inferior ramus of the ischium and from the ischial tuberosity. The fibers of the muscle extend across the perineum and are inserted into its central tendon, meeting those from the opposite side. Frequently, the muscle fibers from the bulbocavernosus, the puborectalis, the superficial transverse perinei, and occasionally the external anal sphincter will interdigitate. The blood supply is from a perforating branch of the perineal division of the internal pudendal artery, and the nerve supply is from the perineal division of the pudendal nerve.

D. Sensory Corpuscles

In the cavernous substances of both the bulbocavernosus and ischiocavernosus muscles, Vater-Pacini corpuscles (corpuscula lamellosa) and Dogiel and Krause corpuscles (corpuscula bulboidea) are present.

E. Inferior Layer of Urogenital Diaphragm

The inferior layer of urogenital diaphragm is a potential space depending upon the size and development of the musculature, the parity of the female, and the pelvic architecture. It contains loose areolar connective tissue interspersed with fat. The bulbocavernosus muscles, with the support of the superficial transverse perinei muscles and the puborectalis muscles, act as a point of fixation on each side for support of the vulva, the external genitalia, and the vagina.

F. Surgical Considerations

A midline perineotomy is most effective to minimize trauma to vital supports of the vulva, bulbocavernosus, and superficial transverse perinei muscles. Overdistention of the vagina caused by the presenting part and body of the infant forms a temporary sacculation. If distention occurs too rapidly or if dilatation is beyond the resilient capacity of the vagina, rupture of the vaginal musculature may occur, often demonstrated by a cuneiform groove on the anterior wall and a tonguelike protrusion on the posterior wall of the vagina. Therefore, return of the vagina and vulva to the nonpregnant state is dependent upon the tonus of the muscle and the degree of distention of the vagina during parturition.

BONY PELVIS

The pelvis (Fig 2–14) is a basin-shaped ring of bones that marks the distal margin of the trunk. The pelvis rests upon the lower extremities and supports the spinal column. It is composed of 2 innominate bones, one on each side, joined anteriorly and articulated with the sacrum posteriorly. The 2 major pelvic divisions are the pelvis major (upper or false pelvis) and the pelvis minor (lower or true pelvis). The pelvis major consists primarily of the space superior to the iliopectineal line, including the 2 iliac fossae and the region between them. The pelvis minor, located below the iliopectineal line, is bounded anteriorly by the pubic bones, posteriorly by the sacrum and coccyx, and laterally by the ischium and a small segment of the ilium.

Innominate Bone

The innominate bone is composed of 3 parts: ilium, ischium, and pubis.

A. Ilium

The ilium consists of a bladelike upper part or ala (wing) and a thicker, lower part called the body. The body forms the upper portion of the acetabulum and unites with the bodies of the ischium and pubis. The medial surface of the ilium presents as a large concave area: The anterior portion is the iliac fossa; the smaller posterior portion is composed of a rough upper part, the iliac tuberosity; and the lower part contains a large surface for articulation with the sacrum. At the inferior medial margin of the iliac fossa, a rounded ridge, the arcuate line, ends anteriorly in the iliopectineal eminence. Posteriorly, the arcuate line is continuous with the anterior margin of the ala of the sacrum across the anterior aspect of the sacroiliac joint. Anteriorly, it is continuous with the ridge or pecten on the superior ramus of the pubis. The lateral surface or dorsum of the ilium is traversed by 3 ridges: the posterior, anterior, and inferior gluteal lines. The superior border is called the crest, and at its 2 extremities are the anterior and posterior superior iliac spines. The principal feature of the anterior border of the ilium is the heavy anterior inferior iliac spine. Important aspects of the posterior border are the posterior superior and the inferior iliac spines and, below the latter, the greater sciatic notch, the inferior part of which is bounded by the ischium. The inferior border of the ilium participates in the formation of the acetabulum.

The main vasculature (Fig 2–15) of the innominate bone appears where the bone is thickest. Blood is supplied to the inner surface of the ilium through twigs of the iliolumbar, deep circumflex iliac, and obturator arteries by foramens on the crest, in the iliac fossa, and below the terminal line near the greater sciatic notch. The outer surface of the ilium is supplied mainly below the inferior gluteal line through nutrient vessels derived from the gluteal arteries. The inferior branch of the deep part of the superior gluteal artery forms the external nutrient artery of the ilium and continues in its course to anastomose with the lateral circumflex artery. Upon leaving the pelvis below the piriform muscle, it divides into a number of branches, a group of which passes to the hip joint.

B. Ischium

The ischium is composed of a body, superior and inferior rami, and a tuberosity. The body is the heaviest part of the bone and is joined with the bodies of the ilium and pubis to form the acetabulum. It presents 3 surfaces: (1) The smooth internal surface is continuous

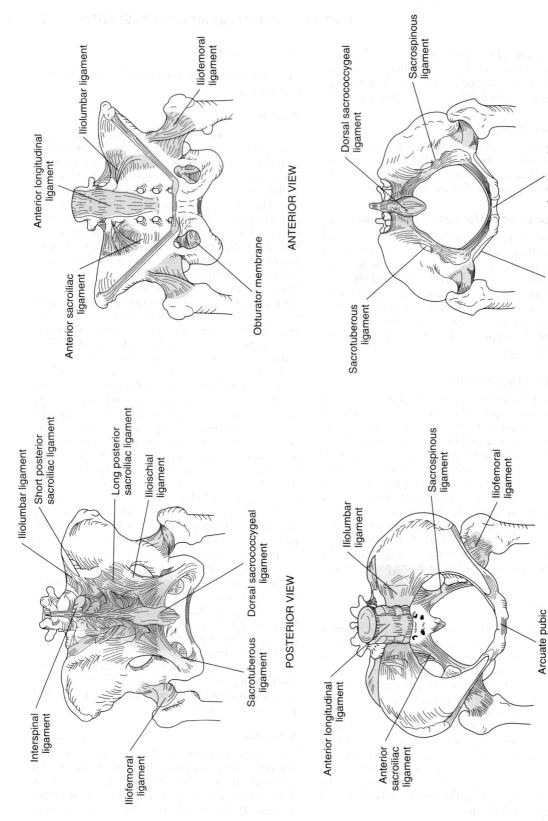

ANTERIOR VIEW

Anterior longitudinal ligament

Iliolumbar ligament

Iliofemoral ligament

Anterior sacroiliac ligament

Obturator membrane

INFERIOR VIEW

Dorsal sacrococcygeal ligament

Sacrospinous ligament

Arcuate pubic ligament

Sacrotuberous ligament

Inguinal ligament

POSTERIOR VIEW

Iliolumbar ligament

Short posterior sacroiliac ligament

Long posterior sacroiliac ligament

Ilioischial ligament

Dorsal sacrococcygeal ligament

Interspinal ligament

Iliofemoral ligament

Sacrotuberous ligament

SUPERIOR VIEW

Iliolumbar ligament

Sacrospinous ligament

Iliofemoral ligament

Anterior longitudinal ligament

Anterior sacroiliac ligament

Arcuate pubic ligament

Figure 2–14. **The bony pelvis.** (Reproduced, with permission, from Benson RC: *Handbook of Obstetrics & Gynecology,* 8th ed. Lange, 1983.)

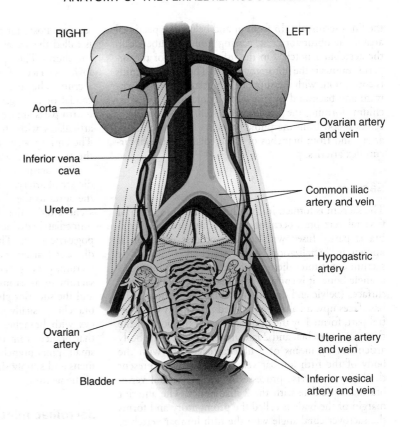

RIGHT

LEFT

Aorta

Ovarian artery
and vein

Inferior vena
cava

Common iliac
artery and vein

Ureter

Hypogastric
artery

Ovarian
artery

Uterine artery
and vein

Bladder

Inferior vesical
artery and vein

Figure 2–15. Blood supply to
pelvis.

above with the body of the ilium and below with the inner surface of the superior ramus of the ischium. Together, these parts form the posterior portion of the lateral wall of the pelvis minor. (2) The external surface of the ischium is the portion that enters into the formation of the acetabulum. (3) The posterior surface is the area between the acetabular rim and the posterior border. It is convex and is separated from the ischial tuberosity by a wide groove. The posterior border, with the ilium, forms the bony margin of the greater sciatic notch. The superior ramus of the ischium descends from the body of the bone to join the inferior ramus at an angle of approximately 90 degrees. The large ischial tuberosity and its inferior portion are situated on the convexity of this angle. The inferior portion of the tuberosity forms the point of support in the sitting position. The posterior surface is divided into 2 areas by an oblique line. The lesser sciatic notch occupies the posterior border of the superior ramus between the spine and the tuberosity. The inferior ramus, as it is traced forward, joins the inferior ramus of the pubis to form the arcus pubis (ischiopubic arch).

The ischium is supplied with blood from the obturator medial and lateral circumflex arteries. The largest vessels are situated between the acetabulum and the sciatic tubercle.

C. PUBIS

The pubis is composed of a body and 2 rami, superior and inferior. The body contributes to the formation of the acetabulum, joining with the body of the ilium at the iliopectineal eminence and with the body of the ischium in the region of the acetabular notch. The superior ramus passes medially and forward from the body to meet the corresponding ramus of the opposite side at the symphysis pubica. The medial or fore portion of the superior ramus is broad and flattened anteroposteriorly. Formerly called "the body," it presents an outer and an inner surface, the symphyseal area, and an upper border or "crest." Approximately 2 cm from the medial edge of the ramus and in line with the upper border is the prominent pubic tubercle, an important landmark. Below the crest is the anterior surface and the posterior or deep surface. The medial portion of the superior ramus is continuous below with the inferior ramus, and the lateral part presents a wide, smooth area anterosuperiorly, behind which is an irregular ridge, the pecten ossispubis. The pecten pubis forms the anterior part of the linea terminalis. In front of and below the pectineal area is the obturator crest, passing from the tubercle to the acetabular notch. On the inferior aspect of the superior ramus is the obturator sulcus. The inferior ramus is continuous with the superior ramus and passes downward and backward to join the inferior ramus of the ischium, forming the "ischiopubic arch." The pubis receives blood from the pubic branches of the obturator artery and from branches of the medial and lateral circumflex arteries.

Sacrum

The sacrum is formed in the adult by the union of 5 or 6 sacral vertebrae; occasionally, the fifth lumbar vertebra is partly fused with it. The process of union is known as "sacralization" in the vertebral column. The sacrum constitutes the base of the vertebral column. As a single bone, it is considered to have a base, an apex, 2 surfaces (pelvic and dorsal), and 2 lateral portions. The base faces upward and is composed principally of a central part, formed by the upper surface of the body of the first sacral vertebra, and 2 lateral areas of alae. The body articulates by means of a fibrocartilage disk with the body of the fifth lumbar vertebra. The alae represent the heavy transverse processes of the first sacral vertebra that articulate with the 2 iliac bones. The anterior margin of the body is called the promontory and forms the sacrovertebral angle with the fifth lumbar vertebra. The rounded anterior margin of each ala constitutes the posterior part (pars sacralis) of the linea terminalis. The pelvic surface of the sacrum is rough and convex. In the midline is the median sacral crest (fused spinal processes), and on either side is a flattened area formed by the fused laminae of the sacral vertebrae. The laminae of the fifth vertebra and, in many cases, those of the fourth and occasionally of the third are incomplete (the spines also are absent), thus leaving a wide opening to the dorsal wall of the sacral canal known as the sacral hiatus. Lateral to the laminae are the articular crests (right and left), which are in line with the paired superior articular processes above. The lateral processes articulate with the inferior articular processes of the fifth lumbar vertebra. The inferior extensions of the articular crests form the sacral cornua that bind the sacral hiatus laterally and are attached to the cornua of the coccyx. The cornua can be palpated in life and are important landmarks indicating the inferior opening of the sacral canal (for sacral-caudal anesthesia). The lateral portions of the sacrum are formed by the fusion of the transverse processes of the sacral vertebrae. They form dorsally a line of elevations called the lateral sacral crests. The parts corresponding to the first 3 vertebrae are particularly massive and present a large area facing laterally called the articular surface, which articulates with the

sacrum. Posterior to the articular area, the rough bone is called the sacral tuberosity. It faces the tuberosity of the ilium. The apex is the small area formed by the lower surface of the body of the fifth part of the sacrum. The coccyx is formed by 4 (occasionally 3 or 5) caudal or coccygeal vertebrae. The second, third, and fourth parts are frequently fused into a single bone that articulates with the first by means of a fibrocartilage. The entire coccyx may become ossified and fused with the sacrum (the sacrococcygeal joint).

The sacrum receives its blood supply from the middle sacral artery, which extends from the bifurcation of the aorta to the tip of the coccyx, and from the lateral sacral arteries that branch either as a single artery that immediately divides or as 2 distinct vessels from the hypogastric artery. The lowest lumbar branch of the middle sacral artery ramifies over the lateral parts of the sacrum, passing back between the last vertebra and the sacrum to anastomose with the lumbar arteries above and the superior gluteal artery below. The lateral sacral branches (usually 4) anastomose anteriorly to the coccyx with branches of the inferior lateral sacral artery that branch from the hypogastric artery. They give off small spinal branches that pass through the sacral foramens and supply the sacral canal and posterior portion of the sacrum.

Sacroiliac Joint

The sacroiliac joint is a diarthrodial joint with irregular surfaces. The articular surfaces are covered with a layer of cartilage, and the cavity of the joint is a narrow cleft. The cartilage on the sacrum is hyaline in its deeper parts but much thicker than that on the ilium. A joint capsule is attached to the margins of the articular surfaces, and the bones are held together by the anterior sacroiliac, long and short posterior sacroiliac, and interosseous ligaments. In addition, there are 3 ligaments (Fig 2–16), classed as belonging to the pelvic girdle itself, which also serve as accessory ligaments to the sacroiliac joint: the iliolumbar, sacrotuberous, and sacrospinous ligaments. The anterior sacroiliac ligaments unite the base and the lateral part of the sacrum to the ilium, blending with the periosteum of the pelvic surface and, on the ilium, reaching the arcuate line to attach in the paraglenoid grooves. The posterior sacroiliac ligament is extremely strong and consists essentially of 2 sets of fibers, deep and superficial, forming the short and long posterior sacroiliac ligaments, respectively. The short posterior sacroiliac ligament passes inferiorly and medially from the tuberosity of the ilium, behind the articular surface and posterior interior iliac spine, to the back of the lateral portion of the sacrum and to the upper sacral articular process, including the area between it and the first sacral foramen. The long

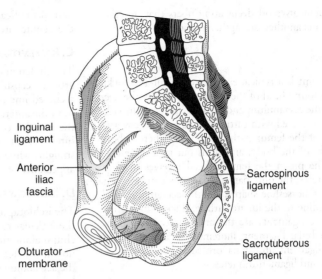

Inguinal
ligament

Anterior
iliac
fascia

Sacrospinous
ligament

Obturator
membrane

Sacrotuberous
ligament

Figure 2–16. Ligaments of the pelvis.

posterior sacroiliac ligament passes inferiorly from the posterior superior iliac spine to the second, third, and fourth articular tubercles on the back of the sacrum. It partly covers the short ligament and is continuous below with the sacrotuberous ligament. The interosseous ligaments are the strongest of all and consist of fibers of different lengths passing in various directions between the 2 bones. They extend from the rough surface of the sacral tuberosity to the corresponding surface on the lateral aspect of the sacrum, above and behind the articular surface.

Ligaments

The sacrotuberous ligament, in common with the long posterior sacroiliac ligament, is attached above to the crest of the ilium and posterior iliac spines and to the posterior aspect of the lower 3 sacral vertebrae. Below, it is attached chiefly to the medial border of the ischial tuberosity. Some of the fibers at the other end extend forward along the inner surface of the ischial ramus, forming the falciform process. Other posterior fibers continue into the tendons of the hamstrings.

The sacrospinous ligament is triangular and thin, extending from the lateral border of the sacrum and coccyx to the spine of the ischium. It passes medially (deep) to the sacrotuberous ligament and is partly blended with it along the lateral border of the sacrum.

The iliolumbar ligament connects the fourth and fifth lumbar vertebrae with the iliac crest. It originates from the transverse process of the fifth lumbar vertebra, where it is closely woven with the sacrolumbar ligament. Some of its fibers spread downward onto the body of the fifth vertebra and others ascend to the disk

above. It is attached to the inner lip of the crest of the ilium for approximately 5 cm. The sacrolumbar ligament is generally inseparable from the iliolumbar ligament and is regarded as part of it.

Pubic Symphysis

The pubic symphysis is a synarthrodial joint of the symphyseal surfaces of the pubic bones. The ligaments associated with it are (1) the interpubic fibrocartilage, (2) the superior pubic ligament, (3) the anterior pubic ligament, and (4) the arcuate ligament. The interpubic fibrocartilage is thicker in front than behind and projects beyond the edges of the bones, especially on the posterior aspect, blending intimately with the ligaments at its margins. Sometimes it is woven throughout, but often the interpubic fibrocartilage presents an elongated, narrow fissure with fluid in the interspace, partially dividing the cartilage into 2 plates. The interpubic cartilage is intimately adherent to the layer of hyaline cartilage that covers the symphyseal surface of each pubic bone. The superior pubic ligament extends laterally along the crest of the pubis on each side to the pubic tubercle, blending in the middle line with the interpubic cartilage. The thick and strong anterior pubic ligament is closely connected with the fascial covering of the muscles arising from the conjoined rami of the pubis. It consists of several strata of thick, decussating fibers of different degrees of obliquity, the superficial being the most oblique and extending lowest over the joint. The arcuate ligament is a thick band of closely connected fibers that fills the angle between the pubic rami to form a smooth, rounded top to the pubic arch. Both on the anterior and posterior aspects of the joint, the ligament gives off decussating fibers that, interlacing with one another, strengthen the joint.

Hip Joint

The hip joint is a typical example of a ball-and-socket joint, the round head of the femur received by the deep cavity of the acetabulum and glenoid lip. Both articular surfaces are coated with cartilage. The portion covering the head of the femur is thicker above, where it bears the weight of the body, and thins out to a mere edge below. The pit in the femoral head receives the ligamentum teres, the only part uncoated by cartilage. The cartilage is horseshoe-shaped on the acetabulum and, corresponding to the lunate surface, thicker above than below. The ligaments are the articular capsule, transverse acetabular ligament, iliofemoral ligament, ischiocapsular ligament and zona orbicularis, pubocapsular ligament, and ligamentum teres.

A. Articular Capsule

The articular capsule is one of the strongest ligaments in the body. It is attached superiorly to the base of the anterior inferior iliac spine at the pelvis, posteriorly to a point a few millimeters from the acetabular rim, and inferiorly to the upper edge of the groove between the acetabulum and tuberosity of the ischium. Anteriorly, it is secured to the pubis near the obturator groove, to the iliopectineal eminence, and posteriorly to the base of the inferior iliac spine. At the femur, the articular capsule is fixed to the anterior portion of the superior border of the greater trochanter and to the cervical tubercle. The capsule runs down the intertrochanteric line as far as the medial aspect of the femur, where it is on a level with the inferior part of the lesser trochanter. It then runs superiorly and posteriorly along an oblique line, just in front of and above the lesser trochanter, and continues along the back of the neck of the femur nearly parallel to and above the intertrochanteric crest. Finally, the capsule passes along the medial side of the trochanteric fossa to reach the anterior superior angle of the greater trochanter. Some of the deeper fibers, the retinacula, are attached nearer the head of the femur. One corresponds to the upper and another to the lower part of the intertrochanteric line; a third is present at the upper and back part of the trochanteric neck.

B. Transverse Acetabular Ligament

The transverse ligament of the acetabulum passes across the acetabular notch. It supports the glenoid lip and is connected with the ligamentum teres and the capsule. The transverse ligament is composed of decussating fibers that arise from the margin of the acetabulum on either side of the notch. Those fibers coming from the pubis are more superficial and pass to form the deep

part of the ligament at the ischium; those superficial at the ischium are deep at the pubis.

C. Iliofemoral Ligament

The iliofemoral ligament is located at the front of the articular capsule and is triangular. Its apex is attached to a curved line on the ilium immediately below and behind the anterior inferior spine; its base is fixed beneath the anterior edge of the greater trochanter and to the intertrochanteric line. The upper fibers are almost straight, while the medial fibers are oblique, giving the appearance of an inverted Y.

D. Ischiocapsular Ligament

The ischiocapsular ligament, on the posterior surface of the articular capsule, is attached to the body of the ischium along the upper border of the notch. Above the notch, the ligament is secured to the ischial margin of the acetabulum. The upper fibers incline superiorly and laterally and are fixed to the greater trochanter. The other fibers curve more and more upward as they pass laterally to their insertion at the inner side of the trochanteric fossa. The deeper fibers take a circular course and form a ring at the back and lower parts of the capsule, where the longitudinal fibers are deficient. This ring, the zona orbicularis, embraces the neck of the femur.

E. Pubocapsular Ligament

The pubocapsular ligament is fixed proximally to the obturator crest and to the anterior border of the iliopectineal eminence, reaching as far down as the pubic end of the acetabular notch. Below, the fibers reach to the neck of the femur and are fixed above and behind the lowermost fibers of the iliofemoral band, blending with it.

F. Ligamentum Teres

The ligamentum teres femoris extends from the acetabular fossa to the head of the femur. It has 2 bony attachments, one on either side of the acetabular notch immediately below the articular cartilage, with intermediate fibers springing from the lower surface of the transverse ligament. At the femur, the ligamentum teres femoris is fixed to the anterior part of the fovea capitis and to the cartilage around the margin of the depression.

Outlets of the True Pelvis

The true pelvis is said to have an upper "inlet" and a lower "outlet." The pelvic inlet to the pelvis minor is bounded, beginning posteriorly, by (1) the promontory of the sacrum; (2) the linea terminalis, composed of the anterior margin of the alasacralis, the arcuate line of the ilium, and the pecten ossis pubis; and (3) the upper border or crest of the pubis, ending medially at the symphysis. The conjugate or the anteroposterior diameter is drawn from the center of the promontory to the symphysis pubica, with 2 conjugates recognized: (1) the true conjugate, measured from the promontory to the top of the symphysis, and (2) the diagonal conjugate, measured from the promontory to the bottom of the symphysis. The transverse diameter is measured through the greatest width of the pelvic inlet. The oblique diameter runs from the sacroiliac joint of one side to the iliopectineal eminence of the other. The pelvic outlet, which faces downward and slightly backward, is very irregular. Beginning anteriorly, it is bounded by (1) the arcuate ligament of the pubis (in the midline), (2) the ischiopubic arch, (3) the ischial tuberosity, (4) the sacrotuberous ligament, and (5) the coccyx (in midline). Its anteroposterior diameter is drawn from the lower border of the symphysis pubica to the tip of the coccyx. The transverse diameter passes between the medial surfaces of the ischial tuberosities.

Musculature Attachments

A. ILIUM

The crest of the ilium gives attachment to the external oblique, internal oblique, transversus (anterior two-thirds), latissimus dorsi and quadratus lumborum (pos-

teriorly), sacrospinalis (internal lip, posteriorly), and tensor fasciae latae and sartorius muscles (anterior superior iliac spine) (Fig 2–17). The posterior superior spine of the ilium gives attachment to the multifidus muscle. The rectus femoris muscle is attached to the anterior inferior iliac spine. The iliacus muscle originates on the iliac fossa. Between the anterior inferior iliac spine and the iliopectineal eminence is a broad groove for the tendon of the iliopsoas muscle. A small portion of the gluteus maximus muscle originates between the posterior gluteus line and the crest. The surface of bone between the anterior gluteal line and the crest gives origin to the gluteus medius muscle. The gluteus minimus muscle has its origin between the anterior and inferior gluteal lines.

B. ISCHIUM

The body and superior ramus of the ischium give rise to the obturator internus muscle on the internal surface. The ischial spine provides, at its root, attachments for the coccygeus and levator ani muscles on its internal surface and for the gemellus superior muscle externally. The outer surface of the ramus is the origin of the adductor magnus and obturator externus muscles. The transversus perinei muscle is attached to the lower border of the ischium. The ischial tuberosity gives rise on its posterior surface to the semimembranosus muscles, the common tendon of the biceps, and semitendinosus muscles and on its inferior surface to the adductor magnus muscle. The

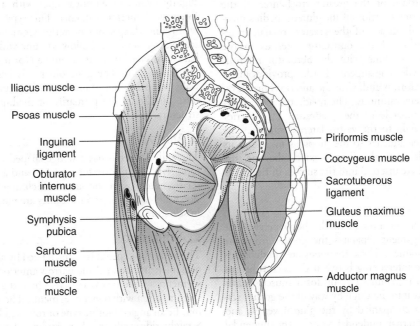

Figure 2–17. Pelvic muscles.

superior border is the site of origin of the inferior gemellus and the outer border of the quadratus femoris muscle. The superior ramus of the pubis gives origin to the adductor longus and obturator externus muscles on its anterior surface and to the levator ani and obturator internus muscles. The superior border provides attachment for the rectus abdominis and pyramidalis muscles. The pectineal surface gives origin at its posterior portion to the pectineus muscle. The posterior surface of the superior ramus is the point of attachment of a few fascicles of the obturator internus muscle. The anterior surface of the inferior ramus attaches to the abductor brevis, adductor magnus, and obturator externus muscles, and its posterior surface attaches to the sphincter urogenitalis and the obturator internus.

C. SACRUM

The pelvic surface of the sacrum is the origin of the piriform muscle. The lateral part of the fifth sacral vertebra is the point of insertion of the sacrospinalis and gluteus maximus muscles. The ala is attached to fibers of the iliacus muscle.

D. COCCYX

The dorsal surface of the coccyx is attached to the gluteus maximus muscle and the sphincter ani externus muscle. The lateral margins receive parts of the coccygeus and of the iliococcygeus muscles.

E. GREATER TROCHANTER

The lateral surface of the greater trochanter of the femur receives the insertion of the gluteus medius muscle. The medial surface of the greater trochanter receives the tendon of the obturator externus in the trochanteric fossa, along with the obturator internus and the 2 gemelli. The superior border provides insertion for the piriformis and, with the anterior border, receives the gluteus minimus. The quadratus femoris attaches to the tubercle of the quadratus. The inferior border gives origin to the vastus lateralis muscle. The lesser trochanter attaches to the iliopsoas muscle at its summit. Fascicles of the iliacus extend beyond the trochanter and are inserted into the surface of the shaft.

Foramens

Several foramens are present in the bony pelvis. The sacrospinous ligament separates the greater from the lesser sciatic foramen. These foramens are subdivisions of a large space intervening between the sacrotuberous ligament and the femur. The piriform muscle passes out of the pelvis into the thigh by way of the greater sciatic foramen, accompanied by the gluteal vessels and nerves. The internal pudendal vessels, the pudendal nerve, and the nerve to the obturator internus muscle

also leave the pelvis by this foramen, after which they then enter the perineal region through the lesser sciatic foramen. The obturator internus muscle passes out of the pelvis by way of the lesser sciatic foramen.

The obturator foramen is situated between the ischium and the pubis. The obturator membrane occupies the obturator foramen and is attached continuously to the inner surface of the bony margin except above, where it bridges the obturator sulcus, converting the latter into the obturator canal, which provides passage for the obturator nerve and vessels.

On either side of the central part of the pelvic surface of the sacrum are 4 anterior sacral foramens that transmit the first 4 sacral nerves. Corresponding to these on the dorsal surface are the 4 posterior sacral foramens for transmission of the small posterior rami of the first 4 sacral nerves.

Types of Pelves

Evaluation of the pelvis is best achieved by using the criteria set by Caldwell and Moloy, which are predicated upon 4 basic types of pelves: (1) the gynecoid type (from Greek *gyne* woman); (2) the android type (from Greek *aner* man); (3) the anthropoid type (from Greek *anthropos* human); and (4) the platypelloid type (from Greek *platys* broad and *pella* bowl) (Fig 2–18).

A. GYNECOID

In pure form, the gynecoid pelvis provides a rounded, slightly ovoid, or elliptical inlet with a well-rounded forepelvis (anterior segment). This type of pelvis has a well-rounded, spacious posterior segment, an adequate sacrosciatic notch, a hollow sacrum with a somewhat backward sacral inclination, and a Norman-type arch of the pubic rami. The gynecoid pelvis has straight side walls and wide interspinous and intertuberous diameters. The bones are primarily of medium weight and structure.

B. ANDROID

The android pelvis has a wedge-shaped inlet, a narrow forepelvis, a flat posterior segment, and a narrow sacrosciatic notch, with the sacrum inclining forward. The side walls converge, and the bones are medium to heavy in structure.

C. ANTHROPOID

The anthropoid pelvis is characterized by a long, narrow, oval inlet; an extended and narrow anterior and posterior segment; a wide sacrosciatic notch; and a long, narrow sacrum, often with 6 sacral segments. The subpubic arch may be an angled Gothic type or rounded Norman type. Straight side walls are characteristic of the anthropoid pelvis, whose interspinous and intertuberous diameters

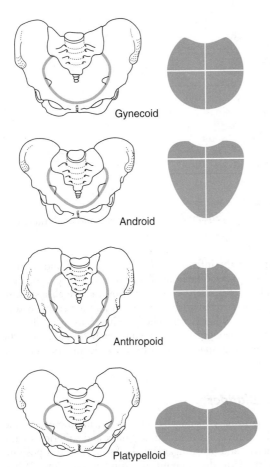

Figure 2–18. Types of pelves. White lines in the diagrams at right (after Steele) show the greatest diameters of the pelves at left. (Reproduced, with permission, from Benson RC: *Handbook of Obstetrics & Gynecology,* 8th ed. Lange, 1983.)

are less than those of the average gynecoid pelvis. A medium bone structure is usual.

D. Platypelloid

The platypelloid pelvis has a distinct oval inlet with a very wide, rounded retropubic angle and a wider, flat posterior segment. The sacrosciatic notch is narrow and has a normal sacral inclination, although it is often short. The subpubic arch is very wide and the side walls are straight, with wide interspinous and intertuberous diameters.

The pelvis in any individual case may be one of the 4 "pure" types or a combination of mixed types. When one discusses the intermediate pelvic forms, the posterior segment with its characteristics generally is de-

scribed first and the anterior segment with its characteristics next, eg, anthropoid-gynecoid, android-anthropoid, or platypelloid-gynecoid. Obviously, it is impossible to have a platypelloid-anthropoid pelvis or a platypelloid-android pelvis.

Pelvic Relationships

Several important relationships should be remembered, beginning with those at the inlet of the pelvis. The transverse diameter of the inlet is the widest diameter, where bone is present for a circumference of 360 degrees. This diameter stretches from pectineal line to pectineal line and denotes the separation of the posterior and anterior segments of the pelvis. In classic pelves (gynecoid), a vertical plane dropped from the transverse diameter of the inlet passes through the level of the interspinous diameter at the ischial spine. These relationships may not hold true, however, in combination or intermediate (mixed type) pelves. The anterior transverse diameter of the inlet reaches from pectineal prominence to pectineal prominence; a vertical plane dropped from the anterior transverse passes through the ischial tuberosities. For good function of the pelvis, the anterior transverse diameter should never be more than 2 cm longer than the transverse diameter (Fig 2–19).

A. Obstetric Conjugate

The obstetric conjugate differs from both the diagonal conjugate and the true conjugate. It is represented by a line drawn from the posterior superior portion of the pubic symphysis (where bone exists for a circumference of 360 degrees) toward intersection with the sacrum. This point need not be at the promontory of the sacrum. The obstetric conjugate is divided into 2 segments: (1) the anterior sagittal, originating at the intersection of the obstetric conjugate with the transverse diameter of the inlet and terminating at the symphysis pubica, and (2) the posterior sagittal, originating at the transverse diameter of the inlet to the point of intersection with the sacrum.

B. Interspinous Diameter

A most significant diameter in the midpelvis is the interspinous diameter. It is represented by a plane passing from ischial spine to ischial spine. The posterior sagittal diameter of the midpelvis is a bisecting line drawn at a right angle from the middle of the interspinous diameter, in the same plane, to a point of intersection with the sacrum. This is the point of greatest importance in the midpelvis. It is sometimes said that the posterior sagittal diameter should be drawn from the posterior segment of the intersecting line of the interspinous diameter, in a plane from the inferior surface of the symphysis, through the interspinous diameter to the sacrum. However, this

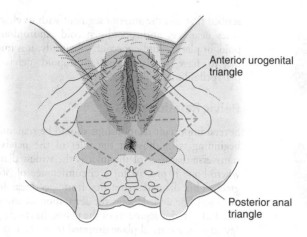

Anterior urogenital triangle

Posterior anal triangle

Figure 2–19. Urogenital and anal triangles.

configuration often places the posterior sagittal diameter lower in the pelvis than the interspinous diameter. It is the interspinous diameter, together with the posterior sagittal diameter of the midpelvis, that determines whether or not there is adequate room for descent and extension of the head during labor.

C. INTERTUBEROUS DIAMETER

The intertuberous diameter of the outlet will reflect the length of the anterior transverse diameter of the inlet, ie, the former cannot be larger than the latter if convergent or straight side walls are present. Therefore, the intertuberous diameter determines the space available in the anterior segment of the pelvis at the inlet, and, similarly, the degree of convergence influences the length of the biparietal diameter at the outlet.

D. POSTERIOR SAGITTAL DIAMETER

The posterior sagittal diameter of the outlet is an intersecting line drawn from the middle of the intertuberous diameter to the sacrococcygeal junction and reflects the inclination of the sacrum toward the outlet for accommodation of the head at delivery. It should be noted that intricate measurements of the pelvis are significant only at minimal levels. Evaluation of the pelvis for a given pregnancy, size of the fetus for a given pelvis, and conduct of labor engagement are far more important.

CONTENTS OF THE PELVIC CAVITY

The organs that occupy the female pelvis (Figs 2–20 to 2–22) are the bladder, the ureters, the urethra, the uterus, the uterine (fallopian) tubes or oviducts, the ovaries, the vagina, and the rectum.* With the excep-

tion of the inferior portion of the rectum and most of the vagina, all lie immediately beneath the peritoneum. The uterus, uterine tubes, and ovaries are almost completely covered with peritoneum and are suspended in peritoneal ligaments. The remainder are partially covered. These organs do not completely fill the cavity; the remaining space is occupied by ileum and sigmoid colon.

1. Bladder

The urinary bladder is a muscular, hollow organ that lies posterior to the pubic bones and anterior to the uterus and broad ligament. Its form, size, and position vary with the amount of urine it contains. When empty, it takes the form of a somewhat rounded pyramid, having a base, a vertex (or apex), a superior surface, and a convex inferior surface that may be divided by a median ridge into 2 inferolateral surfaces.

Relationships

The superior surface of the bladder is covered with peritoneum that is continuous with the medial umbilical fold, forming the paravesical fossae laterally. Posteriorly, the peritoneum passes onto the uterus at the junction of the cervix and corpus, continuing upward on the anterior surface to form the vesicouterine pouch. When the bladder is empty, the normal uterus rests upon its superior surface. When the bladder is distended, coils of intestine may lie upon its superior surface. The base of the bladder rests below the peritoneum and is adjacent to the cervix and the anterior fornix of the vagina. It is separated from these structures by areolar tissue containing plexiform veins. The area over the vagina is extended as the bladder fills. The inferolateral surfaces are separated from the wall of

* The rectum is not described in this chapter.

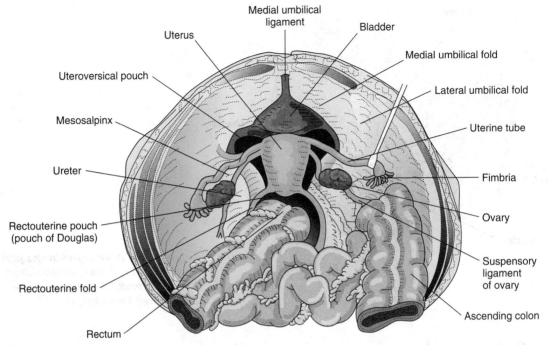

Figure 2-20. Female pelvic contents from above.

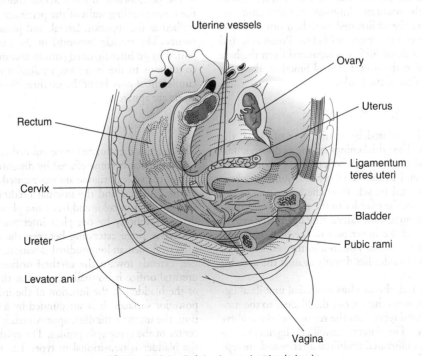

Figure 2-21. Pelvic viscera (sagittal view).

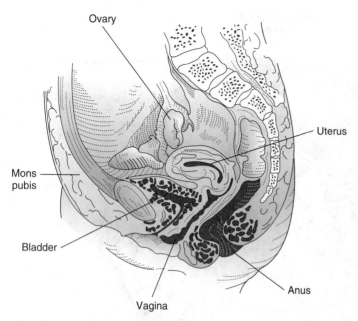

Figure 2–22. Pelvic organs (midsagittal view). (Reproduced, with permission, from Benson RC: *Handbook of Obstetrics & Gynecology*, 8th ed. Lange, 1983.)

the pelvis by the potential prevesical space, containing a small amount of areolar tissue but no large vessels. This surface is nonperitoneal and thus suitable for operative procedures. Posterolateral to the region facing the symphysis, each of the inferolateral surfaces is in relation to the fascia of the obturator internus, the obturator vessels and nerve, the obliterated umbilical artery above, and the fascia of the levator ani below. Posteriorly and medially, the inferior surface is separated from the base by an area called the urethrovesical junction, the most stationary portion of the bladder.

Fascia, Ligaments, & Muscle

The bladder is enclosed by a thin layer of fascia, the vesical sheath. Two thickenings of the endopelvic fascia, the medial and lateral pubovesical or puboprostatic ligaments, extend at the vesicourethral junction abutting the levator ani muscle from the lower part of the anterior aspect of the bladder to the pubic bones. Similar fascial thickenings, the lateral true ligaments, extend from the sides of the lower part of the bladder to the lateral walls of the pelvis. Posteriorly, the vesicourethral junction of the bladder lies directly against the anterior wall of the vagina.

A fibrous band, the urachus or medial umbilical ligament, extends from the apex of the bladder to the umbilicus. This band represents the remains of the embryonic allantois. The lateral umbilical ligaments are formed by the obliterated umbilical arteries and are represented by fibrous cords passing along the sides of the

bladder and ascending toward the umbilicus. Frequently, the vessels will be patent, thus forming the superior vesical arteries. The peritoneal covering of the bladder is limited to the upper surface. The reflections of the peritoneum to the anterior abdominal wall and the corresponding walls of the pelvis are sometimes described as the superior, lateral, and posterior false ligaments. The muscle (smooth) of the bladder is represented by an interdigitated pattern continuous with and contiguous to the inner longitudinal and anterior circumferential muscles of the urethra. No distinct muscle layers are apparent.

Mucous Membrane

The mucous membrane is rose-colored and lies in irregular folds that become effaced by distention. The 3 angles of the vesical trigone are represented by the orifices of the 2 ureters and the internal urethral orifice. This area is redder in color and free from plication. It is bordered posteriorly by the plica interureterica, a curved transverse ridge extending between the orifices of the ureters. A median longitudinal elevation, the uvula vesicae, extends toward the urethral orifice. The internal urethral orifice is normally situated at the lowest point of the bladder, at the junction of the inferolateral and posterior surfaces. It is surrounded by a circular elevation, the urethral annulus, approximately level with the center of the symphysis pubica. The epithelial lining of the bladder is transitional in type. The mucous membrane rests on the submucous coat, composed of areolar tissue superficial to the muscular coat. There is no evidence of a specific smooth muscle sphincter in the vesical neck.

Arteries, Veins, & Lymphatics

The blood supply to the bladder comes from branches of the hypogastric artery. The umbilical artery, a terminal branch of the hypogastric artery, gives off the superior vesical artery prior to its obliterated portion. It approaches the bladder (along with the middle and inferior vesical arteries) through a condensation of fatty areolar tissue, limiting the prevesical "space" posterosuperiorly, to branch out over the upper surface of the bladder. It anastomoses with the arteries of the opposite side and the middle and inferior vesical arteries below. The middle vesical artery may arise from one of the superior vessels, or it may come from the umbilical artery, supplying the sides and base of the bladder. The inferior vesical artery usually arises directly from the hypogastric artery–in common with or as a branch of the uterine artery–and passes downward and medially, where it divides into branches that supply the lower part of the bladder. The fundus may also receive small branches from the middle hemorrhoidal, uterine, and vaginal arteries.

The veins form an extensive plexus at the sides and base of the bladder from which stems pass to the hypogastric trunk.

The lymphatics, in part, accompany the veins and communicate with the hypogastric nodes (Table 2–2). They also communicate laterally with the external iliac glands, and some of those from the fundus pass to nodes situated at the promontory of the sacrum. The lymphatics of the bladder dome are separate on the right and left sides and rarely cross; but extensive anastomoses are present among the lymphatics of the base, which also involve those of the cervix.

Nerves

The nerve supply to the bladder is derived partly from the hypogastric sympathetic plexus and partly from the second and third sacral nerves (the nervi erigentes).

2. Ureters

Relationships

The ureter is a slightly flattened tube that extends from the termination of the renal pelvis to the lower outer corner of the base of the bladder, a distance of 26–28 cm. It is partly abdominal and partly pelvic and lies entirely behind the peritoneum. Its diameter varies from 4 to 6 mm, depending on distention, and its size is uniform except for 3 slightly constricted portions. The first of these constrictions is found at the junction of the ureter with the renal pelvis and is known as the upper isthmus. The second constriction–the lower isthmus–is at the point where the ureter crosses the brim of the pelvis minor. The third (intramural) constriction is at the terminal part of the ureter as it passes through the bladder wall. The pelvic portion of the ureter begins as the ureter crosses the pelvic brim beneath the ovarian vessels and near the bifurcation of the common iliac artery. It conforms to the curvature of the lateral pelvic wall, inclining slightly laterally and posteriorly until it reaches the pelvic floor. The ureter then bends anteriorly and medially at about the level of the ischial spine to reach the bladder. In its upper portion, it is related posteriorly to the sacroiliac articulation; then, lying upon the obturator internus muscle and fascia, it crosses the root of the umbilical artery, the obturator vessels, and the obturator nerve. In its anterior relationship, the ureter emerges from behind the ovary and under its vessels to pass behind the uterine and superior and middle vesical arteries. Coursing anteriorly, it comes into close relation with the lateral fornix of the vagina, passing 8–12 mm from the cervix and vaginal wall before reaching the bladder. When the ureters reach the bladder, they are about 5 cm apart. They pass through the bladder wall on an oblique course (about 2 cm long) and in an anteromedial and downward direction. The ureters open into the bladder by 2 slitlike apertures, the urethral orifices, about 2.5 cm apart when the bladder is empty.

Wall of Ureter

The wall of the ureter is approximately 3 mm thick and is composed of 3 coats: connective tissue, muscle, and mucous membrane. The muscular coat has an external circular and an internal longitudinal layer throughout its course and an external longitudinal layer in its lower third. The mucous membrane is longitudinally plicated and covered by transitional epithelium. The intermittent peristaltic action of the ureteral musculature propels urine into the bladder in jets. The oblique passage of the ureter through the bladder wall tends to constitute a valvular arrangement, but no true valve is present. The circular fibers of the intramural portion of the ureter possess a sphincterlike action. Still, under some conditions of overdistention of the bladder, urine may be forced back into the ureter.

Arteries, Veins, & Lymphatics

The pelvic portion of the ureter receives its blood supply from a direct branch of the hypogastric artery, anastomosing superiorly in its adventitia with branches from the iliolumbar and inferiorly with branches from the in-

Table 2–2. Lymphatics of the female pelvis.

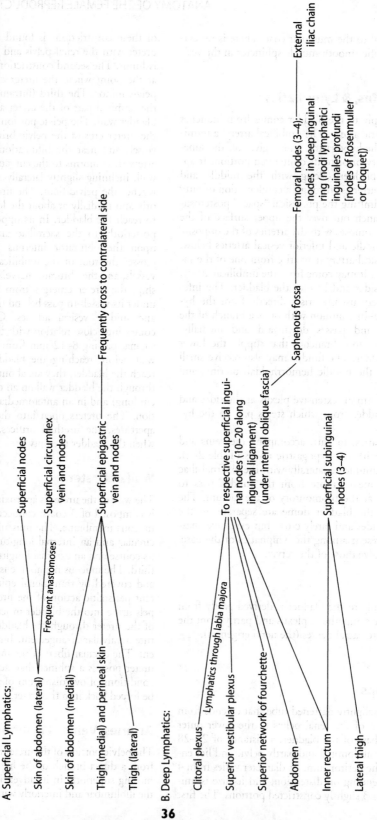

A. Superficial Lymphatics:

Skin of abdomen (lateral) —————— Superficial nodes

Skin of abdomen (medial) —————— Superficial circumflex
                                              vein and nodes
        Frequent anastomoses

Thigh (medial) and perineal skin ——— Superficial epigastric
                                              vein and nodes —— Frequently cross to contralateral side

Thigh (lateral)

B. Deep Lymphatics:

Clitoral plexus

        Lymphatics through labia majora

Superior vestibular plexus ——— To respective superficial ingui-
                                       nal nodes (10–20 along
                                       inguinal ligament)
Superior network of fourchette   (under internal oblique fascia) ——— Saphenous fossa ——— Femoral nodes (3–4); ——— External
                                                                                                        nodes in deep inguinal   iliac chain
                                                                                                        ring (nodi lymphatici
                                                                                                        inguinales profundi
                                                                                                        [nodes of Rosenmuller
                                                                                                        or Cloquet])

Abdomen

Inner rectum ——— Superficial subinguinal
                         nodes (3–4)

Lateral thigh

Vagina

Mucosal plexus ── Inferiorly ────── Introitus ──────────── Superficial ──────── Femoral external iliac chain
                                    Superficial vestibular   subinguinal nodes
                                    plexus

            └─ Superiorly ────── Superficial ── Anastomose with those
                                 inguinal nodes   of cervix (see below)

Muscular plexus ──── Laterally 4 trunks: ──── Hypogastrics
                     2 posterior trunks,   ── External iliac chain
                     2 anterior trunks

              ──── Upper part of vagina ──── Lateral sacral nodes

              ──── Posterior wall (intertwine ──── Rectal stalk
                   with those of rectum)

Cervix

Vaginal plexus ──── Cervical plexus ──── Lateral sacral nodes
                    3 trunks   ── Broad ligament, ── Lumbar chain
                                         uterine pedicle

              ──── Uterine plexus ──── Isthmus ──── External iliac chain
                                       (portio of cervix)

                    Lower portion of corpus
                    of uterus

(continued)

Table 2-2. Lymphatics of the female pelvis. (continued)

Uterus

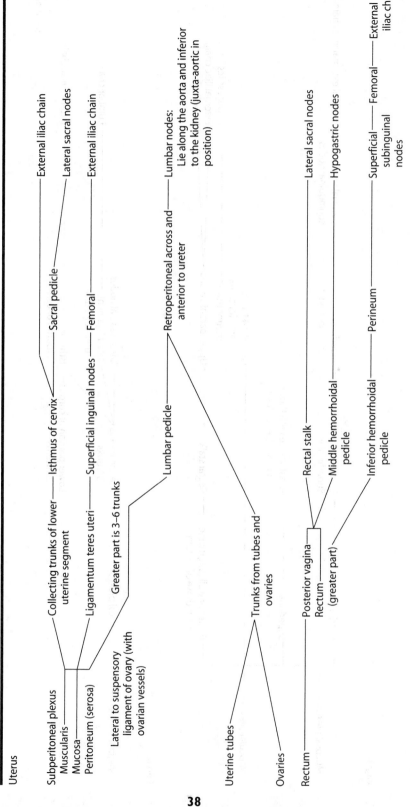

Subperitoneal plexus ——— Collecting trunks of lower ——— Isthmus of cervix ——— Sacral pedicle ——— Lateral sacral nodes
Muscularis   uterine segment
Mucosa ——————————————————————————————— Isthmus of cervix ——— Sacral pedicle ——— External iliac chain
Peritoneum (serosa) ——— Ligamentum teres uteri ——— Superficial inguinal nodes ——— Femoral ——— External iliac chain

Lateral to suspensory
ligament of ovary (with
ovarian vessels)

Greater part is 3–6 trunks

Lumbar pedicle ——— Retroperitoneal across and
                          anterior to ureter

Lumbar nodes:
Lie along the aorta and inferior
to the kidney (juxta-aortic in
position)

Uterine tubes

Ovaries

Trunks from tubes and
ovaries

Rectum ——— Posterior vagina ——— Rectal stalk ——— Lateral sacral nodes
              Rectum
              (greater part) ——— Middle hemorrhoidal ——— Hypogastric nodes
                                  pedicle

Inferior hemorrhoidal ——— Perineum ——— Superficial ——— Femoral ——— External
pedicle   subinguinal   iliac chain
                                     nodes

38

Ureters

Lower third ——— Along hypogastric vessels ——— Along common iliac vessels ——— Large nodes, sacral group on promontory ——— Periaortic chain

——— Obliterated hypogastrics ——— External iliac group (a node is often present on umbilical artery)

——— Up the ureters to the middle portion ——— Periaortic nodes interaorticocaval nodes

Middle third, right ——— Ureteral arteries depend on origin of vessel ———
- Common iliac
- Hypogastric
- Aorta
- Ovarian

——— Lateral sacral nodes
——— Hypogastric node
——— Interaorticocaval chain (on top of vena cava) (near origin of ovarian artery)

——— Along ureter ——— External iliac chain

Middle third, left ——— Similar to right except across sacral promontory ——— Right iliac chain

——— Along ureteral arteries (more extensive spread) ——— Ovarian artery ——— Lumbar chain ——— Preaortic chain (at origin of inferior mesenteric artery)

——— Left lateral lumbar

Upper third ——— Upward on the ureter to the hilum of the kidney to 3 nodes ——— Renal pedicle

Lateral lumbar nodes ——— Above kidney ——— Thoracic duct ——— Node ——— Heart, etc.

Interaorticocaval nodes

(continued)

Table 2-2. Lymphatics of the female pelvis. (continued)

Urethra

Anterior urethra	Vestibular plexus	Superficial inguinal nodes	Superficial subinguinal nodes	Femoral	External iliac chain

Posterior urethra

1. Anterior superior part	Trunks	Interior bladder wall	Lateral inferior border of umbilical artery		Middle chain, external iliacs
2. Anterolateral	Trunks	Lateral bladder wall			Internal chain, external iliac group at the obturator nerve (obturator node)
Posteriorly along internal pundental artery					Hypogastrics at bifurcation of external and internal iliacs
Ischiorectal fossa	Canalis pudendalis (Alcock's canal)	3 nodes	Greater sciatic foramen	Along inferior gluteal artery — Onto obturator artery	Lateral sacral nodes, hypogastric nodes

3. Posterior aspect

Urethrovaginal septum	Cervix	Uterine plexus	Over ureter	Along unmbilical ligaments — Lower uterine pedicle	Middle chain, external iliac nodes, hypogastric nodes

Bladder

Right and left sides remain separate	1. Anterior bladder wall	(Laterally along umbilical ligaments)	One trunk near ureter	(Frequent anastomoses between cervix, vagina, and fundus; large vessels upper third, medium middle third, small lower third)	Nodes of posterior abdominal group
	2. Posterior bladder wall				

ferior vesical and middle hemorrhoidal arteries. Lymphatic drainage passes along the hypogastric vessels to the hypogastric and external iliac nodes, continuing up the ureters to their middle portion where drainage is directed to the periaortic and interaorticocaval nodes (Table 2–2).

Nerves

The nerve supply is provided by the renal, ovarian, and hypogastric plexuses. The spinal level of the afferents is approximately the same as the kidney (T12, L1, L2). The lower third of the ureter receives sensory fibers and postganglionic parasympathetic fibers from the Frankenhauser plexus and sympathetic fibers through this plexus as it supplies the base of the bladder. These fibers ascend the lower third of the ureter, accompanying the arterial supply. The middle segment appears to receive postganglions of sympathetic and parasympathetic fibers through and from the middle hypogastric plexus. The upper third is supplied by the same innervation as the kidney.

3. Urethra

Relationships

The female urethra is a canal 2.5–5.25 cm long. It extends downward and forward in a curve from the neck of the bladder (internal urethral orifice), which lies nearly opposite the symphysis pubica. Its termination, the external urethral orifice, is situated inferiorly and posteriorly from the lower border of the symphysis. Posteriorly, it is closely applied to the anterior wall of the vagina, especially in the lower two-thirds, where it is actually integrated with the wall, forming the urethral carina. Anteriorly, the upper end is separated from the prevesical "space" by the pubovesical (puboprostatic) ligaments, abutting against the levator ani and vagina and extending upward onto the pubic rami.

Anatomy of Walls

The walls of the urethra are very distensible, composed of spongy fibromuscular tissue containing cavernous veins and lined by submucous and mucous coats. The mucosa contains numerous longitudinal lines when undistended, the most prominent of which is located on the posterior wall and termed the crista urethralis. Also, there are numerous small glands (the homologue of the male prostate, para- and periurethral glands of Astruc, ducts of Skene) that open into the urethra. The largest of these, the paraurethral glands of Skene, may open via a pair of ducts beside the external urethral orifice in the vestibule. The epithelium begins as transitional at the upper end and becomes squamous in the lower part. External to the urethral lumen is a smooth muscle coat composed of an outer circular layer and an inner longitudinal layer in the lower two-thirds. In the upper third, the muscle bundles of the layers interdigitate in a basketlike weave to become continuous with and contiguous to those of the bladder. The entire urethral circular smooth muscle acts as the involuntary sphincter. In the region of the juncture of the middle and lower thirds of the urethra, decussating fibers (striated in type) form the middle heads of the bulbo- and ischiocavernosus muscles and encircle the urethra to form the sphincter urethrae (voluntary sphincter).

Arteries & Veins

The arterial supply is intimately involved with that of the anterior vaginal wall, with cruciate anastomoses to the bladder. On each side of the vagina are the vaginal arteries, originating in part from the coronary artery of the cervix, the inferior vesical artery, or a direct branch of the uterine artery. In the midline of the anterior vaginal wall is the azygos artery, originating from the coronary or circular artery of the cervix. Approximately 5 branches traverse the anterior vaginal wall from the lateral vaginal arteries to the azygos in the midline, with small sprigs supplying the urethra. A rich anastomosis with the introitus involves the clitoral artery (urethral branches) as the artery divides into the dorsal and superficial arteries of the clitoris, a terminal branch of the internal pudendal artery. The venous drainage follows the arterial pattern, although it is less well defined. In the upper portion of the vagina, it forms an extensive network called the plexus of Santorini (Table 2–3).

Lymphatics

The lymphatics are richly developed (Fig 2–23). Those of the anterior urethra drain to the vestibular plexus, the superficial inguinal nodes, the superficial subinguinal nodes, and the femoral and external iliac chain. The lymphatic drainage of the posterior urethra can be divided into 3 aspects: the anterior superior, anterolateral, and posterior. The anterior superior portion drains to the anterior bladder wall and up the lateral inferior border of the umbilical artery to the middle chain of the external iliacs. The anterolateral portion drains in several directions. Part extends to the lateral bladder wall and onto the internal chain of the external iliacs at the obturator nerve or to the hypogastrics at the bifurcation of the external and internal iliacs. Another part drains into the ischiorectal fossa and through the canalis pudendalis (Alcock's canal), following the inferior gluteal artery and obturator artery to the lateral sacral and hypogastric nodes. The posterior aspect of the drainage is into the urethrovaginal septum, onto the cervix and the uterine plexus, over the ureter, and along

Table 2–3. Arterial supply to the female pelvis.

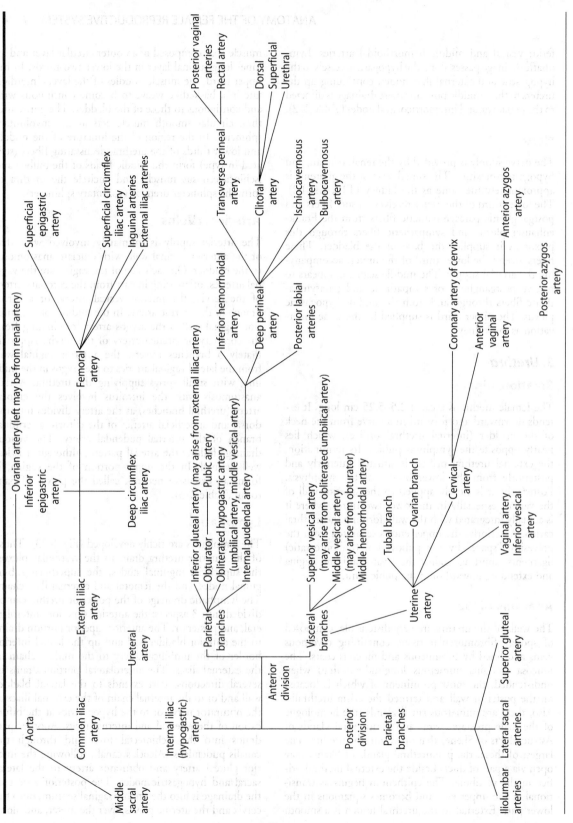

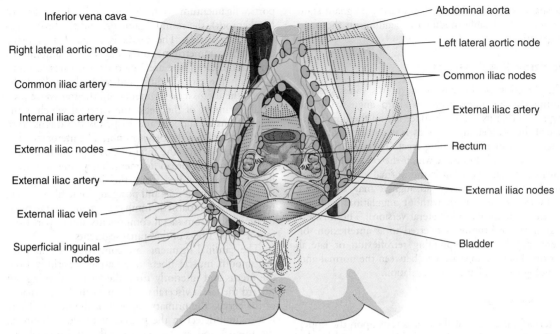

Figure 2–23. Lymphatic drainage of pelvis.

the umbilical ligaments to the middle chain of the external iliacs or to the lower uterine pedicle and the hypogastrics.

Nerves

The nerve supply is parasympathetic, sympathetic, and spinal. The parasympathetic and sympathetic nerves are derived from the hypogastric plexus; the spinal supply is via the pudendal nerve.

4. Uterus

Anatomy

The uterus is a pear-shaped, thick-walled, muscular organ, situated between the base of the bladder and the rectum. Covered on each side by the 2 layers of the broad ligament, it communicates above with the uterine tubes and below with the vagina. It is divided into 2 main portions, the larger portion or body above and the smaller cervix below, connected by a transverse constriction, the isthmus. The body is flattened so that the side-to-side dimension is greater than the anteroposterior dimension and larger in women who have borne children. The anterior or vesical surface is almost flat; the posterior surface is convex. The uterine tubes join the uterus at the superior (lateral) angles. The round

portion that extends above the plane passing through the points of attachment of the 2 tubes is termed the fundus. This portion is the region of greatest breadth. The cavity of the body, when viewed from the front or back, is roughly triangular with the base up. The communication of the cavity below with the cavity of the cervix corresponds in position to the isthmus and forms the internal orifice (internal os uteri). The cervix is somewhat barrel-shaped, its lower end joining the vagina at an angle varying from 45 to 90 degrees. It projects into the vagina and is divided into a supravaginal and a vaginal portion by the line of attachment. About one-fourth of the anterior surface and half of the posterior surface of the cervix belong to the vaginal portion. At the extremity of the vaginal portion is the opening leading to the vagina, the external orifice (external os uteri), which is round or oval before parturition but takes the form of a transverse slit in women who have borne children. It is bounded by anterior and posterior labia. The cavity of the cervix is fusiform in shape, with longitudinal folds or furrows, and extends from the internal to the external orifice.

The size of the uterus varies, under normal conditions, at different ages and in different physiologic states. In the adult who has never borne children, it is approximately 7–8 cm long and 4–5 cm at its widest point. In the prepubertal period, it is considerably smaller. In women who have borne children, it is larger.

Its shape, size, and characteristics in the pregnant state become considerably modified depending on the stage of gestation.

Position & Axis Direction

The direction of the axis of the uterus varies greatly. Normally, the uterus forms a sharp angle with the vagina, so that its anterior surface lies on the upper surface of the bladder and the body is in a horizontal plane when the woman is standing erect. There is a bend in the area of the isthmus, at which the cervix then faces downward. This position is the normal anteversion or angulation of the uterus, although it may be placed backward (retroversion), without angulation (military position), or to one side (lateral version). The forward flexion at the isthmus is referred to as anteflexion, or there may be a corresponding retroflexion or lateral flexion. There is no sharp line between the normal and pathologic state of anterior angulation.

Relationships

Anteriorly, the body of the uterus rests upon the upper and posterior surfaces of the bladder, separated by the uterovesical pouch of the peritoneum. The whole of the anterior wall of the cervix is below the floor of this pouch, and it is separated from the base of the bladder only by connective tissue. Posteriorly, the peritoneal covering extends down as far as the uppermost portion of the vagina; therefore, the entire posterior surface of the uterus is covered by peritoneum, and the convex posterior wall is separated from the rectum by the rectouterine pouch (cul-de-sac or pouch of Douglas). Coils of intestine may rest upon the posterior surface of the body of the uterus and may be present in the rectouterine pouch. Laterally, the uterus is related to the various structures contained within the broad ligament: the uterine tubes, the round ligament and the ligament of the ovary, the uterine artery and veins, and the ureter. The relationships of the ureters and the uterine arteries are very important surgically. The ureters, as they pass to the bladder, run parallel with the cervix for a distance of 8–12 mm. The uterine artery crosses the ureter anterosuperiorly near the cervix, about 1.5 cm from the lateral fornix of the vagina. In effect, the ureter passes under the uterine artery "as water flows under a bridge."

Ligaments

Although the cervix of the uterus is fixed, the body is free to rise and fall with the filling and emptying of the bladder. The so-called ligaments supporting the uterus consist of the uterosacral ligaments, the transverse ligaments of the cervix (cardinal ligaments, cardinal supports, ligamentum transversum colli, ligaments of Mackenrodt), the round ligaments, and the broad ligaments (Fig 2–24). The cervix is embedded in tissue called the parametrium, containing various amounts of smooth muscle. There are 2 pairs of structures continuous with the parametrium and with the wall of the cervix: the uterosacral ligaments and the transverse (cardinal) ligament of the neck, the latter of which is the chief means of support and suspends the uterus from the lateral walls of the pelvis minor. The uterosacral ligaments are, in fact, the inferior posterior folds of peritoneum from the broad ligament. They consist primarily of nerve bundles from the inferior hypogastric plexus and contain pre- and postganglionic fibers and C fibers of the sympathetic lumbar segments, parasympathetic in part from sacral components and in part from sensory or C fibers of the spinal segments.

The cardinal ligaments are composed of longitudinal smooth muscle fibers originating superiorly from the uterus and inferiorly from the vagina, fanning out toward the fascia visceralis to form, with the internal os of the cervix, the primary support of the uterus. There is a natural defect in the muscle at its sides (hilum of the uterus) and at the cervical isthmus (internal os), where the vasculature and nerve supply enter the uterus. The round ligaments of the uterus, although forming no real support, may assist in maintaining the body of the uterus in its typical position over the bladder. They consist of fibrous cords containing smooth muscle (longitudinal) from the outer layer of the corpus. From a point of attachment to the uterus immediately below that of the ovarian ligament, each round ligament extends downward, laterally, and forward between the 2 layers of the mesometrium, toward the abdominal inguinal ring that it traverses and the inguinal canal, to terminate in a fanlike manner in the labia majora and become continuous with connective tissue. The round ligament is the gubernaculum (ligamentum teres uteri), vestigial in the female. It is accompanied by a funicular branch of the ovarian artery, by a branch from the ovarian venous plexus, and, in the lower part of its course, by a branch from the inferior epigastric artery, over which it passes as it enters the inguinal ring. Through the inguinal canal, it is accompanied by the ilioinguinal nerve and the external spermatic branch of the genitofemoral nerve.

The broad ligament, consisting of a transverse fold of peritoneum that arises from the floor of the pelvis between the rectum and the bladder, provides minimal support. In addition to the static support of these ligaments, the pelvic diaphragm (levator ani) provides an indirect and dynamic support. These muscles do not actually come in contact with the uterus, but they aid in supporting the vagina and maintain the entire pelvic floor in resisting downward pressure. The effectiveness of

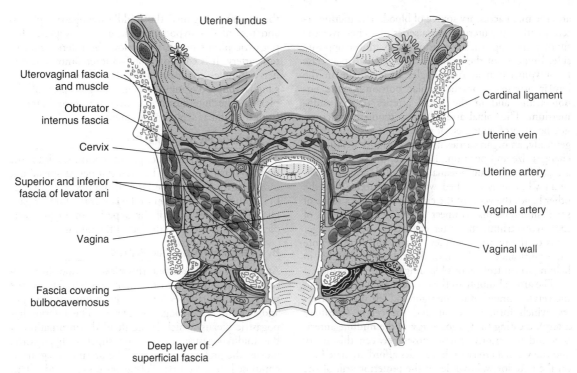

Figure 2–24. Ligamentous and fascial support of pelvic viscera. (Redrawn from original drawings by Frank H. Netter, MD, that first appeared in *Ciba Clinical Symposia,* Copyright ©1950. Ciba Pharmaceutical Co. Reproduced with permission.)

these muscles depends on an intact perineum (perineal body, bulbocavernsous muscle and body), for if it is lacerated or weakened the ligaments will gradually stretch and the uterus will descend. The uterus and its components and the vagina are, in fact, one continuous unit.

Layers of Uterine Wall

The wall of the uterus is very thick and consists of 3 layers: serous, muscular, and mucous. The serous layer (perimetrium) is simply the peritoneal covering. It is thin and firmly adherent over the fundus and most of the body, then thickens posteriorly and becomes separated from the muscle by the parametrium. The muscular layer (myometrium) is extremely thick and continuous with that of the tubes and vagina. It also extends into the ovarian and round ligaments, into the cardinal ligaments at the cervix, and minimally into the uterosacral ligaments. Two principal layers of the muscular coat may be distinguished: (1) the outer layer, which is weaker and composed of longitudinal fibers; and (2) a stronger inner layer, the fibers of which are interlaced and run in various directions, having intermingled within them large venous plexuses. The muscle

layer hypertrophies with the internal os to form a sphincter. The cervix, from the internal os distally, progressively loses its smooth muscle, finally to be entirely devoid of smooth muscle and elastic in its distal half. It is, in fact, the "dead-end tendon" of the uterus, at which point, during the active component of labor, both the uterus and the vagina direct their efforts. The mucous layer (endometrium) is soft and spongy, composed of tissue resembling embryonic connective tissue. The surface consists of a single layer of ciliated columnar epithelium. The tissue is rather delicate and friable and contains many tubular glands that open into the cavity of the uterus.

Arteries

The blood supply to the uterus is from the uterine and ovarian arteries. As a terminal branch of the hypogastric artery, the uterine artery runs downward and medially to cross the ureter near the cervix. It then ascends along the lateral border of the uterus in a tortuous course through the parametrium, giving off lateral branches to both uterine surfaces. Above, it anastomoses to join with the ovarian artery in the mesometrium, which creates the main accessory source of blood. The uterine arteries within the uterus form a series of arches over the fundus, creating cruciate anastomoses with the opposite side. Branches of the arcuate arteries (radial) penetrate the myometrium at right angles to terminate in the basilar arterioles for the basilar portion of the endometrium and in the spinal arteries of the endometrium. The spinal arteries are tortuous in structure, not because of endometrial growth but because, ontogenically, an organ carries its arterial supply with it as it changes size and position. Therefore, the spiral arteries are able to maintain adequate arterial flow to the placenta while it is attached within the uterus. On the other hand, the veins of the endometrium are a series of small sinusoids that connect to the larger sinusoids of the myometrium, the latter coalescing into the larger veins of the uterine complex. It is useful here to note the significance of the muscular role of the uterus in helping to control venous bleeding during parturition.

The arterial supply to the cervix is primarily through the cervical branches of the right and left uterine arteries, which form a rete around the cervix (coronary artery), creating the azygos artery in the midline anteriorly and posteriorly. Anastomoses between this artery and the vaginal artery on both sides afford cruciate flow on the anterior wall, while on the posterior wall of the vagina, anastomoses occur with the right and left middle hemorrhoidal arteries as they supply the wall and the rectum.

Veins

The veins form a plexus and drain through the uterine vein to the hypogastric vein. There are connections with the ovarian veins and the inferior epigastric by way of the vein accompanying the round ligament.

Lymphatics

Lymphatic drainage involves several chains of lymph nodes (Table 2–2). From the subperitoneal plexus, the collecting trunks of the lower uterine segment may drain by way of the cervix to the external iliac chain or by way of the isthmus to the lateral sacral nodes. Drainage along the round ligament progresses to the superficial inguinal nodes, then to the femoral, and finally to the external iliac chain. Drainage laterally to the suspensory ligament of the ovary involves the lumbar pedicle and progresses in a retroperitoneal manner across and anteriorly to the ureter, to the lumbar nodes (interaorticocaval) that lie along the aorta, and inferiorly to the kidney.

Nerves

The pelvic autonomic system can be divided into the superior hypogastric plexus (the presacral plexus and

the uterinus magnus), the middle hypogastric plexus, and the inferior hypogastric plexus. The superior hypogastric plexus begins just below the inferior mesenteric artery. It is composed of 1–3 intercommunicating nerve bundles connected with the inferior mesenteric ganglia, but no ganglia are an integral part of the plexus. The intermesenteric nerves receive branches from the lumbar sympathetic ganglia.

A. Superior Hypogastric Plexus

The superior hypogastric plexus continues into the midhypogastric plexus. The presacral nerves spread out into a lattice-work at the level of the first sacral vertebra, with connecting rami to the last of the lumbar ganglia. The greater part of the superior midhypogastric plexus may be found to the left of the midline.

B. Inferior Hypogastric Plexus

At the first sacral vertebra, this plexus divides into several branches that go to the right and left sides of the pelvis. These branches form the beginning of the right and left inferior hypogastric plexus. The inferior hypogastric plexus, which is the divided continuation of the midhypogastric plexus, the superior hypogastric plexus, the presacral nerve, and the uterinus magnus, is composed of several parallel nerves on each side. This group of nerves descends within the pelvis in a position posterior to the common iliac artery and anterior to the sacral plexus, curves laterally, and finally enters the sacrouterine fold or ligaments. The medial section of the primary division of the sacral nerves sends fibers (nervi erigentes) that enter the pelvic plexus in the sacrouterine folds. The plexus now appears to contain both sympathetic (inferior hypogastric plexus) and parasympathetic (nervi erigentes) components.

C. Nervi Erigentes

The sensory components, which are mostly visceral, are found in the nervi erigentes; however, if one takes into account the amount of spinal anesthetic necessary to eliminate uterine sensation, one must assume that there are a number of sensory fibers in the sympathetic component.

D. Common Iliac Nerves

The common iliac nerves originate separately from the superior hypogastric plexus and descend on the surface of the artery and vein, one part going through the femoral ring and the remainder following the internal iliac, finally rejoining the pelvic plexus.

E. Hypogastric Ganglion

On either side of the uterus, in the base of the broad ligament, is the large plexus described by Lee and Frankenhauser, the so-called hypogastric ganglion. The plexus actually consists of ganglia and nerve ramifications of various sizes as well as branches of the combined inferior hypogastric plexus and the nervi erigentes. It lies parallel to the lateral pelvic wall, its lateral surface superficial to the internal iliac and its branches; the ureter occupies a position superficial to the plexus. The middle vesical artery perforates and supplies the plexus, its medial branches supplying the rectal stalk. The greater part of the plexus terminates in large branches that enter the uterus in the region of the internal os, while another smaller component of the plexus supplies the vagina and the bladder. The branches of the plexus that supply the uterus enter the isthmus primarily through the sacrouterine fold or ligament. In the isthmus, just outside the entrance to the uterus, ascending rami pass out into the broad ligament to enter the body of the uterus at higher levels—besides supplying the uterine tubes. A part of the inferior hypogastric plexus may pass directly to the uterus without involvement in the pelvic plexus.

Ganglia are in close proximity to the uterine arteries and the ureters, in the adventitia of the bladder and vagina, and in the vesicovaginal septum. The nerve bundles entering the ganglia contain both myelinated and unmyelinated elements. Corpuscula lamellosa (Vater-Pacini corpuscles) may be found within the tissues and are often observed within nerve bundles, especially within those in the lower divisions of the plexus. Both myelinated and unmyelinated nerves are present within the uterus. The nerves enter along the blood vessels, the richest supply lying in the isthmic portion of the uterus. The fibers following the blood vessels gradually diminish in number in the direction of the fundus, where the sparsest distribution occurs. The fibers run parallel to the muscle bundles, and the nerves frequently branch to form a syncytium before terminating on the sarcoplasm as small free nerve endings.

Sensory Corpuscles

Vater-Pacini corpuscles (corpuscula lamellosa) are present outside the uterus. Dogiel and Krause corpuscles (corpuscula bulboidea) appear in the region of the endocervix. They may also be found in the broad ligament along with Vater-Pacini corpuscles and at the juncture of the uterine arteries with the uterus. These corpuscles may act to modulate the stretch response that reflexively stimulates uterine contractions during labor.

The innervation of the cervix shows occasional free endings entering papillae of the stratified squamous epithelium of the pars vaginalis. The endocervix contains a rich plexus of free endings that is most pronounced in the region of the internal os. The endocervix and the isthmic portion of the uterus in the nonpregnant state

both contain the highest number of nerves and blood vessels of any part of the uterus. The presence here of a lamellar type of corpuscle has already been noted.

Nerves pass through the myometrium and enter the endometrium. A plexus with penetrating fibers involving the submucosal region is present in the basal third of the endometrium, with branches terminating in the stroma, in the basilar arterioles, and at the origin of the spiral arterioles. The outer two-thirds of the endometrium is devoid of nerves.

5. Uterine (Fallopian) Tubes (Oviducts)

Anatomy

The uterine tubes serve to convey the ova to the uterus. They extend from the superior angles of the uterus to the region of the ovaries, running in the superior border of the broad ligament (mesosalpinx). The course of each tube is nearly horizontal at first and slightly backward. Upon reaching the lower (uterine) pole of the ovary, the tube turns upward, parallel with the anterior (mesovarian) border, then arches backward over the upper pole and descends posteriorly to terminate in contact with the medial surface. Each tube is 7–14 cm long and may be divided into 3 parts: isthmus, ampulla, and infundibulum. The isthmus is the narrow and nearly straight portion immediately adjoining the uterus. It has a rather long intramural course, and its opening into the uterus, the uterine ostium, is approximately 1 mm in diameter. Following the isthmus is the wider, more tortuous ampulla. It terminates in a funnel-like dilatation, the infundibulum. The margins of the infundibulum are fringed by numerous diverging processes, the fimbriae, the longest of which, the fimbria ovarica, is attached to the ovary. The funnel-shaped mouth of the infundibulum, the abdominal ostium, is about 3 mm in diameter and actually leads into the peritoneal cavity, although it is probably closely applied to the surface of the ovary during ovulation.

Layers of Wall

The wall of the tube has 4 coats: serous (peritoneal), subserous or adventitial (fibrous and vascular), muscular, and mucous. Each tube is enclosed within a peritoneal covering except along a small strip on its lower surface, where the mesosalpinx is attached. At the margins of the infundibulum and the fimbriae, this peritoneal covering becomes directly continuous with the mucous membrane lining the interior of the tube. The subserous tissue is lax in the immediate vicinity of the tube. The blood and nerve supply is found within this layer. The muscular coat has an outer longitudinal and an inner circular layer of smooth muscle fibers, more prominent and continuous with that of the uterus at the uterine end of the tube. The mucous coat is ciliated columnar epithelium with coarse longitudinal folds, simple in the region of the isthmus but becoming higher and more complex in the ampulla. The epithelial lining extends outward into the fimbriae. The ciliary motion is directed toward the uterus.

Ligament

The infundibulum is suspended from the pelvic brim by the infundibulopelvic ligament (suspensory ligament of the ovary). This portion of the tube may adjoin the tip of the appendix and fuse with it.

Arteries & Veins

The blood supply to the tubes is derived from the ovarian and uterine arteries. The tubal branch of the uterine artery courses along the lower surface of the uterine tube as far as the fimbriated extremity and may also send a branch to the ligamentum teres. The ovarian branch of the uterine artery runs along the attached border of the ovary and gives off a tubal branch. Both branches form cruciate anastomoses in the mesosalpinx. The veins accompany the arteries.

Lymphatics

The lymphatic drainage occurs through trunks running retroperitoneally across and anterior to the ureter, into the lumbar nodes along the aorta, and inferior to the kidney.

Nerves

The nerve supply is derived from the pelvic plexuses (parasympathetic and sympathetic) and from the ovarian plexus. The nerves of the ampulla are given off from the branches passing to the ovary, while those of the isthmus come from the uterine branches. The nerve fibers enter the muscularis of the tube through the mesosalpinx to form a reticular network of free endings among the smooth muscle cells.

6. Ovaries

Anatomy

The ovaries are paired organs situated close to the wall on either side of the pelvis minor, a little below the brim. Each measures 2.5–5 cm in length, 1.5–3 cm in breadth, and 0.7–1.5 cm in width, weighing about 4–8 g. The ovary has 2 surfaces, medial and lateral; 2 borders, anterior or mesovarian and posterior or free; and 2 poles, upper or tubal and lower or uterine. When the uterus and adnexa are in the normal position, the long axis of the ovary is nearly vertical, but it bends somewhat medially and forward at the lower end so that the lower pole tends to point toward the uterus. The medial surface is rounded and, posteriorly, may have numerous scars or elevations that mark the position of developing follicles and sites of ruptured ones.

Relationships

The upper portion of this surface is overhung by the fimbriated end of the uterine tube, and the remainder lies in relation to coils of intestine. The lateral surface is similar in shape and faces the pelvic wall, where it forms a distinct depression, the fossa ovarica. This fossa is lined by peritoneum and is bounded above by the external iliac vessels and below by the obturator vessels and nerve; its posterior boundary is formed by the ureter and uterine artery and vein, and the pelvic attachment of the broad ligament is located anteriorly. The mesovarian or anterior border is fairly straight and provides attachment for the mesovarium, a peritoneal fold by which the ovary is attached to the posterosuperior layer of the broad ligament. Since the vessels, nerves, and lymphatics enter the ovary through this border, it is referred to as the hilum of the ovary. Anterior to the hilum are embryonic remnants of the male and female germ cell ducts. The posterior or free border is more convex and broader and is directed freely into the rectouterine pouch. The upper or tubal pole is large and rounded. It is overhung closely by the infundibulum of the uterine tube and is connected with the pelvic brim by the suspensory ligament of the ovary, a peritoneal fold. The lower or uterine pole is smaller and directed toward the uterus. It serves as the attachment of the ligament of the ovary proper.

Mesovarium

The ovary is suspended by means of the mesovarium, the suspensory ligament of the ovary, and the ovarian ligament. The mesovarium consists of 2 layers of peritoneum, continuous with both the epithelial coat of the ovary and the posterosuperior layer of the broad ligament. It is short and wide and contains branches of the ovarian and uterine arteries, with plexuses of nerves, the pampiniform plexus of veins, and the lateral end of the ovarian ligament. The suspensory ligament of the ovary is a triangular fold of peritoneum and is actually the upper lateral corner of the broad ligament, which becomes confluent with the parietal peritoneum at the pelvic brim. It attaches to the mesovarium as well as to the peritoneal coat of the infundibulum medially, thus suspending both the ovary and the tube. It contains the ovarian artery, veins, and nerves after they pass over the pelvic brim and before they enter the mesovarium. The ovarian ligament is a band of connective tissue, with numerous small muscle fibers, that lies between the 2 layers of the broad ligament on the boundary line between the mesosalpinx and the mesometrium, connecting the lower (uterine) pole of the ovary with the lateral wall of the uterus. It is attached just below the uterine tube and above the attachment of the round ligament of the uterus and is continuous with the latter.

Structure of Ovary

The ovary is covered by cuboid or low columnar epithelium and consists of a cortex and a medulla. The medulla is made up of connective tissue fibers, smooth muscle cells, and numerous blood vessels, nerves, lymphatic vessels, and supporting tissue. The cortex is composed of a fine areolar stroma, with many vessels and scattered follicles of epithelial cells within which are the definitive ova (oocytes) in various stages of maturity. The more mature follicles enlarge and project onto the free surface of the ovary, where they are visible to the naked eye. They are called graafian follicles. When fully mature, the follicle bursts, releasing the ovum and becoming transformed into a corpus luteum. The corpus luteum, in turn, is later replaced by scar tissue, forming a corpus albicans.

Arteries

The ovarian artery is the chief source of blood for the ovary. Though both arteries may originate as branches of the abdominal aorta, the left frequently originates from the left renal artery; the right, less frequently. The vessels diverge from each other as they descend. Upon reaching the level of the common iliac artery, they turn medially over that vessel and ureter to descend tortuously into the pelvis on each side between the folds of the suspensory ligament of the ovary into the mesovarium. An additional blood supply is formed from anastomosis with the ovarian branch of the uterine artery, which courses along the attached border of the ovary. Blood vessels that enter the hilum send out capillary branches centrifugally.

The veins follow the course of the arteries and, as they emerge from the hilum, form a well-developed plexus (the pampiniform plexus) between the layers of the mesovarium. Smooth muscle fibers occur in the meshes of the plexus, giving the whole structure the appearance of erectile tissue.

Lymphatics

Lymphatic channels drain retroperitoneally, together with those of the tubes and part of those from the uterus, to the lumbar nodes along the aorta inferior to the kidney. The distribution of lymph channels in the ovary is so extensive that it suggests the system may also provide additional fluid to the ovary during periods of preovulatory follicular swelling.

Nerves

The nerve supply of the ovaries arises from the lumbosacral sympathetic chain and passes to the gonad along with the ovarian artery.

7. Vagina

The vagina is a strong canal of muscle approximately 7.5 cm long that extends from the uterus to the vestibule of the external genitalia, where it opens to the exterior. Its long axis is almost parallel with that of the lower part of the sacrum, and it meets the cervix of the uterus at an angle of 45–90 degrees. Because the cervix of the uterus projects into the upper portion, the anterior wall of the vagina is 1.5–2 cm shorter than the posterior wall. The circular cul-de-sac formed around the cervix is known as the fornix and is divided into 4 regions; the anterior fornix, the posterior fornix, and 2 lateral fornices. Toward its lower end, the vagina pierces the urogenital diaphragm and is surrounded by the 2 bulbocavernosus muscles and bodies, which act as a sphincter (sphincter vaginae). In the virginal state, an incomplete fold of highly vascular tissue and mucous membrane, the hymen, partially closes the external orifice.

Relationships

Anteriorly, the vagina is in close relationship to the bladder, ureters, and urethra in succession. The posterior fornix is covered by the peritoneum of the recto-vaginal pouch, which may contain coils of intestine. Below the pouch, the vagina rests almost directly on the rectum, separated from it by a thin layer of areolar connective tissue. Toward the lower end of the vagina, the rectum turns back sharply, and the distance between the vagina and rectum greatly increases. This space, filled with muscle fibers, connective tissue, and fat, is known as the perineal body. The lateral fornix lies just under the root of the broad ligament and is approximately 1 cm from the point where the uterine artery crosses the ureter. The remaining lateral vaginal wall is related to the edges of the anterior portion of the levator ani. The vagina is supported at the introitus by the bulbocavernosus muscles and bodies, in the lower third by the levator ani (puborectalis), and superiorly by the transverse (cardinal) ligaments of the uterus. The ductus epoophori longitudinalis (duct of Gartner), the remains of the lower portion of the wolffian duct (mesonephric duct), may often be found on the sides of the vagina as a minute tube or fibrous cord. These vestigial structures often become cystic and appear as translucent areas.

Wall Structure

The vaginal wall is composed of a mucosal and a muscular layer. The smooth muscle fibers are indistinctly arranged in 3 layers: an outer longitudinal layer, circumferential layer, and a poorly differentiated inner longitudinal layer. In the lower third, the circumferential fibers envelop the urethra. The submucous area is abundantly supplied with a dense plexus of veins and lymphatics. The mucous layer shows many transverse and oblique rugae, which project inward to such an extent that the lumen in transverse section resembles an H-shaped slit. On the anterior and posterior walls, these ridges are more prominent, and the anterior column forms the urethral carina at its lower end, where the urethra slightly invaginates the anterior wall of the vagina. The mucosa of the vagina is lined throughout by stratified squamous epithelium. Even though the vagina has no true glands, there is a secretion present. It consists of cervical mucus, desquamated epithelium, and, with sexual stimulation, a direct transudate.

Arteries & Veins

The chief blood supply to the vagina is through the vaginal branch of the uterine artery. After forming the coronary or circular artery of the cervix, it passes medially, behind the ureter, to send 5 main branches onto the anterior wall to the midline. These branches anastomose with the azygos artery (originating midline from the coronary artery of the cervix) and continue downward to supply the anterior vaginal wall and the lower two-thirds of the urethra. The uterine artery eventually anastomoses to the urethral branch of the clitoral artery. The posterior vaginal wall is supplied by branches of the middle and inferior hemorrhoidal arteries, traversing toward the midline to join the azygos artery from the coronary artery of the cervix. These branches then anastomose on the perineum to the superficial and deep transverse perineal arteries.

The veins follow the course of the arteries.

Lymphatics

The lymphatics are numerous mucosal plexuses, anastomosing with the deeper muscular plexuses (Table 2–2). The superior group of lymphatics join those of the cervix and may follow the uterine artery to terminate in the external iliac nodes or form anastomoses with the uterine plexus. The middle group of lymphatics, which drain the greater part of the vagina, appear to follow the vaginal arteries to the hypogastric channels. In addition, there are lymph nodes in the rectovaginal septum that are primarily responsible for drainage of the rectum and part of the posterior vaginal wall. The inferior group of lymphatics form frequent anastomoses between the right and left sides and either course upward to anastomose with the middle group or enter the vulva and drain to the inguinal nodes.

Nerves

The innervation of the vagina contains both sympathetic and parasympathetic fibers. Only occasional free nerve endings are seen in the mucosa; no other types of nerve endings are noted.

STRUCTURES LINING THE PELVIS

The walls of the pelvis minor are made up of the following layers: (1) the peritoneum, (2) the subperitoneal or extraperitoneal fibroareolar layer, (3) the fascial layer, (4) the muscular layer, and (5) the osseoligamentous layer (not further discussed). The anatomy of the floor of the pelvis is comparable to that of the walls except for the absence of an osseoligamentous layer.

1. Peritoneum

The peritoneum presents several distinct transverse folds that form corresponding fossae on each side. The most anterior is a variable fold, the transverse vesical, extending from the bladder laterally to the pelvic wall. It is not the superficial covering of any definitive structure. Behind it lies the broad ligament, which partially covers and aids in the support of the uterus and adnexa.

Ligaments

The broad ligament extends from the lateral border on either side of the uterus to the floor and side walls of the pelvis. It is composed of 2 layers, anterior and posterior, the anterior facing downward and the posterior facing upward, conforming to the position of the uterus. The inferior or "attached" border of the broad ligament is continuous with the parietal peritoneum on the floor and on the side walls of the pelvis. Along this border, the posterior layer continues laterally and posteriorly in an arc to the region of the sacrum, forming the uterosacral fold. Another fold—the rectouterine fold—frequently passes from the posterior surface of the cervix to the rectum in the midline. The anterior layer of the broad ligament is continuous laterally along the inferior border with the peritoneum of the paravesical fossae and continuous medially with peritoneum on the upper surface of the bladder. Both layers of the attached border continue up the side walls of the pelvis to join with a triangular fold of peritoneum, reaching to the brim of the pelvis to form the suspensory ligament of the ovary or infundibular ligament. This ligament contains the ovarian vessels and nerves. The medial border of the broad ligament on either side is continuous with the peritoneal covering on both uterine surfaces. The 2 layers of the ligament separate to partially contain the uterus, and the superior or "free" border, which is laterally continuous with the suspensory ligament of the ovary, envelops the uterine tube.

The broad ligament can be divided into regions as follows: (1) a larger portion, the mesometrium, which is associated especially with the lateral border of the uterus; (2) the mesovarium, the fold that springs from the posterior layer of the ovary; and (3) the thin portion, the mesosalpinx, which is associated with the uterine tube in the region of the free border. The superior lateral corner of the broad ligament has been referred to as the suspensory ligament of the ovary, or infundibulopelvic ligament, because it suspends the infundibulum as well as the ovary.

Fossae & Spaces

Corresponding to the peritoneal folds are the peritoneal fossae. The prevesical or retropubic space is a potential space that is crossed by the transverse vesical fold. It is situated in front of the bladder and behind the pubis. When the bladder is displaced posteriorly, it becomes an actual space, anteriorly continuous from side to side and posteriorly limited by a condensation of fatty areolar tissue extending from the base of the bladder to the side wall of the pelvis. The vesicouterine pouch is a narrow cul-de-sac between the anterior surface of the body of the uterus and the upper surface of the bladder when the uterus is in normal anteflexed position. In the bottom of this pouch, the peritoneum is reflected from the bladder onto the uterus at the junction of the cervix and corpus. Therefore, the anterior surface of the cervix is below the level of the peritoneum and is connected with the base of the bladder by condensed areolar tissue. The peritoneum on the posterior surface of the body of the uterus extends downward onto the cervix and onto the posterior fornix of the vagina. It is then reflected onto the anterior surface of the rectum to form a narrow cul-de-sac continuous with the pararectal fossa of either side. The entire space, bounded anteriorly by the cervix and by the fornix in the midline, the uterosacral folds laterally, and the rectum posteriorly, is the rectouterine pouch or cul-de-sac (pouch of Douglas).

2. Subperitoneal & Fascial Layers

The subperitoneal layer consists of loose, fatty areolar tissue underlying the peritoneum. External to the subperitoneal layer, a layer of fascia lines the wall of the pelvis, covering the muscles and, where these are lacking, blending with the periosteum of the pelvic bones. This layer is known as the parietal pelvic fascia and is subdivided into the obturator fascia, the fascia of the urogenital diaphragm, and the fascia of the piriformis. The obturator fascia is of considerable thickness and covers the obturator internus muscle. Traced forward, it partially blends with the periosteum of the pubic bone and assists in the formation of the obturator canal. Traced upward, it is continuous at the arcuate line with the iliac fascia. Inferiorly, it extends nearly to the margin of the ischiopubic arch, where it is attached to the bone. In this lower region, it also becomes continuous with a double-layered triangular sheet of fascia, the fasciae of the urogenital diaphragm, passing across the anterior part of the pelvic outlet. A much thinner portion of the parietal pelvic fascia covers the piriform and coccygeus muscles in the posterior pelvic wall. Medially, the piriformis fascia blends with the periosteum of the sacrum around the margins of the anterior sacral foramens and covers the roots and first branches of the sacral plexus. Visceral pelvic fascia denotes the fascia in the bottom of the pelvic bowl, which invests the pelvic organs and forms a number of supports that suspend the organs from the pelvic walls. These supports arise in common from the obturator part of the parietal fascia, along or near the arcus tendineus. This arc or line extends from a point near the lower part of the symphysis pubica to the root of the spine of the ischium. From this common origin, the fascia spreads inward and backward, dividing into a number of parts classified as either investing (endopelvic) fascia or suspensory and diaphragmatic fascia.

3. Muscular Layer

The muscles of the greater pelvis are the psoas major and iliacus. Those of the lesser pelvis are the piriformis, obturator internus, coccygeus, and levator ani; they do not form a continuous layer.

Greater Pelvis

A. PSOAS MAJOR

The fusiform psoas major muscle originates from the 12th thoracic to the fifth lumbar vertebrae. Parallel fiber bundles descend nearly vertically along the side of the vertebral bodies and extend along the border of the minor pelvis, beneath the inguinal ligament, and on toward insertion in the thigh. The medial border inserts into the lesser trochanter, while the lateral border shares its tendon with the iliacus muscle. Together with the iliacus, it is the most powerful flexor of the thigh and acts as a lateral rotator of the femur when the foot is off the ground and free, and a medial rotator when the foot is on the ground and the tibia is fixed. The psoas component flexes the spine and the pelvis and abducts the lumbar region of the spine. The psoas, having longer fibers than the iliacus, gives a quicker but weaker pull.

B. Iliacus

The fan-shaped iliacus muscle originates from the iliac crest, the iliolumbar ligament, the greater part of the iliac fossa, the anterior sacroiliac ligaments, and frequently the ala of the sacrum. It also originates from the ventral border of the ilium between the 2 anterior spines. It is inserted in a penniform manner on the lateral surface of the tendon that emerges from the psoas above the inguinal ligament and directly on the femur immediately distal to the lesser trochanter. The lateral portion of the muscle arising from the ventral border of the ilium is adherent to the direct tendon of the rectus femoris and the capsule of the hip joint.

Lesser Pelvis

A. Piriformis

The piriformis has its origin from the lateral part of the ventral surface of the second, third, and fourth sacral vertebrae, from the posterior border of the greater sciatic notch, and from the deep surface of the sacrotuberous ligament near the sacrum. The fiber bundles pass through the greater sciatic foramen to insert upon the anterior and inner portion of the upper border of the greater trochanter. The piriformis acts as an abductor, lateral rotator, and weak extensor of the thigh.

B. Obturator Internus

The obturator internus arises from the pelvic surface of the pubic rami near the obturator foramen, the pelvic surface of the ischium between the foramen and the greater sciatic notch, the deep surface of the obturator internus fascia, the fibrous arch that bounds the canal for the obturator vessels and nerves, and the pelvic surface of the obturator membrane. The fiber bundles converge toward the lesser sciatic notch, where they curve laterally to insert into the trochanteric fossa of the femur. The obturator internus is a powerful lateral rotator of the thigh. When the thigh is bent at a right angle, the muscle serves as an abductor and extensor.

C. Coccygeus

The coccygeus muscle runs from the ischial spine and the neighboring margin of the greater sciatic notch to the fourth and fifth sacral vertebrae and the coccyx.

A large part of the muscle is aponeurotic. It supports the pelvic and abdominal viscera and possibly flexes and abducts the coccyx.

D. Levator Ani

The levator ani muscle forms the floor of the pelvis and the roof of the perineum. It is divisible into 3 portions: (1) the iliococcygeus, (2) the pubococcygeus, and (3) the puborectalis.

1. **Iliococcygeus**—The iliococcygeus arises from the arcus tendineus, which extends from the ischial spine to the superior ramus of the pubis near the obturator canal and for a variable distance downward below the obturator canal. Its insertion is into the lateral aspect of the coccyx and the raphe that extends from the tip of the coccyx to the rectum. Many fiber bundles cross the median line.

2. **Pubococcygeus**—The pubococcygeus arises from the inner surface of the os pubis, the lower margin of the symphysis pubica to the obturator canal, and the arcus tendineus as far backward as the origin of the iliococcygeus. It passes backward, downward, and medially past the urogenital organs and the rectum, inserting into the anterior sacrococcygeal ligament, the deep part of the anococcygeal raphe, and each side of the rectum. The pubococcygeus lies to some extent on the pelvic surface of the insertion of the iliococcygeus.

3. **Puborectalis**—The puborectalis arises from the body and descending ramus of the pubis beneath the origin of the pubococcygeus, the neighboring part of the obturator fascia, and the fascia covering the pelvic surface of the urogenital diaphragm. Many of the fiber bundles interdigitate with those of the opposite side, and they form a thick band on each side of the rectum behind which those of each side are inserted into the anococcygeal raphe.

The levator ani serves to slightly flex the coccyx, raise the anus, and constrict the rectum and vagina. It resists the downward pressure that the thoracoabdominal diaphragm exerts on the viscera during inspiration.

Pelvic Diaphragm

The pelvic diaphragm (Fig 2–25) extends from the upper part of the pelvic surface of the pubis and ischium to the rectum, which passes through it. The pelvic diaphragm is formed by the levator ani and coccygeus muscles and covering fasciae. The diaphragmatic fasciae cloaking the levator ani arise from the parietal pelvic fascia (obturator fascia), the muscular layer lying between the fasciae. As viewed from above, the superior fascia is the best developed and is reflected onto the rectum, forming the "rectal sheath." The coccygeus muscle forms the deeper portion of the posterolateral wall

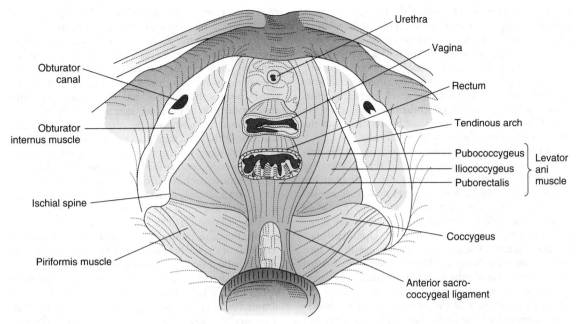

Obturator canal

Obturator internus muscle

Ischial spine

Piriformis muscle

Urethra

Vagina

Rectum

Tendinous arch

Pubococcygeus
Iliococcygeus — Levator ani muscle
Puborectalis

Coccygeus

Anterior sacro-coccygeal ligament

Figure 2–25. Pelvic diaphragm from above.

of the ischiorectal fossa, helping to bound the pelvic outlet. The diaphragm presents a hiatus anteriorly, occupied by the vagina and urethra. The pelvic diaphragm is the main support of the pelvic floor; it suspends the rectum and indirectly supports the uterus.

Arteries & Veins

The blood supply to the muscles lining the pelvis is primarily from branches of the hypogastric artery, accompanied by contributions from the external iliac artery. The iliolumbar branch of the hypogastric artery runs upward and laterally beneath the common iliac artery, then beneath the psoas muscle to the superior aperture of the pelvis minor, where it divides into iliac and lumbar branches. The iliac supplies both the iliacus and psoas muscles. It passes laterally beneath the psoas and the femoral nerve and, perforating the iliacus, ramifies in the iliac fossa between the muscle and the bone. It supplies a nutrient artery to the bone and then divides into several branches that can be traced as follows: (1) upward toward the sacroiliac synchondrosis to anastomose with the last lumbar artery, (2) laterally toward the crest of the ilium to anastomose with the lateral circumflex and gluteal arteries, and (3) medially toward the pelvis minor to anastomose with the deep circumflex iliac from the external iliac. The lumbar branch ascends beneath the psoas and supplies that muscle along

with the quadratus lumborum. It then anastomoses with the last lumbar artery.

Another branch of the hypogastric artery, the lateral sacral artery, may be represented as 2 distinct vessels. It passes medially in front of the sacrum and turns downward to run parallel with the sympathetic trunk. Crossing the slips of origin of the piriform muscle, it sends branches to that muscle. On reaching the coccyx, it anastomoses in front of the bone with the middle sacral artery and with the inferior lateral sacral artery of the opposite side. The obturator artery usually arises from the hypogastric, but occasionally it may stem from the inferior epigastric or directly from the external iliac artery. It runs forward and downward slightly below the brim of the pelvis, lying between the peritoneum and endopelvic fascia. Passing through the obturator canal, it emerges and divides into anterior and posterior branches that curve around the margin of the obturator foramen beneath the obturator externus muscle.

When the obturator artery arises from the inferior epigastric or external iliac artery, its proximal relationships are profoundly altered, the vessel coursing near the femoral ring where it may be endangered during operative procedures. The anterior branch of the obturator artery runs around the medial margin of the obturator foramen and anastomoses with both its posterior branch and the medial circumflex artery. It supplies branches to the obturator muscles. The internal pudendal artery is a terminal branch of the hypogastric artery that arises opposite the piriform muscle and accompanies the inferior gluteal artery downward to the lower border of the greater sciatic foramen. It leaves the pelvis between the piriform and coccygeus muscles, passing over the ischial spine to enter the ischiorectal fossa through the small sciatic foramen. Then, running forward through the canalis pudendalis (Alcock's canal) in the obturator fascia, it terminates by dividing into the perineal artery and the artery of the clitoris.

Within the pelvis, the artery lies anterior to the piriform muscle and the sacral plexus of nerves, lateral to the inferior gluteal artery. Among the small branches that it sends to the gluteal region are those that accompany the nerve to the obturator internus. Another of its branches, the inferior hemorrhodial artery, arises at the posterior part of the ischiorectal fossa. Upon perforating the obturator fascia, it immediately breaks up into several branches. Some of those run medially toward the rectum to supply the levator ani muscle. The superior gluteal artery originates as a short trunk from the lateral and back part of the hypogastric artery, associated in origin with the iliolumbar and lateral sacral and sometimes with the inferior gluteal or with the inferior gluteal and the internal pudendal. It leaves the pelvis through the greater sciatic foramen above the piriform muscle, beneath its vein and in front of the superior gluteal nerve. Under cover of the gluteus maximus muscle, it breaks into a superficial and deep division.

The deep portion further divides into superior and inferior branches. The inferior branch passes forward between the gluteus medius and minimus toward the greater trochanter, where it anastomoses with the ascending branch of the lateral circumflex. It supplies branches to the obturator internus, the piriformis, the levator ani, and the coccygeus muscles and to the hip joint. The deep circumflex iliac artery arises from the side of the external iliac artery either opposite the epigastric or a little below the origin of that vessel. It courses laterally behind the inguinal ligament, lying between the fascia transversalis and the peritoneum or in a fibrous canal formed by the union of the fascia transversalis with the iliac fascia. It sends off branches that supply the psoas and iliacus muscles as well as a cutaneous branch that anastomoses with the superior gluteal artery.

PLACENTA*

At term, the normal placenta is a blue-red, rounded, flattened, meaty discoid organ 15–20 cm in diameter and 2–4 cm thick. It weighs 400–600 g, or about one-sixth the normal weight of the newborn. The umbilical cord arises from almost any point on the fetal surface of the placenta, seemingly at random. The fetal membranes arise from the placenta at its margin. In multiple pregnancy, one or more placentas may be present depending upon the number of ova implanted and the type of segmentation that occurs. The placenta is derived from both maternal and fetal tissue. At term, about four-fifths of the placenta is of fetal origin.

The maternal portion of the placenta amounts to less than one-fifth of the total placenta by weight. It is composed of compressed sheets of decidua basalis, remnants of blood vessels, and, at the margin, spongy decidua. Irregular grooves or clefts divide the placenta into cotyledons. The maternal surface is torn from the uterine wall at birth and as a result is rough, red, and spongy.

The fetal portion of the placenta is composed of numerous functional units called villi. These are branched terminals of the fetal circulation and provide for transfer of metabolic products. The villous surface, which is exposed to maternal blood, may be as much as 12 m^2 (130 square feet). The fetal capillary system within the villi is almost 50 km (27 miles) long. Most villi are free within the intervillous spaces, but an occasional anchor villus attaches the placenta to the decidua basalis. The fetal surface of the placenta is covered by amniotic membrane and is smooth and shiny. The umbilical cord vessels course over the fetal surface before entering the placenta.

Placental Types

A. Circumvallate (Circummarginate) Placentas

In about 1% of cases, the delivered placenta will show a small central chorionic plate surrounded by a thick whitish ring that is composed of a double fold of amnion and chorion with fibrin and degenerated decidua in between. This circumvallate placenta may predispose to premature marginal separation and second-trimester antepartum bleeding (Fig 2–26). This uncommon extrachorial placenta is of uncertain origin. It is associated with increased rates of slight to moderate antepartal bleeding, early delivery, and perinatal death. Older multiparas are more prone to its development. Low-birth-weight infants and extrachorial placentas seem related.

B. Succenturiate Lobe

Occasionally there may be an accessory cotyledon, or succenturiate lobe, with vascular connections to the main body of the placenta. A succenturiate lobe may not always deliver with the parent placenta during the third stage of labor. This leads to postpartal hemorrhage. If a careful examination of the delivered membranes reveals torn vessels, immediate manual exploration of the uterus is indicated for removal of an accessory lobe (Fig 2–27).

---

* This section is contributed by Robert C. Goodlin, MD.

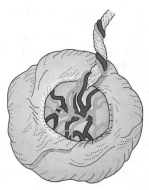

Figure 2–26. Marked circumvallate or extrachorial placenta.

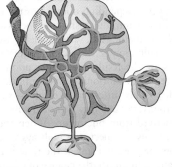

Figure 2–28. Bipartite placenta.

C. BIPARTITE PLACENTA

A bipartite placenta is an uncommon variety. The placenta is divided into 2 separate lobes but united by primary vessels and membranes. Retention of one lobe after birth will cause hemorrhagic and septic complications. Examine the vasculature and note the completeness of membranes of a small placenta for evidence of a missing lobe, and recover the adherent portion without delay (Fig 2–28).

D. MARGINAL INSERTION OF CORD (BATTLEDORE PLACENTA)

The umbilical cord may be found inserted into the chorionic plate at almost any point, but when it inserts at the margin it is sometimes called a battledore placenta (Fig 2–29).

E. PLACENTA MEMBRANACEA

This type of placenta is one in which the decidua capsularis is so well vascularized that the chorion laeve does not atrophy and villi are maintained. Hence, the entire fetal envelope is functioning placenta.

F. PLACENTA ACCRETA

In rare cases, the placenta is abnormally adherent to the myometrium, presumably because it developed where there was a deficiency of decidua. Predisposing factors include placenta previa (one-third of cases), previous cesarean (one-fourth), a prior D&C (one-fourth), and grand multiparity. The adherence may be partial or total. Rarely, the placenta may invade the myometrium deeply (placenta increta) or even perforate the uterus (placenta percreta). When attempts are made to remove a placenta accreta manually, hemorrhage may be severe. The treatment is hysterectomy.

G. PLACENTA PREVIA

This abnormality is discussed in Chapter 20.

H. MULTIPLE PREGNANCY PLACENTA

In fraternal twins, the placentas may be 2 distinct entities or fused. There are 2 distinct chorions and am-

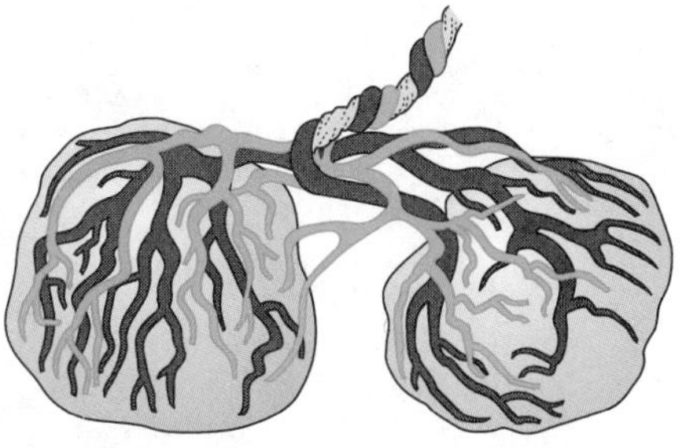

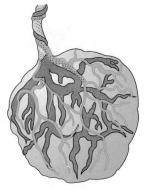

Figure 2–29. Marginal insertion of battledore placenta.

Figure 2–27. Succenturiate placenta.

nions. In the case of identical twins, the picture may be more confusing. Depending upon the time of division of the fertilized ovum, the position of the placentas and number of membranes will vary. If the division occurs soon after fertilization, 2 distinct placentas and sets of membranes are the result. From that point on, many variations (eg monochorionic monoamniotic fused placentas and, possibly, interchange of blood supply) may occur. Further variations may be noted when triplets or more are derived from one ovum. When the presence of identical twins is suspected, it is always wise to clamp the cord on the placental side at the time it is clamped on the infant to minimize the chance of exsanguination of the uterine twin.

REFERENCES

Caldwell WE, Moloy HC: Anatomical variations in the female pelvis. Am J Obstet Gynecol 1933;26:479.

Clemente C: *Gray's Anatomy of the Human Body,* 30th ed. Lippincott Williams & Wilkins, 1985.

Donnelly JE: *Living Anatomy,* 2nd ed. Human Kinetics, 1990.

Harrison RJ, Navarainam V (editors): *Progress in Anatomy.* Vol. 3. Cambridge University Press, 1984.

Junqueira LC, Carneiro J, Kelley RO: *Basic Histology,* 9th ed. McGraw-Hill, 1998.

Moore KL: *Clinically Oriented Anatomy,* 4th ed. Lippincott Williams & Wilkins, 1999.

Netter FH et al: *The Ciba Collection of Medical Illustrations.* Vol. 2: Reproductive System. Novartis Medical Education, 1986.

Schlossberg L, Zuidema GD (editors): *The Johns Hopkins Atlas of Human Functional Anatomy,* 4th ed. Johns Hopkins University Press, 1997.

Scicka D, Murawski E: Tendinous intersections of the rectus abdominis muscle in human fetuses. Folia Morpho 1980;39 427.

Wilson DB, Wilson WJ: *Human Anatomy,* 2nd ed. Oxford University Press, 1983.

The Role of Imaging Techniques in Gynecology

3

Robert A. Graebe, MD

Case Report

C.O. is a 29-year-old white female, who presented with a history of infertility for several years, followed by a history of recurrent pregnancy losses.

Her past medical and surgical histories were negative. Gynecologically, she was remarkable in that she reported severe dysmenorrhea for the previous several years relieved by NSAIDs (nonsteroidal anti-inflammatory drugs). Her gynecologist found a low luteal phase progesterone and treated her with 50 mg of clomiphene citrate (CC) days 5–9 of the cycle.

She responded very well to the medication with a conception. The pregnancy resulted in a spontaneous abortion 5 weeks later. No D&C was required and she recovered well. She was still unable to conceive on her own and was again placed on CC. Again, she conceived and again had a spontaneous abortion—this time at 7 weeks' gestation. No D&C was performed.

The patient was then evaluated for recurrent pregnancy losses. Karyotype was normal for both partners. Hormonal evaluation was normal with the exception of a low mid-luteal phase progesterone. Immunologic and infectious screening also failed to reveal a cause for the recurrent losses. The hysterosalpingogram (HSG) demonstrated a midline filling defect similar to the one seen in Figure 3–1.

The patient was informed of the results and the potential for future miscarriages. The need for further evaluation and possible repair hysteroscopically or abdominally was carefully explained to the patient together with its risks and benefits. She elected to try CC one more time and hoped to avoid surgery.

At 8 weeks' gestation, vaginal ultrasonography revealed positive fetal cardiac activity in a CC-induced ovulation. While still on micronized progesterone, 100 mg 3 times daily, she was referred to her gynecologist for routine obstetric care.

At 12 weeks' gestation, the patient had an incomplete abortion that required a D&C. She recovered uneventfully and later returned to the office for further evaluation and treatment.

Several months were allowed to lapse before a hysteroscopy/laparoscopy revealed a broad-based intrauter-ine septum and stage I endometriosis. To evaluate the depth and width of the septum, a LaparoScan (Endo-Medix, Irvine, CA) laparoscopic 7.5-Hz probe was used during the procedure. The septum was removed with a hysteroscopic resectoscope loop on a 40-watt setting. After the resection had been carried out, the ultrasonic probe was again used to measure the thickness of the myometrium and to verify the resection of the septum. A 30-mL 18F Foley catheter with the distal tip resected was placed in the fundus and inflated. The patient was discharged and placed on a broad-spectrum antibiotic and conjugated estrogen, 2.5 mg daily.

Discussion

As we entered the new millennium, a proliferation of imaging techniques used in medical practice occurred. Research into the development, refinement, and application of imaging in gynecology is very apparent in the literature.

The HSG has been considered the gold standard in the imaging of the uterine corpus for benign disorders (submucous myomas, submucous polyps, localization of tubal occlusion, and evaluation of müllerian fusion defects) and malignant disease (endometrial carcinoma).

In the case reported, the standard scout film was obtained and the cervix was prepared after the following were assured: the position of the uterus, absence of pelvic tenderness, and a negative pregnancy test. The water-soluble contrast medium was injected into the uterine cavity and oblique and anteroposterior films were obtained. These showed a midline uterine filling defect of the type usually seen with septate or bicornuate uteri.

Ultrasonography (US) performed on this patient during her pregnancies failed to show the filling defect. If suspected, the septum might have been encountered by more careful scanning. The scans of the last pregnancy revealed only an eccentrically placed pregnancy that might have been seen ultrasonographically even in normally structured uteri. Although not helpful at this point, ultrasonographic examination of the uterus between conceptions might have been helpful if used with

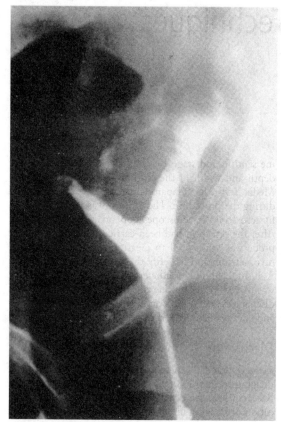

Figure 3–1. Müllerian anomaly as demonstrated by hysterosalpingogram. (Reproduced, with permission, from Doyle MB: Magnetic resonance imaging in müllerian fusion defects. J Reprod Med 1992;37:33.)

a distending medium. This is especially useful in patients allergic to iodine contrast medium (Table 3–1). This technique of ultrasonic HSG is performed by occluding the cervix with a uterine injector and distending the uterus. This method can demonstrate the separate cavities as well as the possible difference between the septate and the bicornuate uterus while demonstrating tubal patency. The technique was adopted for this patient during her uterine septum resection to add ultrasonic contrast between the endometrial cavity and septum and the myometrium. Readers are referred to the many fine texts on diagnostic pelvic ultrasound for instruction and further discussion of these techniques. The development of "sonicated" contrast solutions may add greatly to the usefulness of US.

Using 2 video cameras (one for the resectoscope and the other for the laparoscope and the LaparoScan laparoscopic ultrasound probe), all aspects of the surgery

were evaluated. This setup allowed the operating surgeon adequate visualization of the uterine cavity during the resection and enabled other personnel in the operating room to follow the progress of the surgery. The laparoscopic video allowed the careful monitoring of the uterine surface and assured the surgeon that there would be less likelihood of a uterine perforation. This complication could have resulted in possible bowel injury.

The usefulness of the laparoscopic ultrasound probe with a picture within a picture was that it allowed the visualization of the 2 separate cavities and measurement of the length and width of the septum. It also enabled the operator to demonstrate the complete removal of the septum (Fig 3–2).

Imaging of the Uterus

Pelvic ultrasonography plays a significant role in the diagnosis of uterine leiomyomas (submucous, intramural, and subserosal) and polyps. The laparoscopic probe may be very useful in evaluating myomas during surgery for more accurate assessment of location and vascularity. The feasibility of continuing the procedure may also be assessed by this method intraoperatively.

Occasionally, the detection and localization of myomas, assessment of size, and their differential diagnosis are difficult. In these circumstances it is sometimes useful to perform magnetic resonance imaging (MRI) of the pelvis. MRI can accurately measure the volume of the myoma. This is an aid in determining whether medical management of myomas has resulted in shrinkage or if conservatively treated myomas are growing. Malignant degeneration of myomas visualized by MRI as described by some authors allows for early and appropriate intervention.

MRI also may be useful in the differential diagnosis of myomas and adenomyosis, benign and malignant ovarian pathology, pelvic kidney, and pelvic abscess.

One team of researchers described MRI of müllerian defects as an effective method of discerning between the septate and the bicornuate uterus, thus avoiding the more costly laparoscopy. In patients with very compli-

Table 3–1. Indications for saline infusion sonohysterosalpingogram.

Abnormal x-ray hysterosalpingogram
Abnormal uterine bleeding
Allergies to iodine dyes
Amenorrhea
Infertility

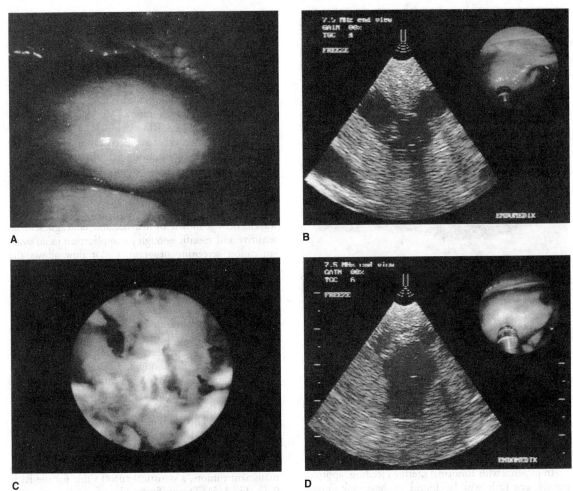

A **B**

C **D**

Figure 3–2. Uterine septum. **A:** Laparoscopic view shows a broad uterine fundus. **B:** Laparoscopic probe on the fundus of the uterus demonstrates the depth and width of the septum. **C:** Hysteroscopic view showing the resection of the uterine septum. **D:** Laparoscopic probe on the fundus of the uterus demonstrates the resected septum. (Note the echogenicity of the debris in the fundus.)

cated müllerian fusion defects (didelphys with transverse vaginal septum or noncommunicating uterine segment), MRI may give a clear anatomic picture of the condition and allow for a properly planned surgical repair. If pelvic MRI had been performed on the patient in the case report that opens this chapter, it would probably have had the same appearance as the MRI in Figure 3–3. (Readers are referred to the review of MRI in müllerian fusion defects in Table 3–2.)

Imaging of the Endometrium

To obtain interobserver consistency in the evaluation of the endometrium, the following guidelines should be

adhered to. Measurements are made in the midfundal region on the sagittal plane. Obtain the maximal double-thickness dimension, remembering to exclude the hypoechoic area between the myometrium and the endometrium and any fluid found between the anterior and posterior walls should be subtracted from the total measurement. The endometrium measures from 4–8 mm in thickness during the follicular phase. The uterine lining ranges from 7–14 mm during the luteal phase and has a uniform echogenic appearance.

Premenopausal women should be evaluated during the early follicular phase, immediately following the menses when the endometrium has a uniform linear appearance.

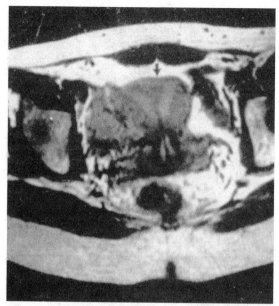

Figure 3–3. Complete uterine septum extending to the cervix. (Reprinted, with permission, from Doyle MB: Magnetic resonance imaging in müllerian fusion defects. J Reprod Med 1992;37:33.)

Menopausal women usually have an endometrial stripe of less than 4 mm. Menopausal women on hormone replacement therapy (HRT) may have endometrial thickness that exceeds 8 mm and a small amount of fluid (< 1 mm).

In patients with abnormal uterine bleeding, approximately one-fifth will be found to have submucous myomas and/or polyps. These may be detected by irregularities in the endometrial stripe or by sonohysterography (SHG). SHG might show polyps to be smooth, surrounded by endometrium, and echogenic, whereas submucous myomas may be seen to be hypo- or heteroechogenic in nature and irregular.

Tissue sampling would be required for definitive diagnosis and to rule out malignancy in any patient not on HRT with a hyperechogenic endometrial stripe > 4 mm.

In the future, three-dimensional ultrasound may be able to improve the diagnosis and staging of endometrial cancer.

Imaging of the Ovaries

About 12,000 women in the United States die annually as a result of ovarian cancer. Unfortunately, the ability of the pelvic examination to detect early ovarian malig-

nancy is low. The same can be said of Ca-125 monoclonal marker for ovarian cancer, which has been found to be a poor predictor of early cases.

The flat plate of the abdomen may still be useful in the diagnosis of dermoid cysts of the ovary. However, cystic and solid structures of the ovary are now better evaluated by transabdominal ultrasonography (TAUS), transvaginal ultrasonography (TVUS), computed tomography (CT), and MRI.

Morphologic criteria have been assigned to increase suspicion concerning ultrasound findings when ovarian cancer is suspected. Cysts > 4 cm, solid and cystic components, septa, and papillary nodules have all been described.

TVUS combined with color flow and Doppler waveform was shown by Kurjak and colleagues to be sensitive and specific enough for application in an ovarian cancer screening program. Color flow allows the identification of vessels not previously identifiable with gray scale. With the use of the Doppler waveform, high- and low-resistance vessels in the ovaries can be distinguished. The resistance index (RI) is the systolic flow velocity peak minus the diastolic trough divided by the systolic peak. Using these techniques in 1000 women, these researchers were able to identify 83 women with the ultrasonographic signs or symptoms that led to surgery (Fig 3–4). Twenty-nine tumors were malignant, 4 from the asymptomatic group (Table 3–3). Color flow was not seen in only 2 of the malignant tumors. This demonstrates a sensitivity of 93% (Table 3–4). With a specificity of 65% for color flow alone, Doppler measurements are needed (Table 3–5). On the basis of distribution of RI values in benign and malignant tumors, a statistical cutoff value for the RI is 0.41 (Fig 3–5). The ability to identify malignant ovarian tumors with a combination of the above-mentioned techniques rather than the simpler laparoscopic approaches to benign adnexal disease may allow for more timely referral to gynecologic oncologists.

Not all studies are in agreement. A more recent evaluation of 47 patients with histologically proven ovarian cancer found that transvaginal color Doppler analysis of intratumoral blood flow didn't provide additional information concerning discriminatory characteristics when scanning individual tumors.

In an attempt to discriminate between malignant and benign adnexal masses in patients having color Doppler and serum Ca-125, one team of researchers developed a complementary multivariate logistic regression analysis. It was determined that the most useful variables among the 31 studied were the menopausal status, the serum Ca-125 level, the presence of one or more papillary growth (> 3 mm in length), and a color score indicative of tumor vascularity and blood flow.

Table 3–2. Types of müllerian anomalies and associated MRI findings.

Class and Type	No.	Finding
I: Segmental agenesis/hypoplasia	7 (24%)	Agenesis: no identifiable organ or small amorphous tissue remnant. Hypoplasia: uterus small for patient's age, maintains adult body/cervix ratio of 2:1, reduced intercornual distance (< 2 cm), low signal intensity on T_2-weighted images with poor zonal differentiation, endometrial/myometrial width reduced
A. Vaginal	0	
B. Cervical	0	
C. Fundal	0	
D. Tubal	0	
E. Combined	7	
II: Unicornuate uterus	5 (17%)	Banana-shaped uterus, normal width of endometrium and myometrium, endometrial/myometrial ratio preserved
A1. Rudimentary horn with endometrium		
(A) Communicating with main uterine cavity	0	
(B) Not communicating with main uterine cavity	1	
A2. Rudimentary horn without endometrium	1	
B. No rudimentary horn	3	
III: Didelphys	5 (17%)	Double, separate uterus, cervix and upper vagina; each uterine cavity of normal volume; endometrium and myometrium of normal width; endometrial/myometrial ratio normal
IV: Bicornuate uterus	10 (34%)	Uterine fundus concave or flattened outward, two horns visible with increased intercornual distance (> 4 cm), high-signal-intensity septum myometrium on T_2-weighted images at level of fundus; high-signal-intensity myometrium (7 patients) or low-signal-intensity fibrous tissue at level of lower uterine segment (3 patients)
A. Complete	3	
B. Partial	3	
C. Arcuate	4	
V: Septate	2 (7%)	Uterine fundus convex outward, normal intercornual distance (2–4 cm), each uterine cavity reduced in volume, endometrial/myometrial width and ratio normal, low-signal-intensity septum on T_1- and T_2-weighted images
A. Complete	1	
B. Incomplete	1	

Because of rounding, the percentages do not add up to 100.
Reprinted, with permission, from Doyle MB: Magnetic resonance imaging in müllerian fusion defects. J Reprod Med 1992;37:33.

The model resulted in a sensitivity of 95.9% and a specificity of 87.1%. This team concluded that the use of a combination of diagnostic criteria and clinical information is more accurate than reliance solely on a single type of data.

CT may be useful for staging ovarian cancer preoperatively or for planning second-look procedures. In patients with benign-appearing adnexal masses (ovarian cysts or tubo-ovarian abscesses), CT may be very useful for biopsy and drainage. The contraindications to needle biopsy and drainage include lack of a safe unobstructed path for the needle, bleeding disorders, and lack of a motivated patient.

Imaging of the Fallopian Tubes

The best direct evaluation of the patency and architecture of the fallopian tubes is by means of endoscopic techniques. The best evaluation of tubal function indirectly is with HSG. This method allows demonstration of tubal patency and visualization of tubal rugations while avoiding the more costly laparoscopic surgery. Some disadvantages of HSG are pelvic infection, dye allergies, failure to detect adnexal adhesions, and false-positives for tubal occlusion. Hysterosalpingo-contrast sonography and MRI are also alternatives to laparoscopy, since women with normal findings probably have a normal pelvis.

The reader is referred to the sections on pelvic inflammatory disease and tubo-ovarian abscess elsewhere in this text for more on the radiographic diagnosis and management of these conditions.

Imaging in Ectopic Pregnancy

One team found that when human chorionic gonadotropin (hCG) levels reach 6500 mIU/mL, most normal intrauterine pregnancies can be detected as a gestational sac by TAUS. The value of adnexal sonography in the management of ectopic pregnancies was demonstrated by another set of researchers. They showed that if no gestational sac was seen on TAUS by 28 days and

OVARIAN TUMOR ULTRASOUND-DOPPLER CLASSIFICATION
Circle all characteristics seen and add numbers in parentheses for a score.

Patient name _____ Date _____ Institution _____

	FLUID			INTERNAL BORDERS		SIZE
UNILOCULAR	Clear	(0)	Smooth	(0)		
	Internal echoes	(1)	Irregular	(2)		
MULTILOCULAR	Clear	(1)	Smooth	(1)		
	Internal echoes	(1)	Irregular	(2)		
CYSTIC-SOLID	Clear	(1)	Smooth	(1)		
	Internal echoes	(2)	Irregular	(2)		

PAPILLARY PROJECTIONS	Suspicious	(1)	Definite	(2)	
SOLID	Homogenous	(1)	Echogenic	(2)	
PERITONEAL FLUID	Absent	(0)	Present	(1)	
LATERALITY	Unilateral	(0)	Bilateral	(1)	

ULTRASOUND SCORE

≤ 2 Benign
3–4 Questionable
> 4 Suspicious

COLOR DOPPLER		**RI (resistance index)**	
No vessels seen	(0)		(0)
Regular separate vessels	(1)	> 0.40	(1)
Randomly dispersed vessels	(2)	< 0.41	(2)

If suspected corpus luteum, repeat in next menstrual cycle in proliferative phase.

COLOR DOPPLER SCORE

≤ 2 Benign
3–4 Questionable

Figure 3–4. Scoring system used to evaluate the morphology of adnexal tumor. RI = resistance index. (Reprinted, with permission, from Kurjak A et al: Transvaginal ultrasound, color flow, and Doppler waveform of the postmenopausal adnexal mass. Obstet Gynecol 1992;80:917.)

the hCG level was greater then 7500 mIU/mL, an ectopic gestation should be suspected. In a second related report, another team stated that the presence of fluid in the cul-de-sac and a noncystic adnexal mass had a predictive value of 94% in the diagnosis of ectopic pregnancy. However, the sonographic appearance of a pseudogestational sac should not be confused with the gestational sac. In the latter, a double-ring sign caused by the decidua parietalis is seen abutting the decidua capsularis.

TVUS, on the other hand, has the advantage of earlier and improved localization of the pregnancy with less pelvic discomfort since the bladder is not painfully distended. An hCG level of 1000 to 1500 mIU/mL (based on the International Reference Preparation) is the discriminatory zone in which an intrauterine pregnancy can be detected by TVUS. One must identify the double-ring sign of the intrauterine pregnancy and/or the yolk sac to ensure that the pregnancy is intrauterine. When an intrauterine pregnancy is not visualized on TVUS and the hCG level exceeds 1000–2000 mIU/mL, then suspicion for an ectopic pregnancy should be high. Also, multiple gestations may take several more days to be identified, and heterotopic pregnancies will be encountered more frequently in the patients using assisted reproductive

Table 3–3. Histology and blood flow characteristics.

Histology	N	Flow Detected	RI
Malignant			
Papillary adeno-carcinoma	13	12	0.39 ± 0.04
Serous cystadeno-carcinoma	3	3	0.30 ± 0.04
Endometrioid adeno-carcinoma	4	4	0.38 ± 0.02
Metastatic carcinoma	7	7	0.37 ± 0.07
Theca-granulosa cell	2	1	0.37
Total	29	27	0.37 ± 0.08
Benign			
Simple cyst	25	5	0.75 ± 0.17
Papillary serous cyst	4	1	0.6
Mucinous cyst	5	3	0.62 ± 0.09
Inflammatory mass	2	1	0.62
Parasitic cyst	1	0	0
Fibroma	4	3	0.56 ± 0.03
Thecoma	2	2	0.60
Cystadenofibroma	1	1	0.56
Endometrioma	4	1	0.56
Cystic teratoma	1	1	0.36
Pseudo- and parovar-ian cyst	4	0	0
Brenner tumor	1	1	0.50
Total	54	19	0.62 ± 0.11[1]

RI = resistance index.
Data are presented as N or mean ± SD.
[1]$P < .001$.
Reprinted, with permission, from Kurjak A et al: Transvaginal ultrasound, color flow, and Doppler waveform of the post-menopausal adnexal mass. Obstet Gynecol 1992;80:917.

Table 3–4. Color flow in ovarian masses.

	Present	Absent
Benign	19	35
Malignant	27	2

Fisher exact two-tailed test: $< 1 \times 10^{-7}$. Sensitivity = 93%; specificity = 65%; positive predictive value = 59%; negative predictive value = 95%.
Reprinted, with permission, from Kurjak A et al: Transvaginal ultrasound, color flow, and Doppler waveform of the post-menopausal adnexal mass. Obstet Gynecol 1992;80:917.

is calculated. This ever-improving technology is beginning to produce excellent imaging to detect uterine structural abnormalities. The precise size and location of polyps and myomas, as well as complete delineation of müllerian fusion defects have been reported. The 3-D measurements of ovarian pathology (with or without color Doppler) offers improved detection of early ovarian cancers with a greater degree of accuracy than the imaging techniques discussed here. Unfortunately, these techniques require a great deal of time and skill to produce these images, and they will require more refinement before they replace the widely used 2-D images.

Conclusion

The imaging techniques prevalent today have proven to be valuable tools in the diagnosis and early treatment of benign and malignant gynecologic disorders. To provide the patient with the highest level of medical care, the contemporary practicing gynecologist must constantly keep abreast of the new developments and applications of diagnostic imaging.

techniques. The reader is referred to the section on ectopic pregnancy for a more complete discussion of this topic.

In a study of 71 patients with suspected ectopic pregnancies, one team failed to find an improvement in the diagnostic results when color Doppler imaging was used versus TVUS.

In the past decade, three-dimensional ultrasound has shown great promise in both obstetrics and gynecology. The technology is based on computer-generated three-dimensional images from a series of two-dimensional slices through the arc of tissue under the transducer. The resulting display shows longitudinal, transverse, and horizontal planes from which the 3-D image

Table 3–5. Flow pattern in benign and malignant ovaries.

Vessel Type	RI Benign	RI Malignant
Peripheral	0.56 (0.48–1.0)	0.40 (0.31–0.61)[1]
Central	0.54 (0.46–0.62)	0.38 (0.27–0.41)[1]
Septal	0.48 (0.47–0.50)	0.37 (0.32–0.42)[1]

RI = resistance index.
Data are pesented as mean (range).
[1]$P < .01$.
Reprinted, with permission, from Kurjak A et al: Transvaginal ultrasound, color flow, and Doppler waveform of the post-menopausal adnexal mass. Obstet Gynecol 1992;80:917.

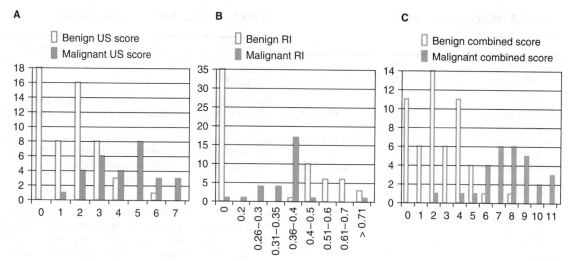

Figure 3–5. Distribution of data results in this study. **A:** The ultrasound (US) score; **B:** resistance index (RI); and **C:** combination of the two. In (**B**), an RI of zero means that no flow was seen. (Reprinted, with permission from Kurjak A et al: Transvaginal ultrasound, color flow, and Doppler waveform of the postmenopausal adnexal mass. Obstet Gynecol 1992;80:917.)

No matter what technology is used today and in the future, the goal will always be the same: to provide quick, low-risk, accurate diagnosis of gynecologic conditions, while keeping in mind the cost-effectiveness of the care delivered.

REFERENCES

Abramowicz JS: Ultrasound contrast media and their use in obstetrics and gynecology. Ultrasound Med Biol 1997;23:1287.

Ayida G et al: Is routine diagnostic laparoscopy for infertility still justified? A pilot study assessing the use of hystersalpingo-contrast sonography and magnetic resonance imaging. Hum Reprod 1997;12:1436.

DePriest PD, Gallion HH, Pavlik EJ: Transvaginal sonography as a screening method for the detection of early ovarian cancer. Gynecol Oncol 1997;65:408.

Karlan BY: The status of ultrasound and color Doppler imaging for the early detection of ovarian carcinoma. Cancer Invest 1997;15:265.

Krampl E et al: Transvaginal ultrasonography, sonohysterography and operative hysteroscopy for the evaluation of abnormal uterine bleeding. Acta Obstet Gynecol Scand 2001;80:616.

Kurjak A et al: Transvaginal ultrasound, color flow, and Doppler waveform of the postmenopausal adnexal mass. Obstet Gynecol 1992;80:917.

Laing FC: *Update on Ultrasonography, The Radiologic Clinics of North America.* WB Saunders, 2001;39:3, 499, 523.

Merz E: Three-dimensional transvaginal ultrasound in gynecological diagnosis. Ultrasound Obstet Gynecol 1999;14:81.

Ohishi H et al: Three-dimensional power Doppler sonography of tumor vascularity. J Ultrasound Med 1998;11:133.

Soper JT: Radiographic imaging in gynecologic oncology. Clin Obstet Gynecol 2001;44:3, 485.

Embryology of the Urogenital System & Congenital Anomalies of the Female Genital Tract

Catherine Marin, MD, & Joseph D. Bast, PhD

The adult genital and urinary systems are distinct both in function and in anatomy, with the exception of the male urethra. During development, however, these 2 systems are closely associated. Primordial elements in the urinary system participate in the formation of genital structures; this requisite initial developmental overlap of the 2 systems occurs during the 4–12 weeks after fertilization. The complexity of developmental events in these systems is evident by the incomplete separation of the 2 systems found in some congenital anomalies (eg, female pseudohermaphroditism with persistent urogenital sinus). For the sake of clarity, this chapter describes the embryology of each system separately, rather than following a strict developmental chronology.

This chapter also presents descriptive overviews of some congenital malformations of the female genital tract and, when possible, an explanation of their embryonic origins. In view of the complexity and duration of differentiation and development of the genital and urinary systems, it is not surprising that the incidence of malformations involving these systems is one of the highest (10%) of all body systems. Etiologies of congenital malformations are sometimes categorized on the basis of genetic, environmental, or genetic-plus-environmental (so-called polyfactorial inheritance) factors. Known genetic and inheritance factors reputedly account for about 20% of anomalies detected at birth, aberration of chromosomes for nearly 5%, and environmental factors for nearly 10%. The significance of these statistics must be viewed against reports that (1) an estimated one-third to one-half of human zygotes are lost during the first week of gestation and (2) the cause of possibly 70% of human anomalies is unknown. Even so, congenital malformations remain a matter of concern because they are detected in nearly 6% of infants, and 20% of perinatal deaths are purportedly due to congenital anomalies.

The inherent pattern of normal development of the genital system can be viewed as one directed toward somatic "femaleness," unless development is directed by factors for "maleness." The presence and expression of a Y chromosome (and its testis-determining genes) in a normal 46, XY karyotype of somatic cells directs differentiation toward a testis, and normal development of the testis makes available its steroidal and proteinaceous hormones for the selection and differentiation of the genital ducts. In the normal absence of these testicular products, the "female" paramesonephric (müllerian) ducts persist. Normal feminization or masculinization of the external genitalia is also a result of the respective timely absence or presence of androgen.

An infant usually is reared as female or male according to the appearance of the external genitalia. However, genital sex is not always immediately discernible, and the choice of sex of rearing can be an anxiety-provoking consideration. Unfortunately, even when genital sex is apparent, later clinical presentation may unmask disorders of sexual differentiation that can lead to problems in psychological adjustment. Whether a somatic disorder is detected at birth or later, investigative backtracking through the developmental process is necessary for proper diagnosis and treatment.

OVERVIEW OF THE FIRST FOUR WEEKS OF DEVELOPMENT*

The transformation of the bilaminar embryonic disk into a trilaminar disk composed of **ectoderm, mesoderm,** and **endoderm** (the 3 embryonic germ layers) occurs during the third week by a process called **gastrulation** (Fig 4–1). All 3 layers are derived from epiblast. During this process, a specialized longitudinal thickening of epiblast, the **primitive streak,** forms near the margin (future caudal region) of the bilaminar disk and eventually elongates cephalad through the midline of the disk and extends to the central region. Some epi-

---

* Embryonic or fetal ages given in this chapter are relative to the time of fertilization and should be considered estimates rather than absolutes.

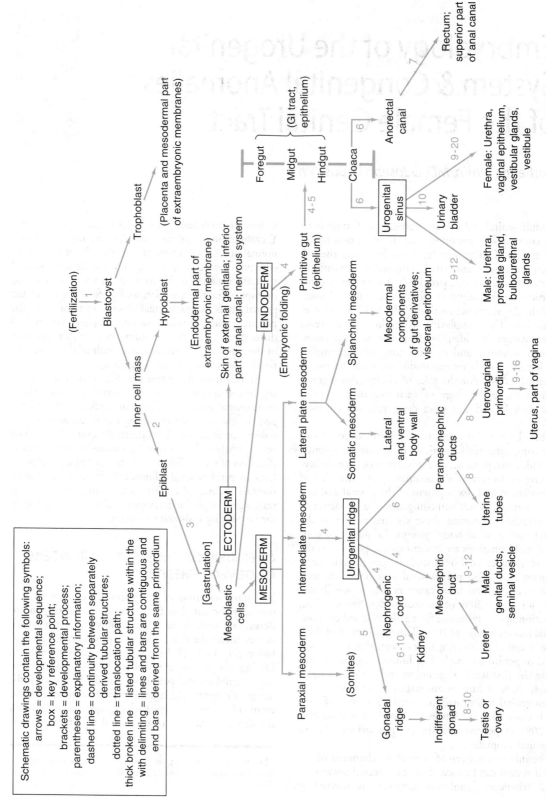

Figure 4–1. Schematic overview of embryonic development of progenitory urinary and genital tissues and structures considered to be derivatives of embryonic ectoderm, mesoderm, or endoderm. Numbers indicate the weeks after fertilization when the indicated developmental change occurs.

Schematic drawings contain the following symbols:
  arrows = developmental sequence;
  box = key reference point;
  brackets = developmental process;
  parentheses = explanatory information;
  dashed line = continuity between separately
      derived tubular structures;
  dotted line = translocation path;
  thick broken line   listed tubular structures within the
  with delimiting = lines and bars are contiguous and
  end bars   derived from the same primordium

blastic cells migrate medially through a midline depression of the streak, to the ventral aspect of the streak, after which they become **mesoblastic cells.** The mesoblastic cells migrate peripherally between most of the epiblast and the hypoblast, forming the middle layer (**embryonic mesoderm**) of the now trilaminar disk. Other mesoblastic cells migrate into the hypoblastic layer, causing lateral displacement of most, if not all, of the hypoblastic cells. This new ventral layer of the disk becomes the **embryonic endoderm.** With formation of the new mesodermal layer, the overlying epiblast becomes the **embryonic ectoderm,** of which the medial part gives rise to **neuroectoderm,** the forerunner of the neural tube and neural crest (ie, the nervous system). By the end of the third week, 3 clusters of embryonic mesoderm are organized on both sides of the midline-developing notochord and neural tube.

The medial cluster is a thickened longitudinal column of mesoderm called **paraxial mesoderm,** from which **somites,** and in turn much of the axial skeleton, will form. The lateralmost cluster is called **lateral plate mesoderm,** in which a space (or coelom) develops, creating dorsal and ventral mesodermal layers (Fig 4–2). The **intermediate mesoderm** is located between the paraxial and lateral plate mesoderm and is the origin of the **urogenital ridge** and, hence, much of the reproductive and excretory systems (Fig 4–3). The primitive streak regresses after the fourth week. Rarely, degeneration of the streak is incomplete and presumptive rem-

nants form a teratoma in the sacrococcygeal region of the fetus (more common in females than in males).

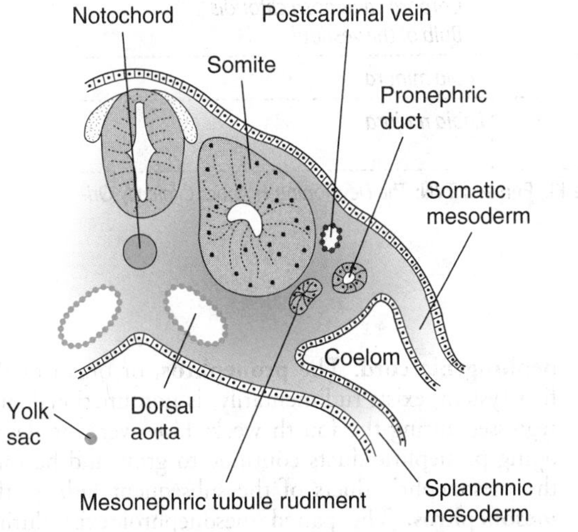

Weeks 4 through 8 of development are called the **embryonic period** (the **fetal period** is from week 9 to term) because formation of all major internal and external structures, including the 2 primary forerunners of the urogenital system (urogenital ridge and urogenital sinus), begins during this time. During this period the embryo is most likely to develop major congenital or acquired morphologic anomalies in response to the effects of various agents. During the fourth week, the shape of the embryo changes from that of a trilaminar disk to that of a crescentic cylinder. The change results from "folding," or flexion, of the embryonic disk in a ventral direction through both its transverse and longitudinal planes. Flexion occurs as midline structures (neural tube and somites) develop and grow at a faster pace than more lateral tissues (ectoderm, 2 layers of lateral plate mesoderm enclosing the coelom between them, and endoderm). Thus, during transverse folding, the lateral tissues on each side of the embryo curl ventromedially and join the respective tissues from the other side, creating a midline ventral tube (the endoderm-lined **primitive gut**), a mesoderm-lined coelomic cavity (the **primitive abdominopelvic cavity**), and the incomplete ventral and lateral body wall. Concurrent longitudinal flexion ventrally of the caudal region of the disk establishes the pouch-like distal end, or **cloaca,** of the primitive gut as well as the distal attachment of the cloaca to the yolk sac through the allantois of the sac (Fig 4–4).

A noteworthy point (see The Gonads, in text that follows) is that the primordial germ cells of the later-developing gonad initially are found close to the allantois and later migrate to the gonadal primordia. Subsequent partitioning of the cloaca during the sixth week results in formation of the anorectal canal and the **urogenital sinus,** the progenitor of the urinary bladder, urethra, vagina, and other genital structures (Fig 4–1 and Table 4–1; see Subdivision of the Cloaca & Formation of the Urogenital Sinus in following text).

Another consequence of the folding process is the repositioning of the intermediate mesoderm, the forerunner of the urogenital ridge. Laterally adjacent to developing somites (from paraxial mesoderm) before flexion, the intermediate mesoderm is located after flexion just lateral to the dorsal mesentery of the gut and in the dorsal wall of the new body cavity. Thickening of this intermediate mesoderm with subsequent bulging into the cavity will form the longitudinal **urogenital ridge** (Figs 4–1 and 4–4). Thus, by the end of the fourth week of development, the principal structures (urogenital ridge and cloaca) and tissues that give rise to the urogenital system are present.

Tables 4–1 and 4–2 provide a general overview of urogenital development.

Labels: Notochord · Postcardinal vein · Somite · Pronephric duct · Somatic mesoderm · Coelom · Yolk sac · Dorsal aorta · Mesonephric tubule rudiment · Splanchnic mesoderm

Figure 4–2. Cross section of embryo at the level of the rudimentary mesonephros. The tubule will form a lumen, grow, and connect with the duct. About 4 weeks' gestation, during embryonic flexion.

Table 4–1. Adult derivatives and vestigial remains of embryonic urogenital structures.[1,2]

Embryonic Structure	Male	Female
Indifferent gonad Cortex Medulla	*Testis* *Seminiferous tubules* *Rete testis*	*Ovary* *Ovarian follicles* *Medulla* *Rete ovarii*
Gubernaculum	*Gubernaculum testis*	*Ovarian ligament* *Round ligament of uterus*
Mesonephric tubules	*Ductus efferentes* Paradidymis	Epoophoron Paroophoron
Mesonephric duct	Appendix of epididymis *Ductus epididymidis* *Ductus deferens* *Ureter, pelvis, calices, and collecting tubules* *Ejaculatory duct and seminal vesicle*	Appendix vesiculosa Duct of epoophoron Duct of Gartner *Ureter, pelvis, calices, and collecting tubules*
Paramesonephric duct	Appendix of testis	Hydatid (of Morgagni) *Uterine tube* *Uterus* *Vagina (fibromuscular wall)*
Urogenital sinus	*Urinary bladder* *Urethra* (except glandular portion) Prostatic utricle *Prostate gland* *Bulbourethral glands*	*Urinary bladder* *Urethra* *Vagina* *Urethral* and *paraurethral glands* *Greater vestibular glands*
Müllerian tubercle	Seminal colliculus	Hymen
Genital tubercle	*Penis* *Glans penis* *Corpora cavernosa penis* *Corpus spongiosum*	*Clitoris* *Glans clitoridis* *Corpora cavernosa clitoridis* *Bulb of the vestibule*
Urogenital folds	*Ventral aspect of penis*	*Labia minora*
Labioscrotal swellings	*Scrotum*	*Labia majora*

[1]Modified and reproduced, with permission, from Moore KL, Persaud TVN: *The Developing Human: Clinically Oriented Embryology,* 5th ed. Saunders, 1993.
[2]Functional derivatives are in italics.

THE URINARY SYSTEM

Three excretory "systems" form successively, with temporal overlap, during the embryonic period. Each system has a different excretory "organ," but the 3 systems share anatomic continuity through development of their excretory ducts. The 3 systems are mesodermal derivatives of the urogenital ridge (Figs 4–3 and 4–4), part of which becomes a longitudinal mass, the nephrogenic cord. The **pronephros,** or organ of the first system, exists rudimentarily, is nonfunctional, and regresses during the fourth week. However, the developing pronephric ducts continue to grow and become the mesonephric ducts of the subsequent kidney, the **mesonephros.** The paired mesonephroi exist during 4–8 weeks as simplified morphologic versions of the third, or permanent, set of kidneys, and they may have transient excretory function. The permanent kidney,

Table 4–2. Developmental chronology of the human urogenital system.[1]

Age in Weeks[2]	Size (C–R)[3] in mm	Urogenital System
2.5	1.5	Allantois present.
3.5	2.5	All pronephric tubules formed. Pronephric duct growing caudad as a blind tube. Cloaca and cloacal membrane present.
4	5	Primordial germ cells near allantois. Pronephros degenerated. Pronephric (mesonephric) duct reaches cloaca. Mesonephric tubules differentiating rapidly. Metanephric bud pushes into secretory primordium.
5	8	Mesonephros reaches its caudal limit. Ureteric and pelvic primordia distinct.
6	12	Cloaca subdividing into urogenital sinus and anorectal canal. Sexless gonad and genital tubercle prominent. Paramesonephric duct appearing. Metanephric collecting tubules begin branching.
7	17	Mesonephros at peak of differentiation. Urogenital sinus separated from anorectal canal (cloaca subdivided). Urogenital and anal membranes rupturing.
8	23	Earliest metanephric secretory tubules differentiating. Testis (8 weeks) and ovary (9–10 weeks) identifiable as such. Paramesonephric ducts, nearing urogenital sinus, are ready to unite a uterovaginal primordium. Genital ligaments indicated.
10	40	Kidney able to excrete urine. Bladder expands as sac. Genital duct of opposite sex degenerating. Bulbourethral and vestibular glands appearing. Vaginal bulbs forming.
12	56	Kidney in lumbar location. Early ovarian folliculogenesis begins. Uterine horns absorbed. External genitalia attain distinctive features. Mesonephros and rete tubules complete male duct. Prostate and seminal vesicle appearing. Hollow viscera gaining muscular walls.
16	112	Testis at deep inguinal ring. Uterus and vagina recognizable as such. Mesonephros involuted.
20–38 (5–9 months)	160–350	Female urogenital sinus becoming a shallow vestibule (5 months). Vagina regains lumen (5 months). Uterine glands begin to appear (5 months). Scrotum solid until sacs and testes descend (7–8 months). Kidney tubules cease forming at birth.

[1]Modified and reproduced, with permission, from Arey LB: *Developmental Anatomy*, 7th ed. Saunders, 1965.
[2]After fertilization.
[3]C–R, crown-rump length.

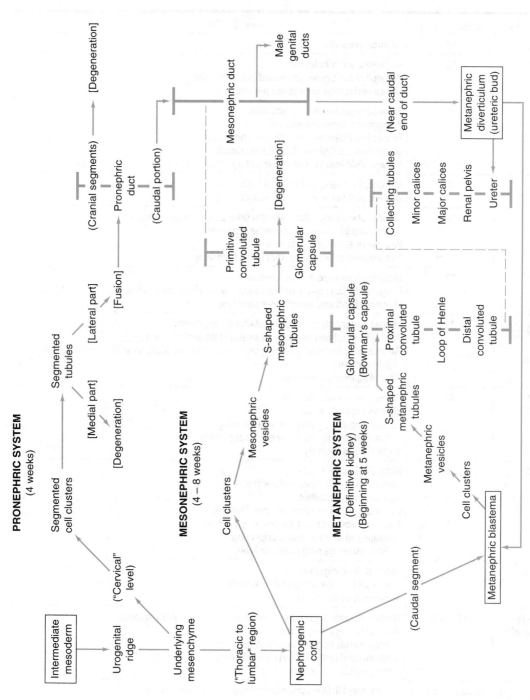

Figure 4–3. Schematic drawing of formation of the definitive kidney and its collecting ducts. The pronephric duct is probably the only structure that participates in all 3 urinary systems, as its caudal portion continues to grow and is called the mesonephric duct when the mesonephric system develops. (Explanatory symbols are given in Fig 4–1.)

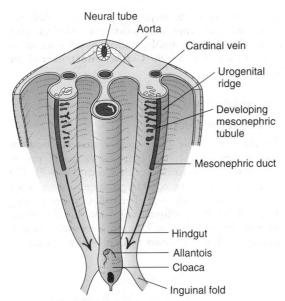

Figure 4–4. Early stage in the formation of the mesonephric kidneys and their collecting ducts in the urogenital ridge. The central tissue of the ridge is the nephrogenic cord, in which the mesonephric tubules are forming. The mesonephric ducts grow toward (arrows) and will open into the cloaca. About 5 weeks' gestation.

the **metanephros,** begins to form in response to an inductive influence of a diverticulum of the mesonephric ducts during the fifth week and becomes functional at 10–13 weeks. During nephric differentiation, the urogenital mass becomes suspended from the dorsal wall by a double-layered urogenital mesentery.

Pronephros

Segmented clusters of cells form in each urogenital ridge opposite the cervical somitic region and give rise to **pronephric tubules.** The lateral end of a tubule in one segment of the ridge grows caudally to fuse with the end of the pronephric tubule in the next segment, thus initiating the cephalic portion of each of the bilateral **pronephric ducts** (Fig 4–3). The pronephroi degenerate by the end of the fourth week, but, by initiating formation of pronephric ducts, they set in motion the developmental sequence for the formation of the permanent excretory ducts and kidneys. The pronephric ducts continue to grow caudally until week 5, when they contact and open into the lateral posterior wall of the cloaca.

Mesonephros

Development of the mesonephric glomerulotubular units begins while the pronephric tubules are regressing. Cells in each nephrogenic cord condense to form cell clusters just caudal to the pronephros and adjacent to the caudally growing pronephric duct (now called the **mesonephric duct**). Each cluster differentiates into a hollow **mesonephric vesicle** and then a **mesonephric tubule.** Subsequently, the lateral end of a tubule joins the mesonephric duct (Figs 4–4 and 4–5), while the medial end of the tubule expands into a double-layered, cup-shaped primitive glomerular capsule (**Bowman's capsule;** Fig 4–6). The capsule is vascularized by a capillary tuft, the **glomerulus,** derived from the aorta. Proliferation of the tubule's midportion produces a primitive version of a convoluted tubule.

While differentiation of the mesonephros is taking place in the caudal region, regression of mature tubules in the cranial region is also occurring (Fig 4–7). This craniocaudal gradient of differentiation followed by regression can give the impression that the relatively

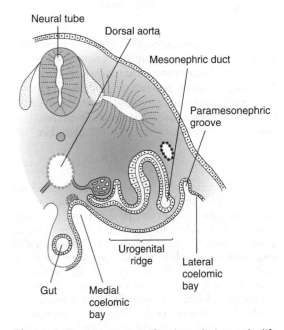

Figure 4–5. Cross section of embryo during early differentiation of the Y-shaped mesonephric tubule. A primitive glomerular unit is forming, and the tubule has opened into the duct. Note the invagination of coelomic epithelium, a very early stage of formation of the paramesonephric duct. Between 5 and 6 weeks' gestation.

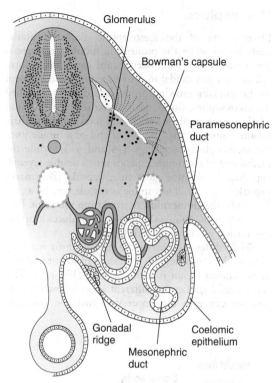

Figure 4–6. Cross section of embryo after formation of the mesonephric excretory unit (a simplified depiction of the primitive convoluted tubule is presented). The collection of cells beneath the epithelium of the urogenital ridge facing the medial coelomic bay is part of the developing gonadal ridge, from which the gonad will differentiate. About 6 weeks' gestation.

large, ovoid mesonephric kidney "descends" along the posterior wall of the body cavity during the embryonic period. By the end of this period, most remaining mesonephric tubules and glomeruli have begun to degenerate. Some of these tubules (descriptively called **epigenital mesonephric tubules**) persist in the mesonephric region laterally adjacent to the developing gonad and will participate in formation of the gonad and the male ductuli efferentes (Fig 4–8). A few tubules at other levels may persist as vestigial remnants near the gonad and sometimes become cystic (see Figs 4–14 and 4–15).

Differentiation of the caudal segment of the mesonephric ducts results in (1) incorporation of part of the ducts into the wall of the urogenital sinus (early vesicular trigone, see following text), and (2) formation of a ductal diverticulum, which plays an essential role in formation of the definitive kidney. If male sex differ-

entiation occurs, the major portion of each duct becomes the epididymis, ductus deferens, and ejaculatory duct. Only small vestigial remnants of the duct sometimes persist in the female (**Gartner's duct; duct of the epoophoron**).

Metanephros (Definitive Kidney)

A. COLLECTING DUCTS

By the end of the fifth week, a **ureteric bud,** or metanephric diverticulum, forms on the caudal part of the mesonephric duct close to the cloaca (Fig 4–7). The bud gives rise to the collecting tubules, calices, renal pelvis, and ureter (Fig 4–3). The stalk of the elongating bud will become the **ureter** when the ductal segment between the stalk and the cloaca becomes incorporated into the wall of the urinary bladder (which is a deriva-

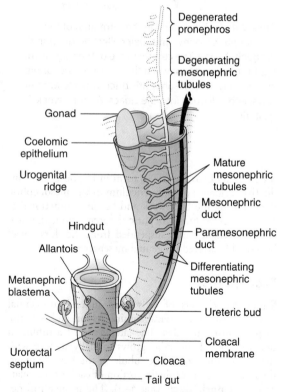

Figure 4–7. Metanephric diverticulum (ureteric bud) and blastema and the relationships between the mesonephric and genital structures in the urogenital ridge. The paramesonephric duct crosses ventral to the mesonephric duct and grows toward the cloaca. The urorectal septum begins to subdivide the cloaca. About 6 weeks' gestation.

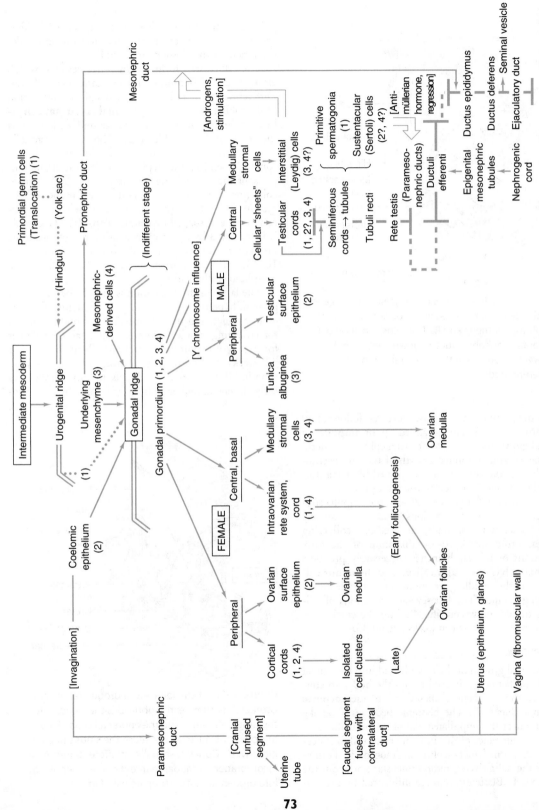

Figure 4–8. Schematic drawing of the formation of the gonads and genital ducts. Numbers in parentheses by tissues after the indifferent stage indicate the presumed cellular origin from the urogenital ridge (see text for details; explanatory symbols are given in Fig 4–1).

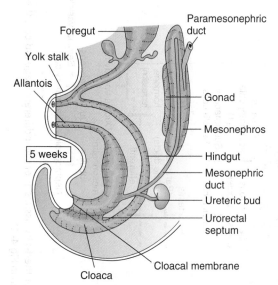

Figure 4–9. Left-side view of urogenital system and cloacal region prior to subdivision of cloaca by urorectal septum (Tourneux and Rathke folds). Position of future paramesonephric duct is shown (begins in the sixth week). Gonad is in the indifferent stage (sexually undifferentiated).

tive of the partitioned cloaca, see text that follows; Figs 4–9 through 4–12). The expanded tip, or **ampulla,** of the bud grows into the adjacent metanephric mesoderm (**blastema**), and continued growth of the bud eventually relocates the ampulla and associated blastema dorsal to the mesonephros (ie, "retroperitoneal").

Between week 6 and weeks 20–24, the ampulla subdivides, and successive divisions yield approximately 12–15 generations of buds, or eventual **collecting tubules.** From weeks 10–14, dilatation of the early generations of tubular branches successively produces the **renal pelvis,** the **major calices,** and the **minor calices,** while the middle generations form the medullary collecting tubules. The last several generations of collecting tubules grow centrifugally into the cortical region of the kidney between weeks 24 and 36.

B. Nephrons

Dorsocranial growth of the ureteric bud into the caudal end of the nephrogenic cord brings the bud into contact with the metanephric mesoderm, or **metanephric blastema** (Fig 4–7). The blastema becomes a caplike structure over the ampullated end of the bud, and continued maintenance of this intimate relationship is necessary for normal metanephric organogenesis. Formation of the definitive excretory units starts at about the eighth week. Blastemic cells are influenced by the am-

pulla to form clusters. Subsequent early stages of differentiation of the blastema are similar to those in the development of the mesonephric tubule.

The cell clusters form **metanephric vesicles, which elongate and differentiate into metanephric tubules.** Differential proliferation of segments of the midportion of the tubule produces the **proximal** and **distal convoluted tubules,** whereas the central midportion forms the **loop of Henle** (Fig 4–3). The loops eventually grow centripetally toward the developing medullary zone. The end of the nephric tubule nearest the ampulla of the subdividing bud joins the newly formed collecting duct of that bud. The other end of the metanephric tubule expands, infolds somewhat, and becomes the cup-shaped **Bowman's capsule.** The capsule is invaginated by a tuft of capillaries, the **glomerulus.** Formation of urine purportedly begins at about weeks 10–13, when an estimated 20% of the nephrons are morphologically mature.

The last month of gestation is marked by interstitial growth, hypertrophy of existing components of uriniferous tubules, and the disappearance of bud primordia for collecting tubules. Opinions differ about whether formation of nephrons ceases prenatally at about 28 or 32 weeks or, postnatally, during the first several months. If the ureteric bud fails to form, undergoes early degeneration, or fails to grow into the nephro-

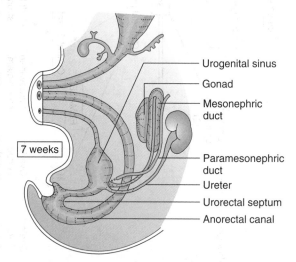

Figure 4–10. Left-side view of urogenital system. Urorectal septum nearly subdivides the cloaca into the urogenital sinus and the anorectal canal. Paramesonephric ducts do not reach the sinus until the ninth week. Gonad is sexually undifferentiated. Note incorporation of caudal segment of mesonephric duct into urogenital sinus (compare with Fig 4–9).

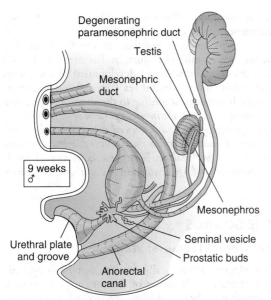

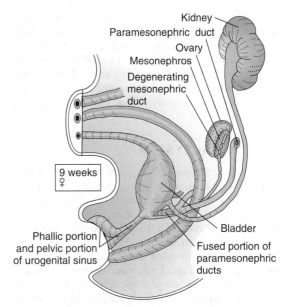

Figure 4–11. Left-side view of urogenital system at an early stage of male sexual differentiation. Phallic part of urogenital sinus is proliferating anteriorly to form the urethral plate and groove. Seminal vesicles and prostatic buds are shown at a more advanced stage (about 12 weeks) for emphasis.

Figure 4–12. Left-side view of urogenital system at an early stage of female sexual differentiation. Paramesonephric (müllerian) ducts have fused caudally (to form uterovaginal primordium) and contacted the pelvic part of the urogenital sinus.

genic mesoderm, aberrations of nephrogenesis result. These may be nonthreatening (**unilateral renal agenesis**), severe, or even fatal (**bilateral renal agenesis, polycystic kidney**).

C. POSITIONAL CHANGES

Figure 4–13 illustrates relocation of the kidney to a deeper position within the posterior body wall, as well as the approximately 90-degree medial rotation of the organ on its longitudinal axis. Rotation and lateral positioning are probably facilitated by the growth of midline structures (axial skeleton and muscles). The "ascent" of the kidney between weeks 5 and 8 can be attributed largely to differential longitudinal growth of the rest of the lumbosacral area and to the reduction of the rather sharp curvature of the caudal region of the embryo. Some migration of the kidney may also occur. Straightening of the curvature may be attributable also to relative changes in growth, especially the development of the infraumbilical abdominal wall. As the kidney moves into its final position (lumbar 1–3 by the 12th week), its arterial supply shifts to successively higher aortic levels. Ectopic kidneys can result from abnormal "ascent." During the seventh week, the "ascending" metanephroi closely approach each other near

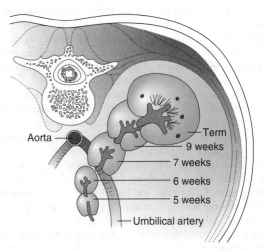

Figure 4–13. Positional changes of the definitive kidney at 5 different stages but projected on one cross-sectional plane. (Redrawn and modified, with permission, from Kelly HA, Burnam CF: *Diseases of Kidneys, Ureters and Bladder.* Appleton-Century-Crofts, 1972.)

the aortic bifurcation. The close approximation of the 2 developing kidneys can lead to fusion of the lower poles of the kidneys, resulting in formation of a single **horseshoe kidney,** the ascent of which would be arrested by the stem of the interior mesenteric artery. Infrequently, a **pelvic kidney** results from trapping of the organ beneath the umbilical artery, which restricts passage out of the pelvis.

THE GENITAL SYSTEM

Sexual differentiation of the genital system occurs in a basically sequential order: genetic, gonadal, ductal, and genital. **Genetic sex** is determined at fertilization by the complement of sex chromosomes (ie, XY specifies a genotypic male and XX a female). However, early morphologic indications of the sex of the developing embryo do not appear until about the eighth or ninth week after conception. Thus, there is a so-called **indifferent stage,** when morphologic identity of sex is not clear or when preferential differentiation for one sex has not been imposed on the sexless primordia. This is characteristic of early developmental stages for the gonads, genital ducts, and external genitalia. When the influence of genetic sex has been expressed on the indifferent gonad, **gonadal sex** is established. The **SRY (sex-determining region of the Y chromosome)** gene in the short arm of the Y chromosome of normal genetic males is considered the best candidate for the gene encoding for the **testis-determining factor (TDF).** TDF initiates a chain of events that results in differentiation of the gonad into a testis with its subsequent production of anti-müllerian hormone and testosterone, which influences development of somatic "maleness" (see Testis, in following text). Normal genetic females do not have the SRY gene, and the early undifferentiated medullary region of their presumptive gonad does not produce the TDF (see Ovary).

The testis and ovary are derived from the same primordial tissue, but histologically visible differentiation toward a testis occurs sooner than that toward an ovary. An "ovary" is first recognized by the absence of testicular histogenesis (eg, thick tunica albuginea) or by the presence of germ cells entering meiotic prophase between the eighth and about the 11th week. The different primordia for male and female genital ducts exist in each embryo during overlapping periods, but establishment of male or female **ductal sex** depends on the presence or absence, respectively, of testicular products and the sensitivity of tissues to these products. The 2 primary testicular products are androgenic steroids (**testosterone** and nonsteroidal **anti-müllerian hormone** (see Testis). Stimulation by testosterone influences the persistence and differentiation of the "male" mesonephric ducts (**wolffian ducts**), whereas anti-mül-

lerian hormone influences regression of the "female" paramesonephric ducts (**müllerian ducts**). Absence of these hormones in a nonaberrant condition specifies persistence of müllerian ducts and regression of wolffian ducts, ie, initiation of development of the uterus and uterine tubes. **Genital sex** (external genitalia) subsequently develops according to the absence or presence of androgen. Thus, *the inherent pattern of differentiation of the genital system can be viewed as one directed toward somatic "femaleness" unless the system is dominated by certain factors for "maleness" (eg, gene expression of the Y chromosome, androgenic steroids, and anti-müllerian hormone).*

THE GONADS

Indifferent (Sexless) Stage

Gonadogenesis temporally overlaps metanephrogenesis and interacts with tissues of the mesonephric system. Formation of the gonad is summarized schematically in Fig 4–8.

About the fifth week, the midportion of each urogenital ridge ventromedially adjacent to the mesonephros thickens as cellular condensation forms the **gonadal ridge** (Fig 4–6). For the next 2 weeks, this ridge is an undifferentiated cell mass, lacking either testicular or ovarian morphology. As shown in Fig 4–8, the cell mass consists of (1) **primordial germ cells,** which translocate into the ridge, and a mixture of **somatic cells** derived by (2) proliferation of the **coelomic epithelial cells,** (3) condensation of the **underlying mesenchyme** of part of the urogenital ridge, and (4) ingrowth of **mesonephric-derived cells.** The epithelial cells are not confined to the coelomic surface because the basal lamina of the coelomic epithelium is discontinuous in the area of the gonadal ridge.

The **mesonephric-derived cells** enter the basal aspect of the undifferentiated gonad, and some of these cells move peripherally, while some epithelial cells penetrate the mesenchyme and move centrally. During the indifferent stage, the germ cells and different somatic cells "intermingle" in the compact mass of the primordium. Later differentiation of the gonadal primordium results from interaction of the germ cells and the 3 types of somatic cells listed above. The end of the gonadal indifferent stage in the male is near the middle of the seventh week, when a basal lamina delineates the coelomic epithelium and the developing tunica albuginea separates the coelomic epithelium from the developing testicular cords. The indifferent stage in the female ends around the ninth week, when the first oogonia enter meiotic prophase.

Primordial germ cells, presumptive progenitors of the gametes, become evident in the late third to early fourth week in the dorsocaudal wall of the yolk sac and the mesenchyme around the allantois. The **allantois** is a caudal diverticulum of the yolk sac that extends distally into the primitive umbilical stalk and, after embryonic flexion, is adjacent proximally to the cloacal hindgut. The primordial germ cells are translocated from the allantoic region (about the middle of the fourth week) to the urogenital ridge (between the middle of the fifth week and late in the sixth week). The mechanism of translocation is uncertain (perhaps partially by ameboid movement and also passively owing to positional change of tissues). It is not known whether primordial germ cells must be present in the gonadal ridge for full differentiation of the gonad to occur. The initial stages of somatic development appear to occur independently of the germ cells. Later endocrine activity in the testis, but not in the ovary, is known to occur in the absence of germ cells. The germ cells appear to have some influence on gonadal differentiation at certain stages of development.

Testis

During early differentiation of the testis, there are condensations of germ cells and somatic cells (see previous text), which have been described as platelike groups, or sheets. These groups are at first distributed throughout the gonad and then become more organized as primitive **testicular cords.** The cords begin to form centrally and are somewhat arranged perpendicular to the long axis of the gonad. In response to testis-determining factor (TDF), these cords will differentiate into Sertoli cells (see following text). The first characteristic feature of male gonadal sex differentiation is evident around week 8, when the **tunica albuginea** begins to form in the mesenchymal tissue underlying the coelomic epithelium. Eventually, this thickened layer of tissue causes the developing testicular cords to be separated from the surface epithelium and placed deeper in the central region of the gonad. The surface epithelium reforms a basal lamina and later thins to a mesothelial covering of the gonad. The testicular cords coil peripherally and thicken as their cellular organization becomes more distinct. A basal lamina eventually develops in the testicular cords, although it is not known if the somatic cells, germ cells, or both are primary contributors to the lamina.

Throughout gonadal differentiation, the developing testicular cords appear to maintain a close relationship to the basal area of the mesonephric-derived cell mass. An interconnected network of cords, **rete cords,** develops in this cell mass and gives rise to the **rete testis.** The rete testis joins centrally with neighboring epigenital mesonephric tubules, which become the **efferent ductules** linking the rete testis with the epididymis, a

derivative of the mesonephric duct. With gradual enlargement of the testis and regression of the mesonephros, a cleft forms between the 2 organs, slowly creating the mesentery of the testis, the **mesorchium.**

The differentiating testicular cords are made up of primordial germ cells (primitive spermatogonia) and somatic "supporting" cells (**sustentacular cells,** or **Sertoli cells**). Some precocious meiotic activity has been observed in the fetal testis. Meiosis in the germ cells usually does not begin until puberty; the cause of this delay is unknown. Besides serving as "supporting cells" for the primitive spermatogonia, Sertoli cells also produce a glycoprotein, **anti-müllerian hormone (AMH;** also called **müllerian-inhibiting substance**). Anti-müllerian hormone causes regression of the para-mesonephric (müllerian) ducts, apparently during a very discrete period of ductal sensitivity in male fetuses. At puberty, the seminiferous cords mature to become the seminiferous tubules, and the Sertoli cells and spermatogonia mature.

Shortly after the testicular cords form, the steroid-producing **interstitial (Leydig) cells** of the extracordal compartment of the testis differentiate from stromal mesenchymal cells, probably due to anti-müllerian hormone. Mesonephric-derived cells may also be a primordial source of Leydig cells. Steroidogenic activity of Leydig cells begins near the tenth week. High levels of testosterone are produced during the period of differentiation of external genitalia (weeks 11–12) and maintained through weeks 16–18. Steroid levels then rise or fall somewhat in accordance with changes in the concentration of Leydig cells. Both the number of cells and the levels of testosterone decrease around the fifth month.

Ovary

A. DEVELOPMENT

In the normal absence of the Y chromosome or the sex-determining region of the Y chromosome (SRY gene; see The Genital System, above), the somatic sex cords of the indifferent gonad do not produce testis-determining factor (TDF). In the absence of TDF, differentiation of the gonad into a testis and its subsequent production of anti-müllerian hormone and testosterone do not occur (see Testis, above). The indifferent gonad becomes an ovary. Complete ovarian differentiation seems to require 2 X chromosomes (XO females exhibit ovarian dysgenesis, in which ovaries have precociously degenerated germ cells and no follicles and are present as gonadal "streaks"). The first recognition of a developing ovary around weeks 9–10 is based on the temporal absence of testicular-associated features (most prominently, the tunica albuginea) and on the presence of early meiotic activity in the germ cells.

Early differentiation toward an ovary involves mesonephric-derived cells "invading" the basal region (adjacent to mesonephros) and central region of the gonad (central and basal regions represent the primitive "medullary" region of the gonad). At the same time, clusters of germ cells are displaced somewhat peripherally into the "cortical" region of the gonad. Some of the central mesonephric cells give rise to the rete system that subsequently forms a network of cords (**intraovarian rete cords**) extending to the primitive cortical area. As these cords extend peripherally between germ clusters, some epithelial cell proliferations extend centrally, and some mixing of these somatic cells apparently takes place around the germ cell clusters. These early cordlike structures are more irregularly distributed than early cords in the testis and not distinctly outlined. The cords open into clusters of germ cells, but all germ cells are not confined to cords. The first oogonia that begin meiosis are located in the innermost part of the cortex and are the first germ cells to contact the intraovarian rete cords.

Folliculogenesis begins in the innermost part of the cortex when the central somatic cells of the cord contact and surround the germ cells and an intact basal lamina is laid down. These somatic cells are morphologically similar to the mesonephric cells that form the intraovarian rete cords associated with the oocytes and apparently differentiate into the presumptive granulosa cells of the early follicle. Folliculogenesis continues peripherally. Between weeks 12 and 20 of gestation, proliferative activity causes the surface epithelium to become a thickened, irregular multilayer of cells, and in the absence of a basal lamina, the cells and apparent epithelial cell cords mix with underlying tissues. These latter cortical cords often retain a connection to and appear similar to the surface epithelium. The epithelial cells of these cords probably differentiate into granulosa cells and contribute to folliculogenesis, although this is after the process is well under way in the central region of the gonad. Follicles fail to form in the absence of oocytes or with precocious loss of germ cells, and oocytes not encompassed by follicular cells degenerate.

Stromal mesenchymal cells, connective tissue, somatic cells of cords not participating in folliculogenesis, and a vascular complex form the **ovarian medulla** in the late fetal ovary. Individual **primordial follicles** containing diplotene oocytes populate the inner and outer cortex of this ovary. The rete ovarii may persist, along with a few vestiges of mesonephric tubules, as the vestigial epoophoron near the adult ovary. Finally, similar to the testicular mesorchium, the **mesovarium** eventually forms as a gonadal mesentery between the ovary and old urogenital ridge. Postnatally, the epithelial surface of the ovary consists of a single layer of cells continuous with peritoneal mesothelium at the ovarian hilum. A thin, fibrous connective tissue, the tunica albuginea, forms beneath the surface epithelium and separates it from the cortical follicles.

B. Anomalies of the Ovaries

Anomalies of the ovaries encompass a broad range of developmental errors from complete absence of the ovaries to supernumerary ovaries. The many variations of gonadal disorders usually are subcategorized within classifications of disorders of sex determination. Unfortunately, there is little consensus for a major classification, although most include pathogenetic consideration. Extensive, excellent summaries of the different classifications are offered in the references to this chapter.

Congenital absence of the ovary (no gonadal remnants found) is very rare. Two types have been considered, agenesis and agonadism. By definition, **agenesis** implies that the primordial gonad did not form in the urogenital ridge, whereas **agonadism** indicates the absence of gonads that may have formed initially and subsequently degenerated. It can be difficult to distinguish one type from the other on a practical basis. For example, a patient with female genital ducts and external genitalia and a 46, XY karyotype could represent either gonadal agenesis or agonadism. In the latter condition, the gonad may form but undergo early degeneration and resorption before any virilizing expression is made. *Whenever congenital absence of the ovaries is suspected, careful examination of the karyotype, the external genitalia, and the genital ducts must be performed.*

Descriptions of agonadism have usually indicated that the external genitalia are abnormal (variable degree of fusion of labioscrotal swellings) and that either very rudimentary ductal derivatives are present or there are no genital ducts. The cause of agonadism is unknown, although several explanations have been suggested, such as (1) failure of the primordial gonad to form, along with abnormal formation of ductal anlagen, and (2) partial differentiation and then regression and absorption of testes (accounting for suppression of müllerian ducts but lack of stimulation of mesonephric, or wolffian, ducts). Explanations that include teratogenic effects or genetic defects are more likely candidates in view of the associated incidence of nonsexual somatic anomalies with the disorder. The **streak gonad** is a product of primordial gonadal formation and subsequent failure of differentiation, which can occur at various stages. The gonad usually appears as a fibrous-like cord of mixed elements (lacking germ cells) located parallel to a uterine tube. Streak gonads are characteristic of **gonadal dysgenesis** and a 45, XO karyotype (**Turner's syndrome;** distinctions are drawn between

Turner's syndrome and **Turner's stigmata** when consideration is given to the various associated somatic anomalies of gonadal dysgenesis). However, streak gonads may be consequent to genetic mutation or hereditary disease other than the anomalous karyotype.

Ectopic ovarian tissue occasionally can be found as **accessory ovarian tissue** or as **supernumerary ovaries.** The former may be a product of disaggregation of the embryonic ovary, and the latter may arise from the urogenital ridge as independent primordia.

SUBDIVISION OF THE CLOACA & FORMATION OF THE UROGENITAL SINUS

The endodermally lined urogenital sinus is derived by partitioning of the endodermal cloaca; it is the precursor of the urinary bladder in both sexes and the urinary and genital structures specific to each sex (see Fig 4–1). The cloaca is a pouch-like enlargement of the caudal end of the hindgut and is formed by the process of "folding" of the caudal region of the embryonic disk between 4 and 5 weeks' gestation (see Overview of the First Four Weeks of Development, above; Figs 4–1 and 4–4). During the "tail-fold" process, the posteriorly placed allantois, or allantoic diverticulum of the yolk sac, becomes an anterior extension of the cloaca (Figs 4–4 and 4–9). Soon after the cloaca forms, it receives posterolaterally the caudal ends of the paired mesonephric ducts and hence becomes a junctional cistern for the allantois, the hindgut, and the ducts (Fig 4–7). A **cloacal membrane,** composed of ectoderm and endoderm, is the caudal limit of the primitive gut and temporarily separates the cloacal cavity from the extraembryonic confines of the amniotic cavity (Figs 4–7 and 4–9).

Between weeks 5 and 7, 3 wedges of splanchnic mesoderm, collectively called the **urorectal septum,** proliferate in the coronal plane in the caudal region of the embryo to eventually subdivide the cloaca (Figs 4–9 through 4–12). The superior wedge, called the **Tourneux fold,** is in the angle between the allantois and the primitive hindgut, and it proliferates caudally into the superior end of the cloaca (Fig 4–9). The other 2 mesodermal wedges, called the **Rathke folds,** proliferate in the right and left walls of the cloaca. Beginning adjacent to the cloacal membrane, these laterally placed folds grow toward each other and the Tourneux fold. With fusion of the 3 folds creating a urorectal septum, the once single chamber is subdivided into the primitive **urogenital sinus** (ventrally) and the **anorectal canal** of the hindgut (dorsally; see Figs 4–10 through 4–12). The mesonephric ducts and allantois then open into the sinus. The uterovaginal primordium of the fused paramesonephric ducts will contact the sinusal wall between the mesonephric ducts early in the ninth week of development. Formation of the external genitalia is discussed below. However, it can be noted that the junctional point of fusion of the cloacal membrane and urorectal septum forms the **primitive perineum** (later differentiation creates the so-called perineal body of tissue) and subdivides the cloacal membrane into the **urogenital membrane** (anteriorly) and the **anal membrane** (posteriorly; Figs 4–9, 4–12, 4–14, and 4–24).

THE GENITAL DUCTS

Indifferent (Sexless) Stage

Two pairs of genital ducts are initially present in both sexes: (1) the **mesonephric (wolffian) ducts,** which give rise to the male ducts and a derivative, the seminal vesicles; and (2) the **paramesonephric (müllerian) ducts,** which form the oviducts, uterus, and part of the vagina. When the adult structures are described as derivatives of embryonic ducts, this refers to the epithelial lining of the structures. Muscle and connective tissues of the differentiating structures originate from splanchnic mesoderm and mesenchyme adjacent to ducts. Mesonephric ducts are originally the excretory ducts of the mesonephric "kidneys" (see previous text), and they develop early in the embryonic period, about 2 weeks before development of paramesonephric ducts (weeks 6–10). The 2 pairs of genital ducts share a close anatomic relationship in their bilateral course through the urogenital ridge. At their caudal limit, both sets contact the part of the cloaca that is later separated as the urogenital sinus (Figs 4–9, 4–10, and 4–14). *Determination of the ductal sex of the embryo (ie, which pair of ducts will continue differentiation rather than undergo regression) is established initially by the gonadal sex and later by the continuing influence of hormones.*

Formation of each paramesonephric duct begins early in the sixth week as an invagination of coelomic epithelium in the lateral wall of the cranial end of the urogenital ridge and adjacent to each mesonephric duct (Fig 4–5). The free edges of the invaginated epithelium join to form the duct except at the site of origin, which persists as a funnel-shaped opening, the future **ostium of the oviduct.** At first, each paramesonephric duct grows caudally through the mesenchyme of the urogenital ridge and laterally parallel to a mesonephric duct. More inferiorly, the paramesonephric duct has a caudomedial course, passing ventral to the mesonephric duct (Fig 4–7). As it follows the ventromedial bend of the caudal portion of the urogenital ridge, the paramesonephric duct then lies medial to the mesonephric duct, and its caudal tip lies in close apposition to its counterpart from the opposite side (Fig 4–14). At approximately the eighth week, the caudal segments of the right and left ducts fuse medi-

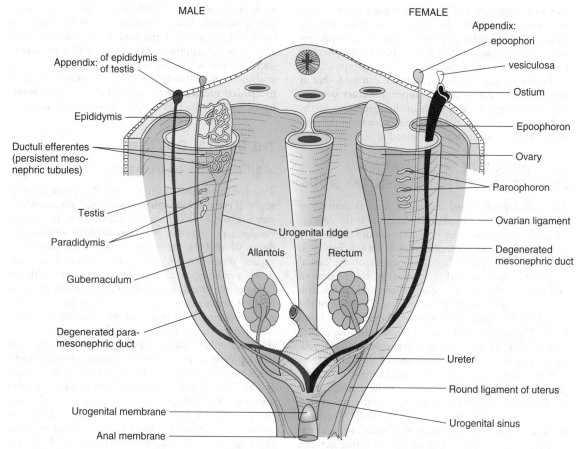

MALE

FEMALE

Appendix:
- of epididymis
- of testis

Epididymis

Ductuli efferentes
(persistent meso-
nephric tubules)

Testis

Paradidymis

Gubernaculum

Degenerated para-
mesonephric duct

Urogenital membrane

Anal membrane

Appendix:
- epoophori
- vesiculosa

Ostium

Epoophoron

Ovary

Paroophoron

Ovarian ligament

Degenerated
mesonephric duct

Ureter

Round ligament of uterus

Urogenital sinus

Urogenital ridge

Allantois

Rectum

Figure 4–14. Diagrammatic comparison between male and female differentiation of internal genitalia.

ally and their lumens coalesce to form a single cavity. This conjoined portion of the Y-shaped paramesonephric ducts becomes the uterovaginal primordium, or canal.

Male: Genital Ducts

A. MESONEPHRIC DUCTS

The mesonephric ducts persist in the male and, under the stimulatory influence of testosterone, differentiate into the internal genital ducts (epididymis, ductus deferens, and ejaculatory ducts). Near the cranial end of the duct, some of the mesonephric tubules (epigenital mesonephric tubules) of the mesonephric kidney persist lateral to the developing testis. These tubules form a connecting link, the **ductuli efferentes,** between the duct and the rete testis (Fig 4–14). The cranial portion of each duct becomes the convoluted **ductus epididymis.** The **ductus deferens** forms when smooth

muscle from adjacent splanchnic mesoderm is added to the central segment of the mesonephric duct. The seminal vesicle develops as a lateral bud from each mesonephric duct just distal to the junction of the duct and the urogenital sinus (Fig 4–11). The terminal segment of the duct between the sinus and seminal vesicle forms the **ejaculatory duct,** which becomes encased by the developing prostate gland early in the 12th week (see Differentiation of the Urogenital Sinus later in chapter). A vestigial remnant of the duct may persist cranially near the head of the epididymis as the **appendix epididymis,** whereas remnants of mesonephric tubules near the inferior pole of the testis and tail of the epididymis may persist as the **paradidymis** (Fig 4–14).

B. PARAMESONEPHRIC DUCTS

The paramesonephric ducts begin to undergo morphologic regression centrally (and progress cranially and caudally) about the time they meet the urogenital sinus caudally (approximately the start of the ninth week).

Regression is effected by nonsteroidal anti-müllerian hormone produced by the differentiating Sertoli cells slightly before androgen is produced by the Leydig cells (see Testis). Anti-müllerian hormone is produced from the time of early testicular differentiation until birth (ie, not only during the period of regression of the paramesonephric duct). However, ductal sensitivity to anti-müllerian hormone in the male seems to exist for only a short "critical" time preceding the first signs of ductal regression. Vestigial remnants of the cranial end of the ducts may persist as the **appendix testis** on the superior pole of the testis (Fig 4–14). Caudally, a ductal remnant is considered to be part of the prostatic utricle of the seminal colliculus in the prostatic urethra.

C. Relocation of the Testes and Ducts

Around weeks 5–6, a bandlike condensation of mesenchymal tissue in the urogenital ridge forms near the caudal end of the mesonephros. Distally, this gubernacular precursor tissue grows into the area of the undifferentiated tissue of the anterior abdominal wall and toward the genital swellings. Proximally, the **gubernaculum** contacts the mesonephric duct when the mesonephros regresses and the gonad begins to form. By the start of the fetal period, the mesonephric duct begins differentiation and the gubernaculum adheres indirectly to the testis via the duct, which lies in the mesorchium of the testis. The external genitalia differentiate over the seventh to about the 19th week. By the 12th week, the testis is near the deep inguinal ring, and the gubernaculum is virtually at the inferior pole of the testis, proximally, and in the mesenchyme of the scrotal swellings, distally.

Although the testis in early development is near the last thoracic segment, it is still close to the area of the developing deep inguinal ring. With rapid growth of the lumbar region and "ascent" of the metanephric kidney, the testis remains relatively immobilized by the gubernaculum, although there is the appearance of a lengthy transabdominal "descent" from an upper abdominal position. The testis descends through the inguinal canal around the 28th week and into the scrotum about the 32nd week. Testicular blood vessels form when the testis is located on the dorsal body wall and retain their origin during the transabdominal and pelvic descent of the testis. The mesonephric duct follows the descent of the testis and hence passes anterior to the ureter, which follows the retroperitoneal ascent of the kidney (Fig 4–14).

Female: Uterus and Uterine Tubes

A. Mesonephric Ducts

Virtually all portions of these paired ducts degenerate in the female embryo, with the exception of the most cau-

dal segment between the ureteric bud and the cloaca, which is later incorporated into the posterior wall of the urogenital sinus (Figs 4–9 and 4–10) as the **trigone of the urinary bladder.** Regression begins just after gonadal sex differentiation and is finished near the onset of the third trimester. Cystlike or tubular vestiges of mesonephric duct (Fig 4–15) may persist to variable degrees parallel with the vagina and uterus (**Gartner's cysts**). Other mesonephric remnants of the duct or tubules may persist in the broad ligament (**epoophoron**).

B. Paramesonephric Ducts

Differentiation of müllerian ducts in female embryos produces the uterine tubes, uterus, and probably the fibromuscular wall of the vagina. In contrast to the ductal/gonadal relationship in the male, ductal differentiation in the female does not require the presence of ovaries. Formation of the bilateral paramesonephric ducts during the second half of the embryonic period has been described (see Indifferent Stage, in previous text). By the onset of the fetal period, the 2 ducts are joined caudally in the midline, and the fused segment of the new Y-shaped ductal structure is the **uterovaginal primordium** (Fig 4–12). The nonfused cranial part of each paramesonephric duct gives rise to the **uterine tubes** (oviducts), and the distal end of this segment remains open and will form the **ostium of the oviduct.**

Early in the ninth week, the uterovaginal primordium contacts medianly the dorsal wall of the urogenital sinus. This places the primordium at a median position between the bilateral openings of the mesonephric ducts, which joined the dorsal wall during the fifth week before subdivision of the urogenital sinus from the cloaca occurred (Figs 4–12 and 4–13). A ventral protrusion of the dorsal wall of the urogenital sinus forms at the area of contact of the uterovaginal primordium with the wall and between the openings of

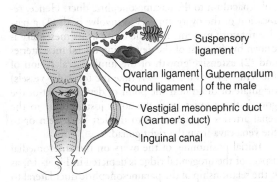

Figure 4–15. Female genital tract. Gubernacular derivatives and mesonephric vestiges are shown.

the mesonephric ducts. In reference to its location, this protrusion is called the **sinusal tubercle (sinus tubercle, paramesonephric tubercle, müllerian tubercle).** This tubercle may consist of several types of epithelia derived from the different ducts as well as from the wall of the sinus.

Shortly after the sinusal tubercle forms, midline fusion of the middle and caudal portions of the paramesonephric ducts is complete, and the vertical septum (apposed walls of the fused ducts) within the newly established uterovaginal primordium degenerates, creating a single cavity or canal (Fig 4–19). The solid tip of this primordium continues to grow caudally, while a mesenchymal thickening gradually surrounds the cervical region of the uterovaginal primordium. The primordium gives rise to the fundus, body, and isthmus of the uterus, specifically the endometrial epithelium and glands of the uterus. The endometrial stroma and smooth muscle of the myometrium are derived from adjacent splanchnic mesenchyme. The epithelium of the cervix forms from the lower aspect of the primordium. Development of the various components of the uterus covers the 3 trimesters of gestation. The basic structure is generated during the latter part of the first trimester. The initial formation of glands and muscular layer occurs near midgestation, whereas mucinous cells in the cervix appear during the third trimester.

The formation of the vagina is discussed below with differentiation of the urogenital sinus, even though it has not been resolved whether the vaginal epithelium is a sinusal or paramesonephric derivative (or both). The fibromuscular wall of the vagina is generally considered to be derived from the uterovaginal primordium (Fig 4–18).

C. RELOCATION OF THE OVARIES AND FORMATION OF LIGAMENTS

Transabdominal "descent" of the ovary, unlike that of the testis, is restricted to a relatively short distance, presumably (at least partly) because of attachment of the gubernaculum to the paramesonephric duct. Hence, relocation of the ovary appears to involve both (1) a passive rotatory movement of the ovary as its mesentery is drawn by the twist of the developing ductal mesenteries and (2) extensive growth of the lumbosacral region of the fetus. The ovarian vessels (like the testicular vessels) originate or drain near the point of development of the gonad, the arteries from the aorta just inferior to the renal arteries and the veins to the left renal vein or to the vena cava from the right gonad.

Initial positioning of the ovary on the anteromedial aspect of the urogenital ridge is depicted in Fig 4–14, as is the relationship of the paramesonephric duct lateral to the degenerating mesonephros, the ovary, and the urogenital mesentery. The urogenital mesentery between the

ridge and the dorsal body wall represents the first mesenteric support for structures developing in the ridge.

Alterations within the urogenital ridge eventually result in formation of contiguous double-layered mesenteries supporting the ovary and segments of the paramesonephric ducts. Enlargement of the ovary and degeneration of the adjacent mesonephric tissue bring previously separated layers of coelomic mesothelium into near apposition, establishing the mesentery of the ovary, the **mesovarium.** Likewise, mesonephric degeneration along the region of differentiation of the unfused cranial segment of the paramesonephric ducts establishes the **mesosalpinx.** Caudally, growth and fusion ventromedially of these bilateral ducts "sweep" the once medially attached mesenteries of the ducts toward the midline. These bilateral mesenteries merge over the fused uterovaginal primordium and extend laterally to the pelvic wall to form a continuous double-layered "drape," the **mesometrium of the broad ligament,** between the upper portion of the primordium and the posterolateral body wall. This central expanse of mesentery creates the rectouterine and vesicouterine pouches. The midline caudal fusion of the ducts also alters the previous longitudinal orientation of the upper free segments of the ducts (the oviducts) to a near transverse orientation. During this alteration, the attached mesovarium is drawn from a medial relationship into a posterior relationship with the paramesonephric mesentery of the mesosalpinx and the mesometrium.

The **suspensory ligament of the ovary,** through which the ovarian vessels, nerves, and lymphatics traverse, forms when cranial degeneration of the mesonephric tissue and regression of the urogenital ridge adjacent to the ovary reduce these tissues to a peritoneal fold.

The **round ligament of the uterus** and the **proper ovarian ligament** are both derivatives of the **gubernaculum,** which originates as a mesenchymal condensation at the caudal end of the mesonephros and extends over the initially short distance to the anterior abdominal wall (see Relocation of the Testes and Ducts in previous text). As the gonad enlarges and the mesonephric tissue degenerates, the cranial attachment of the gubernaculum appears to "shift" to the inferior aspect of the ovary. Distally, growth of the fibrous gubernaculum continues into the inguinal region. However, the midportion of the gubernaculum becomes attached, inexplicably, to the paramesonephric duct at the uterotubal junction. Formation of the uterovaginal primordium by caudal fusion of the paramesonephric ducts apparently carries the attached gubernaculum medially within the cover of the encompassing mesentery of the structures (ie, the parts of the developing broad ligament). This fibrous band of connective tissue eventually becomes 2 ligaments.

Cranially, the band is the proper ligament of the ovary, extending between the inferior pole of the ovary and the lateral wall of the uterus just inferior to the oviduct. Caudally, it continues as the uterine round ligament from a point just inferior to the proper ovarian ligament and extending through the inguinal canal to the labium majus.

D. ANOMALIES OF THE UTERINE TUBES (OVIDUCTS, FALLOPIAN TUBES)

The uterine tubes are derivatives of the cranial segments of the paramesonephric (müllerian) ducts, which differentiate in the urogenital ridge between the sixth and ninth weeks (Figs 4–7 and 4–14). Ductal formation begins with invagination of the coelomic epithelium in the lateral coelomic bay (Fig 4–5). The initial depression remains open to proliferate and differentiate into the ostium (Fig 4–14). Variable degrees of **duplication of the ostium** sometimes occur; in such cases, the leading edges of the initial ductal groove presumably did not fuse completely or anomalous proliferation of epithelium around the opening occurred.

Absence of a uterine tube is very rare when otherwise normal ductal and genital derivatives are present. This anomaly has been associated with (1) ipsilateral absence of an ovary and (2) ipsilateral unicornuate uterus (and probable anomalous broad ligament). Bilateral absence of the uterine tubes is most frequently associated with lack of formation of the uterus and anomalies of the external genitalia. Interestingly, absence of the derivatives of the lower part of the müllerian ducts with persistence of the uterine tubes occurs more frequently than the reverse condition. This might be expected, as the müllerian ducts form in a craniocaudal direction.

Partial absence of a uterine tube (middle or caudal segment) also has been reported. The cause of partial absence is unknown, although several theories have been advanced. One theory holds that when the unilateral anomaly coincides with ipsilateral ovarian absence, a "vascular accident" might occur following differentiation of the ducts and ovaries. Obviously, various factors resulting in somewhat localized atresia could be proposed. From a different perspective, bilateral absence of the uterine tubes as an associated disorder in a female external phenotype is characteristic of **testicular feminization syndrome** (nonpersistence of the rest of the paramesonephric ducts, anomalous external genitalia, hypoplastic male genital ducts, and testicular differentiation with usual ectopic location).

E. ANOMALIES OF THE UTERUS

The epithelium of the uterus and cervix and the fibromuscular wall of the vagina are derived from the paramesonephric (müllerian) ducts, the caudal ends of which fuse medially to form the uterovaginal primordium. Most of the primordium gives rise to the uterus (Fig 4–18). Subsequently, the caudal tip of the primordium contacts the pelvic part of the urogenital sinus, and the interaction of the sinus (sinovaginal bulbs) and primordium leads to differentiation of the vagina. Various steps in this sequential process can go awry, such as (1) complete or partial failure of one or both ducts to form (agenesis), (2) lack of or incomplete fusion of the caudal segments of the paired ducts (abnormal uterovaginal primordium), or (3) failure of development *after* successful formation (aplasia or hypoplasia). Many types of anomalies may occur because of the number of sites for potential error, the complex interactions necessary for the development of the müllerian derivatives, and the duration of the complete process.

Complete **agenesis of the uterus** is very rare, and associated vaginal anomalies are usually expected. Also, a high incidence of associated structural or positional abnormalities of the kidney has been reported; there has been speculation that the initial error in severe cases may be in the development of the urinary system and then in the formation of the paramesonephric ducts.

Aplasia of the paramesonephric ducts (**müllerian aplasia**) is more common than agenesis and could occur after formation and interaction of the primordium with the urogenital sinus. A rudimentary uterus or a vestigial uterus (ie, varying degrees of fibromuscular tissue present) is most frequently accompanied by partial or complete absence of the vagina (see text that follows). As in uterine agenesis, ectopic kidney or absence of a kidney is frequently associated with uterine aplasia (in about 40% of cases). **Uterine hypoplasia** variably yields a rudimentary or infantile uterus and is associated with normal or abnormal uterine tubes and ovaries. Unilateral agenesis or aplasia of the ducts gives rise to **uterus unicornis,** whereas unilateral hypoplasia may result in a rudimentary horn that may or may not be contiguous with the lumen of the "normal" horn (**uterus bicornis unicollis** with one unconnected rudimentary horn; Fig 4–16). The status of the rudimentary horn must be considered for potential hematometra at puberty.

Anomalous **unification** caudally of the paramesonephric ducts results in many uterine malformations (Fig 4–16). The incidence of defective fusion is estimated to be 0.1–3% of females. Furthermore, faulty unification of the ducts has been cited as the primary error responsible for most anomalies of the female genital tract. Partial or complete retention of the apposed walls of the paired ducts can produce slight (**uterus subseptus unicollis**) to complete (**uterus bicornis septus**) septal defects in the uterus. Complete failure of unification of the paramesonephric ducts can result in a

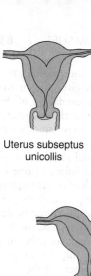
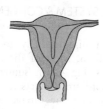
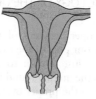
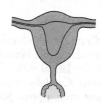

Uterus subseptus
unicollis

Uterus septus
duplex

Uterus septus
duplex with
double vagina

Herniated level
of cervix

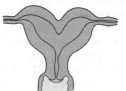
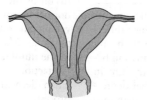
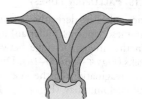

Uterus bicornis
unicollis

Uterus didelphys with
double vagina

Uterus bicornis
septus

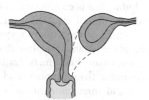

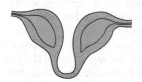

Uterus bicornis unicollis
with one unconnected
rudimentary horn

Uterus unicornis

Uterus acollis with
absence of vagina

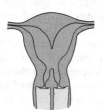
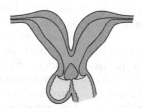
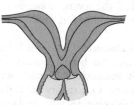

Uterus communicans septus,
cervix septa, vagina septa*

Uterus communicans bicornis,
cervix duplex, vagina septa
unilateralis atretica*

Uterus communicans bicornis,
cervix duplex, vagina septa*

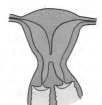
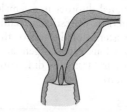

Uterus communicans septus,
cervix duplex, vagina septa*

Uterus communicans bicornis,
cervix septa, vagina simplex*

Figure 4–16. **Uterine anomalies.** (*Redrawn and reproduced, with permission, from Toaff R: A major genital malformation: Communicating uteri. Obstet Gynecol 1974;43:221.)

double uterus (**uterus didelphys**) with either a single or double vagina.

F. ANOMALIES OF THE CERVIX

Because the cervix forms as an integral part of the uterus, cervical anomalies are often the same as uterine anomalies. Thus, absence or hypoplasia of the cervix is rarely found with a normal uterovaginal tract. The cervix appears as a fibrous juncture between the uterine corpus and the vagina.

DIFFERENTIATION OF THE UROGENITAL SINUS

Until differentiation of the genital ducts begins, the urogenital sinus appears similar in both sexes during the middle and late embryonic period. For purposes of describing the origin of sinusal derivatives, the sinus can be divided into 3 parts: (1) the **vesical part,** or the large dilated segment superior to the entrance of the mesonephric ducts; (2) the **pelvic part,** or the narrowed tubular segment between the level of the mesonephric ducts and the inferior segment; and (3) the **phallic part,** often referred to as the definitive urogenital sinus (the anteroposteriorly elongated, transversely flattened inferiormost segment) (Fig 4–12). The **urogenital membrane** temporarily closes the inferior limit of the phallic part. The superior limit of the vesical part becomes delimited by conversion of the once tubular allantois to a thick fibrous cord, the **urachus,** by about 12 weeks. After differentiation of the vesical part of the sinus to form the epithelium of the **urinary bladder,** the urachus maintains its continuity between the apex of the bladder and the umbilical cord and is identified postnatally as the **median umbilical ligament.** Various anomalies of urachal formation can present as **urachal fistula, cyst,** or **sinus,** depending on the degree of patency that persists during obliteration of the allantois.

In both sexes, the caudal segments of each mesonephric duct between the urogenital sinus and the level of the ureter of the differentiating metanephric diverticulum (or ureteric bud) become incorporated into the posterocaudal wall of the vesical part (ie, urinary bladder) of the sinus (Figs 4–9 and 4–10). As the dorsal wall of the bladder grows and "absorbs" these caudal segments, the ureters are gradually "drawn" closer to the bladder and eventually open directly and separately into it, dorsolateral to the mesonephric ducts (Figs 4–10 and 4–11). The mesodermal segment of mesonephric duct incorporated into the bladder defines the epithelium of the **trigone of the bladder,** although this mesodermal epithelium is secondarily replaced by the endodermal epithelium of the sinusal bladder. After formation of the trigone, the remainder of each meso-

nephric duct (ie, the portion that was cranial to the metanephric diverticulum) is joined to the superior end of the pelvic part of the urogenital sinus. Thereafter, the ducts either degenerate (in females) or undergo differentiation (in males), as already discussed.

Male: Urinary Bladder and Urethra (Fig 4–17)

The urogenital sinus gives rise to the endodermal epithelium of the **urinary bladder,** the prostatic and membranous urethra, and most of the spongy (penile) urethra (except the glandular urethra). Outgrowths from its derivatives produce epithelial parts of the prostate and bulbourethral glands (Fig 4–17). The **prostatic urethra** receives the ejaculatory ducts (derived from the mesonephric ducts) and arises from 2 parts of the urogenital sinus. The portion of this urethral segment superior to the ejaculatory ducts originates from the inferiormost area of the vesical part of the sinus. The lower portion of the prostatic urethra is derived from the pelvic part of the sinus near the entrance of the ducts and including the region of the sinusal tubercle—the latter apparently forming the seminal colliculus. Early in the 12th week, endodermal outgrowths of the prostatic urethra form the prostatic anlage, the **prostatic buds,** from which the glandular epithelium of the **prostate** will arise. Differentiation of splanchnic mesoderm contributes other components to the gland (smooth muscle and connective tissue), as is the case also for mesodermal parts of the urinary bladder. The pelvic part of the sinus also gives rise to the epithelium of the **membranous urethra,** which later yields endodermal buds for the **bulbourethral glands.** The phallic, or inferior, part of the urogenital sinus proliferates anteriorly as the external genitalia form (during weeks 9–12) and results in incorporation of this phallic part as the endodermal epithelium of the **spongy (penile) urethra** (the distal glandular urethra is derived from ectoderm; see below).

Female: Urinary Bladder, Urethra, and Vagina

A. DEVELOPMENT

Differentiation of the female sinus is schematically presented in Fig 4–18 and illustrated in Figs 4–12 and 4–19 through 4–21. In contrast to sinusal differentiation in the male, the vesical part of the female urogenital sinus forms the epithelium of the **urinary bladder** and entire **urethra.** Derivatives of the pelvic part of the sinus include the epithelium of the **vagina,** the **greater vestibular glands,** and the **hymen.** Controversy exists about how the vagina is formed, mainly because of a lack of consensus about the origin and degree of inclu-

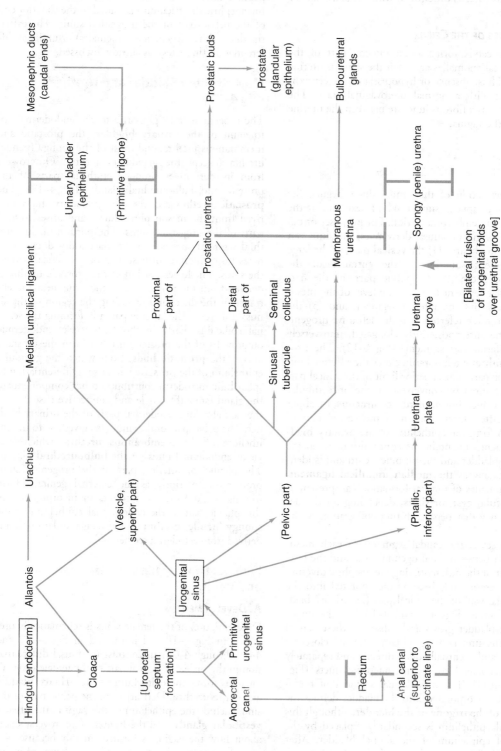

Figure 4–17. Schematic drawing of male differentiation of the urogenital sinus; formation of urinary bladder and urethra. (Explanatory symbols are given in Fig 4–1.)

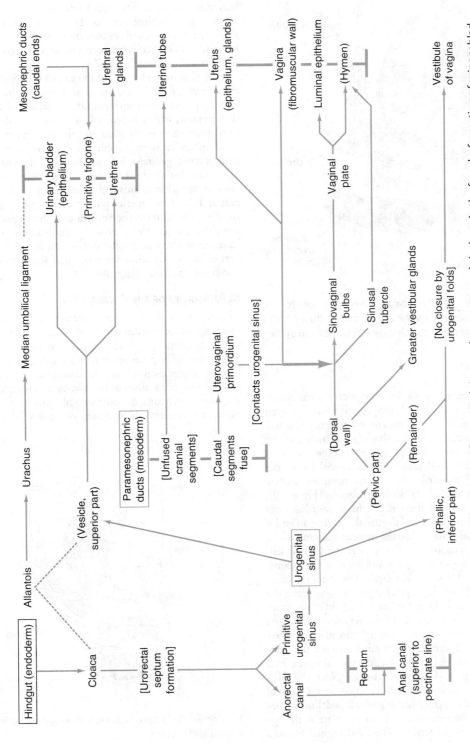

Figure 4–18. Schematic drawing of differentiation of urogenital sinus and paramesonephric ducts in the female; formation of urinary bladder, urethra, uterine tubes, uterus, and vagina. (Explanatory symbols are given in Fig 4–1.)

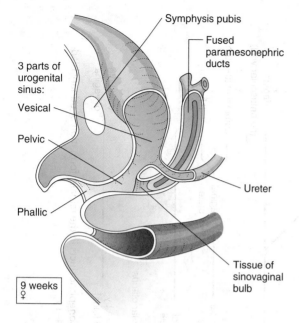

Figure 4–19. Sagittal cutaway view of female urogenital sinus and uterovaginal primordium (fused paramesonephric ducts). Sinovaginal bulbs form in the tenth week.

sion of its precursory tissues (mesodermal paramesonephric duct, endodermal urogenital sinus, or even mesonephric duct). The most common theory is that 2 endodermal outgrowths, the **sinovaginal bulbs,** of the dorsal wall of the pelvic part of the urogenital sinus form bilateral to and join with the caudal tip of the uterovaginal primordium (fused paramesonephric ducts) in the area of the sinusal tubercle (Fig 4–19). This cellular mass at the end of the primordium occludes the inferior aspect of the canal, creating an endodermal **vaginal plate** within the mesodermal wall of the uterovaginal primordium. Eventually, the vaginal segment grows, approaching the vestibule of the vagina. The process of growth has been described either as "down-growth" of the vaginal segment away from the uterine canal and along the urogenital sinus or, more commonly, as "up-growth" of the segment away from the sinus and toward the uterovaginal canal. In either case, the vaginal segment is extended between the paramesonephric-derived cervix and the sinus-derived vestibule (Figs 4–19 through 4–21). Near the fifth month, the breakdown of cells centrally in the vaginal plate creates the vaginal lumen, which is delimited peripherally by the remaining cells of the plate as the epithelial lining of the vagina. The solid vaginal fornices

become hollow soon after canalization of the vaginal lumen is complete. The upper one-third to four-fifths of the vaginal epithelium has been proposed to arise from the uterovaginal primordium, while the lower two-thirds to one-fifth has been proposed as a contribution from the sinovaginal bulbs.

The fibromuscular wall of the vagina is derived from the uterovaginal primordium. The cavities of the vagina and urogenital sinus are temporarily separated by the thin **hymen,** which is probably a mixture of tissue derived from the vaginal plate and the remains of the sinusal tubercle. With concurrent differentiation of female external genitalia, inferior closure of the sinus does not occur during the 12th week of development, as it does in the male. Instead, the remainder of the pelvic part and all of the inferior phallic part of the urogenital sinus expand to form the **vestibule of the vagina.** Presumably, the junctional zone of pigmentation on the labia minora represents the distinction between endodermal derivation from the urogenital sinus (medially) and ectodermal skin (laterally).

B. ANOMALIES OF THE VAGINA

The vagina is derived from interaction between the uterovaginal primordium and the pelvic part of the urogenital sinus (Fig 4–18; see previous section above). The causes of vaginal anomalies are difficult to assess because integration of the uterovaginal primordium and the urogenital sinus in the *normal* differentiation of the vagina remains a controversial subject. Furthermore, an accurate breakdown of causes of certain

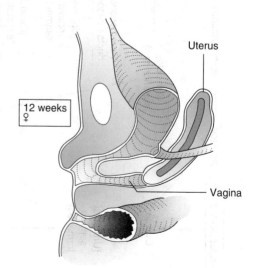

Figure 4–20. Sagittal cutaway view of developing vagina and urethra.

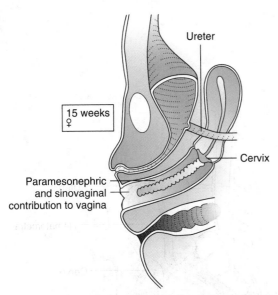

Figure 4–21. Sagittal cutaway view of differentiated urogenital sinus and precanalization stage of vaginal development. The drawing depicts one of several theories about the relative contributions of paramesonephric ducts and sinovaginal bulbs to the vagina (there is little consensus of opinion [see text]).

anomalous vaginal presentations, as with many anomalies of the external genitalia, would have to include potential moderating factors of endocrine and genetic origin as well.

The incidence of absence of the vagina due to suspected **vaginal agenesis** is about 0.025%. Agenesis may be due to failure of the uterovaginal primordium to contact the urogenital sinus. The uterus is usually absent (Fig 4–22). Ovarian agenesis is not usually associated with vaginal agenesis. The presence of greater vestibular glands has been reported with presumed vaginal agenesis; their presence emphasizes the complexity of differentiation of the urogenital sinus.

Vaginal atresia, on the other hand, is considered when the lower portion of the vagina consists merely of fibrous tissue while the contiguous superior structures (the uterus, in particular) are well differentiated (perhaps because the primary defect is in the sinusal contribution to the vagina). In **müllerian aplasia** almost all of the vagina and most of the uterus are absent (Rokitansky-Küster-Hauser syndrome, with a rudimentary uterus of bilateral, solid muscular tissue, was considered virtually the same as this aplasia). Most women with absence of the vagina (and normal external genitalia) are considered to have müllerian aplasia rather than vaginal atresia.

Other somatic anomalies are sometimes associated with müllerian aplasia, suggesting multiple malformation syndrome. Associated vertebral anomalies are much more prevalent than middle ear anomalies, eg, müllerian aplasia associated with **Klippel-Feil syndrome** (fused cervical vertebrae) is more common than müllerian aplasia associated with Klippel-Feil syndrome plus middle ear anomalies ("conductive deafness"). **Winter's syndrome,** which is thought to be autosomal recessive, is evidenced by middle ear anomalies (somewhat similar to those in the triad above), renal agenesis or hypoplasia, and vaginal atresia (rather than aplasia of the paramesonephric ducts). **Dysgenesis** (partial absence) of the vagina and **hypoplasia** (reduced caliber of the lumen) have also been described.

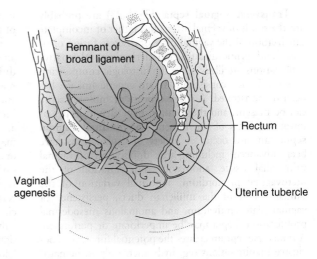

Figure 4–22. Midsagittal view of vaginal agenesis and uterine agenesis with normal ovaries and oviducts. (Reproduced, with permission, from Ingram JM: The Ingram technique for the management of vaginal agenesis and stenosis. The Pelvic Surgeon 1981;2:1.)

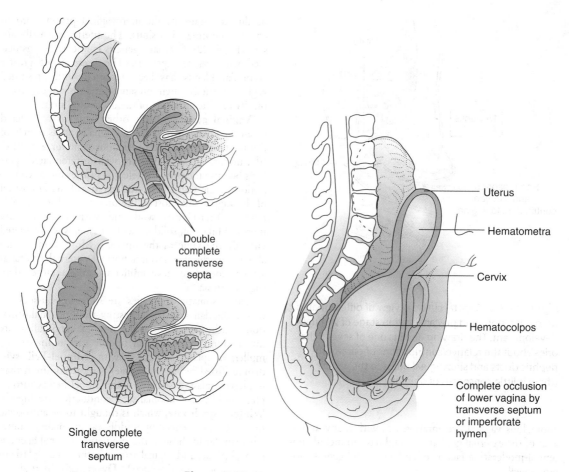

Figure 4–23. Transverse vaginal septa.

Transverse vaginal septa (Fig 4–23) are probably not the result of vaginal atresia but rather of incomplete canalization of the vaginal plate or discrete fusion of sinusal and primordial (ductal) derivatives. Alternative explanations are likely since the histologic composition of septa is not consistent. A rare genetic linkage has been demonstrated. A single septum or multiple septa can be present, and the location may vary in upper or lower segments of the lumen. **Longitudinal vaginal septa** can also occur. A variety of explanations have been advanced, including true duplication of vaginal primordial tissue, anomalous differentiation of the uterovaginal primordium, abnormal variation of the caudal fusion of the müllerian ducts, persistence of vaginal plate epithelium, and anomalous mesodermal proliferation. Septa may be imperforate or perforated. A transverse septum creates the potential for various occlusive manifestations (eg, hydrometrocolpos, hemato-

metra, or hematocolpos, depending on the composition of the trapped fluid). (See Chapter 31.)

Abnormalities of the vagina are often associated with anomalies of the urinary system and the rectum because differentiation of the urogenital sinus is involved in formation of the bladder and urethra as well as the vagina and vestibule. Furthermore, if partitioning of the cloaca into the sinus and anorectal canal is faulty, then associated rectal defects can occur. Compound anomalies may affect the urinary tract or rectum. The urethra may open into the vaginal wall; even a single vesicovaginal cavity has been described. On the other hand, the vagina can open into a persistent urogenital sinus, as in certain forms of female pseudohermaphroditism. Associated rectal abnormalities include vaginorectal fistula, vulvovaginal anus, rectosigmoidal fistula, and vaginosigmoidal cloaca in the absence of the rectum (see also Cloacal Dysgenesis, below).

C. Anomalies of the Hymen

The hymen is probably a mixture of tissue derived from remains of the sinusal tubercle and the vaginal plate. Usually, the hymen is patent, or perforate, by puberty, although an **imperforate hymen** is not rare. The imperforate condition can be a congenital error of lack of central degeneration or a result of inflammatory occlusion after perforation. Obstruction of menstrual flow at puberty may be the first sign (Fig 4–23).

D. Cloacal Dysgenesis (Including Persistence of the Urogenital Sinus)

Anomalous partitioning of the cloaca by the abnormal development of the urorectal septum is rare, at least based on reported cases in the literature. As anticipated from a developmental standpoint, the incidence of associated genitourinary anomalies is high. Five types of cloacal or anorectal malformations are summarized in Table 4–3.

Rectocloacal fistula with a persistent cloaca provides a common canal or outlet for the urinary, genital, and intestinal tracts. The distinction between a canal and an outlet is one of depth (deep versus very shallow, respectively) of the persistent lower portion of the cloaca and, thus, the length of the individual urethral and vaginal canals emptying into the cloaca. The inverse relationship between depth (or length) of the cloaca and length of the vaginal and urethral canals is probably a reflection of the time when arrest of formation of the urorectal septum occurs. Although the bladder, the vagina, and the rectum can empty into a common cloaca as just described, other unusual variations of persistent cloaca can also occur.

For example, the vagina and rectum develop, but the urinary bladder does not develop as a separate entity from the cloaca. Instead, the vagina and rectum open separately into a "urinary bladder," which has ureters entering posterolaterally to the vagina (vaginal orifice is in the "anatomic trigone" of the bladder-like structure). The external orifice from the base of this cloacal "bladder" is a single narrow canal. One explanation for this variant might be that arrest of formation of the urorectal septum occurs much earlier than does the separate development of distal portions of the 3 tracts (urethra, vagina, and anorectum) to a more advanced (but still incomplete) stage before urorectal septal formation ceases. The anomaly is probably rare.

With a **rectovaginal fistula,** the vestibule may appear anatomically normal but the anus does not appear in the perineum. The defect probably results from anorectal agenesis due to incomplete subdivision of the cloaca (similar agenesis in the male could result in a rectourethral fistula). The development of the anterior aspect of the vagina completes the separation of the urethra from the vagina, so there is not a persistent urogenital sinus. **Anorectal agenesis** is reputedly the most common type of anorectal malformation, and usually a fistula occurs. Rectovaginal, anovestibular (or rectovestibular; Table 4–3), and anoperineal fistulas account for most anorectal malformations.

In the absence of the anorectal defect (normal anal presentation) but presence of a **persistent urogenital sinus** with a single external orifice, various irregularities of the urethra and genitalia can appear. The relative positions of urethral and vaginal orifices in the sinus can even change as the child grows. In the discussion of anomalies of the labia majora (see following text), note is made of the association of a persistent urogenital sinus in female pseudohermaphroditism due to congenital adrenal hyperplasia. The vagina opens into the persisting pelvic part of the sinus, which extends with the phallic part of the sinus to the external surface at the urogenital opening. The sinus can be deep and narrow in the neonate, approximating the size of a urethra, or it can be relatively shallow.

Urinary tract disorders associated with persistent urogenital sinus include duplication of the ureters, unilateral ureteral and renal agenesis or atresia, and lack of or abnormal ascent of the kidneys. Variations in the anomalies of derivatives of the urogenital sinus appear to be related in part to the time of arrest of normal differentiation and development of the urogenital sinus, as well as to the impact of other factors associated with abnormal sexual differentiation, such as the variable degrees of response to adrenal androgen in congenital adrenal hyperplasia.

THE EXTERNAL GENITALIA

Undifferentiated Stage

The external genitalia begin to form early in the embryonic period, shortly after development of the cloaca. The progenitory tissues of the genitalia are common to both sexes, and the early stage of development is virtually the same in females and males. Although differentiation of the genitalia can begin around the onset of the fetal period if testicular differentiation is initiated, definitive genital sex is usually not clearly apparent until the 12th week. Formation of external genitalia in the male involves the influence of androgen on the interaction of subepidermal mesoderm with the inferior parts of the endodermal urogenital sinus. In the female, this androgenic influence is absent.

The external genitalia form within the initially compact area bounded by the umbilical cord (anteriorly), the developing limb buds (laterally), the embryonic tail (posteriorly), and the cloacal membrane (centrally). Two of the primordia for the genitalia first appear bilat-

Table 4–3. Cloacal malformations.[1]

	Rectocloacal Fistula
Vestibule	Deformed; flanked by labia; clitoris in front, fourchette behind; anterior vestibule short, shallow, and moist; single external orifice in posterior half of vestibule (common conduit for urine, cervical mucus, and feces).
Bladder/urethra	Anterior; directed cranially and ventrally.
Vagina	Opens into the vault of cloaca.
Anus/rectum	Enters at highest and most posterior point; orifice is in midline and stenotic.
Disposition	Lengths of urethra and vagina are inversely proportionate to length of cloacal canal.
	Rectovaginal Fistula
Vestibule	Normal anatomy (2 orifices: urethral & vaginal).
Bladder/urethra	Normal.
Vagina	May be septate or normal.
Anus/rectum	Internal in the midposterior vaginal wall.
Disposition	Anus absent from perineum.
	Rectovestibular Fistula
Vestibule	Contains rectum, otherwise normal.
Urethra	Normal.
Vagina	Normal.
Anus/rectum	Small, sited at the fossa navicularis.
Disposition	Rectum is parallel with both vagina and urethra.
	Covered Anus
Vestibule	Normal.
Urethra	Normal.
Vagina	(Probably normal.)
Anus	At any point between the normal site and the fourchette; anocutaneous; anovulvar.
Disposition	Genital folds are abnormally fused anterior and posterior to common orifice and give rise to hypertrophied perineal raphe.
	Ectopic Anus
Vestibule	Normal.
Urethra	Normal.
Vagina	Normal.
Anus	Anterior to the normal site; normal function.
Disposition	Fault lies in the development of the perineum.

[1]Modified and reproduced, with permission, from Okonkwo JEN, Crocker KM: Cloacal dysgenesis. Obstet Gynecol 1977; 50:97.

erally adjacent to the cloacal membrane (a medial pair of cloacal folds and a lateral pair of genital [labioscrotal] swellings). The **cloacal folds** are longitudinal proliferations of caudal mesenchyme located between the ectodermal epidermis and the underlying endoderm of the phallic part of the urogenital sinus. Proliferation and bilateral anterior fusion of these folds create the **genital tubercle,** which protrudes near the anterior edge of the cloacal membrane by the sixth week (Figs 4–24 to 4–26). Extension of the tubercle forms the phallus, which at this stage is the same size in both sexes.

By the seventh week, the urorectal septum subdivides the bilayered (ectoderm and endoderm) cloacal membrane into the **urogenital membrane** (anteriorly) and the **anal membrane** (posteriorly). The area of fusion of the urorectal septum and the cloacal membrane becomes the **primitive perineum,** or **perineal body.** With formation of the perineum, the cloacal folds are divided transversely as **urogenital folds** adjacent to the urogenital membrane and **anal folds** around the anal membrane. As the mesoderm within the urogenital folds thickens and elongates between the perineum and the phallus, the urogenital membrane sinks deeper into the fissure between the folds. Within a week, this membrane ruptures, forming the **urogenital orifice** and, thus, opening the urogenital sinus to the exterior. Similar thickening of the anal folds creates a deep anal pit, in which the anal membrane breaks down to establish the **anal orifice** of the anal canal (Figs 4–24 and 4–25).

Subsequent masculinization or feminization of the external genitalia is a consequence of the respective presence or absence of androgen and the androgenic sensitivity or insensitivity of the tissues. The significance of both of these factors (availability of hormone and sensitivity of target tissue) is exemplified by the rare condition (about 1 in 50,000 "females") of **testicular feminization,** wherein testes are present (usually ectopic) and produce testosterone and anti-müllerian hormone. The anti-müllerian hormone suppresses formation of the uterus and uterine tubes (from the paramesonephric ducts), whereas testosterone supports male differentiation of the mesonephric ducts to form the epididymis and ductus deferens. The anomalous feminization of the external genitalia is considered to be due to androgenic insensitivity of the precursor tissues consequent to an abnormal androgen receptor or postreceptor mechanism set by genetic inheritance.

Male

Early masculinization of the undifferentiated or indifferent genitalia takes place during the first 3 weeks of the fetal period (weeks 9–12) and is caused by androgenic stimulation. The phallus and urogenital folds gradually elongate to initiate development of the **penis.**

The subjacent endodermal lining of the inferior part (phallic) of the urogenital sinus extends anteriorly along with the urogenital folds, creating an endodermal plate, the **urethral plate.** The plate deepens into a groove, the **urethral groove,** as the urogenital folds (now called **urethral folds**) thicken on each side of the plate. The urethral groove extends into the ventral aspect of the developing penis, and the bilateral urethral folds slowly fuse in a posterior to anterior direction over the urethral groove to form the **spongy (penile) urethra,** thereby closing the urogenital orifice (Figs 4–17 and 4–24). The line of fusion becomes the **penile raphe** on the ventral surface of the penis.

As closure of the urethral folds approaches the glans, the external urethral opening on this surface is eliminated. Concurrently, an **ectodermal glandular plate** invaginates the tip of the penis. Canalization of the plate forms the distal end of the penile urethra, the **glandular urethra.** Thus, the external urethral meatus becomes located at the tip of the glans when closure of the urethral folds is completed (Fig 4–24). The **prepuce** is formed slightly later by a circular invagination of ectoderm at the tip of the **glans penis.** This cylindric ectodermal plate then cleaves to leave a double-layered fold of skin extending over the glans.

While the cloacal folds and phallic urogenital sinus were differentiating into the penis and the urethra, the **genital (labioscrotal) swellings** of the undifferentiated stage were enlarging lateral to the cloacal folds. Medial growth and fusion of the scrotal swellings to form the **scrotum** and **scrotal raphe** around the 12th week virtually complete the differentiation of the male external genitalia (Figs 4–24 and 4–26).

Female

A. DEVELOPMENT OF EXTERNAL GENITALIA

Feminization of the external genitalia proceeds in the absence of androgenic stimulation (or nonresponsiveness of the tissue). The 2 primary distinctions in the general process of feminization versus masculinization are (1) the lack of continued growth of the phallus and (2) the near absence of fusion of the urogenital folds and the labioscrotal swellings. Female derivatives of the indifferent sexual primordia for the external genitalia are virtually homologous counterparts of the male derivatives. Formation of the female genitalia is schematically presented in Fig 4–25.

The growth of the phallus slows relative to that of the urogenital folds and labioscrotal swellings and becomes the diminutive **clitoris.** The anterior extreme of the urogenital folds fuses superior and inferior to the clitoris, forming the **prepuce** and **frenulum of the clitoris,** respectively. The midportions of these folds do

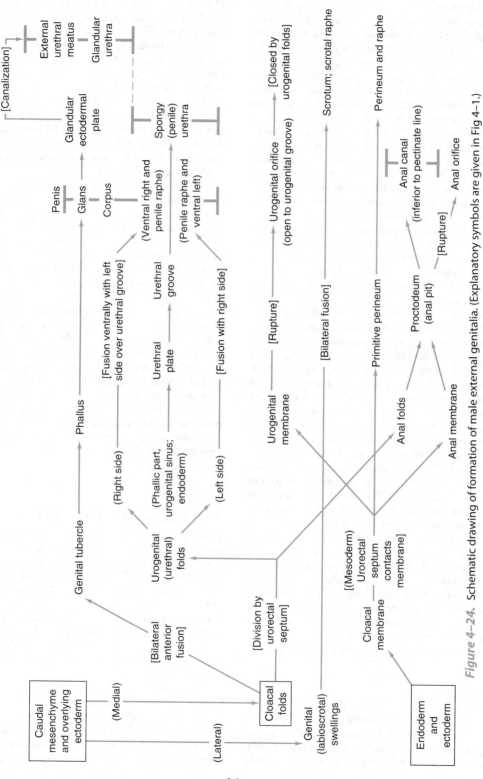

Figure 4-24. Schematic drawing of formation of male external genitalia. (Explanatory symbols are given in Fig 4-1.)

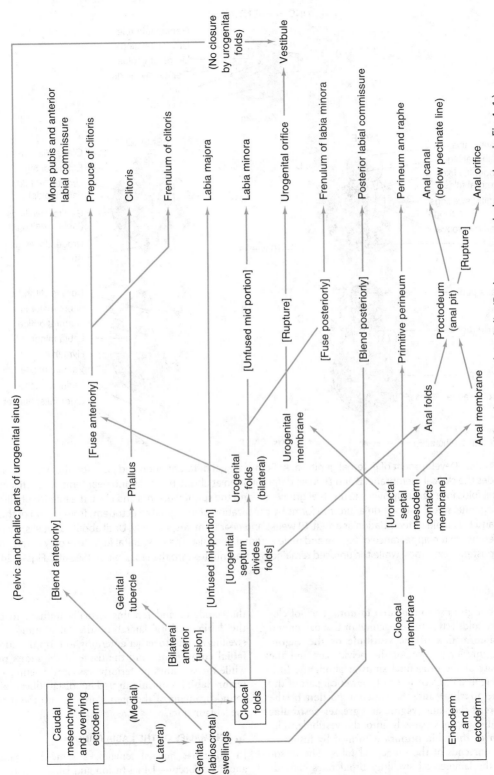

Figure 4-25. Schematic drawing of formation of female external genitalia. (Explanatory symbols are given in Fig 4-1.)

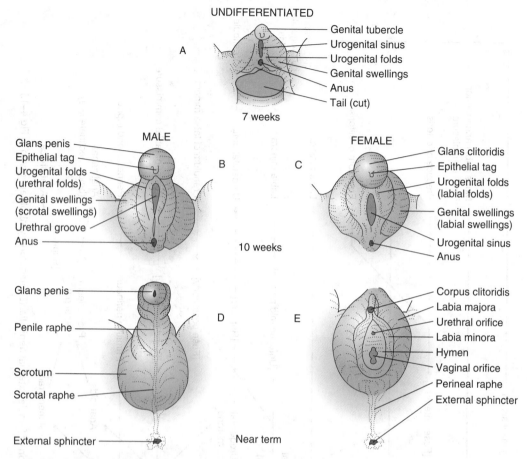

UNDIFFERENTIATED

A

— Genital tubercle
— Urogenital sinus
— Urogenital folds
— Genital swellings
— Anus
— Tail (cut)

7 weeks

MALE

Glans penis
Epithelial tag
Urogenital folds (urethral folds)
Genital swellings (scrotal swellings)
Urethral groove
Anus

B

C

FEMALE

— Glans clitoridis
— Epithelial tag
— Urogenital folds (labial folds)
— Genital swellings (labial swellings)
— Urogenital sinus
— Anus

10 weeks

Glans penis

Penile raphe

Scrotum
Scrotal raphe

D

E

— Corpus clitoridis
— Labia majora
— Urethral orifice
— Labia minora
— Hymen
— Vaginal orifice
— Perineal raphe
— External sphincter

External sphincter

Near term

Figure 4–26. Development of external genitalia. **A:** Before sexual differentiation and just after the urorectal septum divides the cloacal membrane. **B** and **D:** Male differentiation at about 10 weeks and near term, respectively. The urogenital folds fuse ventrally over the urethral groove to form the spongy urethra and close the inferior phallic part of the urogenital sinus. The glandular urethra forms by canalization of invaginated ectoderm from the tip of the glans. **C** and **E:** Female differentiation at about 10 weeks and near term, respectively. Until about 12 weeks, there is little difference in the appearance of female and male external genitalia. The urogenital folds fuse only at their anterior and posterior extremes, while the unfused remainder differentiates into the labia minor. (See also Figs 4–24 and 4–25.)

not fuse but give rise to the **labia minora.** Lack of closure of the folds leaves the urogenital orifice patent and results in formation of the **vestibule of the vagina** from the inferior portion of the pelvic part and the phallic part of the urogenital sinus at about the fifth month (Fig 4–25). Derivatives of the vesical part of the sinus (the **urethra**) and the superior portion of the pelvic part of the sinus (**vagina** and **greater vestibular glands**) then open separately into the vestibule. The **frenulum of the labia minora** is formed by fusion of the posterior ends of the urogenital folds. The mesoderm of the labioscrotal swellings proliferates beneath

the ectoderm and remains virtually unfused to create the **labia majora** lateral to the labia minora. The swellings blend together anteriorly to form the **anterior labial commissure** and the tissue of the **mons pubis,** while the swellings posteriorly less clearly define a **posterior labial commissure.** The distal fibers of the round ligament of the uterus project into the tissue of the labia majora.

B. ANOMALIES OF THE LABIA MINORA

In otherwise normal females, 2 somewhat common anomalies occur—labial fusion and labial hypertrophy.

True labial fusion as an early developmental defect in the normally unfused midportions of the urogenital folds is purportedly less frequent than "fusion" due to inflammatory-type reactions. **Labial hypertrophy** can be unilateral or bilateral and may require surgical correction in extreme cases.

C. ANOMALIES OF THE LABIA MAJORA

The labia majora are derived from the bilateral genital (labioscrotal) swellings, which appear early in the embryonic period and remain unfused centrally during subsequent sex differentiation in the fetal period. Anomalous conditions include **hypoplastic** and **hypertrophic labia** as well as different gradations of fusion of the labia majora. Abnormal fusion (masculinization) of labioscrotal swellings in genetic females is most commonly associated with ambiguous genitalia of female pseudohermaphroditism consequent to **congenital adrenal hyperplasia (adrenogenital syndrome).** Over 90% of females with congenital adrenal hyperplasia have a steroid 21-hydroxylase deficiency (autosomal recessive), resulting in excess adrenal androgen production. This enzyme deficiency has been reported to be "the most common cause of ambiguous genitalia in genetic females." Associated anomalies include clitoral hypertrophy and persistent urogenital sinus. Formation of a penile urethra is extremely rare.

D. ANOMALIES OF THE CLITORIS

Clitoral agenesis is extremely rare and is due to lack of formation of the genital tubercle during the sixth week. Absence of the clitoris could also result from **atresia** of the genital tubercle. The tubercle forms by fusion of the anterior segments of the cloacal folds. Very rarely, these anterior segments fail to fuse, and a **bifid clitoris** forms. This anomaly also occurs when unification of the anterior parts of the folds is restricted by exstrophy of the cloaca or bladder. Duplication of the genital tubercle with consequent formation of a **double clitoris** is equally rare. **Clitoral hypertrophy** alone is not common but may be associated with various intersex disorders.

E. ANOMALIES OF THE PERINEUM

The primitive perineum originates at the area of contact of the mesodermal urorectal septum and the endodermal dorsal surface of the cloacal membrane (at 7 weeks). During normal differentiation of the external genitalia in the fetal period, the primitive perineum maintains the separation of the urogenital folds and ruptured urogenital membrane from the anal folds and ruptured anal membrane, and later develops the perineal body. Malformations of the perineum are rare and usually associated with malformations of cloacal or anorectal development consequent to abnormal devel-opment of the urorectal septum. **Imperforate anus** has an incidence of about 0.02%. The simplest form (rare) is a thin membrane over the anal canal (the anal membrane failed to rupture at the end of the embryonic period). **Anal stenosis** can arise by posterior deviation of the urorectal septum as the septum approaches the cloacal membrane, causing the anal membrane to be smaller (with a relatively increased anogenital distance through the perineum). **Anal agenesis** with a fistula detected as an ectopic anus is considered to be a urorectal septal defect. The incidence of agenesis with a fistula is only slightly less than that without a fistula. In females, the fistula commonly may be located in the perineum (**perineal fistula**) or may open into the posterior aspect of the vestibule of the vagina (**anovestibular fistula;** see Cloacal Dysgenesis).

REFERENCES

Alatas C et al: Evaluation of intrauterine abnormalities in infertile patients by sonohysterography. Hum Reprod 1997;12(3): 487.

Alvarez-Nava F et al: Mixed gonadal dysgenesis: A syndrome of broad clinical, cytogenetic and histopathologic spectrum. Genet Couns 1999;10(3):233.

Bacsko G: Uterine surgery by operative hysteroscopy. Eur J Obstet Gynecol Reprod Biol 1997;71(2):219.

Banerjee R, Laufer MR: Reproductive disorders associated with pelvic pain. Semin Pediatr Surg 1998;7(1): 52.

Breech LL, Laufer MR: Obstructive anomalies of the female reproductive tract. J Reprod Med 1999;44(3):233.

Cadeddu JA, Watumull L, Corwin TS: Laparoscopic gonadectomy and excision of müllerian remnant in an adult intersex patient. Urology 2001;57(3):554.

Cho S, Moore SP, Fangman T: One hundred three consecutive patients with anorectal malformations and their associated anomalies. Arch Pediatr Adolesc Med 2001;155(5):587.

Coloia DV, Morris H, Rahmani MR: Congenital transverse vaginal septum: Vaginal hydrosonic diagnosis. J Ultrasound Med 1998;17(4):261.

Cook CL, Siow Y, Taylor S: Serum müllerian-inhibiting substance levels during normal menstrual cycles. Fertil Steril 2000; 73(4):859.

Di Lorenzo C: Pediatric anorectal disorders. Gastroenterol Clin North Am 2001;30(1):269.

Donnez J, Nisolle M: Endoscopic laser treatment of uterine malformations. Hum Reprod 1997;12(7):1381.

Drews U: Local mechanisms in sex-specific morphogenesis. Cytogenet Cell Genet 2000;91(1-4):72.

Edmonds DK: Congenital malformations of the genital tract. Obstet Gynecol Clin North Am 2000;27(1):49.

Folch M, Pigem I, Konje JC: Müllerian agenesis: Etiology, diagnosis, and management. Obstet Gynecol Surv 2000;55(10):644.

Hiort O: Neonatal endocrinology of abnormal male sexual differentiation: Molecular aspects. Horm Res 2000;53(supp1):38.

Jacobsen LJ, DeCherney A: Results of conventional and hysteroscopic surgery. Hum Reprod 1997;12(7):1376.

Larsen WJ: Development of the urogenital system. In: Sherman (editor): *Human Embryology.* Churchill Livingstone, 2001, p. 235.

Letterie GS: Combined congenital absence of the vagina and cervix. Diagnosis and magnetic resonance imaging and surgical management. Gynecol Obstet Invest 1998;46(1):65.

Levy G, Warren M, Maidman J: Transverse vaginal septum; case report and review of the literature. Int Urogynecol J Pelvic Floor Dysfunct 1997;8(3):173.

Malasanos TH: Sexual development of the fetus and pubertal child. Clin Obstet Gynecol 1997;40(1):153.

Malik E et al: Reproductive outcome of 32 patients with primary or secondary infertility and uterine pathology. Arch Gynecol Obstet 2000;264(1):24.

McElreavy K, Fellous M: Sex determination and the Y chromosome. Am J Med Genet 1999;89(4):176.

Metts JC III et al: Genital malformations and coexistent urinary tract or spinal anomalies in patients with imperforate anus. J Urol 1997;158:1298.

Mittwoch U: Genetics of sex determination: Exceptions that prove the rule. Mol Genet Metab 2000;71(1-2):405.

Muller J et al: Management of males with 45X/46XY gonadal dysgenesis. Horm Res 1999;52:11.

Nef S, Parada LF: Hormones in male sexual development. Genes Dev 2000;14(24):3075.

Neri G, Opiz J: Syndromal and nonsyndromal forms of male pseudohermaphrodism. Am J Med Genet 1999;89(4):201.

O'Neil MJ, O'Neil RJ: Whatever happened to SRY? Cell Mol Life Sci 1999;56(11-12): 883.

Ostrer H: Sexual differentiation. Semin Reprod Med 2000; 18(1):41.

Resendes BL, Sohn SH, Stelling JR: Role for anti-müllerian hormone in congenital absence of the uterus and vagina. Am J Med Genet 2001;98(2):129.

Salas-Cortes L et al: SRY protein is expressed in ovotestis and streak gonads from human sex reversal. Cytogenet Cell Genet 2000;91(1-4):212.

Shimanda K, Hosokawa S, Matsumoto F: Urological management of cloacal anomalies. Int J Urol 2001;8(6):282.

Spence JE: Vaginal and uterine anomalies in the pediatric and adolescent patient. J Pediatr Adolesc Gynecol 1998;11(1):3.

Stelling J et al. Müllerian agenesis: An update. Obstet Gynecol 1997;90(6):1024.

Vendeland LL, Shehadeh L: Incidental finding of an accessory ovary in a 16 year old at laparoscopy. A case report. J Reprod Med 2000;45(5):435.

Vilain E, McCabe ER: Mammalian sex determination: From gonads to brain. Mol Genet Metab 1998;65(2):74.

Warne GL: Disorders of sexual differentiation. Endocrinol Metab Clin North Am 1998;27(4):945.

Genetic Disorders & Sex Chromosome Abnormalities

5

Donelle Laughlin, MD

■ GENETIC DISORDERS

MENDELIAN LAWS OF INHERITANCE

1. Types of Inheritance

Autosomal Dominant

In autosomal dominant inheritance, it is assumed that a mutation has occurred in one gene of an allelic pair and that the presence of this new gene produces enough of the changed protein to give a different phenotypic effect. Environment must also be considered because the effect may vary under different environmental conditions. The following are characteristic of autosomal dominant inheritance:

(1) The trait appears with equal frequency in both sexes.

(2) For inheritance to take place, at least one parent must have the trait unless a new mutation has just occurred.

(3) When a homozygous individual is mated to a normal individual, all offspring will carry the trait. When a heterozygous individual is mated to a normal individual, 50% of the offspring will show the trait.

(4) If the trait is rare, most persons demonstrating it will be heterozygous (see Table 5–1).

Autosomal Recessive

The mutant gene will not be capable of producing a new characteristic in the heterozygous state in this circumstance under customary environmental conditions—ie, with 50% of the genetic material producing the new protein, the phenotypic effect will not be different from that of the normal trait. When the environment is manipulated, the recessive trait occasionally becomes dominant. The characteristics of this form of inheritance are as follows:

(1) The characteristic will occur with equal frequency in both sexes.

(2) For the characteristic to be present, both parents must be carriers of the recessive trait.

(3) If both parents are homozygous for the recessive trait, all offspring will have it.

(4) If both parents are heterozygous for the recessive trait, 25% of the offspring will have it.

(5) In pedigrees showing frequent occurrence of individuals with rare recessive characteristics, consanguinity is often present (see Table 5–2).

X-Linked Recessive

This condition occurs when a gene on the X chromosome undergoes mutation and the new protein formed as a result of this mutation is incapable of producing a change in phenotype characteristic in the heterozygous state. Because the male has only one X chromosome, the presence of this mutant will allow for expression should it occur in the male. The following are characteristic of this form of inheritance:

(1) The condition occurs more commonly in males than in females.

(2) If both parents are normal and an affected male is produced, it must be assumed that the mother is a carrier of the trait.

(3) If the father is affected and an affected male is produced, the mother must be at least heterozygous for the trait.

(4) A female with the trait may be produced in one of 2 ways: (a) She may inherit a recessive gene from both her mother and her father; this suggests that the father is affected and the mother is heterozygous. (b) She may inherit a recessive gene from one of her parents and may express the recessive characteristic as a function of the Lyon hypothesis; this assumes that all females are mosaics for their functioning X chromosome. It is theorized that this occurs because at about the time of implantation each cell in the developing female embryo selects one X chromosome as its functioning X and that all progeny cells thereafter use this X chromosome as their functioning X chromosome. The other X chromosome becomes inactive. Since this selection is done on a random basis, it is conceivable that

Table 5–1. Examples of autosomal dominant conditions and traits.

Achondroplasia
Acoustic neuroma
Aniridia
Cataracts, cortical and nuclear
Chin fissure
Color blindness, yellow-blue
Craniofacial dysostosis
Deafness (several forms)
Dupuytren's contracture
Ehlers-Danlos syndrome
Facial palsy, congenital
Huntington's chorea
Hyperchondroplasia
Intestinal polyposis
Keloid formation
Lipomas, familial
Marfan's syndrome
Mitral valve prolapse
Muscular dystrophy
Neurofibromatosis (Recklinghausen's disease)
Night blindness
Pectus excavatum
Adult polycystic renal disease
Tuberous sclerosis
Von Willebrand's disease
Wolff-Parkinson-White syndrome (some cases)

---

some females will be produced who will be using primarily the X chromosome bearing the recessive gene. Thus, a genotypically heterozygous individual may demonstrate a recessive characteristic phenotypically on this basis (see Table 5–3).

X-Linked Dominant

In this situation, the mutation will produce a protein that, when present in the heterozygous state, is sufficient to cause a change in characteristic. The following are characteristic of this type of inheritance:

(1) The characteristic occurs with the same frequency in males and females.

(2) An affected male mated to a normal female will produce the characteristic in 50% of the offspring.

(3) An affected homozygous female mated to a normal male will produce the affected characteristic in all offspring.

(4) A heterozygous female mated to a normal male will produce the characteristic in 50% of the offspring.

(5) Occasional heterozygous females may not show the dominant trait on the basis of the Lyon hypothesis (see Table 5–4).

2. Applications of Mendelian Laws

Identification of Carriers

When a recessive characteristic is present in a population, carriers may be identified in a variety of ways. If the gene is responsible for the production of a protein (eg, an enzyme), the carrier often possesses 50% of the amount of the substance present in homozygous normal persons. Such a circumstance is found in galactosemia, where the carriers will have approximately half as much galactose-1-phosphate uridyl transferase activity in red cells as do noncarrier normal individuals.

Table 5–2. Examples of autosomal recessive conditions and traits.

Acid maltase deficiency
Albinism
Alkaptonuria
Argininemia
Ataxia-telangiectasia
Bloom's syndrome
Cerebrohepatorenal syndrome
Chloride diarrhea, congenital
Chondrodystrophia myotonia
Color blindness, total
Coronary artery calcinosis
Cystic fibrosis
Cystinosis
Cystinuria
Deafness (several types)
Dubowitz's syndrome
Dysautonomia
Fructose-1,6-diphosphatase deficiency
Galactosemia
Gaucher's disease
Glaucoma, congenital
Histidinemia
Homocystinuria
Laron's dwarfism
Maple syrup urine disease
Mucolipidosis I, II, III
Mucopolysaccharidosis I-H, I-S, III, IV, VI, VII
Muscular dystrophy, autosomal recessive type
Niemann-Pick disease
Phenylketonuria
Sickle cell anemia
17α-Hydroxylase deficiency
18-Hydroxylase deficiency
21-Hydroxylase deficiency
Tay-Sachs disease
Wilson's disease
Xeroderma pigmentosum

Table 5–3. Examples of X-linked recessive conditions and traits.

Androgen insensitivity syndrome (complete and incomplete)
Color blindness, red-green
Diabetes insipidus (most cases)
Fabry's disease
Glucose-6-phosphate dehydrogenase deficiency
Gonadal dysgenesis (XY type)
Gout (certain types)
Hemophilia A (factor VIII deficiency)
Hemophilia B (factor IX deficiency)
Hypothyroidism, X-linked infantile
Hypophosphatemia
Immunodeficiency, X-linked
Lesch-Nyhan syndrome
Mucopolysaccharidosis II
Muscular dystrophy, adult and childhood types
Otopalatodigital syndrome
Reifenstein's syndrome

At times, the level of the affected enzyme may be only slightly below normal, and a challenge with the substance to be acted upon may be required before the carrier can be identified. An example is seen in carriers of phenylketonuria, in whom the deficiency in phenylalanine hydroxylase is in the liver cells and serum levels may not be much lower than normal. Nonetheless, when the individual is given an oral loading dose of phenylalanine, plasma phenylalanine levels may remain high because the enzyme is not present in sufficient quantities to act upon this substance properly.

In still other situations where the 2 alleles produce different proteins that can be measured, a carrier state will have 50% of the normal protein and 50% of the other protein. Such a situation is seen in sickle cell trait, where one gene is producing hemoglobin A and the other hemoglobin S. Thus, the individual has half the amount of hemoglobin A as a normal person and half the hemoglobin S of a person with sickle cell anemia. An interesting but important problem involves the detection of carriers of cystic fibrosis. This is the most common autosomal recessive disease in Caucasian populations of European background, occurring in 1 in 2500 births in such populations, but being found in the carrier state in 1 in 25 Americans. By 1990, over 230 alleles of the single gene responsible have been discovered. The gene is known as the cystic fibrosis transmembrane conductance regulator (CFTR) and the most common mutation, delta F508, accounts for about 70% of all mutations, with 5 specific point mutations accounting for over 85% of cases. Because so many alleles are present, population screening poses

logistical problems that have yet to be worked out. Most programs screen for the most common mutations using DNA replication and amplification studies.

Expressivity & Penetrance

Expressivity and penetrance are examples of how an autosomal characteristic may not be expressed in quite the form that it ordinarily would be. With regard to expressivity, while the gene is present, the entire genome of the individual must be taken into consideration. Other genetic influences may be operating—even environmental ones—that may modify the manner in which the gene expresses itself. Penetrance, on the other hand, involves the expression of a dominant gene and takes into consideration the fact that while the gene may express itself in most individuals in a similar fashion, there may be some circumstance of environment or other gene activity during the development of the individual that may modify its action so that the phenotypic factor is not seen. Thus, one could state that during embryonic development, there is a requirement of some environmental factor to allow the gene to express itself, and, in an occasional rare case, this may not take place. Hence, the gene is not allowed to operate at its specific time.

3. Polygenic Inheritance

Polygenic inheritance is defined as the inheritance of a single phenotypic feature as a result of the effects of many genes. Most physical features in humans are determined by polygenic inheritance. Many common malformations are determined in this way also. For example, cleft palate with or without cleft lip, clubfoot, anencephaly, meningomyelocele, dislocation of the hip, and pyloric stenosis each occur with a frequency of 0.5–2 per 1000 in white populations. Altogether, these anomalies account for slightly less than half of single primary defects noted in early infancy. They are present in siblings of affected infants—when both parents are normal—at a rate of 2–5%. They are also found more commonly among relatives than in the general population. The increase in incidence is not environmentally induced because the frequency of such abnormalities in

Table 5–4. Examples of X-linked dominant conditions and traits.

Acro-osteolysis, dominant type
Cervico-oculo-acoustic syndrome
Hyperammonemia
Orofaciodigital syndrome I

monozygotic twins is 4–8 times that of dizygotic twins and other siblings. The higher incidence in monozygotic twins is called concordance.

Sex also plays a role. Certain conditions appear to be transmitted by polygenic inheritance and are passed on more frequently by the mother who is affected than by the father who is affected. Cleft lip occurs in 6% of the offspring of women with cleft lip, as opposed to 2.8% of offspring of men with cleft lip.

There are many racial variations in diseases believed to be transmitted by polygenic inheritance, making racial background a determinant of how prone an individual will be to a particular defect. In addition, as a general rule, the more severe a defect, the more likely it is to occur in subsequent siblings. Thus, siblings of children with bilateral cleft lip are more likely to have the defect than are those of children with unilateral cleft lip.

Environment undoubtedly plays a role in polygenic inheritance, because seasonal variations alter some defects and their occurrence rate from country to country in similar populations.

CYTOGENETICS

1. Identification of Chromosomes

In 1960, 1963, 1965, and 1971, international meetings were held in Denver, London, Chicago, and Paris, respectively, for the purpose of standardizing the nomenclature of human chromosomes. These meetings resulted in a decision that all autosomal pairs should be numbered in order of decreasing size from 1 to 22. Autosomes are divided into groups on the basis of their morphology, and these groups are labeled by the letters A–G. Thus, the A group is comprised of pairs 1–3; the B group, pairs 4 and 5; the C group, pairs 6–12; the D group, pairs 13–15; the E group, pairs 16–18; the F group, pairs 19 and 20; and the G group, pairs 21 and 22. The sex chromosomes are labeled X and Y, the X chromosome being similar in size and morphology to the number 7 pair and thus frequently included in the C group (C-X) and the Y chromosome being similar in morphology and size to the G group (G-Y) (Fig 5–1).

The short arm of a chromosome is labeled p and the long arm q. If a translocation occurs in which the

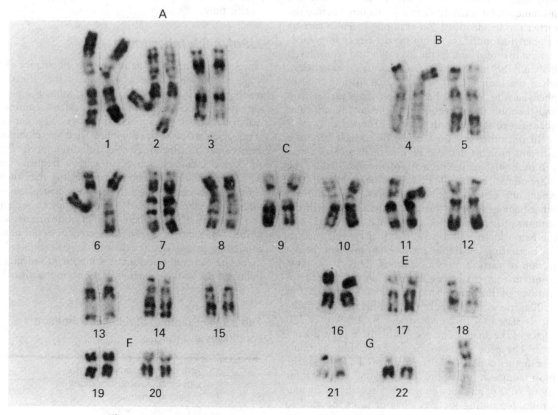

Figure 5–1. A karyotype of a normal male demonstrating R banding.

short arm of a chromosome is added to another chromosome, it is written p+. If the short arm is lost, it is p–. The same can be said for the long arm (q+ and q–).

It has been impossible to separate several chromosome pairs from one another on a strictly morphologic basis because the morphologic variations have been too slight. However, there are other means of identifying each chromosome pair in the karyotype. The first of these is the incorporation of ^{3}H-thymidine, known as the autoradiographic technique. This procedure involves the incorporation of radioactive thymidine into growing cells in tissue culture just before they are harvested. Cells that are actively undergoing DNA replication will pick up the radioactive thymidine, and the chromosomes will demonstrate areas of activity. Each chromosome will incorporate thymidine in a different pattern, and several chromosomes can therefore be identified by their labeling pattern. Nonetheless, with this method it is not possible to identify each chromosome, although it is possible to identify chromosomes involved in pathologic conditions, eg, D_1 trisomy and Down's syndrome.

Innovative staining techniques have made it possible to identify individual chromosomes in the karyotype and to identify small anomalies that might have evaded the observer using older methods. These involve identification of chromosome banding by a variety of staining techniques, at times with predigestion with proteolytic agents. Some of the more commonly used techniques are the following:

Q banding: Fixed chromosome spreads are stained without any pretreatment using quinacrine mustard, quinacrine, or other fluorescent dyes and observed with a fluorescence microscope.

G banding: Preparations are incubated in a variety of saline solutions using any one of several pretreatments and stained with Giemsa's stain.

R banding: Preparations are incubated in buffer solutions at high temperatures or at special pH and stained with Giemsa's stain. This process yields the reverse bands of G banding (see Fig 5–1).

C banding: Preparations are either heated in saline to temperatures just below boiling or treated with certain alkali solutions and then stained with Giemsa's stain. This process causes prominent bands to develop in the region of the centromeres.

2. Cell Division

Each body cell goes through successive stages in its life cycle. As a landmark, cell division may be considered as the beginning of a cycle. Following this, the first phase, which is quite long but depends on how rapidly the particular cell is multiplying, is called the G_1 stage. During this stage, the cell is primarily concerned with

carrying out its function. Following this, the S stage, or period of DNA synthesis, takes place. Next there is a somewhat shorter stage, the G_2 stage, during which time DNA synthesis is completed and chromosome replication begins. Following this comes the M stage, when cell division occurs.

Somatic cells undergo division by a process known as **mitosis** (Fig 5–2). This is divided into 4 periods. The first is the **prophase,** during which the chromosome filaments shorten, thicken, and become visible. At this time they can be seen to be composed of 2 long parallel spiral strands lying adjacent to one another and containing a small clear structure known as the **centromere.** As prophase continues, the strands continue to unwind and may be recognized as chromatids. At the end of the prophase, the nuclear membrane disappears and **metaphase** begins. This stage is heralded by the formation of a spindle and the lining up of the chromosomes in pairs on the spindle. Following this, **anaphase** occurs, at which time the centromere divides and each daughter chromatid goes to one of the poles of the spindle. **Telophase** then ensues, at which time the spindle breaks and cell cytoplasm divides. A nuclear membrane now forms, and mitosis is complete: Each daughter cell has received chromosome material equal in amount and identical to that of the parent cell. Because each cell contains 2 chromosomes of each pair and a total of 46 chromosomes, a cell is considered to be **diploid.** Occasionally, an error takes place on the spindle, and instead of chromosomes dividing, with identical chromatids going to each daughter cell, an extra chromatid goes to one daughter cell and the other lacks that particular member. After the completion of cell division, this leads to a trisomic state (an extra dose of that chromosome) in one daughter cell and a monosomic state (a missing dose of the chromosome) in the other daughter cell. Any chromosome in the karyotype may be involved in such a process, which is known as mitotic nondisjunction. If these cells thrive and produce their own progeny, a new cell line is established within the individual. The individual then has more than one cell line and is known as a **mosaic.** A variety of combinations and permutations have occurred in humans.

Germ cells undergo division for the production of eggs and sperm by a process known as **meiosis.** In the female it is known as oogenesis and in the male as spermatogenesis. The process that produces the egg and the sperm for fertilization essentially reduces the chromosome number from 46 to 23 and changes the normal diploid cell to an anaploid cell, ie, a cell that has only one member of each chromosome pair. Following fertilization and the fusion of the 2 pronuclei, the diploid status is reestablished.

Meiosis can be divided into several stages (Fig 5–3). The first is **prophase I.** Early prophase is known as the

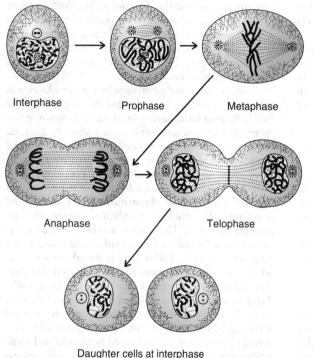

Interphase

Prophase

Metaphase

Anaphase

Telophase

Daughter cells at interphase

Figure 5–2. Mitosis of a somatic cell. (Reproduced, with permission, from Stenchever MA: *Human Cytogenetics: A Workbook in Reproductive Biology.* The press at Case Western Reserve University, 1972.)

leptotene stage, during which chromatin condenses and becomes visible as a single elongated threadlike structure. This is followed by the **zygotene stage,** when the single threadlike chromosomes migrate toward the equatorial plate of the nucleus. At this stage, homologous chromosomes become arranged close to one another to form **bivalents** that exchange materials at several points known as **synapses.** In this way, genetic material located on one member of a pair is exchanged with similar material located on the other member of a pair. Next comes the **pachytene stage** in which the chromosomes contract to become shorter and thicker. During this stage, each chromosome splits longitudinally into 2 chromatids united at the centromere. Thus, the bivalent becomes a structure composed of 4 closely opposed chromatids known as a **tetrad.** The human cell in the pachytene stage demonstrates 23 tetrads. This stage is followed by the **diplotene stage,** in which the chromosomes of the bivalent are held together only at certain points called bridges or chiasms. It is at these points that crossover takes place. The sister chromatids are joined at the centromere so that crossing-over can only take place between chromatids of homologous chromosomes and not between identical sister chromatids. In the case of males, the X and Y chromosomes are not involved in crossing-over. This stage is followed by the last stage of prophase, known as **diakinesis.**

Here the bivalents contract, and the chiasms move toward the end of the chromosome. The homologs pull apart, and the nuclear membrane disappears. This is the end of prophase I.

Metaphase I follows. At this time, the bivalents are now highly contracted and align themselves along the equatorial plate of the cell. Paternal and maternal chromosomes line up at random. This stage is then followed by **anaphase I** and **telophase I,** which are quite similar to the corresponding events in mitosis. However, the difference is that in meiosis the homologous chromosome of the bivalent pair separates and not the sister chromatids. The homologous bivalents pull apart, one going to each pole of the spindle, following which 2 daughter cells are formed at telophase I.

Metaphase, anaphase, and telophase of meiosis II take place next. A new spindle forms in metaphase, the chromosomes align along the equatorial plate, and, as anaphase occurs, the chromatids pull apart, one each going to a daughter cell. This represents a true division of the centromere. Telophase then supervenes, with reconstitution of the nuclear membrane and final cell division. At the end, a haploid number of chromosomes is present in each daughter cell (see Fig 5–3). In the case of spermatogenesis, both daughter cells are similar, forming 2 separate sperms. In the case of oogenesis, only one egg is produced, the nuclear material of the

FIRST MEIOTIC DIVISION

Prophase

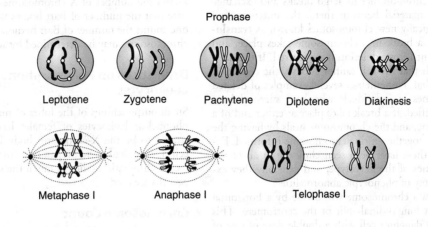

Leptotene   Zygotene   Pachytene   Diplotene   Diakinesis

Metaphase I   Anaphase I   Telophase I

SECOND MEIOTIC DIVISION

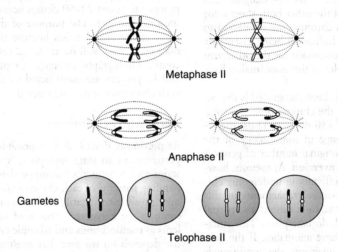

Metaphase II

Anaphase II

Gametes

Telophase II

Figure 5–3. **Meiosis in the human.** (Reproduced, with permission, from Stenchever MA: *Human Cytogenetics: A Workbook in Reproductive Biology.* The press at Case Western Reserve University, 1972.)

other daughter cell being present and intact but with very little cytoplasm, this being known as the **polar body.** A polar body is formed at the end of meiosis I and the end of meiosis II. Thus, each spermatogonium produces 4 sperms at the end of meiosis, whereas each oogonium produces one egg and 2 polar bodies.

Nondisjunction may also occur in meiosis. When it does, both members of the chromosome pair go to one daughter cell and none to the other. If the daughter cell that receives the entire pair is the egg, and fertilization ensues, a triple dose of the chromosome, or trisomy, will occur. If the daughter cell receiving no members of the pair is fertilized, a monosomic state will

result. In the case of autosomes, this is lethal, and a very early abortion will follow. In the case of the sex chromosome, the condition may not be lethal, and examples of both trisomy and monosomy have been seen in humans. Any chromosome pair may be involved in trisomic or monosomic conditions.

3. Abnormalities in Chromosome Morphology & Number

As has been stated, nondisjunction may give rise to conditions of trisomy. In these cases, the morphology of the chromosome is not affected, but the chromosome number is. Be this as it may, breaks and rearrangements in chromosomes may have a variety of results. If 2 chromosomes undergo breaks and exchange chromatin material between them, the outcome is 2 morphologically new chromosomes known as **translocations.** If a break in a chromosome takes place, and the fragment is lost, **deletion** has occurred. If the deletion is such that the cell cannot survive, the condition may be lethal. Nonetheless, several examples of deleted chromosomes in individuals who have survived have been identified. If a break takes place at either end of a chromosome, and the chromosome heals by having the 2 ends fuse together, a ring chromosome is formed. Examples of these have been seen clinically in all of the chromosomes of the karyotype, and generally they exhibit a variety of phenotypic abnormalities.

At times a chromosome will divide by a horizontal rather than longitudinal split of the centromere. This leaves each daughter cell with a double dose of one of the arms of the chromosome. Thus, one daughter cell receives both long arms and the other both short arms of the chromosome. Such a chromosome is referred to as an **isochromosome,** the individual being essentially trisomic for one arm and monosomic for the other arm of the chromosome. Examples of this abnormality have been seen in humans.

Another anomaly that has been recognized is the occurrence of 2 breaks within the chromosome and rotation of the center fragment 180 degrees. Thus, the realignment allows for a change in morphology of the chromosome although the original number of genes is preserved. This is called an **inversion.** At meiosis, however, the chromosome has difficulty in undergoing chiasm formation, and abnormal rearrangements of this chromosome, leading to partial duplications and partial losses of chromatin material, do take place. This situation may lead to several bizarre anomalies. If the centromere is involved in the inversion, the condition is called a **pericentric inversion.**

Breaks occasionally occur in 2 chromosomes, and a portion of one broken chromosome is inserted into the body of another, leading to a grossly abnormal chromosome. This is known as an **insertion** and generally leads to gross anomalies at meiosis.

4. Methods of Study

Sex Chromatin (X-Chromatin) Body (Barr Body)

The X-chromatin body was first seen in the nucleus of the nerve cell of a female cat in 1949 by Barr and Bertram. It has been found to be the constricted, nonfunctioning X chromosome. As a general rule, only one X chromosome functions in a cell at a given time. All other X chromosomes present in a cell may be seen as X-chromatin bodies in a resting nucleus. Thus, if one knows the number of X chromosomes, one can anticipate that the number of Barr bodies will be one less. If one counts the number of Barr bodies, the number of X chromosomes may be determined by adding one.

Drumsticks on Polymorphonuclear Leukocytes

Small outpouchings of the lobes of nuclei in polymorphonuclear leukocytes of females have been demonstrated to be the X-chromatin body in this particular cell. Hence, leukocyte preparations may be used to detect X-chromatin bodies in much the same way as buccal cells are used.

Chromosome Count

In the karyotypic analysis of a patient, it is the usual practice to count 20–50 chromosome spreads for chromosome number. The purpose of this is to determine whether mosaicism exists because if a mosaic pattern does exist, there will be at least 2 cell lines of different counts. Photographs are made of representative spreads, and karyotypes are constructed so the morphology of each chromosome may be studied.

Banding Techniques

As previously described, it is possible after appropriate pretreatment to stain metaphase spreads with special stains and construct a karyotype that demonstrates the banding patterns of each chromosome. In this way, it is now possible to identify with certainty every chromosome in the karyotype. This is of value in such problems as translocations and trisomic conditions. Another use depends on the fact that most of the long arm of the Y chromosome is heterochromic and stains deeply with fluorescent stains. Thus, the Y chromosome may be identified at a glance, even in the resting nucleus.

APPLIED GENETICS & TERATOLOGY

1. Chromosomes & Spontaneous Abortion

An entirely new approach to reproductive biology problems became available with the advent of tissue culture and cytologic techniques that made it possible to culture cells from any tissue of the body and produce karyotypes that could be analyzed. In the early 1960s, investigators in a number of laboratories began to study chromosomes of spontaneous abortions and demonstrated that the earlier the spontaneous abortion occurred, the more likely it was to be due to a chromosomal abnormality. It is now known that in spontaneous abortions occurring in the first 8 weeks, the fetuses have about a 50% incidence of chromosome anomalies.

Of abortuses that are abnormal, approximately one-half are trisomic, suggesting an error of meiotic nondisjunction. One-third of abortuses with trisomy have trisomy 16. While this abnormality does not occur in liveborn infants, it apparently is a frequent problem in abortuses. The karyotype 45, X occurs in nearly one-fourth of chromosomally abnormal abortuses. This karyotype occurs about 24 times more frequently in abortuses than in liveborn infants, a fact that emphasizes its lethal nature. Over 15% of chromosomally abnormal abortuses have polyploidy (triploidy or tetraploidy). These lethal conditions are seen only in abortuses except in extremely rare circumstances and are due to a variety of accidents, including double fertilization and a number of meiotic errors. Finally, a small number of chromosomally abnormal abortuses have unbalanced translocations and other anomalies.

Recurrent Pregnancy Loss

Couples who experience habitual abortion make up about 0.5% of the population. The condition is defined as 2 or more spontaneous abortions. Several investigators have studied groups of these couples using banding techniques and have found that 10–25% of them will have a chromosome anomaly in either the male or female partner. Those seen are 47,XXX, 47,XYY, and a variety of balanced translocation carriers. Those with sex chromosome abnormalities will frequently demonstrate other nondisjunctional events. Chromosome anomalies are thus a major cause of habitual abortion, and the incorporation of genetic evaluation into such a work-up is potentially fruitful.

Lippman-Hand and Bekemans reviewed the world literature and studied the incidence of balanced translocation carriers among 177 couples who had 2 or more spontaneous abortions. These studies suggest that in 2–3% of couples experiencing early fetal loss, one partner will have balanced translocations. This percentage is not markedly increased when more than 2 abortions occur. Females had a somewhat higher incidence of balanced translocations than did males.

2. Chromosomal Disorders

This section will be devoted to a brief discussion of various autosomal abnormalities. Table 5–5 summarizes some of the autosomal abnormalities that have been diagnosed. These are represented as syndromes, together with some of the signs typical of these conditions. In general, autosomal monosomy is so lethal that total loss of a chromosome is rarely seen in an individual born alive. Only a few cases of monosomy 21–22 have been

reported to date, which attests to the rarity of this disorder. Trisomy may occur with any chromosome. The 3 most common trisomic conditions seen in living individuals are trisomies 13, 18, and 21. Trisomy of various C group chromosomes has been reported sporadically. The most frequently reported is trisomy 8. Generally, trisomy of other chromosomes must be assumed to be lethal, because they occur only in abortuses, not in living individuals. To date, trisomy of every autosome except chromosome 1 has been seen in abortuses.

Translocations can occur between any 2 chromosomes of the karyotype, and a variety of phenotypic expressions may be seen after mediocre arrangements. Three different translocation patterns have been identified in Down's syndrome: 15/21, 21/21, and 21/22.

Deletions may also occur with respect to any chromosome in the karyotype and may be brought about by a translocation followed by a rearrangement in meiosis, which leads to the loss of chromatin material, or by a simple loss of the chromatin material following a chromosome break. Some of the more commonly seen deletion patterns are listed in Table 5–5.

The most frequent abnormality related to a chromosome abnormality is Down's syndrome. Down's syndrome serves as an interesting model for the discussion of autosomal diseases. The 21 trisomy type is the most common form and is responsible for approximately 95% of Down's syndrome patients. There is a positive correlation between the frequency of Down's syndrome and maternal age. Babies with Down's syndrome are more often born to teenage mothers, and even more frequently to mothers over 35. Although it is not entirely clear why this is so, it may be that in older women at least, the egg has been present in prophase of the first meiotic division from the time of fetal life and that as it ages there is a greater tendency for nondisjunction to occur, leading to trisomy. A second theory is that coital habits are more erratic in both the very young and the older mothers, and this may lead to an increased incidence in fertilization of older eggs. This theory maintains that these eggs may be more likely to suffer nondisjunction or to accept abnormal sperm. Be this as it may, the incidence of Down's syndrome in the general population is approximately 1 in 600 deliveries and at age 40 approximately 1 in 100 deliveries. At age 45, the incidence is approximately 1 in 40 deliveries (Table 5–6). The other 5% of Down's syndrome patients are the result of translocations, the most common being the 15/21 translocation, but examples of 21/21 and 21/22 have been noted. In the case of 15/21, the chance of recurrence in a later pregnancy is theoretically 25%. In practice, a rate of 10% is observed if the mother is the carrier. When the father is the carrier, the odds are less, because there may be a selection not favoring the sperm carrying both the 15/21 translocation

Table 5–5. Autosomal disorders.

Type	Synonym	Signs
Monosomy		
Monosomy 21–22		Moderate mental retardation, antimongoloid slant of eyes, flared nostrils, small mouth, low-set ears, spade hands.
Trisomy		
Trisomy 13	Trisomy D: the "D₁" syndrome	Severe mental retardation, congenital heart disease (77%), polydactyly, cerebral malformations (especially aplasia of olfactory bulbs), eye defects, low-set ears, cleft lip and palate, low birthweight. Characteristic dermatoglyphic pattern.
Trisomy 18	Trisomy E: the "E" syndrome, Edward's syndrome	Severe mental retardation, long narrow skull with prominent occiput, congenital heart disease, flexion deformities of fingers, narrow palpebral fissures, low-set ears, harelip and cleft palate. Characteristic dermatoglyphics, low birthweight.
Trisomy 21	Down's syndrome	Mental retardation, brachycephaly, prominent epicanthal folds. Brushfield spots, poor nasal bridge development, congenital heart disease, hypotonia, hypermobility of joints, characteristic dermatoglyphics.
Translocations		
15/21	Down's syndrome	Same as trisomy 21.
21/21	Downs' syndrome	Same as trisomy 21.
21/22	Down's syndrome	Same as trisomy 21.
Deletions		
Short arm chromosome 4(4p–)	Wolf's syndrome	Severe growth and mental retardation, midline scalp defects, seizures, deformed iris, beak nose, hypospadias.
Short arm chromosome 5(5p–)	Cri du chat syndrome	Microcephaly, catlike cry, hypertelorism with epicanthus, low-set ears, micrognathism, abnormal dermatoglyphics, low birthweight.
Long arm chromosome 13(13q–)	...	Microcephaly, psychomotor retardation, eye and ear defects, hypoplastic or absent thumbs.
Short arm chromosome 18(18p–)	...	Severe mental retardation, hypertelorism, low-set ears, flexion deformities of hands.
Long arm chromosome 18(18q–)	...	Severe mental retardation, microcephaly, hypotonia, congenital heart disease; marked dimples at elbows, shoulders, and knees.
Long arm chromosome 21(21q–)	...	Associated with chronic myelogenous leukemia.

and the normal 21 chromosome. In the case of 21/21 translocation, there is no chance for a normal child to be formed, because the carrier will contribute either both 21s or no 21 and, following fertilization, will produce either a monosomic 21 or trisomic 21. With regard to 21/22 translocation, the chance of producing a baby with Down's syndrome is 1 in 2.

In general, other trisomic states occur with greater frequency in older women, and the larger the chromosome involved, the more severe the syndrome. Since trisomy 21 involves the smallest of the chromosomes, the phenotypic problems of Down's syndrome are the least severe, and a moderate life expectancy may be anticipated. Even these individuals will be grossly abnormal,

Table 5–6. Estimates of rates per thousand of chromosome abnormalities in live births by single-year interval.[1]

Maternal Age	Down's Syndrome	Edward's Syndrome (Trisomy 18)	Patau's Syndrome (Trisomy 13)	XXY	XYY	Turner's Syndrome Genotype	Other Clinically Significant Abnormality[2]	Total[3]
< 15	1.0[4]	< 0.1[4]	< 0.1–0.1	0.4	0.5	< 0.1	0.2	2.2
15	1.0[4]	< 0.1[4]	< 0.1–0.1	0.4	0.5	< 0.1	0.2	2.2
16	0.9[4]	< 0.1[4]	< 0.1–0.1	0.4	0.5	< 0.1	0.2	2.1
17	0.8[4]	< 0.1[4]	< 0.1–0.1	0.4	0.5	< 0.1	0.2	2.0
18	0.7[4]	< 0.1[4]	< 0.1–0.1	0.4	0.5	< 0.1	0.2	1.9
19	0.6[4]	< 0.1[4]	< 0.1–0.1	0.4	0.5	< 0.1	0.2	1.8
20	0.5–0.7	< 0.1–0.1	< 0.1–0.1	0.4	0.5	< 0.1	0.2	1.9
21	0.5–0.7	< 0.1–0.1	< 0.1–0.1	0.4	0.5	< 0.1	0.2	1.9
22	0.6–0.8	< 0.1–0.1	< 0.1–0.1	0.4	0.5	< 0.1	0.2	2.0
23	0.6–0.8	< 0.1–0.1	< 0.1–0.1	0.4	0.5	< 0.1	0.2	2.0
24	0.7–0.9	0.1–0.1	< 0.1–0.1	0.4	0.5	< 0.1	0.2	2.1
25	0.7–0.9	0.1–0.1	< 0.1–0.1	0.4	0.5	< 0.1	0.2	2.1
26	0.7–1.0	0.1–0.1	<0.1–0.1	0.4	0.5	< 0.1	0.2	2.1
27	0.8–1.0	0.1–0.2	< 0.1–0.1	0.4	0.5	< 0.1	0.2	2.2
28	0.8–1.1	0.1–0.2	< 0.1–0.2	0.4	0.5	< 0.1	0.2	2.3
29	0.8–1.2	0.1–0.2	< 0.1–0.2	0.5	0.5	< 0.1	0.2	2.4
30	0.9–1.2	0.1–0.2	<0.1–0.2	0.5	0.5	< 0.1	0.2	2.6
31	0.9–1.3	0.1–0.2	<0.1–0.2	0.5	0.5	< 0.1	0.2	2.6
32	1.1–1.5	0.1–0.2	0.1–0.2	0.6	0.5	< 0.1	0.2	3.1
33	1.4–1.9	0.1–0.3	0.1–0.2	0.7	0.5	< 0.1	0.2	3.5
34	1.9–2.4	0.2–0.4	0.1–0.3	0.7	0.5	< 0.1	0.2	4.1
35	2.5–3.9	0.3–0.5	0.2–0.3	0.9	0.5	< 0.1	0.3	5.6
36	3.2–5.0	0.3–0.6	0.2–0.4	1.0	0.5	< 0.1	0.3	6.7
37	4.1–6.4	0.4–0.7	0.2–0.5	1.1	0.5	< 0.1	0.3	8.1
38	5.2–8.1	0.5–0.9	0.3–0.7	1.3	0.5	< 0.1	0.3	9.5
39	6.6–10.5	0.7–1.2	0.4–0.8	1.5	0.5	< 0.1	0.3	12.4
40	8.5–13.7	0.9–1.6	0.5–1.1	1.8	0.5	< 0.1	0.3	15.8
41	10.8–17.9	1.1–2.1	0.6–1.4	2.2	0.5	< 0.1	0.3	20.5
42	13.8–23.4	1.4–2.7	0.7–1.8	2.7	0.5	< 0.1	0.3	25.5
43	17.6–30.6	1.8–3.5	0.9–2.4	3.3	0.5	< 0.1	0.3	32.6
44	22.5–40.0	2.3–4.6	1.2–3.1	4.1	0.5	< 0.1	0.3	41.8
45	28.7–52.3	2.9–6.0	1.5–4.1	5.1	0.5	< 0.1	0.3	53.7
46	36.6–68.3	3.7–7.9	1.9–5.3	6.4	0.5	< 0.1	0.3	68.9
47	46.6–89.3	4.7–10.3	2.4–6.9	8.2	0.5	< 0.1	0.3	89.1
48	59.5–116.8	6.0–13.5	3.0–9.0	10.6	0.5	< 0.1	0.3	115.0
49	75.8–152.7	7.6–17.6	3.8–11.8	13.8	0.5	< 0.1	0.3	149.3

[1]Reproduced with permission, from Hook EB: Rates of chromosome abnormalities at different maternal ages. *Obstet Gynecol* 1981;58:282.
[2]XXX is excluded.
[3]Calculation of the total at each age assumes rate for autosomal aneuploidies is at the midpoints of the ranges given.
[4]No range may be constructed for those under 20 years by the same methods as for those 20 and over.

however, because of mental retardation and defects in other organ systems. The average life expectancy of patients with Down's syndrome is much lower than for the general population.

3. Prenatal Diagnosis

Currently the most common use for applied genetics in obstetrics and gynecology is in the use of prenatal counseling, screening, and diagnosis. Prenatal diagnosis first came into use in 1977 with the discovery of the significance of serum alpha-fetoprotein (AFP). The United Kingdom Collaboration Study found that elevated AFP in maternal serum drawn between 16 and 18 weeks of gestation correlated with an increased incidence of neural tube defects. Since that time much research effort has been aimed at perfecting the technique. We now can screen not only for neural tube defects, but also for trisomy 21 and trisomy 18. In addition, cystic fibrosis, sickle cell disease, and Huntington's disease, as well as many inborn errors of metabolism and other genetic disorders can now be identified prenatally.

Neural Tube Disease

Most neural tube diseases, eg, anencephaly, spina bifida, and meningomyelocele, are associated with a multifactorial inheritance pattern. The frequency of their occurrence varies in different populations (eg, rates as high as 10 per 1000 births in Ireland and as low as 0.8 per 1000 births in the western U.S.). Ninety percent are index cases, ie, they occur spontaneously without previous occurrence in a family. In general, if a couple has a child with such an anomaly, the chance of producing another affected child is 2–5%. If they have had 2 such children, the risk can be as high as 10%. However, other diagnostic possibilities involving different modes of inheritance should be considered. Siblings also run greater risks of having affected children, with the highest risk being to female offspring of sisters and the lowest to male offspring of brothers. Maternal serum screening is now available to all mothers between 16 and 20 weeks gestation. If an elevation of 2.5 or more standard deviations above the mean is noted, amniocentesis for AFP should be done along with a careful ultrasound study of the fetus for structural anomalies. Evidence for a neural tube defect noted on ultrasound and suspected by amniotic fluid AFP elevation of 3.0 or more standard deviations indicates a diagnosis of a neural tube defect and allows for appropriate counseling and decision making for the parents.

Maternal serum AFP screening detects about 85% of all open neural tube defects (NTDs). This detection rate allows 80% of all open NTDs and 90% of all anencephalic infants to be detected. Serum AFP does not detect skin-covered lesions or the closed form of neural tube defects. Thus, most encephaloceles may be missed.

Approximately 5–5.5% of women screened will have abnormally elevated values ($\geq$ 2.5 times the mean). Most of these will be false-positive results (a repeat test should determine this) due to inaccurate dating of gestational age, multiple gestation, fetal demise or dying fetus, or a host of other structural abnormalities. In most cases, repeat AFP testing and ultrasound examination will identify the problem. If serum AFP remains elevated and ultrasound examination does not yield a specific diagnosis, amniotic fluid AFP levels should be measured as well as amniotic fluid acetylcholinesterase levels. Further testing and counseling may be necessary before a final diagnosis can be made. When the correct gestational age is utilized, the false positive rate for second trimester maternal screening is 3–4%.

Chromosomal Abnormalities

In 1984, maternal serum AFP levels were found to be lower in patients who delivered infants with Down's syndrome. Using the AFP value with maternal age, 25–30% of fetuses with Down's syndrome were detected prenatally. In 1988, two additional tests were added to the maternal AFP; human chorionic gonadotropin (hCG) and unconjugated estriol (UE3). Using the "triple screen" a 60% detection rate for Down's syndrome was accomplished. In addition, the use of UE3 allowed for the detection of trisomy 18.

Fetuses with Down's syndrome have low maternal AFP, low UE3, and high hCG. Fetuses with trisomy 18 have low values across all serum markers. The false-positive rate for women less than 35 years of age is 5%. Above this age cutoff the false-positive rate is increased. The definitive diagnosis of a chromosomal abnormality must be confirmed with a fetal karyotype.

The risk of fetal trisomies increases with increasing maternal age. At age 35 the risk of a trisomy is approximately 1 in 200. At age 40 the risk is 1 in 20 (see Table 5–6). Prior to the discovery of serum markers advanced maternal age was utilized to guide which women received fetal karyotyping. Trisomies, however, are not the only abnormality increased in this population of women. Sex chromosome aneuploidies (47,XXY and 47,XXX) also occur at an increased rate in women 35 years of age and older. Despite the advances in serum screening, in this group of women, fetal karyotyping continues to be the gold standard for prenatal testing. The use of maternal serum screening in this subset of women is hindered by a high false-positive rate, less than 100% detection rate for trisomy 18 and 21, and lack of ability to screen for the sex chromosome aneuploidies.

Cystic Fibrosis

Cystic fibrosis affects 1/3300 individuals of European descent in the United States. The carrier frequency is 1/29 for North Americans of European descent and Ashkenazi Jewish descent and 1/60 for African Americans. A deletion of phenylalanine at position 508 of the cystic fibrosis transmembrane regulator on chromosome 7 leads to the disease. All individuals with a family history of cystic fibrosis or a high carrier frequency should be offered carrier testing. For couples who are both carriers of the defective allele fetal testing may be provided.

Future Advances in Prenatal Screening

Though the triple marker screen provides better sensitivity for detection of certain trisomies than any single marker alone, the detection rate for trisomy 18 and trisomy 21 still remains quite low. Recently, various investigators have been combining additional serum markers and reporting sensitivities near 90% for Down's syndrome. In addition, the measurement of fetal nuchal translucency via ultrasound at 10–13 weeks appears to have a high correlation with fetal chromosomal abnormalities.

The area of prenatal diagnostics continues to evolve. In the future we should expect higher detection rates with lower false-positive rates. Screening may move into the first trimester, could remain in the second trimester, or may even involve markers taken in both the first and second trimesters.

Fetal Karyotyping

A. Amniocentesis

Amniocentesis for prenatal diagnosis of genetic diseases is an extremely useful tool in the following circumstances or classes of patients:

(1) Maternal age 35 years or above.
(2) Previous chromosomally abnormal child.
(3) Three or more spontaneous abortions.
(4) Patient or husband with chromosome anomaly.
(5) Family history of chromosome anomaly.
(6) Possible female carrier of X-linked disease.
(7) Metabolic disease risk (because of previous experience or family history).
(8) Neural tube defect risk (because of previous experience or family history).
(9) Positive second trimester maternal serum screen.

Currently, so many metabolic diseases may be diagnosed prenatally by amniocentesis that when the history elicits the possibility of one being present, it is prudent to check with a major center to ascertain the availability of a diagnostic method.

Amniocentesis generally is carried out at the 15th to 17th weeks of gestation but can be offered earlier (12–14 weeks). The underlying risk of amniocentesis when performed 15 weeks of gestation and beyond is increased risk of miscarriage. This risk is estimated at 1 in 200, or 0.5%, which is roughly the risk of Down's syndrome of a 35-year-old female. When amniocentesis is performed prior to 15 weeks the miscarriage rate is slightly increased. Table 5–7 lists some of the conditions that now can be diagnosed prenatally by biochemical means.

B. Chorionic Villus Sampling

Chorionic villus sampling (CVS) is a technique used in the first trimester to obtain villi for cytogenetic testing. Most commonly, it is performed transcervically; however, transabdominal routes may also be attempted. The value of CVS is that it can be performed earlier in the pregnancy, and thus the decision of pregnancy termination can be made earlier. The downfall of CVS, however, is a slightly higher miscarriage rate of 1–5% and an association with distal limb defects. These risks appear to be dependent on operator experience and lower numbers have been reported when it is performed between 10 and 12 weeks gestation.

Karyotyping & FISH Analysis

Once the fetal cells are obtained they must be processed. Formal karyotyping should be performed on all specimens. This involves culturing the cells, replication, and eventually karyotyping. The entire process often takes 10–14 days until the final report becomes available. Fortunately, a quicker analysis may be obtained for some of the most common chromosomal anomalies.

Table 5–7. Examples of hereditary diseases diagnosable prenatally.

Lipidoses: Gaucher's, Tay-Sachs, Fabry's, etc.
Mucopolysaccharidoses: Hurler's, Hunter's, etc.
Aminoacidurias: Cystinosis, homocystinuria, maple syrup urine disease, etc.
Diseases of carbohydrate metabolism: Glucose-6-phosphate dehydrogenase deficiency, glycogen storage disease, etc.
Miscellaneous: Adrenogenital syndrome, Lesch-Nyhan syndrome, sickle cell disease, cystic fibrosis, Huntington's disease, etc.

The fluorescence in situ hybridization (FISH) study is a rapid assay for the detection of specific chromosomal aneuploidies using fluorescent-labeled DNA probes. Currently, probes exist for chromosomes 13, 18, 21, and 22, as well as the X and Y sex chromosomes among others. The average time to obtain a result is 24 hours. However, certain chromosomal probes may return as quickly as 4 hours. The more rapid turnaround time can be attained because the probes are mixed with uncultured amniocytes obtained from amniotic fluid or cells from CVS. If a patient is late in gestation or if the ultrasound is highly suggestive of a certain chromosomal composite, FISH analysis may be an appropriate study.

Single Gene Defects

If one parent is affected and the condition is caused by an autosomal dominant disorder, the chances are 1 in 2 that a child will be affected. If both parents are carriers of an autosomal recessive condition, the chances are 1 in 4 that the child would be affected and 1 in 2 that the child would be a carrier. Carrier status of both parents can be assumed if an affected child has been produced or if a carrier testing program was available and both parents were discovered to be carriers by this means. Tay-Sachs disease and sickle cell disease detection programs are examples of the latter possibility.

When carrier testing is available and the couple is at risk, as with Tay-Sachs disease in Jewish couples and sickle cell disease in blacks, the physician should order these tests before pregnancy is undertaken, or immediately if the patient is already pregnant. When parents are carriers and pregnancy has been diagnosed, prenatal diagnostic testing is indicated if there is a test available. If a physician does not know whether or not a test exists or how to obtain one, the local genetic counseling program, local chapter of the National Foundation/March of Dimes, or state health department should be called for consultation. These sources may be able to inform the physician about new research that may have produced a prenatal test. A new test may be likely, because this area of research is very dynamic. If genetic counseling services are readily available, patients with specific problems should be referred to those agencies for consultation. It is impossible for a physician to keep track of all of the current developments in the myriad conditions caused by single gene defects.

X-linked traits are frequently amenable to prenatal diagnostic testing. When such tests are not available, the couple has the option of testing for the sex of the fetus. If a fetus is noted to be a female, the odds are overwhelming that it will not be affected, although a carrier state may be present. If the fetus is a male, the chances are 1 in 2 that it will be affected. With this in-

formation, the couple can decide whether or not to continue the pregnancy in the case of a male fetus. Again, checking with genetic counseling agencies may reveal a prenatal diagnostic test that has only recently been described, or information such as gene linkage studies that may apply in the individual case.

All options should be presented in a nonjudgmental fashion with no attempt to persuade, based on the best information available at the time. The couple should then be encouraged to decide on a course of action that suits their particular needs. If the decision is appropriate, it should be supported by the physician and the genetic counselor. Very rarely, the patient will make a decision the physician regards as unwise or unrealistic. Such a decision may be based on superstition, religious or mystical beliefs, simple naivete, or even personality disorder. The physician should make every attempt to clarify the issues for the patient. Rarely, other resources such as family members or spiritual leaders may be consulted in strict confidence. The physician and the genetic counselor must clearly set forth the circumstances of the problem in the record, in case the patient undertakes a course of action that ends in tragedy and perhaps attempts to blame the professional counselors for not preventing it. Fortunately, these problems occur infrequently. In most instances, the physician, genetic counselor, and couple working together can arrive at a solution in keeping with the family's best interests.

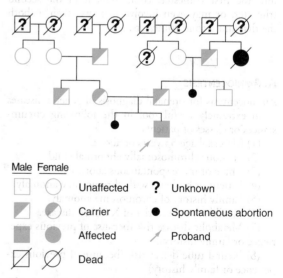

Male Female

☐ ○	Unaffected	**?** Unknown
◨ ◔	Carrier	● Spontaneous abortion
◼ ●	Affected	╱ Proband
⊠ ⊘	Dead	

Figure 5–4. Pedigree showing unaffected offspring, carrier offspring, and affected offspring in a family with an autosomal recessive trait (sickle cell anemia).

Genetic Counseling

Genetic counseling involves interaction between the physician, the family, and the genetic counselor. It is the physician's responsibility to utilize the services of the genetic consultant in the best interest of the patient. The genetic counselor will take a formal family history and construct a family tree (Fig 5–4). The assessment of the underlying general population risk of a disease and the specific family risk should be provided. When a specific diagnosis is known in the proband and the relatives are dead or otherwise not available, the counseler may ask to see photographs, which may show characteristics of the suspected condition. In many cases, when the pedigree is constructed, the inheritance pattern can be determined. If this can be done, the relative risks that future progeny will be affected can be estimated. This pedigree information is also useful in discussing the case with a genetic counselor.

■ GYNECOLOGIC CORRELATES

THE CHROMOSOMAL BASIS OF SEX DETERMINATION

Syngamy

The sex of the fetus is normally determined at fertilization. The cells of normal females contain two X chromosomes; those of normal males contain one X and one Y. During meiotic reduction, half of the male gametes receive a Y chromosome and the other half an X chromosome. Since the female has two X chromosomes, all female gametes contain an X chromosome. If a Y-bearing gamete fertilizes an ovum, the fetus is male; conversely, if an X-bearing gamete fertilizes an ovum, the fetus is female.

Arithmetically, the situation described previously should yield a male:female sex ratio of 100—the sex ratio being defined as 100 times the number of males divided by the number of females. However, for many years, the male:female sex ratio of the newborns in the white population has been approximately 105. Apparently the sex ratio at fertilization is even higher than at birth: most data on the sex of abortuses indicate a preponderance of males.

Abnormalities of Meiosis-Mitosis

The discussion in this section will be limited to anomalies of meiosis and mitosis that result in some abnormality in the sex chromosome complement of the embryo.

Chromosome studies in connection with various clinical conditions suggest that errors in meiosis and mitosis do indeed occur. These errors result in any of the following principal effects: (1) an extra sex chromosome, (2) an absent sex chromosome, (3) 2 cell lines having different sex chromosomes and arising by mosaicism, (4) 2 cell lines having different sex chromosomes and arising by chimerism, (5) a structurally abnormal sex chromosome, and (6) a sex chromosome complement inconsistent with the phenotype.

By and large, an extra or a missing sex chromosome arises as the result of an error of disjunction in meiosis I or II in either the male or the female. In meiosis I, this means that instead of each of the paired homologous sex chromosomes going to the appropriate daughter cell, both go to one cell, leaving that cell with an extra sex chromosome and the daughter cell with none. Failure of disjunction in meiosis II simply means that the centromere fails to divide normally.

A variation of this process, known as anaphase lag, occurs when one of the chromosomes is delayed in arriving at the daughter cell and thus is lost. Theoretically, chromosomes may be lost by failure of association in prophase and by failure of replication, but these possibilities have not been demonstrated.

Persons who have been found to have 2 cell lines apparently have had problems in mitosis in the very early stage of embryogenesis. Thus, if there is nondisjunction or anaphase lag in an early (first, second, or immediately subsequent) cell division in the embryo, mosaicism may be said to exist. In this condition, there are 2 cell lines; one has a normal number of sex chromosomes, and the other is deficient in a sex chromosome or has an extra number of sex chromosomes. A similar situation exists in chimerism, except that there may be a difference in the sex chromosome: one may be an X and one may be a Y. This apparently arises by dispermy, by the fertilization of a double oocyte, or by the fusion, very early in embryogenesis, of 2 separately fertilized oocytes. Each of these conditions has been produced experimentally in animals.

Structural abnormalities of the sex chromosomes—deletion of the long or short arm or the formation of an isochromosome (2 short arms or 2 long arms)—result from injury to the chromosomes during meiosis. How such injuries occur is not known, but the results are noted more commonly in sex chromosomes than in autosomes—perhaps because serious injury to an autosome is much more likely to be lethal than injury to an X chromosome, and surviving injured X chromosomes would therefore be more common.

The situation in which there is a sex chromosome complement with an inappropriate genotype arises in special circumstances of true hermaphroditism and XX males (see later sections).

The X Chromosome in Humans

At about day 16 of embryonic life, there appears on the undersurface of the nuclear membrane of the somatic cells of human females a structure 1 μm in diameter known as the X-chromatin body. There is genetic as well as cytogenetic evidence that this is one of the X chromosomes (the only chromosome visible by ordinary light microscopy during interphase). In a sense, therefore, all females are hemizygous with respect to the X chromosome. However, there are genetic reasons for believing that the X chromosome is not entirely inactivated during the process of formation of the X-chromatin body. In normal females, inactivation of the X chromosome during interphase and its representation as the X-chromatin body are known as the Lyon phenomenon (for Mary Lyon, a British geneticist). This phenomenon may involve, at random, either the maternal or the paternal X chromosome. Furthermore, once the particular chromosome has been selected early in embryogenesis, it is always the same X chromosome that is inactivated in the progeny of that particular cell. Geneticists have found that the ratio of maternal to paternal X chromosomes inactivated is approximately 1:1.

The germ cells of an ovary are an exception to the X inactivation concept in that X inactivation does not characterize the meiotic process. Apparently, meiosis is impossible without 2 genetically active X chromosomes. While random structural damage to one of the X chromosomes seems to cause meiotic arrest, oocyte loss, and therefore failure of ovarian development, an especially critical area necessary for oocyte development has been identified on the long arm of the X. This essential area involves almost all of the long arm and has been specifically located from Xq13 to Xq26. If this area is broken in one of the X chromosomes as in a deletion or translocation, oocyte development does not occur. However, a few exceptions to this rule have been described.

It is a curious biologic phenomenon that if one of the X chromosomes is abnormal, it is always this chromosome that is genetically inactivated and becomes the X-chromatin body, regardless of whether it is maternal or paternal in origin. While this general rule seems to be an exception to the randomness of X inactivation, this is more apparent than real. Presumably, random inactivation does occur, but the disadvantaged cells—ie, those left with a damaged active X—do not survive. Consequently, the embryo develops only with cells with a normal active X chromosome (X-chromatin body) (Fig 5–5).

If there are more than two X chromosomes, all X chromosomes except one are genetically inactivated and become X-chromatin bodies; thus, in this case, the number of X-chromatin bodies will be equal to the

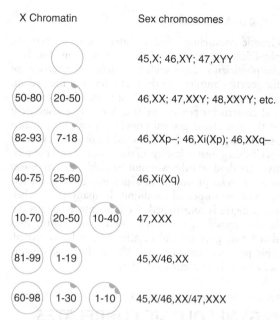

X Chromatin	Sex chromosomes
	45,X; 46,XY; 47,XYY
50-80 20-50	46,XX; 47,XXY; 48,XXYY; etc.
82-93 7-18	46,XXp–; 46,Xi(Xp); 46,XXq–
40-75 25-60	46,Xi(Xq)
10-70 20-50 10-40	47,XXX
81-99 1-19	45,X/46,XX
60-98 1-30 1-10	45,X/46,XX/47,XXX

Figure 5–5. Relation of X-chromatin body to the possible sex chromosome components.

number of X chromosomes minus one. This type of inactivation applies to X chromosomes even when a Y chromosome is present, eg, in Klinefelter's syndrome.

Although the X chromosomes are primarily concerned with the determination of femininity, there is abundant genetic evidence that loci having to do with traits other than sex determination are present on the X chromosome. Thus, in the catalog of genetic disorders given in the 10th edition of *Mendelian Inheritance in Man*, 320 traits are listed as more or less definitely X-linked. Substantial evidence for X linkage has been found for about 160 of these traits; the rest are only suspected of having this relationship. Hemophilia, color blindness, childhood muscular dystrophy (Duchenne's dystrophy), Lesch-Nyhan syndrome, and glucose-6-phosphate dehydrogenase deficiency are among the better known conditions controlled by loci on the X chromosome. These entities probably arise from the expression of a recessive gene due to its hemizygous situation in males.

X-linked dominant traits are infrequent in the human. Vitamin D–resistant rickets is an example.

There is at least one disorder that can be classified somewhere between a structural anomaly of the X chromosome and a single gene mutation. X-linked mental retardation in males is associated with a fragile site at q26, but a special culture medium is required for its demonstration. Furthermore, it has been shown that heterozygote female carriers for this fragile site have low IQ test scores.

The Y Chromosome in Humans

Just as the X chromosome represents the only chromosome visible by ordinary light microscopy in interphase, the Y chromosome is the only chromosome visible in interphase, after exposure to quinacrine compounds, by the use of fluorescence microscopy. This is a very useful diagnostic method.

In contrast to the X chromosome, few traits have been traced to the Y chromosome except those having to do with testicular formation and those at the very tip of the short arm, homologous with those at the tip of the short arm of the X. Possession of the Y chromosome alone, ie, without an X chromosome, apparently is lethal, because such a case has never been described.

Present on the Y chromosome is an area that produces a factor which allows for testicular development. This factor is termed testis determining factor (TDF). Without the presence of TDF normal female anatomy will develop. When it is present testicular development occurs with subsequent differentiation of Sertoli cells. The Sertoli cells in turn produce a second factor central to male differentiation, müllerian inhibiting factor (MIF), also termed antimüllerian factor (AMF). The presence of MIF causes the regression of the müllerian ducts, and thereby allows for the development of normal internal male anatomy.

ABNORMAL DEVELOPMENT

1. Ovarian Agenesis-Dysgenesis

In 1938, Turner described 7 girls 15–23 years of age with sexual infantilism, webbing of the neck, cubitus valgus, and retardation of growth. A survey of the literature indicates that "Turner's syndrome" means different things to different writers. After the later discovery that ovarian streaks are characteristically associated with the clinical entity described by Turner, "ovarian agenesis" became a synonym for Turner's syndrome. After discovery of the absence of the X-chromatin body in such patients, the term ovarian agenesis gave way to "gonadal dysgenesis," "gonadal agenesis," or "gonadal aplasia."

Meanwhile, some patients with the genital characteristics mentioned previously were shown to have a normally positive X-chromatin count. Furthermore, a variety of sex chromosome complements have been found in connection with streak gonads. As if these contradictions were not perplexing enough, it has been noted that streaks are by no means confined to patients with Turner's original tetrad of infantilism, webbing of the neck, cubitus valgus, and retardation of growth, but may be present in girls with sexual infantilism only. Since Turner's original description, a host of additional somatic anomalies (varying in frequency) have been associated with his original clinical picture; these include shield chest, overweight, high palate, micrognathia, epicanthal folds, low-set ears, hypoplasia of nails, osteoporosis, pigmented moles, hypertension, lymphedema, cutix laxa, keloids, coarctation of the aorta, mental retardation, intestinal telangiectasia, and deafness.

For our purposes, the eponym Turner's syndrome will be used to indicate sexual infantilism with ovarian streaks, short stature, and 2 or more of the somatic anomalies mentioned earlier. In this context, such terms as ovarian agenesis, gonadal agenesis, and gonadal dysgenesis lose their clinical significance and become merely descriptions of the gonadal development of the person. At least 21 sex chromosome complements have been associated with streak gonads (Fig 5–6), but only about 9 sex chromosome complements have been associated with Turner's syndrome. However, approximately two-thirds of patients with Turner's syndrome have a 45,X chromosome complement, whereas only one-fourth of patients without Turner's syndrome but with streak ovaries have a 45,X chromosome complement.

```
                45,X
                46,XX
                46,XY
                46,XXp–
                46,XXq–
                46,Xi(Xp)
                46,Xi(Xq)
                46,XXq–?
                45,X/46,XX
                45,X/46,XY
                45,X/46,Xi(Xq)
                45,X/46,XXp–
                45,X/46,XXq–
                45,X/46,XXq–?
                45,X/46,XX            ⎫
                45,X/46,Xi(Xq)        ⎬
                45,X/46,XX/47,XXX     ⎫
                45,X/47,XXX           ⎬
                45,X/46,XX/47,XXX     ⎫
                45,X/46,Xi(Xq)/47,XXX ⎬
                45,X/46,XXr(X)
                45,X/46,XX/46,XXr(X)
                45,X/46,XXr(X)/47,XXr(X)r(X)
                45,X/46,XX/47,XXX     ⎫
                45,X/46,XXq–          ⎬
```

Figure 5–6. The 21 sex chromosome complements that have been found in patients with streak gonads.

Karyotype/phenotype correlations in the syndromes associated with ovarian agenesis are not completely satisfactory. Nonetheless, if gonadal development is considered as one problem and if the somatic difficulties associated with these syndromes are considered as a separate problem, one can make certain correlations.

With respect to failure of gonadal development, it is important to recall that diploid germ cells require 2 normal active X chromosomes. This is in contrast to the somatic cells, where only one sex chromosome is thought to be genetically active, at least after day 16 of embryonic life in the human, when the X-chromatin body first appears in the somatic cells. It is also important to recall that in 45,X persons no oocytes persist, and streak gonads are the rule. From these facts, it may be inferred that failure of gonadal development is not the result of a specific sex chromosome defect but rather of the absence of two X chromosomes with the necessary critical zones.

Karyotype/phenotype correlations with respect to the somatic abnormalities are even sketchier than the correlations with regard to gonadal development. However, there is good evidence to show that monosomy for the short arm of the X chromosome is related to somatic difficulties, although some patients with long-arm deletions have somatic abnormalities.

History of Gonadal Agenesis

The histologic findings in these abnormal ovaries in patients with gonadal streaks are essentially the same regardless of the patient's cytogenetic background (Fig 5–7).

Fibrous tissue is the major component of the streak. It is indistinguishable microscopically from that of the normal ovarian stroma. The so-called germinal epithelium, on the surface of the structure, is a layer of low cuboid cells; this layer appears to be completely inactive.

Tubules of the ovarian rete are invariably found in sections taken from about the midportion of the streak.

In all patients who have reached the age of normal puberty, hilar cells are also demonstrated. The number of hilar cells varies among patients. In those with some enlargement of the clitoris, hilar cells are present in large numbers. It may be that these developments are causally related. Nevertheless, hilar cells are also found in many normal ovaries. The origin of hilar cells is not precisely known, but they are associated with development of the medullary portion of the gonad. Their presence lends further support to the concept that in ovarian agenesis the gonad develops along normal lines until just before the expected appearance of early oocytes. In all cases in which sections of the broad ligament have been available for study, it has been possible to identify the mesonephric duct and tubules—broad ligament structures found in normal females.

Clinical Findings

A. Symptoms and Signs

1. In newborn infants—The newborn with streak ovaries often shows edema of the hands and feet. Histologically, this edema is associated with large dilated vascular spaces. With such findings, it is obviously desir-

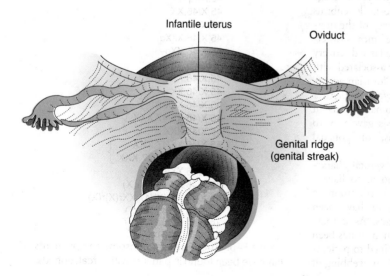

Infantile uterus

Oviduct

Genital ridge
(genital streak)

Figure 5–7. Gonadal streaks in a patient with the phenotype of Turner's syndrome. (Redrawn and reproduced, with permission, from Jones HW Jr, Scott WW: *Hermaphroditism, Genital Anomalies and Related Endocrine Disorders,* 2nd ed. Williams & Wilkins, 1971.)

able to obtain a karyotype. However, some children with streak ovaries—particularly those who have few or no somatic abnormalities—cannot be recognized at birth.

2. In adolescents—The arresting and characteristic clinical finding in many of these patients is their short stature. Typical patients seldom attain a height of 1.5 m (5 ft) (Fig 5–8). In addition, sexual infantilism is a striking finding. As was mentioned earlier, a variety of somatic abnormalities may be present; by definition, if 2 or more of these are noted, the patient may be considered to have Turner's syndrome. Most of these patients have only one normal X chromosome, and two-thirds of them have no other sex chromosome. Patients of normal height without somatic abnormalities may also have gonadal streaks. Under these circumstances, there is likely to be a cell line with 2 normal sex chromosomes but often a second line with a single X. The internal findings are exactly the same as in patients with classic Turner's syndrome, however.

B. LABORATORY FINDINGS

An important finding in patients of any age—but especially after that of expected puberty, ie, about 12

years—is elevation of total gonadotropin production. From a practical point of view, ovarian failure in patients over age 15 cannot be considered as a diagnostic possibility unless the serum FSH is more than 50 mIU/mL and LH is more than 90 mIU/mL.

Nongonadal endocrine functions are normal. Urinary excretion of estrogens is low, and the maturation index and other vaginal smear indices are shifted well to the left.

Treatment

Substitution therapy with estrogen is necessary for development of secondary characteristics.

Therapy with growth hormone will increase height. There remain some uncertainties over whether ultimate height will be greater than it otherwise would be. Current evidence suggests that it will be.

The incidence of malignant degeneration is increased in the gonadal streaks of patients with a Y chromosome, as compared with normal males. Surgical removal of streaks from all patients with a Y chromosome is recommended.

2. True Hermaphroditism

By classic definition, true hermaphroditism exists when both ovarian and testicular tissue can be demonstrated in one patient. In humans, the Y chromosome carries genetic material that is normally responsible for testicular development; this material is active even when multiple X chromosomes are present. Thus, in Klinefelter's syndrome, a testis develops with up to 4 Xs and only 1 Y. Conversely (with rare exceptions), a testis has not been observed to develop in the absence of the Y chromosome. The exceptions are found in true hermaphrodites and XX males, in whom testicular tissue has developed in association with an XX sex chromosome complement.

Clinical Findings

A. SYMPTOMS AND SIGNS

No exclusive features clinically distinguish true hermaphroditism from other forms of intersexuality. Hence, the diagnosis must be entertained in an infant with any form of intersexuality, except only those with a continuing virilizing influence, eg, congenital adrenal hyperplasia. Firm diagnosis is possible after the onset of puberty, when certain clinical features become evident, but the diagnosis can and should be made in infancy.

In the past, most true hermaphrodites have been reared as males because they have rather masculine-

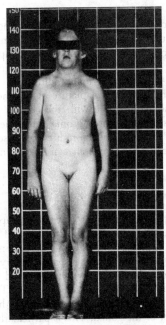

Figure 5–8. Patient with Turner's syndrome. (Reproduced, with permission, from Jones HW Jr, Scott WW: *Hermaphroditism, Genital Anomalies and Related Endocrine Disorders,* 2nd ed. Williams & Wilkins, 1971.)

appearing external genitalia (Fig 5–9). Nevertheless, with early diagnosis, most should be reared as females.

Almost all true hermaphrodites develop female-type breasts. This helps to distinguish male hermaphroditism from true hermaphroditism, because few male hermaphrodites other than those with familial feminizing hermaphroditism develop large breasts.

Many true hermaphrodites menstruate. The presence or absence of menstruation is partially determined by the development of the uterus; many true hermaphrodites have rudimentary or no development of the müllerian ducts (Fig 5–10).

A few patients who had a uterus and menstruated after removal of testicular tissue have become pregnant and delivered normal children.

B. Sex Chromosome Complements

Most true hermaphrodites have X-chromatin bodies and karyotypes that are indistinguishable from those of normal females. In contrast to these, a few patients who cannot be distinguished clinically from other true hermaphrodites have been reported to have a variety of other karyotypes—eg, several chimeric persons with karyotypes of 46,XX/46,XY have been identified.

In true hermaphrodites, the testis is competent in its müllerian-suppressive functions, but an ovotestis may behave as an ovary insofar as its müllerian-suppressive function is concerned. The true hermaphroditic testis or ovotestis is as competent to masculinize the external genitalia as is the testis of a patient with the virilizing type of male hermaphroditism. This is unrelated to karyotype.

Deletion mapping by DNA hybridization has shown that most (but not all) XX true hermaphrodites

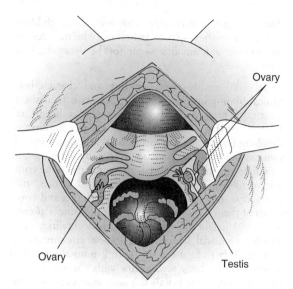

Figure 5–10. Internal genitalia of a patient with true hermaphroditism. (Reproduced, with permission, from Jones HW Jr, Scott WW: *Hermaphroditism, Genital Anomalies and Related Endocrine Disorders,* 2nd ed. Williams & Wilkins, 1971.)

have Y-specific sequences. Abnormal crossing-over of a portion of the Y chromosome to the X in meiosis may explain some cases. This latter is further supported by the finding of a positive H-Y antigen assay in some patients with 46,XX true hermaphroditism.

In general, the clinical picture of true hermaphroditism is not compatible with the clinical picture in other kinds of gross chromosomal anomalies. For example, very few true hermaphrodites have associated somatic anomalies, and mental retardation almost never occurs.

Treatment

The principles of treatment of true hermaphroditism do not differ from those of the treatment of hermaphroditism in general. Therapy can be summarized by stating that surgical removal of contradictory organs is indicated, and the external genitalia should be reconstructed in keeping with the sex of rearing. The special problem in this group is how to establish with certainty the character of the gonad. This is particularly difficult in the presence of an ovotestis, because its recognition by gross characteristics is notoriously inaccurate, and one must not remove too much of the gonad for study. In some instances the gonadal tissue of one sex is com-

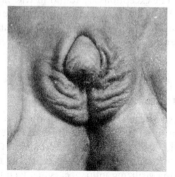

Figure 5–9. External genitalia of a patient with true hermaphroditism. (Reproduced, with permission, from Jones HW Jr, Scott WW: *Hermaphroditism, Genital Anomalies and Related Endocrine Disorders,* 2nd ed. Williams & Wilkins, 1971.)

pletely embedded within a gonadal structure primarily of the opposite sex.

3. Klinefelter's Syndrome

This condition, first described in 1942 by Klinefelter, Reifenstein, and Albright, occurs only in apparent males. As originally described, it is characterized by small testes, azoospermia, gynecomastia, relatively normal external genitalia, and otherwise average somatic development. High levels of gonadotropin in urine or serum are characteristic.

Clinical Findings

A. SYMPTOMS AND SIGNS

By definition, this syndrome applies only to persons reared as males. The disease is not recognizable before puberty except by routine screening of newborn infants (see below). Most patients come under observation at 16–40 years of age.

Somatic development during infancy and childhood may be normal. Growth and muscular development may also be within normal limits. Most patients have a normal general appearance and no complaints referable to this abnormality, which is often discovered in the course of a routine physical examination or an infertility study.

In the original publication by Klinefelter and coworkers, gynecomastia was considered an essential part of the syndrome. Since then, however, cases without gynecomastia have been reported.

The external genitalia are perfectly formed and in most patients are quite well developed. Erection and intercourse usually are satisfactory.

There is no history of delayed descent of the testes in typical cases, and the testes are in the scrotum. Neither is there any history of testicular trauma or disease. Although a history of mumps orchitis is occasionally elicited, this disease has not been correlated with the syndrome. However the testes are often very small in contrast to the rest of the genitalia (about 1.5×1.5 cm).

Psychologic symptoms are often present. Most studies of this syndrome have been done in psychiatric institutions. The seriousness of the psychological disturbance seems to be partly related to the number of extra X chromosomes—eg, it is estimated that about one-fourth of XXY patients have some degree of mental retardation.

B. LABORATORY FINDINGS

One of the extremely important clinical features of Klinefelter's syndrome is the excessive amount of pituitary gonadotropin found in either urine or serum assay.

The urinary excretion of neutral 17-ketosteroids varies from relatively normal to definitely subnormal levels. There is a rough correlation between the degree of hypoleydigism as judged clinically and a low 17-ketosteroid excretion rate.

C. HISTOLOGIC AND CYTOGENETIC FINDINGS

Klinefelter's syndrome may be regarded as a form of primary testicular failure.

Several authors have classified a variety of forms of testicular atrophy as subtypes of Klinefelter's syndrome. Be this as it may, Klinefelter believed that only those patients who have a chromosomal abnormality could be said to have this syndrome. Microscopic examination of the adult testis shows that the seminiferous tubules lack epithelium and are shrunken and hyalinized. They contain large amounts of elastic fibers and Leydig cells are present in large numbers.

Males with positive X-chromatin bodies are likely to have Klinefelter's syndrome. The nuclear sex anomaly reflects a basic genetic abnormality in sex chromosome constitution. All cases studied have had at least two X chromosomes and one Y chromosome. The most common abnormality in the sex chromosome constitution is XXY, but the literature also records XXXY, XXYY, XXXXY, and XXXYY, and mosaics of XX/XXY, XY/XXY, XY/XXXY, and XXXY/XXXXY. In all examples except the XX/XXY mosaic, a Y chromosome is present in all cells. From these patterns, it is obvious that the Y chromosome has a very strong testis-forming impulse, which can operate in spite of the presence of as many as four X chromosomes.

Thus, patients with Klinefelter's syndrome will have not only a positive X-chromatin body but also a positive Y-chromatin body.

The abnormal sex chromosome constitution causes differentiation of an abnormal testis, leading to testicular failure in adulthood. At birth or before puberty, such testes show a marked deficiency or absence of germinal cells.

By means of nursery screening, the frequency of males with positive X-chromatin bodies has been estimated to be 2.65 per 1000 live male births.

Treatment

There is no treatment for the 2 principal complaints of these patients: infertility and gynecomastia. No pituitary preparation has been effective in the regeneration of the hyalinized tubular epithelium or the stimulation of gametogenesis. Furthermore, no hormone regimen is effective in treating the breast hypertrophy. When the breasts are a formidable psychologic problem, surgical removal may be a satisfactory procedure. In patients who have clinical symptoms of hypoleydigism, substitution therapy with testosterone is an important physiologic and psychologic aid. Donor sperm may be offered for the treatment of the infertility.

4. Double-X Males

A few cases have been reported of adult males with a slightly hypoplastic penis and very small testes but no other indication of abnormal sexual development. These males are sterile. Unlike those with Klinefelter's syndrome, they do not have abnormal breast development. They are clinically very similar to patients with Del Castillo's syndrome (testicular dysgenesis). Nevertheless, the XX males have a positive sex chromatin and a normal female karyotype. These may be extreme examples of the sex reversal that is usually partial in true hermaphroditism.

5. Multiple-X Syndromes

The finding of more than one X-chromatin body in a cell indicates the presence of more than two X chromosomes in that particular cell. In many patients, such a finding is associated with mosaicism, and the clinical picture is controlled by this fact—eg, if one of the strains of the mosaicism is 45,X, gonadal agenesis is likely to occur. There also are persons who do not seem to have mosaicism but do have an abnormal number of X chromosomes in all cells. In such persons, the most common complement is XXX (triplo-X syndrome), but XXXX (tetra-X syndrome), and XXXXX (penta-X syndrome) have been reported.

An additional X chromosome does not seem to have a consistent effect on sexual differentiation. The body proportions of these persons are normal, and the external genitalia are normally female. A number of such persons have been examined at laparotomy, and no consistent abnormality of the ovary has been found. In a few cases, the number of follicles appeared to be reduced, and in at least one case the ovaries were very small and the ovarian stroma poorly differentiated. About 20% of postpubertal patients with the triplo-X syndrome report various degrees of amenorrhea or some irregularity in menstruation. For the most part, however, these patients have a normal menstrual history and are of proved fertility.

Almost all patients known to have multiple-X syndromes have some degree of mental retardation. A few have mongoloid features. (The mothers of these patients tended to be older than the mothers of normal children, as is true also in Down's syndrome.) Perhaps these findings are in part circumstantial, since most of these patients have been discovered during surveys in mental institutions. The important clinical point is that mentally retarded infants should have chromosomal study.

Uniformly, the offspring of triplo-X mothers have been normal. This is surprising, because theoretically in such cases meiosis should produce equal numbers of ova containing one or two X chromosomes, and fertilization of the abnormal XX ova should give rise to XXX and XXY individuals. Nevertheless, the triplo-X condition seems selective for normal ova and zygotes.

The diagnosis of this syndrome is made by identifying a high percentage of cells in the buccal smear with double X-chromatin bodies and by finding 47 chromosomes with a karyotype showing an extra X chromosome in all cells cultured from the peripheral blood. It should be noted that in the examination of the buccal smear, some cells have a single X-chromatin body. Hence, on the basis of the chromatin examination, one might suspect XX/XXX mosaicism. Actually, in triplo-X patients, only a single type of cell can be demonstrated in cultures of cells from the peripheral blood. The absence of the second X-chromatin body in some of the somatic cells may result from the time of examination of the cell (during interphase) and from the spatial orientation, which could have prevented the two X-chromatin bodies (adjacent to the nuclear membrane) from being seen. In this syndrome, the number of cells containing either 1 or 2 X-chromatin bodies is very high—at least 60–80%, as compared with an upper limit of about 40% in normal females.

6. Female Hermaphroditism Due to Congenital Adrenal Hyperplasia

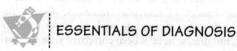

ESSENTIALS OF DIAGNOSIS

- Female pseudohermaphroditism, ambiguous genitalia with clitoral hypertrophy, and, occasionally, persistent urogenital sinus.

- Early appearance of sexual hair; hirsutism, dwarfism.

- Urinary 17-ketosteroids elevated; pregnanetriol may be increased.

- Elevated serum 17-hydroxyprogesterone.

- Occasionally associated with water and electrolyte imbalance—particularly in the neonatal period.

General Considerations

Female hermaphroditism due to congenital adrenal hyperplasia is a clearly delineated clinical syndrome. The syndrome has been better understood since the discovery that cortisone may successfully arrest virilization. The problem is usually due to a deficiency of a gene required for 21 hydroxylation in the biosynthesis of cortisol.

If the diagnosis is not made in infancy, an unfortunate series of events ensues. Because the adrenals secrete an abnormally large amount of virilizing steroid even during embryonic life, these infants are born with abnormal genitalia (Fig 5–11). In extreme cases, there is fusion of the scrotolabial folds and, in rare instances, even the formation of a penile urethra. The clitoris is greatly enlarged, so that it may be mistaken for a penis (Fig 5–12). No gonads are palpable within the fused scrotolabial folds, and their absence has sometimes given rise to the mistaken impression of male cryptorchidism. Usually, there is a single urinary meatus at the base of the phallus and the vagina enters the persistent urogenital sinus as noted in Figure 5–13.

During infancy, provided there are no serious electrolyte disturbances, these children grow more rapidly

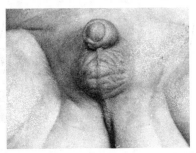

Figure 5–12. External genitalia of a female patient with congenital virilizing adrenal hyperplasia. This is a more severe deformity than that shown in Fig 5–11.

than normal. For a time, they greatly exceed the average in both height and weight. Unfortunately, epiphyseal closure occurs by about age 10, with the result that as adults these people are much shorter than normal (Fig 5–14).

The process of virilization begins at an early age. Pubic hair may appear as early as age 2 years but usually somewhat later. This is followed by growth of axillary hair and finally by the appearance of body hair and a beard, which may be so thick as to require daily shaving. Acne may develop early. Puberty never ensues. There is no breast development. Menstruation does not occur. During the entire process, serum adrenal androgens and 17-hydroxyprogesterone are abnormally high.

Although our principal concern here is with this abnormality in females, it must be mentioned that adrenal hyperplasia of the adrenogenital type may also occur in males, in whom it is called macrogenitosomia precox. Sexual development progresses rapidly, and the sex organs attain adult size at an early age. Just as in the female, sexual hair and acne develop unusually early, and the voice becomes deep. The testes are usually in the scrotum; however, in early childhood they remain small and immature, although the genitalia are of adult dimensions. In adulthood, the testes usually enlarge and spermatogenesis occurs, allowing impregnation rates similar to those of a control population. Somatic development in the male corresponds to that of the female; as a child, the male exceeds the average in height and strength, but (if untreated) as an adult he is stocky, muscular, and well below average height.

Both the male and the female with this disorder—but especially the male—may have the complicating problem of electrolyte imbalance. In infancy, it is manifested by vomiting, progressive weight loss, and dehydration and may be fatal unless recognized promptly. The characteristic findings are an exceedingly low serum sodium level and low CO_2 combining power

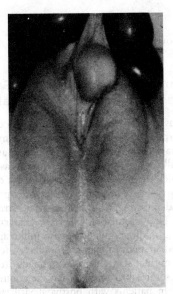

Figure 5–11. External genitalia of a female patient with congenital virilizing adrenal hyperplasia. Compare with Fig 5–12. (Reproduced, with permission, from Jones HW Jr, Scott WW: *Hermaphroditism, Genital Anomalies and Related Endocrine Disorders,* 2nd ed. Williams & Wilkins, 1971.)

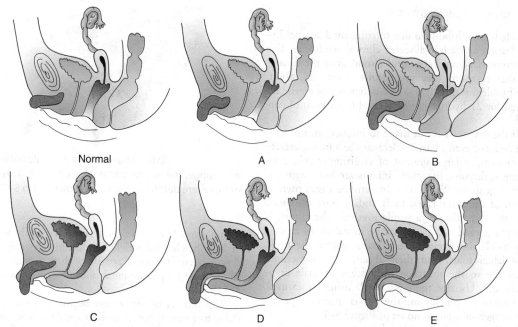

Figure 5–13. Sagittal view of genital deformities of increasing severity (A–E) in congenital virilizing adrenal hyperplasia. (Redrawn and reproduced, with permission, from Verkauf BS, Jones HW Jr: Masculinization of the female genitalia in congenital adrenal hyperplasia. South Med J 1970;63:634.)

level and a high potassium level. The condition is sometimes misdiagnosed as congenital pyloric stenosis.

A few of these patients have a deficiency in 11-hydroxylation which is associated with hypertension in addition to virilization.

Adrenal Histology

The adrenal changes center on a reticular hyperplasia, which becomes more marked as the patient grows older. In some instances, the glomerulosa may participate in the hyperplasia, but the fasciculata is greatly diminished in amount or entirely absent. Lipid studies show absence of fascicular and glomerular lipid but an abnormally strong lipid reaction in the reticularis (Fig 5–15).

Ovarian Histology

The ovarian changes may be summarized by stating that in infants, children, and teenagers, there is normal follicular development to the antrum stage but no evidence of ovulation. With increasing age, less and less follicular activity occurs, and primordial follicles disappear. This disappearance must not be complete, however, because cortisone therapy, even in adults, usually

results in ovulatory menstruation after 4–6 months of treatment.

Developmental Anomalies of the Genital Tubercle & Urogenital Sinus Derivatives

The phallus is composed of 2 lateral corpora cavernosa, but the corpus spongiosum is normally absent. The external urinary meatus is most often located at the base of the phallus (Fig 5–11). An occasional case may be seen in which the urethra does extend to the end of the clitoris (Fig 5–12). The glans penis and the prepuce are present and indistinguishable from these structures in the male. The scrotolabial folds are characteristically fused in the midline, giving a scrotumlike appearance with a median perineal raphe; however, they seldom enlarge to normal scrotal size. No gonads are palpable within the scrotolabial folds. When the anomaly is not severe (eg, in patients with postnatal virilization), fusion of the scrotolabial folds is not complete, and by gentle retraction it is often possible to locate not only the normally located external urinary meatus but also the orifice of the vagina.

An occasional patient has no communication between the urogenital sinus and the vagina. In no case does the vagina communicate with that portion of the

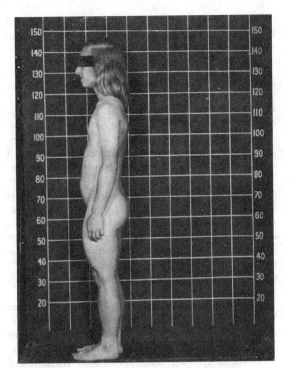

Figure 5–14. An untreated adult with virilizing adrenal hyperplasia. Note the short stature and the relative shortness of the limbs. (Reproduced, with permission, from Jones HW Jr, Scott WW: *Hermaphroditism, Genital Anomalies and Related Endocrine Disorders*, 2nd ed. Williams & Wilkins, 1971.)

urogenital sinus that gives rise to the female urethra or the prostatic urethra. Instead, the vaginal communication is via caudal urogenital sinus derivatives; thus, fortunately, the sphincter mechanism is not involved, and the anomalous communication is with that portion of the sinus that develops as the vaginal vestibule in the female and the membranous urethra in the male. From the gynecologist's point of view, it is much more meaningful to say that the vagina and (female) urethra enter a persistent urogenital sinus than to say that the vagina enters the (membranous [male]) urethra. This conclusion casts some doubt on the embryologic significance of the prostatic utricle, which is commonly said to represent the homologue of the vagina in the normal male.

Hormone Changes

Important and specific endocrine changes occur in congenital adrenal hyperplasia of the adrenogenital type. The ultimate diagnosis depends on demonstration of these abnormalities.

A. Urinary Estrogens

The progressive virilization of female hermaphrodites caused by adrenal hyperplasia would suggest that estrogen secretion in these patients is low, and this hypothesis is further supported by the atrophic condition of both the ovarian follicular apparatus and the estrogen target organs. Actually, the determination of urinary estrogens, both fluorometrically and biologically, indicates that it is elevated.

B. Serum Steroids

The development of satisfactory radioimmunoassay techniques for measuring steroids in blood serum has resulted in an increased tendency to measure serum steroids rather than urinary metabolites in diagnosing the condition and monitoring therapy. Serum steroid profiles of many patients with this disorder show that numerous defects in the biosynthesis of cortisol may occur. The most common defect is at the 21-hydroxylase step. Less frequent defects are at the 11-hydroxylase step and the 3β-ol-dehydrogenase step. Rarely, the defect is at the 17-hydroxylase step. In the most common

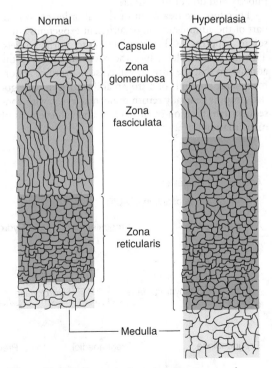

Figure 5–15. Normal adrenal architecture and adrenal histology in congenital virilizing adrenal hyperplasia. Note the great relative increase in the zona reticularis.

form of the disorder—21-hydroxylase deficiency—the serum 17-hydroxyprogesterone level, and to a lesser extent the serum progesterone level, are elevated. This is easily understandable when it is recalled that 17-hydroxyprogesterone is the substrate for the 21-hydroxylation step (Fig 5–16). Likewise, in the other enzyme defects, the serum steroid substrates are greatly elevated.

Pathogenesis of Virilizing Adrenal Hyperplasia

The basic defects in congenital virilizing adrenal hyperplasia are one or more enzyme deficiencies in the biosynthesis of cortisol (Fig 5–16). With the reduced production of cortisol, normal feedback to the hypothalamus fails, with the result that increased amounts of ACTH are produced. This excess production of ACTH stimulates the deficient adrenal gland to produce relatively normal amounts of cortisol—but also stimulates production of abnormally large amounts of estrogen and androgens by the zona reticularis. In this overproduction, a biologic preponderance of androgens causes virilization. These abnormal sex steroids suppress the gonadotropins, so that untreated patients never reach puberty and do not menstruate.

Therefore the treatment of this disorder consists in part of the administration of sufficient exogenous cortisol to suppress ACTH production to normal levels. This in turn should reduce the overstimulation of the adrenal, so that the adrenal will cease to produce abnormally large amounts of estrogen and androgen. The gonadotropins generally return to normal levels, with consequent feminization of the patient and achievement of menstruation.

The pathogenesis of the salt-losing type of adrenal hyperplasia involves a deficiency in aldosterone production.

Diagnosis

Hermaphroditism due to congenital adrenal hyperplasia must be suspected in any infant born with ambiguous or abnormal external genitalia. It is exceedingly important that the diagnosis be made at a very early age if undesirable disturbances of metabolism are to be prevented.

All patients with ambiguous external genitalia should have an appraisal of their chromosomal characteristics. In all instances of female pseudohermaphroditism due to congenital hyperplasia, the chromosomal composition is that of a normal female. A pelvic ultrasound in the newborn to determine the presence of a uterus is very helpful and, if positive, strongly suggests a female infant.

The critical determinations are those of the urinary 17-ketosteroid and serum 17-hydroxyprogesterone levels. If these are elevated, the diagnosis must be either congenital adrenal hyperplasia or tumor. In the newborn, the latter is very rare, but in older children and adults with elevated 17-ketosteroids the possibility of tumor must be considered. One of the most satisfactory methods of making this different diagnosis is to attempt to suppress the excess androgens by the administration of dexamethasone. In an adult or an older child, a suitable test dose of dexamethasone is 1.25 mg/45 kg (100 lb) body weight, given orally for 7 consecutive days. In congenital adrenal hyperplasia, there should be suppression of the urinary 17-ketosteroids on the sev-

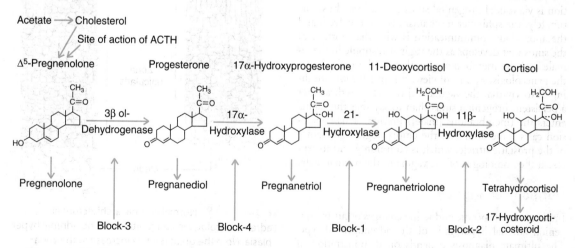

Figure 5–16. Enzymatic steps in cortisol synthesis. Localization of defects in congenital adrenal hyperplasia.

enth day of the test to less than 1 mg/24 h; in the presence of tumor, either there will be no effect or the 17-ketosteroid levels will rise.

Determination of urinary dehydroepiandrosterone (DHEA) or serum dehydroepiandrosterone sulfate (DHEA-S) levels can also be helpful in differentiating congenital adrenal hyperplasia from an adrenal tumor. Levels in patients with congenital adrenal hyperplasia may be up to double the normal amount, whereas an adrenal tumor is usually associated with levels that are much higher than double the normal level.

Determination of the serum, potassium, and CO_2 combining power is also important to ascertain whether electrolyte balance is seriously disturbed.

Treatment

The treatment of female hermaphroditism owing to congenital adrenal hyperplasia is partly medical and partly surgical. Originally, cortisone was administered; today, it is known that various cortisone derivatives are at least as effective. It is most satisfactory to begin treatment with relatively large doses of hydrocortisone divided in three doses orally for 7–10 days to obtain rapid suppression of adrenal activity. In young infants, the initial dose is about 25 mg/d; in older patients, 100 mg/d. After the output of 17-ketosteroids has decreased to a lower level, the dose should be reduced to the minimum amount required to maintain adequate suppression. This requires repeated measurements of plasma 17α-hydroxyprogesterone in order to individualize the dose.

It has been found that even with suppression of the urinary 17-ketosteroids to normal levels, the more sensitive serum 17-hydroxyprogesterone may still be elevated. It seems difficult and perhaps undesirable to suppress the serum 17-hydroxyprogesterone values to normal, because to do so may require doses of hydrocortisone which tend to cause cushingoid symptoms.

In the treatment of newborns with congenital adrenal hyperplasia who have a defect of electrolyte regulation, it is usually necessary to administer sodium chloride in amounts of 4–6 g/d, either orally or parenterally, in addition to cortisone. Furthermore, fludrocortisone acetate usually is required initially. The dose is entirely dependent on the levels of the serum electrolytes, which must be followed serially, but it is generally 0.05–0.1 mg/d.

In addition to the hormone treatment of this disorder, surgical correction of the external genitalia is usually necessary.

During acute illness or other stress, as well as during and after an operation, additional hydrocortisone is indicated to avoid the adrenal insufficiency of stress. Doubling the maintenance dose is usually adequate in such circumstances.

7. Female Hermaphroditism Without Progressive Masculinization

Females with no adrenal abnormality may have fetal masculinization of the external genitalia with the same anatomic findings as in patients with congenital virilizing adrenal hyperplasia. Unlike patients with adrenogenital syndrome, patients without adrenal abnormality do not have elevated levels of serum steroids or urinary 17-ketosteroids, nor do they show precocious sexual development or the metabolic difficulties associated with adrenal hyperplasia as they grow older. At onset of puberty, normal feminization with menstruation and ovulation may be expected.

The diagnosis of female hermaphroditism not owing to adrenal abnormality depends on the demonstration of a 46,XX karyotype and the finding of normal serum steroids or normal levels of 17-ketosteroids in the urine. If fusion of the scrotolabial folds is complete, it is necessary to determine the exact relationship of the urogenital sinus to the urethra and vagina and to demonstrate the presence of a uterus by rectal examination or ultrasonography or endoscopic observation of the cervix. When there is a high degree of masculinization, the differential diagnosis between this condition and true hermaphroditism may be very difficult; an exploratory laparotomy may be required in some cases.

Classification

Patients with this problem may be seen because of a variety of conditions.

1. Exogenous androgen:
   a. Maternal ingestion of androgen.
   b. Maternal androgenic tumor.
   c. Luteoma of pregnancy.
   d. Adrenal androgenic tumor.
2. Idiopathic: No identifiable cause.
3. Special or nonspecific: The same as (2) except that it is associated with various somatic anomalies and with mental retardation.
4. Familial: A very rare anomaly.

8. Male Hermaphroditism

Persons with abnormal or ectopic testes may have external genitalia so ambiguous at birth that the true sex is not identifiable (Fig 5–17). At puberty, these persons tend to become masculinized or feminized depending on factors to be discussed below. Thus, the adult habitus of these persons may be typically male, ie, without breasts, or typically female, with good breast development. In some instances, the external genitalia may be

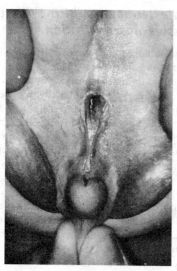

Figure 5–17. External genitalia in male hermaphroditism. (Reproduced, with permission, from Jones HW Jr, Scott WW: *Hermaphroditism, Genital Anomalies and Related Endocrine Disorders,* 2nd ed. Williams & Wilkins, 1971.)

indistinguishable from those of a normal female; in others, the clitoris may be enlarged; and in still other instances there may be fusion of the labia in the midline, resulting in what seems to be a hypospadiac male. A deep or shallow vagina may be present. A cervix, a uterus, and uterine tubes may be developed to varying degrees; however, müllerian structures are often absent. Mesonephric structures may be grossly or microscopically visible. Body hair may be either typically feminine in its distribution and quantity or masculine in distribution and of sufficient quantity as to require plucking or shaving if the person is reared as a female. In a special group, axillary and pubic hair is congenitally absent. Although there is a well-developed uterus in some instances, all patients so far reported have been amenorrheic—in spite of the interesting theoretic possibility of uterine bleeding from endometrium stimulated by estrogen of testicular origin. There is no evidence of adrenal malfunction. In the feminized group, and less frequently in the nonfeminized group, there is a strong familial history of the disorder. Male hermaphrodites reared as females may marry and be well adjusted to their sex role. Others, especially when there has been equivocation regarding sex of rearing in infancy, may be less than attractive as women because of indecisive therapy. Psychiatric studies indicate that the best emotional adjustment comes from directing endocrine, surgical, and psychiatric measures toward improving the person's basic characteristics. Fortunately, this is consonant with the surgical and endocrine possibilities for

those reared as females, because current operative techniques can produce more satisfactory feminine than masculine external genitalia. Furthermore, the testes of male hermaphrodites are nonfunctional as far as spermatogenesis is concerned. Only about one-third of male hermaphrodites are suitable for rearing as males.

Classification

Since about 1970, considerable progress has been made in identifying specific metabolic defects that are etiologically important for the various forms of male hermaphroditism. Details are beyond the scope of this text. Nevertheless, it is important to point out that all cases of male hermaphroditism have a defect in either the biologic action of testosterone or the müllerian inhibiting factor of the testis. Furthermore, it now seems apparent that nearly all—if not all—of these defects have a genetic or cytogenetic background. The causes and pathogenetic mechanisms of these defects may vary, but the final common pathway is one of the 2 problems just mentioned; in the adult a study of the serum gonadotropins and serum steroids, including the intermediate metabolites of testosterone, can often pinpoint a defect in the biosynthesis of testosterone. In other cases, the end organ action of testosterone may be defective. In children, the defect is sometimes more difficult to determine before gonadotropin levels rise at puberty, but one may suspect a problem by observing abnormally high levels of steroids that act as substrates in the metabolism of testosterone. A working classification of male hermaphroditism is as follows:

I. Male hermaphroditism due to a central nervous system defect.
   A. Abnormal pituitary gonadotropin secretion.
   B. No gonadotropin secretion.
II. Male hermaphroditism due to a primary gonadal defect.
   A. Identifiable defect in biosynthesis of testosterone.
      1. Pregnenolone synthesis defect (lipoid adrenal hyperplasia).
      2. 3β-Hydroxysteroid dehydrogenase deficiency.
      3. 17α-Hydroxylase deficiency.
      4. 17,20-Desmolase deficiency.
      5. 17β-Ketosteroid reductase deficiency.
   B. Unidentified defect in androgen effect.
   C. Defect in duct regression (Figs 5–18 and 5–19).
   D. Familial gonadal destruction.
   E. Leydig cell agenesis.
   F. Bilateral testicular dysgenesis.

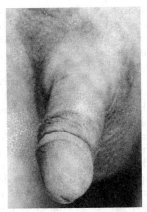

Figure 5–18. External genitalia in male hermaphroditism. (Reproduced, with permission, from Jones HW Jr, Scott WW: *Hermaphroditism, Genital Anomalies and Related Endocrine Disorders*, 2nd ed. Williams & Wilkins, 1971.)

III. Male hermaphroditism due to peripheral end organ defect.
   A. Androgen insensitivity syndrome (Fig 5–20).
      1. Androgen binding protein deficiency.
      2. Unknown deficiency.
   B. 5α-Reductase deficiency.

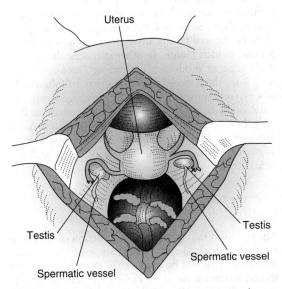

Figure 5–19. Internal genitalia of the patient whose external genitalia are shown in Fig 5–18. (Reproduced, with permission, from Jones HW Jr, Scott WW: *Hermaphroditism, Genital Anomalies and Related Endocrine Disorders*, 2nd ed. Williams & Wilkins, 1971.)

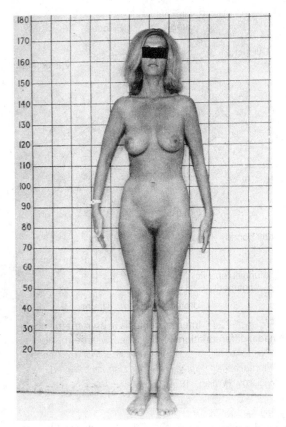

Figure 5–20. Androgen insensitivity syndrome.

   C. Unidentified abnormality of peripheral androgen effect.
IV. Male hermaphroditism due to Y chromosome defect.
   A. Y chromosome mosaicism (asymmetric gonadal differentiation) (Fig 5–21).
   B. Structurally abnormal Y chromosome.
   C. No identifiable Y chromosome.

9. Differential Diagnosis in Infants With Ambiguous Genitalia

Accurate differential diagnosis is possible in most patients with ambiguous genitalia (Table 5–8). This requires a complex history of the mother's medication, a complex sex chromosome study, rectal examination for the presence or absence of a uterus, measurement of serum steroid levels, pelvic ultrasonography, and information about other congenital anomalies. The following disorders, however, do not yield to differentiation

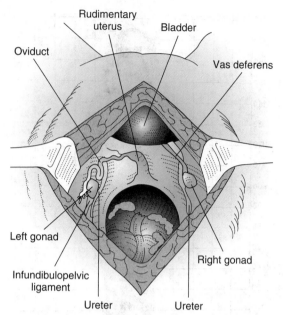

Figure 5–21. Internal genitalia in asymmetric gonadal differentiation. (Reproduced, with permission, from Jones HW Jr, Scott WW: *Hermaphroditism, Genital Anomalies and Related Endocrine Disorders,* 2nd ed. Williams & Wilkins, 1971.)

by the parameters given in Table 5–8: (1) idiopathic masculinization, (2) the "special" forms of female hermaphroditism, (3) 46,XX true hermaphroditism; and occasionally (4) the precise type of male hermaphroditism. For these differentiations, laparotomy may be necessary for diagnosis and also for therapy.

10. Treatment of Hermaphroditism

The sex of rearing is much more important than the obvious morphologic signs (external genitalia, hormone dominance, gonadal structure) in forming the gender role. Furthermore, serious psychologic consequences may result from changing the sex of rearing after infancy. Therefore, it is seldom proper to advise a change of sex after infancy to conform to the gonadal structure of the external genitalia. Instead, the physician should exert efforts to complete the adjustment of the person to the sex role already assigned. Fortunately, most aberrations of sexual development are discovered in the newborn period or in infancy, when reassignment of sex causes few problems.

Regardless of the time of treatment (and the earlier the better), the surgeon should reconstruct the external genitalia to correspond to the sex of rearing. Any con-

tradictory sex structures that may function to the patient's disadvantage in the future should be eradicated. Specifically, testes should always be removed from male hermaphrodites reared as females, regardless of hormone production. In cases of testicular feminization, orchiectomy is warranted because a variety of tumors may develop in these abnormal testes if they are retained, but the orchiectomy may be delayed until after puberty in this variety of hermaphroditism.

In virilized female hermaphroditism due to adrenal hyperplasia, the suppression of adrenal androgen production by the use of cortisone from an early age will result in completely female development. It is no longer necessary to explore the abdomen and the internal genitalia in this well-delineated syndrome. The surgical effort should be confined to reconstruction of the external genitalia along female lines.

Patients with streak gonads or Turner's syndrome, who are invariably reared as females, should be given exogenous estrogen when puberty is expected. Those hermaphrodites reared as females who will not become feminized also require estrogen to promote the development of the female habitus, including the breasts. In patients with a well-developed system, cyclic uterine withdrawal bleeding can be produced even though reproduction is impossible. Estrogen should be started at about age 12 and may be given as conjugated estrogens, 1.5 mg/d orally (or its equivalent). In some patients, after a period of time this dosage may have to be increased for additional breast development. In patients without ovaries who have uteri and in male hermaphrodites in the same condition, cyclic uterine bleeding can often be induced by the administration of estrogen for 3 weeks of each month. In other instances, this may be inadequate to produce a convincing "menstrual" period; if so, the 3 weeks of estrogen may be followed by 3–4 days of progestin (eg, medroxyprogesterone acetate) orally or a single injection of progesterone. Prolonged estrogen therapy increases the risk of subsequent development of adenocarcinoma of the corpus, so periodic endometrial sampling is mandatory in such patients.

Reconstruction of Female External Genitalia

The details of the operative reconstruction of abnormal external genitalia are beyond the scope of this chapter. However, it should be emphasized that the procedure should be carried out at the earliest age possible so as to enhance the desired psychologic, social, and sexual orientation of the patient and also to obtain an easier adjustment by the parents. Sometimes the reconstruction can be done during the neonatal period. In any case, operation should not be delayed beyond the first several

Table 5–8. Differential diagnosis of ambiguous external genitalia.[1]

Diagnosis	Karyotype	History	Uterus	Anomalies	17-KS	Sex Chromosomes
Adrenal hyperplasia	46,XX	+	+	–	E	XX
Maternal androgen	46,XX	+	+	–	N	XX
Idiopathic masculinization	46,XX	–	+	–	N	XX
Special or nonspecific	46,XX	–	+	–	N	XX
Female familial	46,XX	+	+	+	N	XX
True hermaphroditism	46,XX; 46,XY; etc	–	+ or –	–	N	XX or other
Male hermaphroditism	46,XY	+	+ or –	–	N	XY or other
Streak gonad	45,X; 46,XX; 46,XY; etc	-	+	+ or –	N	XO or other

[1] + = positive, – = negative, N = normal, E = elevated.
17KS = 17-Ketosteroid level.

months of life. From a technical point of view, early operation is possible in all but the most exceptional circumstances.

REFERENCES

Antonarakis SE et al: Prenatal diagnosis of haemophilia A by factor VIII gene analysis. Lancet 1985;1:1407.

Botto L et al: Neural tube defects. N Engl J Med 1999;341:1509.

Conde-Agudelo A, Kafury-Goeta A: Triple-marker test as a screen for Down's syndrome: A meta-analysis. Obstet Gynecol Surv 1998;53:369.

Eiben B et al: Rapid prenatal diagnosis of aneuploidies in uncultured amniocytes by fluorescence in situ hybridization. Fetal Diagn Ther 1999;14:193.

Feunteun J et al: A breast-ovarian cancer susceptibility gene maps to chromosome 17q21. Am J Hum Genet 1993;52:736.

Golbus MS et al: Prenatal genetic diagnosis in 3000 amniocenteses. N Engl J Med 1979;300:157.

Haddon JE et al: Reducing the need for amniocentesis in women 35 years of age or older with serum markers for screening. New England Journal of Medicine 1994:330;1114–1118.

Hook EB: Rates of chromosome abnormalities at different maternal ages. Obstet Gynecol 1981;58:282.

Jones HW Jr, Ferguson-Smith MA, Heller RH: Pathologic and cytogenetic findings in true hermaphroditism: Report of six cases and review of 23 cases from the literature. Obstet Gynecol 1965;25:435.

Kajii T et al: Anatomic and chromosomal anomalies in 639 spontaneous abortuses. Hum Genet 1980;55:87.

Klinefelter HF Jr, Reifenstein EC Jr, Albright F: Syndrome characterized by gynecomastia, aspermatogenesis without aleydigism and increased excretion of follicle-stimulating hormone. J Clin Endocrinol 1942;2:615.

Lidsky AS, Guttler F, Woo SLC: Prenatal diagnosis of classic phenylketonuria by DNA analysis. Lancet 1985;1:549.

Lippman-Hand A, Bekemans M: Balanced translocations among couples with two or more spontaneous abortions: Are males and females equally likely to be carriers? Hum Genet 1983;68:252.

McKusick VA: *Mendelian Inheritance in Man,* 10th ed. Johns Hopkins Univ Press, 1992.

Menutti MT et al: An evaluation of cytogenetic analysis as a primary tool in the assessment of recurrent pregnancy wastage. Obstet Gynecol 1978;52:308.

Page DC et al: The sex determining region of the human Y chromosome encodes a finger protein. Cell 1987;51:1091.

Park IJ, Aimakhu VE, Jones HW Jr: An etiologic and pathogenetic classification of male hermaphroditism. Am J Obstet Gynecol 1975;123:505.

Raskin S et al: Cystic fibrosis genotyping by direct PCR analysis of Guthrie blood spots. PCR Methods Appl 1992;2:154.

Rose NC et al: Maternal serum alpha-feto protein screening for chromosomal abnormalities: a prospective study in women aged 35 and older. Am J Obstet Gynecol 1999;170:1073.

Sant-Cassia LJ, Cooke P: Chromosomal analysis of couples with repeated spontaneous abortions. Br J Obstet Gynaecol 1981;88:52.

Simpson E et al: Separation of the genetic loci for the H-Y antigen and for testis determination on human Y chromosome. Nature 1987;326:876.

Stoll CG et al: Interchromosomal effect in balanced translocation. Birth Defects 1978;14:393.

Tiepalo L, Zuffardi O: Location of factors controlling spermatogenesis in the nonfluorescent portion of the human Y chromosome long arm. Hum Genet 1976;34:119.

Turner G et al: Heterozygous expression of X-linked mental retardation and X-chromosome marker fra(X)(q27). N Engl J Med 1980;303:662.

Turner HH: A syndrome of infantilism, congenital webbed neck, and cubitus valgus. Endocrinology 1938;23:566.

Wald NJ et al: Maternal serum screening for Down's syndrome in early pregnancy. Br Med J 1988;297:883.

Wald NJ et al: Integrated screening for Down's syndrome based on tests performed during the first and second trimesters. N Engl J Med 1999;341:461.

Physiology of Reproduction in Women*

William F. Ganong, MD

This chapter is concerned with the function of the female reproductive system from birth through puberty and adulthood to the menopause.

PUBERTY

After birth, the gonads are quiescent until they are activated by gonadotropins from the pituitary to bring about the final maturation of the reproductive system. This period of final maturation is known as **adolescence.** It is often called **puberty,** although strictly defined, puberty is the period when the endocrine and gametogenic functions of the gonads first develop to the point where reproduction is possible. In girls, the first event is **thelarche,** the development of breasts, followed by **pubarche,** the development of axillary and pubic hair, and then **menarche,** the first menstrual period. The initial periods are generally anovulatory, and regular ovulation begins about 1 year later. In contrast to the situation in adulthood, removal of the gonads during the period from soon after birth to puberty causes little or no increase in gonadotropin secretion, so gonadotropin secretion is not being held in check by the gonadal hormones. In children between the ages of 7 and 10, a slow increase in estrogen and androgen secretion precedes the more rapid rise in the early teens (Fig 6–1).

The age at the time of puberty is variable; in Europe and the U.S., it has been declining at the rate of 1–3 months per decade for more than 175 years. In the U.S. in recent years, puberty has generally been occurring between the ages of 8 and 13 in girls and 9 and 14 in boys.

Another event that occurs in humans at the time of puberty is an increase in the secretion of adrenal androgens (Fig 6–2). The onset of this increase is called **adrenarche.** It occurs at age 8–10 years in girls and 10–12 years in boys. Dehydroepiandrosterone (DHEA) values peak at about 25 years of age, and are slightly higher in boys. They then decline slowly to low values after the age of 60.

The increase in adrenal androgen secretion at adrenarche occurs without any changes in the secretion of cortisol or adrenocorticotropic hormone (ACTH). Adrenarche may be due to a change in the enzyme systems in the adrenal, so that more pregnenolone is diverted to the androgen pathway, but there is some evidence that it is due to increased secretion of an as yet unisolated **adrenal androgen-stimulating hormone (AASH)** from the pituitary gland.

The adrenal androgens contribute significantly to the growth of axillary and pubic hair. The breasts develop under the influence of the ovarian hormones estradiol and progesterone, with estradiol primarily responsible for the growth of ducts and progesterone primarily responsible for the growth of lobules and alveoli. The sequence of the changes that occur at puberty in girls are summarized in Fig 6–3.

Control of the Onset of Puberty

A neural mechanism is responsible for the onset of puberty. In children, the gonads can be stimulated by gonadotropins, the pituitary contains gonadotropins, and the hypothalamus contains gonadotropin-releasing hormone(GnRH). However, the gonadotropins are not secreted. In immature monkeys, normal menstrual cycles can be brought on by pulsatile injection of GnRH, and the cycles persist as long as the pulsatile injection is continued. In addition, GnRH is secreted in a pulsatile fashion in adults. Thus, it seems clear that during the period from birth to puberty, a neural mechanism is operating to prevent the normal pulsatile release of GnRH. The nature of the mechanism inhibiting the GnRH pulse generator is unknown.

Relation to Leptin

It has been argued for some time that normally there is a critical body weight that must be reached for puberty to occur. Thus, for example, young women who

---

* This chapter is based in large part on Chapter 23 in: Ganong WF: *Review of Medical Physiology*, 20th ed. McGraw-Hill, 2001.

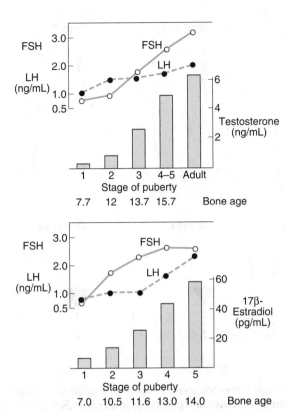

Figure 6–1. Changes in plasma hormone concentrations during puberty in boys (**top**) and girls (**bottom**). Stage 1 of puberty is preadolescence in both sexes. In boys, stage 2 is characterized by beginning enlargement of the testes, stage 3 by penile enlargement, stage 4 by growth of the glans penis, and stage 5 by adult genitalia. The stages of puberty in girls are summarized in Fig 6–3. (Reproduced, with permission, from Grumbach MM: Onset of puberty. In: Berenberg SR [editor]: *Puberty: Biologic and Psychosocial Components.* HE Stenfoert Kroese BV, 1975.)

engage in strenuous athletics lose weight and stop menstruating. So do girls with anorexia nervosa. If these girls start to eat and gain weight, they menstruate again, ie, they "go back through puberty." It now appears that leptin, the satiety-producing hormone secreted by fat cells may be the link between body weight and puberty. Obese ob/ob mice that cannot make leptin are infertile, and their fertility is restored by injections of leptin. Leptin treatment also induces precocious puberty in immature female mice. However, how leptin fits into the overall control of puberty remains to be determined.

Sexual Precocity

The major causes of precocious sexual development in humans are listed in Table 6–1. Early development of secondary sexual characteristics without gametogenesis is caused by abnormal exposure of immature males to androgen or females to estrogen. This syndrome should be called **precocious pseudopuberty** to distinguish it from true precocious puberty due to an early but otherwise normal pubertal pattern of gonadotropin secretion from the pituitary (Fig 6–4).

In one large series of cases, precocious puberty was the most frequent endocrine symptom of hypothalamic disease. It is interesting that in experimental animals and humans, lesions of the ventral hypothalamus near the infundibulum cause precocious puberty. The effect of the lesions may be due to interruption of neural pathways that produce inhibition of the GnRH pulse generator, or to chronic stimulation of GnRH secretion originating in irritative foci around the lesion. Pineal tumors are sometimes associated with precocious puberty, but there is evidence that these tumors are associated with precocious puberty only when there is secondary damage to the hypothalamus. Precocity due to this and other forms of hypothalamic damage probably occurs with equal frequency in both sexes, although the constitutional form of precocious puberty is more common in girls. In addition, it has now been proved that precocious gametogenesis and steroidogenesis can occur

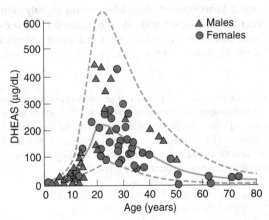

Figure 6–2. Change in serum dehydroepiandrosterone sulfate (DHEAS) with age. The middle line is the mean, and the dashed lines identify ±1.96 standard deviations. (Reproduced, with permission, from Smith MR et al: A radioimmunoassay for the estimation of serum dehydroepiandrosterone sulfate in normal and pathological sera. Clin Chim Acta 1975;65:5.)

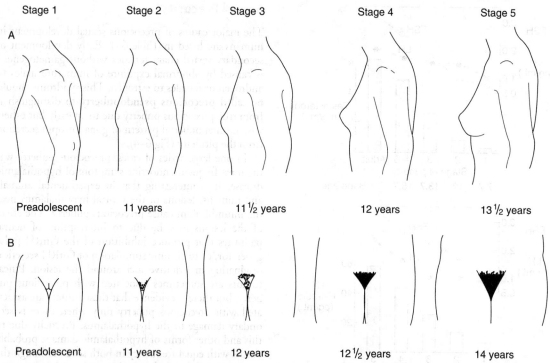

Figure 6–3. Sequence of events at adolescence in girls. **A:** Stage 1: Preadolescent; elevation of papillae only. Stage 2: Breast bud stage (may occur between ages 8 and 13); elevation of breasts and papillae as small mounds, with enlargement of areolar diameter. Stage 3: enlargement and elevation of breasts and areolas with no separation of contours. Stage 4: Areolas and papillae project from breast to form a secondary mound. Stage 5: Mature; projection of papillae only, with recession of areolas into general contour of breast. **B:** Stage 1: Preadolescent; no pubic hair. Stage 2: Sparse growth along labia of long, slightly pigmented, downy hair that is straight or slightly curled (may occur between ages 8 and 14). Stage 3: Darker, coarser, more curled hair growing sparsely over pubic area. Stage 4: Resembles adult in type but covers smaller area. Stage 5: Adult in quantity and type. (Redrawn, with permission, from Tanner JM: *Growth at Adolescence,* 2nd ed. Blackwell, 1962.)

without the pubertal pattern of gonadotropin secretion (gonadotropin-independent precocity). At least in some cases of this condition, the sensitivity of luteinizing hormone (LH) receptors to gonadotropins is increased because of an activating mutation in the G protein that couples receptors to adenylyl cyclase.

Delayed or Absent Puberty

The normal variation in the age at which adolescent changes occur is so wide that puberty cannot be considered to be pathologically delayed until menarche has failed to occur by the age of 17. Failure of maturation due to panhypopituitarism is associated with dwarfing and evidence of other endocrine abnormalities. Patients with the XO chromosomal pattern and gonadal dysgenesis are also dwarfed. In some individuals, pu-

berty is delayed and menarche does not occur (primary amenorrhea), even though the gonads are present and other endocrine functions are normal.

REPRODUCTIVE FUNCTION AFTER SEXUAL MATURITY

Menstrual Cycle

The anatomy of the reproductive system of adult women is described in Chapter 2. Unlike the reproductive system of men, this system shows regular cyclic changes that teleologically may be regarded as periodic preparation for fertilization and pregnancy. In primates, the cycle is a **menstrual cycle,** and its most conspicuous feature is the periodic vaginal bleeding that occurs with the shedding of the uterine mucosa (**men-**

Table 6–1. Classification of the causes of precocious sexual development in humans.[1]

True precocious puberty
Constitutional
Cerebral: Disorders involving posterior hypothalamus
    Tumors
    Infections
    Developmental abnormalities
Gonadotropin-independent precocity
Precocious pseudopuberty
(no spermatogenesis or ovarian development)
    Adrenal
      Congenital virilizing adrenal hyperplasia (without treatment in males; following cortisone treatment in females)
      Androgen-secreting tumors (in males)
      Estrogen-secreting tumors (in females)
    Gonadal
      Interstitial cell tumors of testis
      Granulosa cell tumors of ovary
    Miscellaneous

---

[1](Reproduced, with permission, from Ganong WF: *Review of Medical Physiology*, 20th ed. McGraw-Hill, 2001.)

struation). The length of the cycle is notoriously variable, but an average figure is 28 days from the start of one menstrual period to the start of the next. By common usage, the days of the cycle are identified by number, starting with the first day of menstruation.

Ovarian Cycle

From the time of birth, there are many **primordial follicles** under the ovarian capsule. Each contains an immature ovum (Fig 6–5). At the start of each cycle, several of these follicles enlarge and a cavity forms around the ovum (antrum formation). This cavity is filled with follicular fluid. In humans, one of the follicles in one ovary starts to grow rapidly on about the sixth day and becomes the **dominant follicle.** The others regress, forming **atretic follicles.** It is not known how one follicle is singled out for development during this **follicular phase** of the menstrual cycle, but it seems to be related to the ability of the follicle to secrete the estrogen inside it that is needed for final maturation. When women are given highly purified human pituitary gonadotropin preparations by injection, many follicles develop simultaneously.

The structure of a mature ovarian follicle (**graafian follicle**) is shown in Fig 6–5. The cells of the **theca interna** of the follicle are the primary source of circulating estrogens. The follicular fluid has a high estrogen content, and much of this estrogen comes from the **granulosa cells.**

At about the 14th day of the cycle, the distended follicle ruptures, and the ovum is extruded into the abdominal cavity. This is the process of **ovulation.** The ovum is picked up by the fimbriated ends of the uterine tubes (oviducts) and transported to the uterus. Unless fertilization occurs, the ovum degenerates or is passed on through the uterus and out the vagina.

The follicle that ruptures at the time of ovulation promptly fills with blood, forming what is sometimes called a **corpus hemorrhagicum.** Minor bleeding from the follicle into the abdominal cavity may cause peritoneal irritation and fleeting lower abdominal pain ("mittelschmerz"). The granulosa and theca cells of the follicle lining promptly begin to proliferate, and the clotted blood is rapidly replaced with yellowish, lipid-rich **luteal cells,** forming the **corpus luteum.** This is the **luteal phase** of the menstrual cycle, during which the

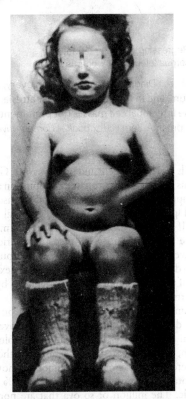

Figure 6–4. Constitutional precocious puberty in a 3½-year-old girl. The patient developed pubic hair and started to menstruate at the age of 17 months. (Reproduced, with permission, from Jolly H: *Sexual Precocity*. Thomas, 1955.)

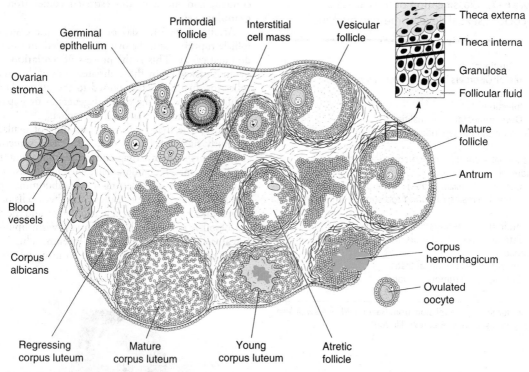

Theca externa
Theca interna
Granulosa
Follicular fluid

Germinal epithelium
Primordial follicle
Interstitial cell mass
Vesicular follicle

Ovarian stroma

Mature follicle

Antrum

Blood vessels

Corpus albicans

Corpus hemorrhagicum

Ovulated oocyte

Regressing corpus luteum
Mature corpus luteum
Young corpus luteum
Atretic follicle

Figure 6–5. Diagram of a mammalian ovary, showing the sequential development of a follicle, formation of a corpus luteum, and in the center, follicular atresia. A section of the wall of a mature follicle is enlarged at the upper right. The interstitial cell mass is not prominent in primates. (After Patten B, Eakin RM. Reproduced, with permission, from Gorbman A, Bern H: *Textbook of Comparative Endocrinology.* Wiley, 1962.)

luteal cells secrete estrogens and progesterone. Growth of the corpus luteum depends on its developing an adequate blood supply, and there is evidence that vascular endothelial growth factor (VEGF) is essential for this process. If pregnancy occurs, the corpus luteum persists, and there are usually no more menstrual periods until after delivery. If there is no pregnancy, the corpus luteum begins to degenerate about 4 days before the next menses (day 24 of the cycle) and is eventually replaced by fibrous tissue, forming a **corpus albicans.**

In humans, no new ova are formed after birth. During fetal development, the ovaries contain over 7 million germ cells; however, many undergo involution before birth, and others are lost after birth. At the time of birth, there are approximately 2 million primordial follicles containing ova, but approximately 50% of these are atretic. The million or so ova that are normal undergo the first part of the first meiotic division at about this time and enter a stage of arrest in prophase in which those that survive persist until adulthood. Atresia continues during development, and the number of ova in both the ovaries at the time of puberty is less than

300,000 (Fig 6–6). Normally, only one of these ova per cycle (or about 500 in the course of a normal reproductive life) is stimulated to mature; the remainder degenerate. Just before ovulation, the first meiotic division is completed. One of the daughter cells, the **secondary oocyte,** receives most of the cytoplasm, while the other, the **first polar body,** fragments and disappears. The secondary oocyte immediately begins the second meiotic division, but this division stops at metaphase and is completed only when a sperm penetrates the oocyte. At that time, the **second polar body** is cast off and the fertilized ovum proceeds to form a new individual. The arrest in metaphase is due, at least in some species, to formation in the ovum of the protein **pp39^{mos},** which is encoded by the *c-mos* proto-oncogene. When fertilization occurs, the pp39^{mos} is destroyed within 30 minutes by **calpain,** a calcium-dependent cysteine protease.

Uterine Cycle

The events that occur in the uterus during the menstrual cycle terminate in the menstrual flow. By the end

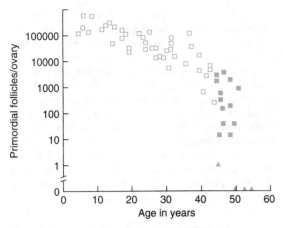

Figure 6–6. Number of primordial follicles per ovary in women at various ages. □, premenopausal women (regular menses); ■, perimenopausal women (irregular menses for at least 1 year); ▲, postmenopausal women (no menses for at least 1 year). Note that the vertical scale is a log scale and that the values are from one rather than two ovaries. (Redrawn by Wise PM and reproduced, with permission, from Richardson SJ, Senikas V, Nelson JF: Follicular depletion during the menopausal transition: evidence for accelerated loss and ultimate exhaustion. J Clin Endocrinol Metab 1987;65:1231.)

6–7), but they do not become convoluted or secrete to any degree. These endometrial changes are called proliferative, and this part of the menstrual cycle is sometimes called the **proliferative phase.** It is also called the preovulatory or follicular phase of the cycle. After ovulation, the endometrium becomes more highly vascularized and slightly edematous under the influence of estrogen and progesterone from the corpus luteum. The glands become coiled and tortuous (Fig 6–7), and they begin to secrete a clear fluid. Consequently, this phase of the cycle is called the **secretory** or **luteal phase.** Late in the luteal phase, the endometrium, like the anterior pituitary, produces prolactin, but the function of this endometrial prolactin is unknown.

The endometrium is supplied by 2 types of arteries. The superficial two-thirds of the endometrium that is shed during menstruation, the **stratum functionale,** is supplied by long, coiled **spiral arteries** (Fig 6–8), whereas the deep layer, the **stratum basale,** that is not shed is supplied by short, straight **basilar arteries.**

When the corpus luteum regresses, hormonal support for the endometrium is withdrawn. The endometrium becomes thinner, which adds to the coiling of the spiral arteries. Foci of necrosis appear in the endometrium, and these coalesce. There is, in addition, necrosis of the walls of the spiral arteries, leading to spotty hemorrhages that become confluent and produce the menstrual flow.

Vasospasm occurs and is probably produced by locally released prostaglandins. There are large quantities of prostaglandins in the secretory endometrium and in menstrual blood, and infusions of $PGF_{2\alpha}$ produce endometrial necrosis and bleeding. One theory of the onset of menstruation holds that in necrotic endometrial cells, lysosomal membranes break down with the release of enzymes that foster the formation of prostaglandins from cellular phospholipids.

of each menstrual period, all but the deep layer of the endometrium has sloughed. Under the influence of estrogens from the developing follicles, the endometrium regenerates from the deep layer and increases rapidly in thickness during the period from the 5th to 16th days of the menstrual cycle. As the thickness increases, the uterine glands are drawn out so that they lengthen (Fig

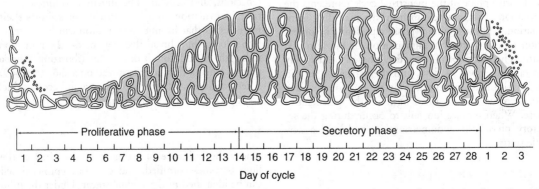

Figure 6–7. Changes in the endometrium during the menstrual cycle. (Reproduced, with permission, from Ganong WF: *Review of Medical Physiology*, 20th ed. McGraw-Hill, 2001.)

Uterine lumen

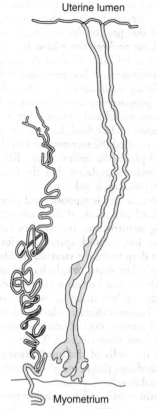

Myometrium

Figure 6–8. Spiral artery of endometrium. Drawing of a spiral artery (**left**) and 2 uterine glands (**right**) from the endometrium of a rhesus monkey; early secretory phase. (Reproduced, with permission, from Daron GH: The arterial pattern of the tunica mucosa of the uterus in the macacus rhesus. Am J Anat 1936;58:349.)

From the point of view of endometrial function, the proliferative phase of the menstrual cycle represents the restoration of the epithelium from the preceding menstruation, and the secretory phase represents the preparation of the uterus for implantation of the fertilized ovum. The length of the secretory phase is remarkably constant, at about 14 days, and the variations seen in the length of the menstrual cycle are due for the most part to variations in the length of the proliferative phase. When fertilization fails to occur during the secretory phase, the endometrium is shed, and a new cycle starts.

Normal Menstruation

Menstrual blood is predominantly arterial, with only 25% of the blood being of venous origin. It contains tis-

sue debris, prostaglandins, and relatively large amounts of fibrinolysin from the endometrial tissue. The fibrinolysin lyses clots, and so menstrual blood does not normally contain clots unless the flow is excessive.

The usual duration of the menstrual cycle is 3–5 days, but flows as short as 1 day and as long as 8 days can occur in normal women. The average amount of blood lost is 30 mL, but may range normally from slight spotting to 80 mL. Loss of more than 80 mL is abnormal. Obviously, the amount of flow can be affected by various factors, including thickness of the endometrium and medications and diseases that affect the clotting mechanism. After menstruation, the endometrium regenerates from the stratum basale.

Anovulatory Cycles

In some instances, ovulation fails to occur during the menstrual cycle. Such anovulatory cycles are common for the first 12–18 months after menarche and again before the onset of menopause. When ovulation does not occur, no corpus luteum is formed, and the effects of progesterone on the endometrium are absent. Estrogens continue to cause growth, however, and the proliferative endometrium becomes thick enough to break down and begin to slough. The time it takes for bleeding to occur is variable, but it usually occurs less than 28 days from the last menstrual period. The flow is also variable and ranges from scanty to relatively profuse.

Cyclic Changes in the Uterine Cervix

Although it is contiguous with the body of the uterus, the cervix of the uterus is different in a number of ways. The mucosa of the uterine cervix does not undergo cyclic desquamation, but there are regular changes in the cervical mucus. Estrogen makes the mucus thinner and more alkaline, changes that promote the survival and transport of sperms. Progesterone makes it thick, tenacious, and cellular. The mucus is thinnest at the time of ovulation, and its elasticity, or **spinnbarkeit,** increases so that by midcycle, a drop can be stretched into a long, thin thread that may be 8–12 cm or more in length. In addition, it dries in an arborizing, fernlike pattern when a thin layer is spread on a slide (Fig 6–9). After ovulation and during pregnancy, it becomes thick and fails to form the fern pattern.

Vaginal Cycle

Under the influence of estrogens, the vaginal epithelium becomes cornified, and cornified epithelial cells can be identified in the vaginal smear. Under the influence of progesterone, a thick mucus is secreted, and the epithelium proliferates and becomes infiltrated with

Normal cycle, 14th day

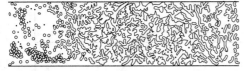

Midluteal phase, normal cycle

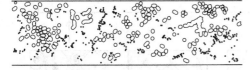

Anovulatory cycle with estrogen present

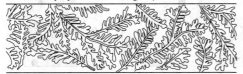

Figure 6–9. Patterns formed when cervical mucus is smeared on a slide, permitted to dry, and examined under the microscope. Progesterone makes the mucus thick and cellular. In the smear from a patient who failed to ovulate (**bottom**), there is no progesterone to inhibit the estrogen-induced fern pattern. (Reproduced, with permission, from Ganong WF: *Review of Medical Physiology*, 20th ed. McGraw-Hill, 2001.)

leukocytes. The cyclic changes in the vaginal smear in rats are particularly well known. The changes in humans and other species are similar but unfortunately not so clear-cut. However, the increase in cornified epithelial cells is apparent when a vaginal smear from an adult woman in the follicular phase of the menstrual cycle is compared, for example, with a smear taken before puberty (Fig 6–10).

Cyclic Changes in the Breasts

Although lactation normally does not occur until the end of pregnancy, there are cyclic changes in the breasts during the menstrual cycle. Estrogens cause proliferation of mammary ducts, whereas progesterone causes growth of lobules and alveoli (see below). The breast swelling, tenderness, and pain experienced by many women during the 10 days preceding menstruation are probably due to distention of the ducts, hyperemia, and edema of the interstitial tissue of the breasts. All of these changes regress, along with the symptoms, during menstruation.

Cyclic Changes in Other Body Functions

In addition to cyclic breast swelling and tenderness, there is usually a small increase in body temperature during the luteal phase of the menstrual cycle. This change in body temperature, which is discussed below, is probably due to the thermogenic effect of progesterone.

Changes During Sexual Intercourse

During sexual excitation, the vaginal walls become moist as a result of transudation of fluid through the mucus membrane. A lubricating mucus is secreted by the vestibular glands. The upper part of the vagina is sensitive to stretch, while tactile stimulation from the labia minora and clitoris adds to the sexual excitement. The stimuli are reinforced by tactile stimuli from the breasts and, as in men, by visual, auditory, and olfactory stimuli; eventually, the crescendo or climax known as orgasm may be reached. During orgasm, there are autonomically mediated rhythmic contractions of the vaginal wall. Impulses also travel via the pudendal nerves and produce rhythmic contractions of the bulbocavernosus and ischiocavernosus muscles. The vaginal contractions may aid in the transport of spermatozoa but are not essential for it, since fertilization of the ovum is not dependent on orgasm.

Indicators of Ovulation

Knowing when during the menstrual cycle ovulation occurs is important in increasing fertility or conversely, in contraception. A convenient but retrospective indicator of the time of ovulation is a rise in the basal body temperature (Fig 6–11). Accurate temperatures can be obtained by use of a thermometer that is able to measure temperature precisely between 96 and 100 °F. The woman should take her temperature orally, vaginally, or rectally in the morning before getting out of bed. The cause of the temperature change at the time of ovulation is unknown, but is probably due to the increase in progesterone secretion, since progesterone is thermogenic. A rise in urinary LH occurs during the rise in circulating LH that causes ovulation, and this increase can be measured as another indicator of ovulation. Kits employing dipsticks or simple color tests for detection of urinary LH are available for home use.

Ovulation normally occurs about 9 hours after the peak of the LH surge at midcycle (Fig 6–11). The ovum lives approximately 72 hours after it is extruded from the follicle, but is probably fertilizable for less than half this time. In a study of the relationship of isolated intercourse to pregnancy, 36% of women had a detected pregnancy following intercourse on the day of

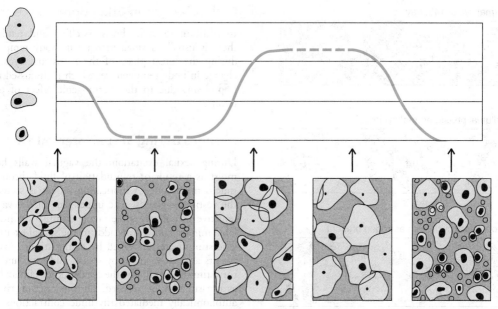

Figure 6–10. Vaginal cytologic picture in various stages of life. **Top:** Graphic representation of the maturation of vaginal epithelium. **Bottom:** Left to right: Epithelial maturation at birth; atrophic cell picture in childhood; beginning of estrogenic influence in puberty; complete maturation in the reproductive period; regression in old age. (Reproduced, with permission, from Beller FK et al: *Gynecology: A Textbook for Students.* Springer-Verlag, 1974.)

ovulation, but with intercourse on days after ovulation, the percentage was zero. Isolated intercourse on the first and second day before ovulation led to pregnancy in about 36% of the women. A few pregnancies resulted from isolated intercourse on day 3, 4, or 5 before ovulation, although the percentage was much lower, eg, 8% on day 5 before ovulation. Thus, some sperms can survive in the female genital tract and produce fertilization for up to 120 hours before ovulation, but the most fertile period is clearly the 48 hours before ovulation. However, for those interested in the "rhythm method" of contraception, it should be noted that there are rare but documented cases in the literature of pregnancy resulting from isolated coitus on every day of the cycle.

OVARIAN HORMONES

Chemistry, Biosynthesis, & Metabolism of Estrogens

The naturally occurring estrogens are **17β-estradiol, estrone,** and **estriol** (Fig 6–12). They are C_{18} steroids, ie, they do not have an angular methyl group attached to the 10 position or a Δ^4-3-keto configuration in the A ring. They are secreted primarily by the granulosa and the thecal cells of the ovarian follicles, the corpus luteum, and the placenta. The biosynthetic pathway in-

volves their formation from androgens. They are also formed by aromatization of androstenedione in the circulation. Aromatase (CYP 19) is the enzyme that catalyzes the conversion of Δ^4-androstenedione to estrone (Fig 6–12). It also catalyzes the conversion of testosterone to estradiol.

Theca interna cells have many LH receptors, and LH acts on them via cyclic AMP (cyclic adenosine 3′, 5′-monophosphate) to increase conversion of cholesterol to androstenedione. Some of the androstenedione is converted to estradiol, which enters the circulation. The theca interna cells also supply androstenedione to the granulosa cells. The granulosa cells only make estradiol when provided with androgens (Fig 6–13), and they secrete the estradiol that they produce into the follicular fluid. They have many follicle-stimulating hormone (FSH) receptors, and FSH facilitates the secretion of estradiol by acting via cyclic AMP to increase the aromatase activity in these cells. Mature granulosa cells also acquire LH receptors, and LH stimulates estradiol production.

The stromal tissue of the ovary also has the potential to produce androgens and estrogens. However, it probably does so in insignificant amounts in normal premenopausal women. 17β-Estradiol, the major secreted estrogen, is in equilibrium in the circulation with estrone. Estrone is further metabolized to **estriol** (Fig

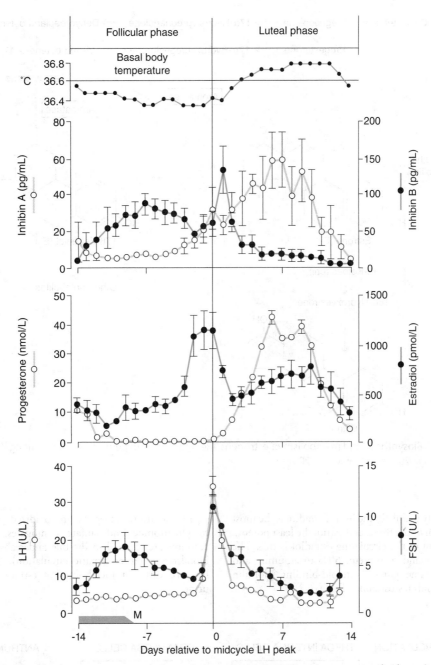

Figure 6–11. Basal body temperature and plasma hormone concentrations (mean ± standard error) during the normal human menstrual cycle. Values are aligned with respect to the day of the midcycle LH peak. (Hormone values from Chabbert Buffet N et al: Regulation of the human menstrual cycle. Front Neuroendocrinol 1998;19:151.)

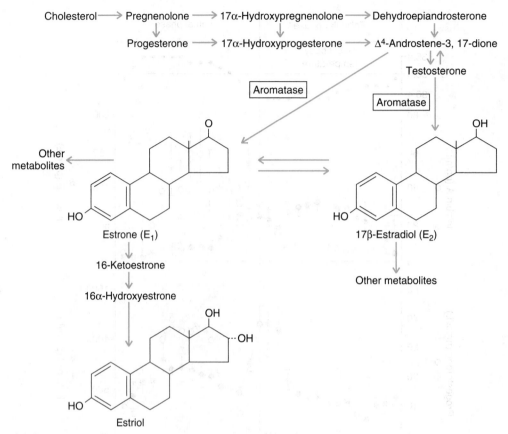

Cholesterol ⟶ Pregnenolone ⟶ 17α-Hydroxypregnenolone ⟶ Dehydroepiandrosterone

Progesterone ⟶ 17α-Hydroxyprogesterone ⟶ Δ⁴-Androstene-3, 17-dione

Testosterone

Aromatase

Aromatase

Other metabolites

Estrone (E₁)

16-Ketoestrone

16α-Hydroxyestrone

17β-Estradiol (E₂)

Other metabolites

Estriol

Figure 6–12. **Biosynthesis and metabolism of estrogens.** (Reproduced, with permission, from Ganong WF: *Review of Medical Physiology,* 20th ed. McGraw-Hill, 2001.)

6–12), probably mainly in the liver. Estradiol is the most potent estrogen of the three, and estriol the least potent.

Two percent of the circulating estradiol is free. The remainder is bound to protein: 60% to albumin, and 38% to the same gonadal steroid-binding globulin (GBG) that binds testosterone (Table 6–2).

In the liver, estrogens are oxidized or converted to glucuronide and sulfate conjugates. Appreciable amounts are secreted in the bile and reabsorbed in the bloodstream (enterohepatic circulation). There are at least 10 different metabolites of estradiol in human urine.

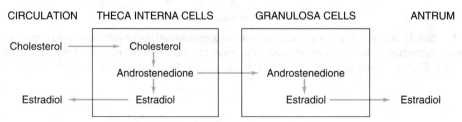

CIRCULATION	THECA INTERNA CELLS	GRANULOSA CELLS	ANTRUM
Cholesterol	Cholesterol		
	Androstenedione ⟶	Androstenedione	
Estradiol ⟵	Estradiol	Estradiol ⟶	Estradiol

Figure 6–13. Interactions between theca and granulosa cells in estradiol synthesis and secretion. (Reproduced, with permission, from Ganong WF: *Review of Medical Physiology,* 20th ed. McGraw-Hill, 2001.)

Table 6–2. Distribution of gonadal steroids and cortisol in plasma.[1]

Steroid	% Free	% Bound to CBG	GBG	Albumin
Testosterone	2	0	65	33
Androstenedione	7	0	8	85
Estradiol	2	0	38	60
Progesterone	2	18	0	80
Cortisol	4	90	0	6

[1]CBG, corticosteroid-binding globulin; GBG, gonadal steroid-binding globulin. (Courtesy of S Munroe.)

Secretion of Estrogens

The concentration of estradiol in plasma during the menstrual cycle is shown in Fig 6–11. Almost all of the estrogen comes from the ovary. There are 2 peaks of secretion: one just before ovulation and one during the midluteal phase. The estradiol secretion rate is 36 μg/d (133 nmol/d) in the early follicular phase, 380 μg/d just before ovulation, and 250 μg/d during the midluteal phase (Table 6–3). After menopause, estrogen secretion declines to low levels. For comparison, the estradiol production rate in men is about 50 μg/d (184 nmol/d).

Effects on Female Genitalia

Estrogens facilitate the growth of the ovarian follicles and increase the motility of the uterine tubes. Their role in the cyclic changes in the endometrium, cervix, and vagina is discussed above. They increase uterine blood flow and have important effects on the smooth muscle of the uterus. In immature and ovariectomized females, the uterus is small and the myometrium atrophic and inactive. Estrogens increase the amount of

uterine muscle and its content of contractile proteins. Under the influence of estrogens, the myometrium becomes more active and excitable, and action potentials in the individual muscle fibers are increased. The "estrogen-dominated" uterus is also more sensitive to oxytocin.

Prolonged treatment with estrogens causes endometrial hypertrophy. When estrogen therapy is discontinued, there is some sloughing and **withdrawal bleeding.** Some "breakthrough" bleeding may also occur during prolonged treatment with estrogens.

Effects on Endocrine Organs

Estrogens decrease FSH secretion. In some circumstances, estrogens inhibit LH secretion (negative feedback), and in others, they increase LH secretion (positive feedback). Estrogens also increase the size of the pituitary. Women are sometimes given large doses of estrogens for 4–6 days to prevent conception during the fertile period (postcoital or "morning-after" contraception). In this instance, pregnancy is probably prevented by interference with implantation of the fertilized ovum rather than by changes in gonadotropin secretion.

Estrogens cause increased secretion of angiotensinogen and thyroid-binding globulin. They exert an important protein anabolic effect in chickens and cattle, possibly by stimulating the secretion of androgens from the adrenal; estrogens have been used commercially to increase the weight of domestic animals. They cause epiphyseal closure in humans.

Effects on the CNS

Estrogens are responsible for estrus behavior in animals, and they may increase libido in humans. They apparently exert this action by a direct effect on certain neurons in the hypothalamus (Fig 6–14).

Table 6–3. Twenty-four-hour production rates of sex steroids in women at different stages of the menstrual cycle.[1]

Sex Steroids	Early Follicular	Preovulatory	Midluteal
Progesterone (mg)	1.0	4.0	25.0
17-Hydroxyprogesterone (mg)	0.5	4.0	4.0
Dehydroepiandrosterone (mg)	7.0	7.0	7.0
Androstenedione (mg)	2.6	4.7	3.4
Testosterone (μg)	144.0	171.0	126.0
Estrone (μg)	50.0	350.0	250.0
Estradiol (μg)	36.0	380.0	250.0

[1]Modified and reproduced, with permission, from Yen SSC, Jaffe RB: *Reproductive Endocrinology*, 3rd ed. Saunders, 1991.

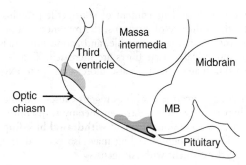

Figure 6–14. Loci where implantations of estrogen in the hypothalamus affect ovarian weight and sexual behavior in rats, projected on a sagittal section of the hypothalamus. The implants that stimulate sex behavior are located in the suprachiasmatic area above the optic chiasm, whereas ovarian atrophy is produced by implants in the arcuate nucleus and surrounding ventral hypothalamus just above the pituitary stalk. MB, **mamillary body.** (Reproduced, with permission, from Ganong WF: *Review of Medical Physiology,* 20th ed. Mc-Graw-Hill, 2001.)

Estrogens increase the proliferation of dendrites on neurons and the number of synaptic knobs in rats. In humans, they have been reported to slow the progression of Alzheimer's disease, but this role of estrogens remains controversial.

Effects on the Breasts

Estrogens produce duct growth in the breasts and are largely responsible for breast enlargement at puberty in girls. Breast enlargement that occurs when estrogen-containing skin creams are applied locally is due primarily to systemic absorption of the estrogen, although a slight local effect is also produced. Estrogens are responsible for the pigmentation of the areolas; pigmentation usually becomes more intense during the first pregnancy than it does at puberty.

Effects on Female Secondary Sex Characteristics

The body changes that develop in girls at puberty—in addition to enlargement of the breasts, uterus, and vagina—are due in part to estrogens, which are the "feminizing hormones," and in part simply to the absence of testicular androgens. Women have narrow shoulders and broad hips, thighs that converge, and arms that diverge (wide **carrying angle**). This body configuration, plus the female distribution of fat in the breasts and buttocks, is also seen in castrated males. In women, the larynx retains its prepubertal proportions

and the voice is high-pitched. There is less body hair and more scalp hair, and the pubic hair generally has a characteristic flattop pattern (**female escutcheon**). Growth of pubic and axillary hair in the female is due primarily to androgens rather than estrogens, although estrogen treatment may cause some hair growth. The androgens are produced by the adrenal cortex and, to a lesser extent, by the ovaries.

Other Actions of Estrogens

Normal women retain salt and water and gain weight just before menstruation. Estrogens can cause some degree of salt and water retention. However, aldosterone secretion is slightly elevated in the luteal phase, and this also contributes to the premenstrual fluid retention.

Estrogens are said to make sebaceous gland secretions more fluid and thus to counter the effect of testosterone and inhibit formation of **comedones** ("blackheads") and acne. The liver palms, spider angiomas, and slight breast enlargement seen in advanced liver disease are due to increased circulating estrogens. The increase appears to be due to decreased hepatic metabolism of androstenedione, making more of this androgen available for conversion to estrogens.

Estrogens have a significant plasma cholesterol-lowering action and they produce vasodilation and inhibit vascular smooth muscle proliferation, possibly by increasing the local production of NO. Estrogen has also been shown to prevent expression of factors important in the initiation of atherosclerosis. These actions may account for the low incidence of myocardial infarction and other complications of atherosclerotic-vascular disease in premenopausal women. There is considerable evidence that small doses of estrogen may reduce the incidence of cardiovascular disease after menopause. However, some recently published data do not support this conclusion, and additional research is needed. Large doses of oral estrogens also promote thrombosis, apparently because they reach the liver in high concentrations in the portal blood and alter hepatic production of clotting factors.

Mechanism of Action

Like other steroids, estrogens combine with protein receptors in the nucleus, and the complexes bind to DNA, promoting formation of mRNAs that in turn direct the formation of new proteins which modify cell function (Fig 16–15). Two estrogen receptors have been cloned: **estrogen receptor α (ERα)** and **estrogen receptor β (ERβ).** Although there is overlap, the distribution of these receptors is different. ERα expression is moderate to high in the uterus, testis, pituitary, kidney, epididymis, and adrenal, whereas ERβ expression

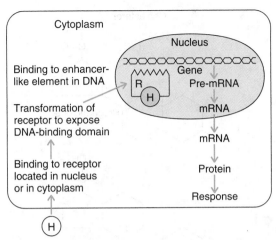

Figure 6–15. Mechanism of action of steroid hormones. H, hormone; R, receptor. The estrogen, progestin, androgen, glucocorticoid, mineralocorticoid, and 1,25-dihydroxycholecalciferol receptors have different molecular weights, but all have a ligand-binding domain and a DNA-binding domain that is exposed when the ligand binds. The receptor-hormone complex then binds to DNA, producing increased transcription. (Reproduced, with permission, from Ganong WF: *Review of Medical Physiology*, 20th ed. McGraw-Hill, 2001.)

is high in the ovary, prostate, lung, bladder, brain, and bone. It has been suggested that the regulation of ovarian function by the pituitary-ovarian axis is primarily ERα-mediated, whereas estrogens secreted into the ovarian follicles act primarily via ERβs. Male and female mice in which the gene for ERα has been knocked out are sterile, develop osteoporosis, and continue to grow because their epiphyses do not close. In contrast, ERβ knockout mice develop normally, reproduce, and lactate, although the females have fewer and smaller litters. However, much additional research is needed to sort out the detailed effects of ERα and ERβ and their interactions.

Most of the actions of estrogens are genomic, ie, mediated via ERα and ERβ. However, a few effects are so rapid that it is difficult to believe they are mediated via increased expression of mRNAs. These include effects on neuronal discharge in the brain and possibly feedback effects on gonadotropin secretion. Their existence has led to the hypothesis that in addition to genomic actions, there are nongenomic effects of estrogens that are presumably mediated by membrane receptors. Similar rapid effects of progesterone, testosterone, and aldosterone may also be produced by membrane receptors.

Synthetic Estrogen

The ethinyl derivative of estradiol (Fig 6–16) is a potent estrogen. Unlike naturally occurring estrogens it is relatively active when given orally, because it has an ethinyl group in position 17, which makes it resistant to hepatic metabolism. Naturally occurring hormones have low activity when given orally, because the portal venous drainage of the intestine carries them to the liver, where they are largely inactivated before they can reach the general circulation. Some nonsteroidal substances and a few compounds found in plants have estrogenic activity. Plant estrogens rarely affect humans but may cause undesirable effects in farm animals. Diethylstilbestrol (Fig 6–16) and a number of related compounds are strongly estrogenic, possibly because they are converted to steroidlike ring structures in the body.

Estradiol reduces the hot flashes and other symptoms of the menopause, and it also prevents the development of osteoporosis. It may reduce the initiation and progression of atherosclerosis and the incidence of heart attack. However, it also stimulates the growth of the endometrium and the breast, and can lead to cancer of the uterus, and probably the breast. Therefore, there has been an active search for "tailor-made" estrogens that have the bone and cardiovascular effects of estradiol but lack its growth-stimulating effects on the uterus and the breast. Two compounds, **tamoxifen** and **raloxifene,** show promise in this regard. Neither combats the symptoms of the menopause but both have the

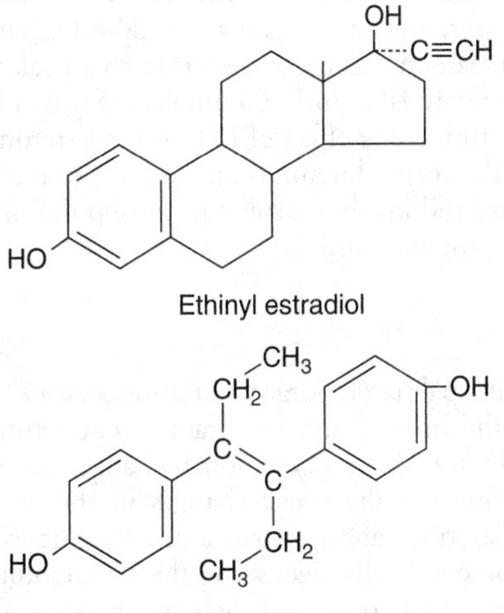

Ethinyl estradiol

Diethylstilbestrol

Figure 6–16. Synthetic estrogens. (Reproduced, with permission, from Ganong WF: *Review of Medical Physiology*, 20th ed. McGraw-Hill, 2001.)

bone-preserving effects of estradiol. They may also have cardioprotective effects, but the clinical relevance of these effects has not been established. In addition, tamoxifen does not stimulate the breast, and raloxifene does not stimulate the breast or uterus. The clinical uses of these two drugs are discussed elsewhere in this book.

Chemistry, Biosynthesis, & Metabolism of Progesterone

Progesterone (Fig 6–17) is a C_{21} steroid secreted in large amounts by the corpus luteum and the placenta. It is an important intermediate in steroid biosynthesis in all tissues that secrete steroid hormones, and small amounts enter the circulation from the testes and adrenal cortex. The 20α- and 20β-hydroxy derivatives of progesterone are formed in the corpus luteum. About 2% of the progesterone in the circulation is free (Table 6–2), whereas 80% is bound to albumin and 18% is bound to corticosteroid-binding globulin. Progesterone has a short half-life and is converted in the liver to pregnanediol, which is conjugated to glucuronic acid and excreted in the urine (Fig 6–17).

Secretion of Progesterone

In women, the plasma progesterone level is approximately 0.9 ng/mL (3 nmol/L) during the follicular phase of the menstrual cycle, whereas in men, the level is approximately 0.3 ng/mL (1 nmol/L). The difference is due to secretion of small amounts of progesterone by cells in the ovarian follicle. During the luteal phase, the large amounts secreted by the corpus luteum cause ovarian secretion to increase about 20-fold. The result is an increase in plasma progesterone to a peak value of approximately 18 ng/mL (60 nmol/L) (Fig 6–11).

The stimulating effect of LH on progesterone secretion by the corpus luteum is due to activation of adenylyl cyclase and involves a subsequent step that is dependent on protein synthesis.

Actions of Progesterone

The principal target organs of progesterone are the uterus, the breasts, and the brain. Progesterone is responsible for the progestational changes in the endometrium and the cyclic changes in the cervix and vagina described above. It has antiestrogenic effects on the myometrial cells, decreasing their excitability, their sensitivity to oxytocin, and their spontaneous electrical activity, while increasing their membrane potential. It decreases the number of estrogen receptors in the endometrium and increases the rate of conversion of 17β-estradiol to less active estrogens.

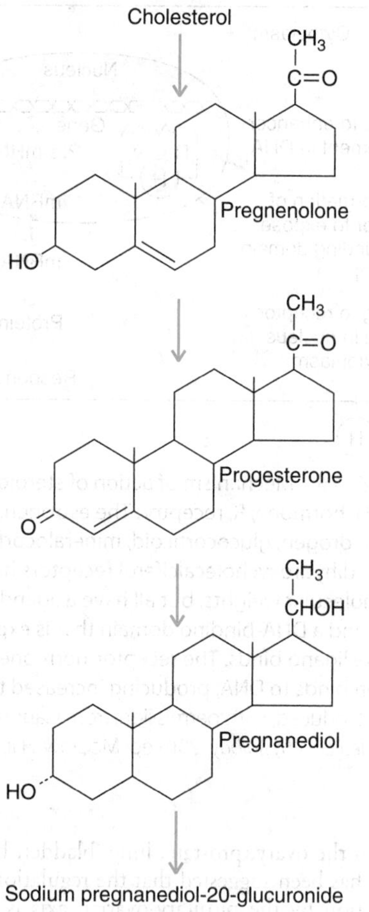

Figure 6–17. Biosynthesis of progesterone and major pathway for its metabolism. Other metabolites are also formed. (Reproduced, with permission, from Ganong WF: *Review of Medical Physiology*, 20th ed. McGraw-Hill, 2001.)

In the breast, progesterone stimulates the development of lobules and alveoli. It induces differentiation of estrogen-prepared ductal tissue and supports the secretory function of the breast during lactation.

The feedback effects of progesterone are complex and are exerted at both the hypothalamic and the pituitary level. Large doses of progesterone inhibit LH secretion and potentiate the inhibitory effects of estrogens, preventing ovulation.

Progesterone is thermogenic and is probably responsible for the rise in basal body temperature at the time of ovulation (Fig 6–11). Progesterone stimulates respiration, and the fact that alveolar PCO_2 in women during the luteal phase of the menstrual cycle is lower than that in men is attributed to the action of secreted progesterone. In pregnancy, alveolar PCO_2 falls as progesterone secretion rises.

Large doses of progesterone produce natriuresis, probably by blocking the action of aldosterone on the kidney. The hormone does not have a significant anabolic effect.

Mechanism of Action

The effects of progesterone, like those of other steroids, are brought about by an action on DNA to initiate synthesis of new mRNA. The progesterone receptor is bound to a heat shock protein in the absence of the steroid, and progesterone binding releases the heat shock protein, exposing the DNA-binding domain of the receptor. The synthetic steroid **mifepristone (RU-486)** binds to the receptor but does not release the heat shock protein, and it blocks the binding of progesterone. Since the maintenance of early pregnancy depends on the stimulatory effect of progesterone on endometrial growth and its inhibition of uterine contractility, mifepristone causes abortion. In some countries, mifepristone combined with a prostaglandin is used to produce elective abortions.

There are two isoforms of the progesterone receptor, produced by differential processing from a single gene. Progesterone receptor A (PR_A) is a truncated form that when activated is capable of inhibiting some of the actions of progesterone receptor B (PR_B). However, the physiologic significance of the existence of the two isoforms remains to be determined.

Substances that mimic the action of progesterone are sometimes called **progestational agents, gestagens,** or **progestins.** They are used along with synthetic estrogens as oral contraceptive agents.

RELAXIN

Relaxin is a polypeptide hormone that is secreted by the corpus luteum in women and the prostate in men. During pregnancy, it relaxes the pubic symphysis and other pelvic joints and softens and dilates the uterine cervix during pregnancy. Thus, it facilitates delivery. It also inhibits uterine contractions and may play a role in the development of the mammary glands. In nonpregnant women, relaxin is found in the corpus luteum and the endometrium during the secretory but not the proliferative phase of the menstrual cycle. Its function in nonpregnant women is unknown.

In most species, there is only one relaxin gene, but in humans there are 2 genes on chromosome 9 that code for 2 structurally different polypeptides with relaxin activity. However, only one of these genes is active in the ovary and the prostate. The structure of the polypeptide produced in these 2 tissues is shown in Fig 6–18.

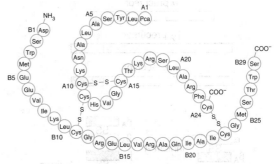

Figure 6–18. Structure of human luteal and prostatic relaxin. Note the A and B chains connected by disulfide bridges. Pca, pyroglutamic acid residue at N terminal of A chain. (Modified and reproduced, with permission, from Winslow JW et al: Human seminal relaxin is a product of the same gene as human luteal relaxin. Endocrinology 1992;130:2660.)

INHIBINS AND ACTIVINS

Polypeptides called **inhibins** that inhibit FSH secretion were first isolated from testes, but it was soon discovered that they were also produced by the ovaries. There are 2 inhibins, and they are formed from 3 polypeptide subunits: a glycosylated α subunit with a molecular weight of 18,000, and 2 nonglycosylated β subunits, β_A and β_B, each with a molecular weight of 14,000. The subunits are formed from precursor proteins (Fig 6–19). The α subunit combines with β_A to form a heterodimer and with β_B to form another heterodimer, with the subunits linked by disulfide bonds. Both $\alpha\beta_A$ (inhibin A) and $\alpha\beta_B$ (inhibin B) inhibit FSH secretion by a direct action on the pituitary, although it now appears that inhibin B is the FSH-regulating hormone in adults. Inhibins are produced by Sertoli cells in males and granulosa cells in females.

The heterodimer $\beta_A\beta_B$ and the homodimers $\beta_A\beta_A$ and $\beta_B\beta_B$ stimulate rather than inhibit FSH secretion and consequently are called **activins.** Their function in reproduction is unsettled. However, the inhibins and activins are members of the TGFβ superfamily of dimeric growth factors that also includes the müllerian inhibitory substance (MIS) that is important in embryonic development of the gonads. Two **activin receptors** have been cloned, and both appear to be serine kinases. Inhibins and activins are found not only in the gonads but also in the brain and many other tissues. In the bone marrow, activins are involved in the development of white blood cells. In embryonic life, activins are involved in the formation of mesoderm. All mice in which a targeted deletion of the α-inhibin gene was produced initially grew in a normal fashion but then

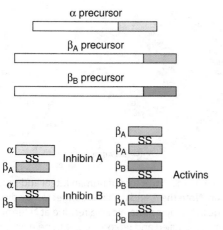

Figure 6–19. Inhibin precursor proteins and the various inhibins and activins that are formed from them. SS, disulfide bonds. (Modified from Ganong WF: *Review of Medical Physiology,* 20th ed. McGraw-Hill, 2001.)

developed gonadal stromal tumors, so the α-inhibin gene is a tumor-suppressor gene.

In plasma, α_2-macroglobulin binds activins and inhibins. In tissues, activins bind to a family of 4 glycoproteins called **follistatins.** Binding of the activins inactivates their biologic activity, but the relation of follistatins to inhibin and their physiologic function are unsettled.

PITUITARY HORMONES

Ovarian secretion depends on the action of hormones secreted by the anterior pituitary gland. The anterior pituitary gland secretes 6 established hormones: adrenocorticotropic hormone (ACTH), growth hormone, thyroid-stimulating hormone (TSH), follicle-stimulating hormone (FSH), luteinizing hormone (LH), and prolactin (Fig 6–20). It also secretes one putative hormone β-lipotropic hormone (β-LPH).

GONADOTROPINS

The gonadotropins FSH and LH act in concert to regulate the cyclic secretion of the ovarian hormones. They are glycoproteins made up of α and β subunits. The α subunits have the same amino acid composition as the α subunits in the glycoproteins TSH and human chorionic gonadotropin (hCG); the specificity of these 4 glycoprotein hormones is imparted by the different structures of their β subunits. The carbohydrates in the gonadotropin molecules increase the potency of the hormones by markedly slowing their metabolism. The half-life of human FSH is about 170 minutes; the half-life of LH is about 60 minutes.

The receptors for FSH and LH are serpentine receptors coupled to adenylyl cyclase through G_S. In addition, each has an extended, glycosylated extracellular domain.

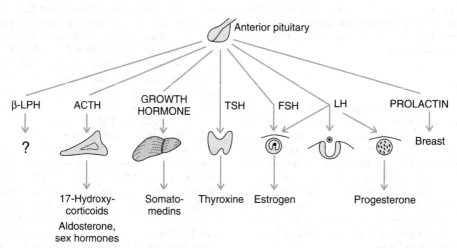

Figure 6–20. Anterior pituitary hormones. In women, FSH and LH act in sequence on the ovary to produce growth of the ovarian follicle, which secretes estrogen, then ovulation, followed by formation and maintenance of the corpus luteum, which secretes estrogen and progesterone. In men, FSH and LH control the functions of the testes. Prolactin stimulates lactation. β-LPH, β-lipotropic hormone; ACTH, adrenocorticotropic hormone; TSH, thyroid-stimulating hormone; FSH, follicle-stimulating hormone; LH, luteinizing hormone. (Reproduced, with permission, from Ganong WF: *Review of Medical Physiology,* 20th ed. McGraw-Hill, 2001.)

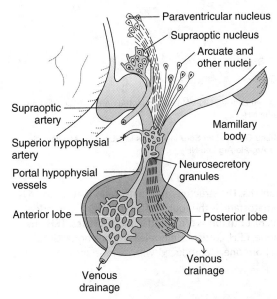

Figure 6–21. Simplified schematic reconstruction of the hypothalamus and the pituitary. (After Hansel; courtesy International Journal of Fertility. Redrawn and reproduced, with permission, from Schally et al: Hypothalamic regulatory hormones. Science 1973;179:341. Copyright 1973 by the American Association for the Advancement of Science.)

Hypothalamic Hormones

The secretion of the anterior pituitary hormones is regulated by the hypothalamic hypophysiotropic hormones. These substances are produced by neurons and enter the portal hypophysial vessels (Fig 6–21), a

special group of blood vessels that transmit substances directly from the hypothalamus to the anterior pituitary gland. The actions of these hormones are summarized in Fig 6–22. The structure of 6 established hypophysiotropic hormones is known (Fig 6–23). No single prolactin-releasing hormone has been isolated and identified. However, several polypeptides that are found in the hypothalamus can increase prolactin secretion, and one or more of these may stimulate prolactin secretion under physiologic conditions.

The posterior pituitary differs from the anterior in that its hormones, oxytocin and arginine vasopressin, are secreted by neurons directly into the systemic circulation. These hormones are produced in the cell bodies of neurons located in the supraoptic and paraventricular nuclei of the hypothalamus and transported down the axons of these neurons to their endings in the posterior lobe of the pituitary. The hormones are released from the endings into the circulation when action potentials pass down the axons and reach the endings. The structures of the hormones are shown in Fig 6–24.

CONTROL OF OVARIAN FUNCTION

FSH from the pituitary is responsible for early maturation of the ovarian follicles, and FSH and LH together are responsible for final follicle maturation. A burst of LH secretion (Fig 6–11) triggers ovulation and the initial formation of the corpus luteum. There is also a smaller midcycle burst of FSH secretion, the significance of which is uncertain. LH stimulates the secretion of estrogen and progesterone from the corpus luteum.

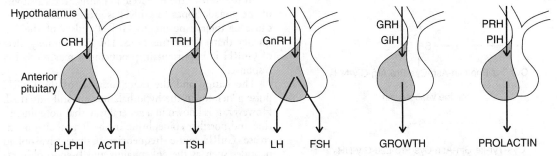

Figure 6–22. Effects of hypophysiotropic hormones on the secretion of anterior pituitary hormones. β-LPH, β-lipotropic hormone; ACTH, adrenocorticotropic hormone; CRH, corticotropin-releasing hormone; TRH, thyroid-releasing hormone; TSH, thyroid-stimulating hormone; GnRH, gonadotropin-releasing hormone; FSH, follicle-stimulating hormone; LH, luteinizing hormone; GRH, growth hormone-releasing hormone; GIH, growth-inhibiting hormone; PRH, prolactin-releasing hormone; PIH, prolactin-inhibiting hormone. (Reproduced, with permission, from Ganong WF: *Review of Medical Physiology*, 20th ed. McGraw-Hill, 2001.)

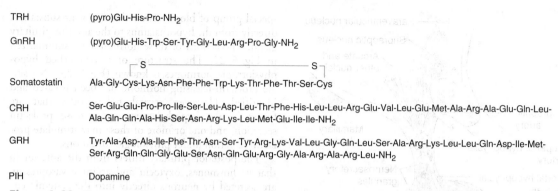

TRH	(pyro)Glu-His-Pro-NH$_2$
GnRH	(pyro)Glu-His-Trp-Ser-Tyr-Gly-Leu-Arg-Pro-Gly-NH$_2$
Somatostatin	Ala-Gly-Cys-Lys-Asn-Phe-Phe-Trp-Lys-Thr-Phe-Thr-Ser-Cys
CRH	Ser-Glu-Glu-Pro-Pro-Ile-Ser-Leu-Asp-Leu-Thr-Phe-His-Leu-Leu-Arg-Glu-Val-Leu-Glu-Met-Ala-Arg-Ala-Glu-Gln-Leu-Ala-Gln-Gln-Ala-His-Ser-Asn-Arg-Lys-Leu-Met-Glu-Ile-Ile-NH$_2$
GRH	Tyr-Ala-Asp-Ala-Ile-Phe-Thr-Asn-Ser-Tyr-Arg-Lys-Val-Leu-Gly-Gln-Leu-Ser-Ala-Arg-Lys-Leu-Leu-Gln-Asp-Ile-Met-Ser-Arg-Gln-Gln-Gly-Glu-Ser-Asn-Gln-Glu-Arg-Gly-Ala-Arg-Ala-Arg-Leu-NH$_2$
PIH	Dopamine

Figure 6–23. Structure of hypophysiotropic hormones in humans. The structure of somatostatin that is shown is the tetradecapeptide (somatostatin 14). In addition, preprosomatostatin is the source of an N-terminal extended polypeptide containing 28 amino acid residues (somatostatin 28). Both forms are found in many tissues. TRH, thyroid-releasing hormone; GnRH, gonadotropin-releasing hormone; CRH, corticotropin-releasing hormone; GRH, growth hormone-releasing hormone; PIH, prolactin-inhibiting hormone. (Reproduced, with permission, from Ganong WF: *Review of Medical Physiology,* 20th ed. McGraw-Hill, 2001.)

Hypothalamic Components

The hypothalamus occupies a key role in the control of gonadotropin secretion. Hypothalamic control is exerted by GnRH secreted into the portal hypophysial vessels. GnRH stimulates the secretion of FSH as well as LH, and it is unlikely that there is an additional separate follicle-stimulating hormone-releasing hormone (FRH).

GnRH is normally secreted in episodic bursts (**circhoral secretion**). These bursts are essential for normal secretion of gonadotropins, which are also exerted in an episodic fashion (Fig 6–25). If GnRH is administered by constant infusion, the number of GnRH receptors in the anterior pituitary decreases (**downregulation**), and LH secretion falls to low levels. However, if GnRH is administered episodically at a rate of 1 pulse per

hour, LH secretion is stimulated. This is true even when endogenous GnRH secretion has been prevented by a lesion of the ventral hypothalamus.

It is now clear not only that episodic secretion of GnRH is a general phenomenon, but that fluctuations in the frequency and amplitude of the GnRH bursts are important in generating the other hormonal changes that are responsible for the menstrual cycle. Frequency is increased by estrogens and decreased by progesterone and testosterone. The frequency increases late in the follicular phase of the cycle, culminating in the LH surge. During the secretory phase, the frequency decreases as a result of the action of progesterone, but when estrogen and progesterone secretion decrease at the end of the cycle, frequency once again increases.

At the time of the midcycle LH surge, the sensitivity of the gonadotropes to GnRH is greatly increased because of their exposure to GnRH pulses of the frequency that exist at this time. This self-priming effect of GnRH is important in producing a maximum LH response.

The nature and the exact location of the GnRH pulse generator in the hypothalamus are still unsettled. However, it is known in a general way that norepinephrine and possibly epinephrine in the hypothalamus increase GnRH pulse frequencies. Conversely, opioid peptides such as the enkephalins and β-endorphin reduce the frequency of GnRH pulses.

The downregulation of pituitary receptors and the consequent decrease in LH secretion produced by constantly elevated levels of GnRH has led to the use of long-acting GnRH agonists to inhibit LH secretion in precocious puberty and cancer of the prostate.

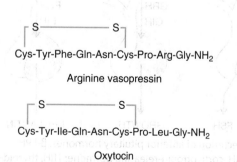

Cys-Tyr-Phe-Gln-Asn-Cys-Pro-Arg-Gly-NH$_2$

Arginine vasopressin

Cys-Tyr-Ile-Gln-Asn-Cys-Pro-Leu-Gly-NH$_2$

Oxytocin

Figure 6–24. Structures of arginine vasopressin and oxytocin. (Reproduced, with permission, from Ganong WF: *Review of Medical Physiology,* 20th ed. McGraw-Hill, 2001.)

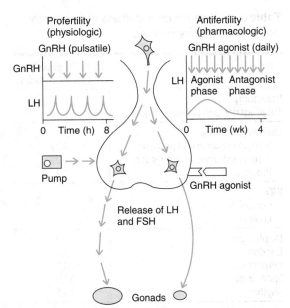

cretion of LH and FSH is low because of the elevated levels of estrogen, progesterone, and inhibin B.

It should be emphasized that a moderate, constant level of circulating estrogen exerts a negative feedback effect on LH secretion, whereas an elevated estrogen level exerts a positive feedback effect and stimulates LH secretion. It has been demonstrated that in monkeys, there is also a minimum time that estrogens must be elevated to produce positive feedback. When circulating estrogen was increased about 300% for 24 hours, only negative feedback was seen; but when it was increased about 300% for 36 hours or more, a brief decline in secretion was followed by a burst of LH secretion that resembled the midcycle surge. When circulating levels of progesterone were high, the positive feedback effect of estrogen was inhibited. There is evidence that in primates, both the negative and the positive feedback ef-

Figure 6–25. Profertility and antifertility actions of GnRH and its agonists. The normal secretion of GnRH is pulsatile, occurring at 30- to 60-minute intervals. This mode, which can be mimicked by timed injections, produces circhoral peaks of LH and FSH secretion and promotes fertility. If GnRH is administered by continuous infusion, or if one of its long-acting synthetic agonists is injected, there is initial stimulation of the pituitary receptors. However, this lasts for only a few days, and is followed by receptor downregulation with inhibition of gonadotropin secretion (antifertility effect). (Reproduced, with permission, from Conn PM, Crowley WF Jr: Gonadotropin-releasing hormone and its analogues. N Engl J Med 1991;324:93.)

Feedback Effects

Changes in plasma LH, FSH, sex steroids, and inhibin B during the menstrual cycle are shown in Fig 6-11, and their feedback relations are diagrammed in Fig 6–26. At the start of the follicular phase, inhibin B is low and FSH is modestly elevated, fostering follicular growth. LH secretion is held in check by the negative feedback effect of the rising plasma estrogen level. At 36–48 hours before ovulation, the estrogen feedback effect becomes positive, and this initiates the burst of LH secretion (LH surge) that produces ovulation. Ovulation occurs about 9 hours after the LH peak. FSH secretion also peaks, despite a small rise in inhibin B, probably because of the strong stimulation of gonadotropes by GnRH. During the luteal phase, the se-

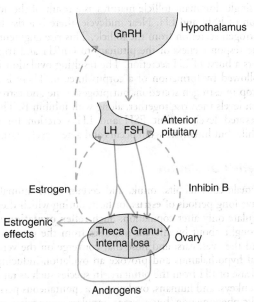

Figure 6–26. Feedback regulation of ovarian function. The cells of the theca interna provide androgens to the granulosa cells, and the thecal cells produce the circulating estrogens, which inhibit the secretion of LH, GnRH, and FSH. Inhibin B from the granulosa cells also inhibits FSH secretion. LH regulates thecal cells, whereas the granulosa cells are regulated by both LH and FSH. The dashed arrows indicate inhibition, and the solid arrows indicate stimulation. GnRH, gonadotropin-releasing hormone; LH, luteinizing hormone; FSH, follicle-stimulating hormone. (Reproduced, with permission, from Ganong WF: *Review of Medical Physiology*, 20th ed. McGraw-Hill, 2001.)

exerted in the mediobasal hypo-
ctly how negative feedback is
feedback and then back to negative
phase remains unknown.

Control of Menstrual Cycle

In an important sense, regression of the corpus luteum
(**luteolysis**) starting 3–4 days before menses is the key
to the menstrual cycle. $PGF_{2\alpha}$ appears to be a physiologic luteolysin, but this prostaglandin is only active
when endothelial cells producing endothelin-1 (ET-1)
are present. Therefore it appears that at least in some
species luteolysis is produced by the combined action of
$PGF_{2\alpha}$ and ET-1. In some domestic animals, oxytocin
secreted by the corpus luteum appears to exert a local
luteolytic effect, possibly by causing the release of
prostaglandins. Once luteolysis begins, the estrogen and
progesterone levels fall and the secretion of FSH and
LH increases. A new crop of follicles develops, and then
a single dominant follicle matures as a result of the action of FSH and LH. Near midcycle, there is a rise in
estrogen secretion from the follicle. This rise augments
the responsiveness of the pituitary to GnRH and triggers a burst of LH secretion. The resulting ovulation is
followed by formation of a corpus luteum. There is a
drop in estrogen secretion, but progesterone and estrogen levels then rise together, along with inhibin B. The
elevated levels inhibit FSH and LH secretion for a
while, but luteolysis again occurs and a new cycle starts.

Reflex Ovulation

Female cats, rabbits, mink, and certain other animals
have long periods of **estrus,** or heat, during which they
ovulate only after copulation. Such **reflex ovulation** is
brought about by afferent impulses from the genitalia
and the eyes, ears, and nose that converge on the ventral hypothalamus and provoke an ovulation-inducing
release of LH from the pituitary. In species such as rats,
monkeys, and humans, ovulation is a spontaneous periodic phenomenon, but afferent impulses converging on
the hypothalamus can also exert effects. Ovulation can
be delayed for 24 hours in rats by administering pento-
barbital or other neurally active drugs 12 hours before
the expected time of follicle rupture. In women, menstrual cycles may be markedly influenced by emotional
stimuli.

Contraception

Methods commonly used to prevent conception are
listed in Table 6–4, along with their failure rates. Once
conception has occurred, abortion can be produced by
progesterone antagonists such as mifepristone.

Table 6–4. Relative effectiveness of frequently
used contraceptive methods.[1]

Method	Failures per 100 Women-Years
Vasectomy	0.02
Tubal ligation and similar procedures	0.13
Oral contraceptive	
> 50 µg estrogen and progestin	0.32
< 50 µg estrogen and progestin	0.27
Progestin only	1.2
IUD	
Copper 7	1.5
Loop D	1.3
Diaphragm	1.9
Condom	3.6
Withdrawal	6.7
Spermicide	11.9
Rhythm	15.5

[1]Data from Vessey M, Lawless M, Yeates D: Efficacy of different
contraceptive methods. Lancet 1982;1:841. Reproduced with permission.

Implantation of foreign bodies in the uterus causes
changes in the duration of the sexual cycle in a number
of mammalian species. In humans, such foreign bodies
do not alter the menstrual cycle, but they act as effective contraceptive devices. Intrauterine implantation of
pieces of metal or plastic (**intrauterine devices; IUDs**)
has been used in programs aimed at controlling population growth. Although their mechanism of action is still
unsettled, they seem in general to prevent sperms from
fertilizing ova. Those containing copper appear to exert
a spermatocidal effect. IUDs that slowly release progesterone or levonorgestrel, the progestin in Norplant implants, have the additional effect of thickening cervical
mucus so that entry into the uterus is impeded. IUDs
can cause intrauterine infections, but these usually
occur in the first month after insertion and in women
exposed to sexually transmitted diseases.

Women undergoing long-term treatment with relatively large doses of estrogen do not ovulate, probably because they have depressed FSH levels and multiple irregular bursts of LH secretion rather than a single midcycle
peak. Women treated with similar doses of estrogen plus
a progestational agent do not ovulate because the secretion of both gonadotropins is suppressed. In addition,
the progestin makes the cervical mucus thick and unfavorable to sperm migration, and it may also interfere
with implantation. For contraception, an orally active estrogen such as ethinyl estradiol (Fig 6–16) is often combined with a synthetic progestin such as norethindrone.

The pills are administered for 21 days, then withdrawn for 5–7 days to permit menstrual flow, and started again. Like ethinyl estradiol, norethindrone has an ethinyl group on position 17 of the steroid nucleus, so it is resistant to hepatic metabolism and consequently is effective when taken orally. In addition to being a progestin, it is partly metabolized to ethinyl estradiol, and for this reason it also has estrogenic activity. It is now clear that small as well as large doses of estrogen are effective (Table 6–4); the use of small doses reduces the risk of thromboses or other complications. Progestins alone can be used for contraception, although they are more effective when combined with estrogens.

Implants made up primarily of progestins are now seeing increased use in some parts of the world. The implants are inserted under the skin and can prevent pregnancy for up to 5 years. They often produce amenorrhea but otherwise appear to be well tolerated.

PROLACTIN

Chemistry of Prolactin

Prolactin is another anterior pituitary hormone that has important functions in reproduction and pregnancy. The prolactin molecule contains 199 amino acid residues and 3 disulfide bridges (Fig 6–27) and has considerable structural similarity to human growth hormone and human chorionic somatomammotropin (hCS). The half-life of prolactin, like that of growth hormone, is about 20 minutes. Structurally similar prolactins are secreted by the endometrium and by the placenta.

Receptors

The human prolactin receptor resembles the growth hormone receptor and is one of the superfamily of receptors that includes the growth hormone receptor and receptors for many cytokines and hematopoietic growth factors. It dimerizes and activates the JAK-Stat and other intracellular enzyme cascades.

Actions

Prolactin causes milk secretion from the breast after estrogen and progesterone priming. Its effect on the breast involves increased action of mRNA and increased production of casein and lactalbumin. However, the action of the hormone is not exerted on the cell nucleus and is prevented by inhibitors of microtubules. Prolactin also inhibits the effects of gonadotropins, possibly by an action at the level of the

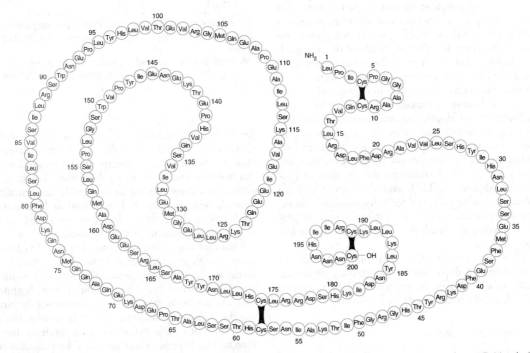

Figure 6–27. Structure of human prolactin. (Reproduced, with permission, from Bondy PK, Rosenberg LE: *Metabolic Control and Disease,* 8th ed. Saunders, 1980.)

ovary. Its role in preventing ovulation in lactating women is discussed below. The function of prolactin in normal males is unsettled, but excess prolactin secreted by tumors causes impotence. An action of prolactin that has been used as the basis for bioassay of this hormone is stimulation of the growth and "secretion" of the crop sacs in pigeons and other birds. The paired crop sacs are outpouchings of the esophagus which form, by desquamation of their inner cell layers, a nutritious material ("milk") that the birds feed to their young. However, prolactin, FSH, and LH are now regularly measured by radioimmunoassay.

Regulation of Prolactin Secretion

The normal plasma prolactin concentration is approximately 5 ng/mL in men and 8 ng/mL in women. Secretion is tonically inhibited by the hypothalamus, and section of the pituitary stalk leads to an increase in circulating prolactin. Thus, the effect of the hypothalamic prolactin-inhibiting hormone dopamine (PIH) is greater than the effect of the putative prolactin-releasing hormone (see above). In humans, prolactin secretion is increased by exercise, surgical and psychological stresses, and stimulation of the nipple (Table 6–5). The plasma prolactin level rises during sleep, the rise starting after the onset of sleep and persisting throughout the sleep period. Secretion is increased during pregnancy, reaching a peak at the time of parturition. After delivery, the plasma concentration falls to nonpregnant levels in about 8 days. Suckling produces a prompt increase in secretion, but the magnitude of this rise gradually declines after a woman has been nursing for more than 3 months. With prolonged lactation, secretion occurs with prolactin levels that are in the normal range.

L-Dopa decreases prolactin secretion by increasing the formation of dopamine, and bromocriptine and other dopamine agonists inhibit secretion because they stimulate dopamine receptors. Chlorpromazine and related drugs that block dopamine receptors increase prolactin secretion. TRH stimulates the secretion of prolactin in addition to TSH, and there are additional prolactin-releasing polypeptides in hypothalamic tissue. Estrogens produce a slowly developing increase in prolactin secretion as a result of a direct action on the lactotropes.

It has now been established that prolactin facilitates the secretion of dopamine in the median eminence. Thus, prolactin acts in the hypothalamus in a negative feedback fashion to inhibit its own secretion.

Hyperprolactinemia

Up to 70% of patients with chromophobe adenomas of the anterior pituitary have elevated plasma prolactin

Table 6–5. Factors affecting the secretion of human prolactin and growth hormone.

Factor	Prolactin[1]	Growth Hormone[1]
Sleep	I+	I+
Nursing	I++	N
Breast stimulation in nonlactating women	I	N
Stress	I+	I+
Hypoglycemia	I	I+
Strenuous exercise	I	I
Sexual intercourse in women	I	N
Pregnancy	I++	N
Estrogens	I	I
Hypothyroidism	I	N
TRH	I+	N
Phenothiazines, butyrophenones	I+	N
Opiates	I	I
Glucose	N	D
Somatostatin	N	D+
L-Dopa	D+	I+
Apomorphine	D+	I+
Bromocriptine and related ergot derivatives	D+	I

[1]I, moderate increase; I+, marked increase; I++, very marked increase; N, no change; D, moderate decrease; D+, marked decrease.
(Modified from Frantz and reproduced with permission from Ganong WF: *Review of Medical Physiology*, 20th ed, McGraw-Hill, 2001.)

levels. In some instances the elevation may be due to damage to the pituitary stalk, but in most cases the tumor cells are actually secreting the hormone. The hyperprolactinemia may cause galactorrhea, but in many individuals there are no demonstrable abnormalities. Indeed, most women with galactorrhea have normal prolactin levels; definite elevations are found in less than a third of patients with this condition.

Another interesting observation is that 15–20% of women with secondary amenorrhea have elevated prolactin levels, and when prolactin secretion is reduced, normal menstrual cycles and fertility return. It appears that the prolactin may produce amenorrhea by blocking the action of gonadotropins on the ovaries, but definitive proof of this hypothesis must await further research. The hypogonadism produced by prolactinomas is associated with osteoporosis due to estrogen deficiency.

Hyperprolactinemia in men is associated with impotence and hypogonadism that disappear when prolactin secretion is reduced.

MENOPAUSE

The human ovary gradually becomes unresponsive to gonadotropins with advancing age, and its function declines, so that sexual cycles and menstruation disappear (menopause). This unresponsiveness is associated with and probably caused by a decline in the number of primordial follicles (Fig 6–6). The ovaries no longer secrete progesterone and 17β-estradiol in appreciable quantities. Estrone is formed by aromatization of androstenedione in the circulation, but the amounts are normally small. The uterus and vagina gradually become atrophic. As the negative feedback effect of the estrogens and progesterone is reduced, secretion of FSH and LH is increased, and plasma FSH and LH rise to high levels. Old female mice and rats have long periods of diestrus and increased levels of gonadotropin secretion, but a clear-cut "menopause" has apparently not been described in experimental animals.

In women, the menses usually become irregular and cease between the ages of 45 and 55. The average age at onset of the menopause has increased since the turn of the century and is currently about 52 years.

Sensations of warmth spreading from the trunk to the face ("hot flushes," also called hot flashes), night sweats, and various psychic symptoms are common after ovarian function has ceased. Hot flushes are said to occur in 75% of menopausal women, and may last as long as 40 years. They are prevented by administration of estrogen. They are not peculiar to the menopause; they also occur in premenopausal women and men whose gonads are removed surgically or destroyed by disease. Their cause is unknown. However, it has been demonstrated that they coincide with surges of LH secretion. LH is secreted in episodic bursts at intervals of 30–60 minutes or more (circhoral secretion), and in the absence of gonadal hormones, these bursts are large. Each hot flush begins with the start of a burst. However, LH itself is not responsible for the symptoms, because they can continue after removal of the pituitary. Instead, it appears that some event in the hypothalamus initiates both the release of LH and the episode of flushing. The menopause and the clinical management of patients with menopausal symptoms are discussed in more detail in Chapter 57.

REFERENCES

Chabbert Buffet N et al: Regulation of the human menstrual cycle. Front Neuroendocrinol 1998;19:151.

Ganong WF: *Review of Medical Physiology,* 20th ed. McGraw-Hill, 2001.

Kelley PA et al: Implications of multiple phenotypes observed in prolactin receptor knockout mice. Front Neuroendocrinol 2001;22:140.

Knobil E, Neill JD (editors): *The Physiology of Reproduction,* 2nd ed, 2 vols. Raven Press, 1994.

Kuiper GGJM et al: The estrogen receptor β: A novel mediator of estrogen action. Front Neuroendocrinol 1998;19:253.

Mather JP, Moore A, Li R-H: Activins, inhibins, and follistatins: Further thoughts on a growing family of regulators. Proc Soc Exper Biol Med 1997;215:209.

Mendelsohn ME, Karas RH: The protective effects of estrogen on the cardiovascular system. N Engl J Med 1999;340:1801.

Ness RB et al: Oral contraceptives, other methods of contraception and risk reduction for ovarian cancer. Epidemiology 2001;12:307.

Palment NR, Boepple PA: Variation in the onset of puberty: clinical spectrum and genetic investigation. J Clin Endocrinol Metab 2001;86:2364.

Reyelli A, Massobrio M, Tesarik J: Nongenomic actions of steroid hormones in reproductive tissues. Endocrinol Rev 1998;19:3.

Wilson JB et al: *William's Textbook of Endocrinology,* 9th ed. Saunders, 1998.

Yen SSC, Jaffe RB, Barbieri RL (editors): *Reproductive Endocrinology,* 4th ed. Saunders, 1999.

Maternal Physiology During Pregnancy

Brian J. Koos, MD, PhD, & Pamela J. Moore, PhD

The physiologic, biochemical, and anatomic changes that occur during pregnancy are extensive and may be systemic or local. However, most systems return to prepregnancy status within 6 weeks postpartum.

Maternal adaptations maintain a healthy environment for the fetus without compromising the mother's health. Thus, in many instances physiologic activity (eg, cardiac output) is increased in pregnant women, but smooth muscle (eg, urinary and gastrointestinal tracts) demonstrates decreased activity. Many laboratory values are dramatically altered from nonpregnant values. An understanding of the normal physiologic changes induced by pregnancy is essential in understanding coincidental disease processes.

GASTROINTESTINAL TRACT

During pregnancy, nutritional requirements, including those for vitamins and minerals, are increased, and several maternal alterations occur to meet this demand. Pregnant women tend to rest more often, conserving their energy and thereby enhancing fetal nutrition. Although the mother's appetite usually increases, so food intake is greater, some women have a decreased appetite or experience nausea and vomiting (see Chapter 9). These symptoms may be related to relative levels of human chorionic gonadotropin (hCG). In rare instances, women may crave bizarre substances such as clay, cornstarch, soap, or even coal.

Oral Cavity

During pregnancy, several changes may occur in the oral cavity. Salivation may seem to increase due to swallowing difficulty associated with nausea. Pregnancy does not predispose to tooth decay or to mobilization of bone calcium.

The gums may become hypertrophic and hyperemic; often, they are so spongy and friable that they bleed easily. This may be due to increased systemic estrogen; similar problems sometimes occur with the use of oral contraceptives. Vitamin C deficiency also can cause tenderness and bleeding of the gums. The gums should return to normal in the early puerperium.

Gastrointestinal Motility

The reduced gastrointestinal motility during pregnancy has been thought to be due to increased circulating levels of progesterone. However, recent evidence suggests that elevated estrogen concentrations mediate the effect by enhancing nitric oxide release from the nonadrenergic noncholinergic nerves that modulate gastrointestinal motility. Gastric emptying has generally been considered to be slowed during pregnancy; however, via indirect methods some researchers have shown no changes in gastric emptying rates in women in the first or second trimesters or at term. Transit time of food through the gastrointestinal tract may be slowed so much that more water than normal is reabsorbed, leading to constipation.

Stomach & Esophagus

Gastric production of hydrochloric acid is variable and sometimes exaggerated, especially during the first trimester. More commonly, gastric acidity is reduced. Production of the hormone gastrin increases significantly, resulting in increased stomach volume and decreased stomach pH. Gastric production of mucus may be increased. Esophageal peristalsis is decreased, and is accompanied by gastric reflux because of the slower emptying time and dilatation or relaxation of the cardiac sphincter. Gastric reflux is more prevalent in later pregnancy due to elevation of the stomach by the enlarged uterus. These conditions may simulate hiatal hernia. Besides leading to heartburn, all of these alterations (increased stomach acidity, slower emptying time, and increased intragastric pressure caused by the enlarged uterus), as well as lying supine, make the use of anesthesia more hazardous because of the increased possibility of regurgitation and aspiration.

Small & Large Bowel & Appendix

As the uterus grows and the stomach is pushed upward, most parts of the large and small bowel move upward and laterally. The appendix is displaced superiorly in the right flank area. These organs return to their normal positions in the early puerperium. As noted previously, gastrointestinal tone and motility are generally decreased.

Gallbladder

Gallbladder function is also altered during pregnancy because of hypotonia of the smooth muscle wall. Emptying time is slowed and emptying often incomplete. Thus at the time of cesarean delivery, the gallbladder often appears dilated and atonic. Bile can become thick, and bile stasis may lead to gallstone formation. The chemical composition of bile is not appreciably altered. Plasma cholinesterase activity is decreased during normal pregnancy.

Liver

There are no apparent morphologic changes in the liver during normal pregnancy, but there are functional alterations. Serum alkaline phosphatase activity can double, probably because of increased placental alkaline phosphatase isozymes. There is also a decrease in plasma albumin and a slight decrease in plasma globulins. Thus a decrease in the albumin:globulin ratio normally occurs in pregnancy. In nonpregnant patients, such a decrease could be an indication of liver disease.

KIDNEYS & URINARY TRACT

Renal Dilatation

During pregnancy, each kidney increases in length by 1–1.5 cm, with a concomitant increase in weight. The renal pelvis is dilated up to 60 mL (10 mL is the normal volume in nonpregnant women). The ureters are dilated above the brim of the bony pelvis, more so on the right side than on the left. The ureters also elongate, widen, and become more curved, although kinking is rare. Thus there is an increase in urinary stasis. As much as 200 mL of residual urine may be present in the dilated collecting system.

Although the cause of hydronephrosis and hydroureter in pregnancy is not known beyond doubt, there may be several contributing factors: (1) Elevated progesterone levels may contribute to hypotonia of smooth muscle in the ureter. However, high progesterone levels do not cause hydroureter in nonpregnant women. (2) The ovarian vein complex in the suspensory (infundibulopelvic) ligament of the ovary may enlarge enough to compress the ureter at the brim of the bony pelvis, thus causing dilatation above that level. (3) Dextrorotation of the uterus during pregnancy may explain why the right ureter is usually dilated more than the left. (4) Hyperplasia of smooth muscle in the distal

one-third of the ureter may cause reduction in luminal size, leading to dilatation in the upper two-thirds. Whatever the cause of dilatation, the effect is stasis of urine. This may lead to infection and may make tests of renal function difficult to interpret.

Renal Function

The changes in renal function that occur during pregnancy are probably due to increased maternal and placental hormones, including adrenocorticotropic hormone (ACTH), antidiuretic hormone (ADH), aldosterone, cortisol, human chorionic somatomammotropin (hCS), and thyroid hormone. An additional factor is the increase in plasma volume. The glomerular filtration rate (GFR) increases during pregnancy by about 50%; the increase begins early in pregnancy, and levels remain relatively high until term, with normal values returning by 20 weeks postpartum. The renal plasma flow (RPF) rate increases by as much as 25–50% throughout early and mid pregnancy (Table 7–1). Differences exist in observations of RPF in late pregnancy. One researcher suggested that the maximum rate of RPF occurs by the end of the second trimester, with the rate remaining constant until term. Posture has little effect on the rate. Urinary flow and sodium excretion rates in late pregnancy can be altered by posture, being twice as great in the lateral recumbent position as in the supine position. Thus posture must be taken into account whenever measurements of urinary function are taken. Collection periods should be at

Table 7–1. Changes in kidney function during pregnancy.[1]

Time	Renal Plasma Flow (mL/min)	Glomerular Filtration Rate (mL/min)
Pregnancy		
13 weeks	805	161
20.8 weeks	749	157
38 weeks	589	146
Postpartum		
20 weeks	491	100
80 weeks	549	97

[1]Reproduced, with permission, from Sims EAH, Krantz KE: Serial studies of renal function during pregnancy and the puerperium in normal women. *J Clin Invest* 1958;37:1764. Copyright permission from the American Society for Clinical Investigation. Tabulation from Danforth DN (editor): Page 334 in: *Obstetrics and Gynecology,* 4th ed. Harper & Row, 1982.

least 12–24 hours to allow for errors caused by the greatly dilated areas of the urinary tract.

At rest, 20% of the cardiac output is delivered to the kidneys. As much as 80% of the filtrate is resorbed by the proximal tubules independent of hormonal control. If this were not so, urine volume would be approximately 150 L/d. Aldosterone regulates sodium resorption in the distal tubules, and arginine vasopressin activity determines the ultimate urine concentration. Even though the GFR increases dramatically during pregnancy, the volume of urine passed each day is not increased. Thus the urinary system appears to be even more efficient during pregnancy.

With the increase in GFR, there is an increase in endogenous clearance of creatinine; the peak increase at 50% above nonpregnant levels occurs at about 32 weeks' gestation, after which creatinine clearance decreases as term approaches. The concentration of creatinine in serum is reduced in proportion to the increase in GFR, and the concentration of blood urea nitrogen is similarly reduced. A nonpregnant woman excretes an average of 0.7–1 g/24 h of creatinine. In pregnant women, serum creatinine is 0.46 ± 0.13 mg/100 mL (nonpregnant values, 0.67 ± 0.14 mg/100 mL). Blood urea nitrogen is also reduced in pregnancy (8.17 ± 1.5 mg/100 mL; nonpregnant values, 13 ± 3 mg/100 mL).

Glucosuria during pregnancy is not necessarily abnormal; glucose is excreted in the urine at some point during pregnancy in more than 50% of women. Glucosuria may be explained by the increase in GFR with impairment of tubular resorption capacity for filtered glucose. Glucose is excreted in varying amounts and in a random pattern unrelated to blood glucose levels. Glucosuria during pregnancy, though common, should be monitored closely because it may also be a sign of diabetes mellitus. Increased levels of urinary glucose also contribute to increased susceptibility of pregnant women to urinary tract infection. For unknown reasons, normal pregnant women demonstrate increased loss of nutrients in the urine (eg, amino acids, water-soluble vitamins).

Proteinuria changes little during pregnancy; 200–300 mg/24 h of protein is normally excreted. A loss of more than 300 mg/24 h suggests a disease process.

Levels of the enzyme renin, which is produced in the kidney, increase early in the first trimester, and continue to rise until term. This enzyme acts on its substrate angiotensinogen, which is formed in the liver, to first form angiotensin I and then angiotensin II, which acts as a vasoconstrictor. Levels of angiotensin I and angiotensin II also increase, but the vasoconstriction that might be expected does not occur, and there is no subsequent rise in blood pressure. Normal pregnant

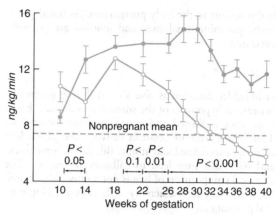

Figure 7–1. Comparison of mean angiotensin II doses required to evoke a pressor response in 120 primigravidas who remained normotensive (●) and 72 primigravidas who ultimately developed preeclampsia (O). (Reproduced, with permission, from Gant NF et al: A prospective study of angiotensin II pressor response throughout primigravid pregnancy. J Clin Invest 1973; 52:2682. Copyright permission from the American Society for Clinical Investigation.)

women are resistant to the pressor effect of elevated levels of angiotensin II (Fig 7–1), which appears to be mediated by increased synthesis of nitric oxide. Angiotensin II is also a major stimulus for adrenocortical secretion of aldosterone, which in conjunction with arginine vasopressin, encourages salt and water retention in pregnancy.

Bladder

As the uterus enlarges, the urinary bladder is displaced upward and flattened in the anteroposterior diameter. Pressure from the uterus leads to increased urinary frequency. Bladder vascularity increases and muscle tone decreases, increasing capacity up to 1500 mL.

HEMATOLOGIC SYSTEM

Blood Volume

Perhaps the most striking maternal physiologic alteration occurring during pregnancy is the increase in blood volume. The magnitude of the increase varies according to the size of the woman, the number of pregnancies she has had, the number of infants she has delivered, and the number of fetuses (one or multiple). A small woman may have an increase in blood volume of only 20%, whereas a large woman may have an increase of 100%. The increase progresses until term (Fig 7–2);

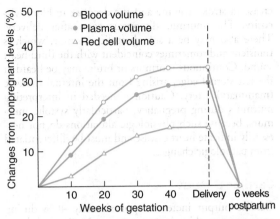

Figure 7–2. Changes in total blood volume, plasma volume, and red cell volume during pregnancy and the postpartum period. Graph constructed from several reports in the literature. (Reproduced, with permission, from Peck TM, Arias F: Hematologic changes associated with pregnancy. Clin Obstet Gynecol 1979; 22:785.)

the average increase in volume at term is 45–50%. Hypervolemia begins in the first trimester, increases rapidly in the second trimester, and plateaus at about the 30th week; some studies have demonstrated a slight decline in the last 10 weeks of gestation.

The mechanisms responsible for increased blood volume are not completely understood. Aldosterone, which is elevated during pregnancy, may contribute to this effect, as may elevated levels of estrogen and progesterone. The increase is needed for extra blood flow to the uterus, extra metabolic needs of the fetus, and increased perfusion of other organs, especially the kidneys. There is also extra blood flow to the skin, allowing dissipation of heat caused by the increased metabolic rate. Extra volume also compensates for maternal blood loss at delivery. The average blood loss with vaginal delivery is 500–600 mL, and with cesarean section 1000 mL.

A. Red Blood Cells

The increase in red blood cell mass is about 33%, or approximately 450 mL of erythrocytes. Erythrocyte volume increases steadily whether or not iron supplementation is given, but the increase is greater with supplementation. Since plasma volume increases earlier in pregnancy and faster than red blood cell volume, the hematocrit falls until the end of the second trimester, when the increase in red blood cells is synchronized with the plasma volume increase. The hematocrit then stabilizes or may increase slightly near term.

B. Iron

With the increase in red blood cells, the need for iron for the production of hemoglobin naturally increases. If supplemental iron is not added to the diet, **iron deficiency anemia** will result (see Chapter 22). Maternal requirements can reach 6–7 mg/d in the latter half of pregnancy. If iron is not readily available, the fetus uses iron from maternal stores. Thus, the production of fetal hemoglobin is usually adequate even if the mother is severely iron-deficient. Therefore, anemia in the newborn is rarely a problem; instead, maternal iron deficiency more commonly may cause preterm labor and late spontaneous abortion, increasing the incidence of infant wastage and morbidity.

C. White Blood Cells

The total blood leukocyte count increases during normal pregnancy from a prepregnancy level of 4300–4500/μL to 5000–12,000/μL in the last trimester, although counts as high as 16,000/μL have been observed in the last trimester. Counts as high as 25,000–30,000/μL have been noted in normal patients during labor. The cause of the rise in the leukocyte count, which primarily involves the polymorphonuclear forms, has not been established, although it seems likely to be caused by increased demargination of white cells. Studies by some researchers indicate an impairment in polymorphonuclear leukocyte chemotaxis that appears to be a cell-associated defect. Pregnant women in the third trimester demonstrated a decrease in polymorphonuclear leukocyte adherence. These results may explain the increased incidence of infection in pregnant women that has been reported by other investigators. Basophils decrease slightly. There is controversy about whether eosinophil numbers increase, decrease, or remain the same as pregnancy advances. There is no apparent explanation for these discrepancies. Levels are only ±2–3% from normal prepregnancy levels.

D. Platelets

Some studies have reported an apparent increase in the production of platelets (thrombocytopoiesis) during pregnancy that is accompanied by progressive platelet consumption. Levels of prostacyclin (PGI_2), a platelet aggregation inhibitor, and thromboxane A_2, an inducer of platelet aggregation and a vasoconstrictor, both increase during pregnancy.

E. Clotting Factors

During pregnancy, levels of several essential coagulation factors increase. There are marked increases in fibrinogen (factor I) and factor VIII. Factors VII, IX, X, and XII also increase but to a lesser extent.

Plasma fibrinogen concentrations begin to increase from normal, nonpregnant levels (1.5–4.5 g/L) during the third month of pregnancy and progressively rise until late pregnancy (4–6.5 g/L). Indeed, with the increase in plasma volume, circulating fibrinogen levels toward the end of pregnancy approach twice those of the nonpregnant state. Fibrinogen synthesis may be increased because of its utilization in the uteroplacental circulation, or it may be the result of hormonal changes, particularly high levels of estrogen.

Prothrombin (factor II) is only slightly affected by pregnancy, if at all. Some investigators have noted small increases; others have reported normal values. Recent studies have also noted mild increases in factor V, and suggest a thrombinlike influence on the activity of factor V. Factor XI decreases slightly toward the end of pregnancy, and factor XIII (fibrin-stabilizing factor) is appreciably reduced, up to 50% at term.

Fibrinolytic activity is depressed during pregnancy and labor, although the precise mechanism is unknown. The placenta may be partially responsible for this alteration in fibrinolytic status. Plasminogen levels increase concomitantly with fibrinogen levels, causing an equilibration of clotting and lysing activity.

Clearly, coagulation and fibrinolytic systems undergo major alterations during pregnancy. Understanding these physiologic changes is necessary to manage two of the more serious problems of pregnancy—hemorrhage and thromboembolic disease—both caused by disorders in the mechanism of hemostasis (see Chapter 59).

CARDIOVASCULAR SYSTEM

Position & Size of Heart

As the uterus enlarges and the diaphragm becomes elevated, the heart is displaced upward and somewhat to the left with rotation on its long axis, so that the apex beat is moved laterally. Cardiac capacity increases by 70–80 mL; this may be due to increased volume or to hypertrophy of cardiac muscle. The size of the heart appears to increase by about 12%.

Heart Rhythms & Murmurs

With the anatomic changes in the heart, there may also be alterations in heart rhythm and electrocardiographic findings, and nonpathologic murmurs may occur. Electrocardiographic changes are probably due to the change in position of the heart and may include a 15- to 20-degree shift to the left in the electrical axis. There may be reversible ST, T, and Q wave changes. The first heart sound may be split, with increased loudness of both portions, and the third heart sound may also be louder. As many as 90% of pregnant women may have a late systolic or ejection murmur attributable to the increase in stroke volume and the decrease in blood viscosity. This murmur disappears soon after delivery. There also may be a soft diastolic murmur, which is transient and sometimes coincident with the third heart sound. Continuous murmurs or bruits may be heard at the left sternal edge, arising from the internal thoracic (mammary) artery. Caution is needed in interpreting murmurs during pregnancy, particularly systolic murmurs, because such physiologic alterations do not necessarily indicate heart disease and must be differentiated from pathologic changes.

Cardiac Output

Cardiac output increases approximately 40% during pregnancy, reaching its maximum at 20–24 weeks' gestation and continuing at this level until term. The increase in output can be as much as 1.5 L/min over the nonpregnant level. Cardiac output is very sensitive to changes in body position. This sensitivity increases with lengthening gestation, presumably because the uterus impinges upon the inferior vena cava, thereby decreasing blood return to the heart.

Cardiac output is the product of **stroke volume** and **heart rate.** In early pregnancy, increased stroke volume accounts for nearly all of the increase in cardiac output. The heart rate increases with lengthening gestation and by term is 15 beats/min higher than the nonpregnant rate. The heart rate is variable and can be affected by exercise, emotional stress, or heat.

Stroke volume increases 25–30% during pregnancy, reaching its maximum at 12–24 weeks' gestation. Stroke volume is very sensitive to positional alterations. For example, in the supine position stroke volume decreases after 20 weeks, reaching normal, nonpregnant levels by term; in the lateral recumbent position, stroke volume remains the same from 19 weeks' gestation until term.

Blood Pressure

Systemic blood pressure declines slightly during pregnancy. There is little change in systolic blood pressure, but diastolic pressure is reduced (5–10 mm Hg) from about 12–26 weeks. Diastolic pressure increases thereafter to prepregnancy levels by about 36 weeks.

Venous pressure in the upper body is basically unchanged during pregnancy, but pressure increases significantly in the lower extremities as pregnancy progresses, particularly when the patient is supine, sitting, or standing. The compression of the inferior vena cava by the uterus and the pressure of the fetal presenting part on the common iliac veins can result in decreased blood return to the heart. This decreases cardiac output, leads to a fall in blood pressure, and causes edema in the lower extremities. The elevated venous pressure returns to near normal if the woman lies in the lateral recumbent position. Venous pressure also falls immediately following cesarean delivery.

Peripheral Resistance

Peripheral vascular resistance equals systemic arterial pressure minus venous pressure divided by cardiac output. Pregnancy-induced changes in maternal arterial pressure (decreased or unchanged) and cardiac output (increased) contribute to the approximately 20% reduction in maternal systemic vascular resistance.

Blood Flow

As in the kidneys, blood flow to the uterus and breasts increases during gestation, but the amount of increase depends on the stage of gestation (Fig 7–3). The increase in uterine blood flow is probably about 500 mL/min but may be as high as 700–800 mL/min. The uterus and placenta have increased blood flow because their vascular resistance is lower than that of the systemic circulation.

Renal blood flow increases approximately 400 mL/min above nonpregnant levels, and blood flow to the breasts increases approximately 200 mL/min. Blood flow to the skin also increases, particularly in the feet and hands. Heat produced by increased maternal metabolism and heat produced by the fetus are dissipated via increased blood flow to the skin.

Physical exercise, which diverts blood flow to large muscles, has the potential to decrease uteroplacental perfusion and thus O_2 delivery to the fetus. This concern mainly applies to unconditioned women who begin a vigorous exercise program while pregnant. Such

women should confine themselves to exercise no more strenuous than walking. Well-conditioned pregnant women generally are able to continue their exercise routines (eg, aerobics, running) if their pregnancy is uncomplicated, and such exercise may even enhance early neonatal behavior.

Effects of Labor on the Cardiovascular System

When a patient is in the supine position, uterine contractions can cause a 25% increase in maternal cardiac output, a 15% decrease in heart rate, and a resultant 33% increase in stroke volume. However, when the laboring patient is in the lateral recumbent position, the hemodynamic parameters stabilize, with only a 7.6% increase in cardiac output, a 0.7% decrease in heart rate, and a 7.7% increase in stroke volume. These significant differences are attributable to inferior vena caval occlusion caused by the gravid uterus. During contractions, pulse pressure increases 26% in the supine position but only 6% in the lateral recumbent position. Central venous pressure increases in direct relationship to the intensity of uterine contraction and increased intra-abdominal pressure. Additionally, cardiopulmonary blood volume increases 300–500 mL during contractions. At the time of delivery, hemodynamic alterations vary with the method of anesthesia used (see Chapter 26).

PULMONARY SYSTEM

Anatomic & Physiologic Changes

Pregnancy produces anatomic and physiologic changes that affect respiratory performance. Early in pregnancy, capillary dilatation occurs throughout the respiratory tract, leading to engorgement of the nasopharynx, larynx, trachea, and bronchi, which can make breathing difficult. Chest x-rays reveal increased vascular markings in the lungs.

As the uterus enlarges, the diaphragm is elevated as much as 4 cm, and the rib cage is displaced upward and widens, increasing the lower thoracic diameter by 2 cm and the thoracic circumference by up to 6 cm. Elevation of the diaphragm does not impede its movement. Abdominal muscles have less tone and are less active during pregnancy, causing respiration to be more diaphragmatic.

Lung Volumes & Capacities

In respiration physiology, there are 4 defined lung "volumes" and 4 "capacities." The 4 volumes do not overlap. They are defined as follows: **Tidal volume** is the volume of gas inspired or expired during each respira-

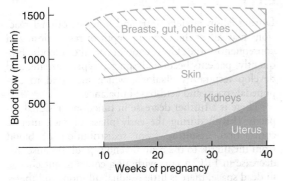

Figure 7–3. The distribution of cardiac output during pregnancy. (Reproduced, with permission, from Hytten FE, Leitch I: *The Physiology of Human Pregnancy.* Blackwell, 1964.)

tion. It varies with body requirements, but the term usually refers to quiet respiration at rest. The position of the chest at the end of quiet expiration is known as the end-expiratory position. **Inspiratory reserve volume** is the maximum amount of air that can be inspired beyond normal tidal inspiration. **Expiratory reserve volume** is the maximum amount of air that can be expired from the resting end-expiratory position. **Residual volume** is the volume of gas remaining in the lungs at the end of maximal expiration.

The 4 "capacities" each include 2 or more of the "volumes" defined above. **Total lung capacity** includes them all; it is the total amount of gas in the lung at the end of maximum inspiration. **Vital capacity** includes all but residual volume; it is the maximum volume of gas that can be expired after a maximum inspiration. **Inspiratory capacity** is tidal volume plus inspiratory reserve volume; it is the maximum volume of gas that can be inspired from the resting end-expiratory position. **Functional residual capacity** is expiratory reserve volume plus residual volume; it is the amount of gas remaining in the lungs at the resting end-expiratory position and the volume of gas with which the tidal air must mix.

Alterations occurring in lung volumes and capacities during pregnancy include the following (Fig 7–4). Dead space volume increases due to relaxation of the musculature of conducting airways. Tidal volume increases gradually (35–50%) as pregnancy progresses. Total lung capacity is reduced (4–5%) by the elevation of the diaphragm. Functional residual capacity, residual volume, and expiratory reserve volume all decrease by about 20%. Larger tidal volume and smaller residual volume cause increased alveolar ventilation (about 65%) during pregnancy. Inspiratory capacity increases 5–10%, reaching a maximum at 22–24 weeks' gestation.

Functional respiratory changes include a slight increase in respiratory rate, a 50% increase in minute ventilation, a 40% increase in tidal volume, and a progressive increase in oxygen consumption of up to 15–20% above nonpregnant levels by term. The increase in oxygen consumption is caused by the increased metabolic needs of the mother (cardiac and respiratory muscles) and fetus (Fig 7–5).

With the increase in respiratory tidal volume associated with a normal respiratory rate, there is an increase in respiratory minute volume of approximately 26%. As the respiratory minute volume increases, **hyperventilation of pregnancy** occurs, causing a decrease in alveolar CO_2. This decrease lowers the maternal blood CO_2 tension; however, alveolar oxygen tension is maintained within normal limits. Maternal hyperventilation is probably due to the action of progesterone on brain neurons that regulate respiration. Maternal hyperventi-

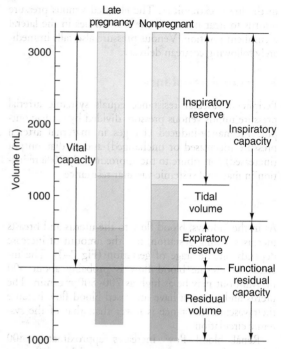

Figure 7–4. The components of lung volume in late pregnancy compared with those in nonpregnant women. (Reproduced, with permission, from Hytten FE, Leitch I: *The Physiology of Human Pregnancy.* Blackwell, 1964.)

lation is considered a protective measure that prevents the fetus from being exposed to excessive levels of CO_2.

Effects of Labor on the Pulmonary System[*]

During labor, anxiety, fear, and other emotional reactions may affect the rate and depth of respiration, and consequently the CO_2 content of the blood. Frequently, patients become dyspneic, hyperventilate, and develop respiratory alkalosis, which may lead to carpopedal spasm and acid-base imbalance.

There is a further decrease in functional residual capacity (FRC) during the early phase of each uterine contraction, resulting from redistribution of blood from the uterus to the central venous pool. Because this decrease in FRC occurs without a concomitant change in dead space, there is little residual dilution, and therefore presumably more efficient gas exchange. Adminis-

---

[*] This section is contributed by Martin L. Pernoll, MD.

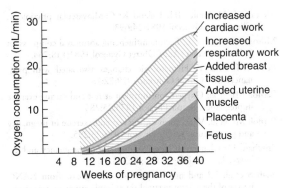

Figure 7–5. Components of increased oxygen consumption during pregnancy. (Reproduced, with permission, from Hytten FE, Leitch I: *The Physiology of Human Pregnancy.* Blackwell, 1964.)

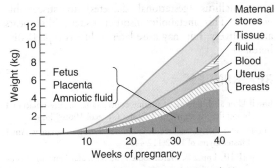

Figure 7–6. Components of weight gain during pregnancy. (Reproduced, with permission, from Hytten FE, Leitch I: *The Physiology of Human Pregnancy.* Blackwell, 1964.)

tration of anesthesia must be adjusted accordingly, because of the more rapid changes in the concentration of gas in the lungs. Oxygen saturation decreases with each contraction and then returns to precontraction levels. During labor, the increase in ventilation, decrease in FRC, and increase in cardiac output significantly influence the induction of and emergence from inhalation anesthesia. The increase in cardiac output increases the uptake of soluble anesthetics by the blood and retards the rate at which alveolar concentration approaches inspired concentration, which delays the induction of anesthesia.

METABOLISM

As the fetus and placenta grow and place increasing demands on the mother, phenomenal alterations in metabolism occur. The most obvious physical changes are weight gain and altered body shape. Weight gain is due not only to the uterus and its contents but also to increased breast tissue, blood volume, and water volume (about 6.8 L) in the form of extravascular and extracellular fluid. Deposition of fat and protein and increased cellular water are added to maternal stores. The average weight gain during pregnancy is 12.5 kg (27.5 lb). Distribution of weight gain is shown in Fig 7–6 and distribution of extracellular and intracellular water in Table 7–2.

During normal pregnancy, approximately 1000 g of the weight gain is attributable to protein. Half of this is found in the fetus and the placenta, with the rest being distributed as uterine contractile protein, breast glandular tissue, plasma protein, and hemoglobin. Plasma albumin levels are decreased and fibrinogen levels increased.

Total body fat increases during pregnancy, but the amount varies with the total weight gain. During the second half of pregnancy, plasma lipids increase (plasma cholesterol increases 50%, plasma triglyceride concentration may triple), but triglycerides, cholesterol, and lipoproteins decrease soon after delivery. The ratio of low-density lipoproteins (LDLs) to high-density lipoproteins (HDLs) increases during pregnancy. It has been suggested that most fat is stored centrally during midpregnancy and that as the fetus demands more nutrition in the latter months, fat storage decreases.

Metabolism of carbohydrates and insulin during pregnancy is discussed in Chapter 18. Pregnancy is associated with insulin resistance which can lead to dia-

Table 7–2. Estimate of extracellular and intracellular water added during pregnancy.[1]

	Total Water (mL)	Extracellular (mL)	Intracellular (mL)
Fetus	2343	1360	983
Placenta	540	260	280
Amniotic fluid	792	792	…
Uterus	743	490	253
Mammary glands	304	148	156
Plasma	920	920	…
Red cells	163	…	163
Extracellular, extra-vascular water	1195	1195	…
Total	7000	5165	1835

[1]Reproduced, with permission, from Hytten FE, Leitch I: *The Physiology of Human Pregnancy.* Blackwell, 1964.

betes mellitus (gestational diabetes) in susceptible women. This metabolic disorder usually disappears after delivery, but may arise later in life as type II diabetes.

REFERENCES

Borell U et al: Influence of uterine contractions on uteroplacental blood flow at term. Am J Obstet Gynecol 1965;93:44.

Chesley LC: Plasma and red cell volumes during pregnancy. Am J Obstet Gynecol 1972;112:440.

Clapp JF III, Lopez B, Harcar-Sevcik R: Neonatal behavioral profile of the offspring of women who continue to exercise regularly throughout pregnancy. Am J Obstet Gynecol 1999;180:91.

Fainstat T: Ureteral dilation in pregnancy: A review. Obstet Gynecol Surv 1963;18:845.

Gant NF et al: A prospective study of angiotensin II pressor response throughout primigravid pregnancy. J Clin Invest 1973;52:2682.

Gibbs CP: Maternal physiology. Clin Obstet Gynecol 1981;24:525.

Metcalfe J, McAnulty JH, Ueland K: Cardiovascular physiology. Clin Obstet Gynecol 1981;24:693.

Milsom I, Forssman L: Factors influencing aortocaval compression in late pregnancy. Am J Obstet Gynecol 1984;148:764.

Peck TM, Arias F: Hematologic changes associated with pregnancy. Clin Obstet Gynecol 1979;22:785.

Pernoll ML et al: Oxygen consumption at rest and during exercise in pregnancy. Respir Physiol 1975;25:285.

Pernoll ML et al: Ventilation during rest and exercise in pregnancy and postpartum. Respir Physiol 1975;25:295.

Pritchard JA: Changes in blood volume during pregnancy and delivery. Anesthesiology 1965;26:393.

Shah S et al: E2 and not P4 increases NO release from NANC nerves of the gastrointestinal tract: implications in pregnancy. Am J Physiol 2001;280:R1546.

Sims EAH, Krantz KE: Serial studies of renal function during pregnancy and the puerperium in normal women. J Clin Invest 1985;37:1764.

Tygart SG et al: Longitudinal study of platelet indices during pregnancy. Am J Obstet Gynecol 1986;154:883.

Maternal-Placental-Fetal Unit; Fetal & Early Neonatal Physiology

Donelle Laughlin, MD, & Robert A. Knuppel, MD, MPH

Fetal genetics, physiology, anatomy, and biochemistry can now be studied with the use of ultrasonography, fetoscopy, chorionic villus sampling, amniocentesis, and fetal cord and scalp blood sampling. Embryology and fetoplacental physiology must now be considered when providing direct patient care.

■ THE PLACENTA

A **placenta** may be defined as any intimate apposition or fusion of fetal organs to maternal tissues for the purpose of physiologic exchange. The basic parenchyma of all placentas is the **trophoblast;** when this becomes a membrane penetrated by fetal **mesoderm,** it is called the **chorion.**

In the evolution of viviparous species, the yolk sac presumably is the most archaic type of placentation, having developed from the egg-laying ancestors of mammals. In higher mammals, the **allantoic sac** fuses with the chorion, forming the chorioallantoic placenta, which has mesodermal vascular villi. When the trophoblast actually invades the maternal endometrium (which in pregnancy is largely composed of decidua), a deciduate placenta results. In humans, maternal blood comes into direct contact with the fetal trophoblast. Thus, the human placenta may be described as a discoid, deciduate, hemochorial chorioallantoic placenta.

DEVELOPMENT OF THE PLACENTA

Soon after ovulation, the endometrium develops its typical secretory pattern under the influence of progesterone from the corpus luteum. The peak of development occurs at about 1 week after ovulation, coinciding with the expected time for implantation of a fertilized ovum.

Pregnancy occurs when healthy spermatozoa in adequate numbers penetrate receptive cervical mucus, ascend through a patent uterotubal tract, and fertilize a healthy ovum within about 24 hours following ovulation. The spermatozoa that penetrate favorable mucus travel through the uterine cavity and the uterine tubes

at a rate of about 6 mm/min. During this transit, an enzymatic change occurs that renders the spermatozoa capable of fertilizing the ovum. This process is called **capacitation.** The cellular union between the sperm and the egg is referred to as **syngamy.** The tip of the sperm head (**acrosome**) loses its cell membrane and probably releases a lytic enzyme that facilitates penetration of the zona pellucida surrounding the ovum.

Once the sperm head containing all of the paternal genetic material enters the cytoplasm of the ovum, a **zona reaction** occurs that prevents the entrance of a second sperm. The first cleavage occurs during the next 36 hours. As the conceptus continues to divide and grow, the peristaltic activity of the uterine tube slowly transports it to the uterus, a journey that requires 6–7 days. Concomitantly, a series of divisions creates a hollow ball, the **blastocyst,** which then implants within the endometrium. Most cells in the wall of the blastocyst are trophoblastic; only a few are destined to become the embryo.

Within a few hours after implantation, the trophoblast invades the endometrium and begins to produce **human chorionic gonadotropin** (**hCG**) which is thought to be important in converting the normal corpus luteum into the corpus luteum of pregnancy. As the cytotrophoblasts (**Langhans' cells**) divide and proliferate, they form transitional cells that are ultrastructurally more mature and a likely source of hCG. Next, these transitional cells fuse, lose their individual membranes, and form the multinucleated **syncytiotrophoblast.** Mitotic division then ceases. Thus, the syncytial layer becomes the front line of the invading fetal tissue. Maternal capillaries and venules are tapped by the invading fetal tissue to cause extravasation of maternal blood and the formation of small lakes (lacunae), the forerunners of the intervillous space. These lacunae fill with maternal blood by reflux from previously tapped veins. An occasional maternal artery then opens, and a sluggish circulation is established (hematotropic phase of the embryo).

The lacunar system is separated by trabeculae, many of which develop buds or extensions. Within these branching projections, the cytotrophoblast forms a mesenchymal core.

The proliferating trophoblast cells then branch to form secondary and tertiary villi. The **mesoblast,** or central stromal core, also formed from the original trophoblast, invades these columns to form a supportive structure within which capillaries are formed. The **embryonic body stalk** (later to become the umbilical cord) invades this stromal core to establish the fetoplacental circulation. If this last step does not occur, the embryo will die. Sensitive tests for hCG suggest that at this stage, more embryos die than live.

Where the placenta is attached, the branching villi resemble a leafy tree (the **chorion frondosum**), whereas that portion of the placenta covering the expanding conceptus is smoother (**chorion laeve**). When the latter is finally pushed against the opposite wall of the uterus, the villi atrophy, leaving the amnion and chorion to form the 2-layered sac of fetal membranes (Fig 8–1).

About 40 days after conception, the trophoblast has invaded approximately 40–60 spiral arterioles, of which 12–15 may be called major arteries. The pulsatile arterial pressure of blood that spurts from each of these major vessels pushes the chorionic plate away from the decidua to form 12–15 "tents," or maternal **cotyledons.** The remaining 24–45 tapped arterioles form minor vascular units that become crowded between the larger units. As the chorionic plate is pushed away from the basal plate, the anchoring villi pull the maternal

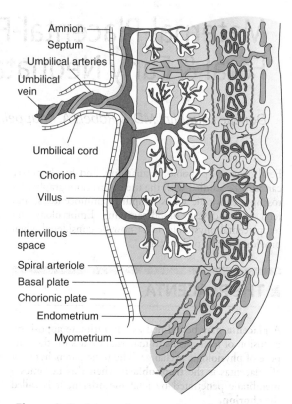

Figure 8–2. Schematic cross section of the circulation of the mature placenta. (Reproduced, with permission, from Benson RC: *Handbook of Obstetrics & Gynecology,* 8th ed. Lange, 1983.)

basal plate up into septa (columns of fibrous tissue that virtually surround the major cotyledons). Thus, at the center of each maternal vascular unit there is one artery that terminates in a thin-walled sac, but there are numerous maternal veins that open through the basal plate at random. The human placenta has no peripheral venous collecting system. Within each maternal vascular unit is the fetal vascular "tree," with the tertiary free-floating villi (the major area for physiologic exchange) acting as thousands of baffles that disperse the maternal bloodstream in many directions. A cross-sectional diagram of the mature placenta is shown in Fig 8–2.

Table 8–1 summarizes the major morphologic-functional correlations that take place during placental development.

FUNCTIONS OF THE MATERNAL-PLACENTAL-FETAL UNIT

The placenta is a complex organ of internal secretion, releasing numerous hormones and enzymes into the

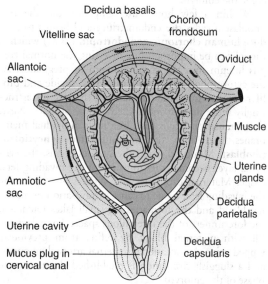

Figure 8–1. Relationships of structures in the uterus at the end of the seventh week of pregnancy. (Reproduced, with permission, from Benson RC: *Handbook of Obstetrics & Gynecology,* 8th ed. Lange, 1983.)

Table 8–1. Development of the human placenta.[1]

Days After Ovulation	Important Morphologic-Functional Correlations
6–7	Implantation of blastocyst.
7–8	Trophoblast proliferation and invasion. Cytotrophoblast gives rise to syncytium.
9–11	Lacunar period. Endometrial venules and capillaries tapped. Sluggish circulation of maternal blood.
13–18	Primary and secondary villi form; body stalk and amnion form.
18–21	Tertiary villi, 2–3 mm long, 0.4 mm thick. Mesoblast invades villi, forming a core. Capillaries form in situ and tap umbilical vessels, which spread through blastoderm. Fetoplacental circulation established. Sluggish lacunar circulation.
21–40	Chorion frondosum; multiple anchored villi, which form free villi shaped like "inverted trees." Chorionic plate forms.
40–50	Cotyledon formation: (1) Cavitation. Trophoblast invasion opens 40–60 spiral arterioles. Further invasion stops. Spurts of arterial blood form localized hollows in chorion frondosum. Maternal circulation established. (2) Crowning and extension. Cavitation causes concentric orientation of anchoring villi around each arterial spurt, separating chorionic plate from basal plate. (3) Completion. Main supplying fetal vessels for groups of second-order vessels are pulled from the chorioallantoic mesenchyme to form first-order vessels of fetal cotyledons. (4) About 150 rudimentary cotyledons with anchoring villi remain, but without cavitation and crowning ("tent formation"). Sluggish, low-pressure (5–8 mm Hg) flow of maternal blood around them.
80–225	Continued growth of definitive placenta. Ten to 12 large cotyledons form, with high maternal blood pressures (40–60 mm Hg) in the central intervillous spaces; 40–50 small to medium-sized cotyledons and about 150 rudimentary ones are delineated. Basal plate pulled up between major cotyledons by anchoring villi to form septa.
225–267 (term)	Cellular proliferation ceases, but cellular hypertrophy continues.

[1]Adapted from Reynolds SRM: Formation of fetal cotyledons in the hemichorial placenta. Am J Obstet Gynecol 1966;94:425. (Reproduced, with permission, from Page EW, Villee CA, Villee DB: *Human Reproduction.* Saunders, 1976.)

maternal bloodstream. In addition, it serves as the organ of transport for all fetal nutrients and metabolic products as well as for the exchange of oxygen and CO_2. Although fetal in origin, the placenta depends almost entirely on maternal blood for its nourishment.

The arterial pressure of maternal blood (60–70 mm Hg) causes it to pulsate toward the chorionic plate into the low-pressure (20 mm Hg) intervillous space. Venous blood in the placenta tends to flow along the basal plate and out through the venules directly into maternal veins. The pressure gradient within the fetal circulation changes slowly with the mother's posture, fetal movements, and physical stress. The pressure within the placental intervillous space is about 10 mm Hg when the pregnant woman is lying down. After a few minutes of standing, this pressure exceeds 30 mm Hg. In comparison, the fetal capillary pressure is 20–40 mm Hg.

Clinically, placental perfusion can be altered by many physiologic changes in the mother or fetus.

When a precipitous fall in maternal blood pressure occurs, increased plasma volume improves placental perfusion. An increased rate of rhythmic uterine contractions benefits placental perfusion, but tetanic labor contractions are detrimental to placental and fetal circulation. An increased fetal heart rate tends to expand the villi during systole, but this is a minor aid in circulatory transfer.

Circulatory Function

A. UTEROPLACENTAL CIRCULATION

The magnitude of the uteroplacental circulation is difficult to measure in humans. The consensus is that total uterine blood flow near term is 500–700 mL/min. Not all of this blood traverses the intervillous space. It is generally assumed that about 85% of the uterine blood flow goes to the cotyledons and the rest to the myometrium and endometrium. One may assume that blood flow in the placenta is 400–500 mL/min in a patient near term who is lying quietly on her side and is not in labor.

As the placenta matures, thrombosis decreases the number of arterial openings into the basal plate. At term, the ratio of veins to arteries is 2:1 (approximately the ratio found in other mature organs).

Near their entry into the intervillous spaces, the terminal maternal arterioles lose their elastic reticulum. Since the distal portions of these vessels are lost with the placenta, bleeding from their source can be controlled only by uterine contraction. Thus, uterine atony causes postpartum hemorrhage.

B. PLASMA VOLUME EXPANSION AND SPIRAL ARTERY CHANGES

Structural alterations occur in the human uterine spiral arteries found in the decidual part of the placental bed. As a consequence of the action of cytotrophoblast on the spiral artery vessel wall, the normal musculoelastic tissue is replaced by a mixture of fibrinoid and fibrous tissue. The small spiral arteries are converted to large tortuous channels, creating low-resistance channels or arteriovenous shunts.

In dogs, when a surgically created arteriovenous shunt is opened, there soon appears a marked increase in plasma volume, cardiac output, and retention of sodium. An apparent anemia occurs, as the red blood cell mass is slower to expand. The reverse happens when the shunt is closed. This situation is similar to that of early normal pregnancy, when there is an early increase in plasma volume and resulting physiologic anemia as the red blood cell mass slowly expands. Immediately after delivery, with closure of the placental shunt, diuresis and natriuresis occur. When the spiral arteries fail to undergo these physiologic changes, fetal growth retardation often occurs with preeclampsia. Campbell (1983) and more recently Voigt and Becker (1992) used gated, pulsed Doppler ultrasound to study the uterine arcuate arteries serving the spiral arteries and placenta in pregnant women. Among the patients who showed evidence of failure of the spiral arteries to dilate and increased vascular resistance, there was subsequently a high frequency of proteinuric hypertension, poor fetal growth, and fetal hypoxia. Voigt and Becker (1992) also noted that Doppler ultrasound profiles correlated well with the histologic findings on subsequent biopsy of the placental bed.

Fleischer and colleagues (1986) reported that normal pregnancy is associated with a uterine artery Doppler velocimetry systolic:diastolic ratio of less than 2:6. With a higher ratio and a notch in the waveform, the pregnancy is usually complicated by stillbirth, premature birth, intrauterine growth retardation, or preeclampsia.

Wells and coworkers (1984) demonstrated that decidual spiral arteries that have been attacked by the cytotrophoblast have a fibrinoid matrix that develops amniotic antigens, apparently to maintain the structural integrity of the vessel wall. Thus, there are histologic and immunologic explanations for the presence or absence of the marked increase in uterine blood flow and plasma volume expansion seen in human pregnancies.

Goodlin and associates (1984) believed that failure of the spiral arteries to dilate and adequately expand plasma volume evokes increased maternal venous reactivity and multiple organ dysfunction. This disorder probably cannot be corrected by medical therapy, but therapy may modify secondary effects.

C. FETOPLACENTAL CIRCULATION

At term, a normal fetus has a total umbilical blood flow of 350–400 mL/min. Thus, the maternoplacental and fetoplacental flows are of a similar order of magnitude.

The villous system is best compared with an inverted tree. The branches pass obliquely downward and outward within the intervillous spaces. This arrangement probably permits preferential currents or gradients of flow and undoubtedly encourages intervillous fibrin deposition, commonly seen in the mature placenta.

Cotyledons (subdivisions of the placenta) can be identified early in placentation. Although they are separated by the placental septa, some communication occurs via the subchorionic lake in the roof of the intervillous spaces.

Prior to labor, placental filling occurs whenever the uterus contracts (*Braxton Hicks contractions*). At these times, the maternal venous exits are closed but the thicker-walled arteries are only slightly narrowed. When the uterus relaxes, blood drains out through the maternal veins. Hence, blood is not squeezed out of the placental lake with each contraction, nor does it enter the placental lake in appreciably greater amounts during relaxation.

During the height of an average first-stage contraction, most of the cotyledons are devoid of any flow and the remainder are only partially filled. Thus, intermittently—for periods of up to a minute—maternoplacental flow virtually ceases. Therefore, it should be evident that any extended prolongation of the contractile phase, as in uterine tetany, could lead to fetal hypoxia.

Maternal Circulation

Aortocaval compression is a common cause of abnormal fetal heart rate during labor. In the third trimester, the contracting uterus obstructs its own blood supply to the level of L3–4 (**Poseiro effect**) when the mother is supine. This obstruction is completely relieved by turning the patient on her side. Although only about 30% of pregnant women will demonstrate aortocaval compression when supine, women in labor (particularly after epidural anesthesia) should not be maintained in a supine position.

In all supine pregnant women at term, obstruction of the inferior vena cava by uterine pressure is relatively complete. However, only about 10% have inadequate collateral circulation (intervertebral venous plexus, lumbar venous plexus, abdominal wall superficial and deep veins, hemorrhoidal plates, vertebral azygous and portal system) and develop **maternal supine hypotension syndrome.** This syndrome is characterized by decreased cardiac output, bradycardia, and hypotension. Relief is obtained when the woman is placed in the lateral position. Most pregnant women near term sleep on their sides instinctively to avoid such problems.

Uterine blood flow and placental perfusion values are directly correlated with the pregnancy-related increase in maternal plasma volume. Relative maternal hypovolemia is found in association with most complications of pregnancy, including preeclampsia, small-for-gestational age (SGA) fetus, premature labor, and various fetal anomalies.

Endocrine Function

A. SECRETIONS OF THE MATERNAL-PLACENTAL-FETAL UNIT

The placenta and the maternal-placental-fetal unit produce increasing amounts of steroids late in the first trimester. Of greatest importance are the steroids required in fetal development from 7 weeks' gestation through parturition. Immediately following conception and until 12–13 weeks' gestation, the principal source of circulating gestational steroids (progesterone is the major one) is the corpus luteum of pregnancy. However, after 42 days, the placenta assumes an increasingly important role in the production of several steroid hormones. Steroid production by the embryo occurs even before implantation is detectable in utero. Prior to implantation, production of progesterone by the embryo may be of importance in ovum transport.

Once implantation occurs, there is secretion of trophoblastic hCG and other pregnancy-related peptides. A more sophisticated array of fetoplacental steroids is produced during organogenesis and with the development of a functioning hypothalamic-pituitary-adrenal axis. Adrenohypophyseal basophilic cells first appear at about 8 weeks in the fetus and indicate the presence of significant quantities of adrenocorticotropic hormone (ACTH). The first adrenal primordial structures are identified at approximately 4 weeks, and the fetal adrenal cortex develops in concert with the adenohypophysis.

The fetus and the placenta acting in concert are the principal steroid regulators controlling intrauterine growth, maturation of vital organs, and parturition.

The fetal adrenal cortex is much larger than its adult counterpart. From midtrimester until term, the large inner mass of the fetal adrenal gland (80% of the adrenal tissue) is known as the **fetal zone.** This tissue is supported by factors unique to the fetal status and regresses rapidly after birth. The outer zone ultimately becomes the bulk of the postnatal and adult cortex.

Trophoblastic mass increases exponentially through the seventh week, after which time the growth velocity gradually increases to an asymptote close to term. The fetal zone and placenta share and exchange steroid precursors to make possible the full complement of fetoplacental steroids. Formation and regulation of steroid hormones also take place within the fetus itself.

In addition to the steroids, another group of placental hormones unique to pregnancy are the polypeptide hormones, each of which has an analogue in the pituitary. These placental protein hormones include hCG and human chorionic somatomammotropin. The existence of placental human chorionic corticotropin also has been suggested.

A summary of the hormones produced by the maternal-placental-fetal unit is shown in Table 8–2.

B. PLACENTAL SECRETIONS

1. Human chorionic gonadotropin—Human chorionic gonadotropin (hCG) was the first of the placental protein hormones to be described. Its molecular weight is 36,000–40,000. It is a glycoprotein that has biologic and immunologic similarities to luteinizing hormone from the pituitary. Recent evidence suggests that hCG is produced by the syncytiotrophoblast of the placenta. hCG is elaborated by all types of trophoblastic tissue, including that of hydatidiform moles, chorioadenoma destruens, and choriocarcinoma. As with all glycoprotein hormones (LH, FSH, TSH), hCG is composed of 2 subunits, alpha and beta. The alpha subunit is common to all glycoproteins, and the beta subunit confers unique specificity to the hormone. Typically, neither subunit is active by itself; only the intact molecule exerts hormonal effects.

Antibodies have been developed to the beta subunit of hCG. This specific reaction allows for differentiation of hCG from pituitary LH. hCG is detectable 9 days after the midcycle LH peak, which occurs 8 days after ovulation and only 1 day after implantation. This measurement is useful because it can detect pregnancy in all patients on day 11 after fertilization. Concentrations of hCG rise exponentially until 9–10 weeks' gestation, with a doubling time of 1.3–2 days. Knowledge of hCG doubling times has important practical applications. Normally, doubling values during early preg-

Table 8–2. Summary of maternal-placental-fetal endocrine-paracrine functions.

Peptides of exclusively placental origin
   Human chorionic gonadotropin (hCG)
   Human chorionic somatomammotropin (hCS)
   Human chorionic corticotropin (hCC)
   SP1—pregnancy specific β-1 glycoprotein
   SP4—pregnancy specific β-1 glycoprotein
   Pregnancy-associated plasma proteins (PAPP)
      PAPP-A
      PAPP-B
      PAPP-C
      PAPP-D (hCS)
   Pregnancy-associated β_1 macroglobulin (β_1 PAM)
   Pregnancy-associated α_2 macroglobulin (α_2 PAM)
   Pregnancy-associated major basic protein (pMBP)
   Placental proteins (PP) 1 through 21
   Placental membrane proteins (MP) 1 through 7.
      MP1 also known as placental alkaline phosphatase
         (PLAP)
   Hypothalamic-like hormone (β-endorphin, ACTH-like)
Steroid of mainly placental origin
   Progesterone
Hormones of maternal-placental-fetal origin
   Estrone
   Estradiol 50% from maternal androgens
Hormone of placental-fetal origin
   Estriol
Hormone of corpus luteum of pregnancy
   Relaxin
Fetal hormones
   Thyroid hormone
   Fetal adrenal zone hormones
   α-Melanocyte-stimulating hormone
   Corticotropin intermediate lobe peptide (CLIP)
   Anterior pituitary hormone
   Adrenocorticotropic hormone (ACTH)
   Tropic hormones for fetal zone of placenta
   β-Endorphin
   β-Lipotropin
   Intermediate pituitary hormones

---

nancy augur well for a successful outcome. Conversely, abnormally slow doubling times are considered a bad prognostic sign indicating an imminent miscarriage or, far worse, an ectopic pregnancy. Concentrations peak at 60–90 days' gestation. Afterwards, hCG levels decrease to a plateau that is maintained until delivery. The half-life of hCG is approximately 32–37 hours, in contrast to that of most protein and steroid hormones, which have half-lives measured in minutes. Structural characteristics of the hCG molecule allow it to interact with the human TSH receptor in activation of the

membrane adenylate cyclase that regulates thyroid cell function. The finding of hCG-specific adenylate stimulation in the placenta may mean that hCG provides "order regulation" within the cell of the trophoblast.

2. Human chorionic somatomammotropin—Human chorionic somatomammotropin (hCS) is a protein hormone with immunologic and biologic similarities to pituitary growth hormone. It has also been designated **human placental lactogen** (**hPL**) and is synthesized in the syncytiotrophoblastic layer of the placenta. It can be found in maternal serum and urine in both normal and molar pregnancies. However, it disappears so rapidly from serum and urine after delivery of the placenta or evacuation of the uterus that it cannot be detected in the serum after the first postpartum day. The somatotropic activity of hCS is 3% or less than that of human growth hormone (hGH). In vitro, hCS stimulates thymidine incorporation into DNA and enhances the action of hGH and insulin. It is present in microgram-per-milliliter quantities in early pregnancy, but its concentration increases as pregnancy progresses, with peak levels reached during the last 4 weeks. Prolonged fasting at midgestation and insulin-induced hypoglycemia are reported to raise hCS concentrations. Amniotic instillation of prostaglandin PGF_2 causes a marked reduction in hCS levels. hCS may exert its major metabolic effect on the mother to ensure that the nutritional demands of the fetus are met.

It has been suggested that hCS is the "growth hormone" of pregnancy. The in vivo effects of hCS owing to its growth hormonelike and anti-insulin characteristics result in impaired glucose uptake and stimulation of free fatty acid release, with resultant decrease in insulin effect. The maternal metabolism appears to be directed toward mobilization of maternal sources to furnish substrate for the fetus.

3. Human chorionic corticotropin—Human chorionic corticotropin (hCC) is another pituitarylike hormone. The physiologic role of hCC and its regulation are unknown.

4. Placental proteins—A number of proteins thought to be specific to the pregnant state have been isolated. The most commonly known are the 4 pregnancy-associated plasma proteins (PAPPs) designated as PAPP-A, PAPP-B, PAPP-C, and PAPP-D. PAPP-D is the hormone hCS (described earlier). All these proteins are produced by the placenta and/or decidua. The physiologic role of these proteins except for PAPP-D are at present unclear. Numerous investigators have postulated various functions ranging from facilitating fetal "allograft" survival and the regulation of coagulation and complement cascades to the maintenance of the placenta and the regulation of carbohydrate metabolism in pregnancy. A host of other pregnancy-specific and pregnancy-associated proteins have since been isolated. The greatest challenge, however, lies in the identification of their function. Such knowledge will provide important insights into placental function and hopefully allow us to understand more completely the pregnant state.

C. Fetoplacental Secretions

The placenta may be an incomplete steroid-producing organ that must rely on precursors reaching it from the fetal and maternal circulations (an integrated maternal-placental-fetal unit). The adult steroid-producing glands can form progestins, androgens, and estrogens, but this is not true of the placenta. Estrogen production by the placenta is dependent upon precursors reaching it from both the fetal and maternal compartments. Placental progesterone formation is accomplished in large part from circulating maternal cholesterol.

In the placenta, cholesterol is converted to pregnenolone and then rapidly and efficiently to progesterone. Production of progesterone approximates 250 mg/d by the end of pregnancy, at which time circulating levels are on the order of 130 mg/mL. To form estrogens, the placenta, which has an active aromatizing capacity, utilizes circulating androgens obtained primarily from the fetus but also from the mother. The major androgenic precursor is **dehydroepiandrosterone sulfate (DHEA-S).**

This compound comes from the fetal adrenal gland. Because the placenta has an abundance of sulfatase (sulfate-cleaving) enzyme, DHEA-S is converted to free unconjugated DHEA when it reaches the placenta, then to androstenedione, testosterone, and finally estrone and 17β-estradiol.

The major estrogen formed in pregnancy is estriol. Ninety percent of the estrogen in the urine of pregnant women is estriol. It is excreted into the urine as sulfate and glucuronide conjugates. Excretion rates increase with advancing gestation, ranging from approximately 2 mg/24 h at 16 weeks to 35–40 mg/24 h at term. Estriol is formed during pregnancy by a unique biosynthetic process that demonstrates the interdependence of the fetus, placenta, and mother. DHEA-S is quantitatively the major steroid produced by the fetal adrenal gland, with most of it being produced in the fetal zone. When DHEA-S of the fetus or mother reaches the placenta, estrone and estradiol are formed. However, little of either is converted to estriol by the placenta; instead, some of the DHEA-S undergoes 16α-hydroxylation, primarily in the fetal liver. When the 16-hydroxydehydroepiandrosterone sulfate (16-OHDHEA-S) reaches the placenta, the placental sulfatase enzyme acts to cleave the sulfate side chain, and the unconjugated 16-OHDHEA-S is aromatized to form estriol. The estriol is then secreted into the maternal circulation. When it reaches the maternal liver, it is conjugated to estriol sulfate and estriol glucosiduronate in a mixed conjugate. These forms are excreted into the maternal urine.

Circulating progesterone and estriol are thought to be important during pregnancy because they are present in such large amounts. Progesterone may play a role in maintaining the myometrium in a state of relative quiescence during much of pregnancy. A high local (intrauterine) concentration of progesterone may block cellular immune responses to foreign antigens. Progesterone appears to be essential for the maintenance of pregnancy in almost all mammals examined. This suggests that progesterone may be instrumental in conferring immunologic privilege to the uterus.

The functional role of estriol in pregnancy is the subject of wide speculation. It appears to be effective in increasing uteroplacental blood flow, as it has a relatively weak estrogenic effect on other organ systems. Indeed, estrogens may exert their effect on blood flow via prostaglandin stimulation.

Placental Transport

The placenta has a high rate of metabolism, with consumption of oxygen and glucose occurring at a faster rate than in the fetus. Presumably, this high requirement is due to multiple transport and biosynthesis activities.

The primary function of the placenta is the transport of oxygen and nutrients to the fetus and the reverse transfer of CO_2, urea, and other catabolites back to the mother. In general, those compounds that are essential for the minute-by-minute homeostasis of the fetus (eg, oxygen, CO_2, water, sodium) are transported very rapidly by diffusion. Compounds required for the synthesis of new tissues (eg, amino acids, enzyme cofactors such as vitamins) are transported by an active process. Substances such as certain maternal hormones, which may modify fetal growth and are at the upper limits of admissible molecular size, may diffuse very slowly, whereas proteins such as IgG immunoglobulins probably reach the fetus by the process of pinocytosis.

This transfer takes place by at least 5 mechanisms: simple diffusion, facilitated diffusion, active transport, pinocytosis, and leakage.

A. Mechanisms of Transport

1. Simple diffusion—Simple diffusion is the method by which gases and other simple molecules cross the placenta. The rate of transport depends on the chemical gradient, the diffusion constant of the compound in question, and the total area of the placenta available for transfer (Fick's law). The chemical gradient—ie, the differences in concentration in fetal and maternal plasma—is in turn affected by the rates of flow of uteroplacental and umbilical blood. Simple diffusion is also the method of transfer for exogenous compounds such as drugs.

2. Facilitated diffusion—The prime example of a substance transported by facilitated diffusion is glucose, the major source of energy for the fetus. The transfer of glucose from mother to fetus occurs more rapidly than can be accounted for by the Fick equation. Presumably, a carrier system operates *with* the chemical gradient (as opposed to active transport, which operates *against* the gradient) and may become saturated at high glucose concentrations. In the steady state, the glucose concentration in fetal plasma is about two-thirds that of the maternal concentration, reflecting the rapid rate of fetal utilization. Substances of low molecular weight, minimal electric charge, and high lipid solubility diffuse across the placenta with ease.

3. Active transport—When compounds such as the essential amino acids and water-soluble vitamins are found in higher concentration in fetal blood than in maternal blood, and when this difference cannot be accounted for by differential protein-binding effects, the presumption is that the placenta concentrates the materials during passage by an active transport system. This has been proved in the case of selected amino acids in human subjects by observing that the natural L forms are transferred with greater rapidity than the unnatural D forms, which are simply optical isomers of identical molecular size. Thus, the selective transport of specific essential nutrients is accomplished by enzymatic mechanisms.

4. Pinocytosis—Electron microscopy has shown pseudopodial projections of the syncytiotrophoblastic layer that reach out to surround minute amounts of maternal plasma. These particles are carried across the cell virtually intact to be released on the other side, whereupon they promptly gain access to the fetal circulation. Certain other proteins (eg, foreign antigens) may be immunologically rejected. This process may work both to and from the fetus, but the selectivity of the process has not been determined. Complex proteins, small amounts of fat, and immune bodies and even viruses may traverse the placenta in this way. For the passage of complex proteins, highly selective processes involving special receptors are involved. For example, maternal antibodies of the IgG class are freely transferred, whereas other antibodies are not.

5. Leakage—Gross breaks in the placental membrane may occur, allowing the passage of intact cells. Despite the fact that the hydrostatic pressure gradient is normally from fetus to mother, tagged red cells and white cells have been found to travel in either direction. Such breaks probably occur most often during labor or with placental disruption (abruptio placentae, placenta previa, or trauma), cesarean section, or intrauterine fetal death. It is at these times that fetal red cells can most often be demonstrated in the maternal circulation. This is the mechanism by which the mother may become sensitized to fetal red cell antigens such as Rh factor.

B. Placental Transport of Drugs

The placental membranes are often referred to as a "barrier" to fetal transfer, but there are few substances (eg, drugs) that will not cross the membranes at all. A few compounds, such as heparin and insulin, are of sufficiently large molecular size or charge that minimal transfer occurs. This lack of transfer is almost unique among drugs. Most medications are transferred from the maternal to the fetal circulation by simple diffusion, the rate of which is determined by the respective gradients of the drugs.

These diffusion gradients are influenced in turn by a number of serum factors, including the degree of drug-protein binding. Since serum albumin concentration is considerably lower during pregnancy, drugs that bind almost exclusively to plasma albumin (eg, warfarin, salicylates) may have relatively higher unbound concentrations and, therefore, an effectively higher placental gradient. By contrast, a compound such as carbon monoxide may attach itself so strongly to the increased total hemoglobin that there will be little left in the plasma for transport.

The placenta also acts as a lipoidal resistance factor to the transfer of water-soluble foreign organic chemicals; as a result, chemicals and drugs that are readily soluble in lipids are transferred much more easily across the placental barrier than are water-soluble drugs or molecules. Ionized drug molecules are highly water soluble and are therefore poorly transmitted across the placenta. Because ionization of chemicals depends in part on their pH-pK relationships, there are multiple factors that determine this "simple diffusion" of drugs across the placenta. *Obviously, drug transfer is not simple, and one must assume that some amount of almost any drug will cross the placenta.*

C. Placental Transfer of Heat

The core temperature of the human fetus is only about 0.5° C above that of the maternal colon (core temperature) and about 0.2° C above that of the amniotic fluid. There is a further temperature gradient of approximately 0.1° C between the amniotic fluid and the uterine wall. Given these low fetal-maternal temperature gradients, it appears that virtually all fetal heat loss is from the umbilical flow through the placenta, as the thermal diffusion capacity of the placental villous surface is considerably greater than that of the fetal body surface.

ANATOMIC DISORDERS OF THE PLACENTA

Observation of structural alterations within the placenta may indicate fetal and maternal disease that otherwise might go undetected.

Twin-Twin Transfusion Syndrome

Nearly all monochorionic twin placentas show an anastomosis between the vessels of the 2 umbilical circulations. These usually involve the major branches of the arteries and veins in the placental surface. Artery-to-artery communications are by far the most common, but the less frequent venovenous anastomosis may also occur. Of great pathologic significance are deep arteriovenous communications between the 2 circulations. This occurs when there are shared lobules supplied by an umbilical arterial branch from one fetus and drained by an umbilical vein branch of the other fetus. Fortunately, one-way flow to the shared lobule may be compensated for by reverse flow through a superficial arterioarterial or venovenous anastomosis, if they coexist.

Twin-twin transfusion syndrome is believed to arise when shared lobules causing blood flow from one twin to the other are not compensated for by the presence of superficial anastomosis or by shared lobules causing flow in the opposite direction. This syndrome occurs in 15–30% of cases of monochorial placentation and is defined in terms of a difference in cord hemoglobin between the pair of greater than 5 dL. The twin receiving the transfusion is plethoric and polycythemic and may show cardiomegaly. The donor twin is pale and anemic and may have organ weights similar to those seen in the intrauterine malnutrition form of SGA.

Placental Infarction

A placental infarct is an area of ischemic necrosis of placental villi resulting from obstruction of blood flow through the spiral arteries as a result of thrombosis. The lesions have a lobular distribution. However, the spiral arteries are not true end arteries, and if there is adequate flow through the arteries supplying adjacent lobules, sufficient circulation will be maintained to prevent necrosis. Thus, ischemic necrosis of one placental lobule probably indicates not only that the spiral artery supplying the infarcted lobule is thrombosed but that flow through adjacent spiral arteries is severely impaired. Placental infarction may serve as a mechanism allowing the fetus to redistribute blood flow to those placental lobules that are adequately supplied by the maternal circulation. The infarct is usually extensive before the fetus is physiologically impaired.

Chorioangioma of the Placenta

A benign neoplasm composed of fetoplacental capillaries may occur within the placenta. It is grossly visible as a purple-red, apparently encapsulated mass, variable in size, and occasionally multicentered. Placental hemangioma, or "chorioangioma," may be linked with maternal, fetal, and neonatal complications. Many placental tumors are accompanied by hydramnios, and some have been associated with preeclampsia-eclampsia. The developing fetus may be subjected to hypoxia, resulting in low birthweight, because blood within the tumor fails to reach the placental villi (and become oxygenated). The tumor may act as an arteriovenous shunt requiring increased fetal cardiac output, with resulting cardiomegaly. Fetal hydrops may occur, as may hypoalbuminemia and a microangiopathic type of hemolytic anemia. Neonatal thrombocytopenia has been associated with disseminated intravascular coagulation secondary to the liberation of thromboplastic substances.

Amniotic Bands

Close inspection of the fetal membranes, particularly near the umbilical cord insertion, may reveal band or stringlike membrane segments that are easily lifted above the placental surface. Such amniotic bands appear to be the result of a tear in the amnion early in pregnancy. They may cause constriction of the developing limbs or other fetal parts. Amputation has been known to result. Syndactyly, clubfoot, and fusion deformities of the cranium and face may also be explained in certain instances on the basis of amniotic bands. Myometrial bands also have been found within the intrauterine cavity but do not appear to place the same amount of tension on fetal anatomy as do amniotic bands.

Amnion Nodosum

Examination of the fetal surface of the placental peripheral membranes after delivery may disclose small elevated nodules several millimeters in diameter. Microscopic examination of these nodules may reveal areas of ulceration of amniotic epithelium covered with deposits of celluloid debris probably representing vernix caseosa. These nodules reflect oligohydramnios regardless of cause. They frequently occur in association with underlying congenital anomalies of the fetal genitourinary system. With this information, one is alerted to the possibility that Potter's syndrome or a variant with pulmonary hypoplasia may affect the infant.

Chronic Intrauterine Infection

Chronic intrauterine infection may have a deleterious effect on organogenesis and interfere with organ development. Infections such as toxoplasmosis, rubella, cytomegalovirus, herpes, and syphilis are seen most frequently. It has been only in the past 2 decades that chronic inflammation within placental villi has been recognized and linked with intrauterine infection. Such inflammatory foci have an incidence of approximately 20% in referral institutions. Usually, no causative organism is found, and the term **chronic villitis of unknown etiology** is used. This is an inflammatory lesion that focuses on placental villi. It has a significant correlation with unexplained stillbirth and a considerable association with fetal morbidity and SGA newborns. An increased risk of recurrence with associated adverse pregnancy outcome is suggested.

The placenta should be sent to the pathology laboratory for examination in the following cases: (1) perinatal death; (2) malformation, edema, or anemia; (3) extremes of amniotic fluid volume; (4) extreme SGA; (5) unexpected severe birth asphyxia; (6) preterm birth; (7) multiple gestation; (8) abnormal placenta; and (9) perinatal infection.

Placental Pathology

Any infant born with a complication may benefit from histologic evaluation of the placenta and umbilical cord. Histopathologic features of a placenta with uteroplacental insufficiency include non-marginal infarcts, shrunken placental villi, increased syncytial knots, increased perivillous fibrin and multifocal and diffuse fibrin deposition. Similarly if the ratio of nucleated red blood cells to leukocytes exceeds 2:3, this indicates fetal hypoxic stress. Chorangiosis is a pathologic change that indicates long-standing placental hypoperfusion or low-grade tissue hypoxia.

The presence of meconium and its location can also give insight into the possible time of the presumed insult. Under gross observation, meconium will stain the placenta and cord after just 3 hours of exposure. Stained infant fingernails indicate meconium exposure for at least 6 hours. Stained vernix equates with exposure of meconium for 15 hours or longer.

Microscopic evaluation also sheds light on the timing of the release of meconium. Meconium-laden macrophages at the chorionic surface of the placenta can be seen when meconium has been present for 2–3 hours. When these macrophages are found deep within the extraplacental membranes, meconium has been present for at least 6–12 hours.

Lastly, when evaluation of the umbilical cord demonstrates necrobiotic and necrotic arterial media with surrounding meconium-laden macrophages, the release of meconium occurred more than 48 hours before delivery.

Abnormalities of Placental Implantation

Normally the placenta selects a location on the endometrium that benefits the growing fetus. However, there are numerous instances when the placental implantation site is not beneficial.

Placenta previa, or the implantation of the placenta over the cervical os, is the most common. This can be seen in as many as 50% of all pregnancies in the second trimester. Fortunately, most previas resolve by the time of delivery. A marginal placenta previa occurs when the edge of the placenta lies within 2–3 cm of the cervical os. The consequences of these abnormal placentation sites is increased risk for bleeding, both for the mother and the fetus, increased need for cesarean delivery, and possible risk of placenta accreta, increta, or percreta. Once the placental edge moves beyond 2–3 cm from the cervical os these risks are minimized.

Placenta accreta is the most dangerous consequence of a placenta previa. It involves abnormal trophoblastic invasion beyond the Nitabuch's layer. Placenta increta is the term used to describe invasion into the myometrium. Placenta percreta describes invasion through the serosa with possible invasion into surrounding tissues such as the bladder. Placenta accreta is associated with life-threatening postpartum hemorrhage and increased need for immediate hysterectomy.

The risk factors for placenta previa and placenta accreta are similar. Advanced maternal age, increased parity, and prior uterine surgery are common risk factors for both entities. The strongest correlation appears to exist with prior uterine surgeries. The prevalence of placenta previa after one prior cesarean delivery reaches 0.65% versus 0.26% in the unscarred uterus. However, after 4 or more cesarean deliveries the prevalence reaches 10%. Similarly, the frequency of accreta in the presence of placenta previa increases as the number of uterine surgeries increases. In patients with one prior uterine surgery, accreta occurs in 24% of placenta previas, whereas after 4 or more surgeries the frequency of placenta accreta may be as high as 67%.

Placenta accreta may be suspected with certain ultrasound findings such as loss of the hypoechoic retroplacental myometrial zone, thinning or disruption of the hyperechoic uterine serosa-bladder interface or with visualization of an exophytic mass. In all cases of placenta previa, and especially if placenta accreta is suspected, the patient must be counseled that hysterectomy may be needed to control excessive postdelivery bleeding. Blood products must be available prior to delivery of the infant to ensure prompt replenishment of lost products and maximize the maternal status.

■ THE UMBILICAL CORD

Development

In the early stages, the embryo has a thick embryonic stalk containing 2 umbilical arteries, one large umbilical vein, the allantois, and primary mesoderm. The arteries carry blood from the embryo to the chorionic villi, and the umbilical vein returns blood to the embryo. The umbilical vein and 2 arteries twist around one another.

In the fifth week of gestation, the amnion expands to fill the entire extraembryonic coelom. This process forces the yolk sac against the embryonic stalk and covers the entire contents with a tube of amniotic ectoderm, forming the umbilical cord. The cord is narrower in diameter than the embryonic stalk and rapidly increases in length. The connective tissue of the umbilical cord is called **Wharton's jelly** and is derived from the primary mesoderm. The umbilical cord can be found in loops around the baby's neck in approximately 23% of normal spontaneous vertex deliveries.

At birth, the mature cord is about 50–60 cm in length and 12 mm in diameter. A long cord is defined as more than 100 cm and a short cord as less than 30 cm. There may be as many as 40 spiral twists in the cord, as well as false knots and true knots. When umbilical blood flow is interrupted at birth, the intra-abdominal sections of the umbilical arteries and vein gradually become fibrous cords. The course of the left umbilical vein is discernible in the adult as a fibrous cord from the umbilicus to the liver (ligamentum teres) contained within the falciform ligament. The umbilical arteries are retained proximally as the internal iliac arteries and give off the superior vesicle arteries and the medial umbilical ligaments within the medial umbilical folds to the umbilicus. When the umbilical cord is cut and the end examined at the time of delivery, the vessels ordinarily are collapsed (Fig 8–3A), but if a segment of cord is fixed while the vessels are distended, the characteristic appearance is as shown in Fig 8–3B.

Analysis of the Umbilical Cord in Fetal Abnormalities

A segment of umbilical cord should be kept available as a source of umbilical cord blood for blood gas measurements at the time of delivery. Cord blood gases are a more objective measure of oxygenation than Apgar scores, especially in dark-skinned babies.

The umbilical cord has recently become a means of evaluating the fetus in utero. Umbilical cord sampling

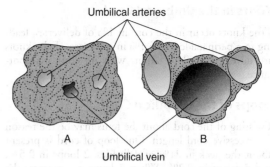

Figure 8–3. Drawings of cross sections of umbilical cord (A) after blood vessels are empty and (B) while they are filled, as in utero. The central vein and 2 arteries occupy most of the space. (Based on photography by SRM Reynolds.)

under ultrasonographic guidance has opened new vistas in perinatal physiology, teratology, genetics, and therapeutic endeavors to correct Rh isoimmunization.

ABNORMALITIES OF THE UMBILICAL CORD

Velamentous Insertion

In velamentous insertion, the umbilical vessels divide to course through the membranes before reaching the chorionic plate. When these vessels present themselves ahead of the fetus (vasa praevia), they may rupture during labor to cause fetal exsanguination. Velamentous insertion occurs in about 1% of placentas, and 25–50% of these infants will have structural defects. Testing of all episodes of painless vaginal bleeding for fetal hemoglobin (Apt test or hemoglobin electrophoresis) will allow detection of this cause of fetal distress or death.

Short Umbilical Cord

It appears from indirect evidence in the human fetus that the length of the umbilical cord at term is determined by the amount of amniotic fluid present during the first and second trimesters and by the mobility of the fetus. If oligohydramnios, amniotic bands, or limitation of fetal motion occur for any reason, the umbilical cord will not develop to an average length. Amniocentesis performed to produce oligohydramnios in pregnant rats at 14–16 days results in significant reduction of umbilical cord length. The length of the umbilical cord does not vary with fetal weight, presentation, or placental size. Simple mechanical factors may determine the eventual length of the cord.

Knots in the Umbilical Cord

True knots occur in the cord in 1% of deliveries, leading to a perinatal loss of 6.1% in such cases. False knots are developmental variations with no clinical importance.

Loops of the Umbilical Cord

Twisting of the cord about the fetus may be the reason for excessive cord length. One loop of cord is present about the neck in 21% of deliveries, 2 loops in 2.5%, and 3 loops in 0.2%. When 3 loops are present, the cord is usually longer than 70 cm. One study of 1000 consecutive deliveries found one or more loops of cord around the neck in approximately 24% of cases. Single or multiple loops of umbilical cord around the neck caused no fetal morbidity or mortality in that series, but Naeye's report (1987) illustrates that cord entanglement may be an important cause of stillbirth.

Torsion of the Umbilical Cord

Torsion of the cord occurs counterclockwise in most cases. If twisting is extreme, fetal asphyxia may result.

Single Artery

A 2-vessel cord (absence of one umbilical artery) occurs about once in 500 deliveries (6% of twins). The cause may be aplasia or atrophy of the missing vessel. The anomaly is more common in blacks than whites but equally frequent in primiparas and multiparas. About 30% of these infants will have structural defects. There is also a strong association between fetal structural anomalies and placental vascular occlusion or thrombosis. Perinatal examination for such vascular defects should be routine.

■ THE FETUS

The human fetus is born about 40 weeks after the first day of the last menstrual period (LMP). The **gestational age** is measured from the first day of the LMP, although obviously conception can not occur until 2 weeks after the beginning of this calculation. The 9.5 calendar months are divided into trimesters for convenient classification of certain obstetric events. The term fetus is born 9.5 lunar cycles (29.53 days each) after conception, and the postconceptional age in weeks is used to denote the stage of development of the embryo.

An estimate of **conceptional age** can be made by measuring the embryo or fetus. Various methods of measurement have been developed, each with its own limitations and inaccuracies. Crown-rump and crown-heel lengths are the most common measurements. Crown-heel lengths are difficult to measure because the legs are often flexed in different positions. Most methods based on measurement are inaccurate because the fetus may move about or stretch while it is being measured. Embryologists most often use the term *conceptual age,* which begins with the date of conception or fertilization. Unfortunately, the confusion in terminology is often transmitted to the patient. It is appropriate to utilize weeks in discussing the length of gestation with the patient, so that communication and understanding is enhanced.

GROWTH & DEVELOPMENT

During the first 8 weeks, the term **embryo** is used to denote the developing organism because it is during this time that all the major organs are formed (Table 8–3). After the eighth week, the word **fetus** is proper; this is a period when further growth and organ maturation occur. The loss of a fetus weighing less than 500 g (about 22 weeks' gestational age) is called a **spontaneous abortion.** A fetus weighing 500–1000 g (22–28 weeks) is called **immature.** From 28–36 weeks, it is referred to as **premature.** A **term fetus** is arbitrarily defined as one that has attained 37 weeks' gestational age.

The growth of the fetus may be conveniently described in units of 4 weeks' gestational age, beginning with the first day of the LMP:

8 weeks: The embryo is 2.1–2.5 cm long and weighs 1 g, and the head makes up almost half the bulk. The hepatic lobes may be recognized. Red blood cells are forming in the yolk sac and liver and contain hemoglobin. The kidneys are beginning to form.

12 weeks: The fetus is 7–9 cm long and weighs 12–15 g. The fingers and toes have nails, and the external genitalia may be recognizable as male or female. The volume of amniotic fluid is about 30 mL. The intestines undergo peristalsis and are capable of absorbing glucose.

16 weeks: The length is 14–17 cm and the weight about 100 g. The sex is discernible. Hemoglobin F is present, and formation of hemoglobin A begins.

20 weeks: The weight is about 300 g. Heart tones may often be detected by stethoscope. Movements have been perceived by the mother for 2–3 weeks. The uterine fundus is near the level of the umbilicus.

24 weeks: The weight is 600 g. Some fat is beginning to be deposited beneath the wrinkled skin. Viability is reached by the 24th week, but survival at this stage is still relatively rare.

28 weeks: The weight is about 1050 g and the length about 37 cm. The lungs are now capable of

Table 8–3. Embryonic and fetal growth and development.

Fertilization Age (weeks)	Crown-Rump Length	Crown-Heel Length	Weight	Gross Appearance	Internal Development
Embryonic stage					
1	0.5 mm	0.5 mm	?	Minute clone free in uterus.	Early morula. No organ differentiation.
2	2 mm	2 mm	?	Ovoid vesicle superficially buried in endometrium.	External trophoblast. Flat embryonic disk forming 2 inner vesicles (amnio-ectomesodermal and endodermal).
3	3 mm	3 mm	?	Early dorsal concavity changes to convexity; head, tail folds form; neural grooves close partially.	Optic vesicles appear. Double heart recognized. Fourteen mesodermal somites present.
4	4 mm	4 mm	0.4 g	Head is at right angle to body; limb rudiments obvious, tail prominent.	Vitelline duct only communication between umbilical vesicle and intestines. Initial stage of most organs has begun.
8	3 cm	3.5 cm	2 g	Eyes, ears, nose, mouth recognizable; digits formed, tail almost gone.	Sensory organ development well along. Ossification beginning in occiput, mandible, and humerus (diaphysis). Small intestines coil within umbilical cord. Pleural pericardial cavities forming. Gonadal development advanced without differentiation.
Fetal stage					
12	8 cm	11.5 cm	19 g	Skin pink, delicate; resembles a human being, but head is disproportionately large.	Brain configuration roughly complete. Internal sex organs now specific. Uterus no longer bicornuate. Blood forming in marrow. Upper cervical to lower sacral arches and bodies ossify.
16	13.5 cm	19 cm	100 g	Scalp hair appears. Fetus active. Arm-leg ratio now proportionate. Sex determination possible.	External sex organs grossly formed. Myelination. Heart muscle well developed. Lobulated kidneys in final situation. Meconium in bowel. Vagina and anus open. Ischium ossified.
20	18.5 cm	22 cm	300 g	Legs lengthen appreciably. Distance from umbilicus to pubis increases.	Sternum ossifies.
24	23 cm	32 cm	600 g	Skin reddish and wrinkled. Slight subcuticular fat. Vernix. Primitive respiratory-like movements.	Os pubis (horizontal ramus) ossifies.
28	27 cm	36 cm	1100 g	Skin less wrinkled; more fat. Nails appear. If delivered may survive with optimal care.	Testes at internal inguinal ring or below. Talus ossifies.
32	31 cm	41 cm	1800 g	Fetal weight increased proportionately more than length.	Middle fourth phalanges ossify.

(continued)

Table 8–3. Embryonic and fetal growth and development. (continued)

Fertilization Age (weeks)	Crown-Rump Length	Crown-Heel Length	Weight	Gross Appearance	Internal Development
Fetal stage (cont.)					
36	34 cm	46 cm	2200 g	Skin pale, body rounded. Lanugo disappearing. Hair fuzzy or wooly. Ear lobes soft with little cartilage. Umbilicus in center of body. Testes in inguinal canals; scrotum small with few rugae. Few sole creases.	Distal femoral ossification centers present.
40	40 cm	52 cm	3200+ g	Skin smooth and pink. Copious vernix. Moderate to profuse silky hair. Lanugo hair on shoulders and upper back. Ear lobes stiffened by thick cartilage. Nasal and alar cartilages distinguishable. Nails extend over tips of digits. Testes in full, pendulous, rugous scrotum (or labia majora) well developed. Creases cover sole.	Proximal tibial ossification centers present. Cuboid, tibia (proximal epiphysis) ossify.

breathing, but the surfactant content is low; survival is possible in level II or level III neonatal centers.

32 weeks: The weight is about 1700 g and the length 42 cm. If born at this stage, about 5 of 6 infants survive.

36 weeks: The weight is about 2500 g and the length about 47 cm. The skin has lost its wrinkled appearance. The chances for survival are good.

40 weeks: The term fetus averages 50 cm in length and 3200–3500 g in weight. The head has a maximal transverse (biparietal) diameter of 9.5 cm, and when the neck is well flexed, the diameter from the brow to a point beneath the occiput (suboccipitobregmatic) is also 9.5 cm. The average fetus, therefore, requires cervical dilatation of almost 10 cm before it can descend into the vagina.

FETAL & EARLY NEONATAL PHYSIOLOGY

During the past 2 decades, improved neonatal care has led to increased survival rates for very low birthweight infants, even those as young as 24 weeks. Obviously, an understanding of fetal and early neonatal physiology is critical in the appropriate management of these babies. The recent introduction of fetoscopy, pulsed Doppler evaluation, and umbilical cord blood sampling allows detection and treatment of fetal disorders in utero. A greater understanding of fetal physiology is needed to perform therapeutic techniques via the umbilical cord or within the intrauterine environment.

Hematology

The fetal circulation is established at about 25 postconceptional days. At that time, the major sources of red blood cells are blood islands in the body stalk. By 10 weeks, the liver assumes the major role in erythropoiesis, but the spleen and bone marrow gradually take over this function. At term, the bone marrow is the source of at least 90% of the red cells. The hormone erythropoietin is produced in considerable quantities by 32 weeks, but levels fall almost to zero during the first week after birth, unless the infant is anemic, in which case the values are higher.

Erythrocytes are the first blood cells produced by the fetus and have a life span of 120 days. The earliest erythrocytes are megaloblastic and circulate as nucleated cells. Mean red cell values change as the fetus grows (Table 8–4).

After the first week of life, erythrocyte concentrations begin to decline gradually, reaching zero by 6–12 weeks after birth. The hemoglobin concentration decreases to about 10 g/dL and by term to as low as 7–8 g/dL (**physiologic anemia of the newborn**).

The synthesis of **hemoglobin** occurs in the proerythroblast, normoblast, and reticulocyte, but not in the mature red blood cell. Types of fetal hemoglobin present prior to 12 weeks are Gower I and II and Portland I. There are at least 7 types of hemoglobin chains. The synthesis of each chain is under the genetic control of a separate structural gene locus. The complete amino acid sequences of the 7 normal globin chains have been

Table 8–4. Mean red cell values during gestation.[1]

Age (weeks)	Hemoglobin (g/dL)	Hematocrit (%)	Red Blood Cells ($10^6/\mu L$)	Mean Corpuscle Volume ($\mu m^3/L$)	Mean Corpuscle Hemoglobin (pg)	Mean Corpuscle Hemoglobin Concentration (g/dL)	Nucleated Red Blood Cells (% or red blood cells)	Reticulocytes (%)	Diameter (μm)
12	8–10	33	1.5	180	60	34	5–8	40	10.5
16	10	35	2	140	45	33	2–4	10–25	9.5
20	11	37	2.5	135	44	33	1	10–20	9
24	14	40	3.5	123	38	31	1	5–10	8.8
28	14.5	45	4	120	40	31	0.5	5–10	8.7
34	15	47	4.4	118	38	32	0.2	3–10	8.5

[1]Reproduced, with permission, from Oskl FA, Naiman JL: *Hematologic Problems in the Newborn*, 3rd ed, Saunders, 1982.

determined. A functional hemoglobin molecule is a tetramer composed of 4 globin chains and 4 heme groups. From the eighth week of gestation to term, **hemoglobin F** is the major hemoglobin in the fetus, but a small amount of hemoglobin A can also be detected. The ratio of beta to gamma synthesis remains approximately 1:10 during this period and until term. The beta to gamma ratio in the fetus is a criterion used for prenatal diagnosis by fetal blood analysis (Fig 8–4). Around the time of birth, the ratio changes because of the gradually decreased synthesis of gamma chains and increased synthesis of beta chains (Table 8–5).

Fortuitously, blood in the fetus has a 50% higher hemoglobin concentration than in the adult and a greater oxygen affinity than maternal blood. Even though fetal oxygen tension is less, fetal blood carries an amount of oxygen comparable to that in maternal blood. The alkali resistance of hemoglobin F makes it possible to demonstrate hemoglobin F-containing cells in the maternal circulation (**Apt test**).

The higher affinity of hemoglobin F for oxygen is accentuated by **2, 3-diphosphoglycerate (2, 3-DPG)**, which is present in adult red cells. Fetal and maternal blood have differing oxygen saturation curves, mostly because 2, 3-DPG competes with oxygen for binding sites on adult cells.

Immunology

There are 3 basic types of leukocytes found in the blood: **granulocytes, monocytes,** and **lymphocytes.** The granular acidic leukocytes are subdivided into 3 types, based on the sustaining characteristics of the acidic plasma granules and their function—eosinophilic, basophilic, and neutrophilic granulocytes. A functional difference also exists among the lymphocytes, which are divided into 2 broad groups designated as **T cells** and **B cells.** The functions of monocytes vary greatly during maturation or with environmental influ-

Table 8–5. Embryonic, fetal, and adult hemoglobin concentrations.

Hemoglobin	Globin Polypeptides	Percent in Cord Blood
Embryo		
Gower I	Zeta-2, epsilon-2	—
Gower II	Alpha-2, epsilon-2	—
Portland I	Zeta-2, gamma-2	—
Portland II	Zeta-4	—
Fetus		
Bart's	Gamma-4	< 1
Hemoglobin F	Alpha-2f, gamma-2	60–85
Adult		
Hemoglobin A	Alpha-2, beta-2	15–40
Hemoglobin A$_2$	Alpha-2, delta-2	< 1

ences; thus, it is not currently possible to divide them into distinct subgroups. Although all these cells are generally regarded as white blood cells, they should be viewed as cell types that merely use the blood as a means of transportation from sites of production to sites of function. Both the sites of production and (for the most part) sites of function are extravascular. The fetus presents with relative leukocytosis, the white count being 15,000–20,000/dL at term.

Circulating white cells constitute the first line of defense against pathogenic bacteria, as outlined in Table 8–6. Leukocytes appear in the fetal circulation after 2 months' gestation. The prothymocytes migrate from the fetal liver or bone marrow to enter the embryonic thymus at approximately 8 weeks' gestation. Soon after, the splenic anlage begins to mature. Both produce lymphocytes, a major source of the antibodies that constitute the second line of defense against harmful foreign antigens. Both antibody-mediated immunity and cell-mediated immunity depend on the activity of small lymphocytes derived from bone marrow precursors.

Table 8–6. Defense mechanisms against infectious pathogens.

	Humoral Defense	Cellular Defense
General	Complement system Properdin system	Granulocytes Monocytes Reticuloendothelial system
Immune	Immunoglobulins	Lymphocytes

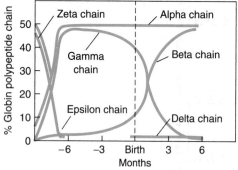

Figure 8–4. Hemoglobin chains.

The stem cells, which during the early embryonic stage originate in the yolk sac, in later stages of development in the liver, and in adults in the bone marrow, differentiate to form 2 distinct lymphocyte populations. One group is **thymus-derived (T lymphocytes)** and the other is **bone marrow-derived (B lymphocytes).** T lymphocytes can be detected in the thymus after 11 weeks' gestation, they appear in the peripheral blood, spleen, and lymph nodes by 16–18 weeks, and by 30–32 weeks the fetus has a near-adult number of circulating T lymphocytes.

The life span of lymphocytes is not uniform. Recent studies suggest that B- and T-cell populations contain similar proportions of long- and short-lived lymphocytes. The T lymphocytes constitute 65–85% of the lymphocytes present in the thoracic duct, blood, and lymph nodes. The long-lived lymphocytes represent the major portion (90%) of the thoracic duct cells, whereas the short-lived lymphocytes are located mainly in the thymus, spleen, and bone marrow. The T cells are effector cells in delayed sensitivity reactions and elimination of foreign tissues. They also play an important role in the expression of some humoral immune responses. The T cells can release a variety of nonspecific chemical mediators called **lymphokines,** eg, **interferon, transfer factor, mitogenic factor, migration** and **inhibition factors,** and **cytotoxic** and **growth inhibitory factors.**

B lymphocytes originate in the bone marrow of most mammals. B cells seem to be more sessile than T cells. B cells are found primarily in the perilymphoid organs, lymph nodes, and the thymic-independent areas around germinal centers. They are also present in very small amounts in the peripheral blood. They seem to be short-lived. B cells differentiate into **plasma cells,** which are ultimately responsible for the synthesis and secretion of all forms of antibody and all circulating immunoglobulins. The average life span of plasma cells is 0.5–2 days.

Immunoglobulins (Ig) are serum globulins with antibody activity as their primary property. The 5 classes of Ig have been designated IgG, IgM, IgA, IgD, and IgE. In the human newborn, plasma cells are absent from the bone marrow and the lamina propria of the ileum and appendix. They appear only 4–6 weeks after birth. However, beginning at 20 weeks' gestation, the fetal spleen synthesizes IgG and IgM but not IgA or IgD (Fig 8–5).

IgG is normally produced only in trace amounts prenatally, its full synthesis beginning 3–4 weeks after birth. **IgM** globulins are also found in small amounts in the fetus, primarily in the circulation but not diffused into extravascular spaces. They are synthesized in lymphocytoid plasma cells and reticular cells of the spleen and lymph nodes. Fetal production of IgG and IgM is

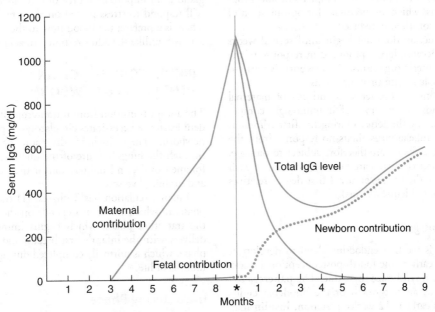

Figure 8–5. Development of IgG levels with age. Relationship of development of normal serum levels of IgG during fetal and newborn stages, and maternal contribution. (Modified from Allansmith M et al: The development of immunoglobulin levels in man. J Pediatr 1968;72:289.)

low, however, in comparison with adult production. The fetal spleen synthesizes relatively more IgM than IgG. IgM is the first class to appear in the circulation after initial immunization and is the predominant class produced by infants in the neonatal period. At birth, the plasma level of IgM is about 5% of the normal adult level, with most, if not all, of this antibody being of fetal origin. Within 2–5 days after birth, the rate of IgM synthesis increases rapidly. IgM, unlike IgG, does not cross the human placenta, and the half-life of IgM is 5 days.

This comparison between IgG and IgM is important in determining possible intrauterine infection. The fetal IgG serum concentration at term equals the maternal concentration because IgG crosses the placenta. IgG constitutes 90% of all serum antibodies in the fetus because of the maternal contribution. IgM is predominantly of fetal origin and, therefore, is used to determine whether fetal infection is present, but there are many false-positive and false-negative results. After birth, the IgG half-life in the newborn circulation is 3–4 weeks. IgE does not cross the placenta, and cord levels are only 10% of maternal levels.

The fetus and newborn are not as well equipped immunologically as the adult to combat infection. The primary deficiency is both cellular and humoral. T lymphocytes do not respond to specific antigens, and B lymphocytes do not develop into plasma cells. This results in IgG levels that are below maternal levels until late in the third trimester, and complement and properdin proteins, which are necessary for opsonization of bacteria, are consistently reduced.

IgA production does not begin until several weeks after birth. Because IgA is produced in response to the antigens of enteric organisms, the newborn is particularly susceptible to intestinal infections.

The response of the fetus to antigens of maternal origin depends on the level of immunologic competence achieved by the fetus. During the first trimester, for example, rubella virus elicits no response from the embryo, whose tissues are therefore subject to damage. Fetal and maternal tissues are no more tolerant of each other than are the tissues of any 2 first-degree relatives (as contrasted to identical twins).

Endocrinology

The thyroid is the first endocrine gland to develop in the fetus. As early as the fourth postconceptional week, the thyroid can synthesize thyroxine. The **pancreas** develops early as an outgrowth of the duodenal endoderm, and as early as 12 weeks' gestation, **insulin** may be extracted from the B cells of the pancreas. Maternal insulin is not transferred to the fetus in physiologic quantities, and the fetus must supply whatever is needed for the metabolism of glucose. Insulin is thus the primary hormone regulating the rate of fetal growth. The B cells of the normal fetus respond poorly to hyperglycemia unless the stimulus is repeated many times, eg, diabetes in the mother may cause hyperplasia of fetal B cells so that larger quantities of insulin will be produced. This may be why some infants of diabetic mothers grow to an excessive size or show evidence of hyperinsulinism immediately after birth.

All the tropic hormones synthesized by the **anterior pituitary gland** are present in the fetus, although the precise role of these protein hormones in fetal growth and metabolism is not well understood. **ACTH** plays a vital role, however, in stimulating growth of the adrenal cortex, because the tropic hormones are too large for placental transfer from the mother in significant quantities.

The fetal **adrenal cortex** consists mainly of a fetal zone that disappears about 6 months after birth. The cortex is an active endocrine organ that produces large quantities of steroid hormones. There is evidence that the steadily increasing activity of the fetal zone triggers the sequence of events that leads to the initiation of labor. Atrophy of the fetal adrenal gland (as in anencephalic fetuses) may result in marked prolongation of pregnancy. The fetal adrenal cortex is larger in premature infants when the cause of labor is unknown than when the pregnancy is terminated by placental abruption or by elective induction of labor. The fetal adrenal gland is an important source of catecholamines, which will respond to stress placed on the fetal myocardium. There is a preferential blood flow to the fetal adrenal in acidosis, unlike the adult response to acidosis.

CIRCULATORY FUNCTION IN THE FETUS & NEWBORN

The abrupt transition from intrauterine life to independent existence necessitates circulatory adaptations in the newborn. These include diversion of blood flow through the lungs, closure of the ductus arteriosus and foramen ovale, and obliteration of the ductus venosus and umbilical vessels.

Infant circulation has 3 phases: (1) the intrauterine phase, in which the fetus depends on the placenta; (2) the transition phase, which begins immediately after delivery with the infant's first breath; and (3) the adult phase, which is normally completed during the first few months of life.

Intrauterine Phase

The umbilical vein carries oxygenated blood from the placenta to the fetus (Figs 8–6 and 8–7). In the abdomen, the vein branches and enters the liver; a small

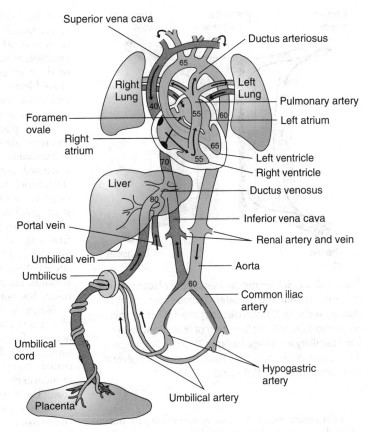

Figure 8–6. The fetal circulation. Numbers represent approximate values of the percentage of oxygen saturation of the blood in utero. (Reproduced, with permission, from Parer JT: *Handbook of Fetal Heart Rate Monitoring*. WB Saunders, 1983.)

branch bypasses the liver as the ductus venosus to enter the inferior vena cava directly.

Almost all the blood from the superior vena cava is directed through the tricuspid valve into the right ventricle, which ejects into the pulmonary trunk. Most of this relatively deoxygenated blood then passes directly through the ductus arteriosus to the descending aorta and on to the placenta. Blood from the inferior vena cava, which includes the oxygenated umbilical venous blood, largely passes directly through the foramen ovale into the left atrium and left ventricle to be ejected into the ascending aorta. The left ventricle ejects about one-third of the combined ventricular output of the fetus. Most of the left ventricular output passes to the fetal head, while the right ventricle, with blood of lower oxygen content, ejects mainly into the descending aorta. The aortic oxygen saturation difference is related not only to superior and inferior vena caval flow patterns but also to flow of the umbilical venous blood as it enters the inferior vena cava. This well-oxygenated blood preferentially passes to the cerebral and coronary circulations. Both ventricles pump in parallel, unlike the situation in adults.

The fetal cardiovascular responses to stress represent a complex interplay between state of arousal, changes in blood gases, hydrogen ion concentration, reflex effects initiated by chemoreceptor or baroreceptor stimulation, and hormonal levels.

Superficially, the fetal hypoxemic-asphyxial response is much like the adult diving response in that they both involve selective vasoconstriction and the baroreceptor reflex, a primitive reflex involving changes in heart rate, arterial and venous dilatation, and cardiac performance. This reflex is evoked by changes in mean blood pressure and is modified by blood gas levels. The ability of some mammals to remain submerged for long periods of time remained a mystery until it was recognized that they become a "heart-brain" preparation through selective vasoconstriction.

In diving mammals, lactic acid is washed out of hypoperfused tissues after relief of the vasoconstriction. The same process occurs with the hypoxic fetus, producing a brief period of acidemia after birth or after oxygenation. While selective vasoconstriction provides a "heart-brain" preparation, at the same time it disturbs the flow of oxygenated blood to other essential organs.

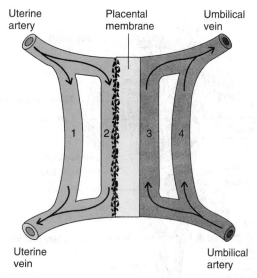

Figure 8–7. Schematic diagram of the placental circulation. (1) Shunting of maternal blood away from exchange surfaces. (2) Intervillous space. (3) Fetal capillaries of chorionic villi. (4) Shunting of fetal blood away from capillary exchange surfaces. (Modified and reproduced, with permission, from Parer JT: *Handbook of Fetal Heart Rate Monitoring.* WB Saunders, 1983.)

A depressed central nervous system often produces a relatively constant heart rate with lack of beat-to-beat variability. Fetal beat-to-beat variability is mediated through autonomic stimulation resulting from the push-and-pull nature of the parasympathetic systems. Such central nervous system activity reflects general fetal arousal levels and is decreased when the fetus is immature, asleep, drugged, or asphyxiated. Lack of fetal heart rate variability plus other signs of fetal stress can be an ominous sign. The central nervous system and cardiovascular system respond differently to hypoxia according to gestational age.

The umbilical vessels are relatively nonreactive, but the systemic and pulmonary circulations respond, when stressed, with vasoconstriction. The fetal pulmonary circulation receives a small portion (8–10%) of the fetal cardiac output, and therefore it does not play a central role in the fetal cardiovascular hypoxia response. Changes in fetal arterial pressure tend to be buffered by the fetal umbilical-placental circulation. Likewise, the decrease in fetal cardiac output seen during bradycardia is modified by the redistribution of cardiac output to vital organs such as the brain, heart, placenta, and adrenal gland, so that the baroreceptor reflex may not be as effective during fetal life. The response of the fetus to hypoxia is even more complex, with chemoreceptor reflex stimulation

from the aortic receptors, baroreceptor reflexes, and direct myocardial depression. Fetal tachycardia may result from sympathetic nervous stimulation and circulating catecholamines. Since the capacity to respond to any one of these different stimuli varies with gestational age, arousal levels, general health, and the presence of drugs and hormones, there are no universal, precise fetal heart rate responses to distress.

When placental transfer of oxygen is inadequate, anaerobic glycolysis leads to the accumulation of excessive amounts of lactic acid in the fetus. There is then an associated accumulation of CO_2 and hydrogen ion (H^+), which results in decreased fetal pH. Although the maternal and fetal H^+ values maintain a relatively constant gradient, differences in the bicarbonate levels allow for variation in fetal pH. Thus, determination of fetal scalp or cord blood gases is useful in the assessment of fetal well-being. During fetal distress (seriously altered homeostasis), fetal blood levels of prostaglandins, catecholamines, steroids, endorphins, and pituitary hormones are often elevated (Table 8–7).

When the fetus shows signs of distress during labor, placental transfer can be improved by use of several maneuvers. First, a vaginal examination should be performed, and if prolapse of the umbilical cord has occurred, compression of the cord should be relieved immediately by lifting the presenting fetal part off the cord. The second maneuver is to roll the mother from one side to the other to check for maternal aortocaval compression. Third, it may be helpful to administer

Table 8–7. Average "normal" fetal scalp[1] and cord acid-base values.[2]

	Before Labor	Second Stage of Labor
Scalp		
pH	7.37	7.3
CO_2 pressure (mm Hg)	38	43
Bicarbonate (mmol/L)	21	21
Base excess (mmol/L)	–3	–5
	Umbilical Vein	**Umbilical Artery**
Cord		
pH	7.32	7.26
P_{O_2}	38.9	17.7
P_{CO_2}	37.1	40
Base deficit	6.8	6.7

[1]Population unrelated to cord sample population.
[2]Related to babies 28–43 weeks with Apgar scores greater than 7 at 1.5 minutes.

oxygen to the mother; however, this only slightly increases the oxygen content of the uterine arterial blood, because the arterial hemoglobin is already nearly saturated. Fourth, discontinue oxytocin and consider administration of a tocolytic agent to inhibit uterine activity. Fifth, rapidly administer 1 L of intravenous fluids to acutely expand the maternal plasma volume; a colloid solution such as 5% albumin is preferred, but a balanced salt solution is acceptable and usually is more readily available.

Transition Phase

At birth, 2 events occur that alter the fetal hemodynamics: (1) ligation of the umbilical cord causes an abrupt though transient rise in arterial pressure, and (2) a rise in plasma CO_2 and fall in blood PO_2 help to initiate regular breathing.

With the first few breaths, the intrathoracic pressure of the newborn remains low (–40 to –50 mm Hg); after distention of the airways, however, the pressure rises to the normal adult level (–7 to –8 mm Hg). The initially high vascular resistance of the pulmonary bed is probably reduced by 75–80%. Pressure in the pulmonary artery falls by at least 50%, whereas pressure in the left atrium doubles.

In the fetus, the high resistance of the pulmonary bed causes most of the deoxygenated blood in the pulmonary artery to enter the descending aorta via the ductus arteriosus. At birth, expansion of the lungs occurs in the newborn, and most of the blood from the right ventricle then enters the lungs via the pulmonary artery. Furthermore, increased systemic arterial pressure reverses the flow of blood through the ductus arteriosus. Neonatal blood flows from the high-pressure aorta to the low-pressure pulmonary artery.

The increased pressure in the left atrium would normally result in backflow into the right heart through a patent foramen ovale. However, the anatomic configuration of the foramen is such that the increased pressure causes closure of the foramen by a valvelike fold situated in the wall of the left atrium.

The neonatal circulation is complete with closure of the ductus arteriosus and foramen ovale, but adjustments continue for 1–2 months, until the adult phase begins.

Adult Phase

The ductus arteriosus usually is obliterated in the early postnatal period, probably by reflex action secondary to elevated oxygen tension and the interaction of prostaglandins. If the ductus remains open, a systolic crescendo murmur that diminishes during diastole (**"machinery murmur"**) is often heard over the second left interspace.

Obliteration of the foramen ovale is usually complete in 6–8 weeks, with fusion of its valve to the left interatrial septum. The foramen may remain patent in some individuals, however, with few or no symptoms. The obliterated ductus venosus from the liver to the vena cava becomes the ligamentum venosum. The occluded umbilical vein becomes the ligamentum teres of the liver.

The hemodynamics of the normal adult differ from those of the fetus in the following respects: (1) venous and arterial blood no longer mix in the atria; (2) the vena cava carries only deoxygenated blood into the right atrium, where it goes to the right ventricle and then is pumped into the pulmonary arteries and finally to the pulmonary capillary bed; and (3) the aorta carries only oxygenated blood from the left heart via the pulmonary veins for distribution to the rest of the body.

RESPIRATORY FUNCTION IN THE FETUS & NEWBORN

Gas exchange in the fetus occurs in the placenta. Transfer of gases is proportionate to the difference in partial pressure of each gas and surface area and inversely proportionate to membrane thickness. Thus, the placenta can be viewed as the fetal "lungs in utero."

Until about 12 weeks, placental permeability is low because of the small surface area of the placental "lake" and the early relative thickness of the trophoblastic membrane. From 12–32 weeks, the membrane thins and the surface area steadily increases. However, placental oxygen utilization makes accurate quantitation of oxygen transfer difficult.

The partial pressure of oxygen (PO_2) of fetal blood is less than that of maternal blood. Although not compatible with extrauterine life, the PO_2 is adequate for the fetus, as there is a higher concentration of hemoglobin in fetal blood, much of which is hemoglobin F. Hemoglobin F has a much greater affinity for oxygen than adult hemoglobin A, resulting in greater fetal oxygen saturation. However, the enhanced ability of the fetus to deliver oxygen to the peripheral tissues seems primarily dependent upon a cardiac output that is 2.5–3 times greater than in the adult.

Both the PCO_2 and the CO_2 content of fetal blood are slightly greater than levels in the mother's blood. As a result, CO_2 diffuses from fetus to mother for elimination.

The central and motor pathways of the fetal respiratory system are active, and respiration at birth is the culmination of in utero processes. Two main types of fetal breathing movements are recognized. One is a paradoxic irregular sequence, in which the abdominal wall moves outward as the chest wall moves inward. The other is a regular gentle movement, in which the chest and abdominal wall move outward and inward together. Fetal respiratory activity permits neuromuscular and skeletal maturation as well as development of the respiratory epithelium. As term approaches, the fetal diaphragm is usually active only during fetal REM sleep. Without such activity, the lungs would be hypoplastic and inadequate for gas exchange. Curiously, the alveolar membrane does excrete chloride into tracheal fluid and perhaps absorbs nutrients from amniotic fluid. Consequently, it has been proposed that, like the fish gill, the fetal alveolar membrane functions as an organ of osmoregulation. In sheep, prolactin has been shown to act on both the fetal lung and amniotic membrane in facilitating sodium transport, and this may be a mechanism of control of fetal blood volume.

Hypoxia or maternal cigarette smoking reduces fetal breathing movements, while hyperglycemia increases fetal breathing movements. In general, these movements are governed by the same central nervous system patterns that control changes in fetal heart rate and body movements. The greatest clinical accuracy in the biophysical identification of the abnormal fetus is achieved when multiple variables are considered, eg, fetal breathing, general movements, heart rate patterns, and response to stimuli. In both sheep and humans, fetal breathing movements diminish or cease 24–36 hours before the onset of true labor. In preterm labor with intact membranes, the presence of fetal breathing movements may indicate that pregnancy will continue, while fetal apnea may indicate early delivery.

The first breath of the newborn normally occurs within the first 10 seconds after delivery. The first breath usually is a gasp, the result of central nervous system reaction to sudden pressure, temperature change, and other external stimuli. With the first breath, the slight increase in PO_2 may activate chemoreceptors to send impulses to the central nervous system respiratory center and then to the respiratory musculature. As a result, a rhythmic but rapid breathing sequence occurs, which persists into the neonatal period. The amniotic fluid usually drains from the respiratory tract or is absorbed. If meconium is present, it may be aspirated, and if not cleared shortly after birth, it will migrate peripherally as continued respiration is established. Complete or partial obstruction of the respiratory tract or chemical pneumonitis may result.

Contrary to popular belief, the fetal lungs are not highly plastic. As development progresses, tissue elastin probably falls as the density of tissue to potential air space decreases. At the same time, liquid and future air space is enriched with phospholipid surfactants secreted by maturing type 2 saccular alveolar cells. When air breathing begins at birth, dispersion of air into the surfactant-rich liquid of the mature lungs results in formation of stable alveoli. Overall, a mature volume-pressure diagram is developed, characterized by relatively low opening pressures, high maximal volume, wide hysteresis, and retention of large volumes at end deflation or expiration.

With the onset of breathing, pulmonary vascular resistance is reduced and the capillaries fill with blood. Normally, the foramen ovale closes and pulmonary circulation is established.

Surfactant-poor lungs do not have the capacity to produce alveolar stability. As a consequence, initial aeration requires greater opening pressure, achieves a smaller maximal volume, and results in little hysteresis and gas retention during deflation. This is the underlying pathophysiologic mechanism of neonatal respiratory distress syndrome. One may anticipate inadequate phospholipid surfactant when the lecithin:sphingomyelin (L:S) ratio is less than 2. Conversely, one can anticipate mature fetal lungs and a 1–2% chance of respiratory distress syndrome if the L:S ratio is greater than 2.

GASTROINTESTINAL FUNCTION IN THE FETUS & NEWBORN

The gastrointestinal tract is not truly functional until after birth, because the placenta is the organ of alimentation during fetal life. Nevertheless, when contrast medium is injected into the amniotic fluid as early as the fourth month of gestation, it may be promptly observed within the stomach and small intestine.

The full development of proteolytic activity does not develop until after birth, but the fetal gastrointestinal tract is quite capable of absorbing amino acids, glucose, and other soluble nutrients.

Meconium is produced during late pregnancy, but the amount is small. Passage of meconium in utero probably occurs with asphyxia, which increases intestinal peristalsis and relaxation of the anal sphincter. Passage of meconium is also seen in increasing frequency as the fetus reaches term and moves beyond term. Meconium is rarely seen in fetuses before 36 weeks. Between 36 and 42 weeks meconium may be found in 25% of births. After 42 weeks meconium may be seen as frequently as 50% of all deliveries. In many circumstances the passage of meconium may simply represent a mature gastrointestinal tract and not be an indicator of an acute hypoxic event.

Intrahepatic erythropoiesis begins during the eighth week in the embryo, and the liver is well developed histologically by midpregnancy. During fetal life, the liver acts as a storage depot for glycogen and iron. Reasonably complete liver function is not achieved until well after the neonatal period has passed. Liver deficiencies at birth are many, including reduced hepatic production of fibrinogen and coagulation factors II, VII, IX, XI, and XII.

Vitamin K stored in the liver is deficient at birth because its formation is dependent upon bacteria in the intestine. These deficiencies predispose the newborn to hemorrhage during the first few days of life.

The formation of glucose from amino acids (gluconeogenesis) in the liver and adequate storage of glucose are not well established in the newborn. Moreover, levels of carbohydrate-regulating hormones such as cortisol, epinephrine, and glucagon may be initially insufficient. As a consequence, neonatal hypoglycemia is common after stressful stimuli such as exposure to cold or malnutrition.

Glucuronidation is limited during the early neonatal period, with the result that bilirubin is not readily conjugated for excretion as bile. After physiologic hemolysis of excess red blood cells in the first week of life or with pathologic hemolysis in isoimmunized newborns, jaundice occurs. If marked hyperbilirubinemia develops, kernicterus may ensue.

Metabolism of drugs by the liver is poor in the newborn period (eg, sulfonamides and chloramphenicol). Moreover, numerous inborn errors of metabolism (eg, galactosemia) may be diagnosed soon after birth. Neonatal liver function gradually improves, assuming proper food, freedom from infection, and a favorable environment.

Secretory and absorptive functions are accelerated after delivery. Most digestive enzymes are present, but the gastric contents are neutral at birth, although acidity soon develops. The initial neutrality may briefly delay the growth in the bowel of bacteria necessary for the formation of vitamin K in the intestine. The newborn can assimilate simple solutions and breast milk immediately after birth but cannot digest cow's milk as well until the second or third day after elimination of excessive gastric mucus. Slow progress of milk through the stomach and upper intestine is usual during the early neonatal period.

Normally, some air enters the stomach during feedings. Pocketing of air in the upper curvature of the stomach occurs when the newborn is lying flat. Hence, turning of the infant and "burping" with the infant upright are necessary.

Large bowel peristalsis promptly increases after delivery, and 1–6 stools per day are passed. Absence of stool within 48 hours after birth is indicative of intestinal obstruction or imperforate anus.

RENAL FUNCTION IN THE FETUS & NEWBORN

During uterine growth and development, the placenta serves as the major regulator of fluid and electrolyte balance. The kidneys are unnecessary for fetal growth and development, as demonstrated by the rare neonate born with renal agenesis. Hence, the placenta and maternal lungs and kidneys normally maintain fetal fluid and electrolyte balance. When the connection between fetal circulation and the placenta is interrupted during delivery, the kidneys are called upon to assume the homeostatic functional demands of extrauterine life.

The placenta (the major homeostatic organ) receives 40–65% of the fetal cardiac output. Renal blood flow in fetal lambs has been shown to be constant when expressed per gram of renal tissue, and renal vascular resistance is maintained at a constant value. Following birth, renal blood flow increases significantly and renal vascular resistance decreases by about 25%. However, renal blood flow is low and vascular resistance high when compared with adult levels.

The high neonatal vascular resistance may be attributable to increased renal adrenergic activity in the newborn. The neonatal renal vasculature has been shown to be sensitive to catecholamines, and the kidneys have been shown to have a high density of high-affinity alpha-adrenoceptors. At birth, a greater percentage of blood perfuses the deeper cortical nephrons. With maturation, the rise in blood flow to the outer cortical region increases faster than the rise to the inner cortex.

The **glomerular filtration rate (GFR)** in fetal animals, particularly lambs, increases proportionately with growth of the kidney (GFR expressed per gram of kidney weight) and rises significantly after birth. Renal blood flow has a similar pattern. During the first 24 hours of life, measurements of the GFR reflect the status of renal function during intrauterine life; at least 24 hours are needed for the GFR to adapt to the extrauterine environment. The GFR and renal blood flow follow a similar postnatal pattern, with values more than doubling during the first 2 weeks of life. This is also true in preterm neonates, although values start at lower levels.

Preterm infants have a negative sodium balance during the first 1–3 weeks of life. The mechanism for sodium wasting in premature infants probably involves proximal and distal tubule function. Preterm infants have a lower rate of sodium resorption in the proximal tubule than term infants. Newborns also have a limited ability to excrete a salt load when compared with adults. The functional tubular immaturity of the kidney in newborns is also demonstrated by increased renal excretion of glucose and amino acids and by decreased ability to concentrate, dilute, and acidify the urine. A normal serum bicarbonate level for a preterm infant may be as low as 14–16 mmol/L, but this level increases to 21 mmol/L during the first week of life (the value is similar in term newborns). Thus, newborn infants have a limited ability to excrete an acid load as well as a lower renal threshold for bicarbonate. Preterm infants do not concentrate urine as well as term infants. Most infants do not concentrate urine as well as adults until

6–12 months of age. Maximal urine osmolality in preterm newborns is 500–600 mOsm/kg water; in term infants, maximum osmolality is 500–700 mOsm/kg water.

Formation of urine is thought to begin at 9–12 weeks' gestation. By 32 weeks, fetal production of urine approaches 12 mL/h, and by term, 28 mL/h. At that point, urine is the major component of amniotic fluid. As mentioned before, the relative amounts of amniotic fluid can provide information on the status of fetal renal function. Oligohydramnios may be associated with renal hypoplasia, dysplasia, or obstructive uropathy. A normal amount of amniotic fluid indicates that there is some function in at least one kidney.

Ninety-three percent of all infants, either term or preterm, will void within the first 24 hours of life; 99% will void within 48 hours. Inadequate urine formation by the neonate can be associated with intravascular volume depletion, hypoxia, congenital nephrotic syndrome, tubular necrosis, renal agenesis, bilateral renal arterial or venous thrombosis, or obstructive uropathy. Normal infants may have transient glycosuria or proteinuria and a urine pH of 6.0–7.0.

Ultrasonography allows diagnosis of hydronephrosis prenatally and has stimulated research into therapeutic use of antenatal urinary aspiration or diversion techniques. A registry has been formed that has compiled data regarding fetal surgery. These attempts continue to be experimental, but the hope is that early "decompression" may prevent renal dysplasia. Prospective studies are warranted to determine whether early neonatal corrective surgery for congenital obstruction (pyeloplasty or ureteral reimplant) is truly worthwhile.

CENTRAL NERVOUS SYSTEM FUNCTION IN THE FETUS & NEWBORN

It has been known for at least a century that the fetus is capable of sustained motor activity well before quickening. Through the eighth week of gestation, nearly 95% of responses are contralateral. Ipsilateral responses (torso stimulus) begin to appear with much greater frequency during the ninth week. By 12–13 weeks, local reflexes have almost completely replaced the total pattern of response. Recent ultrasonographic evaluations have followed motor activity in utero and all confirm a transition from simple whole body movements to complex motor responses. Thus, the sensation of fetal movement is an increasing part of the sensory input to the brainstem.

The cortex begins to develop during the eighth week. The neural maturational events that have been evaluated have emphasized 2 transitional periods: (1) a possible consolidation of brainstem influence over motor activity and sensory input near the end of the first trimester, and (2) establishment of the sensory input channel to the neothalamocortical connection around midgestation. However, it is apparent that the brainstem is only partially developed and functional at term.

The functional development of the human central nervous system is too complex to summarize. Nevertheless, a few clinical correlates must be mentioned. An individual's development neither begins nor ends at birth. Abnormal neuronal migrations in the developing human brain are generally early gestational events induced by genetic factors, teratogens, or infections. Although the major neuronal migrations have formed the cortical plate by 16 weeks' gestation, late migrations from the germinal matrix into the cerebral cortex continue until 5 months postnatally. The external granular layer of the cerebellar cortex continues to migrate until age 1 year. Thus, ample opportunity exists for disturbances of these migratory processes in the postnatal period. Moreover, myelination is only rudimentary in the cerebral cortex of term infants. Axons of the large pyramidal cells of the motor cortex are myelinated only as far cortically as the cerebral peduncles of the midbrain, as demonstrated by light microscopy, and pyramidal tract axons in the medulla oblongata have only 1 or 2 turns of myelin, as seen on electron microscopy.

Neurologic development not only implies acquisition of perceptual, motor, linguistic, and intellectual skills but also signifies progressive organization of the anatomic and physiologic substrates of those achievements. Formation of the nervous system begins with the embryonic neural plate and terminates with completion of the final myelination cycle in the brain, ie, the frontal temporal association bundle at age 32–34 years. It is obvious that there are many things that can interrupt the normal migration, eg, a premature infant who suffers a subependymal hemorrhage affecting the radial glial process that is guiding a neuron to the surface. The neuron may retract from the cortical surface after its cell origin is destroyed. The maturation is in situ, but the migrating neuron is unable to establish the intended synaptic relations with the cortex. Perhaps the faulty synaptic circuitry of this "incidental finding" at autopsy contributes to the development of an epileptic focus. Another mechanism of prenatal or postnatal cerebral dysgenesis involves toxins that destroy the cytoskeletal elements of glial and nerve cells, eg, methylmercury poisoning. Methylmercury chloride abruptly arrests the active movement of migrating neurons in vitro, causing damage to the neural membrane of the growth zone, interferes with DNA synthesis, and ultimately compromises cytoskeletal proteins.

Psychiatrists and psychologists have long recognized in utero modifying influences, and Freud stated that "each individual ego is endowed from the beginning with its own peculiar disposition and tendencies." For example, maternal anxiety levels do affect fetal development, and intrauterine stimuli determine, to a degree, the maturation of nerve cells and structural patterns of the developing brain. Maternal emotional stress can have immediate and long-term effects on fetal development, but it is unclear whether these effects are predictable.

Between 10 and 20 weeks' gestational age, the fetus displays several basic motor patterns that are later integrated into specific actions. The first jerky patterns of the second trimester become the functional movement patterns that allow the fetus to move about in utero. After midpregnancy, these motor patterns mature in a manner similar to the mature repertoire of the newborn. Clues to future central nervous system development may be found in the study of these various fetal motor patterns, and failure to progress at various stages seems to indicate subsequent cerebral dysfunction. Real-time ultrasonic examination of such fetal motor patterns may lead to improved care in high-risk situations.

The fetus demonstrates various sleep-wake patterns throughout its development in utero. During most of its antenatal life, fetal electrocortical activity is of low voltage, associated with rapid eye movements, slow heart rate, and fetal breathing activity. In the third trimester, high-voltage activity is associated with the more lively activity. Finally, near term, the fetus appears to be awake at least 30% of the time. These fetal states may be discerned by ultrasonic study of eye movements, which may be altered by drugs or maternal anxiety levels. These, in turn, affect fetal heart rate responses to stress.

The term fetus has high **endorphin** levels that may modify the behavioral state, including heart rate responses. Endorphin levels may be responsible for the primary apnea of the newborn and for the lack of heart rate reactivity in otherwise normal intrapartum fetuses. The fetus probably suffers pain, as does any other individual, and high endorphin levels may limit pain and other effects of stress. The near-term fetus, then, has nearly all the neurologic attributes of the newborn infant.

■ INTRAUTERINE NUTRITION

Maternal diet among mammals is incredibly varied. For instance, the female black bear hibernates during her pregnancy, but she supplies metabolites to her fetus while neither eating nor drinking. In contrast, the pregnant guinea pig eats continuously. Obviously, forced fasting may have different effects on these different species during pregnancy. As shown in Fig 8–8, many maternal and placental modifications of nutrients occur before the nutrients reach the fetus. The mother and the placenta have first priority in use of these nutrients. Although vitamin B accumulates in greater concentrations in fetal blood than in maternal blood, the placental release of most vitamins to the fetus seems to depend on the degree of saturation of the vitamin reserve in the placenta. Because these nutrient-modifying factors differ markedly in different species, it is hazardous to interpolate data from laboratory animals to humans. The

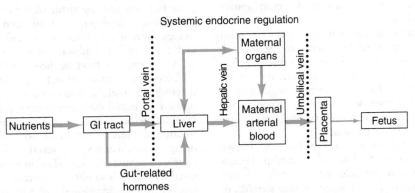

Figure 8–8. Schematic diagram showing the pathway of nutrients in the mother as they are broken down into different concentrations in the maternal portal vein and, finally, the umbilical vein. (Modified and reproduced, with permission, from Battaglia FC: The comparative physiology of fetal nutrition. Am J Obstet Gynecol 1984;148:850.)

human newborn is 16% fat. Normally, the human fetus has a large accumulation of high-calorie fat, which during the last few weeks of gestation represents over 80% of the fetal caloric accretion. There are 2 components of fetal caloric intake: the building-block, or accretion, component and the growth, or heat production, component. Starvation and protein-turnover studies suggest that the fetus uses calories primarily for maintenance rather than growth.

In pregnant sheep at term (pregnancy in sheep and humans is comparable in terms of relative fetal/maternal weights), one-third of the maternal glucose is used by the uterus; of this amount, two-thirds is consumed by the uteroplacental tissue and only one-third by the fetus. In sheep, the placenta rather than the fetus is clearly the primary intrauterine glucose consumer. This large glucose uptake by the placenta is partially explained by its high rate of lactate production. Laboratory studies have shown that when the human fetus is well oxygenated, the umbilical arterial lactate concentration and the umbilical arteriovenous difference are positive, indicating that lactate is also an important nutrient for the human fetus.

Ammonia is another compound produced in large quantities by the placenta and, like lactate, is released into the umbilical circulation. In humans, ketones and free fatty acids play a large role in fetal nutrition. The fetus actively synthesizes fatty acids in the liver, brain, and lung, which have special requirements for myelin and surfactant. Although fatty acids can be transported across the placenta, their oxidation does not seem to add much to the total energy economy of the fetus. The fetus regularly uses protein for oxidative metabolism. The metabolism of the human brain is very active during the perinatal period, and the brain is an obligatory consumer of glucose. Ketone bodies may partially replace glucose during periods of hypoglycemia and may also be a source of carbon for central nervous system lipids and proteins.

The placenta transports more water than any other substance. Since maternal hydrostatic and serum colloid osmotic pressures vary significantly during a normal day, unknown placental mechanisms protect the fetus against rapid shifts of water, which could cause either hydrops or dehydration. It may be that placental water transport is a passive process resulting from active solute transfer, as in the intestine.

The most widely recognized fetal hormone known to modify the rate of fetal growth is insulin. Fetuses with anomalies that preclude the availability of fetal growth hormone, thyroxine, adrenocortical steroids, or sex steroids achieve normal birthweights. Inasmuch as maternal insulin is not transferred to the fetus in physiologic quantities, the fetal pancreas must supply sufficient insulin for the oxidation of glucose. Under the stimulus of recurring hyperglycemia—as with maternal diabetes mellitus—the B cells of the fetal pancreas may become hyperplastic and secrete larger quantities of insulin.

THE AMNIOTIC FLUID

There is a vital need for a nonrestricting intrauterine environment, which develops before the fetus. This environment can only be ensured if it is part of the development of the fetus. Every fetus is surrounded by a protective cushion of amniotic fluid, whether the fetus develops inside the mother as a viviparous species or in an egg. In the first half of pregnancy, amniotic fluid volume appears to increase in association with growth of the fetus, and the correlation between fetal weight and amniotic fluid is very close. The serum osmolality and sodium, urea, and creatinine content of maternal serum and amniotic fluid are not significantly different. This suggests that amniotic fluid is an ultrafiltrate of maternal serum. Ultrasonographic evaluation during the first half of pregnancy reveals that the fetus does empty its bladder during the first half of gestation.

The average volume of amniotic fluid at term is 800 mL, and the sodium concentration is fairly constant. The volume and sodium concentration remain the same in spite of the fact that a normal fetus will swallow some of the fluid and will also contribute urine, which concentrates sodium. Analysis of amniotic fluid provides unique information about the fetus. In the first half of pregnancy, amniotic fluid appears to maintain the extracellular fluid chemistry of the fetus. In the second half, amniotic fluid reflects the development of renal function and, by virtue of the cells it sheds, the morphologic development of skin and mucous membranes. Amniotic fluid has a low specific gravity (1.008) and a pH of 7.2. Pathways of solute and water exchange in amniotic fluid are shown in Fig 8–9.

Diagnostic amniocentesis has provided a means of determining amniotic fluid content. Much of the work initially emanated from amniograms followed by spectrophotometric analysis of amniotic fluid in Rh factor isoimmunization. When an Rh-positive fetus is developing erythroblastosis, the severity of the anemia is closely correlated with the bilirubin concentration. The usual technique is to obtain a spectrophotometric tracing between the wavelengths of 550 nm and 350 nm and then determine the deviation of the optical density (OD) at 450 nm. An illustration of such a determination is shown in Fig 15–2. In this example, the OD 450-nm peak has an OD difference of 0.069, which, if

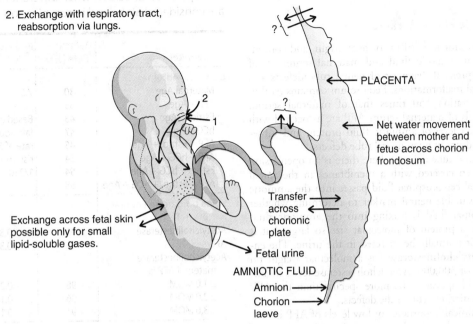

1. Fetal swallowing and reabsorption by intestine.

2. Exchange with respiratory tract, reabsorption via lungs.

PLACENTA

Net water movement between mother and fetus across chorion frondosum

Transfer across chorionic plate

Exchange across fetal skin possible only for small lipid-soluble gases.

Fetal urine

AMNIOTIC FLUID

Amnion

Chorion laeve

Figure 8–9. Solute and water exchange in amniotic fluid.

found at 37 weeks' gestation, would be an indication for immediate cesarean delivery. Further details about the management of the affected fetus are given in Chapter 15.

In the past decade, morphologic chromosomal abnormalities and more than 100 inborn errors of metabolism have been identified. The amniotic fluid collects cells shed from the skin, amnion, and gastrointestinal and genitourinary tracts. In amniotic fluid obtained by amniocentesis at about 16 weeks, 30–80% of these cells are usually alive. Recent cytotechnologic advances may allow karyotyping from amniotic fluid as early as 11 weeks of gestation. The total number of cells increases with the length of gestation, but the proportion of viable cells does not increase, and at about 24 weeks, only 10–15% of the total number of cells are viable. The live cells are induced to adhere to the bottom of a tissue culture vessel after 3–4 days in culture, and they develop either an epithelial or fibroplastic morphology. The cells eventually form a monolayer, and when introduced into a suitable culture medium (containing nutrients and supplied with serum) are induced to divide. The dividing cells are arrested at metaphase with colchicine to prevent formation of the mitotic spindle. The advantage of this method is that a number of slides can be prepared, so that specific stain methods can be used and the chromosome preparation can be banded satisfactorily.

There is no simple or accurate method currently available to measure amniotic fluid volume. **Oligohydramnios** almost always indicates the presence of some abnormality. Polyhydramnios may occur in normal pregnancy but is associated with some abnormality of mother or fetus in approximately 50% of cases. Quantitation of amniotic fluid volume by ultrasound is subjective. The term **polyhydramnios (hydramnios)** has been classically associated with amniotic fluid volume of 2000 mL or more. Oligohydramnios may be more objectively determined by identification of the largest pocket of fluid measuring less than 2 cm × 2 cm or the total of four quadrants less than 5 cm. However, this definition is associated with many false-positive and false-negative readings.

Oligohydramnios is associated with SGA fetus, renal tract abnormalities such as renal agenesis, and urinary tract dysplasia. The clinical manifestation of oligohydramnios is a direct result of the impairment of urine flow to the amniotic fluid in the late part of the first half of pregnancy or during the second and third trimesters.

Amniotic fluid inhibits bacterial growth; the phosphate to zinc ratio is a predictor of inhibitory activity.

In cases of intra-amniotic fluid infection, "inorganic phosphorus" levels in amniotic fluid are often elevated.

Amniotic Fluid Markers

Alpha-fetoprotein (AFP) is of fetal origin, and concentrations in amniotic fluid and maternal serum are of value in prenatal diagnosis of neural tube defects and other fetal malformations. Fetal serum contains AFP in a concentration 150 times that of maternal serum. High levels of maternal serum AFP are associated with an elevated level of amniotic fluid protein and subsequent findings of open neural tube defects.

In neural tube defects where there is an open lesion (even when covered with a membrane) in the spinal canal, fetal cerebrospinal fluid passes into the amniotic fluid. A suitable neural marker to determine whether cerebrospinal fluid is leaking into the amniotic fluid would be a protein of molecular size so large that it would not normally be excreted in the urine. The enzyme **acetylcholinesterase** has a molecular weight on the order of 300,000. Acetylcholinesterase levels in amniotic fluid appear to be more specific than the AFP test in predicting neural tube defects.

The clinical importance of low levels of AFP in maternal serum has also been recognized. Low levels of AFP in conjunction with estriol and comparatively high levels of hCG (roughly twice normal for given gestational age) have been shown to be predictive for Down's syndrome. As an illustration, if one assumes a base rate of diagnostic amniocentesis of 5% (the approximate proportion of pregnancies occurring beyond age 35), the likelihood of detecting Down's syndrome using only maternal age as a risk factor would be only 30%. However, if amniocenteses were to be performed on the basis of age, AFP, estriol, and hCG levels, the yield would rise to almost 60%. Down's syndrome is the most common congenital cause of severe mental retardation, occurring with an incidence of about 1.3 per 1000 live births. Advanced maternal age is the most common consideration in selecting women for diagnostic amniocentesis. This policy derives from the fact that the risk of Down's syndrome rises with advancing maternal age. The greatly improved detection rate (Table 8–8) afforded by combining serum screening and age as screening criteria is fast establishing this method as the screening test of choice in many centers throughout the world.

Other proteins may enter the amniotic fluid from the maternal plasma. Some proteins enter the fluid by transudation of placental components, but they also enter from other sources, including maternal uterine decidua, fetal skin, amnion, chorion, the umbilical cord, amniotic fluid cells, fetal urine, meconium, and fetal nasopharyngeal, oral, and lacrimal secretions. It is

Table 8–8. Detection rate of Down's syndrome and open neural defects when different markers are considered alone and in combination.

Parameter	Detection Rate (%)	False Positive Rate (%)
Down's syndrome		
Maternal Age	30	7.5
AFP + Age	35	
Estriol + Age	43	Based on a
hCG + Age	47	false-positive
AFP + Estriol + Age	45	rate of 5% and
AFP + hCG + Age	54	risk cutoff of
Estriol + hCG + Age	54	1/250
AFP + Estriol + hCG + Age	58	
Spina bifida/open neural tube defects		
Acetylcholinesterase	99	0.34
AFP	85	0.36
Acetylcholinesterase if maternal AFP is		
≥ 1.0 MOM	98	0.29
≥ 2.0 MOM	96	0.14
≤ 3.0 MOM	91	0.11

AFP = Alpha fetoprotein, MOM = multiples of median.
(Adapted from Wald NJ et al: Prenatal biochemical screening for Downs Syndrome and neural tube defects. Curr Opin Obstet Gynecol 1992;4:302.)

assumed that the relative contribution of these tissues will change during pregnancy. The major proportion of soluble proteins in amniotic fluid between 10 weeks' gestation and term is thought to be (1) of serum type and (2) of maternal origin entering the fluid by diffusing through the amniotic chorion. The observed concentration gradient for AFP between fetal serum and amniotic fluid should not be taken to imply that AFP's presence in amniotic fluid is explained largely by permeation. Indeed, the concentration of AFP in fetal urine during the second trimester is comparable with levels of AFP in amniotic fluid at this time.

The amniotic fluid serves a number of important functions besides being a valuable source for analysis of fetal tissues and fluids. It cushions the fetus against severe injury; provides a medium in which the fetus can move easily; may be a source of fetal nutrients; and, in early pregnancy, is essential for fetal lung development. The amniotic fluid is continuously exchanged at a rapid rate. Indeed, it is possible, at least on a temporary basis, to increase amniotic fluid volume by rapid expansion of maternal plasma volume with an intravenous infusion of colloid fluid such as 5% albumin. After 34–36 weeks, determination of amniotic fluid volume becomes even more complicated because the larger fetus swallows more fluid, upsetting the relationship between fetal size and fluid volume. After 38 weeks, both amniotic fluid and maternal plasma volume decrease. These relative decreases are even more apparent in postmature pregnancy.

Studies have shown that the fetus near term drinks 400–500 mL of amniotic fluid per day; this is about the same as the amount of milk consumed by a newborn infant. To maintain a reasonable stability of volume, the fetus must excrete about the same volume of urine into the amniotic fluid each day.

During late pregnancy, the amniotic fluid contains increasing quantities of particulate material, including desquamated cells of fetal origin; lanugo and scalp hairs; vernix caseosa; a few leukocytes; and small quantities of albumin, urates, and other organic and inorganic salts. The calcium content of amniotic fluid is low (5.5 mg/dL), but the electrolyte concentration is otherwise equivalent to that of maternal plasma. As mentioned previously, meconium is ordinarily absent but is excreted by the fetus in response to vagal activity.

REFERENCES

Altshuler G: Role of the placenta in perinatal pathology revisited. Pediatr Pathol Lab Med 1996;16:207.

Battaglia FC: The comparative physiology of fetal nutrition. Am J Obstet Gynecol 1984;148:850.

Bonds DR et al: Fetal weight/placental weight ratio and perinatal outcome. Am J Obstet Gynecol 1984;149:195.

Bonds DR et al: Human fetal weight and placental weight growth curves: A mathematical analysis from a population at sea level. Biol Neonate 1984;45:261.

Campbell S et al: New Doppler technique for assessing uteroplacental blood flow. Lancet 1983;1:675.

Castle BM, Turnbull AC: The presence or absence of fetal breathing movements predicts the outcome of preterm labour. Lancet 1983;2:471.

Dawes GS: The central control of fetal breathing and skeletal muscle movements. J Physiol 1984;346:1.

Farmakides G et al: Prenatal surveillance using non stress testing and Doppler velocimetry. Obstet Gynecol 1988;71:184.

Finberg HJ et al: Placenta accreta: Prospective sonographic diagnosis in patients with placenta previa and prior cesarean section. J Ultrasound Med 1992;11:333.

Fisher DJ: Oxygenation and metabolism in the developing heart. Semin Perinatol 1984;8:217.

Fleischer A et al: Uterine artery Doppler velocimetry in pregnant women with hypertension. Am J Obstet Gynecol 1986;154:806.

Fritz MA, Guo SM: Doubling time of human chorionic gonadotrophin (hCG) in normal early pregnancy: relationship to hCG concentration and gestational age. Fertil Steril 1987;47:584.

Goldenberg RL, Huddleston JF, Nelson KG: Apgar scores and umbilical arterial pH in preterm newborn infants. Am J Obstet Gynecol 1984;149:651.

Goodlin RC: Expanded toxemia syndrome or gestosis. Am J Obstet Gynecol 1986;154:1227.

Goodlin RC, Anderson JC, Gallagher TF: Relationship between amniotic fluid volume and maternal plasma volume expansion. Am J Obstet Gynecol 1984;146:505.

Harris R, Andrews T: Prenatal screening for Down's syndrome. Arch Dis Child 1988;63:705.

Hustin J, Foidart JM, Lambote R: Maternal vascular lesions in preeclampsia and intrauterine growth retardation. Placenta 1983;4:489.

Jaffe RB: Fetoplacental endocrine and metabolic physiology. Clin Perinatol 1983;10:669.

Juchau MR, Faustman-Watts E: Pharmacokinetic considerations in the maternal-placental-fetal unit. Clin Obstet Gynecol 1983;26:379.

Kauaauapaua P: Prostanoids in neonatology. Ann Clin Res 1984; 16:330.

Longo LD: Maternal blood volume and cardiac output during pregnancy: A hypothesis of endocrinologic control. Am J Physiol 1983;245(5-Part 1):R720.

Miller PW et al: Dating the time interval from meconium passage to birth. Obstet Gynecol 1985;66:459.

Naeye RL: Functionally important disorders of the placenta, umbilical cord, and fetal membranes. Hum Pathol 1987;18: 680.

Rosenfeld CR: Consideration of the uteroplacental circulation in intrauterine growth. Semin Perinatol 1984;8:42.

Reed KL: Fetal pulmonary artery and aorta: Two-dimensional Doppler echocardiography. Obstet Gynecol 1987;69:175.

Sarnat HB: Disturbances of late neuronal migrations in the perinatal period. Am J Dis Child 1987;141:969.

Scarpelli EM: Perinatal lung mechanics and the first breath. Lung 1984;162:61.

Silverman F et al: The Apgar score: Is it enough? Obstet Gynecol 1985;66:331.

Suidan JS, Wasserman JF, Young BK: Placental contribution to lactate production by the human fetoplacental unit. Am J Perinatol 1984;1:306.

Voigt HJ, Becker V: Doppler flow measurements and histomorphology of the placental bed in uteroplacental insufficiency. J Perinat Med 1992;20:139.

Wald NJ, Cuckle HS, Nanchahal K: Amniotic fluid acetylcholinesterase measurement in the prenatal diagnosis of open neural tube defects: Second report of the Collaborative Acetylcholinesterase study. Prenat Diagn 1989;9:813.

Wasmoen TL: Placental Proteins. In Polin RA, Fox WW (editors): *Fetal and Neonatal Physiology.* WB Saunders, 1992.

Wells M et al: Spiral (uteroplacental) arteries of the human placental bed show the presence of amniotic basement membrane antigens. Am J Obstet Gynecol 1984;150:973.

SECTION II
Normal Obstetrics

Normal Pregnancy & Prenatal Care 9

Suzanne Bovone, MD, & Martin L. Pernoll, MD

■ NORMAL PREGNANCY

Pregnancy (gestation) is the maternal condition of having a developing fetus in the body. The human conceptus from fertilization through the eighth week of pregnancy is termed an **embryo;** from the eighth week until delivery, it is a **fetus.** For obstetric purposes, the duration of pregnancy is based on **gestational age:** the estimated age of the fetus calculated from the first day of the last (normal) menstrual period (LMP), assuming a 28-day cycle. Gestational age is expressed in completed weeks. This is in contrast to **developmental age (fetal age),** which is the age of the offspring calculated from the time of implantation.

The term **gravid** means pregnant, and **gravidity** is the total number of pregnancies (normal or abnormal). **Parity** is the state of having given birth to an infant or infants weighing 500 g or more, alive or dead. In the absence of known weight, an estimated duration of gestation of 20 completed weeks or more (calculated from the first day of the LMP) may be used. From a practical clinical viewpoint, a fetus is considered viable when it has reached a gestational age of 23–24 weeks and a weight of 600 g or more. However, only very rarely will a fetus of 20–23 weeks weighing 500–600 g or less survive, even with optimal care. With regard to parity, a multiple birth is a single parous experience.

Live Birth

Live birth is the complete expulsion or extraction of a product of conception from the mother, regardless of the duration of pregnancy, which, after such separation, breathes or shows other evidence of life (eg, beating of the heart, pulsation of the umbilical cord, or definite movements of the involuntary muscles) whether or not the cord has been cut or the placenta detached. An **infant** is a live-born individual from the moment of birth until the completion of 1 year of life.

In the most recent nomenclature, a **preterm infant** is defined as one born prior to the 37th week of gestation (259 days). Unfortunately, for purposes of evaluating statistical data, this definition does not specify that there are great differences among fetuses in this group. Therefore, it is useful to preserve the classification by weight or duration of gestation still used by many (Fig 9–1). Using the latter system, an **abortion** is the expulsion or extraction of all (complete) or any part (incomplete) of the placenta or membranes, without an identifiable fetus or with a fetus (alive or dead) weighing less than 500 g. In the absence of known weight, an estimated duration of gestation of under 20 completed weeks (139 days) calculated from the first day of the LMP may be used.

An **immature infant** weighs 500–1000 g and has completed 20 to less than 28 weeks of gestation. A **premature infant** is one with a birthweight of 1000–2500 g and a duration of gestation of 28 to less than 37 weeks. A **low-birthweight infant** is any live-born infant weighing 2500 g or less at birth. An **undergrown** or **small-for-date infant** is one who is significantly undersized (< 2 SD) for the period of gestation. A **mature infant** is a live-born infant who has completed 37 weeks of gestation (and usually weighs over 2500 g). A **postmature infant** is one who has completed 42 weeks or more of gestation. The **postmature syndrome** is characterized by prolonged gestation, sometimes an excessive-size fetus (see Large-For-Gestational-Age Pregnancy in Chapter 16), and diminished placental capacity for sufficient exchange, associated with cutaneous and nutritional changes in the newborn infant.

A fetus or infant of **excessive size** (macrosomic) is one who is larger than the gestation would indicate or

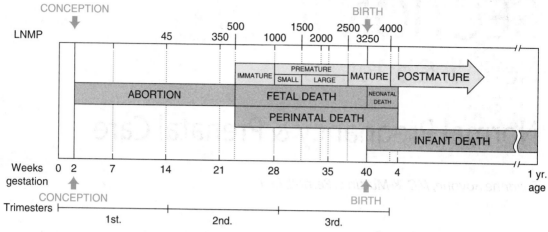

Figure 9–1. Graphic display of perinatal nomenclature.

who at the time of birth weighs over 4500 g. Significantly increased morbidity and mortality rates may be associated with the relative dystocia created by the large fetus. About 10% of newborn infants are **oversized** (> 4000 g), and 2% are of "excessive" size (> 4500 g). With better nutrition and heavier infants, there has not been a commensurate increase in maternal pelvic dimensions. Excessive fetal size should be suspected in large multiparous or obese mothers, those with diabetes mellitus, or those whose weight gain during pregnancy has been greater than anticipated.

Predicting the end of pregnancy constitutes one of the major problems of perinatal care. The factors that lead to the initiation of labor and the subsequent termination of pregnancy remain unknown. This is the case for both late termination and premature termination. A prolonged pregnancy is a gestation that has advanced beyond 2 SD from the mean and with a duration of 42½ weeks or longer (297 days). The perinatal mortality rate at 43 weeks is twice that at 39–42 weeks. The fetus probably develops a relatively restricted placental exchange capability, leading to an increased intrauterine death rate.

Birth Rate & Fertility Rate

Birth rate is commonly expressed in terms of the number of live births per 1000 population. The **fertility rate** is expressed as the number of live births per 1000 women aged 15–44 years and is thus a more sensitive measure of the reproductive activity of a given population. There were an estimated 3,880,894 live births in the United States in 1997. This is the lowest number since 1987. The birth rate of 1997 was 14.5, a record low. Likewise, the fertility rate declined to 65.0, matching the record low of 1976.* Indeed, the fertility rate appears to have peaked in 1990 at 71.1, after having been 67.1 in 1988.

Neonatal Interval

The **neonatal interval** is from birth until 28 days of life. During this interval, the infant is referred to as a newborn infant. The interval may be divided into 3 periods:

Neonatal period I: birth through 23 hours, 59 minutes.

Neonatal period II: 24 hours of life through 6 days, 23 hours, 59 minutes.

Neonatal period III: seventh day of life through 27 days, 23 hours, 59 minutes.

Perinatal Interval

The **perinatal interval** is the span of fetal and neonatal life. It is an important concept because many of the stresses and hazards that affect the fetus have either a direct or an indirect effect in the neonatal period. An arbitrary division of authority (between obstetrician and pediatrician) and attention only to the product of conception at birth may be hazardous and unwarranted. The perinatal interval of life may be divided into 2 periods:

---

* These data are provisional and are from the *Monthly Vital Statistic Report* 1999;47:18, the preeminent source of data concerning births, marriages, divorces, and deaths. It is available on a monthly basis from the National Center for Health Statistics (Centers for Disease Control, Public Health Service), U.S. Department of Health and Human Services.

Perinatal period I: 28 weeks of completed gestation to the first 7 days of life.

Perinatal period II: 20 weeks of gestation through 27 days of life.

Perinatal Mortality Rates

Jeopardy to life is greatest during the perinatal interval than at any subsequent time. Current data indicate that the number of lives lost during the 5-month period from the 20th week of gestation to the seventh day after birth is almost equal to the number lost during the next 40 years of life. Of those deaths occurring in the first year of life, approximately 70% will occur in the first 28 days. If one adds this to the fetal loss, then it is the period of greatest threat to life for a given interval. There are sexual and racial differences in mortality rates; the pertinent data are available through the *Monthly Vital Statistics Report.*

There are many causes of death during the perinatal period. The relative importance of each can only be assessed in the context of overall mortality rates and appraisal of those factors that present the greatest hazard to the fetus and infant. Fetal deaths after 20 weeks account for about 50% of all perinatal deaths.

DIAGNOSIS

The diagnosis of pregnancy is usually made on the basis of a history of amenorrhea, an enlarging uterus, and a positive pregnancy test. Nausea and breast tenderness are also often present. It may be crucial to diagnose pregnancy before the first missed menstrual period to prevent exposure of the fetus to hazardous substances (eg, x-rays, teratogenic drugs), to manage ectopic or nonviable pregnancies, or to provide better health care for the mother.

The manifestations of pregnancy are classified into 3 groups: presumptive, probable, and positive.

Presumptive Manifestations

A. SYMPTOMS

1. Amenorrhea—Cessation of menses is caused by increasing estrogen and progesterone levels produced by the corpus luteum. Thus, amenorrhea is a fairly reliable sign of conception in women with regular menstrual cycles. In women with irregular cycles, amenorrhea is not a reliable sign. Delayed menses may also be caused by other factors such as emotional tension, chronic disease, opioid and dopaminergic medications, endocrine disorders, and certain genitourinary tumors. Spotting due to bleeding at the implantation site may occur from the time of implantation (about 6 days after fertilization) until 29–35 days after the LMP in many women. Some women have unexplained cyclic bleeding throughout pregnancy.

2. Nausea and vomiting—This common symptom occurs in approximately 50% of pregnancies and is most marked at 2–12 weeks' gestation. It is usually most severe in the morning but can occur at any time and may be precipitated by cooking odors and pungent smells. Emotional tension may play a role in the severity of nausea and vomiting. Extreme nausea and vomiting may be a sign of multiple gestation or molar pregnancy. Protracted vomiting associated with dehydration and ketonuria (**hyperemesis gravidarum**) may require hospitalization and relief of symptoms with a droperidol drip.

Treatment for uncomplicated nausea consists of light dry foods, small frequent meals, and emotional support. Some improvement can be seen with the addition of high-dose B_6 therapy and the preconceptional use of prenatal vitamins. Antinauseant drugs are used only as a final measure. The nausea probably results from rapidly rising serum levels of human chorionic gonadotropin (hCG). During the first trimester, serum hCG levels may be as high as 100,000 mIU/mL.

3. Breasts—

a. Mastodynia—Mastodynia, or **breast tenderness,** may range from tingling to frank pain caused by hormonal responses of the mammary ducts and alveolar system. Circulatory increases result in breast engorgement and venous prominence. Similar tenderness may occur just before menses.

b. Enlargement of circumlacteal sebaceous glands of the areola (Montgomery's tubercles)—Enlargement of these glands occurs at 6–8 weeks' gestation and is due to hormonal stimulation.

c. Colostrum secretion—Colostrum secretion may begin after 16 weeks' gestation.

d. Secondary breasts—Secondary breasts may become more prominent both in size and in coloration. These occur along the nipple line. Hypertrophy of axillary breast tissue often causes a symptomatic lump in the axilla.

4. Quickening—The first perception of fetal movement occurs at 18–20 weeks in primigravidas and at 14–16 weeks in multigravidas. Intestinal peristalsis may be mistaken for fetal movement; therefore, perceived fetal movement alone is not a reliable symptom of pregnancy, but may be useful in determining the duration of pregnancy.

5. Urinary tract—

a. Bladder irritability, frequency, and nocturia—These conditions occur because of increased bladder circulation and pressure from the enlarging uterus.

b. Urinary tract infection—Urinary tract infection must always be ruled out because pregnant women are more likely than nonpregnant women to have significant bacteriuria which may be asymptomatic (7% versus 3%).

B. SIGNS

1. Increased basal body temperature—Persistent elevation of basal body temperature over a 3-week period usually indicates pregnancy if temperatures have been carefully charted.

2. Skin—

a. Chloasma—Chloasma, or the **mask of pregnancy,** is darkening of the skin over the forehead, bridge of the nose, or cheekbones and is most marked in those with dark complexions. It usually occurs after 16 weeks' gestation and is intensified by exposure to sunlight.

b. Linea nigra—Linea nigra is darkening of the nipples and lower midline of the abdomen from the umbilicus to the pubis (darkening of the linea alba). The basis of these changes is stimulation of the melanophores by an increase in melanocyte-stimulating hormone.

c. Stretch marks—Stretch marks, or striae of the breast and abdomen, are caused by separation of the underlying collagen tissue and appear as irregular scars. This is probably an adrenocorticosteroid response. These marks generally appear later in pregnancy when the skin is under greater tension.

d. Spider telangiectases—Spider telangiectases are common skin lesions that result from high levels of circulating estrogen. These vascular stellate marks blanch when compressed. Palmar erythema is often an associated sign. Both of these signs are also seen in patients with liver failure.

Probable Manifestations

A. SYMPTOMS

Symptoms are the same as those discussed under Presumptive Manifestations, above.

B. SIGNS

1. Pelvic organs—Many changes in the pelvic organs are perceivable to the experienced physician, including the following.

a. Chadwick's sign—Congestion of the pelvic vasculature causes bluish or purplish discoloration of the vagina and cervix.

b. Leukorrhea—An increase in vaginal discharge consisting of epithelial cells and cervical mucus is due to hormone stimulation. Cervical mucus that has been spread on a glass slide and allowed to dry no longer forms a fernlike pattern but has a granular appearance.

c. Goodell's sign—Cyanosis and softening of the cervix (Fig 9–2) is due to increased vascularity of the cervical tissue. This change may occur as early as 4 weeks.

d. Ladin's sign—At 6 weeks, the uterus softens in the anterior midline along the uterocervical junction (Fig 9–3).

e. Hegar's sign—This is widening of the softened area of the isthmus, resulting in compressibility of the isthmus on bimanual examination. This occurs by 6–8 weeks (Fig 9–4).

f. McDonald's sign—The uterus becomes flexible at the uterocervical junction at 7–8 weeks.

g. Von Fernwald's sign—An irregular softening of the fundus develops over the site of implantation at 4–5 weeks (Fig 9–5). If this occurs in the cornual area (Piskacek's sign), it may be confused with a uterine leiomyoma or abnormal uterine development. By 10 weeks, the uterus becomes symmetrical and doubles its nonpregnant size.

h. Bones and ligaments of pelvis—The bony and ligamentous structures of the pelvis also change during pregnancy. There is slight but definite relaxation of the joints. Relaxation is most pronounced at the pubic symphysis, which may separate to an astonishing degree.

2. Abdominal enlargement—There is progressive abdominal enlargement from 7 to 28 weeks. At 16–22 weeks, growth may appear more rapid as the uterus rises out of the pelvis and into the abdomen (Fig 9–6).

3. Uterine contractions—As the uterus enlarges, it becomes globular and often rotates to the right. Painless

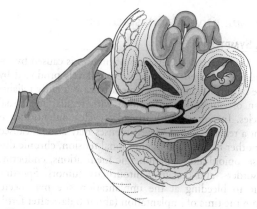

Figure 9–2. Softening of the cervix (Goodell's sign).

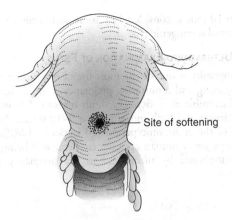

Figure 9–3. Ladin's sign.

Site of softening

uterine contractions (**Braxton Hicks contractions**) are felt as tightening or pressure. They usually begin at about 28 weeks' gestation and increase in regularity. These contractions usually disappear with walking or exercise, whereas true labor contractions become more intense.

4. Ballottement of the uterus—At 16–20 weeks, ballottement of the uterus on bimanual examination may give the impression that a floating object occupies the uterus. This is a valuable sign but is not diagnostic. A similar sign may also be elicited with uterine leiomyomas, ascites, or ovarian cysts.

5. Uterine souffle—Auscultation of the abdomen after 16 weeks often elicits a rushing sound synchro-

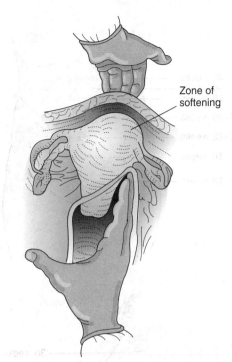

Zone of softening

Figure 9–5. Von Fernwald's sign.

nous with the pulse (caused by the movement of maternal blood filling the placental vessels and sinuses). The intensity may vary from a whisper to a loud rush. With anterior implantation, this sound may mask the fetal heart sounds for several months.

Positive Manifestations

The various signs and symptoms of pregnancy are often reliable, but none is diagnostic. A positive diagnosis must be made upon objective findings, many of which are not produced until after the first trimester. However, more methods are becoming available to diagnose pregnancy at an early stage.

A. FETAL HEART TONES (FHTS)

It is possible to hear FHTs with a fetoscope in a slender woman at 17–18 weeks. The normal fetal heart rate is 120–160 beats per minute. It is best to palpate the maternal pulse for comparison. Doppler devices detect FHTs as early as 10 weeks.

B. PALPATION OF FETUS

After 22 weeks, the fetal outline can be palpated through the maternal abdominal wall. Fetal movements may be palpated after 18 weeks. This may be more easily accomplished by a vaginal examination.

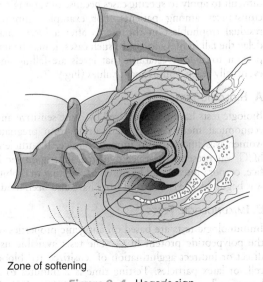

Zone of softening

Figure 9–4. Hegar's sign.

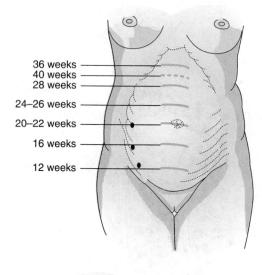

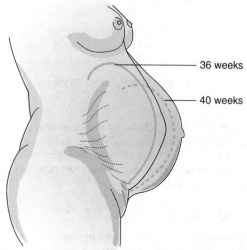

Figure 9–6. Height of fundus at various times during pregnancy.

C. X-Ray of Fetus

X-ray films should be avoided in pregnancy to protect the mother and fetus from possible genetic or oncogenic risk. However, if the potential benefit outweighs the risk, radiographs may be of value. A large body of radiographic data exists about pregnancy. The ossified fetal bones appear at 12–14 weeks. Before 16 weeks, bowel shadows and pelvic bone configuration often conceal a pregnancy in the anteroposterior view. An oblique view of the lower abdomen is most likely to show the fetal skeleton. Diagnostic radiation of less than 10 rads is considered by some authorities to have minimal teratogenic risk.

D. Ultrasound Examination of Fetus

Sonography is one of the most useful technical aids in diagnosing and monitoring pregnancy. Cardiac activity is discernible at 5–6 weeks, limb buds at 7–8 weeks, and finger and limb movements at 9–10 weeks. At the end of the embryonic period (10 weeks by LMP), the embryo has a human appearance. Fetal well-being can be monitored by ultrasound as the pregnancy progresses.

Pregnancy Tests

Sensitive early pregnancy tests measure changes in levels of hCG. There is less cross-reaction with luteinizing hormone (LH) when the β-subunit of hCG is calculated. hCG is produced by the syncytiotrophoblast 8 days after fertilization and may be detected in the maternal serum as early as 9 days. hCG levels peak approximately 65 days after conception. Levels gradually decrease in the second and third trimesters and increase slightly after 34 weeks. Urine values are usually proportionate to serum values if maternal renal function is normal.

The half-life of hCG is 1.5 days. After termination of pregnancy, levels drop exponentially. Normally, serum and urine hCG levels return to nonpregnant values (< 5 mIU/mL) 21–24 days after delivery. The higher the level at pregnancy termination (first-trimester abortion or molar gestation), the longer the time until the return to baseline values. Regression curves have been developed to determine normal hCG disappearance in each of these conditions, but they are difficult to apply to specific cases because of varying circumstances among patients. For example, minimal residual trophoblast in the uterus after a D&C may delay the fall in hCG levels. In such cases, it may be important to at least establish that levels are falling and eventually reach nonpregnant values (Fig 9–7).

A. Biologic Tests

Biologic tests have been replaced by more sensitive and economical methods. In 1928, urine from pregnant women was injected into immature mice. If sufficient hCG was present, the mice ovulated and, upon sacrifice, corpora lutea could be observed. Testing in rabbits was begun in 1931. Rats and frogs have also been used.

B. Immunologic Tests

Immunologic tests are based on antigenic properties of the polypeptide protein hCG. The tests available use direct or indirect agglutination of sensitized red blood cells or latex particles. Testing time is 2 minutes to 2 hours, and sensitivity varies from 250–3500 mIU/mL

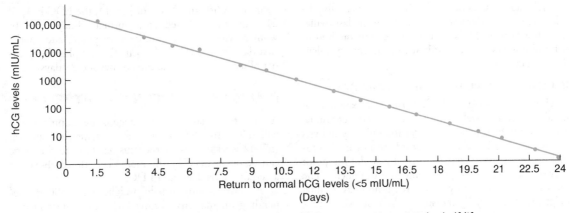

Figure 9–7. Regression of hCG following delivery, assuming a 1.5-day half-life.

of hCG, depending on the product used. Most tests are positive 4–7 days after the first missed period. Test accuracy may be altered by (1) proteinuria, which inactivates anti-hCG agglutination; (2) immunologic disease, which causes false-positive reactions because of IgM interaction with test reagents; and (3) LH levels (the similarity of LH and hCG subunits causes cross-reactivity). Any condition that stimulates release of LH from the anterior pituitary may result in a false-positive reaction. Antipsychotic agents and tranquilizers can cause release of LH. Women who have undergone oophorectomy, who are menopausal, who have hypothyroidism, or who are in renal failure may also have false-positive tests (see Table 9–1).

C. RADIOIMMUNOASSAY FOR HCG

Radioimmunoassay for hCG is a sensitive and specific test for early pregnancy. LH cross-reactivity does not occur when the reagents used are sensitive to the β-sub-

unit of the glycoprotein. Laboratories can detect serum levels as low as 2–4 mIU/mL.

This test requires scintillation counting and 24–48 hours of incubation time. A quantitative analysis of hCG can be obtained and used to determine the normalcy and viability of early pregnancy.

D. RADIORECEPTOR ASSAY

Radioreceptor assay measures receptor sites by a competitive binding mechanism and is capable of measuring levels as low as 200 mIU. This test may be completed in 2–4 hours. Unfortunately, this test also cross-reacts with LH.

E. HOME PREGNANCY TESTS

Home pregnancy tests are immunologic tests and have the same problems mentioned above in addition to the possibility of misinterpretation. hCG is detected in a first-voided morning urine sample. A positive test is indicated by a color change or confirmation mark in the test well. If negative, the test may be repeated in 2 weeks or a radioimmunoassay could be performed. If still negative, amenorrhea due to another condition should be considered.

CALCULATION OF GESTATIONAL AGE & ESTIMATED DATE OF CONFINEMENT

After the diagnosis of pregnancy is made, it is imperative to determine the duration of pregnancy and the estimated date of confinement (EDC).

Calculation of Gestational Age

A. PREGNANCY CALENDAR OR CALCULATOR

Normally, human pregnancy lasts 280 days or 40 weeks (9 calendar months or 10 lunar months) from the last

Table 9–1. Immunologic tests for pregnancy.

Method	Materials	Results
Direct coagulation	Latex particles coated with anti-hCG + serum or urine	Coagulation if hCG is present (pregnant).
Inhibition of coagulation	Anti-hCG + serum or urine **plus** Sensitized red cells **or** Latex particles coated with hCG.	Coagulation if hCG is absent (not pregnant); inhibition if hCG is present (pregnant).

normal menstrual period (LNMP). This may also be calculated as 266 days or 38 weeks from the last ovulation in a normal 28-day cycle. The easiest method of determining gestational age is with a pregnancy calendar or calculator.

B. CLINICAL PARAMETERS OF GESTATIONAL AGE

1. Uterine size—An early first-trimester examination usually correlates well with the estimated gestational age. The uterus is palpable just at the pubic symphysis at 8 weeks. At 12 weeks, the uterus becomes an abdominal organ and at 16 weeks is usually at the midpoint between the pubic symphysis and the umbilicus. The uterus is palpable at 20 weeks at the umbilicus. Fundal height (determined by measuring the distance in centimeters from the pubic symphysis to the curvature of the fundus) correlates roughly with the estimated gestational age at 26–34 weeks (Fig 9–6). After 36 weeks, the fundal height may decrease as the fetal head descends into the pelvis.

2. Quickening—The first fetal movement is usually appreciated at 17 weeks in the average multipara and at 18 weeks in the average primipara.

3. Fetal heart tones—FHTs may be heard by fetoscope at 20 weeks, whereas Doppler ultrasound usually detects heart rates by 10 weeks.

4. X-ray examination—Fetal age can only be approximated by x-ray evaluation of bony calcification. Fortunately, this method has been largely replaced by the use of ultrasound.

5. Ultrasonography—Ultrasonography is now the most widely used technique for determination of gestational age; there is now little or no justification for the use of x-ray for this purpose.

Fetal crown to rump length can be measured at 5–12 weeks and is the most accurate means to determine gestational age. At 20–30 weeks, measurement of fetal biparietal diameter is used. Fetal growth at this time is linear and rapid. After 30 weeks, the accuracy of measurement by ultrasound is much less. Fetal femur length and abdominal circumference are also useful in correlation with biparietal diameter.

Ultrasound is used to measure fetal growth parameters, to estimate fetal weight, to access fetal anatomy, and to measure amniotic fluid volume. Fetal well-being can also be evaluated by measuring biophysical characteristics.

Estimated Date of Confinement (Nägele's Rule)

The EDC can be determined mathematically using Nägele's rule: Subtract 3 months from the month of the LNMP, and add 7 to the first day of the LNMP.

Example: With an LNMP of July 14, the EDC is April 21. This rule is based on a normal 28-day cycle. In women with a longer proliferative phase, add to the first day of the LNMP the usual 7 days plus the number of days that the cycle extends beyond 28 days.

DIAGNOSIS OF PREGNANCY AT TERM

A **term fetus** has reached a stage of development that will allow the best chance for extrauterine survival (37–42 weeks). Whether a fetus has reached this stage can be determined by the methods outlined above for ascertaining fetal age and EDC.

At term, a fetus usually weighs over 2500 g. Depending on maternal factors such as obesity and diabetes, amniotic fluid volume, and genetic and racial factors, the baby may be larger or smaller than expected; therefore, the clinician must rely on objective data to determine fetal maturity. (See also Chapter 16.)

Amniotic Fluid Analysis

The most accurate test of fetal maturity is analysis of amniotic fluid obtained by amniocentesis. The amniotic fluid is evaluated for lecithin:sphingomyelin (L:S) ratio and phosphatidylglycerol content (see also Chapter 13). An L:S ratio of 2:1 usually indicates maturity. Amniotic fluid can also be evaluated for lamellar body count, a more rapid test than those previously mentioned. A count exceeding 30,000/μL indicates pulmonary maturity. The presence of phosphatidylglycerol, one of the last fetal lung surfactants to develop, is the most reliable indicator of lung maturity. Respiratory distress syndrome is not likely to occur following delivery when these values indicate fetal maturity. Values may be less reliable if the mother is diabetic or if amniotic fluid is contaminated by blood, meconium, or other body fluids (eg, urine or vaginal contents).

The **shake test** may be used if biochemical assays are not available. A vial containing 1 mL amniotic fluid mixed with 1 mL 95% ethanol is compared with a second vial containing 1 mL amniotic fluid, 0.5 mL ethanol, and 0.5 mL normal saline solution. If a ring of bubbles appears in the second vial after 30 seconds of vigorous shaking, an L/S ratio of 2 or greater can be assumed. Bubbles in the 1:1 mixture but not in the second vial mean that the fetus is at a borderline stage of development and the pregnancy should be allowed to continue if possible.

Ultrasonography

Multiple early prenatal ultrasound examinations are most accurate in diagnosing fetal maturity. However, a biparietal diameter of 9.8 cm or more late in gestation is usually indicative of fetal maturity.

DIAGNOSIS OF FETAL DEATH

Early in pregnancy, the first sign of fetal death is absence of uterine growth. In such cases, pregnancy testing is initially positive but then negative on 2 subsequent occasions. Descending serial blood hCG values are usually predictive of spontaneous abortion.

In late pregnancy, the first sign of fetal death is usually absence of fetal movement noted by the mother. This is followed by absence of FHTs. Signs and symptoms of pregnancy may subside. A roentgenogram of the fetus may show evidence of fetal death, including overlapping skull bones (**Spalding's sign**), gas in the great vessels (**Robert's sign**), and exaggeration of the fetal spinal curvature or angulation of the spine. These signs are due to postmortem changes in the degenerating fetus.

Real-time ultrasonography is nearly 100% accurate in determining the absence of fetal heart motion. Clot formation in the fetal heart chambers is an early diagnostic sign of fetal death.

Hypofibrinogenemia develops 4–5 weeks after fetal death as thromboplastic substances are released from the degenerating products of conception. Coagulation studies should be started 2 weeks after intrauterine death, and delivery should be attempted by 4 weeks or if serum fibrinogen falls below 200 mg/mL.

DETECTION OF PREVIOUS PREGNANCY

Occasionally, the physician is called on to determine whether a patient has had a previous pregnancy. This diagnosis can rarely be made with certainty, but a reasonably accurate opinion can often be formulated. The appraisal is based on the status of the reproductive organs and the changes that pregnancy usually causes. The breasts of the multiparous patient are in most cases less firm and more pendulous and have increased pigmentation of the areolar areas. A lax abdominal wall may be noted, with separation of the rectus muscles. The scar of a cesarean section may be present. Striae over the abdomen or breasts, although not diagnostic, are suggestive of prior pregnancy. The perineum may reveal the scars of a previous episiotomy or laceration. The vaginal canal may show extreme relaxation. Following delivery, the external cervical os usually appears as a transverse slit or stellate gap, as contrasted with the small circular cervical opening in the nulliparous woman.

■ PRENATAL CARE

Prenatal care as we know it today is a relatively new development in medicine. It originated in Boston in the first decade of this century. Before that time, the patient who thought she was pregnant may have visited a physician for confirmation but did not visit again until delivery was imminent. The nurses of the Instructive Nursing Association in Boston, thinking they might contribute to the health of pregnant mothers, began making house calls on all mothers registered for delivery at the Boston Lying-In Hospital. These visits were so successful that the principle behind them was gradually accepted by physicians, and our present system of prenatal care, which stresses prevention, evolved.

Pregnancy is a normal physiologic event that is complicated by pathologic processes dangerous to the health of the mother and fetus in only 5–20% of cases. The physician who undertakes care of pregnant patients must be familiar with the normal changes that occur during pregnancy, so that significant abnormalities can be recognized and their effects minimized.

Prenatal care should have as a principal aim the identification and special treatment of the high-risk patient—the one whose pregnancy, because of some factor in her medical history or an issue that develops during pregnancy, is likely to have a poor outcome.

The purpose of prenatal care is to ensure, as much as possible, an uncomplicated pregnancy and the delivery of a live healthy infant. There is evidence that mothers and offspring who receive prenatal care have a lower risk of complications. There is also evidence that the mother's emotional state during pregnancy may have a direct effect on fetal outcome. In one study, it was reported that anxiety in labor is positively correlated with plasma epinephrine levels, which in turn seem to result in abnormal fetal heart rate patterns and low Apgar scores. Similarly, another study, that measured anxiety in women in the third trimester, noted that in newborns of anxious women, the 5-minute Apgar score was significantly lower.

Ideally, a woman planning to have a child should have a medical evaluation before she becomes pregnant. This allows the physician to establish by history, physical examination, and laboratory studies the patient's overall fitness for undertaking pregnancy. This is the ideal time to stress the dangers of cigarette smoking, alcohol and drug use, and exposure to teratogens. Instruction on proper diet and exercise habits can also be given. Vitamins, especially folic acid, taken 3 months before conception may be beneficial (decreases incidence of open neural tube defects). Unfortunately, most patients do not seek preconceptional care, and the initial prenatal visit is scheduled well after pregnancy is under way.

Common reasons why pregnant women may not receive adequate prenatal care are inability to pay for health care, fear of or lack of confidence in health care professionals, lack of self-esteem, delays in suspecting pregnancy or in reporting pregnancy to others, different individual or cultural perceptions of the importance of prenatal care, adverse initial feelings about being pregnant, and religious or cultural prohibitions. These factors should be screened for and addressed.

INITIAL OFFICE VISIT

The purpose of the first visit to the physician is to identify all risk factors involving the mother and fetus. Once identified, high-risk pregnancies require individualized specialized care. The diagnosis of pregnancy is made on the basis of physical signs and symptoms and the results of laboratory tests discussed earlier in this chapter.

History

A. PRESENT PREGNANCY

The interview should begin with a full discussion of the symptoms. The patient should have time to express her ideas on childbearing and parenting and to discuss the effect of pregnancy on her life situation.

The patient with regular menses may be able to accurately calculate the EDC using the first day of the LMP and Nägele's rule (LMP – 3 months + 7 days = EDC). Determination of the EDC may be difficult if menses have been irregular or if conception has occurred during use of oral contraceptives. The date of the LNMP may be helpful if there has been some recent irregular bleeding. The EDC may also be determined if the patient knows the probable date of conception.

The common symptoms of pregnancy may be helpful in diagnosing and dating the pregnancy (see previous text).

B. PREVIOUS PREGNANCY

Events of prior pregnancies (regardless of outcome) provide important clues to potential problems in the current one. The following information is necessary: length of gestation, birthweight, fetal outcome, length of labor, fetal presentation, type of delivery, and complications (prenatal, during labor, postpartum). If a cesarean section was performed, an operative report aids in knowing the type of uterine incision and the patient's subsequent risk for dehiscence.

C. MEDICAL HISTORY

Many medical disorders are exacerbated by pregnancy (see Chapter 23). Many cardiovascular, gastrointestinal, and endocrine disorders require careful evaluation and counseling concerning possible deleterious effects on the mother. A history of previous blood transfusion may suggest the rare possibility of associated hemolytic disease of the newborn because of maternal antibodies from a minor blood group mismatch. Knowledge of drug sensitivities is also important.

A history of maternal infections during pregnancy should be obtained. Precautions should be taken to avoid reinfection. If possible, current infections should be treated to prevent hazardous fetal effects. Review of the patient's knowledge about avoiding mutagenic and teratogenic risks (see Chapter 14) is prudent.

The prenatal history should include important social aspects such as the number of sexual partners, the history of sexually transmitted diseases, and possible contact with intravenous drug users. HIV testing should be offered to all patients.

D. SURGICAL HISTORY

Of special importance is a history of previous gynecologic surgery. Prior uterine surgery may necessitate cesarean delivery. A history of multiple induced abortions or midtrimester losses may suggest an incompetent cervix. Patients with previous cesarean deliveries may be candidates for vaginal delivery if they are adequately counseled and meet established guidelines.

E. FAMILY HISTORY

A family history of diabetes mellitus should alert the physician to this disorder, especially if the patient has a history of large or anomalous babies or previous stillbirths. Glucose tolerance testing must be done to determine current endocrine function.

Awareness of familial disorders is also important in pregnancy management. Thus, a brief three-generation pedigree is useful. Antenatal screening tests are available for many hereditary diseases (see Chapter 30).

A history of twinning is important, since dizygotic twinning (polyovulation) may be a maternally inherited trait.

Physical Examination

A. GENERAL EXAMINATION

A complete physical examination must be performed on every new patient. In a young healthy woman, this may be the first complete examination she has ever had.

B. PELVIC EXAMINATION

The pelvic examination is of special importance to the obstetrician.

1. **Pelvic soft tissue**—Any pelvic mass should be described accurately and evaluated by ultrasonography.

2. **Bony pelvis**—The pelvic configuration should be appraised to determine which patients are more likely

to develop cephalopelvic disproportion in labor. X-ray pelvimetry is the most accurate method of assessing the diameters of the vault, midpelvis, and outlet. However, x-ray pelvimetry should be postponed until near term and then used only if the potential benefit exceeds the risk. This technique allows assessment of the fetal head and position as well as the pelvic diameters.

a. Pelvic inlet—Although the transverse diameter of the inlet cannot be measured clinically, the anteroposterior diameter or diagonal conjugate usually can be estimated. For this measurement, the middle finger of the examining hand reaches for the promontory of the sacrum, and the tissue between the examiner's index finger and thumb is pushed against the pubic symphysis while the point of pressure is noted (Fig 9–8). The distance between the tip of the examining finger and this point of pressure measures the **diagonal conjugate** of the inlet. Subtracting 1.5 cm from the diagonal conjugate gives a satisfactory estimate of the **true conjugate** (conjugata vera), or the true anterior diameter of the pelvic inlet.

b. Midpelvis—Precise clinical measurement of the diameter of the midpelvic space is not feasible. With some experience, however, the physician can estimate this distance by noting the prominence and relative closeness of the ischial spines. If the walls of the pelvis seem to converge; if the curve of the sacrum is straight-ened or shallow; or if the sacrosciatic notches are unusually narrow, doubt about the adequacy of the midpelvis is justified.

c. Pelvic outlet—For clinical purposes, the outlet can be adequately estimated by physical examination. The shape of the outlet can be determined by palpating the pubic rami from the symphysis to the ischial tuberosities and noting the angle of the rami. A subpubic angle of less than 90 degrees suggests inadequacy of the outlet. The intertuberous (bi-ischial) diameter can be accurately measured with Thoms' pelvimeter (Fig 9–9). A diameter of more than 8.5 cm usually is adequate for delivery of a term infant. The posterior sagittal diameter can also be measured with Thoms' pelvimeter (Fig 9–10). If the sum of the tuberischial diameter and the posterior sagittal diameter is more than 15 cm, the pelvic outlet is usually adequate. A prominent or angulated coccyx diminishes the anteroposterior diameter of the pelvic outlet.

Martin's pelvimeter or Breisky's pelvimeter may be used to measure the distance from the inferior border of the pubic symphysis to the posterior aspect of the tip of the sacrum (ie, the anteroposterior diameter; normal, 11.9 cm).

On rare occasions, extreme abnormality of the pelvis precludes vaginal delivery. In most cases, below average clinical measurements alert the obstetrician to the pos-

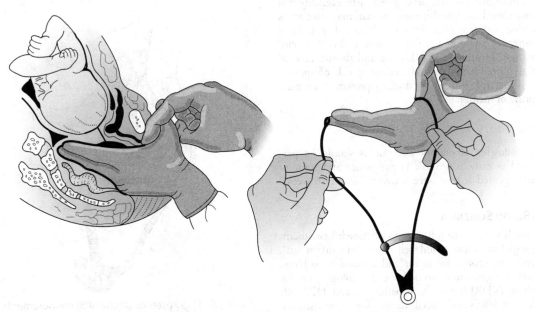

Figure 9–8. Measurement of the diagonal conjugate (DC) (conjugata diagonalis, CD). (Reproduced, with permission, from Benson RC: *Handbook of Obstetrics & Gynecology*, 8th ed. Lange, 1983.)

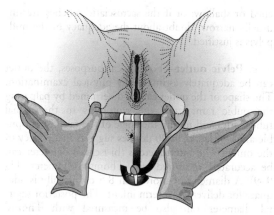

Figure 9–9. Measurement of the bi-ischial (BI) or intertuberous (tuberischial [TI]) diameter with Thoms' pelvimeter. (Reproduced, with permission, from Benson RC: *Handbook of Obstetrics & Gynecology*, 8th ed. Lange, 1983.)

sibility of fetopelvic disproportion, and therefore dystocia. However, an adequate trial of labor is usually the final determinant of true adequacy of the bony pelvis.

d. Cervical length—Assessment should be made by bimanual examination of the cervical length and dilation. Average cervical length is 3–4 cm. A nulliparous woman or one who has never given birth vaginally will have a closed os. A multiparous woman may have an os opening the size of a fingertip, about 1 cm. In a prospective study of healthy women at 24–29 weeks' gestation, greater cervical dilation and shorter cervical length were associated with increased risk of spontaneous preterm delivery, particularly preterm premature rupture of membranes.

Laboratory Tests

The following laboratory assessments should be performed as early as possible in pregnancy and some of these repeated at least once between 24 and 36 weeks' gestation.

A. Blood Screening

At the first visit, the following is obtained: hematocrit, hemoglobin, white blood cell count and differential, blood type group, Rh factor and antibodies to blood group antigens; also needed are a serologic test for syphilis (VDRL), rubella, hepatitis B, and HIV. At-risk individuals may need testing for toxoplasmosis. Women with prior gestational diabetes should be given early 1-hour postglucose testing. The glucose level is checked after ingestion of 50 g of glucose. In a woman

with no increased risk, this is done at 24–28 weeks' gestation. If the test is abnormal, a 3-hour glucose tolerance test is obtained (fasting glucose level, followed by glucose levels 1, 2, and 3 hours after a 100-g glucose load). Hematocrit should be repeated in the third trimester.

Maternal serum testing for hCG, unconjugated estriol, and alpha-fetoprotein (AFP) should be obtained between 15 and 20 weeks' gestation (ideally at 16–18 weeks) to screen for open neural tube defects and chromosomal abnormalities, primarily trisomy 21 and 18. This multiple marker screen has essentially replaced the maternal serum AFP screen because it increases the detection of trisomy 18 and 21 over that achieved with the traditional AFP screen.

In order to allow earlier detection of certain chromosomal abnormalities, first trimester screening utilizing a combination of maternal serum analytes (such as pregnancy-associated plasma protein A [PAPP-A] and free β-hCG) and ultrasound measurement of fetal nuchal translucency is being investigated.

B. Genetics Testing

Genetic studies should be offered to women over age 35 and to those with abnormal pedigrees. Chorionic villus sampling (CVS) is done at 10–12 weeks. It carries a 1–3% risk of fetal loss and is usually offered only at genetic centers. Early amniocentesis may be offered at

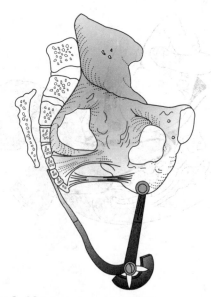

Figure 9–10. Posterior sagittal (PS) measurements with Thoms' pelvimeter. (Reproduced, with permission, from Benson RC: *Handbook of Obstetrics & Gynecology*, 8th ed. Lange, 1983.)

12–14 weeks. Pregnancy loss rates are 1–2% and failed sampling rates are low (1–2%). Standard amniocentesis is offered at 16–18 weeks. With ultrasound guidance, the complication rate is <1%. This is the most likely time to obtain sufficient fetal cells for culture.

C. Urine Testing

Perform urinalysis and screening tests (eg, dipstick nitrite testing) or culture for urinary tract infection. If the bacteria count is over 10^5/mL on a voided sample or if bacteria are noted on a catheterized specimen, perform antibiotic sensitivity testing. Testing for urinary protein, glucose, and ketones should be done at each prenatal visit. Proteinuria of more than 300 mg/24 h ($\geq$ 2+ on standard dipstick testing) may indicate renal dysfunction or, if associated with relative hypertension, the onset or progression of preeclampsia-eclampsia. The presence of glucosuria signifies that the delivery of glucose to the kidneys exceeds renal resorptive capacity. This is not important if blood levels are normal, but elevated blood levels indicate carbohydrate intolerance. The patient should be evaluated for gestational diabetes with the 1- and 3-hour postglucose tests. During pregnancy, the presence of ketones in the urine usually indicates inadequate intake of carbohydrates but not fetal jeopardy or maternal diabetes. The diet should be evaluated in this case to make certain that carbohydrate intake is adequate.

D. Papanicolaou Smear

Papanicolaou smears are performed unless recent results are available. Some obstetricians routinely screen for gonorrhea and chlamydia; others reserve this for high-risk patients. Microscopic examination of vaginal secretions is performed if indicated.

E. Group B Streptococcus

Some authorities currently recommend culture in late pregnancy (at or beyond the 36th week) of the lower vaginal tract for group B streptococcus. The rationale is that if the mother is positive, she may be treated (usually with ampicillin) at the time of admission in labor, thus decreasing the risk of group B streptococcal sepsis in the newborn.

F. Stool Culture

A stool culture for ova and parasites may be indicated in some cases, particularly in recent immigrants from endemic areas such as southeast Asia.

G. Tuberculin Skin Test

A tuberculin skin test is appropriate for high-risk patients.

SUBSEQUENT VISITS

The standard schedule for prenatal office visits is 0–32 weeks: once every 4 weeks; 32–36 weeks: once every 2 weeks; and 36 weeks to delivery: once each week. At each visit, weight gain, blood pressure, fundal height, and findings on abdominal examination by Leopold's maneuvers should be recorded. Additionally, FHTs should be documented and urine should be checked for glucose and protein. These findings should be reviewed and compared with those of previous examinations.

MATERNAL WELL-BEING AS A SIGN OF FETAL WELL-BEING

In modern obstetric practice, fetal well-being has been determined mainly by direct monitoring and testing, but it is important not to overlook the status of the mother when determining fetal well-being. Maternal health is obviously crucial to fetal development and must be continuously assessed during pregnancy.

Maternal Height & Weight

Maternal height and prepregnancy weight along with the rate and amount of weight gain during pregnancy are important in fetal development. Women who are underweight or of short stature tend to have smaller babies, and are at risk for low birthweight and preterm delivery. A teenage mother is compromised if her diet is not adequate to meet her own growth requirements as well as those of her fetus. In such circumstances, women less than 157 cm (5 ft) tall and especially those weighing less than 45 kg (100 lb) should be encouraged to gain at least a minimum of 11–12 kg (25 lb), if not more.

Inadequate progressive weight gain may reflect nutritional deficit, maternal illness, or a hormonal milieu that does not promote proper volume expansion and anabolic state. Often, this is associated with poor fundal growth and a small fetus and placenta, suggesting fetal growth retardation. Weight gain and fundal height should be closely monitored during pregnancy.

Blood Pressure

Blood pressure levels may provide a clue to subtle circulatory compromise. Normally, the mean arterial pressure drops somewhat from prepregnancy or early pregnancy values during the middle trimester. It is important to note this decline so that it does not mask a subsequent rise in blood pressure that may signal the onset of hypertension. In the third trimester, blood pressure recordings taken in the supine position may be higher than those taken in the recumbent position; this may also indicate the onset of hypertension. Normal patients may have a significant drop in blood pressure in the supine position (supine hypotensive syndrome). This is corrected when the patient is in the left lateral position.

Fundal Height

Fundal height should be measured and recorded at each visit after 20 weeks. Measurements should be made with a centimeter tape (**McDonald's technique**) from the pubic symphysis to the top of the uterine mass over the curvilinear abdominal surface. Progress is especially important in the third trimester, when fetal growth retardation is most easily determined.

Fetal Heart Tones

FHTs can usually be heard by 10–12 postmenstrual weeks using a hand-held Doppler device. This may be helpful when gestational age is in doubt or in the presence of threatened abortion or other abnormal observations in the late first trimester. Attention should be paid both to rate and rhythm and to any accelerations, decelerations, or irregularities. Significant abnormalities may be further assessed by ultrasonography, fetal echocardiography, or electronic fetal heart rate monitoring, depending on gestational age. Term gestation can be assumed 18–20 weeks after FHTs have first been heard with the standard unamplified obstetric stethoscope. However, prudence demands use of other clinical landmarks in determining gestational age.

Edema

At each prenatal visit, abnormal or potentially abnormal findings should be noted, and a careful record should be made of any unusual events that have occurred since the last visit. Transient episodes of general edema or swelling should be noted. Lower extremity edema in late pregnancy is a natural consequence of hydrostatic compromise of lower body circulation.

Edema of the upper body (eg, face and hands), especially in association with relative or absolute increases in blood pressure, may be the first sign of preeclampsia. Subtle changes may precede the more obvious picture (eg, finger rings may become too tight; this is a convenient index of early difficulties). A moderate rise in blood pressure without excessive fluid retention may suggest a predisposition to chronic hypertension.

Fetal Size & Position

Manual assessment of fetal size and position is always indicated after about 26 weeks. The fetus may assume a number of positions before late gestation, but persistence of an abnormal lie into late pregnancy suggests abnormal placentation, uterine anomalies, or other problems that should certainly be investigated further. If an abnormal lie persists, consider external version after 37 weeks. Suspected abnormal fetal size should also be investigated, and failure to palpate fetal parts easily may suggest polyhydramnios (also confirmed by uterine measurements that deviate from expectations).

PREPARATION FOR LABOR

As term approaches, the patient must be instructed on the physiologic changes associated with labor. She is usually admitted to the hospital when contractions occur at 5- to 10-minute intervals. She should be told to seek medical advice for any of the following danger signals: (1) rupture of membranes, (2) vaginal bleeding, (3) decreased fetal movement, (4) evidence of preeclampsia (eg, marked swelling of the hands and face, blurring of vision, headache, epigastric pain, convulsions), (5) chills or fever, (6) severe or unusual abdominal or back pain, or (7) any other severe medical problems.

NUTRITION IN PREGNANCY

The mother's nutrition from the moment of conception is an important factor in the development of the infant's metabolic pathways and future well-being. The pregnant woman should be encouraged to eat a balanced diet and should be made aware of special needs for iron, folic acid, calcium, and zinc.

The average woman weighing 58 kg (127 lb) has a normal dietary intake of 2300 kcal/d. An additional 300 kcal/d is needed during pregnancy and an additional 500 kcal/d during breastfeeding (Table 9–2). Consumption of fewer calories could result in inadequate intake of essential nutrients.

WEIGHT GAIN

The American College of Obstetricians and Gynecologists recommends a weight gain of 11.5–16 kg (25–35 lb) during singleton pregnancy. Underweight women may need to gain more, while obese women should gain only 7–11.5 kg (15–25 lb). Heavier women or those with excessive weight gain during pregnancy are likely to have macrosomic infants. Inadequate weight

Table 9–2. Recommended daily dietary allowances for nonpregnant, pregnant, and lactating women.

	Nonpregnant Women (years)				Pregnant Women	Lactating Women
	15–18	19–24	25–50	50+		
Energy (kcal)	2100	2100	2100	2000	+300	+500
Protein (g)	48	46	46	46	+30	+20
Fat-soluble vitamins						
Vitamin A (RE)/(IU)	800	800	800	800	800	1300
Vitamin D (IU)	400	400	200	200	400	400
Vitamin E (IU)	8	8	8	8	10	12
Water-soluble vitamins						
Vitamin C (mg)	60	60	60	60	70	95
Folate (μg)	180	180	180	180	400	280
Niacin (mg)	15	15	15	13	17	20
Riboflavin (mg)	1.3	1.3	1.3	1.2	1.6	1.8
Thiamine (mg)	1.1	1.1	1.1	1.0	1.5	1.6
Vitamin B_6 (mg)	1.5	1.6	1.6	1.6	2.2	2.1
Vitamin B_{12} (μg)	2	2	2	2	2.2	2.6
Minerals						
Calcium (mg)	1300	1000	1000	1200	1000	1000
Iodine (μg)	150	150	150	150	175	200
Iron (mg)	15	15	15	10	30	15
Magnesium (mg)	300	280	280	280	300	355
Phosphorus (mg)	1200	800	800	800	1200	1200
Zinc (mg)	12	12	12	12	15	19

Adapted and modified from American College of Obstetricians and Gynecologists: Nutrition and women. ACOG Educational Bulletin No. 229. ACOG, 1996.

gain is associated with small-for-gestational age (SGA) infant.

The fetus accounts for about one-third of the normal weight gain (3500 g); the placenta, amniotic fluid, and uterus for 650–900 g; interstitial fluid and blood volume for 1200–1800 g each; and breast enlargement for 400 g. The remaining 1640 g or more is largely maternal fat.

NUTRITIONAL REQUIREMENTS

A. PROTEIN

Protein needs in the second half of pregnancy are 1 g/kg plus 20 g per day (approximately 80 g/d for the average woman). Protein intake is essential for embryonic development.

B. CALCIUM

Calcium intake should be increased to 1.5 g/d in the later months and during lactation. If calcium intake is inadequate, fetal needs will be met through demineral-

ization of the maternal skeleton. Maternal calcium stores may be further drained during lactation.

C. IRON

Iron supplements (30–60 mg/d) are currently recommended for pregnant and lactating women. It is estimated that 300–500 mg of iron is transported to the fetus during pregnancy.

D. VITAMINS AND MINERALS

Vitamin and mineral preparations are commonly given but should not be substituted for adequate food intake. Folic acid has been shown to effectively reduce the risk of neural tube defects (NTDs). A daily 4-mg dose is recommended for patients who have had a previous pregnancy affected by NTDs. It should be begun more than 1 month prior to pregnancy (preferably 3 months) and continued through the first 6–12 weeks of pregnancy. Studies show this amount reduces the risk of recurrence by 70%. For all other women a daily intake of at least 0.4 mg taken before conception and through the first 6 weeks of pregnancy is recommended. Patients with insulin-dependent diabetes mellitus and those with seizure disorders treated by valproic acid and carbamazepine are also at greater risk. Vitamin B_{12} supplements are also desirable for vegetarian patients and those with known megaloblastic anemia.

Salt Restriction

Moderate amounts of foods containing sodium are not harmful during normal pregnancy. In fact, sodium restriction may be potentially dangerous. There is no evidence that rapid weight gain in preeclampsia can be controlled with sodium restriction.

COMMON COMPLAINTS DURING PREGNANCY

Most of the minor complaints during pregnancy can be minimized with patient education and prompt treatment. It is best to refrain from using all medications during pregnancy unless they are absolutely essential.

Ptyalism

Excessive salivation (sialism, ptyalism) is an infrequent but troublesome complaint of pregnant women. Belladonna extract, 8–15 mg orally 4 times a day, may be tried.

Pica

Pica (cissa) is the ingestion of substances that have no value as food or are unwholesome. Common examples are clay and laundry starch. This practice probably does not derive from physiologic craving; rather, it seems to be a curious folk custom and is still widespread, especially in the southeastern United States. Pica is harmful because it interferes with good nutrition by substituting nonnutritious bulk for nutritionally important foods. The necessity for good nutrition must be explained to these patients.

Abnormal Frequency of Urination

Urinary frequency is a common complaint throughout pregnancy. Vascular engorgement of the pelvis and hormonal changes are responsible for altered bladder function. Late in pregnancy, when pressure on the bladder by the enlarging uterus and the fetal presenting part decreases bladder capacity, urination becomes even more frequent.

Dysuria or hematuria may be signs that infection has developed; diagnostic and therapeutic measures are needed.

Sexually Transmitted Diseases (STDs)

A. SYPHILIS

Syphilis screening tests such as the Venereal Disease Research Laboratory (VDRL) slide test or the rapid plasma reagent (RPR) test are not specific and will remain positive even after disease treatment. Treponemal antibody tests are used to confirm positive cases. Penicillin remains the treatment of choice with treatment protocols correlating with disease severity. Erythromycin or ceftriaxone are treatment alternatives for the pregnant patient. Monthly serologic tests are followed to assess treatment response.

B. CHLAMYDIA

The most effective screening consists of DNA probe analysis for this infection. Treatment usually consists of 7 days of erythromycin in the pregnant woman. Amoxicillin is used for patients with intolerance to erythromycin base or ethylsuccinate.

C. GONORRHEA

Gonorrhea is best detected by cervical culture. Since many strains are penicillin-resistant, ceftriaxone has become the drug of choice. Amoxicillin is used for nonresistant strains and spectinomycin is recommended for the penicillin-allergic patient.

D. HERPES SIMPLEX VIRUS

Tissue culture is the best confirmation of herpes infection. Topical acyclovir may improve symptoms. Oral acyclovir may be utilized for recurrent outbreaks and should be considered after 36 weeks for prophylaxis against outbreaks at the time of delivery. Cultures are recommended when a lesion is suspected. If no lesions are noted, vaginal delivery is recommended. Cesarean delivery is the route of choice for patients with active lesions at the time of delivery or with prodromal symptoms at the time of delivery or rupture of membranes.

Other Infections

A. TRICHOMONIASIS

Trichomonas vaginalis can be found in 20–30% of pregnant patients, but only 5–10% complain of leukorrhea or irritation. This flagellated, pear-shaped, motile organism can be seen under magnification when the vaginal discharge is diluted with warm normal saline solution and examined microscopically. Suspect trichomoniasis when the discharge is fetid, foamy, or greenish, or when there are reddish ("strawberry") petechiae on the mucous membranes of the cervix or vagina.

Treatment is discussed in Chapter 34. Metronidazole, a good trichomonacide, is not recommended during the first trimester of pregnancy because its safety has not been fully established. Other medications may be helpful and safe during pregnancy. Acceptable antitrichomonas therapy can also be afforded by vaginal clindamycin.

B. CANDIDIASIS

Candida albicans can be cultured from the vagina in many pregnant women, but symptoms occur in less than 50%. When symptoms do occur, they consist of severe vaginal burning and itching and a profuse caseous white discharge. Marked inflammation of the vagina and introitus may be noted. The symptoms are likely to be aggravated by intercourse, and the male partner not infrequently develops mild irritation of the penis. Topical miconazole nitrate, nystatin suppository, or oral fluconazole usually relieves the symptoms. The infection often flares up during pregnancy, in which case retreatment is necessary.

C. NONSPECIFIC INFECTIONS

If irritation is obviously present but a pathogen cannot be identified, symptomatic therapy may be of value. This may include application of a cortisone cream to the vulva to alleviate itching or burning.

Varicose Veins

Varicosities may develop in the legs or in the vulva. A family history of varicosities is often present. Pressure by the enlarging uterus on the venous return from the legs is a major factor in the development of varicosities. The physician should warn the patient early in pregnancy of the need for elastic stockings and elevation of the legs if varices develop. Specific therapy (injection or surgical correction) usually is contraindicated during pregnancy. Superficial varicosities may signal deeper venous disease. These patients should be examined carefully for signs of deep vein thrombosis.

Edema

Dependent edema due to impedance of venous return is a common but rarely serious complaint late in pregnancy. Generalized edema is seen in the hands and face and may be an ominous sign of preeclampsia-eclampsia. Edema in pregnancy is due to fluid retention under the influence of ovarian, placental, and steroid hormones. Preeclampsia-eclampsia of pregnancy must be excluded. Dependent edema should be treated only if the patient is uncomfortable. Elevation of the legs (especially in the lateral decubitus position) will improve the circulation. Diuretics (eg, thiazides, ethacrynic acid) are contraindicated and may be hazardous.

Joint Pain, Backache, & Pelvic Pressure

Although the main bony components of the pelvis consist of 3 separate bones, the symphysial and sacroiliac articulations permit practically no motion in the nonpregnant state. In pregnancy, however, endocrine relaxation of these joints permits some movement. The pregnant patient may develop an unstable pelvis, which produces pain. A tight girdle or a belt worn about the hips, together with frequent bed rest, may relieve the pain; however, hospitalization is sometimes necessary.

Improvement in posture often relieves backache. The increasingly protuberant abdomen causes the patient to throw her shoulders back to maintain her balance; this causes her to thrust her head forward to remain erect. Thus, she increases the curvature of both the lumbar spine and the cervicothoracic spine. A maternity girdle to support the abdominal protuberance and shoes with 2-inch heels, which tend to keep the shoulders forward, may reduce the lumbar lordosis and thus relieve backache. Local heat and back rubs may relax the muscles and ease discomfort. Exercises to strengthen the back are most rewarding.

Leg Cramps

Leg cramps in pregnancy may be due to a reduced level of diffusible serum calcium or elevation of serum phosphorus. Treatment should include curtailment of phosphate intake (less milk and nutritional supplements containing calcium phosphate) and increase of calcium intake (without phosphorus) in the form of calcium carbonate or calcium lactate tablets. Aluminum hydroxide gel, 8 mL orally 3 times a day before meals, adsorbs phosphate and may increase calcium absorption. Symptomatic treatment consists of leg massage, gentle flexing of the feet, and local heat. Tell the patient to avoid pointing toes when she stretches her legs (eg, on awakening in the morning); this triggers a gastrocnemius cramp. She should also practice "leading with the heel" in walking.

Breast Soreness

Physiologic breast engorgement may cause discomfort, especially during early and late pregnancy. A well-fitting brassiere worn 24 hours a day affords relief. Ice bags are temporarily effective. Hormone therapy is of no value.

Discomfort in the Hands

Acrodysesthesia of the hands consists of periodic numbness and tingling of the fingers. (The feet are never involved.) It affects at least 5% of pregnant women. It is a brachial plexus traction syndrome due to drooping of the shoulders during pregnancy. The discomfort is most common at night and early in the morning. It may progress to partial anesthesia and impairment of manual proprioception. The condition is apparently not a serious one, but it may persist after delivery as a consequence of lifting and carrying the baby. Carpal tunnel syndrome may also be a source of discomfort in the hands during pregnancy.

Other Common Complaints

See Chapters 23 and 24 for discussions of other common complaints during pregnancy, including abdominal pain, nausea and vomiting, syncope and faintness, heartburn, constipation, hemorrhoids, genital tract complications, headache, and carpal tunnel syndrome.

DRUGS, CIGARETTE SMOKING, & ALCOHOL DURING PREGNANCY

Drugs

Teratogenicity has been established for only a few drugs, but many more are still not proved to be safe for use during pregnancy. The physician should have a good reason for prescribing any drug early in pregnancy, or indeed during the last half of the menstrual cycle, when any fertile, sexually active woman might become pregnant.

Little is known about the effects of marijuana on the fetus, but major deleterious consequences have not been reported. Heroin, cocaine, and methadone, on the other hand, are associated with major problems in the neonate, especially potentially fatal withdrawal symptoms.

Cigarette Smoking

An increased incidence of low-birthweight infants has been ascribed to heavy cigarette smoking by pregnant women. This effect seems to be dose-related. Smoking also increases the risk of fetal death or damage in utero. Smoking similarly increases the risk of abruptio placentae and placenta previa, each of which increases the fetal risk as well as the maternal risk of death or damage. Since there are many potentially hazardous substances in tobacco smoke, the particular one responsible for these adverse effects has not been identified. Pregnant women should be encouraged not to smoke.

If quitting is too stressful, the patient should at least cut down on the number of cigarettes smoked per day.

Alcoholic Beverages

In the past, it was thought that moderate ingestion of alcohol caused no deleterious effects on the uterus or fetus despite the easy passage of alcohol across the placenta. Instances of newborns showing alcoholic withdrawal symptoms have been reported, but usually these infants were born to chronic alcoholics who drank heavily during pregnancy. However, the precise level of alcohol consumption during pregnancy that causes adverse fetal effects has not been established. Moreover, the chronic alcoholic may suffer from malnutrition, to the extent that the craving for alcohol exceeds the desire for food.

A **fetal alcohol syndrome** following maternal ethanol ingestion has been described, with an incidence varying from 1 in 1500 to 1 in 600 live births, depending apparently on variations in drinking practices. The rate of reported cases identified among newborns in the United States during 1979–1992 increased approximately 4-fold. The major features include growth retardation, characteristic facial dysmorphology (including microcephaly and microphthalmia), central nervous system deficiencies, and other abnormalities. In one study, researchers reported a dose-effect relationship, with full-blown fetal alcohol syndrome occurring in those who reported heavy drinking. They further noted an improved neonatal outcome when the mothers were able to reduce maternal alcohol consumption before the third trimester. These researchers believe that counseling to reduce alcohol intake during pregnancy can be integrated into routine prenatal care. Pregnant women should be encouraged to avoid alcohol intake completely during pregnancy. If this is not possible, the intake should be reduced to a minimum.

OTHER MATTERS OF CONCERN DURING PREGNANCY

Intercourse

There has always been a suspicion that intercourse may be responsible for early abortion. Certainly, if cramps or spotting has followed coitus, it should be proscribed. There is also evidence that coitus late in pregnancy may initiate labor, perhaps because of an orgasm that causes a uterine contraction reflex. All in all, it may be best to proscribe intercourse for patients who have had a previous premature delivery or are currently experiencing uterine bleeding.

Bathing

Bath water does not enter the vagina. Even swimming is not contraindicated during normal pregnancy. Diving should be avoided because of possible trauma.

A woman in the last trimester of pregnancy is clumsy and has poor balance. For this reason, she should be cautioned about slipping and falling in the tub or shower.

Douching

Douching, which is seldom necessary, may be harmful.

Dental Care

There may be generalized gum hypertrophy and bleeding during pregnancy. Interdental papillae (epulis) may also form in the upper gingivae, and these rarely resorb and must be excised. Normal dental procedures under local anesthesia (ie, drilling and filling) may be carried out at any time during gestation. Lengthy procedures should be postponed until the second trimester. Antibiotics are given for dental abscesses and in cases of rheumatic heart disease and mitral valve prolapse.

Immunization

All pregnant women should be vaccinated against poliomyelitis if they are not already immune. Polio vaccine may be administered safely during pregnancy. Live virus vaccines should be avoided during pregnancy because of possible deleterious effects on the fetus.

The American College of Obstetricians and Gynecologists recommends that diphtheria and tetanus toxoid be administered in pregnancy if exposure to pathogens is likely. The hepatitis B vaccine series as well as the influenza vaccine may be given during pregnancy to women at risk. Varicella, measles, mumps, and rubella vaccines should be given 3 months prior to pregnancy or immediately postpartum. Viral shedding occurs in children receiving vaccination but they do not transmit the virus; thus vaccination may be safely given to the children of pregnant women. Immune globulin is recommended for pregnant women exposed to measles, hepatitis A, hepatitis B, tetanus, chickenpox, or rabies.

Clothing

Loose-fitting conventional clothing often suffices until late in pregnancy, although maternity garments may be used as desired. A well-fitted brassiere is essential. A maternity girdle is rarely prescribed except for the relief of back pain or for abdominal weakness. Panty girdles and garters should be avoided because they interfere with circulation in the legs. Well-fitted shoes with heels of medium height are best in pregnancy.

Exercise

Exercise in moderation is acceptable during pregnancy, but the patient should also rest an hour or two during the day. Dangerous sports (eg, horseback riding) and undue physical stress should be avoided. Aerobic and exercise classes have to be designed for pregnancy. Target heart rates are adjusted for age and weight, and routines are aimed to protect joints and promote flexibility.

Employment

Women who have sedentary jobs may continue to work throughout the pregnancy. Employment that requires physical exertion calls for a careful evaluation by the obstetrician and an occupational medical practitioner. It is unwise to adopt rigid policies regarding work during pregnancy—each patient has a different level of capability, a different level of prepregnancy conditioning, a different exercise tolerance, and a different physique.

Substantial physical effort increases maternal oxygen consumption and places an increased demand on cardiac reserve that may result in decreased uterine blood flow. There are no studies as yet that prove this theory beyond doubt, but a conservative approach to the problem is recommended.

Travel

Travel (by automobile, train, or plane) does not adversely affect a pregnancy, but separation from the physician may be hazardous. For this reason, instruct patients with a history of spontaneous abortion and those who have experienced vaginal bleeding in the course of the present pregnancy to avoid travel to distant places.

REFERENCES

American College of Obstetricians and Gynecologists: Maternal serum screening. ACOG Technical Bulletin No. 228. ACOG, 1996.

American College of Obstetricians and Gynecologists: Nutrition and women. ACOG Educational Bulletin No. 229. ACOG, 1996.

American College of Obstetricians and Gynecologists: Preconceptional care. ACOG Technical Bulletin No. 205. ACOG, 1995.

Cunningham FG et al: Prenatal care. *Williams Obstetrics*, 21st ed. McGraw-Hill, 2001, p. 221.

Dalence CR et al: Amniotic fluid lamellar body count: a rapid and reliable fetal lung maturity test. Obstet Gynecol 1995; 86:1.

Hartmann K et al: Cervical dimensions and risk of preterm birth: A prospective cohort study. Obstet Gynecol 1999;93:4.

Institute of Medicine: Nutrition During Pregnancy, 1. Weight gain. 2. Nutrient Supplements. National Academy Press, 1990.

Spencer K et al: One-stop clinic for assessment of risk for fetal anomalies: a report of the first year of a prospective screening for chromosomal anomalies in the first trimester. Br J Obstet Gynecol 2000;107:1271.

Scott LL, Sanchez PJ, Jackson GL et al: Acyclovir suppression to prevent cesarean delivery after first-episode genital herpes. Obstet Gynecol 1996;87:69.

Update: Trends in Fetal Alcohol Syndrome—United States, 1979–1993. Morb Mortal Wkly Rep 1995;44:13.

Ventura S et al: Births: Final data for 1997. Natl Vital Stat Rep 1999;47:18.

The Course & Conduct of Normal Labor & Delivery

Carol L. Archie, MD, & Manoj K. Biswas, MD, FACOG, FRCOG

Labor is a sequence of uterine contractions that results in effacement and dilatation of the cervix and voluntary bearing-down efforts leading to the expulsion per vagina of the products of conception. **Delivery** is the mode of expulsion of the fetus and placenta. Labor and delivery is a normal physiologic process that most women experience without complications. The goal of the management of this process is to foster a safe birth for mothers and their newborns. Additionally, the staff should attempt to make the patient and her support person(s) feel welcome, comfortable, and informed throughout the labor and delivery process. Physical contact between the newborn and the parents in the delivery room should be encouraged. Every effort should be made to foster family interaction and to support the desire of the family to be together. The role of the obstetrician/midwife and the labor and delivery staff is to anticipate and manage complications that may occur which could harm the mother or the fetus. When a decision is made to intervene, it must be considered carefully, because each intervention carries not only potential benefits but also potential risks. The best management in the majority of cases may be close observation, and when necessary, cautious intervention.

PHYSIOLOGIC PREPARATION FOR LABOR

Prior to the onset of true labor, several preparatory physiologic changes commonly occur. The settling of the fetal head into the brim of the pelvis, known as **lightening,** usually occurs 2 or more weeks before labor in first pregnancies. In women who have had a previous delivery, lightening often does not occur until early labor. Clinically, the mother may notice a flattening of the upper abdomen and increased pressure in the pelvis. This descent of the fetus is often accompanied by a decrease in discomfort associated with crowding of the abdominal organs under the diaphragm (eg, heartburn, shortness of breath), while increasing pelvic discomfort and frequency of urination.

During the last 4–8 weeks of pregnancy irregular, generally painless uterine contractions occur with slowly increasing frequency. These contractions, known as **Braxton Hicks contractions,** may occur more frequently, sometimes every 10–20 minutes, and with greater intensity during the last weeks of pregnancy. When these contractions occur early in the third trimester, they must be distinguished from true preterm labor. Later, they are a common cause of "false labor," which is distinguished by the lack of cervical change in response to the contractions.

During the course of several days to several weeks before the onset of true labor, the cervix begins to soften, efface, and dilate. In many cases, when labor starts, the cervix is already dilated 1–3 cm in diameter. This is usually more pronounced in the multiparous patient, the cervix being relatively more firm and closed in nulliparous women. With cervical effacement, the mucus plug within the cervical canal may be released. When this occurs, the onset of labor is sometimes marked by the passage of a small amount of blood-tinged mucus from the vagina known as **bloody show.**

In true labor, the woman is usually aware of her contractions during the first stage. The intensity of pain depends on the fetopelvic relationships, the quality and strength of uterine contractions, and the emotional and physical status of the patient. Very few women experience no discomfort during the first stage of labor. With the beginning of true normal labor, some women describe slight low back pain that radiates around to the lower abdomen. Each contraction starts with a gradual build-up of intensity, and dissipation of discomfort promptly follows the climax. Normally, the contraction will be at its height well before discomfort is reported. Dilatation of the lower birth canal and distention of the perineum during the second stage of labor will almost always cause discomfort.

CHARACTERISTICS OF NORMAL LABOR

Normal labor is a continuous process which has been divided into three stages for purposes of study, with the first stage further subdivided into two phases. The first stage of labor is the interval between the onset of labor and full cervical dilatation. The second stage is the interval between full cervical dilatation and delivery of the infant. The third stage of labor is the period between the delivery of the infant and the delivery of the placenta.

In his classic studies of labor in 1967, Friedman presented data describing the process of spontaneous labor over time. The duration of the first stage of labor in primipara patients is noted to range from 6–18 hours, while in multiparous patients the range is reported to be 2–10 hours. The lower limit of normal for the rate of cervical dilatation during the active phase is 1.2 cm per hour in first pregnancies and 1.5 cm per hour in subsequent pregnancies. The duration of the second stage in the primipara is 30 minutes to 3 hours, and is 5–30 minutes for multiparas. For both, the duration of the third stage was reported to be 0–30 minutes for all pregnancies. These data, while extremely helpful as guidelines, should not be used as strict deadlines that trigger interventions if not met. Even if a numerical (statistical) approach is used to define "abnormal," the cutoff figure would not be the average range, but the 5th percentile numbers (eg, 25.8 hours for the first stage of labor in a primipara). The course that is more appropriate is to consider the overall clinical presentation and use the progress of labor to estimate the likelihood that successful vaginal delivery will occur.

Evaluation of Labor Progress

The first stage of labor is evaluated by the rate of change of cervical effacement, cervical dilatation, and descent of the fetal head. The frequency and duration of uterine contractions alone is not an adequate measure of labor progress. The second stage of labor begins after full cervical dilatation. The progress of this stage is measure by the descent, flexion, and rotation of the presenting part.

■ CLINICAL MANAGEMENT OF NORMAL LABOR

Women most likely to have a normal labor and delivery have had adequate prenatal care without significant maternal or fetal complications and are at 36 weeks' gestation or beyond. Whenever a pregnant woman is evaluated for labor, the following factors should be assessed and recorded:

- Time of onset and frequency of contractions, status of membranes, any history of bleeding, and any fetal movement.
- History of allergies, use of medication, and time, amount, and content of last oral intake.

- Maternal vital signs, urinary protein and glucose, and uterine contraction pattern.
- Fetal heart rate, presentation, and clinical estimated fetal weight.
- Status of the membranes, cervical dilatation and effacement (unless contraindicated, eg, by placenta previa), and station of the presenting part.

If no complications are detected during the initial assessment and the patient is found to be in prodromal labor, admission for labor and delivery may be deferred. When a patient is admitted, a hematocrit or hemoglobin measurement should be obtained and a blood clot should be obtained in the event that a crossmatch is needed. A blood group, Rh type, and antibody screen should also be done.

The First Stage of Labor

In the first stage of normal labor, the pregnant woman may be allowed to ambulate or sit in a comfortable chair as desired. When the patient is lying in bed, the supine position should be discouraged. Patients in active labor should avoid ingestion of anything except sips of clear liquids, ice chips, or preparations for moistening the mouth and lips. When significant amounts of fluids and calories are required because of long labor, they should be given intravenously.

Maternal pulse and blood pressure should be recorded at least every 2–4 hours in normal labor, and more frequently if indicated. Maternal fluid balance (ie, urine output and intravenous and oral intake) should be monitored and both dehydration and fluid overload should be avoided.

Management of discomfort and pain during labor and delivery is a necessary part of good obstetric practice. A patient's request is sufficient justification for providing pain relief during labor. Specific analgesic and anesthetic techniques are discussed in Chapter 26. Some patients tolerate the pain of labor by using techniques learned in childbirth preparation programs. The most common methods of preparation are Lamaze and Bradley, and Read. While specific techniques vary, these classes usually teach relief of pain through the application of principles of education, support, touch, relaxation, paced breathing, and mental focus. The staff at the bedside should be knowledgeable about these pain-management techniques and should be supportive of the patient's decision to use them. When such methods fail to provide adequate pain relief, some patients will ask for medical assistance and such requests should be respected. Indeed, the use of appropriate medical analgesic techniques should be explained to the patient and her labor partner and their use encouraged where medically indicated.

Reassurance of fetal well-being is sought through fetal monitoring. In patients with no significant obstetric risk factors, the fetal heart rate should be auscultated or the electronic monitor tracing should be evaluated at least every 30 minutes in the active phase of the first stage of labor, and at least every 15 minutes in the second stage of labor. In patients with obstetric risk factors, the fetal heart rate should be evaluated every 15 minutes during the active phase of the first stage of labor, and at least every 5 minutes during the second stage.

Uterine contractions should be monitored by palpation every 30 minutes to assess their frequency, duration, and intensity. For at-risk pregnancies, uterine contractions should be monitored continuously along with the fetal heart rate. This can be achieved by using either an external tocodynamometer or an internal pressure catheter in the amniotic cavity. The latter method is particularly useful when abnormal progression of labor is suspected or when the patient requires oxytocin for augmentation of labor.

The progress of labor is monitored by examination of the cervix. During the latent phase, especially when the membranes are ruptured, vaginal examinations should be done sparingly to decrease the risk of an intrauterine infection. In the active phase the cervix should be assessed approximately every 2 hours. The cervical effacement and dilatation, and the station and position of the fetal head should be recorded (Fig 10–1). Additional examinations to determine if full dilation has occurred may be required if the patient reports the urge to push, or to search for prolapse of the umbilical cord or perform fetal scalp stimulation if a significant fetal heart rate deceleration is detected.

The therapeutic rupture of fetal membranes (amniotomy) has been largely discredited as a means of induction when used alone. Moreover, artificial rupture of the membranes increases the risk of chorioamnionitis and the need for antibiotics (especially if labor is prolonged), as well as the risk of cord prolapse if the presenting part is not engaged. Amniotomy may, however, provide information on the volume of amniotic fluid and the presence of meconium. In addition, rupture of the membranes may cause an increase in uterine contractility. Amniotomy should not be performed routinely. It should be used when internal fetal or uterine monitoring is required, and may be helpful when enhancement of uterine contractility in the active phase of labor is indicated. Care should be taken to palpate for the umbilical cord and to avoid dislodging the fetal head. The fetal heart rate should be recorded before, during, and immediately after the procedure.

Second Stage of Labor

At the beginning of the second stage of labor the mother usually feels a desire to bear down with each contraction. This abdominal pressure, together with the force of the uterine contractions, expels the fetus. During the second stage of labor the descent of the fetal head is measured to assess the progress of labor. The descent of the fetus is evaluated by measuring the relationship of the bony portion of the fetal head to the level of the maternal ischial spines (station) (Fig 10–1). When the bony portion of the fetal head is at the level of the ischial spines, the station is "0." The ACOG-endorsed method for describing station is to estimate the number of centimeters from the ischial spines, but some practitioners find it useful to refer to station in estimated thirds of the maternal pelvis. An approximate correlation of these two methods would be: 2 cm = +1, 4 cm = +2, and 6 cm = +3.

The second stage generally takes from 30 minutes to 3 hours in primigravid women and from 5–30 minutes in multigravid women. The median duration is 50 minutes in a primipara and 20 minutes in a multipara. These times may vary depending on the pushing efforts of the mother, the quality of the uterine contractions, and the type of analgesia.

Mechanism of Labor

The mechanism of labor in the vertex position consists of engagement of the presenting part, flexion, descent, internal rotation, extension, external rotation, and expulsion (Table 10–1). The progress of labor is dictated by the pelvic dimensions and configuration, the size of

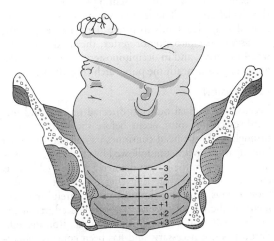

Figure 10–1. Stations of the fetal head. (Reproduced, with permission, from Benson RC: Handbook of Obstetrics & Gynecology, 8th ed. Lange, 1983.)

Table 10–1. Mechanisms of labor: vertex presentation.

Engagement	Flexion	Descent	Internal Rotation	Extension	External Rotation (Restitution)
Generally occurs in late pregnancy or at onset of labor. Mode of entry into superior strait depends on pelvic configuration; posterior occiput is most common position.	Good flexion is noted in most cases. Flexion aids engagement and descent. (Extension occurs in brow and face presentations.)	Depends on pelvic architecture and cephalopelvic relationships. Descent is usually slowly progressive.	Takes place during descent. After engagement, vertex usually rotates to the transverse. It must next rotate to the anterior or posterior to pass the ischial spines, whereupon, when the vertex reaches the perineum, rotation from a posterior to an anterior position generally follows.	Follows distention of the perineum by the vertex. Head concomitantly stems beneath the symphysis. Extension is complete with delivery of the head.	Following delivery, head normally rotates to the position it originally occupied at engagement. Next, the shoulders descend (in a path similar to that traced by the head). They rotate anteroposteriorly for delivery. Then the head swings back to its position at birth. The body of the baby is then delivered.

the fetus, and the strength of the contractions. In essence, delivery proceeds along the line of least resistance, ie, by adaptation of the smallest achievable diameters of the presenting part to the most favorable dimensions and contours of the birth canal.

The sequence of events in vertex presentation is as follows:

A. ENGAGEMENT

This usually occurs late in pregnancy in the primigravida, commonly in the last 2 weeks. In the multiparous patient, engagement usually occurs with the onset of labor. The head enters the superior strait in the occiput transverse position in 70% of women with a gynecoid pelvis (Figs 10–2 and 10–3).

B. FLEXION

In most cases, flexion is essential for both engagement and descent. This will vary, of course, if the head is small in relation to the pelvis or if the pelvis is unusually large. When the head is improperly fixed—or if there is significant narrowing of the pelvic strait (as in the platypelloid type of pelvis)—there may be some degree of deflexion if not actual extension. Such is the case with a brow (deflexion) or face (extension) presentation.

C. DESCENT

Descent is gradually progressive and is affected by the forces of labor and thinning of the lower uterine segment. Other factors also play a part (eg, pelvic configu-

ration and the size and position of the presenting part). The greater the pelvic resistance or the poorer the contractions, the slower the descent. Descent continues progressively until the fetus is delivered; the other movements are superimposed on it (Fig 10–4).

D. INTERNAL ROTATION

With the descent of the head into the midpelvis, rotation occurs so that the sagittal suture occupies the anteroposterior diameter of the pelvis. Internal rotation normally begins with the presenting part at the level of the ischial spines. The levator ani muscles form a V-shaped sling that tends to rotate the vertex anteriorly. In cases of occipitoanterior vertex, the head has to rotate 45 degrees, and in occipitoposterior vertex, 135 degrees, to pass beneath the pubic arch (Fig 10–5).

E. EXTENSION

Because the vaginal outlet is directed upward and forward, extension must occur before the head can pass through it. As the head continues its descent, there is a bulging of the perineum followed by crowning. Crowning occurs when the largest diameter of the fetal head is encircled by the vulvar ring (Fig 10–6). At this time spontaneous delivery is imminent and careful management by the practitioner with controlled efforts of the mother will minimize perineal trauma. Routine episiotomy is not necessary, and has been conclusively associated with increased maternal blood loss, increased risk of disruption of the anal sphincter (third-degree extension) and rectal mucosa (fourth-degree extension),

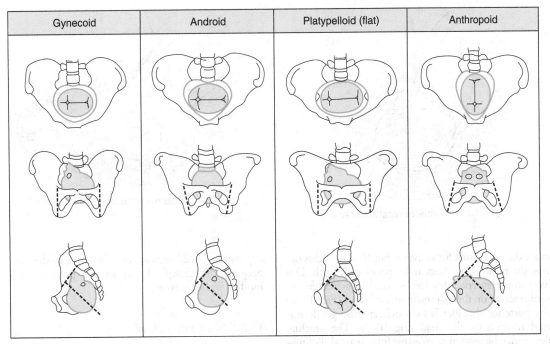

Gynecoid	Android	Platypelloid (flat)	Anthropoid

Figure 10–2. Flexions of the fetal head in the 4 major pelvic types. (Reproduced, with permission, from Danforth DN, Ellis AH: Midforceps delivery: A vanishing art? Am J Obstet Gynecol 1963;86:29.)

as well as delay in the patient's resumption of sexual activity. Further extension follows extrusion of the head beyond the introitus. Once the head is delivered, the airway is cleared of blood and amniotic fluid using a bulb suction device. The oral cavity is cleared initially, followed by clearing of the nares.

After the airway is cleared, an index finger is used to check whether the umbilical cord encircles the neck. If so, the cord can usually be slipped over the infant's head. If the cord is too tight, it can be cut between two clamps.

F. EXTERNAL ROTATION

External rotation (restitution) follows delivery of the head when it rotates to the position it occupied at engagement. Following this, the shoulders descend in a path similar to that traced by the head. The anterior shoulder rotates internally about 45 degrees to come

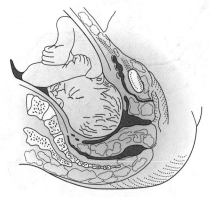

Figure 10–3. Left occipitoanterior engagement.

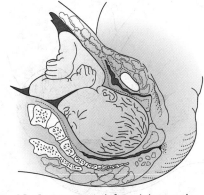

Figure 10–4. Descent in left occipitoanterior position.

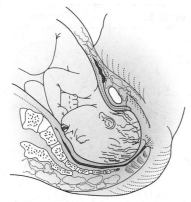

Figure 10–5. Anterior rotation of head.

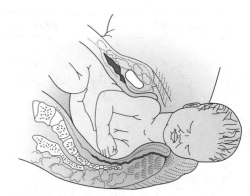

Figure 10–7. External rotation of the head.

under the pubic arch for delivery (Fig 10–7). As this occurs, the head swings back to its position at birth. Delivery of the anterior shoulder is aided by gentle downward traction on the externally rotated head (Fig 10–8). The posterior shoulder is then delivered by gentle upward traction on the head (Fig 10–9). The brachial plexus may be injured if excessive force is used. Following these maneuvers, the body, legs, and feet are delivered with gentle traction on the shoulders.

After delivery, blood will be infused from the placenta into the newborn if the baby is held below the mother's introitus. Delayed cord clamping can result in neonatal hyperbilirubinemia as additional blood is transferred to the newborn infant. Generally, a vigorous newborn can be delivered directly from the introitus to the abdomen and waiting arms of a healthy, alert mother. Placing the child skin to skin (abdomen to abdomen) results in optimum warmth for the newborn. Then the cord, which has been doubly clamped (usu-

ally within 15–20 seconds of delivery) may then be cut between the clamps, by either the practitioner, the mother, or her partner.

Third Stage of Labor

Immediately after the baby is delivered, the cervix and vagina should be thoroughly inspected for lacerations and surgical repair should be performed as needed. Repair of vaginal lacerations should be performed using absorbable suture material, either 2-0 or 3-0. The inspection and repair of the cervix, vagina, and perineum is often easier prior to the separation of the placenta before uterine bleeding obscures visualization.

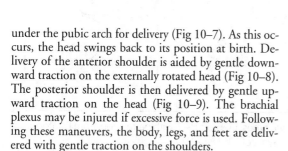

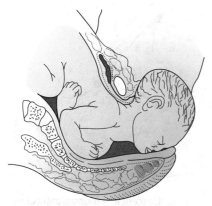

Figure 10–6. Extension of the head.

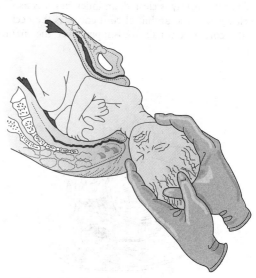

Figure 10–8. Delivery of anterior shoulder.

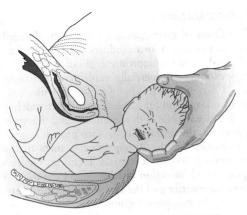

Figure 10–9. Delivery of posterior shoulder.

Separation of the placenta generally occurs within 2–10 minutes of the end of the second stage, but it may take 30 minutes or more to spontaneously separate. Signs of placental separation are: (1) a fresh show of blood from vagina, (2) the umbilical cord lengthens outside the vagina, (3) the fundus of the uterus rises up, and (4) the uterus becomes firm and globular. When these signs appear, it is safe to place traction on the cord. The gentle traction, with or without counterpressure between the symphysis and fundus to prevent descent of the uterus, allows delivery of the placenta.

After the delivery of the placenta, attention is turned to prevention of excessive postpartum bleeding. Uterine contractions which reduce this bleeding may be enhanced with uterine massage and/or the infusion of a dilute solution of oxytocin. The placenta should be examined to ensure complete removal and to detect placental abnormalities.

Puerperium

The puerperium consists of the period following the delivery of the baby and placenta to approximately 6 weeks postpartum. The immediate postpartum period (within the first hour of delivery) is a critical time for both maternal and neonatal physiologic and emotional adjustment. During that hour, the maternal blood pressure, pulse rate, and uterine blood loss must be monitored closely. It is during this time that most postpartum hemorrhage usually occurs, largely due to uterine relaxation, retained placental fragments, or unrepaired lacerations. Occult bleeding (eg, vaginal wall hematoma formation) may manifest as increasing pelvic pain.

At the same time, maternal bonding to the newborn is evolving, and ideally breastfeeding is initiated. Early initiation of breastfeeding is beneficial to the health of both the mother and the newborn. Both benefit because babies are extremely alert and programmed to latch on to the breast during this period. Mother-infant pairs that begin breastfeeding early are most able to continue breastfeeding for longer periods of time. For the mother, nursing accelerates the involution of the uterus, thereby reducing blood loss by increasing uterine contractions. For the newborn, there are important immunologic advantages. For example, various maternal antibodies are present in breast milk, and this provides the newborn with passive immunity against certain infections. Also IgA, a secretory immunoglobulin present in significant amounts in breast milk, protects the infant's gut by preventing attachment of harmful bacteria to cells of the gut mucosal surface. It is also believed that maternal lymphocytes pass through the infant's gut wall and initiate immunologic processes that are not yet fully understood. In addition to the immunologic benefits, breast milk is the ideal nutritional source for the newborn. Moreover it is inexpensive and is usually in good supply. Given all the advantages (the above is only a partial list of the benefits), encouraging successful breastfeeding is an important health goal.

Induction and Augmentation of Labor

Induction of labor is the process of initiating labor by artificial means; augmentation is the artificial stimulation of labor that has begun spontaneously. Labor induction should be performed only after appropriate assessment of the mother and fetus, and after the indications for induction have been explained to the patient. In the absence of medical indications for induction, fetal maturity must be confirmed by either pregnancy dating, ultrasound measurements, and/or amniotic fluid analysis. Evaluation of the cervical status in terms of effacement and softening is important in predicting success of induction and is highly recommended before any elective induction (Table 10–2). Generally, induction should be done in response to specific indications.

A. Indications

The following are common indications for induction of labor:

1. Maternal—Preeclampsia, chronic hypertension, diabetes mellitus, heart disease.

2. Fetal/maternal—Prolonged pregnancy, Rh incompatibility, fetal abnormality, chorioamnionitis, premature rupture of membranes, placental insufficiency, suspected intrauterine growth restriction.

B. Contraindications

Absolute contraindications to induction of labor include: contracted pelvis; placenta previa; uterine scar due to previous classical cesarean section, myomectomy

Table 10–2. Bishop method of pelvic scoring for elective induction of labor.

Examination	Points		
	1	2	3
Cervical dilatation (cm)	1–2	3–4	5–6
Cervical effacement (%)	40–50	60–70	80
Station of presenting part	–1, –2	0	+1, +2
Consistency of cervix	Medium	Soft	...
Position of cervix	Middle	Anterior	...

Modified and reproduced, with permission, from Bishop EH: Pelvic scoring for elective induction. Obstet Gynecol 1964;24:66. Elective induction of labor may be performed safely when pelvic score is 9 or more.

entering the endometrium, hysterotomy, or unification surgery; transverse lie.

Relative contraindications to induction of labor include: breech presentation, oligohydramnios, multiple gestation, grand multiparity, previous cesarean section with transverse scar, prematurity.

Complications of Induction of Labor

A. FOR THE MOTHER

In many cases, induction of labor exposes the mother to more distress and discomfort than judicious delay and subsequent vaginal or cesarean delivery. The following hazards must be kept in mind: (1) failure of induction; (2) uterine inertia and prolonged labor; (3) tumultuous labor and tetanic contractions of the uterus, causing premature separation of the placenta, rupture of the uterus, and laceration of the cervix; (4) intrauterine infection; and (5) postpartum hemorrhage.

B. FOR THE FETUS

An induced delivery exposes the infant to the risk of prematurity if the estimated date of conception has been inaccurately calculated. Precipitous delivery may result in physical injury. Prolapse of the cord may follow amniotomy. Injudicious administration of oxytocin or inadequate observation during induction could lead to fetal demise in utero or delivery of a baby with poor Apgar scores.

Methods of Cervical Ripening

Cervical ripening prior to induction of labor could facilitate the onset and progression of labor and increase the chance of vaginal delivery, particularly in primigravid patients.

A. PROSTAGLANDIN

Two forms of prostaglandins are commonly used for cervical ripening prior to induction at term: misoprostol (PGE_1) and dinoprostone (PGE_2) Though only dinoprostone, commercially available as prostaglandin gel, is currently FDA-approved for this use, off-label use of misoprostol for cervical ripening is widely practiced. Indeed, while both misoprostol and dinoprostone applied locally intravaginally can provide significant improvement in the Bishop score, a meta-analysis of randomized, controlled trials focusing on cervical ripening and induction of labor found the time to delivery was shorter and the rate of cesarean delivery was lower in the misoprostol group.

Dinoprostone comes prepackaged in a single-dose syringe containing 0.5 mg of PGE_2 in 2.5 mL of a viscous gel of colloidal silicon dioxide in triacetin. The syringe is attached to a soft plastic catheter for intracervical administration, and the catheter is shielded to help prevent application above the internal cervical os. Misoprostol is manufactured in 100-µg unscored and 200-µg scored tablets which can be administered orally, vaginally, and rectally. PGE_2 should not be used in patients with a history of asthma, glaucoma, or myocardial infarction. Unexplained vaginal bleeding, chorioamnionitis, ruptured membranes, or previous cesarean section are all relative contraindications to the use of prostaglandins for cervical ripening.

For cervical ripening and induction, misoprostol is given vaginally at a dose of 25 µg every 4–6 hours. With dinoprostone, usually 12 hours should be allowed for cervical ripening, after which oxytocin induction should be started. PGE_1 and PGE_2 have similar side-effect and risk profiles including fetal heart rate deceleration, fetal distress, emergency cesarean section, uterine hypertonicity, nausea, vomiting, fever, and peripartum infection. However, a current literature review does not indicate any significant differences between control and treatment groups with prostaglandin cervical ripening.

B. RELAXIN

Relaxin is a polypeptide hormone that is produced in the human corpus luteum, decidua, and chorion. Purified protein relaxin, 2 mg in tylose gel, given vaginally or intracervically is noted to induce cervical ripening in 80% of cases and labor in about one-third of patients over a 12-hour period.

C. BALLOON CATHETER

A Foley catheter with a 25- to 50-mL balloon is passed into the endocervix above the internal os using tissue forceps. The balloon is then inflated with sterile saline, and the catheter is withdrawn gently to the level of internal cervical os. This method should induce cervical ripening over 8–12 hours. The cervix will be dilated 2–3 cm when the balloon falls out, which will make amniotomy possible, but effacement may be unchanged.

D. HYGROSCOPIC DILATORS

Laminaria tents are made from desiccated stems of the coldwater seaweed *Laminaria digitata* or *L. japonica*. When placed in the endocervix for 6–12 hours, the laminaria increases in diameter three- to fourfold by extracting water from cervical tissues, gradually swelling and expanding the cervical canal. Synthetic dilators like lamicel, a polyvinyl alcohol polymer sponge impregnated with 450 mg of magnesium sulfate, and dilapan, which is made from a stable nontoxic hydrophilic polymer of polyacrylonitrile are also noted to be highly effective in cervical ripening.

Induction of Labor

A. OXYTOCIN

Intravenous administration of a very dilute solution of oxytocin is the most effective medical means of inducing labor. Oxytocin exaggerates the inherent rhythmic pattern of uterine motility, which often becomes clinically evident during the last trimester and increases as term is approached.

The dosage must be individualized. The administration of oxytocin is determined with a biologic assay: the smallest possible effective dose must be determined for each patient and then utilized to initiate and maintain labor. Constant observation by qualified attendants is required when this method is used.

In most cases it is sufficient to add 1 mL of oxytocin (10 units oxytocin to 1 L of 5% dextrose in water [1 mU/mL]). One acceptable oxytocin infusion regimen is to begin induction or augmentation at 1 mU/min, preferably with an infusion pump or other accurate delivery system, and increase oxytocin in 2-mU increments at 15-minute intervals.

When contractions of 50–60 mm Hg (per the internal monitor pressure) or 40–60 seconds (per the external monitor) occur at 2.5- to 4-minute intervals, the oxytocin dose should be increased no further. Oxytocin infusion is discontinued whenever hyperstimulation or fetal distress is identified, but can be restarted when reassuring fetal heart rate and uterine activity patterns are restored.

B. AMNIOTOMY

Amniotomy may be an effective way to induce labor in carefully selected cases with high Bishop scores. Release of amniotic fluid shortens the muscle bundles of the myometrium; the strength and duration of the contractions are thereby increased and a more rapid contraction sequence follows.

The membranes should be ruptured with an amniohook. Make no effort to strip the membranes, and do not displace the head upward to drain off amniotic fluid. Amniotomy has not been proven effective in augmenting labor uniformly; it is probably wise to await the onset of the active phase of labor to perform the procedure. Early and variable deceleration of the fetal heart rate is noted to be relatively common with amniotomy. Amniotomy in selected cases could shorten the course of labor without reducing the incidence of operative delivery.

REFERENCES

Bernal AL: Overview of current research in parturition. Exp Physiol 2000;86:213.

Eason E et al: Preventing perineal trauma during childbirth: A systematic review. Obstet Gynecol 2000;95:464.

El-Turkey M, Grant JM: Sweeping of the membrane is an effective method of induction of labor in prolonged pregnancy: A report of a randomized trial. Br J Obstet Gynaecol 1992;99:455.

Forman A et al: Evidence for a local effect of intracervical prostaglandin E$_2$. Am J Obstet Gynecol 1982;143:756.

Fraser WD, Sokol R: Amniotomy and maternal position in labor. Clin Obstet Gynecol 1992;35:535.

Goldberg AB, Greenberg BS, Darney PD: Misoprostol and pregnancy. N Engl J Med 2001;344:1.

Harbort GM Jr: Assessment of uterine contractility and activity. Clin Obstet Gynecol 1992;35:546.

Kazzi GM, Bottoms SF, Rosen MG: Efficacy and safety of *Laminaria digitata* for preinduction ripening of the cervix. Obstet Gynecol 1982;60:440.

Klein MC et al: Relationship of episiotomy to perineal trauma and morbidity, sexual dysfunction, and pelvic floor relaxation. Am J Obstet Gynecol 1994;171:591.

Laifer SA: Oral intake during labor. Clin Consult Obstet Gynecol 1992;4:206.

Lange AP et al: Prelabor evaluation of inducibility. Obstet Gynecol 1982;60:137.

Martin JN Jr, Morrison JC, Wiser WL: Vaginal birth after cesarean section: The demise of routine repeat abdominal delivery. Obstet Gynecol Clin North Am 1988;15:719.

McColgin SW et al: Stripping membranes at term: Can it safely reduce the incidence of postterm pregnancy? Obstet Gynecol 1990;76:678.

Owen J, Hauth JC: Oxytocin for the induction or augmentation of labor. Clin Obstet Gynecol 1992;35:464.

Renfrew MJ et al: Practices that minimize trauma to the genital tract in childbirth: A systematic review of the literature. Birth 1998;25:143.

Sheiner E et al: The impact of early amniotomy on mode of delivery and pregnancy outcome. Arch Gynecol Obstet 2000;264:63.

Essentials of Normal Newborn Assessment & Care

11

Carla Janzen, MD, & William L. Gill, MD

ESSENTIALS OF DIAGNOSIS

- *Apgar score at 1 and 5 minutes.*
- *Airway patency and adequacy of ventilation.*
- *Maintenance of infant temperature.*
- *Screening physical examination for life-threatening conditions.*
- *Determination of appropriateness for gestational age.*
- *Complete physical examination after infant is stabilized.*
- *Laboratory screening for disease.*
- *Discharge examination.*

General Considerations

Term newborns are defined as those born at 36 weeks' gestation or more. The initial physical examination done as soon as possible after delivery is a rapid screening for life-threatening anomalies that require immediate attention. The most important assessments are airway patency and adequacy of ventilation.

A second and more complete physical examination is performed within 24 hours of birth, given a stable delivery room course during which the infant is observed for stability of temperature and vital signs. The weight, length, and head circumference are carefully recorded and used to classify the neonate as large for gestational age (LGA), appropriate for gestational age (AGA), or small for gestational age (SGA).

Brief examinations should also be performed daily and at the time of discharge. The discharge examination should be performed in the presence of the mother to discuss the findings and review infant care and feeding.

THE INFANT IMMEDIATELY AFTER BIRTH

Apgar Score

The Apgar score, created in 1925 by Virginia Apgar, is a quick method of assessing the clinical status of the newborn at 1 and 5 minutes after birth. A score of 0 through 2 is given for each of 5 components (Table 11–1).

The 1-minute Apgar score is used to evaluate cardiorespiratory function, spontaneous or during resuscitation. A low 1-minute Apgar score may indicate a need for resuscitation but does not correlate with the infant's future outcome.

The 5-minute Apgar score, especially the change in the score between 1 and 5 minutes, is a useful index of the effectiveness of resuscitation. A 5-minute Apgar score of 7 to 10 is normal, while 4 to 7 may require continued resuscitative measures. In full-term infants, an Apgar score of less than 3 at 5 minutes is associated with an increased risk of cerebral palsy (from 0.3% to 1.0%).

Scores are affected by factors such as prematurity, medication, and infection. If hypoxia is likely and rapid positioning, suction, stimulation, and bag ventilation do not improve the infant's heart rate and color, trained personnel should be on hand for immediate intubation.

Caring for the Infant Immediately After Delivery

Newborns should be delivered into a warm room and dried immediately, and sterile equipment should be used to cut the cord. For stable infants, mother is most often the best caregiver and provider of warmth and food. Skin-to-skin contact between mothers and infants immediately after birth correlates with an increased incidence of breastfeeding and longer duration of lactation.

A. DRYING THE SKIN

The skin should be dried with warmed blankets or towels to remove amniotic fluid and to prevent evaporative

Table 11–1. Apgar scoring.

Signs	Points Scored		
	0	1	2
Heartbeats per minute	Absent	Slow (< 100)	Over 100
Respiratory effort	Absent	Slow, irregular	Good, crying
Muscle tone	Limp	Some flexion of extremities	Active motion
Reflex irritability	No response	Grimace	Cry or cough
Color	Blue or pale	Body pink, extremities blue	Completely pink

heat loss and cold stress. This procedure also provides tactile stimulation to the skin, which encourages increased movement.

B. WARMING THE INFANT

The infant should be wrapped in warmed blankets or placed under a radiant heat source. A term infant exposed to cold may exhibit dangerous physiologic responses including vasoconstriction and increased muscular activity and oxygen consumption in order to augment heat production.

C. CLEARING THE AIRWAY

The nose and mouth should be suctioned thoroughly but not more than 5–10 seconds. Suctioning can induce bradycardia via vagal reflexes, especially with deep suctioning in the oropharynx. Gastric suctioning should be abandoned when labor and delivery are uncomplicated.

In the United States, 6% of all newborn infants require basic life support. The most important indication that resuscitation is required is difficulty with breathing after birth. If after quick initial drying, tactile stimulation, positioning, and suctioning, the newborn does not cry or breathe, ventilatory support should be given immediately. If meconium staining is present, endotracheal intubation and suctioning should be done prior to initiation of any ventilation if the particulate meconium is of "pea-soup" thickness or thicker.

Physical Examination

The goal of physical examination in the delivery room is early detection of life-threatening problems.

A. AIRWAY

Since most neonates are obligate nose breathers, it is essential that patency of the nasal passages be confirmed (ie, choanal atresia excluded). If the passages are not patent, insertion and maintenance of an oral airway are essential. Infants with a large protruding tongue may also require insertion of an oral airway.

B. CHEST

Since the tracheobronchial tree is filled with fluid before birth, auscultation of the lungs usually reveals rales with the first few breaths. These should clear within 1 hour. Respiratory rates are 30–60/min for the first 2 hours and are usually irregular. The heart rate is also usually irregular, averaging more than 100 beats/min but sometimes dropping to as low as 80 beats/min in term infants. The maximum systolic blood pressure in a term newborn should not exceed 80 mm Hg, and the diastolic pressure should not exceed 50 mm Hg. A mean arterial blood pressure of less than 30 mm Hg is associated with poor peripheral perfusion and shock.

C. ABDOMEN

The abdomen is usually soft and appears flat at birth. As the bowel fills with gas, abdominal fullness increases. The liver is usually palpable 1.5–2 cm below the right costal margin. The kidneys can be palpated immediately after birth. A scaphoid abdomen associated with increasing respiratory distress suggests diaphragmatic hernia with bowel in the thorax. Marked abdominal distention may indicate abdominal masses, ascites, or bowel obstruction.

D. SKIN

Acrocyanosis of the peripheral extremities is common after birth. Petechiae are usually present over the presenting part and are common over the shoulders and thorax.

Pallor may be indicative of asphyxia, anemia, shock, or edema. Early diagnosis of anemia may lead to recognition of erythroblastosis fetalis, subcapsular hematoma of the liver or spleen, subdural hemorrhage, or fetal-maternal transfusion. Anemia should be corrected to a minimum hematocrit of 40% in any infant requiring oxygen supplementation or having a hematocrit less than 35% at term. This is accomplished with 10–15 mL/kg of packed red blood cells.

Pronounced plethora of the skin suggests the possibility of polycythemia. This occurs frequently in infants of diabetic mothers, SGA infants, and the recipient twin in twin-twin transfusion syndrome. Infants with hematocrits of 70% or more should receive a partial exchange transfusion of plasma protein fraction or fresh-frozen plasma. Jaundice at birth requires immediate evaluation for hemolytic or infectious causes.

E. GENERAL

Malformations and deformations of the extremities, face, and neural tube should be noted. Palsies, asymmetric movements, or other evidence of birth injury should be observed. The infant should be identified by arm and leg bands identical to those placed on the mother.

THE INFANT DURING THE FIRST FEW HOURS AFTER BIRTH

Those providing initial care should observe the infant closely for pallor, cyanosis, respiratory distress, plethora, jaundice, seizures, tremors, abdominal distention, and extreme lethargy or hyperactivity.

The initial assessment by the nursing staff should include vital signs, hematocrit, and peripheral blood sugar in infants of diabetic mothers, LGA and SGA infants, and any infant appearing jittery or having seizures. If close observation or resuscitation is necessary, the infant should be placed under a radiant heat source. The eyes of infants are protected against infection by instilling 1% silver nitrate drops or erythromycin (0.5%) ophthalmic ointment. Vitamin K (phytonadione), 1 mg intramuscularly, is recommended for all infants after birth to prevent vitamin K deficiency as a possible cause of hemorrhagic disease of the newborn.

Once the temperature has stabilized, the infant can be bathed to remove vernix, blood, and debris from the skin and scalp. An initial feeding can also be given during this time.

CLINICAL ESTIMATION OF GESTATIONAL AGE

Estimation of fetal gestational age is based on the date of the last menstrual period, serial fundal height measurements, onset of fetal movement, and detection of fetal heartbeat. Ultrasound measurements of biparietal diameter of the fetal skull, femur length, and abdominal girth may be particularly helpful, especially serial measurements (see Table 13–4.) The lecithin/sphingomyelin (L/S) ratio and phospholipid profile are useful measures of fetal pulmonary maturity. (See also Chapter 9.)

Gestational age can be determined by examination after birth, since physical characteristics and neurologic development progress in a predictable fashion with increasing gestational age.

Table 11–2 shows the clinical criteria used to rate neuromuscular and physical maturity in a shortened version of the Dubowitz estimate of gestational age. These scoring sheets are available in the United States from major infant formula companies. Each aspect of neuromuscular and physical development is scored on a scale from 0 to 5. The total score gives the maturity rating. If

levels of maturity differ for physical and neuromuscular characteristics, problems of intrauterine growth are often present.

Fig 11–1 shows the normal growth curves for fetal length, weight, and head circumference. These measurements are plotted for the gestational age determined in the maturity rating. SGA, LGA, or AGA can then be plotted.

COMPLETE PHYSICAL EXAMINATION OF THE NEWBORN

After a stable delivery room course and within the first 24 hours of life, a more thorough physical examination should be performed.

General Appearance & Vital Signs

The vital signs, physical measurements, and maturity ratings noted during the transition period should be reviewed. Patterns of heart rates and respiratory rates should be evaluated. Normal blood pressures are related to the size and postnatal age of the infant, but in most cases, the mean should be greater than 30 mm Hg. Blood pressures should be determined in both the upper and lower extremities using the Doppler method and a cuff that covers two-thirds of the extremity.

Skin

Vernix caseosa, a whitish cheesy material, normally covers the body of the fetus, increasing in amount as term approaches. The amount may decrease once term is reached, and the substance may be completely absent in postterm infants. Dry skin with cracking and peeling of superficial layers is common in postterm infants and SGA infants. Edema may be generalized, as in renal, cardiac, hematologic, or other systemic disease, or localized, as in Turner's syndrome (dorsum of hands and feet). Meconium staining of the umbilical cord, nails, and skin suggests prior fetal intrauterine stress. The skin of preterm infants is more translucent and may be covered with fine lanugo hair.

Mongolian spots are bluish-black areas of increased pigmentation over the back and buttocks. They are found in over 50% of black and Native American infants and tend to disappear within the first year. **Neonatal pustular melanosis** is also seen in black infants as a small vesicle that leaves a pigmented freckle when the vesicle ruptures. **Erythema toxicum neonatorum** is a benign rash presenting like flea bites, with a raised center on an erythematous base that may progress to vesicles. Wright's stain of the vesicle exudate shows numerous eosinophils. **Milia** are small white papules over the nose and face. **Capillary heman-**

Table 11–2. Newborn maturity rating and classification.

	0	1	2	3	4	5
Neuromuscular maturity						
Posture						
Square window (wrist)	90°	60°	45°	30°	0°	
Arm recoil	180°		100°–180°	90°–100°	< 90°	
Popliteal angle	180°	160°	130°	110°	90°	< 90°
Scarf sign						
Heel to ear						
Physical maturity						
Skin	Gelatinous, red, transparent	Smooth, pink; visible veins	Superficial peeling and/or rash; few veins	Cracking, pale area; rare veins	Parchment, deep cracking; no vessels	Leathery, cracked, wrinkled
Lanugo	None	Abundant	Thinning	Bald areas	Mostly bald	
Plantar creases	No crease	Faint red marks	Anterior transverse crease only	Creases anterior two-thirds	Creases cover entire sole	
Breast	Barely perceptible	Flat areola; no bud	Stippled areola; bud, 1–2 mm	Raised areola; bud, 3–4 mm	Full areola; bud, 5–10 mm	
Ear	Pinna flat; stays folded	Slightly curved pinna; soft; slow recoil	Well-curved pinna; soft; ready recoil	Formed and firm; instant recoil	Thick cartilage; ear stiff	
Genitalia (male)	Scrotum empty; no rugae		Testes descending; few rugae	Testes down; good rugae	Testes pendulous; deep rugae	
Genitalia (female)	Prominent clitoris and labia minora		Majora and minora equally prominent	Majora large; minora small	Clitoris and minora completely covered	

The following information should be recorded: Birth date and Apgar score at 1 and 5 minutes. Two separate examinations should be made within the first 24 hours to determine the estimated gestational age according to maturity rating. Each examination and the age of the infant at each examination should be noted.

Maturity rating:

Score	5	10	15	20	25	30	35	40	45	50
Weeks	26	28	30	32	34	36	38	40	42	44

Reproduced, with permission, from Ballard JL et al: A simplified assessment of gestational age. Pediatr Res 1977;11:374. Figures adapted from Sweet AY: Classification of the low-birth-weight infant. In: Care of the High-Risk Infant, 3rd ed. Klaus MH, Fanaroff AA (editors). Saunders, 1986. This form is available from the Mead Johnson Nutritional Group, Evansville, IN 47721.

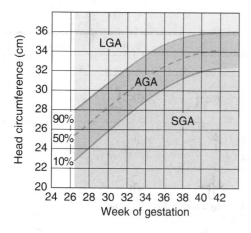

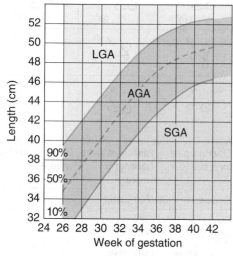

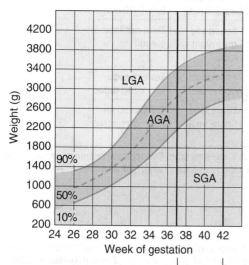

giomas are common over the eyelids, forehead, nares, lips, occiput, and neck.

Staphylococcal or streptococcal infection of the skin may present as vesicles similar to those of erythema toxicum, but Gram's stain shows polymorphonuclear cells with bacteria often visible. Herpesvirus can also present as vesicular lesions, usually in clusters. Tzanck preparation of a scraping from the base of the vesicles shows multinucleated giant cells, which also show fluorescent antibodies to herpesvirus.

Head

The size, shape, and symmetry of the head should be noted. The head circumference should be plotted on the growth curves (Fig 11–1). Molding of the skull in vertex deliveries is due to passage through the birth canal, which causes transient elongation. **Caput succedaneum** is an area of edema over the presenting scalp that extends across suture lines. It is also seen at the application site of vacuum extractors. **Cephalohematomas** represent bleeding in the subperiosteal space of the skull bones; the margins of the hematoma are limited by the edges of the bone involved.

The **anterior fontanelle** varies greatly in size from 1 to 4 cm, and the suture lines vary from palpably open to overriding. The fontanelle is usually concave, pulsates with the infant's heartbeat, may flatten with crying, and becomes slightly depressed when the infant is upright and quiet. The **posterior fontanelle** is usually less than 1 cm in diameter and may not be palpable. A third fontanelle representing a widening of the sagittal suture in the parietal bones may also be palpable, especially in infants with Down's syndrome. **Craniosynostosis** presents as an immobile ridge along one or more sutures and is associated with increasing cranial deformity.

Face, Nose, & Mouth

Symmetry and general appearance of the facial structures should be observed. Unusual facial features may suggest

---

Figure 11–1. Classification of newborns based on gestational age plotted against head circumference, length, and weight. AGA, appropriate for gestational age; LGA, large for gestational age; SGA, small for gestational age. (Adapted and reproduced, with permission, from Lubchenco LO, Hansman C, Boyd E: Intrauterine growth in length and head circumference as estimated from live births at gestational ages from 26 to 42 weeks. Pediatrics 1966;37:403 and Battaglia FC, Lubchenco LO: A practical classification of newborn infants by weight and gestational age. J Pediatr 1967;71:159. This form is available from the Mead Johnson Nutritional Group, Evansville, IN 47721.)

specific syndromes, eg, bushy connected eyebrows in Cornelia de Lange syndrome or widened upper lip frenulum in fetal alcohol syndrome. Detection of one anomaly indicates that others may also be present.

Contusions and localized swelling and asymmetry of facial movement may result from passage through the birth canal or from the use of forceps during delivery. Facial nerve palsy is observed when the infant cries; the unaffected side of the mouth droops downward, giving a distorted facial grimace. With extensive nerve injury, the eyelid will remain partially open on the affected side.

The shape of the nose may be suggestive of specific chromosomal anomalies (eg, the broad beaked nose of trisomy 18). Nose deformity due to intrauterine pressure is common, but nasal fracture is rare. Nasal obstruction not related to structural narrowing or choanal atresia may be caused by congenital infections such as syphilis or cytomegalovirus infection.

Cleft lip and palate may occur as an isolated anomaly or as part of a syndrome such as trisomy 13. A high arched palate may be present as an isolated finding or may be associated with abnormal facies. Most newborns have relatively small mandibles, but micrognathia is seen with Pierre Robin anomaly and may be associated with blockage of the airway by the tongue.

Eyes

The eyes should be examined at least once during the nursery stay. The overall size and shape of the eyes and orbits may suggest chromosomal anomalies. Examination should include the periorbital structures and anterior orbital structures (ie, cornea, iris, and lens). Nerve function and the red light reflex of the retina should be observed. Absence of the red light reflex or detection of a yellowish-white mass in the eye suggests congenital retinoblastoma. Mydriatic and cycloplegic ophthalmic drops, in concentrations not to exceed 0.2% cyclopentolate and 1% phenylephrine, may be instilled to dilate the pupils for a thorough examination. Corneal and lens opacities, pupil size, and iris abnormalities (eg, Brushfield spots and colobomas) should be noted. Congenital glaucoma presents with an enlarged "ox eye" cornea (> 11 mm), which is often cloudy due to edema. Chorioretinitis may result from congenital infection with *Toxoplasma gondii,* cytomegalovirus, rubella virus, or herpesvirus hominis.

Ears

Malformed ears may suggest specific syndromes (eg, Treacher Collins syndrome), and low-set malpositioned ears may be associated with other congenital anomalies, especially of the urinary tract. The tympanic membranes are difficult to visualize before removal of vernix and debris. Fluid may be present in the middle ear for

the first few hours. Otitis media may occur in infants with cleft palate and in those intubated with nasotracheal tubes for long periods.

Congenital deafness may be detected by standardized neonatal screening tests involving infant movement in response to measured levels of sound or by use of scalp electrodes to monitor brainstem-evoked response to sound. If potentially ototoxic drugs were used during pregnancy, screening for hearing deficit is especially important. Brainstem-evoked auditory response (BEAR) screening is also advised in infants < 1500 g birthweight, infants suspected of having congenital infections, those with central nervous system infections, or those with a family history of a syndrome associated with deafness.

Neck

The symmetry, position, range of motion, and muscle tone of the neck should be observed. Webbing or excessive skin folds on the nape of the neck suggest chromosomal abnormalities (eg, Turner's syndrome, Down's syndrome). Torticollis due to shortening or spasm of the sternocleidomastoid may occur if hemorrhage into the body of the muscle occurs at birth. Enlargement of the thyroid may occur, and sinus tracts may be seen as remnants of branchial clefts.

Thorax

The shape and symmetry of the thorax and nipples are noted. Absent clavicles permit unusual anterior movement of the shoulders. Fracture of the clavicle is common in shoulder dystocia and is detected by tenderness and crepitus at the fracture site and decreased movement of the arm. Asymmetry of the chest wall may indicate pulmonary distress, airway obstruction, or air leaks (eg, pneumothorax).

Lungs

Auscultation of the lungs will determine equality of bronchial breath sounds, equal air entry, and the presence of fine rales. In the first few hours of life, rales indicate normal lung expansion. If pneumothorax is present, breath sounds and heart sounds may be distant, percussion may be hyperresonant, and the area lighted on chest transillumination will be larger than the normal 2-cm diameter. Decreased air entry and expiratory grunting are signs of respiratory distress. A chest x-ray must be obtained when abnormal lung findings are suspected. The presence of bowel sounds over the thorax and gas-filled intestinal loops in the chest on x-ray suggest the presence of diaphragmatic hernia.

Heart & Vascular System

Clamping of the umbilical cord and expansion of the lungs initiate the change from fetal circulation to neonatal pulmonary circulation. Fetal shunts at the ductus arteriosus, foramen ovale, and ductus venosus close, and pulmonary blood flow increases as the lungs expand and pulmonary vascular resistance decreases. Because the pressures in the right side of the heart are essentially equal to those in the left in the normal newborn, flow across septal defects does not occur in the immediate newborn period. Cardiac murmurs are heard with valvular narrowing, and abnormal flow patterns cause inequality of pressures in the heart. Clicks are always abnormal in the neonate. General signs of heart disease include tachypnea, cyanosis, and shock or sudden decompensation associated with hypoxemia and metabolic acidosis. The heart size, location and intensity of the cardiac impulse, heart rate and rhythm, peripheral pulse intensity, and blood pressures in the arms and legs should be determined in the cardiovascular evaluation. Further evaluation may require chest x-ray, ECG, M-mode or two-dimensional echocardiography, and possibly cardiac catheterization.

Sudden decompensation of oxygenation accompanied by metabolic acidosis in an infant who had previously been stable is suggestive of a ductal-dependent cardiac anomaly in which closure of the ductus arteriosus leads to a critical decrease in pulmonary or systemic blood flow. 2-D Echocardiography should be done immediately to confirm the presence or absence of a ductal-dependent cardiac lesion.

Abdomen

The abdomen appears flat at birth and becomes more protuberant as the bowel fills with gas. A markedly scaphoid abdomen associated with respiratory distress suggests diaphragmatic hernia (more common on the left side).

Omphalocele is a midline abdominal wall defect that involves the umbilicus and is covered by the yolk sac membrane. **Gastroschisis** is an abdominal wall defect that is distinctly separate from the umbilicus, and the exposed bowel is not covered by a membrane. Complete absence of abdominal musculature (prune-belly syndrome) may occur in association with severe urinary tract anomalies or bladder obstruction. The liver, spleen, and kidneys are easily palpated in the first 24 hours after birth.

Genitalia

A. Male Genitalia

In the term male infant, the testes have descended into the pendulous scrotum, and rugae completely cover the scrotal sac. The size of the scrotum varies, depending on the presence of hydroceles. Inguinal hernias may be present at birth; they are usually reducible and can be distinguished from hydroceles by scrotal transillumination. The foreskin is adherent to the glans and cannot be retracted. The complete formation of the penile shaft and the urethral orifice should be noted. With hypospadias, the urethra may open at any point from the base of the shaft to the corona of the glans.

B. Female Genitalia

In the term female, the labia majora completely cover the labia minora and clitoris. A fully developed hymenal ring is usually visible, often with excess tissue tags. The hymen should be perforate, with a white mucous discharge from the vagina. An imperforate hymen presents as a solid septum sealing the vaginal opening. Persistence of imperforate hymen can lead to the development of hydrometrocolpos. The imperforate hymen is usually easily disrupted with a blunt probe. Within the first 14 days after birth, vaginal bleeding may occur as a result of withdrawal from maternal estrogen. The mother should be reassured that this is normal and will stop within 3 days.

C. Ambiguous Genitalia

If the genitalia appear ambiguous, gender assignment should not be made until a complete evaluation (sometimes including karyotyping) determines the true sex of the infant.

Anus & Rectum

The patency of the rectum and location of the anal opening should be determined, rectal muscle tone should be observed, and passage of meconium should be noted. If an imperforate anus is present, ultrasonography or x-ray will determine the distance between the rectal atresia and the anal surface. Fistulas may open into the vagina or bladder in females or into the bladder or onto the perineum in males.

Hard meconium producing total rectosigmoid blockage is referred to as **meconium plug syndrome**. Abdominal distention is relieved by passage of the plug; a saline enema, 3–5 mL, may be required. Rectal fissures with bleeding can occur in the newborn period.

Extremities

The extremities should be symmetric and equal in size. Hemihypertrophy may be indicative of severe anomalies. Other major abnormalities of the extremities include absence of a bone, clubfoot, syndactyly of digits, extra digits, or absent parts of extremities. Congenital hip dislocation is suspected with limitation of hip abduction or when a "click" can be felt when the femurs are pressed downward and then abducted. Nerve palsies and fractures present as decreased movement of the extremities. Hand and foot deformities are frequent with chromosomal abnormalities.

Central Nervous System

General observations of tone and movement are important in the neonate. Activity may range from complete absence of movement to tremors, jerks, or convulsions as well as opisthotonos and hyperactivity in infants with central nervous system damage. Hypoxic-ischemic central nervous system injury in a term infant is frequently associated with seizures and abnormal tone and reflexes. Intracerebral hemorrhage may be seen in the area of injury, leading to infarction of central nervous system tissue.

Neurologic screening should include the following assessments:

A. MUSCLE TONE

A good test is recoil of the extremities after stretching. The hypertonic baby is frequently jittery, startles easily, and exhibits "tight fisting." The hypotonic infant is "floppy." The extremities fall to the bed loosely when picked up and released.

B. ROOTING REFLEX

The rooting reflex is elicited by stroking the infant at the corners of the mouth and at the midline of the upper and lower lips. The mouth opens, the head turns toward the stimulus, and there is an oral search. Absence of such behavior warrants further investigation.

C. SUCKING REFLEX

This reflex may be observed by placing a finger in the infant's mouth and noting the vigor of movement and suction produced. Hypertonic infants make biting rather than sucking movements.

D. TRACTION RESPONSE

To initiate the traction response, pull the infant to a sitting position by traction on the arms at the wrists. After an initial head lag, active neck muscle flexion normally moves the head and chest into line as the infant reaches the vertical position.

E. GRASP REFLEX

Stroking the palm or sole normally causes active grasping by the involved extremity.

F. BICEPS, TRICEPS, KNEE, AND ANKLE TENDON REFLEXES

Percussion with a finger or thin rubber hammer should elicit the jerk characteristic of deep tendon reflexes. Reflexes should be symmetric.

G. TRUNK INCURVATION

The infant is draped prone over the supporting examiner's hand. Stroking the back parallel with the spine causes the normal infant to twist the pelvis toward the stimulated side.

H. RIGHTING RESPONSE

When the infant is lifted vertically, the legs normally will step. When the soles of the feet are placed on the table, the infant will normally attempt to exhibit upright posture by extension of the leg followed by the trunk and head.

I. PLACING

When the infant is held vertically and the dorsum of the foot is stroked against the edge of the table, the normal infant will flex the knee and attempt to place the foot as though trying to step onto the table.

J. MORO REFLEX (STARTLE REFLEX)

Quick release of traction on the arms or allowing the head to drop suddenly a few centimeters will normally cause a startle reaction. Shoulder abduction and elbow extension will be followed by adduction of the arms associated with spreading and extension of the fingers.

Any abnormal neurologic reactions should be noted and a repeat examination done when the infant is quiet. A Brazelton examination may be indicated to determine a more comprehensive neurologic behavioral status.

CARE OF THE NORMAL NEWBORN

Every effort must be made to allow the mother to see, touch, and examine her infant in the delivery room to begin the bonding process. Some mothers wish to initiate breastfeeding in the delivery room. Although this usually can be easily accomplished, care must be taken to avoid cold stress, since the infant's only source of heat in most air-conditioned delivery rooms will be conduction from the mother's skin.

Duration of Hospitalization Following Delivery

The trend during the past few years has been toward shortened hospital stays after delivery. Most normal newborns who have been delivered vaginally are now discharged with the mother 36–48 hours after delivery. Mothers who have undergone cesarean delivery usually remain in the hospital for an average of 4 days.

Each mother and infant should be evaluated individually to determine the optimal time of discharge from the hospital. The mother and her baby should stay in the hospital long enough to allow identification of early problems and to ensure that the family is able to care for the baby at home. Problems such as jaundice, poor feeding patterns, infection, ductal-dependent cardiac lesions, and gastrointestinal obstruction may require a longer period of observation by experienced personnel. Factors for shortened hospital stay are included in the ACOG Guidelines for perinatal care.

It should be emphasized that the timing of discharge of the mother and newborn from the hospital should be the decision of the physicians caring for them, not by arbitrary policy established by third-party payers.

Infants having a short hospital stay (less than 48 hours) should be examined by experienced health care providers within 48 hours of discharge. The purpose of medical follow-up is to assess the infant's general health, feeding, hydration, and degree of jaundice, and to perform metabolic screening tests in accordance with state regulations.

Screening for Disease

Laboratory testing to screen for potential medical problems is part of routine newborn care. Some tests are required by law. Tests should include the following:

(1) Blood types of mother and infant and direct Coombs' test for the infant (to detect antibody-mediated blood group incompatibilities).

(2) Serologic test for syphilis.

(3) Whole blood screen for phenylalanine (standard requirement in the United States). The Guthrie method on filter paper is usually used. Aminoacidurias, including valine, leucine, isoleucine, and homocystine, can be tested in some states.

(4) Thyroid function tests (T_4 and TSH).

(5) Sickle cell and other hemoglobinopathies.

(6) Hematocrit screening.

(7) Galactosemia in any infant with jaundice (urine test with Clinitest tablets for reducing substances).

Maternal hepatitis B surface antigen status should also be known. If positive, hepatitis B immune globulin as well as hepatitis B vaccine should be given to the infant within 18–24 hours of birth.

Circumcision

Although the American Academy of Pediatrics has stated that there is no longer any medical reason for neonatal circumcision, 1.2 million newborn males are circumcised in the United States each year, at a cost of between $150 and $270 million. Arguments in favor of circumcision include protection against urinary tract infection, and possible protection against sexually transmitted disease, including HIV infection. Arguments against circumcision are that infants are unable to give informed consent, the procedure is painful, and that it is considered elective surgery. Parents must be advised of the risks and benefits of the procedure and be allowed to make an individual choice.

Infant Feeding

A. BREASTFEEDING

Over the past several years, enthusiasm for breastfeeding has grown. Breast milk not only supplies optimal caloric needs in the most digestible form but also offers added protection against infection because of its antibodies (principally secretory IgA) and active macrophages and lymphocytes. These offer protection against gastrointestinal pathogens that cause diarrhea.

Preparation for breastfeeding should begin in the prenatal period. Rolling and stretching the nipple will increase elasticity and "toughen" the nipple to minimize soreness and cracking. Following delivery, production of colostrum begins and continues until the milk "comes in" on approximately the third day. The nursing staff must be supportive of the nursing mother and reassure her that she will be able to supply the baby's needs. They should teach her techniques to minimize nipple trauma and instruct her on infant position and nasal airway maintenance. Supplemental water feedings after breast feedings should be discouraged in the neonatal period unless the infant demonstrates signs of dehydration with urine specific gravity of 1.020 or more and the loss of over 10% of birth weight. Use of artificial nipples for any type of supplementation can lead to "nipple confusion" by the infant, who will begin showing preference for the nipple from which it is easiest to obtain milk. This may lead to decreased interest and difficulty in nursing.

There are relatively few contraindications to breastfeeding. Those that must be considered include active tuberculosis and hepatitis B in the mother and maternal use of certain drugs including tetracyclines, antithyroid medication, and certain antimetabolites. In developed countries, maternal HIV infection is a contraindication to breastfeeding. The risk of vertical transmission is doubled if the infant breastfeeds; it is especially high when women acquire HIV infection during lactation.

B. INFANT FORMULAS

Table 11–3 shows the composition of the major formulas available in the United States. No conclusive data show that any one formula is superior. Selection is often made according to the preference of the mother, the physician, or the current nursery "house formula." All standard formulas contain 20 kcal/oz. Formulas prepared for use in newborn nurseries are ready to feed in 4-oz bottles with disposable nipples. No preparation or sterilization is required, and the formula can be stored and fed at room temperature. Formula prepara-

Table 11–3. Normal and special infant formulas.

Formula	Protein	Fat	Carbohydrate	Osmolality (mOsm/L)	Sodium (mEq/L)	Calcium (mg/L)	Phosphorus (mg/L)
Standard							
Similac (plain, low iron) (Ross)	18% whey, 82% casein	40% coconut oils, 60% soy oils	Lactose	290	11	510	390
Similac with iron (Ross)	18% whey, 82% casein	40% coconut oils, 60% soy oils	Lactose	290	11	510	390
Enfamil (plain, low iron) (Mead Johnson)	60% whey, 40% casein	?45% palm oil, 20% soy oil, 20% coconut oil & 15% high oleic sunflower	Lactose	290	9	440	300
Enfamil with iron (Mead, Johnson)	60% whey, 40% casein	?45% palm oil, 20% soy oil, 20% coconut oil & 15% high oleic sunflower	Lactose	290	9	440	300
Lacto-free (Mead Johnson)	18% whey, 82% casein	45% palm oil, 20% soy oil, 20% coconut oil, 15% high oleic sunflower oil	100% glucose polymers	20	20	550	370
SMA, SMA lo-iron (Wyeth)	60% whey, 40% casein	33% oleo, 27% coconut, 15% soy, 25% safflower oils	Lactose	300	6.5	440	330
Soy							
Isomil (Ross)	Soy protein isolate	60% coconut oils, 40% soy oils	50% corn syrup solids, 50% sucrose	250	13	700	500
Isomil SF (Ross)	Soy protein isolate	60% coconut oils, 40% soy oils	100% corn syrup solids	150	13	700	500
Prosobee (Mead Johnson)	Soy protein isolate	?same % ages as written in	Glucose polymers, corn syrup solids	160	13	630	500
Nursoy (Wyeth)	Soy protein isolate	Oleo, coconut, soy, oleic (safflower) oils	Sucrose	145	13	630	500
Premature							
Special care 24 calorie (Ross)	60% whey, 40% casein	50% MCT, 30% corn oils, 20% coconut oils	50% lactose, 50% polycose	300	15	1440	720
Special Care 20 calorie (Ross)	60% whey, 40% casein	50% MCT, 30% corn oils, 20% coconut oils	50% lactose, 50% polycose	220	13	1200	600

(continued)

Table 11–3. Normal and special infant formulas. (continued)

Formula	Protein	Fat	Carbohydrate	Osmolality (mOsm/L)	Sodium (mEq/L)	Calcium (mg/L)	Phosphorus (mg/L)
Low Birth Weight 24 calorie (Ross)	18% whey, 82% casein	50% MCT, 20% soy oils, 30% coconut oils	50% lactose, 50% polycose	300	16	730	560
Enfamil Premature 24 calorie (Mead Johnson)	60% whey, 40% casein	40% MCT, 40% corn oils, 20% coconut oils	60% polycose, 40% lactose	264	14	940	470
Enfamil Premature 20 calorie (Mead Johnson)	60% whey, 40% casein	40% MCT, 40% corn oils, 20% coconut oils	70% polycose, 30% lactose	300	14	1000	470
SMA "Premie" 24 calorie (Wyeth)	60% whey, 40% casein	Oleo, coconut, soy, and safflower oils, 13% MCT	50% lactose, 50% malto-dextrans	235	15	950	400
Low Mineral							
Similac PM 60/40 (Ross)	60% whey, 40% casein	60% coconut oils	Lactose	260	7	400	200
Carbohydrate Free							
RCF (Ross)	Soy protein isolate	60% coconut oils, 40% soy oils	...	...	13	700	500
Specialty							
Pregestimil (Mead Johnson)	Casein hydrolysates	40% MCT, 60% corn oils	Corn syrup, glucose polymers	348	15	600	400
Alimentum (Ross)	Casein hydrolysates	40% MCT, 60% corn oils	Sucrose, glucose polymers	346	15	600	400
Breast milk	60% whey, 40% casein	Human milk fat	Lactose	300	6.5–10	330	150
Whole cow's milk	18% whey, 82% casein	Butterfat	Lactose	290	22	1230	960

tion after discharge is simplified by the use of formula concentrates that are mixed with equal parts of water. The American Academy of Pediatrics recommends use of a formula containing iron for the first year of life.

Discharge Examination

Since a complete physical examination is performed within the first 24 hours after birth, only supplemental rechecking of heart sounds, vital signs, and weight need be performed at discharge. The discharge examination should ideally be performed in the presence of the mother to discuss any findings, answer any questions, and give instructions about routine care and feeding. Plans for medical follow-up are made at this time.

Car Seats

Safe transportation of infants should begin with the first ride home from the hospital. Most states in the U.S. require safety-approved car seats for children up to 4 years of age. Car seat instructions and literature should be distributed well in advance of discharge and should be discussed in prenatal classes. Many hospitals have a rental or purchase program for infant car seats.

Immunization

The American Academy of Pediatrics now recommends immunization of all newborns with hepatitis B vaccine

in the nursery at discharge or in the physician's office within 2 weeks.

REFERENCES

American Academy of Pediatrics: AAP 2001 Red Book: Report of the Committee on Infectious Diseases, 26th ed, 2001.

American Academy of Pediatrics: Circumcision Policy Statement (1999). Pediatrics 1999;103(3):686.

American Academy of Pediatrics, Committee on Fetus and Newborn and American College of Obstetricians and Gynecologists, Committee on Obstetric Practice. Use and Abuse of the Apgar Score Pediatrics 1996;98(1):141–2.

American Academy of Pediatrics, Committee on Genetics. Newborn screening fact sheets. Pediatrics 1996;98:473–501.

American Academy of Pediatrics, Circumcision Policy Statement (1999). Pediatrics 1999;103(3):686–693.

American Academy of Pediatrics and American Heart Association. Textbook of Neonatal Resuscitation. Elk Grove Village, IL: American Academy of Pediatrics; 1995.

American College of Obstetricians and Gynecologists: Guidelines for Perinatal Care, 4th ed. Washington, DC, ACOG, 1998.

Behrman RE (ed): Nelson Textbook of Pediatrics, Sixteenth Edition. W.B. Saunders Company. 2000.

Laumann EO, Masi CM, Zuckerman EW: Circumcision in the United States. *JAMA* 1997;277:1052–1057.

Websites

American Academy of Pediatrics: http://www.aap.org
Allied Vaccine Group: http://www.vaccine.org
Circumcision: http://www.cirp.org

The Normal Puerperium

Kim Lipscomb, MD, & Miles J. Novy, MD

The puerperium or postpartum period, generally lasts 6–12 weeks and is the period of adjustment after delivery when the anatomic and physiologic changes of pregnancy are reversed and the body returns to the normal nonpregnant state. The postpartum period has been arbitrarily divided into the **immediate puerperium**—the first 24 hours after parturition—when acute postanesthetic or postdelivery complications may occur; the **early puerperium,** which extends until the first week postpartum; and the **remote puerperium,** which includes the period of time required for involution of the genital organs and return of menses, usually by 6 weeks in nonlactating women, and the return of normal cardiovascular and psychological function, which may require months.

ANATOMIC & PHYSIOLOGIC CHANGES DURING THE PUERPERIUM

Uterine Involution

The uterus increases markedly in size and weight during pregnancy (about 10 times the nonpregnant weight, reaching a crude weight of 1000 gm) but involutes rapidly after delivery to the nonpregnant weight of 50 to 100 grams. The gross anatomic and histologic characteristics of this process have been studied through autopsy, hysterectomy, and endometrial specimens. In addition, the decrease in size of the uterus and cervix has been demonstrated by MRI imaging, sonography, and computed tomography.

Immediately following delivery, the uterus weighs about 1 kg and its size approximates that of a 20-week pregnancy (at the level of the umbilicus). At the end of the first postpartum week, it normally will have decreased to the size of a 12-week gestation, and is just palpable at the symphysis pubis (Fig 12–1). Ultrasonography can be used to measure length and width of the uterine cavity. During the first week, there is a 31% decrease in uterine area; during the second and third weeks, a 48% decrease; and subsequently, an 18% decrease. The observed changes in uterine area are mainly due to changes in uterine length, since the transverse diameter remains relatively constant during the puerperium.

Myometrial contractions or **afterpains** assist in involution. These contractions occur during the first 2–3 days of the puerperium and produce more discomfort in multiparas than in primiparas. Such pains are accentuated during nursing as a result of oxytocin release from the posterior pituitary. During the first 12 hours postpartum, uterine contractions are regular, strong, and coordinated (Fig 12–2). The intensity, frequency, and regularity of contractions decrease after the first postpartum day as involutional changes proceed. Uterine involution is nearly complete by 6 weeks, at which time the organ weighs less than 100 g. The increase in the amount of connective tissue and elastin in the myometrium and blood vessels and the increase in numbers of cells are permanent to some degree, so the uterus is slightly larger following pregnancy.

Changes in the Placental Implantation Site

Following delivery of the placenta, there is immediate contraction of the placental site to a size less than half the diameter of the original placenta. This contraction, as well as arterial smooth muscle contractions, leads to hemostasis. Involution occurs by means of the extension and downgrowth of marginal endometrium and by endometrial regeneration from the glands and stroma in the decidua basalis.

By day 16, placental site, endometrial, and superficial myometrial infiltrates of granulocytes and mononuclear cells are seen. Regeneration of endometrial glands and regeneration of endometrial stroma has also begun. Endometrial regeneration at the placental site is not complete until 6 weeks postpartum. In the disorder termed **subinvolution of the placental site,** complete obliteration of the vessels in the placental site fails to occur. Patients with this condition have persistent lochia and are subject to brisk hemorrhagic episodes. This condition can usually be treated with uterotonics. In the rare event uterine curettage is performed, partly obliterated hyalinized vessels can be seen on the histologic specimen.

Normal postpartum discharge begins as **lochia rubra,** containing blood, shreds of tissue, and decidua. The amount of discharge rapidly tapers and changes to a reddish brown color over the next 3–4 days. It is termed **lochia serosa** when it becomes serous to mucopurulent, paler, and often malodorous. During the second or third postpartum week, the lochia becomes thicker, mucoid, and yellowish-white (**lochia alba**), co-incident with a predominance of leukocytes and degenerated decidual cells. Typically during the fifth or sixth week postpartum, the lochial secretions cease as healing nears completion.

Changes in the Cervix, Vagina, & Muscular Walls of the Pelvic Organs

The cervix gradually closes during the puerperium; at the end of the first week, it is little more than 1 cm dilated. The external os is converted into a transverse slit, thus distinguishing the parous woman who delivered vaginally from the nulliparous woman or from one who delivered by cesarean section. Colposcopic examination soon after delivery may reveal ulceration, ecchymosis, and laceration. Complete healing and reepithelialization occur 6–12 weeks later. Stromal edema and round cell infiltration and the endocervical glandular hyperplasia of pregnancy may persist for up to 3 months. Cervical lacerations heal in most uncomplicated cases, but the continuity of the cervix may not be restored, so the site of the tear may remain as a scarred notch.

After vaginal delivery, the overdistended and smooth-walled vagina gradually returns to its antepartum condition by about the third week. Thickening of the mucosa, cervical mucus production, and other estrogenic changes may be delayed in a lactating woman.

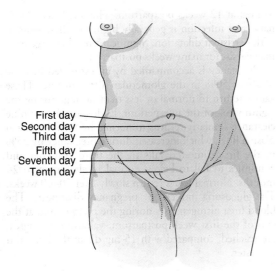

Figure 12–1. Involutional changes in the height of the fundus and the size of the uterus during the first 10 days postpartum.

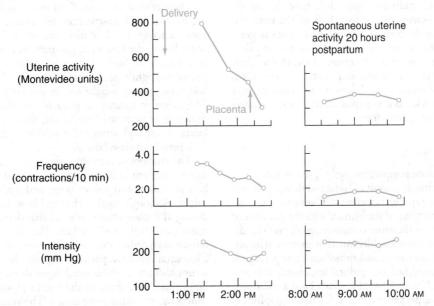

Figure 12–2. Uterine activity during the immediate puerperium (**left**) and at 20 hours postpartum (**right**). (Adapted from Hendricks CH et al: Uterine contractility at delivery and in the puerperium. Am J Obstet Gynecol 1962;83:890.)

The torn hymen heals in the form of fibrosed nodules of mucosa, the **carunculae myrtiformes.**

Two weeks after delivery, the fallopian tube reflects a hypoestrogenic state marked by atrophy of the epithelium. Fallopian tubes removed between postpartum days 5 and 15 demonstrate acute inflammatory changes that have not been correlated with subsequent puerperal fever or salpingitis. Normal changes in the pelvis after uncomplicated term vaginal delivery include widening of the symphysis and sacroiliac joints and occasionally gas in these joints. Gas is often seen by ultrasonography in the endometrial cavity after uncomplicated vaginal delivery and does not necessarily indicate the presence of endometritis.

Ovulation occurs as early as 27 days after delivery, with a mean time of 70–75 days in nonlactating women and 6 months in lactating women. In lactating women the duration of anovulation will ultimately depend on the frequency of breastfeeding, duration of each feed, and proportion of supplementary feeds. Ovulation suppression is due to the high prolactin levels, which remain elevated until approximately 3 weeks after delivery in nonlactating women and 6 weeks in lactating women. However, estrogen levels fall immediately after delivery in all mothers and remain suppressed in lactating mothers. Menstruation returns as soon as 7 weeks in 70% and by 12 weeks in all nonlactating mothers and as late as 36 months in 70% of breastfeeding mothers.

The voluntary muscles of the pelvic floor and the pelvic supports gradually regain their tone during the puerperium. Tearing or overstretching of the musculature or fascia at the time of delivery predisposes to genital hernias. Overdistention of the abdominal wall during pregnancy may result in rupture of the elastic fibers of the cutis, persistent striae, and diastasis of the rectus muscles. Involution of the abdominal musculature may require 6–7 weeks, and vigorous exercise is not recommended until after that time.

Urinary System

In the immediate postpartum period, the bladder mucosa is edematous as a result of labor and delivery. In addition, bladder capacity is increased. Overdistention and incomplete emptying of the bladder with the presence of residual urine are therefore common problems. The diminished postpartum bladder function appears to be unaffected by infant weight and episiotomy, but perhaps is transiently diminished by epidural anesthesia and prolonged labor. Nearly 50% of patients have a mild proteinuria for 1–2 days after delivery. Ultrasonographic examination demonstrates resolution of collecting system dilatation by 6 weeks postpartum in most women. Urinary stasis, however, may persist in more than 50% of women at 12 weeks postpartum. The incidence of urinary tract infection is generally higher in these women with persistent dilatation. Significant renal enlargement may persist for many weeks postpartum.

Pregnancy is accompanied by an estimated increase of about 50% in the glomerular filtration rate. These values return to normal or less than normal during the eighth week of the puerperium. Endogenous creatinine clearance similarly returns to normal by 8 weeks. Renal plasma flow, which increased during pregnancy by 25% in the first trimester, falls in the third trimester and continues to fall to below normal levels for up to 24 months. Normal levels return slowly over 50–60 weeks. The glucosuria induced by pregnancy disappears. The blood urea nitrogen rises during the puerperium; at the end of the first week postpartum, values of 20 mg/dL are reached, compared with 15 mg/dL in the late third trimester.

Fluid Balance & Electrolytes

An average decrease in maternal weight of 10–13 lb occurs intrapartum and immediately postpartum due to the loss of amniotic fluid and blood as well as delivery of the infant and placenta. The average patient may lose an additional 4 kg (9 lb) during the puerperium and over the next 6 months as a result of excretion of the fluids and electrolytes accumulated during pregnancy. Contrary to widespread belief, breastfeeding has minimal effects on hastening weight loss postpartum.

There is an average net fluid loss of at least 2 L during the first week postpartum and an additional loss of approximately 1.5 L during the next 5 weeks. The water loss in the first week postpartum represents a loss of extracellular fluid. A negative balance must be expected of slightly more than 100 mEq of chloride per kilogram of body weight lost in the early puerperium. This negative balance is probably attributable to the discharge of maternal extracellular fluid. The puerperal losses of salt and water are generally larger in women with preeclampsia-eclampsia.

The changes occurring in serum electrolytes during the puerperium indicate a general increase in the numbers of cations and anions compared with antepartum values. Although total exchangeable sodium decreases during the puerperium, the relative decrease in body water exceeds the sodium loss. The diminished aldosterone antagonism due to falling plasma progesterone concentrations may partially explain the rapid rise in serum sodium. Cellular breakdown due to tissue involution may contribute to the rise in plasma potassium concentration noted postpartum. The mean increase in cations, chiefly sodium, amounts to 4.7 mEq/L, with an equal increase in anions. Consequently, the plasma osmolality rises by 7 mOsm/L at the end of the first week postpartum. In keeping with the chloride shift, there is a tendency for the serum chloride concentration to decrease slightly postpartum as serum bicarbonate increases.

Metabolic & Chemical Changes

Total fatty acids and nonesterified fatty acids return to nonpregnant levels on about the second day of the puerperium. Both cholesterol and triglyceride concentrations decrease significantly within 24 hours after delivery, and this change is reflected in all lipoprotein fractions. Plasma triglycerides continue to fall and approach nonpregnant values 6–7 weeks postpartum. By comparison, the decrease in plasma cholesterol levels is slower; LDL cholesterol remains above nonpregnant levels for at least 7 weeks postpartum. Lactation does not influence lipid levels, but, in contrast to pregnancy, the postpartum hyperlipidemia is sensitive to dietary manipulation.

During the early puerperium blood glucose concentrations (both fasting and postprandial) tend to fall below the values seen during pregnancy and delivery. This fall is most marked on the second and third postpartum days. Accordingly, the insulin requirements of diabetic patients are lower. Reliable indications of the insulin sensitivity and the blood glucose concentrations characteristic of the nonpregnant state can be demonstrated only after the first week postpartum. Thus a glucose tolerance test performed in the early puerperium may be interpreted erroneously if nonpuerperal standards are applied to the results.

The concentration of free plasma amino acids increases postpartum. Normal nonpregnant values are regained rapidly on the second or third postpartum day and are presumably a result of reduced utilization and an elevation in the renal threshold.

Cardiovascular Changes

A. BLOOD COAGULATION

The production of both prostacyclin (PGI_2), an inhibitor of platelet aggregation, and thromboxane A_2, an inducer of platelet aggregation and a vasoconstrictor, is increased during pregnancy and the puerperium. Possibly, the balance between thromboxane A_2 and PGI_2 is shifted to the side of thromboxane A_2 dominance during the puerperium, since platelet reactivity is increased at this time. Rapid and dramatic changes in the coagulation and fibrinolytic systems occur after delivery (Table 12–1). A decrease in the platelet count occurs immediately after separation of the placenta, but a secondary elevation occurs in the next few days together with an increase in platelet adhesiveness. The plasma fibrinogen concentration begins to decrease during

Table 12–1. Changes in blood coagulation and fibrinolysis during the puerperium.

	Time Postpartum				
	1 Hour	1 Day	3–5 Days	1st Week	2nd Week
Platelet count	↓	↑	↑↑	↑↑	↑
Platelet adhesiveness	↑	↑↑	↑↑↑	↑	0
Fibrinogen	↓	↓	↑	0	↓
Factor V		↑	↑↑	↑	0
Factor VIII	↓	↓	↑	↑	↓
Factors II, VII, X		↓	↓	↓↓	↓↓
Plasminogen	↓	↓↓	0	↓	
Plasminogen activator	↑↑↑	↑↑	0		
Fibrinolytic activity	↑	↑↑	↑↑	↑	
Fibrin split products	↑	↑↑	↑↑		

The arrows indicate the direction and relative magnitude of change compared with the late third trimester or antepartum values. Zero indicates a return to antepartum but not necessarily nonpregnant values. (Prepared from the data of Manning FA et al: Am J Obstet Gynecol 1971;110:900, Bonnar J et al: Br Med J 1970;2:200; Ygg J: Am J Obstet Gynecol 1969;104:2; and Shaper AG et al: J Obstet Gynaecol Br Commonw 1968;75:433.)

labor and reaches its lowest point during the first day postpartum. Thereafter, rising plasma fibrinogen levels reach prelabor values by the third or fifth day of the puerperium. This secondary peak in fibrinogen activity is maintained until the second postpartum week, after which the level of activity slowly returns to normal nonpregnant levels during the following 7–10 days. A similar pattern occurs with respect to factor VIII and plasminogen. Circulating levels of antithrombin III are decreased in the third trimester of pregnancy. Patients with a congenital deficiency of antithrombin III (an endogenous inhibitor of factor X) have recurrent venous thromboembolic disease, and a low level of this factor has been associated with a hypercoagulable state.

The fibrinolytic activity of maternal plasma is greatly reduced during the last months of pregnancy but increases rapidly after delivery. In the first few hours postpartum, an increase in tissue plasminogen activator (t-PA) develops, together with a slight prolongation of the thrombin time, a decrease in plasminogen activator inhibitors, and a significant increase in fibrin split products. Protein C is an important coagulation inhibitor that requires the nonenzymatic cofactor protein S (which exists as a free protein and as a complex) for its activity. The level of protein S, both total and free, increases on the first day after delivery and gradually returns to normal levels after the first week postpartum.

According to current concepts, the fibrinolytic system is in dynamic equilibrium with the factors that promote coagulation. Thus after delivery, the increased plasma fibrinolytic activity coupled with the consumption of several clotting factors suggests a large deposition of fibrin in the placental bed. Because of the continued release of fibrin breakdown products from the placental site, the concentration of fibrin split products continues to rise even after spontaneous plasma fibrinolytic activity decreases. Increased levels of soluble fibrin monomer complexes are observed during the early puerperium compared with levels at 3 months postpartum.

The increased concentration of clotting factors normally seen during pregnancy can be viewed as teleologically important in providing a reserve to compensate for the rapid consumption of these factors during delivery and in promoting hemostasis after parturition. Nonetheless, extensive activation of clotting factors together with immobility, sepsis, or trauma during delivery may set the stage for later thromboembolic complications (see Chapter 43). The secondary increase in fibrinogen, factor VIII, or platelets (which remain well above nonpregnant values in the first week postpartum) also predisposes to thrombosis during the puerperium. The abrupt return of normal fibrinolytic activity after delivery may be a protective mechanism to combat this hazard. A small percentage of puerperal women who show a diminished ability to activate the fibrinolytic system appear to be at high risk for the development of postpartum thromboembolic complications.

B. Blood Volume Changes

The total blood volume normally decreases from the antepartum value of 5–6 L to the nonpregnant value of 4 L by the third week after delivery. One third of this reduction occurs during delivery and soon afterward, and a similar amount is lost by the end of the first postpartum week. Additional variation occurs with lactation. The hypervolemia of pregnancy may be viewed as a protective mechanism that allows most women to tolerate considerable loss of blood during parturition. The quantity of blood lost during delivery generally determines the blood volume and hematocrit during the puerperium. Normal vaginal delivery of a single fetus entails an average blood loss of about 400 mL, whereas cesarean section leads to a blood loss of nearly 1 L. If total hysterectomy is performed in addition to cesarean

section delivery, the mean blood loss increases to approximately 1500 mL. Delivery of twins and triplets entails blood losses similar to those of operative delivery, but a compensatory increase in maternal plasma volume and red blood cell mass is observed during multiple pregnancy.

Dramatic and rapid readjustments occur in the maternal vasculature after delivery, so that the response to blood loss during the early puerperium is different from that occurring in the nonpregnant woman. Delivery leads to obliteration of the low-resistance uteroplacental circulation and results in a 10–15% reduction in the size of the maternal vascular bed. Loss of placental endocrine function also removes a stimulus to vasodilatation.

A declining blood volume with a rise in hematocrit is usually seen 3–7 days after vaginal delivery (Fig 12–3). In contrast, serial studies of patients after cesarean section indicate a more rapid decline in blood volume and hematocrit and a tendency for the hematocrit to stabilize or even decline in the early puerperium. Hemoconcentration occurs if the loss of red cells is less than the reduction in vascular capacity. Hemodilution takes place in patients who lose 20% or more of their circulating blood volume at delivery. In patients with preeclampsia-eclampsia, resolution of peripheral vasoconstriction and mobilization of excess ex-

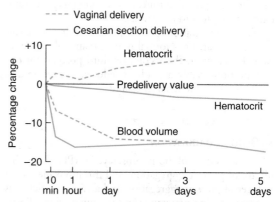

Figure 12–3. Postpartum changes in hematocrit and blood volume in patients delivered vaginally and by cesarean section. Values are expressed as the percentage change from the predelivery hematocrit or blood volume. (From the data of Ueland K et al: Maternal cardiovascular dynamics. 1. Cesarean section under subarachnoid block anesthesia. Am J Obstet Gynecol 1968;100:42; and Ueland K, Hansen J: Maternal cardiovascular dynamics. 3. Labor and delivery under local and caudal analgesia. Am J Obstet Gynecol 1969;103:8.)

tracellular fluid may lead to a significant expansion of the vascular volume by the third postpartum day. Plasma atrial natriuretic peptide levels nearly double during the first days postpartum in response to atrial stretch caused by blood volume expansion and may have relevance for postpartum natriuresis and diuresis. Occasionally, a patient sustains minimal blood loss at delivery. In such a patient, marked hemoconcentration may occur in the puerperium, especially if there has been a preexisting polycythemia or a considerable increase in the red cell mass during pregnancy.

C. HEMATOPOIESIS

The red cell mass increases by about 30% during pregnancy, whereas the average red cell loss at delivery is approximately 14%. Thus, the mean postpartum red cell mass level should be about 15% above nonpregnant values. The sudden loss of blood at delivery, however, leads to a rapid and short-lived reticulocytosis (with a peak on the fourth postpartum day) and moderately elevated erythropoietin levels during the first week postpartum.

The bone marrow in pregnancy and in the early puerperium is hyperactive and capable of delivering a large number of young cells to the peripheral blood. Prolactin may play a minor role in bone marrow stimulation.

A striking leukocytosis occurs during labor and extends into the early puerperium. In the immediate puerperium the white blood cell count may be as high as 25,000/μL, with an increased percentage of granulocytes. The stimulus for this leukocytosis is not known, but it probably represents a release of sequestered cells in response to the stress of labor.

The serum iron level is decreased and the plasma iron turnover is increased between the third and fifth days of the puerperium. Normal values are regained by the second week postpartum. The shorter duration of ferrokinetic changes in puerperal women compared with the duration of changes in nonpregnant women who have had phlebotomy is due to the increased erythroid marrow activity and the circulatory changes described above.

Most women who sustain an average blood loss at delivery and who have had iron supplementation during pregnancy show a relative erythrocytosis during the second week postpartum. Since there is no evidence of increased red cell destruction during the puerperium, any red cells gained during pregnancy will disappear gradually according to their normal life span. A moderate excess of red blood cells after delivery, therefore, may lead to an increase in iron stores. Iron supplementation is not necessary for normal postpartum women if the hematocrit or hemoglobin concentration 5–7 days after delivery is equal to or greater than a normal predelivery value. In the late puerperium, there is a gradual decrease in the red cell mass to nonpregnant levels as the rate of erythropoiesis returns to normal.

D. HEMODYNAMIC CHANGES

The hemodynamic adjustments in the puerperium depend largely on the conduct of labor and delivery, eg, maternal position, method of delivery, mode of anesthesia or analgesia, and blood loss. Cardiac output increases progressively during labor in patients who have received only local anesthesia. The increase in cardiac output peaks immediately after delivery, at which time it is approximately 80% above the prelabor value. During a uterine contraction there is a rise in central venous pressure, arterial pressure, and stroke volume—and, in the absence of pain and anxiety, a reflex decrease in the pulse rate. These changes are magnified in the supine position. Only minimal changes occur in the lateral recumbent position because of unimpaired venous return and absence of aortoiliac compression by the contracting uterus (Poseiro effect). Epidural anesthesia modifies the progressive rise in cardiac output during labor and reduces the absolute increase observed immediately after delivery, probably by limiting pain and anxiety.

Although major hemodynamic readjustments occur during the period immediately following delivery, there is a return to nonpregnant conditions in the early puerperium. A trend for normal women to increase their blood pressure slightly in the first 5 days postpartum reflects an increased uterine vascular resistance and a temporary surplus in plasma volume. A small percentage will have diastolic blood pressures of 100 mm Hg. Cardiac output (measured by Doppler and cross-sectional echocardiography) declines 28% within 2 weeks postpartum from peak values observed at 38 weeks' gestation. This change is associated with a 20% reduction in stroke volume and a smaller decrease in myocardial contractility indices. Postpartum resolution of the pregnancy-induced ventricular hypertrophy takes longer than the functional postpartum changes (Fig 12–4). In fact, limited data support a slow return of cardiac hemodynamics to prepregnancy levels over a 1-year period. There are no hemodynamic differences between lactating and nonlactating mothers.

Respiratory Changes

The pulmonary functions that change most rapidly are those influenced by alterations in abdominal contents and thoracic cage capacity. Lung volume changes in the puerperium are compared with those occurring during pregnancy in Figure 12–5. The residual volume increases, but the vital capacity and inspiratory capacities decrease. The maximum breathing capacity is also re-

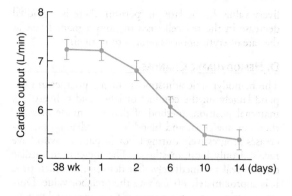

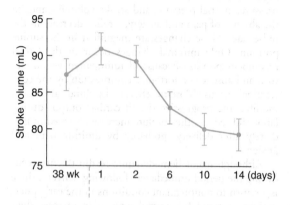

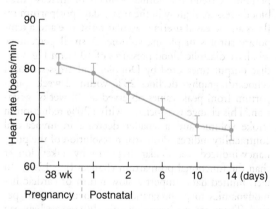

Figure 12–4. Changes in cardiac output, stroke volume, and heart rate during the puerperium after normal delivery. (From Hunter S, Robson SC: Adaptation of the maternal heart in pregnancy. Br Heart J 1992;68:540.)

duced after delivery. An increase in resting ventilation and in oxygen consumption and a less efficient response to exercise may persist during the early postpartum weeks. Comparisons of aerobic capacity prior to pregnancy and again postpartum indicate that lack of activ-

ity and weight gain contribute to a generalized detraining effect 4–8 weeks postpartum.

Changes in acid-base status generally parallel changes in respiratory function. The state of pregnancy is characterized by respiratory alkalosis and compensated metabolic acidosis, whereas labor represents a transitional period. A significant hypocapnia (< 30 mm Hg), a rise in blood lactate, and a fall in pH are first noted at the end of the first stage of labor and extend into the puerperium. Within a few days, a rise toward the normal nonpregnant values of PCO_2 (35–40 mm Hg) occurs. Progesterone influences the rate of ventilation by means of a central effect, and rapidly decreasing levels of this hormone are largely responsible for the increased PCO_2 seen in the first week postpartum. An increase in base excess and plasma bicarbonate accompanies the relative postpartum hypercapnia. A gradual increase in pH and base excess occurs until normal levels are reached at about 3 weeks postpartum.

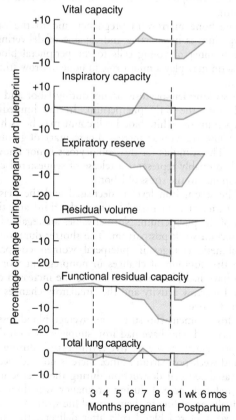

Figure 12–5. Alterations in lung volumes during pregnancy and 1 week and 6 months postpartum. (Modified from Cugell DW et al: Pulmonary function in pregnancy. Am Rev Tuberc 1953;67:568.)

The resting arterial PO$_2$ and oxygen saturation during pregnancy are higher than those in nonpregnant women. During labor, the oxygen saturation may be depressed, especially in the supine position, probably as a result of a decrease in cardiac output and a relative increase in the amount of intrapulmonary shunting. However, a rise in the arterial oxygen saturation to 95% is noted during the first postpartum day. An apparent oxygen debt incurred during labor extends into the immediate puerperium and appears to depend on the length and severity of the second stage of labor. Many investigators have commented on the continued elevation of the basal metabolic rate for a period of 7–14 days following delivery. The increased resting oxygen consumption in the early puerperium has been attributed to mild anemia, lactation, and psychologic factors.

Pituitary-Ovarian Relationships

The plasma levels of placental hormones decline rapidly following delivery. Human placental lactogen has a half-life of 20 minutes and reaches undetectable levels in maternal plasma during the first day after delivery. Human chorionic gonadotropin (hCG) has a mean half-life of about 9 hours. The concentration of hCG in maternal plasma falls below 1000 mU/mL within 48–96 hours postpartum and falls below 100 mU/mL by the seventh day. Follicular phase levels of immunoreactive luteinizing hormone (LH)-hCG are reached during the second postpartum week. Highly specific and sensitive radioimmunoassays for the beta subunit of hCG indicate virtual disappearance of hCG from maternal plasma between the 11th and 16th days following normal delivery. The regressive pattern of hCG activity is slower after first-trimester abortion than it is after term delivery and even more prolonged in patients who have had a suction curettage for molar pregnancy.

Within 3 hours after removal of the placenta, the plasma concentration of estradiol-17β falls to 10% of the antepartum value. The lowest levels are reached by the seventh postpartum day (Fig 12–6). Plasma estrogens do not reach follicular phase levels (> 50 pg/mL) until 19–21 days postpartum in nonlactating women. The return to normal plasma levels of estrogens is delayed in lactating women. Lactating women who resume spontaneous menses achieve follicular phase estradiol levels (> 50 pg/mL) during the first 60–80 days postpartum. Lactating amenorrheic persons are markedly hypoestrogenic (plasma estradiol < 10 pg/mL) during the first 180 days postpartum. The onset of breast engorgement on days 3–4 of the puerperium coincides with a significant fall in estrogens and supports the view that high estrogen levels suppress lactation.

The metabolic clearance rate of progesterone is high, and, as with estradiol, the half-life is calculated in min-utes. By the third day of the puerperium, the plasma progesterone concentrations are below luteal phase levels (< 1 ng/mL).

Prolactin levels in maternal blood rise throughout pregnancy to reach concentrations of 200 ng/mL or more. After delivery, prolactin declines in erratic fashion over a period of 2 weeks to the nongravid range in nonlactating women (Fig 12–6). In women who are breastfeeding, basal concentrations of prolactin remain above the nongravid range and increase dramatically in response to suckling. As lactation progresses, the amount of prolactin released with each suckling episode declines. If breastfeeding occurs only 1–3 times each day, serum prolactin levels return to normal basal values within 6 months postpartum; if suckling takes place more than 6 times each day, high basal concentrations of prolactin will persist for more than 1 year. The diurnal rhythm of peripheral prolactin concentrations (a daytime nadir followed by a nighttime peak) is abolished during late pregnancy but is reestablished within 1 week postpartum in non-nursing women.

Serum follicle-stimulating hormone (FSH) and LH concentrations are very low in all women during the first 10–12 days postpartum whether or not they lactate. The levels increase over the following days and reach follicular phase concentrations during the third week postpartum (Fig 12–6). At this time, a marked LH pulse amplification occurs during sleep, but it disappears as normal ovulatory cycles are established. In this respect, the transition from postpartum amenorrhea to cyclic ovulation is reminiscent of puberty, when gonadotropin secretion increases during sleep. There is a preferential release of FSH over LH postpartum during spontaneous recovery or after stimulation by exogenous gonadotropin-releasing hormone (GnRH). In the early puerperium, the pituitary is relatively refractory to GnRH, but 4–8 weeks postpartum the response to GnRH is exaggerated. The low levels of FSH and LH postpartum are most likely related to an insufficiency of endogenous GnRH secretion during pregnancy and the early puerperium, resulting in the depletion of pituitary gonadotropin stores. The high estrogen and progesterone milieu of late pregnancy is associated with increased endogenous opioid activity, which may be responsible for suppression of GnRH activity in the puerperium. Resumption of FSH and LH secretion can be accelerated by administering a long-acting GnRH agonist during the first 10 days postpartum.

The frequency with which menstruation is reestablished in the puerperium in lactating and nonlactating women is shown in Figure 12–7. The first menses after delivery usually follows an anovulatory cycle or one associated with inadequate corpus luteum function. The ovary may be somewhat refractory to exogenous gonadotropin stimulation during the puerperium in both

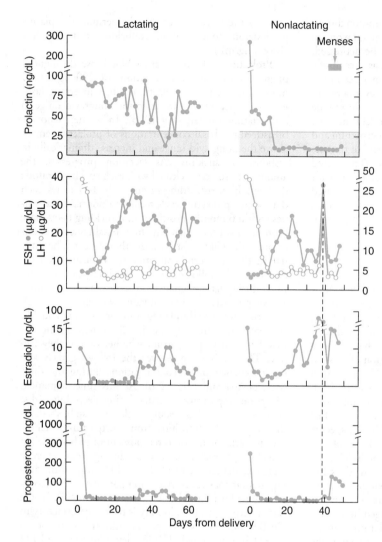

Figure 12–6. Serum concentrations of prolactin, FSH, LH, estradiol, and progesterone in a lactating and nonlactating woman during the puerperium. The hatched bars for the prolactin data represent the normal nongravid range. To convert the FSH and LH to milli-International units per milliliter, divide the FSH values by 2 and multiply the LH values by 4.5. FSH, follicle-stimulating hormone; LH, luteinizing hormone. (From Reyes FI, Winter JS, Faiman C: Pituitary-ovarian interrelationships during the puerperium. Am J Obstet Gynecol 1972;114:589.)

lactating and nonlactating women. When prolactin is suppressed with bromocriptine, postpartum ovarian refractoriness to gonadotropin stimulation persists, suggesting that hyperprolactinemia plays only a partial role in the diminished gonadal response. Lactation is characterized by an increased sensitivity to the negative feedback effects and a decreased sensitivity to the positive feedback effects of estrogens on gonadotropin secretion.

Because ovarian activity normally resumes upon weaning, either the suckling stimulus itself or the raised level of prolactin is responsible for the suppression of pulsatile gonadotropin secretion. Hyperprolactinemia may not entirely account for the inhibition of gonadotropin secretion during lactation, since bromocriptine treatment abolishes the hyperprolactinemia of

suckling but not the inhibition of gonadotropin secretion. Sensory inputs associated with suckling (if sufficiently intense), as well as oxytocin and endogenous opioids that are released during suckling may affect the hypothalamic control of gonadotropin secretion, possibly by inhibiting the pulsatile secretion of GnRH. It appears that by 8 weeks after delivery, while ovarian activity still remains suppressed in fully breastfeeding women, pulsatile secretion of LH has resumed at a low and variable frequency in most women. However, the presence or absence of GnRH or LH pulses at 8 weeks does not predict the time of resumption of ovarian activity.

The time of appearance of the first ovulation is variable, but it is delayed by breastfeeding. Approximately 10–15% of non-nursing mothers ovulate by the time of

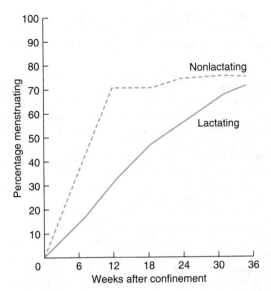

Figure 12–7. Frequency at which menstruation is reestablished in the puerperium in lactating and non-lactating multiparous women. (Adapted from Sherman A: *Reproductive Physiology of the Post-partum Period.* Livingstone, 1966.)

the 6-week postpartum examination, and approximately 30% ovulate within 90 days postpartum. An abnormally short luteal phase is noted in 35% of first ovulatory cycles. The earliest reported time of ovulation as determined by endometrial biopsy is 33 days postpartum. Patients who have had a first-trimester abortion or ectopic pregnancy generally ovulate sooner after termination of pregnancy (as early as 14 days) than do women who deliver at term. Moreover, the majority of these women do ovulate before the first episode of postabortal bleeding—in contrast to women who have had a term pregnancy.

Endometrial biopsies in lactating women do not show a secretory pattern before the seventh postpartum week. Provided that nursing is in progress and that menstruation has not returned, ovulation before the tenth week postpartum is rare. In well-nourished women who breastfed for an extended period of time, less than 20% had ovulated by 6 months postpartum. Much of the variability in the resumption of menstruation and ovulation observed in lactating women may be due to individual differences in the strength of the suckling stimulus and to partial weaning (formula supplementation). This emphasizes the fact that suckling is not a reliable form of birth control. Since the period of lactational infertility is relatively short in Western societies, some form of contraception must be used if

pregnancy is to be avoided. Among women who have unprotected intercourse only during lactational amenorrhea but adopt other contraceptive measures when they resume menstruation, only 2% will become pregnant during the first 6 months of amenorrhea. In underdeveloped countries, lactational amenorrhea and infertility may persist for 1–2 years owing to frequent suckling and poor maternal nutrition. When maternal dietary intake is improved, menstruation resumes at least 6 months earlier.

Other Endocrine Changes

A progressive enlargement of the pituitary gland occurs during pregnancy with a 30–100% increase in weight achieved at term. Magnetic resonance imaging shows a linear gain in pituitary gland height of about 0.08 mm/wk during pregnancy. An additional increase in size occurs during the first week postpartum. Beyond the first week postpartum, however, the pituitary gland returns rapidly to its normal size in both lactating and nonlactating women.

The physiologic hypertrophy of the pituitary gland is associated with an increase in the number of pituitary lactotroph cells at the expense of the somatotropic cell types. Thus, growth hormone secretion is depressed during the second half of pregnancy and the early puerperium. Because levels of circulating insulin-like growth factor (IGF-1) increase throughout pregnancy, a placental growth hormone has been postulated and recently identified. Maternal levels of IGF-1 correlate highly with this distinct placental growth hormone variant but not placental lactogen during pregnancy and in the immediate puerperium.

Late pregnancy and the early puerperium are also characterized by pituitary somatotroph hyporesponsiveness to growth hormone-releasing hormone and to insulin stimulation. Whatever the inhibitory mechanism may be (possibly increased somatostatin secretion), it persists during the early postpartum period.

The rapid disappearance of placental lactogen and the low levels of growth hormone after delivery lead to a relative deficiency of anti-insulin factors in the early puerperium. It is not surprising, therefore, that low fasting plasma glucose levels are noted at this time and that the insulin requirements of diabetic patients usually drop after delivery. Glucose tolerance tests performed in women with gestational diabetes demonstrate that only 30% have abnormal tests 3–5 days after delivery and 20% have abnormal glucose tolerance at 6 weeks postpartum. When the relative hyperinsulinism and hypoglycemia of pregnancy return to the nonpregnant range at 6–8 weeks postpartum, a paradoxical decline in fasting glucagon levels is found. Since the early puerperium represents a transitional period in carbohydrate metabolism, the results of glucose tolerance tests may be difficult to interpret.

The evaluation of thyroid function is also difficult in the period immediately after birth because of rapid fluctuations in many indices. Characteristically, the plasma thyroxine and other indices of thyroid function are highest at delivery and in the first 12 hours thereafter. A decrease to antepartum values is seen on the third or fourth day after delivery. Reduced available estrogens postpartum lead to a subsequent decrease in circulating thyroxine-binding globulin and a gradual diminution in bound thyroid hormones in serum. Serum concentrations of thyroid-stimulating hormone (TSH) are not significantly different postpartum from those of the pregnant or nonpregnant state. Administration of thyroid-releasing hormone (TRH) in the puerperium results in a normal increase in both TSH and prolactin, and the response is similar in lactating and nonlactating patients. Because pregnancy is associated with some immunosuppressive effects, hyperthyroidism or hypothyroidism may recur postpartum in autoimmune thyroid disease. Failure of lactation and prolonged disability may be the result of hypothyroidism postpartum. In Sheehan's syndrome of pituitary infarction, postpartum cachexia and myxedema are seen secondary to anterior hypophyseal insufficiency.

Maternal concentrations of total and unbound (free) plasma cortisol, adrenocorticotropic hormone (ACTH) and immunoreactive corticotropin-releasing hormone (CRH) and β-endorphin rise progressively during pregnancy and increase further during labor. Plasma 17-hydroxycorticosteroids increase from a concentration of 4–14 μg/dL at 40 weeks' gestation. A two- to threefold increase is seen during labor. ACTH, CRH, and β-endorphin decrease rapidly after delivery and return to nonpregnant levels within 24 hours. Prelabor cortisol values are regained on the first day postpartum but a return to normal, nonpregnant cortisol and 17-hydroxycorticosteroid levels is not reached until the end of the first week postpartum.

Much of the rise in total cortisol (but not in the unbound fraction) can be explained by the parallel increase in corticosteroid-binding globulin (CBG) during pregnancy. Displacement of cortisol from CBG by high concentrations of progesterone cannot account for the increased free cortisol levels because saliva progesterone levels (a measure of the unbound hormone) do not fluctuate, whereas a normal diurnal rhythm of saliva cortisol is maintained during pregnancy and postpartum. An extrapituitary source of ACTH, a progesterone-modulated decrease in the hypothalamic-pituitary sensitivity to glucocorticoid feedback inhibition, and an extrahypothalamic (eg, placental) source

of CRH have been suggested as explanations for elevated plasma ACTH levels and the inability of dexamethasone to completely suppress ACTH in pregnant women.

The placenta produces large amounts of CRH in the third trimester, which is released into the maternal circulation and may contribute to the hypercortisolemia of pregnancy. Present evidence suggests that it stimulates the maternal pituitary to produce ACTH while desensitizing the pituitary to further acute stimulation with CRH. Maternal hypothalamic control of ACTH production is retained (perhaps mediated by vasopressin secretion); this permits a normal response to stress and a persistent diurnal rhythm.

Overall, it is most likely that under the influence of rising estrogens and progesterone, there is a resetting of the hypothalamic-pituitary sensitivity to cortisol feedback during pregnancy, which persists for several days postpartum. Several studies have suggested a relationship between peripartum alterations in maternal levels of cortisol and β-endorphin and the development of postnatal mood disturbances.

The excretion of urinary 17-ketosteroids is elevated in late pregnancy as a result of an increase in androgenic precursors from the fetoplacental unit and the ovary. An additional increase of 50% in the amount of excretion occurs during labor. Excretion of 17-ketosteroids returns to antepartum levels on the first day after delivery and to the nonpregnant range by the end of the first week. The mean levels of testosterone during the third trimester of pregnancy range from 3 to 7 times the mean values for nonpregnant women. The elevated levels of testosterone decrease after parturition parallel with the gradual fall in sex hormone-binding globulin (SHBG). Androstenedione, which is poorly bound to SHBG, falls rapidly to nonpregnant values by the third day postpartum. Conversely, the postpartum plasma concentration of dehydroepiandrosterone sulfate (DHEA-S) remains lower than that of nonpregnant women, because its metabolic clearance rate continues to be elevated in the early puerperium. Persistently elevated 17-ketosteroids or androgens during the puerperium are an indication for investigation of ovarian abnormalities. Plasma renin and angiotensin II levels fall during the first 2 hours postpartum to levels within the normal nonpregnant range. This suggests that an extrarenal source of renin has been lost with the expulsion of the fetus and placenta.

There is little direct information about the puerperal changes in numerous other hormones, including aldosterone, parathyroid hormone, and calcitonin. More research should be done on these important endocrine relationships in the puerperium.

CONDUCT AND MANAGEMENT OF THE PUERPERIUM

Most patients will benefit from 2–4 days of hospitalization after delivery. Only 3% of women with a vaginal delivery and 9% of women having a cesarean section have a childbirth-related complication that requires prolonged postpartum hospitalization or readmission. Although a significant amount of symptomatic morbidity may exist postpartum (painful perineum, breastfeeding difficulties, urinary infections, urinary and fecal incontinence, and headache), most women can now return home safely 2 days after normal vaginal delivery if proper education and instructions are given, if confidence exists with infant care and feeding, and if adequate support exists at home. Earlier discharge is acceptable in select mothers and infants who have had uncomplicated labors and deliveries. Discharge criteria should be met and follow-up care provided. Optimal care includes home nursing visits through the fourth postpartum day. Disadvantages of early discharge are the increased risks of rehospitalization of some neonates for hyperbilirubinemia and neonatal infection (eg, from group B streptococci).

Activities & Rest

The policy of early ambulation after delivery benefits the patient. Early ambulation provides a sense of well-being, hastens involution of the uterus, improves uterine drainage, and lessens the incidence of postpartum thrombophlebitis. If the delivery has been uncomplicated, the patient may be out of bed as soon as tolerated. Early ambulation does not mean immediate return to normal activity or work. Commonly mothers complain of lethargy and fatigue. Rest is therefore essential after delivery, and the demands on the mother should be limited to allow for adequate relaxation and adjustment to her new responsibilities. It is helpful to set aside a few hours each day for rest periods. Many mothers do not sleep well for several nights after delivery, and it is surprising how much of the day is occupied with the care of the newborn.

In uncomplicated deliveries, more vigorous activity, climbing stairs, lifting of heavy objects, riding in or driving a car, and performing muscle toning exercises may be resumed without delay. Specific recommendations should be individualized. Current American College of Obstetricians and Gynecologists committee opinions support gradual resumption of exercise routines as soon as medically and physically safe, as detraining may have occurred during pregnancy. No known maternal complications are associated with resumption of exercise, even in women who choose to resume an exercise routine within days. Exercise postpartum does not compromise lactation or neonatal weight gain. It may be beneficial in decreasing anxiety levels and decreasing the incidence of postpartum depression.

Sexual Activity During the Postpartum Period

Establishment of normal prepregnancy sexual response patterns is delayed after delivery. However, it is safe to resume sexual activity when the woman's perineum is comfortable and bleeding is diminished. Although the median time for resumption of intercourse after delivery is 6 weeks and the normal sexual response returns at 12 weeks, sexual desire and activity vary tremendously among women. Most women report low or absent sexual desire during the early puerperium and ascribe this to fatigue, weakness, pain on intromission, irritative vaginal discharge, or fear of injury. Nearly 50% report a return of sexual desire within 2-3 weeks postpartum. In spite of minimal desire in a substantial proportion of women, nearly all resume sexual intercourse by 6–8 weeks after delivery. Roughly 20% of women have no desire for sexual activity at 3 months from delivery and an additional 21% lose the desire completely or develop an aversion. The variation in desire depends on the site and state of perineal or vaginal healing, return of libido, and vaginal atrophy resulting from breastfeeding. Lactating women, however, generally report higher sexual interest than do bottle-feeding mothers.

Sexual counseling is indicated before the mother is discharged from the hospital. A discussion of the normal fluctuations of sexual interest during the puerperium is appropriate, as are suggestions for noncoital sexual options that enhance the expression of mutual pleasure and affection. The importance of sleep and rest and of the partner's emotional and physical support are emphasized. If milk ejection during sexual relations is a concern, nursing the baby prior to sexual intimacy can help. Sexual relations can generally be resumed by the third week postpartum, if desired. A water-soluble lubricant or vaginal estrogen cream is especially helpful in lactating amenorrheic mothers in whom vaginal atrophy occurs, usually because of low circulating estrogen levels. Patients should be informed that roughly 50% of women engaging in sexual intercourse by 6 weeks will experience dyspareunia, which may last for 1 year. Dyspareunia also occurs in women with cesarean sections and in women using oral contraceptives who are not breastfeeding.

Diet

A regular diet is permissible as soon as the patient regains her appetite and is free from the effects of analgesics and anesthetics. Protein foods, fruits, vegetables, milk products, and a high fluid intake are recommended, especially for nursing mothers. However, even lactating women probably require no more than 2600–2800 kcal/d. It may be advisable to continue the daily vitamin-mineral supplement during the early puerperium. Following cesarean section, there is no evidence to support compromise of safety or comfort from the introduction of solid food early and allowing the patient to decide when to eat postoperatively. In fact, early feeding as tolerated by the patient has been shown to be safe and to facilitate a more rapid return to normal diet and bowel function.

Care of the Bladder

Most women empty the bladder during labor or have been catheterized at delivery. Even so, serious bladder distention may develop within 12 hours. A long and difficult labor or a forceps delivery may traumatize the base of the bladder and interfere with normal voiding. In some cases, overdistention of the bladder may be related to pain or spinal anesthesia. The marked polyuria noted for the first few days postpartum causes the bladder to fill in a relatively short time. Hence, obstetric patients require catheterization more frequently than most surgical patients. The patient should be catheterized every 6 hours after delivery if she is unable to void or empty her bladder completely. Intermittent catheterization is preferable to an indwelling catheter because the incidence of urinary tract infection is lower. However, if the bladder fills to more than 1000 mL, 1–2 days of decompression by a retention catheter is usually required to establish voiding without significant residual urine.

The incidence of true asymptomatic bacteriuria is approximately 5% in the early puerperium. Postpartum patients with a history of previous urinary tract infection, conduction anesthesia, and catheterization during delivery and operative delivery, should have a bacterial culture of a midstream urine specimen. In cases of confirmed bacteriuria, antibiotic treatment should be given; otherwise bacteriuria will persist in nearly 30% of patients. Three days of therapy are sufficient and this therapy avoids prolonged antibiotic exposure to the lactating mother.

Bowel Function

Pregnancy itself is associated with increased gastric emptying, but gastrointestinal motility is commonly delayed after labor and delivery. The mild ileus that follows delivery, together with perineal discomfort and postpartum fluid loss by other routes, predisposes to constipation during the puerperium. Obstruction of the colon by a retroverted uterus is a rare complication during the puerperium. If an enema was given before delivery, the patient is unlikely to have a bowel movement for 1-2 days after childbirth. Milk of magnesia, 15–20 mL orally on the evening of the second postpartum day, usually stimulates a bowel movement by the next morning. If not, a rectal suppository such as bisacodyl or a small tap water or oil retention enema may be given. Less bowel stimulation will be needed if the diet contains sufficient roughage. Stool softeners such as dioctyl sodium sulfosuccinate may ease the discomfort of early bowel movements. Hemorrhoidal discomfort is a common complaint postpartum and usually responds to conservative treatment with compresses, suppositories containing corticosteroids, local anesthetic sprays or emollients, and sitz baths. It is rarely necessary to treat hemorrhoids surgically postpartum unless thrombosis is extensive.

Operative vaginal delivery and lacerations involving the anal sphincter increase a woman's risk for anal incontinence. However, 5% of pregnant women overall have some degree of anal incontinence at 3 months postpartum. Complaints of fecal incontinence are often delayed because of embarrassment. Most cases are transient; however, cases persisting beyond 6 months require investigation and probable treatment.

Bathing

As soon as the patient is ambulatory, she may take a shower. Sitz or tub baths are probably safe if performed in a clean environment, because bath water will not gain access to the vagina unless it is directly introduced. Most patients prefer showers to tub baths because of the profuse flow of lochia immediately postpartum. However, sitz baths may be beneficial for perineal pain relief. Vaginal douching is contraindicated in the early puerperium. Tampons may be used whenever the patient is comfortable. However, use should be limited to daylight hours to prevent long hours of use or inadvertent tampon loss.

Care of the Perineum

Postpartum perineal care, even in the patient with an uncomplicated and satisfactorily repaired episiotomy or laceration, usually requires no more than routine cleansing with a bath or shower and analgesia.

Immediately after delivery, cold compresses (usually ice) applied to the perineum decrease traumatic edema and discomfort. The perineal area should be gently cleansed with plain soap at least once or twice a day and after voiding or defecation. If the perineum is kept clean, healing should occur rapidly. Cold or iced sitz baths, rather than hot sitz baths, may provide additional perineal pain relief for some patients. The patient should be put in a lukewarm tub to which ice cubes are added for 20–30 minutes. The cold promotes pain relief by decreasing the excitability of nerve endings, decreased nerve conduction, and local vasoconstriction, which reduces edema, inhibits hematoma formation, and decreases muscle irritability and spasm. Episiotomy pain is easily controlled with nonsteroidal anti-inflammatory agents, which appear to be superior to acetaminophen or proproxyphene.

An episiotomy or repaired lacerations should be inspected daily. A patient with mediolateral episiotomy, a third or fourth degree laceration or extension, or extensive bruising or edema may experience severe perineal pain. In the case of persistent or unusual pain, a vaginal and/or rectal examination should be performed to identify a hematoma, perineal infection, or potentially fatal conditions such as angioedema, necrotizing fasciitis, or perineal cellulitis. Episiotomy wounds rarely become infected, which is remarkable when one considers the difficulty of avoiding contamination of the perineal area. In the event of sepsis, local heat and irrigation should cause the infection to subside. Appropriate antibiotics may be indicated if an immediate response to these measures is not observed. In rare instances, the wound should be opened widely and sutures removed for adequate drainage.

Uterotonic Agents

Prophylactic administration of oxytocin after the second stage of labor and/or after placental delivery is beneficial in the prevention of postpartum hemorrhage and the need for therapeutic uterotonics. The routine use of ergot preparations or prostaglandins may be as effective as oxytocin, but have significantly more side effects. There appear to be no data to support the prophylactic use of oxytocic agents beyond the immediate puerperium. These agents should be limited to patients who have specific indications such as postpartum hemorrhage or uterine atony.

Emotional Reactions

Several basic emotional responses occur in almost every woman who has given birth to a normal baby. A woman's first emotion is usually one of extreme relief followed by a sense of happiness and gratitude that the new baby has arrived safely. A regular pattern of behavior occurs in the human mother immediately after birth of the infant. Touching, holding, and grooming of the infant under normal conditions rapidly strengthen maternal ties of affection. However, not all mothers react in this way, and some may even feel detached from the new baby. These reactions range from the common, physiologic, relatively mild and transient "maternity blues," which affect some 50–70% of postpartum women to more severe reactions including depression and rare puerperal psychosis.

Postpartum blues or maternity blues occurs in up to 70% of postpartum women and appear to be a normal psychological adjustment or response. It is generally characterized by tearfulness, anxiety, irritation, and restlessness. This symptomatology can be quite diverse, and may include depression, feelings of inadequacy, elation, mood swings, confusion, difficulty concentrating, headache, forgetfulness, insomnia, depersonalization, and negative feelings toward the baby. These transient symptoms usually occur within the first few days after delivery and cease by postpartum day 10; although bouts of weeping may occur for weeks after delivery. The blues are self-limiting, but the distress can be diminished by physical comfort and reassurance. Evidence suggests that rooming-in during the hospital stay reduces maternal anxiety and results in more successful breastfeeding.

Prematurity or illness of the newborn delays early intimate maternal-infant contact and may have an adverse effect on the rapid and complete development of normal mothering responses. Stressful factors during the puerperium (eg, marital infidelity or loss of friends as a result of the necessary confinement and preoccupation with the new baby) may leave the mother feeling unsupported and may interfere with the formation of a maternal bond with the infant.

When a baby dies or is born with a congenital defect, the obstetrician should tell the mother and father about the problem together, if possible. The baby's normal, healthy features and potential for improvement should be emphasized, and positive statements should be made about the present availability of corrective treatment and the promises of ongoing research. In the event of a perinatal loss, parents should be assisted in the grieving process. They should be encouraged to see and touch the baby at birth or later, even if maceration or anomalies are present. Mementos such as footprints, locks of hair, or a photograph can be a solace to the parents after the infant has been buried. During the puerperium, the obstetrician has an important opportunity to help the mother whose infant has died work through her period of mourning or discouragement and to assess abnormal reactions of grief that suggest a need for psychiatric assistance. Pathologic grief is characterized by the inability to work through the sense of loss within 3–4 months, with subsequent feelings of low self-esteem.

Postpartum Immunization

A. PREVENTION OF RH ISOIMMUNIZATION

The postpartum injection of Rh_o (D) immunoglobulin* will prevent sensitization in the Rh-negative woman who has had a fetal-to-maternal transfusion of Rh-positive fetal red cells. The risk of maternal sensitization rises with the volume of fetal transplacental hemorrhage. The usual amount of fetal blood that enters the maternal circulation is less than 0.5 mL. The usual dose of 300 μg of Rh_o (D) immunoglobulin is in excess of the dose generally required, because 25 μg of RhoGAM per milliliter of fetal red cells is sufficient to prevent maternal immunization. If neonatal anemia or other clinical symptoms suggest that a large transplacental hemorrhage has occurred, the amount of fetal blood in the maternal circulation can be estimated by the Kleihauer-Betke smear, and the amounts of RhoGAM to be administered can be adjusted accordingly. A dose of 10 mL per estimated mL of whole fetal blood should be administered. An alternative to the acid elution smear is the Du test, which will detect 20 mL or more of Rh-positive fetal blood in the maternal circulation.

Rh_o (D) immunoglobulin is administered after abortion without qualifications or after delivery to women who meet all of the following criteria: (1) The mother must be Rh_o (D)-negative without Rh antibodies; (2) the baby must be Rh_o (D)- or Du-positive; and (3) the cord blood must be Coombs-negative. If these criteria are met, a 1:1000 dilution of Rh_o (D) immunoglobulin is cross-matched to the mother's red cells to ensure compatibility, and 1 mL (300 μg) is given intramuscularly to the mother within 72 hours after delivery. If the 72-hour interval has been exceeded, it is advisable to give the immunoglobulin rather than withhold it, for it may still protect against sensitization 14–28 days after delivery, and the time required to mount a response varies from case to case. The 72-hour time limit for the administration of Rh immune globulin was a study limitation in a study in which patients in prison were allowed to be visited only every 3 days; thus the use of Rh immunoglobulin past the 3-day interval was never studied. Rh_o (D) immunoglobulin should also be given after delivery or abortion when serologic tests of maternal sensitization to the Rh factor are questionable.

The average risk of maternal sensitization after abortion is approximately half the risk incurred by full-term pregnancy and delivery; the latter has been estimated at 11%. Even though mothers have received Rh_o (D) immunoglobulin, they should be screened with each subsequent pregnancy, since postpartum prophylaxis failures still exist. Failures are related to inadequate Rh_o (D) immunoglobulin administration postpartum, an undetected very low titer in the previous pregnancy, and inexcusable oversights. Routine use of postpartum screening protocols to identify excess fetomaternal hemorrhage and strict adherence to recommended protocols for the management of unsensitized Rh-negative women will avoid most of these postpartum sensitizations.

B. RUBELLA VACCINATION

A significant number of women of childbearing age have never had rubella. When tested by the hemagglutination inhibition method, 10–20% of women are seronegative (titer of 1:8 or less). Women who are susceptible to rubella can be vaccinated safely and effectively with a live attenuated rubella virus vaccine (RA 27/3 strain) during the immediate puerperium. It is more immunogenic than earlier forms of the vaccine and is available in monovalent, bivalent (measles-rubella, MR), and the trivalent form (measles-mumps-rubella, MMR). Seroconversion occurs in approximately 95% of women vaccinated postpartum The puerperium is an ideal time for vaccination because there is no risk of inadvertently vaccinating a pregnant woman. Breastfeeding mothers are not excluded from immunization. There is concern, however, that 75% of such women may shed rubella virus in the breast milk, and a persistent rubella carrier state with periodic viral reactivation may rarely occur in the child. The neonate's exposure to the virus in breast milk is not associated with an alteration of responses to subsequent immunization. Women who receive rubella vaccinations are not contagious and cannot transmit infection to other susceptible children or adults. In addition, the serologic response against rubella is satisfactory when given concomitantly with other immunoglobulins such as Rh-immunoglobulin. However, blood transfusions can prevent the success of rubella vaccination if it is performed soon after the transfusion.

Vaccinated patients should be informed that transient side effects can result from rubella vaccination. Mild symptoms such as low-grade fever and malaise may occur in less than 25% of patients, arthralgias and rash in less than 10%, and rarely, overt arthritis may develop. Among adult women there is a 10–15% incidence of acute polyarthritis following immunization. Although the CDC registry of approximately 400 women receiving rubella vaccination within 3 months of conception reports no cases of congenital rubella, the recommendation that secure contraception be used for 3 months after vaccination remains. Rubella virus was, however, isolated from some women who received the vaccination during early pregnancy and elected to terminate. The theoretical maximum theoretical risk of

---

*Trade names include Gamulin Rh, HypRh$_o$-D, and Rh$_o$GAM.

congenital rubella resulting from vaccination during early pregnancy is 1–2%.

Contraception & Sterilization

The immediate puerperium has long been recognized as a convenient time for the discussion of family planning, although these discussions should ideally begin during prenatal care. Pregnancy prevention and birth control decisions should be made prior to discharge with a qualified nurse, physician, or physician's assistant, or with the aid of educational tools. Anovulation infertility lasts only 5 weeks in nonlactating women and greater than 8 weeks in fully lactating women and the lactational pregnancy rate is approximately 1% at 1 year postpartum.

Tubal sterilization is the most common method of contraception used in the United States. It is the procedure of choice for women desiring permanent sterilization. It can be performed easily at the time of cesarean section, 24–48 hours after an uncomplicated vaginal delivery, or immediately postpartum in uncomplicated patients with a labor epidural in place, without prolonging hospitalization or significantly increasing morbidity. Sterilization is not recommended in young women of low parity, or when the neonatal outcome is in doubt and survival of the infant is not assured. Postponing tubal sterilization 6–8 weeks postpartum is desirable for many couples, as it allows time to ensure that the infant is healthy, to fully understand the implications of permanent sterilization, and according to the United States Collaborative Review on Sterilization, to decrease feelings of guilt and regret.

Appropriate counseling regarding risks of failure, permanence of the procedure, the medical risks, and the potential psychosocial reactions to the procedure should be discussed with the patient. Patient ambivalence at the last minute is not unusual, in which case it is advisable to defer the procedure until after the puerperium. The 10-year failure rate of postpartum sterilization is less than 1%, with variations in the rate dependent on the type of sterilization procedure performed. The risks of postpartum or interval tubal ligation are infrequent and deaths from the procedure occur in 2–12/100,000 cases. Long-term complications, such as the posttubal syndrome (irregular menses and increased menstrual pain) have been reported in some 10–15% of women; however, well controlled prospective studies have failed to confirm that these symptoms occur more frequently with sterilization than in controls. A major anesthetic should be initiated only after careful evaluation by the anesthesia service, since the parturient may have an increased risk of regurgitation and aspiration of gastric contents. Postpartum laparoscopic sterilization has not gained popularity because of increased pelvic vascularity, the large size of the uterus, and the risk of visceral injury.

Natural family planning as contraception may begin after normal menses resumes. Breastfeeding with no supplementation will provide 98% contraceptive protection for up to 6 months. When menses returns, natural family planning may begin. This method, which has pregnancy rates comparable to barrier methods, utilizes the detection of the periovulation period by evaluating cervical mucous changes and/or basal body temperature changes. These techniques are often misrepresented by providers who have limited understanding of their use and success in pregnancy prevention.

The use of spermicides, a condom, or both may be prescribed until the postpartum examination; these methods carry a failure rate of 1.6–21 per 100 woman-years. Fitting of a diaphragm is not practical until involution of the reproductive organs has taken place and may be more difficult in lactating women with vaginal dryness. It should always be used in conjunction with a spermicidal lubricant containing nonoxynol-9. The failure rate for the diaphragm varies from 2.4–19.6 per 100 woman-years, with the lowest failure rates (comparable to the IUD) occurring in women who are older, motivated, experienced, or familiar with the technique.

In patients who are not breastfeeding, combination oral contraceptive agents can be taken as early as 2–3 weeks postpartum. They should not be given sooner than this in view of the hypercoagulable state postpartum. The combined estrogen-progestin preparations, which contain 35 µg or less of estrogen and varying amounts of progestin, are associated with pregnancy rates of less than 0.5 per 100 woman-years. In addition, these low-estrogen compounds used in nonsmokers have fewer cardiovascular complications. Lactating women should be given progestin-only oral contraceptives (norethindrone .35 mg a day) as they do not suppress lactation and may enhance it.

The intramuscular injection of a long-acting progestin such as depot medroxyprogesterone acetate (Depo-Provera®), 150 mg given every 3 months, provides effective contraception (> 99% contraceptive efficacy) for the lactating woman without provoking maternal thromboembolism or decreasing milk yield. However, concerns relating to prolonged amenorrhea, the inconvenience of unpredictable and irregular bleeding, as well as reversible bone density reduction and lipid metabolism changes, limit the usefulness of this method.

Levonorgestrel implants placed after establishment of lactation (immediately postpartum or by 6 weeks) provide acceptable contraception with no affect on lactation or infant growth. They have gained little favor, probably due to irregular bleeding, high cost, and difficulty in insertion and removal.

Insertion of an intrauterine device (the copper-containing TCu 380 Ag® and Paraguard T380A®, the progesterone-releasing Progestasert®, or the levonorgestrel-releasing Mirena®) is highly effective in preventing pregnancy (< 2 to 3 pregnancies per 100 woman-years) and is not considered an abortifacient. Ideally, an IUD should be placed at the first postpartum visit; however, it may be placed as early as immediately postpartum. In this latter case, the incidence of expulsion is high. The main side effects include syncope from vagal response to insertion, pelvic infection (relative risk 1.7–9.3), uterine perforation (0–8 per 1000), and abnormal uterine bleeding. The risk of ectopic pregnancy is higher among women using Progestasert as compared to women not using contraception. The risk of uterine perforation during IUD insertion is higher in lactating women, probably because of the accelerated rate of uterine involution. However, the risk of expulsion is not increased. Uterine perforation is highest when insertion is performed in the first 1–8 weeks following delivery.

Discharge Examination & Instructions

Before the patient's hospital discharge, the breasts and abdomen should be examined. The degree of uterine involution and tenderness should be noted. The calves and thighs should be palpated to rule out thrombophlebitis. The characteristics of the lochia are important and should be observed. The episiotomy wound should be inspected to see whether it is healing satisfactorily. A blood sample should be obtained for hematocrit or hemoglobin determination. Unless the patient has an unusual pelvic complaint, there is little need to perform a vaginal examination. The obstetrician should be certain that the patient is voiding normally, has normal bowel function, and is physically able to assume her new responsibilities at home.

The patient will require some advice on what she is allowed to do when she arrives home. Hygiene is essentially the same as practiced in the hospital, with a premium on cleanliness. Upon discharge from the hospital, the patient should be instructed to rest for at least 2 hours during the day, and her usual household activities should be curtailed. Activities, exercise, and return to work will be individualized. Accepted disability following delivery is 6 weeks. Various forms of social support are critical for mothers, especially those employed outside the home: available, high-quality day care; parental leave for both mothers and fathers; and support provided by the workplace such as flexible hours, the opportunity to breastfeed, on-site day care, and care for sick children. The patient who has had frequent prenatal visits to her obstetrician may feel cut off from the doctor during the interval between discharge and the

first postpartum visit. She will feel reassured in this period if she receives thoughtful advice on what she is allowed to do and what she can expect when she arrives home. She should be instructed to take her temperature at home twice daily and to notify the physician or nurse in the event of fever, vaginal bleeding, or back pain. At the time of discharge, the patient should be informed that she will note persistent but decreasing amounts of vaginal lochia for about 3 weeks and possibly for a short period during the fourth or fifth week after delivery.

Postpartum Examination

At the postpartum visit—4–6 weeks after discharge from hospital—the patient's weight and blood pressure should be recorded. Most patients retain about 60% of any weight in excess of 11 kg (24 lb) that was gained during pregnancy. A suitable diet may be prescribed if the patient has not returned to her approximate prepregnant weight. If the patient was anemic upon discharge from the hospital or has been bleeding during the puerperium, a complete blood count should be determined. Persistence of uterine bleeding demands investigation and definitive treatment.

The breasts should be examined, and the adequacy of support, abnormalities of the nipples or lactation, and the presence of any masses should be noted. The patient should be instructed concerning self-examination of the breasts. A complete rectovaginal evaluation is required.

Nursing mothers may show a hypoestrogenic condition of the vaginal epithelium. Prescription of a vaginal estrogen cream to be applied at bedtime should relieve local dryness and coital discomfort without the side effects of systemic estrogen therapy. The cervix should be inspected and a Papanicolaou (Pap) smear obtained. Women whose prenatal smears are normal are still at risk for an abnormal Pap smear at their postpartum visit.

The episiotomy incision and repaired lacerations must be examined and the adequacy of pelvic and perineal support noted. Bimanual examination of the uterus and adnexa is indicated. At the time of the postpartum examination, most patients have some degree of retrodisplacement of the uterus, but this may soon correct itself.

Asymptomatic retroposition of the uterus is not regarded as an abnormal condition. If pain, abnormal bleeding, or other symptoms are present, a vaginal pessary may be inserted as a trial procedure to encourage anteversion of the fundus. However, pessary support for long periods of time is not recommended. In the absence of pelvic disease, uterine retrodisplacement rarely if ever requires surgical correction. If marked uterine descensus is noted or if the patient develops stress incontinence, symptomatic cystocele, or rectocele, surgical correction should be considered if childbearing has been completed. Hysterectomy or vaginal repair is best postponed for at least 3 months after delivery to allow maximal restoration of the pelvic supporting structures.

The patient may resume full activity or employment if her course to this point has been uneventful. Once again, the patient should be advised regarding family planning and contraceptive practices. The postnatal visit is an important opportunity to consider general disorders such as backache and depression and to discuss infant feeding and immunization. The rapport established between the obstetrician and the patient during the prenatal and postpartum periods provides a unique opportunity to establish a preventive health program in subsequent years.

■ LACTATION PHYSIOLOGY

PHYSIOLOGY

The mammary glands are modified exocrine glands that undergo dramatic anatomic and physiologic changes during pregnancy and in the immediate puerperium. Their role is to provide nourishment for the newborn and to transfer antibodies from mother to infant.

During the first half of pregnancy, proliferation of alveolar epithelial cells, formation of new ducts, and development of lobular architecture occur. Later in pregnancy, proliferation declines, and the epithelium differentiates for secretory activity. At the end of gestation, each breast will have gained approximately 400 g. Factors contributing to increase in mammary size include hypertrophy of blood vessels, myoepithelial cells, and connective tissue; deposition of fat; and retention of water and electrolytes. Blood flow is almost double that of the nonpregnant state.

The mammary gland has been called the mirror of the endocrine system, because lactation depends on a delicate balance of several hormones. An intact hypothalamic-pituitary axis is essential to the initiation and maintenance of lactation. Lactation can be divided into 3 stages: (1) mammogenesis, or mammary growth and development; (2) lactogenesis, or initiation of milk secretion; and (3) galactopoiesis, or maintenance of established milk secretion (Table 12–2). Estrogen is responsible for the growth of ductular tissue and alveolar budding, whereas progesterone is required for optimal maturation of the alveolar glands. Glandular stem cells undergo differentiation into secretory and myoepithelial cells under the influence of prolactin, growth hormone, insulin, cortisol, and an epithelial growth factor. Although alveolar secretory cells actively synthesize

Table 12–2. Multihormonal interaction in mammary growth and lactation.

Mammogenesis	Lactogenesis	Galactopoiesis
Estrogens	Prolactin	↓Gonadal hormones
Progesterone	↓Estrogens	Suckling (oxytocin, prolactin)
Prolactin	↓Progesterone	Growth hormone
Growth hormone	↓hPL(?)	Glucocorticoids
Glucocorticoids	Glucocorticoids	Insulin
Epithelial growth factor	Insulin	Thyroxine and parathyroid hormone

Arrows signify that lower than normal levels of the hormone are necessary for the effect to occur.

milk fat and proteins from midpregnancy onward, only small amounts are released into the lumen. However, lactation is possible if pregnancy is interrupted during the second trimester.

Prolactin is an necessary hormone for milk production, but lactogenesis also requires a low-estrogen environment. Although prolactin levels continue to rise as pregnancy advances, placental sex steroids block prolactin-induced secretory activity of the glandular epithelium. It appears that sex steroids and prolactin are synergistic in mammogenesis but antagonistic in galactopoiesis. Therefore, lactation is not initiated until plasma estrogens, progesterone, and human placental lactogen (hPL) fall after delivery. Progesterone inhibits the biosynthesis of lactose and α-lactalbumin; estrogens directly antagonize the lactogenic effect of prolactin on the mammary gland by inhibiting α-lactalbumin production. hPL may also exert a prolactin-antagonist effect through competitive binding to alveolar prolactin receptors.

The maintenance of established milk secretion requires periodic suckling and the actual emptying of ducts and alveoli. Growth hormone, cortisol, thyroxine, and insulin exert a permissive effect. Prolactin is required for galactopoiesis, but high basal levels are not mandatory, because prolactin concentrations in the nursing mother decline gradually during the late puerperium and approach that of the nonpregnant state. However, if a woman does not suckle her baby, her serum prolactin concentration will return to nonpregnant values within 2–3 weeks. If the mother suckles twins simultaneously, the prolactin response is about double that when one baby is fed at a time, illustrating an apparent synergism between the number of nipples stimulated and the frequency of suckling. The mechanism by which suckling stimulates prolactin release probably involves the inhibition of dopamine, which is thought to be the hypothalamic prolactin-inhibiting factor.

Nipple stimulation by suckling or other physical stimuli evokes a reflex release of oxytocin from the neurohypophysis. Because retrograde blood flow can be demonstrated within the pituitary stalk, oxytocin may reach the adenohypophysis in very high concentrations and affect pituitary release of prolactin independently of any effect on dopamine. The release of oxytocin is mediated by afferent fibers of the fourth to sixth intercostal nerves via the dorsal roots of the spinal cord to the midbrain.

The paraventricular and supraoptic neurons of the hypothalamus make up the final afferent pathway of the milk ejection reflex. The central nervous system can modulate the release of oxytocin by either stimulating or inhibiting the hypothalamus to increase or decrease prolactin inhibiting factor (dopamine) and thus the release of oxytocin from the posterior pituitary. Thus positive senses related to nursing, crying of an infant, positive attitudes in pregnancy and toward breastfeeding can improve milk yield and the ultimate success of breastfeeding. Likewise, the expectation of nursing is sufficient to release oxytocin prior to milk let-down but is not effective in releasing prolactin in the absence of suckling. Contrarily, negative stimuli, such as pain, stress, fear, anxiety, insecurity, or negative attitudes may inhibit the let-down reflex. Oxytocin levels may rise during orgasm, and sexual stimuli may trigger milk ejection.

SYNTHESIS OF HUMAN MILK

Prolactin ultimately promotes milk production by inducing the synthesis of mRNAs for the production of milk enzymes and milk proteins at the membrane of mammary epithelial cells (alveolar cells). Milk synthesis and secretion is then initiated via four major transcellular and paracellular pathways. The substrates for milk production are primarily derived from the maternal gut or produced in the maternal liver. The availability of these substrates is aided by a 20–40% increased blood flow to the mammary gland, gastrointestinal tract, and liver, as well as increased cardiac output during breastfeeding. The principal carbohydrate in human milk is lactose. Glucose metabolism is a key function in human milk production, because lactose is derived from glucose and galactose; the latter originates from glucose-6-phosphate. A specific protein, α-lactalbumin, catalyzes lactose synthesis. This rate-limiting enzyme is inhibited by gonadal hormones during pregnancy. Prolactin and insulin, which enhance the uptake of glucose by mammary cells, also stimulate the formation of triglycerides. Fat synthesis takes place in the endoplasmic reticulum.

Most proteins are synthesized de novo in the secretory cells from essential and nonessential plasma amino acids. The formation of milk protein and mammary enzymes is induced by prolactin and enhanced by cortisol and insulin.

Mature human milk contains 7% carbohydrate as lactose, 3–5% fat, 0.9% protein, and 0.2% mineral constituents expressed as ash. Its energy content is 60–75 kcal/dL. About 25% of the total nitrogen of human milk represents nonprotein compounds, eg, urea, uric acid, creatinine, and free amino acids. The principal proteins of human milk are casein, α-lactalbumin, lactoferrin, IgA, lysozyme, and albumin. Milk also contains a variety of enzymes that may contribute to the infant's digestion of breast milk, eg, amylase, catalase, peroxidase, lipase, xanthine oxidase, and alkaline and acid phosphatase. The fatty acid composition of human milk is rich in palmitic and oleic acids and varies somewhat with the diet. The major ions and mineral constituents of human milk are Na^+, K^+, Ca^{2+}, Mg^{2+}, Cl^-, phosphorus, sulfate, and citrate. Calcium concentrations vary from 25–35 mg/dL and phosphorus concentrations from 13–16 mg/dL. Iron, copper, zinc, and trace metal contents vary considerably. All the vitamins except vitamin K are found in human milk in nutritionally adequate amounts. The composition of breast milk is not greatly affected by race, age, parity, normal diet variations, moderate postpartum dieting, weight loss, or aerobic exercise. Volume and caloric density may be reduced in extreme scenarios, such as developing countries where starvation or daily caloric intake is less than 1600 kcal/d. In addition, milk composition does not differ between the two breasts unless one breast is infected. However, the volume and concentration of constituents varies during the day. The volume per feed increases in the late afternoon and evening. Nitrogen peaks in the late afternoon. Fat concentrations peak in the morning and are lowest at night. Lactose levels remain fairly constant.

Colostrum, the premilk secretion, is a yellowish alkaline secretion that may be present in the last months of pregnancy and for the first 2–3 days after delivery. It has a higher specific gravity (1.040–1.060); a higher protein, vitamin A, immunoglobulin, and sodium and chloride content; and a lower carbohydrate, potassium, and fat content than mature breast milk. Colostrum has a normal laxative action and is an ideal natural starter food.

Ions and water pass the membrane of the alveolar cell in both directions. Human milk differs from the milk of many other species by having a lower concentration of monovalent ions and a higher concentration of lactose. The aqueous phase of milk is isosmotic with plasma; thus, the higher the lactose, the lower the ion concentration. The ratio of potassium to sodium is 3:1

in both milk and mammary intracellular fluid. Because milk contains about 87% water and lactose is the major osmotically active solute, it follows that milk yield is largely determined by lactose production.

IMMUNOLOGIC SIGNIFICANCE OF HUMAN MILK

The neonate's secretory immune system and cellular response is immature. In particular, the IgM and IgA responses are poor and cellular immunity is impaired for several months. Maternal transfer of immunoglobulins through breast milk provides support for the infant's developing immune system and thereby enhances neonatal defense against infection. All classes of immunoglobulins are found in milk, but IgA constitutes 90% of immunoglobulins in human colostrum and milk. The output of immunoglobulins by the breast is maximal in the first week of life and declines thereafter as the production of milk-specific proteins increases. Lacteal antibodies against enteric bacteria and their antigenic products are largely of the IgA class. IgG and IgA lacteal antibodies provide short-term systemic and long-term enteric humoral immunity to the breastfed neonate. IgA antipoliomyelitis virus activity present in breastfed infants indicates that at least some transfer of milk antibodies into serum does occur. However, maternal lacteal antibodies are absorbed systemically by human infants for only a very short time after birth. Long-term protection against pathogenic enteric bacteria is provided by the adsorption of lacteal IgA to the intestinal mucosa. In addition to providing passive immunity, there is evidence that lacteal immunoglobulins can modulate the immunocompetence of the neonate, but the exact mechanisms have not been described. For instance, the secretion of IgA into the saliva of breastfed infants is enhanced in comparison with bottle-fed controls.

Breast milk is highly anti-infective, containing more than 4000 cells/mm³, the majority of which are leukocytes. The total cell count is even higher in colostrum. In human milk, the leukocytes are predominantly mononuclear cells and macrophages. Both T and B lymphocytes are present. During maternal infection, antigen-specific lymphocytes can migrate to the breast mucosa or produce immnoglobulins, both of which are key in the fight against infection. Fully functional immunoglobulins are present, primarily as IgA, IgG, and IgM. Polymeric secretory IgA (SIgA) is easily transported across the mucous membrane of the breast, blocking the mucosal receptors of infectious agents.

Elements in breast milk other than immunoglobulins and cells have prophylactic value against infections. The marked difference between the intestinal flora of breastfed and bottle-fed infants is due to a dialyzable ni-

trogen-containing carbohydrate (bifidus factor) that supports the growth of *Lactobacillus bifidus* in breastfed infants. The stool of bottle-fed infants is more alkaline and contains predominantly coliform organisms and *Bacteroides* spp. *L bifidus* inhibits the growth of *Shigella* spp, *Escherichia coli*, and yeast. Human milk also contains a nonspecific antimicrobial factor, lysozyme (a thermostable and acid-stable enzyme that cleaves the peptidoglycans of bacteria), and a "resistance factor," which protect the infant against staphylococcal infection. Lactoferrin, an iron chelator, exerts a strong bacteriostatic effect on staphylococci and *E coli* by depriving the organisms of iron. Both C3 and C4 components of complement and antitoxins for neutralizing *Vibrio cholerae* are found in human milk. Unsaturated vitamin B_{12}-binding protein in milk renders the vitamin unavailable for utilization by *E coli* and *Bacteroides*. Finally, interferon in milk may provide yet another nonspecific anti-infection factor.

Human milk may also have prophylactic value in childhood food allergies. During the neonatal period, permeability of the small intestine to macromolecules is increased. Secretory IgA in colostrum and breast milk reduces the absorption of foreign macromolecules until the endogenous IgA secretory capacity of the newborn intestinal lamina propria and lymph nodes develops at 2–3 months of age. Protein of cow's milk can be highly allergenic in the infant predisposed by heredity. The introduction of cow's milk–free formulas has considerably reduced the incidence of milk allergy. Thus, comparative studies on the incidence of allergy, bacterial and viral infections, severe diarrhea, necrotizing enterocolitis, tuberculosis, and neonatal meningitis in breastfed and bottle-fed infants support the concept that breast milk fulfills a protective function.

ADVANTAGES & DISADVANTAGES OF BREASTFEEDING

For the Mother

A. ADVANTAGES

Breastfeeding is convenient, economical, and emotionally satisfying to most women. It helps to contract the uterus and accelerates the process of uterine involution in the postpartum period, including decreased maternal blood loss. It promotes mother-infant bonding and self-confidence and improves maternal tolerance to stress through an oxytocin-associated antifight/fight response. Maternal gastrointestinal motility and absorption are enhanced. Ovulatory cycles are delayed with nonsupplemented breastfeeding. According to epidemiologic studies, breastfeeding may help to protect against premenopausal cancer and ovarian cancer.

B. DISADVANTAGES

Regular nursing restricts activities and may be perceived by some mothers as an inconvenience. Twins can be nursed successfully, but few women are prepared for the first weeks of almost continual feeding. Cesarean section may necessitate modifications of early breast-feeding routines. Difficulties such as nipple tenderness and mastitis may develop. Compared with nonlactating women, breastfeeding women have a significant decrease (mean, 6.5%) in bone mineral content at 6 months postpartum, but there is "catch-up" remineralization after weaning.

Breastfeeding by a hypoparathyroid mother is undesirable, because adequate calcium supplementation to replace losses in breast milk is difficult in these patients. Furthermore, large amounts of 25-hydroxyvitamin D_3 appear in the milk of mothers receiving therapy for hypoparathyroidism. There are few absolute contraindications to breastfeeding (see below).

Many women with breast implants breastfeed successfully, but reduction mammoplasty involving nipple autotransplantation severs the lactiferous ducts and precludes nursing. Several situations may arise in which a case-by-case assessment will be needed to determine the impact of breastfeeding: environmental exposures, hepatitis C, illicit drugs, metabolic disorders, use of pharmaceutical drugs, and tobacco and alcohol consumption.

For the Infant

A. ADVANTAGES

Breast milk is digestible, of ideal composition, available at the right temperature and the right time, and free of bacterial contamination. Infants of breastfed mothers have a decreased incidence of all of the following: diarrhea, lower respiratory tract infection, otitis media, pneumonia, urinary tract infections, necrotizing enterocolitis, invasive bacterial infection, and sudden infant death. Breastfed infants may also have a decreased risk of developing insulin-dependent diabetes, Crohn's disease, ulcerative colitis, lymphoma, and allergic diseases later in life. Breastfed infants are also less likely to become obese as neonates and adolescents. Suckling promotes infant-mother bonding. Cognitive development and intelligence may be improved.

B. DISADVANTAGES AND CONTRAINDICATIONS

Absolute contraindications to breastfeeding are use of street drugs or excess alcohol; human T-cell leukemia virus type 1; breast cancer; active herpes simplex infection of the breast; active pulmonary tuberculosis in the mother; galactosemia in the infant; maternal intake of cancer chemotherapeutic agents or certain other drugs.

Table 12–3 lists some of the medications that are contraindicated during breast feeding. Additional medications are not recommended during breast feeding. Therefore, specific precautions for individual medications should be reviewed when prescribing to lactating women. Human immunodeficiency virus (HIV) infection in the U.S. is also a contraindication to breastfeeding. Breastfeeding has been recognized as a mode of HIV transmission. Breastfeeding might pose an additional risk (about 15%) for an infant above that already

Table 12–3. Medications contraindicated during breastfeeding.

Medication	Reason
Bromocriptine	Suppresses lactation; may be hazardous to the mother
Cocaine	Cocaine intoxication
Cyclophosphamide	Possible immune suppression; unknown effect on growth or association with carcinogenesis; neutropenia
Cyclosporine	Possible immune suppression; unknown effect on growth or association with carcinogenesis
Doxorubicin[1]	Possible immune suppression; unknown effect on growth or association with carcinogenesis
Ergotamine	Vomiting, diarrhea, convulsions (at doses used in migraine medications)
Lithium	One third to one half of therapeutic blood concentration in infants
Methotrexate	Possible immune suppression; unknown effect on growth or association with carcinogenesis; neutropenia
Phencyclidine	Potent hallucinogen
Phenindione	Anticoagulant; increased prothrombin and partial thromboplastin time in one infant; not used in United States
Radioactive iodine and other radiolabeled elements	Contraindications to breastfeeding for various periods

[1]Medication is concentrated in human milk.
American Academy of Pediatrics, American College of Obstetricians and Gynecologists. Guidelines for perinatal care, 4th ed. Elk Grove Village, Illinois: AAP; Washington, DC: ACOG, 1997.

present at birth because the mother had HIV. The risk of HIV transmission through breast milk is substantially higher among women who become infected during the postpartum lactation period. Most mothers in developed countries who know of their seropositivity choose not to breast feed; in underdeveloped countries where lactation is critical to infant survival, HIV-infected mothers may choose to breast feed their infants.

Breastfeeding does not protect against the deleterious effects of congenital hypothyroidism. The milk of a nursing mother with cystic fibrosis is high in sodium and places the infant at risk for hypernatremia. A woman with clinically infectious varicella should be isolated from the infant and neither breast- or bottle-feed. Once the infant has received varicella zoster immune globulin and there are no skin lesions on the mother's breast, she may provide expressed milk for her infant. A small number of otherwise healthy breastfed infants develop unconjugated hyperbilirubinemia (sometimes exceeding 20 mg/dL) during the first few weeks of life due to the higher-than-normal glucuronyl transferase inhibitory activity of the breast milk. The inhibitor may be a pregnanediol, although increased milk lipase activity and free fatty acids are likely the critical factors.

Breastfeeding is not usually possible for weak, ill, or very premature infants or for infants with cleft palate, choanal atresia, or phenylketonuria. It is common practice in many nurseries to feed premature infants human milk collected fresh from their mothers or processed from donors. The effects of processing and storage on the persistence of viral agents are not well studied. Cytomegalovirus transmission through breast milk has been documented and may pose a significant hazard for preterm infants. It is recommended that seronegative preterm infants receive milk from seronegative donors only. Because maternal antibodies are present in breast milk, an otherwise healthy term infant may do better if breastfed.

PRINCIPLES & TECHNIQUES OF BREASTFEEDING

In the absence of anatomic or medical complications, the timing of the first feeding and the frequency and duration of subsequent feedings largely determine the outcome of breastfeeding. Infants and mothers who are able to initiate breastfeeding within 1–2 hours of delivery are more successful than those whose initial interactions are delayed for several hours. Lactation is established most successfully if the baby remains with the mother and she can feed on demand for adequate intervals throughout the first 24-hour period. The initial feeding should last 5 minutes at each breast in order to condition the let-down reflex. At first, the frequency of feedings may be very irregular (8–10 times a day), but after 1–2 weeks a fairly regular 4- to 6-hour pattern will emerge.

When the milk "comes in" abruptly on the third or fourth postpartum day, there is an initial period of discomfort caused by vascular engorgement and edema of the breasts. The baby does not nurse so much by developing intermittent negative pressure as by a rhythmic grasping of the areola; the infant "works" the milk into its mouth. Little force is required in nursing, because the breast reservoirs can be emptied and refilled without suction. Nursing mothers notice a sensation of drawing and tightening within the breast at the beginning of suckling after the initial breast engorgement disappears. They are thus conscious of the milk ejection reflex, which may even cause milk to spurt or run out.

Some women expend a great deal of emotion on the subject of breastfeeding, and a few are almost overwhelmed by fear of being unable to care for their babies in this way. If attendants are sympathetic and patient, however, a woman who wants to nurse usually can do so. Attendants must be certain that the baby "latches" on (actually over) the nipple and the areola so as to feed properly without causing pain for the mother (Fig 12–8).

The baby should nurse at both breasts at each feeding, because overfilling of the breasts is the main deterrent to the maintenance of milk secretion. Nursing at only one breast at each feeding inhibits the reflex that is provoked simultaneously in both breasts. Thus, nursing at alternate breasts from one feeding to the next may increase discomfort due to engorgement and reduce milk output. It is helpful for the mother to be taught to empty the breasts after each feeding; a sleepy baby may not have accomplished this. The use of supplementary formula or other food during the first 6–8 weeks of breastfeeding can interfere with lactation and should be avoided except when absolutely necessary. The introduction of an artificial nipple, which requires a different sucking mechanism, will weaken the sucking reflex required for breastfeeding. Some groups such as the La Leche League recommend that other fluids be given by spoon or dropper rather than by bottle.

In preparing to nurse, the mother should (1) wash her hands with soap and water, (2) clean her nipples and breasts with water, and (3) assume a comfortable position, preferably in a rocking or upright chair with the infant and mother chest-to-chest. If the mother is unable to sit up to nurse her baby because of painful perineal sutures, she may feel more comfortable lying on her side. An alternative position is the football hold. A woman with large pendulous breasts may find it difficult to manage both the breasts and the baby. If the baby lies on a pillow, the mother will have both hands free to guide the nipple.

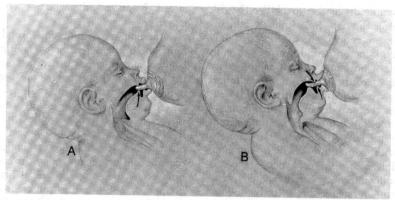

Figure 12–8. Mechanism of suckling in the neonate. **A.** Tongue moves forward to draw nipple in as glottis still permits breathing. **B.** Tongue moves along nipple, pressing it against the palate with the glottis closed. Ductules under the areola are compressed, and milk flow begins. The cheeks fill the mouth and provide negative pressure.

Each baby nurses differently; however, the following procedure is generally successful:

(1) Allow the normal newborn to nurse at each breast on demand or approximately every 3–4 hours, for 5 minutes per breast per feeding the first day. Over the next few days, gradually increase feeding time to initiate the let-down reflex, but do not exceed 10–15 minutes per breast. Suckling for longer than 15 minutes may cause maceration and cracking of the nipples and thus lead to mastitis.

(2) Stimulating the cheek or lateral angle of the baby's mouth should precipitate a reflex turn to the nipple and opening of the mouth. The infant is brought firmly to the breast and the nipple and areola are placed into the mouth as far as the nipple-areola line. Slight negative pressure holds the teat in place and milk is obtained with a peristaltic motion of the tongue. Compressing the periareolar area and expressing a small amount of colostrum or milk for the baby to taste may stimulate the baby to nurse.

(3) Try to keep the baby awake by moving or patting, but do not snap its feet, work its jaw, push its head, or press its cheeks.

(4) Before removing the infant from the breast, gently open its mouth by lifting the outer border of the upper lip to break the suction.

After nursing, gently wipe the nipples with water and dry them.

MILK YIELD

The prodigious energy requirements for lactation are met by mobilization of elements from maternal tissues and from dietary intake. Physiologic fat stores laid down during pregnancy are mobilized during lactation, and the return to prepregnant weight and figure is promoted. A variety of studies suggest that a lactating woman should increase her normal daily food intake by 600 kcal/d but intakes of 2000–2300 calories are sufficient for lactating women. The recommended daily dietary increases for lactation are 20 g of protein; a 20% increase in all vitamins and minerals except folic acid, which should be increased by 50%; and a 33% increase in calcium, phosphorus, and magnesium. There is no evidence that increasing fluid intake will increase milk volume. Fluid restriction also has little effect, because urine output will diminish in preference to milk output.

With nursing, average milk production on the second postpartum day is about 120 mL. The amount increases to about 180 mL on the third postpartum day and to as much as 240 mL on the fourth day. In time, milk production reaches about 300 mL/d.

A good rule of thumb for the calculation of milk production for a given day in the week after delivery is to multiply the number of the postpartum day by 60. This gives the approximate number of milliliters of milk secreted in that 24-hour period.

If all goes well, sustained production of milk will be achieved by most patients after 10–14 days. A yield of 120–180 mL per feeding is common by the end of the second week. When free secretion has been established, marked increases are possible; a wet nurse can often suckle 3 babies successfully for weeks.

Early diminution of milk production often is due to failure to empty the breasts because of weak efforts by the baby or ineffectual nursing procedures; emotional problems, such as aversion to nursing; or medical complications, such as mastitis, debilitating systemic disease, or Sheehan's syndrome. Late diminution of milk production results from too generous complementary feedings of formula, emotional or other illness, and pregnancy.

Adequate rest is essential for successful lactation. Sometimes it is difficult to ensure an adequate milk yield if the mother is working outside the home. If it is not possible to rearrange the nursing schedule to fit the work schedule or vice versa, it may be necessary to empty the breasts manually or by pump. Milk output can be estimated by weighing the infant before and after feeding. If there has been a bowel movement during feeding, the baby should be weighed before the diaper is changed.

It may be necessary to substitute bottle-feeding for breastfeeding if the mother's supply continues to be inadequate (less than 50% of the infant's needs) after 3 weeks of effort, if nipple or breast lesions are severe enough to prevent pumping, or if the mother is either pregnant or severely (physically or mentally) ill. Nourishment from the inadequately lactating breast can be augmented with the Lact-Aide Nursing Trainer, a device that provides a supplemental source of milk via a plastic capillary tube placed beside the breast and suckled simultaneously with the nipple. Disposable plastic bags serve as reservoirs, and the supplemental milk is warmed by hanging the bag next to the mother. The Lact-Aide supplementer has also been used to help nurse premature infants and to reestablish lactation after untimely weaning due to illness. The long-term success of breastfeeding is increased by a structured home support system of postnatal visits by allied health personnel or experienced volunteers.

DISORDERS OF LACTATION

Painful Nipples

Tenderness of the nipples, a common symptom during the first days of breastfeeding, generally begins when the baby starts to suck. As soon as milk begins to flow, nipple sensitivity usually subsides. If maternal tissues are unusually tender, dry heat may help between feedings. Nipple shields should be used only as a last resort, since they interfere with normal sucking. Glass or plastic shields with rubber nursing nipples are preferable to shields made entirely of rubber.

Nipple fissures cause severe pain and prevent normal let-down of milk. Local infection around the fissure can lead to mastitis. The application of vitamin A and D ointment or hydrous lanolin, which do not have to be removed, is often effective. To speed healing, the following steps are recommended. Apply dry heat for 20 minutes 4 times a day with a 60-watt bulb held 18 inches away from the nipple. Conduct prefeeding manual expression. Begin nursing on the side opposite the fissure with the other breast exposed to air to allow the initial let-down to occur atraumatically. Apply expressed breast milk to nipples and let it dry in between feedings. If necessary, use a nipple shield while nursing, and take ibuprofen or acetaminophen with or without codeine just after nursing. On rare occasions, it may be necessary to stop nursing temporarily on the affected side and to empty the breast either manually or by gentle pumping.

A cause of chronic severe sore nipples without remarkable physical findings is candidal infection. Prompt relief is provided by topical nystatin cream. Thrush or candidal diaper rash or maternal candidal vaginitis must be treated as well.

Engorgement

Engorgement of the breasts occurs in the first week postpartum and is due to vascular congestion and accumulation of milk. Vascularity and swelling increase on the second day after delivery; the areola or breast may become engorged. Prepartum breast massage and around-the-clock demand feedings help to prevent engorgement in these patients. When the areola is engorged, the nipple is occluded and proper grasping of the areola by the infant is not possible. With moderately severe engorgement, the breasts become firm and warm, and the lobules may be palpable as tender, irregular masses. Considerable discomfort and often a slight fever can be expected.

Mild cases may be relieved by acetaminophen or other analgesics, cool compresses, and partial expression of the milk before nursing. In severe cases, have the patient empty the breasts manually or with an electric pump.

Mastitis

Mastitis occurs most frequently in primiparous nursing patients and is usually caused by coagulase-positive *Staphylococcus aureus*. High fever should never be ascribed to simple breast engorgement alone. Inflammation of the breast seldom begins before the fifth day postpartum. Most frequently, symptoms of a painful erythematous lobule in an outer quadrant of the breast are noted during the second or third week of the puerperium. Inflammation may occur with weaning when the flow of milk is disrupted, or the nursing mother may acquire the infection during her hospital stay and then transmit it to the infant. The demonstration of antibody-coated bacteria in the milk indicates the presence of infectious mastitis. Many infants harbor an infection and, in turn, infect the mother's breast during nursing. Neonatal streptococcal infection should be suspected if mastitis is recurrent or bilateral.

Infection may be limited to the subareolar region but more frequently involves an obstructed lactiferous duct and the surrounding breast parenchyma. If cellulitis is not properly treated, a breast abscess may develop. When only mastitis is present, it is best to prevent milk stasis by continuing breastfeeding or by using a breast pump. Apply local heat, provide a well-fitted brassiere, and institute appropriate antibiotic treatment. Cephalosporins, methicillin sodium, and dicloxacillin sodium are the antibiotics of choice to combat penicillinase-producing bacteria.

Pitting edema over the inflamed area and some degree of fluctuation are evidence of abscess formation. It is necessary to incise and open loculated areas and provide wide drainage. Unlike with mastitis, continuing breastfeeding is not recommended in the presence of a breast abscess.

Miscellaneous Complications

A galactocele, or milk-retention cyst, is caused by the blockage of a milk duct. It will usually resolve with warm compresses and continuation of breastfeeding. Sometimes the infant will reject one or both breasts. Strong foods such as beans, cabbage, turnips, broccoli, onions, garlic, or rhubarb may cause aversion to milk or neonatal colic. A common cause of nursing problems is maternal fatigue.

INHIBITION & SUPPRESSION OF LACTATION

Despite a recent upsurge in breastfeeding in Western countries, there are many women who will not or cannot breastfeed and others who fail in the attempt. Lactation inhibition is desirable in the event of fetal or neonatal death as well.

The oldest and simplest method of suppressing lactation is to stop nursing, to avoid nipple stimulation, to refrain from expressing or pumping the milk, and to wear a supportive bra. Analgesics are also helpful. Patients will complain of breast engorgement (45%), pain (45%), and leaking breasts (55%). Although the breasts will become considerably engorged and the patient may experience discomfort, the collection of milk in the duct system will suppress its production, and resorption will occur. After approximately 2–3 days, engorgement will begin to recede, and the patient will be comfortable again. Medical suppression of lactation with estrogens or bromocriptine is no longer recommended.

REFERENCES

Anatomy & Physiology of the Puerperium

Allolio B, Hoffmann J, Linton EA et al: Diurnal salivary cortisol patterns during pregnancy and after delivery: Relationship to plasma corticotrophin-releasing-hormone. Clin Endocrinol 1990;33:279.

Bacigalupo G et al: Quantitative relationships between pain intensities during labor and beta-endorphin and cortisol concentrations in plasma: Decline of the hormone concentrations in the early postpartum period. J Perinat Med 1990;18:289.

Battin DA et al: Effect of suckling on serum prolactin, luteinizing hormone, follicle-stimulating hormone, and estradiol during prolonged lactation. Obstet Gynecol 1985;65:785.

Bremme K et al: Enhanced thrombin generation and fibrinolytic activity in normal pregnancy and the puerperium. Obstet Gynecol 1992;80:132.

Brewer MM, Bates RM, Vannoy LP: Postpartum changes in maternal weight and body fat deposits in lactating versus nonlactating women. Am J Clin Nutr 1989;49:259.

Clapp JF III, Capeless E: Cardiovascular function before, during, and after the first and subsequent pregnancies. Am J Cardiol 1997;80:1469.

Coppleson M, Reid BL: A colposcopic study of the cervix during pregnancy and the puerperium. J Obstet Gynaecol Br Commonw 1966;73:575.

Crowell DT: Weight change in the postpartum period: a review of the literature. J Nurse Midwifery 1995;40:418.

Dawood MY et al: Oxytocin release and plasma anterior pituitary and gonadal hormones in women during lactation. J Clin Endocrinol Metab 1981;52:678.

DeAlvarez RR: Renal glomerulotubular mechanisms during normal pregnancy. Am J Obstet Gynecol 1958;75:931.

De Leo V et al: Control of growth hormone secretion during the postpartum period. Gynecol Obstet Invest 1992;33:31.

Elster AD et al: Size and shape of the pituitary gland during pregnancy and postpartum: Measurement with MR imaging. Radiology 1991;181:531.

Gerbasi FR et al: Changes in hemostasis activity during delivery and the immediate postpartum period. Am J Obstet Gynecol 1990;162:1158.

Gray RH et al: Risk of ovulation during lactation. Lancet 1990;335:25.

Hatjis CG et al: Atrial natriuretic factor concentrations during pregnancy and in the postpartum period. Am J Perinatol 1992;9:275.

Hornnes PJ, Kuhl C: Plasma insulin and glucagon responses to isoglycemic stimulation in normal pregnancy and postpartum. Obstet Gynecol 1980;55:425.

Kerr-Wilson RHJ et al: Effect of labor on the postpartum bladder. Obstet Gynecol 1984;64:115.

Kremer JAM et al: Pulsatile secretion of luteinizing hormone and prolactin in lactating and nonlactating women and the response to naltrexone. J Clin Endocrinol Metab 1991;72:294.

Lavery JP, Shaw LA: Sonography of the puerperal uterus. J Ultrasound 1989;8:481.

Lewis PR et al: The resumption of ovulation and menstruation in a well-nourished population of women breastfeeding for an extended period of time. Fertil Steril 1991;55:529.

Liu JH, Park KH: Gonadotropin and prolactin secretion increases during sleep during the puerperium in nonlactating women. J Clin Endocrinol Metab 1988;66:839.

Moore P et al: Insulin binding in human pregnancy: Comparisons to the postpartum, luteal and follicular states. J Clin Endocrinol Metab 1981;52:937.

Oats JN, Beisher NA: The persistence of abnormal glucose tolerance after delivery. Obstet Gynecol 1990;75:397.

Oppenheimer LW et al: The duration of lochia. Br J Obstet Gynecol 1986;93:754.

Robson SC et al: Hemodynamic changes during the puerperium: A Doppler and M-mode echocardiographic study. Br J Obstet Gynecol 1987;94:1028.

Scholl TO et al: Gestational weight gain, pregnancy outcome, and postpartum weight retention. Obstet Gynecol 1995;86:423.

Sheehan KL, Yen SSC: Activation of pituitary gonadotropic function by an agonist of luteinizing hormone-releasing factor in the puerperium. Am J Obstet Gynecol 1979;135:755.

Smith R, Thomson M: Neuroendocrinology of the hypothalamo-pituitary-adrenal axis in pregnancy and the puerperium. Ballieres Clin Endocrinol Metab 1991;5:167.

South-Paul JE, Rajagopal KR, Tenholder MF: Exercise responses prior to pregnancy and in the postpartum state. Med Sci Sports Exerc 1992;24:410.

Tay CCK, Glasier AF, McNeilly AS: The 24 h pattern of pulsatile luteinizing hormone, follicle stimulating hormone and prolactin release during the first 8 weeks of lactational amenorrhoea in breastfeeding women. Hum Reprod 1992;7:951.

Ueland K: Maternal cardiovascular dynamics. VIII. Intrapartum blood volume changes. Am J Obstet Gynecol 1976;126:671.

Visness CM, Kennedy KI, Ramos R: The duration and character of postpartum bleeding among breast-feeding women. Obstet Gynecol 1997;89:159.

Walters BNJ et al: Blood pressure in the puerperium. Clin Sci 1986;71:589.

Wilms AB et al: Anatomic changes in the pelvis after an uncomplicated vaginal delivery: evaluation with serial MRI imaging. Radiology 1995;195:91.

Ylikorkala O, Viinikka L: Thromboxane A$_2$ in pregnancy and puerperium. Br Med J 1980;281:1601.

Conduct of the Puerperium

American College of Obstetricians and Gynecologists: Exercise during pregnancy and the postpartum period. ACOG Committee Opinion No. 267, January 2002.

American College of Obstetricians and Gynecologists: Prevention of RhD alloimmunization. ACOG Practice Bulletin No. 4, 1999.

Aranda C et al: Laparoscopic sterilization immediately after term delivery: preliminary report. J Reprod Med 1963;14:171.

Bart SW et al: Fetal risk associated with rubella vaccine: an update. Rev Infect Dis 1985;7:S95.

Baskett TF, Parsons ML, Peddle LJ: The experience and effectiveness of the Nova Scotia Rh Program, 1964–84. Can Med Assoc J 1986;134:1259.

Bledin KD, Brice B: Psychological conditions in pregnancy and the puerperium and their relevance to postpartum sterilization: a review. Bull WHO 1983;61:533.

Black NA et al: Postpartum rubella immunization: A controlled trial of two vaccines. Lancet 1983;2:990.

Bowman JM: Controversies in Rh prophylaxis. Who needs Rh immune globulin and when should it be used? Am J Obstet Gynecol 1985;151:289.

Britton JR, Britton HL, Gronwaldt V: Early perinatal hospital discharge and parenting during infancy. Pediatrics 1999; 104:1070.

Brumfield CG: Early postpartum discharge. Clin Obstet Gynecol 1998;41:611.

Burrows WR, Gingo AJ Jr., Rose SM: Safety and efficacy of early postoperative solid food consumption after cesarean section. J Reprod Med 1995;40:463.

Chaliha C et al: Antenatal prediction of postpartum fecal incontinence. Obstet Gynecol 1999;94:689.

Chi IC, Gates D, Thapa S: Performing tubal sterilizations during women's postpartum hospitalization: A review of the United States and international experiences. Obstet Gynecol Surv 1992;47:71.

Darney PD: Hormonal implants: contraception for a new century. Am J Obstet Gynecol 1994;170:1536.

Freda VJ et al: Prevention of Rh hemolytic disease: Ten years' clinical experience with Rh-immunoglobulin. N Engl J Med 1975;292:1014.

Glass M, Rosenthal AH: Cervical changes in pregnancy, labor and puerperium. Am J Obstet Gynecol 1950;60:353.

Glazener CMA: Sexual function after childbirth: women's experiences, persistent morbidity and lack of professional recognition. Br J Obstet Gynaecol 1997;104:330.

Goetsch MF : Postpartum dyspareunia. An unexplored problem. J Reprod Med 1999;44:963.

Hale RW, Milne L: The elite athlete and exercise in pregnancy. Semin Perinatol 1996;20:277.

Hebert PR et al: Serious maternal morbidity after childbirth: prolonged hospital stays and readmissions. Obstet Gynecol 1999;94:942.

Hillis SD et al: Poststerilization regret: findings from the United States Collaborative Review of Sterilization. Obstet Gynecol 1999;93:889.

Hume AL, Hijab JC: Oral contraceptives in the immediate postpartum period. J Fam Pract 1991;32:423.

Kazzi A et al: Effectiveness of the lactational amenorrhea method in Pakistan. Fertil Steril 1995;64:717.

Kennedy K, Visness C: Contraceptive efficacy of lactational amenorrhea. Lancet 1992;339:227.

Kennedy KI, Sort RV, Tully MR: Premature introduction of progestin-only contraceptive methods during lactation. Contraception 1997;55:347.

Koetsawang S: The effects of contraceptive methods on the quality and quantity of breast milk. Int J Gynaecol Obstet 1987; 25(Suppl.):115.

Liu LL et al: The safety of early newborn discharge: the Washington state experience. JAMA 1997;278:293.

Koltyn KF, Schultes SS: Psychological effects of an aerobic exercise session and a rest session following pregnancy. J Sports Med Phys Fitness 1997;37:287.

Mandl KD et al: Maternal and infant health: effects of moderate reductions in postpartum length of stay. Arch Pediatr Adolesc Med 1997;151:915.

McCrory MA et al: Randomized trial of the short-term effects of dieting compared with dieting plus aerobic exercise on lactation performance. Am J Clin Nutr 1999;69:959.

O'Hanley K, Huber DH: Postpartum IUDs: Keys for success. Contraception 1992;45:351.

Perez A, Labbok M, Queenan J: Clinical study of the lactational amenorrhea method for family planning. Lancet 1992; 339:968.

Ryding E-L: Sexuality during and after pregnancy. Acta Obstet Gynecol Scand 1984;63:679.

Schanler RJ, Hurst NM, Lau C: The use of human milk and breastfeeding in premature infants. Clin Perinatol 1999; 26:379.

Soriano D, Dulitzki M, Keidar N: Early oral feeding after cesarean delivery. Obstet Gynecol 1996;87:1006.

Stanford JB, Thurnau PB, Lemaire JC: Physician's knowledge and practices regarding natural family planning. Obstet Gynecol 1999;94:672.

Vessey M et al: Tubal sterilization: findings in a large prospective study. Br J Obstet Gynaecol 1983;90:203.

Vessey M, Wiggins P: Use-effectiveness of the diaphragm in a selected family planning clinic population in the United Kingdom. Contraception 1974;9:15.

Windle ML, Booker LA, Rayburn WF: Postpartum pain after vaginal delivery: a review of comparative analgesic trials. J Reprod Med 1989;34:891.

Lactation

American Academy of Pediatrics Committee on Pediatric AIDS: Human milk, breastfeeding, and transmission of human immunodeficiency virus in the United States (RE9542). Pediatrics 1995;96:977.

American Academy of Pediatrics Work Group on Breastfeeding: Breastfeeding and the use of human milk. Pediatrics 1997;100:1035.

American College of Obstetricians and Gynecologists: Breastfeeding: Maternal and infant aspects. ACOG Educational Bulletin No. 258, 2000.

Briggs GG, Freeman RK, Yaffe SJ (editors): *Drugs in Pregnancy and Lactation*, 6th ed. Lippincott Williams & Wilkins, 2002.

Dunn DT et al: Risk of human immunodeficiency virus type 1 transmission through breast-feeding. Lancet 1992;340:585.

Dusdieker LB et al: Effect of supplemental fluids on human milk production. J Pediatr 1985;106:207.

Fowler MG, Bertolli J, Nieburg P: When is breast-feeding not best? The dilemma facing HIV-infected women in resource-poor settings. JAMA 1999;282:781.

Garofalo RP, Goldman AS: Expression of functional immunomodulatory and anti-inflammatory factors in human milk. Clin Perinatol 1999;26:361.

Hayslip CC et al: The effects of lactation on bone mineral content in healthy postpartum women. Obstet Gynecol 1989;73:588.

Labbok MH: Health sequela of breastfeeding for the mother. Clin Perinatol 1999;26:491.

Lawrence RA: A review of the medical benefits and contraindications to breastfeeding in the United States. Maternal and Child Health Technical Information Bulletin. National Center for Education in Maternal and Child Health, 1997, p. 3.

Losh M et al: Impact of attitudes on maternal decisions regarding infant feeding. J Pediatr 1996;126:507.

Neville MC: Physiology of lactation. Clin Perinatol 1999;26:251.

Specker B, Tsang R, Ho M: Changes in calcium homeostasis over the first year postpartum: Effect of lactation and weaning. Obstet Gynecol 1991;78:56.

Van de Perre P et al: Postnatal transmission of HIV type 1 from mother to infant. N Engl J Med 1991;325:593.

West CP: The acceptability of a progestin-only contraceptive during breast-feeding. Contraception 1983;27:563.

Ziegler JB: Breast feeding and HIV. Lancet 1993;342:1437.

Zinaman M et al: Acute prolactin and oxytocin response and milk yield to infant suckling and artificial methods of expression in lactating women. Pediatrics 1992;89:437.

SECTION III
Pregnancy at Risk

Methods of Assessment for Pregnancy at Risk

13

Jonathan Gillen-Goldstein, MD, Michael J. Paidas, MD, Robert J. Sokol, MD, Theodore B. Jones, MD, & Martin L. Pernoll, MD

ESSENTIALS OF DIAGNOSIS

- A careful history to reveal specific risk factors.
- A maternal physical examination organized to identify or exclude risk factors.
- Routine maternal laboratory screening for common disorders.
- Special maternal laboratory evaluations for disorders suggested by any evaluative process.
- Comprehensive fetal assessment by an assortment of techniques over the entire course of the pregnancy.

General Considerations

High-risk pregnancy is broadly defined as one in which the mother, fetus, or newborn is at or may possibly be at increased risk of morbidity or mortality before, during, or after delivery. Many factors are involved, including maternal health, obstetric history, and fetal disease. Obstetric disorders can impose a higher toll on the mother and/or fetus, such as abruptio placentae, prematurity, preeclampsia-eclampsia, and growth restriction, among others (Table 13–1). The purpose of this chapter is to detail essential aspects of the diagnostic modalities available for determination of pregnancies at risk.

The incidence of high-risk pregnancy varies according to the criteria used to define it. A great many factors are involved, and the effects of any given factor differ from patient to patient. Frequently, risk factors are identified only in hindsight and benefit only future pregnancies. Leading causes of maternal death include thromboembolic disease, hypertensive disease, hemorrhage, infection, and ectopic pregnancy. Perinatal death rates can be calculated in a variety of ways, using criteria based on fetal weight, gestational age, or both. Neonatal mortality, which includes infants weighing > 500 grams and up to 28 days of life, have fallen steadily in recent years. However, advancements in neonatal care of severely preterm infants in the 24–26 week range adds to the total of current neonatal mortality statistics, because in the past these infants would never have survived.

In assessing pregnancies to determine risk, several key concepts may offer tremendous insight. Human reproduction is a complex social, biochemical, and physiological process that is not as successful as once thought. Probably less than half of all conceptions are lost before pregnancy is even recognized. Another 15–40% are lost in the first trimester. Of this latter group, more than half have abnormal karyotypes and defy current methodologies for prevention of loss. However, many other causes of reproductive loss are amenable to diagnosis and treatment. In this chapter we will discuss the indications and justifications for antepartum care, intrapartum management, and postpartum follow-up.

PRECONCEPTIONAL EVALUATION

Preconceptional evaluation and counseling of women of reproductive age has gained increasing acceptance as an important component of women's health. Care

Table 13–1. Risk factors related to specific pregnancy problems.

Preterm labor
  Age below 16 or over 35 years
  Low socioeconomic status
  Maternal weight below 50 kg (110 lb)
  Poor nutrition
  Previous preterm birth
  Incomplete cervix
  Uterine anomalies
  Smoking
  Drug addiction and alcohol abuse
  Pyelonephritis, pneumonia
  Multiple gestation
  Anemia
  Abnormal fetal presentation
  Preterm rupture of membranes
  Placental abnormalities
  Infection
Polyhydramnios
  Diabetes mellitus
  Multiple gestation
  Fetal congenital abnormalities
  Isoimmunization (Rh or ABO)
  Nonimmune hydrops
  Abnormal fetal presentation
Intrauterine growth restriction (IUGR)
  Multiple gestation
  Poor nutrition
  Maternal cyanotic heart disease
  Chronic hypertension
  Pregnancy-induced hypertension
  Recurrent antepartum hemorrhage
  Smoking
  Maternal diabetes with vasculopathy
  Fetal infections
  Fetal cardiovascular anomalies
  Drug addiction and alcohol abuse
  Fetal congenital anomalies
  Hemoglobinopathies
Oligohydramnios
  Renal agenesis (Potter's syndrome)
  Prolonged rupture of membranes
  Intrauterine growth restriction
  Intrauterine fetal demise
Postterm pregnancy
  Anencephaly
  Placental sulfatase deficiency
  Perinatal hypoxia, acidosis
  Placental insufficiency
Chromosomal abnormalities
  Maternal age 35 years or more at delivery
  Balanced translocation (maternal and paternal)

given in family planning and gynecology centers provides an opportunity that is rarely seen in the prenatal visits. This valuable opportunity to maximize maternal and fetal health benefits before conception should be taken advantage of. Issues of potential consequence to a pregnancy such as medical problems, lifestyle, or genetic issues should be investigated and interventions devised prior to pregnancy.

■ MATERNAL ASSESSMENT FOR POTENTIAL FETAL OR PERINATAL RISK

INITIAL SCREENING

History

A. MATERNAL AGE

Extremes of maternal age increase risks of maternal or fetal morbidity and mortality. Adolescents are at increased risk for preeclampsia-eclampsia, intrauterine growth restriction (IUGR), and maternal malnutrition.

Women 35 years of age or older at the time of delivery are at higher risk of pregnancy-induced hypertension, diabetes, and obesity as well as other medical conditions. Chromosomal abnormalities are also more common in infants born to older women, as will be discussed in detail later. An increased risk of cesarean section, preeclampsia, and placenta previa is noted in women with advanced maternal age.

B. MODALITY OF CONCEPTION

It is important to differentiate spontaneous pregnancy from that resulting from assisted reproductive technologies (ART). Use of ART increases the risks of multiple gestation, pregnancy-induced hypertension, and preterm delivery.

C. PAST MEDICAL HISTORY

Specific disease states may adversely affect the outcome of pregnancy for the mother or infant. Pregnancy itself may aggravate certain medical disorders and alleviate others. Table 13–2 lists the most important disorders that may complicate pregnancy.

D. FAMILY HISTORY

A detailed family history is helpful in determining any increased risk of heritable disease states (eg, Tay-Sachs, cystic fibrosis, sickle cell disease) which may affect the mother or fetus during the pregnancy or the fetus following delivery.

Table 13–2. Some diseases and disorders complicating pregnancy.

Chronic hypertension
Renal disease
Diabetes mellitus
Heart disease
Previous endocrine ablation (eg, thyroidectomy)
Maternal cancer
Sickle cell trait and disease
Substance use or abuse
Pulmonary disease (eg, tuberculosis, sarcoidosis, asthma)
Thyroid disorders
Gastrointestinal and liver disease
Epilepsy
Blood disorders (eg, anemia, coagulopathy)
Others, including previous pelvic injury or disease producing pelvic deformity, connective tissue disorders, mental retardation, psychiatric disease

---

E. ETHNIC BACKGROUND

Population screening for certain inheritable genetic diseases is not cost effective due to the relative rarity of the gene in the general population. However, many genetic diseases affect certain ethnicities in disproportionate amounts, allowing those groups to be screened in a cost-effective way. Table 13–3 lists several common inheritable genetic diseases for which screening is possible. It includes the group at risk as well as the method of screening.

F. PAST OBSTETRIC HISTORY

1. Habitual abortion—A diagnosis of habitual abortion can be made after 3 or more consecutive spontaneous losses of a previable fetus. Habitual abortion is best investigated before another pregnancy occurs. If the patient is currently pregnant, as much of the workup as possible should be performed.

- Karyotype of abortus specimen
- Parental karyotype
- Survey for cervical and uterine anomalies
- Connective tissue disease work-up
- Screening for hormonal abnormalities (ie, hypothyroidism)
- Acquired and inherited thrombophilias
- Infectious disease evaluation of the genital tract

2. Previous stillbirth or neonatal death—A history of previous stillbirth or neonatal death should trigger an immediate investigation as to the conditions or circumstances surrounding the event. If the demise was the result of a nonrecurring event such as cord prolapse or traumatic injury, then the present pregnancy has a risk approaching a background risk. However, stillbirth or neonatal death may also suggest a cytogenetic abnormality, structural malformation syndrome, fetomaternal hemorrhage or thrombophilia (fetal or maternal), requiring a similar investigation as above.

3. Previous preterm delivery—The greater the number of preterm deliveries, as well as the degree of prematurity, the higher the risk at present for preterm delivery in the index pregnancy. Despite intense investigation, the incidence of preterm delivery has remained unchanged. Two-thirds of preterm deliveries occur near term (34 to 37 weeks), and these carry minimal fetal or neonatal morbidity. The remaining one-third of preterm deliveries accounts for nearly all of the perinatal morbidity and mortality. Approximately 50% of newborns born under 1000 grams suffer from intracranial hemorrhage, retinopathy of prematurity, or bronchopulmonary dysplasia, all of which carry significant long-term consequences. Approximately 40% of preterm delivery is due to spontaneous preterm delivery, another 40% is due to preterm rupture of membranes, and the remaining 20% is due to iatrogenic preterm delivery (eg, delivery due to preeclampsia or deteriorating fetal status). Spontaneous preterm labor is a complex process, but discrete pathophysiological processes have been identified (but may coexist): maternal and/or fetal stress, ascending genital tract infection, abruption (decidual hemorrhage), and uterine distension. Risk factors for preterm labor include prior history of preterm labor, multifetal pregnancy, vaginal bleeding in more than one trimester, in utero exposure to diethylstilbestrol (DES), uterine anomalies, incompetent cervix, and preterm labor in the index pregnancy. Screening for preterm labor in high-risk patients may include cervical length measurements by transvaginal sonography, fetal fibronectin of cervicovaginal secretions, and salivary estriol.

4. Rh isoimmunization or ABO incompatibility—Blood typing of both parents and maternal antibody screening should be performed at the initial prenatal visit. Women at risk for Rh(D) isoimmunization should be screened for anti-Rh(D) antibody at presentation, at 28 weeks gestation, and at delivery.

5. Previous preeclampsia-eclampsia—Previous preeclampsia-eclampsia increases the risk for hypertension in the current pregnancy, especially if there is underlying chronic hypertension or renal disease.

6. Previous infant with genetic disorder or congenital anomaly—A woman with a previously affected infant should be offered genetic counseling. Screening or

Table 13–3. Common inheritable genetic diseases.

Disease	Population at Increased Risk	Method of Testing
Alpha thalassemia	Chinese, Southeast Asian, African	CBC
		Hemoglobin electrophoresis
Beta thalassemia	Chinese, Southeast Asians, Mediterraneans, Pakistanis, Bangladeshis, Middle Easterners, African	CBC
		Hemoglobin electrophoresis
Bloom syndrome	Ashkenazi Jews	Mutation analysis
Canavan disease	Ashkenazi Jews	Mutation analysis
Cystic fibrosis	North American Caucasians of European ancestry, Ashkenazi Jews	Mutation analysis
Familial dysautonomia	Ashkenazi Jews	Mutation analysis
Fanconi anemia	Ashkenazi Jews	Mutation analysis
Gauchers disease	Ashkenazi Jews	Mutation analysis
Niemann-Pick disease	Ashkenazi Jews	Mutation analysis
Sickle cell disease and other structural hemoglobinopathies	African-Americans, Africans, Hispanics, Mediterranean, Middle Easterners, Carribean Indians	CBC
		Hemoglobin electrophoresis
Tay-Sachs	Ashkenazi Jews, French Canadians, Cajuns	Enzyme and mutation analysis

testing is available for some defects using maternal blood samples (eg, alpha-fetoprotein; AFP), ultrasonography, amniocentesis, chorionic villus sampling, and DNA analysis.

7. Teratogen exposure—A teratogen is any substance, agent, or environmental factor that has an adverse affect on the developing fetus. Whereas malformations caused by teratogen exposure are relatively rare, knowledge of exposure can aid in the diagnosis and management.

a. Drugs—Alcohol, anti-seizure medications (phenytoin, valproic acid, etc), lithium, mercury, thalidomide, diethylstilbestrol (DES), coumadin, isotretinoin, etc.

b. Infectious agents—CMV, *Listeria*, rubella, toxoplasmosis, varicella, *Mycoplasma*, etc.

c. Radiation—It is commonly believed that medical diagnostic radiation delivering less than 0.05 Gy to the fetus has no teratogenic risk.

ANTEPARTUM COURSE
Uniform Perinatal Record

A consistent method of recordkeeping which is easily understandable from doctor to doctor and location to location is ideal to manage the high-risk patient. In the event of a transfer of care during a pregnancy, or a review of a previous pregnancy, having a coherent, accessible prenatal record helps avoid duplication of tests and helps to expedite diagnostic confirmation and the onset of treatment. Preprinted records such as American College of Obstetricians and Gynecologists

(ACOG) forms provide uniform data for each patient and are helpful in diagnosis as well as in management decision making.

Prenatal Visits

Every prenatal visit is an opportunity to not only screen for problems that may complicate the course of the pregnancy but also to anticipate any problems before they develop. Several factors should be evaluated at each visit.

A. VITAL SIGNS

Fever (> 100.4° F), even without other subjective complaints may be due to a wide source of infectious etiologies. Urinary, pulmonary, and hematological sources of the fever should be considered. Signs or symptoms of chorioamnionitis should be assessed, and if chorioamnionitis is suspected, amniocentesis for microscopy and culture should be considered. Depending on clinical correlation, delivery may be necessary. Very high fevers (> 103° F) may trigger preterm labor and may also have an adverse effect on the early development of the fetal central nervous system. Antipyretics may be necessary to lower the temperature.

B. PULSE

Maternal tachycardia can be a sign of infection, anemia, or both. Isolated mild tachycardia (> 100 beats per minute [bpm]) should be evaluated and followed up. Moderate to severe tachycardia (> 120 bpm) needs immediate evaluation, including but not limited to a hemogram and an ECG.

C. BLOOD PRESSURE

The normal pattern of maternal blood pressure readings is for a decrease from baseline during the first trimester, reaching its nadir in the second trimester, and slightly rising in the third trimester, although not as high as the baseline levels. Repeated blood pressure readings of 140/90 mm Hg 6 hours apart or a rise of 30 mm Hg systolic pressure or 15 mm Hg diastolic pressure should be considered evidence of pregnancy-induced hypertension. Consideration of the patient's medical history, prepregnancy blood pressure, and gestational age should all be considered in forming a diagnosis and management strategy.

D. URINALYSIS

At the first prenatal visit, a clean-catch urine culture and sensitivity should be performed. Any growth should be treated with the appropriate antibiotics. At all subsequent visits, urine dipstick testing to screen for protein, glucose, leukocyte esterase, blood, or any combination of markers is useful in identifying patients with a change in their baseline urinary composition.

Screening Tests

Screening tests are performed at the appropriate time during the pregnancy.

A. FASTER (FIRST AND SECOND TRIMESTER EVALUATION OF RISK FOR ANEUPLOIDY) TRIAL

Transvaginal sonography between 10⅔ weeks and 13⅔ weeks to visualize and measure nuchal translucency, along with serum measurements of PAPP-A and free β-hCG is currently being studied in several institutions throughout the United States as a screen for Down syndrome, as well as other aneuploidies and malformations.

B. MATERNAL SERUM ANALYTE TESTING

Frequently known as the "triple screen," this test includes maternal serum alpha-fetoprotein (msAFP), β-hCG, and estriol. In some institutions, only the msAFP is used, while in other institutions a fourth test, inhibin, is included, making it a "quad test." The usefulness of this screen is its ability to identify pregnancies at an increased risk for open neural tube defects, as well as for certain chromosomal abnormalities, especially trisomy 21 (75% sensitivity for Down syndrome detection). This test is effective at 15–19 weeks' gestation and can therefore identify an at-risk pregnancy in time to pursue more definitive diagnosis, if desired. It is important to note, however, that the triple screen is not a definitive test and that many positive screens have yielded normal fetuses and many abnormal fetuses have had normal screens.

C. DIABETES SCREEN

Routine screening consists of performing a glucose challenge test between 24 and 28 weeks. The test consists of a 50-g oral glucose load with a plasma glucose level drawn exactly 1 hour after. If the value is over 140 mg/dL, a more specific glucose tolerance test (GTT) should be performed. The GTT involves obtaining a fasting plasma glucose level, giving a 100-g oral glucose load, then drawing plasma levels at 1 hour, 2 hours, and 3 hours after the glucose load. A test is considered positive for gestational diabetes if two out of the four values are elevated.

D. ISOIMMUNIZATION

A patient who is Rh-negative with a pregnancy fathered by an Rh-positive man should be screened for antibodies at the first prenatal visit and again at 24–28 weeks. If there continues to be no antibodies, Rhogam should be administered at 28 weeks to prevent sensitization of the mother during the last trimester and delivery. In the event of a previously isoimmunized patient, the typing and screening performed at the initial visit would detect antibodies, which are reported as a numerical titer. These titers should be followed every 4 weeks to assess for worsening isoimmunization. In the presence of worsening titers, follow-up with amniocentesis may be appropriate. Peak systolic velocity of the fetal middle cerebral artery as determined by sonographic Doppler evaluation has been demonstrated to correlate with degree of fetal anemia, allowing for noninterventional diagnosis and management of fetal isoimmunization; however, the definitive treatment is intrauterine fetal transfusion.

E. BETA HEMOLYTIC STREPTOCOCCUS

This is also known as the group B *Streptococcus* (GBS) test, and between 10% and 30% of pregnant women are colonized with GBS in the vaginal or rectal areas. Whereas they are usually asymptomatic colonizations, perinatal transmission can result in a severe and potentially fatal neonatal infection. Any documented GBS bacteriuria needs to be treated at the time of diagnosis, as well as intrapartum. Intrapartum antibiotic prophylaxis has been shown to decrease the risk of perinatal GBS transmission. There are two approaches to screening: Screen patients at 35–37 weeks' gestation and treat positive cultures with intrapartum antibiotics, or treat patients based on risk factors with intrapartum antibiotic prophylaxis.

Fetal Assessment

Comprehensive fetal assessment begins in the first trimester with nuchal translucency and continues throughout the pregnancy into labor and delivery. Conceptually, antepartum testing in pregnancies at risk falls into one of two categories: assessment of prenatal diagnosis and assessment of fetal well-being.

A. ASSESSMENT OF PRENATAL DIAGNOSIS

Performed during all trimesters, the techniques used are diverse, and the information obtained varies according to the quality of imaging, depth of investigation, and gestational age of pregnancy.

1. Ultrasound—Ultrasound has had a continuous evolution over the last 20 years, with better equipment being produced each year. Real-time sonography allows a 2-D image to demonstrate fetal anatomy, as well as characteristics such as fetal weight, movement, volume of amniotic fluid, and structural anomalies such as myomas or placenta previa which may affect the pregnancy. 3-D sonography allows volume to be ascertained, creating a three-dimensional appearing image on the 2-D screen, which assists in identifying certain anatomical anomalies. Most recently, 4-D machines have been developed, which produce a 3-D image in real time. As the machines become more technically advanced and the computers that run them become faster, the images obtained will continue to improve and push the boundaries of sonographic prenatal diagnosis.

Diagnostic ultrasonography is widely used in the assessment of the pregnancy and the fetus. It is not, however, the standard of care, nor is it recommended by ACOG for every pregnancy. The indications for ultrasonography are multiple and diverse, and the type and timing of the examination varies depending on the information being sought.

A **basic** ultrasound examination should provide such information as fetal number, presentation, documentation of fetal viability, placental location, and assessment of gestational age. A **limited** ultrasound examination is a goal-directed search for a suspected problem or finding. A limited ultrasound may be used for guidance during procedures such as amniocentesis or external cephalic version, assessment of fetal well being, or documentation of presentation or placental location intrapartum. A **comprehensive** ultrasound examination provides information on fetal anatomy, growth, anomalies, and physiologic complications.

Ultrasound evaluation of fetal anatomy may detect some major structural anomalies. Gross malformations such as anencephaly and hydrocephaly are more commonly diagnosed and rarely missed; however, more subtle anomalies such as facial clefts, diaphragmatic hernias, and neural tube defects are more commonly reported to have been missed by ultrasound. The basic fetal anatomy survey should include visualization of the cerebral ventricles, four-chamber view of the heart, and examination of the spine, stomach, urinary bladder, umbilical cord insertion site, and renal region. Any indication of an anomaly should be followed by a more comprehensive sonogram. Typically, the fetal anatomic survey is performed at 17–20 weeks; however, there is controversy surrounding the potential benefits of an earlier sonogram at 14–16 weeks using the transvaginal probe. The earlier scan allows earlier detection of anomalies that are almost always present by the second trimester, as well as allowing greater detailed viewing of the fetal anatomy by using the higher-resolution vaginal transducers.

2. Aneuploidy screening—Multiple sonographic markers for aneuploidy have been identified. The presence of single or multiple markers adjusts the patient's age-related risk of aneuploidy based on the particular markers present. Such sonographic findings include, but are not limited to:

- Echogenic intracardiac focus
- Choroid plexus cysts
- Pyelectasis
- Echogenic bowel
- Short femur
- Hypomineralization of the fifth digit of the fetal hand

3. Amniocentesis—Amniocentesis is frequently performed under the guidance of ultrasonography. A needle is inserted transcutaneously through the abdominal wall into the amniotic cavity, and fluid is removed. There are many uses for this amniotic fluid, including cytology for detection of infection, alpha-fetoprotein evaluation for neural tube defect assessment, assessment of fetal lung maturity (which will be discussed later in the chapter), and the most common indication of cytogenetic analysis. In this case, amniocentesis is often performed between 15 and 20 weeks' gestation and fetal cells from the amniotic fluid are obtained. Risks associated with the procedure are considered to be very low, with the risk of abortion as a result of amniocentesis considered to be between 1 in 200 to 1 in 450 amniocenteses.

4. Chorionic villus sampling—Chorionic villus sampling (CVS) is an alternative to amniocentesis. It is performed between 10 and 12 weeks' gestation, and can be performed either transcervically or transabdominally. CVS is also performed under sonographic guidance, with the passing of a sterile catheter or needle into the placental site. Chorionic villi are aspirated and undergo cytogenetic analysis. The benefit of CVS over amniocentesis is its availability earlier in pregnancy; however, the rate of abortion is higher—as high as 1%. One disadvantage of CVS is that unlike amniocentesis, it does not allow diagnosis of neural tube defects.

5. Fetal blood sampling—Also referred to as cordocentesis or percutaneous umbilical blood sampling (PUBS), this is an option for chromosomal or metabolic analysis of the fetus. Benefits of the procedure include a rapid result turnaround rate and the ability to perform the procedure in the second and third trimester. Intravascular access to the fetus is useful for the assessment and treatment of certain fetal conditions such as Rh sensitization and alloimmune thrombocytopenia. There is a higher risk of fetal death, however, when compared to the other methods. Fetal loss rates are approximately 2%, but can vary depending on the fetal condition involved.

B. Assessment of Fetal Well-Being

1. Fetal monitoring techniques—Assessment of fetal status can be performed using a wide variety of techniques.

a. External fetal monitoring—The external measurement of the fetal heart rate is done by using a continuous beam of ultrasound waves focused on the fetal heart. This ultrasound monitor utilizes Doppler effects to sample the frequency of moving fetal heart valves and the atrial and the ventricular systole. The complex received signal wave is then peak detected and entered into the heart rate monitor. The computer averages several consecutive frequencies, which helps minimize artifact, before the signal is displayed and printed. This process of averaging is called **autocorrelation,** and produces a fetal heart rate pattern which closely resembles that derived from a fetal ECG, although there is more baseline variability inherent in this method.

b. Internal fetal monitoring—The internal measurement of the fetal heart rate is an invasive procedure, utilizing an electrode attached to the fetal scalp. A bipolar spiral electrode is placed transcervically and penetrates the fetal scalp. A reference electrode is placed on the maternal thigh to eliminate electrical interference. The fetal ECG is detected, and the R wave is the signal used for peak detection and for counting. This signal is very clear, and allows accurate beat-to-beat and baseline variability to be measured. Artifact is kept to a minimum, and there is little need for autocorrelation.

c. Sonographic fetal monitoring—There have been reports of a number of sonographically related surveillance techniques for fetal status published in the literature. Such testing techniques as biophysical profile and Doppler velocimetry have been extensively studied and widely used for antepartum evaluation. Doppler velocimetry is a noninvasive technique based on vascular impedance. Most often, the umbilical artery is utilized for this purpose. Both the peak values as well as the actual waveform can be utilized to identify abnormally growing fetuses, or fetuses at risk of cardiac failure or other adverse outcome. Most of the benefit is seen in growth-restricted pregnancies, and use for generalized surveillance is not recommended. Biophysical profile consists of fetal heart rate evaluation combined with sonographically assessed parameters of fetal well being, including fetal breathing movements, fine motor movement, gross fetal tone, and amniotic fluid volume.

2. Fetal heart rate interpretation—

a. Antepartum fetal surveillance—In determining which patients should have antepartum fetal surveillance, a major factor to consider is the lack of evidence that any routine surveillance method results in a decreased risk of fetal death. Therefore, we generally begin monitoring in pregnancies in which the risks of fetal demise are known to be increased. These can include maternal conditions such as antiphospholipid syndrome, lupus, diabetes, or other maternal medical problems. They can also include pregnancy-related conditions such as preeclampsia, IUGR, multiple gestation, poor obstetrical history, or postterm pregnancy.

Antepartum surveillance should include a nonstress test (NST) as a minimum. The addition of sonographic monitoring is common, most often as some variant of the biophysical profile. The criteria for the NST are: baseline between 120 and 160 bpm, the presence of periodic accelerations (ie, two accelerations in 20 minutes) of fetal heart rate of 15 bpm over baseline for 15 seconds, the absence of decelerations of the fetal heart rate, and the subjective assessment of variability of the fetal heart rate. In the case of a nonreassuring NST, further evaluation or delivery depend on the clinical context. In a patient at term, delivery is warranted. Near term, determination of fetal lung maturity can be considered. Remote from term poses a more challenging dilemma to the clinician. If resuscitative efforts are not successful in restoring reactivity to the NST, ancillary tests or testing techniques may prove useful in avoiding a premature iatrogenic delivery for nonreassuring fetal heart rate patterns, since the false-positive rate may be as high as 50–60%.

C. Ancillary Tests

1. Vibroacoustic stimulation—An auditory source, often an artificial larynx, is placed on the maternal abdomen. A short burst of sound is delivered to the fetus. This has proven successful in shortening the duration needed for the test to show reactivity, without compromising the predictive value of the absence of acidosis with a reactive NST.

2. Fetal scalp stimulation—The presence of an acceleration after a vaginal exam where the examiner stimulates the fetal vertex with the examining finger confirms the absence of acidosis (pH > 7.2).

3. Oxytocin challenge test—This may be used to elicit a confirmatory abnormal fetal heart rate response, with one report showing a better correlation with adverse outcome than the NST alone. Other studies, however, have demonstrated no improvement in predicting morbidity over an NST. This is performed by intravenous infusion of dilute oxytocin until three contractions occur in 10 minutes. A positive test indicates decreased fetal reserve, with a 20–40% incidence of abnormal fetal heart rate (FHR) patterns in labor. A positive test is the presence of a late deceleration after each of the three contractions, a negative test shows no decelerations, and anything else is equivocal. Repetitive variable decelerations are termed "suspicious" and are associated with abnormal FHR patterns in labor, particularly in postterm gestations.

Fetal Maturity Tests

Indications for assessing fetal lung maturity— The American College of Obstetricians and Gynecologists has recommended that fetal pulmonary maturity should be confirmed before elective delivery at less than 39 weeks' gestation unless fetal maturity can be inferred from any of these criteria: Fetal heart tones have been documented for 20 weeks by nonelectronic fetoscope or for 30 weeks by Doppler; and 36 weeks have elapsed since a serum or urine hCG-based pregnancy test was reported to be positive.

A. Lecithin:Sphingomyelin Ratio

The lecithin:sphingomyelin (L:S) ratio for assessment of fetal pulmonary maturity was first introduced by Gluck and colleagues in 1971. The test depends upon outward flow of pulmonary secretions from the lungs into the amniotic fluid, thereby changing the phospholipid composition of the latter and permitting measurement of the ratio of lecithin to sphingomyelin in a sample of amniotic fluid. The concentrations of these two substances are approximately equal until 32–33 weeks of gestation, at which time the concentration of lecithin begins to increase significantly while the sphingomyelin concentration remains about the same. The measurement of sphingomyelin serves as a constant comparison for control of the relative increases in lecithin because the volume of amniotic fluid cannot be accurately measured clinically. Determination of the L:S ratio involves thin-layer chromatography after organic solvent extraction. It is a difficult test to perform and interpret; care at each step of sample handling is critical for consistent results. The sample should be kept on ice or refrigerated if transport to a laboratory is required. Improper storage conditions can change the L:S ratio since amniotic fluid contains enzymes that can be affected by temperature. The amniotic fluid samples must be mixed well. The presence of blood or meconium can interfere with test interpretation. Bloody samples give false information due to the presence of sphingomyelin in blood and decreased extraction of lecithin by cold acetone techniques in the presence of red blood cells. Therefore, if blood or other particulate matter is present in the amniotic fluid sample, a low-speed, short centrifugation can be used to remove the cellular component.

Interpretation of the results should be carried out with consideration of the individual clinical circumstances. For example, some physicians require a higher L:S ratio for confirmation of fetal pulmonary maturity in pregnancies complicated by isoimmunization or diabetes mellitus.

A threshold value for prediction of lung maturity should be calculated in individual centers by correlation with clinical outcome, because the variation within and between laboratories can be considerable. Empirically, the risk of respiratory distress syndrome (RDS) is exceedingly low when the L:S ratio is greater than 2.0.

B. Phosphatidylglycerol

Phosphatidylglycerol (PG) is a minor constituent of surfactant. It begins to increase appreciably in amniotic fluid several weeks after the rise in lecithin. Its presence is more indicative of fetal lung maturity as PG enhances the spread of phospholipids on the alveoli; thus, its presence indicates a more advanced state of fetal lung development and function.

PG determination is not generally affected by blood, meconium, or other contaminants; its ability to predict pulmonary maturity is the same whether or not contamination is present. This is an advantage for assessing fetal lung maturity status since these substances are commonly found in amniotic fluid.

PG testing is performed by thin-layer chromatography (as for the L:S measurement), so it may be determined alone or in conjunction with L:S testing. It can be reported qualitatively as positive or negative, where positive represents an exceedingly low risk of RDS, or in a quantitative fashion, in which a value ≥ 0.3 is associated with a minimal rate of respiratory distress.

C. Foam Stability Index

The foam stability index (FSI) is a rapid predictor of fetal lung maturity and is based upon the ability of surfactant to generate stable foam in the presence of ethanol. Ethanol is added to a sample of amniotic fluid to eliminate the effects of nonsurfactant factors on foam formation. The mixture is shaken and will demonstrate generation of a stable ring of foam if surfactant is present in the amniotic fluid. The FSI is calculated by utilizing serial dilutions of ethanol to quantitate the amount of surfactant present.

Amniotic fluid samples should not be collected in silicone tubes when this test is planned, as the silicone will produce "false foam." The discriminating value indicative of lung maturity is usually set at ≥ 47. A positive result virtually excludes the risk of RDS; however, a negative test often occurs in the presence of mature lungs. The presence of blood or meconium interferes with results of the FSI.

D. FLUORESCENCE POLARIZATION

The fluorescence polarization test uses polarized light to quantitate the competitive binding of a probe to both albumin and surfactant in amniotic fluid; thus, it is a true direct measurement of surfactant concentration. It reflects the ratio of surfactant to albumin and is measured by an automatic analyzer, such as the TDx-FLM. An elevated ratio has been correlated with the presence of fetal lung maturity; the threshold for maturity is 55 mg of surfactant per gram of albumin.

Evaluation of the accuracy of TDx measurements has also been studied, specifically in diabetic patients. Despite initial evidence that higher cutoffs were required for diabetics, it is currently believed that the same cutoff for lung maturity can be used for both non-diabetic and diabetic patients.

The accuracy of this test compares favorably with the well-established L:S and PG tests. Blood and meconium contamination interfere with interpretation, although the degree or direction of the interference is unclear. There is insufficient evidence regarding the accuracy of this test for determination of fetal lung maturity in vaginally-collected specimens.

A disadvantage to the TDx-FLM method is the large quantification scale. Values greater than 55 are regarded as mature; however, values of 35–55 are considered borderline. In addition, there is controversy as to whether gestational age should be used in interpreting the TDx for determining the likelihood of RDS. In one report, higher threshold values were needed at earlier gestational ages to determine lung maturity and lower thresholds were required at later gestational ages.

Table 13–4 summarizes the value of these tests of fetal maturity and gives their relative costs.

Intrapartum Fetal Surveillance

Assessment of the fetus in labor is a challenging task. Certain techniques that were useful in the antepartum period are no longer accurate, and certain new techniques have become available. With the presence of contractions, fetal heart rate monitoring is no longer a *nonstress* test. Fetal heart rate assessment is still the initial test of choice. Continuous fetal monitoring and intermittent auscultation have been extensively reviewed, and the evidence does not support one over the other for routine obstetric care. Several reports suggest that continuous monitoring results in higher operative delivery rates without an associated neonatal benefit. For the present, the controversy over routine FHR monitoring remains, but the clinical practice is nearly universal for continuous electronic monitoring of the FHR in hospitals and many birthing centers.

In the intrapartum period, access to the fetus allows for further evaluation in the face of a nonreassuring FHR tracing. Direct measurement of the physiologic status of the fetus is possible after adequate cervical dilation and rupture of the membranes.

A. ANCILLARY TESTS

1. **Fetal scalp blood sampling**—Capillary blood collected from the fetal scalp typically has a pH lower than arterial blood. A pH of 7.20 was initially believed to be

Table 13–4. Fetal Maturity tests.

Test	Positive Discriminating Value	Positive Predictive Value	Relative Cost	Pros and Cons
L:S ratio	> 2.0	95–100%	High	Large laboratory variation
PG	"Present"	95–100%	High	Not affected by blood, meconium. Can use vaginal pooled sample.
FSI	> 47	95%	Low	Affected by blood, meconium, silicone tubes
TDx	> 55	96–100%	Moderate	Minimal inter/intraassay variability. Simple test.
Optical Density	OD 0.15	98%	Low	Simple technique
Lamellar Body Counts	30–40,000	97–98%	Low	Still investigational

the critical value to identify serious fetal stress and an increase in the incidence of low Apgar scores. However, there is much debate over the accuracy of scalp pH in predicting fetal distress with subsequent neurologic sequelae. Continuous scalp pH during labor was highly successful in defining abnormal FHR patterns associated with acidosis, although the advanced technical skill and expense prohibited widespread use. In fact, despite the correlation with FHR, fetal scalp pH is no longer used in many institutions. The only proven benefits reported for scalp pH testing were demonstration of adverse neurologic outcome with pH < 7.1, and fewer cesarean sections for fetal distress.

2. Fetal lactate levels—Collected in the same fashion as scalp pH, lactate levels demonstrated a higher predictive value than pH as markers of neurologic disability.

3. Fetal pulse oximetry—This has been studied over the past 10 years. Controversy exists over its potential clinical value. There is debate about its accuracy in correlating with acidemia. Studies have demonstrated no benefit in relation to FHR patterns, or in detecting neurologically-compromised fetuses. A recent report demonstrating a reduction in the rate of cesarean section for a diagnosis of distress, without an actual decrease in the incidence of cesareans compared with the control group, raised questions about the usefulness of the test, since it was hoped that it could reduce the cesarean section rate in a manner similar to scalp pH and lactate assays. Clearly, more studies need to be initiated to demonstrate a clear benefit to this test.

B. FETAL HEART RATE PATTERNS

1. Reassuring fetal heart rate patterns—Slight deviations from the normal baseline of 120–160 bpm and some periodic changes are innocuous in the continuum of the fetal heart rate pattern. Early decelerations and bradycardia of 100–119 bpm are believed to be vagally mediated due to fetal head compression, and are not associated with fetal acidosis or poor neonatal outcome. Certain cardiac arrhythmias also pose no threat to the fetus while the fetal heart rate pattern deviates from what is considered "normal." In fact, the majority of fetal arrhythmias are benign and spontaneously convert to normal sinus rhythm by 24 hours postpartum. Persistent tachyarrythmias are well tolerated, but may proceed to fetal hydrops if present for many hours to days. Persistent bradyarrhythmias are often associated with fetal heart disease, but are seldom associated with hypoxia or acidosis in fetal life or labor. Accelerations and variable decelerations of variable shape and timing are indicative of a normal autonomic nervous system.

2. Nonreassuring fetal heart rate patterns—This category is of more concern to the clinician, and while there is still evidence that the fetus is not acidotic, continuation or worsening of the clinical situation may result in fetal distress. Late deceleration is a smooth fall in the fetal heart rate beginning after the contraction has started, and ending after the contraction has ended. They are associated with a fall in fetal pH and a potential for perinatal morbidity and mortality. Another nonreassuring pattern is the sinusoidal heart rate. It is best defined as a pattern of regular variability resembling a sine wave with a fixed period of 3–5 cycles per minute and an amplitude of 5–40 bpm. The mechanism for the sinusoidal pattern is believed to be a response to moderate fetal hypoxemia, including secondary to fetal anemia. It was previously thought to carry a high perinatal mortality. However, follow-up with serial scalp pH has been successfully performed with no adverse outcome. The significance of sinusoidal heart rate patterns depends on the clinical setting. Variable decelerations may be divided into categories, with the deciding characteristic being the onset and the timing of the return to baseline. If a variable deceleration, no matter how deep, does not have a late component, then the pattern is benign and at most is mild cord compression not associated with acidosis or low Apgar scores. When there is a late recovery, the fetal pH falls progressively during the period of deceleration.

3. Fetal distress patterns—Considerable confusion surrounds the diagnosis of fetal distress. Fetal distress should be defined operationally as a pathological condition of the fetus that is likely to cause fetal or neonatal death or damage to the newborn if left uncorrected for a period of greater than 1 hour. It is often, but not always, associated with fetal acidemia and hypoxemia. These metabolic changes are highly correlated with a decompensated fetal homeostasis, but not necessarily with all nonreassuring FHR patterns. There are numerous causes and multiple factors associated with fetal distress; however, only a few fetal heart rate patterns are associated with true fetal distress, including:

a. Undulating baseline—Alternating tachycardia and bradycardia with wide swings, often with reduced variability in between.

b. Severe bradycardia—Fetal heart rate below 100 bpm for a prolonged period of time of at least 10 minutes.

c. Tachycardia with diminished variability unrelated to drugs

d. Tachycardia associated with additional nonreassuring periodic patterns such as late decelerations or variable decelerations with late recovery—With careful interpretation, FHR patterns can be a useful screening test for fetal acidemia and hypoxemia. The monitoring and interpretation of the fetal heart rate is ideally used as a screening tool. The presence of a reassuring FHR pattern is just that, reassuring that there is no fetal acidemia *at that time*. The absence of a reassuring tracing is not necessarily problematic, and ancillary testing can be performed to eliminate false positives. However, it must be remembered that a given segment of FHR monitoring is a single point in time. Pregnancy and labor are ongoing dynamic states. Maternal and fetal conditions and the processes of gestation, especially labor, are stresses which challenge fetal homeostasis. Fetal stress may be manifested in the FHR pattern, while the fetus remains compensated. The clinician must discriminate between stress and distress, using interpretation and ancillary testing. All monitoring techniques are to be ultimately used as supplements to clinical judgment, to obtain the best outcome of pregnancy.

CONCLUSIONS

Assessing pregnancy to determine risk as well as carefully monitoring pregnancies with a recognized risk begins early in the gestation. Preconceptual counseling of patients with known medical or genetic disorders helps to optimize outcomes. Early and frequent prenatal care allow the care provider to screen his or her patient population to identify pregnancies at risk and act accordingly. Additionally, pregnancies identified as complicated by one or more issues can be followed by assortments of maternal and fetal surveillance techniques to maximize therapeutic treatment.

As technology advances and our ability to both diagnose and treat improve, the methods for assessment and care of the pregnancy at risk will be a constantly changing field.

REFERENCES

American College of Obstetricians and Gynecologists: Antepartum fetal surveillance. ACOG Practice Bulletin No. 9, 1999.

Ashwood ER: Standards of laboratory practice: Evaluation of fetal lung maturity. Clin Chem 1997;43:211.

Bahado-Singh RO et al: Ratio of nuchal thickness to humerus length for Down syndrome detection. Am J Obstet Gynecol 2001;184:1284.

Bush KD, O'Brien JM, Barton JR: The utility of umbilical artery Doppler investigation in women with the HELLP syndrome. Am J Obstet Gynecol 2001;184:1087.

Chausan SP et al: Intrapartum amniotic fluid index and two dimensional pockets are poor predictors of adverse neonatal outcome. J Perinatology 1997;17:221.

Cunningham FG et al: Intrapartum assessment. *Williams Obstetrics.* Appleton & Lange, 1997.

Garite TJ et al: A multicenter controlled trial of fetal pulse oximetry in the intrapartum management of nonreassuring fetal heart rate patterns. Am J Obstet Gynecol 2000;183:1049.

Gillen-Goldstein J et al: Prediction of respiratory distress syndrome from amniotic fluid surfactant measures: the NACB Fetal Lung Maturity Project. J Soc Gynecol Invest 2001;(Abstract)716:257.

Gluck L et al: Diagnosis of the respiratory distress syndrome by amniocentesis. Am J Obstet Gynecol 1971;109:440.

Jobe AH: Fetal lung development, tests for maturation, induction of maturation and treatment. In: Creasy RK, Resnik R (editors): *Maternal-Fetal Medicine.* WB Saunders, 1999, p. 417.

Kruger K et al: Predictive value of fetal scalp blood lactate concentration and pH as markers of neurologic disability. Am J Obstet Gynecol 1999;181:1072.

Lockwood CJ, Kuczynski E: Risk stratification and pathological mechanisms in preterm delivery. Paediatr Perinat Epidemiol 2001;15(Suppl 2):78.

Low JA, Victory R, Derrick EJ: Predictive value of electronic fetal monitoring for intrapartum fetal asphyxia with metabolic acidosis. Obstet Gynecol 1999;93:285.

Mari G et al: Noninvasive diagnosis by Doppler ultrasonography of fetal anemia due to maternal red cell alloimmunization. Collaborative group for Doppler assessment of the blood velocity in anemic fetuses. N Engl J Med 2000;342:9.

Mires G, Williams F, Howie P: Randomised controlled trial of cardiotocography versus Doppler auscultation of fetal heart at admission in labour in low risk obstetric population. Br Med J 2001;322:1457.

National Center for Health Statistics: March of Dimes Perinatal Data Center, 2000. "Preterm Birth, 1988–1998."

Parer JT: Fetal heart rate. In: Creasy RK, Resnik R (editors): *Maternal-Fetal Medicine: Principles and Practice.* WB Saunders, 1999.

Schmidt S et al: Clinical usefulness of pulse oximetry in the fetus with non-reassuring heart rate pattern? J Perinat Med 2000;28:298.

Snijders RJ et al: UK multicentre project on assessment of risk of trisomy 21 by maternal age and fetal nuchal-translucency thickness at 10–14 weeks of gestation. Lancet 1998;352:343.

Early Pregnancy Risks

14

Sara H. Garmel, MD

SPONTANEOUS ABORTION

ESSENTIALS OF DIAGNOSIS

- Suprapubic pain, uterine cramping, and/or back pain.
- Vaginal bleeding.
- Cervical dilatation.
- Extrusion of products of conception.
- Disappearance of symptoms and signs of pregnancy.
- Negative pregnancy test or quantitative β-hCG that is not properly increasing.
- Abnormal ultrasound findings (eg, empty gestational sac, fetal disorganization, lack of fetal growth).

General Considerations

Spontaneous abortion is the most common complication of pregnancy. It is defined as delivery occurring before the 20th completed week of gestation. It implies delivery of all or any part of the products of conception, with or without a fetus weighing less than 500 grams. **Threatened abortion** is bleeding of intrauterine origin occurring before the 20th completed week, with or without uterine contractions, without dilatation of the cervix, and without expulsion of the products of conception. **Complete abortion** is the expulsion of all of the products of conception before the 20th completed week of gestation, while **incomplete abortion** is the expulsion of some, but not all, of the products of conception. **Inevitable abortion** refers to bleeding of intrauterine origin before the 20th completed week, with dilatation of the cervix without expulsion of the products of conception. In **missed abortion,** the embryo or fetus dies in utero, but the products of conception are retained in utero. In **septic abortion,** infection of the uterus and sometimes surrounding structures occur.

Incidence

Although the true incidence of spontaneous abortion is unknown, approximately 15% of clinically evident pregnancies and 60% of chemically evident pregnancies end in spontaneous abortion. Eighty percent of spontaneous abortions occur prior to 12 weeks' gestation.

The incidence of abortion is influenced by the age of the mother and by a number of pregnancy-related factors, including whether a previous full-term normal pregnancy has occurred, the number of previous spontaneous abortions, whether there has been a previous stillbirth, and whether a previous infant was born with malformations or known genetic defects. Additionally, parental influences, including balanced translocation carriers and medical complications, may influence the rate of spontaneous abortion.

Etiology

In approximately 50% of spontaneous abortions occurring during the first trimester, there is an abnormal karyotype. This incidence decreases to 20–30% in second trimester losses, and 5–10% in third trimester losses. As will be discussed below, the first trimester losses are typically autosomal trisomies or monosomy X, while later losses reflect chromosomal abnormalities seen in neonates.

Other suspected causes of spontaneous abortion account for a smaller percentage of losses. In a significant percentage of spontaneous abortions, the etiology is unknown. Infection, anatomic defects, endocrine factors, immunologic factors, and maternal systemic disease are felt to play a role in spontaneous abortion.

A. MORPHOLOGIC AND GENETIC ABNORMALITIES

Aneuploidy (an abnormal chromosomal number) is responsible for a large percentage of early spontaneous abortions, accounting for at least 50% of these losses.

Autosomal trisomies have been noted for every chromosome except chromosome number 1. Together, the autosomal trisomies make up just over 50% of all aneuploid losses. Trisomy 16 is the most commonly encountered trisomy in spontaneous abortions.

Monosomy X or Turner syndrome is the single most common aneuploidy in spontaneous losses, comprising approximately 20% of these conceptuses.

Polyploidy, usually in the form of triploidy, is found in approximately 20% of all miscarriages. Polyploid conceptions typically result in empty sacs or blighted ovums but occasionally can lead to partial hydatidiform moles.

The remaining half of early abortuses appear to have normal chromosomal complements. Of these, 20% have other genetic abnormalities which may account for the loss. Mendelian or polygenic factors resulting in anatomic defects may play a role. These tend to be more common in later fetal losses.

B. MATERNAL FACTORS

1. Systemic disease

a. Maternal infections—Organisms such as *Treponema pallidum, Chlamydia trachomatis, Neisseria gonorrhoeae, Streptococcus agalactiae,* herpes simplex virus, cytomegalovirus, and *Listeria monocytogenes* have been implicated in spontaneous abortion. Although these agents have been identified in early losses, a causal relationship has not been established.

b. Other diseases—Endocrine disorders such as hyperthyroidism or poorly controlled diabetes mellitus; cardiovascular disorders, such as hypertensive or renal disease; and connective tissue disease, such as systemic lupus erythematosus may also be associated with spontaneous abortion.

2. Uterine defects—Congenital anomalies that distort or reduce the size of the uterine cavity, such as unicornuate, bicornuate, or septate uterus, carry a 25–50% risk of miscarriage. A diethylstilbestrol (DES)-related anomaly, such as a T-shaped or hypoplastic uterus, also carries an increased risk of miscarriage. Acquired anomalies, particularly submucous or intramural myomas, have been associated with spontaneous abortions as well.

Previous scarring of the uterine cavity following dilatation and curettage (Asherman's syndrome), myomectomy, or unification procedures has been implicated in spontaneous miscarriage, as have anatomic or functional incompetence of the uterine cervix.

3. Immunologic disorders—Blood group incompatibility due to ABO, Rh, Kell, or other less common antigens has been associated with spontaneous abortions. Furthermore, similar maternal and paternal HLA may enhance the possibility of abortion by causing insufficient maternal immunologic recognition of the fetus.

4. Malnutrition—Severe malnutrition has been implicated in spontaneous losses.

5. Emotional disturbances—Emotional causes of abortion are speculative. There is no valid evidence to support the concept that abortion may be induced by fright, grief, anger, or anxiety.

C. TOXIC FACTORS

Agents such as radiation, antineoplastic drugs, anesthetic gases, alcohol, and nicotine have been shown to be embryotoxic. Other agents such as lead, ethylene oxide, and formaldehyde may also be toxic.

D. TRAUMA

Direct trauma, such as injury to the uterus from a gunshot wound, or indirect trauma, such as surgical removal of an ovary containing the corpus luteum of pregnancy, may result in spontaneous abortion.

Pathology

In spontaneous abortion, hemorrhage into the decidua basalis often occurs. Necrosis and inflammation appear in the area of implantation. The pregnancy becomes partially or entirely detached. Uterine contractions and dilatation of the cervix result in expulsion of most or all of the products of conception.

Clinical Findings

A. THREATENED ABORTION

At least 20% of pregnant women have some first trimester bleeding. In most cases, this is thought to represent an implantation bleed. The cervix remains closed and slight bleeding with or without cramping may be noted.

B. INEVITABLE ABORTION

Abdominal or back pain and bleeding with an open cervix indicate impending abortion. Abortion is inevitable when cervical effacement, cervical dilatation, and/or rupture of the membranes is noted.

C. INCOMPLETE ABORTION (FIG 14–1)

In incomplete abortion the products of conception have partially passed from the uterine cavity. In gestations of less than 10 weeks' duration, the fetus and placenta are usually passed together. After 10 weeks, they may be passed separately with a portion of the products retained in the uterine cavity. Cramps are usually present. Bleeding generally is persistent and is often severe.

D. COMPLETE ABORTION (FIG 14–2)

Complete abortion is identified by passage of the entire conceptus. Slight bleeding may continue for a short time, although pain usually ceases.

E. MISSED ABORTION

Missed abortion implies that the pregnancy has been retained following death of the fetus. It is not known why the pregnancy is not expelled. It is possible that normal progestogen production by the placenta continues while the estrogen levels fall, which may reduce uterine contractility.

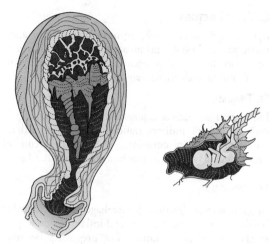

Figure 14–1. Incomplete abortion. **At right:** Product of incomplete abortion. (Reproduced, with permission, from Benson RC: *Handbook of Obstetrics & Gynecology*, 8th ed. Lange, 1983.)

F. Blighted Ovum

Blighted ovum or anembryonic pregnancy represents a failed development of the embryo, so that only a gestational sac, with or without a yolk sac, is present.

Laboratory Findings

A. Complete Blood Count

If significant bleeding has occurred, the patient will be anemic. Both the white blood cell count and the sedimentation rate may be elevated even without the presence of infection.

B. Pregnancy Tests

Falling or abnormally low plasma levels of β-hCG are predictive of an abnormal pregnancy, either a blighted ovum, spontaneous abortion, or ectopic pregnancy.

Ultrasonography

Transvaginal ultrasound is helpful in documenting intrauterine pregnancies as early as 4–5 weeks' gestation. Fetal heart motion should be seen in embryos > 5 mm from crown to rump, or in embryos at least 5–6 weeks' gestation. Ultrasound is useful in determining which pregnancies are viable and which are most likely to miscarry. Perhaps more than any other tool, ultrasound has proven most helpful in the differential diagnosis of early pregnancy complications.

In threatened abortion, ultrasound will reveal a normal gestational sac and viable embryo. However, a large or irregular sac, an eccentric fetal pole, the presence of a large (> 25% of sac size) retrochorionic bleed, and/or a slow fetal heart rate (< 85 bpm) carry a poor prognosis. Miscarriage becomes less and less likely the further the gestation progresses, but most pregnancies are lost weeks before mothers complain of signs or symptoms. If a viable fetus of 6 weeks or less is seen on ultrasound, the risk of miscarriage is approximately 15–30%. This decreases to 5–10% at 7–9 weeks' gestation and less than 5% after 9 weeks' gestation.

In incomplete abortion, the gestational sac is usually deflated, and irregular, echogenic material representing placental tissue is seen in the uterine cavity. In complete abortion, the endometrium appears closely apposed, with no visible products of conception.

An embryo or fetus without heart motion is consistent with a missed abortion, while an abnormal gestational sac, without a yolk sac or embryo, is consistent with a blighted ovum (see Figs 14–3 to 14–6).

Ectopic pregnancy may cause similar symptoms of miscarriage, namely menstrual abnormality and abdominal or pelvic pain. An adnexal mass may or may not be present. Ultrasound can virtually exclude an ectopic pregnancy by documenting an intrauterine pregnancy, as the chance of a simultaneous intra- and extrauterine pregnancy (heterotopic pregnancy) is exceedingly rare in spontaneous pregnancies, occurring in only one in 15,000–40,000 pregnancies.

Hydatidiform mole usually ends in abortion before the fifth month. Theca lutein cysts, when present, cause bilateral ovarian enlargement; the uterus may be unusually large. Bloody discharge may contain hydropic villi.

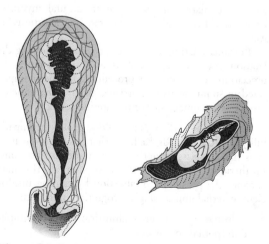

Figure 14–2. Complete abortion. **At right:** product of complete abortion. (Reproduced, with permission, from Benson RC: *Handbook of Obstetrics & Gynecology*, 8th ed. Lange, 1983.)

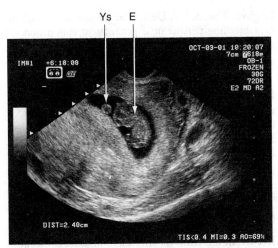

Figure 14–3. Intrauterine pregnancy at 8 weeks' gestation, demonstrating embryo (E) and yolk sac (YS).

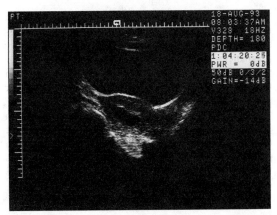

Figure 14–5. Empty gestational sac, consistent with a blighted ovum.

Other entities that may be confused with abortion include cervical infection, extruding pedunculated myoma, and cervical neoplasia. However, the pregnancy test will be negative, unless a pregnancy coexists.

Complications

Severe or persistent hemorrhage during or following abortion may be life threatening. The more advanced the gestation, the greater the likelihood of excessive blood loss. Sepsis develops most frequently after self-induced abortion. Infection, intrauterine synechia, and infertility are other complications of abortion. Perforation of the uterine wall may occur during dilatation and curettage (D&C) because of the soft and vaguely outlined uterine wall and may be accompanied by injury to the bowel and bladder, hemorrhage, infection, and fistula formation.

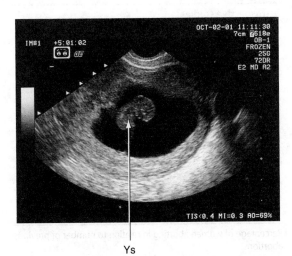

Figure 14–4. Embryonic demise at 8 weeks' gestation, with irregular gestational sac and deflated yolk sac (YS).

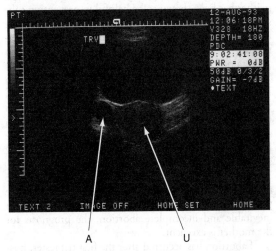

Figure 14–6. Empty uterus (U) with an adnexal mass (A) suspicious for an ectopic pregnancy. β-hCG at the time of transabdominal ultrasound was just over 100 mIU.

Multiple pregnancy with the loss of one fetus and retention of another ("vanishing twin") is not only possible but has been well documented in 20% of early pregnancies closely monitored by ultrasound. Usually the fetus is simply resorbed, but the loss of one fetus in multiple gestation may be accompanied by cramping or vaginal bleeding.

Even with very early miscarriage, a loss can have a significant effect on the family. The fact that most of these losses are unexpected intensifies this grief. Each person responds differently to his or her tragedy. It is the health care worker's responsibility to help parents mourn by acknowledging their loss and identifying potential support systems.

Prevention

Some losses can be prevented by early obstetric care, with adequate treatment of maternal disorders such as diabetes and hypertension, by protection of pregnant women from environmental hazards, and from exposure to infectious diseases.

Treatment

Successful management of spontaneous abortion depends upon early diagnosis. Every patient should receive a general physical examination, and a complete history should be taken. Laboratory studies should include a complete blood count, blood typing, and cervical cultures to determine pathogens in case of infection.

If the diagnosis of threatened abortion is made, bed rest and pelvic rest is typically recommended, although neither has been shown to be helpful in preventing subsequent miscarriage. Prognosis is good when bleeding and/or cramping resolve. D&C may be necessary if significant bleeding persists or if products of conception are retained.

If the diagnosis of inevitable or incomplete abortion is made, evacuation of the uterus by suction D&C should be promptly performed. A type and cross-match for possible blood transfusion and determination of Rh status should be obtained. The prognosis for the mother is excellent if the retained tissue is promptly and completely evacuated.

If the diagnosis of complete abortion is made, the patient should be observed for further bleeding. The products of conception should be examined. As with inevitable and incomplete abortion, the prognosis for the mother is excellent.

If abortion has occurred after the first trimester, hospitalization should be considered. Oxytocics are helpful in contracting the uterus, limiting blood loss, and aiding in expulsion of clots and tissue. Ergot preparations, which contract the cervix as well as the uterus, may also be given if needed. A D&C may be necessary if significant bleeding persists or if products of conception are retained.

Treatment of Complications

Uterine perforation may be manifested by signs of intraperitoneal bleeding, rupture of the bowel or bladder, or peritonitis. Oftentimes, there are no clinical signs and no sequelae. When uterine perforation is suspected, however, laparoscopy and/or laparotomy is indicated to determine the extent of laceration or bowel injury.

RECURRENT ABORTION

General Considerations

Recurrent abortion is defined as 3 or more consecutive pregnancy losses before 20 weeks gestation, each with a fetus weighing less than 500 g. Approximately .4–1% of women are habitual aborters. Recurrence risks are difficult to quantify and studies are conflicting. Although there is an increased risk of abortion after a previous abortion, no generally accepted recurrence risks exist (Table 14–1). The incidence of clinically-evident abortion when there is no previous history is approxi-

Table 14–1. Probability of spontaneous abortion.

Type of Study	Number of Previous Abortions			
	0	1	2	3+
Retrospective studies				
Stevenson et al (1959)		16.3	19.2	26.2
Warburton and Fraser (1964)	12.3	26.2	32.2	30.2
Leridon (1976)	15.2	22.0	35.3	
Poland et al (1977)		19.0	35.0	47.0
Naylor and Warburton (1978)	11.0	20.3	29.2	37.0
Cohort studies				
Shapiro et al (1970)	10.9	18.0		
Awan (1974)	10.4	22.1	27.4	
Prospective studies				
Boué at al (1975)		13.8		
Harger et al (1983)			17.4	29.2
Fitzsimmons et al (1983)			31.3	45.7
Regan (1988)	5.6	11.5	29.4	36.4

Percentage of women aborting in relation to number of previous abortions.

Reproduced, with permission, from Regan L: Prospective study of spontaneous abortion. In: Beard RW, Sharp F (editors). *Early Pregnancy Loss: Mechanisms and Treatment.* Roy Coll Obstet Gynaecol, 1988.

mately 15%. This increases to 25–50% when there have been 3 or more miscarriages.

The recurrence risk is higher if the embryo or fetus has a normal karyotype. It may be that maternal causes are responsible for this higher recurrence risk when the karyotype of the abortus is normal.

Despite these conflicting reports, the prognosis following repeated losses is good, with most couples having an approximately 60% chance of a viable pregnancy.

Etiology & Treatment

Chromosomal abnormalities and uterine malformations have been shown to play a role in repetitive miscarriages. Other causes, including hormonal abnormalities, infection, systemic disease, environmental agents, and/or immunologic factors may also play a role. Table 14–2 summarizes a diagnostic work-up for recurrent abortion.

A. GENETIC ERROR

As described previously, there is a 50–60% incidence of abnormal karyotype in first-trimester spontaneous abortions. Possible causes of genetic errors include balanced rearrangements of parental chromosomes such as translocations, found in approximately 2–5% of patients with repetitive abortions.

A careful reproductive history and pedigree should be taken for both partners, and karyotype screening should be performed. It is also useful to know the kary-

otype of aborted material. If the defect is paternal, artificial insemination is available. For a maternal defect, a donor egg may be fertilized by the husband's sperm. Preimplantation diagnosis is also an option. With this technique, a probe is made for the translocated region. Typically an embryo is allowed to reach the 8-cell stage. A few cells are aspirated and the probe is added. If no translocation is identified in the embryo, it is implanted in the uterus. Table 14–2 details possible therapies for recurrent abortion.

B. UTERINE ABNORMALITIES

Anatomic abnormalities were the first described causes of habitual abortion and account for up to 15% of recurrent pregnancy losses. Defects include congenital uterine anomalies, cervical incompetence, submucous leiomyomas, abnormalities due to diethylstilbestrol exposure in utero, and Asherman's syndrome. A major difficulty in counseling couples is that approximately 50% of women with uterine defects have no reproductive problem. Unicornuate and bicornuate uteri each account for approximately one-third of spontaneous abortions due to anatomic abnormalities, and septate uteri account for another 20–25%. Submucous leiomyomas are responsible for a much smaller percentage of repeated losses. Generally, losses from anatomic abnormalities occur in the second trimester. Interference with implantation, lack of an adequate blood supply, or

Table 14–2. Diagnosis and treatment of recurrent abortion.

Cause	Diagnosis	Treatment
Genetic error	Obtain a 3-generation pedigree and karyotype of both parents and any previously aborted material.	Artificial insemination by donor, embryo transfer, preimplantation diagnosis, or prenatal testing on subsequent conceptions.
Anatomic abnormalities of reproductive tract	Perform hysterosalpingogram or hysteroscopy.	Uterine operation: Jones, Tompkins, Strassman procedure, myomectomy. Cervical cerclage (abdominal or vaginal), reconstruction of cervical isthmus.
Hormonal abnormalities	Perform laboratory studies for T_4 and TSH, serum progesterone or endometrial biopsy during luteal phase, and consider glucose tolerance test.	Thyroid replacement, progesterone or clomiphene citrate, diabetic diet and/or insulin, as indicated.
Infection	Obtain cervical cultures for *Chlamydia* and gonorrhea, and consider cultures for *Mycoplasma* and *Ureaplasma*.	Approriate antibiotics.
Systemic disease	Evaluate blood pressure and kidney function, check for lupus anticoagulant and anticardiolipin antibody.	Low-dose aspirin, heparin, and/or prednisone, as indicated.
Exogenous agents	Patient history and/or drug screen.	Discourage smoking, alcohol, and recreational drug use.
Immunologic factors	Testing not readily available.	Treatment under investigation.

growth restriction are possible mechanisms for recurrent loss.

Diagnosis of uterine anatomic abnormalities is usually accomplished by hysterosalpingography or hysteroscopy. Treatment is primarily surgical, with reported success rates of 70–85% after surgical correction.

Cervical incompetence may be due to congenital abnormalities (eg, DES exposure), trauma from a vigorous D&C or cone biopsy, and/or possibly hormonal influences, and classically presents in mid-second or early third trimester with rapid, painless cervical dilatation. If other causes of recurrent losses are excluded and the presumed etiology is incompetent cervix, a cervical cerclage is recommended between 12 and 14 weeks' gestation. Success rates with cerclage are 85–90%. Complications include risks from anesthesia, bleeding, infection, rupture of membranes, and miscarriage. Contraindications to cerclage placement include bleeding of unknown etiology, infection, labor, ruptured membranes, and congenital anomalies.

C. Hormonal Causes

Possible hormonal causes of habitual abortion include hypothyroidism and hyperthyroidism, progesterone insufficiency, and uncontrolled diabetes mellitus.

Progesterone deficiency or luteal phase defect (LPD) is felt by some to be an important cause of habitual abortion. A defective endometrium resulting in faulty implantation is the proposed mechanism. Inadequate hormonal support of the embryo may also be involved. Diagnosis is usually made by luteal phase endometrial biopsies. However, controlled studies demonstrating an improvement in pregnancy outcome with treatment are lacking, and thus LPD as a cause of recurrent miscarriage remains controversial. If a LPD is diagnosed by endometrial biopsy, however, most physicians advocate treatment with supplemental progesterone.

D. Infection

Infectious agents which have been implicated in repetitive losses include *Mycoplasma, Ureaplasma urealyticum, Toxoplasma gondii, Chlamydia trachomatis, Treponema pallidum, Borrelia burgdorferi, Neisseria gonorrhoeae, Streptococcus agalactiae, Listeria monocytogenes,* herpes simplex, and cytomegalovirus. Although these agents have been identified in early losses, a causal relationship has not been demonstrated.

E. Systemic Disease

Systemic causes of recurrent abortion include uncontrolled diabetes, uncontrolled thyroid disease, and collagen vascular disease. The incidence of systemic disease as a cause of habitual abortion is unknown, but is probably low. Therapy involves treatment of the specific disease.

F. Immunologic Factors

Antiphospholipid antibodies (lupus anticoagulant and anticardiolipin antibodies) may damage platelets and vascular endothelium, resulting in thrombosis. This may account for the relationship to miscarriage when found in combination with clinical features of antiphospholipid syndrome. Low-dose aspirin and/or heparin may be beneficial in this situation.

Compared to women who carry a pregnancy to term, women who are habitual aborters share more HLA antigens with their partners and have blunted responses to paternal antigen with lower levels of blocking antibodies or antileukocytotoxic antibodies. The maternal immunologic response may not be as effective in protecting the pregnancy, resulting in pregnancy loss.

Diagnostic tests for immunologic abnormalities are available in few centers. The efficacy of leukocyte immunotherapy is unknown, and treatment such as paternal leukocyte immunization is still experimental.

In up to 50% of women with recurrent abortion, a definitive cause may not be found. However, although the loss rate may be higher than that in the general population, the majority of these women will have a successful pregnancy in their reproductive lifetime.

SEPTIC ABORTION

General Considerations

Septic abortion is manifested by fever, malodorous vaginal discharge, pelvic and abdominal pain, and cervical motion tenderness. Peritonitis and sepsis may be seen. Trauma to the cervix or upper vagina may be recognized if there has been a criminal abortion.

A complete blood count, urinalysis, endometrial cultures, blood cultures, chest x-ray, and abdominal x-ray to rule out uterine perforation should be obtained. Ultrasound may be helpful in ruling out retained products of conception.

Treatment

Treatment of septic abortion involves hospitalization and intravenous antibiotic therapy. Selection of antibiotic agents should provide for both anaerobic and aerobic coverage. A D&C should be done, and a hysterectomy may have to be performed if the infection does not respond to treatment.

ECTOPIC PREGNANCY

In ectopic pregnancy, a fertilized ovum implants in an area other than the endometrial lining of the uterus (Fig 13–7). More than 95% of extrauterine pregnancies occur in the fallopian tube.

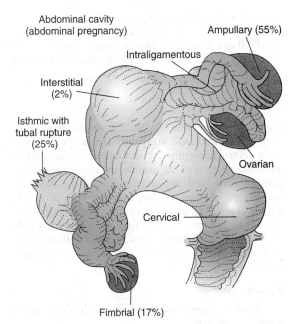

Figure 14–7. Sites of ectopic pregnancies. (Adapted with permission from Benson RC: *Handbook of Obstetrics & Gynecology*, 8th ed. Lange, 1983.)

The incidence of ectopic pregnancy has increased from 4.5/1000 in 1970 to 19.7/1000 in 1992. This may be due, at least in part, to a higher incidence of salpingitis, an increase in ovulation induction, and more tubal sterilizations.

Ectopic pregnancy is a significant cause of maternal morbidity and mortality as well as fetal loss. It is the leading cause of pregnancy-related death in the first trimester, and accounts for 9% of all pregnancy-related deaths. The development of sensitive β-hCG assays, along with the increasing use of ultrasound and laparoscopy, has allowed for earlier diagnosis of ectopic pregnancy. This has resulted in a decrease in both maternal morbidity and mortality.

Classification & Incidence

Ectopic pregnancy may be classified as follows (Fig 14–7).

1. **Tubal** (> 95%)—Includes: ampullary (55%), isthmic (25%), fimbrial (17%), and interstitial (2%).

2. **Other** (< 5%)—Includes: cervical, ovarian, and abdominal (primary abdominal pregnancies have been reported, but most abdominal pregnancies are secondary pregnancies, from tubal abortion or rupture and subsequent implantation in the bowel, omentum, or mesentery).

3. **Intraligamentous**

4. **Heterotopic pregnancy**—An ectopic pregnancy occurs in combination with an intrauterine pregnancy in 1 in 15,000–40,000 spontaneous pregnancies, and in up to 1% of patients undergoing in vitro fertilization.

5. **Bilateral ectopic**—These pregnancies have occasionally been reported.

Etiology

The etiology of ectopic pregnancy is not well understood. However, several risk factors have been found to be associated with ectopic pregnancy (Table 14–3).

A. Tubal Factors

Ectopic pregnancy is 5–10 times more common in women who have had salpingitis. In women with ectopic pregnancies, up to 50% will have had salpingitis previously and in most of these patients, the uninvolved tube is also abnormal. Other tubal factors that interfere with the progress of the fertilized ovum include adherent folds of tubal lumen due to salpingitis isthmica nodosa, developmental abnormalities of the tube or abnormal tubal anatomy due to DES exposure in utero, previous tubal surgery including tubal ligation with a 16–50% ectopic pregnancy rate if pregnancy occurs after tubal ligation, conservative treatment of an unrup-

Table 14–3. Risk factors for ectopic pregnancy.

Risk Factor	Odds Ratio[1]
High risk	
Tubal surgery	21.0
Sterilization	9.3
Previous ectopic pregnancy	8.3
In-utero exposure to diethylstilbestrol	5.6
Use of IUD	4.2–45.0
Documented tubal pathology	3.8–21.0
Moderate risk	
Infertility	2.5–21.0
Previous genital infections	2.5–3.7
Multiple sexual partners	2.1
Slight risk	
Previous pelvic/abdominal surgery	0.9–3.8
Cigarette smoking	2.3–2.5
Vaginal douching	1.1–3.1
Early age at first intercourse (< 18 years)	1.6

[1]Single values indicate common odds ratio from homogeneous studies; point estimates indicate range of values from heterogeneous studies.

Reproduced, with permission, from Pisarska et al: Ectopic pregnancy. Lancet 1998;351:1115.

tured ectopic with a recurrent ectopic rate of 4–16%, and tubal anastomosis with a 4% ectopic rate. Adhesions from infection or previous abdominal surgery, endometriosis, and even leiomyomas have been associated with ectopic pregnancy. Most of these abnormalities are bilateral and irreversible.

B. Zygote Abnormalities

A variety of zygote abnormalities have been reported in ectopic pregnancy, including chromosomal abnormalities, gross malformations, and neural tube defects. The theory is that these abnormal preembryos are more likely to result in abnormal or ectopic implantation.

C. Ovarian Factors

Ovarian factors that may result in the development of an ectopic pregnancy are fertilization of an unextruded ovum, transmigration of the ovum into the contralateral tube with subsequent delayed and faulty implantation, and postmidcycle ovulation and fertilization.

D. Exogenous Hormones

Abnormal hormonal stimulation and/or exogenous hormones may play a role in ectopic gestation. For example, of pregnancies occurring in women taking progestin-only oral contraceptives, 4–6% are ectopic pregnancies. This may be due to progesterone's smooth muscle relaxant effects and subsequent "ovum trapping." Patients with DES exposure are also at risk, as are patients undergoing ovulation induction.

E. Other Factors

Intrauterine device (IUD) users are also at risk for ectopic pregnancy if pregnancy occurs, although the risk of ectopic pregnancy is still lower than if no contraceptive method is used. Whether the IUD prevents intrauterine but not ectopic pregnancy or whether an associated salpingitis is responsible for this increased risk is unclear. Smoking and increasing age are also associated with ectopic pregnancy. Multiple previous elective abortions are also felt to be a risk factor for ectopic pregnancy, as postabortal infection may lead to salpingitis.

Time of Rupture

Rupture is usually spontaneous. Isthmic pregnancies tend to rupture earliest, at 6 to 8 weeks' gestation, due to the small diameter of this portion of the tube. Ampullary pregnancies rupture later, generally at 8–12 weeks. Interstitial pregnancies are the last to rupture, usually at 12–16 weeks, as the myometrium allows more room to grow than the tubal wall. Interstitial rupture is quite dangerous, as its proximity to uterine and ovarian vessels can result in massive hemorrhage.

After rupture, the conceptus may be resorbed or remain as a mass in the abdominal cavity or cul-de-sac. Rarely, if not damaged during rupture, it may implant elsewhere in the abdominal cavity and continue to grow.

Clinical Findings

No specific symptoms or signs are pathognomonic for ectopic pregnancy, and many disorders can present similarly. Normal pregnancy, threatened or incomplete abortion, rupture of an ovarian cyst, ovarian torsion, gastroenteritis, and appendicitis can all be confused with ectopic pregnancy. Since early diagnosis is crucial, a high index of suspicion should be maintained when any pregnant woman in the first trimester presents with bleeding and/or abdominal pain. Fifteen to twenty percent of ectopic gestations will present as surgical emergencies.

A. Symptoms

The following symptoms may assist in the diagnosis of ectopic pregnancy.

1. Pain—Pelvic or abdominal pain is present in close to 100% of cases. Pain can be unilateral or bilateral, localized or generalized. The presence of subdiaphragmatic or shoulder pain is more variable, depending on the amount of intraabdominal bleeding.

2. Bleeding—Abnormal uterine bleeding, usually spotting, occurs in roughly 75% of cases, and represents decidual sloughing.

3. Amenorrhea—Secondary amenorrhea is variable. Approximately half of women with ectopic pregnancies have some spotting at the time of their expected menses, and thus do not realize they are pregnant.

4. Syncope—Dizziness, lightheadedness, and/or syncope is present in one-third to one-half of cases.

5. Decidual cast—A decidual cast is passed in 5–10% of ectopic pregnancies, and may be mistaken for products of conception.

B. Signs

On examination, the following signs are important in the diagnosis of ectopic gestation.

1. Tenderness—Diffuse or localized abdominal tenderness is present in over 80% of ectopic pregnancies. Adnexal and/or cervical motion tenderness is present in over 75% of cases.

2. Adnexal mass—A unilateral adnexal mass is palpated in one-third to one-half of patients. Occasionally, a cul-de-sac mass is present. However, the patient's discomfort may preclude an adequate examination.

3. Uterine changes—The uterus may undergo typical changes of pregnancy, including softening and a slight increase in size.

Laboratory Findings

Hematocrit: The hematocrit will vary depending on the patient population and the degree, if any, of intra-abdominal bleeding.

White blood count: The white blood count is variable, and it is not uncommon to see a leukocytosis.

Pregnancy tests: The β-hCG is positive in virtually 100% of ectopic pregnancies. However, a positive test only confirms pregnancy and does not indicate whether it is intrauterine or extrauterine. In normal pregnancy, β-hCG should double every 2 days. However, while two-thirds of ectopic pregnancies have abnormal serial titers, the remaining third show a normal progression. Ultrasound is often helpful in differentiating ectopic from intrauterine pregnancy.

Special Examinations

Several special procedures are helpful in diagnosing ectopic pregnancy.

1. Ultrasound—Ultrasound is useful in evaluating patients at risk for ectopic pregnancy, namely by documenting the presence or absence of an intrauterine pregnancy (IUP). β-hCG titers and ultrasound complement one another in detecting ectopic pregnancy, and have led to earlier detection with a subsequent decrease in adverse outcome. By correlating β-hCG titers with ultrasound findings, an ectopic pregnancy can often be differentiated from an IUP. Furthermore, ultrasound can help distinguish a normal intrauterine pregnancy from a blighted ovum, incomplete abortion, or complete abortion.

A normal intrauterine sac appears regular and well-defined on ultrasound. It has been described as a "double ring," which represents the decidual lining and the amniotic sac. In ectopic pregnancy, ultrasound may reveal only a thickened, decidualized endometrium. With more advanced ectopics, decidual sloughing with resultant intracavitary fluid or blood may create a so-called "pseudogestational sac." This sac is small and irregular as compared to a true gestational sac, but at times can be confused with a normal sac.

An intrauterine sac should be visible by transvaginal ultrasound when the β-hCG is approximately 1000 mIU/mL, and by transabdominal ultrasound approximately 1 week later, when the β-hCG is 1800–3600 mIU/mL. Thus, when an empty uterine cavity is seen with a β-hCG titer above this threshold, the patient is likely to have an ectopic pregnancy. An empty cavity is less of a concern when a β-hCG below the threshold is

obtained, as this may be associated with an ectopic pregnancy, but may also be seen with an early IUP.

The presence of an adnexal mass with an empty uterus is also of concern. If the β-hCG is low, this may represent an early IUP with a corpus luteum cyst. However, if the β-hCG is above the discriminatory value, an ectopic is likely. A "tubal ring" seen on ultrasound may represent an unruptured ectopic, with a gestational sac and sometimes embryo surrounded by a distorted fallopian tube. This complex is seen adjacent to but separate from both the uterus and ovary. If rupture has occurred, ultrasound may reveal a dilated fallopian tube with fluid in the cul-de-sac.

2. Laparoscopy—The need for laparoscopy in the diagnosis of ectopic pregnancy has declined with the increasing use of ultrasound. It is still useful, however, in certain situations when a definitive diagnosis is difficult, especially in the case of a desired, potentially viable intrauterine pregnancy when a D&C is contraindicated. Laparoscopy may also be used as definitive management in early ectopic gestation.

3. D&C—D&C may confirm or exclude intrauterine pregnancy in the case of an undesired pregnancy. D&C may interrupt an intrauterine gestation and should not be performed if the pregnancy is desired, unless the β-hCG titers have plateaued or fallen and the pregnancy is definitely abnormal. When chorionic villi are recovered, the diagnosis of an intrauterine pregnancy is confirmed. On the other hand, if only decidua is obtained on D&C, ectopic pregnancy is highly likely.

4. Laparotomy—Laparotomy is indicated when the presumptive diagnosis of ectopic pregnancy in an unstable patient necessitates immediate surgery, or when definitive therapy is not possible by medical management or laparoscopy.

5. Culdocentesis—Culdocentesis is the transvaginal passage of a needle into the posterior cul-de-sac in order to determine whether free blood is present in the abdomen (Fig 14–8). The procedure is simple and safe and may be useful in the diagnosis of intraperitoneal bleeding. It is generally accomplished with the unanesthetized patient in the dorsal lithotomy position. A speculum is placed in the vagina and the posterior lip of the cervix grasped with a tenaculum. The vagina is cleansed. An 18-gauge spinal needle is attached to a 10-mL syringe, and with gentle traction on the cervix, the needle is passed into the cul-de-sac.

This procedure will reveal nonclotting blood if intra-abdominal bleeding has occurred. If the blood clots, it is likely from a punctured vessel in the vaginal wall. Usually, the cul-de-sac will contain some straw-colored fluid, and this may be used to determine if the needle has been properly placed when there is no bleed-

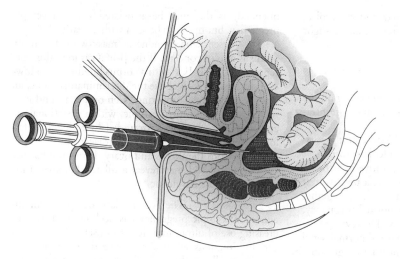

Figure 14–8. Culdocentesis.

ing. If culdocentesis is positive, laparoscopy or laparotomy should be performed immediately. Indeed, some argue that the main purpose of culdocentesis is to better prioritize patients so that those with positive culdocenteses are taken immediately to the operating room.

Although nonclotting blood is assumed to be from a ruptured ectopic, similar results can also be obtained under other circumstances (eg, a hemorrhagic corpus luteum), and thus a positive result is not diagnostic of a ruptured ectopic pregnancy. Furthermore, a negative result may rule out a ruptured or leaking ectopic but not an intact one.

Pathology

In tubal ectopic pregnancy, implantation is typically in the wall of the tube, in the connective tissue beneath the serosa. There may be little or no decidual reaction and minimal defense against the permeating trophoblast. The trophoblast invades blood vessels to cause local hemorrhage. A hematoma in the subserosal space enlarges as pregnancy progresses. Distention of the tube then predisposes to rupture.

Bleeding is of uterine origin and is caused by endometrial involution and decidual sloughing. Atypical changes in the endometrium may be suggestive of ectopic pregnancy. The Arias-Stella reaction consists of hyperchromatic, hypertrophic, irregularly-shaped nuclei, and foamy, vacuolated cytoplasm. These changes can also be seen in normal pregnancy and in miscarriage, and are therefore not diagnostic of ectopic pregnancy.

Occasionally, endometrial tissue may be passed as a so-called decidual cast. Superficial secretory endometrium usually is present, but no trophoblastic cells

are seen. Grossly, this can be confused with passage of products of conception and spontaneous abortion.

Prevention

Prevention of sexually transmitted disease, with early and vigorous treatment of cases that do occur, may avoid tubal damage with subsequent ectopic pregnancy. Other risk factors for ectopic pregnancy are more difficult to control. Early diagnosis of unruptured tubal pregnancy by maintaining a high index of suspicion, and liberally using β-hCG titers, ultrasound, and laparoscopy will minimize potential problems from hemorrhage, infertility, and extensive surgery.

Treatment

A. EXPECTANT MANAGEMENT

Because many ectopic pregnancies resolve spontaneously, it may be reasonable to manage an asymptomatic, compliant patient expectantly if β-hCG titers are low (< 200 mIU/mL) or decreasing, and the risk of rupture is low.

B. SURGICAL TREATMENT

The extent of surgery depends on the degree of damage to the uterus and adnexae. Preservation of the ovary should be attempted if feasible. Conservative surgery (ie, preservation of the fallopian tube) may be indicated in the hemodynamically stable patient with an ampullary pregnancy who wishes to preserve fertility.

A linear salpingostomy may be performed with a small (< 3 cm), intact ampullary pregnancy. The linear incision is allowed to heal by secondary intention. A linear salpingotomy involves closure of the incision and may be recommended in similar situations. Subsequent reproductive performance is comparable, with intrauterine pregnancy rates of 40–90%, but recurrent ectopic rates may be higher, up to 16%.

If the physician is competent in operative laparoscopy, both of these procedures can be performed through the laparoscope, assuming the pregnancy is < 3 cm, unruptured, and easily accessible. With both salpingostomy and salpingotomy, a β-hCG titer should be obtained weekly after surgery to ensure adequate removal of trophoblast and rule out a persistent ectopic. In stable patients, laparoscopy is preferred over laparotomy because of the associated reduction in morbidity and cost.

"Milking" the pregnancy out of the distal end of the tube is often tempting, but this has been associated with persistent trophoblast and need for reexploration, as well as increased risks of recurrent ectopic pregnancy.

With an isthmic ectopic pregnancy, segmental resection with subsequent anastomosis (usually at a later date) is typically recommended. As opposed to ampullary ectopics, the muscularis is well-developed, forcing the pregnancy to grow in the lumen. More conservative treatment such as salpingostomy or salpingotomy would likely cause scarring and compromise of the lumen. Furthermore, a tubal fistula may result if the tube were allowed to heal by secondary intention.

With fimbrial pregnancy, products of conception are often visible at the most distal end of the tube, which may be "plucked out." As with ampullary ectopics, "milking" should be avoided.

Interstitial pregnancies require at least a cornual wedge resection, with uterine reconstruction and sometimes salpingectomy on the affected side. If there has been extensive tissue damage or if the patient is unstable, a hysterectomy may be needed.

Cervical ectopics may be associated with massive hemorrhage and may mandate hysterectomy. Attempts at medical management with methotrexate should be considered. Ovarian pregnancy requires oophorectomy and sometimes salpingectomy on the affected side. Abdominal pregnancy involves delivery of the fetus (sometimes at term) with ligation of the umbilical cord close to the placenta. The placenta is usually left in place to avoid hemorrhage following removal.

C. Emergency Treatment

Immediate surgery is indicated when the diagnosis of ectopic pregnancy with hemorrhage is made. Blood products should be available as transfusion is often necessary. There is no place for conservative therapy in a hemodynamically unstable patient.

D. Medical Management

Methotrexate (MTX), a folinic acid antagonist, has been shown to destroy proliferating trophoblast and may be effective in the medical management of small, unruptured ectopic pregnancies in asymptomatic women. Exclusion criteria include a noncompliant patient, peptic ulcer disease, immunodeficiency, pulmonary disease, liver disease, renal disease, blood dyscrasias, hemodynamic instability, free fluid in the cul-de-sac plus pelvic pain, or known sensitivity to MTX. Relative contraindications include an adnexal mass ≥ 3.5 cm or an extrauterine gestation with fetal heart motion, because of the higher failure rate. In select cases, approximately 90% of ectopics resolve, taking on average just under 1 month. Protocols vary from single to multiple injections, typically given systemically. The dose of MTX depends on the patient's body surface area, and nomograms are available for determining the correct dose. Follow-up β-hCG levels, along with a complete blood count, serum creatinine, and serum aspartate transaminase are obtained, for comparison with baseline values. β-hCG levels should decrease by at least 15% 4–7 days after MTX administration. Failure of MTX therapy is suggested by a persistent rise or plateau in β-hCG titer, worsening pain in conjunction with a hemoperitoneum on ultrasound, and/or hemodynamic instability, and demands either another dose of MTX or surgery. Available studies comparing MTX to traditional surgical management report similar subsequent tubal patency and fertility rates. Arguments against its use include its toxicity, namely marrow suppression, dermatitis, and stomatitis, as well as potential for treatment failure and tubal rupture.

Chronic ectopics, with decreasing but persistent β-hCG titers, pose a management dilemma. Some will resolve on their own, while others will require surgery. Unfortunately, at present it is impossible to predict which patients will fail expectant management.

Rho (D) immune globulin should be given to any Rh-negative mother with the diagnosis of ectopic pregnancy, as sensitization can occur just as with intrauterine pregnancy.

EXPOSURE TO FETOTOXIC AGENTS

Many variations occur in the complex process of human development. Although population heterogeneity is based on such events, some deviations from the usual developmental process result in aberrations of normal structure and function. These adverse alterations have been scrutinized in an effort to determine their cause. The clinician investigating the effects of exposure to fetotoxic agents must consider whether the patient is known to have reproductive risks, whether there has been exposure to fetotoxic agents during pregnancy, and whether structural or functional abnormalities are likely to develop in the fetus.

Many harmful agents are responsible for altering the biologic process of human development (eg, radiation, viruses, medications, and drugs). Aberrations that result from fetal exposure to harmful agents is especially tragic because such exposure is often preventable. However, even the most careful investigation will fail to reveal the cause in the majority of developmental handicaps.

Approximately 3–5% of newborns in the United States have abnormalities at birth that are serious enough to require some form of treatment. Moreover, full recognition of malformations, anomalies, or defects may take years. Thus, estimates that as much as 10% of the total population suffer from some structural or functional developmental disability do not appear unreasonable.

Evaluation

The timing of exposure is crucial, as fetal organs or structures are most vulnerable to adverse influences during organogenesis. Table 14–4 lists some of the potential adverse effects related to the timing of fetotoxic exposure. The route of exposure, the length of time that the exposure occurred, and the total dose received during exposure may also influence the outcome of the pregnancy.

Evaluation of studies of potential toxic exposures is difficult owing to the large number of possible fetotoxic agents and interactive effects of certain agents, the retrospective nature of most studies, the difficulty evaluating damage, the presence or absence of influences that may alter the effects of an agent, and the presence or absence of certain genotypes that might alter an individual's susceptibility. Therefore, specific criteria to recognize teratogens in humans have been defined (Table 14–5). The known mechanisms of abnormal development are summarized in Table 14–6, which also outlines a working hypothesis of the pathogenesis, common pathways, and final manifestations of abnormal development.

Table 14–4. Potential adverse effects of fetotoxic exposure at selected stages of development.

Week Since Ovulation	Potential Adverse Effect
1–8	Miscarriage, structural malformations
9–40	Central nervous system abnormalities, growth restrictions, neurobehavioral abnormalities, reproductive effects

Modified and reproduced, with permission, from Pernoll ML: Abortion induced by chemicals encountered in the environment. Clin Obstet Gynecol 1986;29:955.

Table 14–5. Criteria used to recognize teratogens in humans.

Abrupt increase in the incidence of a particular defect or association of defects
Known environmental change coincident with this increase.
Known exposure to the environmental change early in pregnancy, yielding characteristically affected infants.
Absence of other factors common to all pregnancies, yielding infants with the characteristic defects.

Modified and reproduced, with permission, from Wilson JG: Embryotoxicity of drugs in man. In: *Handbook of Teratology.* Vol 1. Wilson JG, Fraser FC (editors). Plenum Press, 1977.

Counseling of the parents should include review of the exposure history and discussion of the particular agent involved, as well as possible sequelae. In some cases, intervention may be possible. In other cases, if an abnormal pregnancy is found, the parents may elect to abort an affected fetus. Effective counseling should pro-

Table 14–6. General principles of teratology.

Mechanisms	Mutation
	Chromosome disruption
	Mitotic interference
	Altered nucleic acid integrity or function
	Precursor or substrate deprivation
	Altered energy sources
	Changed membrane characteristics
	Altered osmolar balance
	Enzyme inhibition
Pathogenesis	Excessive or reduced cell interactions
	Failed cell interactions
	Reproduced biosynthesis
	Impeded morphogenetic movement
	Mechanical disruption of tissues
Common pathways	Too few cells or cell products to affect localized morphogenesis or functional maturation
	Other imbalances in growth and differentiation
Final defects	Malformation
	Growth retardation
	Functional disorder
	Death

Modified and reproduced, with permission, from Wilson JG: Current status of teratology: General principles and mechanisms derived from animal studies. In: *Handbook of Teratology.* Vol 1. Wilson JG, Fraser FC (editors): Plenum Press, 1977.

Table 14–7. Teratogenicity drug labeling now required by FDA.[1]

Category A: Well-controlled human studies have not disclosed any fetal risk.

Category B: Animal studies have not disclosed any fetal risk; or have suggested some risk not confirmed in controlled studies in women; or there are not adequate studies in women.

Category C: Animal studies have revealed adverse fetal effects; there are no adequate controlled studies in women.

Category D: Some fetal risk, but benefits may outweigh risk (eg, life-threatening illness, no safer effective drug).

Category X: Fetal abnormalities in animal and human studies; risk not outweighed by benefit. *Contraindicated in pregnancy.*

----

[1]The FDA has established 5 categories of drugs based on their potential for causing birth defects in infants born to women who use them during pregnancy. By law, the label must provide available information on teratogenicity.

vide the best information available to assist the parents in what is always a very difficult decision.

The FDA standards for drug labeling with regard to teratogenicity are listed in Table 14–7.

REFERENCES

American College of Obstetricians and Gynecologists: ACOG Technical Bulletin No. 212. Early pregnancy loss. September 1995.

American College of Obstetricians and Gynecologists: ACOG Practice Bulletin No 3. Medical management of tubal pregnancy. December 1998.

Centers for Disease Control and Prevention: Current Trends Ectopic Pregnancy—United States, 1990–1992. MMWR 1995;44:46.

Pisarska MD, Carson SA, Buster JE: Ectopic pregnancy. Lancet 1998;351:1115.

Regan L: Prospective study of spontaneous abortion. In: Beard RW, Sharp F (editors). *Early Pregnancy Loss: Mechanisms and Treatment.* Roy Coll Obstet Gynaecol, 1988.

Tulandi T: New protocols for ectopic pregnancy. Contemp Ob-Gyn 1999;44:42.

Yao M, Tulandi T: Current status of surgical and nonsurgical management of ectopic pregnancy. Fertil Steril 1997;67:421.

Late Pregnancy Complications

Ashley S. Roman, MD, MPH, & Martin L. Pernoll, MD

PRETERM LABOR

ESSENTIALS OF DIAGNOSIS

- *Estimated gestational age of greater than 20 weeks and less than 37 weeks.*
- *Regular uterine contractions at frequent intervals.*
- *Documented cervical change or appreciable cervical dilation or effacement (at least 2 cm without previous examination).*

General Considerations

Labor is the process of coordinated uterine contractions leading to progressive cervical effacement and dilatation by which the fetus and placenta are expelled. Preterm labor is defined as labor occurring after 20 weeks' but before 37 weeks' gestation. Although there is no strict definition in the literature regarding the amount of uterine contractions required for preterm labor, there is consensus that contractions need to be regular and at frequent intervals. Generally, more than 4 contractions an hour are needed to cause cervical change. Furthermore, there must be demonstrated cervical effacement or dilation. The uterine contractions need not be painful to cause cervical change and may manifest themselves as abdominal tightening, lower back pain, or pelvic pressure.

It is important to distinguish preterm labor from other similar clinical entities such as cervical incompetence (cervical change in the absence of uterine contractions) and preterm uterine contractions (regular contractions in the absence of cervical change) because the treatment for these situations differs vastly. Cervical incompetence may require cerclage placement, and preterm uterine contractions without cervical change is generally a self-limited phenomenon that resolves spontaneously and requires no intervention. If ruptured membranes accompany preterm labor, these cases are classified as preterm premature rupture of membranes, a diagnosis that will be discussed later in this chapter.

Preterm labor complicates 10–15% of all pregnancies. It is the number one cause of neonatal morbidity and mortality and causes 75% of neonatal deaths that are not due to congenital anomalies.

Rates of morbidity and mortality in premature infants are high (80% of all perinatal deaths in some institutions). Thirteen percent of infants are classified as having low birthweight (< 2500 g). Three percent of these are mature low-birthweight infants, and about 10% are truly premature. The latter group accounts for nearly two-thirds of infant deaths (approximately 25,000 in the United States annually). One to three percent of premature births are due to miscalculation of gestational age or to medical intervention needed by the mother or fetus.

The care of premature (birthweight 1000–2500 g) and immature (birthweight < 1000 g) infants is costly. Compared with term infants, those born prematurely suffer greatly increased morbidity and mortality (eg, functional disorders, abnormalities of growth and development). Thus, every effort is made to prevent or inhibit premature labor. If preterm labor cannot be inhibited or is best allowed to continue, it should be conducted with the least possible trauma to the mother and infant.

Pathogenesis

Many obstetric, medical, and anatomic disorders are associated with preterm labor. Some of these are shown in Table 15–1. Detailed discussions of these conditions are given in other chapters. The cause of preterm labor in 50% of pregnancies, however, is idiopathic. Although several prospective risk-scoring tools are in use, they have not been convincingly demonstrated to be of value.

Clinical Findings

A. SYMPTOMS AND SIGNS

1. **Uterine contractions**—Regular uterine contractions at frequent intervals as documented by tocometer or uterine palpation, generally more than two in one-half hour.

2. **Dilatation and effacement of cervix**—Documented cervical change in dilation or effacement of at

Table 15–1. Risk factors associated with preterm labor.

Obstetric complications
In previous or current pregnancy
    Severe hypertensive state of pregnancy
    Anatomic disorders of the placenta (eg, abruptio placentae, placenta previa, circumvallate placenta)
    Placental insufficiency
    Premature rupture of membranes
    Polyhydramnios or oligohydramnios
Previous premature or low-birth-weight infant
Low socioeconomic status
Maternal age < 18 years or > 40 years
Low prepregnancy weight
Non-Caucasian race
Multiple pregnancy
Short interval between pregnancies (< 3 months)
Inadequate or excessive weight gain during pregnancy
Previous abortion
Previous laceration of cervix or uterus
Medical complications
Pulmonary or systemic hypertension
Renal disease
Heart disease
Infection: pyelonephritis, acute systemic infection, urinary tract infection, genital tract infection (eg, gonorrhea, herpes simplex, mycoplasmosis), feto-toxic infection (eg, cytomegalovirus infection, toxoplasmosis, listeriosis), maternal systemic infection (eg, pneumonia, influenza, malaria), maternal intra-abdominal sepsis (eg, appendicitis, cholecystitis, diverticulitis)
Heavy cigarette smoking
Alcoholism or drug addiction
Severe anemia
Malnutrition or obesity
Leaking benign cystic teratoma
Perforated gastric or duodenal ulcer
Adnexal torsion
Maternal trauma or burns
Surgical complications
Any intra-abdominal procedure
Conization of cervix
Previous incision in uterus or cervix (eg, cesarean delivery)
Genital tract anomalies
Bicornuate, subseptate, or unicornuate uterus
Congenital cervical incompetency

least 1 cm or a cervix that is well-effaced and dilated (at least 2 cm) on admission is considered diagnostic.

3. Vaginal bleeding—Many patients present with bloody mucous vaginal discharge or "bloody show." More significant vaginal bleeding should be evaluated for abruptio placentae or placenta previa.

B. Evaluation

Evaluation should include determination of the following:

1. Gestational age—Gestational age must be between 20 and 37 weeks' estimated gestational age (EGA) which should be calculated by the patient's last menstrual period or date of conception, if known, or by previous sonographic estimation if these dates are uncertain.

2. Fetal weight—Care must be taken to determine fetal size by ultrasonography.

3. Presenting part—The presenting part must be noted because abnormal presentation is more common in earlier stages of gestation.

4. Fetal monitoring—Continuous fetal monitoring should be performed to ascertain fetal well-being.

C. Laboratory Studies

1. Complete blood count with differential.

2. Urine obtained by catheter for urinalysis, culture, and sensitivity testing.

3. Ultrasound examination for fetal size, position, and placental location.

4. Amniocentesis may be useful to ascertain fetal lung maturity in instances where EGA is uncertain, the size of the fetus is in conflict with the estimated date of conception (EDC) (too small, suggesting IUGR, or too large, suggesting more advanced EGA), or the fetus is more than 34 weeks' EGA. Specifically, the amniotic fluid should be tested for L/S ratio, phosphatidylglycerol levels, and lamellar body count. Amniocentesis should also be performed in instances in which chorioamnionitis is suspected, and the fluid should be tested for Gram's stain, bacterial culture, glucose levels, cell count, and IL-6 level.

5. Speculum examination should be performed. Cervical cultures should be sent for gonorrhea and chlamydia. A wet mount should be performed to look for signs of bacterial vaginosis. Group B streptococcus cultures should be taken from the vaginal and rectal mucosa.

6. Hematologic work-up in cases associated with hemorrhage (see Chapter 20).

7. Fetal fibronectin enzyme immunoassay kits have been approved by the FDA as a means to predict preterm birth in patients with preterm labor. A cervical swab is taken to look for fetal fibronectin. A negative test is effective at ruling out imminent delivery (within 2 weeks). A positive test, however, is less sensitive at predicting preterm birth.

Because of this limitation, the fibronectin swab is not in wide use.

Treatment

The patient diagnosed with preterm labor should be observed for 30–60 minutes to determine appropriate management. A longer period of observation is not desirable, because the effectiveness of therapy diminishes as labor advances. Decisions regarding management are made based on estimated gestational age, estimated weight of the fetus, and whether contraindications exist to suppressing preterm labor. Table 15–2 shows factors indicating that preterm labor should be allowed to continue. Once it has been determined that the patient does not have any of these contraindications, the management of preterm labor depends on fetal age and size. Generally, management falls into one of two categories: expectant management (observation) or intervention. In pregnancies between 24 and 34 weeks' EGA or estimated fetal weight (EFW) between 600 and 2500 g, intervention with corticosteroids and tocolysis has been shown to be of benefit in reducing fetal morbidity and mortality rates.

Extremes of preterm gestational age pose special problems. Fetuses of very preterm pregnancies, 20–24 weeks EGA or EFW less than 600 g, are not considered to be viable. If these pregnancies can be continued for several more weeks, the fetuses will become viable, but they have a high risk of significant morbidity if they survive. Furthermore, intervention carries significant risks to the mother, including the risks of prolonged bed rest and potentially toxic side effects of tocolysis. Given these risks, expectant management is an acceptable and, in certain instances, preferable alternative to intervention. Mothers who choose intervention as opposed to expectant management should be extensively counseled by a multidisciplinary team, including the neonatologist, obstetrician, and social worker.

Conversely, once a pregnancy has continued beyond 34–37 weeks' EGA or EFW greater than 2500 g, the fetal survival rate is within 1% of the survival rate at 37 weeks. Fetal morbidity is less severe and is rarely a cause of long-term sequelae. Furthermore, corticosteroids have not been shown to be of benefit in fetuses of this age or size. Therefore expectant management is usually the recommended course of action. Several factors should be considered when deciding between intervention and expectant management, including the certainty of the patient's dates, estimated fetal weight, the presence of maternal problems that could delay fetal lung maturity such as diabetes mellitus, and a family history of late-onset respiratory distress syndrome (RDS).

There are other cases in which maternal or fetal factors indicate that preterm labor should be allowed to continue regardless of gestational age. Table 15–2 lists these in detail.

The following is a protocol for management of pregnancies with preterm labor between 24 and 34 weeks' gestation or EFW 600–2500 g:

A. HYDRATION AND BED REST

A regimen of hydration and bed rest should be instituted immediately upon presentation.

B. CORTICOSTEROIDS

The administration of corticosteroids to accelerate fetal lung maturity has become the standard of care in the United States for all women at risk of preterm delivery between 24 and 34 weeks' EGA. It has been shown to decrease the incidence of neonatal respiratory distress, intraventricular hemorrhage, and neonatal mortality. Steroids can be given according to one of two protocols: (1) Betamethasone 12 mg IM every 24 hours for a total of 2 doses; or (2) dexamethasone 6 mg IM every 12 hours for a total of 4 doses.

The optimal benefits of antenatal corticosteroids are seen 24 hours after administration, peak at 48 hours, and continue for approximately 7 days. If therapy for preterm labor is successful and the pregnancy continues beyond 1 week, there appears to be no added benefit with repeated courses of corticosteroids. In fact, multiple courses may be associated with delayed psychomotor development in the infant. In terms of safety of a single course of antenatal steroids, there does not ap-

Table 15–2. Some cases in which preterm labor should not be suppressed.

Maternal factors
Severe hypertensive disease (eg, acute exacerbation of chronic hypertension, eclampsia, severe preeclampsia)
Pulmonary or cardiac disease (eg, pulmonary edema, adult respiratory distress syndrome, valvular disease, tachyarrhythmias)
Advanced cervical dilation (> 4 cm)
Maternal hemorrhage (eg, abruptio placentae, placenta previa, disseminated intravascular coagulation)
Fetal factors
Fetal death or lethal anomaly
Fetal distress
Intrauterine infection (chorioamnionitis)
Therapy adversely affecting the fetus (eg, fetal distress due to attempted suppression of labor)
Estimated fetal weight ≥ 2500 g
Erythroblastosis fetalis
Severe intrauterine growth retardation

---

pear to be an increased risk of infection or suppression of the fetal adrenal glands with steroid administration, and long-term follow-up of fetuses who received antenatal steroids shows no sequelae that can be attributed directly to steroid administration.

C. Tocolysis

If the patient continues to contract despite hydration and bed rest, tocolytic therapy should be initiated. When using tocolysis to treat preterm labor, it is important to keep the following goals in mind. The short-term goal is to continue the pregnancy for 48 hours after steroid administration, after which the maximum effect of the steroids can be achieved. The long-term goal is to continue the pregnancy beyond 34–37 weeks (depending on the institution), at which point fetal morbidity and mortality is dramatically reduced and tocolysis can be discontinued.

Tocolytic therapy should be considered in the patient with cervical dilation less than 5 cm. Successful tocolysis is generally considered fewer than 4–6 uterine contractions per hour without further cervical change.

Compared with 10 years ago, there are twice as many different kinds of effective tocolytics in routine use today. The beta-mimetics and magnesium sulfate are the most commonly used tocolytic agents. The decision to use a specific tocolytic should be carefully considered because there are contraindications and side effects associated with each agent (Table 15-3).

1. Beta-mimetic adrenergic agents—Beta-mimetic adrenergic agents act directly on beta receptors (β_2) to relax the uterus and uterine vessels. Their use is limited by dose-related major cardiovascular side effects, including pulmonary edema, adult respiratory distress syndrome, elevated systolic and reduced diastolic blood

Table 15–3. Side effects and complications of common tocolytics.

Tocolytic	Maternal Effects	Fetal/Neonatal Effects
Beta-mimetics (ritodrine, terbutaline)	Pulmonary edema Hypotension Tachycardia Nausea/vomiting Hyperglycemia Hypokalemia Cardiac arrhythmias	Tachycardia Hyperglycemia Hypoglycemia Ileus Possible increased risk for intraventricular hemorrhage
Magnesium sulfate	Flushing Nausea/vomiting Headache Generalized muscle weakness Shortness of breath Diplopia Pulmonary edema Chest pain Hypotension Tetany Respiratory depression	Lethargy Hypotonia Respiratory depression
Indomethacin	Gastrointestinal effects: Nausea/vomiting, heartburn, bleeding Coagulation disturbances Thrombocytopenia Renal failure Hepatitis Elevated blood pressure in hypertensive patients	Renal dysfunction Oligohydramnios Pulmonary hypertension Postpartum patent ductus arteriosus Premature constriction of ductus arteriosus in utero Increased risk for necrotizing enterocolitis and intraventricular hemorrhage
Nifedipine	Hypotension Tachycardia Headache Flushing Dizziness Nausea/vomiting	Tachycardia Hypotension

pressure, and both maternal and fetal tachycardia. Other dose-related effects are decreased serum potassium and increased blood glucose, plasma insulin, and lactic acidosis. Maternal medical contraindications to the use of beta-adrenergic agents include cardiac disease, hyperthyroidism, uncontrolled hypertension or pulmonary hypertension, asthma requiring sympathomimetic drugs or corticosteroids for relief, uncontrolled diabetes, and chronic hepatic or renal disease. Commonly observed effects during intravenous administration are palpitations, tremors, nervousness, and restlessness. Beta-mimetics in common use are ritodrine and terbutaline.

a. Ritodrine—Ritodrine is the standard by which other agents are judged because it is the most studied beta-mimetic. Ritodrine has largely fallen out of use, however, as terbutaline, a very similar medication, has grown in popularity. Terbutaline has replaced ritodrine as the beta-mimetic of choice in the treatment of preterm labor because of its ease of administration.

b. Terbutaline—Although not approved by the FDA, terbutaline has been studied in the United States and used widely as a tocolytic agent. The mode of action is similar to that of ritodrine, and the precautions and contraindications are the same. It can be administered intravenously, subcutaneously, or by mouth. But unlike ritodrine, there are no manufacturer's guidelines for its use as a tocolytic. A bolus of 250 µg followed by 10–80 µg/min until labor stops may be effective. The drug is then administered subcutaneously, 0.25–0.5 mg every 2–4 hours for 12 hours. A maintenance dose of 2.5–5 mg may be given orally 4–6 times a day.

2. Magnesium sulfate—Although its exact mechanism of action is unknown, magnesium sulfate appears to inhibit calcium uptake into smooth muscle cells, reducing uterine contractility. Apparently less effective than ritodrine or terbutaline, magnesium sulfate is better tolerated than beta-mimetics and, as a result, has become the first-line agent for tocolysis in many institutions. A protocol for use of magnesium sulfate is shown in Table 15–4. Magnesium sulfate may appear less likely to cause serious side effects than the beta-mimetics, but its therapeutic range is close to the range in which it will cause respiratory and cardiac depression. Therefore, patients on magnesium sulfate should be monitored closely for signs of toxicity with frequent checks of deep tendon reflexes, pulmonary exams, and strict calculations of the patient's fluid balance. These effects may be reversed by calcium gluconate (10 mL of a 10% solution given intravenously), and this antidote should be kept at the bedside when magnesium sulfate is used.

Table 15–4. Protocol for use of magnesium sulfate in suppression of preterm labor.

Criteria for admission to protocol

Preterm labor has been confirmed.

Gestational age of 20–34 weeks has been confirmed.

Examinations and tests have ruled out any cases of maternal or fetal diseases or disorders in which it would be best to allow labor to continue.

Any specific contraindications to magnesium sulfate therapy have been ruled out.

Protocol

Begin intravenous infusion of magnesium sulfate, 4 g (40 mL of 10% solution). The rate of infusion should be slow enough to prevent flushing or vomiting. Then, continuous infusion of magnesium sulfate should be started at 2 g per hour (magnesium sulfate 10% solution, 200 mL, in 5% dextrose, 800 mL, at a rate of 100 mL/h). This infusion can be titrated up by increments of 0.5 g per hour to a maximum of 4.0 g per hour until adequate tocolysis is achieved (< 4–6 uterine contractions per hour). Infusion should be continued until labor subsides or progresses to an irreversible stage (cervical dilation of 5 cm).

Reduce the rate of infusion if magnesium toxicity is observed.

Protocol for recurrent preterm labor

If contraindications recur after discontinuation of the infusion, the procedure may be repeated.

3. Calcium channel blockers—Calcium channel blockers such as nifedipine work as tocolytics by inhibiting calcium uptake into uterine smooth muscle cells via voltage-dependent channels, thereby reducing uterine contractility. Many studies have shown nifedipine to be equally or more efficacious than beta-mimetics in preterm labor. Other advantages are its low incidence of maternal side effects and ease of administration. Nifedipine can be given by mouth or sublingually. A common regimen for tocolysis is nifedipine 20 mg by mouth then 10–20 mg by mouth every 6 hours until the patient is well tocolyzed.

4. Prostaglandin synthetase inhibitors—Prostaglandin synthetase inhibitors such as indomethacin have been shown to be as effective as ritodrine for tocolysis, but their use has been limited by potentially serious fetal effects. Indomethacin works as a tocolytic by inhibiting prostaglandin synthesis, an important mediator in uterine smooth muscle contractility. The advantages of indomethacin are its ease of administration (it can be given by rectum or by mouth) and its potent tocolytic activity. But it has been shown to cause oligohydramnios, premature closure of the ductus arteriosus, and in preterm infants delivered at less than 30 weeks' EGA, an increased risk of intracranial hemorrhage, necrotizing enterocolitis, and patent ductus arteriosus after birth. A common regimen for tocolysis is indomethacin 100 mg per rectum loading dose (or 50 mg by mouth), then 25–50 mg by mouth or rectum every 4–6 hours. Ultrasound should be performed every 48–72 hours to check for oligohydramnios. Because of the potentially serious fetal effects, many centers limit its use to infants less than 32 weeks' EGA and its duration of use to less than 48 hours.

5. Treatment with multiple tocolytics—All tocolytics have significant failure rates, therefore if one tocolytic appears to be failing, that agent should be stopped and another agent should be tried. The use of multiple tocolytics at the same time appears to have an additive tocolytic effect but also appears to increase the risk of serious side effects. For example, magnesium sulfate used in combination with nifedipine can cause serious maternal hypotension. Likewise, magnesium sulfate supplemented by 1–2 doses of subcutaneous terbutaline can be safe and effective, but sustained treatment with the two can increase the patient's risk of pulmonary edema. It should be remembered that the patient who is difficult to tocolyze may have an unrecognized chorioamnionitis or placental abruption, conditions which may be contraindications to any tocolysis at all.

6. Results of tocolytic therapy—With all tocolytics, a point may be reached where further therapy is not indicated. This may be due to adverse maternal or fetal response to the progress of labor. Thus, if cervical dilatation reaches 5 cm, the treatment should be considered a failure and abandoned. If labor resumes after a period of quiescence, treatment may be reinstituted using the same or a different drug.

D. ANTIBIOTICS

Antibiotic therapy as a treatment for preterm labor has been studied extensively and, for the most part, has shown no benefit in delaying preterm birth in this population of patients. Patients with preterm labor should be started on antibiotics for prevention of neonatal group B streptococcal infection. Penicillin or ampicillin are used as first-line agents; clindamycin should be used if the patient is penicillin-allergic. If the patient is well-tocolyzed and there is no sign of imminent delivery, the group B *Streptococcus* prophylaxis can be discontinued.

Conduct of Labor & Delivery

Small premature infants should be delivered in a hospital equipped for neonatal intensive care whenever possible, because transfer following birth is more hazardous. Premature breech infants weighing less than 1500–2000 g are generally delivered by cesarean section. If the presentation is cephalic, vaginal birth is preferred in the absence of fetal distress.

Every effort should be made to avoid fetal hypoxia and intraventricular hemorrhage. Adequate hydration should assist in preventing maternal acidosis. Internal fetal monitoring or scalp sampling, or both, for blood pH should be done if hypoxia is suspected. Sedative and analgesic drugs in reduced dosages should be used sparingly. Paracervical block should be avoided because of potential adverse fetal effects.

Conduction anesthesia (particularly epidural) may be the best choice because it provides maximum relaxation of the birth canal and reduces transplacental transfer of agents potentially capable of depressing the fetus. Pudendal block anesthesia is also satisfactory if the pelvic floor and perineum are pliable or relaxed. A generous episiotomy should be made to further reduce the risk of injury. Delivery can be aided by forceps with a short cephalic curve (eg, Tucker-McLean forceps) serving as a sort of helmet to protect and guide the fetal head over the perineum. Before clamping the cord, wait 45–60 seconds—while holding the neonate below placental level—to ensure that adequate blood is received from the placental circulation.

If a cesarean section is indicated, the decision to operate is based on maturity of the fetus and prognosis for survival. In borderline cases, good criteria on which to base a decision are lacking. When performing a cesarean section, it is important to ascertain that the uterine incision is adequate for extraction of the fetus without delay or unnecessary trauma. This often requires a vertical incision when the lower uterine segment is incompletely developed.

In managing the premature newborn infant, the avoidance of heat loss is of critical importance. When birth follows the unsuccessful use of parenteral tocolytic agents, keep in mind the potential residual adverse effects of these drugs. Beta-adrenergic agents may cause neonatal hypotension, hypoglycemia, hypocalcemia, and ileus. Magnesium sulfate may be responsible for respiratory and cardiac depression. In addition, oral maintenance doses of a beta-adrenergic agent can produce hypoglycemia in the newborn.

Cord pH & Blood Gases

Apgar scores are often low in low-birthweight babies. This does not indicate asphyxiation or compromised status but merely reflects the immaturity of the physiologic systems. Therefore it is crucial to obtain cord pH and blood gas measurements for premature (and other high-risk) infants in order to document the status at birth. These measurements can also be correlated with intrapartum fetal heart rate monitoring, scalp sampling, and Apgar scores. Cord pH and blood gas measurements may also be helpful in reconstructing intra-partum events; auditing fetal acidemia; evaluating the efficacy of the clinical diagnosis, detection, and therapy; clarifying resuscitative measures; and determining the need for more intensive neonatal care.

Prognosis

Excellent neonatal care in the delivery room and nurs-ery will do much to ensure a good prognosis for the preterm infant (see Chapter 29). Lower-birthweight ba-bies have a lesser chance of survival and a greater chance of permanent sequelae in direct relationship to size. It is difficult to make generalizations regarding survival rates and sequelae because of the many causes of preterm de-livery, the different levels of perinatal care, and the in-stitutional differences in reported series. However, in-fants weighing 2000–2500 g usually have survival rates of more than 97%; those weighing 1500–2000 g, more than 90%; and those weighing 1000–1500 g, 65–80%. Two-thirds of infants weighing 800–1350 g survive, and handicaps occur in fewer than 20%. Mortality and morbidity rates are much higher in smaller fetuses.

PREMATURE RUPTURE OF MEMBRANES (PROM)

 ESSENTIALS OF DIAGNOSIS

- *History of a gush of fluid from the vagina or watery vaginal discharge.*
- *Demonstration of amniotic fluid leakage from the cervix.*

General Considerations

Rupture of the membranes may happen at any time during pregnancy. It becomes a problem if the fetus is preterm (preterm premature rupture of membranes) or, in the case of a term fetus, if the period of time between rupture of the membranes and the onset of labor is pro-longed. If 24 hours elapse between rupture of the mem-branes and the onset of labor, the problem is one of prolonged premature rupture of the membranes.

The exact cause of rupture is not known, although there are many associated conditions (Table 15–5). Pre-mature rupture of the membranes (PROM) occurs in approximately 10.7% of all pregnancies. In approxi-mately 94% of cases, the fetus is mature (approximately 20% of these are cases of prolonged rupture). Prema-

Table 15–5. Diseases and disorders associated with premature rupture of the membranes.

Maternal infection (eg, urinary tract infection, lower genital tract infection, sexually transmitted diseases)
Intrauterine infection
Cervical incompetency
Multiple previous pregnancies
Hydramnios
Nutritional deficit
Decreased tensile strength of membranes
Familial history of premature rupture of membranes

ture fetuses (1000–2500 g) account for about 5% of the total number (about 50% of cases are prolonged), while immature fetuses (< 1000 g) account for less than 0.5% (about 75% of cases are prolonged).

Pathology & Pathophysiology

Premature rupture of the membranes is an important cause of preterm labor, prolapse of the cord, placental abruption, and intrauterine infection. Amnionitis is an important cause of endomyometritis and puerperal sepsis.

In extremely prolonged rupture of the membranes, the fetus may have an appearance similar to that of Pot-ter's syndrome (eg, extraordinary flexion, wrinkling of the skin). It has been reported, but not confirmed, that various anomalies may result from chronically de-creased amniotic fluid volume.

If rupture of membranes occurs early in pregnancy at less than 26 weeks' EGA, it can cause pulmonary hy-poplasia and limb positioning defects in the newborn.

Clinical Findings

A. SYMPTOMS

The diagnostic evaluation must be efficient and impec-cably conducted to minimize the number of vaginal ex-aminations and the risk of chorioamnionitis. Symp-toms are the key to diagnosis; the patient usually reports a sudden gush of fluid or continued leakage. Additional symptoms that may be useful include the color and consistency of the fluid and the presence of flecks of vernix or meconium, reduced size of the uterus, and increased prominence of the fetus to palpa-tion.

B. STERILE SPECULUM EXAMINATION

A most important step in accurate diagnosis is examina-tion with a sterile speculum. This examination is the key to differentiating PROM from hydrorrhea gravidarum, vaginitis, increased vaginal secretions, and urinary incontinence. The examiner should look for the three hallmark confirmatory findings associated with PROM:

1. Pooling—the collection of amniotic fluid in the posterior fornix.
2. Nitrazine test—a sterile cotton-tipped swab should be used to collect fluid from the posterior fornix and apply it to nitrazine paper. In the presence of amniotic fluid, the nitrazine paper will turn blue, demonstrating an alkaline pH (7.0–7.25).
3. Ferning—a drop of fluid from the posterior fornix should be placed on a slide and allowed to air-dry. Amniotic fluid will form a fernlike pattern of crystallization.

Together, these three findings confirm rupture of membranes. The absence of one of the above findings is an indication for further testing because other factors can produce false-positive results. Alkaline pH on nitrazine test can also be caused by vaginal infections or the presence of blood or semen in the sample. Cervical mucus can cause ferning. During the speculum exam, the patient's cervix should be visually inspected to determine the degree of dilation and effacement and whether there is cord prolapse. If there is a significant vaginal pool, this pool can be collected and sent for fetal lung maturity determination. Cervical secretions should also be sent for culture, and a wet mount should be performed.

If no free fluid is found, a dry pad should be placed under the patient's perineum and observed for leakage. Other confirmatory tests for PROM include observed loss of fluid from the cervical os when the patient coughs or performs a Valsalva maneuver during speculum exam and oligohydramnios on ultrasound exam. If the examiner still cannot confirm rupture of membranes and the patient's history is highly suspicious for PROM, it may be necessary to perform amniocentesis and inject a dilute solution of Evans blue or indigo carmine dye. This is done following removal of amniotic fluid for physiologic maturity testing, analysis for white blood cells or bacteria, and possible culture and sensitivity testing. After 15–20 minutes, insertion of a vaginal speculum will reveal blue dye in the vagina if the membranes are ruptured.

C. PHYSICAL EXAMINATION

Once PROM is confirmed, a careful physical examination should be done to search for other signs of infection. Given the risk of infection, there is no indication for digital cervical examination if the patient is in early labor. The sterile speculum exam is sufficient to distinguish between early and advanced labor.

D. LABORATORY STUDIES

Initial laboratory studies should include a complete blood count with differential. In preterm pregnancies, evaluation should also include urine collected by catheterization for urinalysis, culture, and sensitivity testing; ultrasound examination for fetal size and amniotic fluid index; and amniocentesis in some cases to determine fetal lung maturity and the presence of infection.

E. AMNIONITIS

In all cases of amnionitis, it is safer for the fetus to be delivered than to be retained in utero. The most common organisms causing amnionitis are those that ascend from the vagina (eg, streptococci B and D and anaerobes). The most reliable signs of infection include the following: (1) Fever—the temperature should be checked every 4 hours. (2) Maternal leukocytosis—a daily leukocyte count and differential should be obtained. If any abnormalities are encountered, this may be repeated more frequently. In most laboratories, a white blood cell count of more than 16,000/μL is considered alarming. (3) Uterine tenderness—check every 4 hours. (5) Tachycardia—either maternal pulse > 100 beats/min or fetal heart rate > 160 beats/min—is worrisome. (6) Foul-smelling amniotic fluid.

A number of confounding factors may complicate the diagnosis of amnionitis. For example, frequent fundal examinations may cause uterine tenderness. Corticosteroid administration may cause mild leukocytosis (increase of 20–25%), and labor is associated with leukocytosis. If the diagnosis of amnionitis is equivocal, amniocentesis may be performed to search for bona fide evidence (eg, amniotic fluid containing numerous leukocytes or bacteria on Gram's stain or anaerobic or aerobic culture).

Treatment

The management of PROM depends on several factors, including gestational age and the presence or absence of amnionitis.

A. AMNIONITIS

If amnionitis is present in the patient with PROM, the patient should be actively delivered *regardless of gestational age*. Broad-spectrum antibiotics should be started to treat the amnionitis. If the patient is not in labor, labor should be induced to expedite delivery.

B. TERM PREGNANCY WITHOUT AMNIONITIS

The term pregnancy (EGA greater than 37 weeks) with PROM in the absence of amnionitis can be managed expectantly or actively. Expectant management entails nonintervention while waiting for the patient to go into labor spontaneously, whereas active management entails induction of labor with an agent such as pitocin. Nonintervention is an acceptable initial course of treatment, but if the patient does not go into labor within 6–12 hours after PROM, labor should be induced to minimize the risk of infection.

C. PRETERM PREGNANCY WITHOUT AMNIONITIS

The principles of managing the preterm PROM patient are similar to those of the preterm labor patient. The key difference is the much increased risk of developing amnionitis associated with preterm PROM. Pregnancies beyond 33–34 weeks' EGA can be managed as a term pregnancy because there is no evidence that antibiotics, corticosteroids, or tocolytics improve outcome in these patients. As long as these patients show no signs of amnionitis, they can be managed expectantly.

Pregnancies prior to 24 weeks' EGA with PROM have extremely low rates of fetal salvage with considerable maternal risk. Furthermore, at this early gestational age, steroids, tocolytics, and antibiotics have no proven benefit. These patients should be managed with expectant management or active termination.

For pregnancies with PROM between 24 and 32 weeks' EGA, several interventions have been shown to prolong pregnancy and improve outcome. After amnionitis has been ruled out and a specimen of amniotic fluid from vaginal pool collection or amniocentesis is sent for determination of fetal lung maturity, management should consist of the following interventions.

1. Antibiotics—Over the past decade, antibiotics have emerged as an important treatment for preterm PROM. In contrast to preterm labor where antibiotics have shown no benefit in prolonging pregnancy, antibiotics appear to be effective in prolonging the latency period in patients with preterm PROM. They have also been shown to decrease the infection rate in these patients. A number of well-designed studies have shown improved neonatal outcomes with antibiotics alone and with antibiotics combined with corticosteroid therapy. Table 15–6 describes one recommended protocol for antibiotic use in preterm PROM.

2. Corticosteroids—The NIH consensus development panel recommends the use of steroids in PROM patients prior to 32 weeks' EGA in the absence of intra-amniotic infection. In this patient population, corticosteroids have been shown to decrease the rate of respiratory distress syndrome, necrotizing enterocolitis, and intraventricular hemorrhage.

3. Tocolytics—The role of tocolytics in the preterm PROM patient is controversial. No study has shown that tocolytics alone improve fetal outcome. In general, the use of tocolytics in the preterm PROM patient

Table 15–6. Antibiotic therapy for preterm premature rupture of membranes.[1]

Once preterm PROM is confirmed, start:
Ampicillin 2 g IV every 6 hours
plus
Erythromycin 250 mg IV every 6 hours
After 48 hours, if the patient is still undelivered, this regimen should be changed to:
Amoxicillin 250 mg by mouth every 8 hours
plus
Erythromycin 333 mg by mouth every 8 hours
These antibiotics should be continued for 7 days if the patient remains undelivered. Women with GBS-positive cultures should receive prophylaxis intrapartum.

[1]From Mercer BM et al: Antibiotic therapy for reduction of infant morbidity after preterm premature rupture of the membranes. JAMA 1997;278:989.

should be limited to 48 hours' duration, to permit administration of corticosteroids and antibiotics.

If after starting these interventions the fetal lung profile returns as mature, they should be abandoned and the patient should be delivered. Again, if at any time the patient shows signs of chorioamnionitis, she should be delivered.

D. ROLE OF OUTPATIENT MANAGEMENT

In rare selected cases, patients who remain undelivered may be candidates for outpatient management. If leakage of fluid stops and the patient remains afebrile without evidence of increasing uterine irritability, she may be discharged home. These patients should be monitored very closely on an outpatient basis. They must be reliable and compliant with follow-up appointments. They also must take their temperature 4 times a day and be counseled on the warning signs of amnionitis. These patients should also be monitored with frequent biophysical profiles; some sources recommend daily testing.

PROLONGED PREGNANCY

 ESSENTIALS OF DIAGNOSIS

• *Confirmation of gestational age greater than 42 completed weeks.*

General Considerations

Prolonged pregnancy is defined as pregnancy that has reached 42 weeks of completed gestation from the first day of the last menstrual period (LMP) or 40 weeks' gestation from the time of conception. Most fetuses will show effects of impairment of the nutritional supply (weight loss, reduced subcutaneous tissue, scaling, parchmentlike skin). This condition is referred to as dysmaturity. The most common causes of prolonged pregnancy are incorrect dating due to incorrect LMP and variable length of the menstrual cycle. The cause of most cases of true prolonged pregnancy remains unknown, but anencephalic fetuses and those with placental sulfatase deficiency are often associated with it.

At least 3% of infants are born after 42 completed weeks' gestation (in some series, as many as 12%). Because of the potential risks of dysmaturity, these infants deserve particular attention.

The maternal risks usually relate to extraordinary fetal size (ie, dysfunctional labor, arrested progress of labor, fetopelvic disproportion). Extraordinary fetal size may result in birth injury (eg, shoulder girdle dystocia). Placental insufficiency is thought to be associated with aging of the placenta; this is the basis for another group of fetal problems. Oligohydramnios, which is more common in postterm gestation, may lead to cord compromise.

Complications resulting from prolonged pregnancy result in a sharp rise in perinatal mortality and morbidity rates (2–3 times those of infants born at 37–42 weeks). Complications in the survivors increase the chance of mental retardation and neurologic sequelae.

Diagnosis

The diagnosis of prolonged pregnancy is made by confirmation of the gestational age by referring to records of early pregnancy tests and ultrasound examinations, the exact time of conception (if known), and clinical parameters (eg, LMP, quickening, early examination, sequential fundal measurements).

To adequately assess the risk of fetal compromise, the following is a useful protocol for pregnancies beyond 41 weeks' gestation:

1. Perform nonstress testing 2–3 times weekly. (Some authorities believe that contraction stress testing, a biophysical profile, or both are necessary to detect the jeopardized fetus and recommend weekly or biweekly testing.)

2. Perform ultrasonic monitoring at least twice weekly to assess amniotic fluid volume (biophysical profiles may be obtained at the same time).

3. Have the mother count fetal movements each day.

Treatment

Many authorities will not allow a gestation to progress beyond 41 completed weeks and nearly all agree with delivery by 42½ weeks, believing that risks to the infant exceed the risks associated with induced labor. Furthermore, some recent studies suggest that there is an increased risk of cesarean section with induction after 41 weeks as opposed to induction at 41 weeks. If the choice is to continue the pregnancy, it may be advisable to have the patient monitor fetal activity. The following precautions should be taken:

1. Decreased fetal movement warrants an immediate biophysical profile evaluation. Despite the concerns of some authorities, many continue to use the nonstress test as their primary screening device.

2. Abnormalities in the nonstress test mandate an immediate contraction stress test.

3. An abnormal contraction stress test, decreased amniotic fluid volume, abnormal biophysical profile, or detection of meconium or other signs of fetal compromise warrant serious consideration of delivery.

4. A large or compromised fetus may require cesarean delivery.

5. In the absence of fetopelvic disproportion or fetal distress, labor may be induced. Fetal monitoring should be continuous.

Rh ISOIMMUNIZATION & OTHER BLOOD GROUP INCOMPATIBILITIES

 ESSENTIALS OF DIAGNOSIS

- *Maternal Rh-negativity and presence of antibody on indirect Coombs' test.*
- *Rh or other antibody titer posing fetal risk.*
- *May have a previous infant with hemolytic disease of the newborn.*
- *Postnatal fetal cord blood findings of Rh-positivity and anemia (hemoglobin < 10 g).*

General Considerations

A fetus receives half of its genetic components from its mother and half from its father and may therefore have different blood groups than those of its mother. Some blood groups may act as antigens in individuals not possessing those blood groups. The antigens reside on red blood cells. If enough fetal cells leak into the maternal blood, a maternal antibody response may be provoked. Some blood types specifically produce antibodies capable of crossing the placenta. They then enter the fetal circulation and destroy the fetal erythrocytes, causing hemolytic anemia. This leads to responses in the fetus to meet the challenge of enhanced blood cell breakdown. These changes in the fetus and newborn are called erythroblastosis fetalis. As noted below, several blood groups are capable of producing fetal risk, but those in the Rh group have caused the overwhelming majority of cases of erythroblastosis fetalis, so the Rh group will be used as the example.

The Rh blood group is the most complex human blood group. The Rh antigens are grouped in 3 pairs: Dd, Cc, and Ee. The major antigen in this group, Rh_o (D), or Rh factor, is of particular concern. A woman who is lacking the Rh factor (Rh-negative) may carry an Rh-positive fetus. If fetal red blood cells pass into the mother's circulation in sufficient numbers, maternal antibodies to the Rh-positive antigen may develop and cross the placenta, causing hemolysis of fetal blood cells (Fig 15–1). Hemolytic disease of the newborn may occur, and severe disease may cause fetal death.

In standard testing when the father is Rh-positive, 2 possibilities exist, ie, he may be homozygous or heterozygous. Forty-five percent of Rh-positive persons are homozygous for D, and 55% are heterozygous. If the father is homozygous, all of his children will be Rh-positive; if he is heterozygous, his children will have a 50% chance of being Rh-positive. By way of contrast, the Rh-negative individual is always homozygous.

Incidence

Basque populations have the highest incidence of Rh-negativity (30–35%). Caucasian populations in general have a higher incidence (15–16%; Finland, 10–12%).

Blacks in the United States have a rate of 8%; African blacks, 4%; Indoeurasians, 2%; and North American Indians, 1%. The incidence among mongoloid races is nil.

In mothers who do not receive prophylaxis with Rh immunoglobulin, the overall risk of isoimmunization for an Rh-positive ABO-compatible infant with an Rh-negative mother is about 16%. Of these, 1.5–2% of reactions will occur antepartum, 7% within 6 months of delivery, and the remainder (7%) early in the second pregnancy, most likely as the result of an amnestic response. ABO incompatibility between an Rh-positive fetus and an Rh-negative mother provides some protection against Rh isoimmunization; the overall incidence is 1.5–2% in these cases. In mothers who receive prophylaxis with Rh immunoglobulin, the risk of isoimmunization is reduced to 0.2%.

Pathogenesis

A. MATERNAL RH ISOIMMUNIZATION

Rh antigens are lipoproteins that are confined to the red cell membrane. Isoimmunization may occur by 2 mechanisms: (1) following incompatible blood transfusion or (2) following fetomaternal hemorrhage between a mother and an incompatible fetus. Fetomaternal hemorrhage may occur during pregnancy or at delivery. With no apparent predisposing factors, fetal red cells have been detected in maternal blood in 6.7% of women during the first trimester, 15.9% during the second trimester, and 28.9% during the third trimester. There are a number of predispositions to fetomaternal hemorrhage, including spontaneous or induced abortion, amniocentesis, chorionic villus sampling, abdominal trauma (eg, due to motor vehicle accidents or external version), placenta previa, abruptio placentae, fetal death, multiple pregnancy, manual removal of the placenta, and cesarean section.

Although the exact number of Rh-positive cells necessary to cause isoimmunization of the Rh-negative

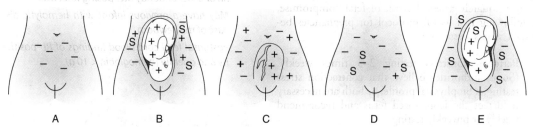

Figure 15–1. **A:** Rh-negative woman before pregnancy. **B:** Pregnancy occurs. The fetus is Rh-positive. **C:** Separation of the placenta. **D:** Following delivery, Rh isoimmunization occurs in the mother, and she develops antibodies (S) to the Rh-positive antigen. **E:** The next pregnancy with an Rh-positive fetus. Maternal antibodies cross the placenta, enter the fetal bloodstream, and attach to Rh-positive red cells, causing hemolysis.

pregnant woman is unknown, as little as 0.1 mL of Rh-positive cells will cause sensitization. Even with delivery, this amount occurs in less than half of cases.

Fortunately, there are other mitigating factors to Rh isoimmunization. A very important one is that about 30% of Rh-negative persons never become sensitized (nonresponders) when given Rh-positive blood. As noted above, ABO incompatibility also confers a protective effect.

The initial maternal immune response to Rh sensitization is low levels of IgM. Within 6 weeks to 6 months, IgG antibodies become detectable. In contrast to IgM, IgG (7S immunoglobulins) is capable of crossing the placenta and destroying fetal Rh-positive cells.

B. OTHER BLOOD GROUP ISOIMMUNIZATION

Of the other blood groups that may evoke immunoglobulins capable of crossing the placenta (often called atypical or irregular immunizing antibodies), those that may cause severe fetal hemolysis (listed in descending order of occurrence) are Kell, Duffy, Kidd, MNSs, and Diego; P. Lutheran, and Xg groups may also cause fetal hemolysis, but it is usually less severe.

C. FETAL EFFECTS

Hemolytic disease of the newborn occurs when the maternal antibodies cross the placenta and destroy the Rh-positive fetal red blood cells. Fetal anemia results, stimulating extramedullary erythropoietic sites to produce high levels of nucleated red cell elements. Immature erythrocytes are present in the fetal blood due to poor maturation control. Hemolysis produces heme, which is converted to bilirubin; both of these substances are neurotoxic. However, while the fetus is in utero, heme and bilirubin are effectively removed by the placenta and the mother metabolizes them.

When fetal red blood cell destruction far exceeds production and severe anemia occurs, erythroblastosis fetalis may occur. This is characterized by extramedullary hematopoiesis, heart failure, edema, ascites, and pericardial effusion. Tissue hypoxia and acidosis may result. Normal hepatic architecture and function may be disturbed by extensive liver erythropoiesis, which may lead to decreased protein production, portal hypertension, and ascites.

D. NEONATAL EFFECTS

In the immediate neonatal interval, the primary problem may relate to anemia and the sequelae mentioned above. However, hyperbilirubinemia may also pose an immediate risk and certainly poses a risk as further red cell breakdown occurs. The immature (and often compromised) liver, with its low levels of glucuronyltransferase, is unable to conjugate the large amounts of bilirubin. This results in high serum bilirubin, with resultant kernicterus (bilirubin deposition in the basal ganglia).

Management of the Unsensitized Rh-Negative Pregnancy

A. PREPREGNANCY OR FIRST PRENATAL VISIT

On the first prenatal visit, all pregnant women should be screened for the ABO blood group and the Rh group, including Du. They should also undergo antibody screening (indirect Coombs' test). If the woman is Rh-negative, testing for paternal ABO and Rh blood groups may be useful. Unless the father of the baby is known to be Rh-negative, all Rh-negative mothers should receive prophylaxis according to the protocol described below.

B. VISIT AT 28 WEEKS

Antibody screening is performed. If negative, 300 µg of Rh immuneglobulin (RhIgG) is given. If positive, the patient should be managed as Rh-sensitized.

C. VISIT AT 35 WEEKS

Antibody screening is repeated. If it is negative, the patient is merely observed. If screening is positive, the patient is managed as Rh-sensitized.

D. POSTPARTUM

If the infant is Rh-positive or Du-positive, 300 µg of RhIgG is administered to the mother (provided maternal antibody screening is negative). Although RhIgG should generally be given within 72 hours after delivery, it has been shown to be effective in preventing isoimmunization if given up to 28 days after delivery. If the antibody screen is positive, the patient is managed as if she will be Rh-sensitized during the next pregnancy.

E. SPECIAL FETOMATERNAL RISK STATES

Several circumstances may occur during pregnancy that mandate giving RhIgG to the unsensitized patient outside the above protocol.

1. Abortion—Sensitization will occur in 2% of spontaneous abortions and 4–5% of induced abortions. In the first trimester, due to the small amount of fetal blood, 50 µg of RhIgG is apparently enough to prevent sensitization. After the first trimester, the 300-µg dose is recommended. The risk of Rh isoimmunization after threatened abortion is less well understood, but many experts agree that RhIgG should also be given to these patients.

2. Amniocentesis, chorionic villus sampling, and cord blood sampling—If the placenta is traversed by the needle, there is up to an 11% chance of sensitization. It is recommended that 300 μg of RhIgG be administered when these procedures are performed in the unsensitized patient.

3. Antepartum hemorrhage—In cases of placenta previa or abruptio placentae, it is recommended that 300 μg of RhIgG be given. If the pregnancy is carried more than 12 weeks from the time of RhIgG administration, it is recommended that the prophylactic dose be repeated.

4. External cephalic version—Patients who undergo external cephalic version, either failed or successful, have fetomaternal hemorrhage in 2–6% of cases and therefore should also receive 300 μg of RhIgG.

F. Delivery With Fetomaternal Hemorrhage

In only about 0.4% of patients will fetomaternal hemorrhage be so great that it cannot be managed with 300 μg of RhIgG. There are a number of studies to determine if this has occurred (eg, Kleihauer-Betke test); however, these are not commonly employed as screening tests because of the rarity of the circumstance and because fetomaternal hemorrhage rarely occurs without antecedent clinical evidence (eg, precipitous delivery, anemic neonate, abruptio placentae, placenta previa, tetanic labor, manual removal of the placenta).

Evaluation of the Pregnancy With Isoimmunization

Evaluation of the pregnancy complicated by isoimmunization is guided by two factors: whether the patient has a history of an affected fetus in a previous pregnancy and maternal antibody titers.

A. No History of Previous Fetus Affected by Rh Isoimmunization

Once the antibody screen is positive for isoimmunization, these patients should be followed by antibody titers at intake, 20 weeks' EGA, and then every 4 weeks. As long as antibody titers remain less than 1:32 by indirect Coombs' test, there is no indication for further intervention. Once antibody titers reach 1:32, amniocentesis should be performed because a titer of 1:32 puts the fetus at significant risk for demise before 37 weeks.

B. History of a Prior Fetus Affected by Rh Isoimmunization

It is not necessary to follow antibody titers in these pregnancies because amniocentesis is indicated by the history of prior affected fetus. Amniocentesis should be performed 4–8 weeks earlier than the gestational age in the previous pregnancy when Rh-associated morbidity was first identified.

When it is determined that amniocentesis is indicated, it should be performed under ultrasound guidance to minimize the risk of transplacental hemorrhage.

The amniotic fluid is analyzed by spectrophotometry and by the amount of light absorbed by the blood breakdown products plotted on a semilogarithmic scale versus gestational age. It is known that the concentration of these pigments in the unsensitized case gradually decreases as pregnancy progresses. Thus the severity of fetal affliction may be approximated (Fig 15–2) and this information used as a guide for further studies and treatment.

In recent years, cordocentesis or percutaneous umbilical cord sampling has emerged as an alternative to amniocentesis in evaluating these patients. The primary advantage of cordocentesis is its ability to evaluate the fetus more precisely by checking the fetal hematocrit. Conversely, the fetal loss rate with cordocentesis is higher than that associated with amniocentesis, therefore it should only be used in experienced hands.

Ultrasound plays an important role in evaluating the isoimmunized patient for hydrops. Ultrasound should

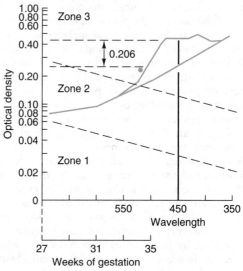

Figure 15–2. Amniotic fluid spectrophotometric reading (Liley method) is 0.206 in this example. The value falls into zone 3, indicating impending fetal death. This first affected infant was delivered at 35 weeks' gestation with a cord hemoglobin level of 4.7 g/100 mL and a cord bilirubin level of 8 mg/100 mL and required 5 exchange transfusions to survive. (Reproduced, with permission, from Creasy RK, Resnick R: *Maternal-Fetal Medicine: Principles and Practice.* Saunders, 1984, p. 575.)

look for fetal heart size, edema, pericardial effusion, ascites, and amniotic fluid index. Serial ultrasounds can document the progression or reversal of disease. Doppler ultrasonography of the fetus's middle cerebral artery is currently being studied as a noninvasive means to predict significant fetal anemia.

Management of the Pregnancy With Isoimmunization

Management of these patients is dictated by amniocentesis results (Fig 15–2).

A. MILDLY AFFECTED FETUS

The unaffected or mildly affected fetus will fall into zone 1. Amniocentesis should be repeated every 2–3 weeks, and delivery should be near term and certainly after the fetus has achieved pulmonary maturity.

B. MODERATELY AFFECTED FETUS

The moderately affected fetus will fall into zone 2. It will be necessary to repeat amniocentesis every 1–2 weeks. Delivery generally is required prior to term, and the fetus is delivered as soon as pulmonary maturity is reached. In some cases, it may be necessary to enhance pulmonary maturity by the use of betamethasone.

C. SEVERELY AFFECTED FETUS

The severely affected fetus falls into zone 3. Intervention is usually needed to allow the fetus to reach a gestational age at which delivery and neonatal risks are fewer than the risks of in utero therapy. Amniocentesis will generally have to be repeated weekly. Ultrasound is used to search for fetal ascites or edema.

Intrauterine transfusion may be necessary to prevent the fetus from dying. This is performed using O-negative, cytomegalovirus-negative, washed, irradiated packed red cells. The volume to be transfused is roughly approximated by the following formula: (Weeks of gestation – 20) × 10 mL.

The fetal heart rate is closely monitored during the procedure, and if tachycardia occurs, the transfusion is stopped. Although the intraperitoneal technique was used in years past, intravascular fetal transfusion has largely replaced it secondary to its more predictable absorption.

After transfusion, repeat transfusions or delivery will be necessary as production of fetal blood markedly decreases or ceases. Timing of these transfusions may be assisted by ultrasonic determination of increasing or decreasing fetal peritoneal fluid. When the fetus has sufficient pulmonary maturity for survival, delivery should take place.

ABO HEMOLYTIC DISEASE

ABO hemolytic disease is much milder than the isoimmunization evoked by Rh_o and the other antigens noted above. The reason for this difference is poorly understood, because both IgG and IgM are produced antenatally. Although 20–25% of pregnancies have potential maternal-infant ABO incompatibility, a recognizable process in the neonate occurs in only 10% of those cases. Those affected are almost always group A (especially A1) or B infants of group O mothers. The neonatal direct Coombs' test may be positive or negative, and maternal antibodies are also variable.

In Rh isoimmunization, only 1–2% of cases occur in the first-born infant, whereas 40–50% of ABO incompatibilities occur in the first-born infant. Serious fetal sequelae (eg, stillbirth, hydrops) almost never occur, and severe fetal anemia is also rare.

ABO hemolytic disease is primarily manifest following birth, with early neonatal onset of jaundice (at < 24 hours) and variable elevation of the indirect bilirubin. The management of ABO incompatibility relates to bilirubin surveillance and phototherapy (required in 10% of cases). The infants may have hepatosplenomegaly. Exchange transfusion is necessary in only 1% of cases, and the incidence of late anemia is rare. Sequelae such as kernicterus almost never occur.

REFERENCES

American College of Obstetricians and Gynecologists: Premature Rupture of Membranes. ACOG Practice Bulletin No. 1, 1998.

American College of Obstetricians and Gynecologists: Prevention of Rh D Alloimmunization. ACOG Practice Bulletin No. 4, 1999.

American College of Obstetricians and Gynecologists: Fetal Fibronectin Preterm Labor Risk Test. ACOG Committee Opinion No. 187, 1997.

American College of Obstetricians and Gynecologists: Antenatal Corticosteroid Therapy for Fetal Maturation. ACOG Committee Opinion No. 210, 1998.

Elimian A et al: Effectiveness of multidose antenatal steroids. Obstet Gynecol 2000;95:34.

How HY et al: Preterm premature rupture of membranes: aggressive tocolysis versus expectant management. J Maternal-Fetal Med 1998;7:8.

Huang WL et al: Effect of corticosteroids on brain growth in fetal sheep. Obstet Gynecol 1999;94:213.

Kenyon SL et al: Broad-spectrum antibiotics for preterm, prelabour rupture of fetal membranes: The ORACLE I randomised trial. Lancet 2001;357:979.

Lo YM et al: Prenatal diagnosis of fetal RhD status by molecular analysis of maternal plasma. N Engl J Med 1998;339:1734.

Macones GA et al: Predicting delivery within 48 hours in women treated with parenteral tocolysis. Obstet Gynecol 1999; 93:432.

Mari G et al: Noninvasive diagnosis by doppler ultrasonography of fetal anemia due to maternal red-cell alloimmunization. N Engl J Med 2000;342:9.

Mercer MD et al: Antibiotic therapy for reduction of infant morbidity after preterm premature rupture of the membranes: a randomized controlled trial. JAMA 1997;278:989.

Queenan JT et al: Management of the Rh-isoimmunized pregnancy. Postgrad Obstet Gynecol 1998;18:1.

Saade GR: Noninvasive testing for fetal anemia. N Engl J Med 2000;342:52.

Seaward PG et al: International multicentre term prelabor rupture of membranes study: evaluation of predictors of clinical chorioamnionitis and postpartum fever in patients with prelabor rupture of membranes at term. Am J Obstet Gynecol 1997;177:1024.

Disproportionate Fetal Growth

16

Jeannine Rahimian, MD, MBA,
& Michael W. Varner, MD

Weight at delivery was once considered evidence of prematurity (birthweight < 2500 g) or postmaturity (macrosomia; birthweight > 4500 g). These criteria were later revised when it was realized that abnormal growth was reflected in factors other than birthweight. Normative standards were developed that include birthweight, length, and head circumference according to gestational age. Abnormal fetal growth is now defined according to percentiles: Infants classified as intrauterine growth restricted (IUGR) are in the 10th percentile or below, and those classified as large for gestational age (LGA) are in the 90th percentile or above. Standards now also vary among different populations.

Both IUGR and LGA fetuses have an increased risk of perinatal morbidity and mortality (Tables 16–1 and 16–2). The pathogenesis, differential diagnosis, and treatment are different for the two extremes of growth.

INTRAUTERINE GROWTH RESTRICTED PREGNANCY

Terminology

Many terms have been used to describe fetuses with disproportionately small growth. These include small for gestational age, intrauterine growth retardation, intrauterine growth restriction, and small for dates. Most often, small for gestational age is used to refer to the infant, while intrauterine growth restriction refers to the fetus. Intrauterine growth restriction is defined as estimated fetal weight at or below the 10th percentile for gestational age. By definition, 10% of infants in any population will be at or below the 10th percentile. Approximately 70% of fetuses with estimated fetal weight below the 10th percentile are simply constitutionally small and it can often be difficult to distinguish between normal and pathologic growth. Some nonpathologic factors affecting fetal and birthweight include maternal height, paternal height, parity, ethnicity, and fetal sex.

Pathophysiology

When compared with average-for-gestational-age (AGA) fetuses, the IUGR fetus has altered body composition (including decreased body fat, total protein, whole body DNA and RNA, glycogen, and free fatty acids), altered distribution of weight among organs, and altered body proportions. About 20% of IUGR infants are symmetrically small, with a relatively proportionate decrease in many organ weights. Eighty percent are asymmetrically small, with relative sparing of brain weight, especially when compared with that of the liver or thymus.

In asymmetric IUGR infants, brain weight is decreased only slightly compared with that of AGA controls, primarily owing to decreased brain cell size and not to decreased brain cell numbers. Cerebral abnormalities include decreased myelination, decreased utilization of metabolic substrates other than glucose, and altered protein synthesis. At least in experimental animals, these changes are more likely to produce adverse effects in the brainstem and cerebellum. This differential sparing is particularly prominent when deprivation occurs in the latter half of pregnancy. Deprivation early in pregnancy is associated with less cerebral sparing and diffusely slowed brain growth.

Symmetric IUGR infants have proportionately small brains, usually because of a decreased number of brain cells. Although this may be the result of early, severe nutritional deprivation, the cause is more often a genetic disorder, infection, or other problem. The thymus is usually small, being decreased by an average of 25%. This may in part explain the decreased cellular immunity seen in IUGR infants.

The liver is also frequently affected, at least partly because of diminished glycogen deposition. The liver may also have functional (metabolic) abnormalities, as manifested by abnormal cord blood and neonatal serum chemistries. Such abnormalities often reflect the underlying cause of decreased size.

Blood flow to the lungs may be decreased, lessening the pulmonary contribution to amniotic fluid volume; this may be partly responsible for the often-encountered oligohydramnios. Decreased pulmonary blood flow may also be associated with accelerated functional pulmonary maturity.

Renal blood flow is frequently reduced in asymmetric IUGR pregnancies. The resultant diminished glomerular filtration rate may further contribute to oligohydramnios.

Table 16–1. Some complications of IUGR pregnancy.

Maternal Complications
  Complications due to underlying disease, preeclampsia, premature labor, cesarean delivery
Fetal Complications
  Stillbirth, hypoxia and acidosis, malformations
Neonatal Complications
  Hypoglycemia, hypocalcemia, hypoxia and acidosis, hypothermia, meconium aspiration syndrome, polycythemia, congenital malformations, sudden infant death syndrome
Long-Term Complications
  Lower IQ, learning and behavior problems, major neurologic handicaps (seizure disorders, cerebral palsy, severe mental retardation, hypertension)

Differential Diagnosis

A classification of IUGR pregnancy according to cause is shown in Table 16–3. Any inference of suboptimal growth requires, by definition, serial observations. It cannot be emphasized too strongly that a pregnancy cannot be described as IUGR unless the gestational age is known with certainty (see Chapter 9).

Numerous authors have differentiated between symmetric and asymmetric IUGR pregnancy regarding cause and prognosis. Briefly stated, symmetric IUGR infants are more likely to have an endogenous defect that may preclude normal development. Asymmetric IUGR infants are more likely to be normal, but small in size owing to intrauterine deprivation. Although this classification is helpful in establishing a differential diagnosis and framework for discussion, it is not sufficiently precise to serve as a basis for decisions regarding intervention or viability.

Table 16–2. Some complications of LGA pregnancy.

Maternal Complications
  Cesarean section, postpartum hemorrhage, shoulder dystocia, perineal trauma, operative vaginal delivery
Fetal Complications
  Stillbirth, anomalies, shoulder dystocia
Neonatal Complications
  Low Apgar score, hypoglycemia, birth injury, hypocalcemia, polycythemia, jaundice, feeding difficulties
Long-Term Complications
  Obesity, type II diabetes, neurologic or behavioral problems, childhood onset of cancer

Table 16–3. Pathogenic classification of IUGR pregnancy.

A. Fetoplacental Causes
  Genetic disorders
    Autosomal: trisomy 13, 18, 21; ring chromosomes; chromosomal deletions; partial trisomies
    Sex chromosomes: Turner syndrome, multiple chromosomes (XXX, XYY)
    Neural tube defects
    Dysmorphic syndromes: achondroplasia, chondrodystrophies, osteogenesis imperfecta
    Abdominal wall defects
    Other rare syndromes
  Congenital infection
    Viral: cytomegalovirus, rubella, herpes, varicella zoster
    Protozoan: toxoplasmosis, malaria
    Bacterial: listeriosis
  Placental disorders: placenta previa, placental infarction, chorionic villitis, chronic partial separation, placental malformations (circumvallate placenta, battledore placenta, placental hemangioma, twin-twin transfusion syndrome)
  Multiple gestation
B. Maternal Factors
  Co-existent maternal disease: hypertension, anemia (hemoglobinopathy, decreased normal hemoglobin [especially <12 g/dL]), renal disease (hypertension, protein loss), malnutrition (inflammatory bowel disease [ulcerative colitis, regional enteritis], pancreatitis, intestinal parasites), cyanotic pulmonary disease
  Substance abuse/drugs: alcohol, cigarette smoking, cocaine, heroin, warfarin, folic acid antagonists (methotrexate, aminopterin), anticonvulsants
  Maternal features, small maternal stature
  Sex of fetus

A. Fetoplacental Causes

1. Chromosomal abnormalities—Genetic disorders account for 10–15% of IUGR infants. Data from the Metropolitan Atlanta Congenital Defects Program suggest that 38% of chromosomally abnormal infants are IUGR and that the risk of an IUGR infant having a major congenital anomaly is 8%. Infants with autosomal trisomies are more likely to be IUGR, the most common being **trisomy 21 (Down's syndrome)**, with an incidence of 1.6 per 1000 live births. At term, such infants weigh an average of 350 g less than comparable normal infants and are 4 times more likely to be IUGR. This decrease is apparent only in the last 6 weeks of pregnancy. A similar decrease in birthweight occurs in translocation Down's syndrome, whereas mosaic Down's syndrome is associated with an intermediate decrease in birthweight.

The second most common autosomal trisomy is **trisomy 18 (Edwards' syndrome)**, which occurs in 1 in 6000–8000 live births. Eighty-four percent of these infants are IUGR. Ultrasound evaluation may reveal associated anomalies. There is an increased likelihood of polyhydramnios plus fetal neural tube defects and visceral anomalies. Fetuses are frequently in breech presentation. The average birthweight in trisomy 18 infants is almost 1000 g less than that of controls. In contrast to that seen in infants with trisomies 13 and 21, the placental weight in trisomy 18 infants is also markedly reduced.

Trisomy 13, the third most common autosomal trisomy, occurs in 1 in 5000–10,000 live births. Over 50% of affected infants are IUGR. Birthweights average 700–800 g less than those of controls. Trisomy 13 is also more common with older mothers. As in trisomy 18, there may be associated abnormalities, including cleft lip and palate, urinary tract abnormalities, central nervous system abnormalities, and polydactyly.

Other autosomal chromosome abnormalities (eg, other trisomies, ring chromosomes, deletions, partial trisomies) are clinically uncommon but associated with an increased likelihood of the fetus being IUGR. Sex chromosome abnormalities may also be associated with lower birthweight. The XYY configuration is the most common of these, but is probably not associated with an increased incidence of IUGR pregnancy. Extra X chromosomes (more than two) are associated with a decrease in birthweight of 200–300 g for each extra X. **Turner's syndrome** is associated with an average birthweight of approximately 400 g below average. Fetuses with mosaic Turner's syndrome are intermediately affected.

Statistically, the growth impairment seen with fetal chromosome abnormalities occurs earlier than that which is of placental origin. However, there is considerable clinical overlap, and this observation is not always of clinical value.

Fetuses with neural tube defects are frequently IUGR. Anencephalic fetuses are IUGR, even considering the absent brain and skull, with average third trimester birthweights of approximately 1000–1100 g less than matched controls. The birthweight difference is less prominent with fetal spina bifida, averaging 250 g less than that of controls.

Certain dysmorphic syndromes are associated with an increased incidence of IUGR fetuses. **Achondroplasia** may be associated with low birthweight (average decrease, 300–600 g) if either parent is affected, but if spontaneous mutation is the cause, infants are generally of normal birthweight. All chondrodystrophies are frequently associated with polyhydramnios.

Osteogenesis imperfecta consists of a spectrum of diseases with different genetic transmissions and prognoses, all of which result in IUGR fetuses. Shortening or fractures of the long bones help determine the diagnosis.

Infants born with abdominal wall defects are characteristically IUGR, particularly those with gastroschisis.

Numerous other autosomal recessive syndromes are associated with IUGR fetuses. Included among these are **Smith-Lemli-Opitz syndrome, Meckel's syndrome, Robert's syndrome, Donohue's syndrome,** and **Seckel's syndrome.** All these conditions are rare and are most likely to be diagnosed prenatally in families where a child has already been affected.

Maternal neurofibromatosis has been associated with IUGR outcome.

Infants with renal anomalies of any nature are often IUGR. Renal agenesis (**Potter's syndrome**) and complete urinary tract outflow obstruction are the two most common examples. A dysmature infant may be IUGR and may have associated oligohydramnios. The presence of oligohydramnios in any infant makes prenatal diagnosis by ultrasonography or amniocentesis much more difficult. Oligohydramnios is relatively more likely to be associated with a small fundal height measurement, which may indicate that the fetus is IUGR in ultrasound evaluation.

Other congenital anomalies associated with an increased incidence of IUGR outcome are gastroschisis, duodenal atresia, and pancreatic agenesis.

2. Congenital infections—Chronic intrauterine infection may be responsible for 5–10% of IUGR pregnancies (Table 16–3). The most commonly identified pathogen is cytomegalovirus. Although cytomegalovirus can be isolated from 0.5–2% of all newborns in the United States, clinically obvious infection at the time of birth affects only 0.2–2 in 1000 live births. Active fetoplacental infection is characterized by cytolysis, followed by secondary inflammation, fibrosis, and calcification. Only infants with clinically apparent infection at the time of birth are likely to be IUGR due to the infection. Signs of congenital infection are nonspecific but include central nervous system involvement (eg, microcephaly), chorioretinitis, and intracranial (periventricular) calcifications. Other signs include pneumonitis, hepatosplenomegaly, and thrombocytopenia.

Congenital rubella infection also increases the likelihood of an IUGR fetus. Infection during the first trimester results in the most severely affected and therefore smallest fetuses, primarily as a result of microvascular endothelial damage. Such infants are likely to have structural cardiovascular defects and central nervous system defects that include microcephaly, deafness, glaucoma, and cataracts.

Other viruses implicated in IUGR pregnancy include herpesvirus, varicella-zoster virus, influenza virus, and poliovirus. However, the number of cases is small, and it is unknown whether specific congenital syndromes can be attributed to these agents.

By virtue of their chronic, indolent nature, protozoan infections would be expected to be associated with IUGR pregnancies. The most commonly associated infection is toxoplasmosis, which is caused by the tissue-bound protozoan *Toxoplasma gondii* and is transmitted by ingesting the oocyte in raw meat or the excrement of infected animals. The infection is acquired transplacentally, and only women with parasitemia (ie, primary infection) are at risk for having an affected infant. The average incidence is 1 in 1000 live births in the United States, although the incidence varies widely among locations and social populations. About 20% of newborns with congenital toxoplasmosis will be sufficiently involved to be IUGR. Malaria is another protozoan infection associated with IUGR pregnancy.

Although bacterial infections occur commonly in pregnancy and are frequently implicated in premature delivery, they are not commonly associated with IUGR infants, because the infections are not usually chronic or subacute. Chronic infection due to *Listeria monocytogenes* is an exception. Infants are usually critically ill at the time of delivery and have encephalitis, pneumonitis, myocarditis, hepatosplenomegaly, jaundice, and petechiae.

3. Placental factors—The placenta plays an important role in normal fetal growth. Several placental abnormalities are associated with an increased likelihood of an IUGR fetus. **Placenta previa** is associated with an increased incidence of IUGR fetuses, probably owing to the unfavorable site of placental implantation. Complete placenta previa is associated with a higher incidence of IUGR than is partial placenta previa. Decreased functional exchange area due to **placental infarction** is also associated with an increased incidence of IUGR fetuses. **Premature placental separation** may occur at any time during pregnancy, with variable effects. When not associated with fetal death, premature labor, or exsanguination, it may be associated with an increased likelihood of IUGR. Malformations of the placenta or cord are associated with an increased incidence of IUGR. Such malformations include **circumvallate placenta, placental hemangioma, battledore placenta,** and **twin-twin transfusion syndrome. Chronic villitis** is also seen with increased frequency when the placentas of IUGR pregnancies are examined histologically. This problem may recur with subsequent pregnancies. Finally, **uterine anomalies** may also result in impaired fetal growth, primarily because of the likelihood of suboptimal uterine blood flow.

4. Multiple Gestations—Multiple gestation has long been associated with premature delivery. However, it is also associated with a 20–30% increased incidence of IUGR fetuses. This may be due to placental insufficiency, twin-twin transfusion syndrome or anomalies. IUGR fetuses can be determined by 32 weeks in twins, 30 weeks in triplets, and 28 weeks in quadruplets. Serial ultrasound estimates of fetal weights should be considered in a multiple gestation pregnancy.

B. MATERNAL FACTORS

Numerous maternal diseases are associated with suboptimal fetal growth via various mechanisms, including any that interfere with uptake or delivery of nutrients or oxygen to the fetus. Any woman who has had one IUGR infant is at increased risk of having another. There is a twofold and fourfold increase in risk for IUGR birth after 1 and 2 IUGR births, respectively.

1. Hypertension—Hypertension is the most common maternal complication causing IUGR pregnancies. With systemic hypertension, there is decreased blood flow through the spiral arterioles perfusing the placenta, resulting in decreased delivery of oxygen and nutrients to the placenta and fetus. Hypertension may also be associated with placental infarction.

2. Drugs—Both social drugs and prescribed medications can affect fetal growth. **Alcohol** use has long been known to be associated with impaired fetal growth. Virtually all infants with fetal alcohol syndrome exhibit signs of growth restriction.

Cigarette smoking is much more common among women of childbearing age in the United States than is alcoholism. It is the single most preventable cause of IUGR pregnancy in the United States today. Women who smoke have a three- to fourfold increase in IUGR infants. Birthweight is reduced by about 200 g in infants of mothers who smoke, with the amount of growth restriction being related to the number of cigarettes smoked per day. Women who quit at 7 months have mean birthweights higher than those who smoke throughout the entire pregnancy, and those who stop smoking before 16 weeks are not at increased risk for an IUGR infant.

Other social drugs have been associated with an increased incidence of IUGR pregnancies. Heroin and cocaine addicts have an increased incidence of IUGR infants, but they have so many other confounding variables that it cannot be said with certainty that the increased incidence is due to their drug use. Studies of pregnant women maintained on methadone have not shown an increased incidence of IUGR infants.

Certain pharmacologic agents have also been associated with an increased incidence of IUGR pregnancies, primarily as a result of teratogenic effects. Warfarin has been associated with an increased incidence of IUGR fetuses, primarily due to the sequelae of intrauterine hemorrhage. The folic acid antagonists are associated with an increased risk of spontaneous abortion and stillbirth, severe malformations, and IUGR infants.

IUGR fetuses are also more common with maternally administered immunosuppressive drugs (eg, cyclosporine, azathioprine, corticosteroids), but when controlled for the underlying maternal diseases for which these medications are indicated, the medications per se probably have little effect on fetal growth.

3. Malnutrition and malabsorption—Poor maternal weight gain is associated with an increased risk of having an IUGR infant. Studies of infants of pregnant women during the Siege of Leningrad during World War II showed that daily intake must be reduced to below 1500 kcal/d before a measurable effect on birthweight becomes evident. Maternal **malabsorption** may predispose to IUGR pregnancy. The most common clinical situations are inflammatory bowel disease (ulcerative colitis or regional enteritis), pancreatitis, and intestinal parasites.

4. Vascular disease—Other diseases that affect maternal microvascular perfusion can be associated with IUGR. These include collagen vascular disease, insulin-dependent diabetes mellitus associated with microvasculopathy, and preeclampsia.

5. Maternal features—A small woman may have a smaller-than-normal infant because of reduced uterine growth potential. These mothers and infants are completely normal and healthy but are small in size because of genetic variation. The infants are described by the ponderal index (PI), calculated from the following formula:

$$PI = \text{Birthweight} \times 1000/(\text{crown-heel length})^3$$

Asymmetric IUGR infants will have a low ponderal index (ie, they will be long, lightweight infants), whereas small normal infants will have a normal index. (A normal index at 28 weeks is 1.8. This increases by 0.2 every 4 weeks to reach 2.4 at 40 weeks.) Errors in cubing of the crown-heel length will skew the measurements greatly.

Maternal parity exerts a modest effect on birthweight. First-born infants tend to be smaller and more often categorized as IUGR. This effect decreases with successive deliveries and is not seen beyond the third birth.

6. Sex of fetus—At term, female fetuses are on average 5% (150 g) smaller and 2% (1 cm) shorter than male fetuses. Referring to separate norms for male and female fetuses may increase the power of biometry in assessing IUGR.

Antenatal Diagnosis

In any pregnancy at risk for IUGR outcome, baseline studies should be obtained early in gestation. These should always include careful attention to gestational dating (menstrual history, serial examinations, biochemical pregnancy testing, quickening, ultrasound). An IUGR outcome may also develop in pregnancies without identified risk factors. Careful attention to fundal height measurements is associated with a diagnostic sensitivity of 46–86%.

Ultrasound examination early in pregnancy is accurate in establishing the estimated date of confinement (EDC) and may sometimes identify genetic or congenital causes of IUGR pregnancy. Serial ultrasound examinations are important in documenting growth and excluding anomalies. Antenatal diagnosis of intrauterine growth restriction is not precise given that estimated fetal weight cannot be measured directly and must be calculated from a combination of directly measured parameters. Overall the predictive accuracy of birthweight formulas have an error of within 10–20%. Selection of the most useful biometric parameter depends on the timing of measurements. The crown-rump length (CRL) is the best parameter for early dating of pregnancy. The biparietal diameter (BPD) and head circumference (HC) are most accurate in the second trimester, with a margin of error of 7–11 days for BPD and 3–5 days for HC. Head circumference is more useful in establishing gestational age in the third trimester because the BPD loses its accuracy secondary to variations in shape. Abdominal circumference measurements are less accurate than BPD, HC, and femur length (FL), but is the most useful measurement to evaluate fetal growth. The fetal abdominal circumference also reflects the volume of fetal subcutaneous fat and the size of the liver which, in turn, correlates with the degree of fetal nutrition. The femur length is not helpful in the identification of the IUGR baby but can identify skeletal dysplasia. Since the definition of IUGR ultimately depends on birthweight and gestational age criteria, the employment of formulas that optimally predict birthweight in a given population will be the most important ultrasonographic criteria.

Fetuses from different populations show different growth patterns. The growth curves developed by Battaglia and Lubchenco in the 1960s do not reflect the variation in birthweight for various ethnic populations. The growth curves used today also do not reflect the median birthweight increase over the last 3 decades. Racial and ethnic anthropometric variations may suggest a need for specific charts for different communities. Ultrasound evaluation should also be used to identify the development of oligohydramnios in fetuses at risk for or with the diagnosis of IUGR. Decreased amniotic fluid volume is clinically associated with IUGR and may be the earliest sign detected on ultrasound. This finding is thought to be a result of decreased perfusion of the fetal kidneys, thereby resulting in decreased urine production. Oligohydramnios is present in the majority of IUGR infants (approximately 80–90%), but the presence of a normal amniotic fluid index (AFI) should not preclude the diagnosis of IUGR.

In fetuses already known to be IUGR, umbilical artery Doppler velocimetry can estimate the likelihood of adverse perinatal outcome and may be useful in determining the intensity of fetal surveillance. Placental circulatory insufficiency is associated with an increase in placental resistance, which causes a fall in umbilical flow and therefore hypoxia. During the compensated stage, diastolic flow in the umbilical artery is reduced or absent. Retrograde diastolic flow in the umbilical artery is a sign that severe hypoxemia and acidemia are present. However, the utility of umbilical artery Doppler velocimetry remains unproven for general population screening. Although not useful for screening, Doppler studies can be helpful in following IUGR pregnancies once they have been identified. Using Doppler flow studies helps reduce intervention and improves overall fetal outcome in IUGR pregnancies. A recent study showed that of fetuses with suspected IUGR evaluated by Doppler studies, none of those with normal Doppler flow measurements (umbilical artery systolic:diastolic [S:D] ratio) were delivered with metabolic acidemia. This suggests that intense antenatal surveillance may be unnecessary in fetuses with normal umbilical artery S:D ratios and normal AFI.

Abnormal umbilical artery flow is associated with a higher risk of fetal growth restriction and an increased likelihood of requiring cesarean or operative delivery. In fetuses with suspected IUGR, abnormal middle cerebral artery (MCA) and umbilical artery (UA) S:D ratios are strongly associated with low gestational age at delivery, low birthweight, and low umbilical artery pH. Also, mean birthweight, interval to delivery, and occurrence of fetal distress are all related to the severity of abnormal Doppler findings after correction for gestational age. Abnormal MCA and UA S:D ratios are also significantly associated with shorter interval to delivery and need for emergent delivery. Respiratory distress syndrome and intracranial hemorrhage are not associated with abnormal Doppler studies.

In addition to the UA and MCA, the descending aorta is also found to have altered perfusion in fetuses with growth restriction. It is thought that the redistribution of systemic blood flow to maintain perfusion to the brain at the expense of abdominal organs results in increased vascular resistance in the perfusion area of the descending aorta and decreased vascular resistance in the cerebrum. Recent studies of the uterine artery early diastolic notch have demonstrated its usefulness as another marker for fetal well-being.

Baseline laboratory studies should also be obtained early in pregnancy. Studies vary from patient to patient, but most patients at risk for IUGR should have a complete blood count, as well as tests for electrolytes, liver function, uric acid, and renal function (including serum blood urea nitrogen and creatinine), plus a 24-hour urine determination for creatinine clearance and total protein.

Maternal serum alpha-fetoprotein (MS-AFP) elevations predict increased risk for IUGR outcome, regardless of maternal weight. Elevated MS-AFP also predicts an increased risk of other obstetric problems including preeclampsia, placental abruption, preterm labor, and stillbirth.

In some centers, severe fetal growth restriction has become an important indication for fetal blood sampling via cordocentesis. These procedures can provide useful information on fetal karyotype, acid-base balance, fetal metabolism, and possible fetal infection. Gestational age-specific values now exist for most hematologic and metabolic parameters.

If clinically indicated, studies should be done to exclude infection. Initially this usually involves determination of immune status (IgG antibodies against cytomegalovirus, rubella virus, and *T gondii*). If the IgG titer is high, specific IgM antibodies should be measured. If these are present in significant quantity, primary infection may be present. A careful targeted ultrasound examination should be performed to determine the degree of fetal involvement, particularly of the central nervous system. Fetal involvement may be further investigated by direct fetal blood sampling for organism-specific IgM assays, cultures, or electron microscopy for direct visualization of viral particles.

Complications

Numerous maternal and perinatal complications occur more frequently in IUGR pregnancy. Underlying maternal disease is more likely to be present (see Table 16–3), and these women require more intensive prenatal care. Premature labor or preeclampsia is more common. IUGR fetuses at any gestational age are less likely to tolerate labor well, and the need for operative delivery is increased.

Perinatal morbidity and mortality is significantly increased with low-birthweight infants, especially those with weights at or below the 3rd percentile. Increased risk of mortality is affected by gestational age and primary etiology of growth restriction and may be modified by the severity and progression of maternal factors (eg, hypertension control). With the advent of fetal surveillance, the perinatal mortality rate decreased to 2–3 times that of the AGA population. With continued improvements in antenatal surveillance and neonatal care, the perinatal mortality rate for IUGR pregnancies in most centers is now 1.5–2 times that of the AGA population. Unfortunately, it is unlikely that this rate will reach in the near future that of the AGA population, because of the persistent occurrence of lethal anomalies and severe congenital infections. The past decade has witnessed increased attention to minimizing the perinatal complications of surviving IUGR neonates.

IUGR fetuses are at risk for in utero complications including hypoxia and metabolic acidosis, which may occur at any time but are likely to occur during labor, with up to 50% of growth-restricted fetuses exhibiting abnormal fetal heart rate patterns, most often variable decelerations. Hypoxia is the result of increasing fetal oxygen requirements during pregnancy with a rapid increase during the third trimester. If the fetus receives inadequate oxygen, for whatever reason, hypoxia and subsequent metabolic acidosis will ensue. If undetected or untreated, this will lead to decreased glycogen and fat stores, ischemic end-organ damage, meconium-stained amniotic fluid, and oligohydramnios, with eventual vital organ damage and intrauterine death.

IUGR infants are at increased risk for neonatal complications, including meconium aspiration syndrome, apneic episodes, low Apgar scores, umbilical artery pH less than 7.0, need for intubation in the delivery room, seizures, sepsis, polycythemia, hypoglycemia, hypocalcemia, temperature instability, and neonatal death. All IUGR infants need thorough evaluation for congenital anomalies.

Prevention

Since many of the causes of IUGR are nonpreventable, there are few interventions that have been shown to be effective for prevention. Interventions which have been shown to be beneficial include smoking cessation, antimalarial chemoprophylaxis, and balanced protein and energy supplementation. Smoking is the single most common preventable cause of IUGR infants in the United States As mentioned earlier, women who quit smoking at 7 months have mean birthweights higher than those who smoke throughout the pregnancy. Those who quit smoking before 16 weeks are not at any increased risk for an IUGR infant. A recent review of trials on **antimalarial drug chemoprophylaxis** showed higher maternal Hb levels and higher birthweights. These effects were more pronounced in primigravidas. There are limited data that suggest that **balanced**

nutritional supplementation improves mean birthweight. As expected, such supplementation is more likely to be beneficial in those with poor nutrition or adolescent pregnancies. Avoidance of factors associated with an increased likelihood of neural tube defects (eg, maternal hyperthermia at the time of neural tube closure) should be encouraged in all pregnancies.

Pregnant women should avoid close contact with individuals known to be infected or colonized with rubella virus or cytomegalovirus. Nonpregnant women of reproductive age should be tested for immunity to rubella virus and, if susceptible, should be immunized. Unfortunately, no vaccine currently exists for cytomegalovirus.

If it is clinically suspected, women of childbearing age should be tested for immunity to *T. gondii*. If the woman is immune, her risk of having an affected infant is remote, but if she is susceptible, she should be cautioned to avoid animal excrement (especially that of domestic cats) and uncooked meat.

Therapeutic medications are not a major cause of IUGR pregnancy, but benefits and risks should be weighed whenever medications are prescribed. Any woman of childbearing age should be questioned about the possibility of pregnancy before receiving therapeutic or diagnostic radiation to the pelvis.

Placental factors causing IUGR pregnancies are not generally preventable. However, low-dose aspirin and dipyridamole may increase prostacyclin production in certain patients and thus prevent idiopathic uteroplacental insufficiency. Aspirin therapy has not been shown to have any significant effect on prevention of IUGR infants in the general population, however.

Preventive measures for the maternal diseases listed in Table 16–3 are too complex to be discussed in this chapter. Treatment of many of these conditions may decrease the likelihood of IUGR pregnancy. Treatment of hypertension has a positive effect on birthweight, at least in the third trimester. However, strict bed rest and hospitalization do not seem to have any beneficial effects for patients with a history of hypertension. Although a complex issue, protein supplements for patients with significant proteinuria may increase the amount of protein available for placental transfer. Correction of maternal anemia (of whatever cause) improves oxygen delivery to the fetus and thus improves fetal growth. However, routine supplements, such as iron supplements, have not been shown to be associated with any altered clinical outcomes other than a lower cesarean section rate.

Treatment of malabsorption syndrome (of whatever cause) can be expected to improve nutrient absorption and subsequent transfer to the fetus. Inflammatory bowel disease should be treated if required, but if possible, pregnancy should be deferred until the disease has been quiescent for approximately 6 months. Intestinal parasites should be appropriately treated and negative cultures confirmed prior to pregnancy.

Treatment

Treatment of IUGR pregnancy presupposes an accurate diagnosis. Even with the history, physical examination, and ultrasound examination, diagnosis remains difficult, and some IUGR pregnancies will not be detected.

All pregnant women should discontinue cigarette smoking as well as use of alcohol and all recreational drugs. This should be done before conception to allow time for clearance of toxins, particularly if the woman has had a previous IUGR infant. Adequate nutrition must also be emphasized.

Controversy exists concerning the role of bed rest in IUGR pregnancy. Its value has not been proved in women with symmetric IUGR fetuses, because the most common causes are not correctable by increased uterine blood flow. However, asymmetric IUGR pregnancies may benefit from the increased uterine blood flow that occurs when the patient is in the lateral recumbent position. Although bed rest may do little to prolong the duration of pregnancy, it probably is associated with increased birthweight per week of gestation, and thus is of value in asymmetric IUGR pregnancy.

Low-dose aspirin may also be of value in selected cases of IUGR pregnancy. This regimen decreases thromboxane A_2 synthesis, with resultant predominance of prostacyclin, a potent vasodilator.

Since IUGR fetuses are at risk for antepartum or intrapartum compromise, they should be followed up carefully. Weekly prenatal visits should include an interview and examination with attention to frequency and intensity of fetal movements, presence or absence of contractions, and signs of rupture of membranes. Physical examination should always include the mother's weight, fundal height, fetal heart rate, assessment of presentation, and maternal blood pressure and urinalysis. Maternal girth at the umbilicus may also be helpful in assessing uterine growth.

Electronic fetal monitoring should be performed at least weekly on all potentially viable IUGR babies. The nonstress test is usually a satisfactory initial choice. Some authorities believe the nonstress test is less sensitive to fetal compromise than the contraction stress test, but if care is taken to note the baseline fetal heart rate (normal on monitoring is 110–150/min) and to allow for small variable decelerations, the 2 tests are probably equally sensitive and useful.

Ultrasound examinations to assess adequacy of fetal growth should be performed at least every 4–6 weeks. Measurements should include biparietal diameter, head circumference, and femur length, especially in those in whom an asymmetric IUGR fetus is suspected. Probably the most sensitive indices of an asymmetric IUGR fetus are abdominal circumference and total intrauterine volume, although both require a definite EDC for optimum interpretation. The femur length:abdominal circumference ratio is a gestational age-independent ratio, with normal being 0.20–0.24. Asymmetric IUGR fetuses generally have a ratio greater than 0.24.

Amniotic fluid volume should also be assessed at least weekly in at-risk pregnancies, because the likelihood of a fetus being small because of nutritional deprivation is much less when normal amniotic fluid volume is present.

Ultrasonography can determine fetal biophysical profiles (see Chapter 13). If a nonstress test is nonreactive or if variable or spontaneous decelerations are seen, further assessment of fetal well-being is immediately indicated. Either a contraction stress test or a fetal biophysical profile can be performed. To date, there have been no randomized prospective evaluations of the relative efficacy of either procedure in an at-risk IUGR population. The presence of late decelerations with more than 50% of contractions (regardless of frequency of contractions) constitutes a positive contraction stress test and is an indication to proceed with delivery unless there is an obvious, easily treatable maternal problem such as dehydration or hyperthermia. The fetal biophysical profile is discussed in more detail in Chapter 13; it provides evidence about fetal well-being and has the additional advantage of assessing fetal anatomy.

In selected cases, ultrasound-directed amniocentesis may be indicated (for determination of fetal pulmonary maturity with an uncertain EDC or for assessment of fetal karyotype, certain biochemical disorders, or AFP levels).

Every IUGR pregnancy must be individually assessed for the optimal time of delivery (ie, the point at which the baby will do as well outside as inside the uterus). This would be whenever surveillance indicates fetal maturity, fetal compromise, or gestational age of 38 weeks (beyond which time there is no advantage to an IUGR fetus remaining in utero). There are conflicting data as to whether IUGR accelerates pulmonary maturity. Therefore, the current recommendation is to administer glucocorticoids to women likely to deliver before 34 weeks as would be done with any other pregnancy.

IUGR pregnancies are at increased risk for intrapartum problems, and whenever possible, delivery should take place in a center where appropriate obstetric care, anesthesia, and neonatal care are readily available. Cesarean delivery may be necessary, and the presence of meconium-stained amniotic fluid or a compromised infant should be anticipated.

The type of delivery depends on the individual case. Cesarean section delivery is often indicated, especially when fetal monitoring reveals fetal compromise, malpresentation, or situations in which traumatic vaginal delivery might be expected.

Continuous electronic fetal heart rate monitoring should be performed during labor in all cases, even if recent antepartum testing has been reassuring. Scalp pH or oxygen saturation determinations (see Chapter 13) should be performed readily if the fetal heart tracing is nonreassuring, especially in preterm IUGR pregnancies. Arteriovenous cord blood gas determinations are also useful in all cases. As many as 50% of IUGR infants have some degree of metabolic acidosis. If metabolic acidosis is present, prompt evaluation by a neonatologist is necessary.

Minimization of anesthesia is generally preferable, but controlled epidural anesthesia is usually safe. Maternal hypotension or hypovolemia must be avoided.

Prognosis

IUGR pregnancy per se is not considered life-threatening for the mother. However, she may be at risk for significant morbidity or even death if she has an underlying condition that predisposes to an IUGR fetus (eg, hypertension or renal disease). Most women who deliver IUGR infants can be expected to have long-term prognoses equivalent to women delivering AGA infants. Infants with low birthweights have relatively high morbidity and mortality. There is no specific birthweight percentile at which morbidity and mortality are increased. Nonetheless, it has been shown that the rate of neonatal death, Apgar at 5 minutes < 3, umbilical artery pH < 7.0, seizures during the first day of life, and incidence of intubation are significantly increased at or below the 3rd percentile for birthweight.

The long-term prognosis is less benign for the IUGR infant. IUGR infants tend to remain physically small, particularly symmetric infants (with normal PI), since these infants are likely either to have significant intrinsic problems that will not improve following birth or to be constitutionally small infants born of constitutionally small mothers. Asymmetric infants (with low PI) tend to have accelerated growth for the first 6 months after birth, particularly if intrauterine deprivation was a major factor.

Taken as a group, IUGR infants also have more neurologic and intellectual deficits than do their AGA peers. IUGR infants have lower IQs as well as a higher incidence of learning and behavioral problems. Major neurologic handicaps such as severe mental retardation, cerebral palsy, and seizures are more common in IUGR infants. IUGR infants are more likely to have hypertension early in life, reflecting the fact that many hypertensive diseases are inheritable. In addition, the incidence of sudden infant death syndrome (SIDS) is increased in IUGR infants, who account for 30% of all SIDS cases. All these problems are more frequent and more severe in infants with small head circumferences, again emphasizing that symmetrically small infants have a worse prognosis than asymmetrically small infants.

LARGE-FOR-GESTATIONAL-AGE PREGNANCY

Terminology

Although LGA pregnancy is defined according to the same concept as IUGR pregnancy (LGA = heaviest 10% of newborns), LGA pregnancy has received substantially less attention. Large for gestational age is defined as above the 90th percentile of weight for any specific gestational age. **Macrosomia** is generally used to refer to fetuses with an estimated fetal weight greater than or equal to 4000 g. However, some feel that macrosomia should be defined as greater than 4500 g, greater than 90th percentile, or greater than 2 standard deviations above the mean for weight at any particular gestational age. Although there are numerous reports and studies regarding macrosomia, there are few data regarding large for gestational age as defined here. Therefore, this section will concentrate on fetal macrosomia, with additional comments regarding LGA pregnancies.

Pathophysiology

Numerous endocrinologic changes occur during pregnancy to ensure an adequate fetal glucose supply. In the second half of pregnancy, increased concentrations of human placental lactogen, free and total cortisol, and prolactin combine to produce modest maternal insulin resistance, which is countered by postprandial hyperinsulinemia. In those who are unable to mount this hyperinsulinemic response, relative hyperglycemia may develop (ie, gestational diabetes). Because glucose crosses the placenta by facilitated diffusion, fetal hyperglycemia ensues. This in turn produces fetal hyperinsulinemia with resultant intracellular transfer of glucose, leading to fetal macrosomia.

Differential Diagnosis

Factors that predispose to LGA pregnancy are listed in Table 16–4. As with IUGR pregnancy, diagnosis of LGA pregnancy depends on knowing with certainty the duration of the pregnancy (see Chapter 9).

A. MATERNAL DIABETES

Maternal diabetes, whether it is gestational, chemical, or insulin-dependent, is the condition classically associ-

Table 16–4. Factors that may predispose to fetal macrosomia or LGA pregnancy.

Maternal Factors
Diabetes (gestational, chemical, or insulin-dependent), obesity, postdatism, multiparity, advanced age, previous LGA infant, large stature
Fetal Factors
Genetic or congenital disorders, male sex

ated with fetal macrosomia. It was long assumed that fetal macrosomia could be accounted for by the "Pedersen hypothesis"—ie, that the condition was due to inadequate management of diabetes during pregnancy. Initial reports suggested that careful control of blood glucose in insulin-dependent diabetic women would prevent fetal macrosomia, but recent studies have suggested that the problem is not so simple and that the incidence may correlate better with cord blood concentrations of maternally acquired anti-insulin IgG antibodies, and/or increased serum levels of free fatty acids, triglycerides, and the amino acids alanine, serine, and isoleucine.

It has also been found that there is a significant correlation between plasma leptin levels and neonatal birthweight, which suggests that leptin levels are directly related to the quantity of body fat tissue in fetal macrosomia.

B. MATERNAL OBESITY

Maternal obesity is associated with a three- to fourfold increased likelihood of fetal macrosomia. This may be due in part to associated gestational or chemical diabetes, although these disorders are not present in most obese women who deliver macrosomic babies.

C. POSTDATISM

Prolonged pregnancy is more likely to result in a macrosomic fetus, presumably due to continued delivery of nutrients and oxygen to the fetus. Placental sulfatase deficiency or congenital adrenal hypoplasia should also be considered in the evaluation.

D. GENETIC AND CONGENITAL DISORDERS

Several genetic and congenital syndromes are associated with an increased incidence of LGA fetuses. **Beckwith-Wiedemann syndrome** is frequently associated with fetal macrosomia, usually because of pancreatic islet cell hyperplasia (nesidioblastosis). Affected infants usually have hypoglycemia, macroglossia, and omphalocele. They may also have intestinal malrotation or visceromegaly. Although usually a sporadic event, in a few families other inheritance patterns have been suggested.

Other rare syndromes include **Weaver's syndrome, Sotos' syndrome, Nevo syndrome, Ruvalcaba-Myhre syndrome,** and **Marshall's syndrome. Carpenter's syndrome** and the **fragile X syndrome** may also be associated with an increased incidence of LGA infants.

E. CONSTITUTIONALLY LARGE FETUS

Fetuses who are suspected to be large for gestational age may simply be large secondary to constitutional factors. **Large maternal stature** should be considered as contributing to macrosomia because birthweight tends to correlate more closely with maternal height than even maternal weight. **Male sex fetuses** are more likely to be considered LGA because male fetuses are an average of 150 g heavier than appropriately matched female fetuses at each gestational week during late pregnancy. Series addressing fetal macrosomia generally report an increased incidence of male fetuses, usually about 60–65%.

Complications

As seen in Table 16–2, there are many complications for which the LGA pregnancy is at increased risk. Macrosomic pregnancies are more likely to require cesarean delivery. Women with diabetes predating pregnancy in particular have rates of cesarean section ~40–80%. By far the most common indication for cesarean delivery is failure to progress in labor. In particular, primigravidas delivering a macrosomic infant (defined as > 4500 g in this instance) are at increased risk for complications such as prolonged labor, operative vaginal delivery, and emergency cesarean section as compared to delivering a normal weight infant. Fetal distress, as determined by electronic fetal monitoring, is not more common in macrosomic pregnancies.

Postpartum hemorrhage is more common in macrosomic pregnancies and presumably in LGA pregnancies as well. Both conditions are associated with a distended uterus, inadequate labor progress, and reproductive tract injury.

Shoulder dystocia occurs in 6–23.6% of vaginally delivered macrosomic fetuses (compared with 0.3–1% of nonmacrosomic controls). The incidence of shoulder dystocia correlates not only with progressive fetal weight but also with increasing chest-to-head circumference. Up to one-fourth of infants with shoulder dystocia experience brachial plexus injury, facial nerve injury, and fractures of the humerus or clavicle. The risk of brachial plexus injury with shoulder dystocia is ~7% in infants whose birthweights exceed 4000 g, but is 14% for mothers with gestational diabetes. This doubled risk may be secondary to increased abdominal obesity in diabetic mothers. There is direct correlation in diabetic patients with the level of fetal truncal asymmetry (abdominal circumference:biparietal diameter [AC:BPD] ratio) measured by ultrasound and the incidence and severity of shoulder dystocia. Risk factors for shoulder dystocia should be assessed prior to delivery. In addition to macrosomia, other risk factors for shoulder dystocia include previous shoulder dystocia, maternal diabetes (three to fourfold increase compared to nondiabetic mothers), previous delivery of a large fetus, and excessive maternal weight gain during pregnancy. The risk of shoulder dystocia is similar in primigravidas and multigravidas delivering macrosomic infants. Frequent clinical estimations of fetal weight may help to select appropriate candidates for cesarean section delivery without a trial of labor.

Perineal trauma is more likely with a macrosomic pregnancy and is related to increased incidence of shoulder dystocia and operative vaginal delivery. Vaginal delivery of a macrosomic infant increases the risk of third- or fourth-degree laceration fivefold.

Although gestational diabetes and postdatism predispose to fetal macrosomia, there is no evidence that fetal macrosomia or an LGA fetus predisposes to gestational diabetes or postdatism.

The incidence of stillbirth remains higher in macrosomic fetuses than in controls of average weight. This problem has persisted even with the availability of fetal monitoring and presumably reflects the increased incidence of maternal diabetes and postdatism. Stillbirths are known to be increased in diabetic mothers, the majority of which are thought to be secondary to lethal congenital malformations. Additionally, excessive prepregnancy weight is an independent risk factor for unexplained death. In fact, large-for-gestational-age is statistically associated with unexplained fetal death even after controlling for maternal age, diabetes, and hypertension.

Many of the neonatal complications of fetal macrosomia are the result of underlying maternal diabetes or birth trauma and include low Apgar scores, hypoglycemia, hypocalcemia, polycythemia, jaundice, and feeding difficulties. Macrosomic infants are also at risk for subsequent Erb's palsy, cerebral palsy, mental retardation, and seizures.

Large-for-gestational-age infants have significantly higher absolute nucleated red blood cell counts, lymphocyte counts, and packed cell volumes. These hematologic abnormalities are the same for all LGA infants regardless of whether they are infants of nondiabetic mothers, insulin-dependent diabetic mothers, or non-insulin-dependent gestational diabetics. It is believed that this reflects a compensatory increase in erythropoiesis as a result of chronic intrauterine hypoxia resulting from increased placental oxygen consumption and decreased fetal oxygen delivery.

LGA infants of diabetic mothers have an increased incidence of asymmetric cardiac septal hypertrophy and interventricular septum.

Prevention

Prevention of macrosomia and ensuing complications requires early detection of risk factors. Risk factors for having an LGA or macrosomic infant include multiparity, advanced maternal age, and previous delivery of an LGA or macrosomic infant. When controlled for gestational age and fetal gender, the average birthweight with successive pregnancies increases by 80–120 g up to the fifth pregnancy. Multiparity is also associated with other risk factors (ie, obesity, diabetes) and may therefore be a confounding variable. Progressive maternal age also contributes to increased birthweight. However, as with multiparity, it is also associated with obesity and diabetes.

Patients with the risk factors noted in Table 16–4 should be evaluated for possible fetal macrosomia with ultrasound estimates of fetal size and weight at regular intervals, and the EDC in each case should be confirmed both clinically and with ultrasonography.

Estimated fetal weight (EFW) by ultrasound is not very accurate. Even in skillful hands, the error of fetal weight estimates by ultrasound is 10–15%. A recent review of ultrasonographic diagnosis of macrosomia shows a sensitivity ranging from 24–88% and specificity from 60–98%. The margin of error in estimating fetal weight means that the EFW by ultrasound must be at least 4750 g in order to predict a birthweight of 4000 g with a confidence interval of 90%. The best single measurement in evaluating macrosomia in diabetic mothers is abdominal circumference. An initial abdominal circumference above the 70th percentile is significantly associated with subsequent delivery of an LGA infant. Cheek-to-cheek diameter and humeral soft tissue thickness can be added to AC to improve diagnosis. However, fetal body composition and fetal shoulder width cannot be accurately assessed by ultrasound.

Adequate control of maternal glucose levels is thought to prevent the development of macrosomia in gestational diabetics, although there have been reports of neonatal complications despite excellent metabolic control. Prepregnancy weight and degree of weight gain are strong indicators for macrosomia regardless of glycemic control. However, there is an overall reduced rate of macrosomia and complications when postprandial levels are monitored. Studies have shown that the risk of macrosomia is reduced to near normal in diabetic women who monitored 1-h postprandial glucose levels and that 1-h postprandial glucose levels are directly related to fetal abdominal circumference values. One study showed that when postprandial glucose levels were kept below 104, macrosomia rates were similar to those of nondiabetics. Furthermore, high carbohydrate intake is associated with decreased incidence of newborn macrosomia. Essential management principles in known diabetics include nutrition and exercise counseling starting in the preconception period. Furthermore, euglycemia is crucial in the first trimester, a period when insulin requirements are frequently less than prepregnancy, and intake can be altered by nausea and vomiting. Insulin adjustments are frequently necessary.

Infants of women who participate in regular aerobic exercise programs have lower average birthweights than the general population, but there are no demonstrable adverse effects. To date, no studies have been done to evaluate the potential efficacy of exercise programs as a means of decreasing birthweight in women at risk for LGA pregnancy.

Treatment

Although widely recommended, labor induction in at-risk pregnancy for reduction in the incidence of fetal macrosomia and/or intrapartum complications remains an unproven hypothesis. Intrapartum treatment considerations center on the increased likelihood of traumatic vaginal delivery.

Several published reviews of fetal macrosomia suggest routine cesarean delivery for fetuses with estimated weights of 5000 g or more. This is based in part on the data given in Table 16–2 and in part on anthropometric studies, suggesting that very macrosomic fetuses have bisacromial circumferences in excess of head circumferences. Because of current limitations in the sensitivity and specificity of ultrasound-derived fetal weight calculations, decisions regarding scheduled abdominal delivery must be partially based on clinical grounds. Such considerations are particularly warranted in women who are obese or are diabetic or in postdate pregnancies. Maternal age and maternal preference should also be taken into consideration when deciding on delivery method. Vacuum-assisted vaginal delivery can be attempted; however, it should be taken into consideration that vacuum assistance is less likely to be successful in the delivery of infants who weigh more than 4000 g. Prolonged second stage of labor or arrest of descent of a fetus with an estimated fetal weight greater than 4500 g is an indication for cesarean delivery. Labor and attempted vaginal delivery is contraindicated for women with estimated fetal weights greater than 5000 g.

Because of these factors, women at risk for macrosomic or LGA babies should deliver in facilities where adequate obstetric care, pediatric care, and anesthesia are present. Large-bore intravenous access must be established, and blood must be available. Delivery should take place in a setting where immediate operation can be accomplished. In many situations, this should occur in a delivery room.

Prognosis

Any woman who delivers an LGA baby should be informed that the risk of her having another LGA baby is increased by 2.5- to 4-fold. Such women should be screened for previously undiagnosed chemical or insulin-dependent diabetes and, even if screening is negative, should be followed carefully in any subsequent pregnancy to rule out gestational diabetes.

Obese women should be strongly encouraged to lose weight prior to becoming pregnant. Any woman who has delivered an LGA infant should also be encouraged to seek early care for any subsequent pregnancy, if for no other reason than early confirmation of the EDC, which can minimize the likelihood of subsequent postdatism. Women who deliver an LGA infant with an underlying genetic or congenital disorder should receive genetic counseling regarding recurrence risks and the feasibility of antepartum diagnosis.

Besides the many neonatal complications previously noted, infants of mothers with gestational or chemical diabetes are at increased risk for subsequent obesity, type 2 diabetes, or both. Infants who suffer from neonatal complications are at increased risk for subsequent neurologic or behavioral problems.

LGA infants have an increased incidence of subsequent neoplasia when compared with AGA controls. This association is not surprising, since rapidly dividing cells are prerequisites for both processes. The risk for childhood leukemia is directly related to birthweight. Likewise, Wilms' tumor and osteosarcoma are associated with increased birthweight. Other neoplasms seen with increased frequency in LGA syndromes are nephroblastoma, adrenal cortical carcinoma, and hepatoblastoma.

It is interesting that diabetic macrosomia is not associated with an increased incidence of neoplasms, probably because the macrosomia is mediated normally rather than by intrinsic cellular hyperplasia.

FUTURE DIAGNOSIS OF IUGR & LGA PREGNANCIES

Although much more is known about the risks of IUGR than of LGA pregnancy, both are known to be associated with increased risks of in utero, intrapartum, neonatal, or long-term compromise. The ability to diagnose and optimally manage these pregnancies remains poor. Further effort must be directed toward precise diagnosis at a point in the pregnancy at which intervention can still be effective.

REFERENCES

Terminology

American College of Obstetricians and Gynecologists: Clinical management guidelines for obstetrician-gynecologists. ACOG Practice Bulletin No. 12, January 2000.

Chatfield J: Practice guidelines. ACOG issues guidelines on fetal macrosomia. Am Fam Physician 2001;64:169.

Degani S: Fetal biometry: Clinical, pathological, and technical considerations. Obstet Gynecol Surv 2001;56:159.

Jovanovic L: What is so bad about a big baby? Diabetes Care 2001;24;1317.

Schwartz R et al: What is the significance of macrosomia? Diabetes Care 1999;22;1201.

Differential Diagnosis

American College of Obstetricians and Gynecologists: Clinical management guidelines for obstetrician-gynecologists. ACOG Practice Bulletin No. 12, January 2000.

Clausson B et al: Perinatal outcome in SGA births defined by customized versus population-based birthweight standards. Br J Obstet Gynecol 2001;108:830.

Degani S: Fetal biometry: Clinical, pathological, and technical considerations. Obstet Gynecol Surv 2001;56:159.

Wiznitzer A et al: Cord leptin level and fetal macrosomia. Obstet Gynecol 2000;96;707.

Wolfe H: High prepregnancy body-mass index—a maternal-fetal risk factor. N Engl J Med 1998;338;191.

Antenatal Diagnosis

Aardema M et al: Uterine artery doppler flow and uteroplacental vascular pathology in normal pregnancy and pregnancies complicated by preeclampsia and small for gestational age fetuses. Placenta 2001;22:405.

American College of Obstetricians and Gynecologists: Clinical management guidelines for obstetrician-gynecologists. ACOG Practice Bulletin No. 12, January 2000.

Baschat A et al: Umbilical artery Doppler screening for detection of the small fetus in need of antepartum surveillance. Am J Obstet Gynecol 2000;182:154.

Bush K et al: The utility of umbilical artery Doppler investigation in women with the HELLP (hemolysis, elevated liver enzymes, and low platelets) syndrome. Am J Obstet Gynecol 2001;184:1087.

Degani S: Fetal biometry: Clinical, pathological, and technical considerations. Obstet Gynecol Surv 2001;56:159.

Fouron J et al: Correlation between prenatal velocity waveforms in the aortic isthmus and neurodevelopmental outcome between the ages of 2 and 4 years. Am J Obstet Gynecol 2001; 184:630.

Goffinet F et al: Screening with a uterine Doppler in low risk pregnancy women followed by low dose aspirin in women with abnormal results: a multicenter randomized control trial. Br J Obstet Gynecol 2001;108:510.

Mandruzzano G et al: Antepartal assessment of IUGR fetuses. J Perinatal Med 2001;29:227.

Maruyama K et al: Superior mesenteric artery blood flow velocity in small for gestational age infants of very low birth weight during the early neonatal period. J Perinat Med 2001;29:64.

Park Y et al: Clinical significance of early diastolic notch depth: Uterine artery Doppler velocimetry in the third trimester. Am J Obstet Gynecol 2000;182:1204.

Sterne G et al: Abnormal fetal cerebral and umbilical Doppler measurements in fetuses with intrauterine growth restriction predicts the severity of perinatal morbidity. J Clin Ultrasound 2001;29:146.

Complications

Bloomgarden Z: American Diabetes Association 60th Scientific Sessions, 2000: Diabetes and pregnancy. Diabetes Care 2000; 23;1699.

Cohen B et al: The incidence of shoulder dystocia correlates with a sonographic measurement of asymmetry in patients with diabetes. Am J Perinatol 1999;16:197.

Cundy T et al: Perinatal mortality in type 2 diabetes mellitus. Obstet Gynecol Surv 2000;55:538.

Dollberg S et al: Normoblasts in large for gestational age infants. Arch Dis Child Fetal Neonatal Ed 2000;83:148.

Gherman R et al: Obstetric maneuvers for shoulder dystocia and associated fetal morbidity. Am J Obstet Gynecol 1998; 178:1126.

Lindley A et al: Maternal cigarette smoking during pregnancy and infant ponderal index at birth in the Swedish Medical Birth Register. Am J Public Health 2000;90:420.

Mocanu E et al: Obstetric and neonatal outcome of babies weighing more than 4.5 kg: an analysis by parity. Eur J Obstet Gynecol 2000;92:229.

Schwartz R et al: What is the significance of macrosomia? Diabetes Care 1999;22:1201.

Vela-Huerta, M: Asymmetrical septal hypertrophy in newborn infants of diabetic mothers. Am J Perinatol 2000;17:89.

Prevention

Bloomgarden Z: American Diabetes Association 60th Scientific Sessions, 2000: Diabetes and pregnancy. Diabetes Care 2000;23:1699.

Gulmezoglu M et al: Effectiveness of interventions to prevent or treat impaired fetal growth. Obstet Gynecol Surv 1999; 54:58.

Holcomb W: Parity and maternal age affect excess fetal growth contrariwise in diabetes. Am J Obstet Gynecol 2000;182:83.

Jovanovic L: What is so bad about a big baby? Diabetes Care 2001; 24:1317.

Kjos S: Prediction of large for gestational age infants in gestational diabetes with moderate fasting hyperglycemia. Am J Obstet Gynecol 2000;182:79.

Lindley A et al: Maternal cigarette smoking during pregnancy and infant ponderal index at birth in the Swedish Medical Birth Register. Am J Public Health 2000;90:420.

Romon M et al: Higher carbohydrate intake is associated with decreased incidence of newborn macrosomia in women with gestational diabetes. J Am Diet Assoc 2001;101:897.

Schwartz R et al: What is the significance of macrosomia? Diabetes Care 1999;22:1201.

Treatment

Chatfield J: Practice Guidelines. American College of Obstetricians and Gynecologists issues guidelines on fetal macrosomia. Am Fam Physician 2001;64:169.

Degani S: Fetal biometry: Clinical, pathological, and technical considerations. Obstet Gynecol Surv 2001;56:159.

Gulmezoglu M et al: Effectiveness of interventions to prevent or treat impaired fetal growth. Obstet Gynecol Surv 1999; 54:58.

Owen P et al: Interval between fetal measurements in predicting growth restriction. Obstet Gynecol 2001;97:499.

Parretti E et al: Third-trimester maternal glucose levels from diurnal profiles in nondiabetic pregnancies: Correlation with sonographic parameters of fetal growth. Diabetes Care 2001;24:1319.

Sheiner E et al: Failed vacuum extraction: Maternal risk factors and pregnancy outcome. Am J Obstet Gynecol 2001; 184:165.

Prognosis

Barker DJP: Fetal growth and adult disease. Br J Obstet Gynaecol 1992;99:275.

Bloomgarden Z: American Diabetes Association 60th Scientific Sessions, 2000: Diabetes and pregnancy. Diabetes Care 2000;23:1699.

Bos AF et al: Intrauterine growth retardation, general movements, and neurodevelopmental outcome: a review. Dev Med Child Neurol 2001;43:61.

Georgieff MK: Intrauterine growth retardation and subsequent somatic growth and neurodevelopment. J Pediatr 1998; 133:3.

Hediger M et al: Growth and fatness at three to six years of age of children born small- or large-for-gestational age. Pediatrics 1999;104:555.

Hediger ML et al: Growth of infants and young children born small or large for gestational age: Findings from the Third National Health and Nutrition Examination Survey. Arch Pediatr Adolesc Med 1998;152:1225.

Leitner Y et al: Six-year follow-up of children with intrauterine growth retardation: Long-term prospective study. J Child Neurol 2000;15:781.

McIntire D et al: Birth weight in relation to morbidity and mortality among newborn infants. N Engl J Med 1999; 340:1234.

Weinerroither H et al: Intrauterine blood flow and long-term intellectual, neurologic and social development. Obstet Gynecol 2001;91:449.

Multiple Pregnancy

Melissa Bush, MD, & Martin L. Pernoll, MD

ESSENTIALS OF DIAGNOSIS

- *Demonstration of 2 or more fetuses (eg, ultrasonography, fetal heartbeats, multiplicity of fetal parts).*
- *Disproportionately large uterus for dates.*
- *Increased fetal activity.*
- *Greater-than-expected maternal weight gain.*
- *Maternal hypochromic normocytic anemia.*

Monozygotic twins ("identical twins") are the result of the division of a single fertilized ovum. Monozygotic twinning occurs in about 2.3–4 of 1000 pregnancies in all races. The rate is remarkably constant and is not influenced by heredity, age of the mother, or other factors. Dizygotic twins ("fraternal twins") are produced from separately fertilized ova. Slightly more than 30% of twins are monozygotic; nearly 70% are dizygotic. Although monozygotism is random—ie, it does not fit any discernible genetic pattern—dizygotism has hereditary determinants.

In North America, dizygotic twinning occurs about once in 83 conceptions and triplets about once in 8000 conceptions. A traditional approximation of the incidence of multiple pregnancies is as follows:

Twins	1:80
Triplets	$1:80^2 = 1:6400$
Quadruplets (Etc)	$1:80^3 = 1:512,000$

The incidence of twin and higher-order multiple gestations has increased significantly over the past 15 years primarily because of the availability and increased use of ovulation-inducing drugs and assisted reproductive technology (ART). Multiple gestations now comprise 3% of all pregnancies, and twins comprise 25–30% of deliveries resulting from ART. Significant maternal and neonatal effects are felt from this increase in multiple births. The financial costs are also staggering, with combined costs of ART plus pregnancy care and delivery averaging $39,249.

Maternal morbidity and mortality rates are much higher in multiple pregnancy than in singleton pregnancy due to preterm labor, hemorrhage, urinary tract infection, and pregnancy-induced hypertension. Approximately two-thirds of twin pregnancies end in a single birth; the other embryo is lost from bleeding, is absorbed within the first 10 weeks of pregnancy, or becomes mummified (fetus papyraceous). Moreover, the perinatal mortality rate of twins is 3–4 times higher—and for triplets much higher still—than in singleton pregnancies as a result of chromosomal abnormalities, prematurity, anomalies, hypoxia, and trauma. This is particularly true of monozygotic twins.

Pathogenesis

A. MONOZYGOTIC MULTIPLE GESTATION

Monozygotic twins, resulting from the fertilization of a single ovum by a single sperm, are always of the same sex. However, the twins may develop differently depending on the time of preimplantation division. Normally, monozygotic twins share the same physical characteristics (skin, hair and eye color, body build) and the same genetic features (blood characteristics: ABO, M, N, haptoglobin, serum group; histocompatible genes; skin grafting possible), and they are often mirror images of one another (one left-handed, the other right-handed, etc). However, their fingerprints differ.

The paradox of "identical" twins is that they may be the antithesis of identical. The very earliest splits are sometimes accompanied by a simultaneous chromosomal error, resulting in heterokaryotypic monozygotes, one with Down's syndrome and the other normal.

Monozygotic triplets result from repeated twinning (also called supertwinning) of a single ovum. Trizygotic triplets develop by individual fertilization of 3 simultaneously expelled ova. Triplets may also be produced by the twinning of 2 ova and the elimination of 1 of the 4 resulting embryos. Similarly, quadruplets may be monozygotic, paired dizygotic, or quadrizygotic (ie, they may arise from 1 to 4 ova).

B. DIZYGOTIC MULTIPLE GESTATION

Dizygotic twins are the product of 2 ova and 2 sperms. The 2 ova are released from separate follicles (or, very rarely, from the same follicle) at approximately the same time. Dizygotic (fraternal) twins may be of the same or different sexes. They bear only the resemblance of brothers or sisters and may or may not have the same blood type. Significant differences usually can be identified over time.

About 75% of dizygotic twins are the same sex. Both twins are males in about 45% of cases (a lesser preponderance of males in twins than in singletons) and both females in about 30%.

Many factors influence dizygotic twinning. Race is a factor, with multiple pregnancy most common in blacks, least common in Asians, and of intermediate occurrence in whites. The incidence of dizygotic twinning varies from 1.3 in 1000 in Japan to 49 in 1000 in western Nigeria. The rate in the United States is about 12 in 1000.

Dizygotic multiple pregnancy tends to be recurrent. Women who have borne dizygotic twins have a 10-fold increased chance of subsequent multiple pregnancy. Dizygotic twinning probably is inherited via the female descendants of mothers of twins; the father's genetic contribution plays little or no part. White women who are dizygotic twins or who are siblings of dizygotic twin mothers have a higher twinning rate among their offspring than women in the general population.

Parity does not influence the incidence of dizygotic twinning, but aging does, with the rate of dizygotic twinning peaking between 35 and 40 years of age and then declining sharply. In women who are twins or daughters of twins, the twinning rate peaks at about age 35, at which time it plateaus until almost age 45 and then declines. Black women, whether or not they are twins or siblings of twins, have a prolonged period of dizygotic twinning from 35 to 45 years of age.

Women of increased height and weight have a higher incidence of twinning, but the rate does not vary among social classes. Blood groups O and A are more prevalent in white mothers of twins than in the general population, for unknown reasons.

High fertility (polyovulation) is associated with multiple pregnancy. Excessive production of pituitary gonadotropins, relatively high frequency of coitus, and inability of one graafian follicle to inhibit others have been postulated as reasons for a higher incidence of dizygotic twinning. Undernutrition appears to be a negative factor. Women who conceive late in an ovulatory cycle have a greater chance of multiple pregnancy, perhaps owing to ovular "overripeness."

Dizygotic twinning is more common among women who become pregnant soon after cessation of long-term oral contraception. This may be a reflection of high "rebound" gonadotropin secretion. Induction of ovulation with human pituitary gonadotropin in previously infertile patients has resulted in many multiple pregnancies—even the gestation of septuplets and octuplets. The estrogen analog clomiphene citrate increases the incidence of dizygotic pregnancy to about 5–10%.

C. OTHER FORMS OF MULTIPLE GESTATION

Other kinds of twinning are theoretically possible in humans. Dispermic mosaicism may result from fertilization of 2 ova that have not been independently released but have instead developed from the same oocyte. Another possibility is the fertilization of 1 ovum by 2 sperms. Twinning of discordant twins may be explained by meiotic abnormalities, including polar body twinning, delayed implantation of the embryo, retarded or arrested intrauterine development, or superfetation.

Superfecundation is the fertilization of 2 ova, released at about the same time, by sperm released at intercourse on 2 different occasions. The rare cases in which the fetuses are of disparate size or skin color and have blood groups corresponding to those of the mother's 2 male partners lend credence to (but do not conclusively validate) this possibility.

Superfetation is the fertilization of 2 ova released in different menstrual cycles. This is virtually impossible in humans, because the initial corpus luteum of pregnancy would have to be suppressed to allow for a second ovulation about 1 month later.

Pathologic Factors Associated with Twinning

Although the blood volume is increased in multiple pregnancy, maternal anemia often develops because of greater demand for iron by the fetuses. However, prior anemia, poor diet, and malabsorption may precede or compound iron deficiency during multiple pregnancy. Respiratory tidal volume is increased, but the woman pregnant with twins often is "breathless" (possibly due to increased levels of progesterone).

Marked uterine distention and increased pressure on the adjacent viscera and pelvic vasculature are typical of multiple pregnancy. Lutein cysts and even ascites are the result of abnormally high levels of chorionic gonadotropin in occasional multiple pregnancies. Placenta previa develops more frequently because of the large size of the placenta or placentas.

The maternal cardiovascular, respiratory, gastrointestinal, renal, and musculoskeletal systems are especially subject to stress in multiple pregnancy, combined with greater maternal-fetal nutritional requirements. Multiple pregnancy is classified as high-risk because of the increased incidence of maternal anemia, urinary tract infection, preeclampsia-eclampsia, hemorrhage (before, during, and after delivery), and uterine inertia.

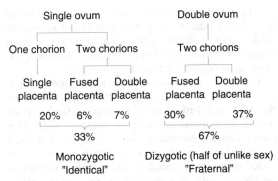

Figure 17–1. Placental variations in twinning. (After Potter. Reproduced, with permission, from Benson RC: *Handbook of Obstetrics & Gynecology*, 8th ed. Lange, 1983.)

A. PLACENTAL AND CORD

The placenta and membranes of monozygotic twins may vary considerably (Fig 17–1), depending on the time of initial division of the embryonic disk. Variations are noted below.

(1) Division prior to the morula stage and differentiation of the trophoblast (third day) results in separate or fused placentas, 2 chorions, and 2 amnions. (This process grossly resembles dizygotic twinning and accounts for almost one-third of monozygotic twinning.)

(2) Division after differentiation of the trophoblast but before the formation of the amnion (fourth to eighth days) yields a single placenta, a common chorion, and 2 amnions. (This accounts for about two-thirds of monozygotic twinning.)

(3) Division after differentiation of the amnion (8th–13th days) results in a single placenta, 1 (common) chorion, and 1 (common) amnion. This is rare.

(4) Division later than day 15 may result in incomplete twinning. Just prior to that time (day 13–15), division may result in conjoined twins.

At delivery, the membranous T-shaped septum or dividing membrane of the placenta between the twins must be inspected and sectioned for evidence of the probable type of twinning (Fig 17–2). Monozygotic twins most commonly have a transparent (< 2 mm) septum made up of 2 amniotic membranes only (no chorion and no decidua). Dizygotic twins almost always have an opaque (thick) septum made up of 2 chorions, 2 amnions, and intervening decidua.

A monochorionic placenta can be identified by stripping away the amnion or amnions to reveal a single chorion over a common placenta. In virtually every case of monochorionic placenta, vascular communications between the 2 parts of the placenta can be identified by careful dissection or injection. In contrast, dichorionic placentas (of dizygotic twinning) only rarely have an anastomosis between the fetal blood vessels.

Placental and membrane examination is a certain indicator of zygosity in twins with monochorionic placentas because these are always monozygotic. Overall, approximately 1% of twins are monoamniotic and these too are monozygotic. Determination of zygosity is clinically significant in case intertwin organ transplantation is needed later in life, as well as for assessing obstetrical risks. Monozygotic twins can rarely be discordant for phenotypic sex when one twin is phenotypically female due to Turner syndrome (45,XO) and its sibling is male, 46,XY.

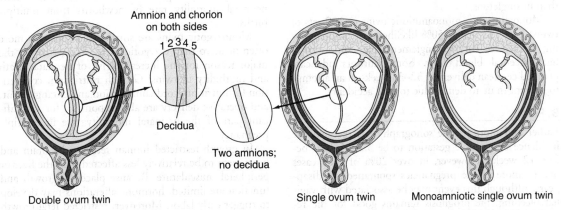

Figure 17–2. **Amniotic membranes of twins.** (Reproduced, with permission, from Benson RC: *Handbook of Obstetrics & Gynecology*, 8th ed. Lange, 1983.)

Monochorionic placentation is associated with more disease processes as a result of placental vascular problems. Inequities of the placental circulation in one area (marginal insertion, partial infarction, or thinning) may lead to growth discordance between the twins. Due to vascular anastomoses in monochorionic placentation, multifetal reduction can only be performed with dichorionic placentation.

The most serious problem with monochorionic placentas is local shunting of blood—also called **twin-to-twin transfusion syndrome.** This occurs because of vascular anastomoses to each twin that are established early in embryonic life. The possible communications are artery to artery, vein to vein, and combinations of these. Artery-to-vein communication is by far the most serious; it is most likely to cause twin-to-twin transfusion. In uncompensated cases, the twins, although genetically identical, differ greatly in size and appearance. The recipient twin is plethoric, edematous, and hypertensive. Ascites and kernicterus are likely. The heart, liver, and kidneys are enlarged (glomerulotubal hypertrophy). Hydramnios follows fetal polyuria. Although ruddy and apparently healthy, the recipient twin with hypervolemia may die of heart failure during the first 24 hours after birth. The donor twin is small, pallid, and dehydrated (from growth restriction, malnutrition, and hypovolemia). Oligohydramnios may be present. Severe anemia, due to chronic blood loss to the other twin, may lead to hydrops and heart failure.

Both twins are threatened by prolapse of the cord. The second twin may be harmed by premature separation of the placenta, hypoxia, constriction ring dystocia, operative manipulation, or prolonged anesthesia.

Velamentous insertion of the cord occurs in about 7% of twins but in only 1% of singletons. There is a corresponding increase in the potentially catastrophic vasa previa. The incidence of 2-vessel cord (single umbilical artery) is 4–5 times higher in monozygotic twins than in singletons.

Monochorionic, monoamniotic twins (1:100 sets of twins) have less than a 50% likelihood of both surviving because of cord entanglement that compromises fetal-placental blood flow. Some authors advocate planned cesarean delivery at 32–34 weeks in an attempt to prevent in utero demise due to cord accidents.

B. Fetal

Earlier and more precise sonography has revealed the incidence of multiple gestation to be 3.29–5.39% before 12 weeks. However, in over 20% of such cases one or more of the pregnancies spontaneously disappears. Although this event may be associated with vaginal bleeding, the prognosis remains good for the remaining twin. This loss has been termed the "vanishing twin."

Major malformations are present in approximately 2% of twin infants, compared with 1% of singletons, while minor malformations are found in 4% of twins compared with about 2.5% in singletons. Monozygotic twins are at higher risk than dizygotic twins.

Conjoined or Siamese twins result from incomplete segmentation of a single fertilized ovum between the 13th and 14th days; if cleavage is further postponed, incomplete twinning (2 heads, 1 body) may occur. Lesser abnormalities are also noted, but these occur without regard to specific organ systems. Conjoined twins are described by site of union: pygopagus (at the sacrum); thoracopagus (at the chest); craniopagus (at the heads); and omphalopagus (at the abdominal wall). Curiously, conjoined twins usually are female. Numerous conjoined twins have survived separation.

Each twin and its placenta generally weigh less than the newborn and placenta of a singleton pregnancy after the 30th week, but near term the aggregate weight may approach twice that of a singleton. In general, the larger the number of fetuses, the greater the degree of growth restriction. Interestingly, multifetal reduction of triplets to twins before 12 weeks results in a growth pattern typical of twins rather than triplets, who are growth restricted compared with twins. Thus the number of fetuses residing in the uterus later in pregnancy, and not their embryonic potential, seems to govern growth. Normal-weight twins that differ considerably in birthweight commonly have diamniotic-dichorionic placentas. This suggests independent intrauterine growth of co-twins. The converse is true of twins with fused diamniotic-dichorionic placentas. Low-birthweight monochorionic twins are the rule rather than the exception. Low birthweight in the various types of multiple pregnancy probably is evidence of growth restriction due to inadequate nutrition. This is at least partially responsible for the much higher early neonatal mortality rate of newborns from multiple births.

Monozygotic twins are smaller and succumb more often in utero than dizygotic twins. Prematurity is the major reason for the increased risk of neonatal death and morbidity in twins. Growth restriction, competition for nutrition, cord compression and entanglement, and operative delivery are also responsible for a significant part of the perinatal mortality rate in multiple pregnancy.

In growth-restricted human fetuses, the brain and heart seem to be relatively less affected than the liver or peripheral musculature. Because placental growth and function are limited, hormone alterations may develop to trigger early labor. Moreover, restricted fetal growth has a small but lasting effect on postnatal physical development.

In late pregnancy, the fetus is jeopardized by the frequency of premature delivery, abnormal presentation and position, and hydramnios.

A fetus acardiacus is a parasitic monozygotic fetus without a heart. It is thought to develop from reversed circulation, perfused by 1 arterial-arterial and 1 venous-venous anastomosis. This represents TRAP, the twin reversed arterial perfusion syndrome. The otherwise normal donor twin is at risk for cardiac hypertrophy and failure, and has a 35% mortality. Various methods of cord occlusion are being studied as in utero therapy.

Fetus papyraceous is a small, blighted, mummified fetus usually discovered at the delivery of a well-developed newborn. This occurs once in 17,000–20,000 pregnancies. The cause is thought to be death of one twin, amniotic fluid loss, or reabsorption and compression of the dead fetus by the surviving twin.

Clinical Findings

With the ready availability of ultrasound, fewer than 10% of twin gestations are undiagnosed before labor and delivery. Early diagnosis facilitates appropriate prenatal care.

A. SYMPTOMS AND SIGNS

All of the common annoyances of pregnancy are more troublesome in multiple pregnancy. The effects of multiple pregnancy on the patient include earlier and more severe pressure in the pelvis, nausea, backache, varicosities, constipation, hemorrhoids, abdominal distention, and difficulty in breathing. A "large pregnancy" may be indicative of twinning (distended uterus). Fetal activity is greater and more persistent in twinning than in singleton pregnancy. The median weight of twins at birth is just over 2270 g in the United States. Male infants weigh slightly more than females.

Considering the possibility of multiple pregnancy is essential to early diagnosis. If one assumes that all pregnancies are multiple until proved otherwise, physical examination alone will identify most cases of twinning before the second trimester. Indeed, diagnosis of twinning is possible in over 75% of cases by physical examination. The following signs should alert the physician to the possibility or definite presence of multiple pregnancy:

(1) Uterus larger than expected (> 4 cm) for dates.

(2) Excessive maternal weight gain that is not explained by edema or obesity.

(3) Polyhydramnios, manifested by uterine size out of proportion to the calculated duration of gestation, is almost 10 times more common in multiple pregnancy.

(4) History of assisted reproduction.

(5) Elevated MSAFP values (see Laboratory Findings, below).

(6) Outline or ballottement of more than one fetus.

(7) Multiplicity of small parts.

(8) Simultaneous recording of different fetal heart rates, each asynchronous with the mother's pulse and with each other and varying by at least 8 beats per minute. (The fetal heart rate may be accelerated by pressure or displacement.)

(9) Palpation of one or more fetuses in the fundus after delivery of one infant.

Some of the common complications in early pregnancy may also occur as a result of multiple gestation. For example, maternal bleeding in the first trimester can indicate threatened or spontaneous abortion; however, the dead fetus may be one of twins, as demonstrated by real-time ultrasonography (one anechoic or hypoechoic amniotic sac and one normal sac). In the second and third trimester, the demise of one fetus in a multiple gestation may trigger disseminated intravascular coagulation ("dead fetus syndrome"), just as a singleton intrauterine demise might. This generally becomes a problem only 3 weeks or more after fetal demise. Preeclampsia-eclampsia is a common complication of multiple pregnancy.

B. LABORATORY FINDINGS

The majority of multiple pregnancies are currently identified by using maternal serum alpha-fetoprotein (MSAFP) screening or ultrasound. Indeed, identification of multiple gestation is so important for the institution of appropriate care that many authorities recommend routine ultrasonic scanning at 18–20 weeks. First-trimester ultrasonography is even more helpful for determining chorionicity.

The hematocrit and hemoglobin values and the red cell count usually are considerably reduced, in direct relationship to the increased blood volume. Indeed, maternal hypochromic normocytic anemia occurs so frequently in multiple pregnancy that it has been suggested that all patients with the process be suspected of having a multiple gestation. Fetal demand for iron increases beyond the mother's ability to assimilate iron in the second trimester.

Glucose tolerance tests demonstrate that both gestational diabetes mellitus and gestational hypoglycemia are much higher in multiple gestation compared with findings in singleton pregnancy. Glucose screening is the standard of care in multiple pregnancy.

C. PRENATAL DIAGNOSIS

The usual indications for prenatal diagnosis and counseling in a singleton pregnancy also apply to twin and higher-order gestations. Because the incidence of twin gestation increases with maternal age, women with multiple gestations are often candidates for prenatal genetic diagnosis. As the risk of aneuploidy is increased, some centers offer invasive testing to all patients carrying multiple gestations who will be over age 33 at delivery. Genetic counseling should make clear to the patient the need to obtain a sample from each fetus, the risk of a chromosomal abnormality, potential complications of the procedure, the possibility of discordant results, and the ethical and technical concerns when one fetus is found to be abnormal.

In twin pregnancies not accompanied by neural tube defects, the median MSAFP level will be 2.5 that of the median level for singleton pregnancies at 14–20 weeks' gestation. The levels in triplets and quadruplets are 3 and 4 times as high, respectively. A value greater than 4.5 times the median is considered abnormal, and requires a targeted ultrasound and possible amniocentesis for the determination of amniotic fluid alpha-fetoprotein and acetylcholinesterase.

Both amniocentesis and chorionic villus sampling (CVS) can safely be performed in multiple gestations in experienced centers. Documentation of the location of the fetuses and the membrane separating the sacs is important in case there is discordance for aneuploidy. Selective termination of an aneuploid fetus can be performed via ultrasound-guided intracardiac injection of potassium chloride. The pregnancy can then continue carrying the normal twin only. Multifetal reduction may be performed to decrease the risk of serious perinatal morbidity and mortality associated with preterm delivery by reducing the number of fetuses from 3 or more to twins.

D. ULTRASOUND FINDINGS

Ultrasonography is the preferred imaging modality for diagnosis of multiple gestation, and is potentially able to differentiate multiple gestation as early as 4 weeks (by intravaginal probe). Dichorionicity is suggested by fetuses of different genders, separate placentas, a thick (> 2 mm) dividing membrane, or a "twin peak sign" in which the membrane inserts into two fused placentas. In the absence of these findings, monochorionicity is likely.

Both twins present as vertex in almost 50% of cases. Twin A will be vertex and twin B a breech in slightly more than 33% of cases (Fig 17–3). Both fetuses will be breech presentations in 10% of cases, and almost that many will be single (or double) transverse presentations. Approximately 70% of first twins present by the vertex. Breech presentation occurs in slightly more than 25%. Overall, nonvertex presentation occurs 10 times more often in multiple pregnancy than in singleton pregnancy.

Differential Diagnosis

Multiple pregnancy must be distinguished from the following conditions.

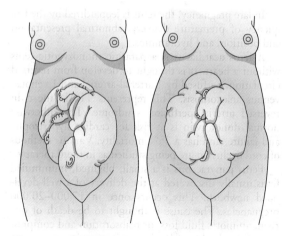

Figure 17–3. **Left:** Both twins presenting by the vertex. **Right:** One vertex and one breech presentation. (Reproduced, with permission, from Benson RC: *Handbook of Obstetrics & Gynecology,* 8th ed. Lange, 1983.)

A. SINGLETON PREGNANCY

Inaccurate dates may give a false impression of the duration of the pregnancy, and the fetus may be larger than expected.

B. POLYHYDRAMNIOS

Either single or multiple pregnancy may be associated with excessive accumulation of fluid.

C. HYDATIDIFORM MOLE

Although usually easily distinguished from multiple gestation, this complication must be considered in diagnosis early in pregnancy.

D. ABDOMINAL TUMORS COMPLICATING PREGNANCY

Fibroid tumors of the uterus, when present in great numbers, are readily identified. Ovarian tumors are generally single, discrete, and harder to diagnose. A distended bladder or full rectum may elevate the pregnant uterus.

E. COMPLICATED TWIN PREGNANCY

If one dizygotic twin dies early in pregnancy and the other lives, the dead fetus may become flattened and mummified (fetus papyraceous; see earlier section on fetal pathologic factors). Its portion of a fused placenta will be pale and atrophic, but remnants of 2 sacs and 2 cords may be found. If one twin dies in late pregnancy, considerable enlargement of the uterus persists, although the findings on palpation may be unusual and only one fetal heartbeat will be heard. Ultrasonography can confirm the diagnosis. The living fetus generally presents first.

Prevention

A. MULTIPLE PREGNANCY

Although human pituitary gonadotropin and other ovulation induction agents result in fewer multiple pregnancies when used by experts, even in the best of hands it is inevitable that some multiple pregnancies will occur. For example, clomiphene citrate induction of multiple ovulation increases the rate of dizygotic pregnancy to 5–10%.

With many forms of assisted reproductive technology (eg, ovulation induction, in vitro fertilization), iatrogenic multiple pregnancies regularly occur in which the number of fetuses is so great that they may preclude any being carried to the point of viability. When this occurs, many authorities recommend multifetal pregnancy reduction by transabdominal intracardiac potassium injection.

B. COMPLICATIONS OF MULTIPLE PREGNANCY

To prevent the complications of multiple pregnancy, it is imperative to make the diagnosis as early in pregnancy as possible. Fortunately, ultrasonography can be safely used at any time during pregnancy, is highly accurate, and may be used as early as the fourth week. Later in pregnancy, ultrasonography is useful to monitor the growth of the fetuses and to detect gross anomalies. It is recommended to perform routine growth scans on twins every 4 weeks in the third trimester, or more frequently if growth restriction is detected. Recall that the risk of fetal abnormality in twins is approximately 3 times that in singleton pregnancy.

There is little question that enhancing antenatal care assists in improving outcome. The most commonly used techniques are iron supplementation, vitamin and folic acid administration (in an attempt to avoid anemia), a high-protein diet, and more weight gain than usual (ideal weight for height plus 35–45 lb). There is not enough evidence to suggest a policy of routine hospitalization for bed rest in multiple pregnancy because no reduction in the risk of preterm birth or perinatal death is evident. There is also no evidence that prophylactic cerclage improves outcome. More frequent antenatal visits are scheduled and several authorities recommend closely following cervical length by ultrasound. Emergency cerclage can be offered for a short cervix or a large funnel of membranes prior to 24 weeks. Early and prompt therapy for any complications (eg, vaginal infections, preeclampsia-eclampsia) should be instituted.

Tocolytic drugs may suppress premature labor and extend gestation 48 hours so that the effects of steroids may be realized. There is no evidence that long-term oral or intravenous tocolysis improves outcome. Most authorities recommend starting with intravenous magnesium sulfate. If terbutaline is used, very close monitoring for pulmonary edema must be maintained, because this complication is much more likely with administration of beta-mimetic agents in multiple gestation. Also, remember that indomethacin may influence fetal ductal constriction and should not be used after 32 weeks' gestation.

In cases of antepartum bleeding or hydramnios, try to delay the delivery until each twin weighs at least 2000 g, or after 34 weeks' gestation.

All patients with multiple pregnancy should be delivered in a well-equipped hospital by an experienced physician who has adequate assistance. It is desirable to have a pediatrician (or neonatologist) in attendance. Delivery must be done in the operating room in case an emergent cesarean section is needed for twin B. An early epidural is recommended; in case of emergent cesarean section, anesthesia is already established and general anesthesia can be avoided. Prematurity, trauma of manipulative delivery, and associated asphyxia are the major preventable causes of morbidity and mortality in twins, especially the second twin.

Treatment

A. LABOR AND DELIVERY

Admit the patient to the hospital at the first sign of labor, if there is leakage of amniotic fluid, or if significant bleeding occurs. An ultrasound evaluation should be performed to ascertain the presentation of each fetus and its estimated fetal weight. Routine, continuous electronic fetal heart rate monitoring is recommended. Labor should be conducted so that immediate cesarean section can be performed if required. A pediatric nurse team for each infant plus obstetric and anesthesiologic attendants should be present. Insert an intravenous line and send a specimen of blood for typing, antibody screening, and complete blood count.

If either twin shows signs of persistent compromise, proceed promptly to cesarean section delivery. Other indications for primary cesarean section include (but are not limited to) compound or monoamniotic twins and probable twin-twin transfusion syndrome (gross disparity in fetal size) and placenta previa. Nearly all (> 85%) triplets warrant cesarean section delivery.

In a woman with a previous lower-segment cesarean scar, limited literature suggests that delivery of twins does not mandate a repeat cesarean section in the absence of other complications. Management of twins that are candidates for vaginal delivery may proceed as outlined below. Intrapartum twin presentations may be classified as follows: (1) twin A and twin B vertex (slightly > 40% of all twins); (2) twin A vertex and twin

B nonvertex (almost 40%); (3) twin A nonvertex and twin B vertex, breech, or transverse (about 20%).

The current intrapartum management of twins is summarized in Fig 17–4. For vertex-vertex presentations in labor (category 1 above), vaginal delivery of both twins may be chosen in the absence of standard indications for cesarean section delivery. Of course, if either twin develops fetal distress, cesarean section delivery should be performed.

Category 2 twins, each weighing more than 2000 g, can usually be managed successfully by vaginal delivery of both. This is generally accomplished by external version of twin B immediately after the delivery of twin A. Recent literature suggests that total breech extraction may be preferable to external cephalic version of twin B. If twin B weighs less than 2000 g and external version is unsuccessful, cesarean section for this infant is warranted (as opposed to breech vaginal birth). When either twin A or both twins are nonvertex (category 3), primary cesarean section should be performed.

Difficult forceps operation or rapid extraction should be avoided, but forceps to protect the aftercoming premature head may be useful. The umbilical cord should be clamped promptly to prevent the second twin of a monozygotic twin pregnancy from exsanguinating into the first born.

Perform a vaginal examination immediately after delivery of twin A to note the presentation of the second twin, the presence of a second sac, an occult cord prolapse, or cord entanglement.

Cut the cord as far outside the vagina as possible so that it can hang loose to permit vaginal examination or manipulation. This eliminates inadvertent cord traction on the placenta. Tag and label the cords (twin A and B) so that they may be associated with the proper placenta or placentas.

Use external version whenever possible for conversion of twin B from breech to vertex. Cautious rupture of the second sac will allow slow loss of fluid while twin B's vertex is being gently guided into the inlet. The amount of time between delivery of twin A and B is still a matter of controversy. If estimated fetal weight suggests fetal well being, it is not necessary to deliver twin B within 30 minutes.

One twin may obstruct the delivery of both fetuses in locked twins. In this circumstance twin A is always a breech and twin B a vertex presentation. The heads become impacted in the pelvis. Locked twins can be avoided by cesarean delivery in all cases in which twin A is not vertex. However, if the obstetrician is presented with a case of locked twins (Fig 17–5), having an assistant support the twin already partially delivered as a

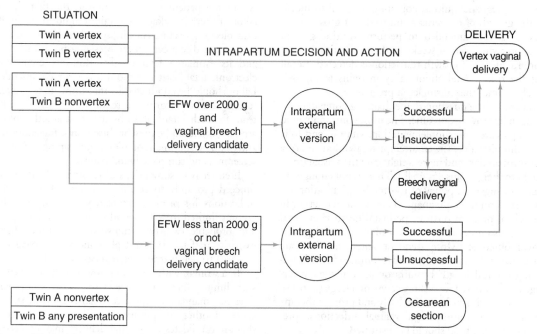

Figure 17–4. Management of twin gestation, intrapartum protocol. EFW, estimated fetal weight. (Modified and reproduced, with permission of the American College of Obstetricians and Gynecologists, from Chervenak FA et al: Intrapartum management of twin gestation. Obstet Gynecol 1985;65:120.)

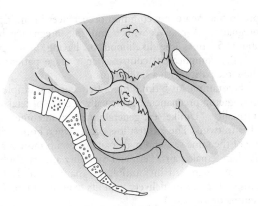

Figure 17–5. **Locked twins.** (Reproduced, with permission, from Benson RC: *Handbook of Obstetrics & Gynecology*, 4th ed. Lange, 1971.)

breech while pushing both heads upward out of the pelvis with rotation of both fetuses may accomplish delivery of the first. This may require deep anesthesia. If this cannot be done, cesarean with abdominal delivery of both fetuses may be the safest route. An alternative while cesarean preparations are underway is to elevate the partially delivered twin, establish an airway, and protect the cord.

Postpartum hemorrhage is common in multiple pregnancy. Increased intravenous oxytocin, elevation, and light massage of the fundus and an intravenous ergot or prostaglandin product (only after the last fetus is delivered) may be required.

After delivery, if separation of the placenta is delayed or bleeding is brisk, manual extraction of the placenta may be necessary. Send the placenta, cord, and membranes to the pathology laboratory to assist in determining whether the fetuses are mono- or dizygotic.

Preeclampsia-eclampsia, premature labor and delivery, etc, are managed as outlined elsewhere in this book.

Complications

A. MATERNAL

The incidence of spontaneous abortion of at least one of several fetuses is increased in multiple pregnancy. Stillbirth occurs twice as often among twins as among singleton pregnancies. Premature labor and delivery as well as premature rupture of the membranes are also greatly increased. The average gestational age at delivery is 36–37 weeks for twins, 33 weeks for triplets, and 31 weeks for quadruplets. Efforts to reduce the incidence of prematurity have thus far been unsuccessful.

Placenta previa may be responsible for antepartum bleeding, malpresentation, or unengagement of the first

fetus. A large placenta (or placentas) and possibly fundal scarring or tumor may lead to low implantation of the placenta. Premature separation of the placenta may occur antepartum, perhaps in association with preeclampsia-eclampsia or with rupture of membranes of twin A and the initiation of strong uterine contractions, or after the delivery of the first twin. Careless traction on the first cord may encourage early partial separation of the placenta.

Hypochromic normocytic anemia is 2–3 times more common in multiple pregnancy than in singleton pregnancy. Urinary tract infection is at least twice as frequent in multiple pregnancy as in singleton pregnancy due to increased ureteral dilatation secondary to higher serum progesterone and uterine pressure on the ureters. Preeclampsia-eclampsia occurs about 3 times more often in multiple pregnancy than in a singleton pregnancy.

A thinned uterine wall, secondary to unusually large uterine contents, is associated with hypotonic uterine contractions and a longer latent stage of labor. However, prolonged labor is uncommon in multiple pregnancy because rupture of the membranes generally is followed by improvements in the uterine contraction pattern. Uterine atony often is accompanied by excessive loss of blood postpartum owing to inability of the overdistended uterus to contract well and remain contracted after delivery.

If the amniotic sac of the second twin ruptures before that of the first and if the cord prolapses, cesarean section usually is indicated.

When there are 2 separate placentas, one of them may deliver immediately after the first twin. Although the second twin may not be compromised, it is best to proceed with its delivery, both for its protection and to conserve maternal blood.

Operative intervention is more likely in multiple pregnancy because of increased obstetric problems such as malpresentation, prolapsed cord, and fetal distress.

B. FETAL

Fetal death is about 3 times more common in multiple pregnancy than in singleton pregnancy. Death may be due to developmental anomalies, cord compression, or placental disorders. The greatest hazard from cord compression is cord entanglement of monozygotic twins with only one amniotic sac. Developmental anomalies and polyhydramnios are common in monozygotic twins.

Almost twice as many monozygotic as dizygotic twins die in the perinatal period. Attrition is even greater for triplets, quadruplets, and higher order pregnancies. Even so, preterm delivery and intrapartum complications are the most common causes of fetal loss in multiple pregnancy. All too frequently preterm delivery is occasioned by premature rupture of the membranes, which occurs in about 25% of twin, 50% of triplet, and 75% of quadruplet pregnancies.

Abnormal and breech presentation, circulatory interference by one fetus with the other, and operative delivery all increase fetal loss. Prolapse of the cord occurs 5 times more often in multiple than in singleton pregnancy. Premature separation of the placenta before delivery of the second twin may cause death of the second twin by hypoxia.

Neonatal outcome is very much dependent on gestational age at delivery. In general, morbidity and mortality rates are similar for twins and singletons of equivalent gestational ages. Many outcome data are stratified according to birthweight. Therefore, the slowing of growth in the third trimester can give twin fetuses the advantage of increased gestational age for weight. Advances in neonatal intensive care have made survival possible even at 23 weeks' gestation, although usually with considerable morbidity, including but not limited to intraventricular hemorrhage, chronic lung disease, and necrotizing enterocolitis. Because intact survival is much more likely after 34 weeks, it is desirable to prolong gestation at least to this point when possible. The adage "one day in utero saves two days in intensive care" applies to the economic as well as the emotional costs of caring for premature infants.

It is imperative that an experienced physician be present for resuscitation and stabilization of each infant born premature. Antenatal diagnosis of multiple gestation facilitates delivery at an appropriate center. Delivery before the 36th week is twice as frequent in twin pregnancies as in singleton pregnancies. Intracranial injury is more common in premature infants, even those delivered spontaneously. An increased risk of cerebral palsy is found in twins, especially very low-birthweight babies, and also in liveborn co-twins of fetuses who died in utero.

Treatment of twin-to-twin transfusion syndrome in utero remains experimental. After delivery, therapy includes replacing blood in the donor twin to correct fluid and electrolyte imbalance. In the recipient twin, phlebotomy is necessary until normal venous pressure is restored. Often, other therapy for cardiac failure (eg, digitalis) is necessary.

Prognosis

The U.S. maternal mortality rate for multiple pregnancy is only slightly higher than for singleton. A history of previous dizygotic twins increases the likelihood of subsequent multiple pregnancy 10-fold. Hemorrhage is about 5 times as frequent in multiple as in single pregnancies. The probability of abnormal presentation and of operative delivery and its complications is increased in multiple pregnancy. Premature rupture of the membranes and premature labor, often with a long prodromal phase, are common occurrences in multiple pregnancy. A gravida with a multiple pregnancy has about 5 times the likelihood of having a morbid (febrile, complicated) course as an average patient of the same parity with a single fetus.

Hydramnios is 5 times more frequent in multiple as in singleton pregnancies, principally because of fetal abnormality. "Unlike sex, generally unlike outcome" applies to twins. The greatest loss occurs when both twins are of the same sex, and male pairs succumb more readily than female pairs. Perinatal mortality and morbidity rates are increased in multiple pregnancy, mainly because of preterm delivery and its complications (ie, trauma or asphyxia).

Almost 50% of twins weigh < 2500 g, but the majority of these are of 36 weeks' gestational age or more. Directly or indirectly, multiple pregnancies are responsible for around 15% of premature births and around 9% of perinatal deaths, a rate 7 times that of single births. Approximately 55% of twins are premature; 80% of perinatal deaths occur in those born before 31 weeks' gestation, and 93% of deaths are in those with birthweight below 1500 g. The incidence of intrauterine growth restriction is increased in multiple gestation, and multiple gestations account for 17% of infants with intrauterine growth restriction. Congenital malformations and abnormal presentation are more serious in monozygous twins. Preeclampsia-eclampsia, diabetes mellitus, and other disorders may further jeopardize the fetuses.

Efforts to reduce the incidence of prematurity have not met with much success in singletons or in multiple gestations. In order to maximize fetal growth, good nutrition, frequent rest periods, and cessation of smoking are encouraged. Approximately 90% of twins born at greater than 28 weeks survive.

A recent study found that neonatal morbidity is reduced when delivery is accomplished between 37 and 38 weeks and routine induction at that time was recommended.

The comparative occurrence of perinatal death (per 1000) for single and multiple pregnancy are as follows: singletons, 39; twins, 152; triplets, 309; and quadruplets, 509. The rates are proportionately higher for higher-order pregnancies.

The best outlook is for both twins to present by vertex. Twins and other multiple fetuses delivered by spontaneous means do better than those extracted by forceps or after version. Internal podalic version is especially dangerous. Hypoxia and trauma of operative delivery are the primary causes of death of the second twin. Central nervous system disease and hyaline membrane disease are frequently diagnosed in the surviving second twin.

Discordance noted at birth is associated with a slower weight gain during extrauterine life. A twin whose birthweight is less than 20% of that of its partner will not gain as rapidly and may never catch up with the other twin in weight and height. The IQ of the larger monozygotic twin is likely to be higher than that of the smaller twin if the weight difference is more than 300 g at birth. The female twin of a female-male pair who survives cross-transfusion is not sterile (in contrast to the situation encountered in the bovine free-martin).

Concordance of placental examination, clinical comparisons, and hematologic and serologic tests provides presumptive evidence of monozygotic twinning. The total probability of diagnosis of zygosity is over 95% using ABO, MNSs, Rh, Kell, Kidd, Duffy, and Lewis A and B antigens, and approaches 100% using chromosomal analysis.

In comprehensive perinatal care centers, morbidity and mortality rates decrease greatly. In one report of triplets receiving optimal care, the mean weight at delivery was 1779 g and the incidence of neonatal mortality was only 23 in 1000. First twins have about a 3% greater chance of survival than second twins. Breech presentation of the second twin carries higher mortality and morbidity rates.

REFERENCES

Alexander GR et al: What are the fetal growth patterns of singletons, twins, and triplets in the United States? Clin Obstet Gynecol 1998;41:114.

American College of Obstetricians and Gynecologists: Special problems of multiple gestations. ACOG Educational Bulletin No. 253. ACOG, 1998.

Blickstein I: Cesarean section for all twins? J Perinat Med 2000; 28:196.

Brambati B et al: Outcome of first-trimester chorionic villus sampling for genetic investigation in multiple pregnancy. Ultrasound Obstet Gynecol 2001;17:209.

Brown JE, Carlson M: Nutrition and multifetal pregnancy. J Am Diet Assoc 2000;100:343.

Crowther CA: Hospitalization and bed rest for multiple pregnancy (Cochrane Review). Cochrane Database Sys Rev 2001;1: CD000110.

Evans MI et al: Selective termination for structural, chromosomal, and mendelian anomalies: International experience. Am J Obstet Gynecol 1999;181:893.

Gaziano EP, De Lia JE, Kuhlmann RS: Diamniotic monochorionic twin gestations: an overview. J Matern Fetal Med 2000;9:89.

Guzman ER et al: Use of cervical ultrasonography in prediction of spontaneous preterm birth in twin gestations. Am J Obstet Gyencol 2000;183:1103.

Hartely RS, Emanuel I, Hitti J: Perinatal and neonatal morbidity rates among twin pairs at different gestational ages: Optimal delivery timing at 37 to 38 weeks' gestation. Am J Obstet Gynecol 2001;184:451.

Kaufman GE et al: Neonatal morbidity and mortality associated with triplet pregnancy. Obstet Gynecol 1998;91:342.

Kinzler WL, Ananth CV, Vintzileos AM: Medical and economic effects of twin gestations. J Soc Gynecol Invest 2000;7:321.

Lynch A et al: Assisted reproductive interventions and multiple birth. Obstet Gynecol 2001;97:195.

Malone FD, D'Alton ME: Management of multiple gestations complicated by a single anomalous fetus. Curr Opin Obstet Gynecol 1997;9:213.

Pharoah POD, Adi Y: Consequences of in-utero death in a twin pregnancy. Lancet 2000;355:1597.

Stone J, Eddleman K: Multifetal pregnancy reduction. Curr Opin Obstet Gynecol 2000;12:491.

Stone J, Eddleman K, Patel S: Controversies in the intrapartum management of twin gestations. Obstet Gynecol Clin North Am 1999;26:327.

Tessen JA, Zlatnik FJ: Monoamniotic twins: A retrospective controlled study. Obstet Gynecol 1991;77:832.

Victoria A, Mora G, Arias F: Perinatal outcome, placental pathology, and severity of discordance in monochorionic and dichorionic twins. Obstet Gynecol 2001;97:310.

Diabetes Mellitus & Pregnancy

18

Carla Janzen, MD, Jeffrey S. Greenspoon, MD, & Sue M. Palmer, MD

Diabetes mellitus, a clinical syndrome characterized by deficiency of or insensitivity to insulin and exposure of organs to chronic hyperglycemia, is the most common medical complication of pregnancy. Over 3 million persons in the United States are sufficiently affected by diabetes mellitus to warrant treatment with insulin or oral hyperglycemics. Another 3 million are treated with diet alone in addition to a possible 4 or more million with varying degrees of asymptomatic glucose intolerance.

Preexisting diabetes (ie, diabetes diagnosed prior to pregnancy) affects approximately 1–3 pregnancies per 1000 births. In spite of the goal of preconception counseling for women with preexisting diabetes, many women will present for medical care for the first time during pregnancy. In this light, pregnancy affords a unique opportunity for diabetes screening and may well be the best opportunity in a woman's life to discover or prevent her diabetes. Gestational diabetes mellitus (GDM) is defined as any degree of glucose intolerance with first recognition during pregnancy. GDM complicates approximately 4% of pregnancies (135,000 cases in the United States annually).

Hyperglycemia around the time of conception and early organogenesis results in the developing embryo having a 6-fold increase in midline birth defects. Ketoacidosis is an immediate threat to life and is the leading cause of perinatal morbidity in diabetic pregnancies today, accounting for 40% of perinatal mortality. Complications of GDM include fetal macrosomia, which is associated with increased rates of secondary complications such as operative delivery, shoulder dystocia, and birth trauma. In addition, neonatal complications attributed to gestational diabetes include respiratory distress syndrome (RDS), hypocalcemia, hyperbilirubinemia, and hypoglycemia.

Before the introduction of insulin in 1922, patients often died during the course of their pregnancy. Twenty years ago it was not uncommon to deliver an unexplained stillbirth from a mother with type 1 diabetes mellitus. In an effort to prevent fetal death, deliveries were often performed early. Today, this tragedy is rare, and over the last decade associated perinatal morbidity and mortality have been reduced from 60% to less than 5%. With therapy beginning prior to conception and continuing throughout pregnancy, including nutrition therapy, insulin when necessary, and eventual antepartum fetal surveillance, there is a marked decline in overall morbidity and mortality. Two decades ago, most diabetics required prolonged hospitalization, but today the majority is managed with only brief hospitalizations. This is partly due to the technologic improvements in home reflectance glucose monitors and the beneficial impact they have had in management of the diabetic during pregnancy.

Currently, the major challenges of caring for diabetics in pregnancy are first, to enhance preconceptual glucose control and reduce the risk of associated congenital malformations, second to adequately screen pregnant women, and third, to detail the full impact of milder glucose elevations, not only on maternal risk for developing diabetes, but also on immediate and long-term consequences to the fetus/child.

Metabolism in Normal & Diabetic Pregnancy

Deterioration of glucose tolerance occurs normally during pregnancy. Significant metabolic changes are necessary to provide proper energy delivery to the growing conceptus. Hormones associated with pregnancy such as human placental lactogen (HPL) and cortisol lower glucose levels, promote fat deposition, and stimulate appetite. Rising serum levels of estrogen and progesterone increase insulin production and secretion while increasing tissue sensitivity to insulin. The overall result is a lowering of the fasting glucose levels, reaching a nadir by the 12th week. The decrease is on average 15 mg/dL; thus fasting values of 70–80 mg/dL are normal in a pregnant woman by the 10th week of gestation. There is a comparable decrease in postprandial values. This acts to protect the developing embryo from elevated glucose levels. Indeed, birth defects are noted at a 2- to 3-fold higher rate in women with diabetes without preconception glycemic control. In summary, hormones associated with pregnancy facilitate maternal storage of energy in the first trimester and then assist in the diversion of energy to the fetus in later pregnancy as demand increases.

In the second trimester, higher fasting and postprandial glucose levels are seen. This facilitates the placental transfer of glucose. Glucose transfer is via a carrier-mediated active transport system that becomes saturated at 250 mg/dL. Fetal glucose levels are 80% of maternal values. In contrast, maternal amino acid levels are lowered during the second trimester by active placental transfer to the fetus. Fetal levels of amino acids are 2- to 3-fold higher than maternal levels, but not as high as levels within the placenta. Lipid metabolism in the second trimester shows continued storage until midgestation; then, as fetal demands increase, there is enhanced mobilization (lipolysis).

HPL is the hormone mainly responsible for insulin resistance and lipolysis. HPL also decreases the hunger sensation and diverts maternal carbohydrate metabolism to fat metabolism in the third trimester. HPL is a single-chain polypeptide secreted by the syncytiotrophoblast and has a molecular weight of 22,308 and a half-life of 17 minutes. HPL levels are elevated during hypoglycemia to mobilize free fatty acids for energy for maternal metabolism. HPL levels are low with maternal hyperglycemia. HPL is similar in structure to growth hormone and acts by reducing the insulin affinity to insulin receptors. The effect on the fetus is to allow longer glucose elevations for placental transfer to the developing fetus and minimizing maternal use of glucose for metabolic needs.

During pregnancy, the levels of HPL rise steadily during the first and second trimesters with a plateau in the late third trimester. This plateau is the natural result of decreasing nutrient delivery to the placenta, thus decreasing hormone production. It appears that this is a necessary signal to the developing fetus to initiate fetal cortisol and thyroid hormone release to in turn initiate enzyme development for maturation. In pregnancies with elevated glucose and other nutrients, there is continued placental growth with a delay in fetal organ/hormonal maturation. In short, mother and fetus communicate through nutrient delivery and utilization.

Cortisol levels rise during pregnancy and stimulate endogenous glucose production and glycogen storage and decrease glucose utilization. The "dawn phenomenon" (elevated fasting glucose to facilitate brain metabolism) is marked in normal pregnancies and is even more enhanced in women with polycystic ovarian syndrome (PCOS) who become pregnant. Therefore, early pregnancy glucose screening is advised for the woman with PCOS who becomes pregnant.

Prolactin levels are also increased 5- to 10-fold during pregnancy and may have an impact on carbohydrate metabolism. Thus patients with hyperprolactinemia also deserve early pregnancy glucose screening.

Fetal somatic growth is associated with the anabolic properties of insulin. In that neither maternal nor fetal insulin crosses the placenta, it is known that the release of fetal insulin is stimulated by glucose and amino acids as well as being regulated by genetic potential. The pathophysiologic impact of elevated maternal glucose levels on the fetus is a product of the level of elevation and its duration.

Diagnostic Criteria for Diabetes Mellitus Prior to Pregnancy

There are three ways to diagnose preexisting diabetes mellitus and each way must be confirmed by a follow-up test. Criteria for diagnosing diabetes mellitus include:

(1) Symptoms of diabetes (polyuria, polydipsia, and/or unexplained weight loss) plus a casual plasma glucose concentration of equal to or greater than 200 mg/dL,

(2) Fasting plasma glucose (at least 8 hours without eating) equal to or greater than 126 mg/dL,

(3) Two-hour plasma glucose of equal to or greater than 200 mg/dL after drinking a 75-gram glucose load. A positive value on any of these tests should be confirmed on a subsequent day by repeating any of these tests.

Diagnostic Criteria for Gestational Diabetes Mellitus

The criteria for the diagnosis of GDM are based on the original work of O'Sullivan and Mahan and modified by Carpenter and Coustan (see section on Gestational Diabetes). Risk assessment for GDM is undertaken at the first prenatal visit. Women with risk factors, including marked obesity, personal history of GDM in prior pregnancy, glycosuria, or strong family history, should have a glucose tolerance test (GTT) as soon as feasible. If results of testing do not demonstrate diabetes, they should be retested between 24 and 28 weeks' gestation. A fasting plasma glucose of greater than 126 mg/dL or a casual level of greater than 200 mg/dL meets the criteria for diabetes if confirmed on a subsequent day.

Evaluation of low-risk women during pregnancy takes place between 24 and 28 weeks' gestation and typically follows a two-step approach. An initial screening is a blood glucose concentration 1 hour after the patient takes a 50-gram oral glucose load. A value of greater than 140 mg/dL identifies approximately 80% of women with GDM. If a screening value is greater than 190 mg/dL, a fasting blood glucose should be checked on a subsequent day. A subsequent fasting value of ≥ 95 mg/dL would provide two abnormal values, as described below.

If the result of the 1-hour screening test falls between 141 and 190 mg/dL, a diagnostic 3-hour oral glucose test is performed. The 3-hour 100-gram oral glucose test is done after an overnight fast for at least 8 hours. Abnormal values are:

(1) Fasting ≥ 95 mg/dL
(2) 1-hour ≥ 180 mg/dL
(3) 2-hour ≥ 155 mg/dL
(4) 3-hour ≥ 140 mg/dL

At least two out of four values must be abnormal to diagnose gestational diabetes.

■ PREGESTATIONAL DIABETES

TYPE 1 DIABETES (INSULIN-DEPENDENT)

ESSENTIALS OF DIAGNOSIS

- *Hyperglycemia requiring exogenous insulin.*
- *Onset earlier than 30 years of age.*
- *Profound thirst, increased urination, weight loss.*
- *Ketoacidosis.*

Etiology

Type 1 diabetes, previously known as insulin-dependent diabetes mellitus (IDDM) or juvenile-onset diabetes, results from a cellular-mediated autoimmune destruction of the β cells of the pancreas. Autoantibodies, such as those specific to islet cells or insulin can be found in 85–90% of individuals when fasting hyperglycemia is detected. The rate of β-cell destruction by autoantibodies is variable, but eventually this condition leads to elevated glucose and elevated free fatty acids due to lack of sufficient insulin production in the β islet cells of the pancreas.

Type 1 diabetes has multiple genetic predispositions. Susceptibility to this form of diabetes is noted to be increased by a gene or genes located near or within the HLA locus on the short arm of chromosome 6 (6p). The risk to offspring of developing type 1 diabetes with an affected sibling is 5% if one haplotype is shared, 13% for two haplotypes, and 2% for no shared haplotypes. If both parents are affected, the incidence of type 1 diabetes is 33%.

Incidence

The incidence of type 1 diabetes in the general population is 0.1–0.4% in various age groups under 30 years of age. Diabetes mellitus represents one of the most common maternal illnesses resulting in anomalous offspring. The incidence of major congenital anomalies among infants of type 1 diabetic mothers has been estimated at 6–10%, representing a 2- to 3-fold increase over the incidence in the general population, and accounting for 40% of all perinatal deaths among these infants. The incidence of malformations is directly related to the level of glucose elevation over the embryonic period as measured by a hemoglobin A_{1c} level in the first trimester. In addition, if not well controlled, type 1 DM results in a comparable increase in abortions.

Pathophysiology

Insulin is an anabolic hormone with crucial roles in carbohydrate, fat, and protein metabolism. It promotes uptake and utilization of amino acids, lipogenesis, glucose uptake, and storage as glycogen. Lack of insulin results in elevated levels of glucose, and lipolysis with elevation of free fatty acids leading to increased formation of ketone bodies, acetoacetate and β-hydroxybutyrate. Blood glucose levels exceeding the renal capability of absorption produce an osmotic diuresis with dehydration and electrolyte loss. Ketoacidosis, a life-threatening condition for both mother and fetus, results from a paucity of insulin.

Elevated glucose levels are toxic to the developing fetus, producing an increase in serious midline defects in direct proportion to the elevation. These birth defects (Table 18–1) are fatal or seriously deleterious to

Table 18–1. Congenital anomalies of infants of diabetic mothers.[1]

Skeletal and CNS	Caudal regression syndrome Neural tube defects excluding anencephaly Anencephaly with or without herniation of neural elements Microcephaly
Cardiac	Transposition of the great vessels with or without ventricular septal defect Ventricular septal defects Coarctation of the aorta with or without ventricular septal defect or patent ductus arteriosus Cardiomegaly
Renal anomalies	Hydronephrosis Renal agenesis Ureteral duplication
Gastrointestinal	Duodenal atresia Anorectal atresia Small left colon syndrome
Other	Single umbilical artery

[1]Reprinted with permission from Reece EA, Hobbins JC: Diabetes embryopathy, pathogenesis, prenatal diagnosis and prevention. Obstet Gynecol Surv 1986;41:325.

Table 18–2. The relationship between the initial pregnancy value of glycosylated hemoglobin and the percentage of major fetal congenital malformations.

Initial Maternal Value HbA$_{1c}$	Percentage of Major Congenital Malformity
7.9 or lower	3.2%
8.9–9.9	8.1%
Greater than 10	23.5%

quality of life and are preventable by preconception glucose control. The presence of ketones significantly reduces the hyperglycemia necessary to produce defects. These anomalies occur within the first 8 weeks of gestation, when most women are just initiating prenatal care. Hemoglobin A$_{1c}$, a particular fraction of a glycosylated hemoglobin molecule, when drawn in the first trimester can indicate the risk of fetal anomalies (Table 18–2).

Diagnosis

Type 1 diabetes has an early age of onset with deficient insulin production. Profound thirst, increased urination, and weight loss or even overt diabetic ketoacidosis are the usual symptoms triggering medical evaluation.

Initial evaluation, if the patient was not seen preconceptionally, includes assessment for other organ damage. This allows more individualized and effective prenatal care as well as classification based on White's criteria (Table 18–3). The usual evaluation includes an ophthalmologic examination for evidence of retinopathy. Retinal hemorrhages may increase in the initial stages of improved glucose control as blood flow increases to these terminal vessels, clearing atherosclerotic plaques. The negative impact of this can be controlled by frequent visits with early laser treatment as needed. The renal status is evaluated by a 24-hour urine test for creatinine clearance and total protein. If the protein value is less than 200 mg, a 24-hour urine test for microalbuminuria should be considered, because microalbuminuria is associated with increased future vascular disease. An electrocardiogram should be done on patients with disease duration of 5 years or those who are over the age of 30. Thyroid status should also be evaluated due to the potential multiendocrine impact of diabetes.

All patients should have a detailed ultrasound examination with fetal echocardiography at 18–20 weeks to rule out anomalies, as well as an AFP (alpha-fetoprotein) or TriScreen at 16–18 weeks' gestation due to the increased rate of congenital anomalies in the offspring of diabetics.

Fetal surveillance is increased at 32 weeks' gestation if vascular disease is present. This is accomplished with ultrasound amniotic fluid assessments until 36 weeks, then biweekly unless contraction stress tests are done weekly. Serial ultrasound testing for growth is done at 28–32 weeks and at 36 weeks. Polyhydramnios (AFI ≥ 20) or increased abdominal girth should alert the practitioner to less-than-ideal glucose control. If glucose values remain labile despite all attempts at management, then it is best to deliver the fetus as soon as lung maturity is established by L:S and prostaglandin by amniocentesis at 37 weeks.

Approach to the Type 1 Diabetic

Care of the insulin-dependent diabetic must be intensive. Support personnel should be identified and constructively involved with the therapy wherever possible. However, it is extremely important to stress that the patient herself is solely responsible for her actions. The educational focus is to develop the patient's understanding of her disease to a point at which she can balance activity, diet, and insulin, with further guidance only as needed to assist her to cease self-destructive behaviors.

If not seen preconceptionally, prenatal vitamins should be started and additional folate should be given, 0.5 mg twice daily, due to the interaction of hyperglycemia with folate receptors.

Table 18–3. Modified White's classification of diabetes mellitus.

Class A:	Chemical diabetes diagnosed *before* pregnancy; managed by diet *alone;* any age of onset or duration.
Class B:	Insulin treatment necessary *before* pregnancy; onset after age 20; duration of less than 10 years.
Class C:	Onset at age 10–19; or duration of 10–19 years.
Class D:	Onset before age 10; or duration of 20 or more years; or chronic hypertension; or background retinopathy.
Class F:	Renal disease.
Class H:	Coronary artery disease.
Class R:	Proliferative retinopathy.
Class T:	Renal transplant.

Education

The education necessary to maximize the diabetic's chances for a successful pregnancy is ideally accomplished through a multidisciplinary team of health care professionals consisting of a physician trained in managing diabetes and pregnancy, a dietician, a diabetes educator, and a social worker. The education process is ongoing and carries the committed woman from a dependent state to one of interdependence. Such a program will result in a successful pregnancy outcome in 96% of patients with preconception control.

A careful review of the patient's existing knowledge of diabetes and her care is necessary. This may be accomplished by any knowledgeable member of the health care team, but is ideally done by a diabetes educator. Each step from diet, glucose monitoring, insulin administration, exercise, and self-care during illnesses is reviewed, assessing her knowledge and correcting inappropriate information. Ideally, the patient then identifies areas that she can correct to improve glucose control. These areas are summarized, and the care goals are written in an individualized form with patient input and given to her for review at home as well as remaining in the chart so that progress toward the goals can be monitored.

The patient is thoroughly instructed on how to properly use a home glucose monitor, including running control solutions, cleaning, troubleshooting, and proper technique of sample collection. It is important not to squeeze the area of lancet puncture because the sample may become diluted by tissue fluids, resulting in lowered values. This is so common that the care providers must constantly assess the patient's technique when values vary.

When the team approach is taken, with active patient cooperation, cesarean delivery is rarely necessary, and most patients go into spontaneous labor or are induced at 40 weeks, thus decreasing the cesarean section rate.

It is hoped that educational efforts result in a lifelong program designed to prevent the development of diabetic complications and retard the progression of complications. Indeed, the recent CDDT trials clearly indicate this to be the attainable goal. Some 20 years after the pioneering work of Karlsson and Kjellmer, which showed a linear relationship between glycemic control and perinatal mortality, the same reduction in complications has been seen in patients with new-onset diabetes, as well as those with early organ damage (eg, eye, kidney).

Normalization of Blood Glucose

Prevention of hyperglycemia and ketoacidosis through rigorous control of blood glucose is mandatory in the pregnant woman with type 1 DM. This is best accomplished by careful preconceptual analysis and counseling, achievement of normal levels of glycosylated hemoglobin before pregnancy, frequent (usually 4–5 times a day) home glucose monitoring, thoughtful control of diet (the diabetic should have the usual weight gain of pregnancy), and stabilization of exercise. Obviously this can be accomplished only by focusing the health care team's efforts on education and by including the patient as an active participant in the care of herself and her fetus.

Optimal glucose levels before and during pregnancy are fasting levels of 70–90 mg/dL and 1-hour postprandial values of 100–130 mg/dL, or 2-hour postprandial values of 90–120 mg/dL.

To achieve these levels, the patient must carry a reliable, portable glucose meter at all times to allow independence and to provide protection from adverse outcomes. It is best if the meter has a large-capacity memory. The memory meter not only records times and values but also allows a review of glucose level changes over time. Unfortunately, good glucose levels are invariably associated with being a "good patient" and vice versa. The team, including the patient, must focus on the goal of glucose normalization and assist in changing behavior while always recognizing the difficulties imposed by society on obtaining this goal.

All patients and significant others should be instructed on treatment of hypoglycemia and have symptoms reviewed. Nocturnal hypoglycemia episodes with nightmares, sleep walking, tossing and turning in bed, and waking with headaches are significant and should be asked about during prenatal visits. After a change in the evening intermediate insulin dose, the efficacy of the dose should be checked with a 2 AM glucose reading. If the value is below 90 mg/dL in a patient with type 1 DM, a snack should be taken, and the health care provider should be contacted in the morning to readjust the dose.

As noted previously, women with diabetes may optimize their reproductive outcomes by normalization of glucose before pregnancy. Correction of glucose levels to normal as well as replacement of vitamins and minerals depleted during periods of diuresis result in anomaly rates similar to those seen in the general population. Counseling of the diabetic woman must include the family and the lifestyle changes necessary to attain this goal of normalization of glucose levels.

A. DIET

The patient should be instructed on an ADA diet, with caloric intake of 25–35 kcal/kg body weight, but no greater than 2400 kcal or less than 1800 kcal. Actual weight gain with confirmation of actual caloric intake will further aid in adjusting the patient's caloric needs to allow appropriate weight gain. Women who are under their ideal weight have additional weight to gain in addition to the recommended 11-kg weight gain (a minimum of 7 kg for obese patients). The diet should be 40–50% carbohydrate, 30% fat, and 20–30% protein. Women with renal disease should have protein limited to 90 g of protein to minimize the impact of pregnancy on their disease. The calories are divided into 3 meals and 3 snacks, with the evening snack recommended to be a half-sandwich. The protein in meat provides calories in the early morning hours, when intermediate insulin is peaking and fetal glucose utilization is maximized due to increased movements during sleep.

The snack for hypoglycemia should be milk or peanut butter with crackers. Orange juice should be discouraged unless it is the only food available, because it causes an abrupt rise in glucose that is not sustained. Glucagon emergency kits should be given to all type 1 patients and their spouses taught how to use it if the patient is found unresponsive.

Soluble fiber assists in satiating hunger, but more importantly, it helps reduce glycemic swings. The patient should note exactly what she ate, the amount, and the mode of preparation when she has a postprandial glucose level over 130 mg/dL. Attention should be directed to the bedtime snack when there is elevation or lowering of the fasting glucose.

The dietitian is a crucial team member in the care of a type 1 diabetic pregnant patient. Visits should occur as often as needed to obtain proper compliance. The dietitian should make a concerted effort to individualize the diet, respecting different lifestyles and ethnicity. A minimum of two visits is always necessary, and family involvement is encouraged to improve compliance.

B. INSULIN

All patients should undergo a review of insulin administration technique, including mixing of regular and intermediate insulin, as well as injection. All patients should be started on human insulin or switched from older animal products to reduce antibody formation. Patients should be advised that regular insulin may have a more profound hypoglycemic effect due to a lack of blocking antibodies, but generally only a slight decrease in dose is necessary. Because of the increased purity of the human insulin preparations, the duration of action is shorter, and most patients require three injections daily for ideal glucose control, with the intermediate insulin being given at bedtime.

Initially, the injection sites should be noted, and these should be reevaluated if anomalous glucose readings are seen. The intermediate insulin at bedtime should be given in the fatty area of the thigh for the most prolonged and even absorption. Injections with regular insulin should be given a minimum of 30 minutes prior to a meal.

Although current studies do not support an improvement in glycemic control or outcome in pregnancy using subcutaneous insulin pumps, some experienced investigators advocate their use in selected patients. Indeed, no research has been conducted using the newer improved pumps. Even advocates of the insulin pump note that initiation with appropriate training is tricky during pregnancy and is probably best done prior to conception.

Severe Hyperglycemia & Ketoacidosis

During pregnancy severe hyperglycemia and ketoacidosis are treated exactly the same as in the nonpregnant state. Insulin therapy, careful monitoring of potassium, and fluid replacement are crucial for maternal survival. Fetal status and survival are enhanced by administration of maternal oxygen, lateral recumbency, and slow but decisive lowering of the blood glucose. Fetal heart rate monitoring often demonstrates late decelerations (indicative of uteroplacental insufficiency), in addition to decreased beat-to-beat variability (due to maternal acidosis combined with limited fetal placental clearance and buffering capabilities).

Postpartum

The postpartum patient should be started back on an ADA diet as soon as clinically indicated. The dose of insulin should be reduced because the rapid clearing of HPL results in increased insulin receptor sensitivity. The general rule is two-thirds of the prepregnant dose or one- to two-thirds to one-half of the present dose with careful observation for hypoglycemia. If the patient underwent surgery, the insulin infusion is continued until oral intake can be established. The glucose levels should be kept relatively controlled to assist the patient in healing. Infections should be aggressively treated in the postpartum patient, and she should be mobilized as soon as possible because of an increased risk of thrombotic events.

The patient may experience a "honeymoon" period with a significant reduction in insulin requirement as the energy expenditure of breastfeeding increases. Breastfeeding is encouraged, and insulin is managed accordingly.

Contraception

Use of a reliable form of contraception is necessary for the patient until she desires pregnancy or until glucose values are in the desired range. The choices are limited but should be presented to the patient. Low-dose oral contraceptives cause a minimal increase in thromboembolic events, but much less than that experienced during pregnancy. Their use offers the most complete protection from pregnancy. Barrier contraceptive methods may be useful in the properly motivated patient. Currently, studies do not indicate an added risk of infection in women with diabetes who use an intrauterine device (IUD). Indeed, the IUD may be a good choice in a woman who has vascular complications. However, if the diabetic woman is not in a monogamous relationship, the use of both oral contraception and condoms might be advisable, to decrease the possibility of infection by sexually transmitted diseases such as human papillomavirus, herpes, and HIV.

Prognosis

Prognosis is primarily dependent on the level of glucose control. Good control requires a motivated patient, an active management approach (education, diet, insulin, and exercise) with trained health care providers, and frequent patient-provider interactions. Another factor influencing prognosis is the amount of degenerative changes. With diligent antenatal care, the patient can anticipate a normal labor and delivery experience. Severe hypoglycemia and diabetic ketoacidosis can result in maternal compromise and even death. The fetus, if spared from congenital malformation or death in utero, may suffer significant impairment in the hostile uterine environment, with poor glucose control affecting brain development as well as that of other organs.

Considerations

There are no data to support a shortening of the woman's lifespan or a worsening of renal disease as a result of pregnancy. Retinal complications might be worsened by pregnancy, and there should be no evidence of macular edema or proliferative retinopathy present before proceeding with a pregnancy. Persons in renal failure should be advised to undergo a transplant prior to a pregnancy, because of the impact of elevated creatinine on pregnancy outcome. A history of severe or frequent maternal hypoglycemia is a major concern during pregnancy and should be addressed with the family in detail, since symptoms of hypoglycemia are blunted during pregnancy. It is especially important to establish appropriate guidelines for operating a motor vehicle by advising the patient to use common sense (eg, avoid taking insulin without eating) and evaluate her glucose prior to driving if the level has not been checked recently.

TYPE 2 DIABETES (NON-INSULIN DEPENDENT)

ESSENTIALS OF DIAGNOSIS

- *Hyperglycemia not requiring exogenous insulin.*
- *Onset at over 30 years of age.*
- *"Apple-shaped" body habitus.*
- *Excess appetite and weight gain, but few other symptoms.*
- *Delayed healing or vascular disease.*

Definition

Type 2 (non-insulin dependent) diabetes is characterized by insufficient insulin receptors to effect proper glucose control after insulin is released (insulin resistance). Those affected typically have a body habitus in which there is increased abdominal girth, often described as an "apple" shape. The reason for this is that the highest concentration of insulin receptors is located in the abdominal rectus muscles and the increased layer of fat appears to impair insulin receptor sensitivity.

The patient has increased hunger due to excess insulin release as a result of elevated glucose levels. This insulin release further decreases insulin receptors due to elevated hormonal levels, and thus a vicious cycle begins of excessive appetite with weight gain. Otherwise, these patients exhibit few symptoms, with the possible exception of poor wound healing and fatigue.

Type 2 diabetics are not ketosis-prone due to the presence of insulin, but do develop a condition of hyperglycemic hyperosmolarity during pregnancy, generally after an episode of vomiting and diarrhea in which the patient replaced fluids with glucose solutions. This condition has a high morbidity for the fetus, but can be effectively treated with immediate fluid replacement.

Also included in this classification is "secondary diabetes." Secondary diabetes is carbohydrate intolerance secondary to pancreatic disease, excess production of certain hormones (eg, growth hormone), use of certain drugs (eg, corticosteroids), insulin receptor abnormalities, and certain genetic disorders.

Genetics of Inheritance

Type 2 diabetes is not linked to HLA or genetic markers, but evidence supports a genetic component. With type 2 diabetes, the risk of frank diabetes in a first-degree relative is almost 15%, and about 30% more will have impaired glucose tolerance. If both parents have type 2 diabetes, the incidence of diabetes in the off-spring is 60–75%. Monozygous twins have a much greater propensity for type 2 diabetes (almost 100%) than for type 1 diabetes (20–50%).

Significance

Type 2 diabetes has a major impact on the morbidity and mortality of the individual as well as on the quality of life (eg, amputation of extremities, blindness, strokes). Controlling glucose minimizes the onset of these complications and reduces the progression of existing ones. Education about glucose control has been shown to have a major impact on the patient's overall health.

Treatment

Type 2 diabetes is treated primarily by lifestyle modification. The level of dietary fat is decreased and the ingestion of soluble fiber increased. Increased exercise, with particular attention to the abdominal muscles, is also advised. Oral hypoglycemic agents are used in nonpregnant patients, but are not yet widely used during pregnancy.

If weight loss can be accomplished and pregnancy delayed, maintaining a woman on oral agents can be advantageous preconceptionally to reduce insulin resistance. Preconception evaluation is the same as in type 1 diabetics. It is surprising that the incidence of initial renal disease detected is higher, probably due to a longer asymptomatic period prior to diagnosis. Insulin is generally used during pregnancy and perhaps even during conception. Also during pregnancy, the health care team emphasizes diet and daily exercise.

Soluble fiber is a key in therapy of type 2 diabetes since it reduces the glycemic intake of the diet, thus reducing insulin release, which results in heightened sensitivity of insulin receptors. Fat intake is closely monitored because it reduces insulin sensitivity and often has been the main source of calories for these obese persons. Thus when fat intake is decreased and portion size increased, the patient is unable to maintain weight during the increased metabolic demand of pregnancy. The dietitian must work closely with the individual and monitor actual calorie intake to allow a minimum of 15 pounds of weight gain, even in the massively obese patient, for proper nutrition in pregnancy.

Exercise is initiated, and increased water intake prior to and during the exercise period is stressed. Swimming is the safest exercise for the massively obese to minimize trauma to joints, but walking and/or upper arm ergometrics or stationary bicycling are excellent alternatives.

Insulin therapy is added in small amounts, with emphasis on long-acting insulin. In the past, many type 2 diabetics received very high doses of insulin. This was not only unnecessary but hazardous, because it resulted in significant downregulation of insulin receptors.

The remainder of therapy, such as glucose monitoring and evaluation of the fetus, is similar to that done in type 1 diabetic management. Emphasis is placed on ultrasonography to assess fetal growth due to anatomic limitations in assessing fundal growth. Unfortunately, fetal weight assessment is often inaccurate in this group of individuals, due to the fat distribution in the pannus region.

When the patient is in labor, it is extremely important to administer a controlled glucose infusion to meet the body's energy needs. Yet it is rare to need an insulin infusion due to the high metabolic demand with a limited amount of glucose. For the postpartum patient, early ambulation assists in decreasing thromboembolic risks. Often glucose control is achieved postpartum on no more than an ADA diet. If hypoglycemic agents are necessary postpartum, insulin is continued for those who are breastfeeding, whereas the oral agents may be used in the nonbreastfeeding mothers. Postpartum weight loss is encouraged (see following section on Gestational Diabetes). Preconception evaluation prior to the next pregnancy is stressed.

■ GESTATIONAL DIABETES

ESSENTIALS OF DIAGNOSIS

- *Any degree of glucose intolerance with onset or first recognition during pregnancy.*
- *In the majority of cases of GDM, glucose regulation will return to normal after delivery.*

Definition

The above definition applies regardless of whether insulin or only diet modification is used for treatment or whether the condition continues after pregnancy. It is possible that unrecognized glucose intolerance may have antedated or begun concomitantly with pregnancy.

Gestational diabetes may be screened for by drawing a 1-hour glucose level following a 50-gram glucose load, but is definitively diagnosed only by an abnormal

3-hour GTT following a 100-gram glucose load. Such persons are not within the norm (95%) for pregnancy.

Significance

The growth and maturation of the fetus are closely associated with the delivery of maternal nutrients, particularly glucose. This is most crucial in the third trimester and is directly related to the duration and degree of maternal glucose elevation. Thus the negative impact is as highly diverse as the variety of carbohydrate intolerance that women bring to pregnancy. In those with severe abnormalities, there is an increased rate of miscarriage, congenital malformations, prematurity, pyelonephritis, preeclampsia, in utero meconium, fetal distress, cesarean section deliveries, and stillbirth.

Incidence & Etiology

Inability to maintain glucose levels required by the body for proper functioning is a growing health problem in the United States; thus it is not surprising that more women are found during pregnancy to be unable to attain the low glucose levels required for proper fetal growth. The incidence of gestational diabetes varies from 12% in racially heterogeneous urban regions to 1% in rural areas with a predominantly white population.

Pathophysiology

Gestational diabetes is pathophysiologically similar to type 2 diabetes. Approximately 90% of the persons identified have a deficiency of insulin receptors (prior to pregnancy) or a marked increase in weight in the abdominal region. The other 10% have deficient insulin production and will proceed to develop mature-onset insulin-dependent diabetes.

Similarly to women with type 2 diabetes, the women most likely to develop gestational diabetes are those who are overweight, with a body habitus often described as "apple shaped." HPL blocks insulin receptors and increases in direct linear relation to the length of pregnancy. Insulin release is enhanced in an attempt to maintain glucose homeostasis. The patient experiences increased hunger due to the excess insulin release as a result of elevated glucose levels. This insulin release further decreases insulin receptors due to elevated hormonal levels. Thus the vicious cycle of excess appetite with weight gain occurs. Few other symptoms mark this condition.

Diagnosis

Glucosuria is a common finding in pregnancy due to increased glomerular filtration and is therefore unreli-

able as a means of diagnosis. Glucose screening should be done in every pregnant patient at or no later than 28 weeks' gestation, since risk factors are insufficient to identify all women with gestational diabetes. Ultrasound findings of fetal weight ≥ 70% for gestational age, polyhydramnios (AFI ≥ 20), midline congenital anomalies, or an abdominal circumference measurement that exceeds the femur growth by 2 weeks merit an immediate 3-hour GTT. Other clinical findings indicating possible diabetes are edema developing early in pregnancy and excessive weight gain.

Initial screening is accomplished by ingestion of 50 grams of glucose (usually chilled glucola) at any time of the day and without regard to prior meal ingestion. The sensitivity and specificity are based on the cutoff value used to indicate a positive result (Table 18–4); however, screening is not as reproducible from day to day as would be desired. If screening is positive, the patient is advised to follow a carbohydrate loading diet for 3 days and then have a full 3-hour glucose tolerance test. A simple carbohydrate loading diet is all the pasta and starches she can eat at each meal and one candy bar per day. For the GTT, the patient fasts, then receives 100 grams of glucose after a fasting glucose level is obtained. A blood sample is then taken every hour for 3 hours. The patient is advised to sit quietly during the test to minimize the impact of exercise on glucose levels.

The glucose values initially used to detect gestational diabetes were determined by O'Sullivan and Mahan in a retrospective study designed to detect risk of developing type 2 diabetes in the future. The values were set using whole blood and required two values reaching or exceeding the value to be positive. Subsequent information has led to alteration in O'Sullivan's criteria. For ex-

Table 18–4. Screening glucose related to gestational diabetes.[1]

Screening Test Result (mg/dL)	Incidence of Gestational Diabetes (%)
135–144	14.6
145–154	17.4
155–164	28.6
165–174	20.0
175–184	50.0
> 185	100.0

[1]Modified with permission from: Carpenter MW, Coustan DR: Criteria for screening tests for gestational diabetes. Am J Obstet Gynecol 1982;144:768.

ample, there is growing evidence that one value is sufficient to make an impact on the health of the fetus, and is now the criterion used by most clinicians to initiate treatment. Whole blood glucose values are lower than plasma levels due to glucose uptake by hemoglobin. The present values used by the American College of Obstetricians and Gynecologists are based on a theoretical increase in hemoglobin and plasma with pregnancy. Recently, a study using all three methods of glucose determination on the same samples have disproved the theoretical values and are listed in Table 18–5.

Treatment

The key to therapy in most patients is diet and exercise (because of the paucity of insulin receptors). This makes therapy more difficult than with the insulin-deficient patient, in whom exogenous insulin may be easily administered. Therapy in the type 2 diabetic is based on the patient's motivation and ability to change lifestyle. Exercise of the non-weight-bearing type (noted previously) is encouraged as even short exercise periods have a major benefit.

Every care provider must stress the importance of diet. Soluble fiber is invaluable to provide satiety and improve insulin receptor numbers and sensitivity. Carbohydrate restriction has been shown to improve glycemic control in diet-controlled GDM. Fats must be reduced because of their negative impact on insulin receptors. Calories should be prescribed at 20–25/kcal per kilogram of present body weight (generally 1800–2400 kcal). Massively obese patients have a reduction in their metabolism rate; therefore, it is better to start low and increase the calories as needed. Food records are kept for 1 week, and the content and calories are reviewed by the dietitian with helpful suggestions on improving favorite dishes to be included in the diet. The patient is instructed to particularly note all food taken in when a 1-hour postprandial glucose value

is 130 mg/dL or greater. The memory reflectance glucose meters are invaluable in assisting the patient to learn the proper diet and the impact of her actions on glucose levels. Insulin is added as needed for glucose control only after clear dietary errors are noted and attempts at correction are done. Approaches to initiating insulin therapy vary, but should remain as simple as possible.

A minimum of 2 visits to the dietitian encourages education and interaction over dietary questions. The customization of diet to ethnic foods is often invaluable in obtaining dietary compliance. The encouragement of other family members to participate in dietary counseling assists their support for the patient and is key to making familial dietary changes. The patient often benefits from direct contact with the dietitian when glucose levels are erratic, when her weight fails to meet expected guidelines, when she is having difficulty with calorie counting, or when she increases daily calories more than 300 kcal over guidelines.

The patient checks her glucose 4 times daily (eg, fasting, and 1-hour postprandial breakfast, lunch, dinner). The desired values are a fasting level of 70–90 mg/dL and a 1-hour level of 130 mg/dL. The average glucose levels should be 90 mg/dL.

ANTEPARTUM CARE

Diabetics have triple the normal rate of asymptomatic bacteriuria. Therefore, a urine culture is obtained initially, and appropriate treatment initiated if it is positive. After cessation of therapy, urinary culture is again obtained to confirm elimination of the infection. Protein detected in clean-catch urine specimens should be evaluated by 24-hour urine testing and repeated as needed. In addition to routine prenatal care (see Chapter 10), the development of edema (including carpal tunnel syndrome) is closely monitored. If edema occurs, greater attention to glucose control (eg, returning to daily monitoring) and enhanced bed rest are necessities. There is an increased incidence of preeclampsia in diabetics, which is directly related to glucose control as well as to the presence of preexisting vascular and renal disease.

Assessment of the fetus by glucose memory meters combined with clinical/ultrasound assessment of fetal growth cannot be replaced by other antenatal tests. Fetuses in whom maternal glucose has been well controlled and whose mothers do not smoke or have other organ damage will tolerate pregnancy well. Patients with poor glucose control, fetal macrosomia, and/or polyhydramnios represent the patients at greatest risk for morbidity and mortality. Biweekly nonstress tests (NSTs) or weekly contraction stress tests are begun at 32 weeks for additional monitoring of poorly con-

Table 18–5. Oral glucose tolerance test (100 g) values for the diagnosis of gestational diabetes (mg/dL).

	O'Sullivan & Mahan (1964)	NDDG (1979)	Carpenter & Coustan (1982)	Sacks et al (1989)
Fasting	90	105	95	96
1 Hour	165	190	180	172
2 Hour	145	165	155	152
3 hour	125	145	140	131

trolled patients, patients with complicated vascular disease, or patients who smoke. Weekly NSTs (also from 32 weeks' gestation) are recommended in patients with insulin-requiring gestational diabetes, with an increase to biweekly recommended after 36 weeks as well as the addition of AFI evaluation. For diet-controlled gestational diabetics, weekly NSTs are usually begun at 36 weeks. All patients should be instructed to make daily assessments of fetal movements and to alert the physician if a decrease is noted. A biophysical profile should be done if decreased movement is noted or if a nonreactive NST occurs.

In the case of abnormal fetal testing, the practitioner should assess gestational age and, if the fetus is found to be mature, should proceed to delivery. If the fetus is intermediate in maturity, amniotic fluid assessment for pulmonary maturity may assist in the decision regarding whether delivery should be effected. Lung maturity should also be assessed before elective induction if glucose control is questionable or if the fetus is less than 38 weeks unless fetal jeopardy is suspected. The lecithin:sphingomyelin ratio should be 2.5 or higher due to the higher incidence of respiratory distress in the fetus. If the fetus is immature, further testing such as contraction stress tests or hospitalization with continuous fetal heart rate monitoring is advised.

Preterm labor is increased in patients with diabetes, and they should be treated with magnesium sulfate as the initial tocolytic agent because the beta mimetics markedly influence glucose control. Corticosteroids increase maternal glucose levels, and therapy should be prescribed to keep levels in the desired range. This therapy may consist of continuous insulin infusion in certain cases.

Induction of labor is recommended at 38 weeks in patients with poor glucose control and macrosomia. Glucose control at a level 100 mg/dL for 24 hours prior to delivery will reduce immediate neonatal hypoglycemia. Prostaglandin gel to ripen the cervix reduces the cesarean section rate, but is not advised without a negative contraction stress test if oligohydramnios is the indication for induction. Insulin-requiring diabetics should be induced at 40 weeks' gestation if spontaneous labor has not occurred. In any glucose-intolerant patient, the decision to continue pregnancy longer than 40 weeks' gestation must be carefully considered.

NEONATAL COMPLICATIONS

Early pregnancy exposure to higher glucose levels results in enhanced rates of abortion and an increased incidence of congenital anomalies. Neonates whose mothers have higher glucose levels over a longer duration of pregnancy have higher incidences of macrosomia, hypoglycemia, hypocalcemia, polycythemia, res-

piratory difficulties, cardiomyopathy, and congestive heart failure. Long-term control of maternal glucose is associated with a reduction in all of these complications.

Macrosomic babies have increasing intolerance to intrauterine compromise as well as an enhanced rate of birth trauma. Respiratory distress syndrome and transient tachypnea are increased in infants of poorly controlled diabetics. In fact, all organ maturation is delayed in direct relation to the degree of hyperglycemia. This may be compounded by impairment of maternal vascular flow to the developing fetus. Infants of inadequately controlled diabetic mothers have an increase in cardiomyopathy and congestive heart failure due to excess glycogen deposition and hypertrophy of the heart muscle as a result of intrauterine compensation for maternal hyperglycemia.

The fetal response to the intrauterine environment such as fetal pancreatic hyperplasia with increased basal insulin secretion can make an impact on the child into adulthood with an increased risk of diabetes. The incidence is increased from that of the familial inheritance; for example, a recent study of Pima Indians showed that there was a greater incidence of diabetes in the offspring of women who had type 2 diabetes during pregnancy than in the offspring of those who developed diabetes years after pregnancy (45% vs. 8.6% at age 20–24 years).

INTRAPARTUM & POSTPARTUM MANAGEMENT

Glucose infusion (D5W, lactated Ringer's solution) is given to all patients in labor unless delivery is immediate, but care is taken to control the infusion at 125 mL/h unless the patient needs additional glucose for metabolic demands, in which case the glucose infusion is increased. It may be anticipated that women >160 kg in weight will require more glucose. Glucose-containing fluids should not be used for bolus prior to induction of conduction anesthesia. A bedside glucose reflectance monitor is used to follow glucose levels every 2–4 hours with the goal of maintaining levels at 70–95 mg/dL. In those requiring insulin, regular insulin (25 U/250 mL normal saline, giving a dilution of 0.1 U/mL) is given by continuous infusion at levels of 0.5–2 U/h.

Oxytocin is given for labor induction similarly to normal pregnancies. Continuous fetal heart rate monitoring is required with careful attention to decelerations. Fetal tolerance to intrauterine stress is limited in diabetic pregnancies. Early scalp pH or oxygen saturation monitoring is indicated if worrisome patterns persist. If fetal macrosomia is suspected, forceps should be used with great caution in the second stage and shoulder girdle dystocia anticipated. Additional personnel may be necessary at the time of delivery.

If repeat cesarean section or other indication for elective surgery occurs, the patient should be directed to take the evening insulin dose prior to surgery, but not her morning dose. Showering with a bacterial solution the night before delivery seems reasonable due to the increase in wound infections in this group. The patient is at increased risk of thromboembolic events due to decreased prostacyclin production by the platelets.

Breastfeeding is not affected by diabetes and is generally encouraged.

Prognosis

Women diagnosed with gestational diabetes have an increased risk of developing diabetes mellitus in the future. If they require insulin for their pregnancy, there is a 50% risk of diabetes within 5 years. If dietary control has been sufficient, a 60% risk of developing diabetes mellitus within 10–15 years still persists. However, evidence shows that lifestyle alteration may delay or entirely prevent the onset of diabetes. Thus these patients benefit from a reduction of their risk factors.

Postpartum, the patient should be placed back on an ADA diet (with increased soluble fiber and reduced fat). She should do a lifestyle assessment and attempt to keep her weight near ideal for her height. Weight reduction is generally necessary, and thus, if the patient is not breastfeeding, calories are reduced to 1200–1500 kcal with repeat dietary instruction, and the same calorie ADA diet is continued as the patient is breastfeeding. The caloric demand of breastfeeding increases with neonatal size but can reach 800–1200 kcal per day. Exercise equivalent to expend the energy is to run hard for 1 hour (900 kcal). It takes 3500 kcal expended to reduce weight by 1 pound! She should enter a regular exercise program.

All gestationally diabetic patients should have a 75-g 3-hour glucose tolerance approximately 6 weeks after pregnancy to evaluate for preexisting diabetes. It is important to individualize a prevention program for the 98% who will have a negative test. If the 1-hour value is high, it represents decreased insulin capacity, whereas an elevated 3-hour value reflects decreased insulin re-

ceptors. With an elevated 1-hour level, limiting simple sugars in the diet should become a lifetime goal. With an elevated 3-hour glucose value, weight loss with increased abdominal musculature should significantly reduce the increased risk of diabetes. Lipids should be evaluated in black and Hispanic patients because of a higher incidence of hypercholesterolemia in this group. This is particularly advisable prior to initiation of oral contraceptive agents. Preconception glucose evaluation should be discussed with the patient, and she should be encouraged to have an annual fasting glucose.

REFERENCES

Adams KM et al: Sequelae of unrecognized gestational diabetes. Am J Obstet Gynecol 1998;178:1321.

American College of Obstetricians and Gynecologists: Fetal macrosomia. ACOG Practice Bulletin No. 22, November 2000.

American College of Obstetricians and Gynecologists: Gestational diabetes. ACOG Practice Bulletin No. 30, September 2001.

American Diabetes Association: Clinical practice recommendations 2001. J Clin Applied Res Educ 2001;24(Suppl 1);3.

American Diabetes Association: Gestational diabetes mellitus. Diabetes Care 2001;24(suppl 1):S77.

Casey BM et al: Pregnancy outcomes in women with gestational diabetes compared with the general obstetric population. Obstet Gynecol 1997;90:869.

Cundy T et al: Perinatal mortality in type 2 diabetes. Diabet Med 2000;17:33.

Dang K, Homko C, Reece EA: Factors associated with fetal macrosomia in offspring of gestational diabetic women. J Maternal Fetal Med 2000;9:114.

Expert Committee on the Diagnosis and Classification of Diabetes Mellitus: Report of the Expert Committee on the Diagnosis and Classification of Diabetes Mellitus. Diabetes Care 2000;23(suppl 1):S4.

Major CM et al: The effects of carbohydrate restriction in patients with diet-controlled gestational diabetes. Obstet Gynecol 1998;91:245.

National Diabetes Data Group (NDDG): Classification and diagnosis of diabetes mellitus. National Institutes of Health, 1979.

Rendell M: Dietary treatment of diabetes mellitus. N Engl J Med 2000;342:1440(editorial).

Schaefer-Graf UM et al: Patterns of congenital anomalies and relationship to initial maternal fasting glucose levels in pregnancies complicated by type 2 and gestational diabetes. Am J Obstet Gynecol 2000;182:313.

Hypertensive States of Pregnancy

Courtney Reynolds, MD, William C. Mabie, MD, & Baha M. Sibai, MD

Hypertensive states in pregnancy include preeclampsia-eclampsia, chronic hypertension (either essential or secondary to renal disease, endocrine disease, or other causes), chronic hypertension with superimposed preeclampsia, and gestational hypertension (Table 19–1). **Preeclampsia** is hypertension associated with proteinuria and edema, occurring primarily in nulliparas after the 20th gestational week and most frequently near term. Recent data support the elimination of edema as a diagnostic criterion. **Eclampsia** is the occurrence of seizures that cannot be attributed to other causes in a preeclamptic patient. **Chronic hypertension** is defined as hypertension that is present before conception, before 20 weeks' gestation or that persists for more than 6 weeks postpartum. Hypertension is defined as blood pressure equal to or greater than 140/90 mm Hg or an increase in mean arterial pressure of 20 mm Hg. The use of an increase in blood pressure of 30/15 mm Hg over first-trimester values is controversial. Recent data report no increased adverse events in women with these changes. However, an increase in blood pressure by this amount warrants close observation. Proteinuria is defined as the excretion of 300 mg or more in a 24-hour specimen or 30 mg/dL in a random specimen. Preeclampsia may occur in women with chronic hypertension (**superimposed preeclampsia**); the prognosis is worse for the mother and fetus than with either condition alone. The criteria for superimposed preeclampsia are worsening hypertension (30 mm Hg systolic or 15 mm Hg diastolic above the average of values before 20 weeks' gestation) together with either nondependent edema or proteinuria. **Gestational hypertension** is further divided into transient hypertension of pregnancy if preeclampsia is present at the time of delivery and the blood pressure is normal by 12 weeks postpartum, and chronic hypertension if the elevation in blood pressure persists beyond 12 weeks postpartum. This condition is often predictive of the later development of essential hypertension.

It is frequently difficult to determine whether a patient has preeclampsia, chronic hypertension, or chronic hypertension with superimposed preeclampsia. This is partly because blood pressure normally decreases during the second trimester, and the decrease may mask the presence of chronic hypertension. Renal biopsy studies have shown that only about 70% of primigravidas under 25 years of age with the triad of edema, hypertension, and proteinuria have **glomeruloendotheliosis,** the characteristic lesion of preeclampsia. Twenty-five percent have unsuspected renal disease. In multiparas with chronic hypertension with superimposed preeclampsia, about 3% have glomeruloendotheliosis and 21% have underlying renal disease. Renal biopsy is rarely performed in pregnancy because the benefit usually does not justify the risk. The sensitivity and specificity of biochemical markers such as uric acid and antithrombin III are unknown.

PREECLAMPSIA

Preeclampsia occurs in about 6% of the general population; the incidence varies with geographic location. Predisposing factors are nulliparity, black race, maternal age below 20 or over 35 years, low socioeconomic status, multiple gestation, hydatidiform mole, polyhydramnios, nonimmune fetal hydrops, twins, obesity, diabetes, chronic hypertension, and underlying renal disease.

Classification

There are 2 categories of preeclampsia, mild and severe. Severe preeclampsia is defined as the following: (1) blood pressure greater than 160 mm Hg systolic or 110 mm Hg diastolic on 2 occasions 6 hours apart; (2) proteinuria exceeding 2 g in a 24-hour period or 2–4+ on dipstick testing; (3) increased serum creatinine (> 1.2 mg/dL unless known to be elevated previously); (4) oliguria ≤500 mL/24 h; (5) cerebral or visual disturbances; (6) epigastric pain; (7) elevated liver enzymes; (8) thrombocytopenia (platelet count < 100,000/mm³); (9) retinal hemorrhages, exudates, or papilledema; and (10) pulmonary edema.

Pathogenesis

Preeclampsia has been described as a disease of theories, because the cause is unknown. Some theories include (1) endothelial cell injury, (2) rejection phenomenon (insufficient production of blocking antibodies), (3) compromised placental perfusion, (4) altered vascular reactivity, (5) imbalance between prostacyclin and thromboxane, (6) decreased glomerular filtration rate with retention of salt and water, (7) decreased intravas-

Table 19–1. Hypertensive states of pregnancy other than preeclampsia-eclampsia.

Chronic essential hypertension
Chronic hypertension due to renal disease
   Interstitial nephritis
   Acute and chronic glomerulonephritis
   Systemic lupus erythematosus
   Diabetic glomerulosclerosis
   Scleroderma
   Polyarteritis nodosa
   Polycystic kidney disease
   Renovascular stenosis
   Chronic renal failure with treatment by dialysis
   Renal transplant
Chronic hypertension due to endocrine disease
   Cushing's disease and syndrome
   Primary hyperaldosteronism
   Thyrotoxicosis
   Pheochromocytoma
   Acromegaly
Chronic hypertension due to coarctation of the aorta

cular volume, (8) increased central nervous system irritability, (9) disseminated intravascular coagulation, (10) uterine muscle stretch (ischemia), (11) dietary factors, and (12) genetic factors. The relatively new theory of endothelial injury explains many of the clinical findings in preeclampsia. The theory emphasizes that there is more to preeclampsia than hypertension. The vascular endothelium produces a number of important substances including endothelial-derived relaxing factor or nitric oxide, endothelin-1, prostacyclin, and tissue plasminogen activator. Thus, endothelial cells modify the contractile response of the underlying smooth muscle cells, prevent intravascular coagulation, and maintain the integrity of the intravascular compartment. Several findings suggest endothelial injury in preeclampsia. The characteristic renal lesion of preeclampsia "glomeruloendotheliosis" is manifested primarily by swelling of the glomerular capillary endothelial cells. The hematologic changes of preeclampsia, ie, thrombocytopenia and microangiopathic hemolytic anemia, are similar to those found in thrombotic thrombocytopenic purpura or hemolytic uremic syndrome—disorders in which endothelial dysfunction is thought to be important. Activation of the clotting cascade and increased sensitivity to pressors are compatible with endothelial cell dysfunction. Biochemical evidence includes an imbalance in the prostacyclin:thromboxane ratio and high circulating concentrations of von Willebrand factor, endothelin, and cellular fibronectin. Serum from preeclamptic women, when applied to human umbilical vein en-

dothelial cell cultures, produces no morphologic abnormalities in the cells but releases procoagulants, vasoconstrictors, and mitogens.

In summary, the current hypothesis for the pathogenesis of preeclampsia is that an immunologic disturbance causes abnormal placental implantation resulting in decreased placental perfusion. The abnormal perfusion stimulates the production of substances in the blood that activate or injure endothelial cells. The vascular endothelium provides a single target for these blood-borne products, which explains the multiple organ system involvement in preeclampsia.

Pathophysiology

A. CENTRAL NERVOUS SYSTEM

Tissues are capable of regulating their own blood flow; this process is known as **autoregulation.** Cerebral perfusion is maintained by autoregulation at a constant level of about 55 mL/min/100 g at a wide range of blood pressures (Fig 19–1). However, blood pressure may rise to levels at which autoregulation cannot function. When this occurs, the endothelial tight junctions open, causing plasma and red blood cells to leak into the extravascular space. This may result in petechial hemorrhage or gross intracranial hemorrhage. The upper limit of autoregulation varies from one person to another; eg, chronic hypertension may cause medial hypertrophy of the cerebral vessels, resulting in a shift of the curve to the right (Fig 19–1). This explains the paradox of 2 patients with equally severe hypertension who have markedly different

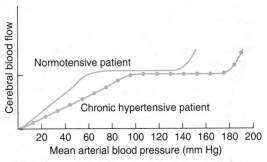

Figure 19–1. Representation of the relationship between cerebral blood flow and mean arterial blood pressure. Cerebral blood flow normally remains constant at mean arterial pressures of 60–140 mm Hg. In chronically hypertensive patients, medial hypertrophy causes the lower and upper limits of autoregulation to be shifted to higher blood pressure values. (Modified and reproduced, with permission, from Donaldson JO: *Neurology of Pregnancy.* Saunders, 1978.)

clinical presentations. The young primigravida whose blood pressure is normally 110/70 mm Hg may convulse with a blood pressure of 180/120 mm Hg, while a chronic hypertensive may be asymptomatic or have only a headache at the same pressure.

The mechanism of the cerebral damage in eclampsia is unclear. The pathologic findings are similar to those of hypertensive encephalopathy. These abnormalities include fibrinoid necrosis and thrombosis of arterioles, microinfarcts, and petechial hemorrhages. In both hypertensive encephalopathy and eclampsia, the lesions are widely distributed throughout the brain, but the brainstem is more severely affected in the former, while the cortex is more severely affected in the latter. Other differences in the two conditions are that eclampsia may be seen in the absence of hypertension and that retinal hemorrhages and infarcts are rare in eclampsia. Two theories have been proposed to explain the pathogenesis of hypertensive encephalopathy, vasospasm, and forced dilation. In the first, vasospasm causes local ischemia, arteriolar necrosis, and disruption of the blood-brain barrier. According to the second, as blood pressure rises above the limit of autoregulation, cerebral vasodilation occurs. Initially, some vessel segments dilate, and some remain constricted. Overdistention of the dilated segments results in necrosis of the medial muscle fibers and damage to the vessel wall. It is possible that both mechanisms are operant.

The presence of cerebral edema in preeclampsia-eclampsia is controversial. One set of researchers stated that cerebral edema was not present in eclamptic patients when autopsy was performed within 1 hour of death and that such edema was a late postmortem change. In contrast, some others found generalized cerebral edema in some autopsy specimens and confirmed increased intracranial pressure in eclamptics with prolonged coma (> 6 hours). Early studies of cerebrospinal fluid opening pressure showed elevated pressures; however, more recent studies have failed to confirm this.

Head computed tomographic (CT) scans in women with eclampsia have shown abnormalities in about one-third. By using fourth-generation equipment and with a short interval from seizure to CT scan, abnormalities may be detected in half the patients. The main findings are focal hypodensities in the white matter in the posterior half of the cerebral hemispheres with occasional lesions in the gray matter, temporal lobes, and brainstem. One researcher suggested that these areas of radiographic hypodensity represented petechial hemorrhages accompanied by local edema. Subarachnoid or intraventricular hemorrhages may be seen in the most severe cases.

Magnetic resonance imaging (MRI) is more sensitive at demonstrating abnormalities than CT scan, but it is not as widely available. T_2-weighed MRI scans show high signal in the cortical and subcortical white matter. Most of the abnormalities lie in the occipital and parietal areas in watershed areas where the anterior, middle, and posterior circulations meet. Basal ganglia and brainstem abnormalities occur in more critically ill patients.

Cerebral angiography has been performed in a few patients with eclampsia, revealing diffuse arterial vasoconstriction.

Electroencephalograms (EEGs) show nonspecific abnormalities in about 75% of patients after eclamptic seizures. The pattern is usually a diffuse slowing of activity (theta or delta waves), sometimes with focal slow activity and occasional paroxysmal spike activity. These abnormalities may be seen in other conditions, such as hypoxia, renal disease, polycythemia, hypocalcemia, and water intoxication. The electroencephalographic pattern is unaffected by magnesium sulfate. It gradually returns to normal 6–8 weeks postpartum. Uncomplicated eclampsia causes no permanent neurologic deficit.

B. Eyes

Both serous retinal detachment and cortical blindness may occur.

C. Pulmonary System

Pulmonary edema may occur with severe preeclampsia or eclampsia. It may be cardiogenic or noncardiogenic and usually occurs postpartum. In some cases it may be related to excessive fluid administration or to delayed mobilization of extravascular fluid. It may also be related to decreased plasma colloid oncotic pressure from proteinuria, use of crystalloids to replace blood loss, and decreased hepatic synthesis of albumin. Pulmonary edema is particularly common in patients with underlying chronic hypertension and hypertensive heart disease, which may be manifested by systolic dysfunction, diastolic dysfunction, or both. Aspiration of gastric contents is one of the most dreaded complications of eclamptic seizures. This may result in death because of asphyxia from particulate matter plugging major airways or in chemical pneumonitis from aspirated gastric acid. Aspiration may cause various types of pneumonia, ranging from patchy pneumonitis to full-blown adult respiratory distress syndrome.

D. Cardiovascular System

Plasma volume is reduced in patients with preeclampsia. Normal physiologic volume expansion does not occur, possibly because of generalized vasoconstriction, capillary leak, or some other factor. Because the cause of the reduced volume is unknown, management is controversial. One theory is that the decreased volume is a primary event causing a chronic shocklike state.

Hypertension is thought to be the result of release of a pressor substance from the hypoperfused uterus or of compensatory secretion of catecholamines. Proponents of this theory advocate avoidance of diuretics and use of volume expanders. Another theory is that decreased volume is secondary to vasoconstriction. Proponents of this theory advocate the use of vasodilators and warn that volume expanders may aggravate hypertension or cause pulmonary edema.

Studies using the Swan-Ganz catheter have demonstrated a spectrum of hemodynamic findings in preeclampsia ranging from a low-output, high-resistance state to a high-output, low-resistance state. One study found a low wedge pressure, low cardiac output, and high systemic vascular resistance in untreated nulliparous preeclamptic women, while patients who received various therapies and were usually referred, a wide range of hemodynamics was found. The conclusion was that the untreated preeclamptic patient was significantly volume-depleted and that the wide spectrum of hemodynamic findings in the treated group resulted from prior therapy and the presence of other variables such as labor, multiparity, and preexisting hypertension.

In another study of a heterogeneous population of pretreated and nonpretreated patients, a generally consistent profile emerged. Preeclampsia was in general a high cardiac output state associated with an inappropriately high peripheral resistance. Although the systemic vascular resistance was within the normal range for pregnancy, it was still inappropriately high for the elevated cardiac output. The failure of the circulation to dilate in the setting of increasing cardiac output appeared to be a characteristic feature of preeclampsia. The normal wedge and central venous pressures found in their study suggested venoconstriction with central relocation of intravascular volume if the generally accepted reports of decreased plasma volume in preeclampsia are correct. They postulated splanchnic venoconstriction as the mechanism of this volume shift.

Normal pregnant women are resistant to the vasoconstrictor effects of angiotensin II. Pregnant women require about 2½ times the amount of angiotensin II required by nonpregnant women to raise the diastolic blood pressure 20 mm Hg. Patients who will develop superimposed preeclampsia lose their refractoriness to angiotensin II many weeks before hypertension develops. These patients may be identified as early as 18–24 weeks' gestation by infusion of angiotensin II.

Normal pregnant women lose their refractoriness to angiotensin II after treatment with prostaglandin synthetase inhibitors such as aspirin or indomethacin; this suggests that prostaglandin is involved in mediating vascular reactivity to angiotensin II in pregnancy. Refractoriness to angiotensin II can be restored in patients with preeclampsia by the administration of theophylline, a phosphodiesterase inhibitor that increases intracellular levels of cAMP. Therefore, prostaglandins synthesized in the arteriole may modulate vascular reactivity to angiotensin II by altering the intracellular level of cAMP in vascular smooth muscle.

E. LIVER

The spectrum of liver disease in preeclampsia is broad, ranging from subclinical involvement with the only manifestation being fibrin deposition along the hepatic sinusoids to rupture of the liver. Within these extremes lie the **HELLP syndrome** (*h*emolysis, *e*levated *l*iver enzymes, and *l*ow *p*latelets) and hepatic infarction.

F. KIDNEYS

The characteristic lesion of preeclampsia, **glomeruloendotheliosis,** is a swelling of the glomerular capillary endothelium that causes decreased glomerular perfusion and glomerular filtration rate. Fibrin split products have been found on the basement membrane by some observers, who have suggested that intravascular coagulation may be secondary to thromboplastin released from the placenta. However, the fibrin split products are found infrequently and only in small amounts. Other investigators have detected IgM, IgG, and complement in the glomeruli of some patients and have suggested an immunologic mechanism. Serial renal biopsies have shown that the lesion is totally reversible over about 6 weeks.

G. BLOOD

Most patients with preeclampsia-eclampsia have normal clotting studies. In some, a spectrum of abnormalities may be found, ranging from isolated thrombocytopenia to microangiopathic hemolytic anemia to disseminated intravascular coagulation (DIC). Thrombocytopenia is the most common abnormality; a count of less than 150,000/μL is found in 15–20% of patients. Fibrinogen levels are actually elevated in preeclamptic women as compared with normotensive patients. Low fibrinogen levels in preeclampsia-eclampsia are usually associated with abruptio placentae or fetal demise. Elevated fibrin split products are seen in 20% of patients (usually in the range of 10–40 μL/mL). Microangiopathic hemolytic anemia without other signs of DIC may be seen in about 5% of patients, and evidence of DIC is also present in about 5%. In the past, DIC was thought to be the cause of preeclampsia; now it is regarded as a sequela of the disease.

The HELLP syndrome describes patients with hemolytic anemia, elevated liver enzymes, and low platelet count. Criteria for the diagnosis at the authors' institution are schistocytes on the peripheral blood smear, lactic dehydrogenase > 600 U/L, total bilirubin > 1.2

mg/dL, aspartate aminotransferase > 70 U/L, and platelet count < 100,000/mm^3. This syndrome is present in about 10% of patients with severe preeclampsia-eclampsia. It is frequently seen in Caucasian patients with delay in diagnosis or delivery and in patients with abruptio placentae. The syndrome may occur remote from term (eg, at 31 weeks) and with no elevation of blood pressure. The syndrome is frequently misdiagnosed as hepatitis, gallbladder disease, idiopathic thrombocytopenic purpura, or thrombotic thrombocytopenic purpura. Most hematologic abnormalities return to normal within 2–3 days after delivery, but thrombocytopenia may persist for a week.

H. ENDOCRINE SYSTEM

The role of the renin-angiotensin-aldosterone system in the regulation of blood pressure during normal and hypertensive pregnancy has not been clearly defined. In normal pregnancy, estrogen's effect on the liver markedly increases production of renin substrate. This increases plasma renin activity, plasma renin concentration, and angiotensin II levels. Plasma aldosterone levels rise even higher than can be accounted for by the prevailing plasma renin activity. Despite the high plasma concentration of aldosterone, there is no blood pressure increase or hypokalemia in normal pregnancy; indeed, blood pressure falls in the midtrimester. This may be due to counterregulatory factors such as the natriuretic effect of progesterone or activation of vasodepressor systems such as kinins or prostaglandins.

Interpreting renin, angiotensin, and aldosterone levels in studies of preeclampsia is difficult because of differences in the definition of preeclampsia (parity, degree of proteinuria, early- or late-onset disease), differences in taking of blood samples (values may be affected by bed rest, sodium intake, labor, etc), and differences in assay techniques. In the majority of studies, renin, angiotensin, and aldosterone are all suppressed in preeclampsia, but they are still above nonpregnant levels. The available evidence suggests that the renin-angiotensin system is only secondarily involved in preeclampsia.

Atrial natriuretic peptide (ANP) is a volume regulatory hormone synthesized by cardiac myocytes, which has potent natriuretic, diuretic, and vasorelaxant properties. ANP secretion is stimulated by increased atrial pressure and alterations in sodium balance. Elevated concentrations of ANP accompany pathologic states characterized by fluid overload such as cirrhosis, congestive heart failure, and chronic renal failure. However, ANP is elevated in preeclampsia, a disorder supposedly characterized by hypovolemia. It is even elevated in the second trimester before the onset of clinical evidence of preeclampsia. The mechanism for the elevation is unknown. It may be that endothelin or another vasoactive peptide is stimulating release of ANP. It may also be that the widely accepted concept of central hypovolemia in preeclampsia is incorrect.

I. CATECHOLAMINES

Urinary and blood catecholamine levels are the same in normotensive pregnant women, women with preeclampsia, and nonpregnant controls. However, it cannot be ruled out that sympathetic activity is of pathogenetic importance for initiation or maintenance of hypertension in patients with preeclampsia. Catecholamine levels increase during labor, presumably owing to stress. The vascular refractoriness to catecholamines is lacking in preeclampsia, as is the refractoriness to other endogenous vasopressors such as antidiuretic hormone and angiotensin II.

J. PROSTACYCLIN

Prostacyclin is a prostaglandin discovered in 1976. It increases intracellular cAMP in smooth muscle cells and platelets resulting in vasodilator and platelet antiaggregatory effects. Its half-life is about 3 minutes, breaking down in plasma to 6-keto-PGF$_{1\alpha}$, which is stable and can be measured as an indication of prostacyclin levels. These plasma levels are low, indicating that prostacyclin acts physiologically at the local level rather than as a circulating hormone.

Prostacyclin is made primarily in the endothelial cell from arachidonic acid, catalyzed by the enzyme cyclooxygenase. Cyclooxygenase can be inhibited by aspirin-like drugs. Mechanical or chemical perturbation of the endothelial cell membrane stimulates formation and release of prostacyclin. For example, pulsatile pressure or chemicals such as bradykinin or thrombin stimulate prostacyclin generation in the vessel wall.

Thromboxane A$_2$ generated by platelets from arachidonic acid via cyclooxygenase induces vasoconstriction and platelet aggregation. Thus, prostacyclin and thromboxane have opposing roles in regulating platelet-vessel wall interaction.

Aspirin irreversibly inhibits cyclooxygenase. Cyclooxygenase must be produced continuously by endothelial cells, because they recover their ability to synthesize prostacyclin within a few hours after a dose of aspirin. On the other hand, platelets do not have a nucleus and therefore cannot make fresh cyclooxygenase. Thromboxane synthesis recovers only as new platelets enter the circulation. Platelet life span is about 1 week. Thus, daily treatment with low-dose aspirin results in chronic inhibition of thromboxane metabolites and decreased excretion of prostacyclin metabolites in preeclamptic patients. Low-dose aspirin therapy is aimed at restoring the presumed thromboxane-prostacyclin imbalance in preeclampsia.

K. Nitric Oxide

Nitric oxide (NO) is an endogenous vasodilator and inhibitor of platelet aggregation and acts synergistically with prostacyclin. It is produced by endothelial cells from L-arginine. Synthesis can be inhibited by arginine analogs such as N^G-monomethyl-L-arginine and N^G-nitro-L-arginine. Intravenous injection of one of these inhibitors into rats, rabbits, or guinea pigs causes an immediate rise in blood pressure that is reversed by L-arginine. This indicates that continual basal release of NO from endothelial cells keeps the vasculature in a dilated state. NO acts only in the immediate vicinity of the cell that releases it. Any that escapes into the bloodstream decays chemically to form nitrite or is immediately inactivated by hemoglobin.

NO plays an important role in several pathologic processes. It is one of the mediators of hypotension in septic shock. A deficiency of NO contributes to the cause of hypertension and atherosclerosis. Currently it is thought that the NO system may be more important than the prostaglandins in the pathogenesis of preeclampsia. Chronic blockade of the endogenous NO system produces a model of hypertension and renal damage in pregnant and nonpregnant rats. Some studies have shown that there is decreased excretion of NO in the urine of pregnant preeclamptic women, but whether NO plays an important pathophysiologic role in the development of preeclampsia remains unknown.

L. Endothelin-1

In addition to the relaxing factors prostacyclin and NO, the vascular endothelium releases vasoconstrictor substances. The vasoconstrictor endothelin was discovered in 1988. There are 3 different isopeptides: endothelin 1, 2, and 3. Endothelin-1 is the only endothelin manufactured by endothelial cells. Endothelins are also synthesized by kidney cells and nervous tissue. There are widespread endothelin-binding sites including those in the brain, lung, kidney, adrenal, spleen, intestine, and placenta. It is thought that endothelins act as endogenous agonists of dihydropyridine-sensitive calcium channels. The most striking property of endothelin-1 is its long-lasting vasoconstrictor action. It is 10 times more potent than angiotensin II. Endothelin may play a role in constriction of placental vessels after delivery and may regulate closure of the ductus arteriosus in the newborn. The mitogenic effects of endothelin-1 may cause vascular wall hypertrophy in atherosclerosis and hypertension. Endothelin-1 may play a role in renal vasoconstriction in acute renal failure. A 3-fold elevation of plasma endothelin 1 and 2 has been found in women with preeclampsia compared with gestation-matched controls.

One hypothesis is that prostacyclin is an antiplatelet and vasodilator mechanism held in reserve to reinforce the NO system when endothelial damage occurs. Lack of NO may be a causative factor in hypertension. Endothelin-1 is released by endothelial cells to constrict the underlying smooth muscle in an emergency such as laceration. Excess endothelin-1 may also be involved in the genesis of hypertension.

M. Placenta

In normal pregnancy, the proliferating trophoblast invades the decidua and the adjacent myometrium in 2 forms: interstitial and endovascular. The role of the interstitial form is not clear but it may serve to anchor the placenta. The endovascular trophoblastic cells invade the maternal spiral arteries, where they replace the endothelium and destroy the medial elastic and muscular tissue of the arterial wall. The arterial wall is replaced by fibrinoid material. This process is complete by the end of the first trimester, at which time it extends to the deciduomyometrial junction. There appears to be a resting phase in the process until 14 to 16 weeks' gestation, when a second wave of trophoblastic invasion extends down the lumen of the spiral arteries to their origin from the radial arteries deep in the myometrium. The same process is then repeated, ie, replacement of the endothelium, destruction of the medial musculoelastic tissue, and fibrinoid change in the vessel wall. The end result is that the thin-walled, muscular spiral arteries are converted to saclike, flaccid uteroplacental vessels, which passively dilate to accommodate the greatly augmented blood flow required in pregnancy (Fig 19–2).

Preeclampsia develops following a partial failure in the process of placentation. First, not all the spiral arteries of the placental bed are invaded by trophoblast. Second, in those arteries that are invaded, the first phase of trophoblastic invasion occurs normally, but the second phase does not occur, and the myometrial portions of the spiral arteries retain their reactive musculoelastic walls.

In addition, acute atherosis (a lesion similar to atherosclerosis) develops in the myometrial segments of the spiral arteries of patients with preeclampsia. The lesion is characterized by fibrinoid necrosis of the arterial wall, the presence of lipid and lipophages in the damaged wall, and a mononuclear cell infiltrate around the damaged vessel. Acute atherosis may progress to vessel obliteration with corresponding areas of placental infarction.

Thus, in preeclampsia there is an area of vascular resistance in the spiral artery because of failure of the second wave of trophoblastic invasion. In addition, acute atherosis further compromises the vascular lumen. Consequently, the fetus is subjected to poor intervillous blood flow from the time of early gestation; this may result in intrauterine growth retardation or stillbirth.

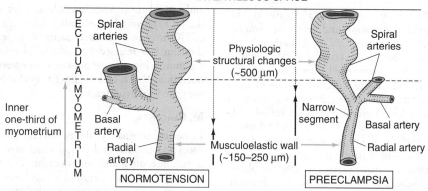

Figure 19–2. The placental bed in normal and preeclamptic pregnancy. In preeclampsia, the physiologic changes in the uteroplacental arteries do not extend beyond the deciduomyometrial junction, leaving a constricting segment between the radial artery and the decidual portions. (Reproduced, with permission, from Brosens IA: Morphological changes in the uteroplacental bed in pregnancy hypertension. Clin Obstet Gynaecol 1977;4:573.)

Antihypertensive therapy may be detrimental because peripheral vasodilatation may further reduce the already compromised placental blood flow.

Clinical Findings

A. SYMPTOMS AND SIGNS

1. Hypertension—Hypertension is the most important criterion for the diagnosis of preeclampsia, and it may occur suddenly. Many young primigravidas have blood pressure readings of 100–110/60–70 mm Hg during the second trimester. An increase of 15 mm Hg in the diastolic or 30 mm Hg in the systolic pressure should be considered ominous. Thus, in these patients, blood pressures of 120/80 mm Hg may be relative hypertension. The blood pressure is often quite labile. It usually falls during sleep in patients with mild preeclampsia and chronic hypertension, but in patients with severe preeclampsia, blood pressure may increase during sleep, eg, the most severe hypertension may occur at 2:00 AM.

2. Proteinuria—Proteinuria is the last sign to develop. Eclampsia may occur without proteinuria. One set of researchers found no proteinuria in 29% of one series of eclamptic patients. Most patients with proteinuria will have glomeruloendotheliosis on kidney biopsy. Proteinuria in preeclampsia is an indicator of fetal jeopardy. The incidence of SGA infants and perinatal mortality is markedly increased in patients with proteinuric preeclampsia.

3. Edema—Previously a weight gain of more than 2 lb/wk or a sudden weight gain over 1 to 2 days was considered worrisome. However, edema is a common occurrence in women with normal pregnancy, and preeclampsia may occur in women with no edema. The use of edema as a defining criterion for preeclampsia is controversial, and most recent reports omit it from the definition.

4. Differing clinical picture in preeclamptic crises—Preeclampsia-eclampsia is a multisystem disease with varying clinical presentations. One patient may present with eclamptic seizures, another with liver dysfunction and intrauterine growth retardation, another with pulmonary edema, still another with abruptio placentae and renal failure, and another with ascites and anasarca.

B. LABORATORY FINDINGS

The hemoglobin and hematocrit may be elevated due to hemoconcentration, or in more severe cases, there may be anemia secondary to hemolysis. Thrombocytopenia is often present. Fibrin split products and decreased coagulation factors may be detected. Uric acid is usually elevated above 6 mg/dL. Serum creatinine is most often normal (0.6–0.8 mg/dL) but may be elevated in severe preeclampsia. Although hepatic abnormalities occur in about 10% of patients, the bilirubin is usually below 5 mg/dL and the aspartate aminotransferase (AST) below 500 IU. Alkaline phosphatase may increase 2- to 3-fold. Lactate dehydrogenase may be quite high (because of hemolysis or liver injury). Blood glucose and electrolytes are normal. Urinalysis reveals proteinuria and occasional hyaline casts.

Differential Diagnosis

See Table 19–1.

Complications

Preeclampsia may be associated with early delivery and fetal complications due to prematurity. Fetal risks include acute and chronic uteroplacental insufficiency. In the most severe cases, this may result in intrapartum fetal distress or stillbirth. Chronic uteroplacental insufficiency increases the risk of intrauterine growth retardation and oligohydramnios.

Prevention

More than 100 clinical, biophysical, and biochemical tests have been reported to predict preeclampsia. Unfortunately, most suffer from poor sensitivity, and none are suitable for routine use as a screening test in clinical practice. As a result, most studies of prevention have used patients with various risk factors for preeclampsia.

A. CALCIUM SUPPLEMENTATION

Several authors have reported reduced urinary excretion of calcium during preeclampsia and for several weeks prior to the onset of clinically apparent disease. In addition, abnormal intracellular calcium metabolism in platelets and red blood cells has been demonstrated in women with preeclampsia as compared with normotensive pregnant women. However, there are no data suggesting that calcium supplementation prevents preeclampsia in women with low-risk pregnancies.

The National Institutes of Health studied 4589 healthy nulliparous women by randomly assigning them to receive 2 g elemental calcium or placebo daily at 13 to 21 weeks' gestation. In this study there was no decrease in the incidence or severity of preeclampsia in the group receiving calcium. However, randomized trials on women considered to be at high risk for developing preeclampsia have suggested a reduction in the incidence of the disease among women receiving supplemental calcium.

B. ASPIRIN

There is evidence to suggest that thromboxane A_2 production is markedly increased, while prostacyclin production is reduced in women with well-established preeclampsia and prior to the onset of preeclampsia. In addition, placental infarcts and thrombosis of the spiral arteries have been demonstrated in pregnancies complicated by preeclampsia, particularly in those with severe fetal growth retardation or fetal demise. As a result of these findings, several authors have used various antithrombotic agents in an attempt to prevent preeclampsia.

Today the prevailing opinion is that aspirin prophylaxis does not benefit most women in the prevention of preeclampsia. Eight large studies have been done worldwide to investigate this treatment. All demonstrated minimal to no reduction in the incidence of preeclampsia. So the place of aspirin in preeclampsia prevention is uncertain. It may be that the benefits are confined to high-risk women. A further matter of concern is the higher incidence of abruptio placentae found in the aspirin-treated patients in one study.

There is currently no proven way to prevent preeclampsia, but good prenatal care and regular visits to the physician will allow for early diagnosis before the condition becomes severe. Pregnant women at high risk for preeclampsia (those with a history of hypertension before conception or in a previous pregnancy, especially before 34 weeks, or multiparity; women with diabetes, collagen vascular disease, or renal disease; and women with multifetal pregnancy) should undergo baseline testing early in the pregnancy. Such tests make it easier later in the pregnancy to determine if preeclampsia is developing. These include hematocrit and hemoglobin, platelet count, serum creatine and uric acid, and 24-hour urine collection for protein and creatinine clearance if 1+ protein is present on dipstick. Women with a preexisting history of hypertension are at increased risk of intrauterine growth retardation and should have early ultrasounds if dating is in question, followed by follow-up scans to monitor growth. The physician must have full knowledge of the patient profile and must maintain a high index of suspicion throughout the pregnancy. Eclampsia cannot always be prevented. Patients may deteriorate suddenly and without warning.

Treatment

A. MILD PREECLAMPSIA

1. **Treatment of mother**—The treatment of preeclampsia is bed rest and delivery. The patient is usually hospitalized upon diagnosis, since this diminishes the possibility of convulsions and enhances the chance of fetal survival. Hospitalization to prevent premature delivery in preeclampsia is far less expensive than the cost of caring for a premature infant.

Women with mild preeclampsia who can be relied on to follow the physician's instructions may be treated as outpatients. A typical home regimen consists of bed rest, daily urine dipstick measurements of proteinuria, and blood pressure monitoring. Patients are seen at least twice weekly for antepartum fetal heart rate testing and periodic 24-hour urine protein measurements. Patients must be warned of danger signals such as severe headache, epigastric pain, or visual disturbances. The occurrence of these signals, increasing blood pressure, or proteinuria mandates communication with the physician and probable hospitalization.

Hospitalized patients are allowed to be up and around as they feel comfortable. The blood pressure is measured every 4 hours, and patients are weighed daily. Urine dipstick testing for protein is performed daily. Twenty-four-hour urine studies for creatinine clearance and total protein are obtained twice weekly. Liver function, uric acid, electrolytes, and serum albumin are determined on admission and weekly. Coagulation studies such as prothrombin clotting time, partial thromboplastin time, fibrinogen, and platelet count should be done in patients with severe preeclampsia. Assessments of gestational age and estimated fetal weight are performed by ultrasonic examination on admission and thereafter as indicated (usually every 2 weeks).

Antihypertensive medications are usually withheld unless the diastolic blood pressure exceeds 100 mm Hg and the gestational age is 30 weeks or less. (Long-term antihypertensive therapy is discussed later under Chronic Hypertension.) Sedatives were used in the past but have become disfavored because they interfere with fetal heart rate testing and because one of them—phenobarbital—impaired vitamin K–dependent clotting factors in the fetus. The usual indications for delivery of patients with preeclampsia are summarized in Table 19–2.

2. Assessment of fetal status—Fetal status is evaluated by twice-weekly nonstress tests and ultrasound assessment of amniotic fluid volume. Nonreactive nonstress tests require further evaluation with either a biophysical profile or an oxytocin challenge test. Amniocentesis to determine the lecithin:sphingomyelin (L:S) ratio is not frequently used in preeclampsia, since early delivery is usually for maternal indications, but it may be useful as the fetus approaches maturity. Corticosteroids should be used to accelerate fetal lung maturity in patients with preeclampsia when there is an im-

Table 19–2. Indications for delivery in patients with preeclampsia.

Blood pressure consistently higher than 100 mm Hg diastolic in a 24-h period or confirmed higher than 110 mm Hg.
Rising serum creatinine.
Persistent or severe headache.
Epigastric pain.
Abnormal liver function tests.
Thrombocytopenia.
HELLP syndrome.
Eclampsia.
Pulmonary edema.
Abnormal antepartum fetal heart rate testing.
SGA fetus with failure to grow on serial ultrasound examinations.

---

mature L:S ratio if it is thought that delivery may occur in the next 2–7 days. With rapidly worsening preeclampsia, fetal monitoring should be continuous because of the risk of abruptio placentae and uteroplacental insufficiency.

B. SEVERE PREECLAMPSIA

The goals of management of severe preeclampsia are (1) prevention of convulsions, (2) control of maternal blood pressure, and (3) initiation of delivery. Delivery is the definitive mode of therapy if severe preeclampsia develops at or beyond 36 weeks' gestation or if there is evidence of fetal lung maturity or fetal jeopardy. If delivery of a preterm infant (< 36 weeks' gestation) is anticipated, maternal transfer to a tertiary care center is advised to ensure proper neonatal intensive care.

Management of patients with severe preeclampsia occurring earlier in pregnancy is controversial. Some institutions use antihypertensive drugs to control maternal blood pressure until fetal lung maturity is reached. Corticosteroids should be used to accelerate lung maturity.

All women at 40 weeks with mild preeclampsia should be delivered. At 38 weeks, women with mild preeclampsia and a favorable cervix should be induced. Anyone at 32–34 weeks with severe preeclampsia should be considered for delivery, and the fetus may benefit from corticosteroids. In patients 23–32 weeks with severe preeclampsia, delivery may be delayed in an effort to reduce perinatal morbidity and mortality. This should be done only at a tertiary care center. The mother should be placed on magnesium sulfate for a minimum of the first 24 hours while the diagnosis is made. Blood pressure should be controlled with the medications to be discussed. The patient should be given corticosteroids to promote fetal lung maturity. The mother may be closely observed with frequent laboratory evaluations. Indications for delivery include development of symptoms, laboratory evidence of organ damage, and fetal deterioration (Table 19–2). If the gestational age is less than 23 weeks, the patient should be offered induction of labor to terminate the pregnancy.

Vaginal delivery is preferable to cesarean section and labor induction should be aggressive. A clear endpoint for delivery should be determined, usually within 24 hours. If delivery is not achieved within the set time frame, cesarean is warranted.

Prognosis

See below, under Eclampsia.

ECLAMPSIA

Eclampsia occurs in 0.2–0.5% of all deliveries, with occurrence being influenced by the same factors as in preeclampsia. In rare instances, eclampsia develops before 20 weeks' gestation. About 75% of eclamptic seizures occur before delivery. About 50% of postpartum eclamptic seizures occur in the first 48 hours after delivery, but they may occur as late as 6 weeks postpartum.

Pathophysiology

The pathogenesis of eclamptic seizures is poorly understood. Seizures have been attributed to platelet thrombi, hypoxia due to localized vasoconstriction, and foci of hemorrhage in the cortex. There is also a mistaken tendency to equate eclampsia with hypertensive encephalopathy. There is a poor correlation between occurrence of seizures and severity of hypertension. Seizures may occur with insignificant blood pressure elevations that are only slightly higher than readings recorded 24 hours previously. The hallmarks of hypertensive encephalopathy (retinal hemorrhages, exudates, and papilledema) are very infrequent in eclampsia, where funduscopic changes are minimal.

Clinical Findings

There is usually no aura preceding the seizure, and the patient may have one, two, or many seizures. Unconsciousness lasts for a variable period of time. The patient hyperventilates after the tonic-clonic seizure to compensate for the respiratory and lactic acidosis that develops during the apneic phase. Fever is rare but is a poor prognostic sign. Seizure-induced complications may include tongue biting, broken bones, head trauma, or aspiration. Pulmonary edema and retinal detachment have also been noted following seizures.

Treatment

A. PRENATAL TREATMENT

1. Control of seizures—In many centers outside the United States, anticonvulsants are not used prophylactically. For example, in the United Kingdom it is thought that the maternal risk of eclampsia, although variable, can be predicted. Anticonvulsant drugs such as diazepam, phenytoin, and chlormethiazole are used sparingly. In the United States, obstetricians believe the risk of eclampsia to be unpredictable and not correlated with symptoms of preeclampsia, blood pressure readings, deep tendon reflexes, or the degree of proteinuria. Most authorities recommend giving anticonvulsants to all patients in labor who have hypertension with or without proteinuria or edema. Since many women will be treated who are at low risk for seizures, the drug must be safe for mother and fetus. Fifty years of experience with magnesium sulfate has shown it to be effective and safe. The

mechanism of the anticonvulsant action of magnesium sulfate is unknown. Its use has been criticized on the grounds that it does not cross the blood-brain barrier and does not have a central nervous system inhibitory effect. While early studies failed to show a significant increase in cerebrospinal fluid (CSF) magnesium concentrations during therapy, more recent studies have shown about a 20% increase in CSF magnesium levels, and these levels parallel those in the serum. Magnesium sulfate decreases the amount of acetylcholine released at the neuromuscular junction, resulting in peripheral neuromuscular blockade at high magnesium concentrations; however, this does not account for its anticonvulsant effect. A recent study demonstrated that magnesium sulfate had a central anticonvulsant effect on electrically-stimulated hippocampal seizures in rats. The researchers speculated that since magnesium ion blocks calcium entry into neurons through the N-methyl-D-aspartate (NMDA) receptor–operated calcium channel, magnesium sulfate might be acting through this mechanism. On the other hand, another study found that magnesium sulfate was ineffective in altering seizure discharge in pentylenetetrazole-induced status epilepticus in rats. These researchers argued that because magnesium blocks calcium entry through the NMDA receptor–operated calcium channel in a voltage-dependent manner, it would be ineffective in neurons that are continuously depolarizing as in status epilepticus. Finally, Doppler studies of brain blood flow in preeclamptic women suggest that magnesium sulfate vasodilates the smaller-diameter intracranial vessels distal to the middle cerebral artery and may exert its main effect in the prophylaxis and treatment of eclampsia by reversing vasospastic cerebral ischemia.

Other actions are transient mild hypotension during intravenous loading, transient mild decrease in uterine activity during active labor, tocolytic effect in premature labor, and potentiation of depolarizing and nondepolarizing muscle relaxants. Magnesium sulfate has unpredictable effects on fetal heart rate variability (increased, decreased, or unchanged).

Maternal dose-related effects at various serum levels are: 10 mg/dL, loss of deep tendon reflexes; 15 mg/dL, respiratory paralysis; and 25 mg/dL, cardiac arrest. The therapeutic level is between 4.8 and 8.4 mg/dL. This range is empiric, based on levels obtained with an intramuscular dose usually found to be effective. Magnesium sulfate is usually given intravenously as a loading dose of 6 g over 20 minutes followed by a constant infusion of 2 g/h. If plasma levels are lower than 5 mg/dL, the maintenance dose is increased to 3 g/h.

Patients may have seizures while receiving magnesium sulfate. If a seizure occurs within 20 minutes after the loading dose, the convulsion is usually short, and no treatment is indicated. If the seizure occurs more than 20 minutes after the loading dose, an additional 2–4 g of magnesium sulfate may be given. Usually a magnesium level drawn acutely reveals subtherapeutic levels, but occasionally this is not so. In such cases, diazepam, 5–10 mg given intravenously, or amobarbital, up to 250 mg given intravenously, may be used. The patient should be checked every 4 hours to be sure that deep tendon reflexes are present, respirations are at least 12/min, and urine output has been at least 100 mL during the preceding 4 hours. The antidote for magnesium sulfate overdose is 10 mL of 10% calcium chloride or calcium gluconate given intravenously. The remedial effect occurs within seconds.

Phenytoin is not as effective as magnesium for the prevention of eclamptic seizures; however, it may be used safely in settings in which there is a risk in using magnesium, such as patients with myasthenia gravis.

Diazepam causes respiratory depression, hypotonia, poor feeding, and thermoregulatory problems in the newborn. Also, the sodium benzoate preservative competes with bilirubin for albumin binding, thus predisposing the infant to kernicterus.

2. Control of hypertension—There is controversy about whether or not uteroplacental blood flow is autoregulated. Most evidence indicates that the uterine vasculature is maximally vasodilated at all times. Therefore, most physicians believe that reductions in maternal blood pressure tend to decrease uteroplacental perfusion and caution against treatments that will cause large, precipitate drops in mean arterial pressure. Antihypertensive drugs are usually given if the diastolic blood pressure exceeds 110 mm Hg. The goal is to bring the diastolic blood pressure into the 90–100 mm Hg range.

a. Hydralazine—The drug of choice is hydralazine, a direct arteriolar vasodilator that causes a secondary baroreceptor-mediated sympathetic discharge resulting in tachycardia and increased cardiac output. This latter effect is important because it increases uterine blood flow and blunts the hypotensive response, making it difficult to give an overdose. If late decelerations of fetal heart rate do occur after hydralazine administration, they usually respond to fluid-loading, administration of oxygen, turning the patient on her side, and discontinuing oxytocin. Hydralazine is metabolized by the liver, and in patients with slow acetylation, it has a longer duration. The dose is 5 mg given intravenously every 15–20 minutes. The onset of action is 15 minutes, the peak effect occurs within 30–60 minutes, and the duration of action is 4–6 hours. Side effects include flushing, headache, dizziness, palpitations, angina, and an idiosyncratic lupuslike syndrome in patients taking more than 200 mg/d chronically. In more than 95% of cases of preeclampsia, hydralazine will be effective in controlling blood pressure. Other agents have been substituted for hydralazine, most commonly labetalol, nifedipine, and diazoxide.

b. Labetalol—Labetalol is a nonselective beta blocker and postsynaptic α_1-adrenergic blocking agent available for both oral and intravenous administration. Intravenous labetalol is given every 10 minutes as follows: the first dose is 20 mg, the second is 40 mg, and subsequent doses are 80 mg—to a maximum cumulative dosage of 300 mg or until blood pressure is controlled. It may also be given as a constant infusion. Onset of action is in 5 minutes, peak effect is in 10–20 minutes, and duration of action ranges from 45 minutes to 6 hours. Uteroplacental blood flow appears to be unaffected by intravenous labetalol. Initial experience indicates it to be well-tolerated by mother and fetus.

c. Nifedipine—Nifedipine, a calcium channel blocker, can be administered in a bite-and-swallow technique to lower blood pressure acutely. It is a powerful arteriolar vasodilator with the main problem being overshoot hypotension. For this reason, it probably should not be used in patients with intrauterine growth retardation or abnormal fetal heart rate patterns. Profound hypotension may be reversed by volume administration or intravenous calcium. Although nifedipine appears to have much potential, it requires further assessment of its use in pregnancy.

d. Sodium nitroprusside—Sodium nitroprusside causes equal degrees of vasodilatation in arteries and veins without autonomic or central nervous system effects. Its onset of action is 1.5–2 minutes, the peak effect occurs in 1–2 minutes, and the duration of action is 3–5 minutes. It is an excellent drug for minute-to-minute control in an intensive care unit setting. It may be titrated against a segmental epidural block for labor or cesarean section. It is recommended that the drug not be administered intravenously over a period longer than 30 minutes in the undelivered mother because of the risk of cyanide and thiocyanate toxicity in the fetus.

e. Trimethaphan—Trimethaphan, a ganglionic blocker, is used acutely by anesthesiologists to lower blood pressure prior to laryngoscopy and intubation for general anesthesia. A reported fetal side effect is meconium ileus.

f. Nitroglycerin—Nitroglycerin given intravenously is a predominantly venular vasodilator that appears to be safe for the fetus. It is only a moderately powerful antihypertensive agent.

Fluids such as 5% dextrose in Ringer's lactate, 125–150 mL/h, are given intravenously. A Swan-Ganz catheter is helpful in patients with pulmonary edema, massive hemorrhage, or oliguria unresponsive to a

1000-mL fluid challenge. Analgesia with intravenous meperidine or butorphanol is given in small doses every 1–2 hours. Local anesthesia with or without pudendal block may be used for vaginal delivery.

The use of epidural anesthesia in patients with preeclampsia is somewhat controversial. The problem is sudden hypotension due to pooling of blood in the venous capacitance vessels secondary to sympathetic blockade. However, with the almost universal use of epidural anesthesia for cesarean section, it has been widely used in preeclamptic patients. If there is no evidence of fetal compromise (by fetal heart rate criteria), if there is no coagulopathy present, if the patient is prehydrated, and if a segmental activation technique is used by an experienced anesthesiologist, epidural anesthesia may be used for labor and delivery or for cesarean section. If these criteria are not met, then balanced general anesthesia is preferred for cesarean section. Spinal anesthesia is considered contraindicated for women with severe preeclampsia.

C. Postpartum Treatment

Some of the constraints of therapy no longer apply once delivery has occurred, eg, sodium nitroprusside or diuretics may be used. Since 25% of eclamptic seizures occur postpartum, patients with preeclampsia are maintained on magnesium sulfate for 24 hours after delivery. Phenobarbital, 120 mg/d, is sometimes used in patients with persistent hypertension in whom spontaneous postpartum diuresis does not occur or in whom hyperreflexia persists after 24 hours of magnesium sulfate. Alternatively, magnesium sulfate may not be continued for 36–48 hours. Hypertension may not resolve until 6 weeks postpartum. If the diastolic blood pressure remains consistently above 100 mm Hg for 24 hours postpartum, any number of antihypertensive agents could be given, including a diuretic, calcium channel blocker, ACE inhibitor, central alpha agonist, or beta-blocker. The blood pressure should be checked in the standing position to avoid the possibility of orthostatic hypotension. At follow-up after 1 week, the need for continuing antihypertensive therapy may be reevaluated.

Prognosis

Maternal deaths due to preeclampsia-eclampsia are rare in the United States, but death may be caused by cerebral hemorrhage, aspiration pneumonia, hypoxic encephalopathy, thromboembolism, hepatic rupture, renal failure, or anesthetic accident. It is important to stress that iatrogenic complications increase if multiple drugs are given. If the patient truly had preeclampsia, the risk of recurrence is less likely (33%) than if she had chronic hypertension mistaken for preeclampsia. In the latter situation, the risk of recurrence is quite high (70%). In studies that include multiparas with preeclampsia, the recurrence rate in the next pregnancy is as high as 70%. In one study of primigravidas with eclampsia, only 33% had some hypertensive disorder in any subsequent pregnancy; in most cases, the condition was not severe, but 2% did have recurrence of eclampsia.

The effect of preeclampsia-eclampsia on subsequent development of chronic hypertension is debatable. Confusion may result from a mistaken diagnosis of preeclampsia in women with underlying renal disease or chronic hypertension. In one study of women with eclampsia during their first pregnancy who were followed for more than 40 years, no increase was seen in the incidence of hypertension or deaths due to cardiovascular disease or other causes. Multiparas with eclampsia had a much higher incidence of subsequent hypertension and deaths due to cardiovascular disease and other causes. It seems reasonable to conclude that the risk of recurrent eclampsia in subsequent pregnancies is not high enough to recommend against future pregnancies. Preeclampsia does not cause permanent damage, predispose to chronic hypertension, or adversely affect the long-term health of the mother.

CHRONIC HYPERTENSION

The incidence of chronic hypertension varies among different populations, ranging from 0.5–4% and averaging 2.5%. Chronic hypertension in pregnancy is usually idiopathic (80%) or due to renal disease (20%), though these figures may reflect insufficient investigation. A number of renal diseases may be causative, the most common being chronic glomerulonephritis, interstitial nephritis, diabetic glomerulosclerosis, IgA nephropathy, and renal artery stenosis.

Clinical Findings

A. Symptoms and Signs

Patients with chronic hypertension tend to be over 30 years of age, obese, and multiparous, with associated medical problems such as diabetes or renal disease. The incidence is higher in black women and in women with a family history of hypertension. A woman who has delivered one or more infants and has hypertension in this pregnancy most likely has chronic hypertension. The typical patient has hypertension without other signs of preeclampsia (eg, proteinuria or nondependent edema). The diagnosis is made on the basis of documented hypertension before conception or before 20 weeks' gestation or persistence of hypertension after the puerperium (6 weeks). The diagnosis of chronic hypertension should be confirmed by multiple measurements including home and/or out-of-office blood pressure readings as recommended in The Sixth Report of the Joint National Committee on Prevention, Detection, Evaluation, and Treatment of High Blood Pressure. If hypertension is severe (stage 3, systolic pressure 180 mm Hg or diastolic pressure 110 mm Hg), the patient should be evaluated for reversible causes. Whether worsening hypertension represents superimposed preeclampsia or hypertension associated with renal disease is sometimes difficult to determine. Preexisting renal disease alone may have all the manifestations of preeclampsia (hypertension, edema, proteinuria, and hyperuricemia). Renal biopsy would confirm the diagnosis but is usually not necessary, because the decision to deliver can be based on difficulty of blood pressure control, renal function, and fetal well-being. For the same reasons, renal biopsy is usually not performed for the work-up of proteinuria or elevated serum creatinine in pregnancy.

B. LABORATORY, X-RAY, AND ELECTROCARDIOGRAPHIC FINDINGS

The ECG may show left ventricular hypertrophy in 5–10% of patients. Elevated serum creatinine, decreased creatinine clearance, and proteinuria are also present in about 5–10% of patients with chronic hypertension. The chest x-ray is usually normal, though it may reveal cardiomegaly. Patients with left ventricular hypertrophy or elevated serum creatinine are at increased risk for developing superimposed preeclampsia. Patients with cardiomegaly due to either hypertensive cardiovascular disease or congestive cardiomyopathy are at increased risk for superimposed preeclampsia, pulmonary edema, and arrhythmias.

Complications

A. MATERNAL COMPLICATIONS

The main complication of chronic hypertension is superimposed preeclampsia, which occurs in about one-third of patients. Patients tend to deteriorate faster with superimposed preeclampsia than with preeclampsia alone. There is an increased risk of abruptio placentae with chronic hypertension (0.4–10%). Associated with this condition is the risk of disseminated intravascular coagulation, acute tubular necrosis, or renal cortical necrosis.

The effect of pregnancy on chronic renal disease is uncertain. Although there are few data for patients with severe disease, limited evidence suggests that if renal function is well preserved (creatinine < 1.5 mg/dL), pregnancy does not change the course of renal disease, but if renal insufficiency exists prior to pregnancy (creatinine > 1.5 mg/dL), the decline in renal function may be more rapid than expected.

B. FETAL COMPLICATIONS

The fetus has a 25–30% risk of prematurity and a 10–15% risk of growth restriction. Preeclampsia tends to occur after 34 weeks' gestation, so that prematurity is not a great concern. Preeclampsia superimposed on chronic hypertension frequently occurs earlier (at 26–34 weeks), and in such cases, fetuses are at double jeopardy for prematurity and intrauterine growth retardation. In addition, there is a risk of stillbirth or intrapartum fetal distress due to abruptio placentae or chronic intrauterine asphyxia.

Treatment

A. CONTROL OF HYPERTENSION

Most authorities agree that antihypertensive therapy will decrease the incidence of stroke and heart failure in pregnant patients with diastolic blood pressures exceeding 110 mm Hg. The real controversy concerns the value of antihypertensive therapy of mild hypertension (approximately 95% of pregnant patients with chronic hypertension have mild hypertension). One study demonstrated that treatment of diastolic blood pressures of 104–115 mm Hg in men decreased cardiovascular morbidity (myocardial infarction, congestive heart failure, and stroke) in just 10 months. Patients with diastolic pressures of 94–104 mm Hg showed benefits of therapy only after 5 years had elapsed. Therefore no benefits of antihypertensive therapy for mild chronic hypertension could be expected during the 9 months of pregnancy, and therapy cannot be justified by the same arguments used in general internal medicine. Some authors claim that antihypertensive therapy for mild chronic hypertension will decrease the incidence or delay the onset of superimposed preeclampsia, thus lowering perinatal mortality and morbidity rates. Others claim there is no benefit and considerable risk. Since this issue is still unresolved, a review of some of the recent clinical studies is helpful (see Reference section).

Several oral agents may be considered if hypertension is to be treated.

1. Thiazide diuretics—Thiazide diuretics have been reported to cause a number of harmful maternal and fetal side effects, the main one being plasma volume contraction. Studies in nonpregnant patients show that thiazides have acute and chronic effects. Acutely, they cause a 5–10% decrease in plasma volume, which lowers cardiac output and blood pressure in the first 3–5 days. Over the next 4–6 weeks, renal compensatory mechanisms return the plasma volume toward normal but not pretreatment levels. At the same time, cardiac output returns to pretreatment levels, but total peripheral resistance stays low. Thus, the acute blood pressure–lowering effect of thiazides is due to volume contraction. The sustained antihypertensive effect is thought to involve mobilization of excess sodium from the arterial wall. This leads to widening of the vascular lumen and possibly to a decrease in the vascular responsiveness to endogenous catecholamines. One set of researchers showed that plasma volume contraction occurs in early pregnancy in hypertensive patients on chronic thiazide therapy. When the thiazide was stopped, normal physiologic volume expansion occurred; if the thiazide was continued, plasma volume expansion was minimal (18% mean increase in patients taking thiazides versus 52% mean increase in patients in whom diuretics were discontinued early in pregnancy). Perinatal outcome was the same in both groups. Another consideration is the volume expansion caused by antihypertensive agents. It may be that the sodium and water retention produced by antihypertensive agents offsets the volume contraction caused by the thiazide. In summary, diuretics do not prevent preeclampsia or eclampsia. Thiazide diuretics are contraindicated in patients with pure preeclampsia. They may have a place in the treatment of patients with chronic hypertension; however, with the availability of more powerful antihypertensive agents such as nifedipine and labetalol, their use is declining.

2. Methyldopa—Methyldopa, a central α-adrenergic agonist, is the only antihypertensive drug whose long-term safety for mother and fetus has been adequately assessed. It reduces total peripheral resistance without causing physiologically significant changes in heart rate or cardiac output. If methyldopa is used alone, fluid retention and loss of antihypertensive effect are frequent. For this reason, methyldopa is usually combined with a diuretic for treatment of nonpregnant patients. It is usually started at a dose of 250 mg 3 times a day and increased to 2 g/d. Peak plasma levels occur 2–3 hours after administration; the plasma half-life is about 2 hours, and the maximum effect occurs 4–6 hours after an oral dose. Most of the agent is excreted via the kidney. The most commonly reported side effects are sedation and postural hypotension. With prolonged therapy, 10–20% of patients develop a positive direct Coombs' test, usually after 6–12 months of therapy. Hemolytic anemia occurs in fewer than 5% of these patients and is an indication to stop the drug. Fever, liver function abnormalities, granulocytopenia, and thrombocytopenia have occurred rarely.

3. Clonidine—Clonidine is another central α-adrenergic agonist. Treatment is usually started at 0.1 mg twice daily and increased in increments of 0.1–0.2 mg/d up to 2.4 mg/d. Blood pressure declines 30–60 mm Hg with use of clonidine, with a maximum effect in 2–4 hours and a duration of action of 6–8 hours. Renal blood flow and the glomerular filtration rate are preserved, but cardiac output falls. This is attributable to a decrease in venous return secondary to systemic vasodilatation and bradycardia. Cardiac output responds normally to exercise. Xerostomia and sedation are the most frequently encountered side effects. Withdrawal of clonidine produces a hypertensive crisis that responds well to reinstitution of the drug. There is not as much information on clonidine in pregnancy as there is on methyldopa; one large study found it to be equivalent to methyldopa.

4. Calcium channel blockers—Currently available calcium channel blockers include nifedipine, verapamil, diltiazem, nicardipine, isradipine, amlodipine, and felodipine. They cause direct arteriolar vasodilation by selective inhibition of slow inward calcium channels in vascular smooth muscle. Since calcium channel blockers affect such a fundamental cellular response, their therapeutic applications are wide-ranging, from angina pectoris to premature labor. Nifedipine is the calcium channel blocker most widely used in pregnancy. Ninety percent of oral nifedipine is absorbed from the gastrointestinal tract. After moderate first-pass liver metabolism, the bioavailability is 65–70%. Onset of action after bite-and-swallow administration is about 3 minutes. The drug has an initial fast half-life of 2.5–3 hours and a terminal slow half-life of 5 hours. It is almost completely metabolized by the liver and excreted 90% by the kidney and 10% by the liver. Side effects include hypotension, headache, flushing, tachycardia, and ankle edema. Since magnesium sulfate is also a calcium channel blocker, the use of both nifedipine and magnesium sulfate together could be potentially hazardous (eg, hypotension). Nifedipine has been used in several human studies comparing its tocolytic effect with ritodrine. It has also been used both acutely and chronically as an antihypertensive agent in pregnancy. In the largest study to date, one set of researchers randomly treated 200 preeclamptic patients with nifedipine and bed rest or bed rest alone. There was no prolongation of pregnancy or improved perinatal outcome in the nifedipine group, but uncontrolled hypertension as an indication for delivery was reduced. Because it is such a powerful and dependable agent, nifedipine is becoming increasingly popular for antihypertensive therapy in pregnancy.

5. Prazosin—Prazosin is a competitive blocker of the postsynaptic α$_1$-adrenergic receptor. It causes vasodilatation of both the resistance and capacitance vessels, reducing cardiac preload and afterload. It lowers blood pressure without significantly lowering heart rate, cardiac output, renal blood flow, or the glomerular filtration rate. It is almost exclusively metabolized in the liver. Approximately 90% of the drug is excreted via bile into the feces. It appears to be more slowly absorbed and its half-life slightly prolonged during pregnancy. In one study, the median time to peak concentration was 165 minutes in pregnant women and 120 minutes in men of similar age. The mean elimination half-life was 171 minutes in pregnant women and 130 minutes in men. Prazosin may cause a first-dose phenomenon characterized by sudden hypotension 30–90 minutes after the initial dose. This can be avoided by limiting the first dose to 1 mg given just prior to bedtime. Animal studies have demonstrated no teratogenic effects. Prazosin is not a very powerful agent and has usually been combined with the beta blocker oxprenolol in obstetric studies. In one study prazosin was used alone or in combination with oxprenolol in 44 pregnant women. No fetal abnormalities or adverse effects were noted. Another set of researchers used prazosin with or without oxprenolol to treat pregnancy hypertension beginning before 34 weeks' gestation. None of the 22 patients had significant maternal or fetal side effects attributable to drug therapy. Although available since 1976, prazosin had not been widely used in pregnancy.

6. Hydralazine—Hydralazine is an excellent drug for intravenous therapy of hypertension in pregnancy. It is an arteriolar vasodilator that causes a secondary baroreceptor-mediated sympathetic response, increasing heart rate and cardiac output. However, it is poorly tolerated orally as a single agent. Prominent side effects are headache, tachycardia, palpitations, fluid retention, and a lupuslike syndrome when chronic dosage exceeds 200 mg/d. Many of the unwanted side effects are minimized when it is used with a diuretic, methyldopa, or a beta blocker; however, use of multiple agents is discouraged in pregnancy. Dosage is initiated at 10 mg 4 times daily and increased to 200 mg/d.

7. Beta blockers—Beta blockers were introduced in the 1960s and have been used in pregnancy to treat migraine headache, hypertrophic obstructive cardiomyopathy, mitral valve prolapse, Graves' disease, and hypertension. Beta blockers are usually not adequate to control severe hypertension and are frequently combined with a diuretic, a vasodilator, or both. Beta blockers have been associated with neonatal bradycardia, hypoglycemia, hyperbilirubinemia, intrauterine growth retardation, respiratory depression, blocking of tachycardiac response to hypoxia, and increase in uterine muscle tone causing decreased uterine blood flow. The frequency of these side effects is unknown. Though clinical experience is accumulating, the safety of beta blockers in pregnancy has not yet been clearly established. Their use requires thoughtful risk-benefit analysis and clinical judgment. Infants of mothers taking beta blockers should be placed in an intermediate care unit after delivery to be monitored for side effects.

8. Labetalol—The low incidence of side effects, lack of teratogenicity, maintenance of uterine blood flow, and low propensity to cross the placenta make labetalol attractive for treatment of pregnant women. One randomized study found it offered no advantages over methyldopa in hypertensive pregnancy. Another study compared the use of labetalol plus hospitalization versus hospitalization alone in the management of 200 mildly preeclamptic women. No benefit was demonstrated in the labetalol-treated group; in addition, the incidence of SGA infants was higher in that group. Labetalol is started at 100 mg 3–4 times daily and increased to a maximum dosage of 2400 mg/d. Side effects are minor and include tremulousness and headache.

9. ACE inhibitors—The FDA-approved angiotensin-converting enzyme inhibitors include captopril, enalapril, lisinopril, fosinopril, ramipril, benazepril, and quinapril. They are widely used as first-line therapy for hypertension because they decrease systemic vascular resistance and have few side effects. Most of the reported experiences with ACE inhibitors in pregnancy are with captopril or enalapril. In human pregnancy these agents have been associated with several fetal and neonatal complications including hypotension, growth retardation, oligohydramnios, anuria, renal failure, malformations, stillbirth, and neonatal death. Although they have been successfully used in pregnancy, they should be avoided in pregnant women.

B. EFFECTS OF ANTIHYPERTENSIVES ON BREASTFEEDING

Little is known about the pharmacokinetics of antihypertensive drugs in human breast milk. In general, drugs that are lipid-soluble, un-ionized, and not protein bound are found in significant levels in breast milk. Specific recommendations concerning some of the more important agents are as follows: Thiazide diuretics should be avoided, since they decrease milk production and have been used in the past to suppress lactation. However, no electrolyte abnormalities have been found in infants of mothers taking thiazides. Methyldopa is probably safe during breastfeeding, since low plasma levels are found in the infants. Except for propranolol, the other beta-blocking agents are found in higher concentrations in breast milk than in maternal plasma. Therefore, propranolol would probably be the drug of choice if a beta blocker was needed. Nevertheless, accumulated experience with various beta blockers has shown only very low drug concentrations in breast milk. Clonidine is found in very small amounts in breast milk. Captopril appears to be safe during breastfeeding because only small amounts are found in breast milk. Data on the other drugs are insufficient to serve as a basis for recommendations.

C. GENERAL OBSTETRIC MANAGEMENT

In taking the medical history of the hypertensive pregnant patient, particular attention should be paid to the duration of hypertension, use of antihypertensive medications, history of renal or heart disease, and the outcome of previous pregnancies. Physical examination should include a careful funduscopic examination, listening for renal artery bruit, and checking the dorsalis pedis pulses for coarctation of the aorta. The blood pressure should be measured in the sitting position. If the bladder of the blood pressure cuff does not completely encircle the arm, a falsely high blood pressure reading may be obtained. In this situation, a thigh cuff should be used.

At the first prenatal visit, baseline laboratory studies should be obtained for organ systems likely to be affected by chronic hypertension or to deteriorate during pregnancy. Tests should include (but are not limited to) urinalysis; complete blood count; measurements of blood urea nitrogen, creatinine, serum electrolytes, uric acid, calcium, and phosphorus; liver function tests; ECG; and 24-hour urine collection for creatinine clearance and total protein. If significant heart disease is suspected, a chest x-ray (with the abdomen shielded) or echocardiogram should be obtained. A 3-hour oral glucose tolerance test is desirable, since as many as one-fourth of patients may have unrecognized diabetes. If hyperglycemia or wide blood pressure swings are evident, 24-hour urine testing for vanillylmandelic acid and metanephrines is recommended to rule out pheochromocytoma. The patient may be given a regular diet without salt restriction and should be followed every 2–3 weeks until 30 weeks' gestation and then weekly thereafter. Gestational age can be documented and an SGA infant detected with serial ultrasound examinations started early in pregnancy. Fetal well-being may also be assessed with the nonstress test and amniotic fluid index starting at 34 weeks or whenever the patient develops superimposed preeclampsia. Superimposed preeclampsia is diagnosed on the basis of worsening hypertension (30 mm Hg systolic or 15 mm Hg diastolic rise) together with either nondependent edema or proteinuria. Some of the more frequent indications for early delivery include superimposed preeclampsia, underlying medical problems such as diabetes or renal insufficiency, abnormal antepartum fetal heart rate, and a growth restricted fetus. A patient with worsening hypertension may be given betamethasone to accelerate fetal lung maturity if the lecithin:sphingomyelin ratio is less than 2 and if delivery can be delayed for 48–72 hours after the first dose.

Prognosis

Pregnancy outcome is usually favorable in patients with mild chronic hypertension, and perinatal survival rates of 95–97% can be expected. The main complications are superimposed preeclampsia, abruptio placentae, prematurity, and intrauterine growth retardation. If the patient has severe hypertension in the first trimester, onset of superimposed preeclampsia before 28 weeks' gestation, renal insufficiency prior to pregnancy, hypertensive cardiovascular disease, or congestive cardiomyopathy, the prognosis is more guarded. These patients require close follow-up of multiple clinical and laboratory parameters. The physician must be certain that these patients can be relied upon to take their medication. They may require a long period of hospitalization and are more likely to require cesarean delivery. Their fetuses are at significant risk for prematurity, growth retardation, and death.

REFERENCES

Bosio PM et al: Maternal central hemodynamics in hypertensive disorders of pregnancy. Obstet Gynecol 1999;94:978.

Brockelsby JC et al: The effects of vascular endothelial growth factor on endothelial cells: a potential role in preeclampsia. Am J Obstet Gynecol 2000;182(1Pt 1):176.

Golding J: A randomized trial of low dose aspirin for primiparae in pregnancy. The Jamaica Low Dose Aspirin Study Group. Br J Obstet Gynaecol 1998;105:293.

Herrera JA, Arevalo-Herrera M, Herrera S: Prevention of preeclampsia by linoleic acid and calcium supplementation: a randomized controlled trial. Obstet Gynecol 1998;91:585.

Levine RJ: Should the definition of preeclampsia include a rise in diastolic blood pressure of 15 mm Hg? Am J Obstet Gynecol 2000;182:225.

Levine RJ et al: Trial of calcium to prevent preeclampsia. N Engl J Med 1997;337:69.

Mills JL et al: Prostacyclin and thromboxane changes predating clinical onset of preeclampsia: a multicenter prospective study. JAMA 1999;282:356.

Morriss MC et al: Cerebral blood flow and cranial magnetic resonance imaging in eclampsia and severe preeclampsia. Obstet Gynecol 1997;89:561.

Ranta V et al: Nitric oxide production with preeclampsia. Obstet Gynecol 1999;93:442.

Report of the National High Blood Pressure Education Program Working Group on High Blood Pressure in Pregnancy. Am J Obstet Gynecol 2000;183:S1.

Rotchell YE et al: Barbados Low Dose Aspirin Study in Pregnancy (BLASP): a randomized trial for the prevention of preeclampsia and its complications. Br J Obstet Gynaecol 1998;105:286.

Sibai BM: Prevention of preeclampsia: a big disappointment. Am J Obstet Gynecol 1998;179:1275.

Sibai BM et al: Risk factors associated with preeclampsia in healthy nulliparous pregnancy. The Calcium for Preeclampsia Prevention (CPEP) Study Group. Am J Obstet Gynecol 1997;177:1003.

The Sixth Report of the Joint National Committee on Prevention, Detection, Evaluation, and Treatment of High Blood Pressure. Arch Intern Med 1997;157:2413.

Taylor RN: Review: immunobiology of preeclampsia. Am J Reprod Immunol 1997;37:79.

Third-Trimester Vaginal Bleeding

20

C.S. Claydon, MD, & Martin L. Pernoll, MD

Third-trimester hemorrhage continues to be one of the most ominous complications of pregnancy. Bleeding in late pregnancy is common; it requires medical evaluation in 5–10% of pregnancies. The seriousness and frequency of obstetric hemorrhage make it one of the 3 leading causes of maternal death and also a major cause of perinatal morbidity and mortality in the United States. Fortunately, most patients have only slight blood loss. However, even minor bleeding may be caused by a life-threatening disorder.

Differentiation must be made between obstetric causes of bleeding (usually more hazardous) and nonobstetric causes (usually less hazardous) (Table 20–1). Nonobstetric causes usually result in relatively little blood loss and little threat to mother or fetus. An exception is invasive carcinoma of the cervix. Obstetric causes are of more concern. Most serious hemorrhages (2–3% of pregnancies) lose more than 800 mL of blood and are due to premature separation of the placenta or placenta previa. Less common but still dangerous causes of bleeding are circumvallate placenta, abnormalities of the blood clotting mechanism, and uterine rupture. Bleeding from the peripheral portion of the intervillous space, or marginal sinus rupture, is a debatable cause of bleeding. Extrusion of cervical mucus ("bloody show") is the most common cause of bleeding in late pregnancy. Enough blood may be lost to cause concern for the mother, but medical intervention is almost never necessary.

This chapter will focus on 3 major causes of hemorrhage: premature separation of the placenta, placenta previa, and uterine rupture. Circumvallate placenta (uncommon in late pregnancy but a major cause of second-trimester hemorrhage and fetal death) and marginal sinus rupture (usually self-limited) will be considered variants of premature separation of the placenta.

Although almost all of the blood loss from placental accidents is maternal, some fetal loss is also possible, particularly if the substance of the placenta is traumatized. Bleeding from vasa praevia is the only cause of pure fetal hemorrhage, but fortunately it is rare. If fetal bleeding is suspected, the presence of nucleated red cells in the vaginal blood may be seen or the presence of fetal hemoglobin may be confirmed by elution or electrophoretic techniques.

INITIAL EVALUATION

Principles of Management

There are 2 principles that must be followed in investigation of third-trimester hemorrhage: (1) Any woman experiencing vaginal bleeding in late pregnancy must be evaluated in a hospital capable of dealing with maternal hemorrhage and a compromised perinate. (2) A vaginal or rectal examination must not be performed until placenta previa has been ruled out and until preparations are complete for management of massive hemorrhage and maternal or perinatal complications. Vaginal or rectal examination is extremely hazardous because of the possibility of provoking an uncontrollable, catastrophic hemorrhage.

Life-Threatening Hemorrhage Associated With Hypovolemic Shock

Early recognition of hypovolemia is essential. Signs and symptoms of hypovolemic shock include pallor, clammy skin, syncope, thirst, dyspnea, restlessness, agitation, anxiety, confusion, falling blood pressure, tachycardia, thready pulse, and oliguria. Nonreassuring fetal heart tracing will occur as the patient decompensates (Table 20–2).

Most healthy gravidas remain hemodynamically stable until approximately 1500 mL (25%) of their blood volume is lost. If adequate treatment is not provided, the patient will rapidly decompensate.

In the unstable patient, the standard ABCDs of resuscitation should be initiated. Guarantee a patent airway. Place the patient in Trendelenburg position with a left tilt. This will maximize venous return by preventing the gravid uterus from compressing the inferior vena cava. Two large-bore (16-gauge or larger) intravenous catheters should be placed and fluid replacement with crystalloid (normal saline or Ringer's lactate) initiated. Hetastarch or other colloid plasma expanders can be given while blood products are being cross-matched. In this case, the "D" in the ABCDs stands for continuous fetal monitoring using Doppler ultrasound while the mother is being stabilized.

Table 20–1. Common causes for third-trimester bleeding.

Obstetric Causes	Nonobstetric Causes
Bloody show	Cervical cancer or dysplasia
Placenta previa	Cervicitis[1]
Abruptio placentae	Cervical polyps
Vasa previa	Cervical eversion
Disseminated intravascular coagulopathy (DIC)	Vaginal laceration
Uterine rupture	Vaginitis
Marginal sinus bleed[2]	

[1]Due to trichomoniasis, *Chlamydia trachomatis, Neisseria gonorrhoeae,* herpes simplex virus, etc.
[2]Marginal sinus bleed is a form of abruptio placentae.
Reproduced, with permission, from Claydon CS, Greenspoon JS: Emergency management of third-trimester vaginal bleeding. Postgrad Obstet Gynecol 2001;21:8.

A. BLOOD TRANSFUSION

The initial hematocrit may be deceptively normal until equilibration occurs in a patient with hemoconcentration. Therefore, the clinical evaluation should be the primary guide in managing the patient with hemorrhage.

When clinically indicated, whole blood or packed red blood cells (PRBCs) should be administered rapidly. When using packed cells, it is important to be aware of the potential for dilution coagulopathy. After 4 units of PRBCs are transfused, a coagulation panel in addition to calcium and potassium levels should be obtained and electrolytes replenished if needed. If fluid overload is a concern, such as in the preeclamptic patient, cryoprecipitate can be used in place of fresh-frozen plasma. In extraordinary cases, invasive hemodynamic monitoring may be necessary.

B. VASOACTIVE DRUGS

Vasoactive drugs should be used only when specific pharmacologic effects are desired (eg, to increase myocardial contractility), when volume expanders are not available, or when volume expansion and other measures are ineffective. Even in these cases, efficacy may be questioned; these agents should be used only when their benefit clearly outweighs their potential risks. The most commonly used agent is dopamine (a mixed alpha- and beta-adrenergic stimulant), 200 mg in 500 mL sodium chloride intravenously, starting at 2–5 μg/kg/min and increasing gradually by 5–10 μg/kg/min to 20–50 μg/kg/min. Other agents that might be given by experienced personnel include levarterenol bitartrate, isoproterenol, metaraminol bitartrate, and phenylephrine.

Nonemergency Bleeding

A. HISTORY AND ABDOMINAL EXAMINATION

Once the patient is evaluated and found to be hemodynamically stable, the cause of bleeding must be quickly identifed. After a brief history is obtained, the patient's

Table 20–2. Clinical picture in hemorrhagic shock and expected response to volume replacement.

Clinical Sign	Primary Shock Early	Primary Shock Late	Secondary Shock
Mental state	Alert and anxious	Confused	Coma
General appearance	Normal and warm	Pale and cold	Cyanotic and cold
Blood pressure	Slightly hypotensive	Moderately hypotensive	Markedly hypotensive
Respiratory system	Slight tachypnea	Tachypnea	Tachypnea and cyanosis
Urinary output	30 to 60 mL/h	< 30 mL/h	Anuria
	(0.5 to 1.0 mL/kg/h)	(<0.5 mL/kg/h)	
Effect of volume challenge on			
Bood pressure	Increased	Slightly increased	No response
Urinary output	Increased	Slightly increased	No response

Reproduced, with permission, from American College of Obstetricians and Gynecologists: Hemorrhagic shock. ACOG Educational Bulletin No 235, April 1997.

abdomen should be examined and a bedside ultrasound performed to evaluate the location of the placenta and the fetal status.

If ultrasound is not immediately available, fetal heart tones should be obtained and the fundal height marked on the abdomen with a ballpoint or other indelible pen. This aids in determining gestational age, and later in ascertaining if the uterus is rapidly expanding from concealed hemorrhage due to abruptio placentae. Leopold's maneuvers assist in determination of fetal size, presentation, position, and engagement. It is crucial to determine whether the presenting part is well engaged in the pelvis. When there is engagement, total placenta previa is unlikely. Palpation for uterine contractions, tone, and tenderness should be conducted. Hemodynamic status can change after initial assessment and therefore should be continuously reevaluated.

B. LABORATORY EVALUATION

Laboratory evaluation should include: blood type and cross-match (give 2–6 units, depending on the hemodynamic status) as well as a complete blood count with platelets and baseline coagulation status (prothrombin time and partial thromboplastin time). D-Dimer or fibrin split products are useful when abruptio placentae is suspected. These are the most sensitive tests to confirm coagulopathy; however, they are qualitative studies and give little information about the severity of abruption. Recent literature has demonstrated a correlation between elevated CA-125 levels and abruption. This assay has little clinical utility, as it usually requires a long turnaround time. A Kleihauer-Betke test may be useful in the Rh-negative patient. The results are useful in calculating the appropriate dose of Rh immune globulin.

C. VAGINAL EXAMINATION

Neither a vaginal examination nor a rectal examination should be performed until placenta previa has been excluded. Once this has been achieved, both a speculum and a manual vaginal examination should be performed to evaluate for the presence of either a nonobstetric etiology or labor. When other causes have been excluded, placental abruption (including marginal sinus bleed) becomes the assumed diagnosis.

D. ULTRASOUND EXAMINATION

The most accurate way to confirm a diagnosis of placenta previa is by ultrasound. A translabial study may better assess the placental location for a posterior placenta than a transabdominal scan. Transvaginal ultrasound is the most accurate means to evaluate for placenta previa. It has been demonstrated to be safe in experienced hands. Finally, the addition of color flow Doppler to real-time ultrasound increases the sensitivity. It has limited sensitivity in diagnosing a retroplacental clot (caused by abruption), even in experienced hands. However, ultrasound may be useful for diagnosis of a concealed hemorrhage when a combination of abnormal findings coexist sonographically.

Ultrasound evaluation should be performed in the labor and delivery suite if possible. Fetal heart rate monitoring should continue at regular intervals throughout the study. Assessment of amniotic fluid volume and confirmation of fetal age should be obtained at time of ultrasound. In addition, an amniocentesis for fetal lung maturity should be performed if indicated.

E. MANAGEMENT OF BLEEDING

At this point, findings regarding the status of the mother, fetus, and placenta and evaluation of labor should be combined to provide a diagnosis and to plan the course of management. The 3 general management options are immediate delivery, continued labor, or expectant management, depending on the diagnosis.

If the fetus is immature, the patient should be treated expectantly unless additional complications appear (eg, continuing bleeding, fetal distress, labor, or spontaneous rupture of the membranes). In about 90% of cases, third-trimester bleeding will subside within 24 hours. If placental studies signify a high placental implantation and bleeding stops, vaginal examination is indicated prior to discharge of the patient to exclude nonobstetric causes of bleeding.

In the past, a **"double setup examination"** was frequently employed for diagnosis of third-trimester bleeding. All preparations were made for cesarean section, except for administering the anesthetic. A careful vaginal examination with a speculum was then conducted. If the placenta was not visualized, it was thought that placenta previa could be ruled out. This proved to be a highly inaccurate, dangerous method of diagnosis as compared with ultrasonic localization of the placenta and cesarean delivery without vaginal examination for placenta previa. Therefore, the double setup examination has largely been abandoned.

Nonobstetric causes of bleeding in late pregnancy usually result only in spotting that does not increase with activity. There are no uterine contractions, and the definitive diagnosis is usually made by speculum examination, Papanicolaou smear, culture, or colposcopy. Only in advanced cancer is there a poor maternal prognosis. Vaginal lacerations and varices may require repair but have a good prognosis. Most infections causing bleeding clear readily when treated with appropriate agents. Benign neoplasias and eversions require simple treatment and have a good prognosis (Fig 20–1).

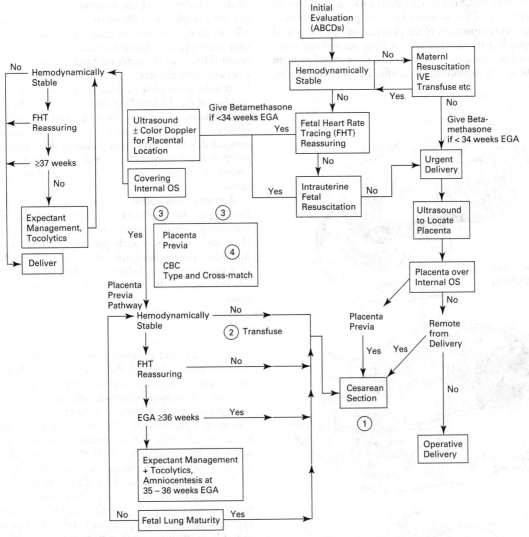

Figure 20–1. Algorithm for evaluation of third-trimester vaginal bleeding.

PREMATURE SEPARATION OF THE PLACENTA (ABRUPTIO PLACENTAE, ABLATIO PLACENTAE, MARGINAL SINUS BLEED)

 ESSENTIALS OF DIAGNOSIS

- Unremittent abdominal (uterine) or back pain.
- Irritable, tender, and often hypertonic uterus.
- Visible or concealed hemorrhage.
- Evidence of fetal distress may or may not be present depending on the severity of the process.

General Considerations

Premature separation of the placenta is defined as separation from the site of uterine implantation before delivery of the fetus (about 1 in 77–89 deliveries). The severe form (resulting in fetal death) has an incidence of about 1 in 500–750 deliveries. Two principal forms of premature separation of the placenta may be recognized depending on whether the resulting hemorrhage is external or concealed (Fig 20–2). In the **concealed form** (20%), the hemorrhage is confined within the uterine

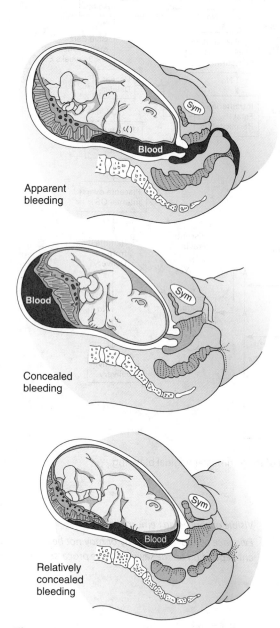

Figure 20–2. Types of premature separation of the placenta. (Redrawn and reproduced, with permission, from Beck AC, Rosenthal AH: *Obstetrical Practice*, 7th ed. Williams & Wilkins, 1957.)

cavity, detachment of the placenta may be complete, and the complications are often severe. Approximately 10% of abruptions are associated with clinically significant coagulopathies (disseminated intravascular coagulation [DIC]). In the **external form** (80%), the blood drains through the cervix, placental detachment is more likely to be incomplete, and the complications are fewer and less severe. Hemorrhage from an incompletely detached placenta may sometimes be concealed by intact membranes, in which case it is said to be **relatively concealed.** Occasionally, the placental detachment involves only the margin or placental rim. Here, the most important complication is the possibility of premature labor.

Approximately 30% of cases of third-trimester bleeding are due to placental separation, with the initial hemorrhage usually encountered after the 26th week. Placental separation in early pregnancy cannot be distinguished from other causes of abortion. About 50% of separations occur before the onset of labor, and 10–15% are not diagnosed before the second stage of labor.

Etiology

The exact causes of placental separation are often difficult to ascertain, although there are a number of predisposing and precipitating factors. A common predisposing factor is previous placental separation. Following one episode, the incidence of recurrence is 10–17%. Following 2 previous episodes, the incidence of recurrence exceeds 20%. The hypertensive states of pregnancy are associated with 2.5–17.9% incidence of placental separation. However, in abruptio placentae extensive enough to cause fetal death, about 50% of cases are associated with hypertensive states of pregnancy. Approximately half of these cases have chronic hypertension and half pregnancy-induced hypertension. Other predisposing factors include advanced maternal age, multiparity, uterine distention (eg, multiple pregnancy, hydramnios), vascular deficiency or deterioration (eg, diabetes mellitus, collagen diseases complicating pregnancy), uterine anomalies or tumors (eg, leiomyoma), cigarette smoking, alcohol consumption (> 14 drinks per week), and possibly maternal type O blood.

Precipitating causes of premature separation of the placenta, although more direct and definable, are no less diverse. All are rare. Included in this category are circumvallate placenta, trauma (eg, external or internal version, automobile accident, abdominal trauma directly transmitted to an anterior placenta), sudden reduction in uterine volume (eg, rapid amniotic fluid loss, delivery of a first twin), abnormally short cord (usually only a problem during delivery, when traction is exerted on the cord as the fetus moves down the birth canal), and increased venous pressure (usually only problematic with abrupt or extreme alterations).

Pathophysiology & Pathology

Several mechanisms are thought to be important in the pathophysiology of premature placental separation. One mechanism is local vascular injury that results in vascular rupture into the decidua basalis, bleeding, and hematoma formation. The hematoma shears off adjacent denuded vessels, producing further bleeding and enlargement of the area of separation. Another mechanism is initiated by an abrupt rise in uterine venous pressure transmitted to the intervillous space. This results in engorgement of the venous bed and the separation of all or a portion of the placenta. Conditions predisposing to vascular injury and known to be associated with an increased incidence of placental separation are preeclampsia-eclampsia, chronic hypertension, diabetes mellitus, chronic renal disease, cigarette smoking, and cocaine use. Factors that may predispose to a disturbed vascular equilibrium and the possibility of passive congestion of the venous bed in response to an abrupt rise in uterine venous pressure are vasodilatation secondary to shock, compensatory hypertension as a result of aortic compression, and the paralytic vasodilatation of conduction anesthesia.

Mechanical factors causing premature separation are rare (1–5%). They include transabdominal trauma, sudden decompression of the uterus such as with the delivery of a first twin or rupture of the membranes in hydramnios, or traction on a short umbilical cord.

Another possible mechanism is initiation of the coagulation cascade. This may occur, for example, with trauma causing release of tissue thromboplastin. These activated coagulation factors in turn may act to initiate clot formation in the relative hemodynamic stasis occurring in the placental pool.

Anatomically, placental abruption may occur by hemorrhage into the decidual basalis, which splits, leaving a thin layer adjacent to the myometrium. This decidual hematoma leads to separation, compression, and further bleeding. Alternatively, a spiral artery may rupture, creating a retroplacental hematoma. In either case, bleeding occurs, a clot forms, and the placental surface can no longer provide metabolic exchange between mother and fetus.

The clot depresses the adjacent placenta. Nonclotted blood courses from the site of injury. In concealed hemorrhage, this effusion may be totally retained behind the placental margins, behind the membrane attachment to the uterine wall, or behind a closely applied fetal presenting part. The blood may rupture through the membranes or placenta and gain access to the amniotic fluid (and vice versa). The tissue disruption by bleeding may allow maternal-fetal hemorrhage, fetomaternal hemorrhage, maternal bleeding into the amniotic fluid, or amniotic fluid embolus, depending on the areas disrupted and their relative pressure differences.

Concealed hemorrhage is more likely to be associated with complete placental detachment. If the placental margins remain adherent, central placental separation may result in hemorrhage that infiltrates the uterine wall. Uterine tetany follows. Occasionally, extensive intramyometrial bleeding results in uteroplacental apoplexy—so-called **Couvelaire uterus,** a purplish and copper-colored, ecchymotic, indurated organ that all but loses its contractile power because of disruption of the muscle bundles.

In the more severe cases of separation, there may be a clinically significant amount of disseminated intravascular coagulation associated with depletion of fibrinogen and platelets as well as other clotting factors. The mother may then develop a hemorrhagic diathesis that is manifested by widespread petechiae, active bleeding, hypovolemic shock, and failure of the normal clotting mechanism. In addition, fibrin deposits in small capillaries (along with the hypoxic vascular damage of shock) can result in potentially lethal complications, including acute cor pulmonale, renal cortical and tubular necrosis, and anterior pituitary necrosis (Sheehan's syndrome).

The likelihood of fetal hypoxia and fetal death depends on the amount and duration of placental separation and, in severe cases, the loss of a significant amount of fetal blood.

Clinical Findings

A. Symptoms and Signs

In general, the clinical findings correspond to the degree of separation. About 30% of separations are small, produce few or no symptoms, and usually are not noted until the placenta is inspected. Larger separations are accompanied by abdominal pain and uterine irritability. Hemorrhage may be visible or concealed. If the process is extensive, there may be evidence of fetal distress, uterine tetany, disseminated intravascular coagulation, or hypovolemic shock. Increased uterine tonus and frequency of contractions may provide early clues of abruption.

About 80% of patients will present with vaginal bleeding, and two-thirds will have uterine tenderness and abdominal or back pain. One-third will have abnormal contractions; about half of these will have high-frequency contractions and half hypertonus. More than 20% of patients with abruptio placentae will be diagnosed erroneously as having idiopathic premature labor. Fetal distress will be present in more than 50% of cases, and 15% will present with fetal demise.

If the placental separation is marginal, there will be only minimal irritability and no uterine tenderness or fetal distress. There may be a limited amount of external bleeding (50–150 mL), either bright or dark red depending on the rapidity of its appearance.

B. Laboratory Findings

The degree of anemia will probably be considerably less than the amount of blood loss would seem to justify, because changes in hemoglobin and hematocrit are delayed during acute blood loss until secondary hemodilution has occurred. A peripheral blood smear may show a reduced platelet count; the presence of schistocytes, suggesting intravascular coagulation; and fibrinogen depletion with release of fibrin split products. If serial laboratory determinations of fibrinogen levels are not available, the clot observation test, a simple but invaluable bedside procedure, can be performed. A venous blood sample is drawn every hour, placed in a clean test tube, and observed for clot formation and clot lysis. Failure of clot formation within 5–10 minutes or dissolution of a formed clot when the tube is gently shaken is proof of a clotting deficiency that is almost surely due principally to a lack of fibrinogen and platelets.

More sophisticated studies should be available on an emergency basis in most hospitals. The following will assist in determination of coagulation status: prothrombin time and partial thromboplastin time, platelet count, fibrinogen, and fibrin split products.

Ultrasonography may be useful but is not totally reliable, because it may not reveal the retroplacental clot in most cases.

Treatment

A. Emergency Measures

If the patient exhibits clinical findings that become progressively more severe or if a major placental separation has already occurred as manifested by hemorrhage, uterine spasm, or fetal distress, an acute emergency exists.

Blood should be drawn for laboratory studies and at least 4 units of packed red blood cells typed and crossed. Two large-bore intravenous catheters should be placed and crystalloid administered.

B. Expectant Therapy

Expectant management is appropriate when the mother is stable, the fetus is immature, and the fetal heart tracing is reassuring. The patient should be observed on the labor and delivery suites for 24–48 hours to ensure that further placental separation is not occurring. Continuous fetal and uterine monitoring should be maintained. Changes in fetal status may be the earliest indication of an expanding abruption.

In retrospective studies of women with placental abruption, tocolytic use is associated with increasing the gestational age at delivery. Tocolytic use did not increase the incidence of hemorrhage, fetal distress, or stillbirth. Currently there are no prospective trials published addressing the efficacy of tocolytic therapy for preventing an abruption from expanding.

Once stable, the decision to manage the patient as an outpatient should be tailored to the clinical situation. If outpatient surveillance is selected, the fetus should be followed closely with nonstress testing.

C. Vaginal Delivery

An attempt at vaginal delivery is indicated if the degree of separation appears to be limited and if the continuous fetal heart rate tracing is reassuring. When placental separation is extensive but the fetus is dead or of dubious viability, vaginal delivery is also indicated. The exception to vaginal delivery occurs when hemorrhage is uncontrollable and operative delivery is necessary to save the life of the fetus or mother.

Induction of labor with an oxytocin infusion should be instituted if active labor does not begin shortly after amniotomy. In practice, augmentation is often not needed, because usually the uterus is already excessively irritable. If the uterus is extremely spastic, uterine contractions cannot be clearly identified unless an internal monitor is used, and the progress of labor must be judged by observing cervical dilatation. Progress in labor is usually so rapid that forceps are not needed to shorten the second stage of labor. Pudendal block anesthesia is recommended. Conduction anesthesia is to be avoided in the face of significant hemorrhage because profound, persistent hypotension may result. However, in the volume-repleted patient in early labor, a preemptive epidural should be considered as rapid deterioration of maternal or fetal status can occur as labor progresses.

D. Cesarean Section

The indications for cesarean section are both fetal and maternal. Abdominal delivery should be selected whenever delivery is not imminent for a fetus with a reasonable chance of survival who exhibits persistent evidence of distress. Cesarean section is also indicated if the fetus is in good condition but the situation is not favorable for rapid delivery in the face of progressive or severe placental separation. This includes most nulliparous patients with less than 3–4 cm of cervical dilatation. Maternal indications for cesarean section are uncontrollable hemorrhage from a contracted uterus, a rapidly expanding uterus with concealed hemorrhage (with or without a live fetus) when delivery is not imminent, uterine apoplexy as manifested by hemorrhage with secondary relaxation of a previously spastic uterus, or refractory uterus with delivery necessary (20%).

Complications

A. Defibrination Syndrome

The mother must be continuously monitored well into the postpartum period for evidence of a clotting deficiency. There may be depletion not only of fibrinogen but also of platelet and of factors II, V, VIII, and X. Treatment will depend not only on the demonstration of hematologic deficiencies but also on the amount of active bleeding and the anticipated route of delivery.

1. Fresh whole blood—Fresh whole blood, although often difficult to obtain, is superior for treating clotting deficiencies and replacing blood loss because all the necessary factors will be present.

2. Packed red blood cells—Packed red blood cells are satisfactory for immediately replacing blood loss, but they do not contain clotting factors.

3. Cryoprecipitate packs—Cryoprecipitate packs contain all the necessary labile coagulation factors and are free of hepatitis B virus.

4. Platelets—During active bleeding, the transfusion of platelets is often the best practical means of counteracting a clotting deficiency. A platelet pack contains about 20% fewer platelets than 1 unit of fresh blood.

5. Fibrinogen—Fibrinogen is rarely indicated. *Do not administer fibrinogen solely on the basis of laboratory tests.* In the absence of active bleeding, fibrinogen deficiency may be corrected spontaneously in a matter of hours. To administer fibrinogen under these circumstances is both unnecessary and likely to make matters worse because the excess fibrinogen may be converted to fibrin emboli. The best source of fibrinogen other than fresh blood is a cryoprecipitated preparation. Concentrated plasma can also be used. Quadruple-strength plasma contains about 4.4 g of fibrinogen per unit. The initial dose of fibrinogen is 4–6 g, but as much as 20–24 g may be required depending on the response.

6. Heparin—The prophylactic administration of heparin to block conversion of prothrombin to thrombin (and thereby reduce the consumption of coagulation factors) has been successfully employed in the management of the defibrination associated with fetal death ("dead fetus syndrome"). The value of heparin in the treatment of acute placental separation has never been established; its use cannot be recommended because of the risks of operative and postoperative hemorrhage if cesarean section is required.

7. Fibrinolysins—Fibrinolysins such as aminocaproic acid should not be given. This drug will complicate the problem by interfering with the mechanism of fibrinolysis.

8. Preparation for surgery—Preparation for surgery must be completed quickly. If cesarean section is indicated, materials to control a clotting deficiency must be on hand before an operation is undertaken, and treatment with coagulants should be underway if a clotting deficiency is already present. Although control of a clotting deficiency before surgery is started is desirable, a rapid rate of blood loss may require earlier intervention. In rare instances, removal of an extensively damaged uterus has been necessary to control hemorrhage—or even the clotting deficiency.

B. Acute Cor Pulmonale

Acute cor pulmonale is always a possibility because of emboli in the pulmonary microcirculation as a result of either defibrination or the escape of amniotic cellular debris into maternal veins. The most important aspect of the immediate treatment of this life-threatening complication is the use of a volume respirator.

C. Renal Cortical and Tubular Necrosis

The possibility of renal cortical or tubular necrosis must be considered if oliguria persists after an adequate blood volume has been restored. An attempt should be made to improve renal circulation and promote diuresis by increasing fluid volume (with the aid of monitoring). If oliguria or anuria persists, renal necrosis is probable and fluid intake and output must be carefully monitored. Continuing impairment of renal function may require peritoneal dialysis or hemodialysis.

D. Uterine Apoplexy

Extensive infiltration of the myometrial wall with blood may result in loss of myometrial contractility. If, as a result, bleeding from the placental bed is not controlled, hysterectomy may be necessary. If future childbearing is an important consideration, bilateral ligation of the ascending branches of the uterine arteries should be accomplished before resorting to hysterectomy. Not only will blood flow be reduced, but the relative ischemia produced may result in a satisfactory contraction of the damaged uterus. If ligation of the uterine vessels proves ineffective, bilateral ligation of the hypogastric arteries, reducing arterial pressure within the uterus to venous levels, may effect hemostasis. Following ligation of either the uterine or hypogastric arteries, collateral circulation should be adequate to preserve uterine function, including subsequent pregnancies.

Prognosis

External or concealed bleeding, excessive blood loss, shock, nulliparity, a closed cervix, absence of labor, and delayed diagnosis and treatment are unfavorable prognostic factors. Maternal mortality rates ranging from 0.5% to 5% are currently reported from various parts of the world. Most women die of hemorrhage (immediate or delayed) or cardiac or renal failure. A high degree of suspicion, early diagnosis, and definitive therapy should reduce the maternal mortality rate to 0.5–1%.

With severe abruption reported fetal mortality rates range from 50% to 80%. In about 15% of cases, no fetal heartbeat can be heard on admission to the hospital, and in another 50% fetal distress is noted early. The fetal distress has several possible causes, eg, decreased metabolic exchange from decreased placental surface, maternal hemorrhage with decreased uterine perfusion, fetal hemorrhage, and uterine hypertonus interfering with proper metabolic exchange. In cases in which transfusion of the mother is urgently required, the fetal mortality rate will probably be at least 50%. Liveborn infants have a high rate of morbidity resulting from predelivery hypoxia, birth trauma, and the hazards of prematurity (40–50%).

PLACENTA PREVIA

ESSENTIALS OF DIAGNOSIS

- Spotting during first and second trimesters.
- Sudden, painless, profuse bleeding in third trimester.
- Initial cramping in 10% of cases.

General Considerations

In placenta previa, the placenta is implanted in the lower uterine segment within the zone of effacement and dilatation of the cervix, thus constituting an obstruction to descent of the presenting part (Fig 20–3). Placenta previa is encountered in approximately 1 in 200 births, but only 20% are total (placenta over the entire cervix). About 90% of patients will be parous. Among grand multiparas the incidence may be as high

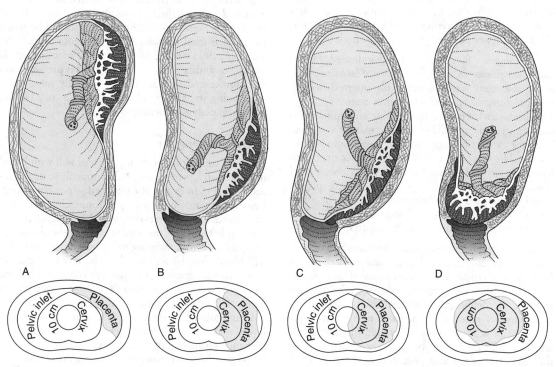

Figure 20–3. **A:** Normal placenta. **B.** Low implantation. **C:** Partial placenta previa. **D:** Complete placenta previa.

as 1 in 20. Placenta previa may also be involved in up to 5% of spontaneous abortions, although its presence usually is not recognized.

Etiology

The incidence of placenta previa is increased by advancing age, multiparity, and previous cesarean delivery. Thus, possible etiologic factors include scarred or poorly vascularized endometrium in the corpus, a large placenta, and abnormal forms of placentation such as succenturiate lobe or placenta diffusa. A large placenta probably accounts for the observation that the incidence of placenta previa is doubled in multiple pregnancy. A low cervical cesarean section scar triples the incidence of placenta previa. Another contributory factor is an increased average surface area of a placenta implanted in the lower uterine segment, possibly because these tissues are less well suited for nidation.

Bleeding in placenta previa may be due to any of the following causes: (1) Mechanical separation of the placenta from its implantation site, either during the formation of the lower uterine segment or during effacement and dilatation of the cervix in labor, or as a result of intravaginal manipulation. (2) Placentitis. (3) Rupture of poorly supported venous lakes in the decidua basalis that have become engorged with venous blood.

Classification

(1) Complete placenta previa: the placenta completely covers the internal cervical os. (2) Partial placenta previa: the placenta partially covers the internal cervical os. (3) Marginal placenta previa: the placenta is implanted at the margin of the internal cervical os.

Diagnosis

Every patient suspected of placenta previa should be hospitalized, and cross-matched blood should be at hand. To avoid provoking hemorrhage, both vaginal and rectal examination should be avoided.

A. SYMPTOMS AND SIGNS

Painless hemorrhage is the cardinal sign of placenta previa. Although spotting may occur during the first and second trimesters of pregnancy, the first episode of hemorrhage usually begins at some point after the 28th week and is characteristically described as being sudden, painless, and profuse. With the initial bleeding episode, clothing or bedding is soaked by an impressive amount of bright red, clotted blood, but the blood loss usually is not extensive, seldom produces shock, and is almost never fatal. In about 10% of cases there is some initial pain because of coexisting placental abruption, and spontaneous labor may be expected over the next few

days in 25% of patients. In a small minority of cases, bleeding will be less dramatic or will not begin until after spontaneous rupture of the membranes or the onset of labor. A few nulliparous patients even reach term without bleeding, possibly because the placenta has been protected by an uneffaced cervix.

The uterus usually is soft, relaxed, and nontender. A high presenting part cannot be pressed into the pelvic inlet. The infant will present in an oblique or transverse lie in about 15% of cases. No evidence of fetal distress is likely unless there are complications such as hypovolemic shock, abruption, or a cord accident.

B. ULTRASONOGRAPHY (FIG 20–4)

The real-time scanner is ideal for screening purposes, because the equipment is portable, the test is rapidly and easily performed, and the accuracy rate is over 95%. During the middle of the second trimester, the placenta will be observed by ultrasound to cover the internal cervical os in about 30% of cases. With development of the lower uterine segment, most of these low implantations will be carried to a higher station. An early ultrasonic diagnosis of placenta previa will require the confirmation of an additional study before definitive action is taken. A second source of error is a blood clot in the lower uterine segment that can be mistaken for placenta if the test has not been carefully performed. The use of color Doppler flow with real-time ultrasound can reduce the incidence of this type of error. In addition, translabial or transvaginal studies are more accurate in diagnosing placenta previa in the posterior lying placenta.

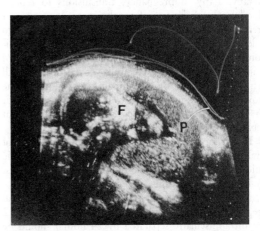

Figure 20–4. Ultrasonogram showing complete placenta previa. The placenta (**P**) is clearly shown implanted on the lower uterine segment. **F,** fetus.

Ultrasonography is an excellent means of identifying those patients who clearly do not have placenta previa and who can thereafter be examined vaginally with impunity. Ultrasonography is also an important method of identifying the low-lying posteriorly implanted placenta. Knowledge of this condition is important for the placenta lying over the sacral promontory may preclude the fetal presenting part from entering the pelvis. Additionally, with long labors or particularly strong contractions the placenta may be traumatized enough to initiate bleeding.

Differential Diagnosis

Placental causes of bleeding other than placenta previa include partial premature separation of the normally implanted placenta or circumvallate placenta.

Treatment

The type of treatment given depends on the amount of uterine bleeding; the duration of pregnancy and viability of the fetus; the degree of placenta previa; the presentation, position, and station of the fetus; the gravidity and parity of the patient; the status of the cervix; and whether or not labor has begun. The patient must be admitted to the hospital to establish the diagnosis and ideally should remain in the hospital once the diagnosis is made. Two or more units of bank blood should be typed, cross-matched, and ready for transfusion.

A. EXPECTANT THERAPY

The initial hemorrhage of placenta previa may occur before pulmonary maturation is established. In such cases, fetal survival can often be enhanced by expectant therapy. Early in pregnancy, transfusions to replace blood loss and the use of tocolytic agents to prevent premature labor are indicated to prolong pregnancy to at least 36 weeks. After 36 weeks, the benefits of additional maturity must be weighed against the risk of major hemorrhage. The possibility that repeated small hemorrhages may be accompanied by intrauterine growth retardation must also be considered. About 75% of cases of placenta previa are now terminated at between 36 and 40 weeks.

In selecting the optimum time for delivery, tests of fetal lung maturation, including assessment of amniotic fluid surfactants and ultrasonic growth measurements, are invaluable adjuvants.

If the patient is between 24 and 34 weeks gestational age, a single course of betamethasone (two doses of 12 mg intramuscularly separated by 24 hours) should be given to promote fetal lung maturity. Clinical judgment should be exercised as to the timing of steroid administration. Recent evidence suggests that multiple courses of antenatal steroids have potentially harmful effects in both the fetus and the mother.

Because of the costs of hospitalization, patients with a presumptive diagnosis of placenta previa are sometimes sent home after their condition has become stable under ideal, controlled circumstances. Such a policy is always a calculated risk in view of the unpredictability of further hemorrhage.

B. DELIVERY

1. Cesarean section—Cesarean section is the delivery method of choice with placenta previa. Cesarean section has proved to be the most important factor in lowering maternal and perinatal mortality rates (more so than blood transfusion or better neonatal care).

If possible, hypovolemic shock should be corrected by intravenous fluids and blood before the operation is started. Not only will the mother be better protected, but an at-risk fetus will also recover more quickly in utero than if born while the mother is still in shock.

The choice of anesthesia depends on current and anticipated blood loss. A combination of rapid induction, endotracheal intubation, succinylcholine, and nitrous oxide is a suitable way to proceed in the presence of active bleeding.

The choice of operative technique is of importance because of the placental location and the development of the lower uterine segment. If the incision passes through the site of placental implantation, there is a strong possibility that the fetus will lose a significant amount of blood—even enough to require subsequent transfusion. With posterior implantation of the placenta, a low transverse incision may be best if the lower uterine segment is well developed. Otherwise, a classic incision may be required to secure sufficient room and to avoid incision through the placenta.

Preparations should be made for care and resuscitation of the infant if it becomes necessary. In addition, the possibility of blood loss should be monitored in the newborn if the placenta has been incised. A fall in hemoglobin to 12 g/dL within 3 hours or to 10 g/dL within 24 hours requires urgent transfusion.

In a small percentage of cases, hemostasis in the placental bed will be unsatisfactory, because of the poor contractility of the lower uterine segment. Mattress sutures or packing may be required in addition to the usual oxytocin, prostaglandins, and methylergonovine. If placenta previa increta is found, hemostasis may necessitate a total hysterectomy.

Puerperal infection and anemia are the most likely postoperative complications.

2. Vaginal delivery—Vaginal delivery is usually reserved for patients with a marginal implantation and a cephalic presentation. If vaginal delivery is elected, the membranes should be artificially ruptured prior to any attempt to stimulate labor (oxytocin given before amniotomy is likely to cause further bleeding). Tamponade of the presenting part against the placental edge usually reduces bleeding as labor progresses.

Because of the possibility of fetal hypoxia either due to placental separation or to a cord accident (as a result of either prolapse or compression of low insertion of the cord by the descending presenting part), continuous fetal monitoring must be employed. If fetal distress develops, a rapid cesarean section should be performed unless vaginal delivery is imminent.

Deliver the patient in the easiest and most expeditious manner as soon as the cervix is fully dilated and the presenting part is on the perineum. For this purpose, a vacuum extractor is particularly valuable because it expedites delivery without risking rupture of the lower uterine segment.

Complications

A. MATERNAL

Maternal hemorrhage, shock, and death may follow severe antepartum bleeding resulting from placenta previa. Death may also occur as a result of intrapartum and postpartum bleeding, operative trauma, infection, or embolism.

Premature separation of a portion of a placenta previa occurs in virtually every case and causes excessive external bleeding without pain; however, complete or wide separation of the placenta before full dilatation of the cervix is uncommon.

Placenta previa accreta is a rare but serious abnormality in which the sparse endometrium and the myometrium of the lower uterine segment are penetrated by the trophoblast in a manner similar to placenta accreta higher in the uterus.

B. FETAL

Prematurity (gestational age < 36 weeks) due to placenta previa accounts for 60% of perinatal deaths. The fetus may die as a result of intrauterine asphyxia or birth injury. Fetal hemorrhage due to tearing of the placenta occurs with vaginal manipulation and especially upon entry into the uterine cavity as cesarean section is done for placenta previa. About half of these cesarean babies lose some blood. Fetal blood loss is directly proportionate to the time that elapses between lacerating the cotyledon and clamping the cord.

Prognosis

A. MATERNAL

With the abandonment of the double setup, use of cesarean section, use of banked blood, and expertly administered anesthesia, the overall maternal mortality has fallen to < 1%.

B. FETAL

The perinatal mortality rate associated with placenta previa is approximately 10%. Although premature labor, placental separation, cord accidents, and uncontrollable hemorrhage cannot be avoided, the mortality rate can be greatly reduced if ideal obstetric and newborn care is given.

RUPTURE OF THE UTERUS

ESSENTIALS OF DIAGNOSIS

- Increased suprapubic pain and tenderness with labor.
- Sudden cessation of uterine contractions with a "tearing" sensation.
- Vaginal bleeding (or bloody urine).
- Recession of the fetal presenting part.
- Disappearance of fetal heart tones.

General Considerations

Rupture of the pregnant uterus is a potential obstetric catastrophe and a major cause of maternal death. The incidence of uterine rupture is reported to be between 1:1148 and 1:2250 deliveries.

Complete rupture includes the entire thickness of the uterine wall and, in most cases, the overlying serosal peritoneum (broad ligament) (Fig 20–5). Occult or incomplete rupture is a term usually reserved for dehiscence of a uterine incision from previous surgery, in which the visceral peritoneum remains intact. Such defects are usually asymptomatic unless converted to complete rupture during the course of pregnancy or labor.

Risk factors for uterine rupture include history of prior hysterotomy (cesarean section, myomectomy, metroplasty, cornual resection), trauma (motor vehicle accident, rotational forceps, extension of a cervical laceration), uterine overdistention (hydramnios, multiple gestation, macrosomia), uterine anomalies, placenta percreta, and choriocarcinoma.

Ruptures usually occur during the course of labor. One notable exception is scars from a classic cesarean section (or hysterotomy), one-third of which rupture during the third trimester before term and before the onset of labor. Other causes of rupture without labor

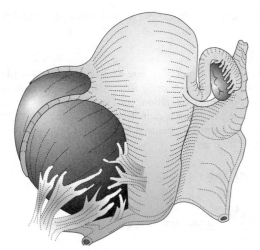

Figure 20–5. Rupture of lower uterine segment into broad ligament.

are placenta percreta, invasive mole, choriocarcinoma, and cornual pregnancy.

Complete ruptures may be classified as traumatic or spontaneous. Traumatic ruptures occur most commonly as a result of motor vehicle accidents, improper administration of an oxytocic agent, or an inept attempt at operative vaginal delivery. Breech extraction through an incompletely dilated cervix is the type of operative vaginal delivery most likely to produce uterine rupture. Other maneuvers that impose risk of rupture are internal podalic version and extraction, difficult forceps, destructive operations, and maneuvers to relieve shoulder dystocia. Tumultuous labor, excessive fundal pressure or violent bearing-down efforts, and neglected obstructed labor may also be responsible for rupture of the uterus. Causes of obstructed labor include contracted pelvis, fetal macrosomia, brow or face presentation, hydrocephalus, or tumors involving the birth canal. Direct abdominal trauma is a rare cause of rupture, but is occasionally encountered in automobile accidents, particularly if the victim was wearing a lap-type seat belt.

Spontaneous rupture is somewhat of a misnomer because most such patients either have a uterine scar or give a history consistent with previous trauma that may have resulted in permanent uterine damage. Previous uterine surgery includes both classic and low cervical section, intramural or submucous myomectomy, resection of the uterine cornu, metroplasty, and trachelectomy. Other operative procedures that may have damaged the uterus are vigorous curettage, induced abortion, and manual removal of the placenta. In contrast, some patients give no history of surgery but may be suspected of having a weakened uterus because of multiparity. Such patients are particularly at risk if they have an old lateral cervical laceration that could extend to involve a uterine artery.

Clinical Findings

There are no reliable signs of impending uterine rupture, although the sudden appearance of gross hematuria is suggestive.

Prior to the onset of labor, a beginning rupture may produce local pain and tenderness associated with increased uterine irritability and, in some cases, a small amount of vaginal bleeding. Premature labor may follow. As the extent of the rupture increases, there will be more pain, more bleeding, and perhaps signs of hypovolemic shock. Exsanguination prior to surgery is unlikely because of the reduced vascularity of scar tissue, but the placenta may be completely separated and the fetus extruded partially or completely into the abdominal cavity.

Rupture of a low cervical scar usually occurs during labor. Clearly identifiable signs and symptoms are often lacking. However 78% of patients will have evidence of fetal distress prior to the onset of pain or bleeding. Thus it is quite possible that labor will progress to the vaginal birth of an unaffected infant. Even so, the rupture may lacerate a uterine artery, producing exsanguination, or the fetus may be extruded into the abdominal cavity. If a defect is palpated in the lower uterine segment following vaginal delivery, laparotomy may be necessary to assess the damage. Laparotomy is mandatory if continuing hemorrhage is present.

The classic findings of spontaneous rupture during labor are suprapubic pain and tenderness, cessation of uterine contractions, disappearance of fetal heart tones, recession of the presenting part, and vaginal hemorrhage—followed by the signs and symptoms of hypovolemic shock and hemoperitoneum. Ultrasound examination might confirm an abnormal fetal position or extension of the fetal extremities. Hemoperitoneum can sometimes be seen on ultrasound.

Uterine rupture due to obstetric trauma is usually not diagnosed until after the infant's birth. The clinical picture depends on the site and extent of rupture. Unfortunately, valuable time is often lost because the rupture was not diagnosed at the time of the initial examination. Whenever a newly delivered patient exhibits persistent bleeding or shock, the uterus must be carefully reexamined for signs of a rupture that may have been difficult to palpate because of the soft, irregular tissue surfaces. Whenever an operative delivery is performed—especially if the past history includes events or problems that increase the likelihood of uterine rupture—the initial examination of the uterus and birth canal must be diligent.

Treatment

Hysterectomy is the preferred treatment for most cases of complete uterine rupture. Either total hysterectomy or the subtotal operation can be employed, depending on the site of rupture and the patient's condition. The most difficult cases are lateral ruptures involving the lower uterine segment and a uterine artery with hemorrhage and hematoma formation obscuring the operative field. These patients may be better saved by ligation of the ipsilateral hypogastric artery for hemostasis, thus avoiding the risk of ureteral drainage by blind suturing at the base of the broad ligament. If there is a question of ureteral occlusion by a suture, it is best to perform cystotomy to observe the bilateral appearance of an intravenously injected dye such as indigo carmine. If doubt still exists, a retrograde ureteral catheter should be passed upward through the cystotomy wound.

If childbearing is important and the risks—both short- and long-term—are acceptable to the patient, rupture repair can be attempted. Many ruptures can be repaired. Successful pregnancies have been reported following uterine repair; however, in this series repeat rupture occurred in approximately 20% of pregnancies.

In long-neglected and badly infected cases, survival may be improved by limiting the surgical procedure to repair of the rupture and by antibiotic therapy.

Occult ruptures of the lower uterine segment encountered at repeat section may be treated by freshening the wound edges and secondary repair, but the newly repaired incision will probably be weak.

Prevention

Most of the causes of uterine rupture can be avoided by good obstetric assessment and technique. Probably the most common error in judgment leading to rupture is underestimation of fetal weight, resulting in traumatic delivery. The most common technical error is the poorly supervised administration of oxytocin during labor. A frequent deficiency in operative technique is poor closure of a cesarean section incision.

Complications

The complications of ruptured uterus are hemorrhage, shock, postoperative infection, ureteral damage, thrombophlebitis, amniotic fluid embolus, disseminated intravascular coagulation, pituitary failure, and death. If the patient survives, infertility or sterility may result.

Prognosis

The maternal mortality rate is 4.2%. The perinatal mortality rate is approximately 46%.

REFERENCES

Adams DM, Druzin ML, Cederqvist LL: Intrapartum uterine rupture. Obstet Gynecol 1989;73:471.

Ali AF et al: Idiopathic abruptio placentae is associated with a molecular variant in the cholesteryl ester transfer protein gene. Obstet Gynecol 2000;95(4 Suppl 1):S37.

Ananth CV, Smulian JC, Vintzileos AM: Incidence of placental abruption in relation to cigarette smoking and hypertensive disorders during pregnancy: a meta-analysis of observational studies. Obstet Gynecol 1999;93:622.

Beck WW: Uterine rupture. Postgrad Obstet Gynecol 1997;17:25.

Benedetti TJ: Obstetric hemorrhage. In Gabbe SG, Niebyl JR, Simpson JL (editors): *Obstetrics Normal & Problem Pregnancies.* Churchill Livingstone, 1996, p. 515.

Besinger RE: The effect of tocolytic use in the management of symptomatic placenta previa. Am J Obstet Gynecol 1995; 172:1770.

Bond AL et al: Expectant management of abruptio placentae before 35 weeks gestation. Am J Perinatol 1989;6:121.

Brenner WE, Edelman DA, Hendricks CH: Characteristics of patients with placenta previa and results of "expectant management." Am J Obstet Gynecol 1978;132:180.

Cho JH, Jun HS, Lee CN: Hemostatic suturing technique for uterine bleeding during cesarean delivery. Obstet Gynecol 2000;96:129.

Clark SL: Placenta previa and abruptio placentae. In: Creasy RK, Resnik R (editors): *Maternal-Fetal Medicine,* 4th ed. WB Saunders, 1999, p. 616.

Clark SL: Rupture of the scarred uterus. Obstet Gynecol Clin North Am 1988;15:737.

Claydon CS, Greenspoon JS: Emergency management of third trimester vaginal bleeding. Postgrad Obstet Gynecol 2001; 21:8.

Comeau J et al: Early placenta previa and delivery outcome. Obstet Gynecol 1983;61:557.

Cotton DB et al: The conservative aggressive management of placenta previa. Am J Obstet Gynecol 1980;137:687.

Darby MJ, Caritis SN, Shen-Schwarz S: Placental abruption in preterm gestation: An association with chorioamnionitis. Obstet Gynecol 1989;74:88.

Eden RD, Parker RT, Stanley AG: Rupture of the pregnant uterus: a 53 year review. Obstet Gynecol 1986;68:671.

Hurd WW et al: Selective management of abruptio placentae: A prospective study. Obstet Gynecol 1983;61:467.

Jaffe MH et al: Sonography of abruptio placenta. Am J Roentgenol 1981;137:1049.

Kay H et al: Antenatal steroid treatment and adverse fetal effects: What is the evidence? J Soc Gynecol Invest 2000;7:269.

McGee S, Abernethy WB III, Simel DL: Is this patient hypovolemic? JAMA 1999;281:1022.

McKenna DS et al: The effects of repeat doses of antenatal corticosteroids on maternal adrenal function. Am J Obstet Gynecol 2000;183:669.

Naeye RL, Harkness WL, Utts J: Abruptio placentae and perinatal death: A prospective study. Am J Obstet Gynecol 1977; 128:740.

NIH Consensus Panel: NIH Consensus Development Panel on the Effect of Corticosteroids for Fetal Maturation on Perinatal

Outcomes. Effect of corticosteroids for fetal maturation on perinatal outcomes. JAMA 1995;273:413.

Paterson MEL: The aetiology and outcome of abruptio placentae. Acta Obstet Gynecol Scand 1979;58:31.

Pritchard JA, et al: Genesis of severe placental abruption. Am J Obstet Gynecol 1970;108:22.

Rasmussen S et al: The occurrence of placental abruption in Norway 1967–1991. Acta Obstet Gynecol Scand 1996;75:222.

Rasmussen S et al: Perinatal mortality and case fatality after placental abruption in Norway 1967–1991. Acta Obstet Gynecol Scand 1996;75:229.

Sholl JS: Abruptio placentae: clinical management on nonacute cases. Am J Obstet Gynecol 1987;156:40.

Spinillo A et al: Early morbidity and neurodevelopmental outcome in low-birthweight infants born after third trimester bleeding. Am J Perinatol 1994;11:85.

Suner S et al: Fatal spontaneous rupture of a gravid uterus: a case report and literature review of uterine rupture. J Emerg Med 1996;14:181.

Towers CV, Pircon RA, Heppard M: Is tocolysis safe in the management of third-trimester bleeding? Am J Obstet Gynecol 1999;180(6 Pt 1):1572.

Wing DA, Richard PH, Lynnae MK: Management of the symptomatic placenta previa: A randomized, controlled trial of inpatient versus outpatient expectant management. Am J Obstet Gynecol 1996;175:806.

Witt BR et al: CA 125 levels in abruptio placentae. Am J Obstet Gynecol 1991;164(5 Pt 1):1225.

Malpresentation & Cord Prolapse

Karen Kish, MD, & Joseph V. Collea, MD

◼ BREECH PRESENTATION

Breech presentation occurs when the fetal pelvis or lower extremities engage in the maternal pelvic inlet, and complicates 3–4% of all pregnancies. Three types of breech are distinguished, according to fetal **attitude** (Fig 21–1). In **frank breech,** the hips are flexed with extended knees bilaterally. In **complete breech,** both hips and knees are flexed. In **footling breech,** one (single footling breech) or both (double footling breech) legs are extended below the level of the buttocks.

In singleton breech presentations in which the infant weighs less than 2500 g, 40% are frank breech, 10% complete breech, and 50% footling breech. With birthweights of more than 2500 g, 65% are frank breech, 10% complete breech, and 25% footling breech. The incidence of singleton breech presentations is shown in Table 21–1.

Fetal **position** in breech presentation is determined by using the sacrum as the fetal point of reference to the maternal pelvis. This is true for frank, complete, and footling breeches. Eight possible positions are recognized: sacrum anterior (SA), sacrum posterior (SP), left sacrum transverse (LST), right sacrum transverse (RST), left sacrum anterior (LSA), left sacrum posterior (LSP), right sacrum anterior (RSA), and right sacrum posterior (RSP).

The **station** of the breech presenting part is the location of the fetal sacrum with regard to the maternal ischial spines.

Causes

Before 28 weeks, the fetus is small enough in relation to intrauterine volume to rotate from cephalic to breech presentation and back again with relative ease. As gestational age and fetal weight increase, the relative decrease in intrauterine volume makes such changes more difficult. In most cases, the fetus spontaneously assumes the cephalic presentation to better accommodate the bulkier breech pole in the roomier fundal portion of the uterus.

Breech presentation occurs when spontaneous version to cephalic presentation is prevented as term approaches or if labor and delivery occur prematurely before cephalic version has taken place. Some causes include oligohydramnios, hydramnios, uterine anomalies such as bicornuate or septate uterus, pelvic tumors obstructing the birth canal, abnormal placentation, advanced multiparity, and contracted maternal pelvis.

In multiple gestations, each fetus may prevent the other from turning, with a 25% incidence of breech in the first twin, nearly 50% for the second twin, and higher percentages with additional fetuses. Additionally, 6% of breech presentations are found to have congenital malformations. This includes congenital hip dislocation, hydrocephalus, anencephalus, familial dysautonomia, spina bifida, meningomyelocele, and chromosomal trisomies 13, 18, and 21. Thus, those conditions that alter fetal muscular tone and mobility increase the likelihood of breech presentation.

Diagnosis

A. PALPATION AND BALLOTTEMENT

Performance of Leopold's maneuvers and ballottement of the uterus may confirm breech presentation. The softer, more ill-defined breech may be felt in the lower uterine segment above the pelvic inlet. Diagnostic error is common, however, if these maneuvers alone are used to determine presentation.

B. PELVIC EXAMINATION

During vaginal examination, the round, firm, smooth head in cephalic presentation can easily be distinguished from the soft, irregular breech presentation if the presenting part is palpable. However, if no presenting part is discernible, further studies are necessary.

C. X-RAY STUDIES

X-ray studies will differentiate breech from cephalic presentations and also help determine the type of breech by locating the position of the lower extremities. X-ray can also reveal multiple gestation and skeletal defects. Fetal attitude may be seen, but fetal size cannot readily be determined by x-ray. Because of the risks of radiation exposure to the fetus with this technique, ultrasonography is now often used instead to determine fetal presentation or malformations.

D. ULTRASOUND

Ultrasonographic scanning by an experienced examiner will document fetal presentation, attitude, and size;

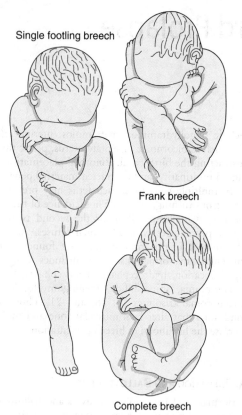

Single footling breech

Frank breech

Complete breech

Figure 21–1. **Types of breech presentations.** (Reproduced, with permission, from Pernoll ML: *Benson and Pernoll's Handbook of Obstetrics and Gynecology*, 10th ed. McGraw-Hill, 2001.)

multiple gestation; location of the placenta; and amniotic fluid volume. Ultrasound will also reveal skeletal and soft tissue malformations of the fetus.

Management

A. ANTEPARTUM MANAGEMENT

Following confirmation of breech presentation, the mother must be closely followed to see if spontaneous version to cephalic presentation occurs. If breech presentation persists beyond 36 weeks, external cephalic version should be considered (see below).

Radiographic pelvimetry using x-ray, computed tomography, or magnetic resonance imaging should be done to rule out women with a borderline or contracted pelvis. Attempts at vaginal delivery with an inadequate pelvis are associated with a high rate of difficulty and significant trauma to mother and fetus. Difficult vaginal delivery may still occur in women with adequate pelvic measurements.

B. MANAGEMENT DURING LABOR

1. Examination—Patients with singleton breech presentations are admitted to the hospital with the onset of labor or when spontaneous rupture of membranes occurs because of the increased risk of umbilical cord complications. Upon admission, a repeat ultrasound is obtained to confirm the type of breech presentation and to ascertain head flexion. The fetus is again scrutinized for lethal congenital malformations, such as anencephaly, which would preclude cesarean delivery for fetal indications. A thorough history is taken, and a physical examination is performed to evaluate the status of mother and fetus. Based on these findings, a decision must be made regarding the route of delivery (see below).

2. Electronic fetal monitoring—Continuous electronic fetal heart rate monitoring is essential during labor. If a fetal ECG electrode is needed, care should be taken to avoid injury to the fetal anus, perineum, and genitalia when attaching the electrode to the breech presenting part. An intrauterine pressure catheter may be used to assess the frequency, strength, and duration of uterine contractions. With the catheter in place, fetal distress or dysfunctional labor can easily be identified and the decision to proceed with a cesarean section made expeditiously to optimize fetal outcome.

3. Oxytocin—The use of oxytocin in the management of breech labor is controversial. Although some obstetricians condemn its use, others employ oxytocin with benefit and without complications. Generally, oxytocin should be administered only if uterine contractions are insufficient to sustain normal progress in labor. Continuous fetal and uterine monitoring should be employed whenever oxytocin is administered.

C. DELIVERY

The decision regarding route of delivery must be made carefully on an individual basis. Criteria for vaginal or cesarean delivery are outlined in Table 21–2.

Table 21–1. **Incidence of singleton breech presentations by birthweight and gestational age.**

Birthweight (g)	Gestational Age (weeks)	Incidence (%)
1000	28	35
1000–1499	28–32	25
1500–1999	32–34	20
2000–2499	34–36	8
2500	36	2–3
All weights		3–4

Table 21–2. Criteria for vaginal or cesarean delivery in breech presentation.

Vaginal Delivery	Cesarean Delivery
Frank breech presentation	**Estimated fetal weight of 3500 g or more or < 1500 g.**
Gestational age of 34 weeks or more.	**Contracted or borderline maternal pelvic measurements.**
Estimated fetal weight of 2000–3500 g.	Deflexed or hyperextended fetal head.
Flexed fetal head.	Prolonged rupture of membranes.
Adequate maternal pelvis as determined by x-ray pelvimetry (pelvic inlet with transverse diameter of 11.5 cm and anteroposterior diameter of 10.5 cm; midpelvis with transverse diameter of 10 cm and anteroposterior diameter of 11.5 cm).	Unengaged presenting part.
	Dysfunctional labor.
	Elderly primigravida.
	Mother with infertility problems or poor obstetric history.
No maternal of fetal indications for cesarean section.	Premature fetus (gestational age of 25–34 weeks).
Previable fetus (gestational age < 25 weeks and weight < 700 g).	Most cases of complete or footling breech over 25 weeks gestation without detectable lethal congenital malformations (to prevent umbilical cord prolapse).
Documented lethal fetal congenital anomalies.	
Presentation of mother in advanced labor with no fetal or maternal distress, even if cesarean delivery was originally planned (a carefully performed, controlled vaginal delivery is safer in such cases than a hastily executed cesarean section).	Fetus with variable heart rate decelerations on electric monitoring
	Footling presentation

Prior to 1975, virtually all viable singleton breech presentations were delivered vaginally. Cesarean section was reserved for specific fetal indications such as unremitting distress or prolapsed umbilical cord, or maternal indications such as placenta previa, abruptio placentae, or failure of progress in labor. However, breech infants delivered vaginally had a 5-fold higher mortality rate in comparison to cephalic presentations.

Cesarean delivery has now become much more common in breech presentation, with lower rates of perinatal morbidity and mortality. However, many breech presentations can be safely delivered vaginally without significant risk of injury or death. Recent data show that the route of delivery has no influence on the long-term morbidity of breech fetuses. Risks to the mother with cesarean section (anesthesia, blood loss, infection) must be weighed against risks to the fetus with vaginal delivery (asphyxia, trauma). Decisions must be made with the utmost care to prevent unnecessary cesarean section or inadvertent vaginal delivery. Only obstetricians skilled in breech techniques should attempt any breech delivery, whether vaginal or cesarean.

1. Cesarean delivery—The type of incision chosen is extremely important. If the lower uterine segment is well developed as is usually the case in women at term in labor, a transverse "lower segment" incision is adequate for easy delivery. In premature gestations, in an unlabored uterus, or in many cases of malpresentation, the lower uterine segment may be quite narrow, and a low vertical incision is almost always required for atraumatic delivery.

2. Vaginal delivery—Obstetricians who contemplate performing a vaginal breech delivery should be experienced in the maneuver and should be assisted by 3 physicians: (1) an experienced obstetrician who will assist with delivery; (2) a pediatrician capable of providing total resuscitation of the newborn; and (3) an anesthesiologist, to ensure that the mother is comfortable and cooperative during labor and delivery. The type of anesthesia required depends on the type of breech delivery. Multiparous women undergoing spontaneous breech delivery may require only intravenous analgesia for pain relief during labor and a pudendal anesthetic during delivery. Epidural anesthesia may also be administered during labor or during partial breech extraction, including application of Piper forceps to the aftercoming head. In emergency circumstances, complete relaxation of the perineum and uterus is essential for a successful outcome. This is accomplished by immediate induction of inhalation anesthesia or by administering intravenous nitroglycerin.

a. Spontaneous vaginal delivery—During spontaneous delivery of an infant in the frank breech position, delivery occurs without assistance, and no obstetric maneuvers are applied to the body. The fetus negotiates the maternal pelvis as outlined below, while the operator simply supports the body as it delivers.

Engagement occurs when the bitrochanteric diameter of the fetus has passed the plane of the pelvic inlet. As the fetus descends into the pelvis (Fig 21–2), the buttocks reach the levator ani muscles of the maternal pelvis. At this point, internal rotation occurs, whereby the anterior hip rotates beneath the pubic symphysis, resulting in a sacrum transverse position. The bitrochanteric diameter of the fetal pelvis is now in an anteroposterior position within the maternal pelvis.

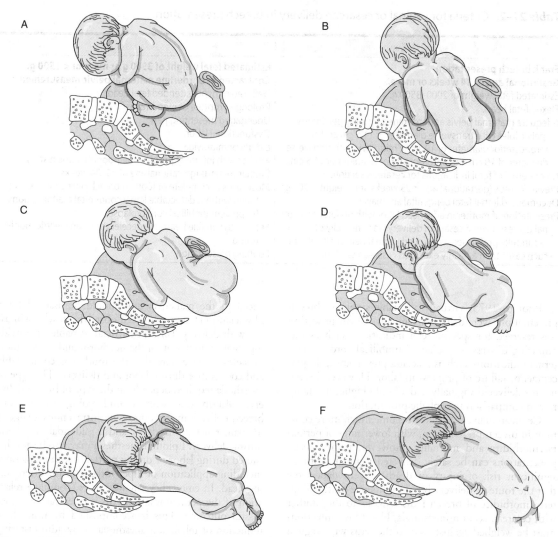

Figure 21–2. Mechanism of labor in breech delivery. **A:** Mechanism of breech delivery. Right sacrum transverse (RST) at the onset of labor; engagement of the buttocks usually occurs in the oblique or transverse diameter of the pelvic brim. **B:** Early second stage. The buttocks have reached the pelvic floor and internal rotation has occurred so that the bitrochanteric diameter lies in the AP diameter of the pelvic outlet. **C:** Late second stage. The anterior buttock appears at the vulva by lateral flexion of the trunk around the pubic symphysis. The shoulders have not yet engaged in the pelvis. **D:** The buttocks have been delivered, and the shoulders are adjusting to engage in the transverse diameter of the brim. This movement causes external rotation of the delivered buttocks so that the fetal back becomes uppermost. **E:** The shoulders have reached the pelvic floor and have undergone internal rotation so that the bisacromial diameter lies in the AP diameter of the pelvic outlet. Simultaneously, the buttocks rotate anteriorly through 90 degrees. This is called **restitution.** The head is engaging in the pelvic brim, and the sagittal suture is lying in the transverse diameter of the brim. **F:** The anterior shoulder is born from behind the pubic symphysis by lateral flexion of the delivered trunk. (Redrawn and reproduced, with permission, from Llewellyn-Jones D: *Fundamentals of Obstetrics and Gynecology,* Vol. 1. Faber & Faber, 1969.)

The breech then presents at the pelvic outlet and upon emerging, rotates from sacrum transverse to sacrum anterior. Crowning occurs when the bitrochanteric diameter passes under the pubic symphysis. As this occurs, the shoulders enter the pelvic inlet with the bisacromial diameter in the transverse position. As descent occurs, the bisacromial diameter rotates to an oblique or anteroposterior diameter, until the anterior shoulder rests beneath the pubic symphysis. Delivery of the anterior shoulder occurs as it slips beneath the pubic symphysis. Upward flexion of the body allows for easy delivery of the posterior shoulder over the perineum.

As the shoulders descend, the head engages the pelvic inlet in a transverse or oblique position. Rotation of the head to the occiput anterior position occurs as it enters the midpelvis. The occiput then slips beneath the pubic symphysis, and the remainder of the head is delivered by flexion as the chin, mouth, nose, and forehead slip over the maternal perineum.

As delivery of the breech occurs, increasingly larger diameters (bitrochanteric, bisacromial, biparietal) of the body enter the pelvis, whereas in cephalic presentation, the largest diameter (biparietal diameter) enters the pelvis first. Particularly in preterm labors, the head is considerably larger than the body and provides a better "dilating wedge" as it passes through the cervix and into the pelvis. The smaller bitrochanteric and bisacromial diameters may descend into the pelvis through a partially dilated cervix, but the larger biparietal diameter may be trapped. Delivery in these cases is described below.

b. Partial breech extraction—Partial breech extraction (assisted breech extraction) is employed when the operator discerns that spontaneous delivery will not occur or that expeditious delivery is indicated for fetal or maternal reasons. The body is allowed to deliver spontaneously up to the level of the umbilicus (Fig 21–3). The operator then assists in delivery of the legs, shoulders, arms, and head (Fig 21–4).

As the umbilicus appears at the maternal perineum, the operator places a finger medial to one thigh and then the other, pressing laterally as the fetal pelvis is rotated away from that side by an assistant. Thus, the thigh is externally rotated at the hip and results in flexion of the knee and delivery of one, then the other, leg (Fig 21–5). The fetal trunk is then wrapped in a towel to support the body. When both scapulae are visible, the body is rotated counterclockwise. The operator locates the right humerus and laterally sweeps the arm across the chest and out the perineum. In a similar fashion, the body is rotated clockwise to deliver the left arm. The head then spontaneously delivers by gently lifting the body upward and applying fundal pressure to

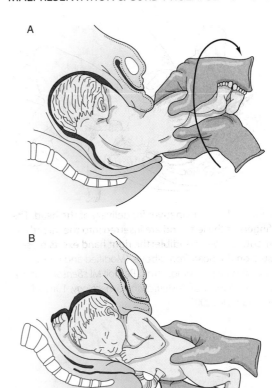

Figure 21–3. Assisted delivery of the shoulders. **A:** Shoulders engaged, posterior (left) shoulder at lower level in pelvis than anterior shoulder. **B:** Rotation of trunk causing posterior shoulder to rotate to anterior and slip beneath the pubic symphysis. (Redrawn and reproduced, with permission, from Lovset J: Shoulder delivery by breech presentation. J Obstet Gynaecol Br Commonw 1937;44:696.)

maintain flexion of the fetal head. During partial breech extraction, the anterior shoulder may be difficult to deliver if it is impacted behind the pubic symphysis. In this event, the body is gently lifted upward toward the pubic symphysis, and the operator inserts one hand along the hollow of the maternal pelvis and identifies the posterior humerus of the fetus. By gentle downward traction on the humerus, the posterior arm can be easily delivered, thus allowing for easier delivery of the anterior shoulder and arm.

The operator may elect to manually assist in delivery of the head by performing the **Mauriceau-Smellie-Veit maneuver** (Fig 21–6). In this procedure, the index and middle fingers of one of the operator's hands are ap-

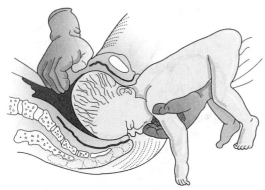

Figure 21–4. Maneuver for delivery of the head. The fingers of the left hand are inserted into the infant's mouth or over mandible; the right hand exerts pressure on the head from above. (Modified and reproduced, with permission, from Pernoll ML: *Benson and Pernoll's Handbook of Obstetrics and Gynecology,* 10th ed. McGraw-Hill, 2001.)

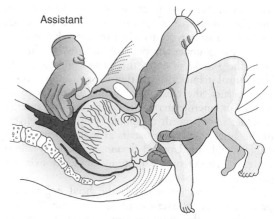

Assistant

Figure 21–6. Mauriceau-Smellie-Veit maneuver for delivery of the head. The fingers of the left hand are inserted into the infant's mouth or over the mandible; the fingers of the right hand curve over the shoulders. An assistant exerts suprapubic pressure on the head. (Reproduced, with permission, from Pernoll ML: *Benson and Pernoll's Handbook of Obstetrics and Gynecology,* 10th ed. McGraw-Hill, 2001.)

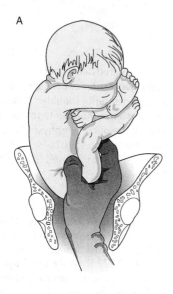

A

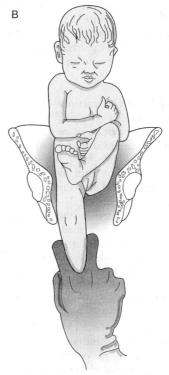

B

Figure 21–5. Extraction of breech. **A:** Abduction of thigh and pressure in popliteal fossa causes the knee to flex and become accessible. **B:** Delivery of leg by traction on the foot.

plied over the maxilla as the body rests on the palm and forearm of the operator. Two fingers of the operator's other hand are applied on either side of the neck with gentle downward traction. At the same time, the body is elevated toward the pubic symphysis, allowing for controlled delivery of the mouth, nose, and brow over the perineum. Likewise, Piper forceps may be used electively or when the Mauriceau-Smellie-Veit maneuver fails to deliver the aftercoming head. Piper forceps may only be used when the cervix is completely dilated and the head is engaged in the pelvis. Ideally, the head is in a direct occiput anterior position, but left or right occiput anterior positions are acceptable. Piper forceps should not be attempted in the occiput transverse positions, since this may result in significant fetal and maternal injury. An assistant supports and slightly elevates the fetal trunk while the operator places each forceps blade alongside the fetal parietal bones (Fig 21–7). After proper placement is confirmed, the forceps are locked and gentle traction is applied to flex and deliver the head over the perineum. A midline episiotomy is often indicated to allow for easier application of the forceps and for delivery.

If, after delivery of the body, the spine remains in the posterior position and rotation is unsuccessful, extraction of the head in a persistent occiput posterior position may be accomplished by the **modified Prague maneuver.** One hand of the operator supports the shoulders from below, while the other hand gently elevates the body upward toward the maternal abdomen.

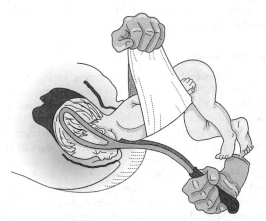

Figure 21–7. Application of Piper forceps, employing towel sling support. The forceps are introduced from below, left blade first, aiming directly at intended positions on sides of the head. (Reproduced, with permission, from Pernoll ML: *Benson and Pernoll's Handbook of Obstetrics and Gynecology,* 10th ed. McGraw-Hill, 2001.)

This flexes the head within the birth canal and results in delivery of the occiput over the perineum.

In premature breech presentations, the incompletely dilated cervix may allow delivery to the smaller body, but the relatively larger aftercoming head may be entrapped. Prompt delivery is mandatory because severe asphyxia leading to death may rapidly ensue. Gentle downward traction on the shoulders combined with fundal pressure applied by an assistant may effect delivery. If this fails, the anesthesiologist should administer nitroglycerin or inhalation anesthesia to obtain complete relaxation of the lower uterine segment and pelvic floor with reattempt at delivery.

If delivery is still not accomplished, **Dührssen's incisions** must be considered to preserve fetal life. Incisions are made in the posterior cervix at 6 o'clock to loosen the entrapped head. Occasionally, additional incisions are necessary at 2 and 10 o'clock. Dührssen's incisions invariably release the fetal head, but the maternal consequences may be severe with resultant hemorrhage. Thus, this procedure should only be performed in an emergent situation. Prevention of head entrapment can be accomplished by delivering viable premature breech gestations by cesarean section.

c. Total breech extraction—In total breech extraction (Fig 21–8), the entire body is manually delivered. This procedure is employed only occasionally when fetal distress is encountered and an expeditious delivery is indicated, and under certain conditions in the setting of delivery of a second twin in a nonvertex position following successful vaginal delivery of a first twin. Total breech extraction has been virtually replaced by cesarean delivery in modern obstetrics.

For complete or footling presentation, total breech extraction is accomplished by initially grasping both feet and applying gentle downward pressure until the buttocks are delivered. A generous midline or mediolateral episiotomy is then performed. The operator gently grasps the fetal pelvis, with both thumbs placed directly on either side of the sacrum. The spine is rotated, if necessary, until it rests under the pubic symphysis. Gentle, firm downward pressure is applied to the body until both scapulas are visible. The shoulders, arms, and head are delivered as in partial breech extraction.

If the fetus is in frank breech presentation, the index finger of the right hand must initially be placed into the anterior groin of the fetus and gentle downward pressure applied (Fig 21–9). As the fetus descends further into the birth canal, the left index finger is inserted into the posterior groin, and additional gentle downward traction is applied, until the buttocks are delivered through the vaginal introitus (Fig 21–10). The fetus is gently rotated until the spine rests directly under the pubic symphysis. To deliver the extended legs from the

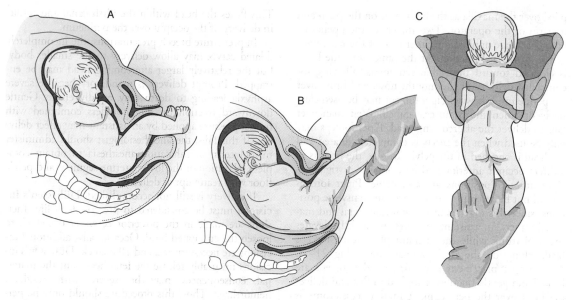

Figure 21–8. Extraction of breech. **A:** Buttocks brought to hollow of sacrum. **B:** Traction on anterior leg causes buttocks to advance and rotate into direct AP diameter of pelvis. Continued downward traction causes the back to rotate anteriorly. **C:** Further downward traction causes the shoulders to engage in the transverse diameter of the inlet. (Redrawn and reproduced, with permission, from Caldwell WE, Studdiford WE: A review of breech deliveries during a 5-year period at the Sloane Hospital for Women. Am J Obstet Gynecol 1929;18:623.)

birth canal, the operator places the index finger in the popliteal fossa of one leg and applies pressure upward and outward, causing the knee to flex. As the knee flexes, the foot is often seen or easily palpated. The lower leg is grasped firmly and gently delivered (Fig 21–7), and the opposite leg is then delivered. The rest of the body is extracted as previously described for footling presentation.

Complications of Breech Delivery

A. Birth Anoxia

Umbilical cord compression and prolapse may be associated with breech delivery, particularly in complete (5%) and footling (15%) presentations. This is due to the inability of the presenting part to fill the maternal pelvis, either due to prematurity or poor application of the presenting part to the cervix, so that the umbilical cord is allowed to prolapse below the level of the breech (see below). Frank breech presentation offers a contoured presenting part, which is better accommodated to the maternal pelvis and is usually well applied to the cervix. The incidence of cord prolapse in frank breech is only 0.5% (the same as for cephalic presentations).

Compression of the prolapsed cord may occur during uterine contractions, causing moderate to severe variable decelerations in the fetal heart rate, leading to fetal anoxia or death. Continuous electronic monitoring is thus mandatory during labor in these cases to detect ominous decelerations. If they occur, immediate cesarean delivery must be performed.

B. Birth Injury

The incidence of birth trauma during vaginal breech delivery is 6.7%, 13 times that of cephalic presentations (0.51%). Only high forceps and internal version and extraction procedures have higher rates of birth injury than vaginal breech deliveries. The types of perinatal injuries reported in breech delivery include tears in the tentorium cerebellum, cephalohematomas, disruption of the spinal cord, brachial palsy, fracture of long bones, and rupture of the sternocleidomastoid muscles. Vaginal breech delivery is also the main cause of injuries to the fetal adrenal glands, liver, anus, genitalia, spine, hip joint, sciatic nerve, and musculature of the arms, legs, and back.

Factors contributing to difficult vaginal breech delivery include a partially dilated cervix, unilateral or bilateral nuchal arms, and deflexion of the head. The type

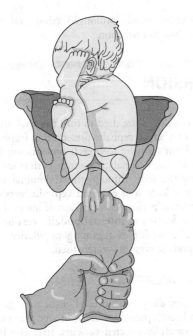

Figure 21–9. Delivery of breech with one finger in the groin. The wrist is supported with the other hand. When the posterior groin is accessible, the index finger of the other hand is placed in it to complete delivery of the breech. (Redrawn and reproduced, with permission, from Greenhill JP: *Obstetrics*, 12th ed. Saunders, 1960.)

of procedure used may also affect the neonatal outcome.

1. Partially dilated cervix—Delivery of a breech fetus may progress even though the cervix is only partially dilated, since the bitrochanteric and bisacromial diameters are smaller than the biparietal diameter. This is true especially in prematurity. The hips and shoulders may negotiate the cervix, but the aftercoming head becomes entrapped, resulting in difficult delivery and birth injury.

2. Nuchal arms—During partial breech extraction and more often in total breech extraction, excessive downward traction on the body results in a single or double nuchal arm. This occurs because of the rapid descent of the body, leading to extension of one or both arms, which become lodged behind the neck. When delivery of the shoulder is difficult to accomplish, a nuchal arm should be suspected. To dislodge the arm, the operator rotates the body 180 degrees to bring the elbow toward the face. The humerus can then be identified and delivered by gentle downward traction. In cases of double nuchal arm, the fetus is rotated counter-

clockwise to dislodge and deliver the right arm and rotated clockwise to deliver the left arm. If this is unsuccessful, the operator must insert a finger into the pelvis, identify the humerus and possibly extract the arm, resulting in fracture of the humerus or clavicle. Nuchal arms cause a delay in delivery and increase the incidence of birth asphyxia.

3. Deflexion of the head—Hyperextension of the head is defined as deflexion or extension of the head posteriorly beyond the longitudinal axis of the fetus (5% of all breech deliveries). Causes of hyperextension include neck cysts, spasm of the neck musculature, and uterine anomalies, but over 75% have no known cause. Although deflexion may be documented by ultrasonographic or x-ray studies weeks before delivery, there is little apparent risk to the fetus until vaginal delivery is attempted. At that time, deflexion causes impaction of the occipital portion of the head behind the pubic symphysis, which may lead to fractures of the cervical vertebrae, lacerations of the spinal cord, epidural and medullary hemorrhages, and perinatal death. If head deflexion is diagnosed prior to delivery, cesarean section should be performed to avert injury. Cesarean section cannot prevent injuries such as minor meningeal hemorrhage or dislocation of the cervical vertebrae; these may develop in utero secondary to longstanding head deflexion.

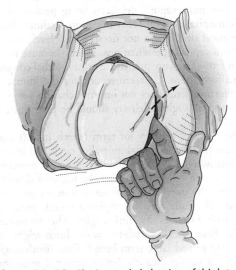

Figure 21–10. Flexion and abduction of thigh to deliver extended leg. (Redrawn and reproduced, with permission, from Llewellyn-Jones D: *Fundamentals of Obstetrics and Gynecology*, Vol. 1. Faber & Faber, 1969.)

4. Type of delivery—More complex delivery procedures have a higher rate of birth trauma. While few infants are injured during spontaneous breech births, as many as 6% are injured during partial breech extraction and 20% during total breech extraction. Injuries associated with total breech extraction are usually extensive and severe, and this procedure should never be attempted unless fetal survival is in jeopardy and cesarean section cannot be immediately performed.

An additional important factor in breech injury and perinatal outcome is the experience of the operator. Inexperience may lead to hasty performance of obstetric maneuvers. Delay in delivery may result in birth asphyxia due to umbilical cord compression, but haste in the management of breech delivery results in application of excessive pressure on the fetal body, causing soft tissue damage and fracture of long bones. Too-rapid extraction of the body from the birth canal causes the arms to extend above the head, resulting in unilateral or bilateral nuchal arms and difficult delivery of the aftercoming head. All breech deliveries should be carried out slowly and methodically by experienced obstetricians who execute the maneuvers with gentleness and skill—not speed.

Prognosis

The incidence of cesarean section for breech delivery has been steadily increasing, from approximately 30% in 1970 to 84% in 1997. A recent review of breech deliveries in California revealed an 88% cesarean section rate, with more vaginal deliveries being performed in public hospitals and far fewer in private facilities. Rates of perinatal death have not decreased to levels associated with cephalic presentations, mainly because many breech fetuses are very premature or have lethal congenital malformations. Cesarean section for the immature or malformed fetus does not improve chances for perinatal survival; vaginal delivery should be performed in these cases.

The route of delivery for term breech infants does not seem to affect neonatal mortality rates. For infants with birthweights of 2000–3500 g, neonatal mortality rates approach zero regardless of the route of delivery. However, the impact of cesarean section on perinatal outcome is clearly seen in singleton breech presentations with extremes in birthweight. The premature breech fetus (25–34 weeks with birthweight of 700–2000 g) and large term breech fetus (birthweight 3500 g) have significantly better neonatal outcomes when delivered by cesarean section. For a tiny premature fetus, cesarean delivery avoids umbilical cord prolapse, entrapment of the aftercoming head by a partially dilated cervix, and birth trauma. For a large fetus, cesarean section avoids prolonged labor and difficult, traumatic breech extraction.

■ VERSION

Version is a procedure used to turn the fetal presenting part from breech to cephalic presentation (cephalic version) or from cephalic to breech presentation (podalic version). Because cephalic version is performed by manipulating the fetus through the abdominal wall, the maneuver is known as **external cephalic version.** Podalic version is performed by means of internal maneuvers and is known as **internal podalic version.** External cephalic version is regaining popularity, whereas internal podalic version is rarely used.

EXTERNAL CEPHALIC VERSION

External cephalic version is used in the management of singleton breech presentations or in a nonvertex second twin. In carefully selected patients, it is safe for both mother and fetus. The goal is to increase the proportion of vertex presentations near term, thus increasing the chance for a vaginal delivery. In the past, external cephalic version was performed earlier in gestation but was accompanied by high reversion rates, making additional procedures necessary. Now it is performed in patients who have completed 36 weeks of gestation so that the risk of spontaneous reversion is decreased, and if complications arise, delivery of a term infant can be accomplished. Current success rates for external cephalic version range from 35–85%, with a mean of 60%.

Indications

Patients with unengaged singleton breech presentations of at least 36 weeks' gestation are candidates for external cephalic version. The procedure is more successful in multigravidas and those with a transverse or oblique lie. Use of fetal heart rate monitoring and real-time ultrasonography are essential to document fetal well-being during the procedure. The use of tocolytics in external cephalic version is controversial. There is recent evidence that in nulliparous women tocolytics offer an advantage, but there are conflicting reports on which type of tocolytic confers the highest success rate. Thus, these agents should be used at the discretion of the physician. Additionally, there is inconsistent evidence regarding the use of regional anesthesia. Recent randomized controlled trials have shown an increased success rate in those with epidural anesthesia. However, the ultimate decision should be based on physician experience.

Contraindications

Contraindications to external cephalic version include engagement of the presenting part in the pelvis, marked oligohydramnios, placenta previa, uterine anomalies, presence of nuchal cord, multiple gestation, premature rupture of membranes, previous uterine surgery (including myomectomy or metroplasty), and suspected or documented congenital malformations or abnormalities (including intrauterine growth retardation).

Complications

Complications are rare, occurring in only 1–2% of all external cephalic versions. Examples include placental abruption, uterine rupture, amniotic fluid embolism, preterm labor, fetal distress, and fetal demise. Thus, given the potential for catastrophic outcome, it is advised that this procedure be performed in a facility where immediate access to cesarean delivery is available.

A. FETAL CARDIAC ABNORMALITIES

Fetal cardiac abnormalities may be readily documented during external cephalic version by intermittent fetal or ultrasonographic surveillance. Fetal bradycardia occurs in 20% of cases, but normal cardiac activity will usually return if the procedure is stopped for a short time. If significant unremitting fetal cardiac alterations occur, the attempt at version should be discontinued, and cesarean delivery performed immediately.

B. FETOMATERNAL TRANSPLACENTAL HEMORRHAGE

Fetomaternal transplacental hemorrhage may occur during version and has been reported to occur in 6–28% of patients undergoing external cephalic version. The **Kleihauer-Betke acid elution test** should be performed if this is suspected. In cases of an Rh-negative-unsensitized woman, Rh immune globulin should be administered after external cephalic version (1 U/100 μg) for prophylaxis.

Technique

External cephalic version is performed as follows:

(1) Obtain informed consent from the patient.

(2) Perform an ultrasound examination to verify presentation and rule out fetal or uterine abnormalities.

(3) Perform a nonstress test. Results must be reactive.

(4) If desired, administer a tocolytic to prevent contractions or irritability.

(5) Administer anesthesia if desired.

(6) Perform external cephalic version. Place both hands on the patient's abdomen, and perform a forward roll by lifting the breech upward while placing pressure on the head downward toward the pelvis. If this is unsuccessful, a backward roll may be attempted.

(7) Fetal well-being should be monitored intermittently with Doppler or real-time ultrasound scanning. The procedure should be abandoned for any significant fetal distress, patient discomfort, or if multiple attempts are unsuccessful.

(8) Following the procedure, external fetal heart rate monitoring should be continued for 1 hour to ensure stability. If the patient is Rh-negative, administer anti-D immune globulin.

(9) If stable, the patient may be sent home to await the onset of spontaneous labor if the version is successful. If unsuccessful, the patient may be scheduled for an elective cesarean section, or plan a trial of labor with a breech vaginal delivery, if the mother is a good candidate.

INTERNAL PODALIC VERSION

Internal podalic version is now rarely used because of the high fetal and maternal morbidity and mortality associated with the procedure. It is occasionally performed as a life-saving procedure or in cases of a noncephalic second twin. (See Chapter 17 for delivery of a second twin.)

Indications

Internal podalic version is the only alternative to cesarean section for the rapid delivery of the second twin in a noncephalic presentation if external cephalic version fails. Thus, when cesarean section is unavailable or when a life-threatening condition arises (maternal hemorrhage due to premature placental separation, fetal distress, prolapsed umbilical cord), internal version may be required.

A life-threatening condition as described above is the only indication for internal podalic version. The cervix must be completely dilated, and the membranes must be intact. A skilled operator is crucial for safe performance of this procedure. In several French studies, internal podalic version was found to be a reliable and effective technique with an excellent long-term maternal and fetal prognosis.

Contraindications

Internal podalic version is contraindicated in cases in which the membranes are ruptured or oligohydramnios is present, precluding easy version. This procedure

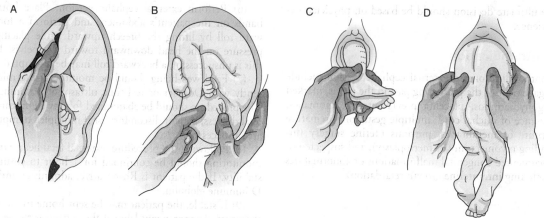

Figure 21–11. Internal podalic version and extraction. **A:** Feet are grasped. **B:** Baby is turned; hand on abdomen pushes head toward uterine fundus. **C:** Feet are extracted. **D:** Torso is delivered. From this point onward, procedure is the same as for uncomplicated breech delivery. (Reproduced, with permission, from DeCosta EL: Cesarean section and other obstetric operations. In: Danforth DN [editor]: *Textbook of Obstetrics and Gynecology,* 2nd ed. Harper & Row, 1972.)

should not be performed through a partially dilated cervix or if the uterus is firmly contracted down on the fetal body. However, recent studies have indicated that intravenous nitroglycerin may be used to provide transient uterine relaxation without affecting maternal or fetal outcome.

Complications

Internal podalic version is associated with considerable risk of traumatic injury to both fetus and mother. Prior to 1950, when this procedure was performed much more frequently than it is today, associated uterine rupture and hemorrhage caused 5% of all maternal deaths. Perinatal mortality rates were 5–25% (primarily due to traumatic intracerebral hemorrhage and birth asphyxia). Considerable birth trauma, including long bone fractures, dislocations, epiphyseal separations, and central nervous system deficits, was also linked to this procedure. For these reasons, internal podalic version has been abandoned with rare exceptions in favor of cesarean section.

Technique

Internal podalic version is performed as follows:

(1) Establish an intravenous line for administration of parenteral fluids, including blood. Cross-matched blood should be available in the hospital blood bank.

(2) Administer anesthesia to achieve relaxation of the uterus.

(3) Place the patient in the dorsolithotomy position. Insert a hand through the fully dilated cervix along the fetal body until both feet are identified and apply traction to bring the feet into the pelvis and out the introitus. Then, grasp both feet firmly. Perform an amniotomy. Apply dorsal traction on both lower extremities until both feet are delivered through the vagina. Then, perform a total breech extraction for delivery of the body (Fig 21–11).

■ COMPOUND PRESENTATION

Compound presentation is prolapse of a fetal extremity alongside the presenting part. Prolapse of the hand in cephalic presentation is most common, followed by prolapse of an upper extremity in breech presentation. Prolapse of a lower extremity in cephalic presentation is relatively rare. Compound presentations are uncommon, occurring in only 1 in 1000 pregnancies.

Causes

Obstetric factors that prevent descent of the presenting part into the pelvic inlet predispose to prolapse of an extremity alongside the presenting part (ie, prematurity, cephalopelvic disproportion, multiple gestation, grand multiparity, and hydramnios). Prematurity occurs in over 50% of compound presentations. In twin gestations, over 90% of compound presentations are associated with the second twin.

Because of poor application of the presenting part to the cervix found in compound presentations, umbilical cord prolapse is common (occurring in 11–20% of cases) and a major contributor to fetal loss during labor.

Diagnosis

The diagnosis of compound presentation is made by palpation of a fetal extremity adjacent to the presenting part on vaginal examination. The diagnosis is usually made during labor; as the cervix dilates, the prolapsed extremity is more easily palpated alongside the vertex or breech. Compound presentation may be suspected if poor progress in labor is noted, particularly when the presenting part fails to engage during the active phase. If the diagnosis of compound presentation is suspected but uncertain, ultrasound or x-ray may be used to locate the position of the extremities and search for malformations.

Management

Management of compound presentation depends on gestational age and type of presentation. Since 50% of compound presentations are associated with prematurity, viability of the fetus should be documented prior to delivery. If the fetus is considered nonviable (< 24 weeks' gestation), labor should be permitted and vaginal delivery anticipated. The small size of the fetus makes dystocia or difficult vaginal delivery uncommon.

Labor may be allowed and vaginal delivery anticipated in viable cephalic presentations with a prolapsed hand. These cases generally pose no difficulty in labor or delivery, since the hand moves upward into the lower uterine segment as the vertex descends into the birth canal.

Umbilical cord prolapse is a risk in all cases of compound presentation, and continuous fetal heart rate monitoring should be done to detect fetal distress or changes in the fetal heart rate. Umbilical cord complications should be managed by immediate cesarean delivery (see below).

Prognosis

Compound presentations are associated with perinatal mortality rates ranging from 9–19%. Contributing significantly to this persistent loss are prematurity, prolapsed umbilical cord complications, and traumatic vaginal delivery.

■ SHOULDER DYSTOCIA

Shoulder dystocia is defined as an inability to deliver the shoulders after the head has delivered. Characteristically, after the head is delivered, the chin presses tightly against the perineum as the anterior shoulder becomes impacted behind the pubic symphysis. It is an acute obstetric emergency requiring prompt, skillful management in order to avoid significant fetal damage or death.

The incidence of shoulder dystocia ranges from 0.15–1.7% of all vaginal deliveries, with increased birthweight imparting a greater risk. The risk also increases dramatically in attempted midpelvic operative deliveries.

Risk Factors

Fetal macrosomia, gestational or overt diabetes mellitus, history of shoulder dystocia in a prior birth, and a prolonged second stage of labor have all been shown to increase the risk of shoulder dystocia. A history of a macrosomic infant, maternal obesity, multiparity, and postterm pregnancy have also been implicated in contributing to shoulder dystocia. However, 50% of patients with shoulder dystocia have no risk factors.

Thus, women at risk for shoulder dystocia should be carefully assessed before labor begins. Ultrasonographic examinations should be performed to evaluate fetal morphology and estimate fetal weight. However, ultrasound has limited accuracy at term.

Complications

Immediate neonatal complications (up to 50% of cases) occur when delivery is delayed or inappropriately performed, resulting in birth asphyxia or traumatic injury. Birth asphyxia may result in fetal death during delivery, neonatal death, or neurologic damage. Short-term neonatal complications of birth asphyxia include metabolic acidosis, shock, renal failure, central nervous system depression, and seizures. Long-term complications include central nervous system damage resulting in mental retardation, cerebral palsy, learning disabilities, seizure disorders, and speech defects.

Traumatic birth injuries include fractures of the humerus or clavicle and injury to the brachial plexus of the anterior shoulder (**Erb's palsy**). Fractures of the humerus and clavicle generally heal without incident, and most traumatic injuries to the brachial plexus resolve with minimal or no neurologic deficit detectable during the neonatal period. However, traumatic injury to the brachial plexus severe enough to cause evulsion of the brachial nerve roots may result in permanent neurologic deficit.

Maternal complications of shoulder dystocia include postpartum hemorrhage and lacerations involving the cervix, vagina, and perineum.

Prevention

Accurate assessment of fetal weight, attention to risk factors associated with shoulder dystocia, and avoidance of midpelvic deliveries in patients with a prolonged second stage of labor should minimize the occurrence of shoulder dystocia. Patients at high risk for shoulder dystocia should be offered a cesarean section, especially if the estimated fetal weight is > 5000 g in a nondiabetic and > 4500 g in a diabetic patient.

Management

Shoulder dystocia should be anticipated when there are any indications of macrosomia. The diagnosis is confirmed when gentle downward pressure on the head fails to deliver the anterior shoulder from behind the pubic symphysis. At this point, the fetus is at risk for asphyxiation, since it cannot expand its chest to breathe, and umbilical cord circulation is compressed within the birth canal. Confronted with this terrifying dilemma, the inexperienced operator often continues to apply downward pressure on the head in a vain attempt to deliver the anterior shoulder. Such action should be avoided, because it is not only ineffective but also potentially damaging to the brachial plexus and may result in permanent Erb's palsy. The following obstetric procedures should be rapidly and skillfully performed to prevent birth anoxia and trauma.

Initially, the operator places a hand in the birth canal to assess the posterior outlet. If inadequate, an episiotomy or a proctoepisiotomy is performed. At the same time, assistants are summoned to aid in the delivery, including a pediatrician and an anesthesiologist.

The **McRoberts manuever** should be used initially because it is simple and resolves shoulder dystocia in 42% of cases. The maternal legs are hyperflexed onto the maternal abdomen, resulting in flattening of the lumbar spine and increasing the size of the posterior outlet. If the shoulders remain undelivered, suprapublic pressure is applied by an assistant to dislodge the anterior shoulder while gentle downward pressure on the head is applied. If these attempts are unsuccessful, the examiner can attempt to rotate the fetal shoulders into the oblique position by placing two fingers against the posterior shoulder and pushing it around toward the fetal chest (**Rubin manuever**) or pushing the posterior

shoulder around toward the fetal back (**Woods manuever**) in a corkscrew fashion.

If the maneuvers to this point fail, delivery of the posterior arm is indicated. The obstetrician's hand is inserted posteriorly into the hollow of the maternal sacrum, and the posterior arm of the fetus is identified. Gentle pressure by the examiner's forefinger on the fetal antecubital fossa will cause flexion of the arm. As the arm flexes across the chest, the forearm is gently grasped, and the hand and forearm are gently delivered from the birth canal. Combined suprapubic and fundal pressure will usually deliver the posterior shoulder. If not, the trunk can be rotated to bring the free arm anteriorly, resulting in delivery.

Deliberate fracture of the clavicle may also be performed, preferably in a direction away from the fetal lungs. This diminishes the size of the shoulder girdle and often facilitates delivery.

Finally, if all previous techniques have failed, a **Zavanelli manuever** may be performed in which the fetal head is replaced in anticipation of a cesarean delivery. A subcutaneous symphysiotomy can also be done to allow disimpaction of the fetal shoulders. Both these procedures are extremely difficult, associated with high maternal and fetal morbidity and mortality, and should only be performed when other conventional maneuvers have failed.

■ UMBILICAL CORD PROLAPSE

Umbilical cord prolapse is defined as descent of the umbilical cord into the lower uterine segment, where it may lie adjacent to the presenting part (**occult cord prolapse**) or below the presenting part (**overt cord prolapse**) (Fig 21–12). In occult prolapse, the umbilical cord cannot be palpated during pelvic examination, whereas in funic presentation, which is characterized by prolapse of the umbilical cord below the level of the presenting part before the rupture of membranes occurs, the cord often can be easily palpated through the membranes. Overt cord prolapse is associated with rupture of the membranes and displacement of the umbilical cord into the vagina, often through the introitus.

Prolapse of the umbilical cord to a level at or below the presenting part exposes the cord to intermittent compression between the presenting part and the pelvic inlet, cervix, or vaginal canal. Compression of the umbilical cord compromises fetal circulation and, depending on the duration and intensity of compression, may lead to fetal hypoxia, brain damage, and death. In overt cord prolapse, exposure of the umbilical cord to air

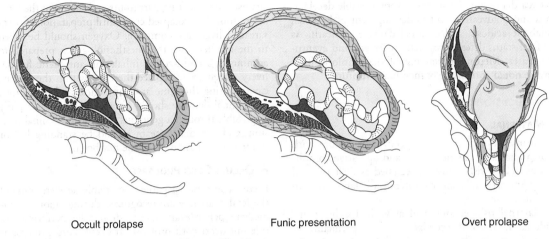

Occult prolapse   Funic presentation   Overt prolapse

Figure 21–12. Types of prolapsed cords.

causes irritation and cooling of the cord, resulting in further vasospasm of the cord vessels.

The incidence of overt umbilical cord prolapse in cephalic presentations is 0.5%; frank breech, 0.5%; complete breech, 5%; footling breech, 15%; and transverse lie, 20%. The incidence of occult prolapse is unknown because it can be detected only by fetal heart rate changes characteristic of umbilical cord compression. However, some degree of occult prolapse appears to be common, since as many as 50% of monitored labors demonstrate fetal heart rate changes compatible with umbilical cord compression. In most cases, the compression is transient and may be rectified simply by changing the position of the patient.

Whether occult or overt, umbilical cord prolapse is associated with significant rates of perinatal morbidity and mortality because of intermittent compression of blood flow and resultant fetal hypoxia. The perinatal mortality rate associated with all cases of overt umbilical cord prolapse approaches 20%. Prematurity, itself a contributor to the incidence of umbilical cord prolapse, accounts for a considerable portion of this perinatal loss.

Causes

Any obstetric condition that predisposes to poor application of the fetal presenting part to the cervix may result in prolapse of the umbilical cord. Cord prolapse is associated with prematurity (< 34 weeks' gestation), abnormal presentations (breech, brow, compound, face, transverse), occiput posterior positions of the head, pelvic tumors, placenta previa, low-lying placenta, and cephalopelvic disproportion. In addition, cord prolapse may occur with hydramnios, multiple gestation, or premature rupture of the membranes occurring before engagement of the presenting part. A recent study revealed that obstetric intervention contributes to nearly half of cases of umbilical cord prolapse. Examples cited include amniotomy, scalp electrode application, intrauterine pressure catheter insertion, attempted external cephalic version, and expectant management of preterm premature rupture of membranes.

Clinical Findings

A. Overt Cord Prolapse

Overt cord prolapse may be diagnosed simply by visualizing the cord protruding from the introitus or by palpating loops of cord in the vaginal canal.

B. Funic Presentation

The diagnosis of funic presentation is also made by pelvic examination if loops of cord are palpated through the membranes.

C. Occult Prolapse

Occult prolapse is rarely palpated during pelvic examination. This condition may be inferred only if fetal heart rate changes (variable decelerations, bradycardia, or both) associated with intermittent compression of the umbilical cord are detected during monitoring.

D. Fetus

The fetus in good condition whose well-being is jeopardized by umbilical cord compression may exhibit violent activity readily apparent to the patient and the obstetrician. Variable fetal heart rate decelerations will occur during uterine contractions, with prompt return of the heart rate to normal as each contraction subsides. If cord compression is complete and prolonged, fetal bradycardia occurs. Persistent, severe, variable decelerations and bradycardia lead to development of hypoxia, metabolic acidosis, and eventual damage or death. As the fetal status deteriorates, activity lessens and eventually ceases. Meconium staining of the amniotic fluid may be noted at the time of membrane rupture.

Complications

A. MATERNAL

Cesarean section is a major operative procedure with known anesthetic, hemorrhagic, and operative complications. These risks must be weighed against the real risk to the fetus of continued hypoxia if labor were to continue.

Maternal risks encountered at vaginal delivery include laceration of the cervix, vagina, or perineum resulting from a hastily performed delivery.

B. NEONATAL

The neonate at delivery may be hypoxic, acidotic, or moribund. A pediatric team should be present to effect immediate resuscitation of the newborn.

Prevention

Patients at risk for umbilical cord prolapse should be treated as high-risk patients. Patients with malpresentations or poorly applied cephalic presentations should be considered for ultrasonographic examination at the onset of labor to determine fetal lie and cord position within the uterine cavity. Because most prolapses occur during labor as the cervix dilates, patients at risk for cord prolapse should be continuously monitored to detect abnormalities of the fetal heart rate. Artificial rupture of membranes should be avoided until the presenting part is well applied to the cervix. At the time of spontaneous membrane rupture, a prompt, careful pelvic examination should be performed to rule out cord prolapse. Should amniotomy be required and the presenting part remains unengaged, careful needling of the membranes and slow release of the amniotic fluid may be performed until the presenting part settles against the cervix.

Management

A. OVERT CORD PROLAPSE

The diagnosis of overt cord prolapse demands immediate action to preserve the life of the fetus. An immediate pelvic examination should be performed to determine cervical effacement and dilatation, station of the presenting part, and the strength and frequency of pulsations within the cord vessels. If the fetus is viable (> 25 weeks' gestation and normal cardiac activity), the patient should be placed in the knee-chest position, and the examiner should apply continuous upward pressure against the presenting part to lift and maintain the fetus away from the prolapsed cord until preparations for cesarean delivery are complete. Oxygen should be given to the mother until the anesthesiologist is prepared to administer a rapid-acting inhalation anesthetic for delivery. Attempts to replace the cord within the uterine cavity during this time are impractical and ineffective. Abdominal delivery should be accomplished as rapidly as possible through a generous midline abdominal incision, and a pediatric team should be standing by for immediate resuscitation of the newborn.

B. OCCULT CORD PROLAPSE

If cord compression patterns (variable decelerations) of the fetal heart rate are recognized during labor, an immediate pelvic examination should be performed to rule out overt cord prolapse. If occult cord prolapse is suspected, the patient should be placed in the lateral Sims or Trendelenburg position in an attempt to alleviate cord compression. If the fetal heart rate returns to normal, labor may be allowed to continue, provided no further fetal insult occurs. Oxygen should be administered to the mother, and the fetal heart rate should be continuously monitored electronically. Amnioinfusion may be performed via an intrauterine pressure catheter in order to instill fluid within the uterine cavity and possibly decrease the incidence of variable decelerations. If the cord compression pattern persists or recurs to the point of fetal jeopardy (moderate to severe variable decelerations or bradycardia), a rapid cesarean section should be accomplished.

C. FUNIC PRESENTATION

The patient at term with funic presentation should be delivered by an expeditiously performed cesarean section prior to membrane rupture. If the fetus is premature, however, the patient should be hospitalized at bed rest in the Sims or Trendelenburg position in an attempt to reposition the cord within the uterine cavity. Serial ultrasonographic examinations should be performed to ascertain cord position, presentation, and gestational age.

D. ROUTE OF DELIVERY

Vaginal delivery may be successfully accomplished in cases of overt or occult cord prolapse if, at the time of prolapse, the cervix is fully dilated, cephalopelvic disproportion is not anticipated, and an experienced physician determines that delivery is imminent. Internal podalic version, midforceps rotation, or any other operative technique is generally more hazardous to mother and fetus in this situation than is a judiciously performed cesarean delivery. Cesarean section is the preferred route of delivery in most cases. Vaginal delivery is the route of choice for an immature or dead fetus.

Prognosis

A. MATERNAL

Maternal complications include those related to anesthesia, blood loss, and infection following cesarean section or operative vaginal delivery. Maternal recovery is generally complete.

B. NEONATAL

Fetal mortality and morbidity rates are high, and the prognosis depends on the degree and duration of umbilical cord compression occurring before the diagnosis is made and neonatal resuscitation begun. If the diagnosis is made early and the duration of complete cord occlusion is less than 5 minutes, the prognosis is good. Gestational age and trauma at delivery also affect the final neonatal outcome. If complete cord occlusion has occurred for longer than 5 minutes or if intermittent partial cord occlusion has occurred over a prolonged period of time, fetal damage or death may be inevitable.

REFERENCES

Breech Presentation

Albrechtsen S et al: Factors influencing delivery method in breech presentation. Acta Obstet Gynecol Scand 1998;77:416.

De Leeuw JP et al: Indications for cesarean section in breech presentation. Eur J Obstet Gynecol Reprod Biol 1998;79:131.

Demol S et al: Breech presentation is a risk factor for intrapartum and neonatal death in preterm delivery. Eur J Obstet Gynecol Reprod Biol 2000;93:47.

Diro M et al: Singleton term breech deliveries in nulliparous and multiparous women: a 5 year experience at the University of Miami/Jackson Memorial Hospital. Am J Obstet Gynecol 1999;181:247.

Eyraud JL et al: Is the Mauriceau manuever deleterious? Study of 103 cases. J Gynecol Obstet Biol Reprod 1997;26:413.

Fait G et al: Breech delivery: the value of X-ray pelvimetry. Eur J Obstet Gynecol Reprod Biol 1998;78:1.

Gregory KD et al: Variation in vaginal breech delivery rates by hospital type. Obstet Gynecol 2000;97:385.

Hannah M et al: Planned cesarean section versus planned vaginal birth for breech presentation at term: a randomized multicentre trial. Lancet 2000;356:1375.

Irion O et al: Planned vaginal delivery versus elective caesarean section: a study of 705 singleton term breech presentations. Br J Obstet Gynaecol 1998;105:710.

Ismail MA et al: Comparison of vaginal and cesarean section delivery for fetuses in breech presentation. J Perinat Med 1999;27:339.

Makris N et al: The management of breech presentation in the last three decades. Clin Exp Obstet Gynecol 1999;26:1799.

Munstedt K et al: Term breech and long-term morbidity—cesarean section versus vaginal breech delivery. Eur J Obstet Gynecol Reprod Biol 2001;96:163.

Sanchez-Ramos L et al: Route of breech delivery and maternal and neonatal outcomes. Int J Gynaecol Obstet 2001;73:7.

Van Loon AJ et al: A randomised control trial of magnetic-resonance pelvimetry in breech presentation at term. Lancet 1997;350:1799.

Ventura ST et al: Births: final data for 1997. Natl Vital Stat Rep 1999;47:1.

Wolf H et al: Vaginal delivery compared with caesarean section in early preterm breech delivery: a comparison of long term outcome. Br J Obstet Gynaecol 1999;106:486.

Version

Andarsio F, Feng TI: External cephalic version. Nitroglycerin versus terbutaline (Abst). Am J Obstet Gynecol 2000;182:S161.

American College of Obstetricians and Gynecologists: External cephalic version. ACOG Practice Bulletin No. 13, 2000.

Dufour P et al: Intravenous nitroglycerin for internal podalic version of the second twin in transverse lie. Obstet Gynecol 1998;92:416.

Dugoff L et al: The effect of spinal anesthesia on the success rate of external cephalic version: a randomized trial. Obstet Gynecol 1999;93:345.

Ezra Y et al: Significance of success rate of external cephalic versions and vaginal breech deliveries in counseling women with breech presentation at term. Eur J Obstet Gynecol Reprod Biol 2000;90:63.

Fernandez CO et al: A randomized placebo-controlled evaluation of terbutaline for external cephalic version. Obstet Gynecol 1997;90:775.

Impey L, Lissoni D: Outcome of external cephalic version after 36 weeks gestation without tocolysis. J Matern Fetal Med 1999; 8:203.

Lau TK et al: Predictor of successful external cephalic version at term: a prospective study. Br J Obstet Gynaecol 1997; 104:798.

Lau TK, Lo KW, Rogers M: Pregnancy outcome after successful external cephalic version for breech presentation at term. Am J Obstet Gynecol 1997;176:218.

Mancuso KM et al: Epidural anesthesia for cephalic version: a randomized trial. Obstet Gynecol 2000;95:648.

Neiger R, Hennessey MD, Patel M: Reattempting failed external cephalic version under epidural anesthesia. Am J Obstet Gynecol 1998;179:1136.

Schorr SJ et al: A randomized trial of epidural anesthesia to improve external cephalic version success. Am J Obstet Gynecol 1997;177:1133.

Siddiqui D et al: Pregnancy outcome after successful external cephalic version. Am J Obstet Gynecol 1999;181:1092.

Compound Presentation

Goplerud J, Eastman NJ: Compound presentation: Survey of 65 cases. Obstet Gynecol 1953;1:59.

Tebes CC et al: Congenital ischemic forearm necrosis associated with a compound presentation. J Matern Fetal Med 1999;8:281.

Weissberg SM, O'Leary JA: Compound presentation of the fetus. Obstet Gynecol 1973;41:60.

Shoulder Dystocia

American College of Obstetricians and Gynecologists: Shoulder dystocia. ACOG Practice Pattern No. 7, 1997.

Beall MH et al: Objective definition of shoulder dystocia: a prospective evaluation. Am J Obstet Gynecol 1998;179:934.

Bofill JA et al: Shoulder dystocia and operative vaginal delivery. J Matern Fetal Med 1997;6:220.

Gherman RB et al: The McRoberts manuever for the alleviation of shoulder dystocia: how successful is it? Am J Obstet Gynecol 1997;176:656.

Gherman RB, Ouzounian JG, Goodwin TM: Obstetric maneuvers for shoulder dystocia and associated fetal morbidity. Am J Obstet Gynecol 1998;178:1126.

Ginsberg NA, Moisidis C: How to predict recurrent shoulder dystocia. Am J Obstet Gynecol 2001;184:1427.

Goodwin TM et al: Catastrophic shoulder dystocia and emergency symphysiotomy. Am J Obstet Gynecol 1997;177:463.

Lewis DF et al: Can shoulder dystocia be predicted? Preconceptive and prenatal factors. J Reprod Med 1998;43:654.

Nesbitt TS, Gilbert WM, Herrchen B: Shoulder dystocia and associated risk factors with macrosomic infants born in California. Am J Obstet Gynecol 1998;179:476.

Rubin A: Management of shoulder dystocia. JAMA 1964;189:835.

Sandberg EC: The Zavanelli manuever: 12 years of recorded experience. Obstet Gynecol 1999;93:312.

Wagner RK, Nielsen PE, Gonik B: Shoulder dystocia. Obstet Gynecol Clin North Am 1999;26:371.

Woods CE: A principle of physics is applicable to shoulder delivery. Am J Obstet Gynecol 1943;45:796.

Umbilical Cord Prolapse

Dare FO et al: Umbilical cord prolapse: a clinical study of 60 cases seen at Obafemi Awolowo University teaching hospital, Ile-Ife. East Afr Med J 1998;75:308.

Katz Z, Lancet M, Borenstein R: Management of labor with umbilical cord prolapse. Am J Obstet Gynecol 1982;142:239.

Prabulos AM, Philipson EH: Umbilical cord prolapse. Is the time from diagnosis to delivery critical? J Reprod Med 1998;43:129.

Surbek DV et al: Transcervical intrapartum amnioinfusion: a simple and effective technique. Eur J Obstet Gynecol Reprod Biol 1997;75:123.

Usta IM, Mercer BM, Sibai BM: Current obstetrical practice and umbilical cord prolapse. Am J Perinatol 1999;16:479.

Cardiac, Hematologic, Pulmonary, Renal & Urinary Tract Disorders In Pregnancy

22

Michelle Grewal, MD, Manoj K. Biswas, MD, FACOG, FRCOG, & Dorothee Perloff, MD

CARDIOVASCULAR DISORDERS*

CARDIOVASCULAR CHANGES IN NORMAL PREGNANCY

The major cardiocirculatory changes that occur during normal pregnancy include an increase in cardiac output and blood volume and a decrease in peripheral resistance (Table 22–1). During normal pregnancy, 6–8.5 L of fluid and 500–900 mmol of sodium are retained because of the action of progesterone, renin, aldosterone, and prolactin. A dilutional anemia occurs as a result of the greater increase in plasma volume relative to red cell mass. Renal blood flow increases by 30%, the glomerular filtration rate increases by 50%, and uterine blood flow reaches 500 mL/min at term. Hormonal changes include a rise in levels of estrogen and progesterone, renin, angiotensinogen, angiotensin II, and aldosterone and a decreased sensitivity to infused angiotensin II.

Myocardial contractility increases as do heart rate and atrial and ventricle chamber size (Table 22–1). Late in pregnancy, a decrease in cardiac output has been reported when measurements are made with the patient in the supine rather than the lateral recumbent position. This apparent decrease is due to interference with venous return resulting from compression of the inferior vena cava by the gravid uterus. If the drop is dramatic enough, the patient may experience **supine hypotensive syndrome,** which is characterized by dizziness and even syncope on recumbency. However, the profound hypotension may represent a failure of the normal baroreceptor-mediated reflex adaptation to a fall in pressure, inadequate collateral venous circulation, and exaggerated parasympathetic response.

Additional hemodynamic changes occur during the various stages of labor and delivery and depend on the patient's position, the degree of sedation, and the type of anesthesia used. Cardiac output increases by about 20% with each uterine contraction as 300–500 mL of blood is expelled from the contracting uterus. Systolic blood pressure also rises with each contraction, increasing the load on the left ventricle by 10%, while the heart rate falls. Pain, fear, and anxiety contribute further to an increase in cardiac output. These changes are less marked if the patient is in the lateral decubitus position during labor or receiving epidural anesthesia. Following delivery, depending on the amount of blood lost—usually 500 mL during vaginal delivery and 1000 mL or more with cesarean section—the cardiac output and plasma volume increase by 20–60% because of a shift of blood from the uterus and placenta into the vascular space as well as resorption of interstitial fluid. Oxytocic drugs can produce further hemodynamic changes. The hemodynamic changes of pregnancy begin to regress shortly after delivery, and pre-pregnancy levels are usually reached within 2 weeks postpartum, but may take longer.

The hemodynamic changes of normal pregnancy can result in symptoms and signs that mimic those of heart disease, often making it difficult to differentiate the two (Table 22–2). It is the severity and persistence of symptoms that suggest underlying organic heart disease (Table 22–3).

HEART DISEASE

Cardiovascular disease is the most important nonobstetric cause of disability and death in pregnant women, occurring in 0.4–4% of pregnancies. The reported maternal mortality rate ranges from 0.4% in patients with New York Heart Association classifications I and II to 6.8% or higher among patients with class III and IV severity. It is not surprising that the added hemodynamic burden of pregnancy, labor, and delivery can aggravate symptoms and precipitate complications in a

---

* See also Chapter 19, Hypertensive States of Pregnancy.

Table 22–1. Hemodynamic and respiratory changes of normal pregnancy.[1]

Physiologic Variable	Direction and Percent of Change		Time of Onset (Weeks)	Time of Peak Effect (Weeks)
Cardiac output	Increased	30–50	±10	20–30
Heart rate	Increased	10–25	10–14	40
Blood volume	Increased	25–50	6–10	32–36
Plasma volume	Increased	40–50	6–10	32
Red cell mass	Increased	20–40	6–10	40
Blood pressure	Decreased early; increased late	No net change	First trimester	20
			Third trimester	40
Pulmonary and peripheral vascular resistance	Decreased	40–50	6–10	20–24
Oxygen consumption	Increased	15–30	12–16	40
Tidal volume	Increased	40	6–10	40

[1]Greater increase with twin or multiple pregnancy.

woman with preexisting cardiac disease. However, even a previously healthy woman may develop cardiovascular problems specifically related to pregnancy, such as preeclampsia, varicose veins, thromboembolic complications such as pulmonary emboli, aortic dissection, or shock due to hemorrhage, amniotic fluid emboli, disseminated intravascular coagulation, or sepsis. Furthermore, any woman in the childbearing years may develop incidental myocarditis, pericarditis, or infective endocarditis while she is pregnant. Drugs used for obstetric complications such as preterm labor may have adverse effects on the woman with heart disease, and drugs used for the treatment of maternal heart disease may have adverse effects on the fetus.

Heart disease can be classified as congenital (operated or unoperated) or acquired. Acquired diseases can be infectious, autoimmune, degenerative, malignant, or idiopathic. Ideally, the patient with known heart disease should consult her physician before becoming pregnant in order to determine the advisability and optimum timing for pregnancy, the need for and timing of diagnostic procedures, the prospects for corrective or palliative cardiac surgery, the type of prosthetic valve to be used, and the need for discontinuing certain drugs during pregnancy. If a woman with heart disease presents for medical care after she has become pregnant, the obstetrician must be able to recognize the presence of preexisting cardiac disease, assess the degree of disability, and understand the impact of the added hemodynamic changes of pregnancy.

Pre-pregnancy planning might, for instance, include performance of an exercise tolerance test to determine if the woman with severe heart disease can tolerate the added hemodynamic burden of pregnancy as well as a 3D echocardiogram to evaluate potential structural defects and the ejection fraction. The obstetrician must also be able to anticipate, prevent, diagnose, and treat complications such as arrhythmias or congestive heart failure when they arise, and advise the patient regarding discontinuation or continuation of the pregnancy and the risk of future pregnancies. Management of an obstetric patient with heart disease should be carried out by a team consisting of an obstetrician, cardiologist, and anesthesiologist.

Rheumatic heart disease has historically been the most common type of heart disease in pregnant women. However, in countries where infectious causes of heart disease are generally less common, congenital heart disease now represents a larger percentage of diseases encountered. It is therefore especially important that obstetricians understand the late complications of surgically corrected or uncorrected congenital heart disease that are likely to occur during pregnancy, labor, delivery, and lactation. In addition, degenerative diseases such as ischemic heart disease are encountered more frequently due to the longer survival of patients with diabetes mellitus and chronic renal disease, the prevalence of tobacco addiction, cocaine use, and delayed childbearing.

In patients with limited ability to increase cardiac output due to valvular or intrinsic myocardial disease, the added hemodynamic burden leads to symptoms early in pregnancy when blood volume has increased considerably. The normal increase in blood flow to the uterus is limited, resulting in increased incidence of spontaneous

Table 22–2. Symptoms and signs of normal pregnancy mimicking heart disease.

Clinical Manifestations	Mechanisms
Symptoms	
Palpitations/cardiac awareness	Increased heart rate; increased stroke volume, increased ectopy
Nasal stuffiness	Vasodilatation, increased cutaneous blood flow
Dyspnea, shortness of breath; orthopnea	Increased progesterone causing hyperventilation; low alveolar CO_2 tension: upward displacement of diaphragm
Decreased exercise tolerance; easy fatigability	Weight gain; lack of exercise; increased cardiac output at rest, limiting maximum cardiac output increase with exercise
Dizziness; lightheadedness; syncope	Decreased venous return due to compression of inferior vena cava by enlarged uterus and increased venous capacitance
Epigastric or subxiphoid pain; bloating, heartburn	Displacement of diaphragm, stomach, and liver by large uterus; decreased gastrointestinal motility
Heat intolerance, sweating and flushing	Increased cutaneous blood flow and increase metabolic rate
Signs	
Sinus tachycardia; ectopic beats (ventricular, atrial)	Increased cardiac output; increased O_2 demand; decreased threshold for ectopic beats and arrhythmias
Bounding pulses and capillary pulsations	Increased cardiac output; decreased total peripheral resistance; widened pulse pressure; increased cutaneous blood flow
Prominent jugular venous pulsations	Increased cardiac output; decreased venous tone; right ventricular volume overload
Plethoric facies	Increased cutaneous blood flow
Lateral displacement of cardiac apex	Mechanical, high diaphragm; right and left ventricular volume overload
Widely split S_1 and S_2 heart sounds	Increased cardiac output; increased venous return; delayed right ventricular emptying
Third heart sound	Increased cardiac output; rapid filling of ventricles
Systolic murmur (left sternal edge or precordial)	Increased cardiac output; turbulent flow through pulmonary valve; increased venous return; increased mammary flow
Continuous murmurs	Venous hum; mammary souffle; increased venous distensibility
Varicose veins	Obstruction of inferior vena cava by uterus; increased venous distensibility
Capillary telangiectases	Increased estrogen level and increased venous distensibility
Pulmonary rales	Atelectasis due to hypoventilation of lung bases because of displacement of diaphragm
Edema (legs, occasionally hands and face)	Mechanical obstruction of inferior vena cava by uterus; increased venous pressure in legs
Ectopic beats; supraventricular tachycardias	Decreased threshold for ectopic beats and arrhythmias
Electrocardiogram	
Leftward or rightward axis shift; nonspecific ST-T wave changes	Mechanical displacement of diaphragm; right ventricular volume overload; altered sympathetic tone and altered repolarization sequence
Echocardiogram/Doppler ultrasound	
Increased left and right ventricular end diastolic dimensions	Increased blood volume; increased cardiac output
Increased velocity of circumferential fiber shortening increased ejection fraction, hyperdynamic function	Increased myocardial contractility, increased cardiac output, increased sympathetic tone

Table 22–3. Symptoms and signs suggesting significant cardiovascular disease.

Severe or progressive dyspnea and orthopnea, especially at rest.

Paroxysmal nocturnal dyspnea; signs of pulmonary edema; cough, frothy pink sputum

Effort syncope or chest pain

Chronic cough, hemoptysis

Clubbing, cyanosis, or persistent edema of extremities

Increased jugular venous pressure, abnormal venous pulsations

Accentuated or barely audible first heart sound

Fixed or paradoxic splitting of S_2; single S_2

Ejection click or late systolic click, opening snap

Friction rub

Systolic murmur of grade III or grade IV intensity or palpable thrill

Any diastolic murmur

Cardiomegaly with diffuse sustained right or left ventricuar heave

Electrocardiographic evidence of significant arrhythmias

---

abortion, prematurity, and intrauterine growth restriction. In women with cyanotic heart disease, the incidence of spontaneous abortion may be as high as 60%, and preterm delivery and fetal growth restriction are common. Maternal risks increase with increasing age and parity and are greatest after 30 weeks' gestation.

Evaluation of the Patient With Heart Disease

Evaluation of the pregnant woman in whom heart disease is suspected should include a careful medical history, complete physical examination, and noninvasive laboratory tests in order to establish a diagnosis and to determine the severity of the disease in order to facilitate planning the patient's management. The degree of functional disability is graded according to the following New York Heart Association classification:

Class I: No symptoms limiting ordinary physical activity.

Class II: Slight limitation with mild to moderate activity but no symptoms at rest.

Class III: Marked limitation with less than ordinary activity; dyspnea or pain on minimal activity.

Class IV: Symptoms at rest or with minimal activity and symptoms of frank congestive heart failure.

A classification such as this one that is based on symptoms is only a rough guideline and may not accurately reflect the severity of disease, and sudden and unpredictable changes in classification can occur during pregnancy.

A. MEDICAL HISTORY

In patients with a previous diagnosis of heart disease or hypertension, the following information should be obtained: age at diagnosis and circumstances of diagnosis; previous symptoms and complications; previous diagnostic procedures, including cardiac catheterization, exercise testing, and echocardiography; prior drug treatment; timing and exact nature of operative procedures and degree of improvement achieved; residual defects, symptoms, and limitations; current medications and diet; and previously imposed prohibitions regarding activity. Medical records from previous physicians regarding previous hospitalizations, diagnostic and therapeutic procedures, and complications should also be obtained.

In patients without an established diagnosis of heart disease, the intake health provider should routinely inquire about a history of rheumatic fever and other illnesses that may be related to heart disease, such as scarlet fever, systemic lupus erythematosus, pulmonary disease, renal disease, diphtheria, or pneumonia, as well as prior hospitalizations, accidents, and major operations. The physician should elicit a history of signs and symptoms such as cyanosis at birth or with exertion, squatting in childhood, multiple respiratory infections in childhood, prior arrhythmias, dyspnea at rest or on exertion, chronic cough, hemoptysis, asthma, exercise intolerance, headache, dizziness, effort syncope, chest pain, and peripheral edema. Activities or events precipitating these symptoms should be assessed. Finally, the family history of cardiovascular disease or other congenital anomalies should be ascertained, together with a history of prior fetal abnormalities. In patients from developing countries, a history of exposure to tuberculosis, hepatitis, and rickettsial and parasitic infections should also be obtained.

B. PHYSICAL EXAMINATION

On physical examination, note should be made of height, weight, and body build; any facial, digital, or skeletal abnormalities that suggest congenital anomalies; and skin changes such as cyanosis, pallor, angiomas, pigmentation, xanthelasmas, and xanthomas. The blood pressure should be carefully measured with an appropriately sized cuff and, if elevated, repeated measurements should be made in both arms and in several positions. The radial pulses should be carefully palpated. A collapsing pulse of aortic insufficiency, a diminished pulse of low cardiac output, or the absence of a pulse due to prior surgery or thrombosis should be noted.

Inspection of the head should focus on congenital abnormalities such as low hairline or low-set ears, nasal deformities, and high-arched palate, as well as gingival overgrowth, dental caries, or cyanosis. The jugular venous pressure and venous waves in the neck should be inspected with the patient's head elevated at a 30-degree angle above the table, and the carotid pulse and thyroid gland should be palpated. A venous hum should be differentiated from a cardiac murmur or bruit.

Inspection and palpation of the chest should identify the presence of scars and skeletal abnormalities such as pectus excavatum deformity, precordial bulge, left or right ventricular heave, or thrill. The cardiac rhythm (regular or irregular, fast or slow) should be assessed. The first heart sound is often widely split in pregnant women, when listening with the diaphragm. Increased intensity of the first heart sound is the hallmark of mitral stenosis, and decreased intensity suggests first-degree heart block. Fixed splitting of the second heart sound suggests atrial septal defect or right bundle branch block, while paradoxic splitting suggests advanced left ventricular hypertrophy or left bundle branch block. A third heart sound is commonly heard, especially late in pregnancy. However, a fourth heart sound, an opening snap, an ejection click, or a mid- or late systolic click should suggest heart disease. In patients with prosthetic valves, the opening and closing of the valve may produce characteristic metallic clicking sounds.

The systolic murmurs of normal pregnancy must be differentiated from those of underlying heart disease. The murmurs of right or left ventricular outflow tract obstruction may be initiated by an ejection click and are characteristically crescendo-decrescendo, ending before the closing sound of the valve involved, and are usually grade III or IV/VI in intensity, as opposed to the grade II murmurs heard in normal pregnancy. Regurgitant murmurs of the semilunar valves (aortic and pulmonary) are diastolic and decrescendo and are well heard along the left sternal edge when the patient is sitting with held expiration.

Diastolic murmurs are not heard in normal pregnancy. The diastolic murmur of mitral stenosis is characteristically associated with a loud first heart sound and an opening snap, a high-frequency sound that follows the aortic valve closure by 0.07–0.12 second. This low-frequency diastolic rumble of mitral stenosis is best heard when the patient is positioned in the left lateral decubitus position, with the bell of the stethoscope lightly placed upon the skin. The mitral regurgitation murmur is a long holosystolic murmur, which is best heard at the apex radiating into the left axilla, whereas the tricuspid regurgitation murmur is best heard at the lower left sternal edge and increases markedly with inspiration. The murmur of mitral valve prolapse may be musical, and both murmur and click are often inaudible late in pregnancy unless the patient is sitting up or standing.

Patients with atrial septal defect have a pulmonary systolic ejection murmur, often a low-frequency diastolic rumble, which represents a tricuspid flow murmur, and a characteristic widely split second heart sound, which remains widely split even in expiration. Those with a ventricular septal defect have a pansystolic, loud, harsh murmur resembling that of mitral regurgitation, which is heard best along the lower left sternal edge. The systolic murmur of coarctation of the aorta is best heard in the left second interspace and between the scapulae. Patients with an extracardiac shunt (patent ductus arteriosus) usually have a continuous systolic and diastolic murmur. Examination should continue with percussion and auscultation of the lungs and palpation and auscultation of the abdomen to ascertain the presence of hepatosplenomegaly, aortic aneurysm, masses, or bruits. The peripheral pulses should be carefully palpated and the extremities examined for the presence of varices, cyanosis, edema, stasis changes, clubbing, "splinter" hemorrhages, joint deformities, muscle wasting, or skeletal deformities such as arachnodactyly or brachydactyly, which suggest multiple congenital anomalies.

Funduscopic examination should be performed in patients with hypertension to determine the presence of arteriolar narrowing, sclerosis, and arteriovenous compression; these imply long-standing hypertension. The presence of retinal edema, cotton-wool patches, and papilledema suggest preeclampsia or accelerated hypertension. A brief neurologic examination, including examination of the cranial nerves, muscle strength, sensation, and reflexes, should be performed when indicated.

C. Laboratory Tests

In addition to routine laboratory tests, patients with suspected cardiac disease may need the following noninvasive diagnostic procedures:

1. Electrocardiogram—The electrocardiogram (ECG) is useful for determining abnormalities of rhythm and the presence of conduction defects, evidence of chamber enlargement, and signs of myocardial or pericardial disease, ischemia, or infarction. The Holter monitor (24-hour continuous ECG) is occasionally useful for documenting the presence and nature of recurring arrhythmias or heart blocks and for correlating symptoms of palpitations, near syncope, or syncope with concurrent cardiac rhythm.

2. Echocardiogram—The transthoracic (TTE) echocardiogram (both M mode and 2-dimensional sector scan) is a rapid, safe, and reliable tool for differentiating the physiologic murmurs resulting from the increased cardiac output of a normal pregnancy from the murmurs of congenital or acquired heart disease. The echocardiogram can provide information about abnormalities of anatomy and function of the chambers, valves, and pericardium. By inspection of the collapsibility of the inferior vena cava, the echocardiogram can provide information about the patient's volume status and differentiate cardiac from noncardiac causes of pulmonary edema that are important for diagnosis and treatment. The presence, location, and magnitude of intracardiac left-to-right and right-to-left shunts can be approximated by injecting 1–2 mL of normal saline shaken with 1 cc of air into a peripheral vein to produce microbubbles. The microbubbles magnify the reflected echo signal, and the presence of bubbles on the left side or an area of "negative contrast" in the right atrium or ventricle suggest an intracardiac shunt. Echocardiography can also be used to diagnose aortic dissection and coarctation. Transesophageal echocardiography (TEE) has added a new dimension to the evaluation, especially of posterior structures such as the left atrium and the mitral valve. Because of its better resolution, TEE is particularly useful for the detection of left atrial thrombi and evaluation of prosthetic valves, and has been used in place of fluoroscopy for insertion of a pacemaker or even for performing valvuloplasty. TEE is also useful in the operating room and intensive care unit when TTE does not provide adequate resolution.

3. Doppler echocardiography—Pulsed, continuous-wave, and color Doppler echocardiography is combined with 2-dimensional echocardiography for determination of blood flow and velocity, quantitation of pressure gradients and the degree of regurgitation, as well as for measuring intracardiac shunts and estimation of pulmonary pressure.

4. Exercise tolerance test—Exercise studies such as the treadmill test are normally not used during pregnancy, since pregnancy itself is a form of stress test. However, they may be useful in a woman contemplating pregnancy or in early pregnancy if the degree of compensation and ability to carry a pregnancy to term are in doubt, or to investigate the cause of chest pain and certain arrhythmias. In a woman with a prior myocardial infarct who is contemplating becoming pregnant, an exercise study with radionuclide myocardial perfusion would be a useful test to perform to determine the amount of fixed myocardial damage and the presence of reversible ischemia.

5. Miscellaneous—Additional studies for specific conditions include a throat culture to diagnose the presence of beta-hemolytic streptococcal infection and a C-reactive protein and antistreptolysin titer if antecedent streptococcal infection is suspected. Serial blood cultures are indicated if infective endocarditis is suspected. Chest x-rays, cardiac catheterization, and radionuclide scans are generally avoided during pregnancy, since the radiation can be harmful to the fetus, especially early in gestation. However, these tests can be performed with careful shielding of the abdomen and pelvis, if the mother's condition requires it.

RHEUMATIC HEART DISEASE

In developed countries, the incidence and the severity of rheumatic fever have declined progressively since the 1960s because of the widespread, prompt use of penicillin in the treatment of group A beta-hemolytic streptococcal upper respiratory tract infections and because of an apparent decrease in virulence of the organism. However, in Asia and Central and South America, rheumatic heart disease is still prevalent, and valvular abnormalities are common in women of childbearing age.

Active rheumatic carditis, although rare during pregnancy, can be a serious and potentially fatal complication. The diagnosis is based on the Jones criteria: evidence of a preceding group A streptococcal infection (positive throat culture, scarlet fever, or elevated antistreptolysin titer), carditis, chorea, subcutaneous nodules, erythema marginatum, and polyarthritis. The minor criteria included fever, arthralgias, elevated sedimentation rate, and first-degree heart block. Carditis may result in acute congestive heart failure or may aggravate established rheumatic valvular disease. Treatment should consist of specific antistreptococcal antibiotics as well as salicylates and corticosteroids when indicated. Sodium restriction and bed rest are general nonspecific measures.

Continuous prophylaxis against recurring rheumatic fever (secondary prevention) is advised until at least age 30 years in any patient with a history of rheumatic fever or rheumatic heart disease. In areas where rheumatic fever is prevalent, prophylaxis probably should be continued for patients with rheumatic heart disease, especially if they have small or school-aged children. The American Heart Association regimen is as follows:

> Benzathine penicillin G, 1.2 million units intramuscularly at monthly intervals; or
> Penicillin V, 250 mg orally twice daily for compliant patients; or
> Sulfadiazine, 0.5–1 g orally once a day (contraindicated late in pregnancy because of transplacental passage); or
> Erythromycin, 250 mg orally twice daily.

1. Mitral Valve Disease

Mitral stenosis is the most common lesion in young women with rheumatic heart disease, although mitral stenosis can result from Libman-Sacks endocarditis in patients with lupus and can be congenital, especially in association with atrial septal defect (Lutembacher's syndrome). Most patients with mild to moderate stenosis who are in sinus rhythm tolerate pregnancy well, although the risk for superimposed infective endocarditis is ever present even in hemodynamically mild disease. Those with moderate to severe disease are more likely to develop complications such as pulmonary venous congestion or frank pulmonary edema, right ventricular failure, pulmonary vascular hypertension, hemoptysis, atrial fibrillation, and systemic or pulmonary emboli. However, sudden and unexpected deterioration can occasionally occur during pregnancy in patients with any degree of mitral stenosis. New onset of atrial fibrillation in a previously asymptomatic woman can precipitate acute pulmonary edema, which occasionally requires emergency commissurotomy.

The normal hemodynamic changes of pregnancy put patients with mitral stenosis at special risk for developing pulmonary congestion. The increased heart rate with consequent shortening of the diastolic filling period, augmented cardiac output and blood volume, and increased pulmonary venous pressure all contribute to raising left atrial pressure. The increased atrial irritability and increased sympathetic tone predispose to the onset of atrial fibrillation. The pregnant cardiac patient is also at risk for the development of thromboembolic complications, because of the hypercoagulable state of the blood during pregnancy as well as venous stasis in the legs. When right ventricular failure is associated with increased pulmonary vascular resistance, fluctuations in venous return can result in decreased cardiac output, and even syncope. The risk for developing heart failure increases progressively throughout pregnancy and is further increased during labor and delivery and immediately postpartum. Symptoms can also be aggravated by associated anemia, thyrotoxicosis, fever, respiratory infections, and tachycardia resulting from anxiety, stress, and unusual physical exertion, as well as a hot, humid environment. The risk of infective endocarditis remains throughout pregnancy, delivery, and the early puerperium.

Labor imposes an additional load on the pregnant cardiac patient, but congestive failure rarely occurs for the first time during labor in a previously well-controlled patient with mitral stenosis. Postpartum pulmonary edema occurs more frequently, however, because of the abrupt redistribution of blood volume. The mortality rate in women with rheumatic mitral valve disease is 1% overall and reaches 3–4% in women with class III and class IV severity.

Clinical Findings

The symptoms of mitral valve disease are those of pulmonary venous congestion; dyspnea on exertion, and later at rest; right ventricular failure; atrial arrhythmias; and occasionally, hemoptysis. Fatigue and decrease in exercise tolerance are more often manifestations of mitral insufficiency. The characteristic findings on physical examination include a right ventricular lift, a loud first heart sound (S-1), accentuated pulmonic component of the second heart sound (P-2), an opening snap (OS), and a low-frequency diastolic rumble at the apex with presystolic accentuation (if the patient is in sinus rhythm). The murmur is best heard with the bell and should be carefully listened for when the characteristic cadence of S-1, P-2, OS is appreciated. The electrocardiogram is often normal but may indicate left atrial enlargement, right axis deviation, or even right ventricular hypertrophy. The echocardiogram is particularly useful for defining the anatomy of the valve and intravalvular structures, quantitating the degree of stenosis and associated regurgitation, and identifying the presence of abnormalities in other valves and pulmonary artery pressure.

Treatment

The goals of treatment for the patient with mitral stenosis should be to prevent or treat tachycardia and atrial fibrillation, to avoid fluid overload, and to avoid unnecessary increases in oxygen demand such as occur with anxiety or physical activity. Digitalis, quinidine, occasionally beta adrenergic blocking agents, sodium restriction, and diuretics may be necessary for treating congestive failure and atrial arrhythmias. Patients with chronic atrial fibrillation should be anticoagulated with subcutaneous heparin. Anemia, intercurrent infection, and thyrotoxicosis should be corrected. Large fluctuations in hemodynamics due to venous pooling in the legs should be avoided by the use of elastic support hose, especially late in pregnancy.

Cardiac surgery or balloon valvuloplasty, although rarely necessary as an adjunct to careful medical management of patients with chronic rheumatic heart disease, occasionally becomes necessary as a lifesaving maneuver. In patients with severe mitral stenosis, especially if manifested in childhood, mitral valvotomy has often been performed for relief of symptoms before the patient becomes pregnant. Closed surgical mitral commissurotomy can be performed at any time during pregnancy but is rarely necessary as a lifesaving procedure until cardiac output has increased significantly in the late second or early third trimester. Balloon valvuloplasty has become a preferred, less invasive procedure, especially for patients with a noncalcified, pliable valve. In an occasional patient, mitral valve replacement may be necessary as an emergency procedure during pregnancy, as, for instance, in a patient with prior valve replacement whose valve becomes obstructed by pannus or thrombus. Recent reports indicate a low mortality rate for both mother and fetus with cardiopulmonary bypass. However, open heart surgery should be deferred until after the first trimester, if possible.

Patients who have had a valve replaced with a prosthetic valve require anticoagulation and need to be switched from coumadin to heparin during the pregnancy. The teratogenic and fetotoxic effects of warfarin and the risks of bleeding for the mother and fetus during labor and delivery must be balanced against the risks of thromboembolic episodes, especially in patients with earlier-model prosthetic valves. The use of tissue valves obviates the need for anticoagulants, but the life span of bioprosthetic valves is only 8–10 years, and if the patient is in atrial fibrillation, anticoagulation is still required.

Patients with rheumatic valvular disease should be delivered vaginally at term unless cesarean section is indicated for obstetric reasons. Appropriate analgesia should be given during labor, and epidural anesthesia without epinephrine should be used for delivery. Fluid loading for epidural anesthesia must be done gradually. To avoid the added exertion of bearing down during the third stage of labor, outlet forceps may be used. Careful hemodynamic monitoring during labor and delivery is indicated in patients with compromised circulation. Postpartum oxytocics should be given cautiously and blood loss carefully monitored. Redistribution of fluid from the interstitial to the intravascular space immediately postpartum can precipitate pulmonary edema in compromised patients.

2. Mitral Regurgitation

Patients with isolated or predominant **mitral regurgitation** tolerate the physiologic consequences of pregnancy better than do patients with predominant mitral stenosis. The fall in systemic vascular resistance decreases the left ventricular afterload and actually reduces the regurgitant fraction, thus reducing the risk of pulmonary congestion. The risk of atrial fibrillation and of endocarditis, however, is no less in patients with predominant mitral insufficiency. Although mitral regurgitation is frequently the result of rheumatic disease, other causes include: genetic defects in collagen synthesis (such as occur in Marfan's syndrome and Ehlers-Danlos syndrome) or following endocarditis on a previously abnormal valve, late complication of mitral valve prolapse, or papillary muscle infarction or rupture. The clinical course and findings are similar to those of rheumatic mitral insufficiency. The characteristic finding on physical examination is a long systolic murmur that ends with the second heart sound and is best heard at the apex with radiation into the axilla. An associated third heart sound is often present, and with associated mitral valve stenosis an opening snap may be present.

3. Rheumatic Disease in Other Valves

The aortic, pulmonary, and tricuspid valves may also be involved by the rheumatic process, usually in association with mitral valve disease. Involvement of multiple valves compounds the problems of management in these patients. In patients with aortic or pulmonary stenosis who have fixed ventricular outflow obstruction, the gradient across the valve increases with progressive increase in cardiac output during pregnancy, leading to an increased systolic pressure load on the ventricle. Although left ventricular failure is rare, postexertion syncope and angina due to inadequate cardiac output reserve may develop for the first time during pregnancy, especially in the last trimester, when venous return may be abruptly reduced due to compression of the inferior vena cava by the uterus. Patients with severe aortic stenosis should be advised to undergo surgical correction before becoming pregnant. Because patients with high-grade aortic stenosis are unable to maintain normal cardiac output, hypotension, hypertension, and increased cardiac work must be avoided by restricting physical activity and carefully replacing intrapartum blood loss.

Patients with aortic insufficiency—like those with mitral regurgitation—tolerate pregnancy well, since the fall in peripheral resistance favors blood flow and decreases the regurgitant fraction. The risk of endocarditis is present in both stenotic and insufficient valves regardless of severity, and antibiotic prophylaxis during delivery is recommended. Patients with elevated left ventricular end-diastolic pressure, however, are more likely to develop left ventricular failure during pregnancy.

Corrective surgical procedures for rheumatic valve disease include balloon valvuloplasty, surgical commissurotomy, and valve replacement. Two types of valves are available. Heterograft or homograft tissue valves do not require systemic anticoagulation but tend to deteriorate in 8–10 years. Prosthetic valves such as the tilting disc or caged ball valves may last 20 years or longer but always require anticoagulation, complicating the management of pregnancy.

INFECTIVE ENDOCARDITIS

Endocarditis is an acute or subacute inflammatory process resulting from blood-borne infection with *Streptococcus viridans* or other streptococci such as enterococcus (eg, *Streptococcus faecalis*), staphylococci, gram-negative organisms, or fungi. Abnormal heart valves and the endocardium in the proximity of congenital anatomic defects are preferential sites for involvement by blood-borne infections. Progressive involvement of the valve leaflets may result in acute aortic, mitral, or tricuspid valvular regurgitation, which may precipitate cardiac failure. Infected material from vegetations can embolize from right-sided lesions such as the tricuspid valve to the lungs, and from left-sided lesions to the systemic circulation. A focal embolic or immune complex glomerulonephritis may also develop. Untreated endocarditis carries a high mortality rate. Patients with endocarditis often give a history of recent extensive dental work, intravascular or urologic procedures, cardiac surgery, or intravenous illicit drug abuse. Intravenous drug users are at particular risk for developing acute endocarditis, often due to unusual pathogens and often on previously normal valves. Aseptic endocarditis occasionally occurs with rheumatoid arthritis, systemic lupus erythematosus (Libman-Sacks disease), and hypereosinophilic states (Löffler's endocarditis).

Clinical Findings

The diagnosis is based on symptoms such as persistent fever, malaise, chills, sweats, weakness, and embolic phenomena, both to the lungs and to the periphery in an individual with risk factors for endocarditis. Physical findings include petechial hemorrhages, clubbing of the fingers and toes, splenomegaly, Osler's nodes, (septic emboli to the fingertips), the appearance of new murmurs or change in existing murmurs, and manifestations of congestive heart failure. The diagnosis is confirmed by the finding of a positive blood culture or demonstration of vegetations on the valves by echocardiography.

Prevention

Patients at risk for developing infective endocarditis include those with underlying congenital or acquired valvular heart disease and intravenous drug abusers (Table 22–4). Table 22–5 lists the types of procedures for which endocarditis prophylaxis is recommended or discretionary. The currently recommended antibiotic regimens for genitourinary and gastrointestinal procedures are listed in Table 22–6. Patients with underlying heart disease should be advised to maintain good oral hygiene and attend promptly to any infections.

PERICARDIAL DISEASE

Pericardial disease, which is rare during pregnancy, occurs in various forms: as an acute infective process, usually due to a virus; as tamponade due to hemorrhage from trauma, aortic dissection, tumor, or effusion com-

Table 22–4. Cardiac conditions for which endocarditis prophylaxis should be considered.

Endocarditis Prophylaxis Recommended
High-risk category
Prosthetic cardiac valves, including bioprosthetic and homograft valves
Previous bacterial endocarditis
Complex cyanotic congenital heart disease (eg, single ventricle states, transposition of the great arteries, tetralogy of Fallot)
Surgically constructed systemic pulmonary shunts or conduits
Moderate-risk category
Most other congenital cardiac malformations (other than above and below)
Acquired valvular dysfunction (eg, rheumatic heart disease)
Hypertrophic cardiomyopathy
Mitral valve prolapse with valvular regurgitation and/or thickened leaflets[1]
Endocarditis Prophylaxis Not Recommended
Negligible-risk category (no greater risk than the general population)
Isolated secundum atrial spetal defect
Surgical repair of atrial septal defect, ventricular septal defect, or patent ductus arteriosus (without residua beyond 6 months)
Previous coronary artery bypass graft surgery
Mitral valve prolapse without valvular regurgitation[1]
Physiologic, functional, or innocent heart murmurs[1]
Previous Kawasaki disease without valvular dysfunction
Previous rheumatic fever without valvular dysfunction
Cardiac pacemakers (intravascular and epicardial) and implanted defibrillators

Reproduced, with permission, from Dajani AS et al: Prevention of bacterial endocarditis. JAMA 1997;277:1794. This table lists selected conditions but is not meant to be all-inclusive.
[1]Individuals who have a mitral valve prolapse associated with thickening and/or redundancy of the valve leaflets may be at increased risk for bacterial endocarditis, particularly men who are 45 years of age or older.

Table 22–5. Dental or surgical procedures for which endocarditis prophylaxis should be considered.

Endocarditis Prophylaxis Recommended
Respiratory tract
Tonsillectomy and/or adenoidectomy
Surgical operations that involve repsiratory mucosa
Bronchoscopy with a rigid bronchoscope
Gastrointestinal tract[1]
Sclerotherapy for esophageal varices
Esophageal stricture dilation
Endoscopic retrograde cholangiography with biliary obstruction
Biliary tract surgery
Surgical operations that involve intestinal mucosa
Genitourinary tract
Prostatic surgery
Cystoscopy
Urethral dilation

Endocarditis Prophylaxis Not Recommended
Respiratory tract
Endotracheal intubation
Bronchoscopy with a flexible bronchoscope, with or without biopsy[2]
Tympanostomy tube insertion
Gastrointestinal tract
Transesophageal echocardiography[2]
Endoscopy with or without gastrointestinal biopsy[2]
Genitourinary tract
Vaginal hysterectomy[2]
Vaginal delivery[2]
Cesarean section
In uninfected tissue:
Urethral catheterization
Uterine dilation and curettage
Therapeutic abortion
Sterilization procedures
Insertion or removal of intrauterine devices
Other
Cardiac catheterization, including balloon angioplasty
Implanted cardiac pacemakers, implanted defibrillators, and coronary stents
Incision or biopsy of surgically scrubbed skin
Circumcision

[1]Prophylaxis is recommended for high-risk patients; optional for medium-risk patients.
[2]Prophylaxis is optional for high-risk patients.
Reproduced with permission from Dajani AS et al: Prevention of bacterial endocarditis. JAMA 1997;277:1794. This table lists selected procedures but is not meant to be all-inclusive.

plicating collagen vascular disease, acquired immune deficiency syndrome (AIDS), or uremia; or as chronic pericardial constriction secondary to infection, irradiation, or infiltrative process. The symptoms and physical findings, diagnostic approach, and management are the same in the pregnant as in the nonpregnant patient and are well described in standard texts. However, the peripheral edema and increased jugular venous pulsations of normal pregnancy may mask the signs of both tamponade and chronic constrictive pericarditis, leading to frequent delays in diagnosis. Diagnosis can be suspected from the presence of a friction rub, a positive Kussmaul sign (increased jugular venous pressure with inspiration), or a pulsus paradoxus (decreased systolic pressure with inspiration), and confirmed by electrocardiography, echocardiography, and pericardiocentesis. *Acute tamponade is a medical emergency requiring rapid pericardiocentesis or surgical decompression.* Symptomatic treatment with salicylates and corticosteroids may be indicated for acute viral infections. In chronic constrictive pericarditis, surgical decortication may be indicated, but is rarely necessary during pregnancy.

MYOCARDIAL DISEASE

1. Myocarditis

Acute inflammation of the myocardium may be due to rheumatic fever, diphtheria, or viral diseases such as infection with group B coxsackieviruses or protozoal diseases such as toxoplasmosis. Other infectious causes include many other viruses, including the human immunodeficiency virus (HIV), rickettsia (Q fever, Rocky Mountain spotted fever, and scrub typhus), trichinosis, and spirochetal infections (leptospirosis, Lyme disease). In South America, Chagas' disease due to *Trypanosoma cruzi* is common. The myocarditis may be acute or subacute, may be associated with symptoms of systemic illness, and may occur at any time during pregnancy. The clinical manifestations are those of chest pain, fever, pulmonary rales, tachycardia, edema, and systolic murmurs and gallops on physical examination; as well as cardiomegaly, reduced ventricular function, conduction defects, and arrhythmias on electrocardiography and echocardiography. Specific serologic and bacteriologic tests may reveal the identity of the initiating organism. The clinical course is variable, depending on the severity of the infection and the extent of myocardial inflammation. The acute phase of the disease may be subclinical and hence is probably often not recognized as such. The disease may run an acute, subacute, or chronic course; be self-limited with complete recovery; or lead to progressive myocardial fibrosis and eventually to cardiomyopathy. The relationship to peripartum cardiomyopathy is unknown.

Table 22–6. Prophylactic regimens for genitourinary gastrointestinal (excluding esophageal) procedures.

Situation	Agents[1]	Regimen[2]
High-risk patients	Ampicillin plus gentamicin	Adults: ampicillin 2.0 g intramuscularly (IM) or intravenously (IV) plus gentamicin 1.5 mg/kg (not to exceed 120 mg) within 30 min of starting the procedure; 6 h later, ampicillin 1 g IM/IV or amoxicillin 1 g orally
		Children: ampicillin 50 mg/kg IM or IV (not to exceed 2.0 g) plus gentamicin 1.5 mg/kg within 30 min of starting the procedure; 6 h later, ampicillin 25 mg/kg IM/IV or amoxicillin 25 mg/kg orally
High-risk patients allergic to ampicillin/amoxicillin	Vancomycin plus gentamicin	Adults: vancomycin 1.0 g IV over 1–2 h plus gentamicin 1.5 mg/kg IV (not to exceed 120 mg); complete injection/infusion within 30 min of starting the procedure
		Children: vancomycin 20 mg/kg IV over 1–2 h plus gentamicin 1.5 mg/kg IV/IM; complete injection/infusion within 30 min of starting the procedure
Moderate-risk patients	Amoxicillin or ampicillin	Adults: amoxicillin 2.0 g orally 1 h before procedure, or ampicillin 2.0 g IM/IV within 30 min of starting the procedure
		Children: amoxicillin 50 mg/kg orally 1 h before procedure, or ampicillin 50 mg/kg IM/IV within 30 min of starting the procedure
Moderate-risk patients allergic to ampicillin/amoxicillin	Vancomycin	Adults: vancomycin 1.0 g IV over 1–2 h; complete infusion within 30 min of starting the procedure
		Children: vancomycin 20 mg/kg IV over 1–2 h; complete infusion within 30 min of starting the procedure

[1]Total children's dose should not exceed adult dose.
[2]No second dose of vancomycin or gentamicin is recommended.
Reproduced, with permission, from Dajani AS et al: Prevention of bacterial endocarditis. JAMA 1997;277:1794.

Treatment consists of bed rest, digitalis, diuretics, antiarrhythmic agents, and appropriate antibiotics if a specific organism has been identified. Salicylates and corticosteroids are effective in patients with active rheumatic carditis. The incidence of spontaneous abortions in patients with persistent infection is high.

2. Cardiomyopathy

Cardiomyopathy is a rare primary disease of cardiac muscle that presents clinically as heart failure and myocardial dysfunction that probably represent the end stage of various processes that affect the myocardium. Cardiomyopathy is classified broadly as **dilated, restrictive/infiltrative, or hypertrophic.** Restrictive cardiomyopathy is seen as the end stage of amyloidosis, scleroderma, sarcoid, hemochromatosis, or endomyocardial fibroelastosis. Dilated cardiomyopathy may result from excess alcohol consumption (beriberi), thyrotoxicosis, excessive catecholamine levels (pheochromocytoma), cocaine use, and cytotoxic drugs such as doxorubicin. Infectious causes for cardiomyopathy include rheumatic fever, diphtheria, rickettsia (scrub typhus), protozoa (Chagas' disease), spirochetes (Lyme disease), toxoplasmosis, and viral diseases. Lupus erythematosus, hypereosinophilia (Löffler's), ischemia, multiple infarction, and sickle cell disease can also cause a diffuse myocardial process that can lead to congestive heart failure.

Peripartum Cardiomyopathy

Peripartum cardiomyopathy is used to describe this form of cardiac failure when the onset occurs in the last months of pregnancy or within 6 months postpartum, and no specific etiology or prior heart disease is identified. The assumption is that the pregnant condition has somehow predisposed the woman to develop myocardial disease, but the mechanism remains unexplained. It is not understood why the symptoms usually appear following parturition rather than during the late second and third trimesters, when the hemodynamic burden is greatest. It may also be that symptoms of congestive failure are overlooked or misinterpreted as complaints commonly seen late in a normal pregnancy. The incidence appears to be higher in women of African descent, perhaps due to the high prevalence of hypertension, and in women living in warm climates, in twin gestations, and in women with preeclampsia. Cardiomegaly and heart failure may persist or regress postpartum and recur in subsequent pregnancies. The incidence varies from one in 1300 to one in 4000 deliveries, although among the Hausa people in Zaria in northern Nigeria, the incidence may be as high as one in 100–400 deliveries, probably because of the tra-

ditional high postpartum salt intake among these women.

Clinical Findings

The clinical manifestations are those of right and left ventricular failure with pulmonary congestion, hepatomegaly, low cardiac output, chest pain, hemoptysis and cough, fatigue, dyspnea, decreased exercise tolerance, edema, systolic murmurs, third heart sound, elevated jugular venous pressure, pulmonary rales, and cardiomegaly. Arrhythmias and pulmonary as well as systemic emboli are common. The electrocardiographic changes are nonspecific but include arrhythmias, low QRS voltage, left ventricular hypertrophy, abnormal Q waves, nonspecific ST-T wave changes, and conduction defects. On echocardiography, there is evidence of enlargement of all chambers, generalized decrease in wall motion, reduced ejection fraction, and often mural thrombi.

Treatment & Prognosis

The prognosis depends on the degree to which the cardiomegaly is reversible with standard treatment for congestive heart failure, such as digitalis, diuretics, salt restriction, and prolonged bed rest. Afterload reduction with vasodilators, but not converting enzyme inhibitors that are contraindicated in pregnancy, and use of anticoagulants are indicated for patients with intractable heart failure and repeated embolic episodes. Mortality rates of 25–50% have been reported. Patients with persistent cardiomegaly following standard therapy or 6 months after the onset of symptoms have a high incidence of recurrence, progression, and even mortality with subsequent pregnancies and should be cautioned not to become pregnant again.

Hypertrophic Cardiomyopathy

Hypertrophic cardiomyopathy with or without left ventricular outflow tract obstruction (subaortic stenosis) is a developmental abnormality of cardiac muscle that is usually inherited as an autosomal dominant abnormality, although it may occur sporadically. It may result in symptoms within the first 3 decades of life. The asymmetrically hypertrophied septum encroaches on the left ventricular outflow tract, producing an intraventricular pressure gradient and outflow tract obstruction, as well as systolic anterior motion that creates distortion of the mitral valve and mitral insufficiency. The thickened, distorted, abnormally developed, noncompliant muscle causes impaired left ventricular diastolic filling. Decreased cardiac output, atrial and ventricular arrhythmias, and postexertion syncope are common complications.

The diagnosis is suspected on physical examination and must be differentiated from valvular aortic stenosis. Physical findings include a left ventricular heave, an aortic systolic murmur along the lower left sternal edge, and a mitral insufficiency murmur at the apex. A fourth heart sound is common. With increased sympathetic stimulation, the left ventricular outflow gradient, and hence the murmur, increase. A definitive diagnosis is made by echocardiography. The electrocardiogram usually shows left ventricular hypertrophy with septal hypertrophy. The axis and prominent Q waves are often suggestive of prior infarction, but may reflect the electrophysiologic properties of the hypertrophied septum. Management includes use of beta-adrenergic blockers and calcium entry blockers to decrease the vigor of ventricular contraction as well as to manage tachyarrhythmias. Care must be taken to avoid volume depletion. Sympathomimetics should not be used. Careful hemodynamic monitoring during labor and delivery is indicated in symptomatic patients.

ISCHEMIC CORONARY ARTERY DISEASE

The diagnosis of myocardial ischemia due to occlusive coronary artery disease is rarely made in women of childbearing age and is even less frequently made during pregnancy. Nonatherosclerotic causes, such as congenital malformations, Kawasaki disease, vasculitis, endocarditis, emboli and coronary artery spasm as may occur with cocaine use, excessive levels of catecholamines, or bromocriptine used for postpartum suppression of lactation, predominate in young women.

However, the presence of risk factors for accelerated arteriosclerosis such as diabetes mellitus, hyperlipidemia, cigarette smoking, chronic hypertension, and a family history of premature coronary artery disease may combine with delayed childbearing to produce atherosclerotic coronary artery disease even in relatively young pregnant women. In addition, angina pectoris can occur in women with high-grade aortic stenosis, hypertrophic cardiomyopathy, thyrotoxicosis, profound anemia, and increased levels of circulating catecholamines. Myocardial ischemia or reversible ischemia, manifested by chest pain and transient electrocardiographic changes, may also occur during tocolytic therapy for premature labor and in a patient with high levels of circulating catecholamines.

The increases in myocardial oxygen consumption, heart rate, cardiac output, and total blood volume of pregnancy are poorly tolerated by patients with limited coronary artery reserve. Symptoms of ischemia occur at lower levels of exertion than in nonpregnant patients, especially as pregnancy advances. In patients with infarction during pregnancy, the outcome for both mother and fetus depends on the size of the infarct and the presence of complications. Risk to the mother and therefore to the fetus increases near term and especially with the stress of labor and delivery.

In addition to controlling precipitating or aggravating factors, the principles of management of angina pectoris and of myocardial infarction in pregnant women do not differ from those in nonpregnant patients. Patients with angina pectoris should be treated with restriction of activity, avoidance of stress (to reduce oxygen demand), and coronary vasodilators to improve oxygen supply. Nitrates, beta-adrenergic blocking drugs, and calcium channel antagonists should be given. Smoking should be forbidden and other risk factors meticulously controlled. Acute myocardial infarction can be a catastrophic event during pregnancy, especially near term when the hemodynamic load is maximal. Standard therapy to reduce oxygen demands and to improve myocardial perfusion include bed rest, oxygen by nasal cannula, control of hypertension, treatment of hypotension, cautious afterload reduction, intravenous nitroglycerin or other coronary vasodilators, beta receptor antagonists for treatment of tachycardia, and, when indicated, thrombolysis and angioplasty. Women who have had a myocardial infarction before or during pregnancy should be delivered vaginally, if possible, with epidural anesthesia and outlet forceps to shorten the second stage of labor. Careful intrapartum hemodynamic monitoring may be indicated, especially if infarction has occurred in the third trimester.

AORTIC DISSECTION

Aortic dissection is a rare catastrophic event that occurs occasionally during the third trimester of pregnancy or postpartum. It is rare in normotensive patients under age 40. However, chronic hypertension and the effects of estrogen and relaxin may cause degeneration of the arterial media and disruption of elastic tissue in the aorta, thus contributing to the risk of dissection, especially late in pregnancy. Aortic dissection is a much feared potential complication in patients with Marfan's syndrome, unoperated coarctation of the aorta, aortic aneurysm, Ehlers-Danlos syndrome, and myxomatous degeneration and dilatation of the ascending aorta or aortic root.

The diagnosis should be suspected in a woman who has a sudden cardiovascular catastrophe in the third trimester, typically with severe crushing or searing pain in the chest or back, pulmonary edema, neurologic symptoms, evidence of cardiac tamponade, acute aortic insufficiency, and shock. Diagnostic radiologic and echocardiographic studies should be initiated immediately. In patients with a proximal intimal tear (type A), immediate operative intervention, occasionally with aortic valve replacement, can be lifesaving. In patients with a more distal intimal tear (type B), if aortic rupture is not imminent, medical treatment is indicated. This consists of rapid and sustained reduction of blood pressure with intravenous nitroprusside and reduction of the shearing forces on the aortic wall with beta-adrenergic blocking agents. The risk to the fetus is unavoidably high in either case.

Pregnant patients with Marfan's syndrome (a hereditary connective tissue disorder) are at an especially increased risk for aortic dissection. Because of the high risk, many obstetricians counsel these women not to become pregnant. However, in women without aortic root dilatation (less than 4 cm in diameter measured just above the aortic valve by echocardiography), the risk of aortic rupture or dissection is acceptably low.

CONGENITAL HEART DISEASE

Patients with congenital heart disease are surviving to childbearing age in increasing numbers because of the early recognition and treatment of complications that develop in infancy and the availability of palliative and curative operative procedures. Congenital heart disease occurs in approximately 0.9% of liveborn infants in the United States. The prevalence in the population of bicuspid aortic valve, mitral valve prolapse, hypertrophic cardiomyopathy, and ventricular preexcitation (Wolff-Parkinson-White syndrome)—all congenital lesions that usually do not become manifest until later in life—is unknown but may be as high as 2%. Congenital cardiac defects may occur as isolated lesions, as part of a syndrome, associated with other congenital anomalies, and possibly inherited as mendelian dominant or recessive characteristics. The common congenital cardiac anomalies can be broadly grouped under various categories such as cyanotic or acyanotic, simple or complex, mild or severe, and compatible with a normal pregnancy or a contraindication for pregnancy. The following is a simplified classification:

(1) Obstructive lesions of the right or left ventricular outflow tract that result in pressure overload of the ventricle, such as pulmonary stenosis, aortic stenosis, hypertrophic subaortic stenosis, or coarctation of the aorta.

(2) Left-to-right shunts resulting in ventricular volume overload and increased pulmonary blood flow, such as atrial septal defect, atrioventricular canal, ventricular septal defect, endocardial cushion defect, patent ductus arteriosus, and truncus arteriosus.

(3) Cyanotic or hypoxic congenital heart disease in which unoxygenated venous blood enters the systemic circulation, such as tetralogy of Fallot, Eisenmenger's complex, tricuspid atresia, pulmonary atresia, single ventricle, transposition of the great arteries, and Ebstein's anomaly. Complex lesions may combine several of these features.

Operative procedures for correction or palliation are now available for almost all of these defects and are performed even in small infants. However, problems persist in most patients because of residual inoperable lesions, conduction defects, arrhythmias, irreversible pulmonary hypertension, valvular incompetence, ventricular failure, deterioration of prosthetic materials such as valves and conduits, and the need for anticoagulation (Table 22–7). Susceptibility to infective endocarditis persists in all patients except those with corrected uncomplicated secundum atrial septal defects, completely closed ventricular septal defects, and patent ductus arteriosus.

Patients with acyanotic congenital heart disease tolerate pregnancy well, whether the heart disease has been surgically corrected or not, and have a low incidence of spontaneous abortions and premature labor. Induced abortion is rarely indicated for cardiac causes in patients with class I or class II severity. However, patients with class III or class IV severity at the onset of pregnancy have a high incidence of spontaneous abortions and stillbirths, and interruption of pregnancy or postponement until a corrective or palliative procedure can be performed for cardiac indications may be required. In patients with congestive heart failure or large intracardiac shunts, pregnancy is not well tolerated.

Atrial Septal Defect

Ostium secundum atrial septal defect, one of the most common forms of congenital heart disease, is well tolerated by most women, although secondary pulmonary hypertension and right ventricular failure can develop, especially in women with large left-to-right shunts. The characteristic findings on physical examination include a right ventricular lift; a widely split and accentuated second heart sound that does not change with respiration; and a pulmonic systolic ejection murmur, usually considerably louder than the systolic murmur of normal pregnancy. A diastolic tricuspid rumble is often present with large shunts. The electrocardiogram shows an incomplete right bundle branch block and right-axis deviation. The presence, location, and size of the shunt can be identified by echocardiography and color flow Doppler studies. If significant pulmonary hypertension has developed, patients are characterized as having Eisenmenger's syndrome, and the risk of pregnancy rises steeply (see later). Atrial arrhythmias are more likely to occur with advancing age. The risk of infectious endocarditis is low, and paradoxic emboli occur rarely.

Patients with **ostium primum atrial septum defects** (one end of the spectrum of atrioventricular canal defect), who have associated cleft mitral or tricuspid valves with insufficiency, tolerate pregnancy less well

Table 22–7. Late problems to be anticipated in patients with common congenital heart defects.

Defect	Prevalence[1] (Percent)	Surgical Repair	Late Complications
Tetralogy of Fallot	5	Blalock-Taussig, Waterston, or Potts extracardiac shunt, or complete intracardiac repair.	Residual right ventricular outflow obstruction; pulmonary valve insufficiency; conduction defects; right bundle branch block and complete heart block; arrhythmias; late sudden death; ventricular aneurysm; recurring ventricular septal defect; endocardial fibroelastosis.
Transposition of great vessels	5	Mustard or Senning intra-atrial baffle; redirection of venous inflow to ventricles or arterial switch with reimplantation of coronary arteries (Jatene).	Ventricular inflow or outflow obstruction; tricuspid valve insufficiency; decreased right ventricular function; arrhythmias; conduction defects; late sudden death; sinus node dysfunction; calcification, degeneration, or progressive proliferative fibrosis of synthetic or heterograft valves or conduits. Complete heart block, need for pacemaker revision.
Ebstein's anomaly	< 1	Usually not surgically corrected, but occasionally right atrium to pulmonary artery conduit or tricuspid valve replacement with closure of atrial septal defect.	Right ventricular failure; right bundle branch block; recurring supraventricular tachycardia or atrial fibrillation; paradoxic embolization; sudden death; preexcitation (Wolff-Parkinson-White syndrome); intermittent cyanosis.
Atrial septal defect	7	Patch repair potentially "curative" for ostium secundum. Mitral valve replacement may be needed for ostium primum.	Atrial arrhythmias; persistent right ventricular enlargement; persistent or progressive pulmonary vascular hypertension; mitral valve prolapse and mitral regurgitation. Mitral regurgitation in ostium primum defect with cleft mitral valve. Tricuspid regurgitation.
Ventricular septal defect	30	Spontaneous closure common; patch repair potentially "curative."	Persistent or progressive pulmonary vascular disease with hypertension; conduction defects; heart block; aortic insufficiency; persistent or recurring ventricular septal defect; late sudden death; arrhythmias.
Patent ductus arteriosus	9	Ligation and division of ductus potentially "curative."	Persistent or progressive pulmonary vascular disease; associated unoperated intracardiac defects; recanalization of ductus; persistent left ventricular hypertrophy.
Aortic stenosis	5	Valvotomy or valve replacement.	Persistent or recurring stenosis; aortic insufficiency; conduction defects; left ventricular failure; calcification; degeneration, progressive proliferative fibrosis, thrombosis, or dehiscence of synthetic or heterograft valves.
Pulmonic stenosis	7	Valvotomy and infundibulectomy; rarely, valve replacement, balloon valvotomy.	Persistent right ventricular outflow gradient; pulmonary valve insufficiency; atrial arrhythmias; right ventricular failure.
Coarctation of aorta	6	Segmental resection with reanastomosis with or without synthetic graft.	Persistent or recurrent gradient bicuspid aortic valve with insufficiency; cerebral hemorrhage due to rupture of berry aneurysm; proximal aortic dissection or rupture, hypertension.
Complex cyanotic lesions, single ventricle, tricuspid or pulmonary atresia, etc.		Various shunts from systemic venous to pulmonary circulation, Fontan, Glenn, Rastelli, etc.	Inadequate pulmonary perfusion, cyanosis, enlarging bronchial collaterals.

[1]Prevalence in patients with common congenital heart defects.

because of the increased risk of both left or right ventricular failure. If the mitral insufficiency is severe, a mitral prosthesis may have been previously implanted, raising the issue of anticoagulation for a mechanical valve and the risk of deterioration of a tissue valve. Due to the presence of mitral regurgitation, the risk for endocarditis is correspondingly higher, as is the risk for developing atrial arrhythmias. In ostium primum septal defect, the clinical findings include a right ventricular lift and often a left ventricular heave as well, a widely split second heart sound, and a pulmonic ejection murmur as well as the long pansystolic murmur of mitral insufficiency at the apex and occasionally of tricuspid insufficiency at the lower end of the sternum. The electrocardiogram is more likely to show left ventricular hypertrophy, and characteristically left axis deviation, although the incomplete right bundle branch block may be present as well. The echocardiogram and color flow Doppler studies are used to define the location of the atrial septal defect and the degree of involvement of the mitral and tricuspid valves. Transesophageal echocardiography may be needed to evaluate a prosthetic valve.

Ventricular Septal Defect

Isolated **ventricular septal defect,** although common in infancy, is seen less frequently among pregnant women because the ventricular septal defect tends to close spontaneously before the woman reaches adulthood. Women with small to moderate-sized ventricular septal defects tolerate pregnancy well, although they are at risk for developing secondary infectious endocarditis and heart failure. With large ventricular septal defects, the risk of secondary pulmonary hypertension (Eisenmenger's syndrome) increases progressively (see later). Ventricular septal defects are often associated with other intracardiac defects, but large, complicated ones are likely to have been surgically corrected before puberty. Important late complications of ventricular septal defect, operated or unoperated, include ventricular arrhythmias and aortic valve insufficiency. The characteristic findings on examination include a palpable systolic thrill along the left sternal border and a loud pansystolic murmur best heard at the same location. There may be both a left and right ventricular heave or lift. When aortic insufficiency has developed, the presence of a systolic and diastolic murmur can be mistaken for a patent ductus arteriosus. Small ventricular septal defects, such as maladie de Roger may be very noisy but hemodynamically unimportant. The electrocardiogram may appear normal or show biventricular hypertrophy. The echocardiogram and Doppler studies readily identify the location and size of the defect, as well as associated lesions.

Patent ductus arteriosus is now rarely seen in adults because the condition is so readily diagnosed in childhood. Small defects are well tolerated, although patients are at risk for endocarditis, but with large defects, the risk of secondary pulmonary hypertension with shunt reversal and left ventricular failure increases. Patients with a patent ductus characteristically have a palpable left ventricular heave, a loud pulmonic component of the second heart sound, and a systolic/diastolic murmur that is often described as a machinery murmur. However, as pulmonary hypertension develops secondary to a large pulmonary flow, the duration and intensity of the diastolic component decrease. The electrocardiogram may be normal or show left ventricular hypertrophy, while the echocardiogram and Doppler studies identify the magnitude of the shunt and size of the ductus, as well as the degree of ventricular hypertrophy.

Pulmonic Valve Stenosis

Pulmonic valve stenosis is another relatively common congenital cardiac lesion that is well tolerated if the gradient across the pulmonary valve is less than 80 mm Hg, since the valve continues to enlarge in relation to body mass. However, the added hemodynamic load of pregnancy can lead to right ventricular failure in patients with larger gradients. The stenosis can be at the valve, subvalvular, or occasionally supravalvular level. The characteristic physical findings include a right ventricular heave, often with a palpable thrill and a crescendo/decrescendo murmur best heard in the left second intercostal space, radiating to the left side of the neck, initiated by an ejection click, and ending before a delayed and diminished pulmonic component of the second heart sound. The electrocardiogram shows increasing degrees of right ventricular hypertrophy depending on the magnitude of the shunt, which can be quantitated by echo/Doppler. The risk of endocarditis is present, and antibiotic prophylaxis is recommended during delivery. In women with a high transvalvular gradient and right ventricular hypertrophy, the risk of right ventricular failure and atrial arrhythmias is increased, and assisted delivery is recommended. Although pulmonary valvotomy has been successfully carried out during pregnancy, this is rarely necessary. Patients who have previously undergone balloon or operative valvuloplasty often have resulting mild pulmonary valve insufficiency (a high-frequency decrescendo diastolic blow along the left sternal border); this is well tolerated.

AORTIC VALVE DISEASE

Patients with left ventricular outflow obstruction, such as congenital **aortic stenosis,** tolerate pregnancy less well and are more likely to develop left ventricular failure with dyspnea, postexertion syncope, and angina resulting from decreased coronary reserve. They are also at high risk for developing infectious endocarditis. The increased afterload resulting from the hypertension of preeclampsia is poorly tolerated and can contribute to left ventricular failure. The incidence of congenital anomalies in the fetus is relatively high. The physical findings include a diminished carotid pulse with delayed upstroke, a left ventricular heave with lateral displacement of the apex, often a diminished aortic component of the second heart sound, and a crescendo/decrescendo murmur, initiated by an ejection click radiating to the neck. The electrocardiogram is likely to show left ventricular hypertrophy and left atrial enlargement, and echocardiogram/Doppler studies can define the magnitude of the transvalvular gradient, the degree of left ventricular hypertrophy, and adequacy of left ventricular function. Balloon valvuloplasty or even valve surgery is rarely necessary during pregnancy as an emergency measure. Eventually the need for valve replacement must be considered, raising the issue of the choice of valve and the need for anticoagulation and the risk of future pregnancies.

Patients with **bicuspid aortic valve** require no special management during pregnancy except for prophylaxis at the time of delivery, because of their susceptibility for developing infective endocarditis, which can lead to aortic insufficiency. The incidence of congenital bicuspid aortic valve in the population is estimated to be 2%. The murmur of a bicuspid aortic valve can be differentiated from the systolic murmur normally heard in pregnancy in that it is heard better to the right of the sternum in the second interspace, radiating to the right carotid artery, and is usually initiated by an ejection click well heard at the lower left sternal edge and apex.

Aortic insufficiency can be due to rheumatic heart disease, usually in association with mitral valve disease, as an isolated congenital lesion, or it can occur as a manifestation of a dilated aortic ring or myxomatous degeneration of the valve, as a complication of Marfan's syndrome. It may also result from infective endocarditis in a patient with underlying aortic valve disease or secondary to balloon or surgical commissurotomy of a stenotic valve or aortic dissection. In patients with acute infective endocarditis or aortic dissection and acute development of aortic insufficiency, left ventricular failure occurs rapidly and operation is often lifesaving. Chronic aortic insufficiency, however, is well tolerated in pregnancy, because of the reduced peripheral resistance and hence reduced afterload of pregnancy. However, antibiotic prophylaxis is recommended at the time of delivery. The characteristic clinical findings include a wide pulse pressure, sometimes with an elevated systolic pressure, readily collapsing peripheral pulses, prominent carotid arterial pulsations, a left ventricular heave and lateral displacement of the apex, and a high-fre-

quency decrescendo diastolic murmur best heard along the left sternal edge with the patient sitting up and leaning forward. A short aortic systolic murmur is often present. The electrocardiogram is likely to show the voltage criteria for left ventricular hypertrophy, and the regurgitant volume and left ventricular size and function can readily be determined by echocardiogram/Doppler. The presence of early closure of the mitral valve on echocardiogram is a sign of acute massive regurgitation and imminent decompensation.

Coarctation of the Aorta

Coarctation of the aorta results in hypertension of the arms with lower pressures in the legs. Pregnant patients are at increased risk for aortic dissection or rupture and congestive heart failure. The frequently associated bicuspid aortic valve increases the risk of infective endocarditis even in operated patients, and aneurysms in the circle of Willis may lead to subarachnoid hemorrhage, especially if the blood pressure rises during pregnancy. Up to 20% of patients with operated coarctation have some residual hypertension and left ventricular hypertrophy. The physical findings include elevated blood pressures in both arms, with diminished and delayed pulses in the lower extremities, bounding arterial pulsation in the neck, usually a systolic aortic murmur of a bicuspid aortic valve, and a characteristically late systolic murmur, which sounds extracardiac and is best heard in the left second intercostal space and between the scapulae in the back. Endocarditis prophylaxis is required for delivery, even in operated cases, and blood pressure control must be carefully maintained.

Mitral Valve Prolapse

Prolapse of the leaflets of the mitral valve into the left atrium during systole is estimated to occur in 5–8% of young women. In some patients, this is due to valvuloventricular disproportion and superior displacement of the mitral valve, a benign variation of normal mitral valve architecture. At the other end of the spectrum are patients with a generalized connective tissue abnormality inherited as an autosomal dominant and characterized by myxomatous degeneration and attenuation of the valve and chordae tendineae, mitral and tricuspid valve insufficiency, dysautonomia, potentially fatal arrhythmias, and transient cerebral ischemic attacks possibly due to platelet emboli. Mitral valve prolapse may be associated with atrial septal defect, hypertrophic subaortic stenosis, Marfan's syndrome, or may result from papillary muscle infarction. A rare patient with mitral valve prolapse develops sudden rupture of the myxomatous chordae, resulting in acute mitral valve insufficiency and pulmonary edema. Urgent surgical therapy (eg, valve plication or replacement) may be required in these patients. Mitral valve prolapse is the usual cause of the nonrheumatic chronic mitral regurgitation that is seen in older patients.

The diagnosis is suspected on the basis of the presence of an apical late systolic murmur or one or more clicks. The diagnosis is confirmed by echocardiography. The auscultatory findings tend to disappear during pregnancy as the augmented cardiac output increases the left ventricular chamber size, resulting in maximal stretching of the mitral valve chordae throughout systole.

Symptoms of mitral valve prolapse are usually nonspecific, including palpitations due to atrial and ventricular ectopic beats and tachyarrhythmias, atypical nonanginal chest pain, vasomotor instability with postural hypotension, and rarely, transient cerebral ischemic attacks. These symptoms also tend to diminish as pregnancy progresses.

Specific therapy is rarely necessary except for treatment of symptomatic tachyarrhythmias. Although patients with mitral valve prolapse are at increased risk for development of infective endocarditis, the routine use of prophylactic antibiotics during uncomplicated vaginal delivery is unnecessary in patients who have only a click but no evidence of valvular insufficiency or valvular thickening.

Cyanotic Congenital Heart Disease

In women with cyanotic congenital heart disease, both maternal and fetal morbidity and mortality rates are high. The incidence of spontaneous abortions, stillbirths, prematurity, and low birthweight is high. The incidence of congenital heart disease in the offspring is also high. Mothers with congenital heart disease are at particular risk for thromboembolic complications, brain abscess, syncope, and even sudden death.

Tetralogy of Fallot

The most common form of cyanotic congenital heart disease in adults is tetralogy of Fallot, which consists of right ventricular outflow obstruction, right ventricular hypertrophy, large ventricular septal defect, and overriding aorta. The increased cardiac output and decreased peripheral resistance of pregnancy increase the right-to-left shunt and hence the degree of cyanosis, desaturation, and secondary polycythemia. These patients tolerate sudden hemodynamic changes (such as occur during labor, parturition, or with positional changes late in pregnancy) poorly and are also at high risk for infective endocarditis. Although spontaneous abortion and premature delivery of small babies are common in women with marked cyanosis, the fetal lungs are often more mature than expected for gestational age because they have adapted to chronic anoxia. In the past, various palliative operative procedures were performed in infants with tetralogy, which were designed to connect a systemic artery to the pulmonary artery, including the Blalock-Taussig, Potts, and Waterston shunts. These are rarely performed now, and most patients undergo a complete repair with closure of the ventricular septal defect and reconstruction of the right ventricular outflow tract. In uncorrected patients the physical findings include cyanosis; clubbing; a right ventricular heave; and a loud, long harsh systolic murmur heard over the entire precordium and also over the back (representing bronchial anastomoses). Because of the pulmonary atresia or stenosis, the second heart sound has only an aortic component.

Tricuspid Atresia, Pulmonary Atresia, & Transposition of the Great Arteries

Tricuspid atresia, pulmonary atresia, and **transposition of the great arteries** are other cyanotic congenital lesions for which various palliative or switch operations are now available in infancy. An increasing number of these infants are maturing to the childbearing age. Decisions about the advisability of pregnancy must be made individually and depend on the degree of residual cyanosis and adequacy of pulmonary blood flow.

Ebstein's Anomaly

Ebstein's anomaly consists of downward displacement of the tricuspid valve that leads in some cases to obstruction of the right ventricular outflow tract. In milder forms, in the absence of an atrial septal defect, there is no cyanosis; only a flare septal leaflet of the tricuspid valve resulting in tricuspid insufficiency, and "atrialization" of a large part of the right ventricle. This form is generally well tolerated, except for the development of atrial arrhythmias, the frequent coexistence of an accessory bypass tract (Wolff-Parkinson-White syndrome) and atrioventricular conduction defects. The condition may be hereditary and the manifestations in the offspring more severe than in the mother. The physical findings include prominent jugular venous pulsations with a large V wave, a murmur of tricuspid insufficiency, and often an early diastolic sound from the motion of the displaced tricuspid leaflet.

Pulmonary Hypertension

The common causes of pulmonary hypertension are as follows: (1) Increased resistance to pulmonary blood flow at any of several sites in the pulmonary vascular bed. This may be due to multiple pulmonary emboli, primary pulmonary vascular disease, Takayasu's arteritis, or infestation with schistosomes or filariae. (2) Increased pulmonary blood flow, as in left-to-right intra- or extracardiac shunts with the development of secondary pulmonary vascular disease. (3) Increased resistance to pulmonary venous drainage, as in increased left ventricular end-diastolic pressure, left ventricular failure, or mitral stenosis. (4) Pulmonary parenchymal disorders such as sarcoid or chronic fibrosis. (5) Hypoventilation syndromes. (6) Chronic hypoxia, as in high-altitude dwellers or heavy cigarette smokers.

Patients with large intracardiac left-to-right shunts eventually develop irreversible structural changes and obliterative pulmonary vascular disease in response to the increased pulmonary flow. In these persons, pressure in the right ventricle approaches systemic levels, and reversal of the shunt may occur, with resulting cyanosis (**Eisenmenger's syndrome**). The term **Eisenmenger's complex** is used specifically for patients with a large ventricular septal defect and with pulmonary hypertension manifest at birth. These patients are considered inoperable because correction of the cardiac defect does not relieve the pulmonary hypertension and because there is a high rate of operative and postoperative mortality due to right ventricular failure. Patients in whom no cardiac or pulmonary cause for pulmonary hypertension is found are considered to have **primary pulmonary hypertension.**

In patients with pulmonary hypertension, either primary or secondary, the right ventricle tends to fail early in pregnancy because of the added hemodynamic load. Later in pregnancy, rapid hemodynamic changes, such as postural hypotension (due to the fall in systemic vascular resistance) or decrease in venous return, result in a sudden decrease in cardiac output with syncope and decreased coronary perfusion, potentially deteriorating to ventricular fibrillation and death. The risk of fetal loss is also high. These patients are at particularly high risk in the last trimester and during parturition.

Patients present clinically with increasing dyspnea, chest pain, edema, and often, syncope. On physical examination patients may be cyanotic at rest or with exercise, and have clubbed fingers and toes and a loud pulmonic component of the second heart sound. The murmur of the primary left-to-right shunt, if present, may be only faint due to reversal of flow through the defect. Because maternal mortality rates as high as 50% have been reported, patients with pulmonary hypertension should be counseled against becoming pregnant or should be advised to have an early induced abortion.

When pregnancy occurs and is continued, patients should avoid all unnecessary exertion, especially in the third trimester, when the risk of complications is highest. Prolonged bed rest, sodium restriction, digitalis, oxygen, maintenance of blood pressure, and close su-

pervision in a hospital setting are mandatory. Close hemodynamic monitoring, meticulous avoidance of hypotension and volume depletion, and maintenance of adequate preload are important concerns in the management. Patients should be delivered vaginally under epidural anesthesia, with close and continued hemodynamic monitoring in an intensive care unit. Close observation must continue for at least 3–5 days postpartum, although complications and even death can occur as late as 2–3 weeks after delivery, as the normal postpartum hemodynamic changes occur.

ARRHYTHMIAS

Rhythm disturbances are common in pregnancy, and most are well tolerated in the absence of underlying heart disease unless the ventricular rate is ≥ 180/min and the episodes are prolonged. In patients with heart disease, especially those with mitral stenosis and hypertrophic cardiomyopathy, tachycardia is poorly tolerated and can lead to rapid decompensation. Cardiac arrhythmias may also be the first manifestation of serious cardiac problems in patients in whom heart disease was not previously suspected. The diagnosis can be readily made with an electrocardiogram or, if intermittent, with a Holter monitor or event recorder. Life-threatening arrhythmias should be treated promptly with standard therapy. *Diagnosis and treatment of arrhythmias may require the attention of a skilled internist or cardiologist.*

Sinus Tachycardia

Sinus tachycardia is a common finding in pregnancy. There is a 10–25% increase in heart rate during normal pregnancy and a greater increase during twin gestations. Conditions such as anxiety, pain, exercise, anemia, fever, and thyrotoxicosis further increase the heart rate. Treatment is usually not necessary other than that directed at underlying or complicating conditions.

Premature Beats

Premature beats, both atrial and ventricular, are common in nonpregnant patients but appear to occur more frequently during pregnancy. Unless associated with underlying heart disease or tachyarrhythmias, treatment is generally not required. Digitalis or beta-adrenergic blocking agents may be effective in suppressing premature beats if the patient is particularly symptomatic or anxious.

Atrial Arrhythmias

Atrial arrhythmias are common in young women, and during pregnancy there is increased atrial irritability. A wandering or shifting atrial pacemaker or accelerated junctional rhythm usually requires no specific intervention if the rate is under 100 beats/min. More serious atrial arrhythmias such as supraventricular tachycardia (reentrant or from an ectopic focus), atrial fibrillation, and atrial flutter occur in patients with atrial septal defects, accessory bypass tracts as in Wolff-Parkinson-White syndrome, AV-node reentrant tachycardia, and rheumatic heart disease. Profound hemodynamic alterations may result. Atrial arrhythmias are identified by electrocardiography and should be treated promptly. Maneuvers that stimulate the vagus nerve, such as carotid sinus massage or the Valsalva maneuver, should be tried first. If these are not effective, verapamil, 5 mg given intravenously (cautiously) over 1–5 minutes, is often effective in converting the rhythm to a sinus rhythm. This dose may be repeated. Because of the potential for hypotension with intravenous verapamil, intravenous adenosine, which has a very brief duration of action, has been used with increasing frequency. The initial dose is 6 mg given rapidly intravenously; rarely is a repeat dose of 12 mg necessary. When given through a central venous line, a starting dose of 3 mg is recommended. Digoxin, 0.25 mg given orally or intravenously, may also be effective. DC cardioversion is reserved for refractory cases. In patients with Wolff-Parkinson-White syndrome with atrial fibrillation and conduction over the bypass tract (broad complex rhythm), both digitalis and verapamil are contraindicated, and DC cardioversion may be required. Digitalis, quinidine, and verapamil have all been used to prevent recurring tachyarrhythmias. In patients with recurring, incapacitating episodes of supraventricular tachycardia, it is often possible to ablate the accessory bypass tract or intranodal reentry with radiofrequency waves delivered via a catheter. The electrophysiologic testing, however, requires fluoroscopy and hence is best deferred until after pregnancy, but can be performed in critical situations with careful abdominal and pelvic shielding.

Ventricular Tachycardia

Ventricular tachycardia is a rare but usually serious tachyarrhythmia that results in rapid hemodynamic deterioration. Prompt recognition and specific therapy, including intravenous lidocaine or procainamide, and occasionally even DC cardioversion, are indicated; a cardiologist should be consulted. Procainamide, quinidine, disopyramide, and amiodarone have all been used to prevent recurring ventricular tachycardia, although they may all have proarrhythmic effects. Patients with congenital (Romano-Ward or Jervelle and Lange-Nielson syndromes) or acquired long QT syndrome are particularly prone to recurring attacks of syncope and sud-

den death because of a peculiar form of ventricular tachycardia known as **torsade de pointes.** These patients may be controlled with beta-adrenergic blocking drugs but may require an automatic implantable defibrillator. Ventricular tachycardia may be a late complication from scars in the myocardium such as occur in operated congenital heart disease, especially in patients with tetralogy of Fallot or right ventricular dysplasia. In some of these situations, ablation of the ectopic focus can be accomplished via a catheter electrode. An occasional patient may have a repetitive ventricular tachycardia (recurring short runs of 5–10 ventricular beats) in the absence of underlying heart disease. This is a relatively benign condition that does not require therapy unless the patient is frightened by the symptoms.

Heart Block

First-degree heart block is a benign condition, diagnosed by the presence of diminished intensity of the first heart sound on physical examination and confirmed by electrocardiogram. It may, however, be associated with acute carditis. **Second-degree heart block** is classified as Mobitz type I or Mobitz type II block. Type I may indicate digitalis intoxication or increased vagal tone, whereas type II usually indicates serious underlying heart disease. Complete heart block may be congenital or acquired, especially after surgery for congenital heart disease. The diagnosis is suspected in the presence of a slow heart rate (30–40/min), cannon venous waves in the neck, and variable intensity of the first heart sound, and is confirmed by electrocardiography. In occasional patients, continuous electrocardiographic (Holter) monitoring is required if the heart block is intermittent. Decisions regarding the need for pacemaker insertion and maintenance should be referred to a cardiologist. Successful pregnancies have been reported in patients with implanted artificial pacemakers, and emergency implantation during pregnancy can be accomplished with echocardiographic guidance.

CARDIOVASCULAR DRUGS IN PREGNANCY

Since many drugs cross the placenta, their use during pregnancy has potential for being teratogenic or directly harmful to the fetus. Table 22–8 lists the drugs most commonly used for the treatment of cardiac disease and their potential side effects. Several newer drugs have been used in pregnant women, including the calcium channel entry blockers and the antiarrhythmic drug amiodarone.

Tocolytic agents, including the sympathomimetic β_2 agonists such as terbutaline and ritodrine, are used as uterine relaxants in the treatment of premature labor.

Table 22–8. Use of cardiovascular drugs in pregnancy.

Drug	Maternal Indications	Maternal Complications	Fetal Complications
Beta-adrenergic blocking agents	Arrhythmias, thyrotoxicosis, hypertrophic cardiomyopathy, angina pectoris. Widely used for treatment of hypertension and mitral stenosis with tachycardia.	Bradycardia, asthma, congestive heart failure, hyperglycemia, and hypoglycemia (in insulin-dependent diabetics).	Fetal bradycardia, rarely heart block, neonatal hypoglycemia, and hyperbilirubinemia.
Coumarin derivatives	Anticoagulant contraindicated in pregnancy because of teratogenic effects.	Hemorrhage.	Teratogenic: causes fetal warfarin syndrome. First trimester: nasal hypoplasia, chondrodysplasia punctata, brachydactyly. Second trimester: optic nerve atrophy, mental retardation, microcephaly. High incidence of spontaneous abortion, stillbirths, deformed offspring. Fetal hemorrhage.
Digoxin	Congestive heart failure, atrial fibrillation or flutter, paroxysmal atrial tachycardia. Prevention of atrial arrhythmias.	Avoid in patients with Wolff-Parkinson-White syndrome and atrial fibrillation. Obtain plasma levels for titration of dosage. Reduce dosage when given with verapamil or quinidine and postpartum.	Negligible.
Disopyramide	Ventricular arrhythmias.	Probably safe, although little experience reported. May be oxytocic and negative inotrope.	Probably safe.
Diuretics (oral)	Hypertension and congestive heart failure. Should not be started after 20 weeks gestation unless required for treatment of heart failure. May be continued in hypertensive patients if used before onset of pregnancy.	Hypercalcemia, hyperuricemia, hyperglycemia, hypokalemia, hyponatremia, hypotension, alkalosis may occur.	Rarely, fetal distress due to abrupt profound volume depletion and blood pressure reduction. Risk of neonatal hypoglycemia and hyperbilirubinemia.
Heparin	Anticoagulant of choice in patients with prosthetic valves, thromboembolic disease, or mitral stenosis with atrial fibrillation.	Hemorrhage.	Does not cross placenta. No teratogenic effects. Risks of premature labor, stillbirths, and hemorrhage during labor and delivery persist.
Phenytoin	Antiepileptic, antiarrhythmic. (Contraindicated in pregnancy because of teratogenic effects.)	Drowsiness, gingival overgrowth, diplopia, ataxia.	Teratogenic: causes fetal hydantoin syndrome: intrauterine growth restriction, microcephaly, mental retardation, ptosis, depressed nasal bridge.
Procainamide	Ventricular arrhythmias.	May cause positive antinuclear antibody reaction and hypotension. Obtain plasma levels for titration of dosage.	Relatively safe.
Quinidine	Atrial or ventricular arrhythmias.	Hypotension and premature labor may occur. Obtain blood levels for titration of dosage. Potentially proarrhythmic, ie, torsade de pointes.	Relatively safe.

Continued

Table 22–8. Use of cardiovascular drugs in pregnancy. (Continued)

Drug	Maternal Indications	Maternal Complications	Fetal Complications
Verapamil	Supraventricular tachycardias, hypertrophic cardiomyopathy, and hypertension.	Heartblock, hypotension, acceleration of rate in Wolff-Parkinson-White syndrome with atrial fibrillation.	No major abnormalities reported.
Nifedipine	Preterm labor and hypertension.	Headache, flushing, tachycardia, hypotension, edema.	None reported.
Amiodarone	Antiarrhythmic, atrial fibrillation, ventricular tachycardia.	Pulmonary fibrosis, hyper- or hypothyroidism.	Fetal or neonatal hypothyroidism.
Adenosine	Antiarrhythmic, supraventricular tachycardia.	Fleeting flush, hypotension.	None reported.

These are often given in conjunction with glucocorticoids such as betamethasone or dexamethasone, which accelerate maturation of fetal lungs. The use of sympathomimetics alone—but especially together with glucocorticoids given in large volumes of fluid—has resulted in pulmonary edema in a small percentage of women with normal hearts. Furthermore, although these drugs are primarily β_2 agonists, they do produce some β_1 stimulation, leading to increased heart rate, cardiac output, cardiac work, increase in systolic blood pressure, and decreased diastolic pressure and systemic vascular resistance. These drugs can also cause a rise in serum glucose, free fatty acids, and lactate, as well as a fall in serum potassium. Experience with the calcium channel antagonists verapamil and nifedipine is growing, and these drugs also have cardiovascular effects. In patients with underlying heart disease, the likelihood of precipitating myocardial ischemia or pulmonary edema with the use of tocolytics is increased, especially in patients with aortic stenosis, hypertrophic subaortic stenosis, or mitral stenosis. Therefore tocolytics must be used with great caution in patients with underlying heart disease, especially in those conditions where tachycardia is not well tolerated.

GENERAL MANAGEMENT OF HEART DISEASE IN PREGNANCY

General principles for management of patients with heart disease can be summarized as follows:

(1) Establish a diagnosis of heart disease, and assess the severity and functional status with appropriate noninvasive diagnostic studies, preferably those that do not involve ionizing radiation.

(2) Establish a method of regular follow-up, close surveillance, and consultation with a cardiologist and other supporting personnel.

(3) Reduce unnecessary cardiac work by ensuring regular rest and by avoidance of excess exertion, heat, and humidity.

(4) Make certain that the patient receives an adequate diet, avoids excessive weight gain, and complies with a regimen of moderate sodium restriction when indicated.

(5) Treat intercurrent infections, anemia, fevers, thyrotoxicosis, and other disorders.

(6) Treat paroxysmal arrhythmias with appropriate drugs or DC cardioversion; prevent recurring arrhythmias with approved antiarrhythmic drugs.

(7) In patients with chronic atrial fibrillation, large left atrium, prosthetic valves, or recurring thromboembolism who require anticoagulant therapy, switch from oral anticoagulants containing coumarin-type drugs to subcutaneous heparin.

(8) Treat chronic venous insufficiency with well-fitting elasticized support hose.

(9) Treat congestive heart failure with bed rest, digitalis, and diuretics, and treat precipitating factors if recognized.

(10) Provide prophylaxis against infective endocarditis at the time of delivery.

(11) In women with compromised cardiac function, provide careful hemodynamic monitoring of both the mother and the fetus during labor and delivery and in the postpartum period. In patients with pulmonary hypertension, heart failure, or major arrhythmias, continue postpartum monitoring for 4–5 days to avoid late complications.

(12) To decrease the work of bearing down and associated pain and anxiety, provide epidural anesthesia for delivery and use outlet forceps to shorten the third stage of labor.

(13) Operative valvotomy or valve replacement is rarely necessary during pregnancy and may be fore-

stalled with the less invasive technique of balloon valvotomy, but should be considered at any time during pregnancy (in consultation with a cardiologist and cardiac surgeon) if rapid deterioration occurs, if a prosthetic valve fails, or if an emergency complication develops.

Fetal echocardiography after 20 weeks of gestation is a useful technique for detecting fetal cardiac abnormalities, especially in women with congenital heart disease or prior offspring with anomalies. The finding of an abnormality can be helpful in planning perinatal management of the fetus, while the assurance of a normal offspring provides great peace of mind to a woman who has cardiac problems.

VARICOSE VEINS

Varicosities are particularly a problem for the multipara and may cause severe complications. They are caused by congenital weakness of the vascular walls, with superimposed increased venous stasis in the legs because of the hemodynamics of pregnancy, extensive collateral circulation in the pelvis, inactivity and poor muscle tone, and obesity.

The vulvar, vaginal, and even the inguinal veins may be markedly enlarged during pregnancy. Damaged vulvovaginal vessels give rise to hemorrhage at delivery. Large vulvar varices cause pudendal discomfort. A vulvar pad wrapped in plastic film, snugly held by a menstrual pad belt or T-binder, and elastic leotards are helpful.

Injection treatment of varicose veins during pregnancy is futile and hazardous. Varicose veins secondary to causes other than pregnancy, eg, deep vein thrombosis or congenital arteriovenous fistula, are difficult to control.

Vascular surgery can be performed during the first or second trimester, but vein stripping is best delayed until after the puerperium. In all other respects, management is the same as in nonpregnant women.

■ HEMATOLOGIC DISORDERS

ANEMIA

Anemia is a significant maternal problem during pregnancy. A hemoglobin of less than 11 g/dL or a hematocrit of less than 33% should be investigated and treated to avoid blood transfusion and its related complications. A pregnant woman will lose blood during delivery and the puerperium, and an anemic woman is therefore at increased jeopardy. During pregnancy, the blood volume increases by about 50% and the red blood cell mass by about 25%. This physiologic hydremia of pregnancy will lower the hematocrit but does not truly represent anemia.

Nutritional anemia is the most common form. It results from deficiency of iron, folic acid, or vitamin B_{12}. Pernicious anemia due to vitamin B_{12} deficiency almost never occurs during pregnancy. Other anemias occurring during pregnancy are aplastic anemia and drug-induced hemolytic anemia.

1. Iron Deficiency Anemia

Iron deficiency is responsible for about 95% of the anemias during pregnancy, reflecting the increased demands for iron. The total body iron consists mostly of (1) iron in hemoglobin (about 70% of total iron; about 1700 mg in a 56-kg woman) and (2) iron stored as ferritin and hemosiderin in reticuloendothelial cells in bone marrow, the spleen, and parenchymal cells of the liver (about 300 mg). Small amounts of iron exist in myoglobin, plasma, and various enzymes. Hemosiderin contains 37% more iron than does ferritin. Absence of hemosiderin in the bone marrow indicates that iron stores are exhausted. This is both diagnostic of anemia and one of the earliest signs of iron deficiency. This will be followed by a decrease in serum iron and an increase in serum total iron binding capacity and anemia.

During the first half of pregnancy, iron requirements may not be increased significantly, and iron from food (10–15 mg/d) is sufficient to cover the basal loss of 1 mg/d. However, in the second half of pregnancy, iron requirements increase due to expansion of red blood cell mass and rapid growth of the fetus. Increased numbers of red blood cells and a greater hemoglobin mass require about 500 mg of iron. The iron needs of the fetus average 300 mg. Thus, the total amount of iron necessary over the course of a normal pregnancy is approximately 800 mg; this cannot be supplied in the diet, and iron supplementation must be given. Data published by the Food and Nutrition Board of the National Academy of Sciences show that pregnancy increases a woman's iron requirements to approximately 3.5 mg/d. This need can be met by iron supplements exceeding 40 mg/d of elemental iron.

Iron deficiency anemia normally does not endanger the pregnancy unless it is severe, in which case intrauterine growth retardation and preterm labor may result.

Clinical Findings

A. SYMPTOMS AND SIGNS

The symptoms may be vague and nonspecific, including pallor, easy fatigability, palpitations, tachycardia, and dyspnea. Angular stomatitis, glossitis, and koilony-chia may be present in long-standing severe anemia.

B. LABORATORY FINDINGS

The hemoglobin may fall as low as 3 g/dL, but the red cell count is rarely below $2.5 \times 10^6/mm^3$. The red cells are usually microcytic, with mean corpuscular volumes of less than 79 fL, and hypochromic. The reticulocyte count is low for the degree of anemia. Platelet counts are frequently increased, but white cell counts are normal. Occasional hypersegmented neutrophils are seen. Serum iron levels are usually less than 60 μg/dL. The total iron-binding capacity is elevated to 350–500 μg/dL, transferrin saturation is less than 16%, and the serum ferritin concentration is less than 10 μg/dL. The amount of stainable iron (hemosiderin) in the marrow aspirate is a reasonably accurate indication of stored iron.

Differential Diagnosis

Anemia due to chronic disease or an inflammatory process (eg, rheumatoid arthritis) may be hypochromic and microcytic. A similar type of anemia in thalassemia trait can be differentiated from iron deficiency anemia by normal serum iron levels, the presence of stainable iron in the marrow, and elevated levels of hemoglobin A_2.

Complications

Angina pectoris or congestive heart failure may develop as a result of marked iron deficiency anemia. **Sidero-penic dysphagia (Paterson-Kelly syndrome, Plummer-Vinson syndrome)** due to long-standing severe iron deficiency anemia is rare in women of childbearing age.

Prevention

During the course of pregnancy and the puerperium, at least 60 mg/d of elemental iron should be prescribed to prevent anemia.

Treatment

In an established case of anemia, prompt adequate treatment is necessary.

A. ORAL IRON THERAPY

Ferrous sulfate, 300 mg (containing 60 mg of elemental iron of which about 10% is absorbed), should be given 3 times a day. If this is not tolerated, ferrous fumarate or gluconate should be prescribed. Therapy should be continued for about 3 months after hemoglobin values return to normal in order to replenish iron stores. He-moglobin levels should increase by at least 0.3 g/dL/wk if the patient is responding to therapy.

B. PARENTERAL IRON THERAPY

The indication for parenteral iron is intolerance of or refractoriness to oral iron. In most cases of moderate iron deficiency anemia, the total iron requirements equal the amount of iron needed to restore hemoglobin levels to normal or near normal plus 50% of that amount to replenish iron stores.

Imferon is a mixture of ferric hydroxide in a 0.9% sodium chloride solution for injection. It contains the equivalent of 50 mg/mL of elemental iron as an iron dextran complex. Imferon may be given intramuscularly or intravenously. Intramuscular injection must always be given into the muscle mass of the upper outer quadrant of the buttock with a 2-inch, 20-gauge needle, using the Z technique (ie, pulling the skin and superficial musculature to one side before inserting the needle to prevent leakage of the solution and subsequent tattooing of the skin). A test dose of 0.5 mL is administered and the patient watched carefully for anaphylactic reactions. After an hour or longer, 2.5 mL of dextran is given in each buttock for a total of 5 mL (total dose of 250 mg of elemental iron). This should be repeated every week until the total dosage has been given. Imferon may also be given intravenously after testing for anaphylaxis has been done with 0.5 mL of dextran. Excessive dosage must be avoided to prevent hemosiderosis.

2. Folic Acid Deficiency Anemia (Megaloblastic Anemia of Pregnancy)

Megaloblastic anemia of pregnancy is caused by folic acid deficiency and is common where nutrition is inadequate. Based on bone marrow studies, the incidence is 25–60%, depending upon the population studied; peripheral blood examination shows a much lower incidence. The incidence of folate deficiency in the United States is 0.5–15%, depending on the population studied and the diagnostic methods used.

The minimum daily intake of folate necessary to maintain stores and adequate hematopoiesis is 50 μg. This is increased during pregnancy (National Academy of Sciences recommendation) to 800 μg. Folic acid deficiency anemia is more common in multiple pregnancy and in multigravid patients. It may recur in subsequent pregnancies.

Folic acid absorption or metabolism may be impaired during use of oral contraceptives, pyrimethamine, trimethoprim-sulfamethoxazole, primidone, phenytoin, or barbiturates. Jejunal bypass surgery for obesity or the malabsorption syndrome (sprue) may also impair folic acid absorption. Folic acid is necessary for the DNA synthesis of erythropoiesis; thus, sickle cell anemia, a chronic hemolytic state, requires increased folate. Other hemolytic states are also commonly complicated by folic acid deficiency, including hereditary spherocytosis and malarial infestation. Alcohol consumption has been known to interfere with folate metabolism.

Megaloblastic anemia should be suspected if iron deficiency anemia fails to respond to iron therapy. Diagnosis of folic acid deficiency anemia is usually made late in pregnancy or in the puerperium. Low birthweight as well as fetal neural tube defects are known to be associated with maternal folic acid deficiency; however, an association with placental abruption, spontaneous abortion, and preeclampsia-eclampsia is not universally accepted.

Clinical Findings

A. SYMPTOMS AND SIGNS

The symptoms are nonspecific (eg, lassitude, anorexia, nausea and vomiting, diarrhea, and depression). Pallor often is not marked. Rarely, a sore mouth or tongue may be present. An accompanying urinary tract infection is common. Occasionally, purpura may be a clinical manifestation.

B. LABORATORY FINDINGS

Folic acid deficiency results in a hematologic picture similar to that of true pernicious anemia (due to vitamin B_{12} deficiency), which is extremely rare in women of childbearing age. Indeed, megaloblastic anemia in pregnancy almost always implies folate deficiency. The hemoglobin may be as low as 4–6 g/dL, and the red cell count may be less than 2 million/μL in severe cases. Extreme anemia often is associated with leukocytopenia and thrombocytopenia. The red cells are macrocytic (mean corpuscular volume usually > 100 fL), and megaloblastic changes are present in the marrow. However, in pregnancy, macrocytosis may be concealed by accompanying iron deficiency or thalassemia. Serum folate levels of less than 4 ng/mL are suggestive of folic acid depletion in nonpregnant patients, but in otherwise normal pregnant patients, folate tends to fall slowly to low levels (3–6 ng/mL) with advancing gestation. The red cell folate level in megaloblastic patients is lower, but in 30% of patients the values overlap. The peripheral white blood cells are hypersegmented. Seventy-five percent of folate-deficient patients have more than 5% of neutrophils with 5 or more lobes, but this may also be true for 25% of normal pregnant patients.

Urinary excretion of formiminoglutamic acid (FIGLU) has been used to diagnose folate deficiency, but levels are abnormal only in severe megaloblastic anemia. Bone marrow aspirate will be helpful in the diagnosis, as well as a positive hematologic response to folate. Serum iron and vitamin B_{12} levels should be normal.

Treatment

Folic acid, 1–5 mg/d orally or parenterally, continued for several weeks after delivery or for several weeks in patients diagnosed in the puerperium, produces the maximum hematologic response, replaces body stores, and provides the minimum daily requirements. The hematocrit should rise about 1% each day beginning at day 5–6 of therapy. The reticulocyte count should become elevated after 3–4 days of therapy and is the earliest morphologic sign of remission. Iron should be administered orally or parenterally as indicated.

Prognosis

Megaloblastic anemia due to folate deficiency during pregnancy carries a good prognosis if adequately treated. The anemia is usually mild unless associated with multifetal pregnancy, systemic infection, or hemolytic disease (eg, sickle cell anemia). The disorder usually disappears after delivery and is likely to recur only when the patient becomes pregnant again. For complete hematologic response during pregnancy, both folic acid and iron must be given because 70% of folate-deficient patients also lack iron stores.

3. Aplastic Anemia

Aplastic anemia with primary bone marrow failure during pregnancy is fortunately rare. The anemia may be secondary to exposure to known marrow toxins such as chloramphenicol, phenylbutazone, mephenytoin, alkylating chemotherapeutic agents, and insecticides. In most cases, no obvious cause is detected. Idiopathic aplastic anemia in pregnancy may have a spontaneous remission following delivery but may recur in subsequent pregnancies. This suggests that the cause is a disorder of the immune mechanism.

Clinical Findings

The rapidly developing anemia causes pallor, fatigue, tachycardia, painful ulceration of the throat, and fever. The diagnostic criteria are pancytopenia and empty bone marrow on biopsy examination. Patients with aplastic anemia are at increased risk for infection and hemorrhage.

Complications

Aplastic anemia in pregnancy may cause increased fetal wastage, prematurity, intrauterine fetal demise, and increased maternal morbidity and death.

Treatment

The patient must avoid any toxic agents known to cause aplastic anemia. Prednisolone should be given, 10–20 mg 4 times a day. A transfusion of packed red blood cells and platelets may be needed. In some cases, termination of pregnancy may be necessary. Bone marrow transplantation is performed if remission does not occur following delivery or termination of pregnancy. Infection must be treated aggressively with appropriate antibiotics, but most authorities do not recommend giving prophylactic antibiotics.

4. Drug-Induced Hemolytic Anemia

Drug-induced hemolytic anemia often occurs in individuals with inborn errors of metabolism. In the United States, blacks are frequently affected. Glucose-6-phosphate dehydrogenase (G6PD) deficiency in erythrocytes is the most common cause, but catalase and glutathione deficiency may also be associated with this disorder. The traits are X-linked. About 12% of black males and 3% of black females are affected.

Clinical Findings

There is decreased G6PD activity in one-third of patients in the third trimester, causing an increased risk of hemolytic episodes. About two-thirds of pregnant patients with this disorder will have a hematocrit of less than 30%. Urinary tract infections are more common in these patients; use of sulfonamides will precipitate hemolysis. Overexposure of the G6PD-deficient fetus to maternally ingested oxidant drugs (eg, sulfonamides) may produce fetal hemolysis, hydrops fetalis, and fetal death. A black pregnant woman should probably be screened for G6PD deficiency before starting sulfonamide therapy for urinary tract infection.

The red blood cell count and morphology are normal until challenged by noxious drugs. Over 40 substances toxic to susceptible people are recognized, including sulfonamides, nitrofurans, antipyretics, some analgesics, sulfones, vitamin K analogues, uncooked fava beans, some antimalarials, naphthalene, and nalidixic acid.

Specific laboratory tests to identify susceptible individuals include a glutathione stability test and cresyl blue dye reduction test.

Treatment

Management includes immediate discontinuation of any suspected medications, treatment of intercurrent illness, and blood transfusion where indicated.

SICKLE CELL DISEASE

Sickle cell disease is a genetic disorder almost always occurring in blacks. It is characterized by an abnormal hemoglobin molecule, hemoglobin S, which causes red blood cells to become sickle-shaped. Sickle cell hemoglobin results from a genetic substitution of valine for glutamic acid in the sixth position from the N-terminal end of beta chains. The autosomal recessive sickle cell gene is passed to both sexes. Patients homozygous for the hemoglobin S gene have **sickle cell anemia,** and those who are heterozygous have **sickle cell trait.** About 10% of blacks in the United States carry sickle cell trait, and 1 in 500 has sickle cell anemia. Women who are heterozygous for both the S and C genes have **hemoglobin S/C disease;** maternal mortality rates are as high as 2–3%. Hemoglobin S/C disease is peculiarly associated with embolization of necrotic fat and cellular bone marrow with resultant respiratory insufficiency. Neurologic symptoms from fat embolism have also been reported with sickle cell disease. In **hemoglobin S/beta thalassemia disease,** the patient is heterozygous for both hemoglobin S and beta thalassemia; the severity of complications during pregnancy is related to hemoglobin S concentrations in this particular trait.

Prenatal genetic counseling is of great importance. If both partners have the gene for S hemoglobin, their offspring have a 1 in 4 chance of having sickle cell anemia. Restrictive nuclease techniques using DNA isolated from amniotic fluid cells are most useful for prenatal diagnosis of hemoglobinopathy in cases at risk.

Clinical Findings

Sickle cell disease is characterized by chronic hemolytic anemia and intermittent crises of variable frequency and severity. While persons with sickle cell trait are not anemic and are usually asymptomatic, they have twice as many urinary tract infections as normal women. Additionally, their red blood cells tend to sickle when oxygen tension is significantly lowered; thus, hypoventilation during general anesthesia may be fatal.

A. SYMPTOMS AND SIGNS

1. Chronic anemia—Chronic anemia results from the shortened survival time of the homozygous S red blood cells due to circulation trauma and intravascular hemolysis or phagocytosis by reticuloendothelial cells in the spleen and liver.

2. Sickling of red blood cells—Intravascular sickling leads to vaso-occlusion and infarction. Small blood vessels supplying various organs and tissues can be partially or completely blocked by sickled erythrocytes, resulting in ischemia, pain, necrosis, and organ damage.

3. Crises—Crises of variable frequency and severity occur. **Pain crises** involve the bones and joints. These are usually precipitated by dehydration, acidosis, or infection. An **aplastic crisis** is characterized by rapidly developing anemia. The hemoglobin is 2–3 g/dL due to cessation of red blood cell production. An **acute splenic sequestration** crisis is associated with severe anemia and hypovolemic shock, resulting from sudden massive trapping of red blood cells within the splenic sinusoids.

4. Other manifestations—Other manifestations include increased susceptibility to bacterial infection; bacterial pneumonia, segmental bronchopneumonia, and pulmonary infarction; myocardial damage and cardiomegaly; and functional and anatomic renal abnormalities in the form of sickle cell nephropathy or papillary renal necrosis, resulting in hematuria. Central nervous system manifestations include headache, convulsions, hemorrhage, or thrombosis (from vasoocclusion). Ophthalmologic abnormalities include anoxic retinal damage, retinal detachments, vitreous hemorrhages, and proliferative retinopathy. Hepatosplenomegaly or cholelithiasis may also occur.

B. LABORATORY FINDINGS

Sickle cell anemia is associated with high risks for mother and fetus. Screening for abnormal hemoglobin is imperative in the population at risk. Two screening tests are in common use. The sodium metabisulfite test uses 1 drop of fresh 2% reagent mixed on a slide with 1 drop of blood. Sickling of most red cells will occur in a few minutes with both sickle cell trait and sickle cell disease. The Sickledex test is a simple solubility test that uses 20 μL of blood mixed with 2 mL of sodium dithionite reagent. Clouding of the solution indicates the presence of hemoglobin S. If the test is positive, the homozygous and heterozygous states must be differentiated by hemoglobin electrophoresis.

C. EFFECTS ON PREGNANCY

Pregnancy has deleterious effects on sickle cell disease. There are increased rates of maternal mortality and morbidity from hemolytic and folic acid deficiency anemias, frequent crises, pulmonary complications, congestive heart failure, infection, and preeclampsia-eclampsia. It is encouraging, however, that the maternal mortality has decreased to 1% since 1972. There is an increased incidence of early fetal wastage, stillbirth, preterm delivery, and intrauterine growth restriction.

Treatment

Good prenatal care, avoidance of complications, and prompt effective treatment for complications are necessary for a good outcome of pregnancy. Folic acid, 1

mg/d, will prevent megaloblastic anemia. Ultrasonic evaluations adequately assess fetal growth, but biophysical monitoring is necessary for antepartum fetal surveillance. Adequate pain relief must be given during labor. Close intrapartum electronic monitoring of labor is indicated. Prevent hypoxia during general anesthesia by maintaining adequate oxygenation and ventilation. Cesarean section should be done at the earliest sign of fetal compromise for the best perinatal outcome.

In the management of crises, predisposing factors should be searched for and eliminated, if possible. Symptomatic treatment for pain crisis consists of intravenous fluid and adequate analgesics (eg, meperidine or codeine). Bacterial pneumonia or pyelonephritis must be treated rigorously with blood culture and intravenous antibiotics. Streptococcal pneumonia is common and is an ominous complication. Pneumococcal polyvalent vaccine has been shown to reduce the incidence of pneumococcal infection in adults with sickle disease, and therefore it is highly recommended. This vaccine is not contraindicated in pregnancy. In all cases, adequate oxygenation must be maintained by face mask as necessary.

The concentration of hemoglobin S should be less than 50% of the total hemoglobin to prevent crisis. Blood transfusion should be considered in cases of a fall in hematocrit to less than 25%; repeated crisis; symptoms of tachycardia, palpitation, dyspnea, or fatigue; or evidence of inadequate or retarded intrauterine growth.

The immediate risk of transfusion (eg, congestive cardiac failure) must be avoided. Prophylactic hypertransfusion or exchange transfusion to prevent maternal complications, improve uteroplacental perfusion, and achieve a better perinatal outcome has been advocated by some, but these methods are not universally accepted. Transfusion always carries a risk of allergic reaction, delayed hemolytic reaction with rapid fall in hemoglobin A, and transmission of hepatitis virus or the AIDS virus. Isoimmunization may also occur. The antibodies most commonly found are Rh, Kell, Duffy, and Kidd; all pregnant patients with sickle cell trait or disease should be tested for these antigens plus ABO type. Hemolytic disease of the newborn or transfusion reactions due to improper cross-matching of blood may occur if careful blood typing is not done. The use of fresh buffy coat–poor washed packed cells for exchange transfusion will help in avoiding transfusion reactions. (See also Chapter 15.) Induction of nonsickling red blood cells (RBCs) from bone marrow has been considered. The use of erythropoietin was found to increase production of hemoglobin F in baboons; however, it stimulated hemoglobin S production in humans. Hemoglobin F synthesis by stimulating Y-chain production appears to be a promising form of therapy for the sickle cell disease and thalassemia syndrome. Y-chains of hemoglobin F inhibit polymerization of hemoglobin S and therefore inhibit sickling. Recombinant erythropoietin and hydroxyurea have been used together recently with elevation of hemoglobin F. More recently intravenous arginine butyrate has been used with the increase in fetal globin synthesis, production of F reticulocytes, and the level of Y-globin. Bone marrow transplant has been limited by the complications of infection and graft-versus-host disease. Prenatal diagnosis of sickle cell disease might encourage in utero stem cell therapy with normal hemoglobin stem cells.

Sterilization should be considered if maternal complications are too threatening. Oral contraceptives are avoided because of the risk of thromboembolism.

THALASSEMIA

The thalassemias are genetically determined disorders of reduced synthesis of one or more of the structurally normal globin chains in hemoglobin. Thalassemia is found throughout the world but is concentrated in the Mediterranean coastal areas, central Africa, and parts of Asia. The high incidence in these regions may represent a balanced polymorphism due to heterozygous advantage.

All thalassemias are inherited as an autosomal recessive trait. The 2 major groups are the alpha and beta thalassemias, both of which affect the synthesis of hemoglobin A, which contains 2 alpha and 2 beta chains. The severity of the anemia varies with the type of hemoglobin abnormality. In beta thalassemia, the beta hemoglobin chains are defective, but the alpha chains are normal; in alpha thalassemia, the reverse is true. The unbalanced synthesis results in precipitation of the normal chains. If the beta chains are impaired, the alpha chains are produced at a normal rate but in relative excess. The alpha chains then form tetramers that precipitate within red blood cell precursors in the bone marrow, resulting in ineffective erythropoiesis, red cell sequestration and destruction, and hypochromic anemia. The most severe forms of this disorder may cause intrauterine or childhood death. A person who is heterozygous, or a carrier, for a thalassemia trait may be asymptomatic.

The most severe form of alpha thalassemia compatible with extrauterine life is **hemoglobin H (beta4) disease,** which results from deletion of 3 genes. In patients with this disease, abnormal quantities of both hemoglobin H and hemoglobin B accumulate. In **alpha thalassemia minor,** 2 genes are deleted, causing a mild hypochromic, microcytic anemia that must be differentiated from iron deficiency anemia.

In beta thalassemia, no gene deletions have been demonstrated. There are 2 forms of beta thalassemia, beta⁺ and beta⁰, depending on whether beta chain production is reduced or entirely absent. **Beta thalassemia major** is the homozygous state, in which there is little or no production of beta chains. **Beta thalassemia minor,** the heterozygous state, is frequently diagnosed only after the patient fails to respond to iron therapy or delivers a baby with homozygous disease. Such patients usually suffer from hypochromic microcytic anemia, with increased red blood cell count, elevated hemoglobin A2 concentrations, increased serum iron levels, and iron saturation greater than 20%.

The fetus is protected from severe disease because fetal hemoglobin (alpha22) contains no beta globin chain. However, this protection disappears at birth, when fetal hemoglobin production terminates. At about 1 year of age, a baby with defective beta globin production usually begins to show signs of thalassemia (anemia, hepatosplenomegaly) and requires frequent blood transfusions. Victims of severe thalassemia often die in their late teens or early twenties because of congestive heart failure, often related to myocardial hemosiderosis, liver failure, or diabetes mellitus. During pregnancy, iron supplementation should be given only following assessment of iron stores to prevent hemosiderosis. Suspected cases of thalassemia must be diagnosed by means of hemoglobin electrophoresis.

Antenatal diagnosis of thalassemia is now possible. A technique known as molecular hybridization measures the number of intact alpha globin structural genes in fetal cells obtained by amniocentesis. In antepartum diagnosis of beta thalassemia, hemoglobin A is measured in fetal blood obtained via fetoscopy or sonographically directed placental aspiration of fetal blood.

LEUKEMIA & LYMPHOMA

Leukemia is a neoplastic process affecting the leukopoietic tissues of the body. Acute leukemia has a short and fulminant clinical course, whereas chronic leukemia may have a prolonged course lasting several years. Depending on the type of leukocyte affected, leukemia may be lymphatic, myeloid, or monocytic. Lymphomas result from proliferation of cells of the lymphoreticular system. Two types are known: **Hodgkin's disease** and **non-Hodgkin's lymphoma.** Fortunately, these diseases are uncommon in pregnancy. The peak incidence of chronic lymphocytic leukemia and non-Hodgkin's lymphoma occurs after childbearing age, so the association of pregnancy with these diseases is extremely rare.

Clinical Findings

Pregnancy does not affect the course of these diseases, but several complications should be anticipated. Chemotherapy may cause fetal death or malformation or intrauterine growth restriction. The teratogenic and mutagenic effects of ionizing radiation in the first trimester have long been known. More than 10 rads of irradiation to the pelvis during the first trimester in Hodgkin's disease can have deleterious effects on the fetus. The carcinogenic potential and alteration in intelligence and behavior in fetuses exposed to chemotherapy and radiation in utero are uncertain. Intrauterine growth restriction and preterm labor, both iatrogenic and spontaneous, are not uncommon in maternal leukemia. Perinatal mortality rates are increased considerably. Several cases of possible transfer of leukemia and Hodgkin's disease to offspring have been reported.

Splenomegaly, a common manifestation, may cause abdominal discomfort. Severe anemia may cause marked weakness and heart failure. The patient may need multiple blood transfusions. Thrombocytopenia may lead to bruising of the skin and bleeding from the mucous membranes, necessitating platelet transfusion. Postpartum hemorrhage occurs in about 20% of cases. In acute leukemia, severe infection with organisms of usually low virulence is common. Patients with Hodgkin's disease may have complications of irradiation, including pneumonitis causing restrictive lung disease, pericarditis leading to congestive heart failure, various neurologic symptoms, nephritis, and ovarian failure. The risk of a second cancer is substantially increased in patients with Hodgkin's disease. The risk for leukemia has been reported to have increased almost 100-fold if chemotherapy has been given.

Treatment

Management is difficult. Therapy must be individualized if pregnancy is allowed to continue. The obstetrician and a hematologic oncologist should work together. Treatment will require chemotherapy, correction of anemia, and prevention of, or aggressive therapy for, infection. Induced abortion should be considered if chemotherapy is given early in pregnancy.

Effective agents in acute leukemia include prednisone, vincristine, asparaginase, daunorubicin, doxorubicin, mercaptopurine, methotrexate, cyclophosphamide, and cytarabine. Major drugs for chronic leukemia include busulfan, hydroxyurea, and cyclophosphamide. Although chemotherapy entails a risk to the fetus, it often cannot be deferred. In acute leukemia, the median maternal survival rate is only 2.5 months without chemotherapy.

Termination of pregnancy does not seem to affect the course of Hodgkin's disease or the length of survival. Interruption of the pregnancy is recommended if irradiation or chemotherapy is given early in pregnancy. However, neither chemotherapy during second and third trimesters nor irradiation to the mediastinum and neck appears to adversely affect the fetus or neonate. The chemotherapeutic agents normally used in Hodgkin's disease include mechlorethamine, vincris-

tine, procarbazine, and prednisone. If local radiation therapy to the liver, spleen, or lymph nodes is indicated, the uterus should be shielded. Agents used in non-Hodgkin's lymphoma include cyclophosphamide, doxorubicin, vincristine, and prednisone.

Fetal status should be monitored with periodic ultrasonic examination and biophysical monitoring. Delivery should be accomplished when fetal lung maturation is evident on amniotic fluid phospholipid study, and ideally, when the mother is in complete remission.

Prognosis

The prognosis of pregnant patients with these disorders is not significantly different from that for nonpregnant patients. However, since 85% of relapses in Hodgkin's disease occur within 2 years, it is generally accepted that pregnancy should be deferred for 2 years following remission.

The newborn should be carefully evaluated periodically to note any immediate or delayed toxic effects of maternal chemotherapy.

HEMORRHAGIC DISORDERS

Although hemorrhagic disorders (eg, immune thrombocytopenic purpura, disseminated intravascular coagulation, circulating anticoagulants) are not common during pregnancy, these conditions could cause significant risks for both mother and fetus.

Immune Thrombocytopenic Purpura

In immune thrombocytopenic purpura, platelet destruction is secondary to a circulating IgG antibody that crosses the placenta and may also affect fetal platelets. The maternal clinical picture varies from asymptomatic to minor bruises or petechiae, bleeding from mucosal sites, or fatal intracranial bleeding. There may be splenomegaly. The marrow aspirate demonstrates hyperplasia of megakaryocytes. In the peripheral circulation, the platelet count will be 80,000–160,000/μL.

Maternal morbidity and mortality rates are low, but the perinatal mortality rate is around 20%, mostly related to intracranial bleeding. Differences of opinion exist regarding antepartum and intrapartum management of the pregnant woman. Steroids should be given. In refractory cases, splenectomy should be performed in the second trimester if possible. Immunosuppressive agents should be used with great caution and only in extraordinary cases of immune thrombocytopenic purpura in pregnancy. Transfusion of platelets and whole blood may be necessary to restore losses from acute hemorrhage or to normalize low perioperative platelet counts

(<50,000/mL). More recently, maternal infusion of gamma globulin during pregnancy has been used in an attempt to block placental transfer of maternal IgG.

Fifty percent of thrombocytopenic mothers have babies with low platelet counts during the first week of neonatal life. Maternal levels of circulating IgG correlate well with the presence of neonatal thrombocytopenia.

Intrapartum management includes avoidance of traumatic vaginal delivery and maternal soft tissue injury. However, delivery by cesarean section is not universally accepted. Fetal scalp blood sampling to determine the fetal platelet count has been recommended in the past to determine the mode of delivery. However, fetal scalp sampling is fraught with technical difficulties and inaccuracies. Furthermore, there is overall a very low incidence of neonatal morbidity and neonatal outcome does not seem to differ between vaginal and cesarean deliveries. Therefore it is the general opinion that fetal scalp blood sampling is not warranted in the setting of immune thrombocytopenic purpura. However, a small minority still recommend assessment of fetal platelet counts (either through cordocentesis or fetal scalp sampling) to identify the small percentage of fetuses with severe thrombocytopenia.

Circulating Anticoagulants

Circulating anticoagulants, mainly inhibitors of factor VIII, an IgG immunoglobulin, can cause minor to severe bleeding from various sites. Bleeding may be spontaneous or due to trauma, surgery, or sometimes delivery. Treatment may include exchange transfusion with replacement of specific factors or use of corticosteroids or immunosuppressive agents.

THROMBOEMBOLIZATION

Thromboembolization denotes all vascular occlusive processes, including thrombophlebitis, phlebothrombosis, septic pelvic thrombophlebitis, and embolization of venous clots to the lungs. The incidence of thromboembolism is 0.2% in the antepartum period and 0.6% in the postpartum period. Cesarean section increases the incidence to 1–2%. Pulmonary embolism, with a mortality rate of 15%, occurs in 50% of patients with documented deep vein thromboses; only 5–10% of these are symptomatic. Early diagnosis and adequate treatment drastically reduce the incidence of pulmonary embolism and death.

Pathophysiology

Vascular clotting develops mainly due to circulatory stasis, infection, vascular damage, or increased coagulability of blood. All the elements of **Virchow's triad** (circula-

tory stasis, vascular damage, and hypercoagulability of blood) are present during pregnancy. Increase in caliber of capacitance vessels produces vascular stasis, and blood hypercoagulability is due to increased amounts of factors VII, VIII, and X. Thrombin-mediated fibrin generation is increased many times during pregnancy. Significant vascular damage occurs during delivery. Venous return from the lower extremities is reduced by the pressure of the gravid uterus on both the iliac veins and the inferior vena cava. Other important predisposing factors include heavy cigarette smoking, obesity, previous thromboembolism, anemia, hemorrhage, heart disease, hypertensive disorders, prolonged labor, operative delivery, and postpartum endomyometritis.

The venous thrombi may develop first in the relatively small veins of the calf muscle and extend proximally as far as the femoral or iliac veins or, rarely, even into the inferior vena cava. Another common site of postpartum thrombosis is the pelvic veins due to diminished blood flow in the hypertrophied uterine veins. Thrombi may extend into the iliac veins and may produce pelvic venous thrombosis. Fatal pulmonary embolism may follow. Septic emboli are usually from the uterine, ovarian, or iliac veins. Partial liquefaction of the infected thrombus creates showers of bacteria-laden emboli. Although the lungs are almost always involved, secondary abscesses may occur in the brain or the heart, or a mycotic aneurysm may develop in one of the great vessels.

Phlebothrombosis is coagulation of blood in the veins without apparent antecedent inflammation. The clot is usually loosely adherent and causes incomplete occlusion. When thrombosis of a vein is secondary to inflammation of the wall of the vein, the condition is known as **thrombophlebitis.** This pathologic difference has little significance so far as the management is concerned because both disorders can cause pulmonary embolism. Superficial thrombophlebitis is the most common venous thrombosis associated with pregnancy. It usually occurs in varicose veins in the calf and is most frequent after delivery. Deep vein thrombophlebitis may be a sequela of the superficial form; this is an ominous condition. It is more common during the third trimester and the first few days of the puerperium.

Clinical Findings

A. SYMPTOMS AND SIGNS

Superficial thrombophlebitis is suspected when an erythematous tender, firm cordlike superficial vein is palpated. Clinical diagnosis of deep vein thrombophlebitis is neither sensitive nor specific; the false-positive rate is as high as 50%. Most deep vein thrombi are completely asymptomatic. Symptoms may be subtle or classic, depending upon the site and extent of the thrombus and the status of the collateral venous circulation. Classic features include swelling of the affected site of the legs, pain, tenderness, local cyanosis, and fever. These features are common if the proximal veins are involved. Pain in the calf muscle with dorsiflexion of the foot on the affected leg (**Homans' sign**) has little value in diagnosis. Moreover, embolic risk cannot be correlated with the severity of the pain. Most patients with pulmonary emboli do not have prior evidence of venous thrombosis. Iliofemoral venous thrombophlebitis causes acute swelling in the leg, pain above the hip, tenderness over the femoral triangle, and vaginal bleeding.

B. DIAGNOSTIC STUDIES

Ideally, the diagnosis should be objectively confirmed prior to initiation of treatment. Objective tests may be noninvasive (eg, Doppler ultrasound) or invasive (eg, venography). There are limitations to both the performance and interpretation of the objective tests, eg, an antepartum venogram exposes the fetus to radiation. The safest method of diagnosing venous thrombosis in pregnancy is use of impedance plethysmography, Doppler ultrasonography, and limited venography.

1. **Impedance plethysmography**—Impedance plethysmography measures the volume changes within the veins of the leg. Thrombotic and nonthrombotic occlusions cannot be differentiated by this method. The pressure by the gravid uterus on the common iliac vein or inferior vena cava (particularly after 20 weeks' gestation) can produce false-positive results. A normal result excludes proximal venous thrombosis but does not exclude calf vein thrombosis.

2. **Directional Doppler ultrasound**—Directional Doppler ultrasound can detect the presence or absence of venous flow. Damping of pulsatile flow is consistent with nonocclusive thrombus. This test is also insensitive to calf vein thrombosis and could be influenced by the pressure of the gravid uterus on the pelvic veins. Real-time sonography coupled with duplex and color Doppler ultrasound have been found to be useful in the diagnosis of deep venous thrombosis of the lower extremities, but its role in the evaluation of pelvic vein thrombosis is less clear. During pregnancy thrombosis frequently originates in the iliac veins. Magnetic resonance imaging allows for excellent delineation of anatomic detail above the inguinal ligaments, and phase images can be used to diagnose the presence or absence of flow in the pelvic veins. Computed tomographic scanning requires contrast agent and ionizing radiation, and is therefore avoided in favor of magnetic resonance imaging.

3. **Venography**—Venography allows the entire lower extremity, including the external and common iliac veins, to be evaluated. It is the most definitive method for diagnosis of venous thrombosis. Unfortunately, 1–2% of patients develop clinically significant phlebitis following venography. This risk can be minimized by flushing the dye with saline and elevating the legs. If the pelvic veins are not well visualized by ascending venography, femoral venography should be done. The abdomen must be shielded during venography.

4. **^{125}I-fibrinogen scanning**—^{125}I-fibrinogen is absorbed by the thrombus following intravenous injection. A hand-held probe is placed over the affected area. Unbound ^{125}I-fibrinogen scanning is contraindicated during pregnancy and breastfeeding. Leg scanning should not be used when proximal vein thrombosis (iliac or femoral vein) is suspected.

Prevention

The indications for preventive therapy include previous documented deep vein thrombosis or pulmonary embolism or antithrombin III deficiency. Heparin is the drug of choice; give 5000–7500 U subcutaneously twice a day during the first and second trimesters. Around the beginning of the third trimester, increase the dosage by approximately one-third to provide additional anticoagulation for the increased coagulation factors in late pregnancy. Prophylaxis should be stopped with the onset of labor and started again following delivery and continued for at least 2 weeks.

Treatment

A. SUPERFICIAL VENOUS THROMBOPHLEBITIS

Treatment of superficial venous thrombophlebitis consists of elevation of the involved leg and local application of moist heat. In resistant cases in nonpregnant patients, nonsteroidal anti-inflammatory agents may be used, but these should be avoided in pregnant women after 30 weeks' gestation because they may cause premature closure of the ductus arteriosus in the fetus. In high-risk patients with varicose veins, custom-made support panty hose should be worn.

B. DEEP VEIN THROMBOSIS

1. **Heparin**—Heparin is the drug of choice. It is a naturally occurring, negatively charged polysaccharide with an average molecular weight of 16,000 found in the mast cells of most mammals. It is effective intravenously or subcutaneously. It exerts its anticoagulant effect in the presence of a plasma cofactor, antithrombin III. The activity of antithrombin III is markedly increased by heparin.

Heparin may be given by continuous intravenous infusion; an initial loading dose of 5000 U is followed by 25,000–30,000 U given over a 24-hour period.

Heparin may also be given subcutaneously, 15,000 U twice daily. With intermittent intravenous infusion, 5000 U is given every 4 hours. For prevention of post-operative thrombosis, 5000 U of heparin is given subcutaneously 2 hours before surgery; this dose should be repeated 12 hours after operation and then twice daily until the patient is ambulatory. The anticoagulant action of heparin occurs within 10–15 minutes of injection, but the effect disappears in about 2 hours.

Tests used to monitor heparin therapy include coagulation time, activated partial thromboplastin time, thrombin clotting time, and heparin assay. Heparin should not be given if the platelet count is below 50,000/μL. The partial thromboplastin time should be 1.5–2 times the control value during heparin therapy.

The major side effect is bleeding in about 5% of cases. Other complications include thrombocytopenia, osteoporosis, and fat necrosis. Protamine sulfate is the antidote for heparin. Protamine, 1 mg per 100 U of heparin, will quickly shorten the partial thromboplastin time. Care must be taken not to give too much protamine, since it can induce bleeding.

The more recent availability of low-molecular-weight heparin has provided an attractive alternative to traditional unfractionated heparin for thromboprophylaxis and treatment of venous thrombosis and thromboembolism. Low molecular weight heparin does not cross the placenta and in not teratogenic, similarly to unfractionated heparin. However, it has a longer half-life and bioavailability, a more predictable dose-response relationship, and decreased risk of thrombocytopenia and hemorrhagic complications when compared to traditional heparin. Because of these characteristics, low-molecular-weight heparin may be administered subcutaneously once or twice daily without laboratory monitoring. Widespread use of low-molecular-weight heparin may be limited, however, by its cost, which exceeds that of unfractionated heparin by about 4–6 times.

2. Oral anticoagulants—Oral anticoagulants such as warfarin, a coumarin derivative, are usually contraindicated during pregnancy and breastfeeding. The teratogenic effects of warfarin (warfarin embryopathy) include nasal hypoplasia, skeletal abnormalities, and multiple central nervous system abnormalities. Fetal and placental bleeding leading to intrauterine fetal demise has been described with the use of warfarin. Its therapeutic effect depends on its ability to inhibit the action of vitamin K. The usual dose of warfarin is 10–15 mg/d until the therapeutic level of prothrombin time is achieved (1.5–2.5 times the control value). Thereafter, a maintenance dose is given based on prothrombin time, which should be checked twice daily. Vitamin K_1 (phytonadione), 5 mg given intravenously, is the specific antidote for warfarin.

SEPTIC PELVIC THROMBOPHLEBITIS

Septic pelvic thrombophlebitis is clotting in the veins of the pelvis due to infection. This may occur following vaginal or cesarean delivery. Predisposing factors include cesarean section after a long labor, premature rupture of the membranes, difficult delivery, anemia, malnourishment, and systemic disease. Septic pelvic thrombophlebitis occurs in 1 in 2000 deliveries. The pathologic process involves bacterial invasion of the intimal lining of the veins. The clotting process is initiated by the damaged intima, and the clot is invaded by microorganisms. Suppuration follows, with liquefaction, fragmentation, and finally, septic embolization. Thirty to 40% of untreated patients will have septic pulmonary emboli.

Clinical Findings

Both the uterine and ovarian veins are involved, as well as the common iliac, hypogastric, and vaginal veins and the inferior vena cava. The ovarian vein is the most common site (40% of cases). The onset may be as early as 2–3 days postpartum or as late as 6 weeks following delivery. The condition is suspected when fever persists in the puerperium in spite of adequate antibiotic therapy for aerobic and anaerobic organisms and there is no other discernible cause of fever. A picket-fence fever curve with wide swings from normal to as high as 41 °C (105.8 °F) is seen in 90% of cases. The pulse rate is rapid and sustained in most cases. The respiratory rate is increased, but there is no indication of pulmonary disease. There are no typical x-ray signs, because the emboli are small, multiple, and infected, but around 46% of cases show some x-ray abnormality due to abscess or infarct. The pelvic examination may be normal; however, hard, tender, wormlike thrombosed veins are palpable in the vaginal fornices or in one or both parametrial areas in about 30% of cases. Abdominal examination may occasionally reveal thrombosed ovarian veins. A temperature spike may be noted following examination because of disturbance of infected pelvic veins; this may be considered one diagnostic indication. Resolution of fever with heparin anticoagulation will help in the presumptive diagnosis. Blood for culture should be drawn during fever spikes; cultures are positive more than 35% of the time.

Differential Diagnosis

The differential diagnosis includes pyelonephritis, meningitis, systemic lupus erythematosus, tuberculosis, malaria, typhoid, sickle cell crisis, appendicitis, and torsion of the adnexa.

Treatment

Heparin and broad-spectrum antibiotics should be given (eg, penicillin and gentamicin with clindamycin or metronidazole; ampicillin may be added to clindamycin and gentamicin to cover enterococci). Within 48–72 hours of initiation of heparin therapy, fever should resolve. Heparin should be continued for 7–10 days.

■ PULMONARY DISORDERS

ASPIRATION PNEUMONITIS

Aspiration of gastric contents is the most common cause of maternal death due to anesthetic complications. With superimposed infection, mortality rates are even higher. In 1946, Curtis Mendelson showed that 96% of 66 cases of aspiration involved acidic gastric contents. The primary causative factor in aspiration pneumonitis is the acidity of the aspirate; a pH less than 2.5 is required to produce clinical manifestations.

Predisposing factors for aspiration include recent ingestion of food, delayed gastric emptying, relaxation of the gastroesophageal sphincter, raised intragastric pressure, use of general anesthesia, and a less experienced anesthesiologist.

Clinical Findings

The pathologic mechanism and clinical manifestations of aspiration pneumonitis will depend on the volume and composition of the aspirate. Aspiration of solid particulate matter may occlude parts of the tracheobronchial tree, causing collapse of the lungs. Aspiration of liquid material will produce cyanosis, tachycardia, dyspnea, and expiratory wheezing. The patient will be hypoxic, hypercapnic, and acidotic. The chest x-ray reveals interstitial pulmonary edema. With aspiration of acidic material, such a clinical picture may be delayed.

Prevention

If one considers the high rate of maternal death associated with aspiration pneumonitis, every effort should be made to prevent this catastrophic condition. Oral intake during labor must be prohibited. All anesthetized obstetric patients should be intubated, and regional anesthesia should be used as often as possible during labor and delivery. Any method that effectively reduces the volume of gastric contents to less than 25 mL or raises the gastric pH to more than 2.5 reduces the risk. Antacids must be given for resorption and buffering of acids and to inhibit further gastric acid production. Administration of 30 mL of nonparticulate systemic alkalizer, a mixture of sodium citrate and citric acid, effectively neutralizes gastric acidity. It should be given every 3 hours and 1 hour prior to elective cesarean section. The physician administering a regional block should also have expertise in intubation and ventilation.

Treatment

If aspiration occurs during anesthesia, immediate intubation and suction of the trachea should be carried out, followed at once by ventilation with oxygen. The patient should be turned onto her right side. Bronchoscopic suction should be done as soon as possible if solid material has been aspirated. A chest x-ray should be taken and blood gas determinations made; these may be repeated periodically. Arterial oxygenation is improved by decreasing the intrapulmonary shunt, and ventilation-perfusion inequalities are improved with positive end-expiratory pressure, which expands collapsed and fluid-filled airways, thereby increasing the functional residual capacity. If the gastric fluid sample has a pH of less than 3.0, the patient should be treated with endotracheal intubation, sedatives, muscle relaxants, and ventilation. If the gastric fluid pH is more than 3.0 and the patient appears to be well oxygenated, she may be followed carefully with periodic chest x-rays and blood gas determinations. The use of corticosteroids and prophylactic broad-spectrum antibiotics is debatable. Gram-stained smears and cultures of the tracheal aspirate should be taken daily, and antibiotics should be given when clinical evidence and culture indicate bacterial pneumonitis.

BRONCHIAL ASTHMA

Asthma is obstructive disease of the large or small airways. It may reverse spontaneously or may require treatment. It is the most common form of obstructive lung disease in pregnancy (0.4–1.3% of pregnancies). Fortunately, severe asthma (status asthmaticus, persistent or recurring asthma) occurs in only a few pregnancies.

Etiology

Based on the etiology, there are several types of asthma.

A. EXTRINSIC ASTHMA

Extrinsic asthma is IgE-mediated. The symptoms of bronchospasm are triggered shortly after inhalation of a specific allergen (eg, ragweed pollen).

B. INTRINSIC ASTHMA

Intrinsic asthma occurs when no specific allergens can be detected.

C. Mixed Asthma

Mixed asthma occurs when both IgE-mediated and non-IgE-mediated factors are present.

D. Aspirin-Intolerant Asthma

Aspirin-intolerant asthma occurs when aspirin and other nonsteroidal anti-inflammatory drugs inhibit prostaglandin synthesis, thereby precipitating bronchospasm.

E. Exercise-Induced Asthma

Asthma induced by exercise occurs when patients who are asymptomatic develop bronchospasm soon after a period of exercise.

F. Occupational Asthma

Persons exposed to allergens on the job may develop occupational asthma.

The course of asthma in pregnancy is unpredictable; disease may improve, remain the same, or worsen. Increased circulating free cortisol, decreased bronchomotor tone and airway resistance, and increased serum levels of cyclic AMP could each be responsible for the improvement of asthma in pregnancy. Exposure to fetal antigens, alterations in cell-mediated immunity (with an increase in viral upper respiratory tract infections), and hyperventilation could precipitate or worsen bronchospasm. In a study of more than 1000 pregnant asthmatics, 48% had no change, 29% improved, and 23% deteriorated. The changes in the course of asthma that women attribute to pregnancy generally revert to the prepregnant course in the 3 months postpartum. It is also interesting to note that the course in a particular patient during a pregnancy tends to repeat in her future pregnancies. Upper respiratory tract infection appears to be the most common precipitating factor of severe asthma during pregnancy.

Mild asthma imposes little, if any, risk to the mother and fetus. Severe asthma is associated with increased perinatal mortality and morbidity rates related to hypoxemia, alkalosis, reduced uterine blood flow, and teratogenic effects of drugs used for treatment. A slightly increased incidence of prematurity and low birthweight has been suggested in severe cases of asthma, but the cause-and-effect relationship is not clear.

Complications

Acute complications include physical exhaustion, progressive hypoxemia or hypercarbia, atelectasis, pneumothorax, pneumomediastinum, pulsus paradoxus, and drug hypersensitivity reactions. Chronic complications are pulmonary emphysema and cor pulmonale.

Treatment

A. General Measures

The general principles of management for pregnant asthmatic patients are similar to those for nonpregnant patients. The following steps should be taken:

1. Prevent exposure to known allergens.
2. Treat sinusitis.
3. Avoid antiprostaglandin drugs (eg, aspirin) in aspirin-intolerant asthma.
4. Avoid strenuous exercise and exposure to cold.
5. Treat viral infections rigorously.
6. Treat reflux esophagitis to avoid induction of bronchospasm.
7. Stop cigarette smoking.
8. Depending on the severity of disease, give a prophylactic short course of prednisone, 30–50 mg/d for 4–7 days, at the onset of a viral upper respiratory tract infection. This often prevents the need for emergency management of asthma.

B. Acute Exacerbations

The patient must be hospitalized. Oxygen may be administered by mask or nasal catheter. Correction of dehydration and electrolyte imbalance is achieved by adequate intravenous fluids. Blood gas determinations are mandatory. Inhaled β_2 agonists (albuterol or metaproterenol) have become the agents of choice to treat acute exacerbations of asthma. Treatments can be repeated every 20–30 minutes unless adverse side effects occur. Subcutaneous terbutaline can be used in place of inhaled agents, but inhalation therapy is favored. Hydrocortisone sodium succinate or equivalent is given intravenously every 2–4 hours as necessary if the exacerbation is severe. If the patient fails to improve clinically with the previous measures and there is evidence of progressive hypoxemia and hypercapnia, intubation and controlled ventilatory assistance may be required.

C. Interim Therapy

The main drugs used in long-term management of asthma include methylxanthines, β-adrenergic agonists, glucocorticoids, and cromolyn sodium. The methylxanthines, anhydrous theophylline and aminophylline, are widely used drugs. β-Adrenergic agonists such as terbutaline can be used for asthma uncontrolled with chronic theophylline. If wheezing persists despite these medications and other diagnoses are unlikely, a short course of prednisone may be indicated to reverse ongoing asthma. Cromolyn sodium or beclomethasone dipropionate by inhalation may be instituted once the acute episode has resolved.

Medications should generally be added one by one until adequate control is achieved. It is important to maintain a high index of suspicion for bacterial respiratory infections during pregnancy, particularly for bacterial sinusitis, which has been estimated to be 6 times more common during pregnancy.

Allergic immunotherapy is effective for allergic rhinitis and possibly for allergic asthma. It may be continued during pregnancy, but caution should be exercised to reduce the risk of anaphylaxis.

Cough preparations with iodides and dextromethorphan should be avoided because of the risks of fetal goiter and malformation, respectively. Antihistamines should be avoided during the first trimester. Pseudoephedrine decongestants can be used when necessary.

D. Management of Labor and Delivery

Vaginal delivery is best for asthmatic patients unless obstetric indications demand cesarean section. During normal labor, minute ventilation can approach or exceed 20 L/min; therefore, the therapeutic goal should be stable pulmonary function without bronchospasm. For patients who have received systemic or inhaled corticosteroids during pregnancy, hydrocortisone, 100 mg intravenously, is given immediately and every 8 hours until delivery has occurred. Paracervical, pudendal, or epidural block is preferable to general anesthesia. Meperidine, 50–100 mg given intramuscularly, usually will relieve bronchospasm while providing adequate pain relief.

TUBERCULOSIS

Tuberculosis in adults is a disease of the pulmonary parenchyma caused by *Mycobacterium tuberculosis,* a nonmotile, acid-fast aerobic rod. Foci of infection are usually widespread, with dissemination occurring early in the course of disease, before sites are walled off by granulomatous inflammation. In the early 1900s, tuberculosis was the leading cause of death in the United States (200 deaths per 100,000 persons per year). As therapy has steadily improved, the incidence of disease progressively declined until recently when the disease made a startling comeback in the underprivileged.

Clinical Findings

Most cases of tuberculosis (77%) can be diagnosed on the basis of a history of cough and weight loss, positive tuberculin skin test, and chest x-ray.

A. Symptoms and Signs

Typical symptoms include cough, weight loss, fatigue, and anorexia. Occasionally, patients are asymptomatic.

B. Laboratory Findings

Laboratory studies are needed for definitive diagnosis. Ziehl-Neelsen staining should be performed. *M. tuber-*

culosis can be distinguished from other organisms by culture (production of niacin in vitro).

C. Tuberculin Skin Test

The tuberculin skin test is the most important screening test for tuberculosis. It should be performed early in pregnancy, especially in high-risk populations. The test is positive with induration at the test site of 10 mm or more.

D. Chest X-Ray

Chest x-ray is not done routinely in pregnancy because of risk to the fetus. With the abdomen shielded, a chest x-ray should be taken in patients in whom skin testing is positive following an earlier negative test and in patients with a suggestive history or physical examination even though skin testing is negative.

E. Congenital Tuberculosis

Congenital tuberculosis is rare. The criteria for diagnosis include positive bacteriologic studies, primary disease complex in the liver, disease occurring within the first few days of life, and exclusion of extrauterine infection. The most common signs are nonspecific, including fever, failure to thrive, lymphadenopathy, hepatomegaly, and splenomegaly. Disease is usually miliary or disseminated. Effective treatment depends on early diagnosis.

Treatment

A. Medical Therapy

Treatment of active tuberculosis during pregnancy is only slightly different from that in nonpregnant patients. A year-long course of isoniazid is given to those with a positive skin test and no radiologic or symptomatic evidence of active disease. Such therapy perhaps could be withheld during pregnancy and started in the postpartum period, although most studies have shown no teratogenic effects of isoniazid. Immigrants and refugees who have received bacillus Calmette-Guérin (BCG) vaccine for prevention of tuberculosis still need chemoprophylaxis if the skin test is positive.

Active tuberculosis should be treated with a 2-drug regimen, usually isoniazid, 5 mg/kg/d (total of 300 mg/d), and ethambutol, 15 mg/kg/d, continued for at least 18 months to prevent relapse. Two-drug regimens are not recommended if isoniazid resistance is suspected. If a third drug or a more potent drug is necessary due to extensive or severe disease, rifampin could be added. Because of the risk of ototoxicity, streptomycin should not be used. Isoniazid has many therapeutic advantages (eg, high efficacy, patient acceptability, and low cost) and appears to be the safest drug during pregnancy.

The major side effects of isoniazid are hepatitis, hypersensitivity reactions, peripheral neuropathy, and gastrointestinal distress. A baseline liver function test should be obtained and then repeated periodically. *Pyridoxine, 50 mg/d, should be administered to prevent isoniazid-induced neuritis due to vitamin B_6 deficiency.* Optic neuritis has been the rare complication described with use of ethambutol. Rifampin may cause hepatitis, hypersensitivity reactions, occasional hematologic toxicity, a flulike syndrome, abdominal pain, acute renal failure, and thrombocytopenia. The role of rifampin in congenital malformations is not clear. Limb reduction defect in the neonate has been suspected, but the number of pregnancies studied is too small for any conclusions to be drawn.

B. OBSTETRIC MANAGEMENT

Routine antepartum obstetric management includes adequate rest, nutritious diet, family support, correction of anemia, and appropriate follow-up.

Immediate neonatal contact is allowed if the mother has received treatment for inactive disease and there is no evidence of reactivation. In cases of inactive disease for which prophylactic isoniazid was not given or of active disease for which adequate treatment was given, early neonatal contact may be allowed, provided the mother is reliable in continuing therapy. A mother with active disease should receive at least 3 weeks of treatment before coming into contact with her baby, and the baby must also receive prophylactic isoniazid.

There are no absolute contraindications to breastfeeding once the mother is noninfectious. Although antituberculosis drugs are found in breast milk, the concentrations are so low that the risk of toxicity in the infant is minimal. However, each case should be judged individually if the mother wishes to breastfeed her infant.

Immunization of the newborn with BCG vaccine remains controversial. If prompt use of isoniazid as prophylaxis is unlikely or if the mother has isoniazid-resistant disease, BCG vaccination of the infant should be considered.

Prognosis

If the pregnant patient is adequately treated with antitubercular chemotherapy for active disease, tuberculosis generally has no deleterious effect on the course of pregnancy or the puerperium or on the fetus. Pregnant women have the same prognosis as nonpregnant women. Therapeutic abortion is no longer recommended for most tuberculosis patients.

■ RENAL & URINARY TRACT DISORDERS

For a discussion of renal and urinary tract function in normal pregnancy, see Chapter 7.

URINARY TRACT INFECTION

Asymptomatic bacteriuria, acute cystitis, and acute pyelonephritis are common renal disorders in pregnancy.

Asymptomatic Bacteriuria

Asymptomatic bacteriuria is defined as the presence of actively multiplying bacteria in the urinary tract excluding the distal urethra in a patient without any obvious symptoms. The incidence during pregnancy is 2–7%. Asymptomatic bacteriuria is twice as common in pregnant women with sickle cell trait and 3 times as common in pregnant women with diabetes as in normal pregnant women. If asymptomatic bacteriuria is untreated in pregnancy, about 25–30% of women will develop acute pyelonephritis. With treatment, the rate is only 10%. The diagnosis of asymptomatic bacteriuria is based upon isolation of microorganisms with a colony count of more than 10^5 organisms per milliliter of urine in 2 consecutive clean-catch specimens. The patient should be instructed to clean the vulvar area from front to back to avoid contamination of the urine sample. *Escherichia coli* is the most common offending organism for asymptomatic bacteriuria (about 80% of cases). The *Klebsiella-Enterobacter-Serratia* family and *Proteus* are responsible for the remainder of cases. Acute cystitis is rare in pregnancy (about 1%).

Acute Cystitis

The bacterial flora in acute cystitis are similar to those in asymptomatic bacteriuria. Clinically, the patient will present with symptoms of urinary frequency, urgency, dysuria, and suprapubic discomfort. An acute febrile illness with nausea, vomiting, and chills is usually absent. The characteristic cloudy, malodorous urine should be cultured for confirmation of the diagnosis.

Acute Pyelonephritis

Acute pyelonephritis occurs in 1–2% of all pregnant women (usually, although not invariably, in those with previous asymptomatic bacteriuria) and is associated with risk to the mother and fetus. Maternal effects include fever, bacterial endotoxemia, endotoxic shock, renal dysfunction leading to acute renal failure, leukocytosis, thrombocytopenia, and elevated fibrin split products. There is an increased incidence of anemia; this may be due to marrow suppression, increased erythrocyte destruction, or diminished red cell production. Pulmonary dysfunction has been described in association with acute pyelonephritis; symptoms and signs may range from minimal (mild cough and slight pulmonary infiltrate) to severe (acute respiratory distress syndrome requiring intensive therapy). Neonatal effects include prematurity and small-for-gestational-age babies.

Clinical manifestations of acute pyelonephritis include fever, shaking chills and flank pain, nausea and vomiting, headache, increased urinary frequency, and dysuria. Urine examination will reveal significant bacteriuria, with pyuria and white blood cell casts in the urinary sediment. A count of 1–2 bacteria per high-power field in unspun urine or more than 20 bacteria in the sediment of a centrifuged specimen of urine collected by bladder catheterization will help in the bedside diagnosis. The diagnosis should be confirmed by culture of urine. Associated hematuria may indicate urinary calculi.

Treatment

A midstream urine specimen should be collected for culture at the initial prenatal visit and repeated later in pregnancy. At each prenatal visit, dipstick testing should be done, and if proteinuria is present, urinalysis, culture, or both should be done. A pregnant woman with sickle cell trait should have urine culture and sensitivity testing every 4 weeks. Pregnant women should be encouraged to maintain adequate fluid intake and to void frequently.

The initial antibiotic selection should be empiric. Based on the fact that the most common offending pathogen is *E. coli,* sulfonamides, nitrofurantoin, ampicillin, or cephalosporins could be selected. These antibiotics should be safe for the mother and fetus, with minimal side effects. A 10- to 14-day course of one of these agents will effectively eradicate asymptomatic bacteriuria in about 65% of pregnant patients. Culture of urine should be done 1–2 weeks after therapy is begun and then monthly for the remainder of pregnancy.

Sulfa drugs must be avoided in mothers with glucose-6-phophatase deficiency. Additionally, sulfa drugs are best avoided late in pregnancy because of the increased likelihood of neonatal hyperbilirubinemia. Trimethoprim is a folic acid antagonist, so trimethoprim-sulfamethoxazole should be avoided in pregnancy. Nitrofurantoin should be avoided at term or before (when labor is imminent) because it may induce hemolytic anemia in the newborn.

Any woman with acute pyelonephritis in pregnancy should be admitted to the hospital for therapy. Antibiotics should be given parenterally and dehydration corrected. Antipyretic agents are given where indicated, and vital signs and urinary output are closely monitored. Ampicillin or a cephalosporin is usually administered intravenously in doses of 1–2 g every 6 hours.

If there is no appropriate response in 48–72 hours, an aminoglycoside (eg, gentamicin or tobramycin, 3–5 mg/kg/24 h in 3 divided doses) is administered. With persistent flank pain and fever despite proper therapy, perinephric abscess must be ruled out with ultrasound examination. This is generally a complication of obstruction associated with infection. With confirmation of the diagnosis, the abscess must be drained to avoid maternal death. An intravenous pyelogram may also be useful in evaluating patients who do not improve despite adequate therapy. A preliminary film and a 15-minute film are usually adequate for the diagnosis of urinary tract obstruction. In selected cases of persistent infection, cystoscopy and retrograde pyelographic studies may be useful.

Cunningham noted that 28% of women with pyelonephritis developed recurrent bacteriuria and 10% had recurrent acute pyelonephritis during the same pregnancy. Such women should be given long-term prophylactic treatment. Nitrofurantoin, 100 mg every night, has been suggested, although the efficacy of such therapy is questionable.

Periodic culture of the urine will assist in detecting recurrence. Relapse is defined as recurrent infection due to the same species and type-specific strain of organism present before treatment; this represents a treatment failure. Most relapses occur less than 2 weeks after completion of therapy. Reinfection is recurrent infection due to a different strain of bacteria following successful treatment of the initial infection, occurring more than 3 weeks after completion of therapy.

URINARY CALCULI

The incidence of urinary calculi is not altered by pregnancy (overall incidence is 0.24% [1 in 425 persons]). This condition predisposes pregnant women to urinary tract infection, recurrent hospitalization, premature labor, and operative intervention. The causes of urinary calculi in pregnant women are the same as in nonpregnant women, ie, chronic urinary tract infection, hyperparathyroidism, congenital or familial cystinuria (or oxaluria), gout, and obstructive uropathy. Most stones are composed of calcium, and they are more common as pregnancy progresses, being rare during the first trimester. Although physiologic hydroureter is more pronounced on the right side, stones occur with equal frequency in both tracts.

Clinical Findings

Patients may present with a variety of symptoms, including classic renal or ureteric colic or vague abdominal or back pain. The differential diagnosis must include other acute abdominal conditions, ie, acute appendicitis, biliary colic, adnexal torsion, preterm labor, and placental abruption. The patient may present with fever, bacteriuria, flank pain, and nausea and vomiting suggestive of acute pyelonephritis. The persistence of fever after 48 hours of parenteral antibiotics is strongly suggestive of urinary tract obstruction with calculus. Although hematuria (varying from gross to microhematuria) may be present, it is not always pathognomonic of calcular disease. A high index of suspicion will help in the diagnosis, particularly in cases with negative culture of urine in suspected pyelonephritis, persistent hematuria, and recurrent urinary tract infection.

Clinical diagnosis may be difficult. In most cases, diagnostic imaging is necessary. For preliminary screening, an ultrasonic examination could be useful. In selected cases, excretory urography (a single film taken 20 minutes after infusion) should be done. This exposes the fetus to only 0.2 rad.

Treatment

Treatment consists of admission to the hospital, hydration, culture of urine, appropriate intravenous antibiotic therapy, correction of electrolyte imbalance, and analgesics. Fortunately, most stones are passed spontaneously. Surgical intervention (ureteral stenting, cystoscopic extraction, open surgery) will be needed in a few cases with persistent severe pain, infection not responding to antibiotics, and obstructive uropathy.

ACUTE RENAL FAILURE

Acute renal failure in pregnancy is rare but carries a high mortality rate and therefore must be prevented where possible and treated aggressively. Most cases are due to acute hypovolemia. Clinically, acute renal failure is a condition in which the kidneys are temporarily unable to perform their excretory and regulatory functions. Urine output is usually less than 40 mL/24 h, and blood urea nitrogen and serum creatinine levels are elevated. Acute renal failure during pregnancy may result in abortion, low birthweight, premature labor, and stillbirth. Hypotension and vaginal hemorrhage may occur during dialysis, although successful outcomes without adverse effects have been reported.

Based on the cause, acute renal failure may be classified as prerenal, renal, or postrenal. In the prerenal type, acute renal failure occurs due to renal hypoperfusion secondary to maternal hypovolemia (eg, hemorrhage, dehydration, abruptio placentae, septicemia), circulating nephrotoxins (eg, aminoglycosides), mismatched blood transfusion, preeclampsia-eclampsia, disseminated intravascular coagulation, and hypoxemia (eg, chronic lung disease and heart failure). In the renal type, a variety of intrinsic renal diseases such as acute glomerulonephritis, acute pyelonephritis, and amyloidosis are responsible for acute renal failure. The postrenal type is caused by urinary obstruction from ureteric stone, retroperitoneal tumor, or other diseases. Bilateral ureteral obstruction due to polyhydramnios is fortunately rare.

The state of renal hypoperfusion is reversible within 24–36 hours with volume restoration and treatment of the precipitating factors. Acute tubular necrosis may develop following reduction of the outer cortical blood flow in the absence of such treatment. The most serious condition arising secondary to acute renal failure is **acute cortical necrosis** in damaged glomerular capillaries and small kidney vessels. Acute cortical necrosis is rare but carries a poor prognosis; partial recovery may be anticipated in patients with patchy lesions.

Clinical Findings

The clinical course has been divided into an oliguric phase, a diuretic phase, and a recovery phase. In the oliguric phase, urine output drops below 30 mL/h, with accumulation of blood urea nitrogen and potassium. The patient becomes acidotic with the increase in hydrogen ion and loss of bicarbonate. In the diuretic phase, large volumes of dilute urine are passed, with loss of electrolytes due to absence of function of the renal tubules. As tubular function returns to normal in the recovery phase, the normal volume and composition of urine returns. Clinical manifestations and complications include anorexia, nausea and vomiting, lethargy, cardiac arrhythmia (secondary to electrolyte disturbance), anemia, renal or extrarenal infection, thrombocytopenia, metabolic acidosis, and electrolyte imbalance (hyperkalemia, hyponatremia, hypermagnesemia, hyperphosphatemia, hypocalcemia).

Infection in an operative site or the respiratory or urinary tract remains the main cause of death. Other causes of death include azotemia, pulmonary edema, and cardiac arrhythmia (induced by hyperkalemia).

Treatment

In obstetric practice, prevention of acute renal failure should be the aim, with appropriate volume replacement to maintain urine output of 60 mL/h or more. Proper management of high-risk obstetric conditions (eg, preeclampsia-eclampsia, abruptio placentae, chorioamnionitis), careful typing and cross-matching of blood, and avoidance of nephrotoxic antibiotics are also important.

Specific treatment includes the following:

A. EMERGENCY TREATMENT

Underlying causes of acute renal failure (eg, hemorrhagic shock) may require emergency treatment.

B. SURGICAL MEASURES

Surgical measures include determination of any obstructive uropathy or sepsis due to infected products of conception. Such problems should be treated appropriately.

C. ROUTINE MEASURES

Routine measures include achieving fluid and electrolyte balance. Fluid intake may be calculated from the urinary output, loss of fluid from other sources (eg, diarrhea, vomiting), and insensible loss of about 500 mL/d (correcting for fever may be necessary). Intake and output must be recorded carefully. The patient should be weighed daily and should maintain a constant weight or lose weight slowly (250 g/d, if one assumes a room temperature of 22–23 °C [71–73 °F]). Hyperkalemia is a significant problem that can be controlled by giving glucose and insulin. The diet should be high in calories, low in protein and electrolytes, and high in carbohydrates. Parenteral feeding may be given in cases of nausea and vomiting. Prophylactic antibiotics should not be used, but infections may be treated with antibiotics without renal toxicity. Indwelling bladder catheters are to be avoided.

D. DIALYSIS

Dialysis is indicated if serum potassium levels rise to 7 mEq/L or more, serum sodium levels are 130 mEq/L or less, the serum bicarbonate is 130 mEq/L or less, blood urea nitrogen levels are more than 120 mg/dL or there are daily increments of 30 mg/dL in patients with sepsis, and dialyzable poisons or toxins are present.

GLOMERULONEPHRITIS

Acute glomerulonephritis during pregnancy is rare. There is increased perinatal loss with this condition. The clinical course is variable during pregnancy. In some patients, the condition may resolve early in pregnancy, with return to normal renal function. These cases may be mistaken for preeclampsia. Microscopic hematuria with red blood cell casts, low serum complement, and a rising antistreptolysin O titer indicate acute glomerulonephritis. Treatment consists of control of blood pressure, prevention of congestive heart failure, administration of fluids and electrolytes, and close follow-up.

The outcome of pregnancy with chronic glomerulonephritis will depend on the degree of functional impairment of the kidneys, blood pressure levels prior to conception, and the exact histology of the glomerulonephritis. Patients are more likely to develop superimposed preeclampsia or hypertensive crisis earlier in pregnancy. Successful pregnancy should be anticipated, although renal function is expected to decrease. The incidence of fetal intrauterine growth retardation, premature labor, abruptio placentae, and intrauterine fetal demise is significantly high. Routine prenatal care must include periodic renal function tests, control of blood pressure, ultrasonic evaluation of fetal growth, and biophysical monitoring of fetal well-being. Early delivery is indicated after evaluation of pulmonary maturity with lecithin:sphingomyelin ratios and phosphatidylglycerol levels in amniotic fluid. Nephrotoxic drugs must be avoided, and acute renal failure should be anticipated, particularly during the postpartum period.

SOLITARY KIDNEY

A solitary kidney may be the result of developmental aberration or disease requiring removal of one kidney. A single kidney may be abnormally developed or it may be placed low, perhaps even within the true pelvis. A second small, virtually functionless kidney may not be discovered by the usual diagnostic tests. Anatomic and functional hypertrophy of the kidney usually occurs and is augmented by pregnancy. There is no medical contraindication to pregnancy with a solitary kidney. However, if infection occurs in a solitary kidney and does not respond to antibiotics quickly, consideration must be given to termination of the pregnancy to preserve renal function.

RENAL TRANSPLANTATION

Successful renal transplantation has not prevented pregnancy in the limited number of cases to date. Patients with adequate renal function prior to pregnancy will experience little if any deterioration in graft function during pregnancy. The likelihood of graft rejection during pregnancy remains the same as in nonpregnant graft recipients. The spontaneous abortion rate is not increased, but many patients choose to terminate the pregnancy. Pregnancy-induced hypertension occurs in about 30% of patients with renal transplant, and there is a 60% incidence of proteinuria in the third trimester.

The risk of infection is considerably higher during pregnancy in renal transplant patients. Primary or reactivated herpesvirus infection is a significant risk. The incidence of hepatitis B surface antigenemia has been noted to be about 50% among patients receiving dialysis.

Prematurity with its related complications, intrauterine growth restriction, and fetal abnormalities caused by immunosuppressive agents taken by the mother may occur. The route of delivery depends primarily on obstetric indications. A transplanted kidney in the false pelvis does not usually cause obstruction leading to dystocia. In patients with aseptic necrosis of the hip joints or other bony dystrophy secondary to long-term use of immunosuppressive agents, cesarean section may be required.

ECTOPIC KIDNEY

An ectopic kidney in the true pelvis with an aberrant blood supply may cause obstruction interfering with delivery. Cesarean section should be done in this situation with great caution to avoid injury to the kidney or its blood supply.

REFERENCES

Cardiovascular Disorders

Ayan A et al: Feto-maternal morbidity and mortality after cardiac valve replacement. Acta Obstet Gynecol Scand 2001;80:713.

Bernstein PS, Magriples U: Cardiomyopathy in pregnancy: a retrospective study. Am J Perinatol 2001;18:163.

Chan WS: What is the optimal management of pregnant women with valvular heart disease in pregnancy? Haemostasis 1999;29(Suppl S1):105.

Cole WC et al: Peripartum cardiomyopathy: echocardiogram to predict prognosis. Tenn Med 2001;94:135.

Connolly HM, Grogan M, Warnes CA: Pregnancy among women with congenitally corrected transposition of great arteries. J Am Coll Cardiol 1999;33:1692.

Dajani AS et al: Prevention of bacterial endocarditis. Recommendations by the American Heart Association. JAMA 1997; 277:1794.

Easterling TR et al: Treatment of hypertension in pregnancy: effect of atenolol on maternal disease, preterm delivery, and fetal growth. Obstet Gynecol 2001;98:427.

Elkayam U et al: Maternal and fetal outcomes of subsequent pregnancies in women with peripartum cardiomyopathy. N Engl J Med 2001;344:1567.

Gei AF, Hankins GD: Cardiac disease and pregnancy. Obstet Gynecol Clin North Am 2001;28:465.

Joglar JA, Page RL: Antiarrhythmic drugs in pregnancy. Curr Opin Cardiol 2001;16:40.

Kansaria JJ, Salvi VS: Eisenmenger syndrome in pregnancy. J Postgrad Med 2000;46:101.

Ramsey PS, Ramin KD, Ramin SM: Cardiac disease in pregnancy. Am J Perinatol 2001;18:245.

Siu SC, Cofman JM: Heart disease and pregnancy. Heart 2001; 85:710.

Smith GC, Pell JP, Walsh D: Pregnancy complications and maternal risk of ischaemic heart disease: a retrospective cohort study of 129,290 births. Lancet 2001;357:2002.

Therrien J, Barnes I, Somerville J: Outcome of pregnancy in patients with congenitally corrected transposition of the great arteries. Am J Cardiol 1999;84:820.

Veille JC, Zaccaro D: Peripartum cardiomyopathy: summary of an international survey on peripartum cardiomyopathy. Am J Obstet Gynecol 1999;181:315.

Weiss BM, Hess OM: Pulmonary vascular disease and pregnancy: current controversies, management strategies, and perspectives. Eur Heart J 2000;21:104.

Hematologic Disorders

Alfirevic Z et al: Postnatal screening for thrombophilia in women with severe pregnancy complications. Obstet Gynecol 2001; 97:753.

American College of Obstetricians and Gynecologists: Anticoagulation with low-molecular-weight heparin during pregnancy. ACOG Committee Opinion No. 211, November 1998.

American College of Obstetricians and Gynecologists: Thrombocytopenia in pregnancy. ACOG Practice Bulletin No. 6, September 1999.

Bazzan M, Donvito V: Low-molecular-weight heparin during pregnancy. Thromb Res 2001;101:V175.

Burlingame J et al: Maternal and fetal outcomes in pregnancies affected by von Willebrand disease type 2. Am J Obstet Gynecol 2001;184:229.

Burns MM: Emerging concepts in the diagnosis and management of venous thromboembolism during pregnancy. J Thromb Thrombolysis 2000;10:59.

Burrows RF: Platelet disorders in pregnancy. Curr Opin Obstet Gynecol 2001;13:115.

Choi JW, Pai SH: Change in erythropoiesis with gestational age during pregnancy. Ann Hematol 2001;80:26.

Greer IA: The challenge of thrombophilia in maternal-fetal medicine. N Engl J Med 2000;342:424.

Kadir RA: Women and inherited bleeding disorders: pregnancy and delivery. Semin Hematol 1999;36(3 Suppl 4):28.

Lockwood CJ: Heritable coagulopathies in pregnancy. Obstet Gynecol Surv 1999;54:754.

Nizzi FA Jr, Mues G: Hemorrhagic problems in obstetrics, exclusive of disseminated intravascular coagulation. Hematol Oncol Clin North Am 2000;14:1171.

Rai R, Regan L: Thrombophilia and adverse pregnancy outcome. Semin Reprod Med 2000;18:369.

Rand JH, Luong TH: Thrombophilias: diagnosis and treatment of thrombophilia relating to contraception and pregnancy. Semin Hematol 1999;36(3 Suppl 4):2.

Spina V, Aleandri V, Morini F: The impact of the factor V Leiden mutation in pregnancy. Hum Reprod Update 2000;6:301.

Sun PM et al: Sickle cell disease in pregnancy: twenty years of experience at Grady Memorial Hospital, Atlanta, Georgia. Am J Obstet Gynecol 2001;184:1127.

Ziong X et al: Anemia during pregnancy and birth outcome: a meta-analysis. Am J Perinatol 2000;17:137.

Pulmonary Disorders

American College of Obstetricians and Gynecologists: Pulmonary diseases in pregnancy. ACOG Technical Bulletin No. 224, June 1996.

De Swiet M: Management of pulmonary embolus in pregnancy. Eur Heart J 1999;20:1378.

Hershfield E: Tuberculosis: 9. Treatment. CMAJ 1999;161:405.

Riley LE: Pneumonia, tuberculosis, and urinary tract infections in pregnancy. Curr Clin Top Infect Dis 1999;19:181.

Renal & Urinary Tract Disorders

Chan WS, Okun N, Kjellstrand CM: Pregnancy in chronic dialysis: a review and analysis of the literature. Int J Artif Organs 1998;21:259.

Julkunen H: Renal lupus in pregnancy. Scand J Rheumatol 1998;107(Suppl):80.

Lauszus FF, Gron PL, Klebe JG: Pregnancies complicated by diabetic proliferative retinopathy. Acta Obstet Gynecol Scand 1998;77:814.

Nzerue CM, Hewan-Lowe K, Nwawka C: Acute renal failure in pregnancy: a review of clinical outcomes at an inner-city hospital from 1986–1996. JAMA 1998;90:486.

Wing DA: Pyelonephritis. Clin Obstet Gynecol 1998;41:515.

General Medical Disorders During Pregnancy

23

Dipika Dandade, MD, L. Wayne Hess, MD, Darla B. Hess, MD, FACC, FAHA, & John C. Morrison, MD

Medical complications of pregnancy may have adverse effects on the mother, fetus, and newborn. The physiologic changes that occur during a normal gestation may aggravate a maternal disease process. The diagnostic and therapeutic acumen of the physician, the severity of the disease, and the stage of gestation at which the complication occurs all have an impact on the outcome of pregnancy. The sum of these variables may cause the complication to improve, equilibrate, or deteriorate during pregnancy. Most of the common medical complications of pregnancy (such as anemia, which affects ~50% of all gestations in the United States) are relatively mild, do not usually affect the pregnancy, and can be managed by the obstetrician-gynecologist.

◾ DISORDERS OF THE NERVOUS SYSTEM

CEREBROVASCULAR DISORDERS

The causes of cerebrovascular disease include insufficiency (**arteriosclerosis, cerebral embolism, vasospasm from hypertensive disease**) and disorders associated with bleeding into the cerebral cortex (**arteriovenous malformation, ruptured aneurysm**). The brain becomes infarcted from lack of blood flow, or intracranial bleeding results in a space-occupying lesion. The severity of such disorders can be affected by blood pressure, oxygen saturation (anemia or polycythemia), hypoglycemia, and adequacy of collateral circulation.

The overall incidence of ischemic cerebrovascular accidents in pregnancy is approximately 1 in 20,000 births, with most occurring in the last trimester or immediately postpartum. Etiologic factors for stroke include cardioembolic disorders, cerebral angiopathies, hematologic disorders, and cerebral vein thrombosis. Causes exclusive to pregnancy are eclampsia, choriocarcinoma, and amniotic fluid embolism. Although cerebral ischemic disease can occur in either the arterial or

venous system, approximately 75% of occlusive cerebral disease is on the arterial side.

Cerebrovascular accidents involving subarachnoid hemorrhage or intraparenchymal hemorrhage similarly occur at a rate of 1 in 20,000 births. These are usually the result of aneurysms or arteriovenous malformations. The most common aneurysm is the saccular (berry) variety, which protrudes from the major arteries in the circle of Willis, particularly at its bifurcations. Aneurysms have an increasing tendency to bleed as the pregnancy progresses, likely due to changes in hemodynamic factors. Rupture of arteriovenous malformations have been found to occur evenly throughout gestation. No consensus has been reached regarding the increased frequency of bleeding from either an aneurysm or arteriovenous malformation during pregnancy or the immediate postpartum period. Rupture of the malformation does appear to be more frequent during pregnancy. Eclampsia can lead to cerebral hemorrhage when elevated blood pressures lead to vasospasm, loss of autoregulatory function, and rupture of the vessel wall.

Clinical Findings

Headaches, visual disturbances, syncope, and hemiparesis are among the most common presenting findings.

Diagnosis

The pattern of clinical signs and symptoms generally allows recognition of the area of the brain involved. CT scan and MRI can be employed in pregnancy to increase the delineation of cerebrovascular involvement. Ultrasonography may be helpful, particularly in hemorrhagic lesions. Arteriography is considered definitive if surgical intervention is being considered, since it can more precisely localize the involved area. Because coagulopathies can also cause intracranial bleeding or may be secondary to the cerebrovascular lesion itself, a coagulation profile should be performed. Additionally, ANA, lupus anticoagulant, factor V Leiden, homocysteine, anticardiolipin, proteins C and S, antithrombin 3, and plasminogen levels should be considered with thrombotic cerebral events.

Treatment

The treatment of ischemic or hemorrhagic cerebrovascular disease is best managed supportively; however, surgery is indicated for the treatment of some aneurysms and arteriovenous malformations. Anticoagulation with heparin may be required depending on the etiology of the infarction. Normalization of blood pressure, adequate respiratory support, therapy for metabolic complications, and treatment of coagulopathies or cardiac abnormalities are crucial. Dexamethasone, 10 mg intravenously initially, followed by 5 mg every 6 hours for 24 hours, may decrease cerebral edema and be of some assistance prior to surgery or in recovery. Additionally, hyperventilation, mannitol infusions, phenobarbital coma, and intracerebral pressure monitoring may be helpful with severe cerebral edema. Once the patient has been stabilized, physical therapy and rehabilitation should begin as soon as possible.

Appropriate surgery for aneurysms and arteriovenous malformations should be carried out with the pregnancy undisturbed unless fetal maturity allows for cesarean birth just prior to the neurosurgical procedure. On the other hand, inoperable lesions during pregnancy are managed by pregnancy conservation until fetal maturity is sufficient to allow abdominal birth. In addition, therapeutic abortion is an option in the first or second trimester. Once a lesion has been surgically corrected, vaginal delivery can be attempted. However, the second stage of labor should be modified by regional anesthesia and forceps delivery to reduce cerebral pressures associated with the Valsalva maneuver.

Complications & Prognosis

The percentage of patients with venous occlusion who recover from the initial episode without neurologic sequelae during rehabilitation is equal to that of patients with arterial occlusion. Thrombosis of the superior sagittal sinus is a rare complication. Its incidence is increased in pregnancy and has a high mortality rate of approximately 55%.

If the cerebral hemorrhagic disorder is operable, the prognosis is quite favorable, with few long-term neurologic deficits. In inoperable lesions or when severe maternal cerebral hemorrhage has occurred, the prognosis—while unfavorable—is better for those with aneurysms than for those with arteriovenous fistulas. If a neurosurgical procedure takes place during pregnancy, the fetus is usually not adversely affected, despite the induced hypotension that is often necessary. The prognosis for the mother and fetus is the same as that in a normal gestation once the condition has been corrected.

CEREBRAL NEOPLASMS

Cerebral neoplasms occur primarily at the extremes of life; thus primary cancer or even metastatic tumors are uncommon during the childbearing years. Although brain tumors are not specifically related to gestation, meningiomas, angiomas, and neurofibromas are thought to grow more rapidly with pregnancy. Of the primary neoplasms (half of all brain tumors), gliomas are the most common (50%), with meningiomas and pituitary adenomas accounting for 35%. Of the metastatic cerebral tumors, lung and breast tumors account for 50%. **Choriocarcinoma** (see Chapter 50) commonly metastasizes to the cerebrum.

Clinical Findings

The clinical manifestations, while dependent on the type and location of the tumor, are generally characterized by a slow progression of neurologic signs with evidence of increased intracranial pressure. One of the most frequent signs is headache, which must be differentiated from that occurring in tension and in vascular or inflammatory conditions. Pain that is not relieved by analgesics or muscle relaxants (as a tension headache would be), the absence of a history of migraine headaches, and the lack of signs of infection or meningeal inflammation all point to increased intracranial pressure as the cause of the headache. Tumors in the pituitary gland or occipital region may be associated with visual deficits. Other presenting signs and symptoms include nausea, vomiting, vertigo, seizures, and altered mental status.

Diagnosis

CT scan and MRI are of greatest assistance in revealing space-occupying lesions. If the cerebrospinal fluid glucose and protein levels are normal, inflammation or infection of the central nervous system are unlikely. Similarly, an increase in the cerebrospinal fluid hCG titer raises the suspicion of metastatic choriocarcinoma. Pleocytosis may be present with cerebral neoplasia, but it is usually lymphocytic or monocytic, without an increase in the number of polymorphonucleocytes. Finally, failure to find blood or xanthochromic fluid in the cerebrospinal fluid helps in differentiating a neoplasm from a hemorrhagic lesion, unless the tumor has undergone hemorrhagic necrosis.

Treatment

The treatment of cerebral neoplasms during pregnancy depends on the type of tumor, its location, and the stage of gestation. Anticonvulsants and steroids may be used to prevent seizure activity and to decrease intracranial pressure. Deterioration of the patient's status in early pregnancy can be managed with therapeutic abortion followed by surgery, chemotherapy, or radiation therapy. During the second trimester, treatment can be started and the pregnancy allowed to continue. Later in gestation, maternal treatment can be delayed until delivery.

Complications & Prognosis

Brain tumors usually do not affect pregnancy or the fetus unless the neoplasm leads to early delivery or maternal death. When diagnosed in the second or third trimester, the outcome for the fetus is excellent, with 95% surviving even though therapy may be initiated during the course of the pregnancy.

MIGRAINE HEADACHE

Chronic migraine headaches decrease during pregnancy in 50–80% of affected patients. Very few women experience initial onset during pregnancy.

Clinical Findings

Most often, the patient has a history of migraine headaches, which are usually described as "pounding" and may settle in the eyes or the temporal region. Frequently, migraines are associated with gastrointestinal complaints (eg, nausea, vomiting, and diarrhea) or with systemic symptoms (eg, vertigo or syncope). An aura may or may not precede the headache, but vision is not usually impaired.

Diagnosis

Migraine headaches are rarely relieved by analgesics and muscle relaxants, a fact that helps differentiate them from tension headaches. If vertigo is associated with migraine headaches, it is important to rule out Meniere's disease (labyrinthitis). In the latter, vertigo is accompanied by tinnitus, a fluctuating sensorineural hearing loss, and nystagmus. If vertigo is associated with ataxia of gait, it is almost always central in origin, in which case head trauma, brain tumors, seizure disorders, and multiple sclerosis need to be excluded. Syncope (fainting) may occur with migraine or vascular headaches and is very common during pregnancy. However, when syncope occurs with migraine headache, it usually is associated with vertigo. Rarely, ocular nerve palsy develops in association with migraine headaches; the third cranial nerve is the most commonly involved, and the palsy usually disappears with abatement of the migraine. It is important to visualize the optic disk to ensure that cerebrospinal fluid pressure

is not increased. In cases in which the disk borders are not sharp, **pseudotumor cerebri** should be considered. When migraine headaches are accompanied by papilledema, visual fields should be assessed.

Treatment

Treatment of migraine headaches initially includes identification of any factor that precipitates attacks, followed by avoidance of those factors. Factors known to precipitate some migraines include the following: cheese, sausage, chocolate, citrus fruit, wine, monosodium glutamate, odors, lights, and inadequate sleep. When this environmental manipulation fails to control migraines, drug therapy is indicated. Migraine therapy is either abortive or prophylactic. Abortive medications include isometheptene, aspirin, naproxen, ibuprofen, ergotamine, acetaminophen and codeine, or sumatriptan. Prophylactic medications include beta mimetic blockers, tricyclic antidepressants, calcium channel blockers, and aspirin. The nonsteroidal anti-inflammatory agents should not be used for prolonged periods and should be avoided in the third trimester to avoid oligohydramnios or premature closure of the ductus arteriosus.

Complications & Prognosis

Migraine headaches usually have no deleterious long-term effect on mother or fetus, and treatment for acute exacerbation is usually successful.

SEIZURE DISORDERS

Seizure disorders during pregnancy are most often generalized and can be either convulsive (tonic-clonic or grand mal) or nonconvulsive (petit mal). Focal motor, sensory, or autonomic seizures are relatively rare during pregnancy. The onset of seizure disorders is not increased during pregnancy. More than 95% of patients who have seizures during pregnancy have a history of a seizure disorder or have been receiving anticonvulsant therapy. Patients whose seizures are adequately controlled are not likely to experience a deterioration of their condition during pregnancy. On the other hand, patients who have had frequent and uncontrolled seizures before pregnancy will likely experience the same pattern, particularly during early pregnancy.

Clinical Findings

It is imperative to distinguish true seizures from other forms of loss of consciousness such as syncopal episodes, hysteric attacks, or hyperventilation. These problems do not commonly involve a postictal state, nor do they usually involve loss of bladder or bowel control. Noncentral nervous system causes, such as hypoxia, hypoglycemia, hypocalcemia, and hyponatremia, also must be excluded. Finally, seizures may result from drug withdrawal, medications, or exposure to toxic substances; thus, appropriate physical examination and screening for toxic substances is important in patients suffering an apparent first seizure during pregnancy.

Diagnosis

Detailed neurologic work-up is required in patients whose first seizure occurs during pregnancy. Skull x-rays, electroencephalogram, CT scan or MRI, and lumbar puncture are useful in detailing the cause of the seizure and are not contraindicated during pregnancy.

Treatment

During pregnancy, the plasma level of anticonvulsants decreases due to increased protein binding, increased plasma volume, and changes in the absorption and excretion of drugs. In addition, phenytoin, phenobarbital, and carbamazepine have an increased plasma clearance that is probably related to high hepatic metabolism. Therefore, blood level measurements of antiseizure medications are used to document a therapeutic range. Phenytoin, 300–400 mg/d in divided doses, is recommended for most generalized seizure disorders. Two weeks of therapy are generally needed to achieve a therapeutic blood level (10–20 μg/mL). For patients with refractory seizures on medication, an attempt should be made to maximize the dosage of one medication before switching to another one. If seizures cannot be controlled with another agent, a second medication should be added to the regimen. Carbamazepine is dosed at 200–400 mg two to four times a day. The therapeutic trough level is 4–12 μg/mL. Phenobarbital is maintained at 100–300 mg a day with a trough level of 15–40 μg/mL. Valproic acid is given at 10–15 mg/kg/d to reach a trough of 50–100 μg/mL. For petit mal seizures, ethosuximide, 250–500 mg one or two times a day, is given instead of trimethadione.

In patients with status epilepticus, control of seizures is mandatory. If delivery is not imminent, 10-mg intravenous doses of diazepam can be slowly administered. If seizures continue, phenytoin (750–1000 mg slow IV push at a rate of 50 mg/min) may be given intravenously. General anesthesia may be considered if seizures persist. In these cases, cerebral edema is almost invariably present and may be reduced with dexamethasone, mannitol, or hyperventilation. Many cases of status epilepticus in pregnancy are due to inadequate treatment with antiepileptic drugs, noncompliance, or failure to monitor serum levels.

Complications & Prognosis

Women with seizure disorders have an increased risk of fetal malformations even without exposure to anticonvulsant medication. The most common defects, whether or not the mother takes medication, include orofacial clefts and congenital heart disease. All therapeutic anticonvulsants cross the placenta, equilibrate rapidly in cord blood, and may have teratogenic effects. The risk of anomalies among infants exposed to anticonvulsants is approximately threefold greater than in the general population. The **fetal hydantoin syndrome** (associated with phenytoin) has been well described and affects 3–5% of exposed offspring. It is characterized by mental retardation, small size for gestational age, craniofacial anomalies, and limb defects. A milder phenytoin-associated syndrome may be present at a greater frequency (8–15%) but is detectable only by careful assessment during the first 3 years of life.

Anomalies associated with trimethadione are similar to those in fetal hydantoin syndrome but are twice as frequent (up to 30%). Affected infants have growth delays, cardiac and ocular defects, microcephaly, hypospadias, low-set ears, and palatal anomalies. The teratogenic potential of ethosuximide and carbamazepine is unclear, but a fetal hydantoin-like syndrome has been described with carbamazepine. There are conflicting data concerning the teratogenesis of primidone. Phenobarbital has been used for many years and appears to be safe for the fetus. Valproic acid has been used for major as well as focal seizures, but several reports have described birth defects (especially neural tube defects [1–2%]) related to use of valproic acid during any pregnancy; thus, it should be avoided if possible.

Women with existing seizure disorders who are contemplating pregnancy should be tested to see whether they still require anticonvulsant therapy—particularly if anticonvulsants were begun during childhood or if the patient has been seizure-free for 2–5 years. If a pregnant woman requires seizure medication, she should be informed of the likelihood of fetal anomalies associated with each drug (eg, phenytoin, 10%; valproic acid, primidone, phenobarbital, and carbamazepine, 3–5%; trimethadione, 25–30%), and informed consent should be obtained. The patient should also be counseled regarding folic acid supplementation (4 mg a day) starting at least 3 months preconceptionally to prevent neural tube defects. Additionally, she should be aware that her baby will receive vitamin K after delivery to prevent hemorrhage.

MULTIPLE SCLEROSIS

Multiple sclerosis is an autoimmune demyelinating process in the white matter of the central nervous system. It affects women twice as often as men and usually has its onset between the ages of 20 and 40. People in the Northern Hemisphere are more commonly affected. The cause is not known, but it is more likely environmental or viral than genetic.

Clinical Findings

Findings include weakness in the extremities, sensory loss, difficulty with coordination, and visual problems. Myasthenia gravis should be ruled out with an anticholinesterase (neostigmine) challenge. A history of recent viral infection may make it important to rule out Guillain-Barré syndrome.

Diagnosis

Laboratory tests and imaging should be done to rule out other possible etiologies. Serum should be checked for vitamin B_{12}, HTLV-1 titer, ESR, and rheumatoid factor. An MRI would reveal involvement of white matter long tracts. Elevated IgG in the cerebrospinal fluid is virtually diagnostic.

Treatment

Treatment options include interferon beta-1A, interferon beta-1B, and glatiramer. These medications decrease relapse rates, decrease disease activity as measured by serial MRIs, and decrease disease progression. No reports of use in human pregnancy have been reported. However, in the Betaseron Multiple Sclerosis trial, spontaneous abortions occurred in 4 patients. At this time, it is recommended that the drug be discontinued prior to conception. Symptomatic treatment of spasticity, pain, fatigue, and bowel and bladder dysfunction will be required as well. IVIG has been used in the postpartum period to decrease the risk of exacerbation with some success. Short courses of corticosteroids may be helpful if the patient has optic neuritis.

Complications & Prognosis

The disease is characterized by exacerbations and remissions, with 70% of patients experiencing slow progression over a number of years. Pregnancy does not appear to exert any deleterious effect on multiple sclerosis, and may improve the rate of exacerbation. There is an increased risk of exacerbations in the first 3 months postpartum. The disease itself may not be an indication for therapeutic abortion or sterilization, but since it is a progressive neurologic disease, the patient's participation in long-term childrearing may be impossible. Average life expectancy after diagnosis is 15–25 years, with death usually resulting from infection.

MYASTHENIA GRAVIS

Myasthenia gravis is a chronic disorder of unknown cause occurring more commonly in females than in males. Its peak occurrence is in the third decade of life. It is characterized by abnormal voluntary muscle function with muscle weakness after repeated effort. Antibodies to acetylcholine receptors are present, but levels do not correlate with the severity of disease. Although some cases of myasthenia gravis appear to be hereditary, most adult cases appear to be acquired.

Clinical Findings

The most common symptom is easily fatigued small muscles, most frequently the ocular muscles. Weakness usually increases as the muscles are used repeatedly. Patients who may not have noticeable symptoms in the morning may be easily diagnosed in the afternoon. Difficulties with swallowing and speech are not uncommon, and the facial muscles are almost always affected.

Diagnosis

The diagnosis may be confirmed by administering edrophonium (Tensilon), a total of 10 mg: 2 mg followed by 8 mg 45 seconds later, to assess improvement in muscular weakness. A radioimmunoassay for the acetylcholine receptor antibody can be done. Repetitive nerve stimulation would show a decrement of greater than 15% if positive.

Treatment

Treatment with anticholinesterases (eg, neostigmine) is the same as in the nonpregnant state, although dosages need to be administered more frequently during pregnancy. Other treatment options include thymectomy, steroids, plasma exchange, and IVIG. During labor, anticholinesterases should be administered parenterally rather than orally. Parenteral and regional anesthesia are not contraindicated in labor. Curare-like agents and magnesium sulfate, as well as the older general anesthetics such as ether and chloroform, should be avoided. Women taking anticholinesterase drugs are advised not to breastfeed.

Complications & Prognosis

One-third of pregnant patients with myasthenia experience exacerbation, one-third do not change, and one-third have a remission. The disease does not affect uterine activity because the uterus consists of smooth muscle. The length of labor is not affected. However, an assisted second stage might be considered due to maternal fatigue. Exacerbations are most common during the postpartum period. Placental transfer of the acetylcholine receptor antibodies can occur. The fetus should thus be monitored at frequent intervals during pregnancy with fetal kick counts and ultrasound. A rare finding in neonates is arthrogryposis multiplex congenita, congenital contractures secondary to lack of movement in utero. Also, antibodies may affect the fetal diaphragm and lead to pulmonary hypoplasia and polyhydramnios. Twelve to fifteen percent of newborns will be affected with transient myasthenia gravis. The mean duration of neonatal symptoms is 3 weeks to 3 months.

SPINAL CORD DISORDERS

Spinal cord lesions that are caused by trauma, tumor, infection, or vascular disorders usually do not prevent conception. Diagnosis and therapy should be carried out without regard to pregnancy. In general, pregnancy coexisting with trauma to the spinal cord from any cause, even paraplegia, proceeds unremarkably with the exception of an increased frequency of urinary tract infections and sepsis from pressure necrosis of the skin. Fetal growth usually is unimpeded even though initial maternal weight is frequently less than 100 pounds because of muscular wasting. Radiographs to assess pelvic deformities may be helpful, but generally labor proceeds without evidence of fetopelvic disproportion. Women whose paraplegia is related to anterior horn cell damage or to cord lesions below the tenth thoracic level have appropriate perception of labor contractions and may need analgesia or anesthesia. In most patients, rapid, painless labors are the rule, with the only abnormality being a prolonged second stage because of decreased muscular effort. Paraplegic patients may develop autonomic hyperreflexia during labor due to loss of central regulation of the sympathetic nervous system below the level of the lesion. This is best managed with an epidural, continuous monitoring of the cardiac rhythm and blood pressures, and an assisted second stage.

DISORDERS OF CRANIAL NERVES

Palsies of the facial nerve due to inflammation are called **Bell's palsy.** Although patients may complain of paresthesia over the area of paralysis, this is strictly a motor disorder involving paralysis of the facial nerve. Since approximately one-fifth of cases of Bell's palsy occur during pregnancy or shortly thereafter, it has been suggested that pregnancy increases the frequency of this disorder, although viral infections have also been causally related. Treatment with corticosteroids (pred-

nisone, 40–60 mg/d) is helpful if given within 1 week of onset. However, Bell's palsy is usually self-limited, and simple therapy such as closure of the affected eye suffices during the 1- to 5-week course. Rarely is surgical decompression of the nerve indicated.

GUILLAIN-BARRÉ SYNDROME

Guillain-Barré syndrome is related to a viral respiratory infection and causes a relapsing idiopathic polyneuritis of unusually rapid onset. Most frequently, weakness of the face and extremities and respiratory depression occur, and supportive treatment aimed at preventing respiratory failure is mandatory. Hospitalization is required, and if the vital respiratory capacity falls to 800 mL or below, tracheostomy should be performed. Although the role of corticosteroids is not clear, prednisone, 60 mg/d for 5–7 days in the early course of the disease, is recommended. Immunosuppressants are not helpful. Most patients progress normally through pregnancy and deliver at term; thus abortion is not mandated. On the other hand, if respiratory paralysis occurs near term, cesarean delivery may be indicated to improve ventilation.

PERIPHERAL NEUROPATHIES

Carpal tunnel syndrome is a neuropathic disorder related to median nerve compression by swelling of the tissue in the synovial sheaths at the wrist. Symptoms are usually limited to paresthesia over the thumb, index, and middle fingers and the medial portion of the ring finger. Most commonly, symptoms are noted at night and are usually best treated conservatively with elevation of the affected wrist and splinting. The syndrome usually abates postpartum. Surgery and corticosteroids are rarely indicated.

Compression of the obturator nerve is characterized by adduction weakness of the thigh and minimal sensory loss over the medial aspect of the affected limb. This can occur from retraction at the time of cesarean delivery or hysterectomy, but it is most commonly related to pressure of the fetus just before and during vaginal delivery.

Peroneal neuropathy reveals footdrop and weakness on dorsiflexion of the foot, occasionally with paresthesia in the foot and second toes. This disorder usually appears 1–2 days postpartum and may be related to prolonged episiotomy repair and to pressure on the nerve from knee stirrups. Women at risk include small women with relatively large babies, those who have had midforceps rotations, and those who have had prolonged labor, especially with abnormally large infants (owing to compression of the L4–L5 lumbosacral nerve trunk). The prognosis is excellent with conservative therapy, but occasionally a short leg brace may be necessary.

Brachialgia or the **thoracic outlet syndrome** occurs when the brachial plexus and subclavian artery are compressed by the clavicle and first rib. Occurrence in pregnancy is increased because of the greater weight of the breasts and abdomen. The pain is referred to the lateral aspect of the hand and forearm, although motor symptoms are rare. Blanching of the fingers and exacerbation of symptoms when the hands are elevated are diagnostic. The syndrome is usually self-limited; posture instruction and strengthening of shoulder suspension muscles are helpful. Surgical removal of the rib may very occasionally be necessary (as in the nonpregnant patient).

Herniation of intervertebral disks occurs more commonly in the lumbar than the cervical region. There are both motor and sensory findings along the distribution of the sciatic nerve. It is limited to one extremity and must be differentiated from more serious disorders such as spinal cord tumors and hemorrhage. Diagnosis can usually be made by physical examination and history. MRI of the spine is the best diagnostic modality. Conservative management with bedrest and pelvic traction is helpful. The process should cause no problems during pregnancy or vaginal delivery unless there is cervical disk disease. In that event, cesarean delivery is advised to prevent herniation and paralysis. Surgical correction should be avoided during pregnancy if possible.

■ DISORDERS OF THE SKIN

PHYSIOLOGIC CHANGES

Many physiologic changes that occur during pregnancy can be noted in the integumentary system and may be confused with disease processes. For example, the impressive vascular changes during pregnancy lead to **erythema** early in gestation, particularly in the midpalmar and thenar areas. Although this sign could be diagnostic of hyperthyroidism, cirrhosis of the liver, or systemic lupus erythematosus, other signs of disease are not present. Palmar erythema usually vanishes postpartum.

Venous congestion and vascular permeability during pregnancy can lead to varicosities and labial edema. Vascular proliferations such as **capillary hemangiomas** are most commonly seen around the gums, tongue, upper lip, and eyelids, and there is usually a history of preexisting lesions. These usually do not recede completely after pregnancy.

Striae are normal findings during pregnancy but also may be observed with adrenocortical hyperactivity (eg, Cushing's syndrome, exogenous corticosteroid ad-

ministration). Increased activity of the adrenal gland during pregnancy may increase their occurrence. Most physicians think heredity is the most common predictor of the development of these pinkish or purplish lines on the abdomen, buttocks, and breasts. After pregnancy, striae usually become silvery-white and sunken, but they rarely disappear. Many remedies have been proposed (vitamin E oil, lubricants, lotions, etc), but none are effective.

Hyperpigmentation is common in pregnancy and occurs most frequently in the localized areas of hyperpigmentation (eg, nipples, areolae, and axillas). Hyperpigmentation is related to increased melanocyte-stimulating hormone (MSH), as well as elevated levels of estrogen and progesterone. Melasma gravidarum ("mask of pregnancy") has a similar cause but usually develops on the forehead and across the cheeks and nose. It tends to recur and worsen with successive pregnancies and oral contraceptive use. There is no effective treatment during pregnancy, although topical application of hydroquinone 2% after delivery may assist in lightening areas of hyperpigmentation. Preexisting nevi or freckles may increase in pigmentation during pregnancy but usually regress afterward.

Changes in distribution and amount of **hair** are common during pregnancy. Increased hair growth in facial areas and around the breasts is common, particularly during the second and third trimesters. Importantly, there are no signs of virilization, and hirsutism regresses slightly or remains unchanged postpartum. Postpartum loss of hair is fairly common. During pregnancy, the number of hair follicles in the resting phase (telogen) is decreased by about half and then nearly doubles in the first few weeks postpartum. This increased hair loss usually stops in 2–6 months as the hair follicles enter the growing phase (anagen). Thus, no therapy other than reassurance is required.

PRURITIC URTICARIAL PAPULES AND PLAQUES OF PREGNANCY (Polymorphic Eruption of Pregnancy)

Pruritic urticarial papules and plaques of pregnancy (PUPPP syndrome) may be the most common of all the pruritic skin conditions that occur during pregnancy. The lesions usually appear during the third trimester and disappear completely within 2 weeks after delivery.

Clinical Findings

The pruritic papules are generally red, unexcoriated, and found principally on the abdomen. In most lesions a marked halo surrounds the small papules and plaques. Focal lesions are rare and rarely appear on the face or distal extremities. The lesions may be indistinguishable from those of herpes gestationis.

Diagnosis

Immunofluorescence reveals no immunoglobulin or complement.

Treatment

Symptomatic treatment with antihistamines, topical steroids, and antipruritic medications is usually helpful. Occasionally, corticosteroid therapy is necessary.

Complications & Prognosis

This disorder appears to have no ill effect on the mother or the fetus and is self-limiting. It does not tend to recur.

HERPES GESTATIONIS (Pemphigoid Gestationis)

Herpes gestationis has an incidence of 1 per 7000 gestations and usually appears in the second and third trimester. Despite its name, the herpes virus is not the causative agent, and the etiology remains unknown. It is suspected that elevated hormone levels during pregnancy are causative since progestins can induce exacerbations.

Clinical Findings

Systemic signs of herpes gestationis may be severe and include malaise, fever, and chills. The lesion appears as erythematous plaques with vesicles that soon form bullae in the periphery of the lesion. The typical blistering eruption has a herpetiform appearance, but the vesicles are not clustered and are more peripheral than herpes. Lesions usually begin on the trunk and spread to the entire body, including the distal extremities. Lesions on mucous membranes are uncommon.

Diagnosis

Most patients with herpes gestationis have circulating IgG that will fix C3 complement. Immunofluoresence testing of bullous lesions aids in establishing the diagnosis. Pemphigus vulgaris can be differentiated by histologic examination. The pustules, fever, and hypocalcemia of impetigo herpetiformis are not present in herpes gestationis. Dermatitis herpetiformis is excluded because, while it is pruritic, the clusters of vesicles do not form bullae, and there are no plaques. In herpes

gestationis a crust forms, and after the lesion heals there is a hyperpigmented area but little or no scarring.

Treatment

Corticosteroids, administered orally, are the treatment of choice.

Complications & Prognosis

Herpes gestationis is characterized by exacerbations and remissions during pregnancy. While significant exacerbations can occur postpartum, the condition usually abates by the sixth week postpartum. Recurrence is frequent in subsequent pregnancies, and the disorder may appear earlier in pregnancy than the other disorders discussed. Its effect on maternal and fetal morbidity is not clear because it is so rare, but an increase in stillbirths, premature births, and small-for-gestational-age infants has been reported. Five percent of newborns have transient blisters.

IMPETIGO HERPETIFORMIS

Impetigo herpetiformis (also called pustular psoriasis, von Zumbusch's type) is a pustular eruption on an erythematous base with total body distribution. It is rare and probably represents an acute form of psoriasis occurring during pregnancy. Pregnancy may precipitate this acute manifestation, but the disease is not restricted to gestation since it has been documented in nonpregnant women and in males. Most patients with this disease also have chronic psoriasis or a family history of psoriasis.

Clinical Findings

Generalized erythematous patches covered with sterile pustules allow a presumptive diagnosis. Fever, nausea, diarrhea, and malaise often accompany this symptom complex.

Diagnosis

Spongiform pustules noted in the epidermis on biopsy distinguish this disorder from pustular dermatosis or infection. The pustules are usually sterile, but they may become secondarily infected. In addition, pruritus is not a prominent symptom. The disorder is often associated with hypocalcemia and ensuing tetany, seizures, and delirium.

Treatment

Treatment is usually limited to supportive measures, occasional corticosteroids, and appropriate antibiotics for superimposed infection. Methotrexate, vitamin A derivatives, and tetracycline should not be used during pregnancy.

Complications & Prognosis

There are inadequate data on the fetal effects of this disorder. There have been reports of increased maternal and perinatal mortality, but reports of such problems may have been related to secondary infection and sepsis.

■ GASTROINTESTINAL DISORDERS

PEPTIC ULCER DISEASE

Pregnancy usually ameliorates extension of ulceration, and an initial attack rarely occurs during pregnancy. The salutary effect of pregnancy may be related to progesterone's ability to inhibit motility, because acid secretion remains unchanged. The incidence of peptic ulcer disease in pregnancy is rare (1 in 4000 deliveries); it seems to be more common when there is associated preeclampsia. If activation of previously dormant ulcer disease does occur, it is usually in the puerperium.

Clinical Findings

The classic signs of gastric or duodenal ulcer are related to a burning epigastric pain that is relieved by meals or antacids. Peptic ulcer disease must be differentiated from reflex esophagitis or simple heartburn, which commonly occurs during pregnancy. Patients with a gastric or duodenal ulcer most often report discomfort rather than pain and describe this feeling as "acid" or burning or indigestion.

Diagnosis

The above symptoms of peptic ulcer disease are relieved by food and return approximately 1–2 hours later, paralleling gastric acidity. Likewise, antacids may relieve the pain and help confirm the diagnosis. Most commonly, the diagnosis is confirmed by endoscopic visualization of the ulcer crater in the stomach or duodenum. Although gastric carcinoma is rare, many physicians recommend biopsy during the endoscopic procedure. Upper gastrointestinal x-rays with barium studies are usually avoided because of radiation exposure and because endoscopy is a more direct diagnostic method.

Helicobacter pylori is an organism associated with gastritis, ulcers, and possibly gastric adenocarcinoma and lymphoma. Diagnosis is based on biopsy histology, culture, or urease test. Noninvasive testing includes the C-urea breath test, stool antigen, or serology.

Treatment

Documented peptic ulcer disorders are treated symptomatically during pregnancy by avoidance of symptom-provoking foods and use of antacids and sucralfate. Supportive advice may be given regarding cessation of smoking, bed rest, avoidance of stress, and so on. For persistent symptoms, an H_2 antagonist such as cimetidine or ranitidine can be given. As a last resort, a proton pump inhibitor such as lansoprazole can be added to the drug regimen. Eradication of *H. pylori* is 90% successful with an antibiotic such as tetracycline or clarithromycin, a bismuth compound, and a proton pump inhibitor.

Complications & Prognosis

In general, the fetus is not adversely affected by peptic ulcer disease unless maternal compromise, such as perforated ulcer with bleeding, occurs. Particular vigilance in the postpartum period is necessary because ulcers become active again during this time and can become penetrating.

INFLAMMATORY BOWEL DISEASE

Inflammatory bowel disease encompasses regional enteritis (Crohn's disease), ulcerative colitis, and granulomatous colitis. In general, inflammatory bowel disease has no effect on fertility unless colonic disease has resulted in pelvic abscesses. Overall, studies show a reduced relapse rate during pregnancy compared to preconception. Relapse shows a predilection for the first trimester and postpartum. Subsequent pregnancies will not necessarily have the same course.

Clinical Findings

In these conditions, cramping, lower abdominal pain, and diarrhea are the main complaints. Weight loss and anorexia, even during pregnancy, may occur, as may electrolyte imbalance with severe diarrhea.

Diagnosis

Infectious disorders that would cause diarrhea and abdominal pain must be ruled out. A personal or family history of inflammatory bowel disease is helpful in confirming the diagnosis. If the lower intestine is involved, proctoscopy or colonoscopy may be helpful. However, in some cases a small bowel series and barium enema are needed to make the diagnosis. Malignancy and infectious disease such as tuberculosis of the small intestine also must be considered because they have appearances similar to inflammatory bowel disease on x-ray. Finally, a response to trials of medication and a change in diet may be helpful in confirming the diagnosis.

Treatment

Treatment for inflammatory bowel disease usually involves dietary management and use of medications. Sulfasalazine inhibits prostaglandin synthesis, which is thought to be important in bowel disease. Although sulfasalazine and corticosteroids cross the placenta, their use during pregnancy may be preferable to acute exacerbations of disease. If sulfasalazine is used, maternal folic acid should be given daily because it inhibits brush border enzymes. Though sulfasalazine is a sulfa drug, there has been no noted increased risk of neonatal jaundice. Azathioprine has not been associated with congenital malformations. There is an associated increase in fetal growth restriction and prematurity. Mercaptopurine has shown no fetal toxicity after first-trimester exposure. Methotrexate should be avoided in pregnancy. Short-term use of antibiotics such as metronidazole is allowed. Other immunosuppressant drugs have not been shown to be helpful and should not be used during pregnancy.

Complications & Prognosis

Complications during pregnancy are similar to those in the nonpregnant state, eg, abdominal pain, cramping, and rectal bleeding. The risk of abortion and stillbirth is dependent on disease activity. Pregnancy is not contraindicated with inflammatory bowel disease, but when possible the disorder should be controlled by surgery or medication prior to conception. Pregnancy does not exert an adverse effect on inflammatory bowel disease. In most patients, pregnancy and delivery proceed smoothly. Patients with ileostomies should be followed for complications, most importantly intestinal obstruction (8%). If a patient has had a prior bowel resection, total parenteral nutrition may be required during the pregnancy. Women with active perianal disease should be delivered via cesarean section.

CHOLECYSTITIS

Cholecystitis occurs rarely during pregnancy (0.3%) because the gallbladder and biliary duct smooth muscle are relaxed by progesterone. Acute inflammation during pregnancy is treated with intravenous fluids and nasogastric suction. If acute cholecystitis does not resolve or if pancreatitis develops, cholecystectomy should be considered. If this operation can be performed in the second trimester, the fetal loss rate is not increased. Surgery during the first trimester increases the risk of abortion. In the third trimester, surgical intervention can cause preterm delivery. Later in gestation, prolonged IV hyperalimentation can be an option to delay surgery until postpartum.

INTRAHEPATIC CHOLESTASIS OF PREGNANCY

Intrahepatic cholestasis is a condition characterized by accumulation of bile acids in the liver, with subsequent accumulation in the plasma, causing pruritus and jaundice. It is similar to the cholestasis that occasionally occurs during oral contraceptive therapy. Estrogen and progesterone are therefore considered to play a role in its etiology. Ultrasound examination of the gallbladder helps rule out cholelithiasis. If hepatitis is not present, the most likely diagnosis is cholestasis associated with pregnancy. Laboratory values show an increased alkaline phosphatase, bilirubin, and serum bile acids (chenodeoxycholic acid, deoxycholic acid, cholic acid). AST and ALT may be mildly elevated as well.

Symptomatic treatment of pruritus with diphenhydramine is useful. Ursodeoxycholic acid 300 mg twice a day has been shown to inhibit absorption of toxic bile acids and increase their biliary secretion. In doing so, the medication normalizes bile acids, improves liver function tests, and alleviates pruritus. Oral steroids have also been used to relieve symptoms. Cholestyramine is no longer routinely used. Symptoms resolve postpartum.

Controversy surrounds the fetal effects of cholestasis. Most literature quotes a slight increase in preterm births and stillbirth. The etiology is unclear, but some refer to the fetal toxicity of bile acids as a causative factor. Antenatal testing with a modified biophysical profile two times per week starting at the time of diagnosis is suggested. There is no agreement as to whether the pregnancy should be induced at 37–38 weeks or whether to await spontaneous labor.

ACUTE FATTY LIVER OF PREGNANCY

Acute fatty liver of pregnancy is a rare complication (1 in 13,000) of the third trimester. Early recognition and termination of the pregnancy (delivery) and extensive supportive therapy have reduced the mortality rate to approximately 20%. There is no increased risk of recurrence in subsequent pregnancies. Studies suggest an association between acute fatty liver of pregnancy and fetal recessive inheritance of long-chain 3-hydroxyacyl-CoA dehydrogenase deficiency.

Symptoms and signs include nausea and vomiting, malaise, epigastric pain, and jaundice. Lab values show an elevated LDH, AST, ALT, bilirubin, and prolonged prothrombin time. Glucose, platelets, cholesterol, triglycerides, and fibrinogen are notably decreased. Liver biopsy reveals microvesicular hepatic steatosis and mitochondrial disruption on electron microscopy. Complications such as acute renal failure, DIC, encephalopathy, and sepsis can be severe.

HELLP SYNDROME

A disorder that mimics acute fatty liver of pregnancy is the HELLP (**h**emolysis, **l**iver dysfunction, and **l**ow **p**latelets) syndrome. Typically, this liver derangement occurs with severe preeclampsia and eclampsia. The disorder occurs in the last trimester of pregnancy and is characterized by vomiting, upper quadrant pain, and progressive nausea. Liver function deteriorates rapidly, and delivery is essential in treatment. Stillbirth is frequent (10–15%), with a high neonatal loss (20–25%), usually due to prematurity (see also Chapter 19). Corticosteroids and dexamethasone 10 mg IV twice a day have been used to help resolve the HELLP syndrome. Laboratory values have been noted to normalize faster with steroid administration.

VIRAL HEPATITIS

Viral hepatitis complicates 0.2% of all pregnancies. Hepatitis may be caused by numerous viruses, drugs, or toxic chemicals; the clinical manifestations of all forms are similar. The development of specific serologic markers has improved the accuracy of the diagnosis. The most common viral agents causing hepatitis in pregnancy are hepatitis A virus, hepatitis B virus, hepatitis C (non-A, non-B hepatitis virus), hepatitis E, hepatitis G, and Epstein-Barr virus. Delta agent hepatitis has also received increasing attention as a cause of hepatitis.

A. HEPATITIS A

Hepatitis A may occur sporadically or in epidemics. A generalized viremia occurs with the infection that is predominantly hepatic. The primary mode of transmission is the fecal-oral route. Excretion of the virus in stool normally begins approximately 2 weeks prior to the onset of clinical symptoms and is complete within 3 weeks following onset of clinical symptoms. No known carrier state exists for the virus. Both blood and stool are infectious during the 2- to 6-week incubation period. Perinatal transmission does not occur.

The hepatitis A virus belongs to the picornavirus group, which also includes poliomyelitis virus and coxsackievirus. It is a 27-nm RNA virus that is readily deactivated by ultraviolet light or heat.

B. HEPATITIS B

Hepatitis B is usually transmitted by inoculation of infected blood or blood products, or sexual intercourse. The virus is contained in most body secretions. Infection by parenteral and sexual contact has been well documented. Groups at risk for hepatitis B infection are intravenous drug users; homosexuals; medical, hemodialysis, blood bank, and medical laboratory personnel; spouses of hepatitis carriers; prostitutes and others with multiple sexual partners; and Southeast Asian emigrants. Approximately 5–10% of people infected with hepatitis B virus become chronic carriers of the virus. The incubation period of hepatitis B is 6 weeks to 6 months. The clinical features of hepatitis A and B are similar, although hepatitis B is more insidious. Additionally, fulminant hepatitis is very rare with hepatitis A, but occurs in approximately 1% of patients infected with hepatitis B.

The hepatitis B virus is a DNA hepadnavirus. It is pleomorphic, occurring in spherical and tubular forms of different sizes. The largest of these, the 42-nm Dane particle, is the complete infectious agent, which is composed of a surface coat and a 27-nm central core. The surface antigen (HBsAg) of the Dane particle is the marker usually measured in blood. The presence of HBsAg is the first manifestation of viral infection; it usually appears before clinical evidence of the disease and lasts throughout the infection. Persistence of HBsAg after the acute phase of hepatitis is usually associated with clinical and laboratory evidence of chronic hepatitis. The core antibody (HBcAb) is produced against the 27-nm core of the Dane particle. Core particles and antigen are not normally present in blood except in overwhelming infections. HBcAb occurs with acute hepatitis B infection at the onset of clinical illness. Hepatitis Be antigen (HBeAg) is a soluble, nonparticulate antigen that is found only when HBsAg is present. HBeAg probably serves as an accurate indicator of viral replication and infectivity. Pregnant women who are HBeAg-positive in the third trimester frequently transmit this infection to the fetus (80–90%) in the absence of immunoprophylaxis, whereas those who are negative rarely infect the fetus. DNA polymerase activity is usually transient, occurring with peak HBsAg positivity; however, its persistence usually suggests continued infectivity.

C. HEPATITIS C (NON-A, NON-B HEPATITIS)

Up to 80% of infected individuals become chronic carriers. About 90% of posttransfusion hepatitis is now caused by hepatitis C. The incubation period is usually 7–8 weeks but may vary from 3–21 weeks. The course of infection is similar to that of hepatitis B. Hepatitis C antibody is present in approximately 90% of these patients. However, the antibody may not be detectable for weeks after infection. PCR for hepatitis C RNA then becomes useful. Vertical transmission occurs in 7–8% of infected pregnancies and is increased with concomitant HIV infection.

D. EPSTEIN-BARR VIRUS

Epstein-Barr virus causes the clinical picture of infectious mononucleosis with hepatitis. Serologic testing for this agent involves determining antibody titers to latently infected (anti-EGNA), early replication cycle (anti-EA), or late replication cycle (anti-VCA) viral proteins.

E. DELTA AGENT

Hepatitis delta virus is an RNA virus that is smaller than all other known RNA viruses. The agent can cause infection only when HBsAg positivity exists. Delta agent is isolated in up to 50% of cases of fulminant hepatitis B infection. HDAg (hepatitis delta antigen) and HDAb (hepatitis delta antibody) are serologic markers for the disease.

F. HEPATITIS E

Hepatitis E is transmitted via the oral/fecal route. The disease is self-limited. Pregnant patients who are acutely infected have a 15% risk of fulminant liver failure with a 5% mortality rate.

G. HEPATITIS G

Hepatitis G is more likely to be found in people infected with hepatitis B or C or with a history of intravenous drug abuse. There is no chronic carrier state. Vertical transmission has been noted.

Clinical Findings

The clinical picture of hepatitis is highly variable; most patients have asymptomatic infection, while a few may present with fulminating disease and die within a few days. Frequent symptoms include general malaise, myalgia, fatigue, anorexia, nausea and vomiting, right upper quadrant pain, and low-grade fever. Mild hepatomegaly and/or splenomegaly occur in 5–10% of affected patients. The white blood cell count is depressed and mild proteinuria and bilirubinuria occur early in the course of the disease. AST, ALT, bilirubin, and alkaline phosphatase are usually elevated. Prothrombin and partial thromboplastin times may also be prolonged with severe liver involvement.

Diagnosis

The diagnosis is made using serologic markers—anti-HA IgM, HBsAg, HC PCR, anti-HBc IgM, HD PCR, anti-HE IgM, and anti-HG IgM. Liver biopsy shows extensive hepatocellular injury and inflammatory infiltrate. The differential diagnosis of viral hepatitis should include viruses A, B, C, and delta; Epstein-Barr virus; cytomegalovirus infection; cholestasis; preeclampsia; acute fatty liver of pregnancy; TORCH infections; secondary syphilis; autoimmune; and toxic or drug-induced hepatitis. Additionally, intra- or extrahepatic bile duct obstruction should be included.

Treatment

Bed rest should be instituted during the acute phase of the illness. If nausea, vomiting, or anorexia is prominent, intravenous hydration and general supportive measures are instituted. All hepatotoxic agents should be avoided. Antepartum fetal assessment should be instituted in the third trimester because of the increased risks of premature delivery and stillbirth. Gamma globulin prophylaxis should be given to pregnant women within 2 weeks of exposure to hepatitis A or non-A, non-B hepatitis. Two hepatitis A vaccines using inactivated virus are now available and can be used during pregnancy. Hepatitis B immunoglobulin may be given to those parenterally or sexually exposed to blood or secretions from hepatitis B–infected individuals. Hepatitis B vaccine also should be administered to an HBsAg-negative patient. Hepatitis B immunoglobulin, 0.5 mL intramuscularly with a repeat dose at 3 and 6 months, should be administered to neonates born of HBsAg-positive mothers, to decrease the risk of vertical transmission. These infants should also receive hepatitis B vaccine at birth and at 1 and 3 months. Passive and active immunization of the newborn is 85–95% effective in preventing perinatal transmission of hepatitis B virus. Breastfeeding is not contraindicated with hepatitis B as long as the infant has been immunized.

Complications & Prognosis

The acute illness usually resolves rapidly in 2–3 weeks, with complete recovery usually occurring within 8 weeks. In 10% of cases of type B and C hepatitis, chronic persistent or chronic active hepatitis develops. Additionally, 1–3% of patients develop acute fulminant hepatitis.

The maternal course of viral hepatitis is unaltered by pregnancy, but prematurity may be increased. In general, with severe liver disease, infertility results. Chronic active hepatitis does not mandate therapeutic abortion, but there is an increase in fetal loss. All pregnant women should routinely be tested for HBsAg during an early prenatal visit in each pregnancy. Women with cirrhosis of the liver from other causes have an outcome related to the extent of maternal disease. Perinatal loss rates are usually high with a poor maternal prognosis, particularly with poor liver function or esophageal varices. Pregnancy in women with liver transplants has been reported and, in general, has an uncomplicated prenatal and delivery course. Treatment with immunosuppressants and corticosteroids usually does not interdict pregnancy. Interferon therapy improves the prognosis for chronic active hepatitis.

■ DISORDERS OF THE THYROID

In pregnancy, the diagnosis of thyroid disease is difficult because of both normal gravid physiologic changes and the hypertrophy of the thyroid gland encountered in pregnancy. Triiodothyronine (T_3) is the active thyroid hormone resulting from peripheral metabolism of thyroxine (T_4). Thyroid-binding globulin (TBG; the major protein fraction responsible for carrying bound thyroxine), albumin, and prealbumin increase with pregnancy, due to enhanced hepatic synthesis. Though total T_4 and T_3 increase, free T_4 and T_3 values remain within the normal reference range. Values of TSH do not normally change in pregnancy.

HYPOTHYROIDISM

Hypothyroidism affects 0.5–3% of pregnant women. Common causes for primary hypothyroidism include autoimmune thyroiditis such as Hashimoto's thyroiditis, iatrogenic causes such as radiation treatment or surgery, congenital hypothyroidism, medications such as lithium or amiodarone, iodine deficiency, and infiltrative diseases. Secondary hypothyroidism may be caused by pituitary or hypothalamic disease (Sheehan's syndrome, adenomas, trauma).

Clinical Findings

General complaints include skin dryness, weakness, fatigue, hoarseness, yellowing of the skin (especially in the periorbital area), hair loss, cold intolerance, constipation, and sleep disturbances. Physical examination of hypothyroid patients usually reveals a goiter and delayed relaxation of deep tendon reflexes. Anemia, low T_4, and elevated TSH are characteristic laboratory findings. Other laboratory findings include antibodies to thyroid peroxidase, TSH receptor, or thyroglobulin. Subclinical hypothyroidism is associated with an ele-

vated TSH and free T_4 and T_3 values within the normal range.

Treatment

Most patients with early hypothyroidism may be started on 50–100 µg/d of levothyroxine. The dosage is increased by 25 µg per week until the patient is euthyroid. The goal of therapy is to bring TSH into the normal to low normal range. After delivery, the dosage will need to be decreased as necessary.

Complications & Prognosis

Congestive heart failure is the most serious complication of hypothyroidism. Megacolon, adrenal crisis, organic psychosis, and myxedema coma are other complications of hypothyroidism. Hyponatremia secondary to the syndrome of inappropriate secretion of antidiuretic hormone (SIADH) may also occur.

Prognosis for both mother and fetus is excellent when hypothyroidism is corrected in pregnancy. Antepartum fetal assessment in the third trimester is indicated because of a small increase in the stillbirth rate.

Recently, researchers have taken a closer look at the effect of maternal hypothyroidism on the psychomotor development of the euthyroid fetus. Until the fetal thyroid develops at 12–13 weeks, maternal thyroid hormones are needed for neuronal development. Studies have shown that women with hypothyroidism have an increased likelihood of having children with lower IQ scores. This underscores the importance of identifying and treating affected women.

THYROIDITIS

Thyroiditis has been diagnosed with increasing frequency in recent years. This disorder is most commonly autoimmune in etiology; viral infection of the thyroid is the second most common cause.

Acute thyroiditis is caused by bacterial or fungal infections, radiation treatment, or amiodarone treatment. In younger patients, infection of the piriform sinus is causative. Patients experience an abrupt onset of thyroid pain with referral to the ears and throat. Systemic symptoms include fever, lymphadenopathy, and a tender, erythematous, asymmetric goiter. Laboratory findings include normal thyroid function tests, elevated ESR, and leukocytosis. Antibiotic treatment is suggested. The presence of an abscess requires surgical intervention.

Subacute thyroiditis (de Quervain's or granulomatous thyroiditis) includes postpartum thyroiditis and thyroiditis due to bacterial and mycobacterial infections. Patients present with a tender, asymmetrically enlarged thyroid. Thyroid pain may be referred to the throat and ears. Some have a history of antecedent malaise and upper respiratory symptoms. Initially, the patient may exhibit signs of thyrotoxicosis when follicular destruction causes release of thyroglobulin and thyroxine. At this time, TSH would be suppressed and free T_4 elevated. A period of hypothyroidism with an elevated TSH and low free T_4 follows once the thyroid has been depleted of thyroid hormones. The clinical course usually leads to complete resolution. Pain, inflammation, and swelling is controlled with aspirin or nonsteroidal anti-inflammatory drugs. A steroid taper over 6–8 weeks can be implemented if there are persistent symptoms. Levothyroxine treatment may be necessary if there is a prolonged period of hypothyroidism.

Postpartum thyroiditis is a silent thyroiditis that usually presents 3–6 months postpartum. Its course differs from other subacute thyroiditis in that it is painless and is associated with a normal ESR and the presence of thyroid peroxidase antibodies. Treatment is usually not required. However, yearly reassessment for subsequent autoimmune hypothyroidism is suggested.

Chronic thyroiditis includes autoimmune thyroiditis such as Hashimoto's thyroiditis, Riedel's thyroiditis, and parasitic thyroiditis. Hashimoto's thyroiditis is a chronic inflammatory disease caused by antibodies to several components of thyroid tissue. Lymphocytic infiltration leads to a uniform goiter. Eventually hypothyroidism develops and treatment with thyroxine is indicated. Riedel's thyroiditis occurs in middle-aged gravidas. The gland is hard, asymmetric, and fixed. It may cause compressive symptoms affecting the esophagus or trachea. Treatment is surgical.

Complications & Prognosis

Hashimoto's thyroiditis frequently leads to clinical hypothyroidism. Hashimoto's disease may also be associated with Addison's disease, hypoparathyroidism, diabetes, pernicious anemia, collagen vascular disease, and other immune disorders. The incidence of mitral valve prolapse is also increased in patients with thyroiditis.

Spontaneous remissions and exacerbations are common with most forms of thyroiditis. Rarely, lymphoma or carcinoma of the thyroid gland develops. Autoantibodies (IgG variety) rarely cross the placenta to cause thyroiditis in the fetus. In general, the prognosis for mother and fetus is very good in the presence of thyroiditis.

HYPERTHYROIDISM

The incidence of maternal hyperthyroidism ranges from 0.05–0.2% during pregnancy. The most frequent etiologies, in order of frequency, are Graves' disease,

acute (subacute) thyroiditis, toxic nodular goiter, and toxic adenoma.

Graves' disease is more frequent in women and is found most frequently in the third and fourth decades of life. Sera of patients with Graves' disease reveal TSH receptor antibodies. The diagnostic triad for Graves' disease includes hyperthyroidism with diffuse goiter, ophthalmopathy, and dermopathy. However, these 3 major manifestations may not appear together. The disease is characterized by unpredictable intervals of exacerbation and remission, but appears to be precipitated by emotional trauma or by metabolic stress. It may also be associated with other systemic autoimmune disorders such as pernicious anemia, myasthenia gravis, and diabetes mellitus.

Acute (subacute) thyroiditis appears to be viral in origin, with symptoms (asthenia, malaise, and pain due to stretching of the thyroid capsule) usually following an upper respiratory infection. Additionally, pain over the thyroid, or more commonly, referred to the lower jaw or ear, is perceived. These symptoms may be present for many weeks before the diagnosis is clear. Less commonly, the onset is acute with severe pain over the thyroid accompanied by fever and occasionally by symptoms of thyrotoxicosis.

Toxic nodular goiter appears to be an infrequent consequence of long-standing simple goiter. Viral toxicosis may develop spontaneously in multinodular goiters (Plummer's disease) or in single nodular goiters. The syndrome may also be the consequence of exogenous iodide in patients with nodular goiters. Affected individuals are usually over 40 years of age.

True **toxic adenomas** of the thyroid are encapsulated and usually compressed contiguous tissues. They vary greatly in size, histologic characteristics, and ability to concentrate radioiodine. They may be classified into 3 major types: papillary, follicular, and those with Haurthle cells. Adenoma function is independent of TSH stimulation. Clinically, they usually present as a solitary nodule. In time, nodular function increases, with subsequent atrophy and decrease of function in the remainder of the gland. Initially, the patient may not be thyrotoxic, but frank thyrotoxicosis usually develops (thus the term *toxic adenoma*).

Clinical Findings

Symptoms of hyperthyroidism include restlessness, fatigue, weakness, weight loss, diarrhea, and heat intolerance. On examination, a patient may exhibit tachycardia, tremor, goiter, muscle weakness, and lid retraction or lag. The TSH is usually decreased and free T_4 values are elevated. Patients with Graves' disease may have antibodies to thyroid peroxidase or TSH receptor.

Treatment

Treatment of hyperthyroidism in pregnancy focuses on stopping release of T_4 and inhibiting conversion of T_4 to T_3. Propylthiouracil (PTU) is suggested for pregnancy. PTU is initially given in doses of 100 mg three times a day until the patient is euthyroid. The dosage is subsequently decreased. Thyroid function should be assessed every 4–6 weeks. Subtotal thyroidectomy is an option for patients who are noncompliant or refractory to medications. Surgery is best undertaken in the second trimester. Radioiodine treatment is contraindicated in pregnancy.

Thyrotoxicosis or thyroid storm can be precipitated by delivery, acute illness, infection, trauma, or surgery. It is associated with fever, delirium, nausea and vomiting, seizures, and coma. Mortality can be as high as 30% even with treatment. It is important to provide supportive care, identify and treat the cause, and decrease T_4 synthesis. Large doses of PTU (600 mg loading dose, followed by 200–300 mg every 6 hours) should be administered. Potassium iodide should be administered soon after the first dose of PTU. Propranolol is given orally or intravenously to suppress adrenergic output and to block peripheral conversion of T_4 to T_3. In patients with congestive heart failure, beta-blockers also serve to increase stroke volume. Some support the use of steroids (dexamethasone 2 mg every 6 hours) in this setting to block thyroid synthesis and as therapy for autoimmune factors. Intravenous fluids, antibiotics, and cooling blankets are useful as well.

Complications & Prognosis

Ophthalmopathy may require short courses of steroids. Rarely, severe exophthalmos requires surgical decompression to prevent corneal ulceration. Dermopathy can be treated with topical steroids. Cardiac disturbances such as atrial fibrillation require rate control and anticoagulation with coumadin to prevent thromboembolic events.

Graves' disease is a cyclic disease and may subside spontaneously. With adequate treatment and follow-up, the long-term maternal prognosis is excellent. Fetal prognosis with well-controlled hyperthyroidism is also excellent. However, some fetal precautions are necessary. A few studies have reported an increased stillbirth rate with maternal hyperthyroidism; thus, antepartum fetal assessment is probably indicated in the third trimester. A fetal goiter rarely may lead to extension of the head at delivery, necessitating operative delivery. Skilled resuscitation of the newborn after delivery may be needed if the airway is obstructed by a goiter. Transplacental passage of IgG TSH receptor antibody can lead to fetal and neonatal hyperthyroidism. A history of stillbirth, fetal heart rate greater than 160 bpm after 22 weeks gestation, and elevated levels of antibody early in pregnancy are suggestive of transplacental IgG transfer. Treatment is achieved with maternal antithyroid drugs. Without treatment, the fetus can suffer from growth restriction, craniosynostosis, and death. Infants may exhibit signs and symptoms for as long as 10 months after birth.

■ DISORDERS OF THE PARATHYROID

During normal pregnancy, the maternal parathyroid undergoes hyperplasia and increased hormone production. Serum levels of parathyroid hormone (PTH) rise progressively throughout pregnancy. Serum calcitonin is inconsistently elevated during pregnancy (220 ± 60 pg/mL). Calcitonin is important in inhibiting PTH-induced bone resorption. Neither PTH nor calcitonin cross the placenta. Maternal 1,25-dihydroxyvitamin D levels are elevated, allowing for increased intestinal calcium absorption. The total serum calcium begins to fall during the second or third month of gestation and reaches a nadir at 28–32 weeks (5 mEq/L, nonpregnant level; 4.6 mEq/L at term) due to the dilutional hypoalbuminemia (4.3–3.4 g/dL) of pregnancy. The serum ionized calcium remains unchanged or falls slightly secondary to increasing fetal requirements. The normal woman requires 1–2 g/d of calcium in the last half of pregnancy to maintain calcium balance. The fetus requires a total of 25–30 g of calcium in the latter half of gestation. Thus, changes during pregnancy generate increased absorption of calcium for transfer to the fetus while maintaining normal maternal skeletal calcium.

HYPERPARATHYROIDISM

Primary hyperparathyroidism is a generalized disorder, usually chronic in nature, that results from increased PTH secretion. Approximately 8 per 100,000 women of childbearing age are diagnosed yearly. In 80–90% of patients, primary hyperparathyroidism is caused by benign adenomas. Parathyroid hyperplasia is causative in 8–9%. Cancer accounts for 1–2% of cases. Occasionally, primary hyperparathyroidism follows a familial pattern and is associated with other endocrinologic abnormalities.

Clinical Findings

The excessive concentration of PTH leads to hypercalcemia and hypophosphatemia. Symptoms may include fatigue, thirst, constipation, transient depression, hyperemesis, and weakness. Renal involvement presents with recurrent nephrolithiasis. Excessive bone resorption can be detected by x-rays of the hands and skull. Radiography may show resorption of phalangeal tips or "punched out" lesions of the skull (osteitis fibrosa cystica). Pancreatitis is a common presentation as well.

Diagnosis

Radioimmunoassay for PTH is diagnostic. In pregnancy coexisting with hyperparathyroidism, serum calcium levels are generally greater than 12 mg/dL. Hypomagnesemia and hypophosphatemia are common laboratory findings.

Treatment

Mild hyperparathyroidism may be managed by aggressive hydration, diuretic treatment, increasing oral phosphate intake, and decreasing oral calcium intake. If symptoms continue during medical therapy, surgical therapy is indicated. Hyperparathyroidism that is refractory to medical treatment can be managed with surgery. The optimal time for surgery is the second trimester, when the risk of abortion and preterm labor are reduced. A parathyroid adenoma should be removed and the remaining glands biopsied for occult involvement. In the case of parathyroid hyperplasia, all glands except a small amount of tissue should be removed. The remaining tissue is transplanted to the arm for easy access in case of reoperation and to prevent postoperative hypocalcemia.

Complications & Prognosis

Maternal hyperparathyroidism has high fetal morbidity and variable mortality rates. There is a small risk of spontaneous abortion, intrauterine fetal demise, and preterm delivery. Elevated maternal calcium levels lead to a decrease in fetal PTH production and increased calcitonin production. Upon delivery, removal of a maternal source of calcium leads to neonatal hypocalcemia. The neonate should be observed for episodes of tetany or seizures in the first 2 weeks of life. Complete recovery is expected within 3–5 months with treatment with calcium, vitamin D, and phosphate restriction.

Maternal complications of hyperparathyroidism involve the skeletal, renal, and gastrointestinal systems. Pathologic fractures are common in severe hyperparathyroidism. Urinary tract infection due to stones and obstruction may (rarely) lead to uremia. With severe hypercalcemia, severe hypertension with acute cardiac or renal failure and intractable pancreatitis may occur. Postpartum there is an increased risk of hyper-

calcemic crisis. Maternal effects include muscle weakness, fatigue, emesis, confusion, dehydration, coma, and even death.

HYPOPARATHYROIDISM

Normal maintenance of calcium balance depends on adequate PTH levels, and significant hypocalemia occurs in its absence. The most common cause of hypoparathyroidism is iatrogenic ablation during thyroid surgery. Other causes include agenesis or dysgenesis of the parathyroid glands, autoimmune destruction, and impaired PTH secretion. Pseudohypoparathyroidism refers to end-organ unresponsiveness to normal levels of PTH.

Clinical Findings

Patients usually report an increased level of excitability, with numbness and tingling in the extremities, laryngeal spasm, cramps, and carpopedal spasms. Tetany can be induced either by alkalosis, which increases calcium binding, or by a measurable decrease in total serum calcium. Chronic disease may result in basal ganglia calcification, extrapyramidal syndromes, and cataracts.

Diagnosis

Diagnosis is by confirmation of low ionized calcium and PTH levels. Urinary cyclic AMP excretion after administration of PTH is decreased. Additional lab findings include elevated phosphate levels and decreased 1,25-dihydroxyvitamin D.

Treatment

The chief therapeutic goal is to restore normal calcium levels with supplementary dietary calcium and vitamin D or calcitriol.

Complications & Prognosis

The fetal effect of decreased calcium transport across the placenta is increased fetal PTH release and resultant parathyroid hyperplasia. In general, hypoparathyroidism causes no deleterious effects on pregnancy or the newborn. The newborn should be assessed for osteitis fibrosa cystica. Since idiopathic hypoparathyroidism may have an inherited autosomal recessive basis, the neonate needs to be evaluated.

Maternal complications of hypoparathyroidism relate predominantly to the degree of hypocalemia. Acute tetany with stridor may lead to respiratory obstruction requiring tracheostomy. Severe hypocalcemia rarely leads to cardiac dilatation and failure or to cardiac arrhythmias resistant to antiarrhythmic agents.

Permanent brain damage with convulsions or psychosis rarely occurs. The mother, however, should be assessed for osteoporosis. Breastfeeding is not discouraged, even in the presence of osteoporosis.

DISORDERS OF ADRENOCORTICAL FUNCTION

The weight of the adrenal gland does not change significantly in pregnancy, although there is a suggestion of increased thickness of the zona fasciculata. There is an increase in both bound and free cortisol levels throughout gestation.

ADRENOCORTICAL INSUFFICIENCY

Primary adrenal insufficiency (Addison's disease) is caused by the inability of the adrenal gland to elaborate hormones. A variety of causes for primary insufficiency include autoimmune, infectious, vascular, infiltrative, congenital, and iatrogenic. Addison's disease occurs at any age and is found in both sexes with equal frequency. Failure in production of ACTH by the pituitary gland is referred to as secondary adrenal insufficiency. Failure of the hypothalamic-pituitary axis may be due to exogenous or endogenous steroid production.

Clinical Findings

Signs and symptoms include slowly progressive fatigue, weakness, anorexia, nausea, weight loss, abdominal pain, cutaneous pigmentation, hypotension, and hypoglycemia. Some of these symptoms are common complaints during pregnancy.

Diagnosis

Diagnosis is based on cortisol secretion after ACTH infusion (cosyntropin test). Normal cortisol levels should rise to greater than 495 nmol/mL. In adrenal insufficiency, there is subnormal or no increase in cortisol levels. Addison's disease can be differentiated from secondary adrenal insufficiency by measuring aldosterone levels. Secondary adrenal insufficiency has normal aldosterone levels. In more advanced disease, laboratory findings include hyponatremia, hyperkalemia, hypoglycemia, and low levels of bicarbonate and chloride.

Treatment

The treatment of chronic primary adrenocortical insufficiency requires both glucocorticoid and mineralocorticoid replacement. The chronic secondary form usually requires only glucocorticoid replacement.

In times of illness, surgical stress, or crisis, adjustments in steroid dosing are needed. With mild illness, the cortisol dose should be doubled. In more severe illness, hydrocortisone 75–100 mg/d orally is administered. For major surgery, the patient should receive hydrocortisone 100 mg intravenously every 8 hours in the first 24 hours, with the first dose given prior to surgery. In the second 24 hours, hydrocortisone 100 mg IV is given every 12 hours. On the third day, the patient can be switched to oral hydrocortisone 60 mg in divided doses. This is then tapered each day to 40 mg, 20 mg, and 10 mg, and then stopped. For those patients previously on maintenance therapy, their prior dosing can be resumed.

Acute adrenal crisis can be precipitated by sepsis or surgical stress, acute hemorrhagic destruction, rapid withdrawal of steroids, or with use of drugs inhibiting steroid synthesis. Signs and symptoms include fever, lethargy, hypovolemia, nausea and vomiting, abdominal pain, and vascular collapse. Treatment requires intensive care with replacement of sodium, glucose, and fluid. Hydrocortisone can be administered as a continuous infusion or 100 mg IV every 6 hours. Vasoconstrictive agents may be required as well.

Complications & Prognosis

The metabolic effects of insufficient mineralocorticoids are expressed by an inability to retain sodium and to excrete potassium, resulting in a decrease in extracellular electrolytes, renal perfusion, and cardiac output. Rarely, a decrease in intravascular volume with poor vascular tone and, ultimately, vascular collapse occurs. Most of these rare cases develop insidiously, but a few are characterized by acute onset with symptoms of anorexia rapidly progressing to nausea and vomiting, diarrhea, and abdominal pain. In these patients, blood pressure soon plummets, temperature elevates, and severe shock occurs.

In general, however, maternal prognosis is excellent with adequate adrenal steroid replacement therapy. Fetal and neonatal effects are few. A reported increase in low birthweight is perhaps attributable to fetal hypoglycemia. It is rare for the newborn to have adrenal insufficiency.

CUSHING'S SYNDROME

Cushing's syndrome is characterized by chronic glucocorticoid excess. The most common cause is overproduction of ACTH by a pituitary adenoma which results in bilateral adrenal hyperplasia. Additional causes include other sites of ectopic ACTH production, adrenal adenoma or carcinoma, and prolonged exogenous corticosteroid administration. Signs and symptoms include truncal obesity, osteoporosis, diabetes mellitus, diastolic hypertension, fatigue, amenorrhea, hirsutism, and striae. The diagnosis of Cushing's syndrome in pregnancy is made difficult because many of the symptoms normally occur while pregnant.

Laboratory diagnosis starts with a screening test in which dexamethasone 1 mg is administered at midnight. If plasma cortisol and urinary free cortisol are found to be elevated at 8 AM the following morning, a second dexamethasone suppression test is administered. Dexamethasone 2 mg every 6 hours over the next 2 days is given. If there is suppression of cortisol, the patient likely has pituitary secretion of ACTH. If no response is elicited, either an ectopic ACTH-producing tumor or adrenal neoplasia is present. The former is associated with an elevated ACTH and the latter with a low ACTH after dexamethasone suppression. Work-up can then proceed to diagnostic imaging to localize a pituitary tumor with MRI with gadolinium contrast or to localize an adrenal or ectopic cause using CT or MRI.

Treatment of Cushing's disease most commonly involves transsphenoidal selective adenomectomy in an attempt to preserve pituitary function. In cases of refractory disease, radiation, bilateral adrenalectomy, or medical treatment are all options. In cases of ectopic or adrenal hormone production, the tumor is surgically excised. Patients undergoing bilateral adrenalectomy will require lifelong glucocorticoid and mineralocorticoid replacement.

Pregnancy is an unusual occurrence in Cushing's syndrome. There is a reported increase in fetal loss from spontaneous abortion, stillbirth, and preterm labor. Neonates may demonstrate adrenal insufficiency.

CONGENITAL ADRENAL HYPERPLASIA

Congenital adrenal hyperplasia (CAH) is an autosomal recessive inherited enzymatic defect of steroid biosynthesis that interferes with the production of cortisol. Although defective enzymatic activity may occur in each step of cortisol biosynthesis, approximately 95% of patients have 21-hydroxylase deficiency. Deficiency in this specific enzymatic activity results in increased cortisol level and ACTH secretion. The hyperplastic adrenal cells may secrete sufficient cortisol for normal life, but overproduction of other adrenal steroids, usually androgens, cause the characteristic hirsutism and acne. Pregnancy is rare in untreated patients. With adequate corticosteroid replacement, pregnancy appears to proceed normally. Steroid treatment should continue during pregnancy. Dosages should be adjusted to maintain normal pregnancy levels of testosterone and androstenedione. When prenatal diagnosis has identified a female fetus affected with classical CAH, the mother should be treated with dexamethasone. Dexamethasone is not inactivated by the placenta and is able to suppress the fetal adrenal gland to avoid virilization of the female external genitalia. Deficiency of this enzyme also exposes the female fetus to elevated levels of androgen that can lead to virilization of the external genitalia. The parents of affected children have a 25% risk of having another affected child. Women who have undergone extensive genital surgery to correct virilization may require cesarean section.

PHEOCHROMOCYTOMA

Pheochromocytomas are catecholamine-producing tumors of neuroectodermal tissue. They are an uncommon cause of hypertension and are amenable to surgical therapy. The frequency of pheochromocytoma is greater at autopsy (1 in 1000) than clinical recognition of the disorder, emphasizing the problem in making the diagnosis. They are predominantly singular and benign, but 10% are malignant, 10% are extra-adrenal, and 10% are bilateral or multiple. All races are affected, and peak occurrence is in the fourth decade, although a few occur in the newborn. Ten percent are familial and usually associated with other endocrinopathies. The clinical manifestations are predominantly those associated with excessive catecholamine secretion and include severe headache, profuse sweating, palpitation, nausea and vomiting, blurred vision, vertigo, tremulousness, seizures, and general weakness.

A 24-hour urine collection showing elevated catecholamines and metanephrines will make the diagnosis of pheochromocytoma. An MRI should be obtained to localize adrenal and extra-adrenal tumors. Treatment depends on gestational age and control of hypertension. Alpha-adrenergic blockade can be obtained by using phenoxybenzamine, prazosin, or labetalol. For patients with tachycardia or arrhythmias, beta-blockade is achieved with metoprolol. Surgical intervention is recommended in the second trimester. At term, adrenalectomy can be carried out after vaginal delivery or at the time of cesarean section. Throughout pregnancy, the mother and fetus must be observed for signs of hypertensive crisis. Pregnancies are at risk for spontaneous abortion, placental abruption, uteroplacental insufficiency, growth restriction, and fetal death.

■ DISORDERS OF THE PITUITARY

The pituitary gland in normal pregnancy shows a two- to threefold increase in size of anterior lobe from an increase in prolactin-secreting cells. Serum prolactin concentration increases from the fifth to eighth weeks of gestation from a level of 10 ng/mL to 200 ng/mL at term. Serum FSH and LH concentrations are reduced because of high estrogen levels. Growth hormone levels are difficult to measure in the first two trimesters, but a sample obtained 1 hour after nocturnal sleep should be greater than 5 ng/mL. Posterior pituitary function demonstrates an increase in neurophysins, which act as intraneuronal carrier proteins for oxytocin and vasopressin.

PITUITARY TUMORS

Prolactinomas are the most common hormonally-active pituitary tumors. Presenting complaints may include amenorrhea, infertility, and galactorrhea. Dopamine agonist treatment (bromocriptine, cabergoline) can help restore fertility in 90% of patients. Patients are usually counseled to discontinue medication use once pregnant. Bromocriptine has not been shown to cause congenital malformations during first trimester use or with use throughout pregnancy. Pregnant patients should be monitored for symptoms such as headaches or visual changes. Symptomatic patients may require medical or surgical treatment. Long-term effects of hyperprolactinemia include decreased bone mineral density. Most patients have carried to term without significant complications. It is recommended that the patient be monitored closely throughout pregnancy for visual changes and increased number of headaches.

ACROMEGALY

Acromegaly is characterized by excessive growth due to a growth hormone-secreting tumor. Acromegaly occurs equally in men and women. Clinical signs are enlargement of the feet, hands, mandible, nose, and lips (which gives the characteristic coarse facial appearance). Pregnancy with acromegaly is rare due to associated anterior hypopituitarism, elevated prolactin, and menstrual irregularities. The aim of treatment with bromocriptine (dopamine agonist) or octreotide (somatostatin analog) is to normalize prolactin and growth hormone levels and eventually restore fertility. These medications should be discontinued with pregnancy. Patients should be followed for symptoms of headache or visual disturbance. Growth of the pituitary tumor may require surgical excision. Growth hormone can exacerbate gestational diabetes, fluid retention, and hypertension. No fetal effects have been documented.

SHEEHAN'S SYNDROME

Sheehan's syndrome (postpartum pituitary necrosis) is the most common cause of anterior pituitary insufficiency in adult females. Symptoms appear after 75% destruction of the pituitary gland. The cause is believed to be insufficient blood flow to the pituitary, usually as a result of postpartum blood loss and subsequent hypotension. Onset of symptomatology depends on the degree of pituitary necrosis. It may begin early as failure to lactate, with rapid breast involution after delivery, or take several years, at which time the patient will have menstrual irregularities or symptoms of decreased thyroid or adrenal function. In patients with amenorrhea, pregnancy may only be able to be achieved with ovulation induction. Treatment of pituitary hypofunction during pregnancy includes prednisone and thyroxine. Generally, patients carry pregnancy well and without complication once treatment is given.

DIABETES INSIPIDUS

Posterior pituitary hypofunction usually is the result of trauma or tumor that has damaged the hypothalamic-hypophyseal region, but one-third of cases may be idiopathic and less than 1% inherited as an autosomal dominant trait. Symptoms and signs include polydipsia and polyuria with a specific gravity below 1.005. Diagnosis is made by water deprivation followed by increasing serum osmolality but continued low urine osmolality. Treatment is by administration of the synthetic analogue of arginine vasopressin, which can be given intranasally. The disease does not adversely affect pregnancy, nor does pregnancy adversely affect the disease.

■ AUTOIMMUNE DISORDERS

RHEUMATOID ARTHRITIS

Rheumatoid arthritis is a chronic autoimmune disease characterized by symmetric inflammatory synovitis. The prevalence in North America is 0.5–3.8%, and it occurs three times more frequently in women. Symptoms of rheumatoid arthritis are insidious, with a prodrome of fatigue, weakness, generalized joint stiffness, and myalgias preceding the appearance of joint swelling. The course is variable and unpredictable, with spontaneous remissions and exacerbations. Laboratory findings are mild leukocytosis, elevated erythrocyte sedimentation rate (which may not always reflect the activity of the disease), and a positive rheumatoid factor (in the majority of patients).

Treatment is rest, anti-inflammatory drugs, splints, physical therapy, a well-balanced diet, and adequate movement of all joints. Nonsteroidal anti-inflammatory drugs should be discontinued prior to 32 weeks to avoid premature closure of the ductus arteriosus. The amniotic fluid index should be followed for oligohydramnios. Other treatment options during pregnancy include low-dose steroids and hydroxychloroquine. Penicillamine, gold, and methotrexate should be avoided. Symptoms are believed to improve during pregnancy. However, many patients relapse within 6 months postpartum. The activity of the disease during pregnancy is best followed by assessment of duration of morning stiffness and the number of joints involved. $Ro(SS_A)$ and $La(SS_B)$ antibodies should be obtained to determine the fetal risk for complete heart block.

SYSTEMIC LUPUS ERYTHEMATOSUS

Systemic lupus erythematosus (SLE) is an autoimmune disorder having a multiorgan effect. It predominantly affects females (8:1) between the ages of 20 and 30 and has a higher incidence among blacks. The diagnosis can be made when four of the following criteria are present: malar rash, discoid rash, photosensitivity, oral ulcers, serositis, renal disorders, neurologic disorders, hematologic disorders, immunologic disorders, and an abnormal ANA titer.

Management during pregnancy includes a careful history, physical examination, and laboratory evaluation. A history of prior spontaneous abortions or fetal losses should be elicited. Though the fertility rate of patients with SLE is normal, they have a higher percentage of total fetal losses. This may be associated with the presence of antiphospholipid antibodies. Physical exam should focus on signs of active disease. Laboratory evaluation should include a complete blood count, serum chemistries, and liver function tests. ANA, double-stranded DNA, urine protein, C3, C4, and CH50 should be obtained. Subsequent changes in these values may herald a flare of lupus nephritis. The presence of anti-Ro and anti-La is associated with neonatal lupus, manifested by cutaneous lesions or congenital heart block. Anticardiolipin antibody and lupus anticoagulant are associated with antiphospholipid antibody syndrome which predisposes patients to thromboembolic events. Prophylactic treatment with daily baby aspirin or low-dose heparin is an option.

There appears to be no true consensus on the effects of pregnancy on SLE and vice versa. It seems that most patients who become pregnant while their SLE is quiescent usually have no problems with pregnancy. SLE is associated with hypertension, renal disease, preterm delivery, fetal distress, deep venous thrombosis, intrauter-ine growth restriction, and neonatal death. Serial ultrasounds for fetal growth and antenatal testing starting at 32 weeks should be instituted to ensure fetal well-being.

SCLERODERMA & DERMATOMYOSITIS

Pregnancy in patients with scleroderma is rare, since the disorder occurs most frequently in patients beyond reproductive age. Symptoms appear to improve or remain unchanged. One study did show an increase in preterm births. Pregnancy progresses normally in otherwise stable disease.

CARDIAC & PULMONARY DISEASE

(See Chapter 22.)

REFERENCES

Disorders of the Nervous System

Agostoni M, Giorgi E: Combined spinal-epidural anesthesia for cesarean section in a paraplegic woman: difficulty in obtaining the expected level of block. Eur J Anesthesiol 2000;17:329.

Ameri, A, Bousser MG: Cerebral venous thrombosis. Neurol Clin 1992;10:87.

Aube M: Migraine in pregnancy. Neurology 1999;53(4 Suppl): 526.

Briggs GG, Freeman RK, Yaffe SJ: *Drugs in Pregnancy and Lactation,* 5th ed. Williams & Wilkins, 1998.

Daskalakis GJ, Papageorgiou IS, Petrogiannis ND: Myasthenia gravis and pregnancy. Eur J Obstet Gynecol Reprod Biol 2000;89:201.

Gautier PE et al: Intensive care management of Guillain-Barré syndrome during pregnancy. Intensive Care Med 1990;16:460.

Goldberg M, Rappaport ZH: Neurosurgical, obstetric and endocrine aspects of meningioma during pregnancy. Isr J Med Sci 1987;23:825.

Haas J: High dose IVIG in the postpartum period for prevention of exacerbations of MS. Multiple Sclerosis 2000;6:S18, discussion S33.

Harrison's Online: Multiple sclerosis and other demyelinating diseases. Chapter 371. McGraw-Hill, 2001.

Horton JC et al: Pregnancy and the risk of hemorrhage from cerebral arteriovenous malformations. Neurosurgery 1990; 27:867.

Hurley TJ et al: Landry Guillain-Barré Strohl syndrome in pregnancy: Report of three cases treated with plasmapheresis. Obstet Gynecol 1991;78:482.

Isla A et al: Brain tumors and pregnancy. Obstet Gynecol 1997;89:19.

Kammerman S, Wasserman L: Seizure disorder: part 2. Treatment. Western J Med 2001;175:184.

Laughey WF, MacGregor EA, Wilkinson MI: How many different headaches do you have? Cephalalgia 1993;13:136.

May JL, Lamy C: Stroke in pregnancy and the puerperium. J Neurol 1998;245:305.

Nygaard IE et al: Hand problems in pregnancy. Am Fam Physician 1989;39:123.

Orvieto R et al: Pregnancy and multiple sclerosis: a 2-year experience. Eur J Obstet Gynecol Reprod Biol 1999;82:191.

Paonessa K, Fernand R: Spinal cord injury and pregnancy. Spine 1991;16:596.

Polizzi A, Juson SM, Vincent A: Teratogen update: maternal myasthenia gravis as a cause of congenital arthrogryposis. Teratology 2000;62:332.

Roelvink NC et al: Pregnancy-related primary brain and spinal tumors. Arch Neurol 1987;44:209.

Scharff L, Marcus DA, Turk DC: Headache during pregnancy and in the postpartum: a prospective study. Headache 1997;37:203.

Stevens JC et al: Conditions associated with carpal tunnel syndrome. Mayo Clin Proc 1992;67:541.

Swartjes JM, van Geijn HP: Pregnancy and epilepsia. Eur J Obstet Gynecol Reprod Biol 1998;79:3.

Tarascon Pocket Pharmacopoeia, 2001 Classic edition. Tarascon Publishing.

Walling AD: Bell's palsy in pregnancy and the puerperium. J Fam Pract 1993;36:559.

Walther EU, Hohlfeld R: Multiple sclerosis: side effects of interferon beta therapy and their management. Neurology 1999;53:162.

Wand JS: Carpal tunnel syndrome in pregnancy and lactation. J Hand Surg [Br] 1990;15:93.

Wiltin AG, Mattar F, Sibai BM: Postpartum stroke: a twenty-year experience. Am J Obstet Gynecol 2000;183:83.

Disorders of the Skin

Aronson IK et al: Pruritic urticarial papules and plaques of pregnancy: Clinical and immunopathologic observations in 57 patients. J Am Acad Dermatol 1998;39:933.

Garcia-Gonzalez E et al: Immunology of the cutaneous disorders of pregnancy. Int J Dermatol 1999;38:721.

Vaughan Jones SA, Black MM: Pregnancy dermatoses. J Am Acad Dermatol 1999;40:233.

Disorders of the Gastrointestinal Tract

American College of Obstetricians and Gynecologists: Viral hepatitis in pregnancy. ACOG Technical Bulletin No. 248, July 1998.

Berkane N: Ursodeoxycholic acid in intrahepatic cholestasis of pregnancy. Acta Obstet Gynecol Scand 2000;79:941.

Campbell MS, Garcia A: Gastric and duodenal ulcers during pregnancy. Gastroenterol Clin North Am 1998;27:169.

Connell W, Miller A: Treating inflammatory bowel disease during pregnancy: risks and safety of drug therapy. Drug Safety 1999;21:311.

Ibdah JA, Yang Z, Bennett MJ: Liver disease in pregnancy and fetal fatty acid oxidation defects. Mol Genet Metab 2000; 71:182.

Ilnyckyji A, Blanchard JF: Perianal Crohn's disease and mode of delivery. Am J Gastroenterol 1999;94:3274.

Kumar D, Tandon RK: Use of ursodeoxycholic acid in liver diseases. J Gastroenterol Hepatol 2001;16:3.

Mabie WC: Obstetric management of gastroenterologic complications of pregnancy. Gastroenterol Clin North Am 1992; 21:923.

Ryder SO, Beckingham IJ: ABC of diseases of liver, pancreas, and biliary system: Acute hepatitis. Br Med J 2001;322:151.

Subhani JM, Hamilton MI: Review article: The management of inflammatory bowel disease during pregnancy. Aliment Pharmacol Ther 1998;12:1039.

Vigil-de Garcia P: Acute fatty liver and HELLP syndrome: two distinct pregnancy disorders. Int J Gynecol Obstet 2001;73:215.

Disorders of the Thyroid

Buckshee K et al: Hypothyroidism complicating pregnancy. Aust NZ J Obstet Gynecol 1992;32:240.

Burrow GN: Thyroid function and hyperfunction during gestation. Endocrinol Rev 1993;14:194.

Haddow JE et al: Maternal thyroid deficiency during pregnancy and subsequent psychological development in the child. N Engl J Med 1999;341:549.

Hamburger JI: Diagnosis and management of Graves' disease in pregnancy. Thyroid 1992;2:219.

Harrison's Online. Chapter 330: Disorders of the thyroid gland. McGraw-Hill, 2001.

Lazarus JH: Treatment of hyper- and hypothyroidism in pregnancy. J Endocrinol Invest 1993;16:391.

Lazarus JH, Kokandi A: Thyroid disease in relation to pregnancy: A decade of change. Clin Endocrinol 2000;53:265.

Leung AS et al: Perinatal outcome in hypothyroid pregnancies. Obstet Gynecol 1993;81:349.

Smith C et al: Congenital thyrotoxicosis in premature infants. Clin Endocrinol 2001;54:371.

Disorders of the Parathyroid

Beattie GC et al: Rare presentation of maternal primary hyperparathyroidism. Br Med J 2000;321:223.

Kort KC, Schiller HJ, Numann PJ: Hyperparathyroidism and pregnancy. Am J Surg 1999;177:66.

Mestmann JH: Parathyroid disorders and pregnancy. Sem Perinatol 1998;22:485.

Zaloga GP, Chernow B: Hypocalcemia in critical illness. JAMA 1986;256:1924.

Disorders of Adrenocortical Function

Boscaro M et al: Cushing's syndrome. Lancet 2001;357:783.

Brunt LM: Phaeochromocytoma in pregnancy. Br J Surg 2001; 88:481.

Byyny RL: Preventing adrenal insufficiency during surgery. Postgrad Med 1980;65:219.

Chee GH et al: Transsphenoidal pituitary surgery in Cushing's disease: can we predict outcome? Clin Endocrinol 2001;54:617.

Easterling TR et al: Hemodynamics associated with the diagnosis and treatment of pheochromocytoma in pregnancy. Am J Perinatol 1992;9:464.

Goldman DR: Surgery in patients with endocrine dysfunction. Med Clin North Am 1987;71:499.

Grudden C, Lawrence D: Use of error: Addison's in pregnancy. Lancet 2001;357:1197.

Harrington JL et al: Adrenal tumors in pregnancy. World J Surg 1999;23:182.

Kim SS, Brady KH. Dihydroepiandosterone replacement in Addison's disease. Eur J Obstet Gynecol Reprod Biol 2001;97:96.

Krone N et al: Mothers with congenital adrenal hyperplasia and their children: outcome of pregnancy, birth and childhood. Clin Endocrinol 2001;55:523.

Murakami S et al: A case of mid-trimester intrauterine fetal death with Cushing's syndrome. J Obstet Gynecol Res 1998;24:153.

Samaan NA, Hickey RC: Pheochromocytoma. Semin Oncol 1987;14:297.

Seckl JR, Dunger DB: Diabetes insipidus. Current treatment recommendations. Drugs 1992;44:216.

Ten S, New M, Maclaren N: Clinical Review 130: Addison's Disease 2001. J Clin Endocrinol Metab 2001;86:2909.

Disorders of the Pituitary

Herman-Bonert V, Sleiverstor M, Melmed S: Pregnancy in acromegaly: successful therapeutic outcome. J Clin Endocrinol Metab 1998;83:727.

Loucopolo A, Jewelewicz R: Prolactinomas and pregnancies. Sem Reprod Endocrinol 1984;2:83.

Molitch ME: Endocrine emergencies in pregnancy. Baillieres Clin Endocrinol Metab 1992;6:167.

Molitch ME: Management of prolactinomas during pregnancy. J Reprod Med 1999;144:1121.

Nader S: Pituitary disorders and pregnancy. Semin Perinatol 1990;14:24.

Ray JG: DDAVP use during pregnancy: analysis of its safety for mother and child. Obstet Gynecol Surv 1998;53:450.

Rebar R: Following patients under treatment for hyperprolactinemia. J Reprod Med 1999;144:1100.

Uhiara JE, Narayan R, Kumar S: Sheehan's syndrome following eclampsia: A case report. Asia Oceania J Obstet Gynecol 1992;18:121.

Yap AS et al: Acromegaly first diagnosed in pregnancy: The role of bromocriptine therapy. Am J Obstet Gynecol 1990;163:477.

Autoimmune Disorders

Avrech OM et al: Raynaud's phenomenon and peripheral gangrene complicating scleroderma in pregnancy—diagnosis and management. Br J Obstet Gynecol 1992;99:850.

Ben-Chetrit E: Target antigens of the SSA/Ro and SSB/La system. Am J Reprod Immunol 1992;28:256.

Birdsall M, Pattison N, Chamley L: Antiphospholipid antibodies in pregnancy. Aust NZ J Obstet Gynaecol 1992;32:328.

Bowden AP et al: Women with polyinflammatory polyarthritis have babies of lower birth weight. J Rheumatol 2001;28:355.

Branch DW: Antiphospholipid antibodies and pregnancy: Maternal implications. Semin Perinatol 1990;14:139.

Buchanan NM et al: A study of 100 high risk lupus pregnancies. Am J Reprod Immunol 1992;28:192.

Carmma F et al: Obstetric outcome of pregnancy on patients with systemic lupus erythematosus. A study of sixty cases. Eur J Obstet Gynecol Reprod Biol 1999;83:137.

Carpenter AB, Medsger TA Jr: Previous pregnancy outcome is an important determinant of subsequent pregnancy outcome in women with systemic lupus erythematosus. Am J Reprod Immunol 1992;28:195.

Englert H et al: Reproductive function prior to disease onset in women with scleroderma. J Rheumatol 1992;19:1575.

Floyd RC, Roberts WE: Autoimmune diseases in pregnancy. Obstet Gynecol Clin North Am 1992;19:719.

Giacoia GP, Azubuike K: Autoimmune diseases in pregnancy: Their effect on the fetus and newborn. Obstet Gynecol Surv 1991;46:732.

Hayslett JP: The effect of systemic lupus erythematosus on pregnancy and pregnancy outcome. Am J Reprod Immunol 1992;28:199.

Janssen NM, Genta MS: The effects of immunosuppressive and anti-inflammatory medications on fertility, pregnancy and lactation. Arch Intern Med 2000;160;610.

Julkunen H et al: Pregnancies in lupus neuropathy. Acta Obstet Gynecol Scand 1993;72:258.

Lansink M et al: The onset of rheumatoid arthritis in relation to pregnancy and childbirth. Clin Exp Rheumatol 1993;11:171.

Lockshin MD: Antiphospholipid antibody and antiphospholipid antibody syndrome. Curr Opin Rheumatol 1991;3:797.

Lockshin MD: Overview of lupus pregnancies. Am J Reprod Immunol 1992;28:181.

Morgan GJ Jr, Chow WS: Clinical features, diagnosis, and prognosis in rheumatoid arthritis. Curr Opin Rheumatol 1993; 5:184.

Nieuwenhuis HK, Derksen RH: A prospective, controlled multicenter study on the obstetric risks of pregnant women with antiphospholipid antibodies. Am J Obstet Gynecol 1992;167:26.

Ollier WE, Harrison B, Symmons D: What is the natural history of rheumatoid arthritis? Best Pract Res Clin Rheumatol 2001; 15:27.

Ostensen M: The effect of pregnancy on ankylosing spondylitis, psoriatic arthritis, and juvenile rheumatoid arthritis. Am J Reprod Immunol 1992;28:235.

Petri M, Allbritton K: Fetal outcome of lupus pregnancy: A retrospective case-control study of the Hopkins Lupus Cohort. J Rheumatol 1993;20:650.

Petri M et al: The Hopkins Lupus Pregnancy Center. 1987–1991 update. Am J Reprod Immunol 1992;28:188.

Pinheiro G da R et al: Juvenile dermatomyositis and pregnancy: report and literature review. J Rheumatol 1992;19:1798.

Rubbert A et al: Pregnancy course and complications in patients with systemic lupus erythematosus. Am J Reprod Immunol 1992;28:205.

Sampaio-Barrios PD, Samara AM, Marques Neto JF: Gynecologic history in systemic sclerosis. Clin Rheumatol 2000; 19:184.

Samuels P, Pfeifer SM: Autoimmune diseases in pregnancy. The obstetrician's view. Rheum Dis Clin North Am 1989;15:307.

Silman AJ: Pregnancy and scleroderma. Am J Reprod Immunol 1992;28:238.

Silver RM, Branch DW: Autoimmune disease in pregnancy. Baillieres Clin Obstet Gynaecol 1992;6:565.

Spector TD, DaSilva JA: Pregnancy and rheumatoid arthritis: an overview. Am J Reprod Immunol 1992;28:222.

Steen V: Pregnancy in women with systemic sclerosis. Obstet Gynecol 1999;94:15.

Witter FR, Petri M: Antenatal detection of intrauterine growth restriction in patients with systemic lupus erythematosus. Int J Gynecol Obstet 2000;71:67.

Varner MW: Autoimmune disorders and pregnancy. Semin Perinatol 1992;15:238.

Yasmeen S et al: Pregnancy outcomes in women with systemic lupus erythematosus. J Matern-Fetal Med 2001;10:91.

Surgical Diseases & Disorders in Pregnancy

Christine H. Holschneider, MD

Surgical interventions other than cesarean section are performed in 0.2–2.2% of all pregnancies and the incidence is rising. Altered anatomy and physiology and potential risks to the mother and fetus make diagnosis and management of surgical disorders more difficult during pregnancy. Generally, the interests of mother and fetus are best served by active participation of the obstetrician throughout the mother's course of diagnosis and management with a nonobstetric surgical disorder, although the responsibility is usually shared with other specialists. It is imperative that the obstetrician be well informed concerning the ways in which surgical disorders influence pregnancy and vice versa, the risks of diagnostic and therapeutic procedures to the fetus, and appropriate management of preterm labor in the immediate postoperative period.

Surgical disorders may be either incidental to or directly related to the pregnancy. Diagnostic evaluation requires gentle, sensitive elicitation of physical signs, often without resorting to sophisticated diagnostic aids that involve risk to the developing fetus. Use of good judgment is important regarding the timing, methods, and extent of treatment. In the absence of peritonitis, visceral perforation, or hemorrhage, surgical disorders during gestation generally have little effect on placental function and fetal development.

MATERNAL CONSIDERATIONS

Pregnancy is accompanied by physiologic and anatomic changes that alter the evaluation and management of the surgical patient. The 30–50% increase in plasma volume during pregnancy affects cardiac output and may alter drug distribution and laboratory tests. Red cell mass increases but not as much as the plasma volume, resulting in a slight physiologic anemia. Colloid osmotic pressure is decreased during pregnancy. Increased interstitial fluid is seen as mild edema particularly in the lower extremities. Systemic vascular resistance decreases during pregnancy. Systolic and diastolic blood pressures characteristically drop during the early second trimester with a gradual return to baseline by term. Lung tidal volume increases and a compensated mild respiratory alkalosis exist. Increased renal blood flow is evidenced by increased glomerular filtration rate and decreased serum creatinine and blood urea nitrogen values. Gastrointestinal motility is diminished resulting in delayed gastric emptying and constipation. The enlarging uterus may alter the anatomic relation among the different organs. In the supine position the enlarged uterus may compress the vena cava and result in the hypotensive vena cava compression syndrome.

FETAL CONSIDERATIONS

Optimal care of the pregnant surgical patient requires that potential hazards to the fetus be minimized. This includes risks associated with the maternal disease, diagnostic radiological procedures, therapeutic drugs, anesthesia, and surgery. It is relatively easy to assess risks and benefits to the mother but less so for the fetus because of its relative inaccessibility.

A number of imaging modalities are available for diagnosis during pregnancy, including ultrasound (US), magnetic resonance imaging (MRI), and x-ray. While there are no reported harmful effects from the diagnostic use of US and MRI during pregnancy, exposure to radiation is associated with fetal risks. Limited diagnostic x-ray procedures may be undertaken with care in the pregnant patient. Shielding of the fetus should be performed whenever possible. The risk of adverse fetal effects associated with radiation exposure changes with gestational age and is related to the radiation dose to the fetus. For example, an 8- to 15-week embryo is the most susceptible to radiation-induced mental retardation, with the risk being about 4% at 10 rads and 60% at 150 rads exposure. The most common fetal defects seen with direct fetal irradiation of 10 rads or more include microcephaly, mental retardation, intrauterine growth restriction, and eye abnormalities. Current evidence suggests that there is no increased structural or developmental fetal risk with radiation doses less that 5 rads. Concern also exists regarding in utero radiation exposure associated with an increase in childhood neoplasms. The risk again appears dose related. Fetal exposure to 1–2 rads is estimated to translate into a relative risk of 1.5 to 2.0 for leukemia during childhood. Table 24–1 outlines estimates of fetal radiation exposure with

Table 24–1. Estimated radiation dose to the pelvis from common radiologic procedures.

Procedure	Pelvic Dose (millirads)
X-Rays	
Skull (4 views)	< 0.05
Chest radiograph (2 views)	0.02–0.07
Mammogram (4 views)	7–20
Abdominal series (2 views)	122–245
Lumbosacral spine series (3 views)	168–358
Intravenous or retrograde pyelogram (5 views)	407–1398
Hip series (2 views)	103–213
Upper GI series	558
Barium enema	805
Computed Tomography	
Head (10 cuts)	50
Chest (10 cuts)	100
Abdomen (10 cuts)	1700–2600
Pelvimetry (1 cut and scout film)	250

Adapted from Pentel RL, Brown ML: Genetically significant dose to the United States population from diagnostic medical roentgenology. Radiology 1968;90:209 and Cunningham FG et al: General considerations and maternal evaluation. *Williams Obstetrics*, 21st ed, McGraw-Hill, 2001, p. 1148.

various diagnostic procedures. In summary, routine preoperative x-ray procedures are not justified. However, if a significant alteration in clinical management of the patient would result from the findings of a judiciously performed radiological procedure, the limited fetal exposure risk is generally warranted.

Fortunately, most women who require surgery during pregnancy are otherwise relatively healthy and undergo an uneventful postoperative course. Nevertheless, there are increased risks associated with surgery and anesthesia during pregnancy. A population-based study from Sweden compared 5405 patients who underwent nonobstetric surgery using general anesthesia during pregnancy with 720,000 similar patients who did not have general anesthesia. Adverse effects including low birthweight, prematurity, intrauterine growth restriction, and early neonatal death are thought to correlate with the underlying condition that necessitates the surgical procedure. The incidence of congenital anomalies was not increased in women who had general anesthesia. However, another report on 572 women operated at 4–5 weeks' gestation suggests a possible increase in neural tube defects. Thus, despite general safety of anesthetic agents in pregnancy, there remains some concern regarding teratogenicity in early gestation. With the exception of cocaine hydrochloride, which is contraindicated during pregnancy, there is no known reproductive toxicity associated with local anesthetic agents used at recommended dose ranges. Short-term postoperative use of narcotic analgesic agents, frequently used in combination with acetaminophen or nonsteroidal anti-inflammatory agents, generally appears to produce no adverse fetal effects.

Because intrauterine asphyxia is a major risk to the fetus consequent to maternal surgery, it is important to monitor and maintain maternal oxygen-carrying capacity, oxygen affinity, arterial PO_2, and placental blood flow throughout the preoperative, operative, and postoperative periods. Attention should be given to providing uterine displacement to prevent venocaval compression in the supine position. Supplemental oxygen administration and maintenance of circulating volume also assist fetal oxygenation. A reduction in maternal blood pressure can lead directly to fetal hypoxia. Greater reductions in uteroplacental perfusion by direct vascular constriction and an increase in uterine tonus are noted in association with the use of vasopressors, especially those with predominantly alpha-adrenergic activity. Ephedrine, with its peripheral beta-adrenergic effect, produces much less vasospasm and is the vasopressor of choice in the pregnant patient, especially in treating hypotensive complications of regional anesthesia. To detect fetal hypoxia, continuous electronic fetal heart rate monitoring should be used when maternal surgery is performed in the latter half of gestation as long as the monitoring device can function outside the sterile surgical field.

The severity of the inflammatory response associated with the disease treated by the surgery appears to be more important in determining pregnancy outcome than is the use of anesthesia or the surgical procedure itself. Premature labor does not appear to be a common result of procedures such as exploratory celiotomy unless visceral perforation and peritonitis is encountered or a low pelvic procedure is performed with significant uterine manipulation. The prophylactic use of tocolytics in this setting is controversial. Often, a single dose of a beta-adrenergic agent such as terbutaline is sufficient to arrest contraction. If there is significant inflammation, the use of indomethacin may be preferred. If possible, uterine activity should be monitored following surgery to detect preterm labor and allow for early intervention.

DIAGNOSTIC CONSIDERATIONS

Pain

Pain is the most prominent symptom encountered with acute abdominal conditions complicating pregnancy. Generalized abdominal pain, guarding, and rebound strongly suggest peritonitis secondary to bleeding, exudation, or leakage of intestinal contents. Cramping lower central abdominal pain suggests a uterine disorder. Lower abdominal pain on either side suggests torsion, rupture, or hemorrhage of an ovarian cyst or tumor. Right lower or mid-abdominal pain suggests appendicitis. Disorders of the descending and sigmoid colon with left lower-quadrant pain are infrequently encountered because of the relatively young age of obstetric patients. Mid-abdominal pain early in gestation suggests an intestinal origin. Upper abdominal pain is often related to the liver, spleen, gallbladder, stomach, duodenum, or pancreas. Constipation is a common problem but is rarely associated with other symptoms.

Other Symptoms

When abdominal pain is associated with nausea and vomiting after the first trimester, it usually suggests a gastrointestinal disorder. The inability to pass gas or stool more frequently is associated with lower intestinal obstruction. Diarrhea is seldom encountered in association with acute surgical problems except as a symptom of recurrent ulcerative colitis.

Syncope associated with pain and signs of peritoneal irritation usually indicates an acute abdominal emergency with rupture of a viscus, ischemia, or hemorrhage. A temperature of over 38 °C (100 °F) suggests infection, which may be localized by other clinical findings. Vaginal bleeding usually points to an intrauterine problem. Urinary tract infection is often accompanied by urinary frequency and urgency.

History Taking & Examination

Clues to the cause of surgical disorders in pregnancy are often found in a careful review of the medical history. The stage and status of pregnancy are also relevant. The patient with an acute abdomen should undergo careful assessment of the reproductive organs, and her vital signs and general condition should be noted as well as the presence or absence of peristalsis, abdominal rigidity, and rebound tenderness, and the presence or absence of a mass. The fewest possible number of abdominal examinations should be gently performed without haste and with adequate explanation, using the flat part of the hand and starting in an asymptomatic area.

Laboratory Studies

Several laboratory studies routinely used in the evaluation of surgical disease have altered normal values during gestation, which will be discussed below where appropriate for the specific disease entity. The white blood cell count is considered elevated if it is above 16,000/μL in any trimester. An interval of several hours usually passes between onset of hemorrhage and detection of lowered hematocrit values.

GENERAL VERSUS REGIONAL ANESTHESIA

The type of anesthesia is determined primarily by the planned surgical procedure. As a general rule in pregnancy, it seems prudent to choose the anesthetic technique that requires minimal quantities of drugs and minimizes fetal exposure (eg, regional anesthesia) that is appropriate for the surgical procedure and the patient's condition. Advantages of general anesthesia include optimization of maternal and fetal oxygenation, and reduction in intraoperative uterine irritability.

PRINCIPLES OF SURGICAL MANAGEMENT

Delay in diagnosis and performance of surgery is the factor primarily responsible for increased maternal morbidity rates and perinatal loss, especially with maternal abdominal trauma. With unmistakable signs of peritoneal irritation, evidence of strangulating intestinal obstruction with possible gangrene, or intra-abdominal hemorrhage, immediate surgical exploration generally is indicated. In subacute conditions, caution should be used in deciding to proceed with surgery. When surgery is not urgent and can be delayed, it is best deferred until the second trimester or puerperium. Surgical techniques usually are not altered because of the pregnancy. Essentials of good preoperative care include adequate hydration, availability of blood for transfusion, and appropriate preoperative medication that will not decrease oxygenation for mother and fetus.

Gestational age, uterine size, the specific surgical disorder, and the anticipated type of surgery to be performed are important factors in the selection of the abdominal incision. At operation, the least extensive procedure necessary should be performed with as little manipulation of the uterus as possible. Unless there is an obstetric indication or the uterus interferes with performance of a procedure, it is usually best not to perform a cesarean delivery during an abdominal operation.

Postoperative care depends on the gestational age and the operation performed. For patients in the second half of gestation, electronic monitoring of the fetal heart rate and uterine activity should be continued in the immediate postoperative period. Oversedation and fluid or electrolyte imbalance are to be avoided. Encouragement of early maternal activity and resumption of normal food intake are generally recommended.

LAPAROSCOPY IN PREGNANCY

Over the past decade, laparoscopy has been increasingly used during pregnancy in the management of a variety of surgical disorders, most commonly for the exploration and treatment of adnexal masses and for appendectomy and cholecystectomy. The major advantages are decreased postoperative morbidity, less pain, and shorter hospital stay and postoperative recovery time. Possible drawbacks are the risk of injury to the pregnant uterus, technical difficulty with exposure due to the enlarged uterus, increased carbon dioxide absorption, and decreased uterine blood flow secondary to excessive intra-abdominal pressure. The precise effects of laparoscopy on the human fetus are currently unknown. During the first half of pregnancy, the risks inherent to the laparoscopic procedure do not appear to be substantially increased compared to nonpregnant patients. One population-based study of 2181 laparoscopies during pregnancy and 1522 laparotomies did not find any differential impact of laparoscopy versus laparotomy on perinatal outcome.

■ UPPER ABDOMINAL DISEASES & DISORDERS

Early, accurate diagnosis of serious abdominal surgical disease during pregnancy is more difficult for the following reasons: (1) altered anatomic relationships, (2) impaired palpation and detection of nonuterine masses, (3) depressed symptoms, (4) symptoms that mimic the normal discomforts of pregnancy, and (5) difficulty in differentiating surgical and obstetric disorders. In general, elective surgery should be avoided during pregnancy, but operation should be performed promptly for definite or probable acute disorders. The approach to surgical problems in pregnant or puerperal patients should be the same as in nonpregnant patients, with prompt surgical intervention when indicated. The risk of inducing labor with diagnostic laparotomy is low, provided unnecessary manipulation of the uterus and adnexa is avoided. Spontaneous abortion is most likely to occur if surgery is performed before 14 weeks' gestation or when peritonitis is present.

APPENDICITIS

Acute appendicitis is the most common extrauterine complication of pregnancy for which laparotomy is performed. Suspected appendicitis accounts for nearly two-thirds of all nonobstetric exploratory celiotomies

performed during pregnancy; most cases occur in the second and third trimesters.

Appendicitis occurs in 0.1–1.4 per 1000 pregnancies. Although the incidence of disease is not increased during gestation, rupture of the appendix occurs 2–3 times more often during pregnancy secondary to delays in diagnosis and operation. Maternal and perinatal morbidity and mortality rates are greatly increased when appendicitis is complicated by peritonitis.

A. SYMPTOMS AND SIGNS

The diagnosis of appendicitis in pregnancy is challenging. Signs and symptoms are often atypical and not dramatic. Right lower- or middle-quadrant pain is almost always present when acute appendicitis occurs in pregnancy but may be ascribed to so-called round ligament pain or urinary tract infection. In nonpregnant women, the appendix is located in the right lower quadrant (65%), the pelvis (30%), or retrocecally (5%), but in pregnancy, there is upward displacement of the appendix (Fig 24–1). After the first trimester, the appendix is gradually displaced above McBurney's point, with horizontal rotation of its base. The migration continues until the eighth month of gestation, when more than 90% of appendices lie above the iliac crest and 80% rotate upward and toward the right subcostal area.

The most consistent clinical symptom encountered in pregnant women with appendicitis is vague pain in the right side of the abdomen, although atypical pain patterns abound. Muscle guarding and rebound tenderness are much less demonstrable as gestation progresses. Rectal and vaginal tenderness are present in 80% of patients, particularly in early pregnancy. Nausea, vomiting, and anorexia are usually present, as in the nonpregnant patient. During early appendicitis, the tem-

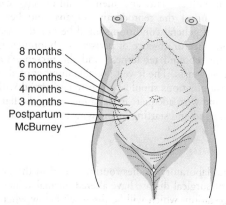

Figure 24–1. Changes in position of the appendix as pregnancy advances.

perature and pulse rate are relatively normal. High fever is not characteristic of the disease, and 25% of pregnant women with appendicitis are afebrile.

B. LABORATORY FINDINGS

The relative leukocytosis of pregnancy (normal, 6000–16,000/μL) clouds interpretation of infection. Although not all patients with appendicitis have white blood cell counts above 16,000/μL, at least 75% show indications of a left shift in the differential. Urinalysis may reveal significant pyuria (20%) as well as microscopic hematuria. This is particularly true in the latter half of pregnancy, when the appendix migrates closer to the retroperitoneal ureter.

C. DIFFERENTIAL DIAGNOSIS

Pyelonephritis is the most common misdiagnosis in patients with acute appendicitis in pregnancy. The differential diagnosis of appendicitis also includes ruptured corpus luteum cyst, adnexal torsion, ectopic pregnancy, abruptio placentae, early labor, round ligament syndrome, chorioamnionitis, degenerating myoma, salpingitis, cholangitis, mesenteric adenitis, neoplasm, diverticulitis, and parasitic infection of the intestine.

D. TREATMENT

The difficult clinical problem in treating appendicitis during pregnancy is making the decision to operate. Most large series report a negative laparotomy rate between 13% and 35%. Diagnostic accuracy is, however, only about 50% at laparotomy due to the many processes that may mimic appendicitis in pregnancy. When the appendix appears normal at laparotomy, it is important to carefully explore for other nonobstetric and obstetric conditions.

Treatment of nonperforated acute appendicitis complicating pregnancy is appendectomy. Prophylactic antibiotic therapy is controversial. However, broad-spectrum intravenous antibiotics are appropriate when there has been perforation, peritonitis, or abscess formation. Induced abortion is rarely indicated. If drainage is necessary for generalized peritonitis, drains should be placed transabdominally and not transvaginally. During the first trimester, a vertical midline or paramedian incision on the right side is generally considered appropriate. Laparoscopy is an alternate surgical approach used with increasing frequency, especially in the first half of pregnancy. In the late second or third trimester, a muscle-splitting incision centered over the point of maximal tenderness usually provides optimal appendiceal exposure. As a rule, appendiceal disease is managed and the pregnancy is left alone. A Smead-Jones closure with secondary wound closure 72 hours later may be advisable when the appendix is gangrenous or perforated or if there is peritonitis or abscess formation.

Depending on the gestational age and expert neonatal care available, abdominal delivery occasionally is performed when there is peritonitis, sepsis, or a large appendiceal or cul-de-sac abscess. Data are limited, so it is difficult to make definitive recommendations regarding the use of prophylactic tocolytics. It appears unnecessary in uncomplicated appendicitis but may be appropriate with advanced disease. Caution is indicated, as there are reports that tocolytics are associated with an increased risk of pulmonary edema in women with sepsis. If labor follows shortly after surgery in the late third trimester, it should be allowed to progress, because it is not associated with a significant risk of wound dehiscence. At times, the large uterus may help wall off an infection, which after delivery may become disrupted, leading to an acute abdomen within hours postpartum.

E. PROGNOSIS

Better fluid and nutritional support, use of antibiotics, safer anesthesia, prompt surgical intervention, and improved surgical technique have been important elements in the significant reduction of maternal mortality from appendicitis during pregnancy. Similarly, the fetal mortality rate has significantly improved over the past 50 years. Perinatal loss may occur in association with preterm labor and delivery or with generalized peritonitis and sepsis; it occurs in 1–5% of uncomplicated appendicitis. With appendiceal rupture, fetal loss rates are reportedly as high as 30%. This is of particular concern because appendiceal rupture occurs most frequently in the third trimester. Thus it is imperative to avoid surgical delay. A higher negative laparotomy rate may be an acceptable trade-off for a lowered fetal mortality rate.

CHOLECYSTITIS & CHOLELITHIASIS

Gallbladder disease represents one of the most common medical conditions and the second most common surgical disorder during pregnancy. Acute cholecystitis occurs in 1 in 1600 to 1 in 10,000 pregnancies. It has been estimated that at least 3.5% of pregnant women harbor gallstones. Multiparas are at increased risk of gallbladder disease. Both an increase in lithogenicity of the bile and a decrease in gallbladder contractility are seen during pregnancy.

A. SYMPTOMS AND SIGNS

These are similar to those seen in the nonpregnant state and include anorexia, nausea, vomiting, dyspepsia, and intolerance of certain foods, particularly those with high fat content. Biliary tract disease may cause epigastric, right scapular, and even left upper-quadrant or lower-quadrant pain that tends to be episodic in nature. Biliary colic attacks are often of acute onset, seemingly triggered by meals, and may last from a few minutes to several hours. Fever, right upper-quadrant pain, and tenderness under the liver with deep inspiration (Murphy's sign) are often present in patients with acute cholecystitis.

B. LABORATORY FINDINGS

An increased white blood cell count with an increase in immature forms is seen with acute cholecystitis. Abnormalities of liver function tests are often encountered, eg, an increase in AST (aspartate transaminase) and ALT (alanine transaminase). Modest increases in the alkaline phosphatase and bilirubin levels are anticipated very early in cholecystitis or common duct obstruction. However, a more characteristic pattern of relatively normal AST and ALT with elevated alkaline phosphatase and bilirubin is generally found after the first day of the attack. These changes are not diagnostic and do not signify common bile duct stone or obstruction alone, but when present serve to support the diagnosis.

C. ULTRASOUND FINDINGS

Ultrasound findings of stones in the gallbladder, a thickened gallbladder wall, fluid collecting around the gallbladder, a dilated common bile duct, or even swelling in the pancreas are suggestive of cholelithiasis and cholecystitis. The diagnostic accuracy of US for detecting gallstones in pregnancy is 95%, making it the diagnostic test of choice.

D. DIFFERENTIAL DIAGNOSIS

The major diagnostic difficulty that pregnancy imposes is differentiating between cholecystitis and appendicitis. In addition to gallstones, cholecystitis can be infectious secondary to *Salmonella typhi* or parasites. A number of other lesions of the biliary tract occur rarely during gestation, including choledochal cysts, which are seen as a spherical dilatation of the common bile duct with a very narrow or obstructed distal end. Associated pancreatitis may be present. Severe preeclampsia with associated right upper-quadrant abdominal pain and abnormal liver function tests, HELLP syndrome, acute fatty liver of pregnancy, and acute viral hepatitis are in the differential. The presence of proteinuria, nondependent edema, hypertension, and sustained increases in AST and ALT compared with alkaline phosphatase are clinical and laboratory features usually associated with preeclampsia.

E. COMPLICATIONS

Pancreatitis may frequently accompany cholecystitis during pregnancy. Removal of the gallbladder and gallstones may be preferred over conservative medical therapy when there is concurrent pancreatitis. Other uncommon complications of cholecystitis during gestation include retained intraductal stones, cholangitis, and rupture of the cystic duct.

F. TREATMENT

The traditional initial management of symptomatic cholelithiasis and cholecystitis in pregnancy is nonoperative. Bowel rest, intravenous hydration, correction of electrolyte imbalances, and intravenous antibiotics result in the resolution of acute symptoms in most patients. Surgical intervention is indicated if symptoms fail to improve with medical management, for recurrent episodes of biliary colic, and complications such as cholecystitis, choledocholithiasis, and gallstone pancreatitis. The majority of patients respond to conservative therapy. Due to the fact that recurrence rates for symptomatic biliary disease during pregnancy may be as high as 60%, active surgical management, especially in the second trimester, has been advocated in recent years. Surgical approaches include open and laparoscopic cholecystectomy. Endoscopic retrograde cholangiopancreatography (ERCP) with endoscopic sphincterotomy may be an alternative for selected patients with common bile duct stones. During the first trimester, a high fetal loss rate has been observed with surgical intervention for gallstone disease. When operative therapy for cholecystitis is effected during the second and third trimesters, there does not appear to be an appreciable increase in morbidity and mortality rates or fetal loss.

G. PROGNOSIS

The outcome for mother and fetus following uncomplicated gallbladder surgery is excellent. Morbidity and mortality rates increase with maternal age and extent of disease.

ACUTE PANCREATITIS

The incidence of acute pancreatitis in pregnancy is reported to range from 1 in 1000 to 1 in 5000 deliveries. Pancreatitis occurs most frequently in the third trimester and puerperium. The mortality rate associated with acute pancreatitis may be higher during pregnancy because of delay in diagnosis. The ultimate cause of pancreatitis is the presence of activated digestive enzymes within the pancreas. Many cases of pancreatitis are idiopathic. As in the nonpregnant state, cholelithiasis is the most commonly identified cause, followed by alcoholism, lipidemia, viral and drug-induced pancreatitis, familial pancreatitis, structural abnormalities of the pancreas or duodenum, severe abdominal trauma, and vascular disease. Some authors have suggested that pregnancy-induced hypertension may lead to pancreatitis.

A. SYMPTOMS AND SIGNS

Gravidas with pancreatitis usually present with severe, steady epigastric pain that often radiates to the back in general approximation of the retroperitoneal location of the pancreas. Often exacerbated by food intake, its onset may be gradual or acute and is frequently accompanied by nausea and vomiting. During gestation, patients may present primarily with vomiting with little or no abdominal pain. Although physical examination is rarely diagnostic, several findings of note may be present, including a low-grade fever, tachycardia, and orthostatic hypotension. The latter finding may be present with hemorrhagic pancreatitis in addition to Cullen's sign (periumbilical ecchymosis) and Turner's sign (flank ecchymosis). Epigastric tenderness and ileus may also be present.

B. Laboratory Findings

The cornerstone of diagnosis is the determination of serum amylase and lipase levels. Interpretation of serum amylase levels in pregnancy is at times difficult due to the physiologic up to twofold rise in serum amylase during pregnancy. A laboratory value of serum amylase that is greater than two times above the upper limit of normal suggests pancreatitis. However, elevated serum amylase is not pancreatitis-specific because cholecystitis, bowel obstruction, hepatic trauma, or a perforated duodenal ulcer can cause similar serum amylase level elevations. Serum lipase is a pancreas-specific enzyme and may be helpful in the differential diagnosis. Serum amylase levels do not correlate with the severity of the disease and usually return to normal within a few days of an attack of uncomplicated acute pancreatitis. In severe pancreatitis, hypocalcemia develops as calcium is complexed by fatty acids liberated by lipase.

C. Ultrasound Diagnosis

Sonographic examination may demonstrate an enlarged pancreas with a blunted contour, peritoneal or peripancreatic fluid, and abscess or pseudocyst formation. Ultrasonography allows for the diagnosis of cholelithiasis, which may be etiologic for pancreatitis. The mere presence of gallstones, however, does not demonstrate etiologic relevance. Ultrasound is also helpful for evaluating other differential diagnostic considerations such as ectopic pregnancy.

D. Differential Diagnosis

Especially pertinent in the differential diagnosis of pancreatitis in pregnancy are hyperemesis gravidarum, preeclampsia, ruptured ectopic pregnancy (often with elevated serum amylase levels), perforated peptic ulcer, intestinal obstruction, acute cholecystitis, ruptured spleen, liver abscess, and perinephric abscess.

E. Complications

Although all of the usual complications of pancreatitis can occur in parturients, there is no special predisposition to complications during pregnancy. Acute complications include hemorrhagic pancreatitis with severe hypotension and hypocalcemia, acute respiratory distress syndrome, pleural effusions, pancreatic ascites, abscess formation, and liponecrosis.

F. Treatment

Treatment of acute pancreatitis is primarily medical and supportive, including bowel rest with or without nasogastric suction, intravenous fluid and electrolyte replacement, and parenteral analgesics. Antibiotics are reserved for cases in which there is evidence of an acute infection. Pancreatic enzyme inhibitors have not been successful. Surgical exploration is reserved for patients with pancreatic abscess, ruptured pseudocyst, or severe hemorrhagic pancreatitis, and for those with pancreatitis secondary to a lesion that is amenable to surgery. Pregnancy does not influence the course of pancreatitis. Pancreatitis in pregnancy is managed as it is in the nonpregnant state, except that parenteral nutritional supplementation is considered at an earlier point in treatment to protect the fetus. In patients with gallstone pancreatitis, consideration is given to cholecystectomy after the acute inflammation subsides.

G. Prognosis

Maternal mortality rates as high as 37% were reported prior to the era of modern medical and surgical management. Respiratory failure, shock, need for massive fluid replacement, and severe hypocalcemia are predictive of severity of disease. Perinatal losses are few, although preterm labor appears to occur in a high proportion of patients with acute pancreatitis in later gestation. Most recent single-institution series reflect a reduced maternal mortality rate of 3.4% and a fetal salvage rate of 89%.

PEPTIC ULCER DISEASE

Pregnancy appears to be somewhat protective against the development of gastrointestinal ulcers as gastric secretion and motility are reduced and mucus secretion increased. Close to 90% of women with known peptic ulcer disease (PUD) experience significant improvement during pregnancy, but more than half will have recurrence of symptoms within 3 months postpartum. Thus, peptic ulcer disease occurring as a complication of pregnancy or diagnosed during gestation is encountered infrequently, although the exact incidence is unknown. Infection with *Helicobacter pylori* is associated with the development of peptic ulcer disease.

A. Clinical Findings

Signs and symptoms of ulcer disease in pregnancy can be mistakenly dismissed as being a normal part of the gravid state. Dyspepsia is the major symptom of ulcers during gestation, although reflux symptoms and nausea are also common. Epigastric discomfort that is temporally unrelated to meals is often reported. Abdominal pain might suggest a perforated ulcer, especially in the presence of peritoneal signs and systemic shock. Endoscopy is the diagnostic method of choice for these patients.

B. Differential Diagnosis

Reflux esophagitis, a common occurrence in pregnancy, and Mallory-Weiss tears may have symptoms very similar to those of peptic ulcer disease. Gastritis and the irritable bowel syndrome must be ruled out. In recent years the diagnosis of persistent hyperemesis gravidarum has been linked to *Helicobacter pylori* infection.

C. Treatment

Dyspepsia during pregnancy first should be treated with dietary and lifestyle changes, supplemented with antacids or sucralfate. When symptoms persist, H_2-receptor antagonists or, in severe cases, proton pump inhibitors may be used. A two-week course of antibiotics covering *Helicobacter pylori* is indicated as in the nonpregnant state.

D. Complications

Fewer than 100 parturients have been reported with complications of peptic ulceration such as perforation, bleeding, and obstruction. Most of these have occurred in the third trimester of pregnancy. Gastric perforation during pregnancy has an exceedingly high mortality rate, partly because of the difficulty in establishing the proper diagnosis. Other causes for upper gastrointestinal bleeding in pregnancy are reflux esophagitis and Mallory-Weiss tears. Surgical intervention is indicated for significant bleeding ulcerations. In patients requiring surgery for complicated peptic ulcers late in the third trimester, concurrent cesarean delivery may be indicated to enhance operative exposure of the upper abdomen and to prevent potential fetal death or damage from maternal hypotension and hypoxemia.

ACUTE INTESTINAL OBSTRUCTION

Intestinal obstruction is an infrequently encountered complication of pregnancy that is estimated to occur in about 1–3 of every 10,000 pregnancies. However, it is the third most common nonobstetric reason for laparotomy during pregnancy (following appendicitis and biliary tract disease). It occurs most commonly in the third trimester. The most common causes of mechanical obstruction are adhesions (60%) and volvulus (25%), followed by intussusception, hernia, and neoplasm.

A. Clinical Findings

The same classic triad of abdominal pain, vomiting, and obstipation is observed in pregnant and nonpreg-

nant women with intestinal obstruction. Pain may be diffuse, constant, or periodic, occurring every 4–5 minutes with small bowel obstruction or every 10–15 minutes with large bowel obstruction. Bowel sounds are of little value in making an early diagnosis of obstruction, and tenderness to palpation is typically absent with early obstruction. Vomiting occurs early with small bowel obstruction. Guarding and rebound tenderness are observed in association with strangulation or perforation. Late in the course of disease, fever, oliguria, and shock occur as manifestations of massive fluid loss into the bowel, acidosis, and infection. The classic findings of bowel ischemia include fever, tachycardia, localized abdominal pain, and a marked leukocytosis.

The diagnosis is usually confirmed by radiologic studies, which should be obtained when intestinal obstruction is suspected. A single abdominal series is nondiagnostic in up to 50% of early cases, but serial films usually reveal progressive changes that confirm the diagnosis. Volvulus should be suspected when there is a single, grossly dilated loop of bowel. A volvulus primarily occurs at the cecum, but may also be seen at the sigmoid colon. Occasionally, radiologic studies following oral or rectal contrast are indicated.

B. Differential Diagnosis

The diagnosis of hyperemesis gravidarum in the second and third trimesters should be viewed with caution and made only after gastrointestinal causes for the symptoms have been excluded. Adynamic ileus of the colon (Ogilvie syndrome) and pseudo-obstruction are included in the differential, but are rarely seen during pregnancy.

C. Treatment

The management of bowel obstruction in pregnancy is essentially no different from treatment of nonpregnant patients. The cornerstones of therapy are bowel decompression, intravenous hydration, and timely surgery. The patient must be rapidly stabilized. The amount of fluid loss is often underestimated and may be 1–6 L by the time obstruction can be identified on a scout film. Aggressive hydration is needed to support both the mother and the fetus. A nasogastric tube should be placed and antibiotic prophylaxis given. A vertical midline incision on the abdomen provides the best operative exposure and can be extended as needed. Surgical principles for intraoperative management apply similarly to pregnant and nonpregnant patients. Cesarean delivery is performed first if the large uterus prevents adequate exposure of the bowel in term pregnancies or if indicated obstetrically. The entire bowel should be examined carefully as there may be more than one area of obstruction or limited bowel viability.

D. PROGNOSIS

Intestinal obstruction in pregnancy is associated with a maternal mortality rate of 6%, with losses occurring secondary to infection and irreversible shock. Early diagnosis and treatment are essential for an improved outcome. Perinatal mortality is about 20% and usually results from maternal hypotension and resultant fetal hypoxia and acidosis.

SPONTANEOUS HEPATIC & SPLENIC RUPTURE

Intra-abdominal hemorrhage during pregnancy has diverse causes, including trauma, preexisting splenic disease, and preeclampsia-eclampsia. Often, the exact cause cannot be determined preoperatively. Spontaneous hepatic rupture associated with severe preeclampsia-eclampsia may be manifested by severe abdominal pain and shock, with thrombocytopenia and low fibrinogen levels. Exploratory celiotomy should be undertaken immediately because early diagnosis, blood transfusion, and prompt operation have been associated with improved survival rates.

Bleeding from a lacerated or ruptured spleen does not cease spontaneously and requires immediate surgical attention. Ultrasound or CT evidence of a hemoperitoneum or a hemorrhagic peritoneal lavage in association with a falling hematocrit and abdominal pain establish the presence of a hemoperitoneum.

SPLENIC ARTERY ANEURYSM

Autopsy data suggest that splenic artery aneurysm occurs in 0.1% of adults. It is estimated that 6–10% of lesions will rupture, with portal hypertension and pregnancy being the main risk factors. Twenty-five to 40% of ruptures occur during gestation, especially in the last trimester. Pregnant women who develop ruptured splenic artery aneurysm have a 75% mortality rate with an even higher fetal mortality rate of up to 95%. Most patients with this condition are thought preoperatively to have placental abruption or uterine rupture.

Spontaneous rupture of a splenic artery aneurysm has been reported as a major cause of intraperitoneal hemorrhage during late gestation. Prior to rupture, the presenting symptoms may be completely absent or vague, with the most common symptom being vague epigastric, left upper-quadrant, or left shoulder pain. In about 25% of patients a two-stage rupture is seen, with a smaller primary hemorrhage into the lesser sac, which may allow for temporary tamponade of the bleeding until complete rupture of the aneurysm into the peritoneal cavity occurs, causing hemorrhagic shock. A bruit may be audible. A highly diagnostic finding on flat x-ray film of the abdomen is the demonstration in the upper left quadrant of an oval calcification with a central lucent area. In stable clinical situations, angiography can provide positive confirmation and is the gold standard for diagnosis. In pregnancy, however, ultrasonography and pulsed-wave Doppler studies are preferred in order to minimize fetal radiation exposure. A splenic artery aneurysm in a woman of childbearing age should be treated electively, even during pregnancy, due to the increased risk of rupture and associated mortality. The elective operative mortality rate is reported to range between 0.5% and 1.3%.

Whenever rupture is suspected, the obstetrician must undertake immediate laparotomy with general surgical assistance. Following ligation of the splenic artery and resection of the aneurysm, the surgeon can choose to retain the spleen if adequate collateral arterial blood supply can be demonstrated, but more usually splenectomy is performed. As in the nonpregnant patient, pneumococcal vaccine should be given 2 weeks prior to elective splenectomy or immediately following emergent splenectomy.

■ PELVIC DISEASES & DISORDERS

OVARIAN MASSES

The incidence of an adnexal mass associated with pregnancy has been reported to range from 1 in 81 to 1 in 2500 pregnancies. Of the adnexal masses diagnosed during pregnancy, 50% will be smaller than 5 cm, 25% will be 5–10 cm, and 25% will be greater than 10 cm in diameter. The majority will be an incidental ultrasonographic finding and resolve spontaneously. In fact, more than 90% of unilateral, noncomplex masses less than 5 cm in diameter that are noticed in the first trimester resolve spontaneously. Patients who undergo assisted reproduction present a special subgroup as their ovaries frequently have ovarian cysts in the first trimester due to ovarian hyperstimulation. More than 90% of these resolve spontaneously as well. However, recent reports associating infertility and ovarian stimulation with an increased incidence of ovarian neoplasms should be kept in mind.

Ovarian masses are usually asymptomatic unless rupture or torsion occurs. Only 2% of such masses will rupture during gestation; however, it is much more likely that torsion will occur, resulting in a 30% emergency laparotomy rate. The most common adnexal mass early in pregnancy is the corpus luteum cyst of gestation, which rarely exceeds 6 cm in diameter. The most common pathologic ovarian neoplasms during pregnancy are benign cystic teratoma (21%), serous cystadenoma (21%), cystic corpus luteum (18%), and mucinous cystadenoma.

Ultrasonography usually facilitates delineation of the size and consistency of adnexal masses. If the mass is unilateral, mobile, and cystic, anaplastic elements are less likely and operation can be deferred until the second trimester. Ovarian enlargement must be differentiated from lesions of the colon, pedunculated leiomyomas, pelvic kidneys, and congenital abnormalities of the uterus. Any adnexal lesion present after 14 weeks' gestation, that is growing in size on serial ultrasonographic evaluations, contains solid and complex components or internal vegetations, is fixed, surrounded by abdominal ascites, or symptomatic warrants surgical exploration and pathologic diagnosis. Asymptomatic ovarian masses that are initially noted in the third trimester of pregnancy may be followed until the onset of labor, because the size of the uterus may present problems of access during laparotomy and because labor may be inadvertently induced.

Solid Ovarian Tumors

Solid ovarian tumors discovered during pregnancy generally should be treated surgically because of the low but significant incidence of cancer (2–5%) and to prevent torsion, rupture, and soft tissue dystocia at the time of labor. Because of these potential hazards, persistent solid or cystic ovarian masses discovered in the first trimester should ideally be removed in the second trimester.

Torsion of the Adnexa

Torsion of the adnexa can involve the ovary, tube, and ancillary structures, either separately or together. The most common time for adnexal torsion to occur is between 6 and 14 weeks and in the immediate puerperium. Although torsion of a normal adnexa has been described, it commonly is associated with a cyst. Symptoms include abdominal pain and tenderness that are usually sudden in onset and result from occulsion of the vascular supply to the twisted organ. Shock and peritonitis may ensue. Ultrasonography frequently demonstrates an adnexal mass and altered blood flow on Doppler studies. The diagnosis of torsion is ultimately made at surgery. Prompt operation is necessary to prevent tissue necrosis, preterm labor, and potential perinatal death. The right ovary is involved more frequently than the left. Benign cystic teratomas and cystadenomas are the most common histologic findings in ovaries that have undergone torsion. Traditional thinking has been that ovarian cysts that have undergone torsion must not be untwisted prior to pedicle clamping, because of the concern for potential fatal thromboembolic complica-

tions. However, recent series on both nonpregnant and pregnant patients demonstrate that adnexae that had undergone torsion can safely be derotated, followed by the appropriate removal of the mass, eg, cystectomy. These adnexae are capable of recovering and being functional. Salpingo-oophorectomy can be reserved for the management of active bleeding or suspicious neoplasms.

Carcinoma of Ovary

Carcinoma of the ovary occurs in less than 0.1% of all gestations and has been encountered in all trimesters. Between 2% and 6% of all ovarian tumors complicating pregnancy are malignant. Consistent with the young age of the pregnant patient population, most neoplasms are germ cell tumors (dysgerminoma, endodermal sinus tumor, malignant teratoma, embryonal carcinoma, and choriocarcinoma) and tumors with low malignant potential, but cystadenocarcinomas do occur.

The treatment for gestational ovarian cancer is no different from that for the nonpregnant patient. A generous surgical incision is important not only to remove the tumor but also to properly explore the abdomen and to reduce uterine manipulation until the definitive surgical course of management is determined. Surgical removal of as much of the cancer as possible is indicated. Staging is accomplished and adequate tissue obtained for histologic diagnosis. Conservative surgery is appropriate for an encapsulated tumor if there is no evidence of uterine or contralateral ovarian involvement. In more advanced stages, the extent of surgery including tumor debulking will depend upon gestational age and the patient's wishes with regard to the pregnancy. Neoadjuvant chemotherapy may offer an interim treatment for selected patients diagnosed at midgestation to allow for fetal maturity prior to extensive surgical cytoreduction. Elevated tumor markers such as alpha-fetoprotein (AFP), lactate dehydrogenase (LDH), beta-human chorionic gonadotropin (β-hCG), and CA-125 may be misleading because pregnancy itself may cause an increase in these values.

If the tumor is benign, residual ovarian tissue is conserved if possible. The contralateral ovary must always be carefully evaluated to rule out disease. Should surgical extirpation of the corpus luteum be required in the first trimester, progestin support is recommended.

LEIOMYOMAS

Uterine leiomyomas occur in 0.3–2.6% of pregnancies and may complicate pregnancy by degeneration, torsion, or mechanical obstruction of labor. A degenerating leiomyoma or one undergoing torsion is characterized by acute abdominal pain with point tenderness over the site of the leiomyoma. Conservative treatment with analgesia, reassurance, and supportive therapy is almost always adequate. The two usual indications for surgery during pregnancy include torsion of an isolated, pedunculated leiomyoma and obstruction of labor. With the exception of a pedunculated leiomyoma on a narrow stalk, myomectomy should not be performed during pregnancy because of the risk of uncontrollable hemorrhage. Disseminated intravascular coagulation has been reported as a complication of leiomyoma degeneration. Although this is certainly a rare occurrence, a coagulation profile may prove useful in selected cases of degeneration.

Ultrasonography is of great value to document the location, size, and consistency of leiomyomas in a pregnant uterus. Cystic changes in leiomyomas are often visualized when there are clinical signs of degeneration. Early in pregnancy, diagnostic laparoscopy may be of value to differentiate leiomyoma from ovarian tumor, especially when ultrasonography is inadequate.

■ BREAST CANCER AND OTHER MALIGNANCIES

BREAST CANCER

Breast cancer is the most common cancer affecting women in the United States. One of every 5 cases occurs in women under 45 years of age; and 2–5% of women are pregnant when diagnosed with breast cancer. The incidence of breast cancer in pregnancy is 3 per 10,000 live births. For this reason, careful breast examination should be performed during the prenatal and postnatal care and a family history should be obtained. Pregnancy- and lactation-related changes in the breast increase the frequency and range of breast problems and make the diagnosis of breast cancer more difficult. Any mass found by the woman or the obstetrician should be fully evaluated without undue delay. The range of differential diagnoses is broad: lactating adenoma, galactocele, milk-filled cyst, fibroadenoma, abscess, and cancer.

Initial management for the pregnant patient with a breast mass does not differ from that for nonpregnant women. When a localized lesion is present, needle aspiration and needle biopsy may be appropriate. Breast ultrasonography during pregnancy is safe and helpful in distinguishing between cystic and solid masses. Although the sensitivity of mammography is diminished by the breast changes in pregnancy, the study may still be helpful for selected patients with inconclusive clinical examinations. With low-dose mammography and appropriate shielding, fetal radiation exposure is minimal. Nonetheless, it is generally recommended that the procedure be avoided during the first trimester. Cystic lesions should be aspirated and the fluid examined for abnormal cytologic characteristics. Malignant cells are rarely found in nonbloody fluid. Surgical excisional biopsy may be more appropriate for clinically suspicious or cytologically equivocal lesions. The increased vascularity of the breasts does not appear to interfere with excisional biopsy in an outpatient setting.

Management of the pregnant woman with breast carcinoma is especially difficult because it requires careful consideration of both mother and fetus. The general approach to treatment for breast cancer in pregnancy should be similar to nonpregnant patients and should not be delayed because of pregnancy. Termination of pregnancy has not been shown to improve survival rates. Modified radical or radical mastectomy is the preferred local management of pregnant patients with breast cancer, with the goal to avoid the need for adjuvant radiation therapy. Breast-conserving surgery, which must be combined with adjuvant radiation, is not feasible unless surgery is performed during late gestation and radiation treatment can be safely postponed until after delivery. Radical mastectomy is well tolerated during pregnancy. The results of treatment are much the same stage for stage as they are in nonpregnant patients, but pregnancy-associated breast cancers tend to be more advanced at diagnosis (larger tumor size, more frequently involved lymph nodes), resulting in an overall worse prognosis for this group of patients as a whole. Adjuvant chemotherapy is frequently recommended for premenopausal women with breast cancer. The recommendation of chemotherapy to a pregnant woman with breast cancer is a complex decision. Cyclophosphamide, doxorubicin, and 5-fluorouracil have been given successfully during the second and third trimester with no increase in congenital malformations. However, there is an increased incidence of prematurity and intrauterine growth restriction. There is no contraindication to breastfeeding after completion of therapy for breast cancer. Breastfeeding should be avoided during chemotherapy, hormone therapy, or radiation. Subsequent pregnancies need not necessarily be discouraged after a suitable period of recuperation and observation, as subsequent pregnancy does not increase the risk of recurrence or death from breast cancer.

BONE TUMORS

Benign bone tumors rarely cause problems in pregnancy. The natural history of malignant bone tumors does not appear to be affected by pregnancy, but treatment can be complicated. The most frequently encountered malignant tumors are Ewing's sarcoma and osteogenic sarcoma. Sites in such areas as the clavicle, sternum, spine, humerus, and femur initially appear as a lump or mass with local pain and disability. In general, pregnancy considerations should not cause postponement of surgery for biopsy and treatment of malignant bone tumors. Osteogenic sarcoma is treated with wide surgical excision followed by adjuvant chemotherapy. Because adjuvant combination chemotherapy considerably enhances the outcome of osteogenic sarcoma, pregnancy should not delay optimum therapy for more than a few weeks. An excellent outcome usually follows wide local excision of giant cell bone tumors.

THYROID CANCER

Although the majority of patients with thyroid carcinoma are in their 50s and 60s, approximately 15% are younger than 30 years of age. Approximately 15% of solitary thyroid nodules are malignant. Thus, prompt investigation of these nodules is indicated. Work-up includes thyroid function tests, ultrasonography, and fine needle aspiration. Radioiodine thyroid scanning is contraindicated in pregnancy. The diagnosis of thyroid cancer in pregnancy is not a reason to delay the necessary surgery. Most thyroid carcinomas are well differentiated and have an indolent course. There are some data to suggest that tumors diagnosed in pregnancy may be more aggressive.

■ CARDIAC DISEASE

Cardiac disease complicates 1–4% of all pregnancies in the United States. Rheumatic and congenital heart disease constitute the majority of cases. Patients requiring cardiac surgery should have the procedure performed prior to becoming pregnant. Nevertheless, the rare patient will require cardiac surgery during pregnancy. Most available reports on cardiac surgery during pregnancy involve closed and open mitral valvotomies and mitral or aortic valve replacement. When valve replacement is necessary, tissue valves rather than artificial valves are generally recommended, so that anticoagulation is not needed. Cardiac surgery can be performed with excellent results, although there is maternal and fetal risk. Operations should generally be performed early in the second trimester when organogenesis is complete and there is comparatively less hemodynamic burden and less risk of preterm labor than later in gestation. The risk for the mother is probably no greater than for the nonpregnant patient and is related to the specific procedure performed and the patient's preoperative cardiovascular status. Fetal risk is substantial due to the nonpulsatile blood flow and

hypotension associated with cardiopulmonary bypass. A fetal mortality rate around 15% is reported. Close fetal surveillance by electronic heart rate and uterine contraction monitoring is essential during any cardiac surgical procedure whether or not cardiopulmonary bypass is used. During bypass, blood flow to the uterus can be assessed indirectly by changes in the fetal heart rate, and alterations in flow can be made accordingly. Closed cardiac surgery techniques appear to be associated with better fetal outcome than open cardiac procedures. Congenital heart defects usually do not require surgery unless cyanotic heart disease is present. Pulmonary hypertension secondary to fixed pulmonary vascular resistance and right-to-left shunting is associated with substantial maternal and perinatal mortality rates. If pulmonary artery hypertension is demonstrated on cardiac catheterization early in pregnancy and is not reactive to oxygen administration, therapeutic abortion is strongly indicated.

■ NEUROLOGIC DISEASE

Intracranial hemorrhage during pregnancy is rare (1–5 per 10,000 pregnancies) but associated with significant maternal and fetal mortality and serious neurologic morbidity in survivors. Rupture of an aneurysm or arteriovenous malformation (AVM) is the most common cause, followed by eclampsia. Other causes include coagulopathy, trauma, and intracranial tumors. The risk of bleeding during pregnancy from an AVM that had not bled previously is 3.5%, which is close to the annual bleeding rate in the nonpregnant patient. However, mortality due to a bleeding AVM in pregnancy is higher (30%) than in the nonpregnant state (10%). Intracranial hemorrhage with associated neurologic damage during pregnancy (limited capacity for decision making, persistent vegetative state, brain death) poses significant medical and ethical challenges in caring for the mother and fetus.

Most commonly, bleeding from an aneurysm is in the subarachnoid space, whereas bleeding from an AVM is located within the brain parenchyma. Symptoms and signs of subarachnoid hemorrhage include headache, nausea and vomiting, stiff neck, photophobia, seizures, and a decreasing level of consciousness. The headache is usually very sudden in onset, whereas the headache associated with intraparenchymal bleeding is usually somewhat less severe and slower in onset. Focal neurologic deficits may be absent in up to 40% of patients. CT or MRI confirm the diagnosis of an intracranial bleed. Cerebral angiography is needed to identify and characterize an aneurysm or AVM.

Early operative intervention after aneurysmal hemorrhage during pregnancy is associated with reduced maternal and fetal mortality. For patients with AVM, the decision to treat the lesion during pregnancy is less clear, but should follow the same guidelines that apply to nonpregnant patients.

■ PHEOCHROMOCYTOMA

Pheochromocytoma is a rare but potentially lethal cause of hypertension in pregnancy. It should be considered in a woman with intermittent labile hypertension or paroxysmal symptoms of anxiety, diaphoresis, headache, and palpitations. Laboratory diagnosis involves biochemical demonstration of elevated vanillylmandelic acid, catecholamine, and metanephrines in a 24-hour urine specimen. Treatment of pheochromocytoma diagnosed in pregnancy is somewhat controversial. When diagnosis is made in the later part of pregnancy, alpha-adrenergic blockade is the treatment to control hypertension. When fetal maturity is achieved, cesarean section should be performed with simultaneous or subsequent excision of the tumor. In cases diagnosed in earlier gestation, surgery during pregnancy has been advocated because elective, nonemergent operative removal of a pheochromocytoma is a life-saving procedure, especially during pregnancy. It has also been associated with a significant reduction in fetal loss. The tumor is best removed in the second trimester, when the patient is optimally prepared and in a stable cardiovascular condition with subsequent progression of the pregnancy to term and with the mode of delivery dependent on obstetric considerations. Vaginal delivery is usually considered only after tumor resection. Later in gestation, the treatment of choice is a combined procedure of tumor resection and cesarean delivery. Despite careful preparations, surgical technique, and timing, the risk of death especially for the fetus still remains high (approximately 15%).

■ HEMORRHOIDS

Pregnancy is the most common cause of symptomatic hemorrhoids. Venous congestion secondary to the enlarging uterus is probably the culprit. The current management approach to hemorrhoid disease is conservative, with simple outpatient treatment preferred, particularly during pregnancy and the puerperium. Medical therapy with dietary changes, avoidance of excessive straining, stool softeners, and hemorrhoidal analgesics often is the only requirement for nonthrombosed hemorrhoids. Rubber-band ligation is a simple, minimally invasive outpatient procedure for the management of hemorrhoids. Hemorrhoidectomy is the best means of definitive therapy for hemorrhoidal disease and should be considered postpartum if the patient continues to fail to respond to conservative measures, if hemorrhoids are severely prolapsed and require manual reduction, or if there is associated pathology such as ulceration, severe bleeding, fissure, or fistula. Thrombosis or clots in the vein lead to severe symptoms. If thrombosed external hemorrhoids remain tender and resist conservative treatment, they can be infiltrated with 1% lidocaine and a small incision made to extract the clot.

■ TRAUMA

Approximately 7% of pregnancies are complicated by trauma, such as motor vehicle accidents (40%), falls (30%), direct assaults to the maternal abdomen (20%), and other causes (10%). Automobile accidents are the most common nonobstetric cause of death during pregnancy. The most common cause of fetal death is death of the mother. The second most common cause of fetal death is abruptio placentae. Pregnant women with traumatic injuries may be victims of physical abuse. A pregnancy may increase family stress, and the practitioner should therefore be alert for signs of abuse.

The primary initial goal in treating a pregnant trauma victim is to stabilize the mother's condition. To optimize maternal and fetal outcome, an organized team approach to the pregnant trauma patient is essential. Maternal assessment and management is similar to the nonpregnant patient, keeping in mind the goal of protecting the fetus from unnecessary drug and x-ray exposure. The fetus should be evaluated early during trauma assessment, and after fetal viability is reached, continuous fetal heart rate and uterine activity monitoring should be instituted, as long as it does not interfere with maternal resuscitative efforts. Much controversy exists regarding the length of fetal monitoring time required subsequent to trauma to identify potential posttraumatic placental abruption. If it is to occur, placental abruption usually occurs quite soon after the injury. It appears that the fetus should be monitored at least 4 hours. Suspicious findings are frequent uterine contractions, vaginal bleeding, abdominouterine tenderness, postural hypotension, or fetal heart rate abnormalities. If any of these signs occur or if the trauma was severe, monitoring should be extended to 24–48 hours. A Kleihauer-Betke test may show evidence of fetomaternal hemorrhage and is recommended for Rh-negative patients. Routine coagulation profiles are not clinically helpful.

REFERENCES

General

Allen JR, Helling TS, Langenfeld M: Intraabdominal surgery during pregnancy. Obstet Gynecol Surv 1990;45:537.

Cunningham FG et al: General considerations and maternal evaluation. In: *Williams Obstetrics,* 21st ed. McGraw-Hill, 2001, p. 1143.

Epstein FB: Acute abdominal pain in pregnancy. Emerg Med Clin North Am 1994;12:151.

Fatum M, Rojansky N: Laparoscopic surgery during pregnancy. Obstet Gynecol Surv 2001;56:50.

Pentel RL, Brown ML: Genetically significant dose to the United States population from diagnostic medical roentgenology. Radiology 1968;90:209.

Anesthesia

Källen B, Mazze RI: Neural tube defects and first trimester operations. Teratology 1990;41:717.

Mazze RI, Källen B: Reproductive outcome after anesthesia and operation during pregnancy: A registry study of 5,405 cases. Am J Obstet Gynecol 1989;161:1178.

Rosen MA: Management of anesthesia for the pregnant surgical patient. Anesthesiology 1999;91:1159.

Appendicitis

Baer JL, Reis RA, Araens RA: Appendicitis in pregnancy with changes in position and axis of the normal appendix in pregnancy. JAMA 1932;98:1359.

Hee P, Viktrup L: The diagnosis of appendicitis during pregnancy and maternal and fetal outcomes after appendectomy. Int J Gynecol Obstet 1999;65:129.

Mazze RI, Källen B: Appendectomy during pregnancy: A Swedish registry study of 778 cases. Obstet Gynecol 1991;77:835.

Mourad J et al: Appendicitis in pregnancy: New information that contradicts long-held clinical beliefs. Am J Obstet Gynecol 2000;182:1027.

Cholecystitis & Cholelithiasis

Cosenza CA et al: Surgical management of biliary gallstone disease during pregnancy. Am J Surg 1999;178:545.

Ghumman E, Barry M, Grace PA: Management of gallstones in pregnancy. Brit J Surg 1997;84:1646.

Lanzafame RJ: Laparoscopic cholecystectomy during pregnancy. Surgery 1995;118:627.

Munford RY, Baron TH: Biliary tract disease in pregnancy. Clin Liver Dis 1999;3:131.

Sungler P et al: Laparoscopic cholecystectomy and interventional endoscopy for gallstone complications during pregnancy. Surg Endoscopy 2000;14:267.

Pancreatitis

Karsenti D et al: Serum amylase and lipase activities in normal pregnancy: A prospective case-control study. Am J Gastroenterol 2001;96:697.

Sakorafas GH, Tsiotou AG: Etiology and pathogenesis of acute pancreatitis: Current concepts. J Clin Gastroenterol 2000;30:343.

Scott LD: Gallstone disease and pancreatitis in pregnancy. Gastroenterol Clin North Am 1992;21:803.

Peptic Ulcer Disease

Brunner G, Meyer H, Athmann C: Omeprazole for peptic ulcer disease in pregnancy. Digestion 1998;59:651.

Cappell MS, Garcia A: Gastric and duodenal ulcers during pregnancy. Gastroenterol Clin North Am 1998;27:169.

Jacoby EB, Porter KB: *Helicobacter pylori* infection and persistent hyperemesis gravidarum. Am J Perinatol 1999;16:85.

Intestinal Tract

Connolly MM, Unti JA, Nora PF: Bowel obstruction in pregnancy. Surg Clin North Am 1995;75:101.

Lord SA, Boswell WC, Hungerpiller JC: Sigmoid volvulus in pregnancy. Am Surgeon 1996;62:380.

Meyerson S et al: Small bowel obstruction in pregnancy. Am J Gastroenterol 1995;90:299.

Perdue PW, Johnson HW Jr, Stafford PW: Intestinal obstruction complicating pregnancy. Am J Surg 1992;164:384.

Splenic/Hepatic Hemorrhage

Fender GRK et al: Management of splenic artery aneurysm during trial of labor with epidural analgesia. Am J Obstet Gynecol 1999;180:1038.

Hillemanns P, Knitza R, Müller-Höcker J: Rupture of splenic artery aneurysm in a pregnant patient with portal hypertension. Am J Obstet Gynecol 1996;174:1665.

Smith LG Jr et al: Spontaneous rupture of liver during pregnancy: current therapy. Obstet Gynecol 1991;77:171.

Adnexal Disease

Bernhard LM et al: Predictors of persistence of adnexal masses in pregnancy. Obstet Gynecol 1999;93:585.

Bromley B, Benacerraf B: Adnexal masses during pregnancy: Accuracy of sonographic diagnosis and outcome. J Ultrasound Med 1997;16:447.

Moore RD, Smith WG: Laparoscopic management of adnexal masses in pregnant women. J Reprod Med 1999;44:97.

Platek DN, Henderson CE, Goldberg GL: The management of a persistent mass in pregnancy. Am J Obstet Gynecol 1995;173:1236.

Whitecar P, Turner S, Higby K: Adnexal masses in pregnancy: A review of 130 cases undergoing surgical management. Am J Obstet Gynecol 1999;181:19.

Breast Cancer

Gemignani ML, Petrek JA, Borgen PI: Breast cancer and pregnancy. Surg Clin North Am 1999;79:1157.

Kouvaris JR et al: Postoperative tailored radiotherapy for locally advanced breast carcinoma during pregnancy: A therapeutic dilemma. Am J Obstet Gynecol 2000;183:498.

Merkel DE: Pregnancy and breast cancer. Sem Surg Oncol 1996;12:370.

Bone Tumors

Simon MA, Phillips WA, Bonfiglio M: Pregnancy and aggressive or malignant primary bone tumors. Cancer 1984;53:2564.

Cardiac Surgery

Chambers CE, Clark SL: Cardiac surgery during pregnancy. Clin Obstet Gynecol 1994;37:316.

Mahli A, Izdes S, Coskun D: Cardiac operations during pregnancy: review of factors influencing fetal outcome. Ann Thorac Surg 2000;69:1622.

Mangione JA et al: Long-term follow-up of pregnant women after percutaneous mitral valvuloplasty. Catheter Cardiovasc Interv 2000;50:413.

Teerlink JR, Foster E: Valvular heart disease in pregnancy. A contemporary perspective. Cardiol Clin 1998;16:573.

Neurologic Disease

Dias MS: Neurovascular emergencies in pregnancy. Clin Obstet Gynecol 1994;37:337.

Finnerty JJ et al: Cerebral arteriovenous malformation in pregnancy: Presentation and neurologic, obstetric, and ethical significance. Am J Obstet Gynecol 1999;181:296.

Stoodley MA, Macdonald RL, Weir BK: Pregnancy and intracranial aneurysm. Neurosurg Clin North Am 1998;9:549.

Tewari KS et al: Obstetric emergencies precipitated by malignant brain tumors. Am J Obstet Gynecol 2000;182:1215.

Trauma

Dahmus MA, Sibai BM: Blunt abdominal trauma: Are there predictive factors for abruptio placentae or maternal-fetal distress? Am J Obstet Gynecol 1993;169:1054.

Fildes J et al: Trauma: The leading cause of maternal death. J Trauma 1992;32:643.

McFarlane J et al: Assessing for abuse during pregnancy: Severity and frequency of injuries and associated entry into prenatal care. JAMA 1992;267:3176.

Moise KJ, Belfort MA: Damage control for the obstetric patient. Surg Clin North Am 1997;77:835.

Stone KI: Trauma in the obstetric patient. Obstet Gynecol Clin 1999;26:459.

Pearlman MD, Tintinallli JE, Lorenz RP: A prospective controlled study of outcome after trauma during pregnancy. Am J Obstet Gynecol 1990;162:1502.

Complications of Labor & Delivery

Ana Polo, MD, Lisbeth Chang, MD, Eduardo Herrera, MD, & Martin L. Pernoll, MD

◼ FETAL BLOOD LOSS IN PREGNANCY

Most blood loss occurring in late pregnancy is of maternal origin, but fetal blood loss may occur from trauma to the placenta or from vasa previa. The fetoplacental vascular volume at term is only 250–500 mL, so what appears to be minor vaginal bleeding could be rapidly fatal to the fetus. Certain fetal heart tracing patterns on electronic monitoring, particularly fetal tachycardia, severe variations, prolonged bradycardia, or a sinusoidal pattern, may signify fetal distress due to bleeding. The Apt test and the Kleihauer-Betke test can both detect fetal hemoglobin. The Kleihauer-Betke test takes about 40 minutes, whereas the Apt test can be performed in 5 minutes, does not require sophisticated equipment, and rarely gives false positive results. However, these tests are only done when there is clinical suspicion of fetomaternal hemorrhage. When significant fetal bleeding is more certain, delivery must be accomplished expeditiously if the infant is to be saved.

TRAUMA TO THE PLACENTA

Trauma to the placenta most commonly occurs with low placental implantation or abruptio placentae. Placenta previa has been documented in about 7% of cases of third trimester bleeding, and significant placental abruption is found in about 15%.

Placenta previa complicates about 0.5% of pregnancies overall. The hallmark of previa is painless vaginal bleeding during the second or third trimester. While it may be possible to carefully induce labor in patients with low-lying placentas, complete previa mandates abdominal delivery.

Abruptio placentae is initiated by bleeding into the decidua basalis, with subsequent development of hematoma formation and placenta separation. Abruption may manifest as heavy vaginal bleeding, bloody fluid at the time of rupture of membranes, abdominal pain, fetal heart tracing abnormalities, or uterine hypertonicity. Risk factors for abruption include trauma, hypertensive disorders, cigarette smoking, antiphospholipid antibody syndrome, grand multiparity, and co-

caine abuse. If bleeding is severe and vaginal delivery is not imminent, cesarean delivery is indicated.

VELAMENTOUS CORD INSERTION & VASA PREVIA

Velamentous Cord Insertion

In velamentous cord insertion, the umbilical cord inserts on some point on the fetal membranes rather than the chorionic plate. It occurs in about 1 in 5000 deliveries. Incidence is 6–9 times higher in twin placentas than in singletons, and even greater in higher orders of multiple birth, as the umbilical vessels often lie within the membranes dividing the fetuses. Although it was earlier thought that velamentous cord insertion did not produce physiological problems, a recent retrospective review noted higher associations with low birthweight, preterm delivery, low Apgar scores, and abnormal intrapartum fetal heart tracings despite normal antenatal Doppler velocimetry. In addition, as umbilical vessels pass through the membranes, the nonvascular matrix of the umbilical cord (Wharton's jelly) and the epithelial surface of the cord are lost, leaving them vulnerable to rupture, shearing, or laceration.

Vasa Previa

In vasa previa, the fetal vessels associated with velamentous insertion of the cord present in advance of the fetal presenting part. In this location, they are likely to be disrupted by labor or at the time of rupture of membranes, with rapid fetal exsanguination occurring in as many as 75% of cases.

Diagnosis & Treatment

Diagnosis of vasa previa or velamentous cord insertion is rarely made before rupture of the membranes. Fetal tachycardia occurring soon after rupture of the membranes may indicate fetal bleeding.

The diagnosis may be difficult, especially during the antenatal period. However, the use of transvaginal color Doppler ultrasound and three-dimensional ultrasonography have increased the recognition of this condition before labor. These diagnostic procedures are especially important in women at risk, such as those with low-lying placentas, multilobed and succenturiate-lobed placentas, multiple pregnancies, and pregnancies resulting from in vitro fertilization. Despite the availability of new tools such as those just mentioned, the diagnosis is often made after the rupture of the membranes by palpation of fetal vessels in the membranes overlying the presenting part through the partially or fully dilated cervix. The usual presentation is sudden-onset bleeding with fetal tachycardia. Sinusoidal fetal heart rate patterns or other signs of fetal distress on electronic fetal monitoring may indicate severe anemia.

If the diagnosis is made before rupture of the membranes or fetal exsanguination occurs, delivery should be by cesarean section. If detected antenatally, the overall fetal outcome is generally favorable. If the diagnosis is made at the time of rupture of the membranes, delivery should be accomplished by the most expeditious method, usually by emergency cesarean section.

▖ DYSTOCIA

DEFINITION & CLASSIFICATION

Dystocia is defined as difficult labor or childbirth. It may be associated with abnormalities involving the maternal pelvis, the fetus, the uterus and cervix, or a combination of these factors.

Abnormalities of the Passage

Abnormalities of the passage constitute pelvic dystocia, ie, aberrations of pelvic architecture and its relationship to the presenting part. Such abnormalities may be related to size or configurational alterations of the bony pelvis, soft tissue abnormalities of the birth canal, reproductive tract masses or neoplasia, or aberrant placental location.

Abnormalities of the Passenger

Abnormalities of the passenger are known as fetal dystocia, ie, difficulties caused by abnormalities of the fetus. Common fetal abnormalities leading to dystocia include excessive fetal size, malpositions, congenital anomalies, and multiple gestation.

Abnormalities of the Powers

Abnormalities of the powers constitute uterine dystocia, ie, uterine activity that is ineffective in eliciting the normal progress of labor. Hypertonic, hypotonic, or discoordinated uterine activity is characteristic of ineffective uterine action. Lack of voluntary expulsive effort during

the second stage may also impede the normal course of delivery.

INCIDENCE

Over the last quarter of a century, the cesarean section rate in the United States has risen to approximately 25% of deliveries done each year. The rise in the number of cesarean sections has been largely attributable to an increase in the number of repeat cesarean sections and in primary cesareans for dystocia.

A trend toward increasing the use of cesarean section was also noted in other countries. The cesarean birth rate in the United Kingdom in 1998 was 18.5%; in Italy it reached 22.4% in 1996, and in China it went up from 11% in 1990 to 29.9% in 1997. The main indications for cesarean section in 1998 were dystocia, followed by prior cesarean delivery, breech presentation, fetal distress, and others, including maternal request.

Dystocia is currently the most common indication for primary cesarean section, and is about three times more common than either nonreassuring fetal status or malpresentation.

The overall incidence of dystocia in women in labor is difficult to determine, in part secondary to ambiguities in definition. In nulliparous patients the incidence of labor disorders is less than 10%. The diagnosis of dystocia is often retrospective; if the outcome is uneventful and spontaneous vaginal delivery occurs, dystocia may go unreported. Failure to progress or cephalopelvic disproportion are most often diagnosed after clinical identification of abnormal labor patterns.

ABNORMAL PATTERNS OF LABOR

Labor is a dynamic process characterized by uterine contractions that increase in regularity, intensity, and duration, causing progressive dilatation and effacement of the cervix and descent of the fetus through the birth canal. The progress of labor is evaluated primarily through estimates of cervical dilatation and descent of the fetal presenting part. Normal labor patterns in primigravidas and multiparas have been described in detail by Friedman and others.

Friedman described four abnormal patterns of labor: (1) prolonged latent phase, (2) protraction disorders (protracted active-phase dilatation and protracted descent), (3) arrest disorders (prolonged deceleration phase, secondary arrest of dilatation, arrest of descent, and failure of descent), and (4) precipitate labor disorders.

1. Prolonged Latent Phase

The latent phase of labor begins with the onset of regular uterine contractions and extends to the beginning of the active phase of cervical dilatation. The duration of the latent phase averages 6.4 hours in nulliparas and 4.8 hours in multiparas. The latent phase is abnormally prolonged if it lasts more than 20 hours in nulliparas or 14 hours in multiparas.

Causes of prolonged latent phase include excessive sedation or sedation given before the end of the latent phase, the use of conduction or general anesthesia before labor enters the active phase, labor beginning with an unfavorable cervix, uterine dysfunction characterized by weak, irregular, uncoordinated, and ineffective uterine contractions, and fetopelvic disproportion.

Treatment options in prolonged latent phase primarily consist of therapeutic rest regimens or active management of labor. After 6–12 hours of rest with sedation and hydration, 85% of patients spontaneously enter the active phase of labor, and further progression in dilatation and effacement may be expected. Ten percent of patients will have been in false labor, and may be allowed to return home to await the onset of true labor if fetal status is reassuring. In the remaining 5% of patients, uterine contractions remain ineffective in producing dilatation; in the absence of any contraindication, active stimulation of labor with oxytocin infusion may be effective in terminating the latent phase of labor.

Some authorities recommend oxytocin infusion as the primary treatment for all patients with prolonged latent phase. If immediate delivery is required for clinical reasons (eg, severe preeclampsia or amnionitis), oxytocin infusion is the treatment of choice.

The prognosis for vaginal delivery after therapeutic measures is excellent. Patients with a prolonged latent phase of labor who respond to rest can be expected to deliver vaginally in nearly all cases. After abnormalities in the latent phase have been corrected, patients are not at any greater risk of developing subsequent labor disorders than are patients who have experienced a normal latent phase.

2. Protraction Disorders

Protracted cervical dilatation in the active phase of labor and protracted descent of the fetus constitute the protraction disorders. Protracted active-phase dilatation is characterized by an abnormally slow rate of dilatation in the active phase, ie, less than 1.2 cm/h in nulliparas or less than 1.5 cm/h in multiparas. Protracted descent of the fetus is characterized by a rate of descent under 1 cm/h in nulliparas or under 2 cm/h in multiparas. The second stage of labor, which normally averages 20 minutes for parous women and 50 minutes in nulliparous women, is protracted when it exceeds 2 hours in nulliparas or 1 hour in multiparas, or 3 and 2 hours respectively in the presence of conduction anesthesia.

The underlying pathogenesis of protracted labor is probably multifactorial. Fetopelvic disproportion is encountered in about one-third of patients. Other factors include minor malpositions such as occiput posterior, improperly administered conduction anesthesia (eg, epidural anesthesia administered above dermatome T10 or given before the onset of the active phase or in the presence of other inhibitory factors), excessive sedation, and pelvic tumors obstructing the birth canal.

Treatment of protraction disorders depends on the presence or absence of fetopelvic disproportion, the adequacy of uterine contractions, and the fetal status. Cesarean section is indicated in the presence of confirmed fetopelvic disproportion. Patients experiencing protraction disorders generally do not respond to oxytocin infusion if adequate uterine contractions are documented by intrauterine pressure catheter monitoring. While it may be possible to enhance uterine contractility, progression of dilatation may not improve. In the absence of fetopelvic disproportion, conservative management, consisting of support and close observation, and therapy with oxytocin augmentation both carry a good prognosis for vaginal delivery (approximately two-thirds of patients) if continued cervical dilation and effacement occur and there is no fetal compromise. The prognosis for the fetus is closely related to the quality of delivery. Spontaneous vaginal delivery or delivery achieved with minimal manipulation is the most crucial factor favoring good fetal outcome.

3. Arrest Disorders

The four patterns of arrest in labor may be characterized as follows: (1) prolonged deceleration, with deceleration phase lasting more than 3 hours in nulliparas or more than 1 hour in multiparas, (2) secondary arrest of dilatation, with no progressive cervical dilatation in the active phase of labor for 2 hours or more, (3) arrest of descent, with descent failing to progress for 1 hour or more, and (4) failure of descent, with descent failing to occur during the deceleration phase of dilatation and during the second stage.

About 50% of patients with arrest disorders demonstrate fetopelvic disproportion. Other causative factors include various fetal malpositions (eg, occiput posterior, occiput transverse, face, or brow), inappropriately administered anesthesia, or excessive sedation.

When an arrest disorder is diagnosed, thorough evaluation of fetopelvic relationships before initiating treatment is crucial. Evaluation should include a careful clinical pelvic examination for pelvic adequacy and estimation of fetal weight. If fetopelvic disproportion is established in the context of an arrest disorder, cesarean section is clearly warranted, since considerable trauma to both mother and baby could otherwise occur. If fetopelvic disproportion is not present and uterine activity is less than optimal, oxytocin stimulation is generally effective in producing further progress.

Arrest disorders generally carry a poor prognosis for vaginal delivery. If allowed to continue, arrest disorders are associated with increased perinatal morbidity. However, if it is possible to establish a postarrest rate of dilatation or descent that is equal to or greater than the prearrest rate, prognosis for vaginal delivery is excellent.

4. Precipitate Labor Disorders

Precipitate dilatation occurs if cervical dilation occurs at a rate of 5 or more centimeters per hour in a primipara or at 10 cm or more per hour in a multipara. Precipitate descent occurs with descent of the fetal presenting part of 5 cm or more per hour in primiparas and 10 cm or more per hour in multiparas.

Precipitate labor may result from either extremely strong uterine contractions or low birth canal resistance. Although the initiating mechanism for extraordinarily forceful uterine contractions is usually not known, abnormal contractions may be associated with administration of oxytocin. Strong uterine contractions (both in force and increased basal tone) may also accompany abruptio placentae. Little is known about causes of low birth canal resistance.

If oxytocin administration is the cause of abnormal contractions, it may simply be stopped. The problem typically resolves in less than 5 minutes. The patient should be placed in the lateral position to prevent any pressure on the inferior vena cava. If excessive uterine activity is associated with fetal heart rate abnormalities, and this pattern persists despite discontinuation of oxytocin, a β-mimetic such as 125–250 μg of terbutaline or ritodrine can be given slowly by intravenous injection if there are no contraindications. Magnesium sulfate has also been recommended to decrease uterine contractions. Physical attempts to retard delivery are absolutely contraindicated.

Maternal complications are rare if the cervix and birth canal are relaxed. However, when the birth canal is rigid and extraordinary contractions occur, uterine rupture may result. Lacerations of the birth canal are common. In addition, precipitate labor is one of the known antecedents of maternal amniotic fluid embolism. Thus enhanced maternal monitoring for this complication is imperative. Furthermore, the uterus that has been hypertonic with labor tends to be hypotonic postpartum, thereby predisposing to postpartum hemorrhage.

Perinatal mortality is increased secondary to hypoxia, possible intracranial hemorrhage, and risks associated with unattended delivery. Impeded placental exchange with resultant hypoxia is created by decreased uteroplacental blood flow as a result of the more frequent and more forceful contractions as well as by increased basal uterine tone. Perinatal intracranial hemorrhage may result from trauma to the fetal head pushing against unyielding maternal tissue with contractions. Resuscitation equipment, baby warmers, and other supportive measures may not be readily available in cases of unattended delivery.

PATHOGENESIS & TREATMENT

Abnormalities of the Passage

Causes of abnormalities of passage include bony abnormalities (pelvic dystocia), soft tissue obstruction of the birth canal, and abnormal placental location. Pelvic dystocia, particularly that due to small bony architecture, is the most common cause of passage abnormalities. The etiology and diagnosis of pelvic abnormalities begins with the shape, classification, and clinical assessment of the adult female pelvis.

Using roentgenographic studies, Caldwell and Moloy classified the 4 major types of adult pelvic types: gynecoid, android, anthropoid, and platypelloid. Pure forms of these pelvic types are rare; mixed elements are more often present in each type of pelvis. The **gynecoid** pelvis is considered the most typically "female" type and is the most favorable for uncomplicated vaginal delivery. Found in about 50% of all women, the pelvic inlet has an oval configuration with a transverse diameter slightly greater than the anteroposterior diameter. Pelvic side walls are straight, the ischial spines are not prominent, the subpubic arch is wide, and the sacrum is concave. The **android,** or male, type of pelvis is found in about 33% of white women and about 15% of black women. The inlet is wedge-shaped with convergent side walls, the ischial spines are prominent, the subpubic arch is narrowed, and the sacrum is inclined anteriorly in its lower third. The android pelvis is associated with persistent occiput posterior position and deep transverse arrest. The **anthropoid** pelvis is present in about 85% of black women and 20% of white women. The inlet is oval, with an anteroposterior diameter greater than the transverse diameter. Pelvic side walls are divergent, and the sacrum is inclined posteriorly. This pelvic type is most often associated with persistent occiput posterior position. The **platypelloid** pelvis is present in fewer than 3% of all women. This pelvis is characterized by a transverse diameter that is wide with respect to the anteroposterior diameter. Deep transverse arrest patterns of labor are commonly associated with this pelvic type.

Disruption of normal female pelvic architecture is an infrequent consideration in the differential diagnosis of the abnormal pelvis. In this category, traumatic pelvic fractures are the most common abnormalities; other possibilities include rachitic pelves, chondrodystrophic dwarf pelves, kyphotic and scoliotic pelves, exostoses, and bony neoplasms.

Ultrasound, magnetic resonance imaging (MRI), and x-rays have been used to investigate pelvic size and shape for evidence of pelvic contraction obstructing the normal progress of labor. Roentgenographic techniques employing the Colcher-Sussman system, which compares average and lower limits of anteroposterior and transverse diameters of the normal female pelvis, have been the most widely used of imaging pelvimetric methods (Table 25–1). X-ray pelvimetry has now fallen into limited use, however, since accumulating evidence suggests that the measurements obtained do not influence the management of labor, and may even increase cesarean section rates. Clinical pelvimetry has largely supplanted imaging studies in the routine evaluation of most obstetric patients because in an era of continuous fetal monitoring and safe protocols for the use of dilute oxytocin to induce labor, trial of labor can be accomplished safely in most patients. The diagnosis of fetopelvic disproportion has generally become a diagnosis of exclusion, after fetal factors and uterine dysfunction have been ruled out. However, x-ray pelvimetry retains a role in the evaluation of a pelvis for the feasibility of vaginal breech delivery and in the assessment of gross bony distortion such as previous pelvic fracture or rachitic deformity.

Contractions of the pelvis are generally classified as contractions of the inlet, midpelvis, or outlet, or as a combination of these elements. Inlet contraction is suspected if the anteroposterior diameter of the pelvis is less than 10 cm, the transverse diameter is under 12 cm, or both. It may present as a floating vertex presentation with no descent during labor, as abnormal presentation, or as a prolapsed cord or extremity. In prolonged labors complicated by inlet contraction, considerable molding of the fetal head, caput succedaneum formation, and prolonged rupture of the membranes are common. If allowed to continue, abnormal thinning of the lower uterine segment may occur, with development of a Bandl's retraction ring, or even frank uterine rupture. Cesarean section is the treatment of choice in true inlet contraction.

Midpelvis contraction is defined as values less than 11.5 cm for the anterior sagittal diameter, 9.5 cm for the interspinous diameter, and 5 cm for the posterior sagittal diameter. Techniques for estimating midpelvic adequacy include the sum of the posterior sagittal diameter and interspinous diameter, which should be greater than 13.5 cm. Criteria for assessing pelvic outlet adequacy include intertuberous diameter greater than 8 cm and a sum of the intertuberous diameter and the anteroposterior diameter greater than 15 cm. Midpelvic outlet obstruction is detected clinically on the basis of convergent side walls, prominent ischial spines, or a narrow pelvic arch. It may present as a prolonged second stage, persistent occiput posterior position, or deep transverse arrest. Molding of the fetal head and caput succedaneum formation are common. Uterine rupture may occur in prolonged labor complicated by midpelvic outlet obstruction, and vesicovaginal or rectovaginal fistula formation may result with pressure necrosis of the surrounding tissues of the birth canal by the fetal head. Poor prognosis for vaginal delivery is typical in midpelvic outlet obstruction, partly due to difficult midforceps rotation and difficult vaginal delivery. Cesarean section is therefore the delivery method of choice in this complication.

Other anatomic abnormalities of the reproductive tract may cause dystocia. So-called soft tissue dystocia may be caused by uterine or vaginal congenital anomalies, scarring of the birth canal, pelvic masses, or low implantation of the placenta.

Abnormalites of the Passenger

Fetal dystocia is abnormal labor caused by malposition or malpresentation, excessive size of the fetus, or fetal malformation.

A. Malposition and Malpresentation

Fetal malpresentations are abnormalities of fetal position, presentation, attitude, or lie. They collectively constitute the most common cause of fetal dystocia, occurring in approximately 5% of all labors. Included in this category are persistent occiput posterior and occiput transverse positions, brow presentation, face presentation, transverse or oblique lies, and breech and compound presentation.

1. Vertex malpositions—

a. Occiput posterior—The occiput posterior position may be normal in early labor, with about 10–20%

Table 25–1. Average and lower limit of normal pelvic diameters.

Diameters	Average (cm)	Lower Limit of Normal (cm)
Inlet		
Anteroposterior	12.5	10
Transverse	13.0	12
Midplane		
Anteroposterior	11.5	Not Critical
Transverse	10.5	9.5

of fetuses in occiput posterior position at onset of labor. In 87% of cases, the head rotates to the occiput anterior position when it reaches the pelvic floor. If the head does not rotate, persistent occiput anterior position may result in dystocia. Interestingly, approximately two-thirds of cases of occiput posterior presentation at delivery occur through malrotation during the active phase of labor. The mechanism of this fetopelvic disproportion is partial deflexion of the fetal head. This partial deflexion increases the diameter that must engage in the pelvis. Occiput posterior presentation may result from a contracted anthropoid or android pelvis or insufficient uterine action. The use of epidural anesthesia and oxytocin augmentation have been associated with higher rates of occiput posterior presentation.

The diagnosis of occiput posterior position is generally made by manual vaginal examination of the orientation of the fetal cephalic sutures. If no gross pelvic contraction is documented on clinical pelvimetry and uterine contractions are inadequate, cautious infusion of oxytocin may be tried. A few authorities advocate midforceps rotation from the occiput posterior to the occiput anterior position. This should only be attempted when macrosomia and gross fetopelvic disproportion have been excluded, other criteria for forceps delivery have been met, and the operator is sufficiently skilled. The prognosis for the infant is excellent when these guidelines are followed; however, maternal morbidity, including extension of episiotomies, higher rates of anal sphincter injury, and other birth canal lacerations, occurs more frequently in occiput posterior deliveries.

b. Occiput transverse—Occiput transverse is also frequently a transient position. In most labors, the fetal head spontaneously rotates to the occiput anterior position. Persistent occiput transverse is associated with pelvic dystocia, uterine dystocia, and platypelloid or android pelves. Diagnosis, management, and prognosis are similar to those of persistent occiput posterior presentation. When the fetal head engages but for various reasons does not rotate spontaneously in the midpelvis as in normal labor, midpelvic transverse arrest is diagnosed. Deep transverse arrest occasionally occurs at the inlet, with molding and caput succedaneum formation falsely indicating a lower descent. Cesarean section is required.

2. Brow presentation—Brow presentations usually are transient fetal presentations with deflexion of the fetal head. During the normal course of labor, conversion to face or vertex presentation generally occurs. If no conversion takes place, dystocia is likely. Brow presentation occurs in approximately 0.06% of deliveries. In approximately 60% of cases, pelvic contraction, prematurity, and grand multiparity are associated findings. The diagnosis is made by vaginal examination. Initial management is expectant, as spontaneous conversion to vertex presentation occurs in more than one-third of all brow presentations. Oxytocin is not recommended, as arrest patterns and uterine inertia are common sequelae because pelvic contraction is often associated with this presentation, and liberal use of cesarean section should be made. Perinatal mortality rates are low when corrected for congenital anomaly, prematurity, and manipulative vaginal delivery.

3. Face presentation—In face presentation, the fetal head is fully deflexed from the longitudinal axis. Face presentation occurs in about 0.2% of all deliveries, and is associated with grand multiparity, advanced maternal age, pelvic masses, pelvic contraction, multiple gestation, polyhydramnios, macrosomia, congenital anomalies including anencephaly and hydrocephaly, prematurity, cornual implantation of the placenta, placenta previa, and premature rupture of the membranes.

Diagnosis of face presentation is most often accomplished by vaginal examination. The prognosis for vaginal delivery is guarded. Complications generally arise with simultaneous pelvic contraction or persistent mentum posterior position. Mentum posterior positions in average-size fetuses are not deliverable vaginally. Arrested labor is typical when spontaneous rotation to the mentum anterior position fails to occur. With mentum anterior presentation, oxytocin augmentation may be considered for arrested labor if cephalopelvic disproportion can be ruled out. Delivery may be accomplished by spontaneous vaginal delivery or cesarean section. There is little or no place for manual flexion of the fetal head or manual rotation from the mentum posterior position to the mentum anterior position.

4. Abnormal fetal lie—In transverse or oblique lie, the long axis of the fetus is perpendicular to or at an angle to the maternal longitudinal axis. Abnormalities in axial lie occur overall in about 0.33% of all deliveries, but may occur 6 times more frequently in premature labors. Causative factors include grand multiparity, prematurity, pelvic contraction, and abnormal placental implantation.

When the diagnosis is made in the third trimester prior to labor, external cephalic version enables a number of these patients to undergo vaginal delivery. Abnormal axial lies have a 20 times greater incidence of cord prolapse than vertex presentations. Thus with onset of labor or when the membranes rupture, prompt cesarean delivery is mandatory. Increased perinatal mortality is associated mainly with prematurity, cord prolapse, and manipulative vaginal delivery. Increased perinatal mortality rates have also been consistently reported secondary to internal podalic version, other birth trauma associated with manipulation, and cord prolapse (11–20% of cases of the latter).

A prolapsed extremity alongside the presenting part constitutes **compound presentation.** Compound presentation complicates about 0.1% of deliveries. Prematurity and a large pelvic inlet are associated clinical findings. Compound presentations are often diagnosed during physical examination and investigation for failure to progress in labor. Most commonly, a hand is palpated beside the vertex. Labor in most of these patients will end in uncomplicated vaginal delivery, but cesarean section should be done in the presence of dystocia or cord prolapse. Attempts to reposition the fetal extremity are discouraged, except for gentle pinching of the digits to determine whether the fetus will retract the extremity.

5. Breech presentation—Breech presentation is a longitudinal lie with the fetal head occupying the fundus. A **frank breech** describes a breech presentation with flexed hips and extended knees. A **complete breech** describes flexion at both hips and knees. An **incomplete (footling) breech** describes extension of one or both hips. Breech presentation at term occurs in about 3–4% of all deliveries. The incidence increases with the degree of prematurity; the incidence at 32 weeks is 7%, and at under 28 weeks the incidence is 25%. Breech presentation is associated with similar causative factors as face presentation, as well as with previous breech presentation, congenital anomalies, and any anomaly that alters the normal piriform shape of the uterus.

Management of breech presentation remains controversial. High perinatal mortality and morbidity rates have been demonstrated retrospectively for term singleton breech fetuses delivered vaginally compared to those delivered by cesarean section, with odds ratios of 2.5 for mortality, 12.2 for birth injury, and 4.1 for convulsions, leading some authors to advocate elective cesarean section for breech presentation. In addition, breech fetuses with congenital anomalies, hyperextended vertex, estimated fetal weight under 1500 g, or those in the footling position have particularly high fetal morbidity and mortality. Indications for cesarean section include contracted pelvis, secondary arrest of dilatation, fetal weight over 3800 g, hyperextended head, floating station, and an inexperienced practitioner.

Prospective studies have identified a subgroup of breech presentations that may be safely delivered vaginally—specifically, near-term frank breeches weighing between 2500 and 3800 g with flexed head and no concurrent congenital anomalies, maternal pelvis of adequate dimensions, and a normal labor pattern without

fetal distress. In addition, women with recurring breech presentation have lower risks of poor perinatal outcome with subsequent breech delivery.

Piper forceps should be available for the delivery of the aftercoming head. Continuous electronic fetal monitoring is essential, and immediate cesarean section should be available.

External cephalic version (ECV) performed after 37 weeks of gestation, usually under tocolysis, may significantly reduce both the incidence of breech presentation in labor and the number of cesarean sections. Success rates range from 35–86%. Predictors of success include prior parity, noncornual placental location, lower uterine tone, and breech location out of the pelvis. While labor after successful ECV demonstrated higher rates of cesarean section and fetal distress on fetal heart rate monitoring, overall cesarean section rates for breech can be lowered.

Recently, a large international multicenter randomized control trial has clearly demonstrated lower rates of fetal morbidity with planned cesarean section rather than planned vaginal delivery for singleton breech fetuses, with relative risk 0.33. In light of these findings, the American College of Obstetricians and Gynecologists (ACOG) Committee on Obstetric Practice issued a formal position that planned vaginal breech delivery may no longer be appropriate for singleton pregnancies. ACOG recommends application of external cephalic version to reduce breech presentation, or cesarean section for persistent singleton presentation.

B. FETAL MACROSOMIA

Excessive fetal size encompasses those fetuses that are large for gestational age (LGA) and those with macrosomia. LGA implies a birthweight greater than the 90th percentile, and macrosomia implies growth beyond a certain size, usually 4000–4500 g, regardless of gestational age. It occurs in about 5% of deliveries. Associated risk factors include maternal diabetes, maternal obesity (> 70 kg), excessive maternal weight gain (> 20 kg), postdate pregnancy, and previous delivery of a macrosomic infant. However, less than 40% of macrosomic infants are born to patients with identifiable risk factors.

Diagnosis by abdominal palpation is notoriously inaccurate. A better estimated weight may be possible with real-time ultrasonography and standard measured parameters, but ultrasound also lacks accuracy, particularly with increased fetal size. While morbidities to infant and mother increase with increasing size between 4000 and 4500 g, perinatal mortality for fetuses weighing more than 4500 g is about fivefold higher than in normal term infants, and incidence of shoulder dystocia is at least 10% in this group.

Shoulder dystocia, or difficult delivery of the shoulders after delivery of the fetal head, is an obstetric emergency, with high risk of fetal brachial plexus injury, hypoxia, or asphyxia. The incidence of shoulder dystocia is 0.15–1.7% of all vaginal deliveries. It is usually heralded by the classic turtle sign. After the fetal head delivers, it retracts back on the maternal perineum. The first thing to do is to call for assistance. Then if gentle posterior and inferior traction of the fetal head is not successful, the McRobert's maneuver may be attempted, which is a rotation of the symphysis pubis. The patient's legs are sharply flexed against her abdomen in an attempt to free the anterior shoulder of the fetus. Application of suprapubic pressure, Wood's screw maneuver, or Reuben's maneuver rotates the shoulder so that it occupies a transverse or oblique diameter of the pelvis, facilitating fetal delivery. Episiotomy may reduce soft tissue dystocia and allow the operator to maneuver more easily. Delivery of the posterior arm or intentional fracture of the clavicle may be required to effect delivery.

If all else fails and there is a chance for a good fetal outcome, a symphysiotomy or the Zavanelli procedure may be performed. This last maneuver consists of a replacement of the fetal head into the vagina in the flexed position, then an urgent cesarean section is performed.

Given the high morbidities associated with shoulder dystocia and the increasing risk of dystocia with larger fetuses, estimated fetal weights of greater than 4500 g in nondiabetic patients and 4250 g in diabetic patients have been suggested as reasonable indications for elective cesarean section for macrosomia. However, because estimations of fetal size are frequently inaccurate, especially in fetuses weighting more than 4000 g, the diagnosis of dystocia secondary to macrosomia requires progression to the active phase of labor and assessment of the adequacy of uterine contractions. In addition, shoulder dystocia cannot be reliably predicted in labor, with over half of cases occurring without identifiable risk factors. Prolonged second stage or arrest of descent in macrosomic infants should be delivered by cesarean section, as rates of shoulder dystocia in infants greater than 4500 g delivered with midforceps have been reported to be above 50%.

C. FETAL MALFORMATION

Fetal malformation may cause dystocia, primarily through fetopelvic disproportion. The most common malformation is hydrocephalus, with an incidence of 0.05%. Management is determined by the severity of the disorder and its prognosis. Other fetal anomalies that may prevent the normal progress of labor include enlargement of the fetal abdomen caused by distended bladder, ascites, or abdominal neoplasms; or other fetal masses, including meningomyelocele or cystosarcoma.

Abnormalities of the Powers

Uterine dystocia denotes any abnormality in the force or coordination of uterine contractility that prevents the normal progress of labor.

Studies of normal uterine activity during labor have revealed the following characteristics: (1) the relative intensity of contractions is greater in the fundus than in the midportion or lower uterine segment (this is termed **fundal dominance**); (2) the average value of the intensity of contractions is more than 24 mm Hg (in the active phase of labor, pressures often increase to 40–60 mm Hg); (3) contractions are well synchronized in different parts of the uterus; (4) the basal resting pressure of the uterus is between 12 and 15 mm Hg; (5) the frequency of contractions progresses from one every 3–5 minutes to one every 2–3 minutes during the active phase; (6) the duration of effective contraction in active labor approaches 60 seconds; and (7) the rhythm and force of contractions are regular.

Quantification of uterine activity during labor uses external tocodynamometry or intrauterine pressure catheter measurement. The external tocodynamometer is a pressure sensor placed over the fundal prominence of the uterus that gives an accurate determination of the frequency and duration of uterine contractions. This technique is not adequate for assessment of the resting tone of the uterus or the intensity of contractions. An internal uterine pressure catheter measures intra-amniotic pressure, which is transmitted through the noncompressible fluid within the catheter to a pressure sensor. This technique shows baseline uterine resting pressure, contraction intensity and duration, and frequency of uterine activity. It is the most accurate method of diagnosing uterine dysfunction and evaluating treatment. The **Montevideo unit** is the most widely used measurement of uterine activity. Defined as the product of the average intensity of uterine contractions (measured from the baseline resting pressure) multiplied by the number of contractions in a 10-minute interval, measurements greater than 200 mm Hg should be adequate to produce normal labor progression in most patients.

Uterine dysfunction generally comprises 3 categories: hypotonic dysfunction, hypertonic dysfunction, and uncoordinated dysfunction. Hypotonic dysfunction is uterine activity characterized by contraction of the uterus with insufficient force (> 24 mm Hg), irregular or infrequent rhythm, or both. Seen most often in primigravidas in the active phase of labor, it may be caused by excessive sedation, early administration of conduction anesthesia, twins, polyhydramnios, or over-distention of the uterus. Hypotonic dysfunction responds well to oxytocin; however, care must be taken to first rule out cephalopelvic disproportion and malpresentation. Active management of labor has been shown to decrease perinatal morbidity and cesarean section rates. Less commonly than hypotonic dysfunction, hypertonic uterine contractions and uncoordinated contraction often occur together and are characterized by elevated resting tone of the uterus, dyssynchronous contractions with elevated tone in the lower uterine segment, and frequent intense uterine contractions. It is generally associated with abruptio placentae, overzealous use of oxytocin, cephalopelvic disproportion, fetal malpresentation, and the latent phase of labor. Treatment may require tocolysis, decrease in oxytocin infusion, or cesarean section as indicated for concomitant malpresentation, cephalopelvic disproportion, or fetal distress. Oxytocin administration is generally of no value. When these patterns occur in the latent phase of labor, sedation may be effective in converting hypertonic contractions to normal labor patterns. Hypertonic labor may also cause precipitate labor disorders, resulting in fetal intracranial hemorrhage, fetal distress, neonatal injury or depression, and birth canal lacerations from rapid delivery.

Inadequate pushing in the second stage of labor is common and may be caused by conduction anesthesia, oversedation, exhaustion, or neurologic dysfunction such as paraplegia or hemiplegia of various causes, or by psychiatric disorders. Mild sedation or a waiting period to permit analgesic or anesthetic agents to wear off may improve expulsive efforts, and outlet forceps or vacuum delivery may be effected in selected cases.

■ FETAL COMPROMISE

Fetal distress may be defined as a complex of signs indicating a critical response in the fetus to stress. It implies metabolic derangements—notably hypoxia and acidosis—that affect the functions of vital organs to the point of temporary or permanent injury or death. Fetal distress may be acute or chronic. Skillful monitoring will detect some degree of fetal compromise in at least 20% of all obstetric patients.

Other available clinical methods for detecting impending or actual fetal asphyxia are quantification of fetal movements, fetal response to a stimulation (fetal scalp stimulation or vibroacoustic stimulation), biophysical profile (BPP), contraction stress test, and fetal scalp blood sampling. The last one can be used only

after rupture of membranes and with an open cervix. Several other techniques have been used to assess fetal acid–base status. These include fetal pulse oximetry, continuous fetal tissue pH measurements in labor, and percutaneous umbilical blood sampling. Fetal pulse oximetry is the most promising minimally invasive adjunctive test, but it also requires ruptured membranes and a dilated cervix.

Prompt recognition of the symptoms of fetal compromise, and when necessary, decisive, well-planned intervention are imperative for the reduction of perinatal mortality and morbidity—especially to prevent permanent damage to the central nervous system.

CHRONIC FETAL COMPROMISE

Chronic fetal compromise implies an interval of fetal deprivation that affects growth and development. It may result from reduced placental perfusion, a placental abnormality, or deficient fetal metabolism. Decreased placental perfusion may reflect any of the following conditions in the mother: (1) vascular abnormality, as in hypertensive disease, preeclampsia-eclampsia, or diabetes with pelvic vascular complications; (2) inadequate systemic circulation, as in congenital or acquired heart disease; and (3) inadequate oxygenation of the blood, as in emphysema or due to residence at high altitude. Chronic fetal compromise due to placental abnormality includes "premature placental aging" and diabetes mellitus. Possible fetal causes of jeopardy include multiple gestations, postmaturity, congenital anomalies, congenital infections, and erythroblastosis fetalis.

The earliest studies involve serial measurements of the height of the uterus or the patient's girth at each antenatal visit. Ultrasonic measurement of the skull, thorax, and placenta provides a more accurate means of determining a decreased fetal growth rate. Antenatal testing may aid in the management of cases of chronic fetal compromise.

ACUTE FETAL COMPROMISE

The differential diagnosis of acute fetal compromise involves 3 possibilities: possible fetal compromise, probable fetal compromise, and certain fetal compromise. No fetal compromise is present when there is absence of any abnormality of fetal heart rate (FHR) or rhythm and no response to uterine contractions other than early decelerations.

Transient acceleration of FHR, in conjunction with uterine contractions, may indicate mild cord occlusion or slight fetal hypercapnia and hypoxia, if normal FHR variability is retained. Variable FHR decelerations in relation to uterine contractions are thought to be due to more severe cord compression. If the variable deceleration is transient and not severe, permanent damage is unlikely.

Lack of FHR short-term variability may be associated with a number of factors (eg, fetal immaturity, effect of drugs) that do not indicate fetal compromise. However, the absence of FHR short-term variability may indicate decreased central nervous system control. Absence of short-term variability of the FHR coupled with acceleration in relation to uterine contractions is a particularly worrisome pattern. Prolonged or increasingly more severe variable decelerations are also concerning. Late decelerations of the FHR, which may or may not be coupled with accelerations, are particularly ominous, as they signify uteroplacental insufficiency.

Maternal causes of fetal compromise include diverse problems such as decreased uterine blood flow (hypotension, shock, sudden heart failure), decreased blood oxygenation (hypoxia-hypercapnia), and uterine hypertonia (injudicious use of oxytocin, tetanic contractions, abruptio placentae). Placenta and cord problems include abruptio placentae, placenta previa, umbilical cord compression (knots, prolapse, or entanglement), lack of sufficient placental reserve to tolerate labor (postmaturity, premature placental aging), and ruptured vasa previa.

Tachycardia, lack of FHR short-term variability, and late FHR decelerations together signify fetal compromise. If severe variable decelerations persist for 30 minutes or more or if late decelerations persist despite attempted therapy, or in cases of refractory bradycardia, fetal compromise is also thought to be present. Concomitantly, the fetal scalp blood pH will probably be 7.20 or less, reflecting fetal hypoxia and acidosis. Prompt evaluation and treatment is mandatory.

MANAGEMENT OF FETAL COMPROMISE

It is important to note that while a reassuring fetal heart tracing carries a high sensitivity and high negative predictive value for a healthy, nonacidotic fetus, the presence of decelerations and decreased variability has a low specificity for asphyxia. Thus except in cases of ominous fetal heart tracing patterns such as refractory bradycardia or a sinusoidal pattern, which mandate prompt delivery, intrauterine resuscitative measures and assessment of fetal status can be accomplished. Scalp sampling of fetal blood has been demonstrated to correlate well with newborn blood acid–base status and Apgar scores. The presence of fetal heart rate accelerations at the time of scalp sampling or elicited by scalp stimulation or fetal acoustic stimulation also strongly correlates with nonacidotic fetal status, suggesting fetal well-being. Preliminary studies show promise for fetal pulse oximetry as an additional tool in the assessment of fetal status. In the presence of continued signs of fetal well-being, it is possible to allow labor to continue.

Intrauterine resuscitation should be tailored to likely underlying causes of fetal compromise. In the presence of a concerning fetal tracing, vaginal examination to assess for rapid progression of labor or cord prolapse should be a part of the initial assessment. A change of the mother's position may relieve pressure on the umbilical cord. Uterine function may also be improved with the patient in a lateral position. Supine hypotension may be corrected by elevation of the maternal legs, application of elastic leg bandages, and rapid administration of fluids intravenously. These help to restore the gravida's arterial pressure and increase the blood flow in the intervillous space and perfusion to the fetus. If drugs are required, cardiotonics (eg, ephedrine) are preferred. Discontinuing the administration of oxytocin may also improve placental perfusion, decreasing the stress of uterine contractions on the fetus. The administration of high concentrations of oxygen (10 L/min by mask) will raise the maternal-fetal P_{O_2} gradient and will increase maternal-fetal oxygen transfer, alleviating fetal hypoxia. However, there is not enough evidence to support the use of prophylactic oxygen therapy for women in the second stage of labor, nor to evaluate its effectiveness for fetal distress. If maternal acidosis is the cause of fetal acidosis, administering bicarbonate to the mother may benefit both patients. However, if acidosis is severe, the infant should be promptly delivered. Hypertonic glucose (usually 50 g intravenously) may be administered when there is maternal deprivation acidosis or hypoglycemia, although there may be only an indirect relationship between the level of fetal blood glucose and the base deficit.

In summary, in cases of possible fetal compromise, vaginal examination should be done to assess for rapid progression or cord prolapse. Intrauterine resuscitation may be accomplished by changing the position of the mother, correcting maternal hypotension by intravenous fluid administration, decreasing uterine activity by stopping the administration of oxytocin or administration of tocolytics, and administering oxygen at 10 L/min by face mask. Labor may be continued in the presence of reassuring signs of fetal status through fetal acoustic stimulation, scalp stimulation, or sampling. If fetal well-being cannot be documented, if the situation worsens, if the signs of probable fetal distress persist for 30 minutes, or if there is continued fetal distress despite conservative treatment, immediate delivery is indicated. Obstetric judgment must dictate how the delivery will be accomplished in accordance with the presentation, station, position, dilatation of the cervix, and presumed fetal status. If cesarean section is chosen, it must be done rapidly.

REFERENCES

Velamentous Insertion of the Cord & Vasa Previa

Lee W et al: Vasa previa: Prenatal diagnosis, natural evolution, and clinical outcome. Obstet Gynecol 2000;95:527.

Oyelese Y et al: Second trimester low-lying placenta and in-vitro fertilization? Exclude vasa previa. J Maternal Fetal Med 2000;9:370.

Dystocia

Abrechtson S et al: Perinatal mortality in breech presentation sibships. Obstet Gynecol 1998;92:775.

American College of Obstetricians and Gynecologists: External cephalic version. ACOG Practice Bulletin No. 13, 2000.

American College of Obstetricians and Gynecologists: Fetal macrosomia. ACOG Practice Bulletin No. 22, 2000.

American College of Obstetricians and Gynecologists: Mode of term singleton breech delivery. ACOG Committee Opinion No. 261, 2001.

American College of Obstetricians and Gynecologists: Shoulder dystocia. ACOG Practice Patterns No. 7, 1997.

Aisenbrey GA et al: External cephalic version: Predictors of success. Obstet Gynecol 1999;94:783.

Caldwell WE, Moloy HC: Anatomical variations in the female pelvis and their effect in labor with a suggested classification. Am J Obstet Gynecol 1933;26:479.

Buist R, Khalid O: Successful Zavanelli manoeuvre for shoulder dystocia with occipitoposterior position. Aust NZ Obstet Gynecol 1999;39:310.

Fitzpatrick M et al: Influence of persistent occiput posterior on delivery outcome. Obstet Gynecol 2001;98:1027.

Friedman EA: The labor curve. Clin Perinatol 1981;8:15.

Gardberg M et al: Intrapartum sonography and the persistent occiput posterior position: a study of 408 deliveries. Obstet Gynecol 1998;91:746.

Gherman RB et al: Analysis of McRoberts' maneuver by x-ray pelvimetry. Obstet Gynecol 2000;95:43.

Hannah ME et al: Planned cesarean section versus planned vaginal birth for breech presentation at term: a randomized multicentre trial. Lancet 2000;356:1375.

Hernandez C, Wendel, GD: Shoulder dystocia. Clin Obstet Gynecol 1990;33:526.

McNiven PS et al: An early labor assessment program: a randomized, controlled trial. Birth 1998;25:5.

Menard MK: Cesarean delivery rates in the United States. Obstet Gynecol Clin 1999;26:275.

Norichi S et al: Efficacy of external cephalic version performed at term. Eur J Obstet Gynecol Reprod Biol 1998;76:161.

Pattison RC: Pelvimetry for fetal cephalic presentations at term. Cochrane Database Syst Rev 2000:CD00161.

Ramsey PS, Ramin KD, Field CS: Shoulder dystocia. Rotational maneuvers revisited. J Reprod Med 2000;45:85.

Roman J et al: Pregnancy outcome by mode of delivery among term breech births: Swedish experience 1987–1993. Obstet Gynecol 1998;92:945.

Sadler LC, Davidson T, McCowan LM: A randomized controlled trial and meta-analysis of active management of labour. Br J Obstet Gynecol 2000;107:909.

Sizer AR, Nirmal DM: Occiput posterior position: Associated factors and obstetric outcomes in nulliparas. Obstet Gynecol 2000;96:749.

Sporri S et al: Pelvimetry by magnetic resonance imaging as a diagnostic tool to evaluate dystocia. Obstet Gynecol 1997; 89:902.

Stubbs TM: Oxytocin for labor induction. Clin Obstet Gynecol 2000;43:489.

Fetal Distress

Hofmeyr GJ, Kulier R: Tocolysis for preventing fetal distress in second stage of labour. Cochrane Database Syst Rev 2000: CD000037.

Huddleston JF: Intrapartum fetal assessment. Clin Perinatol 1999;26:549.

Lindsay MK: Intrauterine resuscitation of the compromised fetus. Clin Perinatol 1999;26:569.

McNamara HM, Dildy GA 3rd: Continuous intrapartum pH, pO_2, pCO_2, and SpO_2 monitoring. Obstet Gynecol Clin North Am 1999;29:671.

Penning S, Garite TJ: Management of fetal distress in labor. Obstet Gynecol Clin North Am 1999;26:259.

Schmidt S et al: Clinical usefulness of pulse oximetry in the fetus with non-reassuring heart rate pattern? J Perinatol Med 2000;28:298.

Obstetric Analgesia & Anesthesia 26

Ralph W. Yarnell, MD, FRCPC, & John S. McDonald, MD

Analgesia is the loss or modulation of pain perception. It may be local and affect only a small area of the body; regional and affect a larger portion; or systemic. Analgesia is achieved by the use of hypnosis (suggestion), systemic medication, regional agents, or inhalational agents.

Anesthesia is the total loss of sensory perception, and may include loss of consciousness. It is induced by various agents and techniques. In obstetrics, **regional anesthesia** is accomplished with local anesthetic techniques (epidural, spinal) and **general anesthesia** with systemic medication and endotracheal intubation.

The terms analgesia and anesthesia are sometimes confused in common usage. Analgesia denotes those states in which only modulation of pain perception is involved. Anesthesia denotes those states in which mental awareness and perception of other sensations are lost. Attempts have been made to divide anesthesia into various components, including analgesia, amnesia, relaxation, and loss of reflex response to pain. Analgesia can be regarded as a component of anesthesia if viewed in this way.

The use of techniques and medications to provide pain relief in obstetrics requires an expert understanding of their effects to ensure the safety of both mother and fetus.

ANATOMY OF PAIN

It may be academic to argue that pain should be defined as the parturient's response to the stimuli of labor, since agreement on a definition of pain has eluded scholars for centuries.

Nevertheless, it should be appreciated that the "pain response" is a response of the total personality and cannot be dissected systematically and scientifically. Physicians are obligated to provide a comfortable or at least tolerable labor and delivery. Many patients are tense and apprehensive at the onset of labor, although there may be little or no discomfort. The physician must be knowledgeable of the options for pain relief and respond to the patient's needs and wishes.

The evolution of the pain in the first stage of labor was originally described as involving spinal segments T11 and T12. Subsequent research has determined that segments T10–L1 are involved. Discomfort is associ-ated with ischemia of the uterus during contraction as well as dilatation and effacement of the cervix. Sensory pathways that convey nociceptive impulses of the first stage of labor include the uterine plexus, the inferior hypogastric plexus, the middle hypogastric plexus, the superior hypogastric plexus, the lumbar and lower thoracic sympathetic chain, and the T10–L1 spinal segments.

Pain in the second stage of labor undoubtedly is produced by distention of the vagina and perineum. Sensory pathways from these areas are conveyed by branches of the pudendal nerve via the dorsal nerve of the clitoris, the labial nerves, and the inferior hemorrhoidal nerves. These are the major sensory branches to the perineum and are conveyed along nerve roots S2, S3, and S4. Nevertheless, other nerves may play a role in perineal innervation; the ilioinguinal nerves, the genital branches of the genitofemoral nerves, and the perineal branches of the posterior femoral cutaneous nerves.

Although the major portion of the perineum is innervated by the 3 major branches of the pudendal nerve, innervation by the other nerves mentioned may be important in some patients. The type of pain reported may be an ache in the back or loins (referred pain, perhaps from the cervix), a cramp in the uterus (due to fundal contraction), or a "bursting" or "splitting" sensation in the lower vaginal canal or pudendum (due to dilatation of the cervix and vagina).

Dystocia, which is usually painful, may be due to fetopelvic disproportion; tetanic, prolonged, or dysrhythmic uterine contractions; intrapartum infection; or many other causes (see Chapter 25).

SAFETY OF OBSTETRIC ANESTHESIA

Substantial advances in the quality and safety of obstetric anesthesia have been made in the past 3 decades. Outdated techniques such as "twilight sleep" and mask anesthesia have been recognized as ineffective or unsafe and have been replaced by epidural infusion of narcotic/local anesthesia mixtures and patient-controlled analgesia during labor and postoperatively. When required, general anesthesia is provided using short-acting drugs with well-known fetal effects, and careful attention is focused on airway management.

Maternal mortality relating to anesthesia has been reduced tenfold since the 1950s, largely due to an enhanced appreciation of special maternal risks associated with anesthesia. The overall anesthesia-related death rate in the United States is now as low as 1.3 per million live births, a fivefold decline in the last decade. Regional anesthesia is now more commonly performed for cesarean delivery, there are fewer births in hospitals performing fewer than 500 deliveries per year, and it is now more common to have both in-house anesthesia and obstetric physician coverage. In the face of these improvements, two distressing statistics have recently emerged. First, the case fatality rate for general anesthesia for cesarean delivery has risen from 20 deaths per million general anesthetics administered in the early 1980s to 32.3 deaths per million general anesthetics administered today. This increase occurred during a period when there was a reduction in the case fatality rate for regional anesthesia in obstetrics from 8.6 per million to 1.9 per million regional anesthetics administered. The increase in the case fatality rate for general anesthesia may have occurred because general anesthesia is now reserved for urgent and critical situations, whereas in the past general anesthesia was more commonly employed for elective obstetric delivery. Difficulty with intubation, aspiration, and hypoxemia leading to cardiopulmonary arrest are the leading causes of anesthesia-related maternal death.

The second point of concern is the increase in overall maternal mortality (not related specifically to anesthesia) in the United States since 1985. This increase in maternal mortality is most pronounced in older parturients (over 35 years of age), particularly in black parturients. Cardiomyopathy, hypertension, and hemorrhage are the principal etiologies associated with these rising mortality rates, and are important factors for the anesthesiologist to consider.

TECHNIQUES OF ANALGESIA WITHOUT THE USE OF DRUGS

Psychophysical Methods
(See also Chapter 10.)

Three distinct psychologic techniques have been developed as a means of facilitating the birth process and making it a positive emotional experience: "natural childbirth," psychoprophylaxis, and hypnosis. So-called natural childbirth was developed by Grantly Dick-Read in the early 1930s and popularized in his book *Childbirth Without Fear.* Dick-Read's approach emphasized the reduction of tension to induce relaxation. The psychoprophylactic technique was developed by Velvovski, who published the results of his work from Russia in 1950. In Russia in the mid-1950s, it became evident that obstetric psychoprophylaxis was a useful substitute for poorly administered or dangerously conducted anesthesia for labor and delivery. This method was later introduced in France by Lamaze. Hypnosis for pain relief has achieved periodic spurts of popularity since the early 1800s and depends on the power of suggestion.

Many obstetricians argue that psychoprophylaxis can largely eliminate the pain of childbirth by diminishing cortical appreciation of pain impulses rather than by depressing cortical function, as occurs with drug-induced analgesia. Relaxation, suggestion, concentration, and motivation are factors that overlap other methods of preparation for childbirth. Some of them are closely related to hypnosis.

These techniques can significantly reduce anxiety, tension, and fear. They also provide the parturient with a valuable understanding of the physiologic changes that occur during labor and delivery. In addition, they provide an opportunity for closer understanding and communication between the patient and her mate, who may be an important source of comfort to the her during the stressful process of childbirth. If psychophysical techniques do no more than this, they deserve the obstetrician's support.

Studies undertaken to assess the effectiveness of psychophysical techniques have reported widely divergent results, with effectiveness ranging from as low as 10–20% to as high as 70–80%. It is clear that the overall benefit is best judged by the parturient herself, with validation by the observations of attendants. As is no doubt true in other aspects of medical practice in which emotional overlay and subjective reporting play a role in the evaluation of specific types of therapy, the personality and level of enthusiasm of the doctor can have a strong influence on the patient's reactions to a given therapy. Practitioners who are skeptical of psychophysical techniques cannot expect to accomplish very much using them.

It should be obvious that none of these psychophysical techniques should be forced on a patient, even by a skillful practitioner. The patient must not be made to feel that she will fail if she does not choose to complete her labor and delivery without analgesic medication. It must be made clear to her from the outset that she is expected to ask for help if she feels she wants or needs it. All things considered, psychophysical techniques should be viewed as adjuncts to other analgesic methods rather than substitutes for them.

The effectiveness of hypnosis is partially due to the well-known although incompletely understood mechanisms by which emotional and other central processes can influence a person's overall responses to the pain experience. Verbal suggestion and somatosensory stimulation may help to alleviate discomfort associated with the first stage of labor. In addition, hypnotic states may provide apparent analgesia and amnesia for distressing, anxiety-provoking experiences. Finally, hypnotic techniques may substantially improve the parturient's outlook and behavior by reducing fear and apprehension. However, there are certain practical points to consider in regard to hypnosis because the time needed to establish a suitable relationship between physician and patient is often more than can be made available in the course of a busy medical practice.

ANALGESIC, AMNESTIC, & ANESTHETIC AGENTS

General Comments & Precautions

1. If the patient is prepared psychologically for her experience, she will require less medication. Anticipate and dispel her fears during the antenatal period and in early labor. Never promise a painless labor.

2. Individualize the treatment of every patient, because each one reacts differently. Unfavorable reactions to any drug can occur.

3. Know the drug you intend to administer. Be familiar with its limitations, dangers, and contraindications as well as its advantages.

4. All analgesics given to the mother will cross the placenta. Systemic medications produce higher maternal and fetal blood levels than regionally administered drugs. Many drugs have central nervous system depressant effects. Although they may have the desired effect on the mother, they may also exert a mild to severe depressant effect on the fetus or newborn.

The ideal drug will have an optimal beneficial effect on the mother and a minimal depressant effect on the offspring. None of the presently available narcotic and sedative medications used in obstetrics has selective maternal effects. The regional administration of local anesthetics accomplished this goal to a large extent because the low maternal serum levels that are produced expose the fetus to insignificant quantities of drugs.

Pharmacologic Aspects

A. Route of Administration

Systemic techniques of analgesia and anesthesia include both oral and parenteral routes of administration. Parenteral administration includes subcutaneous, intramuscular, and intravenous injection. Sedatives, tranquilizers, and analgesics are usually given by intramuscular injection. In some cases, the intravenous route is preferred.

The advantages of intravenous administration are (1) avoidance of variable rates of uptake due to poor vascular supply in fat or muscle; (2) prompt onset of effect; (3) titration of effect, avoiding the "peak effect" of an intramuscular bolus; and (4) smaller effective doses because of earlier onset of action.

The disadvantages of intravenous injection are inadvertent arterial injection and the depressant effect of overdosage, but the advantage of smaller dosage overcomes the disadvantages.

Always administer the lowest concentration and the smallest dose to obtain the desired effect.

B. Physical and Chemical Factors

Anesthetics penetrate body cells by passing through the lipid membrane boundary. This membrane is not permeable to charged (ionized) drugs but is permeable to un-ionized forms of drugs. Much of the total drug transfer is dependent on the degree of lipid solubility, so local anesthetics are characterized by aromatic rings that are lipophilic, and all are lipid-soluble. In addition, the intermediate amine radical of a local anesthetic is a weak base that in aqueous solutions exists partly as undissociated free base and partly as dissociated cation. Figure 26–1 shows the equilibrium for such an existence and the Henderson-Hasselbalch equation, with which the proportion of the anesthetic in the charged and uncharged forms can be determined. The ratio of the cation to the base form of the drug is important, because the base form is responsible for penetration and tissue diffusion of the local anesthetic, whereas the cation form is responsible for local analgesia when the drug contacts the site of action within the sodium channel on the axolemma.

The pK_a of a drug is the pH at which equal proportions of the free base and cation form occur. Most local anesthetics used in obstetric analgesia have pK_a values ranging from 7.7 to 9.1 (Table 26–1). Since the pH of maternal blood is equal to or greater than 7.4, the pK_a of local anesthetics is so close that significant changes in maternal and fetal acid-base balance may result in fluxes in the base versus the cation forms of the drug.

$$R{:}NH^+ + OH^- \longrightarrow R{:}N + HOH$$

$$\text{Cation} \longleftarrow \text{Base}$$

$$pH = pK_a + \log \frac{\text{Base}}{\text{Cation}}$$

Figure 26–1. Local anesthetics are weak bases coexisting as undissociated free base and dissociated cation. Their proportion can be calculated by means of the Henderson-Hasselbalch equation.

Table 26–1. pK$_a$s of the more commonly used local anesthetics.

Drug	Brand Name	pK$_a$
Bupivacaine	Marcaine	8.1
Chloroprocaine	Nesacaine	8.7
Etidocaine	Duranest	7.7
Lidocaine	Xylocaine	7.9
Ropivacaine	Naropin	8.0

For example, a rising pH shifts a given amount of local anesthetic cation to the base form, and conversely a fall in pH will generate more of the cationic form.

Physical factors are also important in drug transfer. Drugs with molecular weights under 600 cross the placenta without difficulty, whereas those with molecular weights of over 1000 do not. A molecule such as digoxin (MW 780.95) crosses the ovine placenta very poorly. Molecular weights of most local anesthetics are in the 200–300 range. From the physical aspect, most local anesthetics cross the maternal-fetal barrier by simple diffusion according to the principles of Fick's law (Fig 26–2), which states that the rate of diffusion of a drug depends on the concentration gradient of the drug between the maternal and fetal compartments and the relationship of the thickness and total surface available for transfer.

C. Placental Transfer

Factors other than the physical or chemical properties of a drug may affect its transfer across the placenta. These factors include the rate and route of drug administration and the distribution, metabolism, and excretion of the drug by the mother and fetus. Fick's law may appear to be a simple method of determining drug transfer, but other complexities exist: differential blood flow on either side of the placenta; volume of maternal and fetal blood; and various shunts in the intervillous space that are important determinants of the final amount of drug a fetus may receive. Certain maternal disorders such as hypertensive cardiovascular disease, diabetes, and preeclampsia-eclampsia may alter placental blood flow and may in some way affect the extent of drug distribution.

As the placenta matures, there is a progressive reduction in the thickness of the epithelial trophoblastic layer. This may cause the thickness of the tissue layers between the maternal and fetal compartments to decrease tenfold (from as much as 25 μm in early gestation to 2 μm at term in some species). As gestation progresses, the surface area of the placenta increases also. At term, these changes in physical structure tend to favor improved transfer of drugs across the placenta.

Placental transfer is also affected by the pH of the blood on both sides of the placenta. The pH of the blood on the fetal side of the placenta is normally 0.1–0.2 U lower than that on the maternal side. Therefore, passage of drug to the fetal unit results in a tendency for more of the drug to exist in the ionized state. Because the maternal/fetal equilibrium is established only between the un-ionized fraction of the drug on either side of the barrier, this physiologic differential will expedite maternal-fetal transfer of drug. With more drug in the ionized form in the fetal unit, the new equilibrium that arises results in a greater total (ionized plus un-ionized) drug load in the fetus. Because the pK$_a$ values of commonly used local anesthetics are closer to the maternal blood pH, these agents tend to accumulate on the fetal side of the placenta. This is also true of other basic drugs such as morphine, meperidine, and propranolol. Further decreases in the fetal pH lead to additional drug entrapment in the fetus. For acidic drugs (eg, thiopental) the shift in total drug concentration is in the opposite direction, ie, toward the maternal side of the placenta.

In summary, the rate of transfer of a drug is governed mainly by (1) lipid solubility, (2) degree of drug ionization, (3) placental blood flow, (4) molecular weight, (5) placental metabolism, and (6) protein binding.

D. Fetal Distribution

After a drug deposited in the maternal compartment passes through the maternal-fetal barrier, the drug must reach the fetus and be distributed (Fig 26–3). The response of the fetus and newborn depends on drug concentration in vessel-rich organs, eg, the brain, heart, and liver. Drugs transferred from the maternal to the fetal compartment of the placenta are then diluted before distribution to the various fetal vital organs. About 85% of the blood in the umbilical vein, which passes from the placenta to the fetus, passes through the fetal liver and then into the inferior vena cava. The remainder bypasses the liver and enters the vena cava primarily via the ductus venosus. The drug concentration is further reduced by an admixture of blood coming from the lower extremities, the abdominal viscera, the upper

$$Q/T = K \left[\frac{A(C_M - C_F)}{D} \right]$$

Figure 26–2. Fick's law. Q/T is rate of diffusion. A, the surface area available for drug transfer; C$_M$, maternal drug concentration; C$_F$, fetal drug concentration; D, membrane thickness; K, the diffusion constant of the drug.

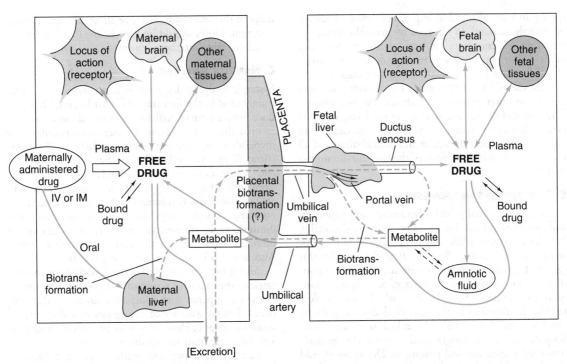

Figure 26–3. Relationship between maternal and fetal compartments and distribution of drugs between them. Drug is passed from the maternal compartment, via the placenta (a partial barrier), to the fetal compartment, where the principles of drug dynamics, ie, distribution, biotransformation, and excretion, determine the eventual specific organ tissue levels. One purely mechanical barrier exists between the maternal and fetal compartments, which attains importance in the late first and second stages of labor—the umbilical cord, which is susceptible to partial and total occlusion. (Reproduced, with permission, from Mirkin BL: Drug distribution in pregnancy. In: Boreus L [editor]: *Fetal Pharmacology*. Raven Press, 1973.)

extremities, and the thorax. Blood from the right atrium shunts from right to left through the foramen ovale into the left atrium, resulting in a final concentration on the left side of the heart, which is only slightly lower than that in the vena cava.

The amount of drug ultimately reaching a vital organ is related to that organ's blood supply. Since the central nervous system is the most highly vascularized fetal organ, it receives the greatest amount of drug. Once the drug reaches the fetal liver, it may either be bound to protein or metabolized.

The uptake of drug by fetal tissues can be very rapid after either intravenous or epidural administration. Measurable concentrations of local anesthetics have been found in fetal tissues as early as 1–2 minutes after injection. Lipid solubility of a drug is important in developing concentrations in certain organs with high lipid content such as the adrenal, ovary, liver, and brain.

Drug metabolism and excretion are the final features of the fetal distribution picture. The fetal liver is able to metabolize drugs and numerous substrates as early as the second trimester, an ability that improves to term. Narcotics and sedatives are metabolized much more slowly by the fetal liver, producing a prolonged effect of these drugs in the newborn who is exposed in utero. Finally, the ability of the fetus to excrete drugs is also reduced by reduced renal function.

Systemic Analgesics & Anesthetics

A. Sedatives (Hypnotics)

The principal use of sedative-hypnotic drugs is to produce drowsiness. For many years, these drugs were the only ones available to reduce anxiety and induce drowsiness. The latent phase of the first stage of labor may be managed by either psychologic support alone or utilization of sedative-hypnotic compounds. Psychologic support may be complemented by the use of sedatives. When properly utilized, these drugs induce tranquility and an enhanced feeling of well-being. They are poor analgesics and do not raise the pain threshold appreciably in conscious subjects. Amnesia does not occur. Labor may be slowed by large doses of sedatives, especially when given too early in the first stage.

The use of barbiturates alone for obstetric analgesia is not common practice and should be discouraged. The required dosage is dangerous to the fetus, which is extremely sensitive to central nervous system depression by these drugs. Periodic apnea and even abolition of all movements outlast the effects of the barbiturates on the mother.

B. Tranquilizers and Amnestics

These drugs are used principally to relieve apprehension and anxiety and produce a calm state. Additionally, they may potentiate the effects of other sedatives. An analgesic-potentiating effect is often claimed for this group of agents, but it has not been definitely demonstrated. Hydroxyzine and diazepam are popular tranquilizer-amnestics. Scopolamine, which was widely popular in obstetrics in the past, produces no analgesia but has a mild sedative and marked amnestic effect. Scopolamine is no longer used because the amnesia produced is excessive and prolonged. Diazepam should also be avoided during labor because it has a long chemical half-life, which is even more prolonged in the neonate. Diazepam readily crosses the placenta and is found in significant concentrations in fetal plasma. At present, diazepam is not recommended if the neonate is premature, because of the threat of kernicterus. Other potential side effects related to the use of diazepam are fetal hypotonia, hypothermia, and a loss of beat-to-beat variability in the fetal heart rate.

One of the controversies over diazepam concerns the content of sodium benzoate and benzoic acid buffers. Both compounds are potent uncouplers of the bilirubin-albumin complex, and some investigators have suggested that the neonate may be more susceptible to kernicterus because of an increase in free circulating bilirubin. However, because injectable diazepam is effective in the treatment of human newborn seizure disorders, opiate withdrawal, and tetanus, and since it is regarded as a useful adjunct in obstetric analgesia, a study was undertaken in animals in which comparable quantities of sodium benzoate were injected to determine whether significant amounts of bilirubin would be made available to the circulation. Midazolam, a short-acting water-soluble benzodiazepine, appears to be devoid of the neonatal effects seen with diazepam and is more rapidly cleared. Midazolam is a relatively new agent with minimal clinical use to date in obstetrics, but in small doses could conceivably become a useful anxiolytic for the laboring patient. Midazolam is 3–4 times more potent than diazepam, and there is a brief delay in the onset of its sedative effect after intravenous injection. Doses should be kept below 0.075 mg/kg to avoid excessive anterograde amnesia.

C. Narcotic Analgesics

Systemic analgesic drugs (including narcotics) are commonly used in the first stage of labor because they produce both a state of analgesia and mood elevation. The favored drugs are codeine, 60 mg intramuscularly, or meperidine, 50–100 mg intramuscularly or 25–50 mg (titrated) intravenously. The combination of morphine and scopolamine was once popular for its "twilight sleep" effect but is rarely used now. Common undesirable effects of this combination of drugs are nausea and vomiting, cough suppression, intestinal stasis, and diminution in frequency, intensity, and duration of uterine contractions in the early first stage of labor. Also, amnesia is excessive for these patients.

Morphine is not used in active laboring patients because of the excessive respiratory depression seen in the neonate compared with equipotent doses of other narcotics. Fetuses who are of young gestational age or are small-for-dates or those who have undergone trauma or long labor are more susceptible to narcosis.

Fentanyl is a popular synthetic narcotic that has been used in obstetrics in both the systemic and epidural compartments. Its use in the epidural compartment has met with good success when combined with small quantities and low concentrations of bupivacaine. Data supporting its use come from both Europe and the U.S.

D. Thiobarbiturates

Intravenous anesthetics such as thiopental and thiamylal are widely used in general surgery. However, less than 4 minutes after injection of a thiobarbiturate into the mother's vein, the concentrations of the drug in the fetal and maternal blood will be equal. The mother will lose consciousness and airway protective reflexes with a thiopental dose of 1.5–2 mg/kg, and therefore it should be used only in association with general endotracheal anesthesia.

E. Ketamine

The phencyclidine derivative ketamine produces anesthesia by a dissociative interruption of afferent pathways from cortical perception. It has become a useful and widely used adjunctive agent in obstetrics, because maternal cardiovascular status and uterine blood flow are well maintained. In low doses of 0.25–0.5 mg/kg intravenously, effective maternal analgesia results but without loss of consciousness or protective reflexes. The margin of safety is narrow, however, and therefore it should be used only by physicians able to easily secure and protect the airway if loss of consciousness occurs.

For cesarean section delivery, general anesthetic induction can be produced with 1–2 mg/kg intravenously and is followed in rapid sequence with a muscle relaxant and endotracheal intubation. Ketamine is therefore useful in the setting of major blood loss, when rapid induction of general anesthesia is required. However, it has significant hallucinogenic effects which limit its utility in obstetrics.

Ketamine stimulates the cardiovascular system to maintain heart rate, blood pressure, and cardiac output, and therefore is useful in complicated situations of maternal hypotension/hemorrhage.

F. INHALATION ANESTHETICS

Inhaled anesthetics are administered as a component of general anesthesia. In the past, inhaled anesthetics were given during labor in subanesthetic concentrations to treat contraction pain, but are no longer used for this indication. The mask administration of these gases to the conscious laboring patient can result in airway obstruction, aspiration, and hypoxia. Also, the labor room environment would become unacceptably contaminated by the vaporized gases because it is not possible to effectively scavenge exhaust gases from the room. Finally, of all the presently used volatile anesthetics, only nitrous oxide has analgesic properties at subanesthetic concentrations.

The most commonly used inhaled anesthetics in pregnancy are nitrous oxide, halothane, and isoflurane. During general anesthesia, 50% nitrous oxide in oxygen is supplemented with either 0.5% halothane or 0.7% isoflurane to provide most of the anesthetic requirements during the maintenance phase of the anesthetic. These drugs all readily cross the placenta and produce significant blood concentration in the fetus. During the brief exposure to maternally administered anesthetic gases, the fetus is not adversely affected. Fetal cardiac output is slightly reduced by these drugs, but critical organ blood flow is unaffected, and fetal acid–base status is unchanged. Exposure to minimum alveolar concentrations of anesthetic gases for more than 15 minutes is associated with reduced Apgar scores, but other parameters of fetal and newborn well-being are unimpaired.

The term parturient is more sensitive to the anesthetic effects of all inhaled anesthetics, presumably as a result of elevated progesterone levels. This increased sensitivity of 20–30% compared to nonpregnant subjects places the patient at increased risk of obtundation and aspiration, and therefore these drugs should not be administered without preparation for endotracheal intubation. Halothane and isoflurane produce uterine relaxation and high concentrations should be avoided during delivery to prevent uterine atony and postpartum hemorrhage. At low concentrations (less than 1%),

they produce amnesia and their tocolytic effects are easily counteracted by standard infusions of pitocin. These gases are both bronchodilators. Halothane has a more depressant effect on the myocardium, and isoflurane produces greater reduction in systemic vascular resistance.

Newer volatile anesthetics (desflurane, sevoflurane) have not been used widely in the parturient. These anesthetic gases are insoluble in blood and tissue and therefore are very short acting. It is not yet clear whether this property is an advantage or disadvantage during cesarean surgery compared to halothane and isoflurane.

REGIONAL ANESTHESIA

Regional anesthesia is achieved by injection of a local anesthetic (Table 26–2) around the nerves that pass from spinal segments to the peripheral nerves responsible for sensory innervation of a portion of the body. More recently, narcotics have been added to local anesthetics to improve analgesia and reduce some side effects of local anesthetics. Regional nerve blocks used in obstetrics include the following: (1) lumbar epidural and caudal epidural block, (2) subarachnoid (spinal) block, and (3) pudendal block.

Infiltration of a local anesthetic drug and pudendal block analgesia carry minimal risks. The hazards increase with the amount of drug used. The safety and suitability of regional anesthesia depend on the proper selection of the drug and the patient and the obstetrician-gynecologist's knowledge, experience, and expertise in the diagnosis and treatment of possible complications. Major conductive anesthesia and general anesthesia in obstetrics require specialized knowledge and expertise in conjunction with close maternal and fetal monitoring. This field of expertise has indeed developed as a subspecialty within anesthesia, reflecting the need for specialized understanding of the obstetric patient and her response and the fetal responses to anesthesia.

Patient Selection

Regional anesthesia is appropriate for labor analgesia, cesarean delivery, and other obstetric operative procedures (eg, postpartum tubal ligation, cervical cerclage). Most patients prefer to remain awake; however, on occasion a choice is made to provide general anesthesia.

The anesthesiologist will assess the patient to determine the relative risks of general versus regional anesthesia. Some forms of valvular heart disease, for example, may contraindicate regional block and general anesthesia may be considered more appropriate. Other contraindications to regional anesthesia include infec-

Table 26–2. Drugs used for local anesthesia.

	Tetracaine (Pontocaine)	Lidocaine (Xylocaine)	Bupivacaine (Marcaine)
Potency (compared to procaine)	10	2–3	9–12
Toxicity (compared to procaine)	10	1–1.5	4–6
Stability at sterilizing temperature	Stable	Stable	Stable
Total maximum dose	50–100 mg	500 mg	175 mg
Infiltration			
Concentration	0.05–0.1%	0.5–1%	0.25%
Onset of action	10–20 min	3–5 min	5–10 min
Duration	1½–3 h	30–60 min	90–120 min
Nerve block and epidural			
Concentration	0.1–0.2%	1–2%	0.5%
Onset of action	10–20 min	5–10 min	7–21 min
Duration	1½–3 h	1–1½ h	2–6 h
Subarachnoid			
Concentration	0.1–0.5%	5%	. . .
Dose	5–20 mg	40–100 mg	. . .
Onset of action	5–10 min	1–3 min	. . .
Duration	1½–2 h	1–1½ h	. . .

Modified and reproduced, with permission, from Guadagni NP, Hamilton WK: Anesthesiology. In: *Current Surgical Diagnosis & Treatment,* 4th ed. Dunphy JE, Way LW (editors). Lange, 1979.

tion, coagulopathy, hypovolemia, progressive neurologic disease, and patient refusal.

Patient Preparation

The woman who is well informed and has good rapport with her physician generally is a calm and cooperative candidate for regional or general anesthesia. The patient and her partner should be well informed early in her pregnancy of the options for labor anesthesia as well as for cesarean section if that circumstance arises. The anesthesiologist can be involved early in pregnancy if the patient has special concerns about anesthesia (family history of anesthetic risk, previous back surgery, coagulation problems). Some hospitals have obstetric anesthesia preassessment clinics organized to deal with these patient concerns.

Local Anesthetic Agents

A local anesthetic drug blocks the action potential of nerves when their axons are exposed to the medication. Local anesthetic agents act by modifying the ionic permeability of the cell membrane to stabilize its resting potential. The smaller the nerve fiber, the more sensitive it is to local anesthetics because the susceptibility of individual nerve fibers is inversely proportional to the cross-sectional diameter of the fibers. Hence, with regional anesthesia, the patient's perception of light touch, pain, and temperature, and her capacity for vasomotor control, are obtunded sooner and with a smaller concentration of the drug than is the perception of pressure or the function of motor nerves to striated muscles. The exception to this rule is the sensitivity of autonomic nerve fibers that are blocked by the lowest concentration of local anesthetic despite being larger than some sensory nerves.

Only anesthetic drugs that are completely reversible and nonirritating and that cause minimal toxicity are clinically acceptable. Other desirable properties of regional anesthetic agents include rapidity of onset, predictability of duration, and ease of sterilization. Table 26–2 summarizes the local anesthetics commonly used in obstetrics and gynecology together with their uses and doses.

All local anesthetics have certain undesirable dose-related side effects when absorbed systemically. All these drugs are capable of stimulating the central nervous system and may cause bradycardia, hypertension, or respiratory stimulation at the medullary level. Moreover, they may produce anxiety, excitement, or convulsions at the cortical or subcortical level. This response stimulates grand mal seizures because it is followed by depression, loss of vasomotor control, hypotension, respiratory depression, and coma. Such an episode of indirect cardiovascular depression often is accentuated by a direct vasodilatory and myocardial depressant effect. The latter is comparable to the action of quinidine. This is why lidocaine is useful for the treatment of certain cardiac arrhythmias.

Chloroprocaine is an ester derivative that was popular in the mid-1960s but fell into disuse clinically. In the 1970s, it enjoyed a resurgence in popularity primarily because of its rapid onset and short duration of action and its low toxicity to the fetus. Its physicochemical properties are imparted by the chloro substitution of the 2-position in the benzene ring of procaine. It is metabolized by plasma cholinesterase and therefore does not demand liver enzyme degradation, as do the more complex and longer-acting amide derivatives. Chloroprocaine has a half-life of 21 seconds in adult blood and 43 seconds in neonatal blood. Direct toxic effects on the fetus are minimized, since less drug is available for transfer in the maternal compartment.

The potency of chloroprocaine is comparable to that of lidocaine and mepivacaine, and the drug is 3 times more potent than procaine. Its average onset of action ranges from 6 to 12 minutes and persists for 30–60 minutes, depending on the amount used. Its use has been severely curtailed because of recent reports of toxicity that include arachnoiditis and associated neuropathies. The new 3% chloroprocaine is less acidic and has a reduced concentration of sodium metabisulfate (0.5 mg/mL) and is safe for epidural use.

Bupivacaine, the amide local anesthetic, is related to lidocaine and mepivacaine but has some very different physicochemical properties. It has a much higher lipid solubility, a higher degree of binding to maternal plasma protein, and a much longer duration of action. More than with other local anesthetics, the concentration of bupivacaine can be reduced to produce sensory block with minimal motor block. Since injection of bupivacaine for labor pain relief is now mostly in the form of continuous small volume and minimal concentration administration via a pump mechanism, the complications previously of concern such as hypotension and convulsions are now rare.

A word of caution must be added regarding the administration of bupivacaine for cesarean section delivery. This drug has been implicated in certain cardiovascular catastrophes associated with initial drug injection, eg, cardiac arrests that were refractory to full and appropriate resuscitative attempts. Although these catastrophes are rare, the practitioner is well advised to inject no more than 5 mL of the drug at any one time, to wait 4–5 minutes, then to repeat the procedure until the desired volume has been delivered. The maximum concentration of bupivacaine now allowed by the FDA for obstetric epidural anesthesia is 0.5%. The toxic dose is now considered 1–2 mg/kg for bupivacaine.

Ropivacaine is a new amide local anesthetic introduced into the United States in the mid-1990s. It is less lipid soluble than bupivacaine, and initial studies suggested that it produced less motor blockade and was less cardiotoxic than its homolog bupivacaine. Later studies have been less convincing in documenting improved efficacy and safety, but ropivacaine has replaced bupivacaine in some institutions. There is ongoing study of the safety and efficacy of levobupivacaine, the levorotatory isomer of bupivacaine, which may also prove less cardiotoxic than its racemic parent molecule. Both of these newer amide local anesthetics are used in doses and concentrations similar to bupivacaine.

Local Infiltration Analgesia

Local tissue infiltration of dilute solutions of anesthetic drugs generally yields satisfactory results because the target is the fine nerve fibers. Nevertheless, one must keep in mind the dangers of systemic toxicity when large areas are anesthetized or when reinjection is required. It is good practice, therefore, to calculate in advance the milligrams of drug and volume of solution that may be required to keep the total dosage below the accepted toxic dose.

Infiltration in or near an area of inflammation is contraindicated. Injections into these zones may be followed by rapid systemic absorption of the drug owing to the increased vascularity of the inflamed tissues. Moreover, the injection may introduce or aggravate infection.

Regional Analgesia

A. LUMBAR EPIDURAL BLOCK

This analgesic technique has become more popular recently, because it is well suited to obstetric anesthesia. Either bolus injections or continuous infusion of local anesthetics is used for labor, vaginal delivery, or cesarean surgery (Fig 26–4). Narcotics are often added to supplement the quality of the block.

After the patient is evaluated, an epidural block may be placed once labor is established. Drug dosages can be adjusted as circumstances change. The catheter can be used for surgery and postoperative analgesia if necessary. The second stage of labor is prolonged by epidural anesthesia; however, the duration of the first stage is unaffected. The use of outlet forceps is increased, but fetal outcome is not adversely affected by epidural block.

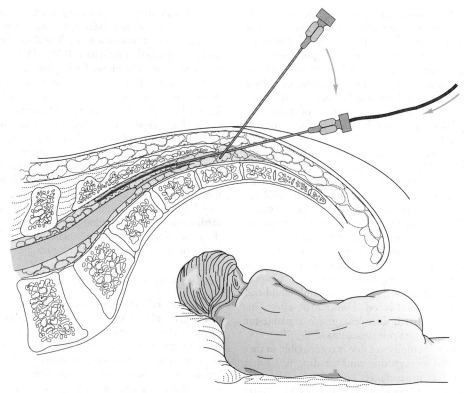

Figure 26–4. Caudal catheter in place for continuous caudal anesthesia.

The epidural block technique must be exact, and inadvertent massive (high) spinal anesthesia occasionally occurs. Other undesirable reactions include the rapid absorption syndrome (hypotension, bradycardia, hallucinations, convulsions), postpartum backache, and paresthesias. Epidural block should eradicate pain between T10 and L1 for first stage, and between T10 and S5 for the second stage of labor.

The procedure is as follows: Inject 3 mL of a 1.5% aqueous solution of lidocaine or similar agent into the catheter as a test dose. If spinal anesthesia does not result after 5–10 minutes, inject an additional 5 mL. Inject 10 mL of the anesthetic solution in total to slowly accomplish an adequate degree and suitable level of anesthesia. Once the block is established, a continuous infusion of 10–12 mL/h will maintain the block for labor. Bupivacaine, 0.125–0.25%, is most often used for an epidural block, with fentanyl 2–5 μg/mL in the epidural mixture.

The mother is nursed in a wedged or lateral position to avoid aortocaval compression. The sympathectomy produced by the block predisposes the patient to venous pooling and reduced venous return. Maternal blood pressure must be measured frequently when the epidural is in effect.

B. CAUDAL BLOCK

Caudal anesthesia is an epidural block approached through the caudal space. It can provide selective sacral block for second-stage labor; however, it is rarely used now because of complications specific to the obstetric patient. The descent of the fetal head against the perineum, in addition to the sacral edema at term, obscures the landmarks of the sacral hiatus. This makes the caudal procedure technically challenging, and reports of transfixing the rectum and fetal skull puncture with the epidural needle have led many anesthesiologists to avoid this technique. Lumbar epidural anesthesia is considered a safer alternative.

C. SPINAL ANESTHESIA

Spinal anesthesia is currently used to alleviate the pain of delivery and the third stage of labor. Short-acting agents (5% lidocaine, 50 mg) or long-acting drugs (0.25% bupivacaine, 2.5 mg) with narcotic (fentanyl, 25 μg) are used. Brief or minimal spinal anesthesia is far safer than prolonged spinal anesthesia, which is not recommended for obstetric use. The advantages of spinal anesthesia are that the mother remains conscious to witness delivery, no inhalation anesthetics or analgesic drugs are required, the technique is not difficult, and good relaxation of the pelvic floor and lower birth canal is achieved. Prompt anesthesia is achieved within 5–10 minutes, and there are fewer failures than with caudal anesthesia. The dosage of spinal anesthetic is small. Complications are fewer and easier to treat. Hypotension is rare with the doses used. However, spinal headache occurs in 1–2% of patients, and operative delivery is more often required because voluntary expulsive efforts are eliminated. Drug reactions (eg, hypotension) may occur. Respiratory failure may occur if the anesthetic ascends within the spinal cord owing to rapid injection or straining by the patient.

The procedure is as follows:

1. Inject 50 mg of lidocaine 5% or 2.5 mg of bupivacaine with 25 μg of fentanyl at the L3–L4 interspace between contractions. Have the patient lying on her side or sitting up. Elevate her head on a pillow immediately after the injection. Tilt the table up or down to achieve a level of anesthesia at or near the umbilicus. Anesthesia will be maximal in 3–5 minutes and will last for 1 hour or longer.

2. Obtain and record the blood pressure and respiratory rate every 3 minutes for the first 10 minutes and every 5 minutes thereafter.

3. Give oxygen for respiratory depression and mild hypotension. In addition, administer a vasopressor such as ephedrine, 5–10 mg intravenously, if blood pressure decreases more than 20% of baseline or to less than 100 mm Hg systolic and is not responsive to intravenous fluids and lateral tilt.

Undesirable Side Effects of Spinal or Epidural Anesthesia

The most serious consequence of spinal or epidural anesthesia has been very rare mortality. Maternal deaths associated with the use of 0.75% bupivacaine for cesarean section delivery and labor were reported in the late 1980s, prompting the FDA to outlaw the use of this drug in obstetrics. These deaths were attributed to venous uptake of the drug and immediate and lasting myocardial depression from the local anesthetic, which did not respond to appropriate cardiac resuscitative efforts. Maternal mortality associated with regional anesthesia is lower today, primarily because bolus dosing of high concentrations of local anesthesia is no longer performed.

Most side effects of spinal or epidural anesthesia are secondary to the block of the sympathetic nerve fibers that accompany the anterior roots of the spinal thoracic and upper lumbar nerves (thoracolumbar outflow). Thus, many physiologic regulating mechanisms are disturbed. The blood lumbar pressure falls as the result of loss of arterial resistance and venous pooling—assuming no compensation is made by change of the patient's position (eg, Trendelenburg position). If high thoracic dermatomes (T1–T5) are blocked, alteration of the cardiac sympathetic innervation slows the heart rate and reduces cardiac contractility. Epinephrine secretion by the adrenal medulla is depressed. Concomitantly, the unopposed parasympathetic effect of cardiac slowing alters vagal stimulations. As a result of these and related changes, shock follows promptly, especially in hypotensive or hypovolemic patients. Moreover, a precipitous fall in the blood pressure of the arteriosclerotic hypertensive patient is inevitable.

Fluids, oxygen therapy for adequate tissue perfusion, shock position to encourage venous return, and pressor drugs given intravenously are recommended.

In the past, postdural puncture headache (PDPH) due to leakage of cerebrospinal fluid through the needle hole in the dura was an early postoperative complication in up to 15% of patients. Small-caliber needles (25F) decrease the incidence of headache to 8–10%. With the introduction of pencil-point Whitacker and Sprotte spinal needles, the incidence of PDPH was reduced to 1–2%. Therapy for PDPH includes recumbent position, hydration, sedation, and in severe cases, epidural injection of 10–20 mL of the patient's fresh blood to "seal" the defect.

Rarely, spinal or epidural anesthesia has caused nerve injury and transient or permanent hypesthesia or paresthesia. Excessive drug concentration, sensitivity, or infection may have been responsible for some of these complications. The incidence of serious complications of spinal or epidural anesthesia is considerably lower than that of cardiac arrest during general anesthesia.

A. PARACERVICAL BLOCK

Paracervical block (Fig 26–5) is no longer considered a safe technique for the obstetric patient. In the past, paracervical anesthesia was used to relieve the pain of the first stage of labor. Pudendal block was required for pain during the second stage of labor. Sensory nerve fibers from the uterus fuse bilaterally at the 4–6 o'clock and 6–8 o'clock positions around the cervix in the region of the cervical-vaginal junction. Ordinarily, when 5–10 mL of 1% lidocaine or its equivalent is injected into these areas, interruption of the sensory input from the cervix and uterus promptly follows.

Many now consider paracervical block to be contraindicated in obstetrics because of the potential ad-

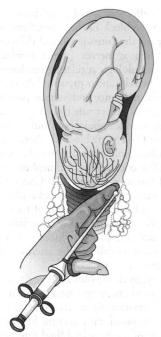

Figure 26–5. Paracervical block. This block is considered by many to be contraindicated in pregnancy.

verse fetal effects. There are many reports in the literature that place the incidence of fetal bradycardia at 8–18%. Recent work with accurate fetal heart rate monitoring associated with continuous uterine contraction patterns, however, suggests that the incidence is closer to 20–25%. Some researchers have attempted to investigate the significance of the bradycardia. One explanation is that an acid-base disturbance in the fetus does not occur unless the bradycardia lasts longer than 10 minutes, and that neonatal depression is rare unless associated with delivery during the period of bradycardia. There seems to be little difference in the incidence and severity of fetal bradycardia by paracervical block between complicated and uncomplicated patients. Other disadvantages of paracervical block include maternal trauma and bleeding, fetal trauma and direct injection, inadvertent intravascular injection with convulsions, and short duration of the block.

B. PUDENDAL NERVE BLOCK

Pudendal block has been one of the most popular of all nerve block techniques in obstetrics. The infant is not depressed, and blood loss is minimal. The technique is simplified by the fact that the pudendal nerve approaches the spine of the ischium on its course to innervate the perineum. Injection of 10 mL of 1% lidocaine on each side will achieve analgesia for 30–45 minutes about 50% of the time.

Both the transvaginal and transcutaneous methods are useful for administering a pudendal block. The transvaginal technique has important practical advantages over the transcutaneous technique. The "Iowa trumpet" needle guide may be used, and the operator's finger should be placed at the end of the needle guide to palpate the sacrospinous ligament, which runs in the same direction and is just anterior to the pudendal nerve and artery. It is usually very difficult to appreciate the sensation of the needle puncturing the ligament. This facet of the technique (no definite endpoint) may make it difficult for the inexperienced clinician to perform. Aspiration of the syringe for possible inadvertent entry into the pudendal artery should be accomplished, and, if no blood is returned, 10 mL of local anesthetic solution should be injected in a fan-like fashion on the right and left sides. The successful performance of the pudendal block requires injection of the drug at least 10–12 minutes before episiotomy. Often, in clinical practice, pudendal block is performed within 4–5 minutes of episiotomy. Hence there may not be adequate time for the local anesthetic to take effect.

1. Advantages and disadvantages—Enthusiasm for pudendal nerve block has been due to its safety and ease of administration and the rapidity of onset of effect. Disadvantages include maternal trauma, bleeding, and infection; rare maternal convulsions due to drug sensitivity; occasional complete or partial failure; and regional discomfort during administration.

The pudendal perineal block, like any other nerve block, demands some technical experience and knowledge of the innervation of the lower birth canal. Nevertheless, in spite of a well-placed bilateral block, skip areas of perineal analgesia may be noted. The reason for this may be that although the pudendal nerve of S2–S4 derivation does contribute to the majority of fibers for sensory innervation to the perineum, other sensory fibers are involved also. For example, the inferior hemorrhoidal nerve may have an origin independent from that of the sacral nerve and therefore will not be a component branch of the pudendal nerve. In this case, it must be infiltrated separately. In addition, the posterior femoral cutaneous nerve (S1–S3) origin may contribute an important perineal branch to the anterior fourchette bilaterally. In instances in which this nerve plays a major role in innervation, it must be blocked separately by local skin infiltration.

Two other nerves contribute to the sensory innervation of the perineum: the ilioinguinal nerve, of L1 origin, and the genital branch of the genitofemoral nerve, of L1 and L2 origin. Both of these nerves sweep superficially over the mons pubis to innervate the skin over the symphysis of the mons pubis and the labium majus. Occasionally, these nerves must also be separately infiltrated to provide optimal perineal analgesic effect. Thus it should be apparent that a simple bilateral pudendal nerve block may not be effective in many cases. For maximum analgesic effectiveness, in addition to a bilateral pudendal block, superficial infiltration of the skin from the symphysis medially to a point halfway between the ischial spines may be necessary. Thus, a true perineal block may be regarded as a regional technique.

Either lumbar epidural or caudal epidural block should eradicate pain between the T10 and S5 level for the second stage. All these nerves are denervated, since they all are derived from L1–S5 segments.

2. Procedure (Fig 26–6)

1. Palpate the ischial spines vaginally. Slowly advance the needle guide toward each spine. After placement is achieved, the needle is advanced through the guide to penetrate approximately 0.5 cm. Aspirate, and if needle is not in a vessel, deposit 5 mL below each spine. This blocks the

right and left pudendal nerves. Refill the syringe when necessary, and proceed in a similar manner to anesthetize the other areas specified. Keep the needle moving while injecting and avoid the sensitive vaginal mucosa and periosteum.

2. Withdraw the needle and guide about 2 cm and redirect toward an ischial tuberosity. Inject 3 mL near the center of each tuberosity to anesthetize the inferior hemorrhoidal and lateral femoral cutaneous nerves.

3. Withdraw the needle and guide almost entirely and then slowly advance toward the symphysis pubica almost to the clitoris, keeping about 2 cm lateral to the labial fold and about 1–2 cm beneath the skin. The injection of 5 mL of lidocaine on each side beneath the symphysis will block the ilioinguinal and genitocrural nerves.

If the procedure explained above is carefully and skillfully done, there will be only slight discomfort during the injections. Prompt flaccid relaxation and good anesthesia for 30–60 minutes can be expected.

Prevention & Treatment of Local Anesthetic Overdosage

The correct dose of any local anesthetic is the smallest quantity of drug in the greatest dilution that will provide adequate analgesia. The pregnant patient is more likely to have an intravascular drug injection because of the venous distention in the epidural space and may be more susceptible to the toxic effects of local anesthetics (Table 26–3). Injection of the drug into a highly vascularized area will result in more rapid systemic absorption than, for example, injection into the skin. To prevent too-rapid absorption, the operator may add epinephrine to produce local vasoconstriction and prolong the anesthetic. A final concentration of 1:200,000 is desirable, especially when a toxic amount is ap-

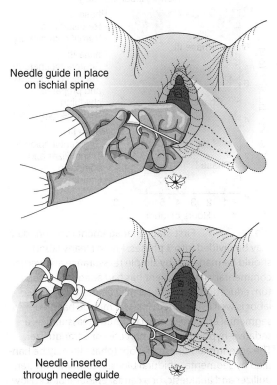

Needle guide in place on ischial spine

Needle inserted through needle guide

Figure 26–6. Use of needle guide ("Iowa trumpet") in pudendal anesthetic block. (Reproduced, with permission, from Benson RC: *Handbook of Obstetrics & Gynecology*, 8th ed. Lange, 1983.)

Table 26–3. Toxic doses of local anesthetics commonly used in obstetrics.

Drug	Toxic Dose
Lidocaine	5 mg/kg, plain 7 mg/kg, with epinephrine
Bupivacaine	1.5 mg/kg[1]
Chloroprocaine	10 mg/kg
Tetracaine	1 mg/kg
Ropivacaine	3 mg/kg

[1]Doses as low as 90 mg have produced cardiac arrest.

proached. Epinephrine is contraindicated, however, in patients with increased cardiac irritability of medical or drug origin.

The treatment of local anesthetic overdosage manifested by central nervous system toxicity (a convulsion) is generally achieved very effectively and without incident. However, the clinician must be aware of certain basic principles. These include the recognition of prodromal signs of a central nervous system toxic reaction and immediate treatment as required. A toxic central nervous system reaction to local anesthetics consists of ringing in the ears, diplopia, perioral numbness, and deep, slurred speech. An adequate airway must be maintained, and the patient should receive 100% oxygen, with respiratory assistance if necessary. Protection of the patient's airway and immediate injection of thiopental, 50 mg, or midazolam, 1–2 mg, usually stop the convulsion immediately. In the past, succinylcholine was recommended, but it is a potent neuromuscular relaxant, which requires placement of an endotracheal tube with positive pressure ventilation. Studies have indicated that cellular metabolism is greatly increased during convulsive episodes, so that a definite increase in cellular oxygenation occurs—hence the use of a depressant selective for the hypothalamus and thalamus, because these sites are the foci of irritation.

ANALGESIA FOR INTRAPARTUM OBSTETRICS

For ideal anesthetic management of intrapartum analgesia, the physician who has an established rapport with the patient should be responsible. Any substitutes should be colleagues who are completely aware of the patient's background, personality, and problems. Current clinical practice is to provide analgesia and not amnesia during the first 2 stages of labor. Most parturients prefer to be awake and help the physician during labor and delivery. The physician must be aware of the patient's attitude and personality during labor. A mother who has been calm and cooperative during the antepartum period may unexpectedly become anxious or distraught once labor progresses. If this occurs, mild sedation with psychologic support may be indicated.

Analgesia management by the physician also requires some basic knowledge of the patient's gestational problems and prognosis. Consequently, the types of analgesic methods available to the patient should be discussed with the patient in the early stages of pregnancy. However, a total commitment on the part of the physician and the patient to a specific analgesia method should be avoided. Both primiparas and multiparas may develop unforeseen complications that could make the method agreed upon undesirable and, in some cases, medically unacceptable.

Management of the First Stage

The management of labor analgesia can be determined only when the patient experiences the pain and decides on options with the help and reassurance of her physician (Fig 26–7).

Management of the Second Stage

A. EPIDURAL BLOCK

If an epidural technique is utilized for first-stage pain relief, it may be extended to cover the second stage. Assuming that a lumbar catheter alone is utilized, the segmental block can be extended to include sacral dermatomes with a larger volume of local anesthetic. Sacral block is present in only 3.5% of patients with the initial epidural dose. This increases to 65% of patients with repeated injections. It is therefore important for the anesthesiologist to assess the degree of sacral anesthesia that is present when a "perineal dose" is requested. No

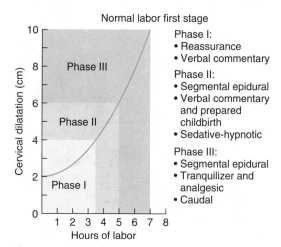

Figure 26–7. First-stage management in a primipara may be divided into 3 phases. Phase I (early labor) should be managed by simple reassurance and verbal commentary if the patient has had adequate antepartum education. An epidural may be performed once labor is well established. Phase II may be handled by a segmental epidural block, continued reassurance, a sedative-hypnotic drug, a narcotic, or a tranquilizer. The accentuated phase of labor (phase III) may be handled by segmental epidural block, a combination tranquilizer and analgesic, or a caudal epidural block. However, use of reassurance and verbal commentary in conjunction with prepared childbirth methods may be adequate for some patients to tolerate the discomfort of phase III labor.

further dosing may be needed, or 10–12 mL of local anesthetic will usually produce sacral block if none is present at the time of delivery.

The timing of second-stage analgesia must be managed carefully because 10–12 minutes are required for a good sacral block to develop after the injection described above. If a caudal catheter is used, 10 mL of 2% lidocaine should be injected into the caudal epidural space; within 5–8 minutes, good sacral analgesia should be present. This technique rarely fails to produce bilateral analgesia, and its onset is more rapid. A 2% solution is preferred for the second stage for a more complete motor block of the pudendum.

B. Subarachnoid Block

Subarachnoid block may also be utilized for good second-stage analgesia and muscle relaxation of the perineum. The technique may be performed with the patient in either the sitting or lateral recumbent position. The latter is the most common position for subarachnoid block and is infinitely more comfortable for the patient. An important feature is the total amount of drug used. Four milligrams of 1% tetracaine, 6–8 mg of 0.75% bupivacaine, or 50 mg of 5% lidocaine are adequate for a low spinal block of dermatomes T10–S5. The block will last only 50–70 minutes and therefore should be used only if delivery is imminent.

One of the advantages of subarachnoid block is the rapid onset of both sensory and motor blockade. Careful attention must be paid to changes in the sensory level and blood pressure. The latter must be recorded every 2–3 minutes for the first 10 minutes to be certain that sudden undetected hypotension does not occur. Thereafter, the blood pressure may be recorded every 5 minutes for 30 minutes.

C. Pudendal Block

Pudendal block, when performed correctly, will suffice also for second-stage pain relief. As outlined above, performance of the pudendal nerve block is not as simple as many physicians believe. Inadequate perineal analgesia often occurs because of lack of knowledge of the sensory distribution to the perineum. Nonetheless, a good bilateral pudendal block combined with superficial injection of the triangular area between the midportion of the symphysis pubica and halfway to a line drawn to the spinous process often will effect complete perineal analgesia. In spite of this, more analgesia is usually needed for an indicated forceps delivery. If forceps extraction is necessary, a caudal or subarachnoid block may be needed to achieve complete perineal anesthesia.

D. Special Problems

1. Midforceps delivery—Each patient's requirements vary and every situation must be evaluated on an individual basis. Midforceps delivery often involves both rotation and traction. Therefore, the anesthetic regimen must provide relaxation as well as analgesia for the perineum, lower vagina, and upper birth canal. In order for the obstetrician to perform the procedures necessary for delivery, it is necessary to provide optimal conditions so that maternal and fetal trauma can be minimized. Regional analgesia with a lumbar, caudal epidural, or subarachnoid block is preferred, since these blocks provide analgesia and optimal relaxation.

2. The trapped head—On the rare occasion when the breech delivery is complicated by a trapped head, the application of forceps or other manipulations may be required urgently. If an epidural block is in place, no further analgesia will be required; however, if one is not in place, immediate anesthesia and pelvic relaxation will be required to facilitate rapid delivery and minimize trauma. The only acceptable technique for this purpose is general anesthesia with halothane after suitable protection of the patient from the hazards of aspiration. Protection should include use of antacid, 30 mL orally, and adequate oxygenation; followed by thiopental, 200 mg intravenously; succinylcholine, 80–100 mg intravenously; and rapid intubation with cricoid pressure.

ANESTHESIA FOR THE FETUS AT RISK

Premature Labor

A. Psychoanalgesia

Familiarize the patient before labor (if possible) with a relaxation technique (Lamaze or Dick-Read) and the use of her delivery powers to reduce tension and pain (psychoprophylaxis). Establish rapport and provide emotional support. Use reassurance and kindly direction. Use suggestion and hypnosis when feasible. Psychoprophylaxis has been quite successful, but fewer than 20% of patients can be carried through labor and delivery with hypnosis alone.

B. Regional Analgesia

Conduction analgesia is usually more desirable than inhalation or parenteral analgesia. All regional blocking agents are rapidly absorbed. These agents may intoxicate the fetus when overdosage occurs, with resultant apnea and vascular collapse due to medullary depression, bradycardia due to the quinidine-like effect on the myocardium, and convulsions due to cortical excitation. These agents with the amide molecular linkage (lidocaine, mepivacaine, and prilocaine) have a stability that resists enzymatic splitting and rapidly cross the placental barrier intact. In contrast, local anesthetics with an ester bond (procaine, 2-chloroprocaine, and tetracaine) are metabolized in the plasma and placenta with only minor transfer to the fetus.

1. Lumbar epidural block—Continuous lumbar epidural block may be a safe method of anesthesia in the delivery of a jeopardized fetus if properly performed by well-trained personnel. It may be selected in maternal complications such as congenital or acquired heart disease, pulmonary disorders, diabetes, preeclampsia-eclampsia, hypertension, and renal or hepatic disease. It may be the best technique for premature or postmature labor, prolonged labor, or cervical dystocia. The low-dosage technique can be augmented to produce anesthesia for cesarean section delivery.

2. Caudal block—Epidural placement of an anesthetic solution in the caudal canal (caudal block), although it involves less risk of dural puncture, requires more medication (with attendant fetal risks), and the procedure blocks a larger nerve distribution, with the hazard of hypotension. The anesthetic may also lead to failure of spontaneous internal rotation.

3. Spinal block—Maternal hypotension with decreased uterine blood flow is the greatest risk to the fetus when subarachnoid (spinal) block is used. It is useful only during delivery because it is a "single shot" technique with a duration of action of only 50–70 minutes.

4. General anesthesia—General anesthetics may be useful adjuncts in certain high-risk patients. It should be stressed, however, that all general anesthetics cross the placenta and can depress the fetus. General anesthetics may be selected if regional anesthetics are contraindicated, if deep uterine relaxation is necessary, for alleviation of constriction rings, for relief of tetanic uterine contractions, or when prompt deep anesthesia is necessary.

Multiple Pregnancy

A. Psychoanalgesia

The psychoprophylactic technique helps to prepare the patient for the intrapartum experience. When the labor progresses normally, psychoanalgesia can effectively reduce apprehension and enhance the pleasurable aspects of childbirth. It may also prepare the patient for an understanding of some of the complications of multiple pregnancy (uterine inertia in the first stage of labor, uterine atony in the third stage, and possible need for cesarean section delivery) and reduce the total amount of drugs required for analgesia.

B. Pudendal Nerve Block

Pudendal nerve block is usually reserved for cases in which epidural block is not available. Analgesia is more limited and does not provide as effective analgesia should version or breech extractions of the second twin be required.

C. Epidural Block

This technique is useful as a first-stage analgesic method, but only a segmental type should be utilized (T10–L2) to prevent the increased hazard of hypotension secondary to a combined large-segment sympathetic block and vena cava occlusion. Ideal management here entails the use of lumbar epidural block for the first stage and low caudal block for the late second stage of labor. Epidural anesthesia does not affect fetal outcome with twin delivery, but has the advantage of enabling the obstetrician to intervene more easily if the second twin presents abnormally. The need for a general anesthetic can be avoided if an epidural is in place and a cesarean section is required urgently for delivery of the second twin.

D. Spinal Block

The low subarachnoid block is rarely used at the end of the second stage for crowning, delivery, and episiotomy. A low spinal block does not provide a high enough block for cesarean section if it is required urgently (eg, in malpresentation or cord prolapse of the second twin). Therefore, an epidural anesthetic is always preferable for the labor and delivery of multiple births.

E. Inhalation Analgesics

The only inhalation anesthetic that is analgesic at low concentration is nitrous oxide. Experience is needed to use this drug safely because the pregnant patient is sensitive to its anesthetic effects and can easily become obtunded. Loss of airway reflexes and aspiration are causes of maternal mortality.

General endotracheal anesthesia can be used for cesarean section delivery of twins. Neonatal depression is more likely if the induction-to-delivery time is long (> 8 minutes), especially if the uterine incision-to-delivery time is also prolonged (> 3 minutes).

ANALGESIA FOR ABNORMAL OBSTETRICS

Abnormal obstetrics may include conditions that compromise both the fetus and the mother. Analgesia management in acute and chronic fetal distress and in maternal complications such as preeclampsia-eclampsia, hypertension, heart disease, and diabetes will be discussed. Finally, the analgesic management of obstetric complications such as placenta previa, cord prolapse, abruptio placentae, and breech presentation will be considered.

Acute Fetal Distress

Acute fetal distress usually occurs intrapartum, without previously suspected fetal compromise. It may be heralded clinically by either the sudden appearance of meconium, the development of bradycardia, or a deceleration pattern detected by fetal monitoring. With continuous heart rate-monitoring equipment, a severe deceleration may be designated as variable or late. In either case, because uterine perfusion presently is correlated with blood pressure, it may be assumed that a maternal pressure fall greater than 20% of the baseline systolic figure will produce a substantial reduction in uterine perfusion. Because this will aggravate any acute intrapartum fetal distress, hypotension should be avoided. Although the incidence and degree of hypotension after sympathetic blockade can be minimized by thorough evaluation, fluid preloading, and patient positioning, it may occur even in the best circumstances. With definite documentation of severe intrapartum distress, therefore, analgesic techniques should be chosen that are not associated with hypotensive sequelae.

Hypotension is more frequent with spinal anesthesia, and therefore this technique is usually contraindicated when fetal distress exists. A systemic technique may be used, but recall that the systemic administration of narcotics and barbiturates may cause neonatal depression after delivery. The use of a narcotic antagonist such as naloxone may reverse the effect of antepartum narcotics. The anesthetic selection during labor with mild fetal distress is usually either a small dose of intravenous tranquilizer and narcotics or a segmental epidural block. If severe fetal distress requires immediate cesarean delivery, time must not be spent placing a regional block. General endotracheal anesthesia is required in this circumstance to enable the most speedy delivery of the distressed fetus. Even the most expeditious spinal procedure will delay the prep and draping of the patient. Therefore, spinal anesthesia should only be preformed with the clear understanding that there will be a few minutes of delay in delivery.

Chronic Fetal Distress

A serious problem in anesthetic management occurs when acute intrapartum distress is superimposed on chronic fetal distress. Underlying chronic distress may be preeclampsia-eclampsia, hypertension, postmaturity, or diabetes. These disorders all reduce fetal reserve. The anesthesiologist must meticulously avoid or manage even mild hypotension, since the primary aim should be maintenance of uterine blood flow. The probable choices are no analgesia, minimal systemic analgesia, or segmental epidural block.

Maternal Complications

A. Preeclampsia-Eclampsia

This syndrome (often called toxemia of pregnancy) is composed of the triad of hypertension, generalized edema, and proteinuria. It accounts for almost 20% of maternal deaths per year in the U.S. The primary pathologic characteristic of this disease process is generalized arterial spasm. As gestation lengthens, there is a tendency toward a fluid shift from the vascular to the extravascular compartment with resultant hypovolemia—in spite of an expanded extracellular fluid space.

It is estimated that nearly 50% of eclamptic patients who die have myocardial hemorrhages or areas of focal necrosis. Major disorders of central nervous system function probably are caused by cerebral vasospasm. It is obvious that optimal anesthetic management of these patients during the intrapartum period must include a careful preanesthetic evaluation of the cardiovascular and central nervous systems.

The physiologic changes of severe preeclampsia-eclampsia are exaggerated by regional block due to a restricted intravascular volume, and this may result in considerable depression of blood pressure. A small subgroup of these patients suffer from a reduced cardiac output (compared to normal pregnancy), decreased intravascular fluid space, and marked increases in systemic vascular resistance (SVR). Patients with severe hemodynamic changes may require direct monitoring of pulmonary artery and wedge pressures to manage labor and the effects of epidural anesthesia. Uterine blood flow is increased with epidural block because of the favorable reduction of SVR, as long as central filling pressures and mean arterial pressure are well maintained.

Regional and general anesthesia is used in the management of preeclamptic patients. Contraindications to regional anesthesia include coagulopathy, and urgency for fetal distress. The latter may mitigate against excessive time being taken for the placement of a spinal or epidural if the baby needs immediate delivery.

Epidural anesthesia is preferred to spinal anesthesia in cases of severe hypertension. The more graduated onset of sympathetic block with this technique is thought to produce less hypotension than would occur with spinal block. However, more recent study suggests that adequate volume preloading of these patients, who by definition are depleted intravascularly, results in similar hemodynamic responses to both regional techniques. More study is required to confirm these findings, but it is clear that more spinal and epidural anesthesia is performed in preeclamptic patients than in the past. Obstetricians have become aware that epidural anesthesia is a valuable adjunct in the management of hypertension as a result of the pain relief as well as the vasodilation produced by epidural block. In the past, epidural anesthesia was avoided because of an exaggerated concern over hypotension; now epidural anesthesia is encouraged if the patient's volume status is well managed and if coagulopathy does not complicate the clinical picture.

B. Hemorrhage and Shock

Intrapartum obstetric emergencies demand immediate diagnosis and therapy for a favorable outcome for the mother and fetus. Placenta previa and abruptio placentae are accompanied by serious maternal hemorrhage. Aggressive obstetric management may be indicated, but superior anesthetic management will play a major role in the reduction of maternal and fetal morbidity and mortality rates. The primary threat to the mother is that of blood loss, which reduces her effective circulating blood volume and her oxygenation potential. Similarly, the chief hazard to the fetus is diminished uteroplacental perfusion secondary to maternal hypovolemia and hypotension. The perinatal mortality rate associated with placenta previa and abruptio placentae ranges from 15–20% in some studies up to 50–100% in others. The overall morbidity and mortality rates for both the fetus and the mother depend on the gestational age and health of the fetus, the extent of the hemorrhage, and the therapy given.

Good anesthetic management demands early consultation. Reliable intravenous lines should be established early. In addition, recommendations for the treatment and control of shock must be formulated. Prompt cesarean section delivery is often indicated. Ketamine can support blood pressure for induction. A modified nitrous oxide-oxygen relaxant method of general anesthesia will provide improved oxygenation for both the mother and the fetus and will have a minimal effect on the maternal blood pressure. As surgery progresses, it may be necessary to administer large volumes of warm blood, intravenous fluids, or even vasopressors when imperative. Regional block is contraindicated in the presence of hypovolemia.

C. Umbilical Cord Prolapse

Umbilical cord prolapse is an acute obstetric emergency that involves a critical threat to the fetus. Often, because of confusion, irrational behavior by the medical staff may threaten the mother's life. For example, a haphazard rapid induction of anesthesia without attention to many of the essential safety details may be attempted. Naturally, prolapse of the umbilical cord is incompatible with fetal survival unless the fetal presenting part is elevated at once and maintained in that position to avoid compression of the cord. There should then be adequate time for a methodical, safe induction of anesthesia. General anesthesia is induced as soon as the abdomen is prepped and draped. In the rush of the emergency situation, the anesthesiologist must remain meticulous in his or her assessment and management of the mother's airway. A failed intubation and its consequent cardiorespiratory arrest constitute the leading cause of anesthetic maternal mortality.

D. Breech Delivery

Epidural anesthesia may be used for the labor patient with a breech presentation. The need for breech extraction is not increased by the use of epidural anesthesia, and a functioning epidural may avoid the need for general anesthesia should an emergency arise at delivery.

If an epidural block is not in place at the time of delivery, the anesthesiologist must be prepared to proceed with an immediate endotracheal general anesthesia if the aftercoming fetal head becomes trapped. Drugs, monitors, and anesthetic equipment must be prepared in anticipation of such an event.

Because breech delivery is associated with a high perinatal mortality rate, excellent communication and cooperation between the obstetrician and the anesthesiologist is greatly needed to effect an atraumatic delivery.

E. Anesthesia for Emergency Cesarean Section

General anesthesia is the technique most suitable for the urgent cesarean section delivery. It entails placement of an endotracheal tube with an inflated cuff to protect the patient from aspiration of gastric contents into the lung after administration of adequate barbiturate and a muscle relaxant to facilitate endotracheal intubation. Several safety measures must be taken: (1) Give 30 mL of a nonparticulate antacid (sodium citrate) within 15 minutes of induction. (2) Accomplish denitrogenation with 100% oxygen by tight mask fit. (3) Inject thiopental, 2.5 mg/kg intravenously. (4) Apply cricoid pressure. (5) Give succinylcholine, 100–120 mg intravenously. (6) Intubate the trachea and inflate the cuff. (7) Give 6–8 deep breaths of 100% oxygen. (8) Continue to administer nitrous oxide 50% with oxygen 50%, 0.5% halothane or isoflurane, and maintain relaxation with vecuronium or atracurium. (9) Supplement with short-acting narcotics and midazolam after the baby is delivered.

The steps just mentioned should be instituted rapidly and with effective communication between the anesthesiologist and the obstetrician, who should be scrubbed and prepared to make the incision. With this technique, anesthesia can be induced and the fetus delivered within 30 minutes from the time cesarean section is ordered. To avoid vena cava occlusion from the gravid uterus, a wedge should be placed under the patient's right hip or the operating table rotated slightly to the left.

ANESTHESIA FOR NONOBSTETRIC COMPLICATIONS

Anesthesiologists use the following classification system developed by the American Society of Anesthesia. It is used in both emergency and nonemergent situations to record physical status and to ascertain that proper materials are available for the anticipated procedure.

Class 1. No organic, physiologic, biochemical, or psychiatric disturbance.

Class 2. Mild to moderate systemic disturbance that may or may not be related to the reason for surgery. (Examples: Heart disease that only slightly limits physical activity, essential hypertension, anemia, extremes of age, obesity, chronic bronchitis.)

Class 3. Severe systemic disturbance that may or may not be related to the reason for surgery. (Examples: Heart disease that limits activity, poorly controlled hypertension, diabetes mellitus with vascular complications, chronic pulmonary disease that limits activity.)

Class 4. Severe systemic disturbance that is life-threatening with or without surgery. (Examples: Congestive heart failure, crescendo angina pectoris, advanced pulmonary, renal, and hepatic dysfunction.)

Class 5. Moribund patient who has little chance of survival but is submitted to surgery as a last resort (resuscitative effort). (Examples: Uncontrolled hemorrhage as from a ruptured abdominal aneurysm, cerebral trauma, pulmonary embolus.)

Emergency operation (E). Any patient in whom an emergency operation is required. (Example: An otherwise healthy 30-year-old female who requires a dilatation and curettage for moderate but persistent hemorrhage [ASA class 1E].)

Hypertension

Preexisting hypertensive cardiovascular disease in a pregnant woman should be differentiated from preeclampsia-eclampsia. Unlike the latter, the manifestations of hypertensive disease usually are present before the 24th week of pregnancy and persist after delivery. The untreated disease by itself presents a serious challenge to the obstetrician and increases maternal and fetal risk. Chronic hypertension does not specifically contraindicate any of the anesthetic options, but the anesthesiologist must assess and manage abnormalities of volume and vascular resistance to avoid hypotension. Systemic analgesia with sedatives and tranquilizers may be selected for first-stage pain relief, but a hazard still remains.

Heart Disease

Pregnancy superimposed on heart disease presents serious problems in anesthetic management. Patients with functional class I or II rheumatic or congenital heart disease usually fare well throughout pregnancy. Except for patients with fixed cardiac output (moderate to severe aortic stenosis or mitral stenosis), regional analgesia epidural block provides ideal management of first-and second-stage pain relief. This avoids undesirable intrapartum problems such as anxiety, tachycardia, increased cardiac output, and the Valsalva maneuver. The lumbar epidural 4 catheter may be activated for first-stage analgesia with sensory levels of T10 through L2 segments. With the restricted epidural technique, wide variations in blood pressure usually will be avoided and adequate analgesia provided.

Patients with valvular heart disease need to be thoroughly assessed prior to the onset of labor so that the anesthesiologist can determine the risks of regional block, tolerance to volume loading, and sympathectomy and determine the need for invasive monitoring. These patients need thorough physical examination, ECG, echocardiography, and Doppler assessment of valve areas and left ventricular function.

Patients with stenotic lesions may not tolerate fluid loading or sympathetic block. Epidural narcotic anesthesia does not provide complete analgesia for labor but may be an appropriate choice if the patient does not tolerate the autonomic effects of local anesthetics. Patients with regurgitant valve lesions generally do well with this afterload reduction of epidural local anesthesia. Central monitoring of preload is indicated with severe lesions.

Marfan's syndrome and ischemic heart disease require early and aggressive management of labor pain to avoid hypertension and tachycardia. Early lumbar epidural anesthesia with narcotic/local anesthetic mixtures is recommended.

Diabetes Mellitus

Diabetes presents unique problems in anesthetic management because of the hazard to the fetus. The patient with diabetes requires a detailed regimen of antepartum care that extends through the intrapartum and the neonatal period. Moreover, hypotension presents an anesthetic hazard in situations of reduced fetal reserve common to diabetes. The latent phase of labor is best managed with psychologic support, mild sedatives, or tranquilizers. The latter part of the first stage may be managed with small intravenous doses of narcotics or epidural block. If labor continues without signs of fetal distress and analgesia for the second stage is desired, either local or pudendal block or epidural or saddle block is appropriate. If a patient is allowed to undergo the stress of labor but fetal decompensation is evident, operative delivery must be performed at once, with emphasis on the avoidance of hypotension. Careful regional block can be used if time permits. If time does not permit placement of a regional block, emergency general endotracheal anesthesia is indicated. Blood glucose levels should be measured intraoperatively because the unconscious patient cannot report hypoglycemia.

Gastrointestinal Difficulties

Gastrointestinal nonstriated muscle has diminished tone and motility during pregnancy. Some medical gastrointestinal difficulties present special problems in management during the intrapartum period. Peptic ulcer often improves during pregnancy, but in some cases the disease worsens in the last trimester and causes serious problems during labor and the immediate postpartum period. Ulcer perforation and hematemesis are rare in labor. Nonetheless, good management of analgesia during delivery is necessary to decrease anxiety and apprehension.

Ulcerative colitis may become worse during pregnancy. Perinatal and maternal mortality rates are not increased, because symptomatic management usually is adequate. Regional ileitis may also become more severe during pregnancy.

Chronic pancreatitis may be reactivated during pregnancy. Acute pancreatitis occasionally occurs in the third trimester. The significant laboratory values are elevated serum amylase and reduced serum calcium, along with typical symptoms of epigastric pain and nausea and vomiting.

Sympathetic blocking techniques are not contraindicated for anesthetic management of the first and second stages of labor in these gastrointestinal disorders that may coincide with pregnancy. It is clinically desirable to alleviate anxiety and apprehension in the first stage of labor, since tension may exacerbate the disease process. Therefore, a tranquilizer/narcotic combination early in the first stage of labor should be considered and then lumbar epidural block for first- and second-stage management. Subarachnoid block may be used to manage the second stage of labor successfully, with use of a true saddle block obtunding chiefly the sacral fibers.

Psychiatric Disorders

Most patients approaching delivery look upon the experience as one of the happiest times of their lives. However, some patients undergo severe emotional stresses during the third trimester and as delivery nears.

The obstetrician and the anesthesiologist should talk openly with a psychiatric patient about problems of labor and delivery management and offer suggestions for management of discomfort so that she will have minimal emotional stress. The ideal technique is the combined use of lumbar epidural block for the first stage and lumbar or caudal epidural block for the second stage. It is best to carefully point out to the patient the reasons for choosing the technique and to review the technical points of the procedure so that she will not be alarmed when the block is attempted. These techniques are preferred because they afford early and continuous analgesia during labor and delivery.

TREATMENT OF COMPLICATIONS OF ANESTHETICS

Resuscitation of the Mother

Anesthesia is responsible for 10% of maternal mortality. The most common cause of maternal death is failure to intubate the trachea at induction of general anesthesia. Less frequently, maternal death is due to inadvertent intravascular injection of local anesthetic (toxic reaction) or inadvertent intrathecal injection of anesthetic (total spinal).

When faced with maternal cardiovascular collapse, full cardiopulmonary resuscitation (CPR) is indicated:

1. Establish a patent airway.
2. Aspirate mucus, blood, vomitus, etc, with a tracheal suction apparatus. Use a laryngoscope for direct visualization of air passages and intubate the trachea.
3. Administer oxygen by artificial respiration if respirations are absent or weak. If high spinal anesthesia has occurred, continue to ventilate the patient until paralysis of the diaphragm has dissipated.
4. Give vasopressors intravenously (ephedrine, 10–20 mg). Place the patient in the wedged supine position with the feet elevated and give transfusions of plasma, plasma expanders, and blood for traumatic or hemorrhagic shock.
5. Specifically treat cardiac arrhythmias in accordance with advanced cardiac life support (ACLS) recommendations.
6. Provide external cardiac massage in the absence of adequate rhythm and blood pressure.
7. Consider immediate cesarean section delivery to salvage fetus and improve venous return if patient does not immediately respond to efforts.

Full cardiopulmonary arrest can be averted if the prodromal symptoms are recognized and immediately treated. A total spinal block is recognized by excessive and dense sensory and motor block to a test injection of local anesthesia through the epidural catheter. Further injections are avoided, and the patient's blood pressure is supported with fluid, positioning, and vasopressors.

An intravascular injection of local anesthetic is recognized early by symptoms of drowsiness, agitation, tinnitus, perioral tingling, bradycardia, and mild hypotension. The patient should be immediately given 100% oxygen and a small dose of diazepam (5 mg), midazolam (1 mg), or pentothal (50 mg). Further treatment may not be needed. The patient must be watched closely and the epidural catheter removed.

ANESTHESIA FOR CESAREAN SECTION DELIVERY

With few exceptions, all cesarean section deliveries in the U.S. are performed with spinal, epidural, or general anesthesia. When these techniques are done effectively, maternal and neonatal outcome is good. In 1982, more than half the cesarean births in the U.S. were carried out under general anesthesia. By 1998, that rate had dropped to less than 10% of all cesarean births. Spinal anesthesia has become more common than epidural for cesarean delivery in the past few years, primarily as a result of the introduction of newer spinal needles that prevent post–lumbar puncture headaches. Although the majority of anesthesia-related maternal mortality is associated with cesarean birth, this rate has continued to dramatically decline over the last few decades, and is now less than 1.5 anesthesia-related deaths per million live births in the United States.

Regional Analgesia

A. LUMBAR EPIDURAL BLOCK

Lumbar epidural blockade may be utilized for cesarean section analgesia and for providing adequate analgesia for operative delivery. As mentioned, the major hazard of the regional analgesic technique is blockade of sympathetic fibers and a decrease in vascular resistance, along with venous pooling and hypotension. However, this can be greatly alleviated by elevation of the patient's right hip to avoid compression of the vena cava by the gravid uterus when the patient is lying on the operating table. In addition, the anesthesiologist may rotate the operating table 15–20 degrees to the left to rotate the uterus away from the vena cava.

An epidural catheter can be placed immediately prior to surgery, or a catheter used to provide pain relief for labor can be reinjected for the surgery. After the catheter is suitably placed and taped in position, the patient should be rotated slightly out of the supine position to remove the hazard of vena cava occlusion when local anesthetic is injected as a test dose. Lidocaine 2% with epinephrine 1:200,000 may be used, or lidocaine 2% without epinephrine if there is cardiovascular instability. Bupivacaine 0.5–0.75% or mepivacaine 1.5% with or without epinephrine (as described above for lidocaine) may also be used. The total dosage for the therapeutic test is approximately 3 mL, which is an adequate amount to ascertain whether or not inadvertent

subarachnoid injection of the drug has occurred. Incremental injections of 5 mL are then titrated to produce a T4–T6 sensory level. Usually a total volume of 18–20 mL of local anesthetic is required.

The blood pressure is monitored every 5 minutes and the dermatome levels examined every 5 minutes for the first 20 minutes to ascertain the height and density of the analgesic block. It is usually necessary to wait only 15–20 minutes for an adequate analgesic block for incision. During this time, the patient's abdomen is surgically scrubbed and prepared and the patient draped for cesarean section delivery. If a brief episode of hypotension occurs, the patient is given a rapid infusion of lactated Ringer's solution. In addition, the uterus must be shifted away from the vena cava. If these measures are not sufficient to relieve a brief episode of hypotension, one may utilize 5–10 mg of ephedrine intravenously for a mild vasopressor effect.

B. SUBARACHNOID BLOCK

Spinal block is now the most common anesthesia for elective cesarean delivery in the U.S. The advantages are the immediate onset of analgesia, so there is no waiting for the block to become effective, and the absence of drug transmission from the maternal to the fetal compartment, because the anesthetic is deposited in the subarachnoid space in such small quantities. In addition, subarachnoid block may be a simpler technique to perform, since the endpoint is definite—the identification of fluid from the subarachnoid space. The disadvantages are a more profound and rapid onset of hypotension and more frequent nausea and vomiting, due either to unopposed parasympathetic stimulation of the gastrointestinal tract or to hypotension. Subarachnoid block is usually achieved via the paramedian or midline technique, details of which are beyond the scope of this text. The agents most commonly used for subarachnoid analgesia are lidocaine 5% (50–75 mg) and bupivacaine (10–12.5%). As with the lumbar epidural technique, the patient is prehydrated with 500–1000 mL of lactated Ringer's solution.

After the technical aspects of the procedure have been completed, the patient is placed in the supine position with the uterus displaced to the left as just described. If hypotension occurs, the uterus should be pushed farther to the left to improve return of blood from the lower extremities into the circulation and increase right atrial pressure and thus cardiac output, and a bolus of Ringer's lactate is given. If these measures are not successful, the patient should receive ephedrine, 5–10 mg intravenously, to sustain a mild vasopressor effect. During a period of hypotension, the mother should receive oxygen by mask to increase oxygen delivery to the uteroplacental bed. Newer spinal needles are associated with a low incidence (1–2%) of spinal headache (PDPH). As a result, spinal anesthesia is becoming more popular for elective cesarean surgery.

General & Local Anesthesia

General anesthesia is indicated for cesarean section delivery when regional techniques cannot be used because of coagulopathy, infection, hypovolemia, or urgency. Some patients prefer to be "put to sleep" and refuse regional techniques.

Ideally, general anesthesia for cesarean section delivery should cause the mother to be unconscious, feel no pain, and have no unpleasant memories of the procedure; the fetus should not be jeopardized, with minimal depression and intact reflex irritability.

General anesthesia for cesarean section delivery is substantially modified from the typical nonobstetric technique. A rapid sequence technique is used with cricoid pressure to prevent aspiration, with recognition that the risks for the term obstetric patient include (1) full stomach (and aspiration), (2) difficulty with laryngoscopy and intubation, and (3) rapid desaturation if intubation is unsuccessful.

A. PATIENT PREPARATION

Preoperative medication is not usually required when the patient is brought to the cesarean section room. Alert the patient preoperatively that she may have a lucid "window" during the operative procedure when she has pain or hears voices. Explain that this is due to the necessity of maintaining a light analgesic state to protect the fetus from large doses of drugs. She should also be prepared with 30 mL of nonparticulate antacid to offset gastric acidity. The patient is then given 100% oxygen with a close-fitting mask for 3 minutes prior to induction.

B. PROCEDURE

When the surgeon is ready to make the incision, thiopental, 2.5 mg/kg, should be injected intravenously and cricoid pressure exerted by an assistant. Immediately, succinylcholine, 120–140 mg intravenously, should be administered, and intubation and inflation of the cuff performed. Intubation is confirmed by auscultation and monitoring end-tidal CO_2 before the cricoid pressure is released and the incision made. After 6–8 breaths of 100% oxygen, the patient should be given

nitrous oxide 50% with oxygen 50% until delivery of the fetus. Low concentrations of halothane or isoflurane (0.5%) will reduce the incidence of awareness. Intermediate-acting muscle relaxants maintain paralysis. An attempt must be made to keep the induction-to-delivery time under 10 minutes. Five minutes are required for redistribution of barbiturate back across the placenta into the maternal compartment. After delivery of the fetus, the nitrous oxide concentration may be increased to 70% if oxygen saturation is more than 98%, and intravenous narcotics and benzodiazepines injected for supplemental anesthesia.

The patient should be fully awakened and on her side before extubation. Postoperative analgesia can be provided by patient-controlled administration of morphine or meperidine.

With this approach, good neonatal outcomes are anticipated if induction-to-delivery times and uterine invasion-to-delivery times are kept to a minimum.

REFERENCES

Breen TW, MacNeil T, Diernenfield L: Obstetric anesthesia practice in Canada: Occasional Survey. Can J Anesth 2000; 47:1230.

Chestnut DH: *Obstetric Anesthesia: Principles and Practice*, 2nd ed. Mosby, 1999.

Chestnut DH et al: Does early administration of epidural analgesia affect obstetric outcome in nulliparous women who are in spontaneous labor? Anesthesiology 1994;80:1201.

Chestnut DH: Anesthesia and maternal mortality (editorial). Anesthesiology 1997;86:273.

Hawkins JL et al: Obstetric anesthesia work force survey, 1981 versus 1992. Anesthesiology 1997;87:135.

Hood DD, Curry R: Spinal versus epidural anesthesia for cesarean section in severely preeclamptic patients: A retrospective survey. Anesthesiology 1999;90:1276.

MacKay AP, Berg CJ, Atrash HK: Pregnancy-related mortality from preeclampsia and eclampsia. Obstet Gynecol 2001; 97:533.

Orlikowski CE, Rocke DA: The coagulopathic parturient: Anesthetic management. Anesth Clin North Am 1998;16:349.

Palmer CM et al: Postcesarean epidural morphine: A dose-response study. Anesth Analg 2000;90:887.

Practice Guidelines for Obstetrical Anesthesia: A Report by the American Society of Anesthesiologists Task Force on Obstetrical Anesthesia. Anesthesiology 1999;90:600.

Santos AC: The placental transfer and effects of levobupivacaine, bupivacaine and ropivacaine on uterine blood flow (abstract). Reg Anesth Pain Med 1998;23:S45.

Operative Delivery

Steven W. Ainbinder, MD

The term **operative delivery** denotes any obstetric procedure in which active measures are taken to accomplish delivery. When discussing operative deliveries, either the vaginal or abdominal route may be considered. The success of these procedures is based on operator skill, proper timing, and clear indications for active intervention.

In former years the ability to perform a difficult vaginal delivery was an essential part of obstetric practice. In current practice one mark of a skilled obstetrician is the ability to avoid difficult vaginal delivery. However, the obstetrician should have sufficient knowledge and experience to be able to intervene vaginally when indicated and to perform the obstetric operation that is safest for mother and baby. This chapter considers the obstetric operations in modern use that should be within the competence of every obstetrician.

■ FORCEPS OPERATIONS

The obstetric forceps is an instrument designed to assist the delivery of the baby's head. It is used either to expedite delivery or to overcome or correct certain abnormalities in the cephalopelvic relationship that interfere with advancement of the head in labor.

The primary functions of the forceps are traction (either for assistance in the terminal phase of labor or to deal with arrest of the head) and rotation (in cases in which there is no disproportion but the head presents with an unfavorable diameter).

Forceps delivery may be indicated in the interests of mother or baby, and when properly performed it may be life-saving. According to a randomized cohort of ACOG (American College of Obstetricians and Gynecologists) fellows, operative vaginal deliveries make up less than 15% of live births in their respective practices.

THE OBSTETRIC FORCEPS

The obstetric forceps consists of 2 matched parts that articulate, or "lock." Each part is composed of a blade, shank, lock, and handle (Fig 27–1). Each blade is so designed that it possesses 2 curves: the cephalic curve, which permits the instrument to be applied accurately to the sides of the baby's head, and the pelvic curve,

which conforms to the curved axis of the maternal pelvis. The tip of each blade is called the toe.

The front of the forceps is the concave side of the pelvic curve. The blades are referred to as left and right according to the side of the mother's pelvis on which they lie after application. According to the rule of the forceps, the handle of the left blade is held in the left hand and the blade is applied to the left side of the mother's pelvis; the handle of the right blade is then held in the right hand and inserted so as to lie on the right side of the mother's pelvis. When the blades are inserted in this order, the right shank comes to lie atop the left so that the forceps articulate, or lock, as the handles are closed.

Physicians have been making modifications in one or more of the 4 basic parts since forceps were first invented. Although more than 600 kinds of forceps have been described, only a few are currently in use.

Obstetric forceps may be divided into 2 groups: classic forceps and special forceps (Fig 27–2). Classic forceps are those with the usual cephalic and pelvic curves and English lock; the Simpson and Elliot forceps are the prototypes. Special forceps are those designed to solve specific problems; those in modern use are the Piper, Kielland, and Barton forceps.

INDICATIONS & CONDITIONS FOR FORCEPS DELIVERY

In each of the following indications for forceps delivery, it should be emphasized that cesarean section is an alternative procedure that should be considered depending on the prevailing circumstances. Recognizing the inherent risks of both procedures, the obstetrician must decide which operation—vaginal delivery or cesarean section—will be safer for mother and baby. In modern obstetrics there is rarely a place for the difficult forceps delivery that endangers either mother or child. Likewise the obstetrician's training and experience must be a primary consideration in deciding between a forceps delivery and a cesarean section.

Prophylaxis

The principle of prophylactic forceps was first enunciated by DeLee in 1920. Although it instantly provoked

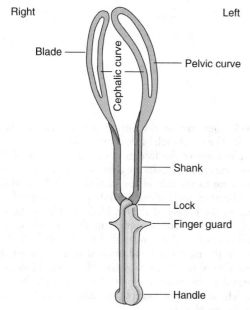

Right   Left

Blade

Cephalic curve

Pelvic curve

Shank

Lock

Finger guard

Handle

Figure 27–1. DeLee modification of Simpson forceps. (Reproduced, with permission, from Benson RC: *Handbook of Obstetrics & Gynecology,* 8th ed. Lange, 1983.)

bitter denunciation as "meddlesome midwifery," it was generally accepted that when the perineum and coccyx offered the only resistance to delivery, the use of episiotomy and outlet forceps was indeed prophylactic because the fetal head was spared unpredictable stress—especially compression against the perineum. The rationale for this acceptance included the belief that the second stage of labor was significantly shortened, greatly minimizing the patient's physical discomfort, and the repair of a cleanly incised wound rather than of a jagged laceration facilitated healing and recovery of the pelvic floor and perineal structures. Episiotomy is still one of the most frequently performed obstetric operations, although it is becoming far less common than in the past and current trends are to use it even less. Today, use of prophylactic forceps has no place in practical routine obstetrics. Any use of a forceps must be predicated on an existing condition for which a forceps is indicated.

Dystocia

During the second stage, when labor fails to progress or a second stage exceeding 2 hours occurs, the use of forceps should be considered. However, good judgment is necessary to decide whether continued labor, forceps delivery, or cesarean section is indicated.

A. UTERINE INERTIA

Uterine inertia may account for both failure to progress and prolongation of the second stage of labor. In such cases, oxytocin should be considered initially if disproportion has been excluded. If the conditions for forceps delivery have not been met, cesarean section may be appropriate. Uterine inertia may also be responsible for failure of the head to rotate to the anterior position. In such cases, artificial rotation is a viable option, but the obstetrician must decide whether cesarean section would be safer. A critical factor is the station of the fetal head when forceps are considered. No rotations should be used at a station above the bispinous level or 0.

B. FAULTY CEPHALOPELVIC RELATIONSHIPS

Despite contractions of good quality, arrest may occur in the following circumstances: (1) if an unfavorable diameter of the head presents to the pelvis (eg, occiput anterior [OA] in a flat pelvis); (2) if the position is such that the head cannot negotiate the pelvic curve (eg, certain cases of occiput posterior [OP]); or (3) if cephalopelvic disproportion exists. In the latter case, molding of the head may overcome minor degrees of disproportion and permit the head to advance without injury. After 1–2 hours of voluntary bearing down in the second stage, the physician should determine whether vaginal delivery by forceps is safe and appropriate or whether true disproportion requiring cesarean section for delivery is present.

Maternal & Fetal Indications for Forceps Delivery

Maternal and fetal indications for forceps delivery include circumstances in which continuation of the second stage of labor would constitute a significant threat to the mother or the baby, as well as those circumstances in which the mother can no longer satisfactorily assist in delivering the infant as with regional anesthesia.

A. MATERNAL INDICATIONS

The second stage can be shortened in cases of exhaustion, severe cardiac or pulmonary problems accompanied by dyspnea, and intercurrent debilitating illness.

B. FETAL INDICATIONS

The primary fetal indication for terminating the second stage prematurely is a nonreassuring fetal heart tracing, as manifested by fetal heart tones (FHTs) with a rate persistently less than 100 or more than 160 beats/min, late deceleration patterns, or gross irregularity.

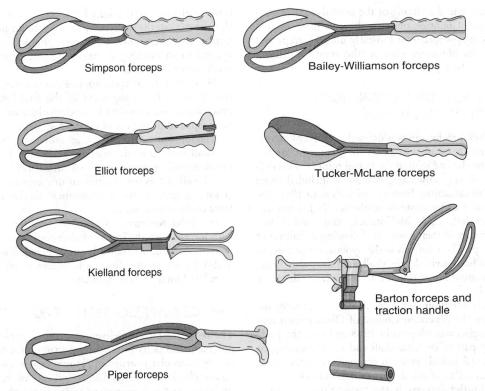

Figure 27–2. Commonly used forceps. (Reproduced, with permission, from Benson RC: *Handbook of Obstetrics & Gynecology*, 8th ed. Lange, 1983.)

Conditions for Forceps Delivery

The use of forceps is permissible *only when all of the following conditions prevail, regardless of the urgent need for delivery.*

(1) **The cervix must be fully dilated.** Extraction of the head through an incompletely dilated cervix invariably produces ragged, bleeding tears that may extend into the broad ligament of the uterus. The uterine support may be damaged also, thus setting the stage for later prolapse.

(2) **The membranes must be ruptured.** Forceps should not be applied before the membranes rupture. If the membranes are intact and forceps are used, they will slip, and traction upon the membranes may detach the edge of the placenta.

(3) **The head must be engaged to a station 0 or below.** Engagement means that the biparietal diameter of the fetal head has passed the plane of the inlet. If the head is not molded, the tip of the vertex at the time of engagement is at 0 station; in extreme molding with a large caput succedaneum, the scalp may be almost at the introitus when the biparietal diameter is still at the level of the inlet. The higher the station of the head, the greater the likelihood of serious damage to mother or baby. One should not apply forceps if the sinciput can be felt above the symphysis.

(4) **The head must present correctly.** All vertex presentations and all face presentations with chin anterior are suitable. Neither brow presentation nor face presentation with chin posterior is suitable for application of forceps. One may apply forceps to the aftercoming head in breech presentation, provided the head is engaged and is in the OA position.

(5) **There must be no significant cephalopelvic disproportion.** In the case of a "tight fit," one may advance the head, provided that only moderate traction is needed. It is potentially severely damaging to use extreme force to drag the head past significant bony resistance.

(6) **The bladder should be empty.** To prevent injury or dystocia, the bladder should be drained by catheterization before forceps are used.

It must be emphasized that merely meeting the foregoing conditions does not justify forceps delivery. A specific indication for the application of forceps must be present, and the timing of the procedure is of vital importance. Countless obstetric disasters have resulted from the inappropriate or too early use of forceps and from the use of forceps when another mode of delivery would have been preferable.

CLASSIFICATION & DEFINITIONS OF FORCEPS DELIVERIES

Until 1949, low forceps was defined as "forceps extraction when the head rests upon the perineum, or lies well below the line joining the ischial spines." This definition was very misleading because it included some formidable extractions from the midpelvis. In 1949, the authors of 4 major obstetric textbooks (N.J. Eastman, J.P. Greenhill, C.O. McCormick, and Paul Titus) agreed to state in their books the following definition of low forceps: "Low forceps is the application of forceps when the head is visible, the skull is on the pelvic floor, and the sagittal suture is in the anteroposterior diameter of the pelvis."

The classification of forceps deliveries currently approved by the American College of Obstetricians and Gynecologists was adopted in 1988 and uses the leading bony part of the fetal skull and its relationship to the maternal ischial spines in centimeters as the point of reference. Part of this definition is as follows:

(1) "**Outlet forceps** is the application of forceps when (a) the scalp is visible at the introitus without separating the labia between contractions, (b) the fetal skull has reached the pelvic floor, (c) the sagittal suture is in the anterior-posterior diameter or in the right or left occiput anterior or posterior position, and (d) the fetal head is at or on the perineum." According to this definition, rotation cannot exceed 45 degrees. There is no difference in perinatal outcome when deliveries involving the use of outlet forceps are compared with similar spontaneous deliveries, and there are no data to support the concept that rotating the head on the pelvic floor 45 degrees or less increases morbidity. Forceps delivery under these conditions may be desirable to shorten the second stage of labor—when indicated.

(2) "**Low forceps** is the application of forceps when the leading point of the skull is at a station +2 cm or more and not on the pelvic floor. Low forceps have 2 subdivisions: (a) rotation 45 degrees or less (eg, left occipitoanterior to occiput anterior, left occipitoposterior to occiput posterior), and (b) rotation more than 45 degrees."

(3) "**Midforceps** is the application of forceps when the head is engaged but the leading point of the skull is above station +2 cm. Under unusual circumstances, such as the sudden onset of severe fetal or maternal compromise or transverse arrest, application of forceps above station +2 may be attempted while simultane-

ously initiating preparations for a cesarean delivery in the event that the forceps maneuver is unsuccessful. Under no circumstances, however, should forceps be applied to an unengaged presenting part or when the cervix is not completely dilated."

(4) **High forceps** is the application of forceps at any time prior to the engagement of the fetal head. This procedure is inappropriate in modern obstetrics and has been replaced by the use of cesarean section.

The foregoing definitions refer only to the station of the head at the time the operation is begun. Two additional definitions apply to special circumstances.

(5) **Failed forceps** denotes an unsuccessful attempt at forceps delivery and abandonment of this effort in favor of cesarean section.

(6) **Trial forceps** is a tentative, cautious traction with forceps with the intent of abandoning attempts at delivery if undue resistance is encountered. Since there is also the intent to deliver with forceps if feasible, the term "trial forceps" is appropriate.

CHOICE & APPLICATION OF FORCEPS

The results of forceps delivery depend far more on the judgment and skill of the operator than on the selection of any particular instrument. However, certain instruments clearly are preferable to others for particular problems, and it is important to know exactly what is to be accomplished and which instrument is safest and most effective for the specific difficulty encountered. Some of the forceps used most frequently are shown in Figure 27–2. It is important for obstetricians in training to become familiar with all the standard instruments and to select the ones that will form the basis of their armamentarium. The obstetrician should generally settle on one instrument for outlet forceps, one instrument for traction in the OA position, one instrument for traction and rotation in the occiput transverse (OT) position, and one instrument for application to the aftercoming head.

(1) **For outlet forceps,** in which no significant traction is needed and there is minimal molding of the fetal head, the Tucker-McLane instrument is preferable. The Tucker-McLane forceps has the advantage of overlapping shanks, which do not spread and extend the perineum as the head is brought through the introitus. The disadvantage is that the blades may not fit the head well, especially if there is extensive molding. If any significant traction is exerted, the fetal cheeks may be marked or cut. Tucker-McLane forceps are most applicable for infants without significant molding (rapid primigravid or multigravid deliveries).

(2) **For traction in the OA** (or in one of the oblique anterior positions or with a fetus with marked molding of the head), the Simpson forceps or one of its modifi-

cations (DeLee-Simpson, DeWeiss, or Elliot) is often used. Moreover, the Simpson and DeLee-Simpson instruments generally cannot be locked or articulated properly except when they are applied accurately—unlike the Tucker-McLane forceps, which usually can be locked regardless of the accuracy of their application.

(3) **For rotation from the OP to the OA,** many obstetricians prefer either the Tucker-McLane or the Luikart forceps. The Kielland forceps is also applicable for rotation from posterior to anterior.

(4) **For transverse arrest,** either the Barton or the Kielland forceps is applicable.

(5) **For application to the aftercoming head,** American obstetricians prefer the Piper forceps. The long-shanked classic forceps is also applicable.

Two methods of application are available:

(1) **Cephalic application** denotes the deliberate and accurate application of the forceps to the sides of the baby's head parallel to a line from the chin to a point between the anterior and posterior fontanelles. The blades should be somewhat closer to the posterior than the anterior. Cephalic application is possible in OA, OT, OP, face presentation with chin anterior, and for the aftercoming head (Fig 27–3).

(2) **Pelvic application** is made by applying the blades and locking the forceps, by force if necessary, without reference to the position of the head. This application is condemned in modern obstetrics because it imposes dangerous (even lethal) stresses that the fetal head can rarely withstand. If a proper cephalic application cannot be made, some other method of management is mandatory.

PREPARATION OF THE PATIENT FOR FORCEPS DELIVERY

The lithotomy position is required, and the patient's buttocks should extend 5 cm beyond the end of the table. The legs should be comfortably placed in stirrups with the hips flexed and abducted. A low position is usually preferable to prevent excessive stretching of the perineum.

If conduction (spinal/epidural) anesthesia is to be used, it must be administered prior to the foregoing steps in delivery. If pudendal block or local infiltration is to be used, it should be administered after the preliminary examination has been made and all is in readiness for delivery. An appropriate and effective anesthetic is essential to the performance of any forceps delivery.

The Preliminary Examination

Before application of the forceps, a careful examination must be made to determine the following:

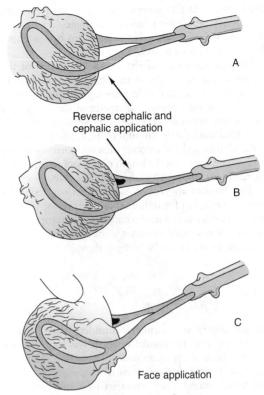

Figure 27–3. Forceps correctly applied along occipitomental diameter of head in various positions of the occiput. **A:** Occiput posterior. **B:** Occiput anterior. **C:** Mentum anterior. (Reproduced, with permission, from Benson RC: *Handbook of Obstetrics & Gynecology,* 8th ed. Lange, 1983.)

(1) **The position of the fetal head,** which is usually easily determined by first locating the lambdoid sutures and then determining the direction of the sagittal suture. The posterior fontanelle is readily evident after the 3 sutures running into it are identified. If the most accessible fontanelle is found to have 4 sutures running into it, it is the anterior fontanelle and the position is usually OP. In the presence of marked edema of the scalp or caput succedaneum, both sutures and fontanelles may be masked, and position can be determined only by feeling an ear and then noting the direction of the pinna. Bedside ultrasound may also prove valuable in this situation.

(2) **The station of the fetal head,** determined by noting the relationship of the presenting bony part to the ischial spines. In labor that proceeds swiftly without complication, such a determination is usually accurate. When the first or, especially, the second stage is pro-

longed and is further complicated by marked molding and a heavy caput, this relation may suggest a false level of the head in the pelvis. If the head can be felt above the symphysis, forceps should not be used.

(3) **The adequacy of the pelvic diameters** of the midpelvis and outlet, determined by noting the following: (a) the prominence of the spines, the degree to which they shorten the transverse diameter of the midpelvis, and the amount of space between the spine and the side of the fetal head; (b) the contour of the accessible portion of the sacrum and the amount of space posterior to the head usually based on the length of the sacrospinous ligament; and (c) the width of the subpubic arch.

This kind of appraisal is not needed or feasible in outlet forceps, but for indicated low forceps or midforceps it is essential to know whether the anteroposterior (AP) or the transverse diameter is the shorter so that the biparietal diameter can be brought through it.

FORCEPS DELIVERY: POSITION OCCIPUT ANTERIOR

An episiotomy was formerly considered an essential part of almost all forceps deliveries. It was usually made after the preliminary examination but before the application of forceps. However, current thought is mixed. The trend among many obstetricians is to perform an episiotomy only as the head is being delivered or not to perform one at all. The individual obstetrician needs to carefully evaluate his or her preference and the current clinical findings before performing "routine episiotomy."

The method of forceps delivery in OA is shown in Figures 27–4 through 27–7. The legends should be given special attention. This technique is applicable to both outlet forceps and low forceps delivery when the head is in the direct OA position or in one of the oblique diameters.

The operator should be seated in front of the patient, and all maneuvers should be made carefully and slowly.

Application of Forceps

The left handle is held between the thumb and fingers of the left hand, and, by means of 2 or 3 fingers of the right hand, the blade is guided to its correct position on the left side of the fetal head. This is repeated with the right hand and the right blade, using the fingers of the left hand to guide the blade. The handles are depressed slightly before locking, in order to place the blades properly along the optimal diameter of the fetal head.

Articulation of Forceps

The forceps are designed such that if the application is accurate they should lock easily as the handles are closed. If the handles are askew or if any force is needed to achieve precise articulation, the application is faulty and the position must be checked again. If simple manipulation of the blades does not permit easy articulation, the forceps should be removed, the position verified (by feeling an ear, if necessary), and the blades reapplied correctly.

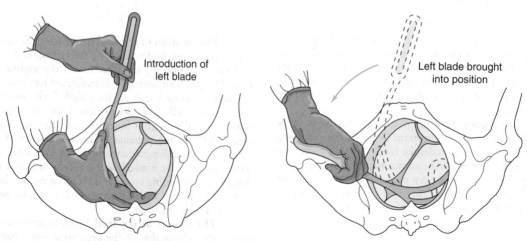

Introduction of left blade

Left blade brought into position

Figure 27–4. Introduction of left blade (left blade, left hand, left side of pelvis). The handle is held with the fingers and thumb, not clenched in the hand. The handle is held vertically. The blade is guided with the fingers of the right hand. Placement of blade is completed by swinging the handle down to the horizontal plane.

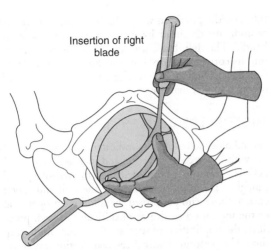

Figure 27–5. Introduction of right blade (right blade, right hand, right side of pelvis). The left blade is already in place. The handle is grasped with the fingers and thumb, not gripped in the whole hand. The handle is held vertically.

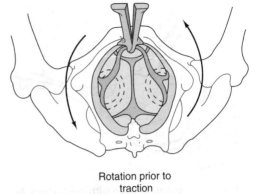

Figure 27–7. Traction on forceps. Some operators prefer to place the fingers of their right hand in the crotch of the instrument to facilitate traction. If heavier traction is needed, no more force should be used than can be exerted by flexed forearms.

Traction

Different obstetricians hold forceps for traction in different ways. One method is to grasp the crossbar of the handle between the index and middle fingers of the left hand from underneath (DeLee-Simpson forceps) and to insert the middle and index finger of the right hand in the crotch of the instrument from above. Another method is to grasp the handles with the fingers on the top of the handles or shanks and the thumbs on the bottom. Traction is made only in the axis of the pelvis along the curve of the birth canal. No more force is applied than can be exerted by the flexed forearms; the muscles of the back must not be used, and the feet must not be braced. If a greater degree of traction is needed, the cause may be either cephalopelvic disproportion or an error in evaluation of the wide and narrow pelvic diameters. The obstetrician should reassess the possibility of successful vaginal delivery.

During normal labor, the head is relieved of pressure between uterine contractions; during a contraction the pressure increases gradually, is sustained at its maximum for 15–30 seconds, and wanes gradually. Similarly, traction on the forceps should also be applied gradually, sustained at its maximum intensity for not more than 30 seconds, and released gradually. When traction ceases, the handles are separated slightly and the head is allowed to recede at will. Traction may be resumed after 15–20 seconds. If time allows, traction is most effectively exerted with contractions.

Delivery of the Head

As the head begins to distend the perineum, both the amount and the direction of traction must be altered. The farther the head advances, the less the resistance offered both by the pelvis and by the soft parts; hence, only minimal traction should be applied as the head is about to be delivered. Unless traction is controlled carefully, the head will "jump" over the coccyx and cause extension of the episiotomy or tearing of the perineum.

The head negotiates the final portion of the pelvic curve by extension, and the physician should simulate this movement by elevating the handles of the forceps

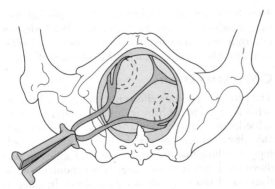

Figure 27–6. Both blades introduced. The 2 handles are brought together and locked. If application is correct, the handles lock precisely, without force.

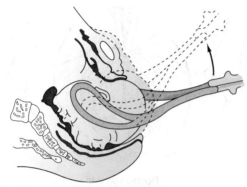

Figure 27–8. Upward traction with low forceps. As the head extends, the handles are raised until they pass the vertical. Little force is needed. One hand suffices; the other hand may support the perineum. (Figures 27–5 through 27–8 are reproduced, with permission, from Benson RC: *Handbook of Obstetrics & Gynecology,* 8th ed. Lange, 1983.)

more and more as the head crowns (Fig 27–8). If the forceps are allowed to remain in place throughout delivery of the head, the handles will have passed the vertical plane as delivery of the head is completed. It is preferable to remove the forceps as the head crowns in the reverse order of their application by first disarticulating the forceps and raising the right handle until the blade is delivered. The left blade is then removed in similar fashion. Early removal of the forceps reduces the size of the spheroid that must pass through the introitus and thus reduces the likelihood of tears or extension of episiotomies.

After removal of the forceps, the head may recede; however, if the forceps have not been removed too soon, the head can be delivered readily by use of the Ritgen maneuver during the next contraction.

The Use of Forceps When Anterior Rotation Is Not Complete

If it is necessary to intervene when the sagittal suture has passed the transverse plane of the pelvis but has not reached the exact anterior position, the physician may obtain a precise cephalic application by "wandering" the appropriate blade of the forceps toward the parietal bone that lies farthest anteriorly and inserting the other blade a little more posteriorly than is done in the direct OA position. For example, if the position is right OA, the left blade is inserted on the left side of the pelvis as if the position were OA; the blade is wandered anteriorly by placing the tips of the right index and middle fingers under the heel of the blade. Using this point as a

fulcrum, the physician wings the blade into the correct position on the head by gentle lever motions of the handle. The right blade usually can be inserted directly into its correct position, but if it skips toward the right lateral aspect of the pelvis it can be wandered posteriorly in a similar manner.

MIDFORCEPS DELIVERY

Several older series of cases indicated increased morbidity, with lowered Apgar scores and increased neurologic deficits, among newborns delivered by midforceps. Although it is not possible to gauge the skill and experience of those who performed the midforceps operations or the indication or degree of difficulty of each procedure, the implication of such studies is that midforceps should be performed only if cesarean section would not offer a better solution to the problem. Trained obstetricians may be able to recognize appropriate midforceps deliveries and perform them safely. In the context of current definitions, forceps delivery from a level higher than station +2 cm is rarely indicated and cesarean section is usually preferable.

Conduct of the Second Stage

The lower the head at the time delivery begins, the less chance of injury to mother and baby. Also, the deeper the head is in the birth canal, the greater the likelihood of spontaneous rotation of the occiput to the anterior. Accordingly, the conduct of the second stage of labor is of special importance.

A. BLADDER

Because a full bladder can impede the second stage of labor, it should be emptied whenever it can be felt abdominally.

B. DEHYDRATION

Most labors are now conducted with an infusion running, which usually prevents dehydration. If dehydration occurs, it can lead to decelerative patterns in the FHTs, maternal exhaustion, and ineffective voluntary effort.

C. VOLUNTARY EFFORTS

The patient's voluntary efforts may not be crucial if the pelvis is large and the baby is small. In contrast, if there is borderline disproportion (a "tight fit"), strong voluntary effort may be essential for safe delivery. Accordingly, anything that impairs the patient's ability to bear down (eg, heavy systemic analgesia or conduction anesthesia used too early) should be avoided. In cases in which voluntary effort is needed, the delivery table should be equipped with handles the patient may pull on while straining, and the knees should be flexed far back on the abdomen so the axis of uterine force is directly into the inlet.

D. UTERINE CONTRACTIONS

Uterine contractions during the second stage normally occur at 2-minute intervals. The contractions are of strong intensity and last 45–50 seconds. A delay in the interval between contractions or in their duration or intensity causes inertia that may be sufficient to delay or even stop progress. The management of second-stage inertia is accomplished by judicious use of oxytocin. An infusion pump designed to administer exact amounts of oxytocin at a preselected rate is essential (a drip should not be used).

E. LENGTH OF THE SECOND STAGE

The length of the second stage is determined by the effectiveness of the contractions and the rate of progress. In the past an active second stage was terminated after 1–2 hours because of the increasing danger of uterine rupture or constriction ring dystocia. However, most of these studies were based on older literature.

With the use of intrapartum monitoring and a fetus that is tolerating labor well, the length of the second stage is no longer a critical indication for operative delivery. If satisfactory but slow progress is occurring, 3 or

more hours may be acceptable. On the other hand, after 2 hours, a thorough evaluation must be made to rule out an unsuspected delaying factor.

F. ANESTHESIA

Anesthesia that is satisfactory for midforceps delivery in most cases is satisfactory for low forceps delivery also.

G. CEPHALOPELVIC RELATIONSHIPS

A knowledge of variations in pelvic architecture and their effect on the mechanism of labor is essential for the proper performance of any midforceps delivery. As a rule, the midpelvis and outlet can be adequately evaluated by digital examination during or before labor. The mechanism of labor that is typical of each of the pure pelvic types is diagrammed in Figure 27–9. Because most pelves are of mixed type, combinations are usually encountered.

Two facts are important in appraising and predicting the mechanism of labor: (1) The biparietal diameter is the shortest diameter of the head; therefore, this diameter should be directed through the narrowest diameter of the pelvis. (2) The occiput tends to rotate to the widest, most ample portion of the pelvis at any given level. Regardless of the position at which arrest occurs, it is essential that the area of greatest narrowing be de-

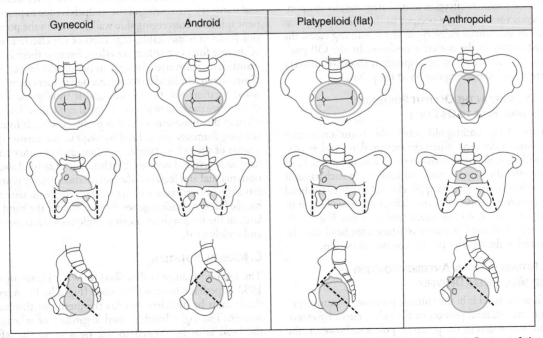

| Gynecoid | Android | Platypelloid (flat) | Anthropoid |

Figure 27–9. Diagrammatic representation of 4 maternal pelvic types (Caldwell-Moloy) and the influence of characteristic pelvic variations on mechanism of labor. (Reproduced, with permission, from Danforth DN, Ellis AH: Midforceps delivery: A vanishing art? Am J Obstet Gynecol 1983;86:29.)

termined, either by palpation or by a trial of traction or both, and that the biparietal diameter of the head be brought through it safely.

Midpelvic Arrest, Position Occiput Anterior

In the presence of uterine contractions of good quality and adequate voluntary effort, arrest in the anterior position most frequently results from the combination of slight transverse narrowing of the midpelvis (caused by either prominent spines or converging side walls) and a slightly forward lower sacrum. Usually, classic forceps are applied to the OA and traction applied as outlined above. If undue resistance is encountered, the head may be elevated slightly, rotated by the forceps to an oblique diameter, and traction repeated. If marked resistance is again encountered, the forceps should be removed and both the position and the pelvic features reevaluated. Cesarean section should be selected in almost all cases of arrest in the anterior or oblique position if heavy resistance is encountered on traction.

Midpelvic Arrest, Position Occiput Posterior

As shown in Figure 27–9, an anthropoid pelvis predisposes to the posterior mechanism of labor. In about 70% of cases, an effective second stage results in spontaneous rotation of the occiput to the anterior position and an uneventful delivery. In the remaining cases, the head arrests in the posterior position. In the OP position, the choice of an appropriate method of delivery depends on the configuration of the pelvis.

A. DELIVERY IN THE OCCIPUT POSTERIOR POSITION, FACE TO OS PUBIS

In the classic anthropoid pelvis, this is the customary method of delivery. When the sacrum flares widely posteriorly and the head is low in the pelvis, the pelvic floor may offer the only resistance to delivery. In such cases, it is entirely appropriate to apply classic forceps to the head in the posterior position and deliver the fetus face to os pubis if there is no significant resistance (see Fig 27–3). On the other hand, if there is resistance, the head must be rotated to the anterior position before extraction.

B. ROTATION TO THE ANTERIOR POSITION AND MIDFORCEPS DELIVERY

When the head is in the anterior position, it must negotiate the terminal portion of the pelvic curve by extension; when it is in the posterior position, however, the chin is already flexed on the thorax as much as possible and cannot advance unless there is virtually no terminal pelvic curve. If the arrest occurs at or above station +2

cm, cephalopelvic disproportion is usually the cause, and delivery should be by cesarean section. However, if the head is well molded, advanced as far as possible by the patient's voluntary effort, and deeply engaged, rotation is almost invariably not only feasible but very easily accomplished. It is emphasized that rotation, either manually or by forceps, is an essential skill required of all obstetricians.

Assisted rotation to the anterior is required in 2 circumstances.

(1) In the patient whose sacrum curves slightly forward, ample space for rotation at the level of arrest exists if the side walls are straight or divergent. If uterine force is sufficient, the occiput should rotate spontaneously away from the forward lower sacrum, and the baby will be delivered in the manner described for the anterior position. The cause of this type of arrest is uterine inertia or inadequate voluntary effort. Rotation in this circumstance is rarely difficult and can usually be facilitated by gently inserting the tips of the fingers of one hand onto the posterior fontanelle against the lambdoid suture that is on the same side as the baby's back. Elevating the head slightly and moving the lambdoid suture toward the side of the baby's back generally will move the head to the anterior position. Delivery may then be accomplished by application of classic forceps as in the anterior position or by voluntary expulsion.

(2) In the presence of a slightly forward lower sacrum and transverse narrowing of the midpelvis (due to prominent spines or converging side walls), arrest in the posterior position is inevitable, regardless of the effectiveness of uterine forces or voluntary effort, because there is an insufficient transverse diameter to permit the longer AP dimension of the head to rotate through it. Generally, assisted rotation will be needed, and it usually must be done above the level of arrest. A "spiral extraction" has no place in the management of this problem, since it forces the long diameter of the head to adapt to the narrow diameter of the pelvis. Irreparable damage to mother and baby may result. There are 2 techniques of assisted rotation: manual and forceps. Manual rotation usually is preferred by obstetricians who have relatively small, narrow hands; forceps rotation generally is selected if the hand is large or the fingers short. Both techniques are acceptable and widely used.

C. MANUAL ROTATION

The rotation maneuver described by W.C. Danforth in 1932 is perhaps most widely used (Fig 27–10). Anesthesia must be sufficient to relax the uterus for this maneuver. The right hand is used regardless of whether the head is to be rotated to the right or to the left. Working on the assumption that the position is right OP, the operator introduces the right hand into the vagina. With the fingers spread widely, the thumb is di-

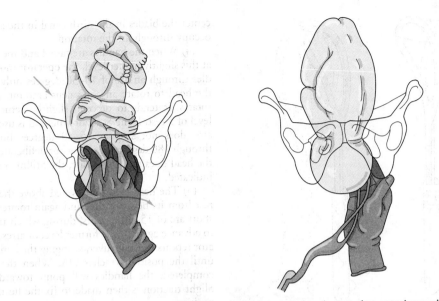

Figure 27–10. Manual rotation. **Left:** Head grasped by whole right hand and rotated to anterior position. Left hand (upper arrow) pushes shoulder toward woman's left, aiding rotation. **Right:** Anterior rotation complete. Right hand maintains head in anterior position while left blade of forceps is applied. (Redrawn and reproduced, with permission, from Danforth WC: The treatment of occiput posterior with special reference to manual rotation. Am J Obstet Gynecol 1932;23:360.)

rected posteriorly in the pelvis and the fingers anteriorly; the head is grasped with the entire hand and turned to the OA position. It is important that the left (external) hand assist in this maneuver by applying pressure on the shoulder through the lower part of the mother's right abdomen. If necessary, the head may be elevated slightly to gain a little more space, but it should not be disengaged. The head is rotated slightly beyond the exact anterior position to allow for the tendency of the presenting part to slip back. The right thumb is now withdrawn from the vagina, leaving the fingers in contact with the side of the infant's face to prevent the head from rotating back to the posterior position. The left blade of the forceps is introduced in the usual manner, using the fingers in the vagina as a guide. The right blade is then introduced, and the delivery proceeds as in the anterior position. If the head lies in the left OP position, the maneuver is reversed, although the right hand is still used. The use of the right hand always makes it possible to introduce the left blade first and obviates the need to readjust the handles for locking, as would be necessary if the right blade were introduced first.

D. FORCEPS ROTATION

Forceps rotation is maligned by many on the grounds that it is likely to produce vaginal tears and severely damage the baby, but if it is performed skillfully, deliberately, and with knowledge of what must be accomplished, it is safe, effective, and extremely simple. In a recent retrospective study done in Texas, no increase in maternal or neonatal morbidity and mortality could be shown with the use of rotational forceps when compared to nonrotational (< 45°) forceps. Many experienced obstetricians prefer it to manual rotation because of its simplicity and safety.

In all operations in which the head is rotated by means of forceps, the operator must clearly understand the movements of the forceps within the birth canal. If any classic forceps with the standard pelvic curve is held horizontally and the instrument rotated while keeping the handles in the same axis, the tips of the blades will describe an arc. Causing the handles to describe a wide arc, however, makes it possible to rotate the forceps so that the tips of the blades remain in the same place (Fig 27–11). The operator who performs a forceps rotation must constantly be aware of the position of each portion of the entire forceps blade and must cause the handles to describe a sufficiently wide arc so that the blades will not deviate from the axis of the pelvis or the space available in the birth canal. Most maternal and fetal injuries result from failure to observe this maxim.

Many techniques of forceps rotation have been described, and several are not recommended either be-

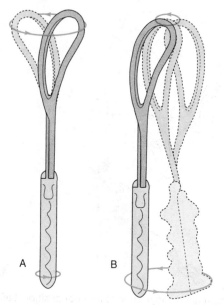

Figure 27–11. Action of forceps in rotation of head in occiput posterior position. **A:** Incorrect technique. If handles are merely turned in the same axis, the tips of the blades swing widely, making rotation impossible and damaging soft parts. **B:** Correct technique. The handles are first elevated and then describe a wide arc; the tips of the blades remain at approximately the same point, and the blades remain in the same axis throughout rotation. (Redrawn and reproduced, with permission, from Douglas RG, Stromme WG: *Operative Obstetrics,* 2nd ed. Appleton-Century-Crofts, 1976.)

cause they are awkward or because the chance of injury to mother and baby seems to be excessive. Included in this category are (1) the spiral extraction using a classic forceps followed by reapplication of the forceps; (2) DeLee's key-and-lock maneuver; and (3) Bill's rotation.

The preferred technique is the Stillman maneuver or the classic Scanzoni maneuver because these 2 procedures are very similar. The steps in the Stillman rotation are as follows (Fig 27–12).

(1) The Tucker-McLane forceps (or equivalent) is placed by an accurate cephalic application with the pelvic curve of the forceps toward the infant's face.

(2) The head is pushed upward gently in the birth canal for a distance of 1–3 cm above the level of arrest, or until an outpouring of amniotic fluid occurs, suggesting that the head has been elevated sufficiently to permit easy rotation.

(3) While the head is held at this slightly higher level, the handles of the forceps are elevated so as to center the blades in the birth canal in the axis they will occupy throughout the rotation.

(4) When the handles are raised and the head is held at this slightly higher level, the operator moves the handles through an arc of 15–30 degrees only; this causes the head to rotate an equivalent amount. As the head rotates, it tends to descend slightly, returning to the level of arrest. If the Scanzoni method is used, the operator does not stop at 15–30 degrees but continues through 180 degrees in a slow but deliberate rotation. If the head does not turn easily, the Stillman maneuver is indicated.

(5) The head is again elevated above the level of arrest from its new position and again rotated through a short arc of 15–30 degrees, during which time it tends to advance again to the former level of arrest. The operator repeats the maneuver, swinging the handles widely, until the position reaches OA. When the rotation is completed, the handles will point toward the floor. Slight traction is then made to fix the head in its new position.

(6) The left blade of the rotating forceps, now lying on the right side of the mother's pelvis, is removed and replaced by the right blade of the DeLee-Simpson forceps. Next, the right blade of the rotating forceps is removed and replaced by the left blade of the DeLee-Simpson (or similar) forceps. (Both blades of the rotating forceps should not be removed at once. If one blade remains in place at all times, the head will be prevented from rotating back to the posterior position.)

(7) Because the right blade of the DeLee-Simpson forceps has been applied first, the handles must be positioned for locking. This done, the extraction is accomplished by intermittent traction as though the position initially had been OA.

The foregoing steps in the rotation should be carried out slowly, deliberately, and with the utmost gentleness. The procedure should require only about 1 minute. The operator's grip on the handles should be sufficiently delicate so that any resistance, however slight, will be perceived immediately. If resistance occurs at any point in the rotation or if the FHTs indicate fetal distress, the head should be returned immediately to its original posterior position and rotation carried out in the opposite direction. During the various steps in the rotation, an assistant may direct the anterior shoulder across the abdomen as described for manual rotation.

Midpelvic Arrest, Position Occiput Transverse

Transverse arrest may result either from failure of the uterine forces of contraction or from borderline cephalopelvic disproportion. It occurs most frequently in the following situations.

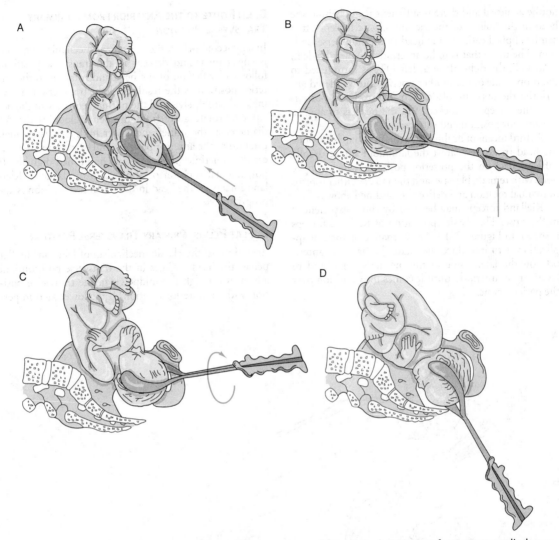

Figure 27–12. Forceps rotation of head in occiput posterior position. **A:** Tucker-McLane forceps are applied accurately to the head. The head is elevated in the axis of the birth canal. **B** and **C:** The handles are elevated and rotated to the right. According to this technique, the head is rotated only through a short arc (during which it advances slightly), elevated again, and so rotated through short arcs until the anterior position is reached. **D:** Rotation complete, handles pointing downward. Forceps are then removed (leaving one blade in place) and replaced by DeLee-Simpson forceps for delivery. (Redrawn and reproduced, with permission, from Danforth DN: A method of forceps rotation in persistent occiput posterior. Am J Obstet Gynecol 1953;65:120.)

A. EN ROUTE TO THE ANTERIOR FROM A PRIMARY OCCIPUT POSTERIOR POSITION

In the presence of an anthropoid inlet, straight or divergent side walls, and a slightly forward lower sacrum or heavy pelvic floor, spontaneous rotation to the anterior position will occur if uterine powers are adequate. If uterine inertia occurs or if the voluntary efforts are insufficient, progress may cease when the head has reached the transverse position but has only partially rotated. In this case, rotation to the anterior position usually can be accomplished digitally by placing 2 fingers against the anterior lambdoid suture and turning the head anteriorly beneath the symphysis. If this cannot be achieved and there is sufficient room behind the head in the hollow of the sacrum, classic forceps often can be applied easily to the head in the transverse position. The blade that is to lie anteriorly (the left blade in right OT, the right blade in left OT) is introduced to the proper side of the mother's pelvis and wandered anteriorly; the opposite blade then is introduced posteriorly, the forceps are locked, and the head is rotated to the anterior position and extracted.

A third means of dealing with this problem is to rotate the head (pressure against the lambdoid suture usually suffices) back to the posterior position, which can be done with remarkable ease, and then to use either forceps or manual rotation and delivery as outlined above.

Kielland forceps may be used by those experienced in their use. The classic application of Kielland forceps is shown in Figure 27–13. An alternative method of application is to introduce the blade that is to lie anteriorly on the lateral side of the mother's pelvis and to "wander" it anteriorly until it comes into position over the parietal bone.

B. En Route to the Anterior from a Primary Transverse Position

In a gynecoid pelvis, the customary mechanism of labor is engagement and descent in the transverse position, followed by flexion of the head and rotation to the anterior position as the result of slight transverse narrowing of the midpelvis and the normal tendency of the occiput to rotate away from the pelvic floor. If the AP diameter at the outlet and lower midpelvis is normal, rotation to the anterior position and extraction are indicated. Sometimes this can be accomplished digitally. If not, manual rotation or application of classic or Kielland forceps to the head in the transverse position is appropriate.

C. Flat Pelvis, Primary Transverse Position

According to the classic mechanism of labor in the flat pelvis, the head engages in the transverse position and advances through the midpelvis in the transverse position without anterior rotation. If the lower sacrum per-

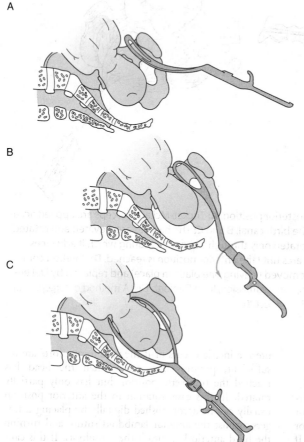

A

B

C

Figure 27–13. Classic application of Kielland forceps. **A:** Introduction of first blade (in this case, left blade, since position is right OT). **B:** Concavity of blade looks upward, and the tip of the blade is rotated toward the patient's right (as shown by arrow) through an arc of 180 degrees until the blade lies in contact with the head. **C:** Instrument applied, right blade having been introduced posteriorly. Note that the buttons point toward the occiput. (Redrawn and reproduced, with permission, from Danforth WC: In: Curtis AH [editor]: *Obstetrics and Gynecology.* Saunders, 1933.)

mits, anterior rotation may occur on the pelvic floor; if the lower sacrum is also forward, the head actually may be born in the transverse position. In this instance, the pelvic curve will be negotiated by lateral flexion of the head.

In the management of transverse arrest of this type, rotation to the anterior and extraction from the anterior position are specifically contraindicated because they would bring the long AP diameter of the head through the shortened AP diameter of the pelvis. The head must be advanced in the transverse position and allowed to rotate to the anterior position only when it has reached a level at which the anteroposterior diameters are favorable. The Barton forceps is preferred for cases of transverse arrest in which the head must be advanced in the transverse position. The Kielland forceps may also be used in this situation, although the application of traction is more difficult and less precise. Application of the Kielland and the Barton forceps is shown in Figures 27–13 and 27–14, respectively. The technique of rotation and delivery with the Barton forceps is shown in Figure 27–15.

Like the Kielland forceps, the Barton forceps should be used only by operators who have experience in its use and are able to predict with confidence that delivery can be safely and easily accomplished by this means. Also, as with Kielland forceps, the position of Barton forceps in the obstetrician's armamentarium is daily becoming more tenuous: If the choice is offered, most problems for which these forceps are really needed are preferably dealt with by cesarean section. With the Barton forceps, traction is made with the head in the transverse position and is continued until the occiput is felt to rotate to the anterior. When the anterior rotation is achieved, the head has passed the area of major obstruction and little force is needed; the traction bar is removed and, with the handles pointing toward one maternal thigh or the other, the delivery is accomplished by continued slight traction.

Forceps Delivery in Face Presentation

If the chin is anterior, the same indications, conditions, and stipulations apply for forceps delivery as in the OA position. The classic forceps are applied to the occipitomental diameter of the head (see Fig 27–3); elevating the handles as the head advances causes the chin to come under the symphysis, and the occiput emerges posteriorly.

If the chin is posterior, rotation of the chin to the anterior position sometimes occurs spontaneously as labor progresses. If not, it is virtually impossible to accomplish artificial rotation safely. Extraction with the chin in the posterior position will almost surely damage the infant regardless of how small it is or how large the

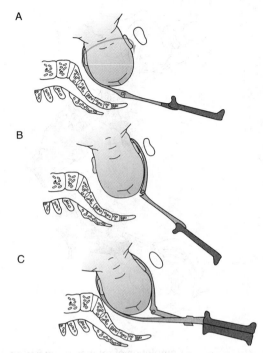

Figure 27–14. Application of Barton forceps for advancement of the head in the transverse position. **A:** Introduction of anterior hinged blade posteriorly, behind the head. **B:** Anterior blade has been wandered to position over anterior parietal bone. **C:** Posterior blade introduced, forceps locked. The traction bar, as shown in Figure 27–2, is now affixed to facilitate traction in the proper pelvic diameter. (Redrawn and reproduced, with permission, from Barton LJ, Caldwell WE, Studdiford WE: A new obstetric forceps. Am J Obstet Gynecol 1928;15:16.)

pelvis is. Forceps delivery is contraindicated, and cesarean section is required.

Forceps Delivery in Brow Presentation

An average-sized fetal head cannot enter even a large pelvic inlet when the brow presents. Some brow presentations convert to an occiput presentation spontaneously during the first stage of labor or can be converted to either occiput or face presentation, in which case labor should be managed accordingly. If a brow presentation fails to convert to a favorable position (chin anterior or occipital presentation) or cannot be converted readily, the infant must be delivered by cesarean section.

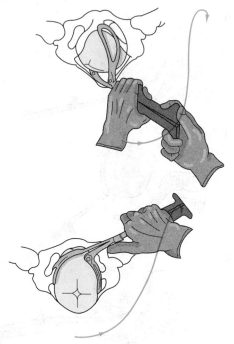

Figure 27–15. Completion of rotation using Barton forceps for advancement of the head in the transverse position. (Redrawn and reproduced, with permission, from Bachman C: The Barton obstetric forceps: A review of its use in 55 cases. Surg Gynecol Obstet 1927;45:805.)

DANGERS & COMPLICATIONS OF FORCEPS DELIVERIES

A number of injuries to both mother and baby can result from the use of forceps, many of them serious and some fatal. With regard to the mother, injuries range from simple extension of the episiotomy to rupture of the uterus or bladder. The baby may sustain transient facial paralysis or irreparable intracranial damage, among other injuries. Almost all of the serious injuries and many of the minor ones inflicted by obstetric forceps result from errors in judgment rather than from lack of technical skill. Such errors include failure to recognize the essential conditions for forceps delivery and lack of an appropriate indication for the operation, as outlined above; intervention too early, before maximal molding and descent have been achieved by the patient's voluntary efforts; relentless traction in the presence of unrecognized cephalopelvic disproportion; errors in diagnosis of the position of the head, with consequent application of forceps to the wrong diameter; and an incomplete knowledge of the architecture of the particular pelvis in question, with an attempt to ad-

vance the head in the wrong diameter. Surprisingly, case-controlled studies have failed to find a higher incidence of urogenital prolapse with operative vaginal deliveries. However, the increase in number of episiotomies has increased long-term maternal morbidity.

Fortunately, most physicians who care for obstetric patients quickly develop respect for the operation of forceps delivery and an intuitive knowledge of when and how a patient can be delivered most safely. It is also essential for physicians to be able to admit an error in judgment and resort to cesarean section when confronted with a forceps delivery of unusual difficulty. Today, the trend is away from forceps delivery. As more and more cesarean sections are performed in order to avoid forceps delivery, fewer obstetricians will gain the skills that are essential to the performance of forceps delivery.

■ THE VACUUM EXTRACTOR

The vacuum extractor, introduced by Malmström in 1954, is designed to assist delivery by applying traction to a suction cup attached to the fetal scalp. The instrument has been widely used with good reported results. The data from reports in which the instrument is used extensively attest to its safety, provided it is used correctly. The instrument lacks the precision of forceps and disregards the finer details of pelvic architecture as well as the mechanism of labor—all essential and traditional parts of skillful forceps delivery.

The vacuum extractor as designed by Malmström has the following components: a specially designed suction cup, a hose connecting the suction cup to a suction pump with intervening trap bottle and manometer, and a chain inside the hose that connects the suction cup to a crossbar for traction (Fig 27–16). The design of the cup, smaller at the rim than above the rim, permits the scalp to be anchored in the peripheral reaches of the cup. A consequence of this construction is a caput succedaneum called a chignon. This usually disappears after a few days. Three sizes (40 mm, 50 mm, and 60 mm) are available. Two important modifications of the device have simplified its use. Bird's modification of the suction cup permits far more efficient traction and also eliminates the need to thread the chain through the hose (Fig 27–17). Use of a soft Silastic cup in preference to a metal cup reportedly simplifies the procedure. The soft cup is easier to manipulate, and a suitable vacuum is attained more quickly. Hand-held vacuum pumps, as well as mechanical pumps with built-in regulators, have added to the safety of the procedure.

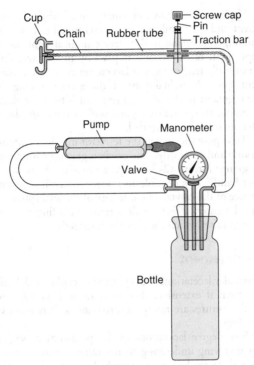

Figure 27–16. Modified Malmström vacuum extractor. (Reproduced, with permission, from Benson RC: *Handbook of Obstetrics & Gynecology,* 8th ed. Lange, 1983.)

The procedure begins with selection of the largest cup that can be easily introduced. The center of the cup should be over the sagittal suture and about 3 cm in front of the posterior fontanelle. Negative pressure is induced until a negative pressure of 0.6 kg/cm² is attained.

Once the cup has been applied, traction is made intermittently, coincident with uterine contractions and supplemented by the mother's bearing-down efforts as needed. The direction of traction is determined with due attention to the pelvic curve of Carus, depending on the station of the head at the time; it should be perpendicular to the cup to prevent the cup from slipping off the scalp. Traction should be sustained and uniform throughout the uterine contraction and should be discontinued between contractions. There is disagreement about the acceptable number of pulls before the procedure is halted. In general, if descent occurs with each episode of traction, 3 to 5 pulls should be sufficient to accomplish delivery. If no descent occurs or the cup slips off after 2 to 3 pulls, cesarean section is the preferable recourse, since failure of vacuum extraction implies cephalopelvic disproportion. The cup should not be allowed to remain in place for more than 30 minutes, because of the possibility of damage to the scalp.

Anesthesia requirements are usually less than for forceps delivery. Pudendal block usually suffices, and in many cases no anesthesia may be needed or local infiltration of the perineum may be sufficient.

Several studies have compared neonatal results by type of delivery—spontaneous vacuum extraction, forceps, or cesarean section. In one study neither perinatal mortality nor serious traumatic complications were attributable to vacuum extraction if the instrument was used judiciously. Apgar scores were similar in each of

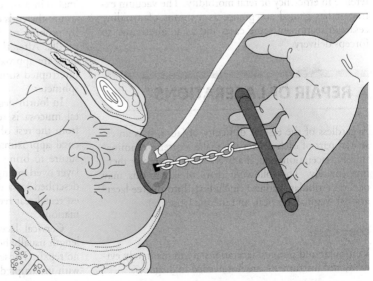

Figure 27–17. Bird's modification of Malmström's vacuum extractor.

the groups. Except for the incidence of chignon, skin bruises and lacerations were less frequent in the group delivered by vacuum extraction than in the group delivered by forceps. Cephalhematoma can be expected in a high percentage of babies delivered by vacuum extraction, but unlike the customary cephalohematomas, they tend to vanish in 2–5 days.

Complications from vacuum extraction include scalp laceration, cephalohematoma, subgaleal hemorrhage, intracranial hemorrhage, neonatal jaundice, retinal hemorrhage, and vaginal lacerations. Complications due to vacuum extraction are usually attributed to improper use, ie, failure to recognize the circumstances in which it is contraindicated, overlong or incorrectly applied traction, use of excessive negative pressure, prolonged application of the suction cup to the scalp, and failure to prevent cervical or vaginal tissue from entering the cup.

Use of the vacuum extractor is obviously contraindicated in the presence of cephalopelvic disproportion; in breech, brow, or face presentation; or if the head of a fetus is not engaged in the pelvis. It should not be used if the membranes are intact. The propriety of its use in preterm delivery is unsettled.

Vacuum extraction technique has been used successfully for delivery of a second twin in preference to version and extraction or cesarean section. Those who are experienced in its use find it to be suitable in occiput posterior presentations. If the interspinous diameter is wide, spontaneous rotation to the anterior usually occurs as the head is advanced. Attempts to rotate the head by turning the instrument may result in a "cookie cutter" type scalp laceration and are not recommended.

One randomized prospective controlled trial compared forceps to the M-cup vacuum and found no difference in efficiency or fetal morbidity. The vacuum extractor has gained acceptance as a means of avoiding cesarean section in some cases and as an alternative to forceps delivery.

■ REPAIR OF LACERATIONS

Regardless of the ease or difficulty of labor, it is an essential part of each delivery to make a careful examination for lacerations and, if any are found, to repair them immediately. The following types of lacerations may occur: vestibular, perineal (including third-degree lacerations), vaginal, cervical, and uterine (rupture).

Diagnosis

Vestibular and perineal lacerations are immediately evident, and instruments are not needed in diagnosis.

Vaginal lacerations can usually be felt digitally, but extent and accessibility can be determined only by examining the vagina under strong surgical light, using appropriate retractors held in place by an assistant. This is especially true of vaginal lacerations over very prominent, spike-like ischial spines. If the laceration is high in the vagina or in the cervix, a retractor is held anteriorly to expose the posterior vaginal wall. A retractor placed laterally may also be needed.

To expose the cervix, the retractor may be used posteriorly and anteriorly. The cervix is grasped with 2 ring or sponge forceps (2–3 cm apart); moving them "hand over hand," it is possible to inspect the entire circumference of the cervix. The integrity of the anal sphincter and the anterior rectal wall is tested by a finger in the rectum (after which the glove is discarded).

Management

Vestibular lacerations usually occur in explosive deliveries. Even if extensive, they tend to heal quickly and neatly. Sutures are rarely required unless there is active bleeding.

First-degree lacerations of the perineum or vagina not involving underlying tissues rarely require sutures. Second-degree lacerations should be repaired. The tissues tend to be frayed and in some cases macerated, making identification more difficult than in episiotomy repair; however, the principles and technique are similar (Fig 27–18). Chromic catgut or polyglycolic sutures should be used.

In third-degree laceration of the perineum (involving the anal sphincter), it is usually difficult to identify the severed ends of the sphincter. However, their position is often marked by a dimple that appears on the anal skin a little anterior to the anal orifice. One may secure the ends of the sphincter with an Allis forceps or by probing to the level of the dimple with the suture needle. After this tissue is secured on both sides, the ends are approximated with a figure-of-eight suture or interrupted suturing of the fibrous sheath encasing the sphincter.

In fourth-degree laceration of the perineum, the rectal mucosa is torn. This must be repaired separately from the rest of the tissue. The usual fashion is a mucosal approximating stitch of chromic or polyglycolic suture to bring the edges together and then a second layer overlapping the first. The repair then continues as described for a third-degree laceration. Even the slightest rectal tear requires careful repair to avoid fistula formation.

Cervical lacerations less than ½ inch (1.5 cm) in length usually heal without leaving a defect and require no repair. Those longer than 1.5 cm should be repaired with interrupted chromic or polyglycolic catgut sutures

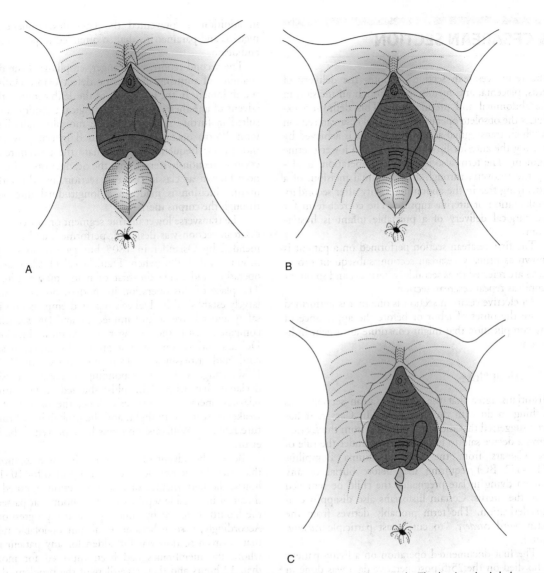

Figure 27–18. After delivery, it is important that the episiotomy be repaired properly. The basic principle is reapproximation of the tissue. **A:** This is accomplished by starting surgical repair 1 cm above the apex of the incision, thereby suturing and ligating any retracted arterial vessels. The suture is then continued in a running fashion to the area of the hymenal ring, reapproximating the mucosa and submucosal tissue. **B:** Once the repair has reached the area of the hymenal ring, the underlying tissue should be reapproximated with either interrupted or running sutures. **C:** After adequate closure of the mucosal, submucosal, and underlying perineal tissue, the perineal skin is reapproximated. This is done by use of subcuticular stitches, although interrupted stitches are occasionally used.

about ¼ in (.5 cm) apart, so placed as to include about 1 cm of tissue lateral to the edge of the tear. The first suture is placed at the exact apex. If this cannot be seen, a suture is placed at the highest accessible point and used for traction to expose the higher reaches of the tear. The same technique is used for high vaginal lacerations.

Uterine rupture must be treated by laparotomy. In some cases, the tear is such that the edges can be accurately apposed in the same way one would repair a cesarean section incision, leaving the uterus fit for future childbearing. If the integrity of the uterus cannot be assured, hysterectomy is appropriate.

■ CESAREAN SECTION

The term "cesarean section" denotes the delivery of fetus, placenta, and membranes through an incision in the abdominal and uterine walls. This definition excludes the obsolete operation of vaginal cesarean section in which transvaginal access to the fetus is achieved by incising the anterior lip of the cervix and lower uterine segment. The term also excludes the operation involving the recovery, through an abdominal incision, of a fetus lying free in the abdominal cavity after secondary implantation or uterine rupture. The correct term for the surgical delivery of a previable infant is hysterotomy.

The first cesarean section performed on a patient is known as primary cesarean section; subsequent procedures are referred to as secondary, tertiary, and so on, or simply as repeat cesarean section.

An elective cesarean section is one that is performed before the onset of labor or before the appearance of any complication that might constitute an urgent indication.

Historical Note

Historians agree that the term "cesarean section" has nothing to do with the birth of Julius Caesar. It has been suggested that the term is derived from the *lex caesarea*, a decree said to have continued under the rule of the Caesars from the time of Numa Pompilius (715–672 BC) requiring that before burial of any women dying in late pregnancy the child be removed from the uterus. Certain historians also disapprove of this derivation. The term probably derives from the Latin word *caedere*, "to cut" (past participle *caesum*, "cut").

The first documented operation on a living patient (who died on the 25th postoperative day) was done in 1610. The first successful cesarean section in the U.S. was done in a cabin near Staunton, Virginia, in 1794; both mother and baby survived.

In early cesarean section, no sutures were placed in the uterus, and sepsis was likely in those who survived the initial hemorrhage from the open uterine sinuses. Two reports, in 1876 and 1882, did much to lower the mortality rate, which theretofore had varied from 50–85%. The first, by Porro, concerned a patient in whom the corpus uteri was excised because of uncontrollable hemorrhage from the uterine wound. He sutured the cervix into the lower angle of the incision for drainage. Although the operation was extremely formidable, it provided a means of controlling hemorrhage;

in addition, it prevented the later development of metritis and parametritis that so often led to peritonitis and death.

The second report, by Scanger, emphasized the desirability of suturing the uterine defect before closing the abdomen. In the latter part of the 19th century, the advent of anesthesia and aseptic surgical techniques resulted in further reduction of the mortality rate. The term "Porro operation" is still used inaccurately (although less frequently) to designate the procedure of cesarean section-hysterectomy; the Scanger operation is now known as classic cesarean section, in which the uterine incision is made in a longitudinal direction through the corpus uteri.

The transverse lower uterine segment or low cervical cesarean section was designed, performed, and recommended by Osiander in 1805 but gained no recognition until 1906, when Frank recalled Osiander's operation and made the first of many modifications. The place of this operation in modern obstetrics was largely established by DeLee's repeated emphasis on its safety and relative lack of immediate and late sequelae compared with the Scanger or classical incision. DeLee's enthusiasm was not greeted by universal accord, and criticism arose from high places. In 1919, J. Whitridge Williams, responding to DeLee's thesis, declared that when "the old-fashioned, conservative (classic) operation is properly done, the danger of a weakened scar is very slight, and the probability of rupture remote." Williams' opinions have proved to be in error.

Before the advent of antibiotics, it was recognized that after the membranes had been ruptured for 10–12 hours, the performance of cesarean section imposed a threat of intractable sepsis; with each hour that passed, the hazard increased by almost geometric progression. Accordingly, it soon became an all but inviolable rule that cesarean section was forbidden for any patient in whom the membranes had been ruptured for more than 12 hours and that, regardless of the problem, delivery was to be accomplished vaginally. This policy saved the lives of many women, but in cases of cephalopelvic disproportion it also imposed a need for craniotomy, sometimes on the living baby, or a technique called **extraperitoneal cesarean section.** This was accomplished by entering the uterus without entering the abdominal cavity. A difficult task, it is rarely used in modern obstetrics.

Today, refinements in surgical technique, asepsis, antibiotic therapy, blood transfusion, and anesthesia have reduced but not eliminated the risks associated with cesarean section. The attainment of good results requires appropriate surgical and perinatal conditions and full knowledge of the possible consequences of deviating from the principles on which this major operation is based.

General Considerations

In the past 20 years, the rate of cesarean section has steadily increased from about 5% to more than 20%. The reasons for this are (1) increasing avoidance of midforceps and vaginal breech deliveries, (2) detection of nonreassuring fetal heart tracings with use of fetal monitoring during labor, and (3) the belief that once a woman has had one cesarean delivery, all subsequent pregnancies must be delivered by cesarean section. In order for the percentage of cesarean deliveries to be reduced, it must be recognized that many women who have had a cesarean delivery can be delivered vaginally in subsequent pregnancies, especially when the indication for the initial procedure is no longer present.

Cesarean section is not to be taken lightly, and unless the indications are unmistakable one should pause to consider its risks versus its benefits. The maternal mortality rate associated with cesarean section varies in different series from 4 per 10,000 to 8 per 10,000. In one series, the risk of death from cesarean section was found to be 26 times greater than with vaginal delivery. As to the fetal effects, it is clear that cesarean section is far preferable to a difficult vaginal delivery, but there is no conclusive proof that liberal use of cesarean section has done anything to improve the mental performance or reduce the incidence of neurologic deficits of children or adults in our population.

Indications

Cesarean section is used in cases in which vaginal delivery either is not feasible or would impose undue risks on mother or baby. Some of the indications are clear and absolute (eg, central placenta previa, obvious cephalopelvic disproportion); others are relative. In some cases, fine judgment is needed to determine whether cesarean section or vaginal delivery would be better. It is not possible to prepare a complete list of indications, for there is hardly an obstetric complication that has not been dealt with by cesarean section. The following indications are the most common.

A. CEPHALOPELVIC DISPROPORTION

Cases in which the head is too large to come through the pelvis should be managed by cesarean section. The term **contracted pelvis** is sometimes listed as an indication; this is not a precise designation, because a small baby can sometimes negotiate a small pelvis, just as a large pelvis may be inadequate for a very large baby.

Extreme cases of cephalopelvic disproportion can sometimes be identified before the onset of labor, whereas in others a test or trial of labor is required. A **test of labor** is defined as 2 hours of good voluntary effort in the second stage of labor with ruptured membranes. If the baby cannot be safely delivered vaginally by this time, cesarean section is elected. In a **trial of labor,** this conclusion is reached either prior to full dilatation of the cervix or before 2 hours of the second stage have elapsed.

Test of labor is now a rarity. If the head fails to descend at an appropriate rate, cesarean section is usually the proper course.

Inlet disproportion can often be diagnosed with reasonable accuracy by careful pelvic examination supplemented by x-ray pelvimetry. However, unless the findings are absolute, it is best to await the onset of labor before making the diagnosis. In the primigravida, inlet disproportion should be suspected if the patient begins labor with the fetal head unengaged; in a significant number of such patients, the head fails to engage and cesarean section is indicated.

Midpelvic disproportion may be suspected if the AP diameter is short, the ischial spines are very prominent, the sacrospinal ligament is less than 5 cm, and the baby is large. Cesarean section should be selected, usually after a trial of labor, if the head can still be felt above the symphysis or if the vertex fails to advance beyond station +2 cm. A trial of forceps may or may not be necessary to make this decision.

Outlet disproportion usually requires a trial of forceps before one can decide definitely that safe vaginal delivery is not possible. In general, x-ray pelvimetry and digital examination are unsatisfactory for assessment of the outlet.

B. UTERINE INERTIA

Uterine inertia (either primary or secondary to abnormal fetal position) is a common indication for cesarean section. A labor curve can be extremely helpful in evaluating the course of labor and in bringing instant attention to the appearance of uterine inertia. If the cervix fails to dilate at a rate of 1 cm/h, one should recognize the possibility of dysfunctional labor. As noted elsewhere in this book (see Chapter 25), many of these cases are resolved by oxytocin infusion, but if not, cesarean section is appropriate.

Failure to progress is a diagnosis that has become more common in the last 10 years. It is a nebulous term that can include inertia or cephalopelvic disproportion. The patient's labor progress becomes stalled during the course of labor and before full dilation. When this has remained unchanged for 2–3 hours, the patient needs a careful reevaluation, including the labor pattern, contractions, and evaluation of the pelvis. The diagnosis invariably results in cesarean section; therefore, all possible factors must be considered before the diagnosis is made.

C. PLACENTA PREVIA

If expectant treatment is not suitable because the pregnancy has proceeded beyond 36 weeks (with a mature fetal lung profile) or because bleeding from the uterus is severe, cesarean section should be performed for placenta previa.

D. PREMATURE SEPARATION OF THE PLACENTA

Cesarean section should be selected (1) if a nonreassuring fetal heart tracing occurs; (2) if effective labor is not achieved; or (3) if the baby or mother show signs of compromise.

E. MALPOSITION AND MALPRESENTATION

Posterior chin position and transverse lie in labor are in themselves indications for cesarean section; attempts to convert these positions to favorable ones are almost invariably futile and may be damaging. Brow presentation during labor warrants cesarean section unless a cautious attempt at conversion to an occipital or anterior chin position is successful. Shoulder presentation and compound presentation are variants of transverse lie and, with few exceptions, are best managed by cesarean section. Planned and appropriately selected vaginal breech deliveries are thought to be equal to cesarean section in maternal and fetal morbidity.

F. PREECLAMPSIA-ECLAMPSIA

Medical management is of course an integral part of the treatment of preeclampsia-eclampsia, but the definitive treatment is delivery. Induction of labor should be initiated in most cases; however, if this is not feasible, the solution is cesarean section.

G. FETAL DISTRESS

Fetal monitoring both before labor (nonstressed and stressed techniques) and during labor may disclose fetal problems that would not otherwise be evident. Consequently, the number of cesarean sections performed for the indication of fetal distress or fetal jeopardy has increased. Cesarean section should only be performed immediately in those with persistent abnormal and ominous patterns.

H. CORD PROLAPSE

This complication must be treated by the most expeditious method. If conditions are such that immediate vaginal delivery would be hazardous to the mother or the baby, the patient should be placed in the Trendelenburg position, with the cord protected by the index and middle fingers inside the cervix between the head and the uterine wall, and cesarean section should be performed without changing this position or altering the digital protection of the cord.

I. DIABETES, ERYTHROBLASTOSIS, AND OTHER THREATENING CONDITIONS

In such conditions as diabetes, Rh incompatibility, or postterm pregnancy, fetal welfare is usually monitored by nonstress or stress testing (contraction stress test, oxytocin challenge test). If the well-being of the fetus seems compromised, it should be decided, first, when to deliver, and, second, how to deliver the fetus. For the most part, a nonreactive nonstress test followed by a positive oxytocin challenge test (late deceleration of FHTs) is an indication for delivery. If the delay involved in induction of labor cannot be justified or if conditions are unfavorable, immediate cesarean section should be chosen. It is usually fruitless to attempt to induce labor without rupturing the membranes simply to avoid a total commitment. The induction is either appropriate or it is not. If it is appropriate, one should proceed by the most effective means; if it is not, no attempt should be made.

J. CARCINOMA OF THE CERVIX

Cesarean section followed by definitive treatment is indicated when invasive carcinoma of the cervix is diagnosed after 28 weeks of gestation.

K. CERVICAL DYSTOCIA

In former years, failure of the cervix to dilate properly was considered to be invariably due to incoordinate uterine action. In fact, most cases do result from uterine inertia, but some are the result of cervical scarring following deep cauterization or conization; some occur following failure of the connective tissue mechanisms normally responsible for effacement of the cervix. Cesarean section may be appropriate for the patient whose cervix remains rigid and fails to dilate more than 3–4 cm despite strong, frequent, first-stage uterine contractions.

L. PREVIOUS UTERINE INCISION

A previous uterine incision such as a myomectomy or a prior cesarean section may weaken the uterine wall or predispose to rupture if labor is permitted. The outmoded but entrenched maxim "Once a cesarean, always a cesarean" still has a few supporters. There is now ample evidence, however, that many uterine scars are indeed firm and that many patients who have had a prior uncomplicated cesarean section can be delivered easily and with less hazard vaginally than by repeat cesarean section. In general, postcesarean section patients who are suitable candidates for vaginal delivery are (1) those whose operation was of the low transverse (not classic) type; (2) those who begin labor at or before the estimated date of confinement; and (3) those with nonrecurring conditions. In such cases it is entirely appropriate to rupture the membranes and await progress. One should be prepared for immediate cesarean section if there is an abnormality of labor or if vaginal bleeding or pain indicates that rupture of the scar is occurring. In general, elective repeat cesarean section is indicated (1) for women whose first cesarean section was done because of cephalopelvic disproportion (although a significant number will deliver vaginally and a trial of labor is acceptable); (2) for those whose labor is likely to be long and tedious (eg, when the patient enters the hospital with ruptured membranes, a high presenting part, and an uneffaced, rigid cervix); (3) for those who have had a prior classic cesarean section or myomectomy in which the uterine cavity was entered; and (4) for those who, after viability is reached, experience persistent pain in the region of the uterine incision. If vaginal delivery is allowed to proceed, alert surveillance is essential, since some cesarean section scars do rupture during labor. In one study 3 scars ruptured in labor among 526 such patients.

The major hazard in the performance of elective repeat cesarean section is miscalculation of dates, with consequent delivery of a premature baby. Amniocentesis with estimation of surfactant, lamellar bodies, or phosphatidyl glycine in amniotic fluid is a definitive method of ascertaining fetal age. Serial ultrasound scans during pregnancy can also be helpful in verifying fetal maturity. Such scans are essential in determining a reasonable date for repeat cesarean section if the menstrual dates are uncertain or if the timing of the pregnancy is uncertain—for example, because of oral contraception or amenorrhea prior to conception.

M. Other Indications

Unusual and infrequent indications for cesarean section include a tumor obstructing the birth canal, a prior extensive vaginal plastic operation, active herpes genitalis, and severe heart disease or other debilitating conditions in which vaginal delivery would impose a greater threat than cesarean section. Interestingly, women impregnated through in vitro fertilization have a higher cesarean rate, although IVF is not an indication for cesarean section.

Contraindications

The major contraindication to cesarean section is absence of an appropriate indication. Pyogenic infections of the abdominal wall, an abnormal fetus, a dead fetus, and lack of appropriate facilities or assistants have been suggested as contraindications. In each instance, the hazard of performing an indicated operation in the face of an alleged contraindication must be weighed against the possible consequence of not performing it.

Preparation for Cesarean Section

A. Ultrasound Scan

If serial scans were not done earlier in pregnancy, a scan is desirable prior to nonemergent operations to determine the position and size of the baby, to rule out gross abnormality or twins, and to determine the location of the placenta.

B. Timing

The low transverse technique, which is preferred for almost all cesarean sections, is simpler to perform if the lower uterine segment changes of early labor have developed and the bladder fold of peritoneum has advanced upward; hence, for elective repeat cesarean section, it may be desirable to await the onset of labor. In addition, the patient may progress rapidly and deliver vaginally. The wait also usually ensures that the baby has attained maximum development before delivery. As to the time of day, no operation should be deliberately undertaken during off hours if it can be safely deferred until full staff and full laboratory facilities are available.

C. Blood for Transfusion

At least 2 units of packed cells should be available before surgery in the following situations: active bleeding, preeclampsia, HELLP, and coagulopathy. In the absence of these indications, the need for transfusion is unlikely. Accordingly, except for these indications, most obstetric services now limit the preoperative blood preparation to "type and screen" (ABO/Rh typing, screen for unexpected antibodies) and cross-match only when blood is actually needed.

D. Preoperative Preparation

Preoperative sedatives should be avoided. A clear antacid (eg, 15 mL of sodium citrate, 0.3 mol/L, in 20% syrup) should be given 1 hour before operation to minimize the effects of aspiration if it should occur during anesthesia. An intravenous 18-gauge needle should be in place and 5% dextrose in lactated Ringer's or similar solution running before the operation begins. A Foley catheter should also be in place. Surgical preparations (shaving, antisepsis) are the same as for other abdominal operations and are used at the surgeon's discretion.

Procedural Details

A. Prophylactic Antibiotics

In patients who are at minimal risk for infection, prophylactic antibiotics are not recommended prior to cesarean section. Such patients include those nonlabored patients having repeat cesarean section and those in whom vaginal examination is not done after admission to the hospital. Women known to be at risk for infection include those who have had premature rupture of the membranes or prolonged labor, those who have undergone invasive methods of monitoring, or those who have undergone trial or failed forceps delivery. Other risk factors that may be sufficient to warrant use of prophylactic antibiotics are anemia and obesity.

Infants of women at risk for postoperative infection are also at risk for infection, and cultures of both mother and baby are required. Many pediatricians believe that early administration of prophylactic antibiotics to the mother produces fetal levels high enough to vitiate neonatal cultures, so that more extensive evaluation for sepsis may be necessary. One researcher suggested that delaying the first dose until after the cord is clamped is just as effective in preventing maternal infection but does not interfere with laboratory work-ups of the baby. Both aerobic and anaerobic coverage are needed. Several agents have proved effective, although the least expensive effective agent should be used.

B. Anesthesia

Anesthesia for cesarean section is discussed in Chapter 26.

C. Position on the Table

Placing the patient in the Trendelenburg position at an angle of 25–30 degrees may be extremely helpful during dissection of the bladder fold and disengagement of the fetal head. If the head is deeply engaged, upward pressure from below by an assistant or use of forceps or vacuum may be needed.

Tilting the patient slightly to the left moves the uterus to the left of the midline and minimizes pressure on the inferior vena cava.

D. Abdominal Incision

Opinions differ regarding the abdominal incision. An increasing number of obstetricians use the transverse incision with or without transection of the rectus muscles because wound dehiscence and postoperative incisional hernia are rare and because the cosmetic result is usually better. In cases of fetal distress or gross obesity, the midline suprapubic incision is preferred because it is much quicker and the exposure for expeditious delivery and dealing with uterine bleeding (by hysterectomy, if needed) is usually better. In the presence of a prior lower abdominal scar, it is important to enter the peritoneal cavity at the upper end of the incision to avoid entering the bladder, which may have been pulled up-

ward on the abdominal wall at the time of closure of the previous incision.

E. Uterine Incision

Before the uterine incision is made, laparotomy pads that have been soaked in warm saline and wrung out may be placed on either side of the uterus to catch the spill of amniotic fluid. The degree of dextrorotation should also be determined by noting the position of the round ligaments so that the uterine incision will be centered. Torsion should not be corrected; instead, access to the midline should be obtained by retraction of the abdominal wall to the patient's right. See below for the different types of uterine incisions.

F. Heavy Bleeding

Heavy bleeding from large sinuses in the uterine incision usually can be controlled with large T clamps (ie, Pennington), but lesser bleeding points should be left to be controlled when closure sutures are placed. It is unwise to routinely place a palisade of clamps on the uterine wall because, even though this may seal the bleeders temporarily, they may begin to bleed again after the patient is in the recovery room.

G. Encountering the Placenta

If the placenta is encountered beneath the uterine incision, the operator must try to avoid perforating it; otherwise serious fetal bleeding may result. A way should be found around the placenta and the membranes then ruptured. If this is impossible, an incision may be made through the placenta. However, the baby must be delivered as quickly as possible and the cord clamped immediately to prevent blood loss.

H. Delivery

The operator delivers the baby and then separates and extracts the placenta. After delivery of the placenta, oxytocin should be administered. Oxytocin should be given by intravenous drip (10 to 20 units in 1000 mL of 5% dextrose in water) at a rate sufficient to maintain a firm contraction. Recent randomized trials have shown no significant difference between exteriorizing the uterus and leaving it in the peritoneal cavity for closure.

I. Suture of the Uterine Incision

Swaged needles cause less bleeding and are useful for placing sutures in the uterine wall. The entire thickness of the myometrium should be closed, and no harm is done if the deep sutures include the edge of the endometrium.

Types of Cesarean Section

The types of cesarean section in modern use are (1) classic cesarean section, (2) low transverse (cervical) cesarean section, and (3) extraperitoneal cesarean section.

A. CLASSIC CESAREAN SECTION

This is the simplest to perform. However, it is also associated with the greatest loss of blood, and it leaves a scar that may rupture in a subsequent pregnancy. Moreover, a loop of small bowel may adhere to the uterine incision and predispose to intestinal obstruction. The currently accepted indications for classic cesarean section are placenta previa (because the incision in the corpus usually avoids the low-lying placenta); transverse lie (in which better access to the baby is provided); and premature delivery (there is little formation of the lower uterine segment). However, some prefer the low transverse operation, if possible, for each of these conditions.

Classic cesarean section may also be preferred if there is need for extreme haste, because it offers the quickest means of delivering the baby. Nonetheless, the hazards of this procedure must be weighed against the additional minute or so needed to dissect the bladder away from the lower uterine segment and to make the transverse semilunar low cervical incision.

In performing the classic procedure, a vertical incision is made in the corpus, a scalpel is used to enter the uterine cavity, and the incision is enlarged with bandage scissors. Since the incision is relatively high in the uterus, the head is rarely accessible. Accordingly, the feet are grasped and brought through the incision. The remainder of the delivery is accomplished using the several maneuvers appropriate for breech delivery (see Chapter 21). After removal of the placenta and membranes, the uterine defect may be repaired with 3 layers of chromic catgut or an absorbable synthetic suture. No. 0 is recommended for the 2 deeper layers and 2-0 for the superficial suture to coapt the serosal edges. In placing the superficial layer, a "baseball stitch" minimizes bleeding from the cut edges: Each suture enters the myometrium on the cut surface, emerging on the serosal surface about $\frac{3}{16}$ inch (5 mm) from the edge, and is so continued side-to-side for the length of the incision.

B. LOW CERVICAL CESAREAN SECTION (LOWER TRANSVERSE UTERINE SEGMENT CESAREAN SECTION OR CERVICAL CESAREAN SECTION)

The confused terminology of this procedure is understandable: Before labor, when the cervix is closed, uneffaced, and located at about the level of the ischial spines, a transverse uterine incision (which is made $\frac{3}{4}$–1 inch [2–3 cm] superior to the symphysis pubica) is needed in the lower uterine segment; when the cervix is fully dilated and retracted, the anterior lip is just superior to the symphysis and the incision just superior to the symphysis is through the cervix. When the operation is performed after the onset of labor but before full dilatation, there is no indication whether the incision is made in the cervix proper or in the lower uterine segment—a detail of only academic interest.

The steps in the operation are shown in Figure 27–19. The bladder fold of peritoneum is picked up with tissue forceps and incised transversely. By means of finger dissection through the loose areolar tissue, the bladder is separated from the anterior aspect of the uterus interiorly for a distance of 3–4 cm. The bladder is held away from this denuded area by a specially designed bladder retractor, and a transverse incision about 2 cm long is made through the anterior uterine wall. The membranes are preferably left intact, but no real damage follows if they should be ruptured. Using bandage scissors or fingers, the operator enlarges the transverse incision in a crescent-shaped path that extends superiorly at the lateral extremities to avoid the uterine vessels.

If it can be readily accomplished, the baby is delivered by elevation with the hand. If it cannot, the baby's face is rotated into the incision, and the left blade of the DeLee cesarean section forceps or the Simpson forceps is introduced and applied to one side of the head. Using this blade as a vectis and combining it with moderate fundal pressure by the assistant, the operator can usually deliver the baby's head with ease; if not, the second blade may be applied. If the face cannot be easily rotated into the incision, the head should be turned to the OA position and delivered using one or both blades of the forceps, as above. Occasionally, with considerable molding and deep engagement, a vertex delivery may be difficult, in which case the baby's feet must be brought down and delivery must be accomplished as in classic cesarean section.

Most obstetricians prefer the transverse semilunar incision. In former years a longitudinal incision, usually extending into the corpus uteri superiorly, was more popular. However, this incision has many of the same complications and risks as those of a classic incision.

The uterine incision generally is repaired using 2 layers of No. 0 or 2-0 chromic catgut or absorbable synthetic suture. (It is helpful, in gaining exposure for subsequent steps, to leave the first suture long at each end of the incision. These function as lifting sutures, and they should not be cut until the peritonization is completed.) The peritoneal reflection can be sutured either to the superior peritoneal flap or to the anterior uterine wall just superior to the uterine incision. Today, closure of the peritoneum is no longer standard. Decreased operating room time with an appropriate de-

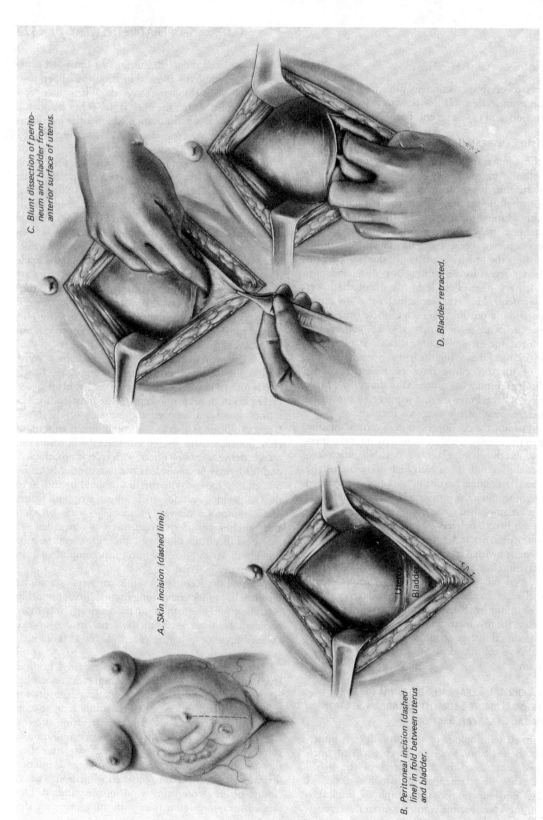

Figure 27–19. **Cesarean section.** (Reproduced, with permission, from Dunn LG: Cesarean section and other obstetric operations. In: Danforth DN, Scott JR [editors]: *Obstetrics and Gynecology,* 5th ed. Lippincott, 1986.)

C. Blunt dissection of peritoneum and bladder from anterior surface of uterus.

D. Bladder retracted.

A. Skin incision (dashed line).

B. Peritoneal incision (dashed line) in fold between uterus and bladder.

Uterus
Bladder

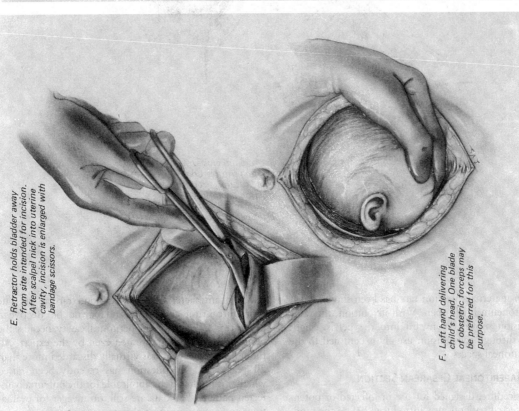

E. Retractor holds bladder away from site intended for incision. After scalpel nick into uterine cavity, incision is enlarged with bandage scissors.

F. Left hand delivering child's head. One blade of obstetric forceps may be preferred for this purpose.

G. Delivery of infant.

Figure 27–19 (cont'd). Cesarean section.

525

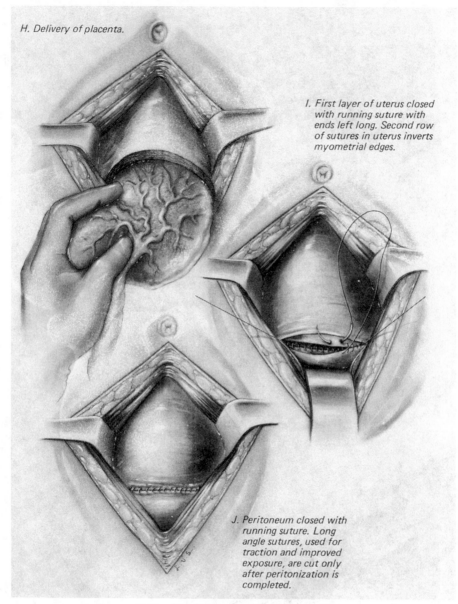

H. Delivery of placenta.

I. First layer of uterus closed with running suture with ends left long. Second row of sutures in uterus inverts myometrial edges.

J. Peritoneum closed with running suture. Long angle sutures, used for traction and improved exposure, are cut only after peritonization is completed.

Figure 27–19 (cont'd). Cesarean section.

crease in maternal infection rate has been shown when the peritoneum is left open. With involution, the uterine incision moves downward into the pelvis. Slight seepage through the incision usually is confined to the retroperitoneal spaces.

C. EXTRAPERITONEAL CESAREAN SECTION

This procedure, designed for use in infected or potentially infected patients, was introduced before the mod-

ern era of antibacterial agents and blood transfusion. The procedure is time-consuming and may not be effective in preventing spillage into the peritoneal cavity, because the peritoneum often is perforated even by the expert. Although the operation was virtually discarded more than 20 years ago, the question has recently been raised whether it might not be applicable for the potentially infected patient. The data are still too meager for evaluation, and at present most obstetricians perform cesarean hysterectomy if the uterus is frankly infected; if it is only potentially infected, they perform low transverse cesarean section with prophylactic antibiotic coverage.

Complications & Prognosis

The major factors affecting healing of the uterine incision are hemostasis, accuracy of apposition, quality and amount of suture material, and avoidance of infection and tissue strangulation. Unfortunately, little information about the integrity of a particular scar in a subsequent pregnancy is gained by inquiry as to the presence or absence of postoperative infection and the location of the incision.

In a later pregnancy, pain in the area of the scar may suggest dehiscence. About 50% of all ruptures of uterine scars occur before the onset of labor. The incidence of rupture is about 4–9% of classic scars and 0.2–1.5% in cases of low transverse cesarean section. Rupture of the classic scar is usually catastrophic, occurring suddenly, totally, and with partial or total extrusion of the fetus into the abdominal cavity. Shock due to internal hemorrhage is a prominent sign. Rupture of the low transverse scar is usually more subtle and is characterized principally by pain and occasionally by evidence of slower internal bleeding. Some ruptures are entirely silent, and during repeat cesarean section myometrial fenestrations covered only by visceral peritoneum may be noted.

A. MATERNAL MORBIDITY AND MORTALITY

Average maternal morbidity and mortality rates after cesarean section suggest that the risk from the operation per se is very small. Some large series with no postoperative deaths have been reported. In other series, incidences of mortality have ranged from 40 to 80 per 100,000 cases. In general, it is reasonable to conclude that the risk of death following cesarean delivery is at least twice the risk following vaginal delivery. Such figures are difficult to interpret, however, because of the great variability of indications and complications. Even in the most favorable cases variable factors exist, including spill of amniotic fluid and blood into the peritoneal cavity; ease or difficulty of delivering the baby through the uterine incision; amount of incisional bleeding; and patient response to anesthesia. Factors contributing heavily to postoperative complications are prior internal monitoring, prolonged rupture of the membranes, unsuccessful prior efforts at vaginal delivery, hemorrhage, uterine rupture, and countless other obstetric problems that may have compromised the patient and for which emergency cesarean section was performed. See Prophylactic Antibiotics, earlier in this chapter, for a discussion of the risk of postoperative infection.

The longer the operative procedure, the greater the likelihood of postoperative complications. As Victor

Bonney noted in an early edition of his classic *Gynecological Surgery*, "An operation rapidly yet correctly performed has many advantages over one technically as correct, yet laboriously and tediously accomplished." Most cesarean sections should be completed in less than 1 hour unless significant technical problems are encountered.

Disasters following cesarean section are rare. Some clearly are not preventable. Others are due directly to faulty surgical technique, especially lack of attention to hemostasis, inept or ill-chosen anesthesia, inadequate blood replacement or transfusion of mismatched blood, and mismanagement of infection.

B. PERINATAL MORBIDITY AND MORTALITY

Perinatal problems are as difficult to assess as maternal ones. Data suggest that spontaneous vaginal delivery in the uncomplicated multipara is less hazardous for the baby than repeat elective cesarean section and that if elective cesarean section is performed, regional anesthesia appears to be less noxious than general anesthesia.

The first conclusion will be acceptable to most: Spontaneous vaginal delivery is usually the most normal of births, whereas repeat cesarean section may entail time-consuming procedures such as dissection of an adherent bladder, aspiration of amniotic fluid during attempts at delivery, fetal hypoxia if the placenta is encountered beneath the prior incision, and the occasional need for version to accomplish delivery.

It must be emphasized that iatrogenic prematurity is still an important consequence of elective cesarean section. Whenever repeat cesarean section is contemplated or whenever risk factors make it necessary to terminate the pregnancy before term, every effort must be made to establish an accurate term date, preferably by ultrasound scans at 20–21 weeks' gestation and again at 30–31 weeks. If gestational age is still in doubt, the lecithin:sphingomyelin ratio or amniotic fluid phosphatidyl glycine concentration should be determined before operation.

Some evidence suggests that cesarean section per se contributes in some unknown way to increased occurrence of respiratory problems in the newborn, and this underscores the desirability of examination of the infant by a pediatrician as soon as possible after delivery.

Elective Procedures Coincidental to Cesarean Section

A. APPENDECTOMY

Appendectomy should not be performed routinely at the time of cesarean section. An appendectomy may seem to be innocuous but can result in obstruction and peritonitis.

B. Myomectomy

Myomectomy is permissible at the time of cesarean section only if the tumor is pedunculated. Extracting intramural tumors can provoke intense and uncontrollable bleeding. Also, myomas almost invariably regress after pregnancy; indeed, even large myomas are sometimes not palpable 3 months after delivery.

C. Tubal Ligation

This procedure is usually offered to the multiparous patient at the time of the cesarean section. If a Pomeroy sterilization procedure is done, the fimbriated end of the tube must first be identified (the round ligament has been mistaken for the tube) and the operation performed at the junction of the middle and outer thirds of the tube. Caution should be used to avoid excessive pulling on the tube, which could rupture veins in the broad ligament.

Cesarean Hysterectomy

A major indication for cesarean hysterectomy is inability to stop bleeding from the uterine incision. Other indications are rupture of the uterus in which repair is impractical, placenta accreta, uterine hemorrhage from uncontrollable atony, and large uterine myomas.

Cesarean hysterectomy should never be done as a means of sterilization. The procedure is too formidable for this purpose alone; postpartum tubal ligation is far less hazardous and is highly effective if done properly.

At the time of cesarean section, it is preferable to remove the cervix if the patient's condition is good and if there is no contraindication to prolonging operating time by 10–15 minutes. Supracervical hysterectomy should be performed only when it is desirable to terminate the operation quickly. A risk of leaving the cervix intact is postoperative hemorrhage, and thus good hemostasis is critical.

The technical aspects of hysterectomy at the time of cesarean section do not differ basically from those of hysterectomy in the nonpregnant patient except that all structures and cleavage planes are highly vascular and the tissues are friable. At least 4 units of matched blood must be at hand. In one study, blood replacement was needed in 98% of the indicated cesarean hysterectomies and in 66% of the elective sterilization group; two-thirds of the patients in the elective group received an average of 1.6 units of blood.

Postmortem Cesarean Section

Postmortem cesarean section is a difficult problem for the following reasons.

(1) The possibility of litigation is introduced if the operation is done without informed consent of the next of kin (usually an impractical detail in these circumstances) or if it is not done in the interests of the baby.

(2) The definition of legal death is not firmly established, but most agree that in the adult, irreversible brain damage results after 5 minutes or more of total anoxia. There is inconclusive evidence that the fetal brain may be more resistant to hypoxia than that of the adult. The prospects for a healthy baby depend to a certain extent on whether the mother's death was instantaneous or whether she was moribund for an extended period.

Regardless of how quickly the operation is done after the mother's death, the outlook for the baby is bleak. Jeffcoate, the preeminent Liverpudlian obstetrician-gynecologist, commented that some "continue to report with misplaced pride the delivery by postmortem caesarean section of babies which have suffered so much cerebral anoxia whilst in utero that they are permanently crippled mentally and physically as well as being motherless."

Arthur has reviewed the subject and suggests that with modern life-support systems, the outlook for the baby may be immeasurably improved if the operation can be performed when death is imminent but has not yet occurred. According to a news release from the Roanoke (Virginia) Memorial Hospital, a brain-dead woman who had been kept breathing by respirator for 84 days was delivered by cesarean section of a 3-lb 11-oz (1.67-kg) apparently normal baby. Life support was withdrawn after delivery.

Fetal Injury

While performing a cesarean section, most emphasis is placed on careful dissection of maternal tissues. The obstetrician must be just as careful with the fetus. The incision in the uterus can lacerate the infant if it is too deep. Although this is an unusual occurrence, it does occur in 0.2–0.4% of all cesarean sections. The usual site is on the face in the area of the cheek. It may also occur on the buttock, ear, head, or any other body site under the incision. To avoid this injury completely is probably impossible. However, careful incision through the uterine layers will minimize any laceration that may occur.

VAGINAL DELIVERY FOLLOWING PREVIOUS CESAREAN SECTION (VBAC)

A marked rise in the incidence of cesarean section deliveries has occurred in the U.S., and rates of 25–70% are common in those hospitals that encourage or require a trial of labor following a previous cesarean section. Factors responsible for the increase include the relative safety of the procedure and concern about malpractice litigation. Vaginal delivery is associated with fewer delivery risks, requires less anesthesia, poses a lower potential for postpartum morbidity, involves a shorter hospital stay, saves money, and encourages earlier and often smoother interaction between mother and infant. Since approximately 30% of cesarean sections are performed solely because of previous cesarean section, a substantial (and beneficial) decrease in incidence would occur if VBAC were more widely adopted in the absence of contraindications. In recent studies 60–80% of all patients who undergo a trial of labor after previous cesarean section have a successful vaginal delivery when the obstetrician actively promotes VBAC. In the case of cesarean delivery performed for malpresentation and other indications not necessarily recurring in subsequent pregnancies, vaginal delivery should occur in 75–80% of subsequent pregnancies. Previous vaginal delivery is an indicator of probable success in future vaginal delivery.

Indications

Criteria for vaginal delivery following previous cesarean section may include the following: (1) The patient agrees to the procedure. (2) A low transverse uterine incision was used. (3) The original indication for cesarean section was a cause not necessarily recurring in subsequent pregnancies. (4) The postoperative course was benign. (5) The current pregnancy is not complicated by macrosomia, malposition, multiple gestation, or other conditions that would be likely to preclude vaginal delivery.

Contraindications

Although authorities agree that a previous classic uterine incision is an absolute contraindication to vaginal delivery in later pregnancies, other contraindications are less clear. For example, there appears to be little increased risk in attempting a trial of labor in the presence of mild macrosomia, and many authors now feel that the occurrence of 2 prior cesarean sections is no longer an absolute contraindication.

Management

A. DEFINITIONS

Dehiscence is the unsuspected and undiagnosed silent separation of a uterine scar from a previous cesarean section; it is usually limited to the immediate area of the scar. **Rupture** is the sudden separation of the scar, usually with hemorrhage; the laceration may be extensive. A rupture is termed **complete** if it communicates with the peritoneal cavity and **incomplete** if the visceral peritoneum is intact. Uterine rupture occurs in 0.2–1.5% of patients following a low transverse incision, and 4–9% after a classical incision. Exact information on the safety of vaginal delivery in the presence of

low vertical cesarean scars is lacking, but rates of rupture have been reported as 1–7%.

B. OXYTOCIN

Judicious use of oxytocin appears to be safe in vaginal delivery following previous cesarean section. Several reports show no greater incidence of necessary cesarean section, dehiscence or rupture of the scar, uterine atony, hemorrhage, transfusion, hysterectomy, birth trauma, or adverse neonatal outcome with carefully controlled infusion of oxytocin. However, there are reports that suggest that induction with oxytocin and/or prostaglandins may be associated with an increased risk of uterine rupture.

C. EPIDURAL ANESTHESIA

The role of epidural anesthesia in vaginal delivery following previous cesarean section remains controversial. Although pain may not be a reliable sign of uterine rupture and epidural anesthesia may not completely block the pain associated with such an event, the concern is that epidural anesthesia could potentially mask the rupture, thereby jeopardizing both mother and infant. On the other hand, epidural anesthesia removes the fear of labor pain and helps the obstetrician encourage VBAC.

D. COMPLICATIONS

The most feared complication is uterine rupture, although 44–60% of these ruptures precede the onset of labor and are most frequently associated with a classic incision. Current studies cite a maternal mortality rate of about 1% and a perinatal mortality rate of about 50% in association with uterine rupture, although exact data are unavailable. The institution in which delivery is to occur must therefore be fully capable of managing possible uterine rupture. Equipment for both maternal and electronic fetal monitoring and appropriate obstetric and neonatal facilities must be available. A large-bore intravenous catheter must be used, and type-specific blood for possible maternal transfusion must be at hand. Appropriate anesthesia, a fully equipped operating room, and obstetric and neonatal staff experienced in emergency care all must be immediately available.

REFERENCES

Forceps Delivery

Hankins GDV et al: The role of forceps rotation in maternal and neonatal injury. Am J Obstet Gynecol 1999;180:231.

Cesarean Section

American College of Obstetricians and Gynecologists: Vaginal birth after cesarean delivery. ACOG Practice Bulletin, July 1999.

Edi-Osagie EC et al: Uterine exteriorization at cesarean section: influence on maternal morbidity. Br J Obstet Gynaecol 1998;105:1070.

Grundsell HS, Rizk DE, Kumar RM: Randomized study of nonclosure of peritoneum in lower segment cesarean section. ACTA Obstet Gynecol Scand 1998;77:110.

Irion O, Hirsbrunner Almagbaly P, Morabia A: Planned vaginal delivery versus elective cesarean section: a study of 705 singleton term breech presentations. Br J Obstet Gynaecol 1998;105:710.

Reubinoff BE et al: Is the obstetric outcome of in vitro fertilized singleton gestations different from natural ones? A controlled study. Fertil Steril 1997;67:1077.

Rizk DE et al: Systemic antibiotic prophylaxis in elective cesarean delivery. Int J Gynaecol Obstet 1998;61:245.

General Operative Vaginal Delivery

Bofill JA et al: Shoulder dystocia and operative vaginal delivery. J Matern Fetal Med 1997;6:220.

Ezenagu LC, Kakaria R, Bofill JA: Sequential use of instruments at operative vaginal delivery: is it safe? Am J Obstet Gynecol 1999;180:1446.

Revah A et al: Failed trial of vacuum of forceps—maternal and fetal outcome. Am J Obstet and Gynecol 1997;176:200.

Postpartum Hemorrhage & the Abnormal Puerperium

28

Sarah B.H. Poggi, MD, & Peter S. Kapernick, MD, MPH

POSTPARTUM HEMORRHAGE

Definition

Postpartum hemorrhage denotes excessive bleeding (> 500 mL in vaginal delivery) following delivery. Hemorrhage may occur before, during, or after delivery of the placenta. Actual measured blood loss during uncomplicated vaginal deliveries has been shown to average 700 mL, and blood loss may often be underestimated. Nevertheless, the criterion of a loss of 500 mL is acceptable on historical grounds.

Blood lost during the first 24 hours after delivery is early postpartum hemorrhage; blood lost between 24 hours and 6 weeks after delivery is late postpartum hemorrhage.

Incidence

The incidence of excessive blood loss following vaginal delivery is 5–8%. Postpartum hemorrhage is the most common cause of excessive blood loss in pregnancy, and most transfusions in pregnant women are performed to replace blood lost after delivery. Hemorrhage is the third leading cause of maternal mortality in the U.S. and is directly responsible for about one-sixth of maternal deaths. In less-developed countries, hemorrhage is among the leading obstetric causes of maternal death.

Morbidity & Mortality

Although any woman may suffer excessive blood loss during delivery, women already compromised by anemia or intercurrent illness are more likely to demonstrate serious deterioration of condition, and anemia and excessive blood loss may predispose to subsequent puerperal infection. Major morbidity associated with transfusion therapy (eg, hepatitis, human immunodeficiency virus infection, transfusion reactions) is infrequent but is not insignificant. Moreover, other types of treatment for anemia may involve some risk.

Postpartum hypotension may lead to partial or total necrosis of the anterior pituitary gland and cause postpartum panhypopituitarism, or Sheehan's syndrome, which is characterized by failure to lactate, amenorrhea, decreased breast size, loss of pubic and axillary hair, hypothyroidism, and adrenal insufficiency. The condition is rare (< 1 in 10,000 deliveries). A woman who has been hypotensive postpartum and who is actively lactating probably does not have Sheehan's syndrome. Hypotension can also lead to acute renal failure and other organ system injury. In extreme hemorrhage, sterility will result from hysterectomy performed to control intractable postpartum hemorrhage.

Etiology

Causes of postpartum hemorrhage include uterine atony, obstetric lacerations, retained placental tissue, and coagulation defects.

A. UTERINE ATONY

Postpartum bleeding is physiologically controlled by constriction of interlacing myometrial fibers that surround the blood vessels supplying the placental implantation site. Uterine atony exists when the myometrium cannot contract.

Atony is the most common cause of postpartum hemorrhage (50% of cases). Predisposing causes include excessive manipulation of the uterus, general anesthesia (particularly with halogenated compounds), uterine overdistention (twins or polyhydramnios), prolonged labor, grand multiparity, uterine leiomyomas, operative delivery and intrauterine manipulation, oxytocin induction or augmentation of labor, previous hemorrhage in the third stage, uterine infection, extravasation of blood into the myometrium (Couvelaire uterus), and intrinsic myometrial dysfunction.

B. OBSTETRIC LACERATIONS

Excessive bleeding from an episiotomy, lacerations, or both causes about 20% of postpartum hemorrhages. Lacerations can involve the uterus, cervix, vagina, or vulva, and they usually result from precipitate or uncontrolled delivery or operative delivery of a large infant; however, they may occur after any delivery. Laceration of blood vessels underneath the vaginal or vulvar epithelium results in hematomas. Bleeding is concealed and can be particularly dangerous, since it may go unrecognized for several hours and only become apparent when shock occurs.

Episiotomies may cause excessive bleeding if they involve arteries or large varicosities, if the episiotomy is large, if there is a delay between episiotomy and delivery, or if there is a delay between delivery and repair of the episiotomy.

Persistent bleeding (especially bright red) and a well-contracted, firm uterus suggests bleeding from a laceration or from the episiotomy. When cervical or vaginal lacerations are identified as the source of postpartum hemorrhage, repair is best performed with adequate anesthesia.

Spontaneous rupture of the uterus is rare. Risk factors for this complication include grand multiparity, malpresentation, previous uterine surgery, and oxytocin induction of labor. Rupture of a previous cesarean section scar after vaginal delivery may be an increasingly important cause of postpartum hemorrhage.

C. RETAINED PLACENTAL TISSUE

Retained placental tissue and membranes cause 5–10% of postpartum hemorrhages. Retention of placental tissue in the uterine cavity occurs in placenta accreta, in manual removal of the placenta, in mismanagement of the third stage of labor, and in unrecognized succenturiate placenta.

Ultrasonographic findings of an echogenic uterine mass strongly support a diagnosis of retained placental products. The technique is probably better used in cases of hemorrhage occurring a few hours after delivery or in late postpartum hemorrhage. Transvaginal duplex Doppler imaging is also effective in evaluating these patients. There is some evidence that sonohysterography may aid in the diagnosis of residual trophoblastic tissue. If the endometrial cavity appears empty, unnecessary dilatation and curettage may be avoided.

D. COAGULATION DEFECTS

Coagulopathies in pregnancy may be acquired coagulation defects seen in association with several obstetric disorders, including abruptio placentae, excess thromboplastin from a retained dead fetus, amniotic fluid embolism, severe preeclampsia, eclampsia, and sepsis (see Chapter 59). These coagulopathies may present as hypofibrinogenemia, thrombocytopenia, and disseminated intravascular coagulation. Transfusion of more than 8 U of blood may in itself induce a dilutional coagulopathy.

Von Willebrand's disease, autoimmune thrombocytopenia, and leukemia may also occur in pregnant women.

Risk Factors

Prevention of hemorrhage is preferable to even the best treatment. All patients in labor should be evaluated for risk of postpartum hemorrhage. Risk factors include coagulopathy, hemorrhage, or blood transfusion during a previous pregnancy; anemia during labor; grand multiparity; multiple gestation; large infant; polyhydramnios; dysfunctional labor; oxytocin induction or augmentation of labor; rapid or tumultuous labor; severe preeclampsia or eclampsia; vaginal delivery after previous cesarean birth; general anesthesia for delivery; and midforceps delivery.

Management

A. PREDELIVERY PREPARATION

All obstetric patients should have blood typed and screened on admission. Patients identified as being at risk for postpartum hemorrhage should have their blood typed and cross-matched immediately. The blood should be reserved in the blood bank for 24 hours after delivery. A large-bore intravenous catheter should be securely taped into place after insertion. Delivery room personnel should be alerted to the risk of hemorrhage. Severely anemic patients should be transfused as soon as cross-matched blood is ready.

With concerns associated with blood transfusion, autologous blood donation in obstetric patients at risk for postpartum hemorrhage has been advocated. Despite careful evaluation for risk factors, with the exception of cases of placenta previa, our ability to predict which patients will have hemorrhage and require blood transfusion remains poor; therefore, the cost of such an approach may not be justified.

B. DELIVERY

Following delivery of the infant, the uterus is massaged in a circular or back-and-forth motion until the myometrium becomes firm and well contracted. Excessive and vigorous massage of the uterus before, during, or after delivery of the placenta may interfere with normal contraction of the myometrium and instead of hastening contraction may lead to excessive postpartum blood loss.

C. THIRD STAGE OF NORMAL LABOR; PLACENTAL SEPARATION

The placenta typically separates from the uterus and is delivered within 5 minutes of delivery of the infant. Attempts to speed separation are of no benefit and may cause harm. Spontaneous placental separation is impending if the uterus becomes round and firm, a sudden gush of blood comes from the vagina, the uterus seems to rise in the abdomen, and the umbilical cord moves down out of the vagina.

The placenta can then be removed from the vagina by gentle traction on the umbilical cord. Prior to placental separation, gentle steady traction on the cord combined with upward pressure on the lower uterine segment (Brandt-Andrews maneuver) ensures that the placenta can be removed as soon as separation occurs and provides a means of monitoring the consistency of the uterus. Adherent membranes can be removed by gentle traction with ring forceps. The placenta is inspected for completeness immediately after delivery.

Manual Removal of the Placenta

Opinion is divided about the timing of manual removal of the placenta. In the presence of hemorrhage, it is obviously unreasonable to wait for spontaneous separation, and manual removal of the placenta should be undertaken without delay. In the absence of bleeding, many would advocate removal of the placenta 30 minutes after delivery of the infant.

Efforts to promote routine manual removal of the placenta were often made in the past. The rationale includes shortening the third stage of labor, decreasing blood loss, developing experience in manual removal as practice for dealing with placenta accreta, and providing a way to simultaneously explore the uterus. There is now evidence that manual removal of the placenta may be a risk factor for postpartum endometritis. These real or potential benefits must be weighed against the discomfort caused to the patient, the risk of infection, and the risk of causing more bleeding by interfering with normal mechanisms of placental separation.

Technique. The uterus is stabilized by grasping the fundus with a hand placed over the abdomen. The other hand traces the course of the umbilical cord through the vagina and cervix into the uterus to palpate the edge of the placenta. The membranes at the placental margin are perforated, and the hand is inserted between the placenta and the uterine wall, palmar side toward the placenta. The hand is then gently swept from side to side and up and down to peel the placenta from its attachments to the uterus. When the placenta has been completely separated from the uterus, it is grasped and pulled from the uterus.

The fetal and maternal sides of the placenta should be inspected to ensure that it has been removed in its entirety. On the fetal surface, incomplete placental removal is manifested as interruption of the vessels on the chorionic plate, usually shown by hemorrhage. On the maternal surface, it is possible to see where cotyledons have been detached. If there is evidence of incomplete removal, the uterus must be re-explored and any small pieces of adherent placenta removed. The uterus should be massaged until a firm myometrial tone is achieved. Depending on the patient's other risk factors for postpartum endometritis, prophylactic antibiotics may be given at the time of manual removal of the placenta.

Immediate Postpartum Period

Uterotonic agents may be administered as soon as the infant's anterior shoulder is delivered. Recent studies show a significantly lowered incidence of postpartum hemorrhage in patients receiving oxytocin (either low-dose IV or IM) at the time of delivery of the anterior shoulder and controlled cord traction, when compared to patients receiving IV oxytocin following placental delivery. There was no greater incidence of placental retention. However, in populations without ultrasound screening for twins, there is a potential risk of entrapment of an undiagnosed second twin and oxytocin should only be given after placental delivery. Routine administration of oxytocics during the third stage reduces the blood loss of delivery and decreases the chances of postpartum hemorrhage by 40%. Oxytocin, 10–20 U/L of isotonic saline, or other intravenous solution by slow intravenous infusion or 10 U intramuscularly can be used. Bolus administration should not be used, since large doses (> 5 U) can cause hypotension. Ergot alkaloids (eg, methylergonovine maleate, 0.2 mg intramuscularly) can also be routinely used but they are not more effective than oxytocin and pose more risk, since they may rarely cause marked hypertension. This occurs most commonly in intravenous administration or when regional anesthesia is used. Ergot alkaloids should not be used in hypertensive women or in women with cardiac disease.

Repair of Lacerations

If bleeding is excessive before placental separation, manual removal of the placenta is indicated. Otherwise, excessive manipulation of the uterus should be avoided.

The vagina and cervix should be carefully inspected immediately after delivery of the placenta, with adequate lighting and assistants available. The episiotomy is quickly repaired after massage has produced a firm, tightly contracted uterus. A pack placed in the vagina above the episiotomy helps to keep the field dry; attaching the free end of the pack to the adjacent drapes reminds the operator to remove it after the repair is completed.

The tendency of bleeding vessels to retract from the laceration site is the reason for one of the cardinal principles of repair. Begin the repair above the highest extent of the laceration. The highest suture is also used to provide gentle traction to bring the laceration site closer to the introitus. Hemostatic ligatures are then placed in the usual manner, and the entire birth canal is carefully inspected to make sure that there are no additional bleeding sites. Extensive inspection also provides time to confirm that prior hemostatic efforts have been effective.

A cervical or vaginal laceration extending into the broad ligament should not be repaired vaginally. Laparotomy with evacuation of the resultant hematoma and hemostatic repair or hysterectomy is required.

Large or expanding hematomas of the vaginal walls require operative management for proper control. The vaginal wall is first exposed by an assistant. If a laceration accompanies the hematoma, the laceration is extended so that the hematoma can be completely evacuated and explored. When the bleeding site is identified, a large hemostatic ligature can be placed well above the site. This ensures hemostasis in the vessel, which is likely to retract when lacerated. The hematoma cavity should be left open to allow drainage of blood and ensure that bleeding will not be concealed if hemostasis cannot be achieved.

If there is no laceration in the vaginal side wall when a hematoma is identified, then an incision must be made over the hematoma to allow treatment to proceed as outlined above.

Following delivery, recovery room attendants should frequently massage the uterus and check for vaginal bleeding.

Evaluation of Persistent Bleeding

If vaginal bleeding persists after delivery of the placenta, aggressive treatment should be initiated. It is not sufficient to perform perfunctory uterine massage, for instance, without searching for the cause of the bleeding and initiating definitive treatment. The following steps should be undertaken without delay:

(1) Manually compress the uterus.

(2) Obtain assistance.

(3) If not already done, obtain blood for typing and cross-matching.

(4) Observe blood for clotting to rule out coagulopathy.

(5) Begin fluid or blood replacement.

(6) Carefully explore the uterine cavity.

(7) Completely inspect the cervix and vagina.

(8) Insert a second intravenous catheter for administration of blood or fluids.

A. MEASURES TO CONTROL BLEEDING

1. Manual exploration of the uterus—The uterus should be explored immediately in women with postpartum hemorrhage. Manual exploration should also be considered after delivery of the placenta in the following circumstances: (1) when vaginal delivery follows previous cesarean section; (2) when intrauterine manipulation, eg, version and extraction, has been performed; (3) when malpresentation has occurred during labor and delivery; (4) when a premature infant has been delivered; (5) when an abnormal uterine contour has been noted prior to delivery; and (6) when there is a possibility of undiagnosed multiple pregnancy—to rule out twins.

Ensure that all placental parts have been delivered and that the uterus is intact. This should be done even in the case of a well-contracted uterus. Exploration performed for reasons other than the evaluation of hemorrhage should also confirm that the uterine wall is intact and should attempt to identify any possible intrauterine structural abnormalities. Manual exploration of the uterus does not increase febrile morbidity or blood loss.

Technique. Place a fresh glove over the glove on the exploring hand. Form the hand into a cone and gently introduce it by firm pressure through the cervix while the fundus is stabilized with the other hand. Sweep the backs of the first and second fingers across the entire surface of the uterus, beginning at the fundus. In the lower uterine segment, palpate the walls with the palmar surface of one finger. Uterine lacerations will be felt as an obvious anatomic defect. All exploration should be gentle, since the postpartum uterus is easily perforated.

Uterine rupture detected by manual exploration in the presence of postpartum hemorrhage requires immediate laparotomy. A decision to repair the defect or proceed with hysterectomy is made on the basis of the extent of the rupture, the patient's desire for future childbearing, and the degree of the patient's clinical deterioration.

2. Bimanual compression and massage—The most important step in controlling atonic postpartum hemorrhage is immediate bimanual uterine compression, which may have to be continued for 20–30 minutes or more. Fluid replacement should begin as soon as a secure intravenous line is in place. Typed and cross-matched blood is given when it is available. Manual compression of the uterus will control virtually all cases of hemorrhage due to uterine atony, retained products of conception, and coagulopathies, and it may even control bleeding from a lacerated cervix.

Technique. Place a hand on the patient's abdomen and grasp the uterine fundus; bring it down over the symphysis pubis. Insert the other hand into the vagina and place the first and second fingers on either side of the cervix and push it cephalad and anteriorly. The pulsating uterine arteries should be felt by the fingertips. Massage the uterus with both hands while compression is maintained. Prolonged compression (20–30 minutes) may be required but is almost always successful in controlling bleeding.

Insert a Foley catheter into the bladder during compression and massage, since vigorous fluid and blood replacement will cause diuresis. A distended bladder will interfere with compression and massage, will contribute to the patient's discomfort, and may itself be a major contributor to uterine atony.

3. Curettage—Curettage of a large, soft postpartum uterus can be a formidable undertaking, since the risk of perforation is high and the procedure commonly results in increased rather than decreased bleeding. The suction curet, even with a large cannula, covers only a small area of the postpartum uterus, and its size and shape increase the likelihood of perforation. A large blunt curet, the "banjo" curet, is probably the safest instrument for curettage of the postpartum uterus. It may be used when manual exploration fails to remove fragments of adherent placenta.

Curettage should be delayed unless bleeding cannot be controlled by compression and massage alone. Overly vigorous puerperal curettage can result in focal complete removal of the endometrium, particularly if the uterus is infected, with subsequent healing characterized by formation of adhesions and **Asherman's syndrome** (amenorrhea and secondary sterility due to intrauterine adhesions and uterine synechiae). If circumstances permit, ultrasonic evaluation of the postpartum uterus may distinguish those patients who will benefit from curettage from those who should be managed without it.

4. Uterine packing—Although once widely used for control of obstetric hemorrhage, uterine packing is no longer favored. The uterus may expand to considerable size after delivery of the placenta, thus accommodating both a large volume of packing material and a large volume of blood. The technique also demands considerable technical expertise because the uterus must be packed uniformly with 5 yards of 4-inch gauze, sometimes with aid of special instrumentation (Torpin packer). However, this method has been used successfully, avoiding conversion to laparotomy in 9 reported cases. As a last resort, uterine packing may be particularly appropriate in centers where an interventional radiologist is not immediately available.

5. Uterotonic agents—Oxytocin 20–40 U/L of crystalloid should be infused, if not already running, at a rate of 10–15 mL/minute. Methylergonovine, 0.2 mg, can be given intramuscularly, but is contraindicated if the patient is hypertensive. Intramyometrial injection of prostaglandin $F_{2\alpha}$ ($PGF_{2\alpha}$) to control bleeding was initially described in 1976. Intravaginal or rectal prostaglandin suppositories, intrauterine irrigation with prostaglandins, and intramyometrial injection of prostaglandins have also been reported to control hemorrhage from uterine atony. Intramuscular administration

of 15-methylprostaglandin analog was successful in treating 85% of patients with postpartum hemorrhage due to atony. Failures in these series occurred in women who had uterine infections or unrecognized placenta accreta. Side effects are usually minimal, but may include transient oxygen desaturation, bronchospasm, and, rarely, significant hypertension. Transient fever and diarrhea may also occur. A recent randomized controlled trial showed excellent efficacy of 800 µg of rectal misoprostol, a prostaglandin E_1 analog, in the treatment of primary postpartum hemorrhage secondary to atony.

6. Radiographic embolization of pelvic vessels—Embolization of pelvic and uterine vessels by angiographic techniques is increasingly common and has success rates from 85–95% in experienced hands. In institutions with trained interventional radiologists, it is certainly worth considering in women of low parity as an alternative to hysterectomy. With the patient under local anesthesia, a catheter is placed in the aorta and fluoroscopy is used to identify the bleeding vessel. Pieces of absorbable gelatin sponge (Gelfoam) are injected into the damaged vessel, or into the internal iliac vessels if no specific site of bleeding can be identified. If bleeding continues, further embolization can be performed. This technique has the advantage of being effective even when the cause of hemorrhage is extrauterine and in the presence or absence of uterine atony. Many authors recommend embolization before internal iliac ligation, because ligation obstructs the access route for angiography. Adequate recanalization can occur to maintain fertility, although fertility rates following embolization are not known.

7. Operative management—The patient's wishes regarding further childbearing should be made clear as soon as laparotomy is contemplated for the management of postpartum hemorrhage. If the patient's wishes cannot be ascertained, the operator should assume that the childbearing function is to be retained. Whenever possible, the spouse or family members should also be consulted prior to laparotomy.

a. Pressure occlusion of the aorta—Immediate temporary control of pelvic bleeding may be obtained at laparotomy by pressure occlusion of the aorta, which will provide valuable time to treat hypotension, obtain experienced assistants, identify the source of bleeding, and plan the operative procedure. In the young and otherwise healthy patient, pressure occlusion can be maintained for several minutes without permanent sequelae.

b. Uterine artery ligation—During pregnancy, 90% of the blood flow to the uterus is supplied by the uterine arteries. Direct ligation of these easily accessible vessels can successfully control hemorrhage in 75–90%

of cases, particularly when the bleeding is uterine in origin. Recanalization can occur, and subsequent pregnancies have been reported.

Technique. The uterus is lifted upward and away from the side to be ligated. Absorbable suture on a large needle is placed around the ascending uterine artery and vein on one side of the uterus, passing through the myometrium 2–4 cm medial to the vessels and through the avascular area of the broad ligament. The suture includes the myometrium to fix the suture and to avoid tearing the vessels. The same procedure is then performed on the opposite side. If the ligation is performed during cesarean section, the sutures can be placed just below the uterine incision under the bladder flap. It is not necessary to mobilize the bladder otherwise. Bilateral utero-ovarian artery ligation can also be performed in an attempt to reduce blood flow to the uterus. This should be performed with absorbable suture near the point of anastomoses between the ovarian artery and the ascending uterine artery at the utero-ovarian ligament.

c. Internal iliac artery ligation—Bilateral internal iliac (hypogastric) artery ligation is the surgical method most often used to control severe postpartum bleeding

(Fig 28–1). Exposure can be difficult, particularly in the presence of a large boggy uterus or hematoma. Failure rates of this technique can range as high as 57%, but may be related to the skill of the operator, the cause of the hemorrhage, and the patient's condition before ligation is attempted.

Technique. The peritoneum lateral to the infundibulopelvic ligament is incised parallel with the ligament, or the round ligament is transected. In either case, the peritoneum to which the ureter will adhere is dissected medially, which removes the ureter from the operative field. The pararectal space is then enlarged by blunt dissection. The internal iliac artery on the lateral side of the space is isolated and doubly ligated (but not cut) with silk ligatures at its origin from the common iliac artery. The operator must be careful not to tear the adjacent thin veins. Blood flow distally to the uterus, cervix, and upper vagina is not occluded, but the pulse pressure is sufficiently diminished to allow hemostasis to occur by in situ thrombosis. Fertility is preserved, and subsequent pregnancies are not compromised.

d. B-Lynch brace suture—An alternative to the vessel ligation techniques is placement of a brace suture to compress the uterus in cases of diffuse bleeding from

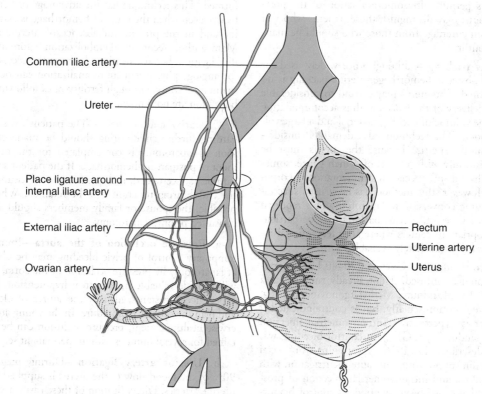

Figure 28–1. Location of ligatures for right internal iliac (hypogastric) artery ligation.

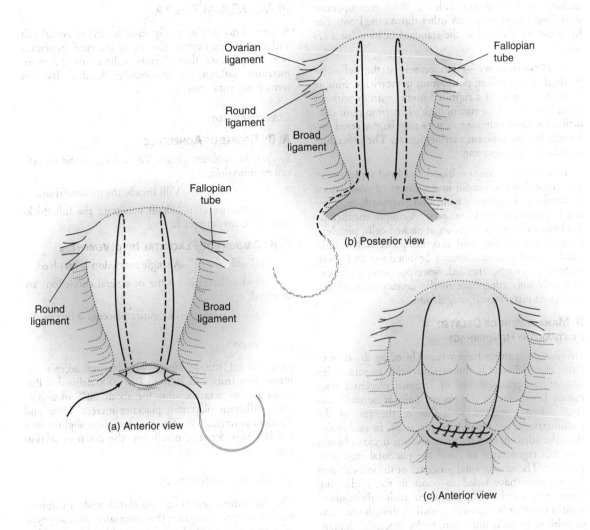

Figure 28–2. B-Lynch brace suture (see text for details).

atony or percreta (Fig 28–2). A small case series shows success and avoidance of hysterectomy using this novel approach.

Technique. Laparotomy is made in the standard way for cesarean section, and a low transverse uterine incision is made after the bladder is taken down. The uterus is exteriorized. To test the effectiveness of the method, the uterus is compressed manually and another operator checks the vagina for decreased bleeding. Using no. 2 catgut, the uterus is punctured 3 cm from the right lower incision and 3 cm from the right lateral border. The suture is threaded to emerge 3 cm above

the upper incision margin and 4 cm from the lateral border. The catgut is now visible anteriorly as it is passed over to compress the uterine fundus approximately 34 cm from the right cornual border. The suture is now fed posteriorly and vertically to enter the posterior wall of the uterine cavity at the same level as the previous entry point. After manual compression, the suture is tightened and then passed posteriorly on the left side and passed around the uterine fundus again, this time on the left. The suture is brought anteriorly to puncture the uterus at the upper part of the left uterine incision and then reemerge below the lower incision in a symmetric fashion. With one operator providing compression, the other throws the knot. The hysterotomy is closed in the standard fashion for a cesarean section.

e. Hysterectomy—Hysterectomy is the definitive method of controlling postpartum hemorrhage. Simple hemostatic repair of a ruptured uterus with or without tubal ligation in a woman of high parity or in poor condition for more extensive surgery may be preferred unless she has intercurrent uterine disease. The procedure is undoubtedly lifesaving.

8. Blood replacement—Blood and fluid replacement are required for successful management of postpartum hemorrhage. In patients with severe hemorrhage, massive transfusions may be necessary. Component therapy is advocated, with transfusion of packed cells, platelets, fresh frozen plasma, and cryoprecipitate when indicated. Blood products should be obtained and given without delay when needed, since postponing transfusion may only contribute to the development of disseminated intravascular coagulation.

B. Management of Delayed Postpartum Hemorrhage

Delayed postpartum hemorrhage (bleeding 2 weeks or more after delivery) is almost always due to subinvolution of the placental bed or retained placental fragments. Involution of the placental site is normally delayed when compared with that of the rest of the endometrium, but for unknown reasons, in subinvolution, the adjacent endometrium and the decidua basalis have not regenerated to cover the placental implantation site. The involutional processes of thrombosis and hyalinization have failed to occur in the underlying blood vessels, so bleeding may occur with only minimal trauma or other (unknown) stimuli. Although the cause of subinvolution is unknown, faulty placental implantation, implantation in the poorly vascularized lower uterine segment, and persistent infection at the implantation site have been suggested as possible factors. Uterine compression and bimanual massage, as previously described, control this type of bleeding, but it may be necessary to continue compression and massage for 30–45 minutes or longer. As previously mentioned, transvaginal ultrasound may aid in diagnosis of retained placental products. If imaging studies suggest intracavitary tissue, curettage is warranted.

Broad-spectrum antibiotics should be started when resuscitation allows. Oxytocin, 10 U intramuscularly every 4 hours or 10–20 U/L intravenous solution by slow continuous infusion, 15-methyl $PGF_{2\alpha}$ (Prostin 15M), 0.25 mg intramuscularly every 2 hours, or ergot alkaloids, eg, methylergonovine maleate, 0.2 mg orally every 6 hours, should be administered for at least 48 hours.

PLACENTA ACCRETA

A layer of decidua normally separates the placental villi and the myometrium at the site of placental implantation. A placenta that directly adheres to the myometrium without an intervening decidual layer is termed placenta accreta.

Classification

A. By Degree of Adherence

1. Placenta accreta vera—Villi adhere to the superficial myometrium.

2. Placenta increta—Villi invade the myometrium.

3. Placenta percreta—Villi penetrate the full thickness of the myometrium.

B. By Amount of Placental Involvement

1. Focal adherence—A single cotyledon is involved.

2. Partial adherence—One or several cotyledons are involved.

3. Total adherence—The entire placenta is involved.

Incidence

Estimates of the incidence of placenta accreta (all forms) vary from 1 in 2000 to 1 in 7000 deliveries. Placenta accreta vera accounts for about 80% of abnormally adherent placentas; placenta increta, 15%; and placenta percreta, 5%. The rate has risen slightly over the last two decades, paralleling the cesarean section rate.

Morbidity & Mortality

The immediate morbidity associated with an abnormally adherent placenta is that associated with any type of postpartum hemorrhage. Massive blood loss and hypotension can occur. Intrauterine manipulation necessary to diagnose and treat placenta accreta may result in uterine perforation and infection. Sterility may occur as a result of hysterectomy performed to control bleeding.

Recurrence may be common with lesser degrees of adherence.

Etiology

Both excessive penetrability of the trophoblast and defective or missing decidua basalis have been suggested as causes of placenta accreta. Histologic examination of the placental implantation site usually demonstrates the absence of the decidua and Nitabuch's layer. Cases of placenta accreta have been seen in the first trimester, suggesting that the process may occur at the time of implantation and not later in gestation.

Although the exact cause is unknown, several clinical situations are associated with placenta accreta, eg, previous cesarean section, placenta previa, grand multiparity, previous uterine curettage, and previously treated Asherman's syndrome.

These conditions share a common possible defect in formation of the decidua basalis. The incidence of placenta accreta in the presence of placenta previa after 1 prior uterine incision is between 14% and 24%, after 2, 23–48%, and after 3 35–50% . The incidence of placenta accreta after successful treatment of Asherman's syndrome may be as high as 15%.

Diagnosis

Adverse effects from placenta accreta in pregnancy or during the course of labor and delivery are uncommon. Rarely, intra-abdominal hemorrhage or placental invasion of adjacent organs prior to labor has occurred, with the diagnosis being made at laparotomy.

The diagnosis of placenta increta prior to delivery based on the lack of the sonolucent area normally seen beneath the implantation site during ultrasonographic examination is a finding confirmed in several reports. Sonographic antenatal diagnosis of the less invasive placental accreta has also been reported. Color Doppler imaging appears to be particularly helpful in diagnosis. MRI has also aided in the diagnosis of placenta accreta. The diagnosis is more often established when no plane of cleavage is found between the placenta or parts of the placenta and the myometrium in the presence of postpartum hemorrhage. Retained placental parts prevent the myometrium from contracting and thereby achieving hemostasis. Bleeding can be brisk. Inspection of the already separated placenta shows that portions are missing, and manual exploration may produce additional placental fragments.

Delayed spontaneous separation of the placenta is also an indication of an unusually adherent placenta. Focal or partial involvement may be manifested as difficulty in establishing a cleavage plane during manual removal of the placenta. Removal of a totally adherent placenta is very difficult. Persistent efforts to manually remove a totally adherent placenta are futile and waste time, and they result in even more blood loss. Preparation for hysterectomy should begin as soon as the diagnosis is suspected.

Management

Fluid and blood replacement should begin as soon as excessive blood loss is diagnosed. It may be necessary to insert a second large-bore intravenous catheter. Evaluation of puerperal hemorrhage should be performed as outlined above.

Conservative treatment of placenta accreta in women of low parity has occasionally succeeded. The placenta (or portions of it) is left in situ if bleeding is minimal and will later slough off. Successful subsequent pregnancies have been reported, although the risk of recurrence of placenta accreta may be high. In up to 72% of cases of placenta accreta, particularly those associated with placenta-previa, hysterectomy is required.

Successful conservative treatment of placenta percreta is rare, but the conservative approach may be a reasonable option if only focal defects are present, blood loss is not excessive, and the patient is interested in preserving fertility. In anticipated cases of severe placenta accreta, preoperative balloon occlusion and embolization of the internal iliac arteries may minimize intraoperative blood losses. There have been several reports of successful embolization in unpredicted cases of placenta accreta as well. However, additional resection of adjacent organs, such as partial cystectomy, may be necessary in placenta percreta.

UTERINE INVERSION

Definition

Uterine inversion is the prolapse of the fundus to or through the cervix so that the uterus is in effect turned inside out. Almost all cases of uterine inversion occur after delivery and may be worsened by excess traction on the cord before placental separation. Nonpuerperal uterine inversion is very rare and is usually associated with tumors (eg, polypoid leiomyomas).

Classification

If the uterus is inverted but does not protrude through the cervix, the inversion is incomplete. In complete inversion, the fundus has prolapsed through the cervix. Occasionally, the entire uterus may prolapse out the vagina.

Puerperal inversion has also been classified on the basis of its duration. Acute inversion occurs immediately after delivery and before the cervix constricts. Once the cervix constricts, the inversion is termed subacute. Chronic inversion is noted more than 4 weeks after delivery. Today, nearly all cases of uterine inversion are of the acute variety and are recognized and treated immediately after delivery.

Incidence

The incidence of uterine inversion has varied in series reported within the past 30 years from 1 in 4000 to 1 in 100,000 deliveries; an incidence of 1 in 20,000 is frequently cited. One worker reported no inversions in over 10,000 personally conducted deliveries. More recent reviews indicate a greater incidence of uterine inversion, approximately 1 in 2000–2500 deliveries.

Morbidity & Mortality

The morbidity and mortality associated with uterine inversion correlate with the degree of hemorrhage, the rapidity of diagnosis, and the effectiveness of treatment.

The immediate morbidity is that associated with any postpartum hemorrhage; however, endomyometritis frequently follows uterine inversion. The intestines and uterine appendages may be injured if they are entrapped by the prolapsed uterine fundus. Death has occurred from uterine inversion, although with prompt recognition, definitive treatment, and vigorous resuscitation, the mortality rate in this condition should be quite low.

Etiology

The exact cause of uterine inversion is unknown, and the condition is not always preventable. The cervix must be dilated and the uterine fundus must be relaxed for inversion to occur. Rapid uterine emptying may contribute to uterine relaxation.

Conditions that may predispose women to uterine inversion include fundal implantation of the placenta, abnormal adherence of the placenta (partial placenta accreta), congenital or acquired weakness of the myometrium, uterine anomalies, protracted labor, previous uterine inversion, intrapartum therapy with magnesium sulfate, strong traction exerted on the umbilical cord, and fundal pressure.

Many cases of uterine inversion result from mismanagement of the third stage of labor in women who are already at risk for developing uterine inversion. The following maneuvers are to be avoided: excessive traction on the umbilical cord, excessive fundal pressure, excessive intra-abdominal pressure, and excessively vigorous manual removal of the placenta.

Diagnosis

The diagnosis of uterine inversion is usually obvious. Shock and hemorrhage are prominent, as is considerable pain. A dark red-blue bleeding mass is palpable and often visible at the cervix, in the vagina, or outside the vagina. A depression in the uterine fundus or even an absent fundus is noted on abdominal examination.

Treatment

Successful management of patients with uterine inversion depends on prompt recognition and treatment. If initial measures fail to relieve the condition, it may progress to the point at which operative treatment or even hysterectomy is necessary. Shock associated with uterine inversion is typically profound. Hemorrhage can be massive, and hypovolemia should be vigorously treated with fluid and blood replacement.

A. Manual Repositioning of the Uterus

Treatment should begin as soon as the diagnosis of uterine inversion is made. Assistance is vital. An initial attempt should be made to reposition the fundus. The inverted fundus, along with the placenta if it is still attached, is slowly and steadily pushed upward in the axis of the uterus (Fig 28–3). If the placenta has not separated, do not remove it until an adequate intravenous infusion has been established.

If the initial attempt fails, induce general anesthesia, preferably with a halogenated agent (eg, halothane) to provide uterine relaxation. Alternatively, 50 μg of IV nitroglycerin may be given as a bolus to relax the uterus and avoid intubation. The dose can be repeated at least once. While awaiting anesthesiology assistance, easily

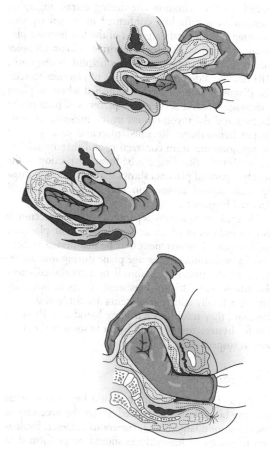

Figure 28–3. Replacement of an inverted uterus.

available tocolytics may be used effectively. Either intravenous magnesium sulfate or terbutaline, 0.25 mg given as a bolus dose intravenously, has been successfully used to achieve uterine relaxation in subacute inversion and neither has been associated with bleeding.

Technique. The operator's fist is placed on the uterine fundus, and the fundus is gradually pushed back into the pelvis through the dilated cervix. The general anesthetic or uterine relaxant is then discontinued. Infusion of oxytocin or ergot alkaloids is started and fluid and blood replacement continued. Alternatively, prostaglandins may be used to effect uterine contraction after repositioning. Bimanual uterine compression and massage are maintained until the uterus is well contracted and hemorrhage has ceased. The placenta can then be removed.

Antibiotics should be started as soon as is practical. Oxytocics or ergot alkaloids are continued for at least 24 hours. Frequent determinations of the hematocrit should be made to ascertain the need for further blood replacement. Iron supplements should begin with resumption of oral intake.

B. Surgical Repositioning of the Uterus

Surgical repositioning of the uterus is rarely necessary in contemporary medical practice in the U.S. However, when all other efforts have failed to reposition the everted uterus, operative intervention may be lifesaving. This is generally accomplished by a vertical incision through the lower uterine segment directly posterior. The uterus is repositioned by either pulling from above or, very rarely, pushing from below (using a sterile glove). The incision is then repaired as would be any uterine incision. Blood replacement, antibiotics, and careful monitoring are necessary for successful perioperative management.

■ ABNORMALITIES OF THE PUERPERIUM

When compared with the dramatic and climactic events of delivery, the puerperium may seem uneventful. Nevertheless, significant physiologic changes occur during this interval, and these undoubtedly influence many of the problems that often arise rapidly and without warning. Hypotension and shock demand urgent treatment and careful follow-up. Cardiac monitoring and insertion of Swan-Ganz or central venous pressure catheters may be prudent to permit rapid evaluation of hemodynamic status. Appropriate medical and surgical consultation is also recommended.

POSTPARTUM & PUERPERAL INFECTIONS

Infections are among the most prominent puerperal complications. An improved understanding of the natural history of female genital infections and the availability of powerful antibiotics may have produced a complacent attitude toward puerperal infections that is as yet unrealistic. Postpartum infections are still costly to both patients and society, and they are associated with an admittedly small but not negligible threat of serious disability and death.

Puerperal morbidity due to infection has occurred if the patient's temperature is higher than 38 °C (100.4 °F) on 2 separate occasions at least 24 hours apart following the first 24 hours after delivery. Overt infections can and do occur in the absence of these criteria, but fever of some degree remains the hallmark of puerperal infection, and the patient with fever can be assumed to have a genital infection until proved otherwise.

Incidence

Puerperal infectious morbidity affects 2–8% of pregnant women and is more common in those of low socioeconomic status, those who have undergone operative delivery, those with premature rupture of the membranes, those with long labors, and those with multiple pelvic examinations.

Morbidity & Mortality

Postpartum infections are responsible for much of the morbidity associated with childbirth, and they either are directly responsible for or contribute to the death of about 8% of all pregnant women who die each year. The costs are also considerable, not only in additional days of hospitalization and medications but also in time lost from work.

Sterility may result from the sequelae of postpartum infections, eg, periadnexal adhesions. Hysterectomy is occasionally required in patients with serious postpartum or postoperative infection.

Pathogenesis

The flora of the birth canal of pregnant women is essentially the same as that of nonpregnant women, although variations in culture techniques and in the study populations have produced markedly different results. The vaginal flora typically includes aerobic and anaerobic organisms that are commonly considered pathogenic (Table 28–1). Several mechanisms appear to prevent overt infection in the genital tract, eg, the

Table 28–1. Percentage of organisms isolated from the vagina or cervix in normal pregnant and nonpregnant women.

Organism	Percentage Isolated
Aerobic bacteria	
Lactobacillus	17–97
Diphtheroids	14–83
Staphylococcus epidermidis	7–67
Staphylococcus aureus	0–12
Alpha-hemolytic streptococci	2–53
Beta-hemolytic streptococci	0–93
Nonhemolytic streptococci	4–37
Group D streptococci	4–44
Escherichia coli	0–28
Gardnerella vaginalis	40–43
Neisseria gonorrhoeae	1–7
Mycoplasma	15–72
Ureaplasma	40–95
Anaerobic bacteria	
Lactobacillis	11–72
Bacteroides fragilis	0–20
Bacteroides species	0–50
Fusobacterium species	0–18
Peptococcus species	0–71
Peptostreptococcus species	12–40
Veillonella species	0–27
Clostridium species	0–17
Bifidobacterium species	0–32
Eubacterium species	0–36

(Reproduced and modified, with permission, from Sweet RL: Perinatal infections: Bacteriology, diagnosis, and management. In: *Principles & Practice of Obstetrics & Perinatology*, 1981. Iffy L, Kaminetzky HA (editors). Copyright © 1981. Reprinted by permission of John Wiley & Sons, Inc.)

acidity of the normal vagina; thick, tenacious cervical mucus; and maternal antibodies to most vaginal flora.

During labor and particularly after rupture of the membranes, some of these protective mechanisms are no longer present. Examinations and invasive monitoring apparatus probably facilitate the introduction of vaginal bacteria into the uterine cavity. Bacteria can be cultured from the amniotic fluid of most women undergoing intrauterine pressure monitoring, but overt postpartum infection is seen in fewer than 10% of these cases. Contractions during labor may spread bacteria present in the amniotic cavity to the adjacent uterine lymphatics and even into the bloodstream.

The postpartum uterus is initially devoid of mechanisms that keep it sterile, and bacteria may be recovered from the uterus in nearly all women in the postpartum period. Whether or not disease is clinically expressed depends on the presence of predisposing factors, the

duration of uterine contamination, and the type and amount of microorganisms involved. The necrosis of decidua and other intrauterine contents (lochia) promotes an increase in the number of anaerobic bacteria, heretofore limited by lack of suitable nutrients and other factors necessary for growth.

Sterility of the endometrial cavity returns by the third or fourth postpartum week. Granulocytes that penetrate the endometrial cavity and the open drainage of lochia are effective in preventing infection in most patients.

Etiology

Almost all postpartum infections are caused by bacteria normally present in the genitalia of pregnant women. The lochia is an excellent culture medium for organisms ascending from the vagina. In women who have undergone cesarean section, more devitalized tissue and foreign bodies (sutures) are present, providing additional fertile ground for possible contamination and subsequent infection. About 70% of puerperal soft tissue infections are mixed infections consisting of both aerobic and anaerobic organisms; infections occurring in women undergoing cesarean section are more likely to be serious.

General Evaluation

The source of infection should be identified, the likely cause determined, and the severity assessed. Most women with fever in the postpartum period have endometritis. Urinary tract infection is the next most common infection. Neglected or virulent endomyometritis may progress to more serious infection. Generalized sepsis, septic pelvic thrombophlebitis, or pelvic abscess may be the end result of an initial infection of the endometrial cavity.

1. Endometritis

Etiology

All of the following circumstances have led to higher than normal postpartum infection rates: prolonged rupture of the membranes (> 24 hours), chorioamnionitis, an excessive number of digital vaginal examinations, prolonged labor (> 12 hours), toxemia, intrauterine pressure catheters (> 8 hours), fetal scalp electrode monitoring, preexisting vaginitis or cervicitis, operative vaginal deliveries, cesarean section, intrapartum and postpartum anemia, poor nutrition, obesity, low socioeconomic status, and coitus near term.

Cesarean section and low socioeconomic class are consistently associated with higher rates of postpartum infection, and cesarean section is easily the most common identifiable risk factor for development of puerperal infection. Some series report an infection rate of 40–80% following cesarean section delivery. Postpartum infection is more likely to be serious after cesarean section than after vaginal delivery. A history of bacterial vaginosis confers a higher risk of postcesarean endometritis.

Clinical Findings

A. SYMPTOMS AND SIGNS

Fever and a soft, tender uterus are the most prominent signs of endometritis. The lochia may or may not have a foul odor. Leukocytosis (white blood cell count > 10,000/(L) is seen. In more severe disease, high fever, malaise, abdominal tenderness, ileus, hypotension, and generalized sepsis may be seen. Movement of the uterus causes increased pain.

1. Fever—Although it is true that the puerperium is a period of high metabolic activity, this factor should not raise the temperature above 37.2 °C (99 °F) and then only briefly in the first 24 hours postpartum. Modest temperature elevations may occur with dehydration. Any woman with a fever over 38 °C (100.4 °F) at any time in the puerperium should be evaluated.

Endometritis results in temperatures ranging from 38 °C to over 40 °C (100.4 °F to over 104 °F), depending on the patient, the causative microorganism, and the extent of infection. The lower range of temperatures is more common. Endometritis usually develops on the second or third postpartum day. Early fever (within hours of delivery) and hypotension are almost pathognomonic for infection with beta-hemolytic streptococci.

2. Uterine tenderness—The uterus is soft and exquisitely tender. Motion of the cervix and uterus may cause increased pain.

Abdominal tenderness is generally limited to the lower abdomen and does not lateralize. A carefully performed baseline examination should include an adnexal evaluation. Adnexal masses palpable on abdominal or pelvic examination are not seen in uncomplicated endometritis, but tubo-ovarian abscess may be a later complication of an infection originally confined to the uterus. Bowel sounds may be decreased and the abdomen distended and tympanitic.

Pelvic examination confirms the findings disclosed by abdominal examination.

B. LABORATORY FINDINGS

1. Hematologic findings—Leukocytosis is a normal finding during labor and the immediate puerperal period. White blood cell counts may be as high as 20,000/μL in the absence of infection; higher counts

may thus be anticipated in infection. Bacteremia is present in 5–10% of women with uncomplicated endometritis. *Mycoplasma* is also frequently recovered from the blood of patients with postpartum fever. Infections with *Bacteroides* as the predominant organism are frequently associated with positive blood cultures.

2. Urinalysis—Urinalysis should be routinely performed in patients thought to have endometritis, since urinary tract infections are often associated with a clinical picture similar to that of mild endometritis. If pyuria and bacteria are noted in a properly collected specimen, appropriate antibiotic therapy for urinary tract infections should be started and a portion of the specimen sent for culture.

3. Lochia cultures—Bacteria colonizing the cervical canal and ectocervix can almost always be recovered from lochia cultures, but these may not be the same organisms causing endometritis. Accurate cultures can be achieved only if specimens obtained transcervically are free from vaginal contamination. Material should be obtained using a speculum to allow direct visualization of the cervix and a gloved culture device (a swab that is covered while it is passed through a contaminated area, then uncovered to obtain a culture from the desired area). Transabdominal aspiration of uterine contents does secure an uncontaminated specimen, but routine use of this technique is probably not justified, and confirmation of placement within the uterine cavity may be difficult. Unless special means are taken to prevent cervical contamination and to ensure the recovery of anaerobic species, results of lochia cultures must be interpreted with great care.

4. Bacteriologic findings—Although the organisms responsible for puerperal infections vary considerably from hospital to hospital, most puerperal infections are due to anaerobic streptococci, gram-negative coliforms, *Bacteroides* species, and aerobic streptococci. *Chlamydia* and *Mycoplasma* are also implicated in many postpartum infections, but clinical isolates are rare because of the difficulty in culturing these organisms. Gonococci are recovered in varying degrees. The percentage of representative microorganisms recovered from women with endometritis is set forth in Table 28–2.

Patterns of bacterial isolates in puerperal infections in the patient's hospital are more important in guiding selection of appropriate antibiotics than are studies from the literature.

a. Aerobic bacteria—Group A streptococci are no longer a major cause of postpartum infection, but infection with these organisms still occurs occasionally. If more than an isolated instance of infection due to these streptococci occurs, immediate measures should be

Table 28–2. Percentage of organisms recovered from women with postpartum endomyometritis.

Organism	Percentage Isolated
Aerobic bacteria	
Group A streptococci	2–6
Group B streptococci	6–21
Group D streptococci	3–14
Enterococcus	12–21
Other streptococci	32
Staphylococcus epidermidis	28
Staphylococcus aureus	10
Escherichia coli	13–36
Gonococci	1–40
Gardnerella vaginalis	16
Anaerobic bacteria	
Bacteriodes fragilis	19–75
Bacteroides species	17–100
Peptococcus	4–40
Peptostreptococcus	15–54
Veillonella species	10
Clostridium species	4–32

taken to halt a potential epidemic. Penicillin is highly effective.

In as many as 30% of women with clinically recognized endometritis, group B streptococci are partly or wholly responsible for the infection. Classic presenting signs are high fever and hypotension shortly after delivery. However, group B streptococci are commonly recovered from the vaginas of pregnant women whether or not they have endometritis. Why some women with positive cultures develop serious illness whereas others do not undoubtedly depends on the presence of predisposing factors as well as other, as yet unknown, elements. It is interesting that positive cultures in women do not correlate well with incidence of streptococcal infection in their newborns. Penicillin is the treatment of choice for patients with endometritis.

Group D streptococci, which include *S faecalis,* are common isolates in endometritis. Ampicillin in high doses is the treatment of choice. Aminoglycosides are also effective against this group.

Staphylococcus aureus is not commonly seen in cultures from women with postpartum infections of the uterus. *S epidermidis* is frequently recovered from women with postpartum infections. These organisms are typically not seen in pure culture. When established staphylococcal infections require treatment, nafcillin, cloxacillin, or cephalosporins should be used.

Among the gram-negative aerobic organisms likely to be recovered in postpartum uterine infections, *Escherichia coli* is the most common. In postpartum uterine infections, *E coli* is more likely to be isolated from seriously ill patients, whereas in urinary tract infections, it is the most commonly isolated organism but is not necessarily found in the sickest patients. Hospital-acquired *E coli* is most susceptible to aminoglycosides and cephalosporins.

The incidence of *Neisseria gonorrhoeae* is 2–8% in pregnant women antepartum. Unless repeat screening examinations and treatment of patients with positive cultures are undertaken in women near term, the incidence of asymptomatic endocervical gonorrhea at delivery is probably only slightly less, and it is reasonable to believe that some cases of puerperal endometritis are gonococcal in origin.

Gardnerella vaginalis, a cause of vaginitis, is seen in isolates from women with postpartum infections, usually in those with a polymicrobial cause, although pure isolates have been reported.

Other gram-negative bacilli that are commonly encountered on medical and surgical wards (eg, *Klebsiella pneumoniae, Enterobacter, Proteus,* and *Pseudomonas* species) are uncommon causes of endometritis.

b. Anaerobic bacteria—Anaerobic bacteria are involved in puerperal infections of the uterus in at least 50% and perhaps as many as 95% of cases. They are much less commonly seen in urinary tract infections. Anaerobic peptostreptococci and peptococci are commonly recovered in specimens from women with postpartum infection, particularly with other anaerobic species. Clindamycin, chloramphenicol, and the newer cephalosporins are active against these organisms.

Bacteroides species and in particular *B fragilis* are commonly found in mixed puerperal infections. These are likely to be the more serious infections (eg, puerperal pelvic abscess, cesarean section wound infections, and septic pelvic thrombophlebitis). When infection with this organism is suspected or confirmed, clindamycin, chloramphenicol, or third-generation cephalosporins should be used.

Gram-positive anaerobic organisms are represented only by *Clostridium perfringens,* which is not infrequently isolated from an infected uterus but which is a rare cause of puerperal infection.

c. Other organisms—*Mycoplasma* and *Ureaplasma* species are common genital pathogens that have been isolated from the genital tract and blood of postpartum women both with and without overt infection. These pathogens are frequently found in the presence of other bacteria. The role of these organisms in puerperal infections is unknown.

Chlamydia trachomatis is now thought to be the leading cause of pelvic inflammatory disease in some populations. Since the population most at risk for pelvic inflammatory disease is the same as that most likely to become pregnant, it is not surprising that *Chlamydia* is in some way involved in puerperal infections, but it is infrequently isolated as a cause of early postpartum endometritis. *Chlamydia* is more frequently associated with mild late-onset endometritis, so cultures for this organism should be obtained from patients with endometritis diagnosed several days after delivery. *Chlamydia* is difficult to culture, and it is possible that as more effective culture techniques become available, the place of this organism in the morbidity associated with postpartum infections may be clarified.

Differential Diagnosis

In the immediate postpartum period, involuntary chills are common and are not necessarily an indication of overt infection. Lower abdominal pain is also common as the uterus undergoes involution with continuing contractions.

Extragenital infections are much less common than endometritis and urinary tract infections. Most of them can be effectively ruled out by history and examination alone. Patients should be asked, at a minimum, about coughing, chest pain, pain at the insertion site of intravenous catheters, breast tenderness, and leg pain. Examination of the breasts, chest, intravenous catheter insertion site, and leg veins should determine whether these areas might be the source of the postpartum fever. Chest x-rays are rarely of benefit unless signs and symptoms point to a possible pulmonary cause of the fever.

Treatment

The choice of antibiotics for treatment of endometritis depends on the suspected causative organisms and the severity of the disease. If the illness is serious enough to require antibiotics, initial therapy should use intravenous antibiotics in high doses. Factors reinforcing the need for this approach include the large volume of the uterus, the expanded maternal blood volume, the brisk diuresis associated with the puerperium, and the difficulty of achieving adequate tissue concentrations of the antibiotic distal to the thrombosed myometrial blood vessels. Clindamycin plus an aminoglycoside is a standard first-line regimen. There is now good evidence that once-a-day dosing of gentamicin is as effective as the traditional thrice-daily regimen. Single-agent therapy with second- or third-generation cephalosporins is an acceptable alternative.

The response to therapy should be carefully monitored for 24–48 hours. Deterioration or failure to respond both clinically and on laboratory test results requires a complete reevaluation. Ampicillin is added when the patient has a less than adequate response to the usual regimen, particularly if *Enterococcus* species are suspected.

Intravenous antibiotics are continued until the patient has been afebrile for 24–48 hours. Randomized and prospective trials have shown that additional treatment with oral antibiotics after intravenous therapy is unnecessary. Patients with documented concurrent bacteremia can be treated similarly, unless the patient has persistently positive blood cultures or a staphylococcal species cultured. If the patient remains febrile despite the standard antibiotic regimens, further evaluation should be initiated to look for abscess formation, hematomas, wound infection, and septic pelvic thrombophlebitis.

For patients known to be infected or at extremely high risk for infection at the time of delivery, initial therapy with 2- or 3-drug regimens in which one of the agents is clindamycin is prudent. Single-agent intravenous infusion of broad-spectrum agents such as piperacillin or cefoxitin appears to be equally effective.

2. Urinary Tract Infection

About 2–4% of women develop a urinary tract infection postpartum. Following delivery, the bladder and lower urinary tract remain somewhat hypotonic, and residual urine and reflux result. This altered physiologic state, in conjunction with catheterization, birth trauma, conduction anesthesia, frequent pelvic examinations, and nearly continuous contamination of the perineum, is sufficient to explain the high incidence of lower urinary tract infections postpartum. In many women, preexisting asymptomatic bacteria, chronic urinary tract infections, and anatomic disorders of the bladder, urethra, and kidneys contribute to urinary tract infection postpartum.

Clinical Findings

A. SYMPTOMS AND SIGNS

Urinary tract infection usually presents with dysuria, frequency, urgency, and low-grade fever; however, an elevated temperature is occasionally the only symptom. White blood cells and bacteria are seen in a centrifuged sample of catheterized urine. A urine culture should be obtained. The history should be reviewed for evidence of chronic antepartum infections. If a woman has had an antepartum urinary tract infection, it is likely that postpartum infection is caused by the same organism. Repeated urinary tract infections call for careful postpartum evaluation. Urethral diverticulum, kidney stones, and upper urinary tract anomalies should be ruled out.

Urinary retention postpartum in the absence of regional anesthesia or well after its effects have worn off almost always indicates urinary tract infection.

Pyelonephritis may be accompanied by fever, chills, malaise, and nausea and vomiting. Characteristic signs of kidney involvement associated with pyelonephritis include costovertebral angle tenderness, dysuria, pyuria, and, in the case of hemorrhagic cystitis, hematuria.

B. LABORATORY FINDINGS

E coli is easily the most common organism isolated from infected urine in postpartum women (about 75% of cases). Other gram-negative bacilli are much less likely to be recovered. *E coli* is less likely to be the causative organism in women who have had repeated urinary tract infections in the recent past.

Treatment

Antibiotics with specific activity against the causative organism are the cornerstone of therapy in uncomplicated cystitis. These include sulfonamides, nitrofurantoin, trimethoprim-sulfamethoxazole, oral cephalosporins (cephalexin, cephradine), and ampicillin. Some hospitals report a high incidence of microbial resistance to ampicillin. The oral combination of amoxicillin-clavulanic acid provides a better spectrum of bacterial sensitivity. Sulfa antibiotics can be used safely in women who are breastfeeding if the infants are term without hyperbilirubinemia or suspected glucose-6-phosphate dehydrogenase deficiency. High fluid intake should be encouraged.

Pyelonephritis requires initial therapy with high doses of intravenous antibiotics, eg, ampicillin, 8–12 g/d, or first-generation cephalosporins (cefazolin, 3–6 g/d; cephalothin, 4–8 g/d). An aminoglycoside can be added when resistant organisms are suspected or when the patient has clinical signs of sepsis. A long-acting third-generation cephalosporin such as ceftriaxone, 1–2 g every 12 hours, may also be used. The response to therapy may be rapid, but some women respond with gradual defervescence over 48 hours or longer. Urine cultures should be obtained to guide any necessary modifications in drug therapy if the patient's response is not prompt. Even with prompt resolution of fever, antibiotic therapy should be continued intravenously or orally for a total of 10 days of therapy. Urine for culture should also be obtained at a postpartum visit after therapy has been completed.

3. Pneumonia

Women with obstructive lung disease, smokers, and those undergoing general anesthesia have an increased risk of developing pneumonia postpartum.

Clinical Findings

A. SYMPTOMS AND SIGNS

Symptoms and signs are the same as those of pneumonia in nonpregnant patients: productive cough, chest pain, fever, chills, rales, and infiltrates on chest x-ray. In some cases, careful differentiation from pulmonary embolus is required.

B. X-RAY AND LABORATORY FINDINGS

Chest x-ray confirms the diagnosis of pneumonia. Gram-stained smears of sputum and material for culture should be obtained.

Streptococcus pneumoniae and *Mycoplasma pneumoniae* are the 2 most likely causative organisms. *S pneumoniae* can easily be identified on gram-stained smears. Infection with *M pneumoniae* can be suspected on clinical grounds.

Treatment

Appropriate antibiotics, oxygen (if the patient is hypoxic), intravenous hydration, and pulmonary toilet are the mainstays of therapy.

4. Cesarean Section Wound Infection

Incidence

Wound infection occurs in 4–12% of patients following cesarean section.

Etiology

The following risk factors predispose to subsequent wound infection in women undergoing cesarean section: obesity, diabetes, prolonged hospitalization before cesarean section, prolonged rupture of the membranes, chorioamnionitis, endomyometritis, prolonged labor, emergency rather than elective indications for cesarean section, and anemia.

Clinical Findings

A. SYMPTOMS AND SIGNS

Fever with no apparent cause which persists to the fourth or fifth postoperative day strongly suggests a wound infection. Wound erythema and tenderness may not be evident until several days after surgery. Occasionally, wound infections are manifested by spontaneous drainage, often accompanied by resolution of fever and relief of local tenderness. Rarely, a deep-seated wound infection becomes apparent when the skin overtly separates, usually after some strenuous activity by the patient.

B. Laboratory Findings

Gram-stained smears and culture of material from the wound may be helpful in guiding selection of the initial antibiotic. Blood cultures may be positive in the patient with systemic sepsis due to wound infection. The organisms responsible for most wound infections originate on the patient's skin. *S aureus* is the organism most commonly isolated. *Streptococcus* species, *E coli,* and other gram-negative organisms that may originally have colonized the amniotic cavity are also seen. Occasionally, *Bacteroides,* which comes only from the genital tract, is isolated from material taken from serious wound infections.

Rarely, necrotizing fasciitis and the closely related synergistic bacterial gangrene can involve cesarean section incisions. They are recognized by their intense tissue destruction and rapid extension. Radical debridement of necrotic and infected tissue is the cornerstone of treatment.

Treatment

A. Initial Evaluation

The incision should be opened along its entire length and the deeper portion of the wound gently explored to determine whether fascial separation has occurred. If the fascia is not intact, the wound is dissected to the fascial level, debrided, and repaired. Wound dehiscence has a high mortality rate and should be treated aggressively. Dehiscence is uncommon in healthy patients and with Pfannenstiel incisions. The skin may be left open to undergo delayed closure or to heal by primary intention.

If the fascia is intact, the wound infection can be treated by local measures.

B. Definitive Measures

Mechanical cleansing of the wound is the mainstay of therapy for cesarean wound infection. Opening the wound encourages drainage of infected material. The wound may be packed with saline-soaked gauze 2–3 times per day, which will remove necrotic debris each time the wound is unpacked. The wound may be left open to heal, or it may be closed secondarily when granulation tissue has begun to form.

Antibiotic Prophylaxis for Cesarean Section

The high rate of infection (averaging 35–40%) following cesarean section is reason enough to consider prophylactic perioperative antibiotic administration in high-risk patients. If possible, a single drug should be used because of the convenience. The drug should have a wide spectrum of activity, including reasonably good activity against pathogens likely to be present at the incision site. The dosage regimen should be designed to ensure adequate tissue levels at the time the operation begins or shortly thereafter. The drug should not be one that is used to treat serious, established infections. The duration of therapy should be short. (Antibiotics administered for more than 48 hours can hardly be called prophylactic.) The drug should be free of major side effects and should be relatively inexpensive.

One drug commonly used is cefazolin, 1 g intravenously, when the umbilical cord is clamped, followed by 2 similar doses at 6-hour intervals. A single dose has been shown to be as effective as a 3-dose regimen. Almost all studies of the use of prophylactic antibiotics in patients with cesarean section deliveries have shown significant reductions in the incidence of infection, regardless of the drugs, doses, and schedules used. However, no regimen has provided total protection against the incidence of fever and associated morbidity, nor has one completely prevented serious postoperative infections. Low-risk women, ie, those undergoing elective cesarean section who are not in active labor, do not benefit to the same degree from prophylactic antibiotics.

5. Episiotomy Infection

It is surprising that infected episiotomies do not occur more often than they do, since contamination at the time of delivery is universal. Subsequent contamination during the healing phase must also be common, yet infection and disruption of the wound are infrequent—0.5–3%. The excellent local blood supply is suggested as an explanation for this phenomenon.

Etiology

In general, the more extensive the laceration or episiotomy, the greater the chances for infection and breakdown of the wound. More tissue is devitalized in a large episiotomy, thereby providing greater opportunity for contamination. Women with infections elsewhere in the genital area are probably at greater risk for infection of the episiotomy.

Clinical Findings

A. Symptoms and Signs

Pain at the episiotomy site is the most common symptom. Spontaneous drainage is frequent, so a mass rarely forms. Incontinence of flatus and stool may be the presenting symptom of an episiotomy that breaks down and heals spontaneously.

Inspection of the episiotomy site shows disruption of the wound and gaping of the incision. A necrotic membrane may cover the wound and should be debrided if possible. A careful rectovaginal examination should be performed to determine whether a rectovaginal fistula has formed. The integrity of the anal sphincter should also be evaluated.

B. LABORATORY FINDINGS

Infection with mixed aerobic and anaerobic organisms is common. *Staphylococcus* may be recovered from cultures of material from these infections. Culture results are frequently misleading, since the area of the episiotomy is typically contaminated with a wide variety of pathogenic bacteria.

Treatment

Initial treatment should be directed toward opening and cleaning the wound and promoting the formation of granulation tissue. Warm sitz baths or Hubbard tank treatments help the debridement process. Attempts to close an infected, disrupted episiotomy are likely to fail and may make ultimate closure more difficult. Surgical closure by perineorrhaphy should be undertaken only after granulation tissue has thoroughly covered the wound site. There is an increasing trend towards early repair of episiotomy wound dehiscence, in contrast to conventional wisdom, which suggests a 3- to 4-month delay. Several large case series show excellent results once initial infection is treated.

6. Mastitis

Congestive mastitis, or breast engorgement, is more common in primigravidas than in multiparas. Infectious mastitis and breast abscesses are also more common in women pregnant for the first time and are seen almost exclusively in nursing mothers.

Etiology

Infectious mastitis and breast abscesses are uncommon complications of breastfeeding. They almost certainly occur as a result of trauma to the nipple and the subsequent introduction of organisms from the infant's nostrils to the mother's breast. *S aureus* contracted by the infant while in the hospital nursery is the usual causative agent.

Clinical Findings

A. SYMPTOMS AND SIGNS

Breast engorgement usually occurs on the second or third postpartum day. The breasts are swollen, tender,

tense, and warm. The patient's temperature may be mildly elevated. Axillary adenopathy can be seen.

Mastitis presents 1 week or more after delivery. Usually only 1 breast is affected and often only 1 quadrant or lobule. It is tender, reddened, swollen, and hot. There may be purulent drainage, and aspiration may produce pus. The patient is febrile and appears ill.

B. LABORATORY FINDINGS

The organism responsible for infectious mastitis and breast abscess is almost always *S aureus*. *Streptococcus* species and *E coli* are occasionally isolated. Leukocytosis is evident.

Treatment

A. CONGESTIVE MASTITIS

The form of treatment depends on whether or not the patient plans to breastfeed. If she does not, tight breast binding, ice packs, restriction of breast stimulation, and analgesics help to relieve pain and suppress lactation. Medical suppression of lactation probably does not hasten involution of congested breasts unless it is begun very early after delivery. Bromocriptine, 2.5 mg twice daily orally for 10 days, is an effective regimen, though concerns about its side-effect profile have curtailed its use. For the woman who is breastfeeding, manually emptying the breasts following infant feeding is all that is necessary to relieve discomfort.

B. INFECTIOUS MASTITIS

Infectious mastitis is treated in the same way as congestive mastitis. Local heat and support of the breasts help to reduce pain. Cloxacillin, dicloxacillin, nafcillin, or a cephalosporin—antibiotics with activity against the commonly encountered causative organisms—should be administered. Infants tolerate the small amount of antibiotics in breast milk without difficulty. It may be prudent to check the infant for possible colonization with the same bacteria present in the mother's breast.

If an abscess is present, incision and drainage are necessary. The cavity should be packed open with gauze, which is then advanced toward the surface in stages daily. Most authorities recommend cessation of breastfeeding when an abscess develops. Antistaphylococcal antibiotics should be prescribed. Inhibition of lactation is also recommended.

DISORDERS OF LACTATION

Inhibition & Suppression of Lactation

Anatomic alteration of the breasts during pregnancy prepares them for sustained milk production shortly after delivery. The rapid decrease of serum estrogen and progesterone levels postpartum does not occur in prolactin levels, which decrease much more slowly. The breast is no longer subject to the inhibitory effects of the steroid hormones and now comes under the influence of high prolactin levels to begin sustained milk production.

Colostrum is secreted in late pregnancy and for the first 2–3 days postpartum. It is higher in protein (much of which may be antibodies) and minerals and lower in carbohydrates and fat than is later breast milk. Prior to full milk production, from the second to the fourth postpartum days, the breasts become enlarged, engorged, and tender. The breast lobules enlarge, and alveoli and blood vessels proliferate. Milk production truly begins around the third or fourth postpartum day. Fortuitously, infants may frequently take this long to feel a sensation of hunger and develop the neuromuscular control necessary to successfully empty the breast.

In spite of the manifold benefits of breastfeeding for both infants and mothers, at least a third of all women who give birth today do not wish to nurse, and perhaps an additional 10–20% discontinue attempts within a few weeks of delivery. For these women, inhibition of lactation for relief of breast congestion and tenderness may be necessary.

A. Physical Methods of Suppression of Lactation

Inhibition of physical stimuli that encourage milk secretion can prevent lactation. Tight breast binding, avoidance of any tactile breast stimulation, ice packs, and mild analgesics (eg, aspirin or ibuprofen) are effective in inhibiting lactation and relieving the symptoms of breast engorgement in 50% of women. Physical methods successfully inhibit lactation and prevent breast engorgement either before the onset of lactation or after it has been established for some time.

B. Hormonal Suppression of Lactation

Large doses of estrogen alone have been used to suppress lactation; they do inhibit milk production, probably by acting directly on the breast. Estrogens are somewhat more successful than physical methods alone. Side effects are tolerable in young women who have had vaginal deliveries, but increased rates of thrombophlebitis and pulmonary embolism are seen in women over age 35, in those who have undergone cesarean section, and in those with difficult deliveries. For these reasons, pure estrogens are no longer used for suppression of lactation as they once were. Furthermore, drug-induced suppression of lactation is not very effective after lactation has been established.

An ergot derivative, bromocriptine, has strong prolactin-inhibiting and thus lactation-inhibiting properties. In the dosage ranges used to suppress lactation, the drug is relatively free of serious side effects. Minor side effects include nausea and nasal congestion. More serious associations with hypertension, cerebrovascular accidents, and myocardial infarction have also been reported. The risks seem to be reported frequently when bromocriptine is used in patients with pregnancy-induced hypertension. Drawbacks of bromocriptine therapy include the necessity for prolonged treatment (10–14 days) and a more rapid resumption of ovulation. A significant number of women have rebound lactation (18–40%). The Food and Drug Administration removed painful breast engorgement as an indication for the use of bromocriptine in 1989. The FDA noted that although there is no clear proof of adverse effects of these medications, there is no proved health benefit, so even minor safety concerns become significant, because of their potential unfavorable effects on the benefit-risk ratio. In women with severe congestive mastitis, bromocriptine may be a reasonable treatment option.

Inappropriate Lactation

Lactation is physiologic in late pregnancy and for a considerable period of time after delivery. In the woman who has not lactated for 1 year or more or who has never been pregnant, lactation may indicate a significant endocrinopathy.

POSTPARTUM MONITORING

Serious and acute obstetric and postanesthetic complications often occur during the first few hours immediately following delivery. The patient should therefore be transferred to a recovery room where she can be constantly attended to and where observation of bleeding, blood pressure, pulse, and respiratory change can be made every 15 minutes for at least 1–2 hours after delivery or until the effects of general or major regional anesthesia have disappeared. On return to the patient's room or ward, the patient's blood pressure should be taken and the measurement repeated every 12 hours for the first 24 hours and daily thereafter for several days. Preeclampsia-eclampsia, infection, or other medical or surgical complications of pregnancy may require more prolonged and intensive postpartum care.

POSTPARTUM COMPLICATIONS

1. Complications of Anesthesia

The most common respiratory complications that follow general anesthesia and delivery are airway obstruction or laryngospasm and vomiting with aspiration of vomitus. Bronchoscopy, tracheostomy, and other related procedures must be done promptly as indicated.

Hypoventilation and hypotension may follow an abnormally high subarachnoid block. Because serum cholinesterase activity is lower during labor and the postpartum period, hypoventilation during the early puerperium may also follow the use of large amounts of succinylcholine during anesthesia for cesarean section. Brief postpartum shivering is commonly seen after completion of the third stage of labor and is no cause for alarm. The cause of the shivering is unknown, but it may be related to loss of heat, or it may be a sympathetic response. Subcutaneous emphysema may make its appearance postpartum after vigorous bearing-down efforts. Most cases resolve spontaneously.

Hypertension in the immediate puerperium is most often due to excessive use of vasopressor or oxytocic drugs. It must be treated promptly with a vasodilator. Hydralazine, 5 mg administered slowly intravenously, usually reduces the blood pressure.

Postanesthetic complications that manifest themselves later in the puerperium include postsubarachnoid puncture headache, atelectasis, renal or hepatic dysfunction, and neurologic sequelae.

Postpuncture headache is usually located in the forehead, deep behind the eyes; occasionally, the pain radiates to both temples and to the occipital region. It usually begins on the first or second postpartum day and lasts 1–3 days. Because new mothers frequently develop various types of headache, the correct diagnosis is essential. An important characteristic of postspinal puncture headache is increased pain in the sitting or standing position and significant improvement when the patient is supine. The mild form is relieved by aspirin or other analgesics. Headache is due to leakage of cerebrospinal fluid through the site of dural puncture into the extradural space. It is advisable to supplement the daily oral intake of fluids with at least 1 L of 5% glucose in saline intravenously. Administration of 7–10 mL of the patient's own blood into the thecal space at the point of previous needle insertion will "patch" the leaking point and relieve the headache in most patients. Subdural hematoma is a rare complication of chronic leakage of cerebrospinal fluid and resultant loss of support to intracranial structures.

A small percentage of women who develop headaches during this time also show symptoms of meningeal irritation. Headache due to aseptic chemical meningitis is not relieved by lying down. Lumbar puncture reveals a slightly elevated pressure and an increase in spinal fluid protein and white blood cells but no bacteria. Symptoms usually disappear 1–3 days later, and the spinal fluid returns to normal within 4 days with no sequelae. Treatment is conservative and includes supportive measures, analgesics, and fluids.

Neurologic problems in the puerperium sometimes follow traumatic childbirth, eg, injury to the femoral nerve caused by forceps when the patient was in the lithotomy position. Such complications are rarely bilateral, which aids in the differential diagnosis of a spinal cord lesion. Evidence of more serious neurologic sequelae following regional or general anesthesia for delivery requires consultation with the anesthesiologist or a neurologist.

2. Postpartum Cardiac Problems

The puerperium is relatively complicated for the patient with congenital or acquired heart disease. Following delivery, the cardiovascular system responds with sharply increased cardiac output as a result of unimpeded venous return from the lower extremities and pelvis. This produces a relative bradycardia that may persist for several days. For the initial few days after delivery, the intracellular water and sodium retained during pregnancy are mobilized and contribute to increasing cardiac output. A concomitant postpartum diuresis gradually mitigates the bradycardia and increases cardiac output (see Chapter 7).

Valvular Heart Disease

The management principles underlying treatment of valvular heart disease in the postpartum period are those begun in the intrapartum period: antibiotic prophylaxis of bacterial endocarditis, careful fluid and electrolyte administration, accurate (often continuous invasive) monitoring, and frequent physical examination to detect changes in cardiovascular status. Return to an ambulatory state soon after delivery reduces the possibility of thrombophlebitis. The postpartum period is also a time for the patient to carefully consider further childbearing options in light of the fetal outcome and the possible progression of heart disease during the antecedent pregnancy.

Women whose valvular heart disease required systemic anticoagulation before delivery should continue the treatment postpartum; however, oral anticoagulants may be used instead of heparin. There are no reports of problems in term breastfed infants of women taking warfarin or dicumarol. Other oral anticoagulants are contraindicated if the patient is breastfeeding.

Postpartum Cardiomyopathy

A cardiomyopathy unique to the latter half of pregnancy and the puerperium has been described by numerous investigators. The incidence is estimated to be 1 in 4000 deliveries. Congestive heart failure, cardiomegaly, and cardiac arrhythmias develop in otherwise healthy young women. A number of causes—viral, immunologic, toxic, and genetic—have been suggested, but none has been confirmed. An incidence of myocarditis between 8% and 29% has been reported. The clinical presentation of disease and the appearance of heart muscle on histologic examination do not differ from those of idiopathic cardiomyopathy.

Patients with postpartum cardiomyopathy are generally in their mid 20s to early 30s. The disease is more common in blacks and parous women. Twin pregnancy is reported in 7–10% of patients with this disorder. Patients usually present a few days to several weeks postpartum in florid congestive heart failure. Treatment with digitalis, diuretics, oxygen, bedrest, and salt restriction relieves symptoms in most cases. Cardiac function returns to normal within 6 months in over 50% of women with this disorder. Slow improvement, continued cardiac symptoms, or deterioration characterizes the course of other patients. Recurrence of disease in a subsequent pregnancy has been described but is not inevitable. Cardiac transplantation has been used successfully in a few women with severe progressive disease. Brown and Bertolet have reviewed the literature on this disorder.

3. Postpartum Pulmonary Problems

Return to nonpregnant pulmonary physiology occurs by 6 weeks after delivery. Except for women undergoing general anesthesia, the puerperium is not a time of special concern. The factors placing pregnant women at risk for highly destructive chemical aspiration pneumonitis (gastric pH < 2.5 and fasting gastric contents > 25 mL) persist for at least 48 hours after delivery. Thus, women undergoing general anesthesia in the puerperium (eg, for tubal ligation) are at a high risk for aspiration. A nonparticulate antacid should be used preoperatively for women undergoing general anesthesia in the puerperal period as well as other anesthetic techniques (rapid sequence induction of anesthesia, endotracheal intubation, and preanesthetic fasting) designed to prevent aspiration of gastric contents.

Pulmonary hypertension, either primary or secondary to congenital heart disease, is an overt threat to the mother's life in the intrapartum and postpartum periods. The most important management principle is to use invasive monitoring to avoid hypovolemia (see Chapter 59).

4. Postpartum Thyroiditis

Thyroid abnormalities, particularly of immunologic origin, are common in the postpartum period. Though there are racial differences, between 3% and 17% of women will develop postpartum thyroiditis, and over half of these women will have positive microsomal antibody titers. Patients with known Graves disease are at

particular risk; even if they are euthyroid at time of delivery, about 10% will experience postpartum hyperthyroidism. Postpartum thyroiditis usually presents with mild transient hyperthyroidism 1–3 months postpartum, followed by mild and transient hypothyroidism. Suppression of hyperthyroid symptoms or temporary thyroid hormone supplementation may be necessary, but most women recover completely and are euthyroid within 6–9 months after delivery. The recurrence risk for postpartum thyroiditis in a subsequent pregnancy is 10–25%.

5. Postpartum Thrombophlebitis & Thromboembolism

Historically, the puerperium has been known as the time when severe thrombophlebitic conditions and pulmonary embolism occur, probably as a result of the once-prevalent recommendation of prolonged bedrest following parturition. Even though contemporary postpartum management encourages early ambulation, puerperal thrombophlebitis and thromboembolism remain a serious problem.

Thrombophlebitis requires careful and prolonged medical management. The risk of recurrence in a subsequent pregnancy is substantial, and a history of thrombophlebitis may prohibit the future use of oral contraceptives and replacement estrogens.

The incidence of thrombophlebitic conditions is difficult to estimate since the clinical diagnosis of these disorders is highly unreliable. One study of venographically confirmed deep venous thrombosis reported 1.3 antepartum cases per 10,000 deliveries and 6.1 postpartum cases per 10,000 deliveries. Most studies confirm that the incidence of superficial thrombophlebitis, deep venous thrombosis, and pulmonary embolism is 2–6 times higher in the postpartum period than in the antepartum period, though these data may be influenced by the effects of the prolonged postpartum bedrest once advocated. (Methods of diagnosis and treatment of thromboembolic conditions are discussed in Chapter 22.)

6. Postpartum Neuropsychiatric Complications

Peripheral Nerve Palsy

Nerve palsies involving pelvic nerves or parts of the lumbosacral plexus result from pressure by the presenting part or trauma by obstetric forceps. Typically, the palsy occurs after prolonged labor in a nullipara, and presents as unilateral footdrop noted when ambulation resumes after delivery. Most cases resolve spontaneously in a matter of days or weeks. A few may have a more protracted course. Electromyography may help in predicting the course of the disorder.

Seizures

Postpartum seizures immediately raise the possibility of eclampsia, but if the interval since delivery is greater than 48 hours, other etiologies should be considered. In the absence of a prior history of epilepsy or signs of pregnancy-induced hypertension, a thorough evaluation to determine the cause of the seizures must be performed.

Postpartum Depression

Considering the excitement, anticipation, and tension associated with imminent delivery; the marked hormonal alterations following delivery; and the substantial new burdens and responsibilities that result from childbirth, it is not surprising that some women experience depression after delivery. The incidence of postpartum depression is difficult to estimate, but the disorder is common. The disorder in its usual form is self-limited and benign. However, hypothyroidism is emerging as a cause for some cases of postpartum depression and screening for this disorder should be considered if suggested by clinical presentation.

In women who suffered from depression before they became pregnant and in those without effective support mechanisms, the severity of depression may be more profound and the consequences far more serious. An openly psychotic state may develop within a few days after delivery and render the woman incapable of caring for herself or her newborn. In some cases she may harm her infant and herself.

Psychiatric consultation should be obtained for the postpartum woman who shows symptoms of severe depression or overt psychosis. Nursery personnel are often the first to notice that the new mother does not devote the usual amount of attention to her newborn (see Chapter 60).

REFERENCES

B-Lynch et al: The B-Lynch surgical technique for the control of massive postpartum hemorrhage: an alternative to hysterectomy? Five cases reported. Br J Obstet Gynecol 1997; 104:372.

Brown CS, Bertolet BD: Peripartum cardiomyopathy: a comprehensive review. Obstet Gynecol 1998;178:408.

Capella-Allouc S et al: Hysteroscopic treatment of severe Asherman's syndrome and subsequent fertility. Hum Reprod 1999;14:1230.

Dubois J et al: Placenta percreta: balloon occlusion and embolization of the internal iliac arteries to reduce intraoperative blood losses. Am J Obstet Gynecol 1997;176:723.

Khan GQ et al: Controlled cord traction versus minimal intervention techniques in delivery of the placenta: a randomized control study. Am J Obstet Gynecol 1997;177:770.

Lokumamage AU et al: A randomized study comparing rectally administered misoprostol versus Syntometrine combined with an oxytocin infusion for the cessation of primary post partum hemorrhage. Acta Obstet Gynecol Scand 2001;80:835.

Miller DA et al: Clinical risk factors for placenta previa-placenta accreta. Am J Obstet Gynecol 1997;177:210.

Pelage J et al: Life-threatening primary postpartum hemorrhage: treatment with emergency selective arterial embolization. Radiology 1998;208:359.

Rogers J et al: Active versus expectant management of the third stage of labour: the Hinchingbrooke randomised controlled trial. Lancet 1998;351:693.

Terry AJ, Hague WM: Postpartum thyroiditis. Semin Perinat 1998;22:497.

Neonatal Resuscitation & Care of the Newborn at Risk

29

Milena Weinstein, MD

PERINATAL RESUSCITATION

When a high-risk mother and fetus are identified, plans for appropriate management must be made immediately. These plans should take into consideration not only the best time and method of delivery, but also the level of care required by both mother and infant. It may be best to transfer the mother to a tertiary care perinatal center well before delivery, particularly if she is to be delivered before term. Such planning requires the combined efforts of obstetricians, pediatricians, perinatologists, neonatologists, and skilled nurses. However, not all high-risk mothers can be transferred prior to delivery, and indeed the delivery of an infant requiring resuscitation cannot always be anticipated. At every delivery, there should be at least one person skilled in all aspects of neonatal resuscitation, and all of the equipment necessary for a complete resuscitation should be present in the delivery room.

Delivery Room Management

Optimal resuscitation of the high-risk, premature, or depressed neonate requires as much notice as possible, and ready communication between the obstetric and pediatric staffs is critical. When a depressed or premature neonate is expected, the resuscitation team should be comprised of a two-person team capable of complete resuscitation. The Apgar score, an objective evaluation of the newborn's condition, is generally assigned at 1 and 5 minutes. Assessment of the infant and necessary interventions should begin immediately at birth, so the Apgar may then be useful as an assessment of the effectiveness of the resuscitation effort.

Figure 29–1 provides an outline that is recommended by the American Academy of Pediatrics (AAP) and the American Heart Association (AHA) for the general care of depressed infants in the delivery room.

A. INITIAL STEPS

The steps in resuscitation begin with preventing heat loss by immediately drying the infant and providing a warm environment (eg, preheated overhead warmer bed), clearing the airway by positioning and suctioning if needed, and assessing adequacy of the infant's breathing. If an infant is not breathing, tactile stimulation while 100% oxygen is administered by face mask is usually sufficient to stimulate breathing. If breathing does not begin within a few seconds, positive pressure ventilation with a bag and mask should be initiated. The pressure required for initial breaths is 30–40 mm Hg. This will expand the lungs, clear fetal lung fluid, and facilitate the increase in pulmonary perfusion that is required in transition from fetal circulation (Fig 29–2). Ventilation should also be initiated if the infant's heart rate (HR) is < 100 beats/min.

B. VENTILATION

Either a small anesthesia bag with a manometer or a small self-inflating bag with an oxygen reservoir may be used, as long as the mask is the proper size to create a seal over the mouth and nose but not over the eyes. A high oxygen concentration (90–100%) should be used. If the infant is profoundly depressed, intubation and ventilation via endotracheal tube may be elected, if staff well-skilled in intubation is present. A respiratory rate of 40–60 breaths/min should be provided at pressures high enough to cause chest wall expansion. The infant's HR should be checked and should be above 100 beats/min. Most infants will respond to adequate expansion of the lung with spontaneous respirations. If not, adequacy of bag and mask ventilation should be checked, or endotracheal intubation should be considered.

C. CHEST COMPRESSIONS

Techniques for infant chest compressions are shown in Figure 29–3. The HR should be 120 beats/min. It is the rare infant that does not respond within 30 seconds of such ventilatory and cardiac resuscitation. If the HR rises, ventilation should continue until regular spontaneous respiration begins. If the infant does not respond, medications should be administered.

D. MEDICATIONS

The use of drugs or volume expansion is rarely needed in the delivery room and should not be given until adequate ventilation and circulation have been established

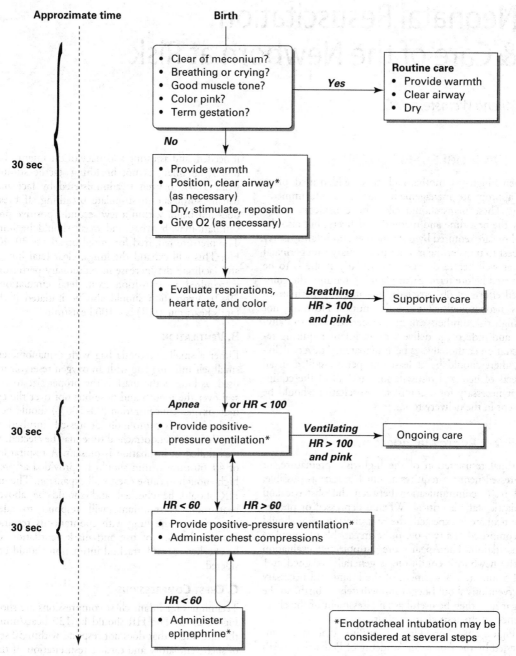

Approximate time

Birth

- Clear of meconium?
- Breathing or crying?
- Good muscle tone?
- Color pink?
- Term gestation?

Yes →

Routine care
- Provide warmth
- Clear airway
- Dry

No

30 sec

- Provide warmth
- Position, clear airway*
  (as necessary)
- Dry, stimulate, reposition
- Give O2 (as necessary)

- Evaluate respirations,
  heart rate, and color

**Breathing
HR > 100
and pink** →

Supportive care

Apnea **or HR < 100**

30 sec

- Provide positive-
  pressure ventilation*

**Ventilating
HR > 100
and pink** →

Ongoing care

HR < 60 **HR > 60**

30 sec

- Provide positive-pressure ventilation*
- Administer chest compressions

HR < 60

- Administer
  epinephrine*

*Endotracheal intubation may be
considered at several steps

Figure 29–1. **Algorithm for resuscitation of the newborn.** (Reproduced, with permission, from *Textbook of Neonatal Resuscitation*, 1987, 1990, 2001. Copyright © American Heart Association.)

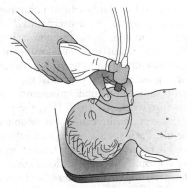

Figure 29–2. The technique of bag and mask ventilation of the newborn. The neck should be slightly extended. An anesthesia bag should have a manometer attached; a self-inflating bag should have an oxygen reservoir attached. (Reproduced, with permission, from *Textbook of Neonatal Resuscitation,* 1987, 1990, 2001. Copyright © American Heart Association.)

Table 29–1. Neonatal resuscitation and newborn infant drug doses.

Epinephrine	(1:10,000) 0.2 mL/kg IV or ET. Give rapidly. Dilute 1:1 with saline for ET use.
Volume Expansion	(whole blood, saline, 5% albumin, Ringer's lactate) 10 mL/kg. Give over 5–10 minutes.
NaHCO₃	(0.5 mEq/mL) 1–2 mEq/kg IV. Give slowly, only if ventilation adequate.
Naloxone	(0.4 mg/mL) 0.1 mg/kg = 0.25 mL/kg IV, ET, IM, SQ. Give rapidly.
Glucose	D₁₀W 2 mL/kg IV. Give over 1–2 minutes.

for a minimum of 30 seconds. Table 29–1 lists the medications used with doses and routes of administration when needed for neonatal resuscitation. The preferred route is intravenously (IV) via the umbilical vein, which can be easily cannulated. However, dilute epinephrine is often effective when given via endotracheal tube (ET), and naloxone can be given IV or ET and may sometimes be effective if given intramuscularly (IM).

Naloxone, a narcotic antagonist, is the first drug to be administered when respiratory depression due to recent maternal narcotic treatment is suspected. Note, however, that naloxone is contraindicated for the infant of a narcotic-addicted mother, since it may elicit imme-

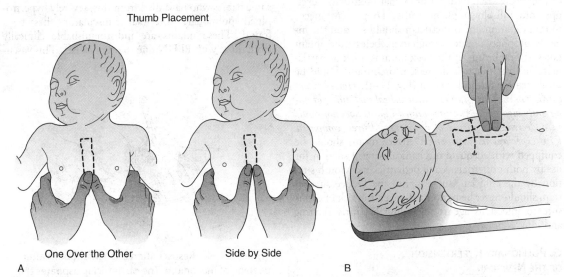

Thumb Placement

One Over the Other   Side by Side

A   B

Figure 29–3. **A.** Thumb technique for performing chest compressions on an infant. The two thumbs, either side by side or overlapping one another, are used to depress the lower third of the sternum, with the hands encircling the torso and the fingers supporting the back. **B.** Two-finger method for performing chest compressions on the infant. The tips of the middle finger and either the index finger or ring finger of one hand are used to compress the lower third of the sternum. (Reproduced, with permission, from *Textbook of Neonatal Resuscitation,* 1987, 1990, 2001. Copyright © American Heart Association.)

diate withdrawal and result in severe seizures. Volume expanders are indicated when acute bleeding and signs of hypovolemia, such as pallor, weak pulses, and hypotension, are present. Sodium bicarbonate may be given when metabolic acidosis is documented or assumed due to prolonged asphyxia, after ventilation is established. Atropine and calcium are not currently thought to be helpful in the acute phase of neonatal resuscitation.

E. INTUBATION

The resuscitator must be skilled in intubation, since failed attempts at intubation may greatly jeopardize an already compromised infant. The heart rate should be constantly monitored during this procedure, since reflex bradycardia resulting from an underlying disorder or stimulation of the hypopharynx may occur. If intubation is unsuccessful within 20–30 seconds or if it is unclear whether the endotracheal tube is in the trachea or the esophagus, ventilation with a bag and mask should be resumed.

F. MECONIUM ASPIRATION

Term and postterm infants who are stressed are likely to pass meconium in utero or during delivery and are at risk of developing meconium aspiration syndrome. Meconium passes slowly from the upper to the lower airways, a pattern that explains the clinical presentation of progressive respiratory distress that eventually develops into full-blown pneumonitis. To prevent meconium aspiration, the obstetrician should suction the infant's oropharynx and nasopharynx before the infant takes its first breath. If the meconium is thick or particulate and the infant is depressed, the infant should be intubated for tracheal suction (Fig 29–4). *However, according to the latest studies, intratracheal suctioning of apparently vigorous meconium-stained infants does not result in a decreased incidence of respiratory distress compared with expectant management.* Delivery rooms should be equipped with adequate mechanical or wall suction for use by both obstetricians and pediatricians. Mouth suction by the clinician, such as into the DeLee suction trap, should never be performed, given the risk of exposure to infectious agents, including hepatitis B virus and HIV.

G. PULMONARY HYPERTENSION OF THE NEWBORN

Perinatal asphyxia as well as meconium aspiration may result in persistent pulmonary hypertension of the newborn (PPHN) (Fig 29–5). Hypoxia, acidosis, and hypercapnia, probably acting through elevated plasma concentrations of potent vasoconstrictors such as thromboxane, prevent the reduction of pulmonary vas-

cular resistance and establishment of pulmonary blood flow that accompany normal delivery. PPHN may also occur in association with sepsis, pulmonary hypoplasia, or congenital diaphragmatic hernia. Treatment consists of vigorous resuscitation and measures to maintain systemic blood pressure with generous use of pressor agents (eg, dopamine and dobutamine) and reduce pulmonary vascular resistance. In PPHN, the pulmonary vasculature is very sensitive to hypoxia and acidosis. When possible, PaO_2 should be maintained in the 80- to 100-mm Hg range. Higher PaO_2 has not been shown to improve outcome and may be detrimental. *The use of inhaled nitric oxide (iNO), a potent and selective pulmonary vasodilator, has improved oxygenation in patients with PPHN and reduced the need for extracorporeal membrane oxygenation (ECMO).* Respiratory acidosis should be corrected, but attempts to induce alkalosis by hyperventilation, although controversial, are no longer standard. Rather, administration of alkali to induce *metabolic* alkalosis can effectively lower pulmonary vascular resistance without contributing to barotrauma and worsening lung disease. Vasodilating agents (eg, tolazoline) can be very useful in lowering pulmonary vascular resistance, but because of potential severe complications are generally reserved for the most refractory pulmonary hypertension. The use of paralytic agents is controversial, but most infants should be sedated with morphine or fentanyl since they are exquisitely sensitive to external stimuli. PPHN can also be idiopathic. In some babies who have died from this, severely hypertrophied pulmonary arteriolar musculature has been found. These infants are indistinguishable clinically from those with PPHN due to other causes. This vascu-

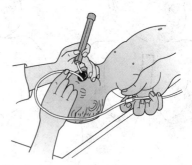

Figure 29–4. Resuscitation of an infant born after passage of meconium. The obstetrician aspirates the oropharynx and nasopharynx with mechanical suction before the infant utters its first cry. The infant is then intubated and the upper airway suctioned. (Reproduced, with permission, from *Textbook of Neonatal Resuscitation,* 1987, 1990, 2001. Copyright © American Heart Association.)

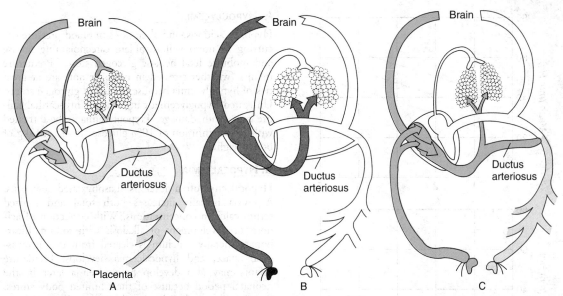

Figure 29–5. **A.** The normal fetal circulation, with saturated blood coursing from the umbilical vein to the right side of the heart. Right-to-left shunting of saturated blood occurs across the ductus arteriosus. **B.** Normal transition to extrauterine life. Some transient left-to-right shunting across the ductus arteriosus may occur. **C.** Persistent pulmonary hypertension. Because of persistence of elevated pulmonary vascular resistance into the neonatal period, little blood flow to the lungs is allowed, and excessive right-to-left shunting of unsaturated blood occurs across the ductus arteriosus.

lar smooth muscle maldevelopment may be a consequence of chronic intrauterine hypoxia or other situations that result in sustained pulmonary hypertension in utero. ECMO is a form of cardiopulmonary bypass that augments systemic perfusion and provides gas exchange. The indications for many of these infants were PPHN with or without meconium aspiration syndrome, pneumonia, or sepsis. Most criteria for treatment with ECMO include failure of conventional medical management such that an 80% chance of death is anticipated. Yet survival rates with ECMO treatment of these patients now exceed 75%. Complications of ECMO include thromboembolism, air embolization, bleeding, stroke, seizures, atelectasis, cholestatic jaundice, thrombocytopenia, neutropenia, hemolysis, infectious complications of blood transfusions, edema formation, and systemic hypertension.

H. METABOLIC ACIDOSIS

As mentioned above, during a resuscitation, bicarbonate should not be given prior to documenting metabolic acidosis with cord blood gas determination and/or arterial blood gas sampled from the infant, and then not until ventilation has been established. After an infant has been resuscitated, stabilization should continue with establishment of venous, and usually arterial, ac-

cess for blood sampling. The base deficit should be calculated, but only a portion ($\frac{1}{4}$–$\frac{1}{2}$) should be given initially. Bicarbonate should always be diluted 1:1 with sterile water (4.2% solution) and given very slowly. Concentrated or rapid doses of bicarbonate, particularly in premature infants, increase the risk of intraventricular hemorrhage. It should not be administered via umbilical venous catheter unless the tip is documented to be in the inferior vena cava, or severe hepatic damage, scarring, and subsequent portal hypertension could result. Frequent arterial blood gases should be followed after treatment.

Blood Pressure

Figure 29–6 shows normal pulse and blood pressure ranges for full term-infants relative to their birthweight. The normal ranges for small preterm infants are generally lower. Infants who have been asphyxiated may be hypovolemic. Hypovolemia may be diagnosed by measuring arterial blood pressure. However, infants who are acidotic may have falsely high arterial blood pressure readings. Noting that the infant is pale with cool extremities and slow capillary filling (> 3 seconds) can help assess the circulatory status. Correction of blood pressure should be achieved slowly unless the infant is

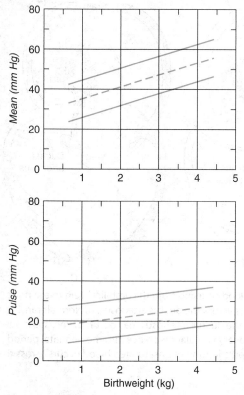

Figure 29–6. Mean and pulse pressures of healthy newborn infants relative to birthweight during the first 12 hours of life. (Reproduced, with permission, from Versmold HT et al: Aortic blood pressure during the first 12 hours of life in infants with birth weight 610–4220 grams. Pediatrics 1981;67:607.)

extremely hypotensive, since premature and term infants have limited autoregulatory capabilities in the cerebrum, and rapid shifts in systemic arterial blood pressure and volume will be immediately reflected in the cerebral vasculature. Such fluctuations may increase the risk of intraventricular hemorrhage in a premature infant and brain damage in a term infant. Hypovolemia is best treated with whole blood; however, 5% albumin or normal saline 10 mL/kg IV can also be used. Uncrossmatched O-negative whole blood or packed red blood cells may also be used in emergencies when the hematocrit is low.

Metabolic Considerations

Infants who are stressed in utero are at increased risk of developing hypoglycemia and hypocalcemia as neonates.

A. Hypoglycemia

Hypoxia, acidosis, and alterations in blood pressure occurring in utero will stimulate catecholamine release and mobilize fetal hepatic glycogen stores. Premature infants (whether stressed in utero or not) are at great risk of hypoglycemia because of limited glycogen stores. Untreated hypoglycemia can result in myocardial failure and brain damage. Hypoglycemia is best treated with a slow infusion of 10% glucose, 10–15 mL/kg of body weight.

B. Hypocalcemia

Hypocalcemia often develops in asphyxiated newborns. Asphyxia initially increases both total and ionized serum calcium concentrations. With correction of acidosis or development of alkalosis with sodium bicarbonate therapy, calcium is cleared from the intravascular space, and hypocalcemia develops. Premature infants may also develop hypocalcemia later in the neonatal period because of their limited body stores. Sustained hypocalcemia may also cause seizures, neuromuscular alterations, and heart failure. Hypocalcemia should be corrected with a slow intravenous infusion of calcium gluconate, 100 mg/kg. Daily maintenance doses of calcium for premature infants should also be provided (100–200 mg/kg/d IV).

C. Heat Loss

Throughout resuscitation, heat loss must be minimized. Initially, the infant should be dried and placed on a warm, dry mattress. The infant's temperature should be maintained with a servomechanism-controlled overhead radiant heater to maintain thermoneutral status. A hat should be placed on the infant's head, and heat loss due to convection should also be minimized.

THE PRETERM INFANT

Resuscitation and care of the infant with respiratory distress syndrome are discussed in other sections of this chapter.

General Fluid Balance

For immediate newborn care, administration of fluids should be based on the degree of prematurity and the severity of illness. Fluid restriction will facilitate closure of the ductus arteriosus and will avoid the numerous problems associated with congestive heart failure due to a patent ductus arteriosus that can complicate the infant's later course. However, enough fluid must be provided for sometimes enormous insensible water losses by evaporation from the skin and respiratory tract, which can be affected by open radiant warmer beds, phototherapy, and humidified ventilatory support. Careful, ongoing clinical evaluation of hydration and close monitoring of urine output and weight changes are required.

Nutritional Considerations

A. PREMATURE INFANTS

Small premature infants (< 1500 grams, < 32 weeks gestation) and all sick premature infants require intravenous glucose initially, 5–7 mg/kg/min, to maintain glucose homeostasis and plasma glucose concentrations of 40–180 mg/dL. Nutrition should then be provided either parenterally or enterally to meet the infant's caloric needs of 100–150 kcal/kg of body weight per day. When enteral feeds are possible, human milk is considered the preferred nutritional source for premature infants because of its unique composition and the well-established immunologic, nutritional, and psychologic advantages. Although it has been suggested that enteral feedings increase the risk of necrotizing enterocolitis, no studies have confirmed this impression. Indeed, early enteral feedings may reduce the risk of hyperbilirubinemia and enhance the infant's ability to tolerate feeding. Parenteral nutrition should be provided whenever enteral feedings are withheld or insufficient for longer than a few days. If possible, prolonged total parenteral nutrition should be avoided since it greatly increases the risk of cholestatic jaundice. Nurseries should follow consistent regimens for providing nutrition, whether enteral or parenteral methods are selected.

B. CARBOHYDRATES

The carbohydrate offered to a neonate should provide about 40% of the total calories administered. Any increase in the rate or concentration of intravenous glucose must be implemented slowly, since the premature infant's ability to modulate insulin and glucagon secretion is quite sluggish when compared with that of older children and adults. Glucose offered enterally should not be hyperosmolar.

C. AMINO ACIDS

Intravenous amino acids should not exceed 3–3.5 g of protein per kilogram of body weight per day, since doses exceeding this amount can cause metabolic acidosis, hepatic and renal damage, and possibly brain damage. Doses exceeding this amount do not improve weight gain. Some amino acids that are nonessential for term infants and older children (eg, cystine, cysteine, tyrosine, and taurine) are essential for premature infants, since the enzymes necessary for synthesis of these amino acids do not appear until late in gestation. With enteral feedings, it should be remembered that milk from the mother who has delivered prematurely offers a greater caloric density and more favorable amino acid and lipid composition than milk from a mother who has delivered at term. Currently-available formulas for premature infants provide proteins and essential amino acids similar to those found in preterm human milk.

D. LIPIDS

Intravenous lipid preparations provide both calories and essential fatty acids with low osmolality. Parenteral lipids should not exceed 40% of the total calories provided in 24 hours. High doses of intravenous lipids have been associated with hypoxia and worsening of the alveolar-arterial oxygen gradient when given over short periods of time. Careful monitoring of respiratory variables is therefore indicated, and lipid emulsions should be administered over prolonged infusion periods. Parenteral lipid solutions are invaluable for the support of very tiny infants who require as many calories as possible with limited fluid administration. Formulas prepared for preterm infants contain up to half of the fat blend as medium-chain triglycerides (MCT), which are more readily absorbed from the premature gut.

E. CALCIUM AND IRON

Fetal stores of iron and calcium are normally established during the third trimester. Premature infants are therefore at great risk of developing osteopenia, since they have limited calcium stores, a higher rate of bone growth and mineralization, and relatively poor absorption of dietary calcium. With either enteral or parenteral nutrition, every attempt should be made to provide a minimum of 130 mg of calcium per 100 kcal consumed. However, this does not approach the amount of calcium normally acquired by the fetus during the third trimester, and careful observation for the possible development of osteopenia is therefore mandatory in premature infants. The available formulas for premature infants offer more calcium than standard formulas. In addition, the presence of MCT oil is believed to enhance calcium absorption by improving fat absorption, and may therefore reduce the risk of osteopenia. If small premature infants are to be provided breast milk, human milk fortifier should be used since prolonged provision of human breast milk alone may not meet the calcium needs of the very premature infant.

Premature infants are born with decreased iron stores because most iron is accumulated toward the end of pregnancy. The exact age at which iron supplementation should be started has not been clearly established. Iron supplementation has been shown to increase the requirements for vitamin E, and thus could increase the risk of hemolysis due to vitamin E deficiency. When erythropoiesis has begun (as evidenced by reticulocytosis), iron supplementation can be provided in some of the preterm formulas or as an additive to human milk-fed babies. Earlier administration of exogenous iron will not stimulate erythropoiesis. The AAP recommends that serum vitamin E levels be closely monitored in preterm infants receiving iron supplementation prior to 2 months of age.

Heat Conservation

The decision to use an open radiant heater bed or closed incubator should be based on the routine operations of the nursery. Both systems offer advantages and disadvantages. Radiant heater beds offer caretakers ready access to unstable infants; however, heat losses due to convection and increased insensible water loss due to evaporation are greater than with incubators. Incubators are particularly useful for very premature infants, whose insensible fluid losses can be considerable. In addition, a heat shield can be placed over the infant in an incubator; this will decrease radiant heat losses even further. Double-walled incubators will also accomplish this purpose. They may also shield the infant from some extraneous noise, light, and air currents. Incubators, however, limit access and may obstruct the care of an acutely ill infant. With either system, skin or environmental temperature should be adjusted to maintain a thermoneutral state and minimize caloric expenditure and oxygen consumption.

Diseases of the Premature Neonate

RESPIRATORY DISTRESS SYNDROME (RDS, HYALINE MEMBRANE DISEASE [HMD])

Respiratory distress syndrome (RDS) is caused by a functional deficiency of the pulmonary surfactant system. Pulmonary surfactant is a surface-active complex of phospholipids and proteins produced by type II cells of alveoli that reduces alveolar surface tension and prevents atelectasis. In addition, inhibitors of surfactant function may limit the surfactant's effectiveness as respiratory distress syndrome progresses. The progressive generalized atelectasis of RDS results in a loss of functional residual capacity and mismatched ventilation and perfusion. Increased alveolar-arterial differences, ventilatory failure with consequent cyanosis, tachypnea, and grunting at end expiration result, the last finding representing the infant's attempt to maintain alveolar distention during exhalation.

Clinical Findings

A. SIGNS

Tachypnea, retractions, and grunting generally begin soon after birth and become progressively more severe,

eventually progressing into cyanosis and respiratory failure. In babies not treated with surfactant replacement therapy, decreased air exchange and cyanosis worsen for the first 24–48 hours. The very premature infant may present with or develop apnea due to RDS. Since it has little chest wall muscularity or stability, the infant is unable to sustain respiration against the generalized atelectasis.

B. LABORATORY FINDINGS

Affected infants are hypoxic and often hypercapnic and acidotic. These stresses may cause hypotension. Chest x-ray shows characteristic low lung volumes and a diffuse ground-glass appearance caused by atelectasis, which develops during the first 6 hours of life (Fig 29–7). Pulmonary function studies demonstrate increased work of breathing and diminished compliance, lung volume, and functional residual capacity.

C. ASSOCIATED DISORDERS

While all premature infants are at great risk of developing RDS (incidence is approximately 60% at 29 weeks gestation), other conditions are also associated with this disorder. Maternal diabetes mellitus increases the risk of RDS because the associated fetal hyperinsulinism limits the induction of enzymes necessary for surfactant production. Acidosis during labor and delivery can cause or worsen RDS by limiting surfactant production. Evaluation of fetal lung maturity by testing amniotic fluid for the presence of surfactant (lecithin:sphingomyelin [L:S] ratio,

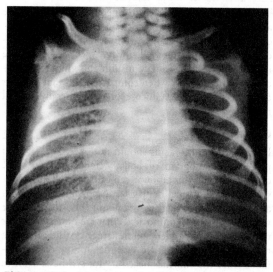

Figure 29-7. Chest x-ray of an infant with respiratory distress syndrome. The ground-glass appearance results from generalized atelectasis.

presence of phosphatidylinositol and phosphatidylglyc-erol, foam stability test) assists both obstetric and neonatal management. Corticosteroids administered to the mother to encourage maturation of the fetal lungs have been clearly shown to reduce the incidence and severity of RDS, as well as bronchopulmonary dysplasia, in infants born prior to 32 weeks gestation.

Differential Diagnosis

The differential diagnosis of RDS includes bacterial and viral pneumonias, transient tachypnea of the newborn (TTN), and aspiration syndromes including meconium and amniotic fluid. TTN is self-limited (by definition resolving within 24 hours of birth) and generally requires minimal oxygen therapy. Viral pneumonias generally manifest streaky infiltrates on x-ray and can thereby be distinguished from RDS. On the other hand, bacterial pneumonias, particularly those caused by group B beta-hemolytic streptococci, often mimic RDS in both their clinical and their radiologic presentation. In fact, they may coexist with RDS, given the higher attack rate of bacterial pathogens in premature infants. For this reason, blood cultures should be obtained, culture of cerebrospinal fluid (CSF) should be considered, and antibiotic therapy should be considered in the initial management of an infant with presumed RDS.

Treatment

For optimal care, a premature infant at risk for RDS should be delivered in a perinatal center with a pediatric resuscitation team in attendance. Early treatment to establish oxygenation, ventilation, and correction of acidosis and hypotension will moderate the clinical course of RDS. This is important, since acidosis and hypotension can destroy surfactant present in the lungs and impede production of surfactant by type II alveolar cells. In addition, early stabilization of the infant may reduce the risk of numerous other complications of prematurity (eg, intraventricular hemorrhage and necrotizing enterocolitis).

Several approaches exist for providing respiratory support to the premature infant with RDS. In general, infants with mild disease may simply be maintained in an environment with increased oxygen. Physical signs of respiratory distress as well as fractional inspired oxygen (FIO_2) and arterial blood gas tensions and pH must be closely monitored so that any worsening of condition—manifested by decreasing arterial oxygen tension (PaO_2) and increasing arterial carbon dioxide tension ($PaCO_2$)—can be quickly detected.

Infants with moderate to severe RDS (inability to maintain $PaO_2 > 50$ mm Hg with FIO_2 of .50–.80 or inability to maintain $PaCO_2 < 50$ mm Hg) require assisted ventilation. Numerous approaches, including continuous positive airway pressure or intermittent mandatory ventilation with either pressure- or volume-limited ventilators, are possible. Continuous positive airway pressure (CPAP) alone is often sufficient, particularly in larger premature infants. CPAP should be started earlier (ie, when FIO_2 reaches 0.5). When intermittent mandatory ventilation is used, positive end-expiratory pressure (4–8 cm water) is necessary in order to limit atelectasis at the end of expiration. Respiratory rate, inspiratory and expiratory time, inspiratory pressure or volume, and end-expiratory pressure can be adjusted to maintain PaO_2 between 50 and 70 mm Hg; $PaCO_2$ up to 50–60 mm Hg can be tolerated and may reduce barotrauma, which is thought to contribute to chronic lung disease. Frequent measurement of arterial blood gas tensions and pH or O_2 saturation is necessary. If transcutaneous or oxygen saturation monitors are used to measure oxygenation, correlation with arterial blood samples is necessary so that use of ventilatory therapy can be minimized to avoid its toxic effects.

Other methods of ventilatory support include high-frequency jet ventilation and oscillators; other experimental modalities are also being studied. The rate ranges of conventional ventilators are 10–80 breaths/min, those of high-frequency jet ventilation (HFJV) are 150–600 pulses of gas/min, and those of oscillators 300–1800 pulses of gas/min. HFJV and oscillators may improve carbon dioxide elimination, lower mean airway pressure, and improve oxygenation in patients who do not respond to conventional ventilators and who have HMD, interstitial emphysema, many pneumothoraces, or meconium aspiration pneumonia. HFJV may cause necrotizing tracheal damage, especially in the presence of hypotension or poor humidification, and oscillator therapy has been associated with an increased risk of air leaks, intraventricular hemorrhage, and periventricular leukomalacia. Both methods may cause gas trapping. Partial liquid ventilation with oxygen-carrying perflubron, administered via the endotracheal tube, has resulted in improvement in oxygenation. Inhaled nitric oxide has also acutely improved oxygenation, but may not improve overall outcome of HMD. These are both experimental therapies.

A number of exogenous surfactant preparations have undergone numerous clinical trials. Two are Federal Drug Administration (FDA) approved for general clinical use in the U.S.: a synthetic surfactant (EXOSURF Neonatal, Burroughs Wellcome Company, Research Triangle Park, NC) and a modified natural bovine surfactant (SURVANTA, Ross Laboratories, Columbus, OH). Additional surfactants undergoing testing include Curosurf and Infasurf (both natural) and ALEC (artificial lung expanding compound). Treatment (rescue) is initiated as soon as possible in the first 24 hours of life; therapy is given via the endotracheal tube every 6–12 hours for a total of 2–4 doses, depending on the preparation. Complications of surfactant therapy include transient hypoxia and hypotension, blockage of the endotracheal tube, and pulmonary hemorrhage. There is now plentiful evidence that surfactant replacement therapy decreases the severity of RDS, decreases neonatal mortality, and increases survival without bronchopulmonary dysplasia. In addition, there is now evidence that replacement surfactant is even more effective in infants that have been treated prenatally with corticosteroids. Dosing variables, including size of dose, method of administration, timing of first dose, and total number of doses, remain active areas of investigation.

Complications

A. RETINOPATHY OF PREMATURITY

Retinopathy of prematurity (ROP, previously called retrolental fibroplasia), is a vasoproliferative retinal disorder that primarily affects premature, very low birthweight (VLBW) infants. It has been associated with prolonged exposure to high concentrations of oxygen in blood, but can develop even in room air, particularly in the most immature infants. Studies indicate that oxygen therapy alone does not cause ROP and that other factors that have not yet been entirely elucidated are associated with its development. The more immature the infant, the greater the risk of ROP. The theory of pathogenesis includes retinal vessel spasm, proliferation, hemorrhage, and fibrosis. ROP may regress spontaneously or progress to complete retinal detachment. It is responsible for producing visual loss or blindness in hundreds of children every year in the U.S. Cryotherapy appears to be a promising means of treating this condition and may reduce the incidence of retinal detachment by up to 50%. Other treatment and prevention approaches under investigation include laser therapy and supplemental oxygen therapy. All infants born at 30 weeks gestation or < 1300 grams and all infants < 35 weeks or < 1800 grams who have received oxygen therapy should be screened for ROP by 4–8 weeks of age.

B. BRONCHOPULMONARY DYSPLASIA (BPD)

Prolonged exposure of the immature lung to high oxygen concentrations and barotrauma pressure can result in BPD, characterized pathologically by scarring of the airways and lung parenchyma, and clinically by supplemental oxygen requirement, increased airway reactivity, and a tendency toward pulmonary edema. It is not yet clear what part is played by the numerous contributing factors in the development of the disorder. The immature lung may lack sufficient antioxidant enzymes to scavenge damaging oxygen radicals; in addition, the ex-

uberant inflammatory response of the immature lung may cause excessive scarring and fibrosis. Infants with BPD often require prolonged ventilatory support and environments with increased oxygen. Patience is required during treatment, since overzealous attempts to reduce supportive therapy will fail and possibly worsen the infant's condition. Bronchospasm, which often occurs with this disorder, can be effectively treated with bronchodilators (eg, theophylline and selective β_2-agonists). Fluid restriction and the use of diuretics may reduce interstitial edema and improve lung function. Excessive osteopenia due to urinary calcium wasting and nephrocalcinosis are two side effects of this therapy. Corticosteroid administration can improve lung function in some infants with BPD, but can have significant side effects including sepsis, hypertension, and adrenal malfunction. Studies of corticosteroids administered locally (ie, inhaled) are in progress, with the hope of providing pulmonary improvements with fewer adverse systemic effects.

C. "AIR LEAKS"

This risk of pulmonary interstitial edema (PIE) pneumothorax, pneumomediastinum, or pneumopericardium exists in any premature infant requiring assisted ventilation. The development of any of these "air leaks" is the result of overdistention and rupture of alveoli and is typically signaled by a decrease in PaO_2 and blood pressure and, in the case of pneumothorax, narrowing of the pulse pressure. PIE is a serious complication with significant mortality in small premature infants. Treatment attempts include positioning and altering mechanical ventilation in an attempt to minimize gas trapping. Pneumothorax can be immediately evacuated with needle and syringe aspiration; however, all symptomatic or "tension" pneumothoraces require placement of a chest tube attached to an underwater seal and suction device, since the likelihood of reaccumulation of gas in the pleural space following needle aspiration is great, especially during positive pressure ventilation. Chest and pericardial tubes should remain in place for at least 24–48 hours so that sufficient healing will occur to prevent recurrence of pneumothorax.

HEART DISEASE

The incidence of congenital heart disease is the same in premature and term infants and ranges from 3–8 per 1000 live births. The incidence of patent ductus arteriosus is greatly increased in premature infants. Premature delivery does not automatically trigger closure of the ductus; continued hypoxia as a result of severe respiratory distress syndrome may maintain ductal patency, possibly because of the continued local production of vasodilator prostanoids such as prostaglandin E.

Early in RDS, when pulmonary vascular resistance is elevated, blood may shunt from right to left through the patent ductus arteriosus. With resolution of RDS, pulmonary vascular resistance decreases and left-to-right shunting develops, both of which can complicate the ventilatory management of an infant with RDS, since the development of congestive heart failure will prolong the need for assisted ventilation. Prolonged ductal patency is also implicated in the etiology of bronchopulmonary dysplasia, necrotizing enterocolitis, and intraventricular hemorrhage.

The diagnosis of congestive heart failure due to patent ductus arteriosus is suggested by a systolic murmur over the precordium, rales at the lung bases, wide pulse pressure, and bounding peripheral pulses. The "machinery murmur" characteristic of patent ductus arteriosus in older children is rarely heard in premature infants. Chest x-ray demonstrates cardiac enlargement and fluid in the lung fields. Echocardiography and Doppler flow methods will delineate the patent ductus.

Closure of the ductus can be achieved in premature infants who have RDS by stringent limitation of fluid administration early in the disease. In symptomatic infants, early administration of indomethacin, a potent inhibitor of prostaglandin synthesis, may close the ductus. The drug may also be used later in the clinical course when congestive heart failure develops or if the duct reopens. Known complications of indomethacin therapy include transient renal failure and gastrointestinal bleeding. Indomethacin has been implicated in increasing the incidence of necrotizing enterocolitis and has been used in research trials for prevention of intraventricular hemorrhage. Congestive heart failure in the premature infant is best treated with fluid restriction and diuretics. Surgical ligation of the ductus is indicated in symptomatic infants if two courses of indomethacin therapy are unsuccessful or if indomethacin is contraindicated.

Preserving the patency of the ductus can be lifesaving in a number of different heart defects, including those with restriction of pulmonary blood flow, transposition of the great vessels, or severe left ventricular outflow obstruction. Infusion of prostaglandin E will maintain ductal patency in preparation for neonatal transport or cardiac surgery.

HYPERBILIRUBINEMIA

Most neonates develop some degree of jaundice (**icterus neonatorum**) during the newborn period; because of the relatively rapid rate of hemolysis of fetal red blood cells, neonatal cells have higher rates of turnover and a shorter life span; neonates also have immature hepatic mechanisms for bilirubin conjugation and excretion. Certain disorders are associated with an increased degree of or prolonged hyperbilirubinemia as a result of altered rates of red cell breakdown, conjugation of bilirubin, and excretion of conjugated bilirubin. It should be noted that in the term infant, the severity of disease (as manifested by the extent of jaundice) correlates reasonably well with plasma bilirubin concentrations. However, this is not the case in premature infants.

Etiology

A. INCREASED RATE OF HEMOLYSIS

These neonates have increased unconjugated bilirubin concentration and an increased reticulocyte count:

1. Newborns with a positive Coombs' test (this category includes all patients with isoimmunization, including ABO incompatibility, Rh incompatibility, etc).
2. Neonates with negative Coombs' test.
   a. Abnormal red cell membrane, including spherocytosis, elliptocytosis, pyknocytosis, and stomatocytosis.
   b. Red cell enzyme abnormalities: glucose 6-phosphate dehydrogenase deficiency, pyruvate kinase deficiency.
   c. Sepsis (eg, due to *Clostridia*).

B. DECREASED RATE OF CONJUGATION

These newborns have elevated levels of unconjugated bilirubin and a normal reticulocyte count:

(1) Immaturity of bilirubin conjugation ("physiologic jaundice").

(2) Congenital familial nonhemolytic jaundice (inborn errors of metabolism affecting glucuronyl transferase system and bilirubin transport).

(3) Breast milk jaundice.

C. ABNORMALITIES OF EXCRETION OR REABSORPTION

These neonates have elevated levels of conjugated and unconjugated bilirubin, negative Coombs' test, and normal reticulocyte count:

1. Hepatitis.
   a. Infection.
   b. Toxic (eg, parenteral nutrition).
2. Metabolic abnormalities.
   a. Galactosemia.
   b. Glycogen storage diseases.
   c. Maternal diabetes.
   d. Cystic fibrosis.
   e. α_1-Antitrypsin deficiency.
3. Obstruction to biliary flow.
   a. Extrahepatic biliary atresia.

b. Choledochal cyst.

c. Alagille syndrome (paucity of intrahepatic bile ducts).

d. Inspissated bile syndrome.

4. Sepsis (eg, due to *E coli*).

5. Gastrointestinal obstruction (due to increased enterohepatic circulation of bilirubin).

The serum concentration of unconjugated bilirubin should be checked in all jaundiced infants, because in some infants hyperbilirubinemia may cause sensorineural hearing loss or kernicterus.

Bilirubin concentrations that pose a definite risk to premature infants have not been established, although it is generally held that the acidosis, hypoxia, and fluid shifts that frequently complicate a premature infant's clinical course greatly increase the risk of central nervous system damage at relatively low bilirubin concentrations.

Treatment

1. Infant approaching phototherapy level (and being fed):

a. Increase frequency of enteral feedings if possible. One study showed that infants fed every 2 hours had increased frequency of defecation and lower bilirubin levels than those fed every 3 or 4 hours. Intake volume and weight gain/loss were similar between the two groups, thus the difference was not due to hydration, but to the increased frequency of defecation, and decreased contribution of the "enterohepatic circulation" of bilirubin.

b. It is not necessary (or advisable) to discontinue breast milk. If the mother's milk has not "come in" yet, or she cannot nurse every 2–3 hours, or the infant seems thirsty, supplement with formula. Water has been shown to *increase* the "enterohepatic circulation" of bilirubin.

2. Phototherapy is an important treatment method that uses radiant energy to isomerize bilirubin to a soluble form that is excreted by both the kidneys and gastrointestinal tract and remains the standard of care for treatment of hyperbilirubinemia. When phototherapy is used, the infant's eyes must be covered to prevent damage to the rods and cones. Phototherapy lessens jaundice, so that skin appearance can no longer be used as a measure of bilirubin concentration. It also substantially increases sensible fluid loss, so that fluid therapy must be managed accordingly. Use of phototherapy in infants with conjugated hyperbilirubinemia may result in bronze baby syndrome. The National Institute of Child Health

and Human Development determined that phototherapy used to control serum bilirubin is safe and as effective in preventing brain injury as exchange transfusion.

3. A double-volume exchange transfusion through an umbilical arterial or venous catheter is performed when serum bilirubin approaches a level at which neurologic damage can occur. This technique rapidly eliminates bilirubin as well as circulating antibodies that target erythrocytes. Fresh O-negative, low-antibody-titer whole blood should be used. The risks of exchange transfusion include catheter accidents, infection, and acute blood pressure changes that can increase the risk of hemorrhage or cause or worsen congestive heart failure.

The American Academy of Pediatrics has published guidelines for phototherapy for full-term infants, however no guidelines are established for preterm infants. The following recommendations are published in the literature: Phototherapy can be discontinued when the serum bilirubin concentration has been reduced by about 4–5 mg/dL. Guidelines for suggested bilirubin levels for phototherapy or exchange transfusion based on birthweight and clinical course of the infant are shown in Table 29–2.

HEMATOLOGIC DISORDERS

Isoimmunization
(See Chapter 15.)

Hemorrhagic Diseases of the Newborn (Hypoprothrombinemia)

Levels of vitamin K–dependent clotting factors (factors II, VII, IX, and X) are normal at birth but decrease within 2–3 days. In vitamin K–deficient infants, these levels may be very low, resulting in prolonged bleeding times. The reported incidence of classic hemorrhagic disease of the newborn ranges from 1.7% of births to 5.4/100,000 births. Bleeding may occur into the skin or gastrointestinal tract, at the site of injection or circumcision, or at internal sites.

Small amounts of vitamin K are generally sufficient to correct clotting factor defects. All newborns should receive vitamin K, 1 mg intramuscularly, on admission to the nursery.

Anemia

Placenta previa, abruptio placentae, velamentous cord insertion, a torn cord or placenta, or twin-to-twin transfusion syndrome may result in hemorrhage and consequent anemia. Anemia may also result from accelerated red cell hemolysis due to isoimmunization,

Table 29–2. Indirect bilirubin concentration (mg/dL).

BW (kg)	5–6	7–9	10–12	13–15	16–20	> 20
<1.0	Phototherapy		Think of exchange		Exchange transfusion	
1.0–1.5		Phototherapy		Think of exchange	Exchange transfusion	
1.5–2.0			Phototherapy		Think of exchange	Exchange transfusion
2.0–2.5				Phototherapy	Think of exchange	Exchange transfusion
> 2.5					Phototherapy	Think of exchange

Guidelines for suggested bilirubin levels for phototherapy or exchange transfusion based on birthweight and clinical course of the infant. (Reproduced, with permission, from Harvey-Wilkes K, 1993).

membrane defects, hemoglobinopathy, enzymopathy or microangiopathic hemolysis. A regenerative anemia is rare. Treatment depends on the severity of anemia. If hypotension or hypoperfusion develops, as characterized by a capillary filling time exceeding 3 seconds, volume expansion is indicated. The asymptomatic term infant with a hematocrit between 20% and 30% may not require transfusion; supplemental iron (3–6 mg/kg/d of elemental iron orally) should be given and the infant followed closely. While transfusions are often required, recombinant human erythropoietin (rHuEpo) has been used to prevent or treat chronic anemia associated with prematurity, chronic lung disease, and the hyporegenerative anemia of erythroblastosis fetalis. Therapy with rHuEpo is given by intravenous or subcutaneous routes and must be supplemented with oral iron and possibly vitamin E. Doses and regimens vary from 100–200 U/kg/dose 5 days/week to 400 U/kg/dose 3 days/week to 150–200 U/kg/dose every 3 days.

Polycythemia

A venous hematocrit exceeding 65% is considered polycythemia in a neonate and is found in 2–6% of newborns. Blood viscosity increases roughly exponentially with increases in hematocrit. Polycythemia is associated with twin-to-twin transfusion and enhanced placental transfusion due to late cord clamping; it is also noted in infants of diabetic mothers, small-for-gestational-age (SGA) infants, and infants with congenital adrenal hyperplasia, thyrotoxicosis, or Down syndrome.

The complications of polycythemia per se are related to volume overload and congestive heart failure. Hyperviscosity, on the other hand, causes sludging in the vascular bed, and complications include infarction of the cerebral, mesenteric, and renal vascular beds. Clinical manifestations include tachypnea, central nervous system disturbances, and hypoglycemia. Current experience suggests that many hyperviscous infants have long-lasting neural pathology.

Phlebotomy alone should never be performed. Intravenous hydration may be sufficient to reduce the hematocrit. It is likely that early partial exchange transfusion will limit or prevent most of the complications of hyperviscosity, although controversy exists over the value of partial exchange transfusion in asymptomatic polycythemic infants.

Current recommendations are that infants with signs of hyperviscous disease, polycythemia, and no other evident explanation for the findings should have their hematocrits reduced promptly by a small exchange transfusion with 4% or 5% albumin in saline, or isotonic saline alone. The albumin solutions were used most commonly in the past, but recent studies suggest that isotonic saline alone is just as effective. The object is to lower the hematocrit to the range of 50–55%. The volume to be exchanged can be estimated as follows:

Volume of exchange (mL) = blood volume × (observed – desired hematocrit)/observed hematocrit

GASTROINTESTINAL DISORDERS

Necrotizing Enterocolitis

Necrotizing enterocolitis occurs mainly in premature infants and is characterized by various degrees of mucosal or transmural necrosis of the intestine. In severe situations, bowel perforation and seepage of gas into the hepatic portal tree can occur. Necrotizing enterocolitis typically develops in the small intestine. Infants will develop feeding intolerance and abdominal distention, pass bloody stools, and demonstrate intramural gas in dilated loops of bowel on x-ray.

The causes of necrotizing enterocolitis are unclear. In relatively large premature infants (about 34 weeks gestation), the period of greatest risk for the development of necrotizing enterocolitis is the first 2 weeks of life. Smaller and more immature infants have a longer risk period, and the onset is often delayed. Necrotizing enterocolitis is known to occur in both sporadic and epidemic patterns. The etiology of necrotizing enterocolitis is felt to be multifactorial. Hypoxic-ischemic states, bacteria, and enteral feeding all have potential roles in mediating bowel injury.

If necrotizing enterocolitis is suspected or diagnosed, feedings should be discontinued and the bowel decompressed with low-pressure suction applied to a soft feeding tube. Blood and stool cultures should be obtained and antibiotics and parenteral nutrition administered. Careful surveillance should be maintained for acidosis and hypovolemia. Surgical consultation should be obtained early. Plain abdominal roentgenograms may demonstrate pneumatosis intestinalis, a finding that is diagnostic of NEC. Frequent abdominal x-rays should be obtained to monitor disease progression. The need for surgical treatment is based on resolution or progression of the disease. The overall survival rate is 70–80%, and approximately 60% will develop sepsis. Of those treated medically, 11–36% will develop strictures.

Diaphragmatic Hernia

Diaphragmatic hernia is a congenital malformation in which herniation of abdominal organs into a hemithorax occurs because of a defect in the diaphragm. Hernias on the left, due to a defect in the foramen of Bochdalek, account for 70% of diaphragmatic hernias. Infants with diaphragmatic hernias present with cyanosis and severe respiratory distress immediately after birth. Because the abdominal viscera are in the chest, the abdominal contour is scaphoid, and breath sounds are diminished or absent. With assisted ventilation, the gastrointestinal tract fills with gas, further compromising ventilation. Successful management depends on early diagnosis, decompression of the stomach and intestines with continuous suction, appropriate ventilation with an endotracheal tube, and circulatory support. Immediate surgical intervention is indicated. Although in the past diaphragmatic hernia was considered a surgical emergency and immediate repair of the diaphragm was thought important, it has been proven that in mild to moderately involved infants, delaying the operation 3–5 days is of great benefit, permitting the pulmonary circulation to adjust.

Prognosis for survival depends on the severity of pulmonary hypoplasia and pulmonary hypertension and on the presence of associated structural or chromosomal abnormalities. Extracorporeal membrane oxygenation has been used successfully for diaphragmatic hernia therapy in selected cases, although the impact on overall survival rates is controversial. While early results of attempts at in-utero repair have been discouraging, active research on fetal surgery techniques continues.

Omphalocele & Gastroschisis

Both omphalocele and gastroschisis require immediate care in the delivery room. In omphalocele, part or all of the intestines as well as the liver and spleen may be visible in a sac protruding through the abdominal wall. In gastroschisis, abdominal organs protrude through a congenital fissure of the abdominal wall. In both disorders, the externalized viscera should be covered with gauze soaked in warm, sterile saline and covered with a sterile plastic bag. Every effort should be made to avoid trauma to the viscera before corrective surgery.

Tracheoesophageal Fistula & Esophageal Atresia

Atresia of the esophagus with an associated fistula between the distal segment of the esophagus and the trachea is the most frequently occurring esophageal anomaly. Less common are esophageal atresia without fistula and the H-type fistula. Esophageal atresia should be suspected in cases of polyhydramnios or absent fetal stomach bubble on prenatal ultrasound. The earliest sign of tracheoesophageal fistula is regurgitation of saliva on the first feeding. Aspiration may occur and cause choking and coughing. As inspired air is drawn through the fistula, abdominal distention may occur.

Tracheoesophageal fistula can be diagnosed by passing a catheter through the nose or mouth down into the fistula and obtaining an x-ray of the upper airway. Contrast studies to determine the type of lesion should be performed only by a skilled pediatric radiologist at a tertiary care hospital.

RENAL FAILURE

Severe perinatal asphyxia, cardiorespiratory arrest, hemorrhage, or other stressors that acutely limit perfusion of the kidneys may cause cortical or medullary necrosis. This is characterized by anuria or oliguria and is followed by polyuria if the infant survives. Decreased urine output also occurs with indomethacin therapy or with clot formation in the renal arteries occurring as a complication of the use of umbilical catheters.

When renal failure is suspected in an infant with decreased urine output (normal, 1–2 mL/kg of body weight per hour), fluid challenge with intravenous fluids, 10–20 mL/kg of body weight, followed by furosemide, 1–2 mg/kg IV should be performed. If urine output increases, fluid administration should be increased. Dopamine, 5 μg/kg/min, may improve renal perfusion and output at this time. If fluid challenge fails to stimulate urine production, fluid administration should be limited to replacement of insensible losses and urine output. Serum electrolyte concentrations should be measured frequently so that metabolic derangements associated with renal failure can be detected. These include hyponatremia, hyperkalemia, hyperphosphatemia, hypocalcemia, and metabolic acidosis. Hypertension may also occur. The characteristic electrocardiographic changes associated with hyperkalemia in adults may not develop in infants. Hyperkalemia may be treated acutely with intravenous sodium bicarbonate, insulin, and glucose, or ion exchange resin enemas (eg, sodium polystyrene sulfonate, 1 g/kg in sorbitol).

In some newborns with acute renal failure, dialysis is considered. Peritoneal dialysis is preferred to hemodialysis in newborns because of less technical difficulty and similar effectiveness. Continuous arteriovenous hemofiltration is an alternative technique for removal of excess fluid without dialysis, and it may also be considered.

Acute oliguric failure in the newborn carries a mortality rate of 50%. Nonoliguric renal failure has a much better prognosis.

CENTRAL NERVOUS SYSTEM DISORDERS

Newborn Encephalopathy

Newborn encephalopathy occurs at a rate of 1–6/1000 term births depending on severity. The use of fetal heart rate monitoring does not seem to have had a major impact on the incidence. This condition has been given a variety of names, including hypoxic-ischemic encephalopathy and postasphyxial encephalopathy. An undefined proportion of newborn encephalopathy is felt to be due to hypoxia and ischemia, which can occur prior to labor or during labor and delivery. Depending on the timing and severity of the insult, the manifestations include irritability, tremor, stupor, seizures, coma, and death.

Supportive care includes maintenance of nutrition, respiratory support, and anticonvulsants for seizures. CT scan, cranial ultrasound, and EEG are useful in determining the site of brain lesions. The prognosis for infants who have suffered hypoxic ischemic encephalopathy is unpredictable. The risk of long-term impairment of cognitive and psychomotor development to survivors is approximately 25%. The prognostic value of measures of intrapartum asphyxia such as Apgar scores is especially poor. Perinatal asphyxia is felt to account for only 8–10% of cases of cerebral palsy, and most survivors of asphyxia do not have cerebral palsy.

Seizures

The cause of seizures must be quickly identified. The infant should be evaluated for treatable causes such as hypoglycemia, hypocalcemia, acidosis, and sepsis. Initial management should ensure adequate ventilation, oxygenation, and perfusion. Phenobarbital, 15–20 mg/kg IV, is the treatment of choice. If seizures continue, a second and third dose (10 mg/kg) may be given, to a maximum of 30–40 mg/kg. With high doses of phenobarbital, the infant should be observed carefully for respiratory depression. If phenobarbital fails to control seizures, phenytoin, 15–20 mg/kg IV, may be administered. The rate of administration should not exceed 1 mg/kg/min to avoid depression of cardiac rhythm. Diazepam, 0.1 mg/kg intravenously, may be administered, but it acts synergistically with phenobarbital to depress respiration. If plasma levels of 30–45 mg/mL of phenobarbital and 10–20 mg/mL of phenytoin fail to control seizures, diazepam, 0.1–0.3 mg/kg IV in repeated doses, or lorazepam, 0.05–0.1 mg/kg/dose IV in repeated doses may be given.

Intracranial Hemorrhage in the Premature Infant

Up to 50% of premature infants develop some degree of intracranial hemorrhage. These hemorrhages most commonly begin in the fragile capillaries of the germinal matrix layer of the subependymal region, the ventricles, and the periventricular white matter. A commonly used grading system defines grade I as germinal matrix hemorrhage, grade II as blood within but not distending the lateral ventricles, grade III as blood distending the ventricles, and grade IV as parenchymal involvement. It is not clear whether low-grade hemorrhage has an impact on long-term outcome, while the more severe grades are associated with a higher incidence of adverse neurologic outcome and posthemorrhagic hydrocephalus.

The development of intraventricular hemorrhage is thought to relate to fluctuation in cerebral blood flow and pressure and is associated with hypercapnia, rapid volume expansion, seizures, and pneumothorax. No specific preventive therapy is presently available. Abrupt increases in blood pressure should be avoided. Blood gas values should be monitored frequently, and coagulopathies should be corrected.

All infants with identified hemorrhage should be followed with serial cranial ultrasounds or CT scans to check for extension of bleeding and the development of posthemorrhagic hydrocephalus. If hydrocephalus progresses, serial lumbar puncture or neurosurgery to drain cerebrospinal fluid may be indicated.

INFECTIONS

Signs of infection in the newborn may be as subtle as slight temperature instability and jaundice or as overt as respiratory distress and shock. Whenever an infection is suspected, samples of blood, urine, and when appropriate cerebrospinal fluid should be obtained for examination and culture. A complete blood count, smear for differential, and platelet count should also be obtained. Thrombocytopenia and both of the extremes of neutrophil count suggest sepsis. Broad-spectrum antibiotics to cover both gram-positive and gramnegative organisms should be initiated. When culture results become available, drugs may be changed as necessary.

In infants born more than 24 hours after rupture of the membranes, white blood cell counts and blood cultures should be obtained. The decision to initiate antibiotic therapy should be based on the infant's clinical status.

Group B streptococcus is the most common cause of neonatal sepsis. Although 15–30% of pregnant women are colonized with these organisms, and there is a 70% rate of vertical transmission of colonization, relatively few infants actually develop sepsis. Those who do often present with respiratory difficulties that mimic RDS. Risk factors for the development of group B streptococcal sepsis include premature delivery, rupture of membranes greater than 18 hours, maternal fever in labor, and multiple gestation. Intrapartum chemoprophylactic strategies have been developed to decrease the risk of sepsis. Treatment consists of intravenous penicillin or ampicillin. A sample of cerebrospinal fluid should be examined to check for signs of meningitis. Other bacteria that cause neonatal sepsis and meningitis include *E coli, Listeria monocytogenes,* and staphylococci.

Infants thought to have viral infections acquired in utero require antibody titers and cultures to confirm the diagnosis. Infants who are shedding virus may require isolation. Evaluation for potential long-term difficulties such as impaired hearing and cognitive development should be carried out (brainstem auditory evoked potentials, neurosonograms, etc).

Infants with herpesvirus infections such as herpes simplex and varicella may require acyclovir therapy. Infants born to mothers who develop chicken pox within 5 days of delivery should be given varicella-zoster immune globulin prophylaxis.

Hepatitis immune globulin and hepatitis vaccine should be given to infants born to mothers with hepatitis B surface antigenemia. Hepatitis vaccine has also been added to the schedule of routine pediatric vaccination. The first dose is given prior to hospital discharge.

Infants delivered of mothers with human immunodeficiency virus (HIV) infection should be identified. The risk of infection for an infant born to an HIV-seropositive mother who did not receive antiretroviral therapy during pregnancy is estimated to be between 13% and 39%. Use of antiretroviral therapy decreases transmission rates by more than 50%. Early initiation of antiviral and antibacterial treatment is of significant benefit to the infant. Breastfeeding is contraindicated when formula feeding is available.

Infection with cytomegalovirus poses a great threat to the fetus and neonate and may even be fatal in utero. Intrauterine infection occurs in 0.5–3% of all live births and is the most common congenital infection. Although infection in most infants is asymptomatic and goes unrecognized, some infants with cytomegalovirus infection are at risk for severe deficits in cognitive and psychomotor development, and they may demonstrate varying degrees of sensorineural hearing loss. Primary maternal infection carries the greatest risk of transmission and of severe sequelae. Recurrent infection is thought rarely to cause congenital infection with an adverse outcome. Cytomegalovirus can be transmitted in breast milk.

Chlamydia trachomatis is a gram-negative bacterium acquired by the newborn at delivery that can cause both conjunctivitis and pneumonitis during the later neonatal period. Conjunctivitis develops 5–12 days after birth and can be severe, resulting in conjunctival scarring if untreated. Pneumonitis develops within the first 3 months of life. The infant is typically afebrile and tachypneic and has a short, abrupt, staccato cough. Treatment of chlamydial conjunctivitis includes oral erythromycin and topical sulfacetamide ointment for the eyes.

DRUG & ALCOHOL ADDICTION

There was a dramatic increase during the 1980s in the number of infants born to mothers using legal and illegal substances that can harm the fetus. However, these numbers slowly declined in the last decade of the 20th century. Even with declining exposure rates, the problem of neonatal drug exposure is unlikely to disappear in the near future. The most commonly used drugs currently are cocaine and other stimulants. Infants born to these women have an increased incidence of prematurity, low birthweight, and congenital infections. Other problems for which they may be at risk include drug withdrawal, visual dysfunction, vascular accidents resulting in cerebral infarcts, necrotizing enterocolitis, and limb anomalies. They also appear to be at greater risk for sudden infant death syndrome (SIDS).

Infants born to narcotic-addicted women are more likely to be born prematurely and intrauterine growth restricted. They may undergo withdrawal and manifest the neonatal abstinence syndrome findings of tremors, irritability, hyperactivity, diarrhea, sweating, sneezing, and possibly seizures. Toxicologic analysis of urine can confirm the in utero exposure to drugs such as cocaine and opiates.

Many passively addicted infants can be treated without medication; holding, rocking, swaddling, and frequent feedings may be sufficient. Infants who fail to respond to symptomatic treatment will require pharmacologic therapy. The AAP recommends that drug selection should match the type of agent causing withdrawal. Thus for opioid withdrawal, dilute tincture of opium is the preferred drug. Other medications include paregoric, clonidine, and chlorpromazine; for sedative-hypnotic withdrawal, phenobarbital is the agent of choice.

Maternal alcohol use during gestation causes a teratogenic syndrome of fetal malformation. The fetal alcohol syndrome includes growth retardation, microcephaly, characteristic facial features, mental retardation, and cardiac and renal abnormalities.

Excessive ingestion of alcohol by the mother during late pregnancy may result in withdrawal symptoms in the infant that generally begin on the first day and may include tremors, hyperactivity, seizures, and hypoglycemia.

Multiple-drug abuse is common among substance-abusing women; simultaneous use of more than one drug should be suspected when fetal exposure to one drug has been identified. Furthermore, IV drug abusers are the second largest risk group for HIV infection. Infants born to substance abusers should be evaluated for HIV infection.

THE INFANT WITH DEVELOPMENTAL ABNORMALITIES

Infants born with developmental abnormalities need prompt evaluation by pediatricians, clinical geneticists, perinatologists, and other clinicians with expertise in dysmorphology. Most of these experts will be found in referral centers, which may necessitate transfer of a child born in a community hospital. The purpose of the following discussion is to outline certain principles of dysmorphology, to define commonly used terminology, and to furnish a method of assessment and a method of counseling for parents of dysmorphic offspring.

Principles of Dysmorphology

(1) Most defects are nonspecific. An isolated defect does not generally allow diagnosis of a specific syndrome. For example, facial clefts occur in trisomy 13 syndrome, but not all infants with facial clefts have trisomy 13 syndrome.

(2) The overall pattern of defects is important for diagnosis. Thus the presence of minor anomalies may be very useful in diagnosis.

(3) Not every malformation reported in a syndrome is necessary for diagnosis. Rarely does a patient exhibit every malformation reported with any given syndrome; and the same patient may exhibit variability from one side of the body to the other in those defects capable of being bilateral. This variance of expression is common to virtually all syndromes. For example, the characteristics of clefting, polydactyly, and cardiac defects form a basis for the diagnosis of trisomy 13 syndrome. However, only 60–80% of patients with this syndrome will have each of these specific anomalies.

(4) Similar phenotypes may mask different syndromes. Individuals with Marfan syndrome appear similar to individuals with homocystinuria; however, genetically, biochemically, and medically, they are dissimilar.

Terminology

An **anomaly** or **malformation** is a primary structural defect that results from a localized developmental error, eg, cleft lip. A **deformation** is an alteration in the structure or shape of a previously normally formed part, eg, clubfoot. A **syndrome** is a recognized pattern of malformations with the same cause and not the result of an isolated morphogenic error. Down syndrome (trisomy 21 syndrome) is an example. A **sequence** is a pattern of malformations caused by a single developmental abnormality that leads to a cascade of defects, eg, Potter's sequence. Anomalies that occur together more frequently than expected by chance but that do not represent a syndrome are known as an **association.**

Assessment of Developmental Defects

A. Thorough Physical Examination

Careful definition and recording of the anomalies and their extent is mandatory. This facilitates categorization of the errors, separation of primary and secondary defects, and definition of problems requiring immediate attention. The temptation to make a diagnosis based on preliminary information must be avoided. The information communicated (to families or other health care providers) should be descriptive and should serve to facilitate any further evaluation.

B. History

If physical examination alone is insufficient for diagnosis, the taking of a detailed history is imperative. The history should include at least the following information: a thorough history of this pregnancy with emphasis on the first trimester, including potential teratogen exposure and illness during pregnancy; a reproductive history; a 3-generation pedigree; and a complete maternal medical history.

C. Genetic or Dysmorphic Consultation

Given the extraordinary emotional impact of most anomalies, it is usually prudent to seek consultation from clinical geneticists, dysmorphologists, or appropriate pediatric subspecialists. With even the most obvious diagnoses it may assist the family in their acceptance of the problem.

D. Photography

Photographs permanently document the findings and may later serve to confirm the diagnosis or assist in study and consultation. They may be crucial should a severely malformed infant die before it can be evaluated by a dysmorphologist.

E. Radiography

Many syndromes have well-defined radiographic findings, but diagnosis may be difficult in certain cases. Selected radiographs, including whole-body radiographs of the infant that has died, may facilitate the diagnosis.

F. Laboratory Evaluation

The need for laboratory evaluation depends on the nature of the defect. In some cases, no laboratory evaluation is necessary. However, in many it is prudent to obtain cytogenetic studies. In other situations, it may be necessary to obtain microbiologic, immunologic, histologic, and metabolic studies.

G. Autopsy

In the event of the infant's death, autopsy may facilitate diagnosis. The type and extent of specific abnormalities must be recorded if the autopsy is to provide meaningful information.

Counseling for Developmental Disabilities

Counseling for developmental disabilities can be difficult, and it may require a significant amount of time. It may be adequately provided by the primary physician who is sufficiently motivated and prepared, although the assistance of specialists can be helpful. Preparation for counseling includes (1) allocating enough time for a meaningful discussion, (2) having adequate information about the abnormality, (3) being comfortable dealing with this type of situation, and (4) being able to listen carefully and be sensitive to the family's needs. Careful attention to questions will generally uncover misinformation.

While counseling for each family must be individualized, certain basic elements of counseling should be included (Table 29–3). Definitive counseling may require several visits, because factors such as stress may preclude normal assimilation of information.

The parents' adjustment to and acceptance of the situation may well depend upon the physician's initial introduction and explanations. Concerned relatives, friends, and medical staff often give the parents well-meaning but misdirected information. Parents frequently attempt to relate something they did or did not do during the course of the pregnancy to the defect. Careful consideration and factual explanation of the perceived relationship between the defect and the time when the event occurred often assist in answering such questions. For example, the mother with a viral illness at 24 weeks gestation may be reassured that this was not the cause of her infant's cleft palate.

Parents and siblings may experience psychologic trauma, which must be recognized in order to be managed effectively. This trauma may be expressed individually or collectively as shame, guilt, anger, denial, intellectualization, fear, depression, and a sense of failure. The family may consider the infant's condition to be retribution for a real or imagined sin. Blame between the parents will require thoughtful exploration and explanation. Sexual dysfunction often develops after the birth of an anomalous child. The entire family constellation must be considered for counseling to be effective.

Table 29–3. Elements of counseling for developmental defects.[1]

Description of the anomalies present
The cause of the condition (if known)
An indication of the prognosis
A discussion of immediate options
Therapeutic means that may be necessary
The potential for recurrence
The mode of inheritance (if known)
Late complications to be expected
In cases of death, the autopsy findings
Thorough answering of questions
Provisions for familial emotional support

[1]Modified and reproduced, with permission, from: Pernoll ML, King CR, Prescott GH: Genetics in Obstetrics and Gynecology. In: Wynn RM (editor): *Obstetrics and Gynecology Annual: 1980,* vol 9. Appleton-Century-Crofts, 1980, p. 31.

REFERENCES

American Academy of Pediatrics: Use of psychoactive medications during pregnancy and possible effects on the fetus and newborn. Pediatrics 2000;105:880.

American Academy of Pediatrics Committee on Drugs: Neonatal drug withdrawal. Pediatrics 1998;101:1079.

American Academy of Pediatrics Committee on Fetus and Newborn: Surfactant replacement therapy for respiratory distress syndrome. Pediatrics 1999;103:684.

American Academy of Pediatrics Committee on Fetus and Newborn: Use of Inhaled Nitric Oxide. Pediatrics 2000;106:344.

American Academy of Pediatrics Committee on Infectious Diseases and Committee on Fetus and Newborn: Revised guidelines for prevention of group B streptococci (GBS) infection by chemoprophylaxis. Pediatrics 1997;99:775.

Andersen CC: Peripheral retinal ablation for threshold retinopathy of prematurity in preterm infants. Cochrane Database Syst Rev 2000;2:CD001693.

Apgar V: A proposal for a new method of evaluation of the newborn infant. Curr Res Anesth Analg 1953;32:260.

Autret-Leca E: Vitamin K in neonates: how to administer, when and to whom. Paediatr Drugs 2001;3:1.

Avery GB et al: Controlled trial of dexamethasone in respiratory-dependent infants with bronchopulmonary dysplasia. Pediatrics 1985;75:106.

Banach MJ: Laser therapy for retinopathy of prematurity. Curr Opin Ophthalmol 2001;12:164.

Bunt JE: Treatment with exogenous surfactant stimulates endogenous surfactant synthesis in premature infants with respiratory distress syndrome. Crit Care Med 2000;28):3383.

Burn J et al: Recurrence risks in offspring of adults with major heart defects: Results from first cohort of British collaborative study. Lancet 1998;351:311.

Cleary GM: Meconium-stained amniotic fluid and the meconium aspiration syndrome: An update. Pediatr Clin North Am 1998;45:511.

Cordero L et al: Management of infants of diabetic mothers. Arch Pediatr Adolesc Med 1998;152:249.

Davidson D, Barefield ES, Kattwinkel J: Inhaled nitric oxide for the early treatment of persistent pulmonary hypertension of the term newborn: A randomized, double-masked, placebo-controlled, dose-response, multicenter study. Pediatrics 1998;101:325.

Davis Eyler F et al: Birth outcome from a prospective, matched study of prenatal crack/cocaine use: I. Interactive and dose effects on health and growth. Pediatrics 1998;101:229.

DeCarvahlo M, Klause MH, Merkatz RB: Frequency of breastfeeding and serum bilirubin concentration. Am J Dis Child 1982;136:737.

Dekowski SA: Surfactant replacement therapy: An update on applications. Pediatr Clin North Am 1998;45:549.

Dennery: Neonatal hyperbilirubinemia. N Engl J Med 2001;8:581.

Dinarevi S: Use of prostaglandins in neonatal cardiology. Med Arh 2000;54:279.

Gourley GR: Neonatal jaundice and diet. Arch Pediatr Adolesc Med 1999;153:184.

Guerra B: Prenatal diagnosis of symptomatic congenital cytomegalovirus infection. Am J Obstet Gynecol 2000; 183:476.

Gunn AJ: Is temperature important in delivery room resuscitation? Semin Neonatol 2001;6:241.

Hegyi T et al: The Apgar score and its components in the preterm infant. Pediatrics 1998;101:77.

Jackson JC: Adverse events associated with exchange transfusion in healthy and ill newborns. Pediatrics 99:http://www.pediatrics.org/cgi/content/full/99/5/e7, 1997.

Janssens HM et al: Outcome for children treated with fetal intravascular transfusions because of severe blood group antagonism. J Pediatr 1997;131:373.

Jona JZ: Advances in neonatal surgery. Pediatr Clin North Am 1998;45:605.

Kaftan H: Early onset neonatal bacterial infections. Semin Perinatol 1998;22:15.

Kluckow M: Low systemic blood flow and hyperkalemia in preterm infants. J Pediatr 2001;139:227.

Ledermann SE: Long-term outcome of peritoneal dialysis in infants. J Pediatr 2000;136:24.

Lotze A et al: Multicenter study of surfactant (beractant) use in the treatment of term infants with severe respiratory failure. Pediatrics 1998;132:40.

Martin RW: Screening for fetal abdominal wall defects. Obstet Gynecol Clin North Am 1998;25:517.

McGettigan MC: New ways to ventilate newborns in acute respiratory failure. Pediatr Clin North Am 1998;45:475.

Milner A: The importance of ventilation to effective resuscitation in the term and preterm infant. Semin Neonatol 2001;6:219.

Mizrah EM: Neonatal seizures and neonatal epileptic syndromes. Neurol Clin 2001;19:427.

Moriette G: High-frequency oscillatory ventilation in the management of respiratory distress syndrome. Biol Neonate 2000;77(Suppl 1):14.

Ohls RK: Erythropoetin to prevent and treat the anemia of prematurity. Curr Opin Pediatr 1999;11:108.

Passmore SJ: Ecological studies of relation between hospital policies on neonatal vitamin K administration and subsequent occurrence of childhood cancer. Br Med J 1998;316:184.

Piazza AJ: Postasphyxial management of the newborn. Clin Perinatol 1999;26:749-65, ix.

Pschirrer ER: Does asphyxia cause cerebral palsy? Semin Perinatol 2000;24:215.

Rais-Bahrami K, Short BL: The current status of neonatal extracorporeal membrane oxygenation. Semin Perinatol 2000; 24:406.

Ramey J: Evaluation of periventricular-intraventricular hemorrhage in premature infants using cranial ultrasounds. Neonatal Netw 1998;17:65.

Rovin J et al: The role of peritoneal drainage for intestinal perforation in infants with and without necrotizing enterocolitis. J Pediatr Surg 1999;34:143.

Saugstad OD: Practical aspects of resuscitating asphyxiated newborn infants. Eur J Pediatr 1998;157(Suppl 1):S11.

Soll R: Consensus and controversy over resuscitation of the newborn infant. Lancet 1999;354:4.

Suda K: Echocardiographic predictors of outcome in newborns with congenital diaphragmatic hernia. Pediatrics 2000; 105:1106.

Supplemental Therapeutic Oxygen for Prethreshold Retinopathy of Prematurity (STOP-ROP), A Randomized, Controlled Trial. I: Primary Outcomes. Pediatrics 2000;105:295.

Sweet DG, Halliday HL: Current perspectives on the drug treatment of neonatal respiratory distress syndrome. Paediatr Drugs 1999;1:19.

Tan KL: Decreased response to phototherapy for neonatal jaundice in breast-fed infants. Arch Pediatr Adolesc Med 1998; 152:1187.

Thilo EH, Rosenberg AA: The newborn infant. In: Way WW Jr et al (editor): *Current Pediatric Diagnosis & Treatment*, 15th ed. McGraw-Hill, 2001.

Toth-Heyn P: The stressed neonatal kidney: From pathophysiology to clinical management of neonatal vasomotor nephropathy. Pediatr Nephrol 2000;14:227.

UK Collaborative ECMO Trial Group: UK collaborative randomised trial of neonatal extracorporeal membrane oxygenation. Lancet 1996;348:75.

Van Overmeire B: Early versus late indomethacin treatment for patent ductus arteriosus in premature infants with respiratory distress syndrome. J Pediatr 2001;138:205.

Vamvakas EC: Meta-analysis of controlled clinical trials studying the efficacy of rHuEPO in reducing blood transfusions in the anemia of prematurity. Transfusion 2001;41:406.

Vermillion ST: Effectiveness of antenatal corticosteroid administration after preterm premature rupture of the membranes. Am J Obstet Gynecol 2000;183:925.

Wiswell TE: Delivery room management of the apparently vigorous meconium-stained neonate: Results of the multicenter, international collaborative trial. Pediatrics 2000;105:1.

Wong W et al: Randomised controlled trial: Comparison of colloid or crystalloid for partial exchange transfusion for treatment of neonatal polycythaemia. Arch Dis Child 1997;77:F115.

Wyckoff MH: Medications during resuscitation—what is the evidence? Semin Neonatol 2001;6:251.

Zipursky A: Vitamin K at birth. Br Med J 1996;313:179.

SECTION IV
General Gynecology

Gynecologic History, Examination, & Diagnostic Procedures

30

Charles Kawada, MD

The gynecologist needs to approach each patient not just as a person needing medical intervention for a specific presenting problem, but also as one that may have variety of factors that may affect her health. The initial approach to the gynecologic patient and the general diagnostic procedures available for the investigation of gynecologic complaints are presented here. Although other aspects of the general medical examination are left to other texts, concern for the patient's total health and well-being is mandatory.

THE PERIODIC HEALTH SCREENING EXAMINATION

It is now a generally accepted part of the physician's responsibility to advise patients to have periodic medical evaluations. The frequency of visits varies according to the patient's problem.

The periodic health screening examination helps detect the following ailments of women that are especially amenable to early diagnosis and treatment: diabetes mellitus; urinary tract infection or tumor; hypertension; malnutrition or obesity; thyroid dysfunction or tumor; and breast, abdominal, or pelvic tumor. These conditions can be detected by a review of systems, with specific questions regarding recent abnormalities or any variation in function. Determination of weight, blood pressure, and urinalysis, which can be done in minutes, may reveal variations from the previous examination. An examination of the thyroid gland, breasts, abdomen, and pelvis, including a Papanicolaou (Pap) smear, should then be performed. A rectal examination is also advisable, and a conveniently packaged test for occult blood (Hemoccult) is recommended for patients over 40 years of age.

The physician should also be concerned about conditions other than purely somatic ones. Unless a patient's problems require the services of a psychiatrist or some other specialist, the doctor should be prepared to act as a counselor and work with the patient during a mutually agreeable time when it is possible to listen to her problems without being hurried and to give support, counsel, and other kinds of help as required.

HISTORY

To adequately evaluate the gynecologic patient, it is important to establish a rapport during the history taking. The patient must be allowed to tell her story to an interested listener who does not allow body language or facial expressions to imply disinterest or boredom. One should avoid cutting off the patient's story, since doing so may obscure important clues or other problems that may have contributed to the reasons for the visit.

The following outline varies from the routine medical history because, in evaluating the gynecologic patient, the problem can often be clarified if the history is obtained in the following order.

Identifying Information

A. AGE

Knowledge of the patient's age sets the tone for the complaint and the approach to the patient. Obviously, the problems and the approach to them vary at different stages in a woman's life (pubescence, adolescence, childbearing years, and pre- and postmenopausal years).

B. LAST NORMAL MENSTRUAL PERIOD

The date of onset of the last normal menstrual period (LNMP) is important to define. A missed period, irregularity of periods, erratic bleeding, or other abnormalities may all imply certain events that are more easily diagnosed when the date of onset of the LNMP is established.

C. GRAVIDITY AND PARITY

The process of taking the patient's obstetric history is detailed in Chapter 9, but the reproductive history should be recorded as part of the gynecologic evaluation. A convenient symbol for recording the reproductive history is a 4-digit code denoting the number of term pregnancies, premature deliveries, abortions, and living children (TPAL); eg, 2-1-1-3 means 2 term pregnancies, 1 premature delivery, 1 abortion, and 3 living children.

Chief Complaint

The chief complaint is usually best elicited by asking "What kind of problem are you having?" or "How can I help you?" It is important to listen carefully to the way the patient responds to this question and to allow her to fully explain her complaint. The patient should be interrupted only to clarify certain points that may be unclear.

Present Illness

Each of the problems the patient describes must be obtained in detail by questioning regarding what exactly the problem is, where exactly the problem is occurring, the date and time of onset, whether the symptoms are abating or getting worse, the duration of the symptoms when they do occur, and how these symptoms are related to or influence other events in her life. For example, the site, duration, and intensity of pain must be accurately described. Often helpful in evaluating the intensity of pain is getting a sense of how the pain affects her life: "Does the pain prevent you from standing or walking?"

It is important to maintain eye contact with the patient and to listen to every word. Do not rely on a patient's sophistication as a measure of her knowledge of anatomy and medical terminology. It is important for the physician to judiciously adjust the level of terminology according to the patient's knowledge and vocabulary. Communicating with the patient in this manner may help the physician obtain an accurate history and establish rapport.

In addition to physiologic events and the life cycle, symptoms described could be related to starting a new job, the beginning of a new relationship or difficulties in the current relationship, an exercise regimen, new medication, and any emotional changes in the patient's life.

Past History

After the physician is satisfied that all possible information concerning the present illness and the important corollaries has been obtained, the past history should be elicited.

A. CONTRACEPTION

Continuing with the history, it is important to elicit whether the patient is using or needs some form of contraception. If she is using contraception, her level of satisfaction with her chosen method should be determined. In patients taking oral contraceptives, the history should reflect the agent and dose, whether there is a great variation in the time of day she takes her pill, and any impact the pill has had on other physiologic functions. It is also extremely important to ask questions during the remainder of the history and to key the physical examination to ascertain whether there are any contraindications to the patient's current form of contraception.

B. MEDICATIONS AND HABITS

Any medications, prescribed or otherwise, that are being taken or that were being taken when symptoms first occurred should be described. Particular attention must be directed to use of hormones, steroids, and other compounds likely to influence the reproductive tract. In addition to medications the patient should be questioned concerning her use of recreational drugs. It must be ascertained whether the patient smokes and, if so, how much and for how long. It is also important to ascertain the amount of alcohol ingested, if any. This questioning provides an ideal time to indicate the health risks of various habits.

C. MEDICAL

It is important to discover any history of prior serious medical and psychiatric illnesses and whether hospitalization was required. Particularly important are illnesses in the major organ systems. It is also important to know whether there is a major endocrinopathy in the patient's history. Notable weight gain or loss prior to the onset of the patient's current symptoms should be detailed. Other important details include when she had her last physical examination, including pelvic examination and Pap smear.

D. SURGICAL

The surgical history includes all operations, the dates performed, and associated postoperative or anesthetic complications.

E. ALLERGIES

Questioning should continue relating any possible allergic reactions to drugs or specific foods. The reaction produced (eg, rash, gastrointestinal upset) must be elicited and the approximate time when it occurred ascertained. Any testing to confirm or deny the observation must be noted.

F. BLEEDING DIATHESES

Determining whether or not the patient bleeds excessively in relation to prior surgery or minor trauma is important. A history of easy bruising or of bleeding from the gums while brushing teeth may be useful in this judgment. Suspicion of a bleeding problem indicates the need for further laboratory evaluation.

G. OBSTETRICS

The obstetric history includes each of the patient's pregnancies listed in chronological order. The date of birth; sex and weight of the offspring; duration of pregnancy; length of labor; type of delivery; type of anesthesia; and any complications should be included.

H. GYNECOLOGIC

The first item in the gynecologic past history is the menstrual history: age at menarche, interval between periods, duration of flow, amount and character of flow, degree of discomfort, and age at menopause. The menstrual history is often an important clue in the diagnosis.

A prior history of sexually transmitted disease (STD) needs to be detailed. Although in the past it was more common to note only gonorrhea and syphilis, it is important to also document exposure to HIV, hepatitis, herpesvirus, chlamydia, and papillomavirus. Any treatment or admissions to the hospital for treatment of salpingitis, endometritis, or tubo-ovarian abscess must be carefully documented. Attempts to assess the impact of these processes in relation to ectopic pregnancy, infertility, and the type of contraception must be elicited.

Although its significance is less than that of the prior stated diseases, the occurrence of episodes of vaginitis should not be dismissed. Their frequency and the medications used to treat them should be discussed. In the case of such infections, it is important to detail whether or not it was a pathologic situation or merely a misinterpreted physiologic circumstance.

I. SEXUAL

The sexual history should be an integral part of any general gynecologic history. In taking a sexual history, the physician must be nonjudgmental and not embarrassed or critical.

Questions that may be covered include the following. Is she currently sexually active? Is the relationship satisfactory to her and, if not, why not? A question regarding whether the patient is heterosexual or lesbian is important but often difficult to ask because the question may be offensive to some patients. It is important, however, not to assume that a relationship is heterosexual because a lesbian woman will lose all rapport with the physician when the physician is insensitive to such issues.

J. SOCIAL

A social history can be an extension of earlier questions pertaining to the marital and sexual history. Knowing the type of work the patient does (including the amount of physical exercise entailed), something of her education, and her community activities may assist in ascertaining the patient's relationship to her entire environment.

The patient's involvement with her own health care should be carefully elicited, including her attention and knowledge concerning diet, health screening examinations, exercise, and recreation.

Family History

The patient's family history must include the state of health of immediate relatives (parents, siblings, grandparents, and offspring). In addition to listing these relatives, it is useful in cases where genetic illnesses may be apparent to record a 3-generation pedigree.

The incidence of familial heart disease, hypertensive renal or vascular disease, diabetes mellitus (insulin-dependent or non-insulin-dependent), vascular accidents, and hematologic abnormalities should be ascertained. If the patient has a problem with hirsutism or if she perceives excessive hair growth, it is important to elicit whether anyone in her family has the same distribution of hair growth. Familial history of breast and ovarian cancers is important to elicit since a close familial history may require additional testing and close follow-up. It is important to relate the time of menopause in the mother or grandmother and to ascertain a history of osteoporosis.

PHYSICAL EXAMINATION

The physical examination is most useful if it is conducted in an environment that is aesthetically pleasing to the patient. Adequate gowning and draping assist in the prevention of embarrassment. Often a physician's assistant conducts the patient to the dressing area and gives explicit instructions about what to take off and how to put on her gown and then may assist in draping the patient.

A physician may have a female assistant remain in the examining room to assist when necessary, but whether or not she remains solely as a chaperone depends on local custom and the preference of the patient and the physician. A chaperone is not customarily or legally required, but the physician, male or female, must be selective in this matter and have an assistant present during the examination of an overly fearful or potentially seductive patient. If the patient wants her partner, relative, or a female friend to be present, the request should be honored unless, in the physician's judgment, some impropriety might result or such an arrangement would interfere with the examination or with obtaining an accurate history.

General Examination

If the gynecologist is the primary care physician for the patient, a general physical examination should be performed yearly or whenever the situation warrants. A complete examination obviously provides more information, demonstrates the physician's thoroughness, and establishes rapport with the patient.

General Evaluation

A. VITAL SIGNS

As part of every examination—whether for a specific problem, routine annual examination, or a return visit for a previously diagnosed problem—the patient should be weighed and her blood pressure taken. Postmenopausal patients should have their height measured to document whether there is loss of height from osteoporosis and vertebral fractures. Before she empties her bladder for the examination, it should be determined whether the urine will need to be sent for urinalysis, culture, or pregnancy testing.

The examination of the chest should include visual examination for any skin lesions and symmetry of movement. Auscultation and percussion of the lungs are important for excluding primary pulmonary problems such as asthma and pneumonia. The examination of the heart includes percussion for size and auscultation for arrhythmias and significant murmurs.

Breast Examination
(See also Chapter 62.)

Breast examination should be a routine part of the physical examination. Breast cancer will occur in 1 in 8 women in the U.S. during her lifetime. Physicians who treat women should educate patients in the technique of self-examination, since the well-prepared patient is one of the most accurate screening methods for breast disease.

The physical examination provides an ideal time to ascertain the frequency and methodology of breast self-examination. It also is an ideal time to teach the patient how to perform breast self-examination. The patient should be advised to examine herself in the mirror, looking for skin changes or dimpling, and then carefully palpate all quadrants of the breast. Most women prefer to do this with soapy hands while showering or bathing. The examination should be repeated at the same time each month, preferably 1 week after the initiation of the menses, when the breasts are least nodular; postmenopausal women should perform self-examination on the same day each month.

The frequency of mammography or the earlier use of mammography depends on both the individual woman and her family history. Patients with a positive family history of breast cancer should have a mammogram at an earlier age, particularly those whose mother, aunt, or sister developed premenopausal breast cancer. In general, a mammogram should be obtained every 1–2 years from ages 40 to 50 and annually thereafter. Ultrasonography can now reliably differentiate solid from cystic lesions; this technique complements but does not supplant mammography. Indeed, breast self-examination, physician examination, mammography, and ultrasonography are complementary and all should be employed in the early detection of breast cancer.

The correct technique for breast examination is demonstrated in Figure 30–1. If abnormalities are encountered, a decision should be reached concerning the need for mammography (or other imaging methods) or direct referral to a breast surgeon unless the gynecologist is trained in performing breast biopsies. Skin lesions, particularly eczematous lesions in the area of the nipple, should be closely observed; if they are not easily cured by simple measures, they should be biopsied. An eczematous lesion on the nipple or areola may represent Paget's carcinoma.

Abdominal Examination

The patient should be lying completely supine and relaxed; the knees may be slightly flexed and supported as an aid to relaxation of the abdominal muscles. Inspection should detect irregularity of contour or color. Auscultation should follow inspection but precede palpation because the latter may change the character of intestinal activity. Palpation of the entire abdomen—gently at first, then more firmly as indicated—should detect rigidity, voluntary guarding, masses, and tenderness. If the patient complains of abdominal pain or if unexpected tenderness is elicited, the examiner should ask her to indicate the point of maximal pain or tenderness with one finger. Suprapubic palpation is designed to detect uterine, ovarian, or urinary bladder enlargements. A painful area should be left until last for deep palpation; otherwise, the entire abdomen may be guarded voluntarily. As a final part of the abdominal examination, the physician should carefully check for any abnormality of the abdominal organs: liver, gallbladder, spleen, kidneys, and intestines. In some instances, the demonstration of an abnormality of the ab-

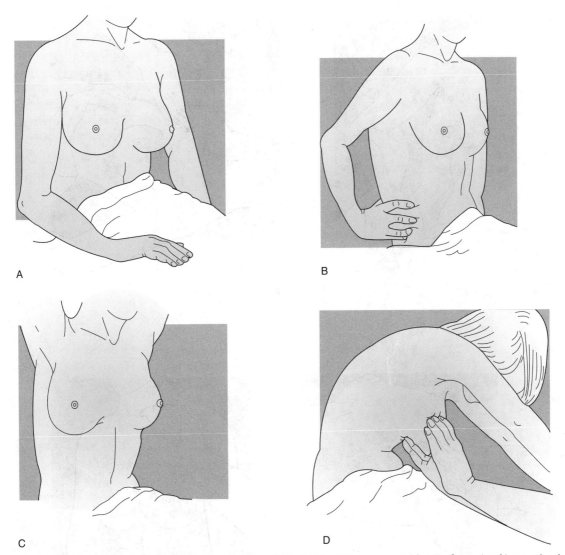

Figure 30–1. Breast examination by the physician. **A:** Patient is sitting, arms at sides. Perform visual inspection in good light, looking for lumps or for dimpling or wrinkling of skin. **B:** Patient is sitting, hands pressing on hips so that pectoralis muscles are tensed. Repeat visual inspection. **C:** Patient is sitting, arms above head. Repeat visual inspection of breasts and also perform visual inspection of axillae. **D:** Patient is sitting and leaning forward, hands on examiner's shoulders, the stirrups, or her own knees. Perform bimanual palpation, paying particular attention to the base of the glandular portion of the breast.

dominal muscle reflexes may be diagnostically helpful. Percussion of the abdomen should be performed to identify organ enlargement, tumor, or ascites.

Pelvic Examination

The pelvic examination is a procedure feared by many women and must be conducted in such a way as to allay her anxieties. A patient's first pelvic examination may be especially disturbing, so it is important for the physician to attempt to allay fear and to inspire confidence and cooperation. The empathic physician usually finds that by the time the history has been obtained and a painless and nonembarrassing general examination performed, a satisfactory gynecologic examination is not a problem. Relaxing surroundings; a nurse or attendant

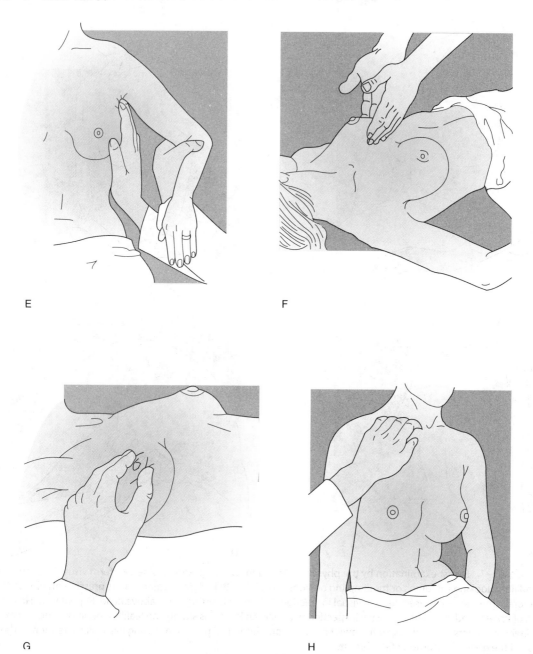

E

F

G

H

Figure 30–1 (cont'd). **E:** Patient is sitting, arms extended 60–90 degrees. Palpate axillae. **F:** Patient is supine, arms relaxed at sides. Perform bimanual palpation of each portion of breast (usually each quadrant, but smaller sections for unusually large breasts). Repeat examinations **C, E,** and **F** with patient supine, arms above head. **G:** Patient is supine, arms relaxed at sides. Palpate under the areola and nipple with the thumb and forefinger to detect a mass or test for expression of fluid from the nipple. **H:** Patient is either sitting or supine. Palpate supraclavicular areas.

chaperone if indicated; warm instruments; and a gentle, unhurried manner with continued explanation and re-assurance are helpful in securing patient relaxation and cooperation. This is especially true with the woman who has never had a pelvic examination before. In these patients a one-finger examination and a narrow specu-lum often are necessary. In some cases, vaginal exami-nation is not possible; palpation of the pelvic structures by rectal examination is then the only recourse. Occa-sionally an ultrasound examination may be helpful in ascertaining whether the pelvic organs are normal in size and configuration in patients from whom adequate relaxation of the abdominal muscles cannot be ob-

tained. If a more definitive pelvic examination is essen-tial, it can be performed with the patient anesthetized.

A. EXTERNAL GENITALIA (FIG 30–2)

The pubic hair should be inspected for its pattern (mas-culine or feminine), for the nits of pubic lice, for in-fected hair follicles, or for any other abnormality. The skin of the vulva, mons pubis, and perineal area should be examined for evidence of dermatitis or discoloration. The glans clitoridis can be exposed by gently retracting the surrounding skin folds. The clitoris is at the ventral confluence of the 2 labia; it should be no more than 2.5 cm in length, most of which is subcutaneous. The

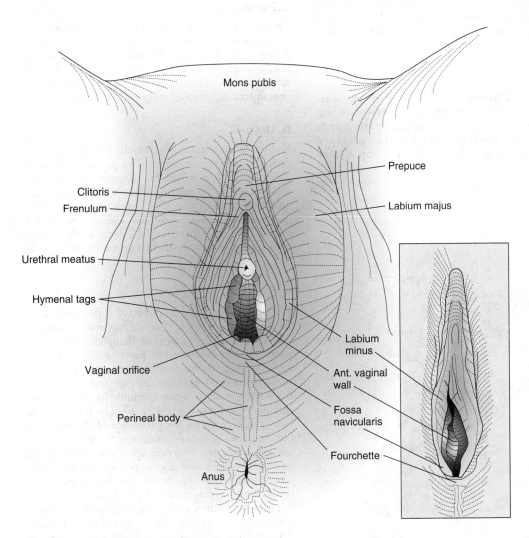

Figure 30–2. **Normal external genitalia in a mature woman.** (Reproduced with permission from Benson RC: *Hand-book of Obstetrics & Gynecology,* 8th ed. Lange, 1983.)

major and minor labia are usually the same size on both sides, but a moderate difference in size is not abnormal. Small protuberances or subcutaneous nodules may be either sebaceous cysts or tumors. External condylomata are often found in this area. The urethra, just below the clitoris, should be the same color as the surrounding tissue and without protuberances. Normally, vestibular (Bartholin's) glands can be neither seen nor felt; thus enlargement may indicate an abnormality of this gland system. The area of vestibular glands should be palpated by placing the index finger in the vagina and the thumb outside and gently feeling for enlargement or tenderness (Fig 30–3). The perineal skin may be reddened as a result of vulvar or vaginal infection. Scars may indicate obstetric lacerations or surgery. The anus should also be inspected at this time for the presence of hemorrhoids, fissures, irritation, or perianal infections (eg, condylomata or herpesvirus lesions).

B. HYMEN

An unruptured hymen may present in many forms, but only a completely imperforate, cribriform, or septate hymen is pathologic. After rupture, it also may be seen in various forms (Fig 30–4). After the birth of several children, the hymen may almost disappear completely.

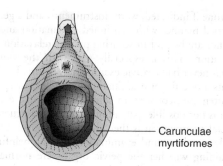

Carunculae myrtiformes

Figure 30–4. Ruptured hymen (parous introitus).

C. PERINEAL SUPPORT

To determine the presence of pelvic relaxation, the physician spreads the labia with 2 fingers and tells the patient to "bear down." This will demonstrate urethrocele, cystocele, rectocele, or uterine prolapse, although sometimes an upright position may be necessary to demonstrate significant prolapse (see Chapter 41).

D. URETHRA

Redness of the urethra may indicate infection or a urethral caruncle or carcinoma. The paraurethral glands are situated below the urethra and empty into the urethra just inside the meatus. With the labia spread adequately for better vision, the urethra may be "stripped" (ie, pressure exerted by the examining finger as it is moved from the proximal to the distal urethra) to express discharge from the urethra or paraurethral glands.

Vaginal Examination

The vagina should first be inspected with the speculum for abnormalities and to obtain a Pap smear before further examination. A speculum dampened with warm water but not lubricated is gently inserted into the vagina so that the cervix and fornices can be thoroughly visualized (Fig 30–5). After the Pap smear is prepared, the vaginal wall is again carefully inspected as the speculum is withdrawn (Fig 30–6). The type of speculum used depends on the preference of the physician, but the most satisfactory instrument for the sexually active patient is the Pederson speculum, although the wider Graves speculum may be necessary to afford adequate visualization (Fig 30–7). For the patient with a small introitus, the narrow-bladed Pederson speculum is preferable. When more than the usual exposure is necessary, an extra large Graves speculum is available. To visualize a child's vagina, a Huffman or nasal speculum, a large otoscope, or a Kelly air cystoscope is invaluable.

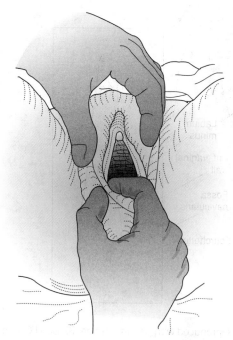

Figure 30–3. Palpation of vestibular glands.

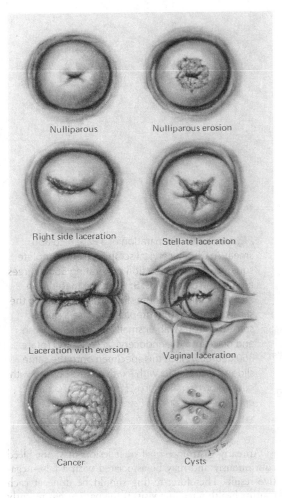

Figure 30–5. The uterine cervix: normal and pathologic appearance.

Next, the vagina is palpated; unless the patient's introitus is too small, the index and middle fingers of either hand are inserted gently and the tissues palpated. The vaginal walls should be smooth, elastic, and nontender.

Bimanual Examination

The uterus and adnexal structures should be outlined between the 2 fingers of the hand in the vagina and the flat of the opposite hand, which is placed upon the lower abdominal wall (Fig 30–8). Gentle palpation and manipulation of the structures will delineate position, size, shape, mobility, consistency, and tenderness of the pelvic structures—except in the obese or uncooperative patient or in a patient whose abdominal muscles are

taut as a result of fear or tenderness. Tenderness can be elicited either on direct palpation or on movement or stretching of the pelvic structures.

A. Cervix

The cervix is a firm structure traditionally described as having the consistency of the tip of the nose. Normally it is round and approximately 3–4 cm in diameter. Various appearances of the cervix are shown in Figure 30–5. The external os is also round and virtually closed. Multiparous women may have an os that has been lacerated. An irregularity in shape or nodularity may be due to one or more nabothian cysts. If the cervix is extremely firm, it may contain a tumor, even cancer. The cervix (along with the body of the uterus) normally is moderately mobile, so that it can be moved 2–4 cm in any direction without causing undue discomfort. (When examining a patient, it is helpful to warn her that she will feel the movement of her uterus but that ordinarily this maneuver is not painful.) Restriction of mobility of the cervix or corpus often follows inflammation, neoplasia, or surgery.

B. Corpus of the Uterus

The corpus of the uterus is approximately half the size of the patient's fist and weighs approximately 70–90 g. It is regular in outline and not tender to pressure or moderate motion. In most women, the uterus is anteverted; in about one-third of women, it is retroverted (see Chapter 41). A retroverted uterus is usually not a pathologic finding. In certain cases of endometriosis or previous salpingitis, it may be that the "tipped" uterus is a result of adhesions caused by the disease process. The uterus is usually described in terms of its size, shape, position, consistency, and mobility.

C. Adnexa

Adnexal structures (fallopian tubes and ovaries) cannot be palpated in many overweight women, because the normal tube is only about 7 mm in diameter and the ovary no more than 3 cm in its greatest dimension. In very slender women, however, the ovaries nearly always are palpable and, in some instances, the oviducts are as well. In the postmenopausal woman usually no adnexal structures can be palpated. Unusual tenderness or enlargement of any adnexal structure indicates the need for further diagnostic procedures; an adnexal mass in any woman is an indication for investigation.

Rectovaginal Examination

At the completion of the bimanual pelvic examination, a rectovaginal examination should always be performed, especially after the age of 40. The well-lubricated middle finger of the examining hand should be inserted

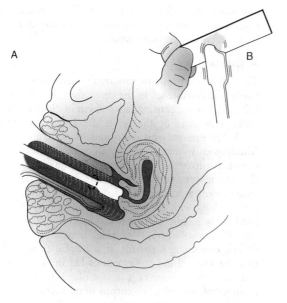

Materials Needed

One cervical spatula, cut tongue depressor, cotton swab, or small
  brush made especially for obtaining endocervical cells.
One glass slide (one end frosted). Identify by writing the patient's
  name on the frosted end with a lead pencil.
One speculum (without lubricant).
One bottle of fixative (75% ethyl alcohol) or spray-on fixative, eg,
  Aqua-Net or Cyto-Spray.

Figure 30–6. Preparation of a Papanicolaou
smear **A:** Obtain cervical scraping from complete
squamocolumnar junction by rotating 360 degrees
around the external os. **B:** Place the material an
inch from the end of the slide and smear along the
slide to obtain a thin preparation. Use a saline-
soaked cotton swab or small endocervical brush
and place into the endocervical canal and rotate
360 degrees. Place this specimen onto the same
slide and quickly fix with fixative. (Reproduced with
permission from Benson RC: *Handbook of Obstetrics
and Gynecology,* 8th ed. Lange, 1983.)

gently into the rectum to feel for tenderness, masses, or
irregularities. When the examining finger has been inserted a short distance, the index finger can then be inserted into the vagina until the depth of the vagina is
reached (Fig 30–9). It is much easier to examine some
aspects of the posterior portion of the pelvis by rectovaginal examination than by vaginal examination alone.
The index finger can now raise the cervix toward the
anterior abdominal wall, which stretches the uterosacral
ligaments. This is not usually painful; if it causes
pain—and especially if the finger in the rectum can palpate tender nodules along the uterosacral ligaments—
endometriosis may be present.

Occult Bleeding Due to Gastrointestinal Cancer

Cancer of the gastrointestinal tract is the third most
common cancer in women, after cancer of the breast,
lung, and reproductive organs. The physician should
check for occult bleeding from the gastrointestinal tract
by performing a guaiac test on feces adhering to the examination glove following the rectovaginal examination. Several commercial test kits are available.

An early gastrointestinal tract lesion may not bleed
continuously and may be associated with a false-negative result. Therefore, testing should be done at each
routine health screening visit. If the patient has recently
eaten a large amount of meat, a false-positive reaction
may result. Therefore, patients with a positive guaiac
test should be placed on a meat-free diet for 3 days, and
the test should then be repeated. Patients can be given a
test kit to take home and mail back to the physician.

DIAGNOSTIC OFFICE PROCEDURES

Certain diagnostic procedures may be performed in the
office because complicated equipment and general
anesthesia are not required. Other office diagnostic procedures useful in specific situations (eg, tests used in infertility evaluation) will be found in appropriate chapters elsewhere in this book.

Tests for Vaginal Infection

If abnormal vaginal discharge is present, a sample of
vaginal discharge should be scrutinized. A culture is obtained by applying a sterile cotton-tipped applicator to

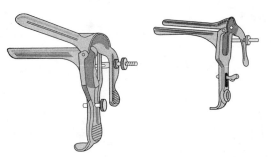

Graves vaginal speculum   Pederson vaginal speculum

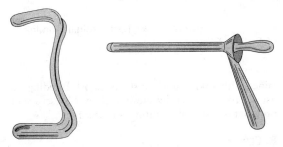

Sims vaginal retractor   Kelly air cystoscope

Figure 30–7. Specula. (Reproduced with permission from Benson RC: *Handbook of Obstetrics & Gynecology*, 8th ed. Lange, 1983.)

the suspect area and then transferring the suspect material to an appropriate culture medium. Since this is inconvenient in the physician's office, most laboratories supply a prepackaged kit that allows the physician to put the cotton-tipped applicator into a sterile container, which is then sent to the laboratory. A chlamydia swab should be obtained from the endocervix and sent for identification. The vaginal discharge can also be tested for the vaginal pH. An acidic pH of 4–5 is consistent with fungal infection, whereas an alkaline pH of 5.5–7 suggests infections such as bacterial vaginosis and *Trichomonas*. Often an endocervical infection may be perceived as a vaginal infection. Obtaining a swab for gonorrhea and chlamydia testing from the endocervix is warranted.

A. Saline (Plain Slide)

To demonstrate *Trichomonas vaginalis* organisms, the physician mixes on a slide 1 drop of vaginal discharge with 1 drop of normal saline warmed to approximately body temperature. The slide should have a coverslip. If the smear is examined while it is still warm, actively motile trichomonads can usually be seen.

The saline slide can also be used to look for the mycelia of the fungus *Candida albicans,* which appear as segmented and branching filaments. The slide can be useful in looking for bacterial vaginosis by looking for "clue cells," epithelial cells covered from edge to edge by short coccobacilli-type bacteria.

B. Potassium Hydroxide

One drop of an aqueous 10% potassium hydroxide solution is mixed with 1 drop of vaginal discharge on a clean slide and covered with a coverslip. The potassium hydroxide dissolves epithelial cells and debris and facilitates visualization of the mycelia of a fungus causing vaginal infection. The slide can be brought near the nose to see if the discharge has a "fishy" odor. This odor is strongly suggestive of bacterial vaginosis, a common vaginal infection associated with a mixed anaerobic bacterial flora. In addition, this same slide with a coverslip can be magnified with a microscope to visualize mycelia that may have been hidden by debris with just the saline smear.

C. Bacterial Infection

Bacterial infection may be present, especially if there is an ischemic lesion such as after radiation therapy for

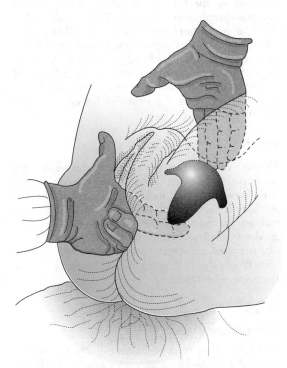

Figure 30–8. Bimanual pelvic examination.

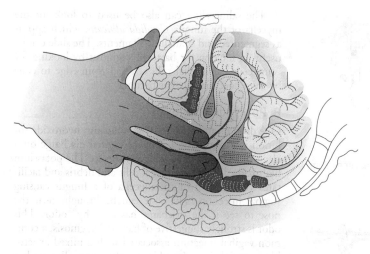

Figure 30–9. Rectovaginal examination.

cervical carcinoma, or if a patient is suspected of having bacterial vaginosis, gonorrhea, or a *Chlamydia trachomatis* infection. Material from the cervix, urethra, or vaginal lesion may be smeared, stained, and examined microscopically, or the material may be cultured.

Fern Test for Ovulation

The fern test can determine the presence or absence of ovulation or the time of ovulation. When cervical mucus is spread upon a clean, dry slide and allowed to dry in air, it may or may not assume a frondlike pattern when viewed under the microscope (sometimes it can be seen grossly). The fern frond pattern indicates an estrogenic effect on the mucus without the influence of progesterone; thus, a non-frondlike pattern can be interpreted as showing that ovulation has occurred (Fig 30–10).

Schiller Test for Neoplasia

Although colposcopy is more accurate, the Schiller test can be performed when cancer or precancerous changes of the cervix or vaginal mucosa are suspected. The suspect area is painted with Lugol's (strong iodine) solution; any portion of the epithelium that does not accept the dye is abnormal because of the presence of scar tissue, neoplasia and precursors, and columnar epithelium. Biopsy should be performed in this area if there is any suspicion of cancer.

Biopsy

A. Vulva and Vagina

For biopsy of the vulva or vagina, a 1–2% aqueous solution of a standard local anesthetic solution can be injected around a small suspicious area and a sample ob-

tained with a skin punch or sharp scalpel. Bleeding can usually be controlled by pressure or by Monsel's solution, but occasionally suturing is necessary.

B. Cervix

Colposcopically directed biopsy is the method of choice for the diagnosis of cervical lesions, either suspected on visualization or indicated after an abnormal Pap smear. Colposcopy should reveal the full columnar-squamous "transformation zone" (TZ) at the juncture of the exocervix and endocervix. In addition, it may be advisable to sample the endocervix by curettage. Specific instruments have been devised for cervical biopsy and endocervical curettage (Fig 30–11). The cervix is less sensitive to cutting procedures than the vagina, so one or more small biopsies of the cervix can be taken with little discomfort to the patient. Bleeding usually is minimal and controlled with light pressure for a few minutes or by the use of Monsel's solution when colposcopy is not available. A "4-quadrant" biopsy of the squamocolumnar junction may be taken at 12, 3, 6, and 9 o'clock if colposcopy is not available. A Schiller test may often more quickly direct the physician to the area that should be biopsied.

C. Endometrium

Endometrial biopsy can be helpful in the diagnosis of ovarian dysfunction (eg, infertility) and as a test for carcinoma of the uterine corpus. The endometrial biopsy may be performed with a Duncan curet (see Fig 30–11) or by passing any of several available hollow endometrial biopsy curets into the uterine cavity and using suction to aspirate fragments of endometrium into the curet (Fig 30–12). Endometrial biopsy may be performed with the newer, flexible disposable cannulas, such as the Pipelle, which have replaced most metal curettes previously used.

Normal cycle, 14th day

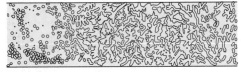

Midluteal phase, normal cycle

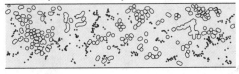

Anovulatory cycle with estrogen present

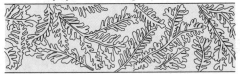

Figure 30–10. Patterns formed when cervical mucus is smeared on a slide, permitted to dry, and examined under a microscope. Progesterone makes the mucus thick and cellular. In the smear from a patient who failed to ovulate (bottom), there is no progesterone to inhibit the estrogen-induced fern pattern. (Reproduced, with permission, from Ganong WF: *Review of Medical Physiology,* 12th ed. Lange, 1985.)

In fact, endometrial biopsies have dramatically reduced the need for doing formal dilatation and curettage since the accuracy of biopsy is nearly the same. Since the procedure causes cramping, the patient should be warned and advised to take a pain medication such as ibuprofen 1 hour prior to the procedure.

DIAGNOSTIC LABORATORY PROCEDURES

Routine procedures that are not discussed here but should be considered with periodic primary care visits include a complete blood count (including differential white cell count), glucose screening, a lipid profile, and thyroid function tests. The frequency with which these tests are given should be at the discretion of the physician, based on risk factors and presenting complaints.

Urinalysis

Urinalysis should be obtained in symptomatic patients and should include both gross and microscopic exami-

nations. A microscopic examination may reveal crystals or bacteria, but unless the specimen is collected in a manner that will exclude vaginal discharge, the presence of bacteria is meaningless (see below).

Urine Culture

Studies have demonstrated that a significant number of women (about 3% of nonpregnant and 7% of pregnant women) have asymptomatic urinary tract infections. Culture and antibiotic sensitivity testing are required for the diagnosis and as a guide to treatment of urinary tract infections.

Reliable specimens of urine for culture often can be obtained by the "clean catch" method: the patient is instructed to cleanse the urethral meatus carefully with soap and water, to urinate for a few seconds to dispose of urethral contaminants, and then to catch a "midstream" portion of the urine. It is essential that the urine not dribble over the labia, but this may be difficult for some patients to accomplish.

A more reliable method of collecting urine for culture is by sterile catheterization performed by the physician or nurse. However, care must be exercised in catheterization to guarantee that infection is not introduced by faulty technique. When correctly performed, catheterization rarely causes infection of the urinary tract.

Other Cultures

A. URETHRAL

Urethral cultures are indicated if a sexually transmitted disease is suspected.

B. VAGINAL

A culture is usually unnecessary for the diagnosis of vaginal infections, since visual inspection or microscopic examination will usually enable the physician to make a diagnosis, eg, curdlike vaginal material that reveals mycelia (candidiasis). However, in questionable cases, a culture should be obtained.

C. CERVICAL

As in the case of the urethra, the usual indication for a culture of cervical discharge is the suspected presence of a sexually transmitted disease.

Specific Tests

A. HERPESVIRUS HOMINIS

Herpesvirus hominis (herpes genitalis, both types 1 and 2) is a frequently seen vulvar lesion (see Chapter 38). It can be diagnosed by the cytopathologist, who finds

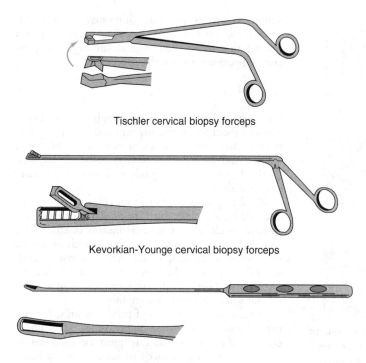

Tischler cervical biopsy forceps

Kevorkian-Younge cervical biopsy forceps

Duncan curet

Figure 30–11. Biopsy instruments.

typical cellular changes. The most accurate method is culturing.

B. Chlamydia and Gonorrheal Infections

These sexually transmitted infections are the two most prevalent infections, with chlamydia being the most common. They are found more often in women who have multiple sexual partners and those who do not use barrier methods of contraception. Fluorescent antibody testing is the most commonly used method of diagnosis, with a sensitivity greater than 90%. Newer tests using polymerase chain reaction may improve the sensitivity.

C. Human Immunodeficiency Virus

Acquired immunodeficiency syndrome (AIDS) has become one of the most difficult issues confronting all kinds of clinicians. The need for screening for human immunodeficiency virus (HIV) for the general population has become more pressing since the largest increase in incidence is in the young heterosexually active female with no other risk factors. An accurate blood test is available for diagnosis. Prior to having the blood drawn, the physician must discuss with the patient the accuracy of the blood test for diagnosing the presence of HIV. The patient must also be made aware that

there are infrequent false-positive tests and a "window" during which the test may be falsely negative prior to the development of antibodies. At present, a written consent must be signed by the patient prior to having the blood drawn.

Other Specific Tests

Specific diagnostic laboratory procedures may be indicated for some of the less common venereal diseases, eg, lymphogranuloma venereum and hepatitis B. These will be indicated in the discussions of the specific diseases in other chapters in this book.

Pregnancy Testing

Pregnancy testing is discussed in Chapter 9.

Papanicolaou Smear of Cervix

The Pap smear is an important part of the gynecologic examination. The frequency of the need for this test is in dispute; epidemiologic statistics have led some physicians to state that for the average woman, a smear test every 2 or 3 years is adequate. This recommendation is based on the observation that most cervical cancers are

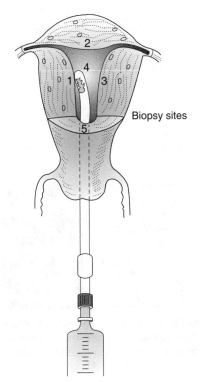

Biopsy sites

Figure 30–12. **Sites of endometrial biopsy.** (Reproduced with permission from Benson RC: *Handbook of Obstetrics & Gynecology*, 8th ed. Lange, 1983.)

slow-growing. However, because rapidly growing cervical cancers are occasionally reported and because there is always a possibility of false-negative laboratory reports, the American College of Obstetricians and Gynecologists continues to advocate annual smears. Even those who advocate less frequent smears generally agree that patients at risk should have annual smear tests. Those at risk include women with multiple sexual partners, a history of sexually transmitted disease, genital condylomata, and prior abnormal Pap smears.

Aside from premalignant and malignant changes, other local conditions can often be suspected by the cytologist. Viral infections such as herpes simplex and condylomata acuminata can be seen as mucosal changes. Actinomycosis and *Trichomonas* infections can be detected on a Pap smear.

The Pap smear is a screening test only; positive tests are an indication for further diagnostic procedures such as colposcopy, cervical biopsy or conization, endometrial biopsy, or D&C. The properly collected Pap smear can accurately lead to the diagnosis of carcinoma of the cervix in about 95% of cases. The Pap smear is also helpful in the detection of endometrial abnormalities such as endometrial polyps, hyperplasia, and cancers, but it picks up less than 50% of cases.

The techniques of collection of a Pap smear may vary, but the following is a common procedure.

The patient should not have douched for at least 24 hours before the examination and should not be menstruating. The speculum is placed in the vagina after being lubricated with water only. With the cervix exposed, either a cotton-tipped applicator slightly dampened with saline solution or a specially designed plastic or wooden spatula is applied to the cervix and rotated 360 degrees to abrade the surface slightly and to pick up cells from the squamocolumnar area of the cervical os. Care should be taken to ascertain that endocervical cells are also obtained. If this is not accomplished with the spatula, a cotton-tipped applicator or small brush is now available for this purpose; it can be inserted into the cervical canal of most women and rotated, picking up endocervical cells more efficiently. These 2 specimens may be mixed or put on the slide separately according to the preference of the examiner. A preservative is applied immediately to prevent air drying, which will compromise the interpretation. The slide is sent to the laboratory with an identification sheet containing pertinent history and findings (see Fig 30–6).

A vaginal smear from the lateral vaginal wall may be obtained for hormonal evaluation, which is a rough indicator of the amount of estrogen stimulation present in a given patient. A vaginal smear is also important in detecting diethylstilbestrol (DES)-related changes of the vagina and also for detecting vaginal malignancies. Figure 30–13 shows vaginal cytology during different stages of life.

The laboratory reports the Pap smear using the Bethesda System which has advocated a standardized reporting system for cytologic reports. See chapter 47 for the recently updated nomenclature.

Alternatives to the traditional Pap smear are being evaluated in an attempt to decrease the false-negative and false-positive Pap smear. There is evidence that the computerized screening of Pap smears can decrease the likelihood of missing significant pathologies. Another method called ThinPrep automates the preparation of the Pap smear slide so that the variability introduced by the clinician in smearing and fixing the slide itself is no longer a factor. In addition, the ThinPrep technique has been shown to decrease the rate of smears showing ASCUS, thereby decreasing the need for colposcopic evaluations. For these reasons, in many parts of the country, the ThinPrep technique has replaced the conventional Pap smear.

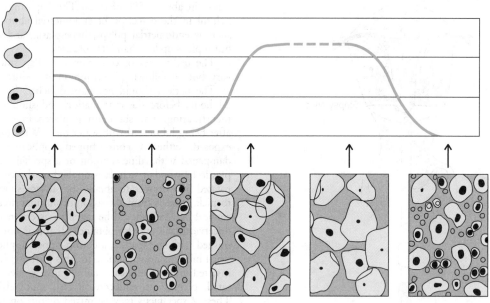

Figure 30–13. Vaginal cytologic picture in various stages of life. **Top:** Graphic representation of the maturation of vaginal epithelium. **Bottom:** Left to right: Epithelial maturation at birth; atrophic cell picture in childhood; beginning of estrogenic influence in puberty; complete maturation in the reproductive period; regression in old age. (Reproduced with permission from Beller FK et al: *Gynecology: A Textbook for Students.* Springer-Verlag, 1974.)

Colposcopy

The colposcope is a binocular microscope used for direct visualization of the cervix (Fig 30–14). Magnification as high as 60x is available, but the most popular instrument in clinical use has 13.5 magnification that effectively bridges the gap between what can be seen by the naked eye and by the microscope. Some colposcopes are equipped with a camera for single or serial photographic recording of pathologic conditions.

Colposcopy does not replace other methods of diagnosing abnormalities of the cervix, but is instead an additional and important tool. The 2 most important groups of patients who can benefit by its use are (1) patients with an abnormal Pap smear and (2) DES-exposed daughters, who may have dysplasia of the vagina or cervix (see Chapter 35).

The colposcopist is able to see areas of cellular dysplasia and vascular or tissue abnormalities not visible otherwise, which makes it possible to select areas most propitious for biopsy. Stains and other chemical agents are also used to improve visualization. The colposcope has reduced the need for doing blind cervical biopsies for which the rate of finding abnormalities was low. In addition, the necessity for doing cone biopsies, a procedure with a high morbidity rate, has been greatly reduced. Thus the experienced colposcopist is able to find focal cervical lesions, obtain directed biopsy at the most appropriate sites, and make decisions about the most appropriate therapy largely based on what is seen through the colposcope.

Hysteroscopy

Hysteroscopy is the visual examination of the uterine cavity through a fiberoptic instrument, the hysteroscope. In order to inspect the interior of the uterus with the hysteroscope, the uterine cavity is inflated with solution such as saline, glycine, or dextran, or by carbon dioxide insufflation. Intravenous sedation and paracervical block are often adequate for hysteroscopy so long as prolonged manipulation is not required.

Hysteroscopic applications include evaluation for abnormal uterine bleeding, resection of uterine synechiae and septa, removal of polyps and IUDs, resection of submucous myomas, and endometrial ablation. Most of these therapeutic maneuvers require extensive manipulation, so regional or general anesthesia is required.

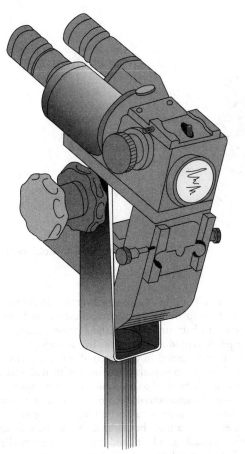

Figure 30–14. Zeiss colposcope.

Hysteroscopy should be performed only by physicians with proper training. The tip of the instrument should be inserted just beyond the internal cervical os and then advanced slowly, with adequate distention under direct vision.

Hysteroscopy is often used in conjunction with another operative procedures such as curettage or laparoscopy.

Failure of hysteroscopy may be due to cervical stenosis, inadequate distention of the uterine cavity, bleeding, or excessive mucus secretion. The most common complications include perforation, bleeding, and infection. Perforation of the uterus usually occurs at the fundus. Unless there is damage to a viscus or internal bleeding develops, surgical repair may not be required. Bleeding generally subsides, but fulguration following attempts to remove polyps or myomas may be required to stop bleeding in some cases. Parametritis or salpingitis, rarely noted, usually necessitates antibiotic therapy.

Intravascular extravasation of fluid or gas from hysteroscopy does not become clinically significant very often, but has been associated with severe consequences such as hyponatremia, air embolism, cerebral edema, and even death.

Culdocentesis

The passage of a needle into the cul-de-sac—culdocentesis—in order to obtain fluid from the pouch of Douglas is a diagnostic procedure that can be performed in the office or in a hospital treatment room (Fig 30–15). The type of fluid obtained indicates the type of intraperitoneal lesion, eg, bloody with a ruptured ectopic pregnancy; pus with acute salpingitis; ascitic fluid with malignant cells in cancer. With refinements in ultrasound technology enabling more definitive evaluation of pelvic pathology, culdocentesis is performed less frequently today.

Radiographic Diagnostic Procedures

There are many common radiologic procedures that may be helpful in the diagnosis of pelvic conditions. The "flat film" will show calcified lesions, teeth, or a ring of a dermoid cyst and will indicate other pelvic masses by shadows or displaced intestinal loops. The use of contrast media is frequently indicated to help delineate pelvic masses or to rule out metastatic lesions. Barium enema, upper gastrointestinal series, intravenous urogram, and cystogram may be helpful.

Hysterography & Sonohysterography

The uterine cavity and the lumens of the oviducts can be outlined by instillation of contrast medium through the cervix, followed by fluoroscopic observations or film. The technique was first widely used for the diagnosis of tubal disease as part of the investigation of infertile women; its use is now being extended to the investigation of uterine disease.

To diagnose tubal patency or occlusion, the medium is instilled through a cervical cannula; the filling of the uterine cavity and the spreading of the medium through the tubes are watched via a fluoroscope, with the radiologist taking spot films at intervals for subsequent, more definitive, scrutiny. If there is no occlusion, the medium will reach the fimbriated end of the tube and spill into the pelvis—evidence of tubal patency. This procedure can reveal an abnormality of the uterus, eg, congenital malformation, submucous myomas, endometrial polyps.

Another technique that is gaining acceptance is sonohysterography, in which the uterine cavity is filled

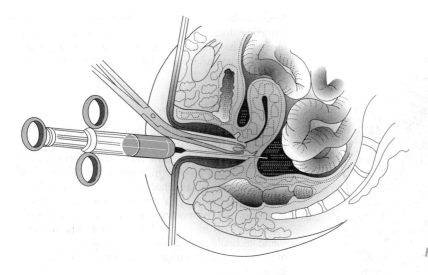

Figure 30–15. Culdocentesis.

with fluid while ultrasound is used to delineate the architecture of the endometrial cavity. Thus it becomes easier to diagnose intrauterine abnormalities such as polyps and fibroids.

Angiography

Angiography is the use of radiographic contrast medium to visualize the blood vascular system. By demonstrating the vascular pattern of an area, tumors or other abnormalities can be delineated. It is also used in delineating continued bleeding from pelvic vessels postoperatively, bleeding from infiltration by cancer in cancer patients, or to embolize the uterine arteries to decrease acute bleeding and/or reduce the size of uterine myomas. These vessels can then be embolized with synthetic fabrics to stop the bleeding or indicate therapy that can be used to avoid the necessity of a major abdominal operation in a very compromised patient.

Computed Tomography (CT)

Computed tomography or CT scan is a diagnostic imaging technique that provides high-resolution two-dimensional images. The CT scan takes cross-sectional images through the body at very close intervals so that multiple "slices" of the body are obtained. The beam transmission is measured and calculated through an array of sensors that are about 100 times more sensitive than conventional x-rays. The computer is able to translate the densities of different types of tissues into gray-scale pictures that can be read on an x-ray film or a television monitor.

Contrast media can be given orally, intravenously, or rectally to outline the gastrointestinal and urinary systems to help differentiate these organ systems from the pelvic reproductive organs. In gynecology, the CT scan is most useful in accurately diagnosing retroperitoneal lymphadenopathy associated with malignancies. It has also been used to determine depth of myometrial invasion in endometrial carcinoma as well as extrauterine spread. It is an accurate tool for locating pelvic abscesses that cannot be located by ultrasonography. Often a needle can be placed into an abscess pocket to both drain the abscess and find out what organism may be involved. Pelvic thrombophlebitis can often be diagnosed by CT scan as an adjunct to clinical suspicion. Common abnormalities such as ovarian cysts and myomas are also easily diagnosed (Fig 30–16).

Magnetic Resonance Imaging (MRI)

Magnetic resonance imaging (MRI) is a diagnostic imaging technique that creates a high-resolution, cross-sectional image of the body like a CT scan. The technique is based on the body absorbing radio waves from the machine. A small amount of this energy is absorbed by the nuclei in the various tissues. These nuclei act like small bar magnets and are influenced by the magnetic field created by the machine. These nuclei then emit some of the radio waves back out of the body and the waves are picked up by sensitive and sophisticated receivers and these signals are then translated into images by computer technology.

The advantages of MRI include the fact that it uses nonionized radiation that has no adverse or harmful ef-

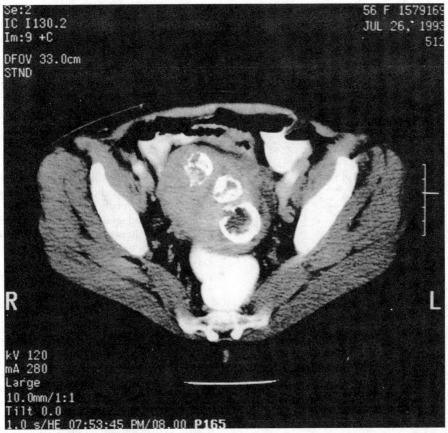

Figure 30–16. CT scan of the pelvis showing a large fibroid uterus with three calcified fibroids in the body of the uterus. (Picture courtesy of Dr. Barbara Carter, New England Medical Center, Boston.)

fects on the body. It is superior to the CT scan in its ability to differentiate different types of tissue, including inflammatory masses, cancers, and abnormal tissue metabolism. Its disadvantages are mainly its high cost and the fact that calcifications are poorly demonstrated. Its main use in gynecology appears to be for staging and following up pelvic cancers. Use of MRI in obstetrics is mainly experimental and may be limited because of fetal movement that makes it unsuitable for most studies.

Other potential uses of MRI include evaluation of placental blood flow and accurately performing pelvimetry.

Ultrasonography

Ultrasonography records high-frequency sound waves as they are reflected from anatomic structures. As the sounds waves pass through tissues, they encounter variable acoustic densities; each of these tissues returns a different echo, depending on the amount of energy reflected. This echo signal can be measured and converted into a two-dimensional image of the area under examination, with the relative densities being shown as differing shades of gray.

Ultrasonography is a simple and painless procedure that has the added advantage of being free of any radiation hazard. It is especially helpful in patients in whom an adequate pelvic examination may be difficult, such as in children, virginal women, and uncooperative patients.

The pelvis and lower abdomen are scanned and recorded at regular intervals of distance, using a sector scanner that provides a better two-dimensional picture than the linear array scanner (Fig 30–17). Generally, the scan is performed with the bladder full; this elevates

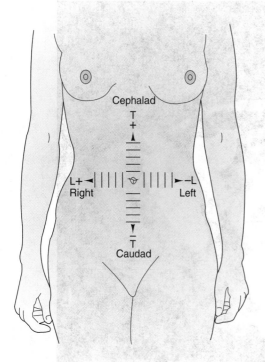

Figure 30–17. Planes of ultrasonograms.

the uterus out of the pelvis, displaces air-filled loops of bowel, and provides the operator with an index of density—a sonographic "window" differentiating the pelvic organs.

Ultrasonography can be helpful in the diagnosis of almost any pelvic abnormality, since all structures, normal and abnormal, can usually be demonstrated. In most instances, a clinical picture has been developed—by history, physical examination, or both—before ultrasonograms are obtained. Thus, the scan often will corroborate the clinical impression, but it may also uncover an unexpected condition that the clinician should be aware of.

There are many indications for ultrasonography. Normal early pregnancy can be diagnosed as can pathologic pregnancies such as incomplete and missed abortions and hydatidiform moles. Ultrasonography can also be extremely helpful in avoiding the placenta and fetus during midtrimester amniocentesis. The uses for ultrasound examination in obstetrics are discussed elsewhere in this book.

Ultrasonography may be used to locate a lost intrauterine device or a foreign body in the vagina of a child. Congenital malformations such as a bicornuate

uterus or vaginal agenesis are sometimes, but not always, detected. Ultrasound examination is useful in the placement of uterine tandems for radiation therapy for endometrial cancer and for guidance during second-trimester abortion procedures.

One of the more common uses for ultrasonography is the diagnosis of pelvic masses. Often because of their location, attachment, and density, myomas can be diagnosed without too much difficulty (Fig 30–18A).

Adnexal masses can also be found with relative ease by ultrasonography, although an accurate diagnosis is more difficult because of the various types of adnexal masses that can be found (Fig 30–18B and C).

Ovarian cysts can be described as being unilocular or multilocular, totally fluid-filled or partially solid. A very common adnexal mass, a dermoid cyst, can have characteristic ultrasound findings because of fat tissue and bone densities seen in these cysts (Fig 30–18D). Pelvic abscesses can be diagnosed by ultrasonography, especially if there is a well-encapsulated large abscess pocket.

In addition to the traditional abdominal scan, the vaginal probe scan has become a useful modality. The vaginal probe is used for determining early gestations and can diagnose a pregnancy as early as 5 weeks from the last normal menstrual period. Ectopic pregnancies can sometimes be seen on vaginal ultrasonography, but it is more useful for excluding an intrauterine gestation when there is a suspicion of an ectopic pregnancy.

Ultrasonography is commonly used to diagnose ovarian cysts, especially in obese patients in whom abdominal scans are of limited use. The vaginal scan is used very often to determine follicular size with in vitro fertilization and to predict the best time for ovum retrieval.

Carbon Dioxide Laser

Controlled tissue vaporization by laser is a modality for the treatment of cervical, vaginal, or perineal condylomata and dysplasia. It also can be used for conization of the cervix for diagnosis of dysplasia or carcinoma within the cervical canal.

The vaporization procedure is not difficult, but training is essential, especially in the physics of laser light and the potential risks of laser therapy not only to the patient but to the operator and others in the immediate vicinity. Antiseptic preparation of the vagina should be gentle to avoid trauma to the tissue that is to be examined histologically. Local anesthesia, with or without preliminary intravenous sedation, is usually adequate.

Advantages of the laser method of cervical conization include little or no pain; a low incidence of infection because the beam sterilizes the tissues; decreased

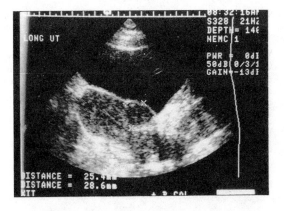 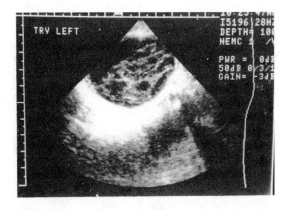

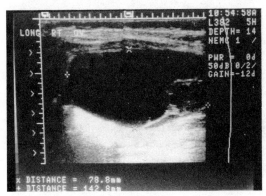 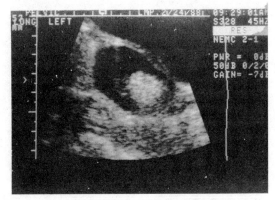

Figure 30–18. **A:** Longitudinal view of the uterus with anterior fibroid outlined by the x's; bladder anterior. **B:** Transverse section through an endometrioma with multiple loculations and debris. **C:** Longitudinal view of large ovarian cyst outlined by the +'s and x's with a focal multicystic area. **D:** Longitudinal view of a dermoid cyst showing areas of fat within the cyst. (Pictures courtesy of Dr. Frederick Doherty, New England Medical Center, Boston.)

blood loss, since the laser instrument—at a decreased energy level—is a hemostatic agent; less tissue necrosis than occurs with electrocautery (but probably the same as with excision by a sharp knife); and a decreased incidence of postoperative cervical stenosis.

Loop Electrosurgical Excision Procedure

Loop electrosurgical excision procedure (LEEP) is another modality of therapy for vulvar and cervical lesions. LEEP uses a low-voltage, high-frequency alternating current that limits thermal damage, and at the same time has good hemostatic properties. It is most commonly used for excision of vulvar condylomata and cervical dysplasias and for cone biopsies of the cervix. It has displaced sharp knife and laser cone biopsies for treatment of most cervical dysplasias.

The technique requires the use of local anesthesia followed by the use of a wire loop cautery unit that cauterizes and cuts the desired tissue. Various sized loops are used for different sized specimens. The major advantages of LEEP include its usefulness in an office setting with lower equipment cost, minimal damage to the surrounding tissue, and low morbidity.

REFERENCES

American College of Obstetricians and Gynecologists: Cervical cytology: Evaluation and management of abnormalities. ACOG Technical Bulletin No. 183, 1999.

Carroll N: Optimal gynecologic and obstetric care for lesbians. Obstet Gynecol 1999;93:611.

Laughead M, Stones L: Clinical utility of saline solution infusion sonohysterography in a primary care obstetric-gynecologic practice. Am J Obstet Gynecol 1997;176:1313.

Leitch A et al: American Cancer Society guidelines for the early detection of breast cancer: update 1997. CA Cancer J Clin 1997;47:150.

Mitchell MF, Schottenfeld D, Tortolero-Luna G et al: Colposcopy for the diagnosis of squamous intraepithelial lesions: a meta-analysis. Obstet Gynecol 1998;91:626.

Perlman S: Pap smear: screening, interpretation, treatment. Adolesc Med 1999;10:243.

Schweickert EA, Heeren AB: Scripted role play: A technique for teaching sexual history taking. J Am Osteopath Assoc 1999; 99:275.

Valle RF: Office hysteroscopy. Clin Obstet Gynecol 1999;42:276.

Vassilakos P et al: Biopsy-based comparison of liquid-based, thin-layer preparations to conventional Pap smear. J Reprod Med 2000;45:11.

Pediatric & Adolescent Gynecology   31

Lisbeth Chang, MD, & David Muram, MD

The field of pediatric and adolescent gynecology has expanded greatly over the last half century, as increased attention has been directed to the complex roles of children and adolescents in society. Today, pediatric and adolescent gynecology has evolved from reviews of developmental physiology and case reports of aberrations to discussions that include not only these topics but also address issues related to adolescent reproductive health.

Gynecologic care begins in the delivery room, with inspection of the external genitalia during routine newborn examination. Evaluation of the external genitalia continues through routine well-child examinations, permitting early detection of infections, labial adhesions, congenital anomalies, and even genital tumors. A complete gynecologic examination is indicated when a child has symptoms or signs of a genital disorder. The American College of Obstetricians and Gynecologists recommends that adolescents should have their first visit to an obstetrician/gynecologist for health guidance, general physical screening, and the provision of preventive health care services at age 13–15 years. A pelvic examination should be performed on adolescents who are sexually active, older than 18 years of age, or when indicated by medical history. Specially designed equipment must be used (eg, vaginoscope, virginal vaginal speculum) to prevent undue discomfort and consequent anxiety about future examinations.

ANATOMIC & PHYSIOLOGIC CONSIDERATIONS

Newborn Infants

During the first few weeks of life, residual maternal sex hormones may produce physiologic effects on the newborn. Breast budding occurs in nearly all female infants born at term. In some cases, breast enlargement is marked, and there may be fluid discharge from the nipples. No treatment is indicated. The labia majora are bulbous, and the labia minora are thick and protruding (Fig 31–1). The clitoris is relatively large, with a normal index of 0.6 cm^2 or less.* The hymen initially is turgid, covering the external urethral orifice. Vaginal discharge

is common, comprised mainly of cervical mucus and exfoliated vaginal cells.

The vagina is approximately 4 cm long at birth. The uterus is enlarged (4 cm in length) and without axial flexion; the ratio between the cervix and the corpus is 3:1. Columnar epithelium protrudes through the external cervical os, creating a reddened zone of physiologic eversion. The ovaries remain abdominal organs in early childhood and should not be palpable on pelvic or rectal examination. Vaginal bleeding may occur as estrogen levels decline following birth and the stimulated endometrial lining is shed. Such bleeding usually stops within 7–10 days.

Young Children

In early childhood, the female genital organs receive little estrogen stimulation. The labia majora flatten and the labia minora and hymen become thin (Fig 31–2). The clitoris remains relatively small, although the clitoral index is unchanged. The vagina, lined with atrophic mucosa with relatively few rugae, offers very little resistance to trauma and infection. The vaginal barrel contains neutral or slightly alkaline secretions and mixed bacterial flora. Since vaginal fornices do not develop until puberty, the cervix in childhood is flush with the vaginal vault, its opening appearing as a small slit. The uterus regresses in size, regaining the size present at birth at around age 6. As the child matures, the ovaries begin to enlarge and descend into the true pelvis. The number and size of ovarian follicles increase. They may attain significant size and then regress.

At laparotomy, the uterus may appear as merely a strip of dense tissue in the anteromedial area of the broad ligaments. Palpation may aid in delineating the uterine outline. The ovaries may appear cystic secondary to follicular development. Biopsy is not warranted.

Older Children

During late childhood (age 7–10 years), the external genitalia again show signs of estrogen stimulation: the mons pubis thickens, the labia majora fill out, and the labia minora become rounded. The hymen thickens (Fig 31–3), losing its thin, transparent character. The

---

* Clitoral index (cm^2) = length (cm) × width (cm), ie, a clitoris 1 cm long and 0.5 cm wide = 0.5 cm^2.

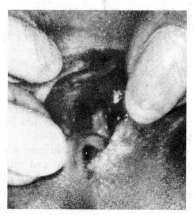

Figure 31–1. External genitalia of a newborn female. Note the hypertrophy and turgor of the vulvar tissues. A small catheter is inserted into the vagina to demonstrate patency. (Reproduced [as are a number of other illustrations in this chapter] from Huffman JW: *The Gynecology of Childhood and Adolescence.* Saunders, 1968.)

vagina elongates to 8 cm, the mucosa becomes thicker, the corpus uteri enlarges, and the ratio of cervix to corpus becomes 1:1. The cervix remains flush with the vault. A maturation index determination at this time will show not only basal cells but also a greater proportion of parabasal cells and superficial cells, in a typical ratio of 75:25:0 or 70:25:5.

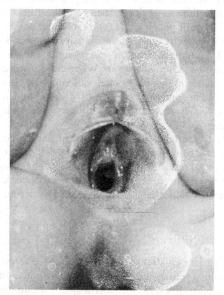

Figure 31–2. External genitalia of a child 3 years of age.

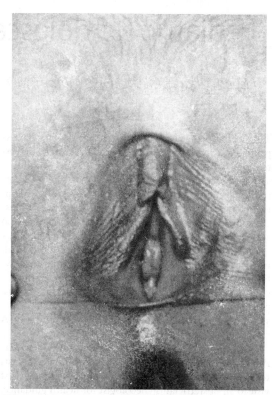

Figure 31–3. External genitalia of a child 11 years of age. Early estrogen response is evidenced by the fuller labia, wrinkling of the vulvar mucosa, and thickening of the hymen.

By the time a girl reaches age 9–10 years of age, uterine growth begins, with alteration in uterine shape resulting primarily from myometrial proliferation. Rapid endometrial proliferation occurs as menarche is imminent. Prior to this time, the endometrium gradually thickens, with modest increases in the depth and complexity of the endometrial glands. As the ovaries enlarge and descend into the pelvis, the number of ovarian follicles increases. Although these follicles are in various stages of development, ovulation generally does not occur.

Young Adolescents

During early puberty (age 10–13 years), the external genitalia take on adult appearance. The major vestibular glands (Bartholin's glands) begin to produce mucus just prior to menarche. The vagina reaches adult length (10–12 cm) and becomes more distensible, the mucosa thickens, vaginal secretions grow more acidic, and lactobacilli reappear. With the development of vaginal fornices, the cervix becomes separated from the vaginal

Table 31–1 Tanner classification of female adolescent development.

Stage	Breast Development	Pubic Hair Development
I	Papillae elevated (preadolescent), no breast buds	None
II	Breast buds and papillae slightly elevated	Sparse, long, slightly pigmented
III	Breasts and areolae confluent, elevated	Darker, coarser, curly
IV	Areolae and papillae project above breast	Adult-type pubis only
V	Papillae projected, mature	Lateral distribution

vault, and the differential growth of the corpus and cervix becomes more pronounced. The corpus grows twice as large as the cervix. The ovaries descend into the true pelvis.

Secondary sexual characteristics develop, often rapidly, during the late premenarcheal period. Body habitus becomes more rounded, especially the shoulders and hips. Accelerated somatic growth velocity (the adolescent growth spurt) occurs. At the same time, estrogen increases adipose tissue deposition and initiates stromal and ductal growth in the breasts. Physiologic leukorrhea often is noted.

Pubic hair growth appears to be under the control of adrenal androgens. Sparse, long, slightly curly, pigmented hair over the pubic area gives way to coarse, pigmented curly hair. The pubic hair pattern assumes the characteristic triangle with the base above the mons pubis. Hair growth in the axilla appears later, also as a result of adrenocorticosteroid stimulation. The development of secondary sexual features described by Marshall and Tanner is summarized in Table 31–1 (see also Fig 6–3).

GYNECOLOGIC EXAMINATION OF INFANTS, CHILDREN, & YOUNG ADOLESCENTS

Examination of the Newborn Infant

Newborns should be examined immediately upon delivery or in the nursery. When an infant is born with ambiguous genitalia, immediate actions should be to counsel the parents and to prevent dehydration, as congenital adrenal hyperplasia accounts for greater than 90% of cases of ambiguous genitalia, and salt-wasting forms may lead to rapid dehydration and fluid imbalances. In most cases, it is unnecessary to perform an internal examination, as most gynecologic abnormalities

that should be recognized at this stage are limited to the external genitalia.

A. GENERAL EXAMINATION

As in adults, the first step in a genital evaluation of the newborn is a careful general examination, which may reveal abnormalities suggesting genital anomaly (eg, webbed neck, abdominal mass, edema of the hands and legs, coarctation of the aorta).

B. CLITORIS

Clitoral enlargement in the newborn is almost always associated with congenital adrenal hyperplasia. Other causes must also be considered (eg, true hermaphroditism, male pseudohermaphroditism).

C. VAGINA

The vaginal orifice should be evident when the labia are separated or retracted. If the vaginal orifice cannot be located, most likely the infant has an imperforate hymen or vaginal agenesis. Inguinal masses suggest the possibility that the child is a genetic male.

D. RECTOABDOMINAL EXAMINATION

Usually, the uterus and adnexa in the newborn cannot be palpated on rectal examination. Occasionally, a small central mass representing the uterine cervix can be felt on examination. When an ovary is palpable, it denotes enlargement and the possibility of an ovarian tumor should be investigated. Rectal examination can confirm patency of the anorectal canal.

Examination of the Premenarcheal Child

The examination of the premenarcheal and peripubertal child should focus on the main symptoms identified in this population: pruritus, dysuria, skin color changes, and discharge.

Parents can be helpful in the examination of a young child because they provide a sense of security and may also distract the patient. Placing a child up to 5 years of age on her parent's lap affords a better opportunity to perform an adequate examination (Fig 31–4). Older children may be placed on the examination table, but the use of stirrups is not generally necessary if the patient is asked to flex her knees and abduct her legs. The knee-chest position is useful in visualizing the upper vagina and cervix.

Studies indicate that young patients and adolescents tend to prefer physicians who wear white coats. As a uniform, the white coat identifies the physician in his or her role, which may involve inspection and occasional palpation of private areas. Explaining procedures to the older child, showing her instruments, and asking

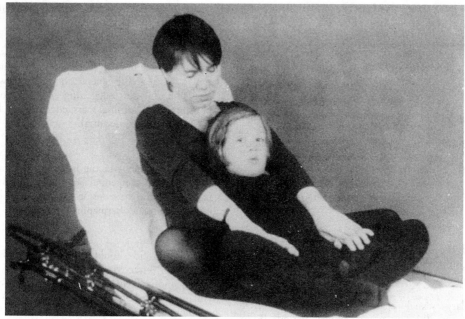

Figure 31–4. Child is positioned on mother's lap and feels secure in mother's arms. The mother can assist by supporting the child's legs, providing an excellent view of the genital area. (Photo courtesy of Dr. T. Anglin.)

her to help with the examination may decrease her apprehension by providing a sense of control.

A. Physical Examination

1. General inspection—The examination begins with an evaluation of the patient's general appearance, nutritional status, body habitus, and any gross congenital anomalies.

2. Breasts—Breast budding usually begins around age 8–9 years. Prominence of the nipple and breast development at an earlier age may be early signs of sexual precocity. Appropriate monitoring may include assessment of bone age, as well following height and breast development at 3-month intervals.

3. Abdomen—Inspection and palpation of the abdomen should precede examination of the genitalia. If the child is ticklish, having her place one hand on or under the examiner's hand usually will overcome the problem.

The ovary of a premenarcheal child is situated high in the pelvis. This location and the small size of the pelvic cavity tend to force ovarian tumors above the true pelvic brim. Thus, large neoplasms of the ovary are likely to be mistaken for other abdominal masses (eg, polycystic kidney). Although inguinal hernias are less common in females than in males (about 1:10), they may occur, usually without discomfort. An excellent

method of demonstrating an inguinal hernia is to have the child stand up and increase the intra-abdominal pressure by blowing up a balloon.

4. Genitalia—The vulva and vestibule may be exposed by light lateral and downward pressure on each side of the perineum. When exposure of the vaginal walls is necessary, the labia may be grasped between the examiner's thumb and forefinger and pulled forward, downward, and sideways. Particular attention should be paid to the adequacy of perineal hygiene, because poor hygiene may predispose a child to vulvovaginitis. The examiner should also look for skin lesions, perineal excoriations, ulcers, and tumors. Signs of hormonal stimulation in early childhood and absence of such signs later in childhood are important signs of endocrine disorders associated with precocious or delayed puberty. Attention should be paid to vulvar inflammation and vulvar and vaginal discharge.

Enlargement of the clitoris is of diagnostic significance. The vestibule may not be visible because of labial adhesions or congenital anomalies. The former condition is frequently mistaken for vaginal agenesis or imperforate hymen. Imperforate hymen can occur in up to 3–4% of patients. Surgical correction is usually not required until puberty, as this condition may spontaneously resolve.

It is extremely difficult to perform a digital vaginal examination in a child whose vagina is normal-sized for her age. Gentle rectal digital examination can be accomplished, but the small size of the uterus and ovaries and the resistance most children offer to the examination render accurate intrapelvic evaluation difficult. If the uterus and ovaries are not palpable, it is unlikely that a child has a genital tumor. If the presence of a pelvic tumor is suspected and the neoplasm cannot be palpated on rectal examination, other diagnostic procedures (eg, sonography, laparoscopy) should be performed.

B. VAGINOSCOPY

Instrumentation is required when it is necessary to carefully visualize the upper third of the vagina for a source of abnormal vaginal bleeding, to confirm patency of the genital tract, to detect and remove foreign bodies, or to exclude penetrating injuries. In the latter case, the examination is often performed under general anesthesia. Figure 31–5 shows the office vaginoscope in use. The water cystoscope allows some distention of the vagina and thus better visualization of the vaginal mucosa while washing away secretions, blood, and debris (Fig 31–6). Alternatively, a urethroscope or laparoscope may be used.

In infancy and childhood, the hymenal orifice normally will admit a 0.5-cm vaginoscope. An instrument 0.8 cm in diameter can be used to examine most older premenarcheal girls. Topical lidocaine solution can be used to anesthetize the vulva prior to insertion of instruments. If the aperture is too small for an instrument to be passed without discomfort, vaginoscopy should not be further attempted without general anesthesia.

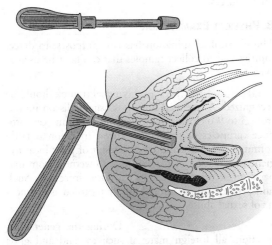

Figure 31–5. Huffman vaginoscope being used for examination of a premenarcheal child.

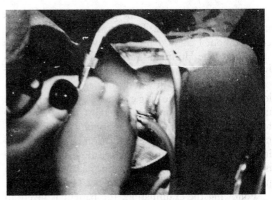

Figure 31–6. Performing vaginoscopy under anesthesia using a water cystoscope.

Examination of the Adolescent

The adolescent's first trip to the gynecologist is often laden with fear and apprehension. Time spent putting the patient at ease and winning her confidence will save time and frustration in the examining room. The physician should make it clear that the adolescent is the patient. She, rather than an accompanying adult, if present, is asked for information that will go on the medical record. Questions about high-risk behaviors, including sexual behavior and sexually transmitted diseases (STDs), should be asked privately.

After the history is taken, the patient should be given a brief description of what the examination entails. She should be assured that the examination should not be painful. The examination is performed in the presence of a female chaperone.

A breast examination is integral in the physical examination of every female patient. Controversy exists over whether self-examination techniques should be taught to adolescents at this time, as the risks of a mass being cancerous in this age group are extremely low and evaluation at the time of routine examination is most likely sufficient.

The examination is also used to provide the patient with health maintenance instructions and explanations about her body and its various functions. Many adolescents are not familiar with the appearance of their own genitalia. Some physicians use mirrors during the examination to show normal anatomic details, to demonstrate abnormalities, to explain treatment plans, and to provide explanations regarding health maintenance. Others use a colposcope attached to a video monitor for the genital examination of young children. This provides an enlarged image seen simultaneously by the examiner and the patient, and permits direct communication, particularly in difficult cases.

Following inspection of the genitalia, a speculum is inserted into the vagina. The introitus of most adolescents is about 1 cm in diameter and will admit a narrow speculum. The Huffman-Graves and Pedersen specula both are designed to allow for easy inspection of the cervix in adolescents, in whom the vagina is 10–12 cm long (Fig 31–7). The larger Graves speculum, while useful in parous women, is generally not appropriate for most younger patients. In a patient with a large hymenal opening, bimanual examination is performed by inserting a finger into the vagina. If the hymenal orifice is too small for digital examination, rectal examination may be performed.

Following the examination, the patient is given an opportunity to talk to the examiner alone. Confidentiality is essential to the physician-patient relationship, and problems may be discussed with the patient's guardians only with the patient's consent. Physical or sexual abuse, however, is a legal issue, requiring breach of confidentiality.

The gynecologic visit also serves as an excellent opportunity to review basic health care maintenance. For example, current recommendations advise universal vaccination for hepatitis B for all adolescents at ages 11–12 years, with immunization for older adolescents based on risk status. Tetanus and measles-mumps-rubella (MMR) vaccinations should also be updated. In addition, screening for eating disorders, depression, and behavioral risks including sexual activity and tobacco, alcohol, and substance abuse should be done routinely. To assist providers of adolescent health care, the American Medical Association has issued recommendations

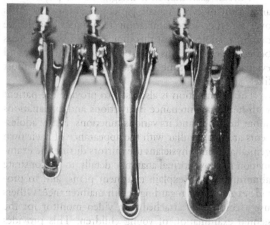

Figure 31–7. The Huffman-Graves speculum (**middle**) is as long as the adult Graves speculum (**right**) and as narrow as the short pediatric Graves speculum (**left**).

based on annual health guidance, screening, and immunization schedules.

Examination of the Young Victim of Sexual Abuse

Studies show that about 38% of girls are sexually victimized before age 18. Many children who are possible victims of sexual abuse are brought to a hospital emergency room or to their physician's office for a comprehensive medical evaluation. Statutes vary from state to state as to the need for legal consent from a parent or guardian to perform a genital examination and collect evidence in cases of suspected abuse.

Among adolescent girls in grades 9–12, 26% report experiencing physical or sexual abuse. Therefore, all adolescents should be asked about history of abuse.

A. History

An account of the incident is extremely valuable, as it can later be used in court as evidence, or it may reveal an unusual area of injury, and thus uncommon sites for collection of evidence. It is important to know how and from whom the patient sustained the injury. The examiner should note the patient's composure, behavior, and mental state, as well as how she interacts with her parents and other persons. Victims of physical or sexual abuse must be removed immediately from an unsafe environment.

The information should be recorded carefully in the patient's own words. Although a detailed history is desirable, the victim should not be made to repeat the account of the incident over and over. When it is impossible to obtain a history from a very young child, the physician should obtain accounts of the incident from other sources.

B. Physical Examination

The physical examination has two purposes: to detect injuries and to collect samples that can later be used as evidence.

1. Detection of injuries—Hymenal trauma should be recognized. A lacerated hymen is usually discontinuous from 3 to 9 o'clock clockwise. Stretch trauma can produce caruncles or remnants. Vulvar irritation is fairly common in small children as a result of poor local hygiene, maceration of the skin due to wetness from diapers, or excoriations caused by local infection. Such nonspecific findings should not be regarded as diagnostic of sexual abuse.

2. Collection of evidence—During the general inspection, all foreign material such as sand and grass should be removed and placed in clearly labeled envelopes. Scrapings from underneath the fingernails and

loose hairs on the skin are collected. Semen can be detected on the skin many hours after the assault. A Wood's lamp can be used to detect the presence of seminal fluid on the patient's body, since the ultraviolet light causes semen to fluoresce. The stain may be lifted off the skin with moistened cotton swabs for further analysis.

If vaginal penetration is suspected, vaginal fluid is collected and sent for sexual disease evaluation, wet mount preparation, cytology, acid phosphatase determination, and enzyme p30. To avoid additional psychological trauma in a prepubescent child, these specimens may be collected without the insertion of a pediatric speculum, via vaginal aspiration using a feeding tube or angiocath. Current data indicate that a prepubertal child with gonorrhea or trichomonas most likely had genital-genital contact. The mode of transmission of other STDs is controversial. Testing for STDs, including HIV, should be offered.

An immediate wet mount preparation done by the examining physician may detect motile sperm. Culture swabs are obtained from the rectum, vagina, urethra, and pharynx. All specimens must be clearly labeled and the containers and envelopes sealed and signed by the examiner. All persons handling the materials must sign for them. Such a system is necessary to maintain the chain of evidence; otherwise, these specimens may not be admissible in court. Many hospitals now offer preassembled "rape kits" that guide the examiner in documenting and collecting specimens in a manner suitable for legal uses.

If a sexually transmitted disease or other signs of abuse are found, all states require the findings to be reported to child protective service agencies for the investigation of sexual abuse. Furthermore, it is important to keep in mind that a normal physical examination does not exclude the possibility of sexual abuse.

■ CONGENITAL ANOMALIES OF THE FEMALE GENITAL TRACT

Congenital anomalies of the genitalia may be divided into those that suggest sexual ambiguity (intersex problems) and those that do not. Intersex individuals have significant ambiguity of the external genitalia such that the true gender cannot be immediately determined.

ANOMALIES OF THE VULVA & LABIA

Minor differences in the contour or size of vulvar structures are not unusual. Often there is considerable variation in the distance between the posterior fourchette and the anus or between the urethra and the clitoris. Rare anomalies of the vulva include bifid clitoris, which occurs in conjunction with bladder exstrophy; a caudal appendage resembling a tail; congenital prolapse of the vagina; and variations in the insertion of the bulbocavernosus muscle, which may alter the appearance of the labia majora and at times obliterate the fossa navicularis. Duplication of the vulva is an extremely rare anomaly, which may be associated with duplication of the urinary or intestinal tracts.

There is considerable variation in the size and shape of the labia minora. One of the labia may be considerably larger than the other, or both labia may be unusually large. These variations usually require no treatment (Fig 31–8). If asymmetry is significant or if large labia are pulled into the vagina during intercourse, the hypertrophied labia may be trimmed surgically to provide a more symmetric appearance or to relieve dyspareunia.

ANOMALIES OF THE CLITORIS

Clitoral enlargement almost invariably suggests exposure to elevated levels of androgens. Such enlargement is often associated with fusion of the labioscrotal folds. Recklinghausen's neurofibromatosis, lymphangiomas, and fibromas may also involve the clitoris and cause enlargement. When an isolated neoplasm causes enlargement of the clitoris, therapy consists of excision of the neoplasm with reduction of the clitoris to normal size.

Clitoral splitting is caused by a midline fusion defect. Bifid clitoris usually occurs in conjunction with bladder exstrophy, epispadias, and absence or cleavage of the symphysis pubis. The labia majora are widely separated, and the labia minora are separated anteriorly but can be traced posteriorly around the vaginal orifice. The uterus often shows a fusion deformity, and the

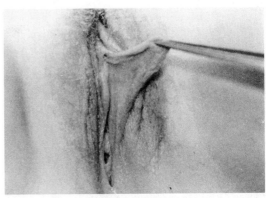

Figure 31–8. Labial asymmetry resulting from enlargement of the left labium minor.

vaginal orifice is narrow. The vagina is shortened and rotated anteriorly. The pelvic floor is incomplete, and uterine prolapse is often observed in these patients. Other congenital anomalies may be present.

Clitoral agenesis is extremely rare.

ANOMALIES OF THE HYMEN

Hymenal anomalies result from incomplete degeneration of the central portion of the hymen. Variations include imperforate, microperforate, septate, and cribriform hymens. Although most of these variants are of no clinical significance, hymenal anomalies require surgical correction if they block vaginal secretions or menstrual fluid, interfere with intercourse, or prevent treatment of a vaginal disorder.

Imperforate Hymen

Imperforate hymen represents a persistent portion of the urogenital membrane, occurring when the mesoderm of the primitive streak abnormally invades the urogenital portion of the cloacal membrane. It is one of the most common obstructive lesions of the female genital tract. When mucocolpos develops from accumulation of vaginal secretions behind the hymen, the membrane is seen as a shiny, thin bulge (Fig 31–9), and the distended vagina forms a large mass that may interfere with urination and at times may be mistaken for an abdominal tumor.

Imperforate hymen often is not diagnosed until an adolescent presents with complaints of primary amenorrhea and cyclic pelvic pain. It may present as back pain or difficulty with defecation or urination secondary to mass effect from vaginal distension. Inspection of the vulva may reveal a purplish-red hymenal membrane bulging outward as a result of accumulation of blood above it (hematocolpos). Blood may fill the

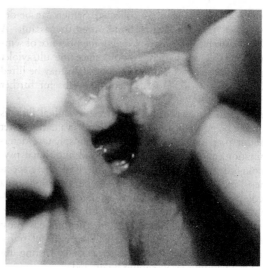

Figure 31–10. Newborn infant following excision of an imperforate hymen. Forward traction on the labia majora provides an unimpaired view of the hymenal ring. Note the large opening created. No bleeding was noted and no sutures were required.

uterus (hematometra) and spill through the fallopian tubes into the peritoneal cavity. Endometriosis and vaginal adenosis are known but not inevitable complications.

Repair of imperforate hymen is facilitated if the tissue has undergone estrogen stimulation. When imperforate hymen is corrected in infants, the central portion of the membrane is excised; sutures usually are not necessary (Fig 31–10). In postmenarcheal girls, a large central portion of the membrane should be removed, as the edges of a small incision may coalesce, allowing the obstructing membrane to reform.

ANOMALIES OF THE VAGINA

1. Transverse Vaginal Septum

Transverse vaginal septa are the result of faulty fusion or canalization of the urogenital sinus and müllerian ducts. The incidence is approximately 1/30,000 to 1/80,000 women. Approximately 46% occur in the upper vagina, 40% in the midportion, and 14% in the lower vagina. When the septum is located in the upper vagina, it is likely to be patent, whereas those located in the lower part of the vagina are more often complete.

A complete septum results in signs and symptoms similar to those of an imperforate hymen. An undiscovered imperforate transverse septum may lead to the formation of a large mucocolpos in infancy. Diagnosis is

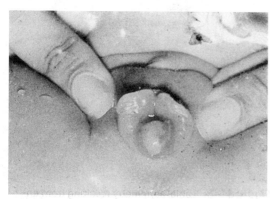

Figure 31–9. Mucocolpos in a newborn infant.

often delayed until after menarche, when menstrual blood is trapped behind an obstructing membrane. An incomplete septum is usually asymptomatic, as the central aperture allows for vaginal secretions and menstrual flow to egress from the vagina. Excision is indicated in the sexually active patient with dyspareunia.

Treatment

If the diagnosis of a complete septum is established prior to menarche, it should be incised, creating an aperture to allow drainage. Incision of a complete septum is most easily accomplished when the upper vagina is distended and the membrane is bulging, reducing the risk of injury to adjacent structures. Because of the technical difficulties in performing intravaginal surgery on immature structures, it is best to limit the procedure only to allow the establishment of vaginal drainage.

Surgical correction of vaginal narrowing should be performed only when the patient is contemplating initiation of sexual activity. The membrane should be excised with its surrounding ring of subepithelial connective tissue at the level of partition. End-to-end reanastamosis of the upper and lower vaginal mucosa, which may be accomplished with the aid of a Lucite bridge, is then undertaken.

2. Longitudinal Vaginal Septum

Duplication of the vagina is an extremely rare condition, often associated with duplication of the vulva, bladder, and uterus. More commonly, a longitudinal vaginal septum forms when the distal ends of the müllerian ducts fail to fuse properly. Both parts of the vagina are encircled by one muscular layer, and a fibrous septum lined with epithelium divides the vagina. The uterus may be bicornuate, with one or two cervices (Fig 31–11).

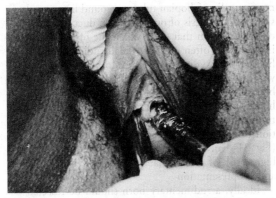

Figure 31–11. Longitudinal septum dividing the vagina.

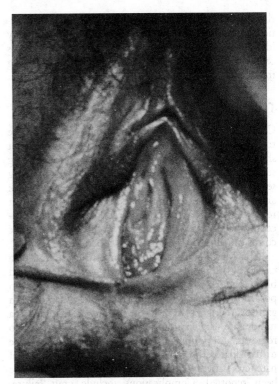

Figure 31–12. Vaginal agenesis in a girl 16 years of age.

Asymptomatic longitudinal septa require no treatment. Division of the septum is indicated when dyspareunia is present, when obstruction of drainage from one half of the vagina is noted, or when it appears that the septum will interfere with vaginal delivery.

3. Vaginal Agenesis

The incidence of vaginal agenesis is approximately 1/5000. The external genitalia of patients with vaginal agenesis (**Mayer-Rokitansky-Kuster-Hauser [MRKH] syndrome**) are normal, with a ruffled ridge of tissue representing the hymen (Fig 31–12). Variable levels of uterine development are present, with most cases accompanied by cervical and uterine agenesis. Other developmental defects are often present, affecting the urinary tract (45–50%), the spine (10%), and, less frequently, the middle ear and other mesodermal structures. Evaluation of the urinary tract and spine, as well as a hearing test, should be done after diagnosis.

Persons with vaginal agenesis typically have normal female karyotypes with normal ovaries and ovarian function; thus, they develop normal secondary sexual attributes. They often present with primary amenorrhea, or with cyclic pelvic pain in women with functioning uteri. Serum testosterone and karyotyping may identify the rare instances in which müllerian agenesis represents the effects of testicular activity, indicating male pseudohermaphroditism.

Treatment

Creation of a satisfactory vagina is the objective in the treatment of patients with vaginal agenesis. Treatment should be deferred until the patient is contemplating sexual activity. Nonoperative creation of a vagina using serial vaginal dilators, in a method described by Frank and later modified by Ingram, is relatively risk-free, but requires patient motivation and cooperation. The procedure takes a few months to complete. Repetitive coitus can also be used to create a functioning vagina.

The McIndoe procedure involves the creation of a cavity by surgical dissection between the urethra and bladder anteriorly and the perineal body and rectum posteriorly. The cavity is lined by a split-thickness skin graft overlying a plastic or soft silicone mold. The labia minora are secured around the mold for 7 days prior to removal, and postoperatively the patient must continue to use dilators for several months to maintain vaginal patency. Patient satisfaction rates of over 80% have been reported. Complications include graft failure, hematoma, fistula formation, and rectal perforation.

The Williams vulvovaginoplasty utilizes the labia majora to construct a coital pouch. Placing the labia under tension, a U-shaped incision is carried from the level of the urethra along the margins of the labia majora to the midpoint between the posterior fourchette and the anus. The vulvar skin is dissected from the subcutaneous fat to allow approximation without tension. The vagina is closed in three layers. This procedure is not performed as often as the McIndoe procedure because the vaginal pouch created is only 4–5 cm in length and positioned at an unusual angle for intercourse.

Alternative procedures, such as sigmoid vaginoplasty and laparoscopic approaches using the Vecchietti procedure and the Davydov procedure, have also been described. Limited data are available on success and complications rates at this time.

4. Partial Vaginal Agenesis

Partial vaginal agenesis occurs when a large portion of the vaginal plate, usually the distal part, fails to canalize. The affected vaginal segment of the vagina is replaced by a soft mass of tissue. The cause of this uncommon anomaly is unknown. Absence of the distal vagina may be identified when the infant is examined at birth, and sonographic visualization of the upper va-

gina, cervix, and uterus serves to distinguish it from Rokitansky syndrome.

If the uterus has developed normally, the upper part of the vagina fills with blood when menstruation begins. The symptoms are similar to those associated with imperforate hymen after the menarche. Vulvar inspection reveals findings identical with those of vaginal agenesis, but rectoabdominal palpation reveals a large, boggy pelvic mass. Diagnostic imaging using sonography, computed tomography, or magnetic resonance imaging will confirm the diagnosis.

Treatment

Surgery is indicated as obstruction to menstrual flow may occur. In some, drainage of the uterus can be achieved through a reconstructed vagina. In others, particularly when the uterus is rudimentary, consideration may be given to performing a hysterectomy.

ANOMALIES OF THE UTERUS

Uterine anomalies result from agenesis of the müllerian duct or a defect in fusion or canalization. These anomalies include bicornuate uterus (37%), arcuate uterus (15%), incomplete septum (13%), uterine didelphys (11%), complete septum (9%), and unicornuate uterus (4%).

Most uterine anomalies are asymptomatic and therefore are not detected during childhood or early adolescence. Symptoms during adolescence are primarily caused by retention of menstrual flow. Asymptomatic abnormalities often escape detection until they interfere with reproduction.

1. Unicornuate Uterus and Rudimentary Uterine Horn

A unicornuate uterus is a single-horned uterus with its corresponding fallopian tube and round ligament. It results from agenesis of one müllerian duct, with absence of structures on that side. When the other hemiuterus is present, it often creates a small rudimentary uterine horn. If this rudimentary horn does not communicate with the other uterine cavity or the vagina, menstrual blood cannot escape, resulting in severe dysmenorrhea, hematometra, or pyometra. If pregnancy occurs in a rudimentary horn, it may result in rupture, a complication that is potentially fatal for both mother and fetus (Fig 31–13). Women with unicornuate uteri are at higher risk of preterm labor, infertility, endometriosis, and malpresentation.

Ideally, a rudimentary horn should be resected before conception. The tube and ovary on the affected

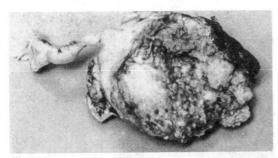

Figure 31–13. Pregnancy in a noncommunicating rudimentary uterine horn that has resulted in rupture.

side can be preserved, provided that the blood supply is not impaired. If the endometrial cavity of the remaining horn is entered during the operation, cesarean section is a reasonable mode of delivery for any subsequent pregnancies.

A unicornuate uterus is occasionally accompanied by an anomaly of the opposite paramesonephric duct, creating a lateral vaginal wall cyst with an endometrial lining. As a result, the cyst fills with blood following menarche and produces a vaginal mass (Fig 31–14). Excision of a small segment of the wall between the cyst and the vagina often provides adequate drainage. Attempts to remove the cyst may involve extensive dissection, with potential damage to the urethra, bladder, or ureter.

2. Uterine Didelphys

Failure of fusion of the müllerian duct may result in two separate uterine bodies. The fusion defect is usually limited to the uterine body and cervix. Duplication of the bladder, urethra, vagina, anus, and vulva may also occur.

Women with uterine didelphys generally have good reproductive outcomes. Vaginal septae may require resection if they cause difficulty with sexual intercourse or vaginal delivery or if pain results from obstructed menstrual flow.

3. Bicornuate Uterus and Septate Uterus

Bicornuate uterus results from partial fusion of the müllerian ducts, leading to varying degrees of separation of the uterine horns. Uterine septa result from failures of canalization or resorption of the midline septum between the two müllerian ducts. While reproductive function is good overall in bicornuate uterus, there is a higher risk of miscarriage with increasing length of septa. Hysteroscopic resection of septa or metroplasty may be considered for infertility.

ANOMALIES OF THE OVARIES

At about the fifth week of gestation, the midportion of the urogenital ridge, close to the mesonephric duct, thickens to form the gonadal ridge. Located along the urogenital ridge, an additional ovary is infrequently found, separated from the normal ovaries (supernumerary ovary). Similarly, excess ovarian tissue may be observed near a normally placed ovary and connected to it (accessory ovary).

During development, the testes are drawn into the scrotum by the gubernaculum testis. Similarly, an ovary may be drawn by the round ligament into the inguinal canal or the labium major. A firm inguinal mass should alert the examiner to the possible presence of an aberrant gonad, possibly containing testicular elements, even in the presence of female external genitalia. A karyotype should be obtained. At the time of hernia repair, the gonad should be biopsied. If it proves to be an ovary, it should be returned to the peritoneal cavity and the hernia repaired. If a testis is identified, the gonad should be removed.

Gonadal dysgenesis may demonstrate typical physical manifestations. These include cutis laxa and edema of the dorsal surfaces of the hands and feet in infants, height and weight below the third percentile, broad

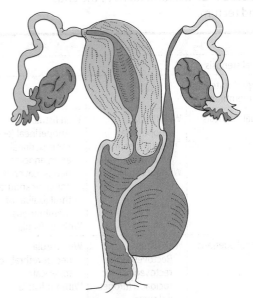

Figure 31–14. Unicornuate uterus with paramesonephric vaginal cyst. The endometrium lining the upper part of the cyst bleeds at menarche, and the blood filling the lower part of the cyst forms a mass protruding into the vagina.

chest and small nipples, webbed neck, coarctation of the aorta, prominent epicanthal folds, nevi, and other somatic anomalies (eg, short fourth metacarpal). In most adults with gonadal dysgenesis, the normal gonad is replaced by a white fibrous streak, 2–3 cm long and about 0.5 cm wide, located in the gonadal ridge. Histologically, the streak gonad is characterized by interlacing waves of dense fibrous stroma, indistinguishable from normal ovarian stroma.

Although oocytes are present in children, they are usually absent in 45,X adults. Increased atresia and failure of germ cell formation deplete oocyte supply, but when atresia is incomplete, pubertal changes, spontaneous menstruation, and even pregnancies have been reported.

ANOMALIES OF THE URETHRA & ANUS

Failure of a newborn infant to pass meconium or urine demands investigation. Passage of feces or urine through the vagina suggests a fistulous communication, and usually either the urethra or the anus is imperforate.

Anal and rectal anomalies are classified according to Ladd and Gross (Table 31–2). In general, anomalies

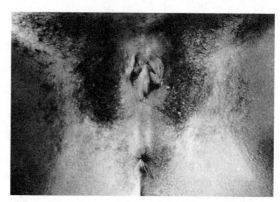

Figure 31–15. An adolescent girl following repair of bladder exstrophy. Note the bifid clitoris and anterior displacement of the vagina.

are divided into 2 major groups: those that form complete obstruction of the intestinal tract and those that are associated with some type of abnormal opening or fistula.

Because findings are so diverse, only broad generalizations can be offered regarding the management of urogenital anomalies of this type. The following principles may serve as guidelines: (1) Obstruction of the intestinal tract must be corrected. (2) Obstruction of the urinary tract must be relieved (this may require an initial ureterostomy or cystostomy). (3) If the urogenital sinus cannot be used later as a urethra, a permanent diversion (eg, ileal conduit) must be created. (4) If fecal contamination of the urinary tract is present, it is essential that it be corrected, usually with a temporary colostomy.

Epispadias & Bladder Exstrophy

Epispadias denotes the failure of normal fusion of the anterior wall of the urogenital sinus, resulting in a urethra that opens cephalad to a bifid clitoris under the symphysis pubis (Fig 31–15). Occasionally, the defect is more extensive, involving the bladder and the anterior abdominal wall, causing exstrophy of the bladder. Both conditions may be associated with defects involving the anterior pelvic girdle, resulting in diminished pelvic support. Uterine and vaginal vault prolapse as well as anterior displacement of the vagina are common gynecologic complications. Rarely, vaginal and uterine prolapse may occur in the absence of other malformations. Major urologic reconstruction is required promptly, although gynecologic defects can be repaired later, usually during adolescence.

Table 31–2. Malformations of the anus and rectum.

	Female	Male
Anal stenosis		
Imperforate anal membrane		
Anal agenesis	With fistula Anoperineal (ectopic perineal anus, anovulvar) Without fistula	With fistula Anoperineal (ectopic perineal anus, anocutaneous [covered anus]) or anourethral (bulbar or membranous) Without fistula
Rectal agenesis	With fistula Rectovestibular, rectovaginal, rectocloacal (urogenital sinus) Without fistula	With fistula Rectourethral, rectovesical Without fistula
Rectal atresia		

Reproduced, with permission, from Ladd WE, Gross RE: Congenital malformations of the anus and rectum: Report of 162 cases. Am J Surg 1934;23:167.

■ GYNECOLOGIC DISORDERS IN PREMENARCHEAL CHILDREN

VULVOVAGINITIS

Pruritus vulvae and vulvovaginitis are common gynecologic disorders in children. Pruritus vulvae refers to itching of the external female genitalia, while vulvovaginitis, though inconsistently delineated in the literature, generally involves prominent vaginal discharge. The child is susceptible to both these conditions as the prepubertal vulva is thin without labial fat pads and pubic hair, as well as anatomically in close proximity to the anus and its contaminants, the unestrogenized vagina is atrophic with pH ranges excellent for bacterial growth, and perineal hygiene is often suboptimal as supervision declines with age. See Table 31–3 for classification.

Clinical Findings

Acute vulvovaginitis may denude the thin vulvar or vaginal mucosa; however, bleeding is usually minimal. Mucopurulent or purulent discharge is usually present. Vaginal discharge may vary from minimal to copious, and at times it is bloodstained. Symptoms vary from minor discomfort to relatively intense perineal pruritus. The child often complains of a burning sensation accompanied by a foul-smelling discharge. The irritating discharge inflames the vulva and often causes the child to scratch the area to the point of bleeding. Inspection of the vagina reveals an area of redness and soreness that may be minimal or may extend laterally to the thighs and backward to the anus. Many patients experience a

Table 31–3. Classification of vulvovaginitis according to cause.

Nonspecific vulvovaginitis
  Polymicrobial infection associated with disturbed homeostasis: secondary to poor perineal hygiene or a foreign body
Vulvovaginitis due to secondary inoculation
  Infection resulting from inoculation of the vagina with pathogens affecting other areas of the body by contact or bloodborne transmission: secondary to upper respiratory tract infection or urinary tract infection
Specific vulvovaginitis
  Specific primary infection, most commonly sexually transmitted: *Neisseria gonorrhoeae, Gardnerella vaginalis,* herpesvirus, *Treponema pallidum,* others

burning sensation when urine flows over the inflamed tissues, and vulvovaginitis should be excluded in children prior to treatment for urinary tract infection.

Diagnosis is suspected by the typical appearance of the inflamed tissue. A wet mount preparation reveals numerous leukocytes and occasional red blood cells. Culture of vaginal secretions will sometimes identify the offending organism.

Evaluation of the vaginal secretions may include smears for Gram's stain, bacterial cultures, cultures for mycotic organisms, wet prep, *Trichomonas,* and parasitic ova.

Improvement of perineal hygiene is important to relieve the symptoms and to prevent recurrences. Most cases of nonspecific pruritus vulvae resolve with improvements in hygiene and avoidance of irritants, including soaps.

Amoxicillin (20–40 mg/kg/d in 3 divided doses) is effective against a variety of potentially pathogenic organisms in nonspecific vulvovaginitis. When the infection is severe and extensive mucosal damage is seen, a short course of topical estrogen cream is given to promote healing of vulval and vaginal tissues. When irritation is intense, hydrocortisone cream may be necessary to alleviate the itch. In recurrent infections refractory to treatment or associated with a foul-smelling, bloody discharge, vaginoscopy is necessary to exclude a foreign body or tumor.

FOREIGN BODIES

Vaginal foreign bodies induce an intense inflammatory reaction and result in blood-stained, foul-smelling discharge. Usually, the child does not recall inserting the foreign object or will not admit to it. Radiographs cannot be depended on to reveal a foreign body, because many objects are not radiopaque. Foreign bodies in the lower third of the vagina can be flushed out with warm saline irrigation. Even after removal, if the vagina cannot be adequately inspected in the office, vaginoscopy is indicated to confirm that no other foreign bodies are present in the upper vagina.

URETHRAL PROLAPSE

Occasionally, vulvar bleeding is the result of urethral prolapse. The urethral mucosa protrudes through the meatus and forms a hemorrhagic, sensitive vulvar mass (Fig 31–16). Prolapse of the urethra is diagnosed when the urethral orifice is identified in the center of the mass and the mass is separated from the vagina. When the lesion is small and urination is unimpaired, a short course of therapy using estrogen cream is beneficial. When urinary retention is present, if the lesion is large and necrotic, if medical therapy fails, or if the child is

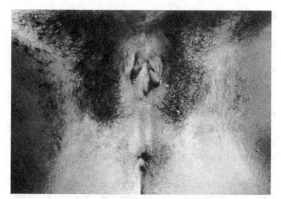

Figure 31–16. Urethral prolapse in a child aged 6 years.

being examined under anesthesia, resection of the prolapsed tissue should be performed and an indwelling catheter inserted for 24 hours.

LICHEN SCLEROSUS

Lichen sclerosus of the vulva is a hypotrophic dystrophy. More common in postmenopausal women, it is occasionally seen in children. Histologically, the findings in both age groups are similar, with flattening of the rete pegs, hyalinization of the subdermal tissues, and keratinization. In children, the lesion has no known malignant potential if only hypoplastic dystrophy is present.

The clinical presentation includes flat papules which may coalesce into plaques or, in extreme cases, involve the entire vulva (Fig 31–17). Usually, the lesion does not extend beyond the middle of the labia majora laterally or into the vagina medially. The clitoris, posterior fourchette, and anorectal areas are frequently involved. Occasionally, there are lesions affecting extragenital areas. Although most lesions are predominantly white, some have pronounced vascular markings. They tend to bruise easily, forming bloody blisters, and they are susceptible to secondary infections. Symptoms consist of vulvar irritation, dysuria, and pruritus. Scratching is common and occasionally may provoke bleeding or lead to secondary infection.

While histologic confirmation is necessary in postmenopausal women, it is not always mandatory in children. Treatment usually consists of improved local hygiene, reduction of trauma, and short-term use of hydrocortisone cream to alleviate the pruritus. Topical testosterone or newer androgen-containing skin patches have also been used, but longer-term exposure may induce androgen-dependent secondary sex characteristics. Over half of children improve significantly or recover during puberty.

LABIAL ADHESION

Labial adhesion is common in prepubertal children. The cause is not known but is probably related to low levels of estrogen. The skin covering the labia is extremely thin, and local irritation may induce scratching, which may denude the labia. The labia then adhere in the midline, and reepithelialization occurs on both sides (Fig 31–18). It is important to differentiate this condition from congenital absence of the vagina.

Most children with small areas of labial adhesions are asymptomatic. When symptoms occur, they usually relate to interference with urination or accumulation of urine behind the adhesion. Dysuria and recurrent vulvar and vaginal infections are cardinal symptoms. Rarely, urinary retention may occur.

Asymptomatic minimal-to-moderate labial fusion does not require treatment. Symptomatic fusion may be treated with a short course of estrogen cream applied twice daily for 7–10 days; this may separate the labia. A new therapeutic alternative is to use estrogen transdermal patches in close proximity to the labia. When medical treatment fails or if severe urinary symptoms exist, surgical separation of the labia is indicated. This can be done as an office procedure using 1–2% topical xylocaine gel.

Because of low levels of estrogen, recurrences of labial adhesion are common until puberty. Following

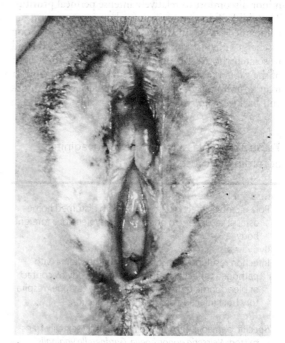

Figure 31–17. Lichen sclerosus of the vulva of 6-year-old child.

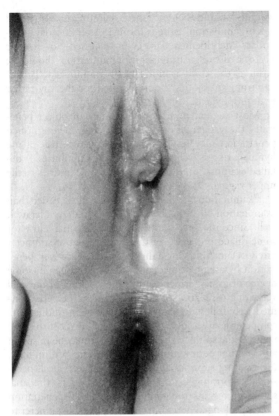

Figure 31–18. Labial adhesion in a young girl. Note the translucent vertical line in the center where the labia are fused together.

puberty, the condition resolves spontaneously. Improved perineal hygiene and removal of vulvar irritants may prevent recurrences.

GENITAL INJURIES

Most injuries to the genitalia during childhood are accidental. Many are of minor significance, but a few are life-threatening and require surgical intervention. The physician must determine how the child sustained the injury, bearing in mind that the child requires protection if she is the victim of physical or sexual abuse.

1. Vulvar Injuries

Contusion of the vulva usually does not require treatment. A hematoma manifests itself as a round, tense, ecchymotic, tender mass (Fig 31–19). A small vulvar hematoma can usually be controlled by pressure with an ice pack. The vulva should be kept clean and dry. A

large hematoma, or one that continues to increase in size, may need to be incised, the clotted blood removed, and the bleeding points ligated. If the source of bleeding cannot be found, the cavity should be packed with gauze and a firm pressure dressing applied. The pack is removed in 24 hours. Prophylactic broad-spectrum antibiotics may be advisable.

When a large hematoma obstructs the urethra, it is necessary to insert a catheter, usually by a suprapubic approach. X-ray of the pelvis may be necessary to rule out pelvic fracture.

2. Vaginal Injuries

Usually, there is only a small amount of bleeding from a hymenal injury. However, when the hymen is lacerated or when there is other evidence that an object has entered the vagina or penetrated the perineum, a detailed examination must be carried out to exclude injuries to the upper vagina or intrapelvic viscera (Fig 31–20).

Most vaginal injuries involve the lateral walls. Generally, there is relatively little blood loss, and the child does not have much pain if only the mucosa is damaged. If the laceration extends beyond the vaginal vault, exploration of the pelvic cavity is necessary to rule out extension into the broad ligament or peritoneal cavity. Bladder and bowel integrity must be confirmed by catheterization and rectal palpation. Because of the small caliber of the organs involved, special instruments, as well as proper exposure and assistance, may be required for repair of vaginal injuries in young girls. Many vaginal lacerations are limited to the mucosal and submucosal tissues and are repaired with fine suture material after complete hemostasis is secured.

A vaginal wall hematoma from a small vessel may stop bleeding spontaneously. Larger vessels may form large, tense hematomas that distend the vagina and re-

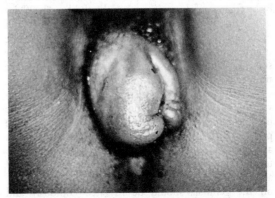

Figure 31–19. A large vulvar hematoma secondary to bicycle injury.

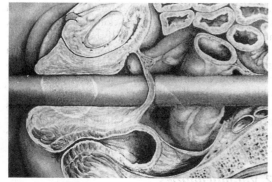

Figure 31–20. Transvaginal perforation of cul-de-sac and penetration of peritoneal cavity by a fall on a mop handle. Scanty bleeding from a hymenal tear was the only symptom on admission.

quire evacuation and ligation of the bleeding vessel. When a vessel is torn above the pelvic floor, a retroperitoneal hematoma may develop. If the hematoma is enlarging, laparotomy must be performed, the clot removed, and the bleeding vessel ligated. Alternatively, the bleeding may be controlled by angiographic embolization of the bleeding vessel.

3. Anogenital Injuries Caused by Abuse

Many children who are victims of sexual abuse do not sustain physical injuries, and an examination is not expected to detect signs of abuse. Even when injured, many of these children may not be seen for weeks, months, or even years after the incident occurred. The delay allows for semen and debris to wash away and for most, if not all, injuries to heal.

Injuries to the vulva may be caused by manipulation of the vulva or introitus, without vaginal penetration, or by friction of the penis against the child's vulva ("dry intercourse"). Erythema, swelling, skin bruising, and excoriations are found on the labia and vestibule. These injuries are superficial and often limited to the vulvar skin; they should resolve within a few days and require no special treatment.

Meticulous perineal hygiene is important in the prevention of secondary infections. Sitz baths should be used to remove secretions and contaminants. In some patients with extensive skin abrasions, broad-spectrum antibiotics should be given as prophylaxis. Large vulvar tears require suturing, which is best done under general anesthesia, using fine absorbable sutures. Bite wounds on the genitalia should be irrigated copiously and necrotic tissue cautiously debrided. A noninfected fresh wound can often be closed primarily, but most bite wounds should be left open. Closure is completed when granulation tissue is formed. After 3–5 days, secondary debridement may be required to remove necrotic tissues. Antitetanus immunization should be given if the child is not already immunized. Broad-spectrum antibiotics should be used for therapy rather than prophylaxis.

Most vaginal injuries occur when an object penetrates the vagina through the hymenal opening. Such penetration may result in a laceration or a tear of the hymenal ring as well as associated vaginal injuries. A detailed examination is necessary to exclude injuries to the upper vagina.

Examination of the anus and rectum is easier than examination of the vagina, and most children tolerate it well. Since the anal sphincter and anal canal allow for some dilatation, a tear of the anal mucosa or sphincter rarely occurs following a digital assault. However, penetration by a larger object almost always results in some degree of injury, which varies from swelling of the anal verge to gross tearing of the sphincter. In the period immediately following penetration, the main findings are sphincter laxity and swelling and small tears of the anal verge. If the sphincter is not severed, it may be in spasm and will not permit a digital examination. Within days, the swelling subsides and the mucosal tears heal, occasionally forming skin tags. If not severed, the anal sphincter regains function. Repeated anal penetration over a prolonged period may cause the anal sphincter to become loose, forming an enlarged opening. The anal mucosa thickens and loses its normal folds.

Occasionally, child victims of abuse contract an STD. Treatment for gonorrhea, chlamydia, and syphilis may be deferred until the results of tests become available. If vulvovaginitis is clinically suspected on the initial visit, appropriate antibiotic therapy is given. If the infection is severe, a short course of topical estrogen cream is given to promote healing of vulval and vaginal tissues. When irritation is intense, hydrocortisone cream may be necessary to alleviate itching. A repeat VDRL to detect seroconversion is required 6 weeks later. Prophylaxis for hepatitis B with hepatitis B vaccination is recommended following sexual assault. For nonimmune victims with a high-risk exposure, practitioners may also consider adding hepatitis B immune globulin to the regimen.

Although the likelihood of a child becoming infected with HIV as a result of sexual abuse is relatively low, many victims and their families are concerned about this possibility. Unfortunately, HIV infection in children can result in a prolonged clinical latency and can masquerade as other pathologic conditions. One study reported that 41 HIV-infected children were identified by HIV antibody tests conducted during sex abuse assessments on 5622 children. Thirteen children had alternative risk factors, but 28 children lacked any alternative transmission route to that of sexual abuse. Eighteen of these 28 victims were female and 20 were African-American. The mean age was 9 years. Coinfection with another STD occurred in 9 (33%) cases. Prophylaxis against HIV is controversial as it remains to be proven that treatment of sexual exposure prevents transmission of HIV. However, sexual assault victims, particularly those who are children, may sustain additional tissue injury which may increase the transmission rate of HIV. Therefore, HIV prophylaxis is offered in certain centers.

Protective Services & Counseling

It is imperative to ensure that the child is being discharged to a safe environment. Sometimes it is advisable to admit the child to the hospital or utilize temporary placement. All patients who are suspected of being victims of child sexual abuse must be referred to child protective services for further evaluation.

In the period immediately following sexual assault or disclosure of sexual abuse, the child and her family often require intensive day-to-day emotional support, counseling, and guidance. Child victims often show signs of depression and have feelings of guilt, fear, and low self-esteem. Appropriate referral for counseling is imperative. The major emphasis of emotional support involves strengthening the child's ego, improving her self-image, and helping her to learn to trust others and feel secure again. To begin the strengthening process, the child needs to realize that she was a victim. She must be encouraged to express her feelings of anger and hurt so that these feelings may be later expressed without experiencing further guilt. Often, the child has both positive and negative feelings toward the perpetrator and may need help in sorting out these feelings. Sometimes the child blames her parents for not protecting her. The child's relationships with her parents and other family members are critical and may need restructuring. Following this crisis intervention phase, a treatment program using individual and peer-group therapy is initiated. The patient and her family should be offered treatment.

GENITAL NEOPLASMS

Genital tumors, although uncommon, must be considered when a girl is found to have a chronic genital ulcer, nontraumatic swelling of the external genitalia, tissue protruding from the vagina, a fetid or bloody discharge, abdominal pain or enlargement, or premature sexual maturation. Virtually every type of genital neoplasm reported in adults has also been found in girls under 14 years of age. About 50% of the genital tumors in children are premalignant or malignant.

1. Benign Tumors of the Vulva & Vagina

Teratomas, hemangiomas, simple cysts of the hymen, retention cysts of the paraurethral ducts, benign granulomas of the perineum, and condylomata acuminata are some of the benign vulvar neoplasms observed in children and adolescents.

Obstruction of a paraurethral duct may form a relatively large cyst distorting the urethral orifice. The recommended treatment is incision and drainage, marsupialization, or excision.

Teratomas usually present as cystic masses arising from the midline of the perineum. Although a teratoma in this area may be benign, local recurrence is likely. To prevent recurrences, a generous margin of healthy tissue is excised about the periphery of the mass.

Capillary hemangiomas usually disappear as the child grows older and thus require no therapy except reassurance. Cavernous hemangiomas, in contrast, are composed of vessels of considerable size, and injury to them may cause serious hemorrhage. They are best treated surgically.

Most benign tumors of the vagina in children are unilocular cystic remnants of the mesonephric duct (Fig 31–21). Small cysts of the mesonephric duct (Gartner's duct) do not require surgery when they are asymptomatic. Large cysts (eg, those that block the vagina) must be treated surgically. The technical difficulties associated with excision of a large mesonephric cyst from the wall of the vagina in an infant may be considerable. Removal of a large portion of the cyst wall

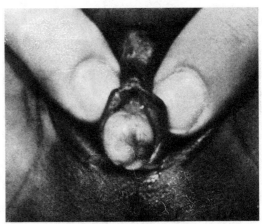

Figure 31–21. Simple vulvar or hymeneal cyst arising posterior to the urethra of a newborn infant.

and marsupialization of the edges, which prevents reaccumulation of fluid, are usually sufficient.

2. Malignant Tumors of the Vagina & Cervix

Embryonal Carcinoma of the Vagina (Botryoid Sarcoma)

Embryonal vaginal carcinomas are most commonly seen in very young girls (< 3 years old). The tumor usually involves the vagina, but the cervix may be affected as well, particularly in an older child. The tumors arise in the submucosal tissues and spread rapidly beneath an intact vaginal epithelium. The vaginal mucosa then bulges into a series of polypoid growths (thus the term botryoid sarcoma; Fig 31–22). The diagnosis is made on the basis of histologic evaluation of a biopsy specimen, but routine microscopic evaluation may lead to an erroneous diagnosis of these lesions as benign. Striated muscle fibers are not always seen, and most of the tumor demonstrates myxomatous changes. Electron microscopy may be required to confirm the diagnosis of embryonal rhabdomyosarcoma.

Combination chemotherapy regimens—often, vincristine, dactinomycin (actinomycin D), and cyclophosphamide—have been used with success. Following a course of chemotherapy lasting for at least 6 months, the tumor is reexamined and rebiopsied. If following chemotherapy no residual tumor is found, surgical extirpation may not be required. If a tumor is present and is amenable to surgical removal, radical hysterectomy and vaginectomy may be performed. The ovaries are preserved, and exenteration is not recommended. If the tumor is unresectable, radiation therapy is used to further shrink and control tumor growth. Following

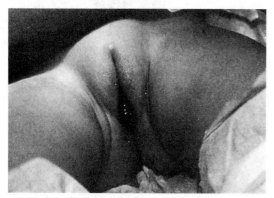

Figure 31–22. Botryoid sarcoma presenting as a hemorrhagic growth extruding from the vagina.

surgery, chemotherapy should be continued for another 6–12 months.

Other Malignant Tumors of the Vagina

Three types of vaginal carcinoma may appear during childhood and the early teens. Endodermal carcinoma occurs most often in young children. Carcinoma arising in a remnant of a mesonephric duct (mesonephric carcinoma) occurs more often in girls 3 years of age or older. Clear cell adenocarcinoma of müllerian origin, often associated with a history of antenatal exposure to diethylstilbestrol (DES), is encountered most frequently in postmenarcheal teenage girls. The clinical features and treatment of malignant lesions of the vagina and cervix are similar to those in adult women.

3. Ovarian Tumors

Even though ovarian tumors are the most common genital neoplasm encountered in children and adolescents, they represent only 1% of all neoplasms in premenarcheal children. Ovarian tumors of all varieties (except Brenner tumors) have been reported in premenarcheal children, with benign cystic teratomas accounting for at least 30%. Seventy percent of ovarian cancers in youth are of germ cell origin. The most common symptoms of ovarian tumors are abdominal pain and an abdominal mass. The small pelvic cavity of a child causes most ovarian tumors to rise above the pelvic inlet and present abdominally. Acute symptoms of severe pain, peritoneal irritation, or intra-abdominal hemorrhage resulting from a tumor accident (torsion, rupture, or perforation) may lead to an erroneous diagnosis of appendicitis, intussusception, or volvulus. At least 25% of all childhood ovarian tumors elude diagnosis until exploratory laparotomy is performed. Tumors of the ovary should be considered in the differential diagnosis of most disorders causing abdominal pain or mass in a child. Pelvic (rectal) examination may be helpful if the tumor is in the pelvis but will not detect most abdominal tumors. Imaging is a critical step in the evaluation of the adolescent or child with an adnexal mass.

The management of ovarian neoplasms in premenarcheal children varies from that in older patients because continued ovarian function is necessary to complete sexual and somatic maturation in children. While laparoscopy is an acceptable option if an adnexal mass is thought to be benign, suspicion for malignancy should prompt laparotomy. Conservative surgery (unilateral salpingo-oophorectomy) is justified for most premenarcheal patients with stage I cancer of the ovary, provided that it can be shown that the tumor is limited to the ovary. If a tumor has extended beyond the ovary, more radical surgery (bilateral salpingo-oophorectomy with hysterectomy) is indicated, regardless of age. Germ cell tumors are highly responsive to chemotherapy, with the exception of dysgerminomas, which respond well to radiation.

DISORDERS OF SEXUAL MATURATION

ACCELERATED SEXUAL MATURATION

Puberty is the process by which sexually immature persons become capable of reproduction. These changes occur largely as the result of maturation of the hypothalamic-pituitary-gonadal axis. As a rule, breast development, cornification of the vaginal mucosa, and growth of genital hair precede uterine bleeding by about 2 years. The normal sequence of events in sexual development is outlined in Fig 31–23. Usually, initial growth acceleration occurs first. Breast budding occurs between ages 9 and 11 years and is followed by pubarche and a marked increase in growth rate, often referred to as the adolescent growth spurt. The first menstrual period occurs at an average age of 12.8 years in girls in the U.S. Regular ovulatory cycles, 20 months later, mark the end of the pubertal changes.

Sexual precocity is the onset of sexual maturation at any age that is 2.5 SD earlier than the normal age. At present, the appearance of any secondary sexual characteristics before 8 years of age or onset of menarche prior to age 10 is considered precocious. Sexual precocity may be classified as gonadotropin-releasing hormone (GnRH)-dependent precocious puberty or GnRH-independent precocious puberty.

GnRH-Dependent Precocious Puberty

GnRH-dependent precocious puberty is normal pubertal development that occurs at an earlier age. Premature activation of the hypothalamic-pituitary axis is followed by gonadotropin secretion, which in turn stimulates the gonads to produce steroid hormones, and subsequently, pubertal changes. GnRH-dependent precocious puberty is seen more frequently in girls than in boys. The cause of such early development often remains unclear and has been labeled as idiopathic.

Occasionally, precocious puberty is associated with central nervous system (CNS) abnormalities, including hypothalamic hamartomas, optic gliomas, and neurofibromas, as well as other CNS neoplasms. Cranial irradiation and CNS injuries may also be associated with precocious puberty. Prolonged excessive therapy with exogenous sex steroids also may accelerate hypothalamic-pituitary axis maturation, resulting in precocious puberty.

GnRH-Independent Precocious Puberty

A. ENDOGENOUS ESTROGENS

The ovary in the newborn female contains 1–2 million primordial follicles, most of which undergo atresia dur-

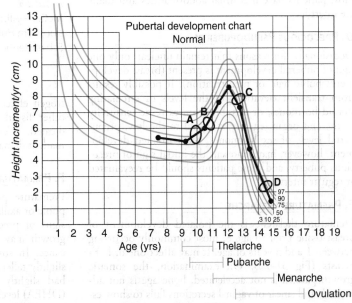

Figure 31–23. A pubertal development chart for a normally-developing female adolescent. Growth data are converted to growth velocity and plotted. The growth velocity curve shows initial acceleration in growth followed by the growth spurt and subsequent deceleration. Superimposed on this curve are the following pubertal events: **A,** thelarche; **B,** pubarche; **C,** menarche; **D,** onset of ovulation. (From Reindollar RH, McDonough PG: Delayed sexual development: Common causes and basic clinical approach. Pediatr Ann 1981;10:178.)

ing childhood without producing significant quantities of estrogen. However, large follicular cysts capable of estrogen production occur occasionally and may cause early feminization. Benign tumors of the ovary (eg, teratoma, cystadenoma) may produce estrogen or may induce surrounding ovarian tissue to produce steroids. Granulosa cell tumors capable of estrogen production are a rare cause of prepubertal feminization. Other rare tumors of extragonadal origin, including adrenal adenomas and hepatomas, may produce estrogens as well.

B. EXOGENOUS ESTROGENS

Ingestion of estrogens or prolonged use of creams containing estrogens is a possible, though uncommon, cause of early feminization. Prompt discontinuation is indicated.

C. MCCUNE-ALBRIGHT SYNDROME

Polyosthotic fibrous dysplasia, irregular cutaneous pigmentation, and precocious puberty occurring together are cardinal signs of McCune-Albright syndrome (Fig 31–24). Affected children usually present at a younger age than those with idiopathic precocious puberty. Vaginal bleeding occurs early and in most is the first sign of puberty. The diagnosis is made on the basis of skin pigmentation and demonstration of bone lesions or pathologic fractures. The exact cause is unknown; a primary ovarian abnormality with premature estrogen production has been suggested.

The prognosis for children with McCune-Albright syndrome is unfavorable. Adult height is significantly reduced, not only because of early epiphyseal closure but also because of pathologic bone fractures. As adults, most patients have menstrual abnormalities and many are infertile.

D. PRECOCIOUS PSEUDOPUBERTY

Occasionally, for reasons that remain unclear, only one sign of pubertal development is present (breast development, pubic hair, or menstruation). It possibly results from transient elevations of the levels of circulating steroid hormones, or possibly from extreme sensitivity of the end organ (eg, breast tissue) to the low, prepubertal levels of sex hormones. Such isolated development, however, may represent the initial sign of precocious puberty, and these patients should be reevaluated at regular intervals.

E. PREMATURE THELARCHE

Premature thelarche is the isolated development of breast tissue prior to age 8, most commonly occurring between 1 and 3 years of age. It may affect one or both breasts (Fig 31–25). On examination, the somatic growth pattern is not accelerated, bone age is not advanced, and smear of vaginal secretions fails to show es-

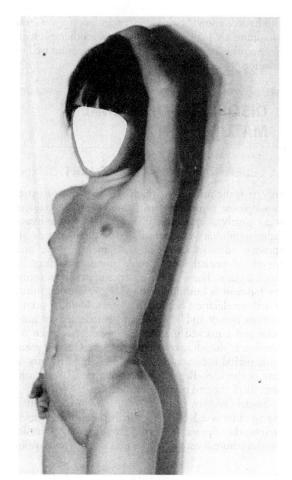

Figure 31–24. Six-and-a-half-year-old child with McCune-Albright syndrome. (Reproduced, with permission, from Huffman JW: *Gynauakologie des Kindes.* Urban & Schwarzenberg, 1975.)

trogen effect. The diagnosis is made by exclusion of other disorders. Surgical biopsy of the breast is not indicated, as extensive excision of tissue may cause permanent damage to the breast.

F. PREMATURE PUBARCHE

Premature pubarche is the isolated development of pubic or axillary hair prior to age 8 years without other signs of precocious puberty (Fig 31–26). Such hair growth may be idiopathic and of no clinical significance. In some studies, these children tended to be slightly taller, had marginally advanced bone age, and had slightly elevated serum dehydroepiandrosterone (DHEA) levels.

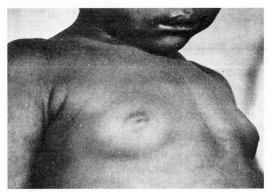

Figure 31–25. Premature thelarche in a child 5 years of age.

Early pubarche may be a sign of excess androgen production due to enzyme deficiency (congenital adrenal hyperplasia) or tumor (Leydig cell tumor). Thorough evaluation of adrenal and gonadal function and assessment of androgen production are necessary to exclude such abnormalities. The diagnosis of idiopathic premature pubarche is made only after such an evaluation fails to detect an abnormality.

G. PREMATURE MENARCHE

Premature menarche denotes the appearance of cyclic vaginal bleeding in children in the absence of other signs of secondary sexual development. The cause is unknown but may be related to increased end organ sensitivity of the endometrium to low prepubertal levels of estrogens. Alternatively, bleeding may be related to transient elevation of estrogens due to premature follicular development. These patients have estradiol levels in the prepubertal range, and cytologic smears of vaginal secretions indicate lack of estrogenic stimulation. When patients are given GnRH, the response of the pituitary gland is similar to that seen in prepubertal children.

The diagnosis of premature menarche is formulated by exclusion following investigation of other causes of vaginal bleeding and is confirmed when the cyclic nature of the bleeding becomes apparent. The prognosis is excellent. Adult height is uncompromised; the menstrual pattern is normal; and fertility potential remains unimpaired.

Evaluation of the Patient with Precocious Puberty

When evaluating the patient with sexual precocity, the age at onset, duration, and progression of signs and symptoms constitute important historical information. Family history and review of systems may add important facts.

A. GENERAL CHANGES

Enhancement of general growth is coincident with the onset of estrogen-stimulated change. The child often exhibits accelerated growth velocity, tall stature for age, and advanced skeletal maturation.

B. SKIN

Additional androgen-dependent findings include acne and adult-type body odor.

C. BREAST DEVELOPMENT

Breast development is at least at Tanner stage II, with the areolae having a broadened, darkened appearance.

D. GENITALIA

Genital changes reflect estrogen-induced thickening of the genital tissues. Increased vaginal secretions may result in leukorrhea. Dark, coarse pubic hair may be present.

Diagnosis

The diagnosis of GnRH-dependent precocity requires demonstration of pubertal gonadotropin secretion. The diagnostic evaluation required to document early pubertal development and differentiate central from peripheral causes includes the determination of serum luteinizing hormone (LH), follicle-stimulating hormone (FSH), and estradiol levels, and a GnRH stimulation test. In patients with GnRH-dependent precocious puberty, the results of these tests will be in the

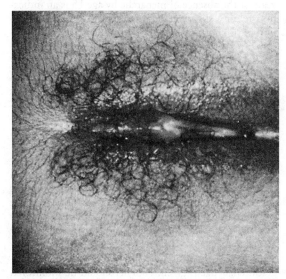

Figure 31–26. Premature pubarche in a child 4 years of age.

normal pubertal range. In addition, these patients will require diagnostic imaging to document skeletal age and the absence of gonadal or CNS lesions.

Treatment of GnRH-Dependent Precocious Puberty

The treatment of choice for GnRH-dependent precocious puberty is with GnRH analogs (GnRHa). Analogs of GnRH are modifications of the native hormone, which have greater resistance to degradation and increased affinity for the pituitary GnRH receptors. They induce downregulation of receptor function, resulting in temporary, reversible inhibition of the hypothalamic-pituitary-ovarian (H-P-O) axis, as reflected by minimal or no response to GnRH stimulation, and regression of the manifestations of puberty.

Treatment with GnRHa decreases gonadotropins and sex steroids to prepubertal levels, which is followed by regression of secondary sexual features. Treatment also causes a deceleration in the skeletal maturation rate, preserving or even improving predicted height, unless bone age is so advanced that further growth is precluded. Treatment is continued until puberty is appropriate based on age, emotional maturity, height, and height potential. Resumption of puberty occurs promptly after discontinuation of GnRHa therapy.

DELAYED SEXUAL MATURATION

Delayed sexual development has been defined as the absence of normal pubertal events at an age 2.5 SD later than the mean. The absence of thelarche by age 13 years or the absence of menarche by age 15 is an indication for investigation. Some degree of sexual maturation occurs in over 30% of patients with gonadal dysgenesis; therefore, a patient who presents following thelarche with a delay in the orderly progression of pubertal development should also undergo investigation. Delayed sexual development may be classified according to gonadal function (Table 31–4).

1. Delayed Menarche with Adequate Secondary Sexual Development

Patients with functioning gonads and delayed sexual maturation usually consult a physician in their midteens because of amenorrhea. Most have well-formed female configuration with adequately developed breasts. Many of these patients suffer from an inappropriate H-P-O feedback mechanism leading to anovulation and androgen excess. Primary amenorrhea may persist until a progestin challenge is given. Patients should be monitored for continued menstrual shedding. Persistent amenorrhea is treated with progestins administered every other

Table 31–4. Classification of patients with delayed sexual maturation.

Delayed Menarche with Adequate Secondary Sexual Development
Anatomic genital abnormalities
Inappropriate positive feedback
Androgen insensitivity syndromes (complete forms)
Delayed Puberty with Inadequate or Absent Secondary Sexual Development
Hypothalamic-pituitary dysfunction (low FSH)
Reversible: Constitutional delay, weight loss due to extreme dieting, protein deficiency, fat loss without muscle loss, drug abuse
Irreversible: Kallmann's syndrome, pituitary destruction
Gonadal failure (high FSH)
Abnormal chromosomal complement (eg, Turner's syndrome)
Normal chromosomal complement: chemotherapy, irradiation, infection, infiltrative or autoimmune disease, resistant ovary syndrome
Delayed Puberty with Heterosexual Secondary Sexual Development (Virilization)
Enzyme deficiency (eg, 21α-hydroxylase deficiency), neoplasm, male pseudohermaphroditism

month to prevent endometrial hyperplasia. A sexually active girl should be given oral contraceptives rather than cyclic progestins. Further evaluation is required in patients with persistent menstrual abnormalities, since similar clinical manifestations are also encountered in adolescents with adult-onset congenital adrenal hyperplasia and those with polycystic ovarian disease.

Most patients with congenital anomalies of the paramesonephric (müllerian) structures present with complaints of primary amenorrhea. The most common defect is congenital absence of the uterus and vagina; other causes are imperforate hymen, transverse vaginal septa, and agenesis of the cervix. Gynecologic examination supplemented by ultrasonography establishes the diagnosis of these congenital anomalies.

The complete forms of androgen insensitivity (Fig 31–27) are also associated with amenorrhea and normal breast development. Affected persons have normal testicular function but are not responsive to male concentrations of testosterone, and the development of breasts is secondary to the small amounts of unopposed estrogens produced by the testis. Pubic and axillary hair is scant or often absent. A short blind vaginal pouch is present. Once pubertal development has been completed, surgical extirpation of the gonads and reconstruction of the vagina are necessary.

The possibility of pregnancy in an adolescent who has not begun to menstruate is highly unlikely, but

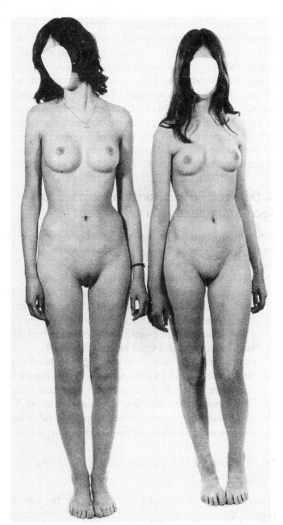

Figure 31–27. XY sisters with androgen insensitivity syndrome. (Courtesy of CJ Dewhurst.)

must be borne in mind when considering causes of delayed menarche in patients with normal pubertal development.

2. Delayed Puberty with Inadequate or Absent Secondary Sexual Development

Hypothalamic-Pituitary Dysfunction

Both reversible and irreversible causes of delayed puberty secondary to lack of maturation or function of the hypothalamus and pituitary have been described.

The onset of puberty depends on an ill-defined stage of maturity that is reflected in skeletal age. Maturation is partly genetically determined but also depends on multiple environmental factors; thus the chronologic age of puberty varies considerably. Statistical limits of normal variation in a defined population group indicate that by definition, 2.5% of all normal adolescents will develop later than the age defined as "normal." This group has been labeled "late bloomers," or having a constitutional delay in the maturation process. Although these patients are normal, absence of signs of puberty (including the growth spurt) often concerns the patient when her adolescent friends have developed secondary sexual features and gained the characteristic increase in height.

The diagnosis of hypothalamic-pituitary dysfunction is made by exclusion of other causes of delayed sexual maturation. The GnRH challenge test differentiates constitutional delay from similar conditions associated with a deficiency of GnRH. Reassurance is the only treatment necessary, but the patient must be kept under observation until regular menstrual cycles are established. Occasionally, an adolescent requires hormonal replacement therapy because of emotional distress over her condition.

Isolated deficiency of GnRH, often associated with intracranial anomalies and anosmia (**Kallmann's syndrome**), is uncommon. These patients fail to develop secondary sexual features, and blood levels of gonadotropins are very low. Following GnRH challenge, a rise in gonadotropin levels is noted. Estrogen replacement therapy is used to initiate and sustain sexual development. Induction of ovulation with human menopausal gonadotropins or GnRH is necessary when pregnancy is desired.

A pituitary or parasellar tumor, particularly craniopharyngioma or pituitary adenoma, must be considered in the evaluation of a patient with delayed sexual maturation. Craniopharyngiomas are rapidly growing tumors that often develop in late childhood. Pituitary adenomas are slow-growing, may become symptomatic during puberty, and may interfere with sexual maturation. An occult pituitary prolactinoma in adolescents with unexplained delayed sexual maturation must also be ruled out. Serum prolactin levels should be measured yearly in patients with unexplained delayed sexual maturation.

Weight loss due to extreme dieting, marked protein deficiency, and fat loss without notable loss of muscle (often seen in athletes) may also delay or suppress hypothalamic pituitary maturation. Heroin addiction may cause amenorrhea, but its effects on sexual maturation have not been documented.

Gonadal Failure

Most patients with gonadal dysgenesis present during adolescence with delayed puberty and primary amenorrhea. If untreated, estrogen and androgen levels are decreased and FSH and LH levels are increased. Estrogen-dependent organs show the predictable effects of hormonal deficiency. Breasts contain little parenchymal tissue, and the areolar tissue is only slightly darker than the surrounding skin; the well-differentiated external genitalia, vagina, and müllerian derivatives remain small. Pubic and axillary hair fail to develop in normal quantity.

However, normal pubertal development, menstruation, and even pregnancies have been reported in adults with gonadal dysgenesis. It is possible that a few of these persons maintain some germ cells into adulthood. Spontaneous development is more commonly observed in patients with mosaicism with a 46,XX line. The rare offspring of these women probably do not have an increased risk for chromosomal abnormalities.

Some patients may have ovarian failure even though they have a normal chromosome complement and two intact sex chromosomes (46,XX). An autosomal recessive form of ovarian failure has been demonstrated in some families. Other causes of follicular depletion include chemotherapy, irradiation, infections (eg, mumps), infiltrative disease processes of the ovary (eg, tuberculosis), autoimmune diseases, and unknown environmental agents.

A karyotype is necessary to rule out the presence of Y chromosome material. DNA probes and assays for the minor histocompatibility antigen, H-Y, have also been used to identify Y chromosome material. A high incidence of neoplastic changes in the gonadal ridge has been reported in the presence of a Y chromosome; thus, prophylactic gonadectomy is recommended (Fig 31–28). Replacement hormonal therapy is then given in a cyclic manner.

The resistant ovary syndrome is characterized by delayed menarche or primary amenorrhea, a 46,XX chromosome complement, high FSH levels, and ovaries

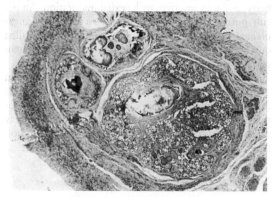

Figure 31–28. Gonadoblastoma developing in a gonadal ridge in a patient with gonadal dysgenesis and 45,XO/46,XY karyotype.

with apparently normal follicular apparatus that do not respond to endogenous gonadotropins. It is assumed that absence of follicular receptors for gonadotropins is responsible for ovarian dysfunction in these patients. These individuals may have normally developed secondary sexual characteristics. Estrogen replacement therapy is required to prevent long-term complications of estrogen deficiency (eg, vaginal dryness, osteoporosis). Pregnancies have been reported in some patients treated with menotropins or following discontinuation of estrogen therapy.

3. Delayed Puberty with Heterosexual Secondary Sexual Development

Virilization refers to the concomitant presentation of hirsutism with various signs of androgen excess, including acne, frontotemporal balding, deepening of the voice, decrease in breast size, clitoral hypertrophy, increase in muscle mass, and amenorrhea. Virilization at puberty is the result of elevated androgens from adrenal or gonadal sources. These may be the result of an enzyme deficiency (eg, late-onset congenital adrenal hyperplasia) or a neoplasm (eg, Leydig cell tumor).

A small group of patients are male pseudohermaphrodites. These are adolescents who are being reared as girls and have female external genitalia, intraabdominal or ectopic malfunctioning testes, and a normal 46,XY chromosomal complement. The diagnosis and treatment of intersex disorders are discussed in Chapter 5.

Evaluation of the Patient with Delayed Sexual Development

Determination of gonadal function can be accomplished by obtaining a medical history and performing a detailed physical examination, supplemented by selected laboratory studies. Historical information should center around previous growth and pubertal development. Linear and velocity growth charts as well as a pubertal development chart clarify previous growth patterns and are useful in subsequent follow-up. Knowledge of previous medical disorders may immediately identify the cause of aberrant puberty.

Physical examination must include height and weight assessments and a careful search for somatic anomalies. Staging of pubertal development by Tanner criteria is most important in the determination of gonadal function. Presence of breast development signifies prior gonadal function. A vaginal smear for cytohormonal evaluation can determine whether the gonad is continuing to produce estrogen. Pelvic and rectal examination will identify patients with an obstructed outflow tract, as well as patients with congenital absence of the vagina and uterus. Further confirmation of patients with Rokitansky sequence is dependent on a karyotype to identify normal 46,XX complement and a pelvic sonogram to confirm uterine absence and ovarian presence.

Absence of pubic hair is suggestive of the androgen insensitivity syndrome. Karyotype will identify the 46,XY cell line in patients with testicular feminization syndrome (Fig. 31–27). Patients with complete pubertal development, evidence of continued estrogen production, and normal müllerian systems probably have inappropriate positive feedback and thus chronic anovulation. Progesterone challenge in such patients is helpful. A withdrawal bleed signifies a normal müllerian system and continued estrogen production.

When breast development is minimal, the usual diagnosis is lack of gonadal function. Serum gonadotropin assays are performed for further elucidation. Elevated FSH levels suggest gonadal failure. Other endocrine profiles should be obtained if hypothyroidism, congenital adrenal hyperplasia, or Cushing's syndrome is suspected. Karyotype is necessary in all patients with gonadal failure and will identify both normal and abnormal chromosome complements. The presence of a Y chromosome in either group dictates gonadal removal.

Low FSH levels suggest an interference with hypothalamic-pituitary maturation and gonadotropin release. Skull films and prolactin assays must be obtained for all patients to rule out the presence of pituitary or hypothalamic tumors. Appropriate endocrine evaluation identifies the occasional patient with hypothyroidism or congenital adrenal hyperplasia and the rare patient with Cushing's syndrome. Diagnosis of Kallmann's syndrome is suspected in hypogonadotrophic patients who have an associated anosmia, and it is confirmed when GnRH challenge tests are performed. The presumed diagnosis of constitutional delay is made by exclusion of all other causes and by the typical GnRH release patterns after GnRH challenge.

Evaluation of the Patient with Vaginal Bleeding

A. VAGINAL BLEEDING IN CHILDREN

When vaginal bleeding occurs in children, two sources generally should be suspected: (1) the endometrium (bleeding is usually a manifestation of precocious puberty) and (2) a local vulvar or vaginal lesion (eg, vulvovaginitis, foreign bodies, urethral prolapse, trauma, botryoid sarcoma, adenocarcinoma of the cervix or vagina, and vulvar skin disorders).

Vaginal bleeding during childhood should always alert the physician to the possibility of a genital tumor. Vaginoscopy and examination under anesthesia are the mainstays of evaluation to exclude the presence of tumors, foreign bodies, and other local lesions. Benign tumors of the vulva and vagina are rare in childhood, and

those that do occur seldom cause bleeding. Malignant neoplasms usually bleed from necrotic or ulcerative areas that appear early in their development. Suspicious lesions require biopsy for diagnosis.

B. BLEEDING DISORDERS IN ADOLESCENTS

One of the most common gynecologic complaints of adolescents is a problem with the menstrual period. In most cases, there is no true medical disorder, especially in the first 2 years after menarche, when 50–80% of periods are anovulatory. Evaluation of abnormal bleeding is indicated if the menstrual interval is less than 22 days or more than 44 days, lasts longer than 1 week, menses is so heavy that anemia develops, or if the cycle interval is still unstable 2 years after menarche. Dysfunctional uterine bleeding accounts for 95% of abnormal vaginal bleeding in teenagers. Screening for inherited coagulation disorders, such as von Willebrand's disease, may be indicated, as 18% of adolescents hospitalized for menorrhagia have an underlying bleeding disorder. When menstrual irregularity is accompanied by such symptoms as acne, hirsutism, and obesity, polycystic ovarian syndrome should be suspected, and treatment may need to address some of these symptoms as well.

Pregnancy should always be considered in a young woman with abnormal bleeding or amenorrhea until proven otherwise. Nonmenstrual causes of bleeding such as hypothyroidism, cervicitis, condylomas, polyps, cervical cancer, estrogen-producing ovarian tumors, and vaginitis also may be considered.

The management of anovulatory bleeding is directed toward controlling symptoms and preventing anemia. Oral contraceptive pill tapers, cyclic oral contraceptives, and medroxyprogesterone acetate have been used to control bleeding. In severe cases hospitalization and intravenous conjugated equine estrogen in doses of 25 mg every 4–6 hours until bleeding stops for 24 hours have been used successfully. If oral contraceptives are given for secondary amenorrhea, they should be continued for at least 9–12 months before attempting to stop. If menses do not resume within 8 weeks, oral contraceptive pills should be resumed for another 9–12 months.

■ SEXUALITY AND PREGNANCY IN CHILDREN AND ADOLESCENTS

PRECOCIOUS (JUVENILE) PREGNANCY

Precocious, or juvenile, pregnancy is rare. The youngest known patient was a Peruvian girl aged 5 years, 8 months, who was delivered at term by cesarean section in 1939 of a healthy male infant weighing 2950 g (6 lb, 8 oz). Both mother and infant survived. In every reported instance, the underage mothers were sexually precocious, most having menstruated for several years before becoming pregnant. Juvenile pregnancy per se does not increase the chance of congenital anomalies in the offspring, but in many cases the mother is a victim of sexual abuse, and if the pregnancy is the result of incest, there is a greater likelihood of genetic malformations carried by recessive genes.

Most precocious mothers and their babies have not done well; there is an increased incidence of spontaneous abortion, pregnancy-induced hypertension, and premature labor and delivery. In patients under 9 years of age, less than 50% have normal labor, and there is a 35% likelihood of neonatal loss.

The underage mother and her family may need psychiatric counseling, both during pregnancy and following delivery. Lessening the emotional, social, and medical trauma associated with such a gestation is an important task for all who assist in the care of the pregnant child.

SEXUALLY TRANSMITTED DISEASES

Sexually transmitted diseases (STDs) are the most common infectious diseases of adolescents today. Approximately 25% of all sexually active adolescents aged 13–19 years become infected each year. By age 15, one in four girls in the United States has sexual relations. The younger the age of first intercourse, the higher the risk for STDs. Chlamydia is the most prevalent of the bacterial STDs, with almost 30% of inner city female adolescents aged 12–19 showing positive cultures in a longitudinal 2-year study of family planning, school-based, and STD clinics. Sequelae of chlamydial infections include pelvic inflammatory disease (PID), ectopic pregnancy, and infertility. This age group accounts for 8% of cases of HIV in females, with the majority of these women asymptomatic at the time of positive testing. In the U.S., 15- to 24-year-olds accounted for about 60% of gonorrhea cases, 25% of syphilis cases, and 17% of hepatitis B cases in 1996. By the time they reach college age, 43% of women are infected with human papillomavirus (HPV).

Nearly 70% of patients with PID are younger than 25 years. The estimated incidence of PID in sexually active females is about 1 in 8 for 15-year-olds, and 1 in 10 for 16-year-olds. PID in adolescents should be treated with hospitalization and intravenous antibiotics. Tubo-ovarian abscess (TOA) has been found in 2–4% of adolescents with adnexal masses. Treatment includes broad-spectrum antibiotics and possible surgical drainage. Patients who have had PID or TOA are at high risk for pelvic pain, pelvic adhesive disease, infertility, and ectopic pregnancy.

CERVICAL CANCER SCREENING IN ADOLESCENTS

Because infection with certain strains of HPV is the most important risk factor for the development of cervical cancer, and HPV infection in women is usually acquired via heterosexual transmission, cervical cancer screening with a Papanicolaou (Pap) test should be initiated soon after the onset of sexual activity. Pap smear screening is underutilized in sexually active adolescents. While measures including teen clinics have increased the rate of surveillance, efforts at both prevention by encouraging condom use and increased availability of services are still needed.

If a Pap smear is abnormal, colposcopic evaluation may be indicated. STD screening should also be incorporated as part of the evaluation. Low-grade lesions can usually be followed with serial Pap smears. Ablative or excisional procedures are indicated for moderate- to high-grade lesions, regardless of age. Cryotherapy offers a 92–95% cure rate for CIN 2–3 in young women. Loop electrosurgical excisional procedure (LEEP) offers similar cure rates, and does not appear to impact cervical competence in future pregnancies with depths of excision of 1.5 cm or less. Teens with abnormal Pap smears should be advised regarding smoking cessation and follow-up.

CONTRACEPTION IN ADOLESCENTS

More than 95% of adolescent pregnancies are unintended. By age 18, one in four experiences a pregnancy. Half of adolescent pregnancies occur in the first 6 months after initiation of sexual activity. Despite a decline in teenage pregnancy rates during the 1990s, teenage pregnancy rates remain higher in the United States than in other Western countries. In addition, teenagers in this country use contraceptives less frequently and use less effective methods of contraception than their European counterparts. While great inroads in adolescent access to healthcare have been made over the last decade, problems of cost and fears of lack of confidentiality still appear to inhibit young women from obtaining contraceptives, ultimately resulting in high teenage pregnancy rates.

Contraception is the voluntary prevention of impregnation. As such, postponing sexual activity is an appropriate option to suggest. If this is not realistic, counseling regarding various methods of contraception requires consideration of not only the side effects and efficacy of the various methods, but must also take into account the personal requirements of each teenager. For example, a teenager who has difficulty remembering to take pills or who has to hide pill packs may be better served by medroxyprogesterone acetate injections. Health benefits of adolescents taking oral contraceptive pills include decreased menstrual pain; increased menstrual regularity; decreased risk of pelvic inflammatory disease, anemia, and fibrocystic breast disease; improved long-term fertility; and treatment of acne and hirsutism. The importance of both contraception and STD prevention should be reviewed, and the use of barrier methods should therefore also be encouraged. Adolescents with chronic medical illnesses represent an especially high-risk group, as issues of both fertility and contraceptive risks and efficacy may be affected by these illnesses.

Emergency contraception regimens with progestin-only regimens or combined estrogens and progestins are highly effective means of preventing pregnancy after intercourse if taken at the appropriate interval. Improving access through education or prescribing pills in advance or over the telephone may give a young woman a second chance at avoiding unintended pregnancy.

PREGNANCY TERMINATION

The rate of teenage abortion remains higher in the United States than in other Western countries for which data are available. The Supreme Court initially ruled in favor of a minor's right to have an abortion in 1976. While this ruling has been amended to allow states to require parental notification before abortion, a system of judicial bypass for minors who do not want parental involvement is required in these states.

ADOLESCENT PREGNANCY

For years it has been accepted that adolescent pregnancy is a high-risk pregnancy. Many pregnant adolescents come from low socioeconomic backgrounds, having poor education and perhaps poor general health due to inadequate nutrition, cigarette smoking, drug abuse, or STDs. Nutrition is an important problem. Bone mineral content, iron stores, and caloric intake are often reduced among adolescent girls, and iron deficiency anemia is frequently found. Proper education and dietary counseling may improve nutritional status and prevent anemia.

Optimal care should be given to teenage mothers not only to improve the pregnancy outcome but also to enhance their social, educational, and emotional adjustment. Complications of labor and delivery are highly dependent on the quality of prenatal care. Preeclampsia-eclampsia, which is more common in a first pregnancy, occurs more frequently among adolescents than among adult women. Prematurity and small-for-dates infants are a major problem in adolescent pregnancies. Predisposing factors are high-risk factors such as low prepregnancy weight, poor weight gain, adverse socioeconomic conditions, cigarette smoking, anemia, first

pregnancy, and deficient prenatal care, all of which occur more commonly in adolescents. To minimize prenatal complications and improve maternal and fetal outcome, the young patient should be enrolled in an aggressive prenatal care program that addresses the unique problems of the adolescent patient.

REFERENCES

Acquavella AP, Braverman P: Adolescent gynecology in the office setting. Pediatr Clin North Am 1999;46:489.

Arbel-DeRowe Y et al: The contribution of pelvic ultrasonography to the diagnostic process in pediatric and adolescent gynecology. J Pediatr Adolesc Gynecol 1997;10:3.

Bamberger J et al: HIV postexposure prophylaxis following sexual assault. Am J Med 1999;106:323.

Bays J, Chadwick D: Medical diagnosis of the sexually abused child. Child Abuse Negl 1993;17:91.

Bechtel K, Podrazik M: Evaluation of the adolescent rape victim. Pediatr Clin North Am 1999;46:809.

Bravender T, Emans SJ: Menstrual disorders. Pediatr Clin North Am 1999;46:545.

Cothran MM, White JP: Adolescent behavior and sexually transmitted diseases: The dilemma of human papillomavirus. Health Care Women Int 2002;3:306.

Craighill MC: Pediatric and adolescent gynecology for the primary care physician. Pediatr Clin North Am 1998;45:1659.

Cutler GB Jr, Laue L: Congenital adrenal hyperplasia due to 21-hydroxylase deficiency. N Engl J Med 1990;323:1806.

Edmonds DK: Congenital malformations in the genital tract. Obstet Gynecol Clin North Am 2000;27:49.

Elster AB, Kuznets NJ: AMA Guidelines for Adolescent Preventative Services (GAPS): recommendations and rationale, 1994:93.

English A: Reproductive health services for adolescents. Obstet Gynecol Clin North Am 2000;27:195-211.

Frank R: Formation of artificial vagina without operation. Am J Obstet Gynecol 1938;35:1053.

Gellert GA et al: Situational and sociodemographic characteristics of children infected with human immunodeficiency virus from pediatric sexual abuse. Pediatrics 1993;91:39.

Gevelber MA, Biro FM: Adolescents and sexually transmitted diseases. Pediatr Clin North Am 1999;46:747.

Gold MA: Prescribing and managing oral contraceptive pills and emergency contraception for adolescents. Pediatr Clin North Am 1999;46:695.

Gordon CM: Menstrual disorders in adolescents. Pediatr Clin North Am 1999;46:519.

Griffin JE et al: Congenital absence of the vagina: The Mayer-Rokitansky-Kuster-Hauser syndrome. Ann Intern Med 1976;85:224.

Hampton HL: Examination of the adolescent patient. Obstet Gynecol Clin North Am 2000;27:1.

Harel Z, Cromer B: The use of long-acting contraceptives in adolescents. Pediatr Clin North Am 1999;46:719.

Heller ME, Dewhurst J, Grant DB: Premature menarche without other evidence of precocious puberty. Arch Dis Child 1979;54:472.

Hewitt G, Cromer B: Update on adolescent contraception. Obstet Gynecol Clin North Am 2000;27:143.

Imperato-McGinley J et al: The diagnosis of 5 alpha-reductase deficiency in infancy. J Clin Endocrinol Metab 1986;63:1313.

Ingram JM: The bicycle seat stool in the treatment of vaginal agenesis and stenosis: A preliminary report. Am J Obstet Gynecol 1981;140:867.

Kahn JA et al: Intention to return for Papanicolaou smears in adolescent girls and young women. Pediatrics 2001;108:333.

Lavery JP et al: Pregnancy outcome in a comprehensive teenage parent program. Adolesc Pediatr Gynecol 1988;1:34.

Lawson MA, Blythe MJ: Pelvic inflammatory disease in adolescents. Pediatr Clin North Am 1999;46:767.

Marshall WA, Tanner JM: Variation in the pattern of pubertal changes in girls. Arch Dis Child 1969;44:291.

McCann J, Voris J: Perianal injuries resulting from sexual abuse: A longitudinal study. Pediatrics 1993;91:390.

McCann J, Voris J, Simon M: Genital injuries resulting from sexual abuse: A longitudinal study. Pediatrics 1992;89:307.

McCann J et al: Comparison of genital examination techniques in prepubertal girls. Pediatrics 1990;85:182.

McCann J et al: Perianal findings in prepubertal children selected for nonabuse: A descriptive study. Child Abuse Negl 1989;13:179.

McCann J et al: Genital findings in prepubertal girls selected for nonabuse: A descriptive study. Pediatrics 1990;86:428.

McDonough PG, Tho PT: The spectrum of 45,X/46,XY gonadal dysgenesis and its implications (a study of 19 patients). Pediatr Adolesc Gynecol 1983;1:1.

Meneses MF, Ostrowski ML: Female splenic-gonadal fusion of the discontinuous type. Hum Pathol 1989;20:486.

Minjarez DA, Bradshaw KD: Abnormal uterine bleeding in adolescents. Obstet Gynecol Clin 2000;27:63.

Moscicki A: Human papillomavirus infection in adolescents. Pediatr Clin North Am 1999;46:783.

Muram D, Dewhurst J: The inheritance of intersexuality. Can Med Assoc J 1984;130:121.

Muram D, Elias S: The treatment of labial adhesions in prepubertal girls. Surg Forum 1988;34:464.

Muram D et al: Ovarian cancer in children and adolescents. Adolesc Pediatr Gynecol 1992;5:21.

Muram D, Grant DB, Dewhurst J: Precocious puberty: A follow-up study. Arch Dis Child 1984;59:77.

Muram D, Rau F: Anatomic variations of the bulbocavernosus muscle. Adolesc Pediatr Gynecol 1991;4:85.

Muram D: Child sexual abuse: Correlation between genital findings and sexual acts. Child Abuse Negl 1989;13:211.

Muram D: Genital tract trauma in pre-pubertal children. Pediatr Ann 1986;15:616.

Neinstein LS: Breast disease in adolescents and young women. Pediatr Clin North Am 1999;46:607.

Nyirjesy P: Vaginitis in the adolescent patient. Pediatr Clin North Am 1999;46:733.

Owens K, Honebrink A: Gynecological care of the medically complicated adolescents. Pediatr Clin North Am 1999;46:631.

Paek SC, Merritt DF, Mallory SB: Pruritus vulvae in prepubertal children. J Am Acad Dermatol 2001;44:795.

Persaud D et al: Delayed recognition of human immunodeficiency virus infection in preadolescent children. Pediatrics 1992;90:688.

Pfeifer SM, Gosman GG: Evaluation of adnexal masses in adolescents: Pediatr Clin North Am 1999;46:573.

Pinsky L, Kaufman M: Genetics of steroid receptors and their disorders. Adv Hum Genet 1987;16:299.

Pinsky L, Kaufman M, Levitsky LL: Partial androgen resistance due to a distinctive qualitative defect of the androgen receptor. Am J Med Genet 1987;27:459.

Pletcher JR, Slap GB: Menstrual disorders. Pediatr Clin North Am 1999;46:505.

Plouffe L: Disorders of excessive hair growth in the adolescent. Obstet Gynecol Clin 2000;27:79.

Pokorny S: Anatomic detail of the prepubertal hymen. Am J Obstet Gynecol 1987;157:950.

Quint EH, Smith YR: Vulvar disorders in adolescent patients. Pediatr Clin North Am 1999;46:593.

Reider J, Coupey SM: The use of nonhormonal methods of contraception in adolescents. Pediatr Clin North Am 1999;46:671.

Reindollar RH, Tho SPT, McFonough PG: Abnormalities of sexual differentiation. Clin Obstet Gynecol 1987;30:697.

Rock JA, Azziz R: Genital anomalies in childhood. Clin Obstet Gynecol 1987;30:682.

Russo JF: Pediatric and adolescent gynecology. Curr Opin Obstet Gynecol 2001;13:449.

Schroeder B: Vulvar disorders in adolescents. Obstet Gynecol Clin North Am 2000;27:35.

Shulman L et al: Marker chromosomes in gonadal dysgenesis: Avoiding unnecessary surgery. Adolesc Pediatr Gynecol 1992;5:39.

Siegel SF et al: Assessment of clinical hyperandrogenism in adolescent girls. Adolesc Pediatr Gynecol 1992;5:13.

Siegel SF et al: Premature pubarche: Etiological heterogeneity. J Clin Endocrinol Metab 1992;74:239.

Templeman C, Hertweck SP: Breast disorders in the pediatric and adolescent patient. Obstet Gynecol Clin North Am 2000;27:19.

Ulloa-Aguirre A et al: Incomplete regression of müllerian ducts in androgen insensitivity syndrome. Fertil Steril 1990;53:1024.

Verp MS, Simpson JL: Abnormal sexual differentiation and neoplasia. Cancer Genet Cytogenet 1987;25:191.

Vermillion ST, Holmes MM, Soper DE: Adolescents and sexually transmitted diseases. Obstet Gynecol Clin 2000;27:163.

Winer-Muram HT et al: The sonographic features of the peripubertal ovaries. Adolesc Pediatr Gynecol 1989;2:158.

Complications of Menstruation; Abnormal Uterine Bleeding

32

Taaly Silberstein, MD

COMPLICATIONS OF MENSTRUATION

PREMENSTRUAL SYNDROME

ESSENTIALS OF DIAGNOSIS

- *Symptoms include edema, weight gain, restlessness, irritability, and increased tension.*
- *Symptoms must occur in the second half of the menstrual cycle.*
- *There must be a symptom-free period of at least 7 days in the first half of the cycle.*
- *Symptoms must occur in at least 2 consecutive cycles.*
- *Symptoms must be severe enough to require medical advice or treatment.*

General Considerations

Premenstrual syndrome (PMS) is a psychoneuroendocrine disorder with biologic, psychologic, and social parameters. It is both difficult to define adequately and quite controversial. Indeed, one major difficulty in detailing whether PMS is a disease or a description of physiologic changes is its extraordinary prevalence. Up to 75% of women experience some recurrent PMS symptoms; 20–40% are mentally or physically incapacitated to some degree, and 5% experience severe distress. The highest incidence is in women in their late 20s to early 30s. PMS is rarely encountered in adolescents.

The symptoms of PMS may include headache, breast tenderness, pelvic pain, bloating, and premenstrual tension. More severe symptoms include irritability, dysphoria, and mood lability. When these symptoms disrupt daily functioning, they are clustered under the name premenstrual dysphoric disorder (PMDD).

Other symptoms commonly included in PMS are abdominal discomfort, clumsiness, lack of energy, sleep changes, and mood swings. Behavioral changes include social withdrawal, altered daily activities, marked change in appetite, increased crying, and changes in sexual desire. In all, more than 150 symptoms have been related to PMS. Thus the symptom complex of PMS has not been clearly defined.

The potential relationship between PMS and antisocial behavior has resulted in successful courtroom defenses of female offenders in England. U.S. courts have not been as accepting of PMS as a defense, but legal argument was incorporated into statute with the Insanity Defense Reform Act of 1985 [18 U.S.C.A. 20 (Supp. 1985)], which provides that PMS may be argued as a mitigating factor in criminal behavior if it is connected with a psychosis. Arguments for and against such defenses have been the subject of a number of publications. Although such controversy is interesting, discussion of it exceeds the scope of this text.

Pathogenesis

The etiology of the symptom complex of PMS is not known, although several theories have been proposed, including estrogen-progesterone imbalance, excess aldosterone, hypoglycemia, hyperprolactinemia, and psychogenic factors. Previously, it was thought that a hormonal imbalance was related to the clinical manifestations of PMS/PMDD, but the most recent consensus is that physiologic ovarian function is the trigger. This is supported by the efficacy of ovarian cyclicity suppression, either medically or surgically, in eliminating premenstrual complaints.

Further research has shown that serotonin (5-HT), a neurotransmitter, is important in the pathogenesis of PMS/PMDD. Both estrogen and progesterone have been shown to influence the activity of serotonin centrally. Many of the symptoms of other mood disorders resembling the features of PMS/PMDD have been associated with serotonergic dysfunction.

Diagnosis

There are no objective screening or diagnostic tests for PMS and PMDD; thus special attention must be paid to the patient's medical history. Because the symptoms of certain medical conditions (such as thyroid disease and anemia) can mimic those of PMS/PMDD, they must be ruled out.

The patient is instructed to chart her symptoms for at least 2 symptomatic cycles. The classic criteria for PMS require that the patient have symptoms in the luteal phase and a symptom-free period of at least 7 days in the first half of the cycle for a minimum of 2 consecutive symptomatic cycles. To meet the criteria for PMDD, in addition to the above, she must have a chief complaint of at least one of the following: irritability, tension, dysphoria, or mood lability; and 5 out of 11 of the following: depressed mood, anxiety, affective lability, irritability, decreased interest in daily activities, concentration difficulties, lack of energy, change in appetite or food cravings, sleep disturbances, feeling overwhelmed, or physical symptoms (eg, breast tenderness, bloating).

Clinical Findings

A careful history and physical examination are most important to exclude organic causes of PMS localized to the reproductive, urinary, or gastrointestinal tracts. Most patients readily describe their symptoms, but careful questioning may be needed with some patients who may be reluctant to do so. Although it is important not to lead a patient to exaggerate her concerns, it is equally important not to minimize them.

Symptoms of PMS may be specific, well-localized, and recurrent. They may be exacerbated by emotional stress. Migraine-like headaches may also occur, often preceded by visual scotomas and vomiting. Symptomatology varies from patient to patient but is often consistent in the same patient.

A psychiatric history should be obtained, with special attention paid to a personal history of psychiatric problems or a family history of affective disorders. A mental status evaluation of affect, thinking, and behavior should be performed and recorded. A prospective diary correlating symptoms, daily activities, and menstrual flow can be very useful to document changes and to encourage patient participation in her care.

If underlying psychiatric illness is suspected, a psychiatric evaluation is indicated. The most common associated psychiatric illness is depression, which generally responds to antidepressant drugs and psychotherapy. It should also be recalled that psychiatric illnesses have premenstrual exacerbations, and medications should be altered accordingly.

Treatment

Treatment of PMS/PMDD depends on the severity of the symptoms. For some women, changes in eating habits—limiting caffeine, alcohol, tobacco, and chocolate intake, and eating small, frequent meals high in complex carbohydrates—may be sufficient. Decreasing sodium intake may alleviate edema. Stress management, cognitive behavioral therapy, and exercise have all been shown to improve symptoms.

Low-risk pharmacologic interventions that may be effective include calcium carbonate (1000–1200 mg daily) for bloating, food cravings, and pain; magnesium (200–360 mg daily) for water retention; vitamins B_6 and E; nonsteroidal anti-inflammatory drugs (NSAIDs); spironolactone for cyclic edema; and bromocriptine for mastalgia.

For symptoms of severe PMS and PMDD, further pharmacologic intervention may be necessary. Psychotropic medications that are effective include selective serotonin reuptake inhibitors (SSRIs), desipramine, and L-tryptophan. SSRIs have minimal side effects, and provide symptom improvement in more than 60% of patients studied. Treatment should be given 14 days prior to the onset of menstruation and continued through the end of the cycle. Anxiolytics such as alprazolam and buspirone have also been shown to be efficacious, but their side effects and potential for dependence must be seriously considered.

Hormonal interventions have also been shown to be effective. Use of gonadotropin-releasing hormone (GnRH) agonists leads to a temporary "medical menopause" and an improvement in symptoms. Their limitations lie in a hypoestrogenic state and a risk for osteoporosis, though "add-back" therapy with estrogen and progesterone may obviate these problems. Danazol may improve mastalgia. Finally, bilateral oophorectomy is a definitive surgical treatment option; again, estrogen replacement would be recommended.

Use of oral contraceptives has been suggested because they suppress ovulation. Studies, however, have found little difference between women taking a low-dose birth control pill and non-pill-takers, and currently oral contraceptives are not recommended for the treatment of PMS/PMDD.

MASTODYNIA

Pain, and usually swelling, of the breasts caused by edema and engorgement of the vascular and ductal systems is termed mastodynia, or mastalgia. Mastodynia specifically refers to a cyclical occurrence of severe breast pain, usually in the luteal phase of the menstrual cycle. Common in women with PMS/PMDD, it may be the primary symptom of this syndrome in some. It has been shown to be related to high gonadotropin levels. An augmented response to prolactin has also been suggested. Examination is always necessary to rule out neoplasm, although most malignant tumors are painless. In postpartum patients, mastitis must be considered.

The presence of solitary or multiple cystic areas suggests fibrocystic change. The diagnosis can usually be confirmed by aspiration, but excisional biopsy is occasionally necessary. Serial mammograms or ultrasound examinations can be used to help monitor these patients. (See also Chapter 62.)

Treatment

Management of painful breasts due to fibrocystic changes consists of support of the breasts, avoidance of methylxanthenes (coffee, tea, chocolate, cola drinks), and occasional use of a mild diuretic. Patients with mastodynia have had improvement with danazol, bromocriptine, oral contraceptives, and vitamins, though with limited success. In one study, lisuride maleate, a dopamine agonist, was associated with a significant decrease in pain.

DYSMENORRHEA

Dysmenorrhea, or painful menstruation, is the most common complaint of gynecologic patients. Many women experience mild discomfort during menstruation, but the term "dysmenorrhea" is reserved for those women whose pain prevents normal activity and requires medication, whether over-the-counter or by prescription.

There are 3 types of dysmenorrhea: (1) primary (no organic cause), (2) secondary (pathologic cause), and (3) membranous (cast of endometrial cavity shed as a single entity). This discussion will focus mainly on primary dysmenorrhea. Secondary dysmenorrhea is discussed elsewhere in this book in association with specific diseases and disorders (eg, endometriosis, adenomyosis, pelvic inflammatory disease [particularly in patients with residua of pelvic infection], cervical stenosis, fibroid polyps, and possibly, uterine displacement with fixation).

Membranous dysmenorrhea is rare; it causes intense cramping pain due to passage of a cast of the endometrium through an undilated cervix. Another cause of dysmenorrhea that should be considered is cramping due to the presence of an intrauterine device (IUD).

Pathogenesis

It has long been known that pain during menstruation is associated with ovulatory cycles. The mechanism of pain has been attributed to prostaglandin activity. Prostaglandins are present in much higher concentrations in women with dysmenorrhea than in those with mild or no pain.

Other studies have confirmed increased leukotriene levels as a contributing factor. Vasopressin was thought to be an aggravating agent, but atosiban, a vasopressin antagonist, has shown no effect on menstrual pain.

Psychologic factors may be involved, including attitudes passed from mother to daughter. Girls should receive accurate information about menstruation before menarche; this can be provided by parents, teachers, physicians, or counselors. Emotional anxiety due to academic or social demands may also be a cofactor.

Clinical Findings

Reactions to pain are subjective, and questioning by the physician should not lead the patient to exaggerate or minimize her discomfort. History taking is most important and should include the following questions: When does the pain occur? What does the patient do about the pain? Are there other symptoms? Do oral contraceptives relieve or intensify the pain? Is the pain becoming more severe over time?

Because dysmenorrhea is almost always associated with ovulatory cycles, it does not usually occur at menarche but rather later in adolescence. As many as 14–26% of adolescents miss school or work as a result of pain. Typically, pain occurs on the first day of the menses, usually about the time the flow begins, but it may not be present until the second day. Nausea and vomiting, diarrhea, and headache may occur. The specific symptoms associated with endometriosis are not present.

The physical examination does not reveal any significant pelvic disease. When the patient is symptomatic, she has generalized pelvic tenderness, perhaps more so in the area of the uterus than in the adnexa. Occasionally, ultrasonography or laparoscopy is necessary to rule out pelvic abnormalities such as endometriosis, pelvic inflammatory disease, or an accident in an ovarian cyst.

Differential Diagnosis

The most common misdiagnosis of primary dysmenorrhea is secondary dysmenorrhea due to endometriosis. With endometriosis, the pain usually begins 1–2 weeks before the menses, reaches a peak 1–2 days before, and is relieved at the onset of flow or shortly thereafter. Severe pain during sexual intercourse or findings of adnexal tenderness or mass or cul-de-sac modularity, particularly in the premenstrual interval, help to confirm the diagnosis. (See also Chapter 40.) A similar pain pattern occurs with adenomyosis, although in an older age group and in the absence of extrauterine clinical findings.

Treatment

NSAIDs or acetaminophen may relieve mild discomfort. For severe pain, codeine or other stronger analgesics may be needed and bedrest may be desirable. Occasionally, emergency treatment with parenteral medication may be necessary. Analgesics may cause drowsiness at the dosages required.

A. ANTIPROSTAGLANDINS

Antiprostaglandins are now used for the treatment of dysmenorrhea. The newer, stronger, faster-acting drugs appear to be more useful than aspirin. Ibuprofen, an NSAID, has been extremely effective in reducing menstrual prostaglandin and relieving dysmenorrhea. Over-the-counter formulations of ibuprofen are available; dosages must be adjusted to compare with prescription products. The drug must be used at the earliest onset of symptoms, usually at the onset of, and sometimes 1–2 days prior to, bleeding or cramping.

Antiprostaglandins work by blocking prostaglandin synthesis and metabolism; once the pain has been established, antiprostaglandins are not nearly as effective as with early use.

A newer class of drugs, cyclooxygenase-2 (COX-2) inhibitors, can also be employed successfully. Their limitation lies in their significantly higher cost.

B. ORAL CONTRACEPTIVES

Cyclic administration of oral contraceptives, usually in the lowest dosage but occasionally with increased estrogen, prevent pain in most patients who do not obtain relief from antiprostaglandins or cannot tolerate them. The mechanism of pain relief may be related to absence of ovulation or to altered endometrium resulting in decreased prostaglandin production. In women who do not require contraception, oral contraceptives are given for 6–12 months. Many women continue to be free of pain after treatment has been discontinued. NSAIDs act synergistically with oral contraceptive pills to improve dysmenorrhea.

C. SURGICAL TREATMENT

In a few women, no medication will control dysmenorrhea. Cervical dilatation is of little use. Laparoscopic uterosacral ligament division and presacral neurectomy are infrequently performed, although some physicians consider these to be important adjuncts to conservative operation for endometriosis.

Adenomyosis, endometriosis, or residual pelvic infection unresponsive to medical therapy or conservative surgical therapy may eventually require hysterectomy

with or without ovarian removal in extreme cases. Very rarely a patient with no organic source of pain may eventually require hysterectomy to relieve symptoms.

D. ADJUVANT TREATMENTS

Continuous low-level topical heat therapy has been shown to be as effective as ibuprofen in treating dysmenorrhea, though its practicality in daily life may be questionable. Many studies have indicated that exercise decreases prevalence and/or improves symptomatology of dysmenorrhea, though solid evidence is lacking.

ABNORMAL UTERINE BLEEDING

Abnormal uterine bleeding includes abnormal menstrual bleeding and bleeding due to other causes such as pregnancy, systemic disease, or cancer. The diagnosis and management of abnormal uterine bleeding present some of the most difficult problems in gynecology. Patients may not be able to localize the source of the bleeding from the vagina, urethra, or rectum. In childbearing women, a complication of pregnancy must always be considered, and one must always remember that more than one entity may be present, eg, uterine myomas and cervical cancer.

Patterns of Abnormal Uterine Bleeding

The standard classification for patterns of abnormal bleeding recognizes 7 different patterns.

(1) **Menorrhagia (hypermenorrhea)** is heavy or prolonged menstrual flow. The presence of clots may not be abnormal but may signify excessive bleeding. "Gushing" or "open-faucet" bleeding is always abnormal. Submucous myomas, complications of pregnancy, adenomyosis, IUDs, endometrial hyperplasias, malignant tumors, and dysfunctional bleeding are causes of menorrhagia.

(2) **Hypomenorrhea (cryptomenorrhea)** is unusually light menstrual flow, sometimes only spotting. An obstruction such as hymenal or cervical stenosis may be the cause. Uterine synechiae (Asherman's syndrome) can be causative and are diagnosed by a hysterogram or hysteroscopy. Patients receiving oral contraceptives occasionally complain of light flow and can be reassured that this is not significant.

(3) **Metrorrhagia (intermenstrual bleeding)** is bleeding occurring at any time between menstrual periods. Ovulatory bleeding occurs at midcycle as spotting and can be documented with basal body temperatures. Endometrial polyps and endometrial and cervical carcinomas are pathologic causes. In recent years, exogenous estrogen administration has become a common cause of this type of bleeding.

(4) **Polymenorrhea** describes periods that occur too frequently. This is usually associated with anovulation and rarely with a shortened luteal phase in the menstrual cycle.

(5) **Menometrorrhagia** is bleeding that occurs at irregular intervals. The amount and duration of bleeding also vary. Any condition that causes intermenstrual bleeding can eventually lead to menometrorrhagia. Sudden onset of irregular bleeding episodes may be an indication of malignant tumors or complications of pregnancy.

(6) **Oligomenorrhea** describes menstrual periods that occur more than 35 days apart. Amenorrhea is diagnosed if there is no menstrual period for more than 6 months. Bleeding is usually decreased in amount and associated with anovulation, either from endocrine causes (eg, pregnancy, pituitary-hypothalamic causes, menopause) or systemic causes (eg, excessive weight loss). Estrogen-secreting tumors produce oligomenorrhea prior to other patterns of abnormal bleeding.

(7) **Contact bleeding (postcoital bleeding)** is self-explanatory but must be considered a sign of cervical cancer until proved otherwise. Other causes of contact bleeding are much more common, including cervical eversion, cervical polyps, cervical or vaginal infection (eg, due to *Trichomonas*), or atrophic vaginitis. A negative cytologic smear does not rule out invasive cervical cancer, and colposcopy or biopsy or both may be necessary.

EVALUATION OF ABNORMAL UTERINE BLEEDING

Endometrial biopsy in the office is usually the first step in evaluation of abnormal uterine bleeding. The time-honored method for the evaluation of abnormal bleeding, however, is dilatation and curettage (D&C) performed under general anesthesia. Although D&C is still essential in some cases, hysteroscopy provides a more precise diagnosis by allowing visualization and directed biopsy. With either modality, most patients can be properly evaluated either in the office or, occasionally, in the outpatient department with local anesthesia.

A. History

Many causes of bleeding are strongly suggested by the history alone. Note the amount of menstrual flow, the length of the menstrual cycle and menstrual period, the length and amount of episodes of intermenstrual bleeding, and any episodes of contact bleeding. Note also the last menstrual period, the last normal menstrual period, age at menarche and menopause, and any changes in general health. The patient must keep a record of bleeding patterns to determine whether bleeding is abnormal or only a variation of normal. How-

ever, most women have an occasional menstrual cycle that is not in their usual pattern. Depending on the patient's age and the pattern of the bleeding, observation may be all that is necessary.

B. Physical Examination

Abdominal masses and an enlarged, irregular uterus suggest myoma. A symmetrically enlarged uterus is more typical of adenomyosis or endometrial carcinoma. Atrophic and inflammatory vulvar and vaginal lesions can be visualized, and cervical polyps and invasive lesions of cervical carcinoma can be seen. Rectovaginal examination is especially important to identify lateral and posterior spread or the presence of a barrel-shaped cervix. In pregnancy, a decidual reaction of the cervix may be the source of bleeding. The appearance is a velvety, friable erythematous lesion on the ectocervix.

C. Cytologic Examination

Although most useful in diagnosing asymptomatic intraepithelial lesions of the cervix, cytologic smears can help screen for invasive cervical (particularly endocervical) lesions. Although cytology is not reliable for the diagnosis of endometrial abnormalities, the presence of endometrial cells in a postmenopausal woman is abnormal unless she is receiving exogenous estrogens. Likewise, women in the secretory phase of the menstrual cycle should not shed endometrial cells. Of course, a cytologic examination that is positive or suspicious for endometrial cancer demands further evaluation.

Tubal or ovarian cancer also can be suspected on a cervical smear. The technique of obtaining a smear is important, since a tumor may be present only in the endocervical canal and may not shed cells to the ectocervix or vagina. Laboratories should report the presence or absence of endocervical cells. The current use of a spatula and endocervical brush has significantly increased the adequacy of cytologic smears from the cervix. Any abnormal smear requires further evaluation. (See also Chapter 47.)

D. Endometrial Biopsy

Methods of endometrial biopsy include use of the Novak suction curet, the Duncan curet, the Kevorkian curet, or the pipelle. Cervical dilatation is not necessary with these instruments. Small areas of the endometrial lining are sampled.

If no cause of bleeding can be found or if the tissue obtained is inadequate for diagnosis, D&C must be performed.

E. Saline Hysterosonogram

Ultrasound following injection of saline into the uterus has been used to evaluate the endometrial cavity for polyps, fibroids, or other abnormalities.

F. HYSTEROSCOPY

Placing an endoscopic camera through the cervix into the endometrial cavity allows direct visualization of the cavity. Resection attachments allow immediate capability to remove or biopsy lesions.

G. DILATATION AND CURETTAGE

D&C is the gold standard for the diagnosis of abnormal uterine bleeding. It can be done under local or general anesthesia, almost always in an outpatient or ambulatory setting. With general anesthesia, relaxation of the abdominal musculature is greater, allowing for a more thorough pelvic examination, more precise evaluation of pelvic masses, and more complete curettage. Curettage of the endocervix should be performed before sounding of the endometrial cavity or dilatation of the cervix is done.

H. OTHER DIAGNOSTIC PROCEDURES

Assay of the beta-subunit of human chorionic gonadotropin (hCG) may be used for complications of pregnancy and trophoblastic disease. Pelvic ultrasonography and laparoscopy may help to evaluate uterine and adnexal masses.

General Principles of Management

In making the diagnosis, it is important not to assume the obvious. A careful history and pelvic examination are vital. The possibility of pregnancy must be considered as well as use of oral contraceptives, IUDs, and hormones. Adequate sampling of the endometrium is essential for a definitive diagnosis.

Improved diagnostic techniques and treatment have resulted in decreased use of hysterectomy to treat abnormal bleeding patterns. If pathologic causes (eg, submucous myomas, adenomyosis) can be excluded, if there is no significant risk of cancer developing (as from atypical endometrial hyperplasia), and if there is no acute life-threatening hemorrhage, most patients can be treated with hormone preparations. Myomectomy can be suggested for myoma if the patient wishes to retain her potential for childbearing. Endometrial ablation and endometrial resection may offer successful outpatient and in-office alternatives.

For menorrhagia, prostaglandin synthetase inhibitors have been shown to significantly decrease blood loss during menses, as has antifibrinolytic therapy. Long-acting intramuscular progestin administration (Depo-Provera) can be given, but may result in erratic bleeding or even amenorrhea. Finally, levonorgestrel-releasing intrauterine devices are effective in decreasing blood loss.

ABNORMAL UTERINE BLEEDING DURING PREGNANCY

See Chapter 20.

ABNORMAL BLEEDING DUE TO NONGYNECOLOGIC DISEASES & DISORDERS

In the differential diagnosis of abnormal bleeding, nongynecologic causes of bleeding (eg, rectal or urologic disorders) must be ruled out, because patients may have difficulty differentiating the source of bleeding. Gynecologic and nongynecologic causes of bleeding may coexist. Systemic disease may cause abnormal uterine bleeding. For example, myxedema usually causes amenorrhea, but less severe hypothyroidism is associated with increased uterine bleeding. Liver disease interferes with estrogen metabolism and may cause variable degrees of bleeding. Both of these conditions are usually clinically apparent before gynecologic symptoms appear. Blood dyscrasias and coagulation abnormalities can also produce gynecologic bleeding. Patients receiving anticoagulants or adrenal steroids may expect abnormalities. Extreme weight loss due to eating disorders, exercise, or dieting may be associated with anovulation and amenorrhea.

DYSFUNCTIONAL UTERINE BLEEDING

Exclusion of pathologic causes of abnormal bleeding establishes the diagnosis of dysfunctional uterine bleeding. Although a persistent corpus luteum cyst or short luteal phase can produce abnormal bleeding associated with ovulation, most patients are anovulatory. The exact cause of anovulation is not truly understood but probably represents dysfunction of the hypothalamic-pituitary-ovarian axis, resulting in continued estrogenic stimulation of the endometrium. The endometrium outgrows its blood supply, partially breaks down, and is sloughed in an irregular manner. Conversion from proliferative to secretory endometrium corrects most acute and chronic bleeding problems. Organic causes of anovulation must be excluded (eg, thyroid or adrenal abnormalities).

Dysfunctional bleeding occurs most commonly at the extremes of reproductive age (20% of cases occur in adolescence and 40% in patients over age 40). Management depends on the age of the patient (adolescent, young woman, or premenopausal woman). The diagnosis is made by history, absence of ovulatory temperature changes, low serum progesterone, and results of endometrial sampling in the older woman.

Treatment

A. ADOLESCENTS

Because the first menstrual cycles are frequently anovulatory, it is not unusual for menses to be irregular, and explanation of the reason is all that is necessary for treatment. Heavy bleeding—even hemorrhage—may occur. Diagnostic procedures are usually not necessary in young patients, but pelvic examination must be performed to exclude pregnancy or pathologic conditions. Estrogens given orally should be adequate for all patients except those requiring curettage to control hemorrhage. Numerous regimens are available, including estrogens followed by progesterone, progesterone alone, or combination oral contraceptives. For acute hemorrhage, high-dose estrogen given intravenously (25 mg conjugated estrogen every 4 hours) gives rapid response. In hemodynamically stable patients, the oral dose of conjugated estrogens is 2.5 mg every 4–6 hours for 14–21 days. Once bleeding has stopped, medroxyprogesterone acetate 10 mg once or twice a day should be given for 7–10 days.

Oral contraceptives, 3–4 times the usual dose, are just as effective and may be simpler to use than sequential hormones. Again, the dose is lowered after a few days and the lower dose is continued for the next few cycles, particularly to raise the hemoglobin levels in an anemic patient. Medroxyprogesterone acetate, 10 mg/d for 10 days, can be used in patients who have proliferative endometrium on biopsy. In patients receiving cyclic therapy, 3–6 monthly courses are usually administered, after which treatment is discontinued and further evaluation is performed if necessary. In adolescents in whom the bleeding is not severe, oral contraceptives may be used as normally prescribed.

B. YOUNG WOMEN

In patients 20–30 years old, pathologic causes are more common and diagnostic procedures are more often necessary, particularly endometrial biopsy or aspiration. Hormonal management is the same as for adolescents.

C. PREMENOPAUSAL WOMEN

In the later reproductive years, even more care must be given to excluding pathologic causes because of the possibility of endometrial cancer. Aspiration, curettage, or both should clearly establish anovulatory or dyssynchronous cycles as the cause before hormonal therapy is started. Recurrences of abnormal bleeding demand further evaluation.

D. SURGICAL MEASURES

For patients whose bleeding cannot be controlled with hormones, who are symptomatically anemic, and whose lifestyle is compromised by persistence of irregular bleeding, D&C may temporarily stop bleeding, but abdominal or vaginal hysterectomy may be necessary. Endometrial ablation techniques are useful in patients who have personal or medical contraindications to hysterectomy. Definitive surgery may also be needed for coexistent endometriosis, myoma, and disorders of pelvic relaxation.

POSTMENOPAUSAL BLEEDING

Postmenopausal bleeding may be defined as bleeding that occurs after 12 months of amenorrhea in a middle-aged woman. When amenorrhea occurs in a younger person for 1 year and premature ovarian failure or menopause has been diagnosed, episodes of bleeding may be classified as postmenopausal, although resumption of ovulatory cycles can occur. Follicle-stimulating hormone (FSH) levels are particularly helpful in the differential diagnoses of menopausal versus hypothalamic amenorrhea. An FSH level greater than 30 mIU/mL is highly suggestive of menopause.

Postmenopausal bleeding is more likely to be caused by pathologic disease than is bleeding in younger women, and it must always be investigated. Nongynecologic causes must be excluded; these are also more likely to be caused by pathologic disease in older women, and the patient may be unable to determine the site of bleeding. The source of bleeding should not be assumed to be nongynecologic unless there is good evidence or proper evaluation has excluded gynecologic causes.

Neither normal ("functional") bleeding nor dysfunctional bleeding should occur after menopause. Although pathologic disorders are more likely, other causes may also occur. Atrophic or proliferative endometrium is not unusual. Secretory patterns should not occur unless the patient has resumed ovulation or has received progesterone therapy.

After nongynecologic causes of bleeding are excluded, gynecologic causes must be considered.

A. EXOGENOUS HORMONES

The most common cause of postmenopausal uterine bleeding is the use of exogenous hormones. In the past, face creams and cosmetics contained homeopathic amounts of estrogens, but this is highly unlikely today. Careful history taking becomes vital, since patients may not follow specific instructions on the use of estrogen and progesterone therapy.

Recent recommendations for long-term estrogen/progesterone administration for prevention of osteoporosis have improved quality of life and caused resumption of regular menstrual bleeding in many patients taking them cyclically. It is not uncommon to present with vaginal bleeding for as long as 6–12 months after initiation of any hormone replacement therapy. If by that time bleeding is still occurring, further investigation is warranted to discover its etiology. If endometrial hyperplasia is found, specific attention must be paid to the presence of atypia and treatment begun by increasing the progesterone component or by hysterectomy.

B. VAGINAL ATROPHY AND VAGINAL AND VULVAR LESIONS

Bleeding from the lower reproductive tract is almost always related to vaginal atrophy, with or without trauma. Examination reveals thin tissue with ecchymosis. Rarely, there will be a tear at the introitus or deep in the vagina requiring suturing. With vulvar dystrophies, there may be a white area and cracking of the skin of the vulva. Cytologic study of material obtained from the cervix and vagina will reveal immature epithelial cells with or without inflammation. After excluding coexisting upper tract lesions, treatment can include local or systemic estrogen therapy for vaginal lesions. Vulvar lesions need further diagnostic evaluation to determine the proper treatment.

C. TUMORS OF THE REPRODUCTIVE TRACT

The differential diagnosis of organic causes of postmenopausal uterine bleeding includes endometrial hyperplasias (simple, complex, and atypical), endometrial polyps, endometrial carcinoma or other more rare tumors such as cervical or endocervical carcinoma, uterine sarcomas (including mixed mesodermal and myosarcomas), and, even more rarely, uterine tube and ovarian cancer. Estrogen-secreting ovarian tumors should also be considered.

Uterine sampling must be done, and tissue must be obtained. Endocervical curettage should be done along with any endometrial sampling technique. If a diagnosis cannot be established or is questionable with office procedures, D&C must be done. Hysteroscopy done in the office or operating room may prove helpful in locating endometrial polyps or fibroids that could be missed even by fractional curettage. Pelvic ultrasonography may be extremely helpful in the diagnosis of ovarian tumors and in evaluation of the thickness of the endometrium, as well as in discerning between uterine myomas and adnexal tumors. Recurring episodes of postmenopausal bleeding may rarely require hysterectomy, even when a diagnosis cannot be established by endometrial sampling.

REFERENCES

Abu JI et al: Leukotrienes in gynaecology: the hypothetical value of anti-leukotriene therapy in dysmenorrhea and endometriosis. Hum Reprod Update 2000;6:200.

Akin MD et al: Continuous low-level topical heat in the treatment of dysmenorrhea. Obstet Gynecol 2000;97:343.

Chan WY et al: Prostaglandins in primary dysmenorrhea. Comparison of prophylactic and nonprophylactic treatment with ibuprofen and use of oral contraceptives. Am J Med 1981;70:535.

Cross GB et al: Changes in nutrient intake during the menstrual cycle of over-weight women with premenstrual syndrome. Br J Nutr 2001;85:475.

Di Carlo C et al: Use of leuprolide acetate plus tibolone in the treatment of severe premenstrual syndrome. Fertil Steril 2001;75:380.

Ecochard R et al: Gonadotropin level abnormalities in women with cyclic mastalgia. Eur J Obstet Gyn 2001;94:92.

Golumb LM et al: Primary dysmenorrhea and physical activity. Med Sci Exerc 1998;30:906.

Jensen JT et al: Health benefits of oral contraceptives. Obstet Gynecol Clin North Am 2000;27:705.

Kaleli S et al: Symptomatic treatment of premenstrual mastalgia in premenopausal women with lisuride maleate: a double-blind placebo-controlled randomized study. Fertil Steril 2001;75:718.

Morrison BW et al: Rofecoxib, a specific cyclooxygenase-2 inhibitor, in primary dysmenorrhea: a randomized controlled trial. Obstet Gynecol 1999;94:504.

Schwayder JM: Pathophysiology of abnormal uterine bleeding. Obstet Gynecol Clin North Am 2000;27:219.

Steiner M: Premenstrual syndrome and premenstrual dysphoric disorder: guidelines for management. J Psychiatry Neuro 2000;25:459.

Valentin L et al: Effects of a vasopressin antagonist in women with dysmenorrhea. Gynecol Obstet Invest 2000;50:170.

Yuk VJ et al: Frequency and severity of premenstrual symptoms in women taking birth control pills. Gynecol Obstet Invest 1991;31:42.

Contraception & Family Planning

Michelle Grewal, MD, & Ronald T. Burkman, MD

■ CONTRACEPTION

One of the most sensitive and intimate decisions made by an individual or by a couple is that of fertility control. This decision is often based on deeply held religious or philosophical convictions. Thus, the clinician must approach the patient's fertility needs with particular sensitivity, empathy, maturity, and nonjudgmental behavior.

However, it must be recognized that there is a considerable need for contraception. The number of births rose 3% between 1999 and 2000. While the birth rate among teenagers fell to a historic low, the fertility rate rose 3% to 67.6 per 1000 women aged 15–44 years. Birth rates increased for all age groups over the age of 20. The number of births among unmarried, older women was also the highest ever reported, with a 3% increase compared to 1999. These numbers reflect the tendency for women to delay childbearing until their 30s or 40s, perhaps when their careers are well established. Thus, health care professionals who provide contraception need to meet the needs of women with diverse social and economic circumstances.

Individual Indications for Birth Control

Contraception is practiced by most couples for personal reasons. Many couples use contraception to space their children or to limit the size of their family. Others desire to avoid childbearing because of the effects of preexisting illness on the pregnancy, such as severe diabetes, or heart disease, such as severe aortic stenosis. For all of these types of decisions, clinicians must provide accurate information about the benefits and risks of both pregnancy and contraception. However, medical conditions that may substantially increase the risk of using some form of birth control usually increase the risks associated with pregnancy to an even greater extent. As a matter of public policy some countries, especially those that are less developed, promote contraception in an effort to curb undesired population growth.

Legal Aspects of Contraception

Contraceptives are prescribed, demonstrated, and sold in most states of the U.S. without restriction.

Despite high rates of unprotected intercourse and unintended pregnancy, the pros and cons of providing contraceptive information and materials to teenagers have been vigorously debated. A regulation proposed in 1982 for federally funded family planning programs in the U.S. would have required personnel at family planning facilities to notify the parent or guardian of any person under the age of 18 years at least 10 working days before the clinic would be able to provide a prescription contraceptive to the teenager. This proposal was declared unconstitutional by the courts. Furthermore, in 1977, the United States Supreme Court ruled that minors have a constitutional right of access to contraceptives. Most states either have legislation that permits access to contraception for persons under 18 or have not addressed the issue legislatively. Most physicians agree that teenagers should be given contraceptive advice and prescriptions within the confines of appropriate legal restraints. However, they must be careful to avoid imposing their own religious or moral views on their patients.

Health care providers must provide all persons requesting contraception with detailed information about the use of the method or methods, benefits, risks, and side effects so that an informed choice can be made relative to a particular method. Not only is the provision of this information of ethical and legal importance, but such counseling is also likely to ensure that the method will be used appropriately with overall improved compliance. Documentation of the discussion with the patient and her understanding of what has been said is of legal importance.

In particular, when using methods that require instrumentation or some type of surgical approach and that also may require intervention by a health care professional for discontinuation (eg, IUD, injectable or implantable progestin, or sterilization), use of signed consent forms that outline the information discussed and the patient's understanding is important. Such a form serves as evidence, if needed, that counseling about use of a particular birth control method was given; that the patient appeared competent to understand what was said to her; and that she consented to receive contraceptive management in the manner specified.

METHODS OF CONTRACEPTION

The available methods of contraception may be classified in many ways. For the sake of this discussion, traditional or folk methods are coitus interruptus, postcoital douche, lactational amenorrhea, and periodic abstinence (rhythm or natural family planning). Barrier methods include condoms (male and female), diaphragm, cervical cap, vaginal sponge, and spermicides. Hormonal methods encompass oral contraceptives and injectable or implantable long-acting progestins. In addition, the intrauterine contraceptive device (IUD) and sterilization (tubal ligation or vasectomy) are also part of the contraceptive armamentarium. However, sterilization is discussed elsewhere in this book (Chapter 45).

COITUS INTERRUPTUS

One of the oldest contraceptive methods is withdrawal of the penis before ejaculation. This results in deposition of the semen outside the female genital tract. It has the disadvantage of demanding sufficient self-control by the man so that withdrawal can precede ejaculation. Although the failure rate is probably higher than that of most methods, reliable statistics are not available. Failure may result from escape of semen before orgasm or the deposition of semen on the external female genitalia near the vagina.

POSTCOITAL DOUCHE

Plain water, vinegar, and a number of "feminine hygiene" products are widely used as postcoital douches. Theoretically, the douche serves to flush the semen out of the vagina, and the additives to the water may possess some spermicidal properties. Nevertheless, sperm have been found within the cervical mucus within 90 seconds after ejaculation. Hence, the method is ineffective and unreliable.

LACTATIONAL AMENORRHEA

The lactational amenorrhea method (LAM) can be a highly efficient method for breastfeeding women to utilize physiology to space births. Suckling results in a reduction in the release of gonadotropin releasing hormone, luteinizing hormone, and follicle-stimulating hormone. Beta-endorphins induced by suckling also in-

duce a decline in the secretion of dopamine, which normally suppresses the release of prolactin. This results in a condition of amenorrhea and anovulation. During the first 6 months, if breastfeeding is exclusive, menses are mostly anovulatory and fertility remains low. A recent WHO Study on LAM revealed that during the first 6 months of nursing, cumulative pregnancy rates ranged from 0.9 to 1.2 percent. However, at 12 months, pregnancy rates rose as high as 7.4 percent. When using lactation as a method of birth control, the mother must provide breastfeeding as the only form of infant nutrition. Supplemental feedings may alter both the pattern of lactation and the intensity of infant suckling, which secondarily may affect suppression of ovulation. Second, amenorrhea must be maintained. Finally, the method should be practiced as the only form of birth control for a maximum of 6 months after birth.

MALE CONDOM

The latex rubber or animal intestine condom, or contraceptive sheath, serves as a cover for the penis during coitus and prevents the deposition of semen in the vagina. The advantages of the condom are that it provides highly effective and inexpensive contraception as well as protection against sexually transmitted diseases (STDs). Some condoms now contain a spermicide, which may offer further protection against failure, particularly if the condom breaks. Given the concern about both STDs and the HIV epidemic, condom use should be a significant consideration for persons who are at risk for contracting such infections.

The condom probably is the most widely used mechanical contraceptive in the world today. Most condoms are made of latex that is 0.3–0.8 mm thick, a membrane that is impervious to both sperm and most bacterial and viral organisms that cause STDs or HIV infection. However, the less commonly used lamb's intestine condom is not impermeable to such organisms. The failure of all condoms is due to imperfections of manufacture (about 3 per 1000); errors of technique, such as applying the condom after some semen has escaped into the vagina; and escape of semen from the condom as a result of failure to withdraw before detumescence. In overall use, failure rates with condoms range from 2–15% in the first year of use.

When greater contraceptive effectiveness is desired, a second method such as contraceptive vaginal jelly or foam should be used in conjunction with the condom. This significantly reduces the chances for condom failure due to mechanical or technical deficiencies. No association has been established between the use of vaginal contraceptives (spermicides) and the occurrence of congenital malformations if a pregnancy occurs.

FEMALE CONDOM

The female condom (Reality Vaginal Pouch) is made of thin polyurethane material with 2 flexible rings at each end. One ring fits into the depth of the vagina, and the other ring sits outside the vagina near the introitus. Female condoms have the advantage of being under the control of the female partner and of offering some protection against STDs. Significant disadvantages may be their cost and overall bulkiness. Comparisons of the female condom with other female barrier methods such as the diaphragm and cervical cap indicate that failure rates are comparable. The 6-month probability of failure during perfect use of the condom is 2.6%, which is much lower than the initial prediction of 15%. Perfect use of the female condom may also reduce the annual risk of acquiring HIV by more than 90 percent.

VAGINAL DIAPHRAGM

The diaphragm is a mechanical barrier between the vagina and the cervical canal. Diaphragms are circular rings ranging from 50–105 mm in diameter, which are designed to fit in the vaginal cul-de-sac and cover the cervix. Although the designs vary, the arcing spring version is probably the easiest to use for most women. A contraceptive jelly or cream should be placed on the cervical side of the diaphragm before insertion, since the device is ineffective without it. This medication also serves as a lubricant for insertion of the device. Additional jelly should be introduced into the vagina on and around the diaphragm after it is securely in place. When the diaphragm is of proper size (as determined by pelvic examination and trial with fitting rings) and is used according to directions, its failure rate is 2–20 pregnancies per 100 women per year of exposure. The diaphragm has the disadvantages of requiring fitting by a physician or a trained paramedical person and the necessity for anticipating the need for contraception. Failures may result from improper fitting or placement and dislodgment of the diaphragm during intercourse. As with condoms, diaphragms also offer some protection against STDs. The only side effects are vaginal wall irritation, usually with initial use or if the device fits too tightly, and an increased risk of urinary tract infections.

CERVICAL CAP

Cervical caps are small cuplike diaphragms placed over the cervix. They are supposed to be held in place by suction. To provide a successful barrier against sperm, they must fit tightly over the cervix. Because of variability in cervical size, individualization is almost essential. This greatly limits the practical usefulness of the method. Tailoring the cap to fit each cervix is difficult.

In addition, many women are unable to feel their own cervix and thus have great difficulty in placing the cap correctly over the cervix. Because of these problems, the cervical cap has few advantages over the traditional vaginal diaphragm. Although some advocates of the cervical cap recommend that it remain in place for 1 or 2 days at a time, a foul discharge often develops after about 1 day's use. With proper use, the efficacy of the cervical cap is similar to that of the diaphragm, with dislodgment being the most frequently cited cause of failure in most reports. In any event, due to the difficulty associated with proper fitting and routine insertion, it is doubtful that the cap in its present state of development will play an important role in contraception.

SPERMICIDAL PREPARATIONS

Spermicidal vaginal jellies, creams, gels, suppositories, and foams, in addition to their toxic effect on sperm, also act as a mechanical barrier to entry of sperm into the cervical canal. The majority of spermicides marketed in the U.S. contain nonoxynol 9, which is a long-chain surfactant that is toxic to spermatozoa. Spermicides may be used alone or in conjunction with a diaphragm or condom. Some of the foam tablets and suppositories require a few minutes for adequate dispersion throughout the vagina, and failures may result if dispersion is not allowed to occur. In general, when used alone, spermicides have a failure rate of about 15% per year. Rarely, these chemical agents may irritate the vaginal mucosa and external genitalia. Recent evidence indicates that spermicides containing nonoxynol-9 (N-9) are not effective in preventing cervical gonorrhea, chlamydia or HIV infection. In addition, frequent use of spermicides containing N-9 has been associated with genital lesions which may be associated with an increased risk of HIV transmission.

NATURAL FAMILY PLANNING METHOD

It has long been known that women are fertile for only a few days of the menstrual cycle. The periodic abstinence or rhythm method of contraception requires that coitus be avoided during the time of the cycle when a fertilizable ovum and motile sperm could meet in the oviduct. Fertilization takes place within the tube, and the ovum remains in the tube for about 1–3 days after ovulation; hence the fertile period is from the time of ovulation to 2–3 days thereafter.

Accurate prediction or indication of ovulation is essential to the success of the rhythm method. Data from surveys in developed and developing countries done during the past decade indicate the use of natural family planning methods varies from 0–11%. Pregnancy rates vary, but most reliable studies report 1-year life table pregnancy rates between 10 and 25 per 100 woman years. Accordingly, the types of periodic abstinence vary in their approaches to determining the fertile period.

(1) The **calendar method** predicts the day of ovulation by means of a formula based on the menstrual pattern recorded over a period of several months. Ovulation ordinarily occurs 14 days before the first day of the next menstrual period. The fertile interval should be assumed to extend from at least 2 days before ovulation to no less than 2 days after ovulation. An overlap of 1–2 days of abstinence either way increases the likelihood of success. Successful use of this approach is based on the knowledge that the luteal phase of a menstrual cycle is relatively constant at 14 days for normal women. Furthermore, for this approach to be successful as the only form of contraception requires regular menstrual cycles so that the various timing schedules retain validity. Although this is the most commonly used method of periodic abstinence, it is also the least reliable with failure rates as high as 35% in 1 year's use.

(2) A somewhat more efficacious approach to periodic abstinence is the temperature method, since more reliable evidence of ovulation may be obtained by recording the basal body temperature (BBT). The vaginal or rectal temperature must be recorded upon awakening in the morning before any physical activity is undertaken. Although it is often missed, there is a slight drop in temperature 24–36 hours after ovulation. The temperature then rises abruptly about 0.3–0.4 °C (0.5–0.7 °F) and remains at this plateau for the remainder of the cycle. The third day after the onset of elevated temperature is considered to be the end of the fertile period. For reliability, care must be taken by the woman to ensure that true basal temperatures are recorded, ie, that hyperthermia due to other causes does not provide misleading information. A distinct limitation of this technique is that prediction of timing of ovulation in any given cycle is retrospective, making it difficult to predict the onset of the fertile period.

(3) The **combined temperature and calendar method** uses features of both the previously mentioned methods to more accurately predict the time of ovulation. Failure rates of only 5 pregnancies per 100 couples per year have been reported in studies of well-motivated couples.

(4) The **cervical mucus (Billings) method** uses changes in cervical mucus secretions as affected by menstrual cycle hormonal alterations to predict ovulation. Starting several days before and until just after ovulation, the mucus becomes thin and watery, whereas at other times the mucus is thick and opaque. Women using this approach are trained to evaluate their mucus on a daily basis. Success rates are similar to those described for the combined temperature and calendar method. Advantages of this approach include relative

simplicity and lack of a requirement for charting; disadvantages include difficulty in evaluating mucus in the presence of vaginal infection and the reluctance of some women to evaluate such secretions.

(5) The **symptothermal method,** if used properly, is probably the most effective of all the periodic abstinence approaches. It combines features of both the cervical mucus and the temperature methods. In addition, symptoms that may occur just prior to ovulation such as bloating and vulvar swelling are used as adjuncts to predict the likely occurrence of ovulation.

The most accurate method of determining ovulation time is to demonstrate the luteinizing hormone (LH) peak in serum specimens. Because of the cost and the time required for the serial measurements of LH that are essential to indicate the abrupt rise, this method is impractical as a method of birth control. It is valuable in the treatment of infertility, however, when the optimal time for coitus or artificial insemination is of great importance.

Figure 33–1 shows the relationships among ovulation, BBT, serum levels of LH and follicle-stimulating hormone (FSH), and menses. At least 20% of fertile women have enough variation in their cycles that reliable prediction of the fertile period is impossible.

Epidemiologic studies of women using the rhythm method have suggested an increased incidence of congenital anomalies such as anencephaly and Down's syndrome among children resulting from unplanned pregnancies. Delayed fertilization has been shown in animal experiments to result in an increased incidence of aneuploidy and polyploidy in offspring, thus suggesting a possible explanation for similar human fetal anomalies. However, despite a theoretical explanation for the occurrence of such birth defects, it is important to recognize that much of the data are subject to bias, and it would be inappropriate to conclude that such associations have been conclusively proved.

ORAL HORMONAL CONTRACEPTIVES

The oral contraceptives in general use are synthetic steroids similar to the natural female sex hormones—the estrogens and progestins. These steroids are used in doses and in combinations that provide contraception by inhibiting ovulation.

When first developed, the 2 principal regimens of oral contraception were combined and sequential. In the combined method, pills containing estrogen and progestin are taken each day for 20–21 days. The sequential method, in which an estrogen pill is taken each day for 15–16 days followed by an estrogen-progestin pill each day for 5 days, has been abandoned in the U.S. because several studies showed a higher than nor-

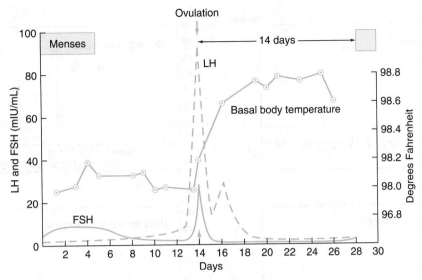

Figure 33–1. Relationship between ovulation and basal body temperature and luteinizing hormone (LH) and follicle-stimulating hormone (FSH) surges in the normal menstrual cycle.

mal incidence of endometrial cancer in women using this method of contraception.

The combined regimen is begun either with the onset of the menstrual cycle or on the Sunday closest to the start of menses. Since most oral contraceptive preparations are packaged in 28-day regimens (the pills taken the last 7 days being placebos), the Sunday start approach may be easier to follow for most women. However, a good practice is to recommend use of an additional form of contraception during the first cycle to maximize efficacy. Withdrawal bleeding can be expected within 3–5 days after completion of the 20- or 21-day regimen.

The serum levels of FSH and LH throughout the normal menstrual cycle are shown in Figure 33–2A. During a typical cycle under the combined oral contraceptive regimen (Fig 33–2B), there is no rise during the first half of the cycle; thus, follicle growth is either not initiated or, if initiated, recruitment does not occur, ovulation does not occur, and consequently there is no FSH and LH surge. During the sequential oral contraceptive regimen (Fig 33–2C), the estrogen stimulates LH secretion in an irregular manner. There is no concomitant early rise in FSH when progestin is added, and another LH surge usually is produced. When a progestin-only regimen (Fig 33–2D) is followed (eg, with the minipill; see Minipill section), there are multiple LH surges but no significant changes in FSH levels. For the reasons given, these oral contraceptive regimens significantly alter the physiologic hormonal balance. The minipill regimen causes the least derangement, but

its efficacy as a contraceptive is less than that of combined oral contraception. Moreover, occasional amenorrhea may occur.

Advantages

Major noncontraceptive advantages derived from use of oral contraceptives in the U.S. alone include approximately 50,000 hospitalizations averted annually for conditions that include benign breast disease, retention cysts of the ovaries, iron deficiency anemia, and pelvic inflammatory disease. Studies in the U.S. and Great Britain showed that users of oral contraceptives have almost complete protection against ectopic pregnancies. Oral contraceptive use is estimated to prevent about 10,000 hospitalizations for this life-threatening complications annually in the U.S. alone.

Oral contraceptives provide a reduction in risk of developing ovarian and endometrial cancer. The data with ovarian cancer are significant enough to recommend oral contraceptive usage to women considered at high risk by family history or BRCA gene status. In one population-based, case-control study to evaluate the impact of dose of oral contraceptives on ovarian cancer risk, the adjusted risk of ovarian cancer was reduced by 40% for oral contraceptive users overall, with longer duration of use affording greater protection.

Other well-established benefits include a reduction in menorrhagia and dysmenorrhea, iron-deficiency anemia, and acne, as well as improvements in hirsutism and symptomatic endometriosis.

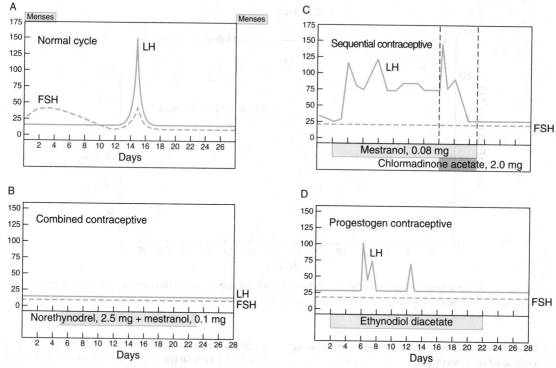

Figure 33–2. Serum levels (in mIU/mL) of follicle-stimulating hormone (FSH) and luteinizing hormone (LH) during the menstrual cycle, with and without oral contraception. **A:** During a normal cycle without medication. **B:** During atypical cycle with combined medication (see text). **C:** During a typical cycle with sequential medication (see text). **D:** During progestin-only medication. (Reproduced, with permission, from Odell WD, Moyer DL: *Physiology of Reproduction.* Mosby, 1971.)

Disadvantages & Side Effects

Much attention has been paid to a possible relationship between the use of oral contraceptives and the incidence of thromboembolic disease, including pulmonary embolism and cerebral thrombosis. Between 1967 and 1969, reports of retrospective studies in Great Britain and the U.S. provided statistically valid data indicating that deep vein thrombosis, pulmonary embolism, and cerebral thrombosis occur 3–6 times more frequently in users of oral contraceptives than in nonusers. However, since those earlier reports were published, the dosages of steroids contained in oral contraceptives have been reduced 3 to 4 times. In particular, ethinyl estradiol, the most widely used estrogen, is now provided in doses of about 20–35 μg in most preparations. More recent publications studying these disorders in association with oral contraceptive use suggest that a significant reduction in risk has occurred in conjunction with dosage reduction. A recent case-control study revealed that current users of low estrogen dose (< 35 μg ethinyl

estradiol) combined oral contraceptives containing desogestrel or gestodene appear to be at higher risk of developing venous thromboembolism than users of combined oral contraceptives containing levonorgestrel, but this remains controversial. Another British study in 1995 concluded that there was a significant association between idiopathic venous thromboembolism and current smoking, body mass index over 35, and asthma. Current users of low estrogen dose oral contraceptives have a small increased risk of ischemic stroke, although most of the risk occurs in women with other risk factors such as smoking, hypertension, and history of migraines.

Some users of oral contraceptives may have a greater risk of developing coronary thrombosis than nonusers. The increased risk, if present, appears to be confined to older users who smoke one or more packs of cigarettes per day. Furthermore, following oral contraceptive use, the Nurses Health Study has shown that past oral contraceptive use, regardless of duration, does not increase the risk of subsequent cardiovascular disease, including myocardial infarction. Although the progestins contained in oral contraceptives may change the lipid/lipoprotein profile in an adverse direction, the advent of new progestins and dosage reductions have led to a reduction in the magnitude of such changes. In addition, estrogen affects such profiles in a favorable direction. Thus, the interaction of the two steroids combined with recent dosage and formulation changes has led to preparations that are essentially neutral relative to their effects on the cardiovascular system.

Although epithelial abnormalities of the uterine cervix among users of oral contraceptives were at one time a matter of concern, the preponderance of evidence cannot demonstrate that the use of oral contraceptives either causes or predisposes to the development of cancer of the cervix. A major problem with studies attempting to examine this relationship is the confounding factors such as multiple sexual partners, age at first intercourse, and frequency of sexual activity.

The association between oral contraceptive use and breast cancer has been extensively studied during the past decade. At this time, it is unclear whether any positive association exists. The data in some studies suggest that long-term oral contraceptive use before childbearing may increase the risk of premenopausal breast cancer. However some data also suggest that use may also offer modest protection against the more common postmenopausal form of this cancer. As with cervical neoplasia, studies attempting to explore this relationship are subject to a number of potential biases such as varying practices of breast disease screening. Other infrequent problems occasionally noted with oral contraceptive use include hypertension, cholelithiasis, and benign liver tumors. However, none of these problems occurs frequently enough to be of significant concern to most users.

Since the current formulations are associated with significant reductions in risk of serious sequelae, side effect control will be of greater importance to most users in the future. Furthermore, studies have also shown that compliance is affected by occurrence of side effects and that such "minor" problems account for about 40% of the discontinuations. Factors affecting compliance are of significance particularly when one studies efficacy. For example, the theoretical failure rate with combination oral contraceptives after 1 year's use is less than 1%. However, the use-effectiveness failure rate in some studies is as high as 4–6%. Intermenstrual bleeding including breakthrough bleeding and spotting may be experienced by about 10–20% of users in the first few months of use. With today's formulations, at about 6 months of use such problems stabilize and are seen in only about 5% of users. Missed menstrual periods or amenorrhea are relatively infrequent and of little clinical significance except that these problems can raise concern as to whether a contraceptive failure has oc-

curred. Nausea may be seen in up to 10% of users; as with intermenstrual bleeding, this is a duration effect that declines rapidly after several months of use. With current formulations, acne tends to improve or show little change. Furthermore, significant headaches and weight gain are far less frequent than reported with higher-dose preparations.

Since compliance and a clear understanding of how to take oral contraceptives are important to their successful use, health care providers should take the time at the initial visit to explain the packaging of the brand being prescribed, discuss the side effects, review how to start the first cycle, and discuss what to do when pills are missed. It should be emphasized that the patient package insert provides useful information on these topics. In addition, users should be encouraged to contact their provider or someone in the office or clinic who is familiar with oral contraceptive health care if problems occur. Finally, users should be advised to use alternate forms of contraception if oral contraceptive use is interrupted because of forgotten pills or the occurrence of side effects.

Table 33–1 lists the currently available oral contraceptives and their contents.

The Minipill or Progestin-Only Pill

The idea of administering small daily amounts of a progestin arose when clinical experience with some of the low-dose combination pills indicated that contraception was being provided even though ovulation was not always inhibited. Subsequent studies demonstrated that a small daily quantity of a progestin alone would provide reasonably good protection against pregnancy without suppressing ovulation. The method has the following advantages: (1) Because no estrogen is given, the side effects attributable to the estrogen component of conventional oral contraceptives are eliminated; (2) the minipill is taken every day; thus no special sequence of pill-taking is necessary. The mechanism of contraceptive action of the microdose nonstop progestins is not known. It has been suggested that the cervical mucus becomes less permeable to sperm and that endometrial activity goes out of phase, so that nidation is thwarted even if fertilization does occur. In clinical tests, the use of microdoses of progestins has resulted in a pregnancy rate of about 2–7 per 100 woman years.

Progestin is associated with some side effects, mainly irregularity of the ovulatory cycle and ectopic pregnancies, and these significantly reduce its contraceptive acceptability. Its overall effectiveness is less than that of combination pills. Currently, the minipill is thought to be useful in only a few patients, ie, in those having a documented hypersensitivity to estrogens and perhaps for the lactating woman.

Table 33–1. Oral contraceptive agents in use. The estrogen-containing compounds are arranged in order of increasing content of estrogen (ethinyl estradiol and mestranol have similar potencies).

	Estrogen (mg)	Progestin (mg)	
Combination tablets			
Loestrin 1/20	Ethinyl estradiol 0.02	Norethindrone acetate	1
Loestrin 1.5/30	Ethinyl estradiol 0.03	Norethindrone acetate	1.5
Ovcon-35	Ethinyl estradiol 0.035	Norethindrone	0.4
Brevicon	Ethinyl estradiol 0.035	Norethindrone	0.5
Modicon			
Nordette	Ethinyl estradiol 0.03	L-Norgestrel	0.15
Ortho-Cept, Desogen	Ethinyl estradiol 0.30	Desogestrel	0.15
Ortho-Cyclen	Ethinyl estradiol 0.35	Norgestimate	0.25
Lo/Ovral	Ethinyl estradiol 0.03	DL-Norgestrel	0.3
Ovral	Ethinyl estradiol 0.05	DL-Norgestrel	0.5
Demulen 1/50	Ethinyl estradiol 0.05	Ethynodiol diacetate	1
Demulen 1/35	Ethinyl estradiol 0.35	Ethynodiol diacetate	1
Ovcon 50	Ethinyl estradiol 0.05	Norethindrone	1
Ovcon 35	Ethinyl estradiol 0.35	Norethindrone	0.4
Norinyl 1/50	Mestranol 0.05	Norethindrone	1
Norinyl 1/35	Ethinyl estradiol 0.35	Norethindrone	1
Ortho-Novum 1/50			
Ortho-Novum 1/35	Ethinyl estradiol 0.35	Norethindrone	0.4
Alesse	Ethinyl estradiol 0.20	Levonorgestrel	0.1
Levlite	Ethinyl estradiol 0.20	Levonorgestrel	0.1
Levlen	Ethinyl estradiol 0.30	Levonorgestrel	0.15
Nordette	Ethinyl estradiol 0.30	Levonorgestrel	0.15
Yasmin	Ethinyl estradiol 0.30	Drosperinone	3
Combination tablets—multidose			
Biphasic			
Ortho-Novum 10/11			
Day 1–10	Ethinyl estradiol 0.035	Norethindrone	0.5
Day 11–21	Ethinyl estradiol 0.035	Norethindrone	1
Jenest-28			
Day 1–7	Ethinyl estradiol 0.35	Norethindrone	0.5
Day 8–21	Ethinyl estradiol 0.35	Norethindrone	1
Mircette			
Day 1–21	Ethinyl estradiol 0.20	Desogestrel	0.15
Day 22–26	Ethinyl estradiol 0.10	None	
Triphasic			
Tri-Norinyl			
Day 1–7	Ethinyl estradiol 0.035	Norethindrone	0.5
Day 8–16	Ethinyl estradiol 0.035	Norethindrone	1
Day 17–21	Ethinyl estradiol 0.035	Norethindrone	0.5
Day 22–28		Placebo	
Triphasil, Trilevlen			
Day 1–6	Ethinyl estradiol 0.030	Levonorgestrel	0.05
Day 7–11	Ethinyl estradiol 0.040	Levonorgestrel	0.075

(continued)

Table 33–1. Oral contraceptive agents in use. The estrogen-containing compounds are arranged in order of increasing content of estrogen (ethinyl estradiol and mestranol have similar potencies). (*continued*)

	Estrogen (mg)	Progestin (mg)	
Triphasic (cont'd)			
Day 12–21	Ethinyl estradiol 0.030	Levonorgestrel	0.125
Day 22–28		Placebo	
Ortho-Novum 7/7/7			
Day 1–7	Ethinyl estradiol 0.035	Norethindrone	0.5
Day 8–14	Ethinyl estradiol 0.035	Norethindrone	0.75
Day 15–21	Ethinyl estradiol 0.035	Norethindrone	1
Day 22–28		Placebo	
Ortho-Tri-Cyclen			
Day 1–7	Ethinyl estradiol 0.35	Norgestimate	0.180
Day 8–14	Ethinyl estradiol 0.35	Norgestimate	0.215
Day 15–21	Ethinyl estradiol 0.35	Norgestimate	0.250
Combination Estrophasic			
Estrostep Fe			
Day 1–5	Ethinyl estradiol 0.20	Norethindrone	1
Day 6–12	Ethinyl estradiol 0.30	Norethindrone	1
Day 13–21	Ethinyl estradiol 0.35	Norethindrone	1
Daily progestin tablets			
Micronor	...	Norethindrone	0.35
Nor-QD	...	Norethindrone	0.35
Ovrette	...	DL-Norgestrel	0.075

Some of the above oral contraceptives are available as generic formulations.

Postcoital or Emergency Contraception

Postcoital or emergency contraception is a therapy used to prevent unwanted pregnancy after unprotected intercourse or after a failure of a barrier method. There are various methods to achieve emergency contraception. The Yuzpe method is the most widely prescribed. It consists of two tablets, each containing ethinyl estradiol 0.05 mg and 0.5 mg norgestrel ingested 12 hours apart for a total of 4 tablets. When the therapy is initiated within 72 hours of intercourse the effectiveness is about 74%. While it is recommended to start therapy within 72 hours, there have been some studies that showed protection up to 120 hours later. Nausea occurs in 30–60% of patients who receive emergency contraception. Emesis occurs in up to 22% of patients. Some prescribers administer antiemetics 1 hour before the pills are taken. Progestin-only post-coital contraception is also available and possibly better tolerated due to less nausea with comparable success rates to combined methods. Levonorgestrel at a dose of .750 micrograms is given by mouth within 72 hours of intercourse and repeated 12 hours later. Patients are also advised to seek medical attention if menses have not begun within 21 days after treatment.

HORMONAL CONTRACEPTION BY INJECTION, IMPLANTATION OR TRANSDERMAL ROUTES

Steroid sex hormones may be injected intramuscularly to provide a depot that, depending on the drug, dosage, and formulation, may provide contraception for 1 month, 6 months, or even 1 year. A pure progestin may be used, or the injection may consist of a combination of a progestin with an estrogen. Most of these regimens prevent ovulation by suppression of anterior pituitary function.

The compound that has been most widely used worldwide for contraception is medroxyprogesterone acetate (Depo-Provera). The most extensively evaluated regimen consists of 150 mg every 90 days. This results in marked interference with the midcycle production of LH. Ovulation is suppressed, although small amounts of FSH may be produced and some ovarian follicle development may occur. Because of the marked imbalance of estrogen and progesterone produced as a consequence of pituitary suppression, the endometrium usually is atrophic, and uterine bleeding is either irregular or absent for months. For example, in sharp contrast to Norplant (an implantable contraceptive that releases levonorgestrel), about 60% of users of the injection method of progestin administration experience amenorrhea after 1 year of use. Nonetheless, contraceptive effectiveness is very high. Published failure rates of 0.3% in the first year of use indicate that this injectable form of birth control is one of the most effective available. After the injections are discontinued, there may be considerable delay in reestablishment of regular ovulation and corresponding true menstrual bleeding. However, fertility rates are essentially normal at about 18 months after discontinuation.

Approximately a twofold increased risk of premenopausal breast cancer among women under 35 years of age using medroxyprogesterone was reported in one study, although the overall risk of breast cancer in older postmenopausal users was not elevated. Whether or not this constitutes a significant risk requires confirmation in other studies.

Bone mineral density may be reduced among those who receive injections of medroxyprogesterone. Changes in bone density appear similar to those seen during lactation. Subgroups of long-term users of Depo-Provera may experience a decrease in spinal bone density that appears to be reversible following discontinuation. Side effects other than irregular bleeding that may be encountered are weight gain, headache, nervousness, abdominal discomfort, dizziness, and fatigue. An advantage of the drug is that its use is independent of coitus or a daily activity like pill taking; a disadvantage is the need for injections every 3 months.

Norplant, which is a system that contains 36 mg of levonorgestrel in each of 6 Silastic rods, is another form of progestin contraception. The Silastic rods, which are placed subdermally in the inner aspect of the upper arm, provide contraceptive protection for up to 5 years. Efficacy is high and first-year pregnancy rates are only 0.2% with cumulative 5-year rates of 3.9%. As with most progestins, pregnancy protection is likely for

many women because of ovulation inhibition. However, since a significant number of women may ovulate while using the Norplant system, other mechanisms such as thickening of the cervical mucus are also of importance.

Major potential health sequelae have not been identified in association with use of Norplant, but side effects are fairly common. Some degree of menstrual irregularity such as increased flow or spotting has been reported in up to 60% of Norplant users in the first year. However, the occurrence of such side effects is time-dependent, with the rate declining by about 50% after 1 year. Headache is cited as the reason for discontinuation of Norplant in about 20% of women. Weight change and mastalgia are also reported with varying frequency among users. Like medroxyprogesterone, a significant advantage of the system is long-term effectiveness in a method that is independent of coitus or a daily activity, eg, taking a pill. The disadvantage is the requirement that a health care provider place and remove the rods via a minor surgical procedure.

In the summer of 2000, the FDA approved a once-a-month injectable combination contraceptive containing 25 mg of medroxyprogesterone acetate and 5 mg estradiol cypionate (Lunelle). This monthly injectable method combines the convenience and contraceptive efficacy of long-acting steroids with cycle control, return to fertility, and a side effect profile more typical of combination low-dose oral contraceptives.

Three additional hormonal contraceptives methods have recently become available: The transdermal patch (Ortho Evra, Ortho-McNeil Pharmaceuticals, Inc.), the vaginal ring, (NuvaRing, Organon, Inc.) and a single rod implant system (Implanon, Organon, Inc.). The patch, measuring 20 cm^2, delivers 150 μg norelgestromin (the primary active metabolite of norgestimate) and 20 μg ethinyl estradiol daily into the circulation. It is applied once per week for 3 consecutive weeks followed by 1 week off. The contraceptive efficacy is similar to that of oral contraceptives, but compliance may be better relative to that with oral contraceptives. One disadvantage is that it may be less effective in women at or above 198 lb.

The vaginal ring is a flexible plastice device, measuring approximatley 2 inches in diameter. It is inserted for a 3 week period, then removed for 1 week during which time withdrawal bleeding is expected. The ring releases 120 μg of the etonogestrel (the major metabolite of desogestrel) and 15 μg of ethinyl estradiol daily into the circulation. The contraceptive efficacy of the ring is comparable to that of combination oral contraceptives. The ring can be expelled if improperly placed, while removing tampons, or during straining. If the ring is left out of the vagina for more than 3 hours,

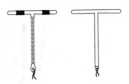

Figure 33–3. Intrauterine contraceptive devices currently available in the U.S.

then adequate protection may not occur and backup protection is required until the ring has been in place continuously for 7 days.

The single rod implant measures 40 mm long and 2 mm in diameter and releases 60 μg of etonogestrel daily. It has been shown to prevent ovulation in most women for 3 years. Adverse effects are similar to those of other progestin only methods. A change in bleeding pattern was the most frequent adverse event causing discontinuation according to one study. Weight gain was also significant in one study where the mean BMI increased by 3.5%. An advantage to the single rod system is that it allows for faster and easier insertion and removal than the six capsule system.

INTRAUTERINE CONTRACEPTIVE DEVICES

The intrauterine device (IUD or IUCD) is made of plastic or metal or a combination of these materials. It is introduced into the endometrial cavity through the cervical canal. A large variety of shapes and sizes have been tried, with varying degrees of contraceptive effectiveness.

At the present time, only 3 IUDs are available for use in the U.S.: the Progestasert, the Copper TCu380A (Paragard), and a levonorgestrel-releasing system (Mirena) (Fig 33–3). The Progestasert is made of a special polymer that contains a reservoir of 38 mg of progesterone, which is released at a rate of 65 g per day. However, due to this design, the useful lifespan of this device is only 1 year. The Paragard is wound with copper wire that creates a surface area of copper of 300 mm^2 on the vertical arms and 40 mm^2 on each of the transverse arms. The lifespan of this device is at least 10 years.

Recently, an intrauterine system containing levonorgestrel (released at 20 μg/d; Mirena) has been approved for use in the U.S. It provides contraception for up to 5 years. When compared to the copper TCu380A and Norplant, it was found to be just as effective for contraception but also more likely to cause amenorrhea, which in some patients is a benefit. Hormonal side ef-

fects such as depression, acne, headache, and weight change may also occur.

Just how IUDs act to prevent conception is not known. The most widely observed phenomenon is mobilization of leukocytes in response to the presence of the foreign body. The leukocytes aggregate around the IUD in the endometrial fluids and mucosa and, to a lesser extent, in the stroma and underlying myometrium. It is hypothesized that the leukocytes produce an environment hostile to the fertilized ovum. In laboratory animals, this leukocytic infiltration apparently is not dependent on microbial invasion. In human beings, the uterine cavity sterilizes itself, usually within 2–4 weeks after the device is inserted. Other theories regarding the mechanism of action are spermicidal activity with copper devices, disruption of endometrial maturation with the progesterone-releasing device, alteration of normal tubal cilial action, and even disruption of normal oocyte maturation. In short, the mechanism of action is not established. Furthermore, there are no data to suggest that a major mechanism of action may be that of an abortifacient.

Efficacy with the Paragard device is high, with a failure rate of less than 1% per year with prolonged use. In contrast, the Progestasert has a failure rate of about 1–1.5% with 25% of the pregnancies being ectopic. These data suggest that the latter device, unlike many contraceptive choices, offers no protection against extrauterine pregnancy.

It is felt by many practitioners that it is best to insert an IUD during a menstrual period because the cervical canal is fully patent then and the patient is least likely to be pregnant (Fig 33–4). Furthermore, the endometrial cavity may be more distensible at this time in the cycle, and uterine cramps, if they occur as a result of insertion, will be less noticeable. However, insertion can be accomplished at any other time if this is desired or more convenient for the patient.

After a pelvic examination has shown that the external and internal genitalia are normal, an antiseptic is used to cleanse the cervix. A single-toothed tenaculum is then placed on the anterior lip of the cervix and gentle traction is applied. This traction tends to reduce the angle between the cervix and the fundus and facilitates introduction of the uterine sound.

After the direction and depth of the uterine cavity have been determined by means of the sound, the device is inserted with the aid of the appropriate insertion tube. Most inserters are equipped with a guide that indicates the direction and the plane in which the device will lie when it emerges from the insertion tube into the cavity. Currently available devices are freed within the uterine cavity by withdrawal of the insertion tube over the plunger rather than by being pushed out of the

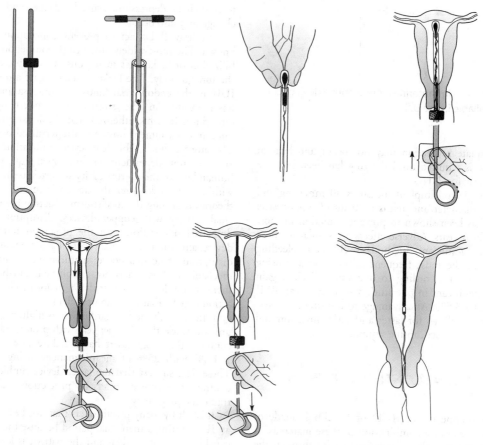

Figure 33–4. Insertion of the Paragard (TCu380A) IUD.

inserted tube and into the uterine cavity by the plunger. This withdrawal technique reduces the chances for perforation of the uterine wall.

Most IUDs have a monofilament plastic tail or strand that extends through the cervix so that the patient can feel the thread and thus be certain the device is staying in place. Moreover, the tail facilitates removal when desired.

Complications of Insertion

There may be moderate discomfort or pain when the uterus is sounded or when the IUD is inserted. In general, the larger the IUD, the more likely it is to cause pain. The pain and occasional syncopal reactions are due to dilatation of the cervical canal and distention of the endometrial cavity. Paracervical anesthesia is desirable, since both pain and syncope are significantly reduced. Mild analgesics may be helpful for several hours following IUD insertion.

Partial or complete perforation of the uterus is a rare complication of IUD insertion. It can be avoided by meticulous care in ascertaining the position and size of the uterus and by strict adherence to the recommended insertion procedure.

The presence of the IUD may elicit uterine cramps (an attempt by the uterus to rid itself of the device) for hours or days after insertion. With larger devices, the intensity of the cramps may require removal of the IUD.

Disadvantages & Side Effects

A. PREGNANCY

If pregnancy occurs and the patient wishes it to continue, the IUD may be removed by traction on the plastic tail. If gentle traction does not effect prompt and easy removal, it is probably best to leave the device in place. However, the incidence of spontaneous abortion with a device in situ is about 50%, whereas the normal incidence is 12% or higher. Removal of the IUD reduces the risk of spontaneous abortion to about 20–25% and virtually eliminates the risk of septic abortion. In patients using the copper IUDs, the risk of ectopic pregnancy is reduced twofold or more relative to patients using no contraception. Although about 5% of the pregnancies that occur with a copper IUD in situ are ectopic, the overall contraceptive action of copper IUDs reduces the risk of all pregnancies and the absolute risk of an ectopic pregnancy. Data involving the Progestasert suggests that ectopic pregnancy protection does not occur with that device; there are even some data that indicate that the risk may be 50% or more greater in comparison with that of no contraception. In large trials of Mirena, half of all pregnancies during the study were ectopic, but the rate of ectopics with Mirena was not significantly different than the rate for sexually active women not using contraception. There is no increased incidence of congenital abnormalities in babies who are conceived with the IUD in utero.

B. Expulsion

Most spontaneous expulsions of IUDs occur in the first few months after their insertion—most frequently during menstruation. The incidence of expulsion varies with the stiffness, size, and shape of the device. In general, the expulsion rate is roughly proportional to the degree of distortion of the endometrial cavity brought about by the presence of the IUD. The patient should examine herself periodically, and routinely after her menses, to be assured that the tail of the device is still present, ie, that the device is in place. If the tail cannot be felt and the patient is unaware of having expelled the device, she should see her physician. Until her appointment, alternate contraception should be used. Expulsion may have gone unnoticed, the plastic filament may have been drawn back into the cervix or endometrial cavity, the device may have perforated the uterine wall at insertion and passed into the peritoneal cavity (< 1 out of 1000 insertions), or the tail may have separated from the device and been expelled unnoticed.

The correct explanation can be found by careful inspection or by exploration of the endometrial cavity with an ultrasound examination or, if necessary, by an x-ray examination that includes an anteroposterior as well as a lateral film and use of a sound to localize the uterine cavity. (All IUDs available in the U.S. are radiopaque because of their metallic components or because they have been impregnated with barium sulfate.)

C. Bleeding or Pain

Either bleeding or pain or both are common reasons for removal of an IUD and discontinuation of this method of contraception. As is the case with expulsions, the incidence of pain or bleeding is more or less proportional to the degree of endometrial compression and myometrial distention brought about by the IUD. Thus, an IUD that conforms to the natural size and shape of the endometrial cavity is likely to cause less pain or bleeding than one that distorts the cavity and the uterine wall. Nevertheless, bleeding may increase with the copper IUD, but decreases with Mirena.

D. Pelvic Infection

A number of epidemiologic studies have documented the association between IUD use and pelvic inflammatory disease or salpingitis. However, more recent studies that have controlled for risk factors associated with salpingitis have better clarified the extent of risk. It appears that the highest risk (3- to 4-fold increase) occurs around the time of insertion, suggesting that endometrial cavity contamination in the presence of a foreign body (the IUD) is the major mechanism. No evidence of an increased risk of salpingitis is found 3–4 months after insertion or thereafter in women who don't have risk factors for STDs or salpingitis. In addition, it appears that women at risk for STDs, ie, those with multiple sexual partners or prior STDs, have a higher risk of infection than other women. However, a recent review of the literature indicates that the evidence concerning IUD-associated infection and infertility may be exaggerated.

Infection with *Actinomyces israelii,* an anaerobic, gram-positive bacteria, has been reported in association with IUD use. Most diagnoses have been made using the appearance of colonies on cervicovaginal Papanicolaou (Pap) smears due to the difficulty of culturing the organism. When *A israelii* is detected on PAP smear, antibiotic treatment is recommended (ampicillin, 250 mg four times a day for 14 days), and if the repeat PAP smear is positive, the IUD should be removed.

Contraindications to the Use of IUDs

Absolute contraindications to IUD use are current pregnancy; undiagnosed abnormal vaginal bleeding; acute cervical, uterine, or salpingeal infection; past salpingitis; and suspected gynecologic malignancy. Relative contraindications include nulliparity or high priority attached to future childbearing; prior ectopic pregnancy; history of STDs; multiple sexual partners; moderate or severe dysmenorrhea; congenital anomalies of the uterus or other abnormalities such as leiomyomas; iron deficiency anemia (for the copper IUD); valvular heart disease; frequent expulsions or problems with prior IUD use; age younger than 25 years (due to higher prevalence of *Chlamydia* infections); and Wilson's disease (if a copper IUD is contemplated).

Suitable Candidates for an IUD

The most suitable candidates for IUD use are parous women in a mutually monogamous relationship who do not have a current or prior history of STDs or salpingitis. Other potential candidates include women desiring a method of high efficacy that is free of daily or coitally related activity and women who cannot use hormonal contraception due to side effects or medical conditions. Studies among diabetic IUD users have shown that use is highly effective with no increase in rate of pelvic infection.

Finally, it should be noted that several surveys of women using contraceptives indicate that IUD users are highly satisfied with their method.

Indications for Removal of an IUD

The major reason for IUD removal is desire for pregnancy. Medical reasons for removal are partial expulsion, usually occurring in the first few months of use; persistent cramping, bleeding, or anemia, accounting for about 20% of removals during the first 3 months; acute salpingitis or *Actinomyces* infection on Pap smear; pregnancy (for the reasons previously cited); intra-abdominal placement/perforation; and significant postinsertion pain, which may indicate improper placement or partial perforation.

■ INDUCED ABORTION

Induced abortion is the deliberate termination of pregnancy in a manner that ensures that the embryo or fetus will not survive. Attitudes of society toward elective abortion have undergone marked changes in the past few decades. In some situations the need for abortion is accepted by most people, but political and medical attitudes regarding induced abortion have continued to lag behind changing philosophies. Some religious concepts remain unchanged, resulting in personal, medical, and political conflicts.

About one-third of the world's population lives in nations with nonrestrictive laws governing abortion. Another third live in countries with moderately restrictive abortion laws, ie, where unwanted pregnancies may not be terminated as a matter of right or personal decision but only on broadly interpreted medical, psychologic, and sociologic indications. The remainder live in countries where abortion is illegal without qualification or is allowed only when the woman's life or health would be severely threatened if the pregnancy were allowed to continue.

An estimated 1 out of every 4 pregnancies in the world is terminated by induced abortion, making it perhaps the most common method of reproduction limitation. In the U.S., estimates of the number of criminal abortions performed prior to legalization of the procedure ranged from 0.25–1.25 million per year. The number of legal abortions now being performed in this country approximates 1 abortion per 4 live births. In 1997, there were 1.33 million induced abortions compared to 3.88 million live births.

The procedures being used in the U.S. for legally induced abortions during the first trimester are relatively safe. Table 33–2 shows that first-trimester legal abortions are consistently safer for the woman than if she used no birth control method and gave birth. Note also in Table 33–2 that whereas the number of maternal deaths related to births steadily increased from 5.6 to 22.6 per 100,000 women as age increased, age-related increase in number of deaths per 100,000 women per year from legal abortions was insignificant.

In general, the risk of death from legal abortion is lowest when it is performed at 8 menstrual weeks or sooner. Table 33–3 shows the relationship between death due to legal abortion and the gestational age at the time of the procedure.

Paracervical anesthesia has replaced general anesthesia in many health settings, resulting in fewer complica-

Table 33–2. Pregnancy-related deaths per 100,000 women per year in developed countries compared with deaths resulting from legal abortion as a means of contraception.

Type of Birth Control	Age Groups (Years)					
	15–19	20–24	25–29	30–34	35–39	40–44
No birth control; birth related	5.6	6.1	7.4	13.9	20.8	22.6
First trimester abortion only; method related	1.2	1.6	1.8	1.7	1.9	1.2

(Adapted from Tietze C: Induced abortion: 1977 supplement, Table 11. Rep Popul Fam Plann 1977; 14[2nd ed. Suppl]:16.)

Table 33–3. Death-to-case for legal abortions by weeks of gestation (USA, 1972–1975).

Weeks of Gestation	Deaths per 100,000 Procedures
8 or less	0.7
9–10	1.9
11–12	4.1
13–15	7.5
16–20	19.6
21 or more	22.9

(Adapted from Tyler CW Jr: In: *Abortion Surveillance, 1975.* Center for Disease Control, United States Department of Health, Education, and Welfare Annual Summary 1975, April 1977, p. 36.)

tions related to anesthesia. Midtrimester abortion techniques are still problematic and are associated with a higher mortality rate. Hysterectomy carries a far greater risk than induction of labor by amnioinfusion or dilatation and evacuation.

Legal Aspects of Induced Abortion in the United States

The United States Supreme Court ruled in 1973 (1) that the restrictive abortion laws in the U.S. were invalid, largely because these laws invaded the individual's right to privacy, and (2) that an abortion could not be denied to a woman in the first 3 months of pregnancy. The Court indicated that after 3 months a state may "regulate the abortion procedure in ways that are reasonably related to maternal health" and that after the fetus reaches the stage of viability (about 24 weeks) the states may refuse the right to terminate the pregnancy except when necessary for the preservation of the life or health of the mother. Still, much opposition is raised by various "right-to-life" groups and religious groups. In spite of this opposition, over 1 million procedures are still performed annually in the United States, with about one-third being performed on teenaged women. This dramatically emphasizes the inadequacy of sex education and the need for greater availability of adequate contraceptive methods in order to avoid such pregnancy wastage.

The patient must be informed regarding the nature of the procedure and its risks, including possible infertility or even continuation of pregnancy. The rights of the spouse, parents, or guardian must also be considered and permission obtained when indicated (until the individual woman's rights are clearly established).

State laws must be obeyed with special reference to residence, duration of pregnancy, indications for abortion, consent, and consultations required.

Evaluation of Patients Requesting Induced Abortion

Patients give varied reasons for requesting abortion. Since in some cases the request is made at the urging of the woman's parents or in-laws, husband, or peers, every effort should be made to ascertain that the patient herself desires abortion for her own reasons. In addition, one should be certain that she knows she is free to choose among other methods of solving the problem of unplanned pregnancy, eg, adoption or single-parent rearing.

Although the majority of abortions are performed as elective procedures, ie, because of social or economic reasons as opposed to medical reasons, some women still request such services for medical or surgical indications. For example, for women with certain medical conditions, such as Eisenmenger's complex and cystic fibrosis, continuation of pregnancy may pose a threat to the life of the mother. Other indications are pregnancy resulting from a rape or pregnancy with a fetus affected with a major disorder, eg, trisomy 13. In any event, the ultimate decision rests with the pregnant woman.

Help from social agencies should be made available as necessary. A complete social history, medical history, and physical examination are required. Particular attention must be given to uterine size and position; the importance of accurate calculation of the duration of pregnancy (within 2 weeks but preferably within 1 week) cannot be overstated. With uncertainty, pelvic sonography should be used liberally. Routine laboratory tests should include pregnancy tests, urinalysis, hematocrit, Rh typing, serologic tests for syphilis, culture for gonorrhea, and Pap smear.

Methods of Induced Abortion

Numerous methods are used to induce an abortion: suction or surgical curettage; induction of labor by means of intra- or extraovular injection of a hypertonic solution or other oxytocic agent; dilatation and evacuation; extraovular placement of devices such as catheters, bougies, or bags; hysterotomy—abdominal or vaginal; hysterectomy—abdominal or vaginal; and menstrual regulation.

The method of abortion used is determined primarily by the duration of pregnancy, with consideration for the patient's health, the experience of the physician, and the available physical facilities.

Suction curettage on an outpatient basis under local or light general anesthesia can be accomplished with a

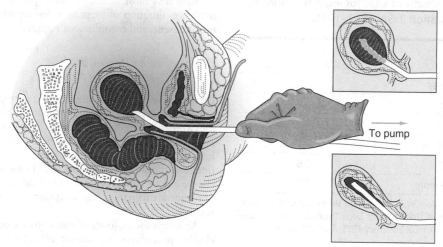

Figure 33–5. Suction method for induced abortion.

high degree of safety. The safety of outpatient abortion and the shortage of hospital beds have led to the development of single-function, "free-standing" abortion clinics. In addition to providing more efficient counseling and social services, these clinics have effectively reduced the cost of abortion. Many hospitals have "short-stay units," that match the efficiency of the outpatient clinics but also offer the back-up facilities of the general hospital.

A. Suction Curettage

Suction curettage is the safest and most effective method to terminate pregnancies of 12 weeks' duration or less. This technique has gained rapid worldwide acceptance, and over 90% of induced abortions in the U.S. are now performed by this method. The procedure involves dilatation of the cervix by instruments or by hydrophilic *Laminaria* tent (see following text), followed by the insertion of a suction cannula of the appropriate diameter into the uterine cavity (Fig 33–5). Standard negative pressures used are in the range of 30–50 mm Hg. Many physicians follow aspiration with light instrumental curettage of the uterine cavity.

The advantages of suction over surgical curettage are that the former empties the uterus more rapidly, minimizes blood loss, and reduces the likelihood of perforation of the uterus. However, failure to recognize perforation of the uterus with a cannula may result in serious damage to other organs. Knowledge of the size and position of the uterus and the volume of the contents is mandatory for safe suction curettage. Moreover, extreme care and slow minimal dilatation of the cervix, with special consideration for the integrity of the internal os, should prevent injury to the cervix or uterus. At-

tention to the decrease in uterine size that occurs with rapid evacuation helps to avoid uterine injury.

When performed in early pregnancy by properly trained physicians, suction curettage should be associated with a very low failure rate; the complication rate should be under 1% for infection, about 2% for excessive bleeding, and under 1% for uterine perforation. The risk of major complications such as persistent fever, hemorrhage requiring transfusion, and unintended major surgery ranges between 0.2% and 0.6% and is proportional to pregnancy duration. The incidence of mortality for suction curettage is about 1 in 100,000 patients.

B. Surgical Curettage

Surgical ("sharp") curettage has been used for first-trimester abortion in the absence of suction curettage equipment. This procedure is performed as a standard D&C, such as for the diagnosis of abnormal uterine bleeding or for the removal of endometrial polyps. The blood loss, duration of surgery, and likelihood of damage to the cervix or uterus are greatly increased when surgical curettage is used. In addition, the risk of uterine synechiae or Asherman's syndrome is also increased with this approach. Accordingly, suction curettage is generally preferred over sharp curettage for carrying out first-trimester termination procedures.

C. Medical Abortion with Methotrexate and Misoprostol

Women with first trimester pregnancies less than 49 days from their first day of the last menstrual period may be eligible for medical abortion. The protocol consists of intramuscular methotrexate (50 mg/m^2) given on day 1 and then misoprostol (prostaglandin E$_1$) 800 μg inserted vaginally on day 5, 6, or 7. Suction curettage may be required if the pregnancy appears viable 2 weeks after methotrexate, if a gestational sac persists 4 weeks after methotrexate, or at any time for excessive bleeding. In a study of 659 women, only 13% required a suction curettage.

D. Induction of Labor
By Intra-Amniotic Instillation

The Japanese developed this technique for induced abortion after the first trimester. Currently, it is used almost exclusively for initiating midtrimester abortion. The original procedure was to perform amniocentesis, aspirate as much fluid as possible, and then instill into the amniotic sac 200 mL of hypertonic (20%) sodium chloride solution. In most (80–90%) cases, spontaneous labor and expulsion of the fetus and placenta would occur within 48 hours. Modifications of this technique have developed, primarily to reduce the injection-abortion interval, and as a result of the development of other agents that initiate labor when instilled intra-amniotically.

Because of the problems associated with hypertonic sodium chloride, many clinicians have used intra-amniotic hyperosmolar (59.7%) urea, usually with oxytocin or prostaglandin or intra-amniotic prostaglandin alone. These approaches result in injection-abortion intervals of 16–17 hours for urea and 19–22 hours for prostaglandin. The urea is instilled in a fashion similar to that described for hypertonic sodium chloride; the prostaglandin, most frequently PGF$_{2\alpha}$, is usually instilled as a single dose of 40–50 mg or as 2 doses of 25 mg instilled 6 hours apart. When using oxytocin to augment these agents, note that because of the relative insensitivity of the myometrium to oxytocin at this stage of pregnancy, doses as high as 332 mU/min are required to produce uterine contractions. To avoid water intoxication, the oxytocin is made up in highly concentrated solutions and given at slow rates.

It is advantageous to soften the unripe cervix with *Laminaria* tents placed in the cervix a few hours before amniocentesis is performed. Such an approach markedly reduces the risk of cervical injury.

Midtrimester induced abortion by this method must be done with scrupulous aseptic surgical technique, and the patient must be monitored until the fetus and placenta are delivered and postabortion bleeding is under control. The complication rate is high—up to 20% in some institutions—and the mortality rate is comparable to that of term parturition. Fortunately, because first-trimester abortion is now more readily available, more women are consulting their physicians early and

thus availing themselves of the much safer suction curettage.

Several types of complications are associated with the use of instillation agents. Retained placenta is the most common problem; rates ranging from 13–46% have been reported. The placenta can usually be removed with ring forceps and large curets without difficulty with the patient under local anesthesia. Hemorrhage may be caused by retained products or atony; coagulopathy is seen in up to 1% of patients in whom hypertonic sodium chloride is used. Infection can also be encountered, but is reduced significantly by the use of prophylactic antibiotics in high-risk situations, eg, in patients with early ruptured membranes and during injection-abortion intervals greater than 24 hours. Cervical laceration can also occur; a complication that is reduced by the use of *Laminaria* tents. Hypernatremia can occur with the use of hypertonic sodium chloride if the drug is absorbed rapidly by the placental bed or if it is given intravascularly by mistake.

Failure of labor to expel the products of conception necessitates either a repetition of the procedure if the membranes are still intact or oxytocin stimulation, usually by intravenous injection or use of the dilatation and evacuation technique.

Emotional stress is an important factor for many women, since they are awake at the time of the expulsion of the fetus and the fetus is well formed. (The emotional stress is also a factor for hospital personnel—a problem impossible to avoid.)

E. Induction of Labor
With Vaginal Prostaglandins

Prostaglandin E$_2$ given intravaginally can also be used to induce midtrimester abortion. Vaginal suppositories containing 20 mg are used every 3–4 hours until abortion occurs; the presence or absence of labor determines whether to stop the prostaglandin E$_2$. Misoprostol, a synthetic prostaglandin E$_1$ analog is also utilized. Treatment-abortion intervals, rates of incomplete abortion, and complications are similar to those described for instillation agents. The major disadvantages are significant gastrointestinal side effects, a higher incidence of live abortion, and a more frequent occurrence of fever.

F. Dilatation and Evacuation

This technique for inducing midtrimester abortion is essentially a modification of suction curettage. Because fetal parts are larger at this stage of pregnancy, serial placement of *Laminaria* tents is used by most operators to effect cervical dilatation with less likelihood of injury. Larger suction cannulas and specially designed forceps are used to extract tissue. In most instances, the operation can be performed in the outpatient setting using paracervical block anesthesia and intravenous sedation on patients with pregnancies of up to 18 weeks' gestation. Complications include hemorrhage (usually due to atony or laceration), perforation, and rarely infection. Retained tissue is uncommon, especially when careful inspection of tissue for completion is carried out at the end of each procedure. Compared with instillation techniques or vaginal prostaglandin, the overall incidence of complications (in pregnancies up to 18 weeks' gestation) is less with dilatation and evacuation. In addition, the technique is preferred by most patients because it is an outpatient procedure and the woman does not undergo labor.

G. HYSTEROTOMY AND HYSTERECTOMY

The use of hysterotomy and hysterectomy is currently reserved for special circumstances such as in failure to complete a midtrimester abortion due to cervical stenosis or in the management of other complications. Both approaches, compared with other techniques discussed, have unacceptably high rates of morbidity and mortality and neither should be used as a primary method.

H. MENSTRUAL REGULATION

Menstrual regulation consists of aspiration of the endometrium within 14 days after a missed menstrual cycle or within 42 days after the beginning of the last menstrual period by means of a small cannula attached to a source of low-pressure suction such as a syringe or other suction machine. This is a simple and safe procedure that can be readily performed in the office or outpatient clinic, usually without any anesthetic, although paracervical block can be used if necessary. Menstrual regulation was used extensively in the 1970s and 1980s before reliable, inexpensive, and sensitive urine pregnancy tests were available. It offered a safe early approach to pregnancy termination; however, about 40% of women were not pregnant at the time of the procedure. With the advent of urine pregnancy tests that have the ability to document pregnancy even before a missed menstrual period, standard first-trimester suction curettage is probably more widely used. Complications are similar to those described for suction curettage except that persistent pregnancy is more common, particularly when very early menstrual regulation procedures are performed.

I. RU-486

RU-486 (mifepristone) is a synthetic drug developed by French pharmacologists, which acts at least partially as an antiprogestational agent. When given orally in conjunction with a prostaglandin such as misoprostol, it effects first-trimester abortion. Complications include failure to terminate a pregnancy, incomplete abortion, and significant uterine cramping.

Follow-up of Patients After Induced Abortion

Follow-up care after all procedures must be ensured. After abortion by all methods, human Rh_o (D) immune globulin (Rh_oGAM) should be administered promptly if the patient is Rh-negative, unless it is known that the male partner was Rh-negative. The patient should take her temperature several times daily and report fever or unusual bleeding at once. She should avoid intercourse or the use of tampons or douches for at least 2 weeks. The physician should discuss with the patient the possibility that emotional depression, similar to that following term pregnancy and delivery, may occur after induced abortion. Follow-up care should include pelvic examination to rule out endo- and parametritis, salpingitis, failure of involution, or continued uterine growth. Finally, effective contraception should be made available according to the patient's needs and desires.

Long-Term Sequelae of Induced Abortion

A large number of studies have been conducted during the past 2 decades to examine the possible long-term sequelae of elective induced abortion. Most of the attention has focused on subsequent reproductive function; unfortunately, many of the studies have had inherent biases and serious methodologic flaws. Despite these problems, enough information is available to provide relative estimates of potential risks. Data from some studies suggest that midtrimester pregnancy loss is more common in women who have undergone 2 or more induced or spontaneous abortions. However, women who have undergone one procedure have essentially the same risk as women who have experienced a single term pregnancy. Regarding low birthweight, only women who have undergone a first-trimester procedure by sharp curettage under general anesthesia appear to have increased risks. The reason for this association might be related to the method of dilatation used. Finally, studies that have examined both ectopic pregnancy and infertility have failed to show any consistent association between these adverse events and prior induced abortion.

REFERENCES

General

Knopp RH, LaRosa JC, Burkman RT: Contraception and dyslipidemia. Am J Obstet Gynecol 1993;(6 pt 2):1994.

Kubba A et al: Contraception. Lancet 2000;356:1913.

Lethbridge DJ: Coitus interruptus. Considerations as a method of birth control. J Obstet Gynecol Neonatal Nurs 1991;20:80.

Loriaux DL, Wild RA: Contraceptive choices for women with endocrine complications. Am J Obstet Gynecol 1993; 168:2021.

Martin JA, Hamilton BE, Ventura SJ: Births: Preliminary data for 2000. Natl Vital Stat Rep 2001;49:1.

Mishell DR: Contraception. N Engl J Med 1989;320:777.

Contraception in the Adolescent

Kahn JG, Brindis CD, Glei DA: Pregnancies averted among U.S. teenagers by the use of contraceptives. Fam Plann Perspect 1999;31:29.

Rosenfeld WD, Bassoon Swedler J: Role of hormonal contraceptives in prevention of pregnancy and sexually transmitted diseases. Adolesc Med 1992;3:207.

Lactational Amenorrhea

Vekeman M: Postpartum contraception: the lactational amenorrhea method. Eur J Contracept Reprod Health Care 1997; 2:105.

World Health Organization Task Force on Methods for the Natural Regulation of Fertility: World Health Organization Multinational Study of Breast-feeding and Lactational Amenorrhea. III. Pregnancy during breastfeeding. Fertil Steril 1999;72:431.

Condom

Smith C et al: Female barrier contraceptive. Lancet 1993;341 (8846):696.

Trussell J et al: Comparative contraceptive efficacy of the female condom and other barrier methods. Fam Plann Perspect 1994;26:66.

Diaphragms

Davidson AJ et al: Barrier contraceptives and sexually transmitted diseases in women: A comparison of female-dependent methods and condoms. Am J Public Health 1992;82:669.

Hooten TM et al: A prospective study of risk factors for symptomatic urinary tract infection in young women. N Engl J Med 1996;335:468.

Spermicidal Preparations

Jick H et al: Vaginal spermicides and congenital disorders. JAMA 1981;245:1329.

Richardson BA: Nonoxynol-9 as a vaginal microbicide for prevention of sexually transmitted infections. JAMA 2002;287: 1171–1172.

Tatum HJ, Connell-Tatum EB: Barrier contraception: a comprehensive overview. Fertil Steril 1981;36:1.

Natural Family Planning

Gray RH, Kambic RT: Epidemiologic studies of natural family planning. Hum Reprod 1988;3:693.

Hormonal Contraceptives

Audet M, Moreau M, Koltun W, Waldbaum AS, Shangold G, Fisher AC, Creasy GW. Evaluation of contraceptive efficacy and cycle control of a transdermal contraceptive patch vs an oral contraceptive. JAMA 2001;285:2347–2354.

Bottiger LE et al: Oral contraceptives and thromboembolic disease: Effects of lowering estrogen content. Lancet 1980;i:1097.

Burkman RT: Cardiovascular issues with oral contraceptives: evidenced-based medicine. Int J Fertil Womens Med 2000; 45:166.

Burkman RT: Lipid and lipoprotein changes in relation to oral contraception and hormonal replacement therapy. Fertil Steril 1988;49:39s.

Burkman RT: Oral contraceptive use and coronary and cardiovascular risk. Med Sci Sports Exerc 1996;28:11.

Cardiovascular risk of oral contraceptives. Low and mainly in women at risk. Prescrire Int 1998;7:118.

Chang CL, Donaghy M, Poulter N: Migraine and stroke in young women: case-control study. The World Health Organization Collaborative Study of Cardiovascular Disease and Steroid Hormone Contraception. Br Med J 1999;318:13.

Clarkson TB et al: Oral contraceptives and coronary artery atherosclerosis of cynomolgus monkeys. Obstet Gynecol 1990;75:217.

Croft P, Hannaford PC: Risk factors for acute myocardial infarction in women: Evidence from the Royal College of General Practitioners' Oral Contraception Study. Br Med J 1989; 298:165.

Croxatto HB, Urbancsek J, Massai R, Coelingh-Bennink H, van Beek A, and the Implanon Study Group. A multicentre efficacy and safety study of the single contraceptive implant Implanon. Hum Reprod. 1999;14:976–981.

Darney PD. Implantable contraception. Eur J Contracept Reprod Health Care. 2000;5(suppl 2):2–11.

Gerstman BB et al: Oral contraceptive estrogen dose and the risk of deep venous thromboembolic disease. Am J Epidemiol 1991;133:32.

Hannaford P: Health consequences of combined oral contraceptives. Br Med Bull 2000;56:749.

Huggins GR, Zucker PK: Oral contraceptives and neoplasia: 1987 update. Fertil Steril 1987;47:733.

Institute of Medicine: *Oral Contraceptives and Breast Cancer*. National Academy Press, 1991.

Kaufman DW et al: Decreased risk of endometrial cancer among oral contraceptive users. N Engl J Med 1980;303:1045.

Kleerekoper M et al: Oral contraceptive use may protect against low bone mass. Arch Intern Med 1991;151:1971.

Le J, Tsourounis C. Implanon: a critical review. Ann Pharmacother. 2001;35:329–336.

Makarainen L, van Beek A, Tuomivaara L, Aplund B, Coelingh-Bennink H. Ovarian function during the use of a single contraceptive implant: Implanon compared with Norplant. Fertil Steril. 1998;69:714–721.

Mulders TMT, Dieben TO. Use of the novel combined contraceptive vaginal ring NuvaRing for ovulation inhibition. Fertil Steril. 2001;75:865–870.

Ory H: The noncontraceptive health benefits for moral contraceptive use. Fam Plann Perspect 1982;14:182.

Rosenberg L et al: Myocardial infarction and cigarette smoking in women younger than 50 years of age. JAMA 1985;253:2965.

Rosenberg L et al: A case-control study of the risk of breast cancer in relation to oral contraceptive use. Am J Epidemiol 1992;136:1437.

Shoupe D et al: The significance of bleeding patterns in Norplant implant users. Obstet Gynecol 1991;77:256.

Stadel BV: Oral contraceptives and premenopausal breast cancer in nulliparous women. Contraception 1988;38:287.

Stampfer MJ et al: Past use of oral contraceptives and cardiovascular disease: A meta-analysis in the context of the Nurses' Health Study. Am J Obstet Gynecol 1990;163:285.

Thomas DB: Oral contraceptives and breast cancer: Review of the epidemiologic literature. Contraception 1991;43:597.

Thorogood M et al: Fatal stroke and use of oral contraceptives: Findings from a case-control study. Am J Epidemiol 1992;136:35.

Yuzpe AA, Lancee WI: Ethinyl estradiol and dl-norgestrel as a post-coital contraceptive. Fertil Steril 1977;28:932.

Intrauterine Contraceptive Devices

Alvarez F et al: New insights on the mode of action of intra-uterine contraceptive devices in women. Fertil Steril 1988; 49:768.

Barbosa I, Olsson SE, Odlind V, Goncalves T, Coutinho E. Ovarian function after seven years' use of a levonorgestrel IUD. Adv Contracept 1995;11:85–95.

Burkman RT et al: The relationship of genital tract *Actinomycetes* and the development of pelvic inflammatory disease. Am J Obstet Gynecol 1982;143:585.

Burkman RT and the Women's Health Study: Association between intrauterine device and pelvic inflammatory disease. Obstet Gynecol 1981;57:269.

Keebler C, Chatwani A, Schwartz R: Actinomycosis infection associated with intrauterine contraceptive devices. Am J Obstet Gynecol 1983;145:596.

Lee NC, Rubin GL, Borucki R: The intrauterine device and pelvic inflammatory disease revisited: New results from the Women's Health Study. Obstet Gynecol 1988;72:1.

Lee NC et al: Type of intrauterine device and the risk of pelvic inflammatory disease. Obstet Gynecol 1983;62:1.

Sivin I, Schmidt F: Effectiveness of IUDs: A review. Contraception 1987;36:55.

Sivin I, Tatum HJ: Four years' experience with the TCU 380A intrauterine contraceptive device. Fertil Steril 1981;36:159.

Tatum HJ, Connell EB: A decade of intrauterine contraception: 1976–1986. Fertil Steril 1986;46:173.

Zinger M, Thomas MA. Using the levonorgestrel IUS. Contemp OB/GYN. May 2001;35–48.

Induced Abortion

Burkman RT et al: Hyperosmolar urea for elective midtrimester abortion: Experience in 1913 cases. Am J Obstet Gynecol 1978;131:10.

Centers for Disease Control: Mortality Vital Statistics. Vol. 37, No. 6 (Suppl). Sept 30, 1988, p. 42. U.S. Dept. of Health and Human Services.

Couzinet B et al: Termination of early pregnancy by the progesterone antagonist RU 486 (mifepristone). N Engl J Med 1986;315:1565.

Grimes DA, Cates W Jr: The comparative efficacy and safety of intraamniotic prostaglandin $F_{2\alpha}$ and hypertonic saline for second-trimester abortion: A review and critique. J Reprod Med 1979;22:248.

Grimes DA, Cates W Jr: Complications from legally-induced abortion: A review. Obstet Gynecol Surv 1979;34:177.

Grimes DA et al: Midtrimester abortion by dilatation and evacuation: A safe and practical alternative. N Engl J Med 1977;296:1141.

Grimes DA et al: Local versus general anesthesia: Which is safer for performing suction curettage abortions? Am J Obstet Gynecol 1979;135:1030.

Hogue CJW, Cates W, Tietze C: The effects of induced abortion on subsequent reproduction. Epidemiol Rev 1982;4:66.

Peyron R et al: Early termination of pregnancy with mifepristone (RU 486) and the orally active prostaglandin misoprostol. N Engl J Med 1993;328:1509.

Segal SJ: Mifepristone (RU 486). N Engl J Med 1990;322:691.

Benign Disorders of the Vulva & Vagina

Tricia E. Markusen, MD, & David L. Barclay, MD

Benign vulvar and vaginal disorders are common in the practice of gynecology. These disorders may present with significant clinical symptoms or may be asymptomatic and noted only during routine examination. A thorough understanding of vulvar and vaginal pathophysiology is therefore of clinical importance in diagnosing and treating these disorders. This chapter reviews the predisposing factors that contribute to the development of these disorders as well as the evaluation, diagnosis, and treatment of the different benign vulvovaginal disorders. The premalignant and invasive vulvar and vaginal disorders are discussed in Chapter 46.

ANATOMY & PHYSIOLOGY

The anatomy of the vagina and vulva is described in Chapter 2. The development of vulvar and vaginal disorders is influenced in part by the presence or absence of endogenous and exogenous estrogen. Estrogen thickens the vaginal epithelium and results in large quantities of glycogen being present in the epithelial cells. The collection of intraepithelial glycogen results in the production of lactic acid. This acid environment (pH of 3.5–4.0) promotes the growth of normal vaginal flora, chiefly lactobacilli and acidogenic corynebacteria. *Candida* organisms may be present, but in small quantities only, due to the preponderance of the bacteria. The absence of endogenous estrogen in prepubertal girls results in a thin vaginal epithelium, which predisposes this age group most commonly to bacterial infections. In the postmenopausal women endogenous estrogen production declines, the cells of the vaginal epithelium and vulvar skin lose glycogen, and the vaginal acidity declines. The resulting atrophic vaginal and vulvar tissue is prone to trauma and infection, and the lactobacilli are replaced by a mixed flora consisting chiefly of pathogenic cocci. Vulvar irritation also occurs with urinary and fecal soiling, which can be an underlying factor in this age group.

EVALUATION

Evaluation of a patient with vulvar and/or vaginal symptoms requires a detailed history and physical exam, including inspection of other mucosal and skin surfaces. Specific questions regarding symptoms of vulvar or vaginal pain, itching, discharge, and previous infections should be elicited. Sexual activity, the use of feminine hygiene products (douching, soaps, perfumes), and medications (oral contraceptive pills, antibiotics) can alter the normal vaginal flora. Any underlying medical conditions, such as diabetes, can impact the development of certain vulvovaginal disorders. Overlying garments made of synthetic fabrics that retain heat and moisture can exacerbate vulvovaginal symptoms.

The first symptom of vaginal irritation is often vulvar pruritus, which often results from contact with vaginal discharge. Any variance from the normal, physiologic milky vaginal discharge should be noted. Before menarche, there may be a scant vaginal discharge that normally does not cause irritation and is not considered abnormal. Inspection in the adolescent girl may reveal a small amount of white mucoid material in the vaginal vault that is the result of normal desquamation and accumulation of vaginal epithelial cells. The most common cause of leukorrhea (vaginal discharge) is a vaginal infection. The presence or absence of odor, pruritus, and the color can help determine the etiology.

A vaginal discharge is considered abnormal by the patient if there is an increase in the volume (especially if there is soiling of the clothing), an objectionable odor, or a change in consistency or color. Specific characteristics depend on the cause (Table 34–1). Secondary irritation of the vulvar skin may be minimal or extensive, causing pruritus or dyspareunia. Ideally, evaluation should occur after the onset of symptoms if the patient is not menstruating. She should be instructed not to douche. After the clinical history is obtained, the vulva, vagina, and cervix should be thoroughly inspected (Table 34–2). The pH of the vaginal secretions in the speculum blade should be determined, and a small amount of secretion should be placed on each of two glass slides. One slide should be treated with 10% room-temperature potassium hydroxide and the other diluted with room-temperature normal saline. A transient "fishy odor" after application of the potassium hydroxide is characteristic of bacterial vaginosis, the "sniff

Table 34–1. Diagnosis of major causes of vaginitis.

	Symptom	pH	Discharge	Wet Smear
Candida	Pruritus	4.0–5.0	Thick, curdy	Hyphae
Tricho-monas	Discharge	5.0–7.0	Thin, copious	Motile pro-tozoa
Bacterial vaginosis	Odor	4.0–6.0	Scant, nonir-ritating	Clue cells

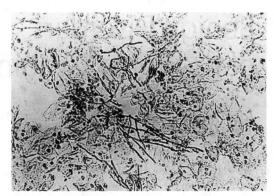

Figure 34–1. Saline wet mount demonstrating *Candida albicans.*

test" or "whiff test." White blood cells and epithelial cells are digested by the potassium hydroxide; therefore, the candidal pseudohyphae and spores are easier to detect (Fig 34–1 and Fig 34–2). Motile trichomonads may be detected under low power on the saline-diluted slide (Fig 34–3). Bacterial vaginosis is diagnosed with the presence of "clue cells," which are epithelial cells that have bacteria attached to their cell membranes (Fig 34–4). The relative number of white blood cells and the maturity of the epithelial cells should be determined. Patients with vaginitis or cervicitis show many white blood cells, and the presence of intermediate or basal cells indicates inflammation of the vaginal epithelium. Selective cultures may be performed for trichomoniasis, bacterial infection, and candidiasis.

VAGINAL DISORDERS (Table 34–3)

Candidiasis

It is estimated that approximately 75% of women will experience an episode of vulvovaginal candidiasis. *Candida albicans* is the most common *Candida* species, causing symptomatic candidiasis in approximately 90% of cases. *C albicans* frequently inhabits the mouth, throat, large intestine, and vagina normally. Clinical infection may be associated with a systemic disorder (diabetes mellitus, HIV, obesity), pregnancy, medication (antibiotics, corticosteroids, oral contraceptives), and chronic debilitation.

Vulvovaginal candidiasis presents with intense vulvar pruritus; a white curdlike, cheesy vaginal discharge;

Table 34–2. Diagnosis of vaginitis.

Obtain history, symptoms.
Examine vulva, vaginal walls, and cervix.
Check pH of discharge.
Prepare wet smear with saline.
Prepare potassium hydroxide smear ("sniff test").

and vulvar erythema. A burning sensation may follow urination, particularly if there is excoriation of the skin from scratching. Widespread involvement of the skin adjacent to the labia may suggest an underlying systemic illness such as diabetes. The labia minora may be erythematous, excoriated, and edematous. Clinical manifestations may worsen just prior to menses. The ubiquitous nature of the organism allows for repeated infections that may be interpreted as a chronic resistant infection. Diagnosis is based on the clinical features of the disease as well as the demonstration of candidal mycelia and a normal vaginal pH, ≤ 4.5. Identification of *C albicans* requires finding filamentous forms (pseudohyphae) of the organism (Fig 34–2) when vaginal secretions are mixed with 10% potassium hydroxide (KOH) solution. Vaginal secretions may also be cultured.

Treatment is reserved for symptomatic patients (Table 34–4). Short-term or erratic therapy is usually

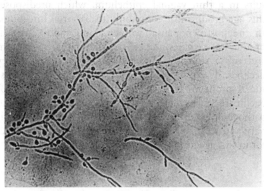

Figure 34–2. KOH preparation showing branched and budding *Candida albicans.*

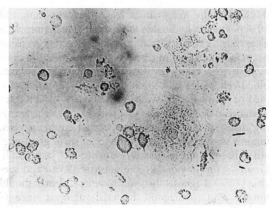

Figure 34–3. Saline wet mount with mobile trichomonads in the center.

Table 34–3. Causes of vaginitis.

Infectious
  Vulvovaginal candidiasis
  Bacterial vaginosis
  Bacterial infections
  Trichomoniasis
  Viral infections
  Desquamative inflammatory vaginitis (clindamycin responsive)
  Secondary bacterial infection associated with foreign body or atrophic vaginitis
  Parasitic
Noninfectious
  Atrophic vaginitis
  Allergic vaginitis
  Foreign body
  Desquamative inflammatory vaginitis (steroid responsive)
  Collagen vascular disease, Behçet's syndrome, pemphigus syndromes

not beneficial. Underlying metabolic illnesses (diabetes) should be well controlled, and complicating medications (antibiotics) should be discontinued if possible. Nonabsorbent undergarments should be avoided as well as douching. Multiple topical medications are available in different forms and lengths of treatment. Inclusion of a topical steroid (Mycolog, Lotrisone) may also be beneficial if the patient remains symptomatic to help decrease inflammation and relieve itching externally. Lotrisone contains a potent corticosteroid, so it should not be used extensively in pregnant women in large amounts or for a prolonged period. A single 150-mg oral dose of fluconazole has also been shown to be effective in treating symptomatic candidiasis in nonpregnant patients.

During pregnancy, vulvovaginal candidiasis may be more difficult to eradicate. The azoles have not been well studied for use during the first trimester; therefore, treatment should be avoided until the second trimester or nystatin 100,000 units, 1 tablet vaginally at night for 2 weeks, may be given during the first trimester.

Chronic or recurrent infections (4 or more infections per year) may occur in 5% of the population. Recurrent disease is more difficult to treat. Treating diges-

Table 34–4. Medications used in the treatment of vulvovaginal candidiasis.

Butoconazole 2% cream, 1 applicator vaginally, for 3–5 days
Clotrimazole 1% cream, 1 applicator (5 g) vaginally, for 7 days (14 days if chronic)
Clotrimazole 100 mg tablet, vaginally, for 7 days
Clotrimazole 100 mg tablets, 2 tablets vaginally, for 3 days
Clotrimazole 500 mg tablet, vaginally, for 1 dose
Miconazole 2% cream, 1 applicator vaginally, for 7 days
Miconazole 100 mg suppository, vaginally, for 7 days
Miconazole 200 mg suppository, vaginally, for 3 days
Tioconazole 2% cream, 1 applicator vaginally, for 3 days
Tioconazole 6.5% cream, 1 applicator vaginally, for 1 dose
Terconazole 0.4% cream, 1 applicator vaginally, for 7 days
Terconazole 0.8% cream, 1 applicator vaginally, for 3 days
Terconazole 80 mg suppository, vaginally, for 3 days
Boric acid 600 mg gelatin capsule, vaginally at night, for 2 weeks or nightly for 1 week then 2 times per week for 3 weeks
Ketoconazole 200 mg, orally 2 times per day for 5 days
Itraconazole 200 mg, orally 2 times per day for 1 day
Fluconazole 150 mg tablet, orally, for 1 day

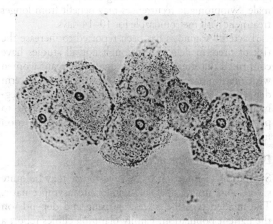

Figure 34–4. Bacterial vaginosis. Saline wet mount of clue cells. Note the absence of inflammatory cells.

tive tract *C albicans* neither improves treatment success nor decreases recurrence. Estrogen treatment as well as oral contraceptive use may precipitate infection. Treatment includes prolonging antifungal therapy from 7 to 14 days, self-medication for 3 to 5 days at the first evidence of symptoms, and prophylactic treatment for several days prior to menstruation or during antibiotic therapy. Ketoconazole 100 mg orally each day for 6 months, fluconazole 150 mg weekly for 6 months, or itraconazole 100 mg orally daily for 6 months may reduce the frequency of recurrence to 10% during maintenance therapy. Liver function tests should be monitored with the prolonged oral therapy. Treatment of the partner may be considered in cases of symptomatic balanitis. Periodic examinations should be performed to verify reinfection. In addition, chronic or recurrent infections may be secondary to *Candida tropicalis* or *Candida glabrata* infections, which are resistant to imidazole medications. In this case oral ketoconazole or fluconazole should be given. Acidification of the vagina may also help.

Bacterial Infections

In the premenarcheal and postmenopausal hypoestrogenic vagina, a mixed bacterial flora may be expected, particularly in the presence of trauma or a foreign body. Specific diagnosis can be made through stained smears and cultures, although culture reports can be misleading in the presence of mixed flora. Bacterial vaginosis, previously referred to as *Gardnerella* vaginitis or nonspecific vaginitis, is the most common cause of symptomatic bacterial infection in reproductive-age women. In bacterial vaginosis the normal vaginal flora is altered. The concentration of the hydrogen peroxide–producing lactobacilli is decreased, and there is an overgrowth of *Gardnerella vaginalis, Mobiluncus* spp., anaerobic gram-negative rods (*Prevotella* spp., *Porphyromonas* spp., *Bacteroides* spp.), and *Peptostreptococcus* spp. Other significant causes of bacterial infections are *Neisseria gonorrhoeae, Chlamydia, Mycoplasma hominis,* and *Ureaplasma urealyticum.*

Each bacterial agent is associated with characteristic symptoms. In the hypoestrogenic vagina, bacterial infection may present as discharge and spotting. Inspection of the vagina will rule out a foreign body. Microscopic examination of the vaginal secretions is necessary to detect the more common causes of vaginitis and will demonstrate intermediate and parabasal epithelial cells.

A. BACTERIAL VAGINOSIS

Bacterial vaginosis presents as a "fishy" vaginal discharge, which is more noticeable following unprotected intercourse. The patient complains of a malodorous, nonirritating discharge, and examination reveals homogeneous, gray-white secretions with a pH of 5.0–5.5. A transient "fishy" odor can be released on application of 10% potassium hydroxide to the vaginal secretions on a glass slide. A wet mount of the vaginal secretions using normal saline under microscopy demonstrates the characteristic clue cells, decreased lactobacilli, and few white blood cells. Clue cells are identified as numerous stippled or granulated epithelial cells (Fig 34–4). This appearance is caused by the adherence of the *G vaginalis* organisms to the edges of the vaginal epithelial cells. Gram's stain reveals a large number of small gram-negative bacilli and a relative absence of lactobacilli. Gram's stain provides a more sensitive (93%) and specific (70%) diagnosis than wet mount. Cultures should not be used to diagnose bacterial vaginosis since *G vaginalis* can be present in asymptomatic women. It is controversial whether bacterial vaginosis is a true sexually transmitted disease, although women who are not sexually active are rarely affected.

Treatment in symptomatic patients should be implemented and should be considered in asymptomatic patients. Treatment regimens in nonpregnant women include metronidazole 500 mg orally twice daily for 7 days, metronidazole gel 0.75% (one full applicator, 5 g) intravaginally once or twice daily for 5 days or clindamycin cream 2% (one full applicator, 5 g) intravaginally at bedtime for 7 days. (Clindamycin is oil based, so patients should be told that condoms or diaphragms might be weakened during treatment.) Alternative regimens include metronidazole 2 g orally in a single dose, clindamycin 300 mg orally twice daily for 7 days or clindamycin ovules 100g intravaginally once at bedtime for 3 days. In pregnant women, the recommended treatment is metronidazole 250 mg orally three times daily for 7 days. Alternatively, clindamycin 300 mg orally twice daily for 7 days, can be given. Existing data do not support the use of topical agents during pregnancy. Treatment of the male does not help in preventing recurrence in the female. Symptomatic recurrences may benefit from longer treatment with metronidazole for 10–14 days.

Bacterial vaginosis has been reported to increase the risk of preterm delivery, although not all studies have confirmed that treating asymptomatic pregnant women with metronidazole reduces the occurrence of preterm delivery or adverse pregnancy outcomes. In nonpregnant women, bacterial vaginosis has been related to post-hysterectomy vaginal cuff cellulitis, post-abortion infection, and pelvic inflammatory disease.

B. NEISSERIA GONORRHOEAE

Symptoms of infection by *N gonorrhoeae* may be quite severe, but up to 85% of women are asymptomatic. The incidence of the disease is rising and depends on the patient population. Family planning clinics report a 10% prevalence; private practitioners report 2–3%. The glandular structures of the cervix, urethra, vulva, perineum, and anus are most commonly infected. Although clinically evident infection of the vagina is only transitory, it can be a common cause of a positive culture in post-hysterectomy patients. In acute disease, patients present with a copious mucopurulent discharge, and Gram's stain will reveal gram-negative diplococci within leukocytes. However, diagnosis should be confirmed with a culture or with nucleic acid amplification. The specimen is collected from the endocervix. Excess cervical mucus should be removed and the swab should be rotated in the endocervix. Cultures may also be taken from the urethra, rectum, and mouth. An estimated 15–20% of women with lower tract disease will develop upper tract disease presenting with salpingitis, tubo-ovarian abscess, and peritonitis. Ectopic pregnancy and infertility may result. If active infection is present during delivery, the newborn may develop conjunctivitis by contamination during vaginal delivery. Treatment for uncomplicated gonococcal infections of the cervix is with ceftriaxone 125 mg IM in a single dose. Cefixime 400 mg orally in a single dose, ciprofloxacin 500 mg orally in a single dose, ofloxacin 400 mg orally in a single dose or levofloxacin 250 mg orally in a single dose are also recommended regimens. Due to quinolone-resistant strains of N. gonorrhaeae in parts of Asia and the Pacific, quinolones are no longer recommended for patients residing in, or who may have acquired infection in Asia and the Pacific (including Hawaii). The prevalence of quinolone resistance is also increasing in California. Therefore the use of fluoroquinolones in California is probably inadvisable. Spectinomycin 2 g IM in a single dose can be given to patients sensitive to cephalosporins and quinolones. Treatment for *Chlamydia trachomatis* should be considered.

C. CHLAMYDIA TRACHOMATIS

C trachomatis infections can also be asymptomatic or present with a mucopurulent cervicitis, dysuria, and/or postcoital bleeding. Sexually active young women should be screened. *C trachomatis* can be identified by culture (50–90% sensitivity), a direct fluorescent antibody (DFA, 50–80% sensitivity) and enzyme immunoassay (EIA, 40–60% sensitivity), or most recently using nucleic acid amplification tests (PCR or LCR, 60–100% sensitivity). All tests have a specificity > 99%. *Chlamydia* can also cause an ascending infection, salpingitis, in 20–40% of untreated cases. More than 50% of upper tract infections may be due to *C trachomatis* leading to tubal occlusion, ectopic pregnancy, or infertility. *C trachomatis* can also cause neonatal conjunctivitis if untreated and atypical cytologic findings on Papanicolaou smear. *C trachomatis* may also present as lymphogranuloma venereum (LGV), which most commonly affects the vulvar tissues. Retroperitoneal lymphadenopathy may be present. The initial lesion in LGV presents as a transient, painless vesicular lesion or shallow ulcer at the inoculation site. More advanced disease is characterized by anal or genital fistulas, stricture, or rectal stenosis. The disease is uncommon in the United States but is endemic in Southeast Asia and Africa.

If *C trachomatis* is suspected or diagnosed, both the patient and partner should be treated. In addition, a concurrent gonococcal infection should be considered. Recommended therapy includes azithromycin 1 g orally in a single dose or doxycycline 100 mg orally twice daily for 7 days. Erythromycin base 500 mg orally four times daily for 7 days, ofloxacin 300 mg orally twice daily or Levofloxacin 50 mg once daily for 7 days are alternative regimens. Doxycycline, levofloxacin, and ofloxacin should be avoided in pregnancy and during lactation. Patients should abstain from intercourse for 7 days. Test of cure is required, in cases of possible reinfection or persistent symptoms and in pregnancy. Repeat testing may be considered 3 weeks after treatment with erythromycin. Women should also be rescreened 3–4 months after treatment. For LGV, the recommended regimen is doxycycline 100 mg twice daily for 21 days.

D. OTHER

Mycoplasma hominis and *Ureaplasma urealyticum* also cause genital disease. Identification using polymerase chain reaction can increase the sensitivity over culture. Mycoplasma infections may cause infertility, spontaneous abortion, postpartum fever, nongonococcal urethritis in men, and possibly salpingitis and pelvic abscess. Treatment is most effective with doxycycline 100 mg orally twice daily for 10 days.

Trichomonas Vaginitis

Trichomonas vaginalis is a unicellular flagellate protozoan (Fig 34–5). *T vaginalis* organisms are larger than polymorphonuclear leukocytes but smaller than mature epithelial cells. *T vaginalis* also infects the lower urinary tract in both women and men. It is a sexually transmitted disease; other forms of transmission are infrequent because large numbers of organisms are required to produce symptoms.

Symptoms associated with trichomoniasis are generally worse just after menstruation or during pregnancy. A persistent vaginal discharge is the principal symptom with or without secondary vulvar pruritus. The discharge is profuse, extremely frothy, greenish, and at times foul-smelling. These characteristics may be altered by prior medication use and/or douching. The pH of the vagina usually exceeds 5.0. Involvement of the vulva may be limited to the vestibule and labia minora, although a profuse discharge often causes inflammation of the labia majora, perineum, and adjacent skin surfaces. The labia minora may become edematous

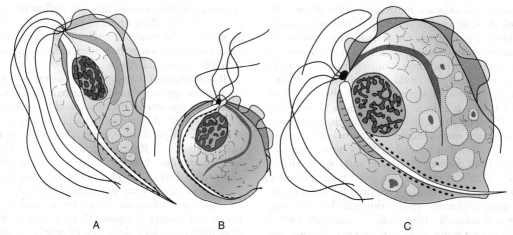

Figure 34–5. Trichomonas vaginalis as found in vaginal and prostatic secretions. **A:** Normal trophozoite. **B:** Round form after division. **C:** Common form seen in stained preparation. Cysts not found. (Reproduced, with permission, from Brooks GF, Butel JS, Ornston LN: *Jawetz, Melinick, & Adelberg's Medical Microbiology,* 19th ed. Appleton & Lange, 1991.)

and tender. Urinary symptoms may occur; however, burning with urination is most often associated with severe vulvitis, particularly if there has been excoriation of the skin from scratching. Examination of the vaginal mucosa and cervix shows generalized vaginal erythema with multiple small petechiae, the so-called strawberry spots, which may be confused with epithelial punctation. Wet mount with normal saline reveals an increase in polymorphonuclear cells and characteristic motile flagellates in 50–70% of culture-confirmed cases (Fig 34–3). Papanicolaou smears have a sensitivity of approximately 60% and may have false positives. Culture is the gold standard and provides 95% sensitivity and 100% specificity. DNA probes and monoclonal antibodies may further provide an accurate diagnosis.

Systemic therapy with metronidazole is the treatment of choice since trichomonads can be present in the urinary tract system. Most men with affected sexual partners also harbor the organism but are asymptomatic. Therefore, partners should be treated simultaneously, with intercourse avoided or a condom used until treatment is completed. Metronidazole is the only FDA-approved treatment in the United States, with cure rates of approximately 90–95%. A single-dose regimen of 2 g may assure compliance. Other regimens include a 500 mg tablet orally 2 times per day for 7 days. In resistant cases, which most likely are related to reinfection, oral metronidazole may be repeated after 4 to 6 weeks if the presence of trichomonads has been confirmed and the white blood cell count and differential are normal. Side effects of metronidazole include nausea or emesis with alcohol consumption. Contraindica-

tions include certain blood dyscrasias (neutropenia) and central nervous system diseases. An oncogenic effect has been demonstrated in animals but not humans. Other treatment options include antitrichomonal suppositories (polyoxyethylene nonyl phenol, aminacrine, sodium edetate, and docusate sodium), 1 suppository inserted deep in the vagina twice daily for 2 weeks and then at least 1 week after no organisms are identified on a vaginal smear. Although temporary relief of symptoms may occur, complete cure is rare. Resistance to metronidazole therapy is rare but is rising and can be confirmed in vitro. A maximal dose of 2 to 4 g daily of metronidazole should be given for 10 to 14 days if the patient tolerates it. If treatment fails, consultation with the Centers for Disease Control is recommended. Nonoxynol 9 and other spermicidal agents have been demonstrated to decrease the transmission of *Trichomonas.*

Trichomoniasis is associated with many perinatal complications and an increased incidence in the transmission of HIV. Women with trichomoniasis should be evaluated for other sexually transmitted diseases, including *N gonorrhoeae, C trachomatis,* syphilis, and HIV.

Viral Infections

The viruses that affect the vulva and vagina are the herpesvirus (herpes simplex, varicella, herpes zoster, molluscum contagiosum, and cytomegalovirus), poxvirus, and papovavirus types.

The viruses that affect the lower genital tract are symptomatic, primarily because of involvement of the vulvar skin. Two exceptions are the herpesvirus hominis and the human papillomavirus (HPV), which may also affect the cervix and vagina.

A. Herpesvirus

The herpesvirus (HSV) may cause superficial ulcerations or an exophytic necrotic mass involving the cervix, which may cause a profuse vaginal discharge. The cervix may be tender to manipulation and bleed easily. The primary lesion lasts 2–6 weeks and heals without scarring. Recurrent infections may also cause cervical lesions. The virus may be cultured from ulcers or ruptured vesicles. Cervical cytologic examination may reveal multinucleated giant cells with intranuclear inclusions. The herpesvirus hominis has two immunologic variants, type I and type II. In general most genital lesions are secondary to the type II virus. The type I virus is responsible for only 10–15% of genital herpes infections. Approximately 83% of patients will develop antibodies to herpesvirus type II in a minimum of 21 days following a primary infection. HSV is responsible for recurrent and disabling symptomatic disease, venereal transmission, and infection to the neonate (ie, herpes encephalitis). Further discussion of HSV is reviewed later in the chapter.

B. Human Papillomavirus

HPV is responsible for condyloma acuminata of the vagina, cervix, vulva, perineum, and perianal areas as well as for dysplasia and cancer. The HPV rate is high and is rising; approximately 30–60% of people may have had HPV infection at some point in their lives, but the gross clinical prevalence of HPV is less than 1%. The virus is small and contains all its genetic material on a single double-stranded molecule of DNA. More than 20 types of HPV have been identified using viral DNA probes that can infect the genital tract. Types 16, 18, 31, 33, and 35 appear to have the most oncogenic potential. Types 6 and 11 are associated with genital condyloma. Most types cause an asymptomatic infection. The viruses are sexually transmitted and infect both partners.

The typical lesion is an exophytic or papillomatous condyloma. Colposcopic examination permits identification of flat, spiked, and inverted condyloma (Fig 34–6). The florid, papillomatous condyloma shows a raised white lesion with fingerlike projections often containing capillaries. Although large lesions may be seen with the naked eye, the colposcope is necessary to identify smaller lesions. The flat condyloma appears as a white lesion with a somewhat granular surface; a mosaic pattern and punctation may also be present, suggesting vaginal intraepithelial neoplasia (VAIN), which

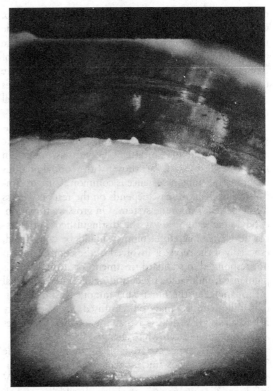

Figure 34–6. Vaginal condylomata acuminata as seen with a colposcope (× 13).

must be excluded by biopsy. Spiked lesions present as a hyperkeratotic lesion, with surface projections and prominent capillary tips. An inverted condyloma grows into the glands of the cervix but has not been identified on the vaginal mucosa. Condylomatous vaginitis causes a rough vaginal surface, demonstrating white projections from the pink vaginal mucosa. Vaginal discharge and pruritus are the most common symptom with florid condylomas. Postcoital bleeding may also occur. No specific symptoms are related to the other types of condylomas. The entire lower tract is usually involved with subclinical or florid lesions when vulvar lesions are present. States of immunosuppression (pregnancy, HIV infection, diabetes, renal transplant) are associated with massive proliferation of condyloma and are often difficult to treat. Laryngeal papilloma and vulvar condylomas in infants delivered through an infected vaginal canal have been reported; however, unlike herpetic lesions, the presence of HPV lesions is not a contraindication to a vaginal delivery.

HPV infection is also associated with dysplasia. The presence of koilocytes is pathognomonic for HPV infection. Koilocytes are superficial or intermediate cells on biopsy characterized by a large perinuclear halo. Colposcopic-directed biopsies must be taken to exclude intraepithelial neoplasia. The chief histologic difference between dysplasia and condyloma is the progression of cellular atypia. In dysplasia, the dysplastic cells move toward the surface, whereas in condyloma the changes progress from the surface inward toward the basal membrane.

Prior to treatment, a colposcope may be used to inspect the lower genital tract. Lesions may extend to the anal canal or urethral meatus. The virus is present in normal cells as well as those with condylomatous changes; therefore, recurrence is common. Cure of clinically identifiable disease depends on the responsiveness of the patient's immune system. On gross examination, condylomas cannot always be distinguished from dysplastic warts. Therefore, biopsy should be considered, especially if the cervix is involved, if the condyloma has not responded to standard treatment, or if the lesion is pigmented, indurated, fixed, and/or ulcerated. Normal micropapillae of the inner labia minora (vestibular micropapillomatosis) may be confused with papillary HPV. True HPV disease is patchy and has koilocytes and more intense acetowhite changes.

Multiple therapies are available for treatment (Table 34–5); however, it is unclear whether treatment actually affects the natural progression or eradicates HPV infection. Coexistent vulvovaginitis should be treated. Treatment should be based on patient preference and convenience. If treatment fails with an initial regimen, a different agent may be used. Patients should be informed that complications with treatment are rare but can result in scarring and pigmentation changes. Rarely

Table 34–5. Treatment of condyloma acuminata.

Applied by Provider
Bichloroacetic acid (BCA) or trichloroacetic acid (TCA), 50–80% solution

A lower percentage solution is generally applied to the cervix and vagina, a higher percentage to the vulva. One should be careful to avoid excessive amounts, which may burn normal skin. Xylocaine 1% gel may be applied around the wart to avoid damage to adjacent skin. Repeat treatments are given weekly as necessary.

Podophyllin 10–25% in tincture of benzoin

Cryosurgery, electrosurgery, simple surgical excision, laser vaporization

Applied by Patient
Podofilox 0.5% solution or gel

Imiquimod 5% cream (topically active immune enhancer that stimulates production of interferon and other cytokines)

---

can dysesthesias develop, resulting in chronic pain and/or dyspareunia.

Prevention of recurrence is difficult in patients who are immunosuppressed or receiving lifelong corticosteroid therapy. Also, examination of sex partners is not necessary as most partners are likely to have subclinical infection. The use of condoms may help in reducing transmission to partners who are not already infected.

Condylomas may also complicate pregnancy. In most cases if the lesions are small, therapy is not necessary. Treatment with trichloroacetic acid (TCA) may be applied in the last 4 weeks of pregnancy to avoid cesarean section with larger lesions. Electrocoagulation, cryotherapy, or laser therapy should be used prior to 32 weeks to avoid post-treatment necrosis, which may last as long as 4–6 weeks. Podophyllin, podofilox, and imiquimod, should not be used during pregnancy.

Atrophic Vaginitis

Prepubertal, lactating, and postmenopausal women lack the vaginal effects of estrogen production. The pH of the vagina is abnormally high, and the normally acidogenic flora of the vagina may be replaced by mixed flora. The vaginal mucosa is thinned, and the vaginal epithelium is more susceptible to infection and trauma. Although most patients are asymptomatic, many postmenopausal women report vaginal dryness, spotting, and/or dyspareunia. Some of the symptoms of irritation are caused by a secondary infection. On exam, the vaginal mucosa is thin, with few or absent vaginal folds. The pH is 5.0 to 7.0. The wet mount shows small, rounded parabasal epithelial cells and an increase in polymorphonuclear cells.

Treatment includes intravaginal application of estrogen cream. Approximately one-third of the vaginal estrogen is systemically absorbed; therefore, this treatment may be contraindicated in women with a history of breast or endometrial cancer. The estradiol vaginal ring, which is changed every 90 days, may provide a more preferable route of administration for some women, or Vagifem, 1 tablet intravaginally daily for 2 weeks and then 2 times per week for at least 3–6 months, may be less messy. Maturation of the vaginal mucosa generally eradicates a bacterial infection but may predispose the patient to a secondary trichomonal or candidal vaginitis. Systemic estrogen therapy should be considered if there are no contraindications.

Foreign Bodies

Foreign bodies commonly cause vaginal discharge and infection in preadolescent girls. Paper, cotton, or other materials may be placed in the vagina and cause secondary infection. Children may require vaginal examination under anesthesia to identify or rule out a foreign body or tumor high in the vaginal vault. The vaginal canal may also be flushed in the office using a small catheter to potentially remove a foreign body. In adults, a forgotten menstrual tampon or contraceptive device may cause a malodorous discharge. The diagnosis can usually be made by pelvic examination.

Clinical symptoms associated with foreign bodies include an abnormal vaginal discharge and intermenstrual spotting. Symptoms are generally secondary to the drying of the vaginal mucosa and micro-ulcerations, which can be detected by colposcopy. Ulcerative lesions, particularly associated with tampon use, are typically located in the vaginal fornices and have rolled, irregular edges with a red granulation tissue base (Fig 34–7). Regenerating epithelium at the ulcer edge may shed cells that may be interpreted as atypical, suggesting dysplasia. The lesions heal spontaneously once tampon use is discontinued. A foreign body retained in the vagina for a prolonged period may erode into the bladder or rectum.

Treatment involves removal of the foreign body. Rarely, antibiotics may be required for ulcerations or cellulitis of the vulva or vagina. Dryness or ulceration of the vagina secondary to use of menstrual tampons is transient and heals spontaneously.

Toxic shock syndrome (see also Chapter 38) is the most serious complication of improper use of vaginal tampons. The syndrome has been linked to staphylococcal vaginal infection in healthy young women using high-absorbency tampons continuously throughout the menstrual period. Symptoms consist of a high fever ≥ 38.9 °C (102 °F) and may be accompanied by severe headache, sore throat, vomiting, and diarrhea. The disease may resemble meningitis or viremia. Palmar erythema and a diffuse sunburn-like rash have also been described. The skin rash usually disappears within 24–48 hours, but on occasion a patient will have a recurrent maculopapular, morbilliform eruption between the sixth and tenth days. Superficial desquamation of the palms and soles often follows within 2–3 weeks. Progressive hypotension may occur and proceed to shock levels within 48 hours. Multisystem organ failure may occur, including renal and cardiac dysfunction. The incidence of toxic shock syndrome was 1 per 100,000 among women ages 15 to 44 years in 1986. Any menstruating woman who presents with sudden onset of a febrile illness should be evaluated and treated for toxic shock syndrome. The tampon should be removed, cultures sent, and the vagina cleansed to decrease the organism inoculum. Appropriate supportive

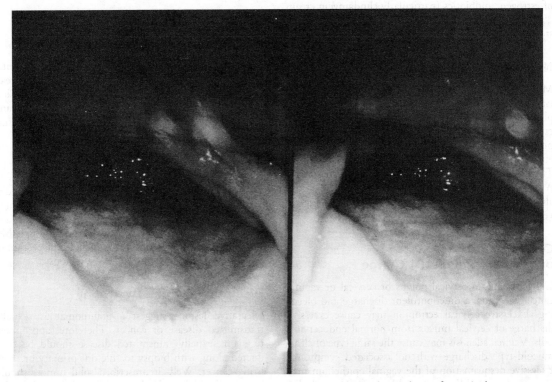

Figure 34–7. Colposcopic view of ulcer anterior to cervix caused by prolonged use of a vaginal tampon.

measures should be provided and β-lactamase-resistant penicillin or vancomycin (if the patient is allergic to penicillin) administered. Women who have been treated for toxic shock syndrome are at considerable risk for recurrence. Therefore, these women should avoid tampon use until *Staphylococcus aureus* has been eradicated from the vagina.

Desquamative Inflammatory Vaginitis

This disorder demonstrates clinical and microscopic features of postmenopausal atrophic vaginitis; however, it presents in premenopausal women with normal estrogen levels. The cause is unknown. Patients complain of a profuse purulent vaginal discharge, vaginal burning or irritation, dyspareunia, and occasional spotting. The process is patchy and usually localized to the upper half of the vagina. The purulent discharge contains many immature epithelial and pus cells not due to any identifiable cause. Vaginal erythema is present and synechiae may develop in the upper vagina, causing partial occlusion. The diagnosis is one of exclusion. Vaginal pH may be elevated, with wet mount and Gram's stain demonstrating an increased number of parabasal cells, an absence of gram-positive bacilli, and presence of gram-positive cocci, usually streptococci. Treatment is often unsatisfactory but has included local application of estrogen, antibiotics (particularly clindamycin cream 2% 5 g intravaginally daily for 7 days), and corticosteroids.

Noninfectious Vaginitis

Multiple irritating offenders, including topical irritants (sanitary supplies, spermicides, feminine hygiene supplies, soaps, perfumes), allergens (latex, antimycotic creams), and possibly excessive sexual activity can cause pruritus, irritation, burning, and vaginal discharge. The etiology may be confused with vulvovaginal candidiasis. The offending agent should be removed for treatment. A short course of corticosteroid treatment may be used along with sodium bicarbonate sitz baths and topical vegetable oils.

Cervical Mucorrhea or Vaginal Epithelial Discharge

Cervicitis due to cervical polyps or cervical or vaginal cancer can cause a mucopurulent discharge and bleeding. Excessive cervical ectropion may cause excessive discharge of cervical mucus from normal endocervical cells. Vaginal adenosis may cause the same type of clear, mucoid-type discharge with no associated symptoms. Excessive desquamation of the vaginal epithelium may also produce a diffuse gray-white pasty vaginal dis-

charge, which may be confused with candidiasis. Vaginal pH is normal with microscopic evaluation showing normal bacterial flora, mature vaginal squamae, and no increase in leukocytes. Excessive but normal vaginal discharge should be treated with reassurance and if required at times with cryosurgery or carbon dioxide treatment of the cervix. Continuous use of a tampon should be avoided.

Parasitic Infection

Parasitic infection with pinworms (*Enterobius vermicularis*) and *Entamoeba histolytica* may cause vaginitis less commonly. Pinworm infection is usually seen in children. Fecal contamination at the introitus is the source of infection. The perineal area is extremely pruritic. The parasite is generally detected by pressing a strip of adhesive cellulose tape to the perineum. The tape is then adhered to a slide, allowing the double-walled ova to be identified under the microscope. *E histolytica* infection of the vagina and cervix is rare in the United States but is quite common in developing countries. Severe infection may resemble cervical cancer, but symptoms generally are due to vulvar involvement. Trophozoites of *E histolytica* may be demonstrated on wet mount preparations or occasionally on a Papanicolaou smear.

PRINCIPLES OF DIAGNOSIS OF VULVAR DISEASES

A complete history of potential causes of vulvar irritation such as creams, powders, soaps, type of underwear, and cleansing techniques should be reviewed. Physical exam should include careful inspection, palpation, and liberal use of colposcopy, followed by biopsy of any suspicious areas, lesions, or discolorations if indicated.

Pruritus

Pruritus is the most common symptom of vulvar disease. The term **pruritus vulvae** denotes intense itching of the vulvar skin and mucous membranes due to any cause. Specific diagnosis depends on a thorough history, a physical examination that includes inspection of all body surfaces, and, in some cases, a biopsy.

Ulceration, Tumor, Dystrophy

Ulcerative lesions suggest a granulomatous sexually transmitted disease or cancer. Therefore, appropriate tests for sexually transmitted disease should be conducted along with biopsy to rule out primary or coexisting cancer. Well-circumscribed solid tumors should be excised widely and submitted for microscopic evaluation. Diffuse, dystrophic white lesions may demonstrate great histologic variability. A colposcope should be used to select the most suitable biopsy site(s). A satisfactory full-thickness biopsy of the skin and tumor can be obtained with a dermatologic punch biopsy of the skin under local anesthesia.

Abnormalities of Pigmentation

A. WHITE

The color of vulvar skin or lesions depends principally on the vascularity of the dermis, the thickness of the overlying epidermis, and the amount of intervening pigment, either melanin or blood pigments. A dystrophic lesion of the vulva may have a white appearance due primarily to a decrease in the vascularity (lichen sclerosus) or an increase in the keratin layer (squamous hyperplasia) that has undergone maceration from the increased moisture in the vulvar area. During the acute phase of lichen sclerosus, the vulvar skin is moderately erythematous. As the lesion matures, it becomes hyperkeratotic and develops a typical white appearance resembling cigarette paper. The epidermal thickening of neoplasia obscures the underlying vasculature and, in conjunction with the macerating effects of the moist environment, usually produces a hyperplastic white lesion. A diffuse white lesion of the vulva is also produced by the loss or absence of melanin pigmentation as with vitiligo, a hereditary disorder. Leukoderma is a localized white lesion resulting from transient loss of pigment in a residual scar after healing of an ulcer.

B. RED

A red lesion results from thinning or ulceration of the epidermis, the vasodilation of inflammation or an immune response, or the neovascularization of a neoplasia. With ulceration of the epithelium, there is loss of areas in the epidermis, and the vascular dermis is apparent. Acute candidal vulvovaginitis, as seen with diabetes, is a typical example of vulvar erythema secondary to inflammation and the local immune response. Paget's disease (adenocarcinoma in situ of the vulva) is characterized by the velvety red lesion that spreads over the vulvar skin. Psoriasis involving the vulva is another lesion that can take on a red appearance.

C. BLUE/BLACK

Dark lesions are due to an increased amount or concentration of melanin or blood pigments. These may occur following trauma. A persistent dark lesion on the vulva skin likely represents a nevus or a melanoma. **Melanosis,** or **lentigo,** is a benign, darkly pigmented flat lesion that may be mistaken for a melanoma. With carcinoma in situ of the vulva, the atypical squamous cells are unable to contain the melanin pigment. It is instead

concentrated in the local macrophages, causing dark coloration of the tumor. Vulvar skin may darken following the use of estrogen cream or oral contraceptive pills.

VULVAR DISORDERS (Table 34–6)
Vascular & Lymphatic Diseases

The vulva and vagina have a rich vascular and lymphatic blood supply. These channels may undergo obstruction, dilatation, rupture, or infection or may develop into tumorous lesions, which are usually malformations rather than true neoplasms.

A. VARICOSITIES

Varicosities of the vulva involve one or more veins. Severe varicosities of the legs and vulva may be aggravated during pregnancy. Symptomatic vulvar varices in a patient who is not pregnant are uncommon and may signify an underlying vascular disease in the pelvis, either primary or secondary to a tumor in the pelvis. Regardless of the cause, varicosities can cause considerable discomfort, consisting of pain, pruritus, and a sense of

Table 34–6. Vulvar disorders.

Vascular and lymphatic diseases
Varicosities, hematoma, edema, granuloma pyogenicum, hemangioma, lymphangioma
Vulvar manifestation of systemic diseases
Leukemia, dermatologic disorders (disseminated lupus erythematosus, pemphigus vulgaris, contact dermatitis, psoriasis), obesity, diabetes mellitus, Behçet's syndrome
Viral infections
Herpes genitalis, herpes zoster, molluscum contagiosum, condyloma acuminatum
Infestations of the vulva
Pediculosis pubis, scabies, enterobiasis
Mycotic infections of the vulva
Candidiasis, fungal dermatitis
Other infections of the vulva
Impetigo, furunculosis, erysipelas, hidradenitis, tuberculosis
Vulvar nonneoplastic epithelial disorders
Lichen sclerosus, squamous cell hyperplasia, other dermatoses (lichen planus, lichen simplex chronicus)
Benign cystic tumors
Epidermal cysts, sebaceous cysts, apocrine sweat gland cysts, Skene duct cyst, urethral diverticulum, inguinal hernia, Gartner's duct cyst, Bartholin's duct cyst and abscess
Benign solid tumors
Acrochordon, pigmented nevi, leiomyoma, fibroma, lipoma, neurofibromas, granular cell myoblastoma

heaviness. On examination a large mass of veins may be apparent, which is best diagnosed with the patient standing to distend the veins. Rupture of a vulvar varicosity during pregnancy may cause profuse hemorrhage. Pain and tenderness may be caused by acute phlebitis or thrombosis.

Treatment of vulvar and vaginal varicosities is seldom necessary, although symptoms might be quite severe during pregnancy. Support clothing such as panty hose or leotards usually provides adequate relief of symptoms. Operative intervention is usually required only in cases of rupture and hemorrhage, which are rare. Management of the pregnancy should be guided by standard obstetric care, with vaginal delivery advised. Persistent postpartum cases may be alleviated with injection of a sclerosing agent.

B. Hematoma

The vulva has a rich blood supply arising predominately from the pudendal vessels. If a vessel is ruptured, especially in a pregnant patient, significant bleeding and hematoma formation can occur due to the distensible nature of the vulvar tissue. Following trauma, an ice pack should be applied. If the hematoma continues to expand, the area should be incised and any bleeders (which may be multiple) ligated. The wound may be packed and left open or closed with a drain in place, if appropriate. Antibiotics should be administered on an individual basis, depending on the initiating event and contamination in the area.

C. Edema

The loose integument of the vulva predisposes to the development of edema. Vascular or lymphatic obstruction may be the result of an underlying neoplasm or infection such as lymphogranuloma venereum (LGV), which can cause extensive lymphatic obstruction and gross deformity of the vulvar tissues. If edema persists following appropriate antibiotic treatment, vulvectomy may be indicated.

Accidental trauma from a bicycle accident (saddle injury) in a young girl or a kick to the pudendum may cause painful swelling. An ice pack applied to the perineum after an acute trauma tends to retard the development of significant edema. Warm packs or warm sitz baths may then be applied after one to two days to help assist in resolution of the associated inflammation and/or hematoma.

Severe generalized vulvar edema may also represent an underlying systemic illness such as congestive heart failure, nephrotic syndrome, preeclampsia, or eclampsia. Acute development of edema may result from a systemic or local allergic reaction. Dependent edema is occasionally seen with prolonged bed rest.

D. Granuloma Pyogenicum

Pyogenic granuloma is considered to be a variant of a capillary hemangioma. It is usually single, raised, and dull red. It seldom exceeds 3 cm in size (Fig 34–8). It is important because it tends to bleed easily if traumatized. Wide excisional biopsy is indicated to alleviate symptoms and to rule out a malignant melanoma.

E. Hemangioma

1. Senile—Senile hemangiomas are usually multiple, small, dark blue, asymptomatic papules discovered incidentally during examination of the older patient. Excision biopsy is needed only if they bleed repeatedly. A cryosurgical probe or carbon dioxide laser may also be used.

2. Childhood—Childhood hemangiomas are usually diagnosed in the first few months of life. They may vary in size from small strawberry hemangiomas to large cavernous ones. They tend to be elevated and bright red or dark, depending on their size and the thickness of the overlying skin. Those that tend to increase in size during the first few months of life often will become static or regress without therapy after about age 18 months.

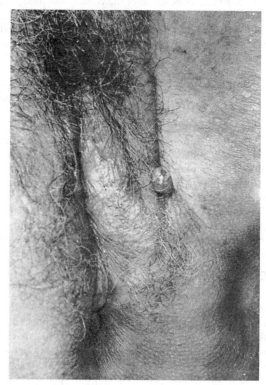

Figure 34–8. Pyogenic granuloma.

Although most of these can be observed without therapy, larger ones may need to be treated using cryosurgery, argon laser therapy, or sclerosing solutions. A dermatology consultation may be required for larger ones.

F. LYMPHANGIOMA

Lymphangiomas are tumors of the lymphatic vessels and may be difficult to differentiate from hemangiomas microscopically unless blood cells are present within the blood vessels. Lymphangioma cavernosum may cause a diffuse enlargement of one side of the vulva and extend down over the remainder of the vulva and perineum. If the tumor is sufficiently enlarged it should be surgically excised. Lymphangioma simplex tumors (circumscription tumors) are usually small, soft, white or purple nodules or small wartlike lesions most commonly seen on the labia majora. They are usually asymptomatic and do not need to be excised unless intense pruritus and excoriation are present and are not alleviated with topical measures.

Vulvar Manifestation of Systemic Diseases

A. LEUKEMIA

Rarely, nodular infiltration and ulceration of the vulva and rectovaginal septum occur with acute leukemia.

B. DERMATOLOGIC DISORDERS

Recurrent ulcerations of the mucous membranes of the mouth and vagina may be a manifestation of **disseminated lupus erythematosus.** Bullous eruptions of apparently normal skin and mucous membrane surfaces of the vulva may be one of the first signs of **pemphigus vulgaris** (a rare, chronic autoimmune disease).

Contact dermatitis is an inflammatory response of the vulvar tissue to agents that may either be locally irritating or induce sensitivity on contact. The local reaction to a systemically administered drug is called **dermatitis medicamentosa.**

Psoriasis is a chronic relapsing dermatosis that may also affect the scalp, the extensor surfaces of the extremities, the trunk, and the vulva. The vulvar skin may be the only body surface affected, and the primary lesions are raised and appear typically erythematous, resembling a candidal infection. Most lesions are sharply demarcated. The silver scaly crusts that are present on other parts of the body are usually absent (Fig 34–9). Treatment includes topical corticosteroids.

C. OBESITY

Acanthosis nigricans is a benign hyperpigmented lesion characterized by papillomatous hypertrophy. It may be associated with an underlying adenocarcinoma. **Pseudoacanthosis nigricans** is a benign process that

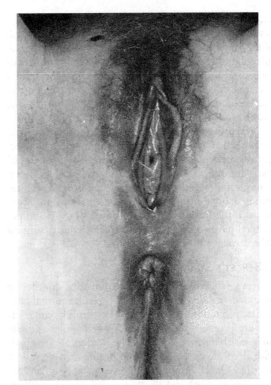

Figure 34–9. Typical lesions of psoriasis with a sharp outline and bright red surface.

may appear on the skin of the vulva and inner thighs in obese and darkly pigmented women. Glucose intolerance, chronic anovulation, and androgen disorders may be associated. **Intertrigo** is an inflammatory reaction involving the genitocrural folds or the skin under the abdominal panniculus. It is common in obese patients and results from persistent moistness of the skin surfaces. An associated superficial fungal or bacterial infection may be present. The area may be either erythematous or white from maceration. Measures to promote dryness such as wearing absorbent cotton undergarments and dusting with cornstarch powder may be helpful.

D. DIABETES MELLITUS

Diabetes mellitus is the systemic disease most commonly associated with chronic pruritus vulvae. The chronic vulvitis that develops may be termed **diabetic vulvitis.** It is due to a chronic vulvovaginal candidiasis. A diagnosis of diabetes should be considered in any patient who responds poorly to antifungal treatment or who has recurrent fungal infections. Glycosuria is not necessary to cause diabetic vulvitis; therefore, asymptomatic patients may require glucose tolerance testing or a 2-hour postprandial blood sugar test to diagnose diabetes. In uncontrolled diabetes, the vulvar skin will often undergo lichenification and secondary bacterial infection. Occasionally, a vulvar abscess, chronic subcutaneous abscesses, and draining sinuses develop from a bacterial infection. Treatment should include controlling the underlying diabetes and specific therapy for the bacterial or fungal infection.

Necrotizing fasciitis is seen most commonly in diabetics. It is an uncommon, acute, rapidly spreading, frequently fatal polymicrobial infection of the superficial fascia and subcutaneous fascia. It may be seen following a surgical procedure such as an episiotomy or after minor trauma. It presents as an extremely painful, tender, and indurated region with central necrosis and peripheral purplish erythema. Treatment requires surgical debridement and systemic antibiotics.

E. Behçet's Syndrome

Behçet's syndrome is a rare inflammatory disorder of unknown cause characterized by recurrent oral and genital ulcerations and uveitis. The painful genital ulcers are preceded by small vesicles or papules and last for a variable period of time. The borders are irregular, with deep ulcers that, following healing, may result in scarring. Ocular lesions begin as superficial inflammation and may proceed to iridocyclitis and even blindness. Monoarticular arthritis and central nervous system symptoms are manifestations of severe disease. Susceptibility to Behçet's disease is strongly associated with the presence of the *HLA-B51* allele and is primarily seen in Eastern Europe and the Mediterranean. The exact etiology is unknown, but it likely represents an underlying autoimmune process. No specific viral infection has been implicated.

Behçet's syndrome, together with disseminated lupus erythematosus and pemphigus, should be included in the differential diagnosis of recurrent aphthous ulcers of the oral and vaginal mucosa. There is no specific therapy—only palliative care. Topical and systemic corticosteroids provide the most consistent relief. Patients with Behçet's syndrome require consultation and long-term management by a dermatologist.

Viral Infections

Systemic infections in children, such as varicella and rubeola, may involve the skin and mucosa of the vulva. The principal viruses that affect the vulva are DNA viruses, primarily of the herpesvirus, poxvirus, and papovavirus types. In adults, the principal viral infections of the lower genital tract are herpes genitalis, herpes zoster, molluscum contagiosum, and condyloma acuminatum.

A. Herpes Genitalis

Herpesvirus hominis infection of the lower genital tract (herpes genitalis) is the most common cause of genital ulcer disease in the United States. In private practice 10% of women demonstrate serologic prior exposure to the virus. Approximately 85% of primary infections are secondary to herpesvirus hominis type II, with the remainder by type I.

Infection occurs through direct contact with secretions or mucosal surfaces contaminated with the virus. The virus enters the skin through cracks or other lesions but can enter through an intact mucosa. The virus initially replicates in the dermis and epidermis. Incubation time is 2–7 days. Prodromal symptoms of tingling, burning, or itching may occur shortly before vesicular eruptions appear. The vesicles erode rapidly, resulting in painful ulcers distributed in small patches, or they may involve most of the vulvar surfaces (Fig 34–10). Dysuria or other urinary symptoms may develop, including urinary retention. In severe infections, fever, malaise, and bilateral inguinal adenopathy can develop. Herpetic cervicitis causes a profuse watery discharge. Rarely a disseminated infection can follow a primary

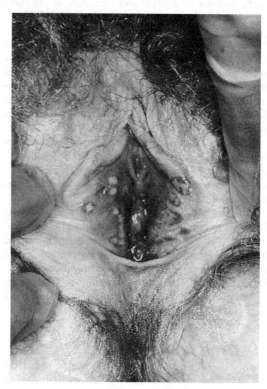

Figure 34–10. Ulcerating vesicles of herpes genitalis.

infection. In other cases the primary infection is asymptomatic. Lesions may persist for 2–6 weeks with no subsequent scarring.

Diagnosis is based on clinical presentation and laboratory results. The virus can be cultured from vesicle fluid during the acute phase. However, organisms usually cannot be cultured after healing of the primary vesicles, which occurs by 2 weeks. A scraping taken from the ulcer and stained as a Papanicolaou smear can also demonstrate the characteristic giant cells indicative of viral infection, although they may also be confused with malignant cells. Other cells demonstrate a homogeneous "ground glass" appearance of cellular nuclei with numerous small intracellular, scattered basophilic particles and acidophilic inclusion bodies. Unsuspected disease is occasionally detected on a cervical or vaginal smear with a sensitivity of 50%. Approximately 85% of patients develop IgM antibodies to type II virus within 21 days of exposure. Serologic tests are best utilized to determine whether the patient has been infected in the past. A 4-fold or higher increase in neutralizing complement fixation antibody titers between acute and convalescent sera may be useful to document a primary infection. Only 5% of patients with recurrent infection demonstrate a 4-fold or higher rise in antibody titer. New type-specific serologic tests for herpes simplex virus are available. The serologic type-specific glycoprotein G-based assays should be specifically requested when serology is performed to distinguish between herpes simplex type 1 and 2.

Despite the presence of adequate humoral and cell-mediated immunity, reactivation of the virus occurs. Following replication in the skin, the viral particles are transported along the peripheral sensory nerves to the dorsal root ganglion, where latent infection is established. Exogenous factors known to contribute to activation of herpesvirus include fever, emotional stress, and menstruation. Immunocompromised patients are prone to develop extensive local disease and systemic dissemination. Whether frequent coitus promotes recurrent disease is unknown. Type II virus is more likely to recur than type I virus, with men more likely to have recurrent symptoms then women. Approximately 50% of patients will have a recurrence within 6 months of the primary infection. The ulcers tend to be smaller, fewer in number, and confined to one area in the vulva, cervix, or vagina. Healing is generally complete in 1–3 weeks. Virus is not recoverable within 7 days after healing of recurrent lesions. Inguinal adenopathy and systemic symptoms generally do not occur. Primary infection can usually be distinguished from secondary infection based on clinical findings. Extragenital sites, such as the fingers, buttocks, and trunk (eczema herpeticum) have been described.

1. Pregnancy—The incidence of neonatal simplex virus infection ranges from 1 in 5000 to 1 in 20,000 live births. Infection in the newborn is associated with a 60% mortality rate, and at least one-half of the survivors have significant neurologic and/or ocular sequelae. The risk of infection to an infant born vaginally in a mother with active primary genital infection is 40–50%; for recurrent infection the risk is 5%. However, most infants who develop herpetic infection are born to women who have no history or clinical evidence of infection during pregnancy. Therefore, it is difficult to identify women whose infants may be in jeopardy. All pregnant women should be asked whether they or their partners have had genital herpetic lesions. In women who have a history of herpes, vaginal delivery can occur if there are no clinical signs or symptoms of infection. It is not standard to obtain routine vaginal cultures to detect herpes. However, suppressive antiviral therapy may be initiated at 36 weeks to decrease the need for cesarean section (Table 34–7).

2. Treatment—The lesions of herpesvirus infection are self-limiting, and they heal spontaneously unless they become infected secondarily. Symptomatic treatment includes good genital hygiene, loose-fitting undergarments, cool compresses or sitz baths, and oral analgesics. Indications for hospitalization for a severe primary infection include urinary retention, severe headache or other systemic symptoms, and temperature greater than 101 °F (38.3 °C). Immunosuppressed patients are more prone to systemic dissemination and should be carefully managed. Treatment includes intravenous acyclovir for hospitalized patients and oral and/or topical antivirals for outpatient treatment. Recurrent herpes should be treated at the onset of prodromal symptoms or vesicle formation. Studies have indicated a decrease in the frequency and

Table 34–7. Oral treatment of herpes genitalis.

First episode of genital herpes	
Acyclovir	400 mg orally three times a day for 7–10 days
Famciclovir	250 mg orally three times a day for 7–10 days
Valacyclovir	1000 mg orally twice a day for 10 days
Recurrent genital herpes	
Acyclovir	400 mg orally three times a day for 5 days
Famciclovir	125 mg orally twice a day for 5 days
Valacyclovir	500 mg orally twice a day for 5 days
Genital herpes prophylaxis	
Acyclovir	400 mg orally twice a day
Famciclovir	250 mg orally twice a day
Valacyclovir	500–1000 mg orally daily

severity of recurrences with antiviral treatment. Once-daily dosing may be considered for frequent recurrent outbreaks with 40–70% of patients being free of recurrence at one year (Table 34–7).

Avoidance of direct contact with active lesions prevents spread of the disease. However, contact with an individual with subclinical disease can result in some primary infections. The general rules for prevention of dissemination are:

1. Precautions are unnecessary in the absence of active lesions.

2. Small lesions situated away from the oral or vaginal orifices may be covered with adhesive or paper tape during coitus.

3. In the presence of active lesions, whether or not the partner contracts the disease depends on previous exposure to herpes. A nonimmune partner usually will be infected. If a regular partner has had genital herpes or has not been infected after prolonged exposure, no precautions are necessary. If a casual partner has had a history of genital herpes, a contraceptive cream or foam should be used, followed by genital cleansing with soap and water. If a partner has no past history of genital herpes, a condom may be used but may be of limited value.

B. HERPES ZOSTER (SHINGLES)

Herpes zoster is an inflammatory disorder in which a painful eruption of groups of vesicles is distributed over an area of skin corresponding to the course of one or more peripheral sensory nerves. The causative agent is varicella zoster virus. The lesion is commonly unilateral and not infrequently attacks one buttock, one thigh, or one side of the vulva. The vesicles may rupture and crust over although they usually dry, forming a scab that ultimately separates. The primary purposes of treatment (antivirals) are alleviation of pain, resolution of vesicles, and prevention of secondary infection and ulceration.

C. MOLLUSCUM CONTAGIOSUM

These benign epithelial virus-induced tumors are dome-shaped, often umbilicated, and vary in size up to 1 cm. The lesions are often multiple and are mildly contagious. The microscopic appearance is characterized by numerous inclusion bodies (molluscum bodies) in the cytoplasm of the cells. Each lesion may be treated by desiccation, freezing, or curettage and chemical cauterization of the base.

D. CONDYLOMA ACUMINATUM

Condylomata acuminata (genital warts) are caused by the papovavirus group. Papillary growths, small at first, tend to coalesce and form large cauliflower-like masses that may proliferate profusely during pregnancy.

Before treatment is undertaken, the entire lower genital tract should be examined with the colposcope and a cytologic smear taken from the cervix. Considering the frequent coexistence of other sexually transmitted diseases, appropriate studies are indicated. There is considerable variation in the oncogenic potential of human papovaviruses; therefore, a biopsy may be indicated. The incubation period for appearance of clinical disease after exposure is 3 months or longer. Apparent clinical disease may represent only a small area of the infected surface. Prompt recurrences after treatment may represent reinfection or clinical manifestation of latent disease. During treatment, the patient should keep the area as clean as possible and abstain from sexual intercourse or have her partner use a condom. If clinical disease recurs, then the sexual partner should be examined and treated as necessary. Penile, urethral, and perianal warts in the male may be overlooked.

Standard treatment is to cover the wart with bichloroacetic or trichloroacetic acid every week until the wart is gone. Alternative forms of treatment include cryosurgery, electrosurgical destruction, excision, and laser vaporization. Some authors recommend laser ablation of all visible lesions plus a margin of normal adjacent skin under colposcopic guidance. Intralesional interferon has been shown to be effective in refractory cases. Self-administered medication includes podofilox 0.5% solution or gel or imiquimod 5% cream (Table 34–5). **Condyloma lata,** a variation of secondary syphilis, should be considered in the differential diagnosis of condyloma acuminata.

Condylomatous warts may grow rapidly during pregnancy. Warts at the vaginal introitus may bleed during delivery and predispose the newborn to genital warts or laryngeal papillomatosis. Condylomata recognized early in pregnancy should be treated early enough to allow healing prior to delivery. If treatment is not successful, delivery by cesarean section should be considered.

Infestations of the Vulva

A. PEDICULOSIS PUBIS

The crab louse (*Phthirus pubis*) is transmitted through sexual contact or from shared infected bedding or clothing. The louse eggs are laid at the base of a hair shaft near the skin. The eggs hatch in 7–9 days, and the louse must attach to the skin of the host to survive. The result is intense pubic and anogenital itching.

Minute pale-brown insects and their ova may be seen attached to terminal hair shafts. Treatment is with Permethrin 1% cream, Lindane 1% shampoo or

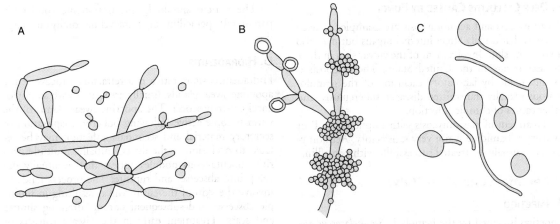

Figure 34–11. *Candida albicans.* **A:** Blastospores and pseudohyphae in exudate. **B:** Blastospores, pseudohyphae, and conidia in culture at 20 °C. **C:** Young culture forms germ tubes when placed in serum for 3 hours at 37 °C. (Reproduced, with permission, from Brooks GF, Butel JS, Ornston LN: *Jawetz, Melinick, & Adelberg's Medical Microbiology,* 19th ed. Appleton & Lange, 1991.)

pyrethrins with piperonly butoxide. Lindane is not recommended for pergnant or lactating women or children < 2 years of age. Treat all contacts and sterilize clothing that has been in contact with the infested area.

B. Scabies

Sarcoptes scabiei causes intractable itching and excoriation of the skin surfaces in the vicinity of minute skin burrows where parasites have deposited ova. The itch mite is transmitted, often directly, from infected persons. The patient should take a hot soapy bath, scrubbing the burrows and encrusted areas thoroughly. Treatment is with Permethrin cream (5%) which should be applied to the entire body from the neck down, with particular attention to the hands, wrists, axillae, breasts, and anogenital region. It should be washed off after 8–14 hours. All potentially infected clothing or bedding should be washed or dry-cleaned. All contacts or persons in the family must be treated in the same way to prevent reinfection. Therapy should be repeated in 10–14 days if new lesions develop.

C. Enterobiasis (Pinworm, Seatworm)

Enterobius vermicularis infection is common in children. Nocturnal perineal itching is described by the patient, and perianal excoriation may be observed. Apply adhesive cellulose tape to the anal region, stick the tape to a glass slide, and examine under the microscope for ova. Patients should wash their hands and scrub their nails following each defecation. Underclothes must be boiled. Apply ammoniated mercury ointment to the

perianal region twice daily for relief of itching. Pinworms succumb to systemic treatment with pyrantel pamoate, mebendazole, or pyrvinium pamoate.

Mycotic Infections of the Vulva*

A. Fungal Dermatitis (Dermatophytoses)

Tinea cruris is a superficial fungal infection of the genitocrural area that is more common in men than in women. The most common organisms are *Trichophyton mentagrophytes* and *Trichophyton rubrum*. The initial lesions are usually on the upper inner thighs and are well circumscribed, erythematous, dry, scaly areas that coalesce. Scratching causes lichenification and a gross appearance similar to neurodermatitis. The diagnosis depends on microscopic examination (as for *Candida*) (Fig 34–11); culture on Sabouraud's medium confirms it. Treatment with 1% haloprogin, tolnaftate, or a similar agent is effective.

Tinea versicolor usually involves the skin of the trunk, although occasionally the vulvar skin is involved. The lesions are usually multiple and may have a red, brown, or yellowish appearance. Diagnosis is as described for other fungal infections. Treatment with selenium sulfide suspension daily for 5–7 days is usually curative. Ketoconazole has been used in recalcitrant cases.

---

* Candidiasis is discussed earlier in this chapter.

B. Deep Cellulitis Caused by Fungi

Blastomycosis and actinomycosis are examples of deep mycoses that usually affect internal organs but may also involve the skin. Involvement of the vulvar skin in these diseases is rare in the United States. The diagnosis is usually made by laboratory exclusion of the granulomatous sexually transmitted diseases, tuberculosis, and other causes of chronic infection.

Treatment of blastomycosis with amphotericin B or hydroxystilbamidine is not very satisfactory. Actinomycosis can usually be treated successfully with penicillin.

Other Infections of the Vulva

A. Impetigo

Impetigo is caused by the hemolytic *Staphylococcus aureus* or streptococci. The disease is autoinoculable and spreads quickly to other parts of the body, including the vulva. Thin-walled vesicles and bullae develop that display reddened edges and crusted surfaces after rupture. The disease is common in children, particularly on the face, hands, and vulva.

The patient must be isolated and the blebs incised or crusts removed aseptically. Neomycin or bacitracin should be applied twice daily for one week. Bathing with an antibacterial soap is recommended.

B. Furunculosis

Vulvar folliculitis is due to a staphylococcal infection of hair follicles. Furunculosis occurs if the infection spreads into the perifollicular tissues to produce a localized cellulitis. Some follicular lesions are palpable as tender subcutaneous nodules that resolve without suppuration. A furuncle begins as a hard, tender subcutaneous nodule that ruptures through the skin, discharging blood and purulent material. After expulsion of a core of necrotic tissue, the lesion heals. New furuncles may appear sporadically over a period of years.

Minor infections may be treated by applications of topical antibiotic lotions. Deeper infections may be brought to a head with hot soaks, after which the pustule should be incised and drained. Appropriate systemic antibiotics are warranted when extensive furunculosis is present.

C. Erysipelas

Erysipelas is a rapidly spreading erythematous lesion of the skin caused by invasion of the superficial lymphatics by β-hemolytic streptococci. Erysipelas of the vulva is exceedingly rare and is most commonly seen after trauma to the vulva or a surgical procedure. Systemic symptoms of chills, fever, and malaise associated with an erythematous vulvitis suggest the diagnosis. Vesicles and bullae may appear, and erythematous streaks leading to the regional lymph nodes are typical.

The patient should be given systemic (preferably parenteral) penicillin or tetracycline orally in large doses.

D. Hidradenitis

Hidradenitis suppurativa is a refractory process of the apocrine sweat glands, usually associated with staphylococci or streptococci. The apocrine sweat glands of the vulva become active following puberty. Inspissation of secretory material and secondary infection may be related to occlusion of the ducts. Initially, multiple pruritic subcutaneous nodules appear that eventually develop into abscesses and rupture. The process tends to involve the skin of the entire vulva, resulting in multiple abscesses and subsequent chronic draining sinuses and scars. Treatment early in the disease consists of drainage and administration of antibiotics based on organism sensitivity testing. Long-term therapy with isotretinoin may be considered. Severe chronic infections may not respond to medical therapy, and the involved skin and subcutaneous tissues must be removed down to the deep fascia. This may necessitate a filet and curettage or a complete vulvectomy. The area generally will not heal after a primary closure; therefore, the wound must be left open and allowed to heal by secondary intention, or a split-thickness graft may be placed. Squamous cell carcinoma is rarely associated with hidradenitis suppurativa.

E. Tuberculosis (Vulvovaginal Lupus Vulgaris)

Pudendal tuberculosis is manifested by chronic, minimally painful, exudative "sores" that are tender, reddish, raised, moderately firm, and nodular, with central "apple-jelly"-like contents. Ulcerative, necrotic discharging lesions develop later. There is some tendency toward healing with heavy scarring. Induration and sinus formation are common in the scrofulous type of infection. Cancer and sexually transmitted disease must be ruled out and evaluation for tuberculosis at other sites carried out.

Wet compresses of aluminum acetate solution (Burow's solution) are helpful. Systemic antituberculosis therapy should be given.

Vulvar Nonneoplastic Epithelial Disorders

The term **vulvar dystrophies** was previously used to define the nonneoplastic epithelial disorders of the vulva. These lesions represent a spectrum of atrophic and hypertrophic lesions caused by a diverse number of stimuli that result in circumscribed or diffuse white lesions of the vulva. As characterized by the International Society for the Study of Vulvovaginal Disease (ISSVD), these lesions include: (1) lichen sclerosus (previously lichen sclerosus et atrophicus), (2) squamous cell hyperplasia (previously hyperplastic dystrophy), and (3) other dermatoses (lichen simplex chronicus, lichen planus). These lesions present classically with intense pruritus with or without pain and vulvar skin changes; differentiation within the disorders and ruling out an underlying malignant process require histopathologic diagnosis. The risk of an underlying malignancy is less than 5%. These patients must be reexamined periodically, and one should not hesitate to take additional biopsy specimens. These lesions have been classified as shown in Table 34–8.

A. LICHEN SCLEROSUS

With aging there is a decrease in endogenous estrogen, and atrophic changes in the vulvar skin and subdermal tissues usually occur some years after advanced atrophy of the vaginal mucous membrane. The result is contracture of the vaginal introitus, thinning of the vulvar skin, skin fragility, and sensitization to trauma. Lichen sclerosus is a benign, chronic, inflammatory process and the most common vulvar dermatologic disorder. The etiology is unknown, but it is likely related to an autoimmune process. Koebner's phenomenon occurs in lichen sclerosus; therefore, scarring or trauma may elicit its development. The skin of the vulva is most commonly involved, although other sites may be affected. White women over age 65 are classically affected, although reported cases occur in the prepubertal population. During the acute phase, the lesion may appear reddish or purple in color and classically involves the

Table 34–8. Nonneoplastic epithelial disorders of the vulva.

Dermatosis	Physical Exam	Histology	Treatment
Lichen sclerosus	Thin, white, wrinkled tissue, with a cigarette-paper appearance Agglutination of the labia minora and prepuce Introital stenosis	*Epidermis*—Hyperkeratosis, epithelial atrophy, and flattening of the rete pegs; cytoplasmic vacuolization of the basal layer of cells *Upper dermis*—Edematous, pale-staining, acellular, homogenous collagen tissue *Deeper dermis*—Inflammatory infiltrate, mainly lymphocytic	Clobetasol propionate 0.05% twice daily for 1 month, then once daily for 2 months Not proven—2% testosterone cream, 1.25% topical progesterone
Squamous cell hyperplasia	Circumscribed, single or multifocal Raised white lesion on vulva or adjacent tissue (generally of labia majora and clitoris)	*Epidermis*—Hyperkeratosis and acanthosis, producing thickening of the epithelium and elongation of the rete pegs *Dermis*—No inflammatory infiltrate present	Medium potency topical steroids twice a day
Lichen simplex chronicus	Thickened white epithelium on vulva Generally unilateral and localized	*Epidermis*—Hyperkeratosis and acanthosis, producing thickening of the epithelium and elongation of the rete pegs *Superficial dermis*—Chronic inflammatory cells, fibrosis, and collagenization Presence of cellular atypia signifies vulvar intraepithelial neoplasia (VIN I–III)	Medium potency topical steroids twice a day
Lichen planus	Erosive lesions at vestibule ± vaginal synechiae resulting in stenosis May have associated oral mucocutaneous lesions and desquamative vaginitis	Mild, localized, lichenoid, chronic inflammatory process at the epidermal-dermis junction to ulcerative process with fibrosis Immunofluorescent staining should be considered to exclude pemphigus and pemphigoid	Vaginal hydrocortisone suppository 25 mg Betamethasone cream 0.1% vaginally at bedtime for 2 weeks Vaginal estrogen cream in cases of atrophic epithelium Vaginal dilators in cases of stenosis
Psoriasis	Red moist lesions ± scales	*Epidermis*—Parakeratosis with clubbing of the rete pegs *Dermis*—Microabscesses of Munro	Topical corticosteroids

non-hair-bearing areas of the vulva, perineum, and perianal area in an hourglass pattern (Fig 34–12). With chronic disease, the skin is thin, wrinkled, and white and has a cigarette-paper appearance. The vulvar structures contract with agglutination of the labia minora and prepuce and introital stenosis. The chief symptom is intense pruritus. This leads to rubbing and scratching, which may lead to areas of hypertrophy and ulceration. Symptoms of pain including dyspareunia may also be present. Although this process is primarily one of atrophy of the skin, areas of dysplasia may develop. Therefore, suspicious areas must be biopsied (Fig 34–13). Repeat biopsies should be taken as indicated since this is a chronic condition. Patients should be monitored for possible malignant changes since there is an estimated 4–6% risk of developing squamous cell carcinoma.

Definitive diagnosis depends on histologic examination of the biopsy; the differential diagnosis includes pemphigoid, pemphigus, advanced scleroderma, lupus erythematosus, advanced lichen planus, and radiation fibrosis. In the well-developed lesion, lichen sclerosus is characterized by hyperkeratosis, epithelial atrophy, and flattening of the rete pegs. The upper dermis is edematous, pale staining with fibrin deposition. The deeper

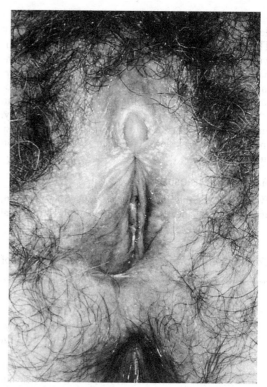

Figure 34–13. Advanced lesion of lichen sclerosus. The labia minora and prepuce of the clitoris have blended into the labial skin. Focal dysplasia was present in the posterior third of the right labium majus.

dermis has an inflammatory infiltrate, mainly monocytic. Beneath the epidermis is a zone of homogenized collagenous tissue that is acellular and pink in appearance (Fig 34–14).

Treatment involves initially stopping the pruritus and building up the epithelium. An oral antihistamine agent can be given at bedtime. Recent studies recommend treatment with very high potency steroid cream or ointment. Clobetasol propionate 0.05%, twice daily for 1 month and then daily for 2 months, has been shown to be most effective in treatment of lichen sclerosus, with approximately 75% success. Subsequent treatment with clobetasol 2–3 times per week or with lower-dose topical steroids as needed is used for maintenance therapy. Atrophic degeneration of the skin secondary to the steroid paradoxically does not occur. Treatment with 2% testosterone cream (twice daily or three times daily for 6–12 weeks) is also beneficial, but its long-term effectiveness may be less than that of clobetasol and testosterone has potential unwanted side ef-

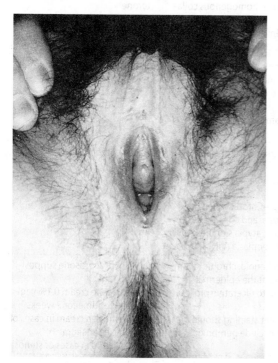

Figure 34–12. Early lesion of lichen sclerosus—typical hourglass configuration.

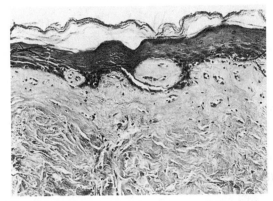

Figure 34–14. Microscopic appearance of lichen sclerosus, characterized by hyperkeratosis, flattened epidermis, and hyalinization of the dermis.

fects, including systemic and local androgen effects (virilization and metabolic changes). Topical progesterone also has been used, but effectiveness is lacking. In addition patients should avoid tight undergarments and cleanse daily with mild soap and use a hair dryer to keep the vulvar skin dry. Surgical excision should be considered only in refractory cases or in cases with associated carcinoma. Vulvar denervation, alcohol injections, laser ablation, and cryotherapy have also been used in refractory cases. Treatment success should be based on symptomatic improvement (ie, decreases in pruritus, pain, and dyspareunia).

B. SQUAMOUS CELL HYPERPLASIA

Vulvar squamous cell hyperplasia is known by various names—hyperplastic dystrophy, atopic dermatitis, atopic eczema, or neurodermatitis. The benign epithelial thickening and hyperkeratosis may be the result of chronic vulvovaginal infections or other causes of chronic irritation. During the acute phase, as in diabetic vulvitis, the lesions may be red and moist and demonstrate evidence of secondary infection. The condition is exacerbated by the accompanying pruritus, which leads to rubbing and scratching. This becomes involuntary over time. As epithelial thickening develops, the environment of the vulva causes maceration, and a raised white lesion may be circumscribed or diffuse and may involve any portion of the vulva, adjacent thighs, perineum, or perianal skin. Biopsy must be performed to eliminate intraepithelial neoplasm or invasive tumor. With squamous cell hyperplasia, histologic examination demonstrates hyperkeratosis and acanthosis, producing thickening of the epithelium and elongation

of the rete pegs. No dermal inflammatory infiltrate is present as with lichen sclerosus. Atypical hyperplasia or cancer is characterized by nuclear pleomorphism and loss of cellular polarity in the epithelium.

Treatment for squamous cell hyperplasia is also to achieve symptomatic relief. Sitz baths and lubricants can help restore moisture to cells and reconstruct the epithelial barrier. Oral antihistamines or antidepressants (ie, selective serotonin reuptake inhibitors) may help relieve pruritus. Local application of medium-potency topical steroids twice a day can also decrease the inflammation and pruritus. Vulvar epithelium takes at least 6 weeks to heal. In intractable cases, subcutaneous intralesional injection of steroids or alcohol could be considered. Differential diagnosis includes lichen simplex chronicus, lichen planus, condyloma acuminatum, psoriasis, and vulvar intraepithelial neoplasia.

C. OTHER DERMATOSES

Lichen planus of the vulva is part of the systemic manifestation of this skin and mucous membrane disease. Pruritus is commonly the presenting symptom. Skin involvement is characterized by small, polygonal violaceous papules. Ulcerations and white patches may be found in both the oral and vaginal/vulvar mucous membranes. Treatment is with topical and systemic corticosteroids.

Lichen simplex chronicus is another chronic inflammatory process of the vulva that presents as a white lesion associated with vulvar pruritus. Biopsy is generally necessary for the diagnosis. Histologically, the features are similar to squamous cell hyperplasia. Again, treatment is with medium-strength topical corticosteroid cream.

Benign Cystic Tumors

The diagnosis of small cystic structures on the vulva is ordinarily made by clinical examination or by excision biopsy, which also serves as treatment.

A. EPIDERMAL CYSTS

Cysts of epidermal origin are lined with squamous epithelium and filled with oily material and desquamated epithelial cells. Epidermal inclusion cysts may result from traumatic suturing of skin fragments during closure of the vulvar mucosa and skin after trauma or episiotomy. However, most epidermal cysts arise from occlusion of pilosebaceous ducts. These cysts are usually small, solitary, and asymptomatic.

B. SEBACEOUS CYSTS

A sebaceous cyst develops when the sebaceous gland's duct becomes occluded and accumulation of the sebaceous material occurs. These cysts are frequently multiple and almost always involve the labia majora. They are generally asymptomatic; however, acutely infected cysts may require incision and drainage.

C. Apocrine Sweat Gland Cysts

Apocrine sweat glands are numerous in the skin of the labia majora and the mons pubis. They become functional after puberty. Occlusion of the ducts with keratin results in an extremely pruritic, microcystic disease called **Fox-Fordyce disease.** Chronic infection in the apocrine glands, usually with staphylococci or streptococci, results in multiple painful subcutaneous abscesses and draining sinuses. This condition is called **hidradenitis suppurativa,** which is generally treated with a broad-spectrum antibiotic. Hidradenoma and syringoma are included in a diverse group of benign cystic or solid tumors of apocrine sweat gland origin present as small subcutaneous and asymptomatic tumors.

D. Bartholin's Duct Cyst and Abscess

Obstruction of the main duct of Bartholin's gland results in retention of secretions and cystic dilatation. Infection is an important cause of obstruction; however, other causes include inspissated mucus and congenital narrowing of the duct. Secondary infection may result in recurrent abscess formation.

The gland and duct are located deep in the posterior third of each labium majus. Enlargement in the postmenopausal patient may represent a malignant process (although the incidence is less than 1%), and biopsy should be considered.

Acute symptoms are ordinarily the result of infection, which results in pain, tenderness, and dyspareunia. The surrounding tissues become edematous and inflamed. A fluctuant, tender mass is usually palpable. Unless there is an extensive inflammatory process, systemic symptoms or signs of infection are less likely.

Primary treatment consists of drainage of the infected cyst or abscess, preferably with insertion of a Word catheter (an inflatable bulb-tipped catheter) or by marsupialization (Fig 34–15). Simple incision and drainage may provide temporary relief. However, the end may become obstructed and recurrent cystic dilatation may recur. Appropriate antibiotics should be given if considerable surrounding inflammation develops. Excision of the cyst may be required in recurrent cases or in the postmenopausal patient.

Recurrent infection resulting in cystic dilatation of the duct is the rule unless a permanent opening for drainage is established.

E. Other

A variety of other infrequent cystic vulvar tumors must be considered in the differential diagnosis. Anteriorly, a

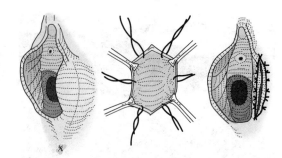

Figure 34–15. Marsupialization of a vestibular duct (Bartholin's) cyst.

Skene duct cyst or **urethral diverticulum** may be visible, suggesting a vulvar tumor. An **inguinal hernia** may extend into the labium majus, causing a large cystic dilatation. Occlusion of a persistent processus vaginalis (canal of Nuck) may cause a cystic tumor or hydrocele. Dilatation of the mesonephric duct vestiges produces lateral vaginal wall cysts, **Gartner's duct cyst.** Supernumerary mammary tissue that persists in the labia majora may form a cystic or solid tumor or even an adenocarcinoma; engorgement of such tissue in the pregnant patient can be symptomatic.

Benign Solid Tumors

A benign solid tumor may be an incidental finding at the time of pelvic examination, or it may be of sufficient size to cause symptoms of irritation and/or bleeding. The diagnosis should be established by excision or biopsy to rule out an underlying malignancy.

A. Acrochordon

An acrochordon is a flesh-colored, soft polypoid tumor of the vulvar skin that has been called a fibroepithelial polyp or simply a skin tag. The tumor does not become malignant and is of no clinical importance, unless it becomes traumatized, causing bleeding. Simple excision biopsy in the office is ordinarily adequate therapy.

B. Pigmented Nevus

Pigmented lesions, suggestive of nevi, should be removed by wide local excision or biopsied to diagnose or exclude a melanoma. A nevus on the vulvar skin may be flat, slightly elevated, papillomatous, dome-shaped, or pedunculated. Melanomas of the vulva are uncommon neoplasms constituting only 1–3% of vulvar cancers. They are extremely aggressive malignant lesions and may arise from pigmented nevi of the vulva. Melanosis of the vaginal mucosa or vulvar skin is a benign, flat, darkly pigmented lesion that usually can be differentiated from a nevus without histologic examination.

C. LEIOMYOMA, FIBROMA, LIPOMA

Tumors of mesodermal origin occur infrequently on the vulva, but they can become extremely large. A **leiomyoma** arises from muscle in the round ligament and appears as a firm, symmetric, freely mobile tumor deep in the substance of the labium majus. **Fibromas** arise from proliferation of fibroblasts and vary in size from small subcutaneous nodules found incidentally to large polypoid tumors. Large tumors often undergo myxomatous degeneration and are very soft and cystic to palpation. **Lipomas** consist of a combination of mature fat cells and connective tissue. They cannot be differentiated from degenerated fibromas except by histopathologic examination.

Small tumors can be removed under local anesthesia in the office; large ones require general anesthesia and operating room facilities. The diagnosis of sarcoma depends on histologic examination.

D. NEUROFIBROMA

Neurofibromas are fleshy polypoid lesions and may be solitary, solid tumors of the vulva or associated with generalized neurofibromatosis (Recklinghausen's disease). They arise from the neural sheath and are usually small lesions of no consequence. Multiple disfiguring tumors of the vulva may interfere with sexual function and require excision or vulvectomy.

E. GRANULAR CELL MYOBLASTOMA (SCHWANNOMA)

Granular cell myoblastoma is usually a solitary, painless, slow-growing, infiltrating but benign tumor of neural sheath origin, most commonly found in the tongue or integument, although about 7% involve the vulva. The usual picture is of small subcutaneous nodules 1–4 cm in diameter. With increasing size, they erode through the surface and result in ulcerations that may be confused with cancer. The margins of the tumor are indistinct, and wide local excision is necessary to completely excise the cells extending into contiguous tissues. The area of resection must then be periodically reexamined and secondary excision performed promptly if recurrence is suspected.

VULVAR PAIN SYNDROME

Vulvodynia, or vulvar pain, is chronic vulvar discomfort characterized by burning, stinging, irritation, and/or rawness. Within this syndrome, several clinical entities are classified, including vulvar vestibulitis, vulvar dermatoses (lichen sclerosus and lichen planus), cyclic vulvovaginitis, and dysesthetic or "essential" vulvodynia (no apparent physical abnormality). These conditions may coexist and are often difficult to distinguish completely from each other. A detailed history and examination are therefore important to help determine the etiology (Table 34–9) and direct the diagnosis and treatment.

The time of onset, the type of pain (burning, stinging, irritation), timing (constant or cyclic), associated activities (eg, intercourse), inciting agents (eg, perfumes, lotions, detergents, clothing), and relieving factors (eg, antifungal medications) should be elicited. In addition, past or current infections (HPV, herpes, *Candida*), medications (eg, trichloroacetic acid, 5-fluorouracil), local and systemic dermatologic disorders, neurologic disorders (eg, herniated discs, herpes zoster, pudendal or genitofemoral neuralgia), urologic disorders (eg, interstitial cystitis and urethral syndrome), and physical trauma (eg, vaginal deliveries, episiotomy, vaginal surgery) should be ascertained. In many cases the vulva appears normal on physical exam. However, careful inspection should be performed to evaluate for discoloration (erythema, hypopigmentation or hyper-

Table 34–9. Etiologies of vulvodynia.

Infections
Bartholin's gland abscess, vulvovaginal candidiasis, herpes, herpes zoster, human papillomavirus, molluscum contagiosum, trichomoniasis
Trauma
Sexual assault, prior vaginal deliveries, hymenectomy
Systemic Illness
Behçet's disease, Crohn's disease, Sjögren's syndrome, systemic lupus erythematosus
Neoplasia
Vulvar intraepithelial neolplasia and invasive squamous cell carcinoma
Allergens/toxic medications
Soaps, sprays, douches, antiseptics, suppositories, creams, laser treatment, podophyllin, trichloroacetic acid, 5-fluorouracil
Dermatologic conditions
Allergic and contact dermatitis, eczema, hidradenitis suppurativa, lichen planus, lichen sclerosus, pemphigoid, pemphigus, psoriasis, squamous cell hyperplasia
Urinary tract syndromes
Interstitial cystitis and urethral syndrome
Neurologic
Referred pain from urethra, vagina, and bladder; dysesthesias secondary to herpes zoster, spinal disc problems; specific neuralgias (pudendal, genitofemoral)
Psychologic
Sexual/physical abuse history

pigmentation), lesions (ulcers and fissures), and atrophy (presence or absence of well-estrogenized tissue). Points of tenderness should be outlined using a cotton-tipped swab and scored (0 for no pain to 10 for severe pain). Vaginal pH and microscopic examination of vaginal secretions with KOH and normal saline can help evaluate for vaginitis. All lesions or discolorations should be further evaluated by colposcopy. Acetowhite changes with application of 5% acetic acid should be biopsied as well as any distinct lesions to evaluate for an underlying dermatosis, infectious, or neoplastic process.

Vulvar Vestibulitis

Vulvar vestibulitis is a subset of vulvodynia. The vestibule is the nonpigmented, nonkeratinized squamous epithelium of the vulva between the labia minora and the hymen. Vulvar vestibulitis is characterized by three criteria: (1) introital pain on vestibular or vaginal entry (entry dyspareunia), (2) vestibular erythema or inflammation of the vestibule, commonly involving the posterior fourchette, and (3) vestibular tenderness—pressure from a cotton-tipped applicator at the vestibule reproduces the pain. This syndrome generally affects women in their twenties and thirties. It may present as persistent vaginal discharge and burning. On biopsy, the subepithelial tissue demonstrates a nonspecific, chronic inflammatory infiltrate, consisting predominately of lymphocytes without direct glandular inflammation. However, the etiology may remain undetermined in up to one-third of cases. It is controversial whether HPV is an important factor in the etiology of vestibulitis. Current studies utilizing molecular techniques have not consistently demonstrated HPV infection, and it is currently not considered a causative agent for vestibulitis.

Treatment

Numerous medical options are available for treatment and depend in part on the etiology (Table 34–10). Supportive measures, including sitz baths and topical 2% lidocaine gel, should initially be utilized. Patients should be instructed on proper vulvar hygiene (cotton underwear, keeping area dry, avoidance of constrictive garments and irritating agents). Although it is not completely clear whether HPV is an inciting agent for vestibulitis, numerous antiviral agents including trichloroacetic acid, interferon, and 5-fluorouracil have often been utilized to treat this disorder, especially when HPV has been identified on biopsy. Vulvovaginal candidiasis has often been implicated in vulvodynia; therefore, antifungals, including fluconazole 150 mg orally once a week for 6 weeks then once a month for 6

Table 34–10. Treatment of vulvodynia.

Supportive measures—warm sitz baths, Burrow's solution, topical anesthetic agents (2% topical xylocaine gel or 5% ointment) and other lubricants with intercourse
Vulvar hygiene—cotton underwear, avoidance of constrictive garments

Treat underlying cause:
Human papillomavirus (HPV)[1]—trichloroacetic acid, topical 5-fluorouracil, interferon 1 million IU per injection site with total of 12 injection sites over 4 weeks, laser, and cream
Candida—fluconazole 150 mg once a week for 6 weeks then once a month for 6 months (for cyclic vulvodynia)
Allergens—avoidance of agent (also of local creams and suppositories containing propylene glycol), hydroxyzine or other antihistamine, hydrocortisone 1% cream twice a day, 5% aspirin cream
Atrophy—topical estrogen vaginal cream, oral hormone replacement therapy
Diet modification—low-oxalate diet with calcium citrate 400 mg orally twice a day
Tricyclic antidepressants—amitriptyline 10–25 mg three times a day (use lowest dose possible)
Psychological and behavioral pain management
Biofeedback
Surgery—vestibuloplasty, partial vestibulectomy with vaginal advancement, total vestibulectomy with vaginal advancement

[1]Current studies do not substantiate HPV as a causative factor in vulvodynia; however, its treatment in particular with interferon is still supported in the literature.

months, may provide relief in certain cases. Allergens may also be an inciting agent for vulvodynia. In addition to avoiding the noxious substance, antihistamines (ie, hydroxyzine) as well as topical corticosteroids (hydrocortisone 1% cream twice daily) may help alleviate the discomfort. Estrogen vaginal cream and/or oral hormone replacement therapy should be given when pain is secondary to atrophied tissue. Tricyclic antidepressants such as amitriptyline, 25–50 mg at night or in divided amounts throughout the day, have been utilized in cases of vulvodynia felt to be secondary to neural dysfunction (dysesthetic vulvodynia). The lowest effective dose should be given to avoid the anticholinergic side effects. Capsaicin is a cream also used in the treatment of neuralgia, most commonly in herpes zoster and diabetic neuropathy. Hyperoxaluria has also been implicated in aggravating vulvar pain through the formation of sharp oxalate crystals, which on contact with the skin causes severe burning. A low-oxalate diet (avoiding such foods as tea, coffee, cocoa, wine, chocolate, peanuts, peanut butter, all berries, prunes, all beans, eggplant, sweet potatoes, spinach, spicy food, vinegar, wheat germ, and tofu) with calcium citrate 400 mg three times daily to inhibit formation of calcium oxalate crystals may improve symptoms. Electromyographic biofeedback may benefit pelvic floor muscle irritability presenting as vaginismus.

The Woodruff procedure, the surgical excision of the vestibule or perineoplasty, is often performed in cases of severe vulvar vestibulitis recalcitrant to medical management. The excision extends from the posterior fourchette to approximately 5 mm beneath and lateral to the urethra to a depth of approximately 2 mm. The adjacent vaginal tissue is then mobilized to cover the excised area. In the literature, success rates based on nonrandomized, retrospective studies range from 47% to 100%. Success diminishes as the length of follow-up increases. Less aggressive surgery (subtotal perineoplasty) with interferon may be as effective as total perineoplasty. Ablative techniques, such as laser therapy, have shown less success in relieving pain secondary to scar formation from third-degree burns.

Up to two-thirds of patients may be cured following a variety of treatments. Recalcitrant cases even subsequent to surgery may occur, resulting in continued dyspareunia. In these cases further medical management should be pursued prior to intervening with additional surgical methods.

REFERENCES

General

Centers for Disease Control and Prevention: Sexually transmitted diseases treatment guidelines 2002. MMWR 51(RR06); 1–80.

Gilson RJ, Mindel A: Recent advances: Sexually transmitted infections. BMJ 2001;322:1160.

Sobel JD: Vaginitis. N Engl J Med 1997;337:1896.

Sobel JD et al: Vulvovaginal candidiasis: Epidemiologic, diagnostic, and therapeutic considerations. Am J Obstet Gynecol 1998;178:203.

Wilkinson EJ: Vulvar nonneoplastic epithelial disorders. ACOG Educational Bulletin 1997;241:1.

Specific

ACOG practice bulletin. Management of herpes in pregnancy. Clinical management guidelines for obstetrician-gynecologists. Int J Gynaecol Obstet 2000;68:165.

Baker DA, Blythe JG, Miller JM: Once-daily valacyclovir hydrochloride for suppression of recurrent genital herpes. Obstet Gynecol 1999;94:103.

Boer J, van Gemert MJ: Long-term results of isotretinoin in the treatment of 68 patients with hidradenitis suppurativa. J Am Acad Dermatol 1999;40:73.

Bornstein J et al: Persistent vulvar vestibulitis: The continuing challenge. Obstet Gynecol Surv 1998;53:39.

Bornstein J et al: Clobetasol dipropionate 0.05% versus testosterone propionate 2% topical application for severe vulvar lichen sclerosus. Am J Obstet Gynecol 1998;178:80.

Braig S et al: Acyclovir prophylaxis in late pregnancy prevents recurrent genital herpes and viral shedding. Eur J Obstet Gynecol Reprod Biol 2001;96:55.

Brocklehurst P, Hannah M, McDonald H: Interventions for treating bacterial vaginosis in pregnancy (Cochrane Review). In: The Cochrane Library. Update Software, 2001, p. 3.

Carey JC et al: Metronidazole to prevent preterm delivery in pregnant women with asymptomatic bacterial vaginosis. N Engl J Med 2000;342:534.

Clavel C et al: Hybrid capture II-based human papillomavirus detection, a sensitive test to detect routine high-grade cervical lesions: A preliminary study on 1518 women. Br J Cancer 1999;80:1306.

Edwards L et al: Self-administered topical 5% imiquimod cream for external anogenital warts. Human Papillomavirus Study Group. Arch Dermatol 1998;134:25.

Forna F, Gülmezoglu AM: Interventions for treating trichomoniasis in women (Cochrane Review). In: The Cochrane Library. Oxford: Update Software, 2001, p. 3.

Goodman A: Role of routine human papillomavirus subtyping in cervical screening. Curr Opin Obstet Gynecol 2000;12:11.

Gülmezoglu AM: Interventions for trichomoniasis in pregnancy (Cochrane Review). In: The Cochrane Library. Update Software, 2001, p. 3.

Hajjeh RA et al: Toxic shock syndrome in the United States: Surveillance update, 1979–1996. Emerg Infect Dis 1999;5:807.

Haley JC, Mirowski GW, Hood AF: Benign vulvar tumors. Semin Cutan Med Surg 1998;17:196.

Handa VL, Stice CW: Fungal culture findings in cyclic vulvitis. Obstet Gynecol 2000;96:301.

Hanson JM et al: Metronidazole for bacterial vaginosis. A comparison of vaginal gel vs. oral therapy. J Reprod Med 2000; 45:889.

Joura EA et al: Short-term effects of topical testosterone in vulvar lichen sclerosus. Obstet Gynecol 1997;89:297.

Kamarashev JA, Vassileya SG: Dermatologic diseases of the vulva. Clin Dermatol 1997;15:53.

Kirschner RE, Low DW: Treatment of pyogenic granuloma by shave excision and laser photocoagulation. Plast Reconstr Surg 1999;104:1346.

Marrazzo JM, Stamm WE: New approaches to the diagnosis, treatment, and prevention of chlamydial infection. Curr Clin Top Infect Dis 1998;18:45.

McGregor JA, French JI: Bacterial vaginosis in pregnancy. Obstet Gynecol Surv 2000;55 (5 suppl 1):S1.

Moraes PS, Taketomi EA: Allergic vulvovaginitis. Ann Allergy Asthma Immunol 2000;85:253.

Morris MC, Rogers PA, Kinghorn GR: Is bacterial vaginosis a sexually transmitted infection? Sex Transm Infect 2001;77:63.

Ninia JG: Treatment of vulvar varicosities by injection—compression sclerotherapy. Dermatol Surg 1997;23:573.

Pandit L, Ouslander JG: Postmenopausal vaginal atrophy and atrophic vaginitis. Am J Med Sci 1997;314:228.

Petrin D et al: Clinical and microbiological aspects of *Trichomonas vaginalis.* Clin Microbiol Rev 1998;11:300.

Powell JJ, Wojnarowska F: Lichen sclerosus. Lancet 1999; 353:1777.

Puranen MH et al: Exposure of an infant to cervical human papillomavirus infection of the mother is common. Am J Obstet Gynecol 1997;176:1039.

Rioux JE et al: 17-beta-estradiol vaginal tablet versus conjugated equine estrogen vaginal cream to relieve menopausal atrophic vaginitis. Menopause 2000;7:156.

Sakane T et al: Behçet's disease. N Engl J Med 1999;341:1284.

Young GL, Jewell D: Topical treatment for vaginal candidiasis in pregnancy (Cochrane Review). In: *The Cochrane Library.* Update Software, 2001, p. 3.

Benign Disorders of the Uterine Cervix

Edward Evantash, MD, Edward C. Hill, MD, & Martin L. Pernoll, MD

35

CONGENITAL ANOMALIES OF THE CERVIX

The cervix develops from the paramesonephric ducts in the sixth week of embryologic development. After fusion of the two müllerian ducts in the midline there is resorption of the septum (Fig. 35–1). In the absence of the development of paramesonephric ducts, there is agenesis of the cervix and uterus. Other anomalies may result from incomplete fusion of these ducts or failure of resorption of the midline septum.

Cervical Agenesis

There are reported cases of an absent uterine cervix with a normal uterine corpus and normal vagina. This is presumably due to either failure of müllerian duct canalization or abnormal epithelial proliferation after canalization. More common is the absence of a cervix along with the absence of a uterine corpus and upper vagina. Since most of the vagina is derived from müllerian ducts, the vagina may be shortened in müllerian aplasia. Women with müllerian aplasia have normal ovaries and are able to contribute oocytes for in vitro fertilization with their partner's sperm. This allows for a transfer to a uterus of a surrogate woman who may carry the pregnancy to term. Female offspring of women with müllerian aplasia have been studied to identify a possible genetic contribution to this disorder. Since no reports have been made of an offspring with müllerian aplasia it is assumed that this disorder is due to a polygenic multifactorial inheritance pattern.

Cervical agenesis with a normal functioning uterine corpus must be differentiated from müllerian aplasia (Figs 35–2 and 35–3). In the former, menstrual blood may accumulate, leading to retrograde flow and development of endometriosis. Ultrasonography, magnetic resonance imaging (MRI), and laparoscopy can help with the diagnosis by defining the anatomy. Many of these patients also have urinary tract abnormalities and require an intravenous pyelogram.

Nonsurgical treatment involves the use of vaginal dilators. Using a bicycle stool designed by Ingram, special dilators are placed that are under constant perineal pressure. The most common surgical approach is the McIndoe technique for creation of a neovagina. The Vecchietti operation combines a surgical and nonsurgical approach to creating a neovagina and has been recently performed by laparoscopy.

Incomplete Müllerian Fusion

If the müllerian ducts fail to completely fuse and canalize, a variety of anomalies may be found. Complete failure of fusion of the ducts results in uterine didelphys; there are two separate uterine horns, each with a distinct cervix and vagina. The two vaginas are separated by a midline septum. If incomplete fusion results in a uterine horn ending blindly, a hematocolpus can develop (Fig 35–4).

Bicornuate uterus and arcuate uterus are due to partial incomplete fusion of the müllerian ducts. In the bicornuate uterus there are two discrete uterine cavities which lead to the same cervix (Fig 35–5). The arcuate uterus may demonstrate minimal depression of the uterine fundus and is often clinically insignificant. Renal abnormalities frequently accompany incomplete fusion of the müllerian ducts and can be diagnosed with radiologic studies.

Failure of Resorption

After fusion of the müllerian ducts, resorption of the intervening septum proceeds both caudal and cephalic. A septate uterus results from failure of resorption of the intervening septum (Fig 35–6). The septum may project from the uterine fundus through the cervical canal, completely dividing the uterine cavity in two, or it may be segmental.

The septum consists of fibromuscular tissue. Failure or incomplete resorption of this septum is associated with reproductive and obstetric complications. First and second trimester spontaneous miscarriages are quite common and usually occur between 8 and 16 weeks of gestation. It is hypothesized that the septum interferes with placental implantation. Obstetric complications can include premature labor, malpresentation, and intrauterine growth restriction. Approximately 15–25%

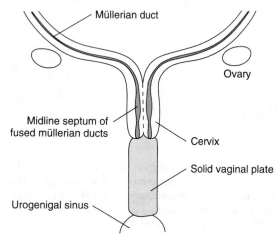

Figure 35–1. Fusion of müllerian ducts to form cervix and corpus uteri.

of spontaneous miscarriages are due to müllerian abnormalities and the majority are associated with the septate uterus (70–88%).

If a septate uterus is identified in association with reproductive or obstetric complications, surgical therapy is recommended. Imaging studies including ultrasound, magnetic resonance imaging, sonohysterography, and hysterosalpingogram provide information to differentiate the septate uterus from other uterine abnormalities. Combined laparoscopy and hysteroscopy remains the most reliable method for accurately differentiating the septate uterus from a bicornuate uterus. Hysteroscopic resection of the uterine septum has been demonstrated to improve reproductive outcome in women with recurrent spontaneous miscarriages. It is controversial whether a hysteroscopic metroplasty may improve fertility in those infertile women.

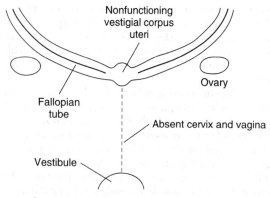

Figure 35–2. Congenital absence of vagina.

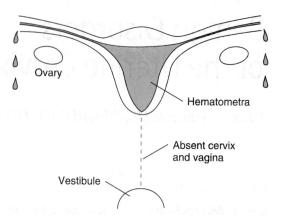

Figure 35–3. Cervical aplasia with hematometra and retrograde menstruation.

CERVICAL ABNORMALITIES DUE TO DIETHYLSTILBESTROL EXPOSURE IN UTERO

Diethylstilbestrol (DES) is a synthetic nonsteroidal estrogen that was first synthesized in 1938. Although the number of pregnant women treated with DES is unknown, estimates range from 2 to 10 million. DES has been shown to cause uterine and cervical abnormalities. Common structural changes of the cervix include collars, hoods, cockscombs, and pseudopolyps (Fig 35–7). Multiple anomalies of the uterus and vagina are also reported in association with DES exposure in utero.

Women who are exposed to DES in utero and have cervical abnormalities are at increased risk for infertil-

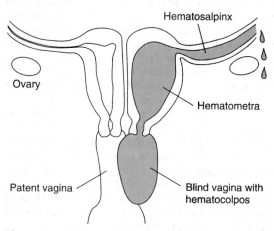

Figure 35–4. Uterus didelphys with blind vagina hematocolpos, hematometra, hematosalpinx, and retrograde menstruation.

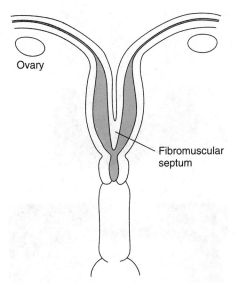

Figure 35–5. Complete bicornuate uterus with fibromuscular septum at level of internal cervical os.

ity. These women are also at increased risk for adverse outcomes in pregnancy, including miscarriage, ectopic pregnancy, and premature delivery. The use of prophylactic cervical cerclage for cervical incompetence related to DES exposure in utero is controversial.

CERVICAL INJURIES

Lacerations

Cervical lacerations most frequently occur after a normal or abnormal vaginal delivery, but can occur in the

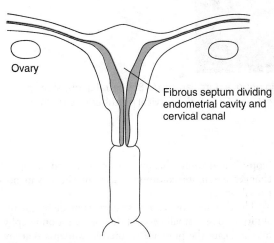

Figure 35–6. Complete septate uterus.

nonobstetric patient as well. With delivery, the most common tears will occur at the 3 and 6 o'clock positions. It is more commonly found after an operative vaginal delivery requiring forceps or vacuum. It is important to carefully inspect the entire cervix after delivery to identify any lacerations. Most lacerations can be easily repaired with suture technique. Oftentimes, a laceration is asymptomatic and does not require repair. More severe lacerations that may extend into the broad ligament have been reported and may require more extensive surgical repair.

Performance of dilation and curettage, particularly on the postmenopausal patient, can result in cervical laceration. The use of cervical laminaria preoperatively may decrease the risk of trauma and laceration of the cervix. There are also reports of preoperative use of misoprostol to reduce the force required to dilate the cervix, potentially reducing the incidence of cervical lacerations.

Cervical lacerations are also reported with the use of the resecting loop in hysteroscopic surgery. The use of the rollerball and other instruments for ablating the endometrium as treatment for menorrhagia have also been found to increase the incidence of cervical lacerations. Additionally, excessive traction on the anterior lip of the cervix with a single-tooth tenaculum may lead to a laceration.

Perforations

Perforation of the cervix may occur during self-induced abortion with sharp objects (eg, wires or darning or knitting needles), or inadvertently during sounding of the uterus, cervical dilation, insertion of radioactive sources, or conization of the cervix. The urinary bladder and the rectum are at risk of injury because of their close proximity to the cervix.

Ulcerations

Ulceration of the cervix may result from pressure necrosis due to a vaginal pessary or a cervical stem pessary. Cervical ulceration may also develop with uterine prolapse when the cervix protrudes through the vaginal introitus.

Cervical Stenosis

Cervical stenosis usually occurs at the level of the internal os and may lead to significant symptoms. In the premenopausal woman, cervical stenosis may be responsible for obstruction of menstrual flow, leading to amenorrhea and pelvic pain. Additionally, infertility may result from cervical stenosis. A postmenopausal woman with cervical stenosis may have pyometria, re-

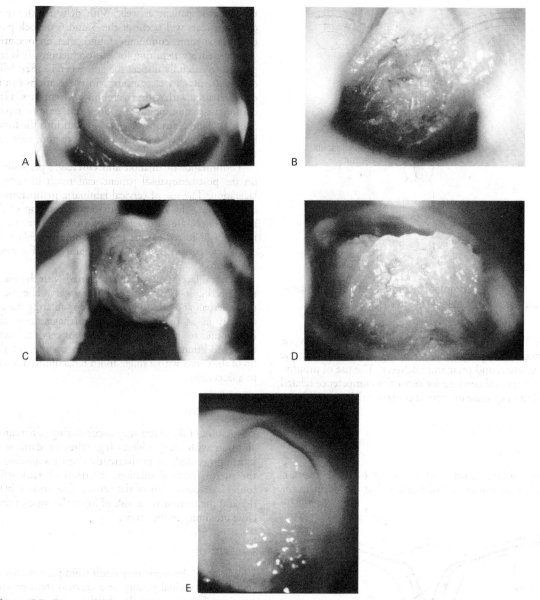

Figure 35–7. Cervical changes in women exposed to DES in utero. **A:** Circular sulcus. **B:** Central depression and ectopy. **C:** Portio vaginalis covered by columnar epithelium (ectopy). **D:** Anterior cervical protuberance (rough). **E:** Anterior cervical protuberance (smooth).

quiring evacuation of uterine contents and biopsy to rule out the possibility of endometrial carcinoma.

Cervical surgery such as cone biopsy, loop excision, or ablative techniques for treatment of dysplasia may lead to cervical stenosis. Excision by loop diathermy tends to remove less cervical stroma and is therefore less likely to cause cervical stenosis than a cold knife cone

biopsy. Radiation therapy, neoplasia, and atrophic changes are more common causes in the postmenopausal woman

The diagnosis of cervical stenosis is made by the inability to pass a small cervical dilator. Ultrasonography may indicate the presence of uterine contents that are obstructed. Treatment is usually with dilators under ultrasound guidance. There are reports of using various techniques such as laser treatment, loop diathermy, and the hysteroscope with resecting loop to remove areas of cervical stenosis. After successful dilation, placing a pediatric Foley catheter in the cervix for a few weeks may be beneficial in order to maintain patency.

Annular Detachment

Annular detachment of the cervix is a rare complication resulting from compression necrosis of the cervix during labor. It occurs when the external os fails to dilate and the blood supply is compromised by pressure of the fetal head. The diagnosis is made when the detached ring or portion of cervix is expelled prior to the delivery of the presenting part of the fetus.

Complications of Cervical Injuries

Hemorrhage is the most immediate and serious complication of cervical laceration. Although external bleeding is usually present, intra- or extraperitoneal hemorrhage may occur when the cervical tear extends into the uterus. The clinical picture is that of hypovolemic shock out of proportion to visible blood loss.

Cervical incompetence results from unrecognized or improperly repaired lacerations at the level of the internal os. Repeated or habitual abortion, often occurring during the second trimester of pregnancy, may be due to cervical incompetence.

CERVICAL INFECTIONS

General Considerations

Advances in colposcopy and sensitive testing for infectious diseases has allowed us to better assess the causes of acute and chronic cervicitis. Hypervascularity, erythema, and ectopy are more consistent with squamous metaplasia than an inflammatory change requiring therapy. Histologic diagnosis of cervicitis is common enough to be considered a normal finding. The cervix is in direct contact with the vagina and is therefore exposed to viral, bacterial, fungal, and parasitic agents. Cervical infections of these types may be found in the absence of vaginal disease. The cervix is a reservoir for infections with *Neisseria gonorrhoeae, Chlamydia trachomatis,* herpes simplex virus, human papillomavirus (HPV), and *Mycoplasma* species. Since many of these women are asymptomatic it is important to screen women at risk.

Etiology and Pathogenesis

C trachomatis is sexually transmitted and invades the columnar epithelium of the cervix. It is thus best cate-

gorized as endocervicitis. With the cervix as a reservoir, the organism may be carried to the eyes, where it causes trachoma and inclusion conjunctivitis. It may infect the fetus during its passage through the birth canal, or it may ascend via the endometrial cavity to the fallopian tubes to cause salpingitis as well as pelvic and perihepatic peritonitis. It has been implicated as the agent responsible for the Fitz-Hugh–Curtis syndrome (violinstring adhesions between the liver and the parietal peritoneum). *C trachomatis* and *N gonorrhoeae* often are coinfecting agents in the etiology of acute and chronic cervicitis and salpingitis.

N gonorrhoeae is a common cause of cervicitis also infecting the columnar epithelium of the endocervix, the mature squamous epithelium of the adult cervix and vagina being resistant to the invading organism. As in the case of *Chlamydia* infections, the cervix acts as a nidus for ascending infection of the endometrium and the fallopian tubes, the upward invasion often occurring after a menstrual period and the loss of the protective mucus plug.

Herpes simplex virus (HSV) infection produces cervical lesions similar to those found on the vulva. Vesicular at first, the lesion becomes ulcerative. Primary infections may be extensive and severe, producing constitutional symptoms of low-grade fever, myalgia, and malaise lasting about 2 weeks. The ulcers eventually heal, but recurrences of lesser severity and duration are common. Herpes simplex type 2 (HSV-2) is the etiologic agent in more than 90% of genital herpes infections, the remainder being due to herpes simplex type 1 (HSV-1), the cause of the common cold sore or fever blister. Orogenital contact is thought to be responsible. After the initial infection has healed, the virus continues to reside in the epithelial cells of the cervix, and viral shedding occurs in asymptomatic patients. Infection of infants during their passage through the birth canal has led to the practice of cesarean section in women who have evidence of active infection at term. Women with the antibodies to HSV-2 have a higher incidence of intraepithelial neoplasia as well as invasive malignancy, although a direct etiologic link has not been established.

The cervical lesions of human papillomavirus (HPV) are also sexually transmitted, and are flatter and moister than the typical genital warts (condylomata acuminata) seen on the vulva and perianal skin. In fact, they are often invisible to the naked eye, becoming visible only after the application of a dilute solution of acetic acid (acetowhite epithelium) or by colposcopic examination (white epithelium, mosaicism, and coarse punctation). More than 65 types of HPV have been identified. Benign lesions of the cervix are associated with types 6, 11, 42, 43, 44, 53, 54, and 55, whereas types 16, 18, 31, 33, 35, 39, 45, and 56 are more often found in association with cervical intraepithelial neoplasia and invasive cancers.

Approximately one-third of women with HPV infection have coexistent cervicitis caused by other organisms. The presence of cervicitis does not significantly affect the clinical course of HPV lesions.

Cytopathology

The Papanicolaou smear often reflects the pathologic changes of cervical infections. A few inflammatory cells are seen normally in the smear, particularly immediately before, during, and immediately after the menses. However, large numbers of polymorphonuclear leukocytes and histiocytes indicate an acute cervicitis. At times the inflammatory exudate may be so dense that it obscures the epithelial cells, in which case the smear should repeated after the inflammatory process has been treated and cleared. Epithelial cell changes are commonly associated with cervical inflammation and must be distinguished from those related to neoplastic disease. Nuclear enlargement, clumping of chromatin, hyperchromatism, and nucleoli, as well as cytoplasmic eosinophilia and poorly defined cell membranes, are often seen. These are the findings of "cytologic atypia" and are nonspecific. Frequently, however, a specific diagnosis can be made either by directly identifying the offending organism or organisms or by noting typical changes in the epithelial cells characteristic of a specific type of infection. For example, the organism of trichomoniasis and moniliasis can be identified directly on the Pap smear. HPV, of course, cannot be seen, but the infection is characterized by squamous epithelial cell enlargement, multinucleation, and the perinuclear "halo" effect of koilocytosis. The so-called "balloon-cell" is almost pathognomonic of this condition. Cellular changes of mild dysplasia (low-grade squamous intraepithelial lesion [SIL]), moderate or severe dysplasia (carcinoma in situ [CIS], high-grade SIL), and even invasive cancer may be associated findings.

Greatly enlarged, multinucleated cells with ground-glass cytoplasm and nuclei containing characteristic inclusion bodies are indicative of infection with HSV.

Histopathology of Cervical Infections

Histopathologic findings of cervical infection also are both nonspecific and specific. Characteristically, both *N gonorrhoeae* and *C trachomatis* infections produce a nonspecific acute inflammatory reaction. Because of edema and increased vascularity, the cervix becomes swollen and reddened. Stromal edema and infiltration by polymorphonuclear leukocytes are seen microscopically, and there may be focal loss of overlying mucous membrane.

As the acute process subsides, the swelling and redness disappear, and the polymorphonuclear leukocytes are replaced by lymphocytes, plasma cells, and macrophages—the histologic picture of chronic cervicitis. Irritation due to infection causes the glandular epithelium to hyperfunction, and mucus mixed with inflammatory cells produces a copious purulent or mucopurulent exudate, which may be clinically apparent only by introducing a cotton swab into the cervical canal. Because the infected clefts and crypts drain poorly, they become dilated and often obstructed, leading to microabscess formation. With longstanding inflammation, proliferation of fibrous connective tissue in the cervical stroma occurs. This results in hypertrophy and elongation of the cervix, and if this process is extreme, the portio vaginalis may actually protrude beyond the vaginal introitus, giving the impression of a prolapse of the uterus.

On numerous occasions a histopathologic diagnosis of chronic cervicitis is made based on the finding of small collections of lymphocytes in the cervical stroma. This is a characteristic of the cervix of almost all parous women, and unless there is some clinical manifestation of cervicitis, it is probably not a significant finding.

The gross appearance of acute cervicitis must be distinguished clinically and at times histologically from the red, granular inflamed-appearing cervix of cervical ectopy, in which variable portions of the cervical portio vaginalis are covered by endocervical, mucus-secreting epithelium or by a thin layer of immature metaplastic epithelium. Particularly in younger women, the squamocolumnar junction, instead of being located at or near the external os, is found on the surface of the portio. Being covered only by a single layer of columnar cells, the underlying vascular stroma is clearly visible, producing a red, granular appearance. In the past this has been called a cervical "erosion." "Erosion" is not a proper term for cervical redness except as an acute, limited denudation of mucous membrane as might be seen with an especially virulent acute cervicitis or following punch biopsy, cauterization, cryotherapy, laser treatment, loop excision, cone biopsy, or radiation therapy.

The location of squamocolumnar tissue of the cervix is not static throughout life, but instead undergoes continuous change. Through the process of squamous metaplasia, columnar epithelium on the portio vaginalis is gradually converted to stratified squamous epithelium. Initially the stratified metaplastic epithelium is thin and immature, but with the passage of time becomes thicker and more mature, eventually taking on the appearance of original squamous epithelium. Microscopically, the squamocolumnar junction rarely demonstrates an abrupt transition from squamous to columnar epithelium, but instead is marked by a zone of immature squamous metaplasia (Figs 35–8 and

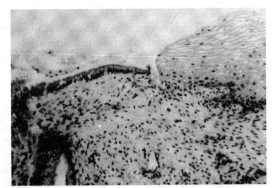

Figure 35–8. Abrupt transition, squamocolumnar junction.

35–9). This change from a mucous membrane covered by a single layer of columnar epithelium to one of the stratified squamous epithelium is not only a continuously ongoing process, but is accelerated during three periods of a woman's life: fetal existence, adolescence, and during the first pregnancy.

By the time a woman reaches her fifth decade, the squamocolumnar junction has receded into the endocervical canal, and the portio vaginalis is completely covered by squamous epithelium. In the process, however, the deeper crypts and clefts of columnar epithelium are bridged over and occluded by metaplastic epithelium, obstructing the egress of mucus, producing the common, typical nabothian cysts of the cervix. To the naked eye, the presence of nabothian cysts indicates that this area at one time was occupied by columnar epithelium which has undergone transformation. Therefore, the nabothian cyst is the hallmark of the "transformation zone," the area in which epithelial neoplasia first appears.

Certain pathologic findings are specific in that they may implicate specific organisms. For example, microscopic examination of a cervical biopsy obtained from a vesicular lesion may demonstrate intraepithelial, multinucleated giant cells containing nuclear inclusions surrounded by a clear halo typical of HSV infection. Colposcopically directed biopsy of an area of white epithelium, coarse punctation, or mosaicism may show a flat, thickened, squamous epithelium whose superficial layers are occupied by cells demonstrating large cytoplasmic vacuoles that are devoid of glycogen, surrounding shrunken, hyperchromatic nuclei and cell membranes that are thickened and eosinophilic. These are the typical histologic findings of HPV infection (Fig. 35–10). They may be associated with the findings of intraepithelial neoplasia (see Chapter 47).

Clinical Findings

A. SYMPTOMS AND SIGNS

1. Acute cervicitis—The primary symptom of acute cervicitis is a purulent vaginal discharge. The appearance of the discharge is variable—often thick and creamy as in gonorrheal infection; foamy and greenish-white as in trichomonal infection; white and curd-like in candidiasis; and thin and gray in bacterial vaginosis. Chlamydia infections often produce a purulent discharge from an angry, reddened, congested cervix. The discharge is often indistinguishable from that due to gonorrheal cervicitis and has been characterized as mucopurulent. Mucopurulent cervicitis, however, may be present in 40–60% of women in whom no infection is identified.

Inspection of the cervix initially infected by *N gonorrhoeae* generally reveals an acutely inflamed, edematous cervix with a purulent discharge escaping from the external os. In trichomonal infection, there might be

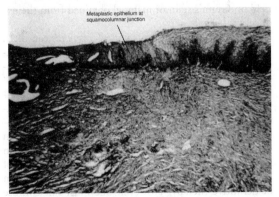

Figure 35–9. Metaplastic epithelium at the squamocolumnar junction.

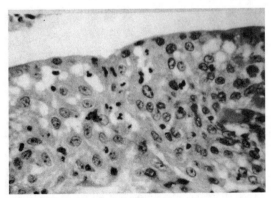

Figure 35–10. Squamous epithelium showing histologic changes of HPV infection.

the classic strawberry-like appearance visible on the squamous epithelial surface of the portio vaginalis as well as the adjacent vaginal mucosa. As noted previously, mucopurulent endocervical exudate is the hallmark of *C trachomatis* infection. In candidiasis, there is likely to be a white cheesy exudate that is difficult to wipe away, and that if scraped off, usually leaves punctate hemorrhagic areas. Colposcopic findings of acute cervicitis are those primarily of an altered microangioarchitecture with marked increase in the surface capillaries, which when viewed end-on may show a pattern of diffuse "punctation." Trichomoniasis is typified by characteristic double-hairpin capillaries. The capillary pattern of inflammation should not be confused with that of neoplasia. In an inflammatory process, the colposcopic picture is diffuse with ill-defined margins in contrast with the localized and sharply demarcated vascular changes associated with intraepithelial neoplasia. It should be emphasized that invasive cancers often are secondarily infected, so that in addition to the colposcopic changes associated with frank malignancy, those related to inflammation are also present. Colposcopy also readily identifies the fine villiform pattern of cervical ectopy (Fig. 35-11).

Infertility may be a consequence of cervicitis. A thick, glutinous, acidic, pus-laden cervical mucus is noxious to sperm and prevents fertilization.

Vulvar burning and itching may be prominent symptoms. Gonorrheal cervicitis may be accompanied by urethritis with frequency, urgency, and dysuria. If associated with acute salpingitis, the symptoms and signs will be those of pelvic peritonitis.

Hyperemia of the infected cervix may be associated with freely bleeding areas. Cervical ooze may account for intermenstrual (often postcoital) spotting. Bleeding commonly occurs due to cervical friability when endocervical smears are obtained.

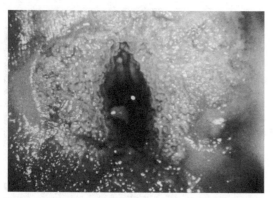

Figure 35–11. Colposcopic view of villiform pattern of cervical ectopy.

2. Chronic cervicitis—In chronic cervicitis, leukorrhea may be the chief symptom. Although it may not be as profuse as in acute cervicitis, this discharge may also cause vulvar irritation. The discharge may be frankly purulent and variable in color, or it may present simply as thick, tenacious, turbid mucus. Intermenstrual bleeding may occur.

Associated eversion may present as a velvety to granular redness or as patchy erythema due to scattered squamous metaplasia (epithelialization or epidermization). Nabothian cysts in the area of the so-called transformation zone often occur. The Schiller test may show poorly staining or nonstaining areas. There is often some tenderness and thickening in the region of the uterosacral ligaments on pelvic examination, and motion of the cervix may be painful.

Lower abdominal pain, lumbosacral backache, dysmenorrhea, or dyspareunia may occur occasionally related to an associated parametritis. Infertility may be due to the inflammatory changes that results in a tacky cervical mucus that is acidic and otherwise hostile (toxic) to sperm. Urinary frequency, urgency, and dysuria may be seen in association with chronic cervicitis. These symptoms are related to an associated subvesical lymphangitis, not to cystitis.

Inspection of the chronically infected cervix often reveals only abnormal discharge. Fibrosis and stenosis of the cervix may follow chronic cervical infection. Patulousness of the deeply lacerated external os often exposes the endocervical canal, which may bleed when wiped with a cotton applicator. The portio and the upper vagina usually appear normal in cervicitis.

B. LABORATORY FINDINGS

1. Stains and smears—Mucopurulent cervicitis is defined as gross evidence of purulent material at an inflamed cervix along with a microscopic presence of ten or more polymorphonuclear leukocytes per microscopic field on Gram's stain of material obtained from the endocervical canal.

Cervicovaginal infections with *T vaginalis* can often be identified on wet smear preparations by identification of the motile flagellated organisms. Bacterial vaginosis can be seen on wet mount by the hallmark trait of a speckled periphery to the epithelial cells. Candidal infections can be seen on potassium hydroxide preparations, with the distinctive presence of hyphae.

In acute cervicitis with *N gonorrhoeae*, a Gram's stain of cervical exudate may show the typical coffee-bean shaped, paired, gram-negative, intracellular diplococci of *N gonorrhoeae*. This finding is adequate for the initiation of definitive therapy. However, one must not confuse this organism with nonpathogenic diplococci, which may also be found in the lower reproductive tract.

2. Detection of *N gonorrhoeae* and *C trachomatis*—Previously, culture of *C trachomatis* was the preferred method for detection of infection, and was considered the gold standard for diagnosis. Although it has excellent specificity, the sensitivity is no higher than 70% in females. There also are variables involved in the testing, such as the manner of specimen collection, transport condition, culture procedures, and identification of a positive culture.

More recently, new techniques for detection of *C trachomatis* include direct fluorescent antibody (DFA), enzyme immunoassay (EIA), polymerase chain reaction (PCR), and ligase chain reaction (LCR). EIA and DFA rely on antigen detection and have a sensitivity ranging from 70–100%. The specimen can be obtained from either a urethral or cervical swab. The benefit of using nucleic acid amplification by LCR or PCR is high sensitivity and specificity. The specimen can be noninvasively obtained from either a vulvar swab or urine. These tests also allow for simultaneous detection of *N gonorrhoeae* from the same specimen.

N gonorrhoeae may also be diagnosed by direct culture of the endocervical mucus. The culture is performed on Thayer-Martin or blood agar medium. Once again, proper transport medium and timing are essential for accurate diagnosis. Most laboratories are moving towards nonculture assays such as LCR, which offer high sensitivity and specificity.

3. Blood studies—In uncomplicated cervicitis not accompanied by salpingitis, the white count may be normal or only a slight leukocytosis sedimentation rate elevation may be present.

Patients with gonorrhea or chlamydia are also at risk for infection with other sexually transmitted diseases. Counseling and testing should be offered for syphilis, hepatitis B, and HIV.

Differential Diagnosis

Noninfectious cervicitis is most commonly due to an increased mucous discharge at the time of ovulation. The mucus is clear and shows only rare leukocytes on microscopic examination. Bimanual examination should be performed to distinguish the signs and symptoms of pelvic tenderness, induration, and mass formation about the cervix when discharge is noted from the cervix.

Cervicitis must be distinguished from early neoplastic processes. This may not be easy because inflammatory conditions may alter the epithelial cells to produce atypia on cytologic examination. Colposcopy is useful (see sections on cervical dysplasia and cervical cancer). Cervical cytology and histologic examination by endocervical curettage and biopsy should be done to help distinguish chronic cervicitis from developing cancer of the cervix.

Consider also the lesions of syphilis and chancroid as well as the chronic granulomatous ulcerations of tuberculosis and granuloma inguinale.

Complications

Leukorrhea, cervical stenosis, and infertility are sequelae of chronic cervicitis. Patients with acute or chronic cervicitis may also complain of vaginal discharge and vaginal bleeding, most frequently after sexual intercourse. With *N gonorrhoeae* or *C trachomatis* cervicitis, salpingitis is a common complication, with long-term consequences including infertility and chronic pelvic pain.

Carcinoma of the cervix usually occurs in sexually active parous women. Examination often reveals neglected cervical lacerations and chronic infection; however, these cannot be implicated as the causes of cervical cancer.

Prevention

Gonorrheal, herpetic, and chlamydial cervicitis can be prevented by education of those at risk about ways to reduce their risk. Avoidance of sexual contact with infected persons or the use of condoms for protection during coitus is the most important recommendation for changing the sexual behaviors of those women at risk for infection. Clinicians should also be aware of the importance of detection in the asymptomatic patient, followed by effective treatment and counseling of the patient and her sexual partners. The avoidance of surgical or obstetric trauma and the prompt recognition and proper repair of cervical lacerations help to prevent the subsequent development of a chronically infected cervix.

When surgical removal of the corpus of the uterus is indicated, the cervix should also be removed if this is feasible. Recommendations to retain the cervix at the time of hysterectomy in order to maintain sexual function or vaginal support are controversial.

Treatment

Selection of the most appropriate treatment depends on the age of the patient and her desire for pregnancy; whether she is presently pregnant or is breastfeeding; the severity of the cervical infection; the presence of complicating factors (eg, salpingitis); and previous treatment. Instrumentation and vigorous topical therapy should be avoided during the acute phase of cervicitis and before the menses, when ascending infection may occur.

A. ACUTE CERVICITIS

When acute cervicitis is associated with vaginitis due to a specific organism, treatment must be directed accordingly. Metronidazole is specific for the treatment of *T vaginalis* infection. This may be administered as 2 g orally in a single dose or alternatively as 500 mg twice a day for 7 days. This has resulted in cure rates of approximately 90–95%. Insuring treatment of sex partners might increase the cure rate. Topical administration of metronidazole appears to be less efficacious than the oral preparations. Candidiasis is most effectively treated with topically applied azole drugs. This will result in relief of symptoms and negative cultures in 80–90% of patients. Treatment may continue for 1, 3, or 7 days, depending on the severity of the infection. Oral fluconazole in a 150-mg oral tablet has also been shown to be effective treatment.

Bacterial vaginosis can be treated with oral metronidazole, 500 mg twice daily for 7 days, or with topical clindamycin cream or metronidazole gel. It is particularly important to treat bacterial vaginosis in pregnancy due to its association with adverse outcomes such as preterm labor and premature rupture of the membranes. Pregnant women without risk of premature delivery should be treated if they have symptomatic bacterial vaginosis. High-risk women should be tested and treated regardless of the presence of symptoms. Treatment in pregnancy is metronidazole 250 mg orally 3 times a day for 7 days. Metronidazole has not been shown to be teratogenic in humans.

C trachomatis can be treated with azithromycin, 1 g orally in a single dose, or alternatively with doxycycline 100 mg, twice a day for 7 days. Alternative treatments with erythromycin or ofloxacin are suggested. In pregnancy, azithromycin may be given. Amoxicillin for 7 days has also been shown to be effective and well tolerated. Cervicitis due to *N gonorrhoeae* can be treated with single oral doses of ofloxacin 400 mg, ciprofloxacin 500 mg, or cefixime 400 mg. An intramuscular injection of ceftriaxone 125 mg may also be used. In pregnancy, fluoroquinolones should be avoided. Fluoroquinolones should also not be used in patients residing in, or who may have acquired infections in, Asia, the Pacific (including Hawaii) or California. This is due to increasing quinolone-resistant N gonorrhoeae (QRNG) in these areas. See chapter 38, and 2002 updated CDC guidelines for treatment of sexually transmitted diseases for full recommendations. Because of the high rate of coinfection with *C trachomatis,* it is recommended that patients also receive treatment for *C trachomatis* when *N gonorrhoeae* infection is found.

B. CHRONIC CERVICITIS

Several studies using more sensitive testing for *N gonorrhoeae* and *C trachomatis* have demonstrated that microscopic findings of 10 or more polymorphonuclear leukocytes per high-power field do not correlate with infection. It is therefore not necessary to treat an asymptomatic patient with chronic cervicitis who does not test positive for a sexually transmitted disease.

Surgical procedures may be useful for treatment of symptomatic chronic cervicitis or in the absence of an infectious pathogen or evidence of dysplasia. Techniques including cryosurgery, electrocauterization, and laser therapy may be of use, although there are significant disadvantages, including the high risk of recurrence and risk of cervical injury.

Treatment of Complications

A. CERVICAL HEMORRHAGE

This may follow electrocauterization, loop excision, cryosurgery, or laser vaporization, and may require suture and ligation of the bleeding vessels. Usually, point coagulation of bleeding areas with monsel solution or silver nitrate applied topically is successful. Repeat electrocauterization may also be beneficial.

B. SALPINGITIS

Inflammation of the uterine tubes usually necessitates the administration of a broad-spectrum antibiotic.

C. LEUKORRHEA

Significant cervical discharge may be due to persistent infection with a pathogen. Appropriate testing should be performed and selective antibiotic treatment administered.

D. CERVICAL STENOSIS

The gentle passage of graduated sounds through the cervical canal at weekly intervals during the intermenstrual phase for 2–3 months following treatment will prevent or correct stenosis.

E. INFERTILITY

The absence of cervical mucus necessary for sperm migration often causes infertility and may be due to extensive destruction (cauterization, freezing, or vaporization) or removal (conization or loop excision) of the endocervical glandular cells. Treatment includes low dose estrogen for 1 week prior to ovulation or intrauterine insemination with washed and incubated sperm.

Prognosis

With conservative, systemic, and persistent therapy, cervicitis can almost always be cured. With neglect or overtreatment, the prognosis is poor.

GRANULOMATOUS INFECTIONS OF THE CERVIX

Tuberculosis, tertiary syphilis, and granuloma inguinale may on rare occasions be manifested by chronic cervical lesions. These lesions usually take the form of nodules, ulcerations, or granulation tissue. They produce a chronic inflammatory exudate characterized histologically by lymphocytes, giant cells, and histiocytes. They may simulate carcinoma of the cervix and must be distinguished from this and other neoplastic diseases.

Tuberculosis

Since 1986, the steadily decreasing incidence of tuberculosis in the U.S. over the previous several decades has recently reversed, and the risk has increased, particularly for blacks, Hispanics, and Asians. Some of this increase has been attributed to the epidemic spread of the human immunodeficiency virus (HIV).

Genitourinary tuberculosis is almost always secondary to infection elsewhere in the body, usually pulmonary, but active pulmonary disease can be documented in only one-third of patients. Vascular dissemination is responsible for infection of the fallopian tubes in almost all patients with genital tuberculosis, and involvement of the endometrium follows in 90%. Cervical disease is thought to be secondary to involvement of the endometrium, but is rare, occurring in only 1% of cases. In the past, genital tuberculosis has accounted for only 1% of patients with pelvic inflammatory disease; however, in European and Asian countries, the occurrence ranges from 2–10%. With increasing numbers of immigrants to the U.S. and with the rise in incidence of AIDS in American women, an increase in the incidence of pelvic tuberculosis can be expected.

The chief clinical manifestations of cervical involvement are a foul-smelling discharge and contact bleeding. The cervix may be hypertrophied and nodular, without any visible lesion on the portio vaginalis, or speculum examination may demonstrate either an ulcerative or a papillary lesion, thus resembling neoplastic disease.

The diagnosis of tuberculosis of the cervix must be made by biopsy. Histologically, the disease is characterized by tubercles undergoing central caseation. Because such lesions may be caused by other organisms, it is necessary to demonstrate the tubercle bacillus by acid-fast stains or culture.

The reader is referred to other texts for the details of medical therapy of genital tuberculosis. Most patients are cured by medical management alone; patients who respond poorly or who have other problems (eg, tumors, fistulas) may require total hysterectomy and bilateral salpingo-oophorectomy after a trial of chemotherapy.

RARE INFECTIOUS DISEASES OF THE CERVIX

Lymphogranuloma venereum, a chlamydial infection, and chancroid, caused by *Haemophilus ducreyi*, may attack the cervix along with other areas of the reproductive tract.

Cervical actinomycosis may occur as a result of contamination by instruments and by intrauterine devices. The cervical lesion may be a nodular tumor, ulcer, or fistula. Prolonged penicillin or sulfonamide therapy is recommended.

Schistosomiasis of the cervix is usually secondary to involvement of the pelvic and uterine veins by the blood fluke *Schistosoma haematobium.* Cervical schistosomiasis may produce a large papillary growth that ulcerates and bleeds on contact, simulating cervical cancer. In other instances, it may be found in endocervical polyps, causing intermenstrual and postcoital bleeding. An ovum can occasionally be identified in a biopsy specimen taken from the granulomatous cervical lesion. The diagnosis is usually made, however, by recovering the parasite from the urine or feces. Chemical, serologic, and intradermal tests for schistosomiasis are also available.

Echinococcal cysts may involve the cervix. Treatment consists of surgical excision.

CYSTIC ABNORMALITIES OF THE CERVIX

Nabothian Cysts

Nabothian cysts develop when a tunnel or cleft of tall columnar endocervical epithelium becomes covered by squamous metaplasia. These appear grossly as translucent or yellow in color and may vary in size from a few millimeters to 3 cm in diameter.

Mesonephric Cysts

Microscopic remnants of the mesonephric (wolffian) duct are often seen deep in the stroma externally in the normal cervix. Occasionally they become cystic, forming structures up to 2.5 mm in diameter, lined by ragged cuboid epithelium. They may be confused with deeply situated nabothian cysts, but their location and the wolffian-type cells lining the cysts serve as useful distinguishing features.

CERVICAL STENOSIS

Cervical stenosis of congenital, inflammatory, neoplastic, or surgical origin may be partially or even completely occlusive. Most cases of cervical stenosis follow extensive surgical manipulation of the cervix (eg, electrocoagulation, cryotherapy, laser vaporization, conization, or cervical amputation) or radiation therapy. Cervical stenosis is not uncommon, however, in postmenopausal women with prolonged estrogen deficiency. Marked to complete obstruction of menstrual drainage will result in hematometra, typified by cryptomenorrhea or amenorrhea; abdominal discomfort; and a soft, slightly tender midpelvic mass. Pyometra may develop in the post-menopausal woman with cervical stenosis and always raises the suspicion of an associated endometrial carcinoma. Both hematometra and pyometra are readily confirmed by pelvic ultrasonography.

Cautious dilatation of the cervix is recommended, with drainage of the entrapped fluid. Cultures and sensitivity tests should be done and, with appropriate antibiotic coverage, cervical endometrial tissue or both should be obtained to rule out cancer. The endocervical canal should receive minimal caustic therapy or electrotherapy for chronic cervicitis to avoid cervical stenosis. Removal of the cicatrix by laser vaporization and loop excision has been effective in cases of postconization stenosis.

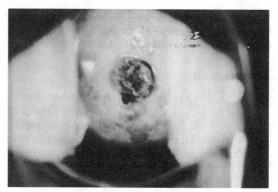

Figure 35–12. Cervical polyp.

BENIGN NEOPLASMS OF THE CERVIX

1. Microglandular Hyperplasia of the Endocervical Mucosa

Microglandular (adenomatous) hyperplasia of the endocervix and abnormal response to the hormonal stimulus of oral contraceptive medication may occur in occasional patients. It may also result from inflammation. Grossly, adenomatous hyperplasia appears as exuberant granular tissue within the cervical canal, often extruding beyond the cervical os. The disorder may be mistaken for cancer, but biopsy should done to make the distinction. Microscopically, it presents as a collection of closely packed cystic spaces lined by nonneoplastic columnar epithelium and filled with mucus.

2. Cervical Polyps

ESSENTIALS OF DIAGNOSIS

- *Intermenstrual or postcoital bleeding.*
- *A soft, red pedunculated protrusion from the cervical canal at the external os.*
- *Microscopic examination confirms the diagnosis of benign polyp.*

General Considerations

Cervical polyps are small pedunculated, often sessile neoplasms of the cervix. Most originate from the endocervix; a few arise from the portio (Fig 35–12). They are composed of a vascular connective tissue stroma and covered by columnar, squamocolumnar, or squamous epithelium. Polyps are relatively common, especially in multigravidas over 20 years of age. They are rare before menarche, but an occasional polyp may develop after menopause. Asymptomatic polyps often are discovered on routine pelvic examination. Most are benign, but all should be removed and submitted for pathologic examination because malignant change may occur. Moreover, some cervical cancers present as a polypoid mass.

Polyps arise as a result of focal hyperplasia of the endocervix. It is not known whether this is due to chronic inflammation, an abnormal local responsiveness to hormonal stimulation, or a localized vascular congestion of cervical blood vessels. They are often found in association with endometrial hyperplasia, suggesting that hyperestrogenism plays a significant etiologic role.

Endocervical polyps are usually red, flame-shaped, fragile growths and may vary in size from a few millimeters in length and diameter to larger tumors 2–3 cm in diameter and several centimeters long. These polyps are usually attached to the endocervical mucosa near the external os by a narrow pedicle, but occasionally the base is broad. On microscopic examination, the stroma of a polyp is composed of fibrous connective tissue containing numerous small vessels in the center. There is often extravasation of blood and marked infiltration of the stroma by inflammatory cells (polymorphonuclear neutrophils, lymphocytes, and plasma cells). The surface epithelium resembles that of the endocervix, varying from typical picket-fence columnar cells to areas that show squamous metaplasia and mature stratified squamous epithelium. The surface often is thrown into folds, as is much of the normal endocervical mucosa.

Ectocervical polyps are pale, flesh-colored, smooth, and rounded or elongated, often with a broad pedicle. They arise from the portio and are less likely to bleed than endocervical polyps. Microscopically, they are more fibrous than endocervical polyps, having few or no mucus glands. They are covered by stratified squamous epithelium.

Metaplastic alteration is common. Inflammation, often with necrosis at the tip (or more extensively), is typical of both polyp types.

The incidence of malignant change in a cervical polyp is estimated to be less than 1%. Squamous cell carcinoma is the most common type, although adenocarcinomas have been reported. Endometrial cancer may involve the polyp secondarily. Sarcoma rarely develops within a polyp.

Botryoid sarcoma, an embryonal tumor of the cervix (or vaginal wall) resembling small pink or yellow grapes, contains striated muscle and other mesenchymal elements. It is extremely malignant.

Most polypoid structures are vascular and often infected, and are subject to displacement or torsion. Discharge commonly results, and bleeding, often metrorrhagia of the postcoital type, follows.

Chronic irritation and bleeding are annoying and cause cervicitis, endometritis, and parametritis; salpingitis may develop if these are not treated successfully.

Because polyps are a potential focus of cancer, they must be examined routinely for malignant characteristics upon removal.

Clinical Findings

A. Symptoms and Signs

Intermenstrual or postcoital bleeding is the most common symptom of cervical polyps. Leukorrhea and hypermenorrhea have also been associated with cervical polyps.

Abnormal vaginal bleeding is often reported. Postmenopausal bleeding is frequently described by older women. Infertility may be traceable to cervical polyps and cervicitis.

Cervical polyps appear as smooth, red, finger-like projections from the cervical canal and are usually about 1–2 cm in length and 0.5–1 cm in diameter. Generally they are too soft to be felt by the examiner's finger.

B. X-Ray Findings

Polyps high in the endocervical canal may be demonstrated by hysterosalpingogram or saline infusion sonohysterography, and often are significant findings in hitherto unexplained infertility.

C. Laboratory Findings

Vaginal cytology will reveal signs of infection and often mildly atypical cells. Blood and urine studies are not helpful.

D. Special Examination

A polyp high in the endocervical canal may be seen with the aid of a special endocervical speculum or by hysteroscopy. Some polyps are found only at the time of diagnostic D&C in the investigation of abnormal bleeding.

Differential Diagnosis

Masses projecting from the cervix may be polypoid but not polyps. Adenocarcinoma of the endometrium or endometrial sarcoma may present at the external os or even beyond. Discharge and bleeding usually occur.

Typical polyps are not difficult to diagnose by gross inspection, but ulcerated and atypical growths must be distinguished from small submucous pedunculated myomas or endometrial polyps arising low in the uterus. These often result in dilatation of the cervix, presenting just within the os and resembling cervical polyps. The products of conception, usually decidua, may push through the cervix and resemble a polypoid tissue mass, but other signs and symptoms of recent pregnancy generally are absent. Condylomata, submucous myomas, and polypoid carcinomas are diagnosed by microscopic examination.

Complications

Cervical polyps may be infected, some by virulent staphylococci, streptococci, or other pathogens. Serious infections occasionally follow instrumentation for the identification or removal of polyps. A broad-spectrum antibiotic should be administered at the first sign or symptom of spreading infection.

Acute salpingitis may be initiated or exacerbated by polypectomy.

It is unwise to remove a large polyp and then do a hysterectomy several days thereafter. Pelvic peritonitis may complicate the latter procedure. A delay of several weeks or a month between polypectomy and hysterectomy is recommended.

Treatment

A. Medical Measures

Appropriate testing for cervical discharge should be performed as indicated and treated if infection is identified.

B. Specific Measures

Most polyps can be removed in the physician's office. This is done with little bleeding by grasping the pedicle with a hemostat or long grasping instrument and twisting it until the growth is avulsed. Large polyps and those with sessile attachments may require excision in an operating room setting. This will allow for anesthesia to be administered for further visualization and treatment using the hysteroscope and control of any hemorrhage.

If the cervix is soft, patulous, or definitely dilated, and the polyp is large, hysteroscopy should be performed, especially if the pedicle is not readily visible. Exploration of the cervical and uterine cavities with the hysteroscope allows for further identification of other polyps. All tissue must be sent to a pathologist to be examined for possible underlying malignant or premalignant conditions.

Prognosis

Simple removal of cervical polyps is usually curative.

3. Papillomas of the Cervix

ESSENTIALS OF DIAGNOSIS

- *Asymptomatic.*
- *Papillary projection from the exocervix.*
- *The presence of koilocytes with or without cytologic atypia.*
- *Colposcopic identification.*

General Considerations

Cervical papillomas are benign neoplasms found on the portio vaginalis of the cervix. They are of two types: (1) The typical solitary papillary projection from the exocervix, composed of a central core of fibrous connective tissue covered by stratified squamous epithelium. This is a true benign neoplasm, and the cause is unknown. (2) Condylomata of the cervix, which may be present in various forms ranging from a slightly raised area on the exocervix that appears white after acetic acid application (on colposcopy) to the typical condyloma acuminatum. These are usually multiple and are caused by HPV infection, a sexually transmitted disease. Similar lesions of the vagina and vulva are often, but not always, present. Evidence of HPV infections can be found in 1–2% of cytologically screened women. The incidence is much higher in women attending STD clinics.

Clinical Findings

A. Symptoms and Signs

There are no characteristic symptoms of cervical papillomas; they are often discovered on routine pelvic ex-

amination or colposcopic examination for dysplasia revealed by Papanicolaou smear.

B. Laboratory Findings

Cytologic findings of koilocytes—squamous cells with perinuclear clear halos—are strongly suggestive of HPV infection. Dysplastic squamous cells are frequently found in association with koilocytes. Biopsy of involved epithelium reveals papillomatosis and acanthosis. Mitoses may be frequent, but in the absence of neoplastic change, the cells are orderly with regular nuclear features. Koilocytes predominate in the superficial cells.

Complications

Intraepithelial neoplasia is associated with certain types of HPV infection (see Cervical Intraepithelial Neoplasia, Chapter 47). The presence of condylomata of the portio vaginalis substantially increases the risk of squamous cell carcinoma of the cervix.

Prevention

Contraception with condoms and possibly other barrier methods may prevent primary infection and reinfection.

Treatment

Solitary papillomas should be surgically excised and submitted for pathologic examination. Likewise, biopsies of flat condylomata should be submitted for histopathologic examination. Flat condylomata may be completely removed with a biopsy instrument if they are small. More extensive lesions may require cryotherapy, loop excision, or laser vaporization. Dysplasia associated with HPV infection should be managed according to the severity and extent of the dysplastic process (see Cervical Intraepithelial Neoplasia, Chapter 47).

Prognosis

Because the entire lower genital tract is a target area for HPV infection, long-term follow-up with attention to the cervix, vagina, and vulva is necessary. Excision of solitary, non-HPV-related papillomas is curative.

4. Leiomyomas of the Cervix

The paucity of smooth muscle elements in the cervical stroma makes leiomyomas that arise in the cervix uncommon. The ratio of corpus leiomyomas to cervical leiomyomas is in the range of 12:1.

Although myomas are usually multiple in the corpus, cervical myomas are most often solitary and may be large enough to fill the entire pelvic cavity, compressing the bladder, rectum, and ureters (Fig. 35–13).

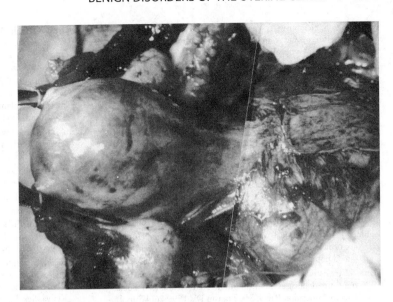

Figure 35–13. Large cervical leiomyoma filling true pelvis.

Grossly and microscopically they are identical with leiomyomas that arise elsewhere in the uterus.

Clinical Findings

A. SYMPTOMS AND SIGNS

Cervical leiomyomas are often silent, producing no symptoms unless they become very large. Symptoms are those due to pressure on surrounding organs such as the bladder, rectum, or soft tissues of the parametrium, or obstruction of the cervical canal. Frequency and urgency of urination are the result of bladder compression. Urinary retention occasionally occurs as a result of pressure against the urethra. Hematometra may develop with obstruction of the cervix.

If the direction of growth is lateral, there may be ureteral obstruction with hydronephrosis. Rectal encroachment causes constipation. Dyspareunia may occur if the tumor occupies the vagina. In pregnancy, because of their location, large cervical leiomyomas, unlike those involving the corpus, are apt to cause soft tissue dystocia, preventing descent of the presenting part in the pelvis. Cervical leiomyomas of significant size can be readily palpated on bimanual examination.

B. IMAGING

A plain film may demonstrate the typical mottled calcific pattern associated with cervical leiomyomas. Hysterography may define distortion of the endocervical canal. Intravenous urography may demonstrate ureteral displacement or obstruction. MRI is diagnostic.

Treatment

Small, asymptomatic cervical leiomyomas do not require treatment. If the leiomyomas become symptomatic, removal may be possible via hysteroscopic resection. If there are additional multiple leiomyomas that cannot be resected with the hysteroscope, uterine artery embolization, abdominal myomectomy, or hysterectomy may be indicated, depending on the patient's desire for preservation of fertility.

Because of the proximity of the pelvic ureter to the cervix, this structure may be in jeopardy in any operation involving a cervical leiomyoma, and precautions should be taken to prevent its injury.

Prognosis

Recurrence of cervical myomas after surgical removal is rare.

REFERENCES

Anomalies of the Cervix

Folch M, Pigem I, Konje JC: Müllerian agenesis: etiology, diagnosis and management. Obstet Gynecol Surv 2000;55:644.

Goldberg JM, Falcone T: Effect of diethylstilbestrol on reproductive function. Fertil Steril 1999;72:1.

Kaufman RH et al: Continued follow-up of pregnancy outcomes in diethylstilbestrol-exposed offspring. Obstet Gynecol 2000; 96:483.

Fujimoto VY et al: Congenital cervical atresia: report of seven cases and review of the literature. Am J Obstet Gynecol 1997; 177:1419.

Preutthipan S, Herabutya Y: Vaginal misoprostol for cervical priming before operative hysteroscopy: a randomized controlled trial. Obstet Gynecol 2000;96:890.

Simpson JL: Genetics of the female reproductive ducts. Am J Med Genet (Semin Med Genet) 1999;89:224.

Cervical Infections

Adair CD et al: Chlamydia in pregnancy: a randomized trial of azithromycin and erythromycin. Obstet Gynecol 1998; 91:165.

Anttila T et al: Serotypes of *Chlamydia trachomatis* and risk for development of cervical squamous cell carcinoma. JAMA 2001;285:47.

Black CM: Current methods of laboratory diagnosis of *Chlamydia trachomatis* infections. Clin Microbiol Rev 1997;10:160.

Bohmer JT et al: Cervical wet mount as a negative predictor for gonococci- and *Chlamydia trachomatis*-induced cervicitis in a gravid population. Am J Obstet Gynecol 1999;181:283.

Cates W Jr: Estimates of the incidence and prevalence of sexually transmitted diseases in the United States. American Social Health Association Panel. Sex Transm Dis 1999;26(4 Suppl): S2.

Centers for Disease Control and Prevention: Sexually transmitted disease treatment guidelines. MMWR 2002;51(RR06); 1–80.

Gaydos CA et al: *Chlamydia trachomatis* infections in female military recruits. N Engl J Med 1998;339:739.

Hook EW III et al: Diagnosis of genitourinary *Chlamydia trachomatis* infections by using the ligase chain reaction on patient-obtained vaginal swabs. J Clin Microbiol 1997;35:2133.

Kaufman RH et al: Human papillomavirus testing as triage for atypical squamous cells of undetermined significance and low-grade squamous intraepithelial lesions: sensitivity, specificity, and cost-effectiveness. Am J Obstet Gynecol 1997; 177:930.

Mehta SD et al: Unsuspected gonorrhea and chlamydia in patients of an urban adult emergency department: a critical population for STD control intervention. Sex Transm Dis 2001; 28:33.

Modarress KJ et al: Detection of *Chlamydia trachomatis* and *Neisseria gonorrhoeae* in swab specimens by the Hybrid Capture II and PACE 2 nucleic acid probe tests. Sex Transm Dis 1999;26:303.

Moore SG et al: Clinical utility of measuring white blood cells on vaginal wet mount and endocervical gram stain for the prediction of chlamydial and gonococcal infections. Sex Transm Dis 2000;27:530.

Myziuk L, Romanowski B, Brown M: Endocervical Gram stain smears and their usefulness in the diagnosis of *Chlamydia trachomatis*. Sex Transm Infect 2001;77:103.

Paavonen J et al: Cost-benefit analysis of first-void urine *Chlamydia trachomatis* screening program. Obstet Gynecol 1998;92:292.

Sellors J et al: Chlamydial cervicitis: testing the practice guidelines for presumptive diagnosis. Can Med Assoc J 1998;158:41.

Stary A: Chlamydia screening: which sample for which technique? Genitourinary Med 1997;73:99.

Tyndall MW et al: Predicting *Neisseria gonorrhoeae* and *Chlamydia trachomatis* infection using risk scores, physical examination, microscopy, and leukocyte esterase urine dipsticks among asymptomatic women attending a family planning clinic in Kenya. Sex Transm Dis 1999;26:476.

Woodman CB et al: Natural history of cervical human papillomavirus infection in young women: a longitudinal cohort study. Lancet 2001;357:1831.

Wright TC Jr et al: Human immunodeficiency virus 1 expression in the female genital tract in association with cervical inflammation and ulceration. Am J Obstet Gynecol 2001;184:279.

Cervical Polyps and Leiomyomas

Ozsaran AA, Itil IM, Sagol S: Endometrial hyperplasia co-existing with cervical polyps. Int J Gynaecol Obstet 1999;66:185.

Tiltman AJ: Leiomyomas of the uterine cervix: a study of frequency. Int J Gynecol Pathol 1998;17:231.

Varasteh NN et al: Pregnancy rates after hysteroscopic polypectomy and myomectomy in infertile women. Obstet Gynecol 1999;94:168.

Benign Disorders of the Uterine Corpus

Sanaz Memarzadeh, MD, Michael S. Broder, MD, MSHS, Alvin S. Wexler, MD, & Martin L. Pernoll, MD

LEIOMYOMA OF THE UTERUS (FIBROMYOMA, FIBROID, MYOMA)

ESSENTIALS OF DIAGNOSIS

- Mass: irregular enlargement of the uterus.
- Bleeding: hypermenorrhea, metrorrhagia, dysmenorrhea.
- Pain: torsion or degeneration.
- Pressure: symptoms from neighboring organs.

General Considerations

Uterine leiomyomas are benign neoplasms composed primarily of smooth muscle. Leiomyomas are present in 20–25% of reproductive-age women, but for an unknown reason, leiomyomas are 3–9 times more frequent in black than in white women. Indeed, by the fifth decade as many as 50% of black women will have leiomyomata.

The etiology of this common tumor is not known. Leiomyomas are not detectable before puberty and, being hormonally responsive, normally grow only during the reproductive years. While they can occur as isolated growths, they are more commonly multiple. They are usually less than 15 cm in size but rarely may reach enormous proportions, weighing more than 45 kg (100 lb).

While usually asymptomatic, leiomyomata can produce a wide spectrum of problems including metrorrhagia and menorrhagia, pain, and infertility. Indeed, excessive uterine bleeding from leiomyomas is one of the most common indications for hysterectomy in the U.S.

Asymptomatic leiomyomas may mask other concomitant and potentially lethal pelvic tumors, so the physician should not be deceived into following "asymptomatic myomas" without verification that an underlying uterine tube, ovarian, or bowel carcinoma does not also exist. Occasionally it is necessary to differentiate leiomyomata from leiomyosarcoma. The latter occurs infrequently and is malignant.

Pathogenesis

The cause of uterine leiomyomata is not known. There is evidence that each individual leiomyoma is unicellular in origin (monoclonal) from glucose-6-phosphate dehydrogenase studies. While there is no evidence to suggest that estrogens cause leiomyomas, estrogens are certainly implicated in growth of myomas. Leiomyomas contain estrogen receptors in higher concentrations than the surrounding myometrium but in lower concentrations than the endometrium. Progesterone increases the mitotic activity of myomas in young women, but the mechanisms and growth factors involved are still not characterized. Progesterone may also allow for tumor enlargement by downregulating apoptosis in the tumor. Estrogens may contribute to tumor enlargement by increasing the production of extracellular matrix. Leiomyomas may increase in size with estrogen therapy and during pregnancy, but don't always do so. They usually decrease in size following menopause.

The hypothesis that human growth hormone (HGH) is related to the development of leiomyomas has been largely dispelled by radioimmunoassay studies of HGH in pregnant patients and in patients taking estrogens, but there is speculation that leiomyoma growth in pregnancy is related to synergistic activity of estradiol and human placental lactogen (HPL).

Pathology

Leiomyomas are usually multiple, discrete, and either spherical or irregularly lobulated. Leiomyomas have a false capsular covering, and they are clearly demarcated from the surrounding myometrium. They can be easily and cleanly enucleated from the surrounding myometrial tissue. On gross examination in transverse section, they are buff-colored, rounded, smooth, and usually firm. Generally, they are lighter in color than the myometrium (Fig 36–1). When a fresh specimen is sectioned, the tumor surface projects above the surface

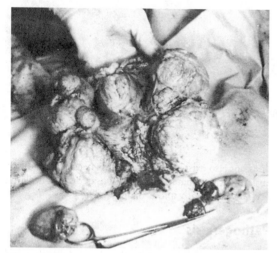

Figure 36–1. Multiple leiomyomas. Cervix is opened at the bottom.

of the surrounding musculature, revealing the pseudocapsule.

A. Classification

Uterine leiomyomas originate in the myometrium and are classified by anatomic location (Fig 36–2). Submucous leiomyomas lie just beneath the endometrium and tend to compress it as they grow toward the uterine lumen. Their impact on the endometrium and its blood supply most often leads to irregular uterine bleeding. Leiomyomata may also develop pedicles and protrude fully into the uterine cavity. Occasionally they may even pass through the cervical canal while still attached within the corpus by a long stalk. When this occurs, leiomyomata are subject to torsion or infection, conditions that must be taken into consideration before treatment.

Intramural or interstitial leiomyomas lie within the uterine wall, giving it a variable consistency. Subserous or subperitoneal leiomyomata may lie just at the serosal surface of the uterus or may bulge outward from the myometrium. The subserous leiomyomata may also become pedunculated. If such a tumor acquires an extrauterine blood supply from omental vessels, its pedicle may atrophy and resorb; the tumor is then said to be parasitic. Subserous tumors arising laterally may extend between the 2 peritoneal layers of the broad ligament to become intraligamentary leiomyomas. This may lead to compromise of the ureter and/or pelvic blood supply.

B. Microscopic Structure

Nonstriated muscle fibers are arranged in interlacing bundles of varying size running in different directions (whorled appearance). Individual cells are spindle-shaped, have elongated nuclei, and are quite uniform in size. Varying amounts of connective tissue are intermixed with the smooth muscle bundles. Leiomyomata are sharply demarcated from surrounding normal musculature by a pseudocapsule of areolar tissue and compressed myometrium. The arterial density of a leiomyoma is less than that of the surrounding myometrium, and the small arteries that supply the tumor are less tortuous than the adjacent radial arteries. The arteries penetrate the myoma randomly on its surface and are oriented in the direction of the muscle bundles; thus, they present no regular pattern. One or 2 major vessels may be found in the base or pedicle. The venous pattern appears to be even more sparse, but this may be in part artifactual because of the difficulty encountered in filling the venous circulation under artificial conditions.

C. Secondary Changes

There may be areas of hyalinization, liquefaction (cystic degeneration), calcification, hemorrhage, fat, or inflammation within leiomyomata. While these secondary alterations are histologically interesting, they usually have

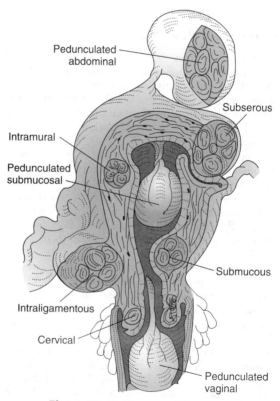

Figure 36–2. Myomas of the uterus.

little clinical significance. Whether or not leiomyosarcomas are a malignant alteration within a mature leiomyoma, as is commonly stated, or arise de novo remains an unsettled issue. Extraordinarily cellular myomas have often been misinterpreted as sarcomas because the criteria used to differentiate leiomyoma from sarcoma are imprecise and often subjective. Ultrastructural studies suggest that leiomyoma and leiomyosarcoma are distinct entities and that the cellular leiomyoma is merely a variety of the common leiomyoma.

1. Benign degeneration—Benign degeneration is of the following types:

a. Atrophic—Signs and symptoms regress or disappear as the tumor size decreases at menopause or after pregnancy.

b. Hyaline—Mature or "old" leiomyomas are white but contain yellow, soft, and often gelatinous areas of hyaline change. These tumors are usually asymptomatic.

c. Cystic—Liquefaction follows extreme hyalinization, and physical stress may cause sudden evacuation of fluid contents into the uterus, the peritoneal cavity, or the retroperitoneal space.

d. Calcific (calcareous)—Subserous leiomyomata are most commonly affected by circulatory deprivation, which causes precipitation of calcium carbonate and phosphate within the tumor.

e. Septic—Circulatory inadequacy may cause necrosis of the central portion of the tumor followed by infection. Acute pain, tenderness, and fever result.

f. Carneous (red)—Venous thrombosis and congestion with interstitial hemorrhage are responsible for the color of a leiomyoma undergoing red degeneration (Fig 36–3). During pregnancy, when carneous degeneration is most common, edema and hypertrophy of the myometrium occur. The physiologic changes in the leiomyoma are not the same as in the myometrium; the resultant anatomic discrepancy impedes the blood supply, resulting in aseptic degeneration and infarction. The process is usually accompanied by pain but is self-limited. Potential complications of degeneration in pregnancy include preterm labor, and rarely, initiation of disseminated intravascular coagulation.

g. Myxomatous (fatty)—This uncommon and asymptomatic degeneration follows hyaline and cystic degeneration.

2. Malignant transformation—Malignant transformation (leiomyosarcomas) are reported to develop with a frequency of 0.1–0.5% that of diagnosed leiomyomata.

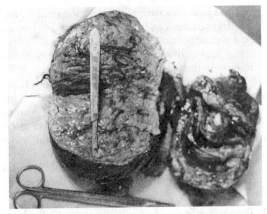

Figure 36–3. Carneous (red) degeneration. Note the congested, dark appearance as compared with Figure 36–1.

Clinical Findings

A. Symptoms

Symptoms are present in only 35–50% of patients with leiomyomas. Thus, most leiomyomata do not produce symptoms, and even very large ones may remain undetected, particularly in the obese patient. Symptoms from leiomyomas depend on their location, size, state of preservation, and whether or not the patient is pregnant.

1. Abnormal uterine bleeding—Abnormal uterine bleeding is the most common and most important clinical manifestation of leiomyomas, being present in up to 30% of patients. The abnormal bleeding commonly produces iron deficiency anemia, which may not be uncontrollable even with iron therapy if the bleeding is heavy and protracted.

Bleeding from a submucous leiomyoma may occur from interruption of the blood supply to the endometrium, distortion and congestion of the surrounding vessels, particularly the veins, or ulceration of the overlying endometrium. Most commonly, the patient has prolonged, heavy menses (menorrhagia), premenstrual spotting, or prolonged light staining following menses; however, any type of abnormal bleeding is possible.

Minor degrees of metrorrhagia (intermenstrual bleeding) may be associated with a tumor that has areas of endometrial venous thrombosis and necrosis on its surface, particularly if it is pedunculated and partially extruded through the cervical canal.

2. Pain—Leiomyomata may cause pain when vascular compromise occurs. Thus, pain may result from degeneration associated with vascular occlusion, infection, torsion of a pedunculated tumor, or myometrial contractions to expel a subserous myoma from the uterine cavity. The pain associated with infarction from torsion or red degeneration can be excruciating and produce a clinical picture consistent with acute abdomen.

Large tumors may produce a sensation of heaviness or fullness in the pelvic area, a feeling of a mass in the pelvis, or a feeling of a mass palpable through the abdominal wall. Tumors that become impacted within the bony pelvis may press on nerves and create pain radiating to the back or lower extremities; however, backache is such a common general complaint that it is usually difficult to ascribe it specifically to myomas.

Pain with intercourse may result, depending on the position of the tumors and the pressure they exert on the vaginal walls.

3. Pressure effects—Pressure effects are unusual and difficult to directly relate to leiomyomata, unless the tumors are very large. Intramural or intraligamentous leiomyomata may distort or obstruct other organs. Parasitic tumors may cause intestinal obstruction if they are large or involve omentum or bowel. Cervical tumors may cause serosanguineous vaginal discharge, vaginal bleeding, dyspareunia, and infertility. Large tumors may fill the true pelvis and displace or compress the ureters, bladder, or rectum.

Compression of surrounding structures may result in urinary symptoms or hydroureter. Large tumors may cause pelvic venous congestion and lower extremity edema or constipation. Rarely, a posterior fundal leiomyoma may carry the uterus into extreme retroflexion, distorting the bladder base and causing urinary retention. This may present as intermittent overflow incontinence produced by elongation of the urethra with loss of sphincter control—a situation identical to sacculation of the uterus during early pregnancy. The condition is relieved by dislodging the uterus from the true pelvis with the patient in the knee-chest position.

4. Infertility—The relationship between fibroids and infertility remains uncertain. Between 27% and 40% of women with multiple leiomyomas are reported to be infertile, but other causes of infertility are present in a majority of cases. When fibroids are entirely or mostly endocavitary, there is a strong rationale supporting the use of surgery to improve fertility.

5. Spontaneous abortion—The incidence of spontaneous abortion secondary to leiomyoma is unknown but is possibly 2 times the incidence in normal pregnant women. For example, the incidence of spontaneous abortion prior to myomectomy is approximately 40% and following myomectomy is approximately 20%.

B. EXAMINATION

Most myomas are discovered by routine bimanual examination of the uterus or sometimes by palpation of the lower abdomen. Uterine retroflexion and retrover-

sion may obscure the physical examination diagnosis of even moderately large leiomyomata. When the cervix is pulled up behind the symphysis, large fibroids are usually implicated. The diagnosis is obvious when the normal uterine contour is distorted by one or more smooth, spherical, firm masses, but often it is difficult to be absolutely certain that such masses are part of the uterus. A pelvic ultrasound generally assists in establishing the diagnosis, as well as excluding pregnancy as a cause of the uterine enlargement. Magnetic resonance imaging (MRI) may better delineate the size and position of myomas but is not always clinically necessary.

C. LABORATORY FINDINGS

As noted earlier, anemia is a common consequence of leiomyomata due to excessive uterine bleeding and depletion of iron reserves. However, occasional patients display erythrocytosis. The hematocrit returns to normal levels following removal of the uterus, and elevated erythropoietin levels have been reported in such cases. Moreover, the recognized association of polycythemia and renal disease has led to speculation that leiomyomas may compress the ureters to cause ureteral back pressure and thus induce renal erythropoietin production.

Leukocytosis, fever, and an elevated sedimentation rate may be present with acute degeneration or infection.

D. IMAGING

Pelvic ultrasound examinations are useful in confirming the diagnosis of leiomyomata. While ultrasound should never be a substitute for a thorough pelvic examination, it can be extremely helpful in identifying leiomyomata, detailing the cause of other pelvic masses, and in the identification of pregnancy. Moreover, ultrasonography is particularly useful in the obese individual. Saline sonohysterography can identify submucosal myomas that may be missed on ultrasound.

Large leiomyomata typically appear as soft tissue masses on x-rays of the lower abdomen and pelvis; however, attention is sometimes drawn to the tumors by calcifications. Hysterosalpingography may be useful in detailing an intrauterine leiomyoma in the infertile patient.

Intravenous urography may be useful in the workup of any pelvic mass, because it frequently reveals ureteral deviation or compression and identifies urinary anomalies. MRI can also be used to evaluate the urinary tract and is highly accurate in depicting the number, size, and location of leiomyomata.

E. SPECIAL EXAMINATIONS

Hysteroscopy may assist in identification, and may also be used for removal, of submucous leiomyomata. Laparoscopy is often definitive in establishing the precise origin of leiomyomata and is increasingly being used for myomectomy (see later).

Differential Diagnosis

The diagnosis of uterine myoma is not usually difficult, although any pelvic mass, including pregnancy, may be mistaken for a leiomyoma. Indeed, leiomyoma is a common preoperative diagnosis for ovarian carcinoma, endolymphatic stromal meiosis, tubo-ovarian abscess, and endometriosis. Modern imaging techniques may clarify the diagnosis, particularly in obese women or when palpation is difficult for other reasons, eg, when the abdominal muscles are tense.

Ovarian cysts or neoplasia must be considered in the differential diagnosis of uterine leiomyomata. Other adnexal considerations include tubo-ovarian inflammatory or neoplastic masses. Uterine enlargement simulating leiomyomata may be due to pregnancy (including subinvolution), endometrial cancer, adenomyosis, myometrial hypertrophy, or congenital anomalies. Adnexa, omentum, or bowel adherent to the uterus also may be erroneously diagnosed as leiomyomata. Because a fetus may exist within an obviously myomatous uterus, a pregnancy test should be obtained in all women of childbearing age with a suspected pelvic mass.

The most common symptom of leiomyomata, recurrent abnormal bleeding, may be caused by any of the numerous conditions that affect the uterus. Adenocarcinoma of the endometrium or uterine tube, uterine sarcomas, and ovarian carcinomas are the most lethal and therefore the most important to be excluded. Hyperplasia, polyps, irregular shedding, dysfunctional (nonorganic) bleeding, ovarian neoplasms, endometriosis, adenomyosis, and exogenous estrogens or steroid hormones may all cause abnormal bleeding.

The definitive diagnosis in cases of uterine bleeding can usually be established by endometrial biopsy or fractional dilatation and curettage (D&C). Some type of endometrial evaluation should be considered essential in the work-up of any patient with abnormal bleeding or a pelvic mass, particularly those over the age of 35, in whom endometrial cancer may be a serious concern. Even in the presence of uterine leiomyomas, other conditions can coexist and must be ruled out before definitive therapy is undertaken.

Complications

A. MYOMAS AND PREGNANCY

Slightly less than two-thirds of women with uterine leiomyomas and otherwise unexplained infertility conceive after myomectomy, and about half of these women go on to deliver term infants. However, comparisons with expectant management are needed before drawing conclusions on the effectiveness of the procedure.

During the second and third trimesters of pregnancy, myomas may rapidly increase in size and undergo vascular deprivation and subsequent degenerative changes. Clinically this most commonly leads to pain and localized tenderness (see carneous degeneration, earlier) but may also initiate preterm labor. Expectant management with bedrest and narcotics is virtually always successful in alleviation of the pain, but tocolytics may be necessary to control the uterine contractions. Once the acute episode is over, most patients can be carried to term without further complications.

During labor, leiomyomas may produce uterine inertia, fetal malpresentation, or obstruction of the birth canal. In general, leiomyomas tend to rise out of the pelvis as pregnancy progresses, and vaginal delivery may be accomplished. Nevertheless, a large cervical or isthmic myoma may be rather immobile and may necessitate cesarean delivery. Leiomyomas may interfere with effective uterine contraction immediately after delivery; therefore, the possibility of postpartum hemorrhage should be anticipated.

B. COMPLICATIONS IN NONPREGNANT WOMEN

As noted previously, heavy bleeding with anemia is the most common complication of myomas. Urinary or bowel obstruction from large or parasitic myomas is much less common, and malignant transformation is rare. Ureteral injury or ligation is a well-recognized complication of surgery for leiomyomas, particularly cervical.

Precautions

Exogenous hormones must be used with caution in postmenopausal patients with leiomyomas. The dose should be the lowest necessary to control symptoms, and the size of the tumors should be closely followed with pelvic examinations (every 6 months) and imaging studies as necessary. No evidence exists linking oral contraceptive use with an increase in myoma size. However, close clinical follow-up of these patients is reasonable given the potential for exogenous hormones to affect growth of myomas.

Treatment

Choice of treatment depends on the patient's age, parity, pregnancy status, desire for future pregnancies, general health, and symptoms, as well as the size, location, and state of preservation of the leiomyomas.

A. EMERGENCY MEASURES

Blood transfusions may be necessary to correct anemia. Transfusion of packed red blood cells is preferred over whole blood. Surgery is usually indicated for these cases when they become hemodynamically stable. Emergency surgery is indicated for infected leiomyomata, acute torsion, or intestinal obstruction caused by a pedunculated or parasitic myoma. Myomectomy is generally contraindicated during pregnancy, except for the rare symptomatic torsion.

B. SPECIFIC MEASURES

1. Nonpregnant women—In most instances, myomas do not require treatment, particularly if there are no symptoms or if the patient is postmenopausal. However, other causes of pelvic masses (see earlier) must be ruled out. The clinical diagnosis of myoma must be unequivocal, and the patient should initially be examined every 6 months after diagnosis to establish the rate of growth of the myomas.

Although no definitive medical therapy is currently available for leiomyomata, the gonadotropin-releasing hormone (GnRH) agonists have proven very useful for limiting growth or to cause a temporary decrease in tumor size. Gonadotropin-releasing hormone agonists induce hypogonadism through pituitary desensitization, downregulation of receptors, and inhibition of gonadotropins. GnRH treatment of uterine fibroids will achieve the following results: (1) maximal shrinkage of the myomatous uterus to approximately 50% of its volume; (2) this shrinkage is achieved within 3 months of treatment; (3) amenorrhea and hypoestrogenic side effects occur; and (4) osteoporosis may occur, especially with treatment lasting longer than 6 months. Examples of clinical situations in which GnRH agonists may be useful include control of bleeding from leiomyomata (except the for the polypoid submucous type, in which it may actually be worsened); the unstable or unsuitable surgical candidate, in whom shrinkage may be sufficient to allow laparoscopically assisted vaginal hysterectomy; standard vaginal hysterectomy; and in certain cases for myomectomy.

It is impossible to precisely define the size to which a myomatous uterus may be safely allowed to grow, and judgment in each case must be individualized. Traditional teaching held that a uterus greater than 12–14 weeks in size should be removed regardless of symptoms, because such size precludes adequate examination of the adnexa. However, this view is unsupported by scientific evidence and is no longer appropriate in light of advances made in imaging studies such as MRI. Because these tumors are benign (except in rare cases) greater weight must be given to symptoms rather than to arbitrary size criteria.

Depending on the size and location of such myomas and the presence of other pelvic disease (such as pelvic inflammatory disease or endometriosis), surgical extirpation may be difficult and challenging.

2. Puerperal—Surgical intervention for properly diagnosed uterine fibroids should normally be avoided in

pregnancy. The only indication for myomectomy in pregnancy is torsion of a pedunculated fibroid in which transection and hemostasis of the stalk can be achieved with relative safety. Similarly, myomectomy is not recommended during cesarean section, except perhaps to facilitate access to the lower uterine segment.

C. SUPPORTIVE MEASURES

All patients should have a cervical Papanicolaou smear and evaluation of the endometrium if bleeding is irregular. Before definitive surgery, necessary blood volume should be replenished, and other measures such as the administration of prophylactic antibiotics or heparin should be considered. Mechanical and antibiotic bowel preparation may be employed when difficult pelvic surgery is anticipated.

D. SURGICAL MEASURES

1. Evaluation for other neoplasia—Imaging most often must be accompanied by endometrial evaluation to rule out other pelvic neoplastic processes. The endometrial evaluation may be accomplished by endometrial biopsy in the uncomplicated patient but may necessitate hysteroscopy in the more complicated case. Occasionally examination under anesthesia is necessary, but this has largely been replaced by the measures noted earlier to rule out coexisting problems, especially cancer.

2. Myomectomy—Myomectomy should be planned for the symptomatic patient who wishes to preserve fertility or conserve the uterus, but one can never be certain before operation that myomectomy can be accomplished easily. Myomectomy is quite successful for control of chronic bleeding associated with leiomyomata. Increasingly myomectomy is being performed through the hysteroscope in cases of submucous leiomyomata and through the laparoscope for subserous leiomyomata. Indeed, these less invasive procedures are liberalizing the surgical indications for myomectomy.

A pedunculated submucous myoma protruding into the vagina can sometimes be removed vaginally with a looped wire snare or by hysteroscopy. This is most useful if other tumors do not obviously require removal. If the pedunculated myoma cannot be removed vaginally, careful biopsy should be performed to rule out leiomyosarcoma or a mixed mesodermal sarcoma. Both of these tumors are known to protrude through the cervix in older women and may be clinically indistinguishable from an infarcted prolapsed myoma (Fig 36–4). Since infection is common in this setting, prophylactic antibiotics should be utilized.

3. Hysterectomy—Uteri with small myomas may be removed by total vaginal hysterectomy, particularly if

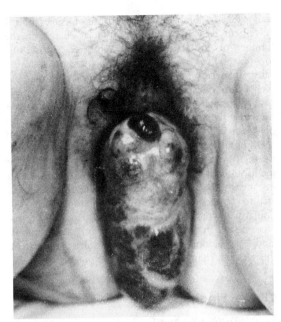

Figure 36–4. Prolapsed and partially infarcted myoma.

vaginal relaxation demands repair of cystocele, rectocele, or enterocele.

When numerous large tumors (especially intraligamentary myomas) are found, total abdominal hysterectomy is indicated. If the ovaries are diseased or if their blood supply has been destroyed, oophorectomy is necessary; otherwise, the ovaries should be preserved. Ovaries generally are preserved in premenopausal women. There is no consensus about the virtue of conserving or removing ovaries in postmenopausal women, with advocates and opponents of such prophylactic castration both relying on hypothetical scenarios and not scientific studies.

4. Investigational techniques—Embolic occlusion of the uterine arteries may successfully treat symptoms of leiomyomas, particularly menorrhagia; however, adequate long-term scientific study of this less invasive treatment is still lacking.

E. SURGICAL TREATMENT OF COMPLICATIONS FROM MYOMAS DURING PREGNANCY

Patients who have undergone previous multiple myomectomy, particularly if the endometrial cavity was entered, have less risk of uterine rupture if delivered by cesarean section. In some cases, cesarean hysterectomy is a sensible solution to the problem of myomas in a pregnant woman who wants no more children.

On the other hand, although rather small myomas may grow appreciably during pregnancy, they usually regress after delivery. Furthermore, one must not overlook the hazards—blood loss and possible urinary tract damage—associated with removal of a huge puerperal uterus. The mere presence of myomas that were not clinically of much significance before pregnancy should not be cited as an indication for cesarean hysterectomy in the absence of compelling reasons for abdominal delivery or for removal of the uterus.

Prognosis

Hysterectomy with removal of all leiomyomas is curative. Following myomectomy, the uterus and its cavity gradually return to normal contour. One major concern is the risk of recurrence after myomectomy. Recent studies suggest a rate of 2–3% per year of symptomatic myomas after myomectomy.

ADENOMYOSIS

ESSENTIALS OF DIAGNOSIS

- *Premenstrual and comenstrual dysmenorrhea.*
- *Diffuse globular uterine enlargement.*
- *Hypermenorrhea.*
- *Softening of areas of adenomyosis just prior to or during the early phases of menstruation.*

General Considerations

Adenomyosis is defined by the presence of endometrial glands and stroma within the myometrium; ie, the endometrium is growing beneath the basement membrane, marking its separation from the myometrium. It is found in 8–40% of extirpated uteri, depending on the number of sections that are taken. Although histologic sections often show direct continuity of ectopic endometrial islands with the mucosal surface, many foci of adenomyosis appear isolated, perhaps because their connections with the surface have been interrupted by fibrosis and areas of musculature. As adenomyosis becomes more advanced, the uterus is diffusely enlarged and globular because of hypertrophy of the smooth muscle elements adjacent to the ectopic glands.

The pathogenesis of adenomyosis is unknown. It is a disease of parous women, and it is thought that postpartum endometritis might cause the initial break in the normal boundary. Other possible causes include an arrest of müllerian cells in the myometrium and the development of endometrial glands in this site.

It causes symptoms in approximately 70% of proved cases; about 30% of cases are asymptomatic and are discovered accidentally. The condition regresses after the menopause. Obviously, the pathologic diagnosis depends on the diligence with which the specimens are assessed and on whether or not examples of minimal muscular invasion (adenomyosis subbasalis) are included.

Pathology

The myometrial thickening produced by adenomyosis is usually diffuse and of uniform consistency rather than irregularly nodular (as with myomas). The fundus generally is the site of adenomyosis. It may involve either or both walls of the uterus, to create a globular enlargement (usually 10–12 cm in diameter; Fig 36–5, left). The consistency of the uterus is irregularly firm, and it has enhanced vascularity. The cut surface appears convex (bulging) and exudes serum. The cut surface may have a whorl-like or granular trabecular pattern, and there may be coarse stippling or granular trabeculation with small yellow or brown cystic spaces containing fluid or blood (Fig 36–5, right). Small hemorrhagic areas represent endometrial islands in which menstrual bleeding has occurred. The endometrial-myometrial juncture is often indiscernible. Leiomyomas and adenomyosis may coexist in the same specimen.

The microscopic pattern is one of endometrial islands scattered throughout the myometrium. Depth of penetration can be graded, and opinion varies about what constitutes true adenomyosis rather than superfi-

cial extension of basal endometrium. Degrees of involvement have been described that are based on the number of endometrial glands observed within one low-power field, but this is somewhat impractical because of variations in the distribution of glandular elements from one area to another.

Myometrial hypertrophy and hyperplasia are almost invariably apparent around the endometrial islets, and phagocytosed hemosiderin occasionally may be seen in the muscularis. If the degree of involvement is marked, the ectopic endometrium may show cyclic changes identical to those of normal endometrium, but in most instances the aberrant tissue appears to respond fairly well to estrogen though not to progesterone. When endometrial hyperplasia involves the mucosal layer, the same histologic pattern may be seen in the ectopic islands. The ectopic endometrium may also participate in the decidual changes characteristic of pregnancy.

Clinical Findings

A. Symptoms and Signs

Significant degrees of adenomyosis are associated with hypermenorrhea in fully 50% of patients, and about 30% have an acquired, increasingly severe form of dysmenorrhea. The classic patient with adenomyosis is a parous middle-aged woman with menorrhagia and dysmenorrhea who has a symmetrically enlarged uterus.

Despite widespread knowledge of the major symptoms of adenomyosis, the correct preoperative diagnosis is made in somewhat less than one-third of all instances. Failure to make the diagnosis preoperatively is largely the consequence of failure to think of it,

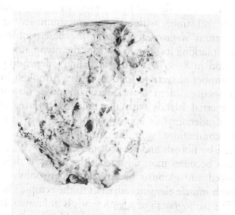 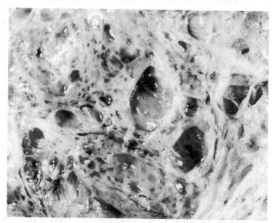

Figure 36–5. Adenomyosis. Left: Gross view showing globular mass. Right: Close-up view showing stippled trabeculation with small cystic spaces containing fluid or blood.

although coexisting lesions such as myomas, endometrial polyps, endometrial hyperplasia, endometrial carcinoma, or endometriosis may disguise the symptomatology.

1. Hypermenorrhea—It is claimed that even adenomyosis subbasalis may produce hypermenorrhea in a high proportion of cases. This would seem to invalidate the contention that increased menstrual flow results from interference with normal myometrial contraction when large areas of musculature are disrupted by numerous endometrial islands. Nevertheless, there is clearly a positive correlation between the degree of involvement (as opposed to depth of penetration), vascularity, and the occurrence of menorrhagia, whatever the precise explanation for the increased bleeding may be.

2. Dysmenorrhea—Dysmenorrhea is directly related to the depth of penetration and degree of involvement, and probably results from myometrial contractions invoked by premenstrual swelling and menstrual bleeding in endometrial islands. The uterus is usually tender and slightly softened under bimanual examination done premenstrually (Halban's sign).

B. IMAGING

Improved ultrasound techniques have made the preoperative diagnosis of adenomyosis more common. MRI can detect adenomyosis in the symptomatic patient with a negative or equivocal sonogram or in the presence of leiomyomas, but the cost of the procedure must be weighed against the information gathered.

Differential Diagnosis

Pregnancy may be ruled out with a pregnancy test.

Submucous leiomyomas may be present in 50–60% of cases of adenomyosis, and the two bear differentiation. Leiomyomas may cause excessive and progressive menorrhagia and pain. The uterus is firm and nontender, even during menstruation, and discomfort occurs if the leiomyoma is pedunculated and in the process of extrusion. Diagnosis is confirmed by hysteroscopy and/or D&C. Endometrial cancer is diagnosed by endometrial biopsy or D&C.

Pelvic congestion syndrome (Taylor's syndrome) is characterized by the chronic complaints of continuous pelvic pain and menometrorrhagia. In some instances, the uterus is enlarged, symmetric, and minimally softened; the cervix may be cyanotic and somewhat patulous. At operation, the pelvic vessels may appear enlarged or tortuous.

Pelvic endometriosis is marked by premenstrual and intramenstrual dysmenorrhea, adherent adnexal masses, and "shotty" cul-de-sac or uterosacral ligament nodulations. The disorder is associated with adenomyosis in about 15% of patients.

Complications

Chronic severe anemia may result from persistent menorrhagia.

Primary adenocarcinoma has rarely been observed in islands of aberrant endometrium within myometrium provided the surface endometrium is normal. On the other hand, endometrial adenocarcinoma is often associated with islands of malignant glands in the muscularis, but it may be impossible to determine whether there has been myometrial metastasis from the primary surface tumor or development of carcinoma within a focus of adenomyosis. However, if the surface tumor is markedly anaplastic and the myometrial islets exhibit well-differentiated glands, it seems reasonable to conclude that the latter are not metastases.

When the stromal component of endometrium, without glands, invades the myometrium, the resulting "tumor" is referred to as endolymphatic stromal myosis, or stromatosis. This entity is not dependent on ovarian hormonal production and therefore is not truly comparable to adenomyosis.

Prevention

Adenomyosis cannot be prevented.

Treatment

A. HYSTERECTOMY

Although focal adenomyomas may occasionally be successfully removed, hysterectomy is the only other definitive treatment for adenomyosis. Hysterectomy is also the only way to establish the diagnosis with certainty. Whether the ovaries should be removed depends, as in many other situations, on the patient's age and the presence of obvious ovarian lesions or generalized pelvic endometriosis.

B. HORMONAL THERAPY

Medical treatment with hormones has not been successful in the treatment of adenomyosis. Some foci of adenomyosis have shown pseudodecidual reaction to progestins with no symptomatic relief. GnRH agonists can provide temporary relief of symptoms if the focus of adenomyosis is estrogen- and progesterone-receptor positive. However, symptoms recur after discontinuation of the medication. Oral contraceptives may exacerbate the symptoms.

Prognosis

Hysterectomy is curative.

ENDOMETRIAL POLYPS

ESSENTIALS OF DIAGNOSIS

- *Menometrorrhagia or postmenopausal bleeding.*
- *Direct visualization and biopsy (hysteroscopy).*

General Considerations

"Polyp" is a general descriptive term for any mass of tissue that projects outward or away from the surface of surrounding tissues. A polyp is grossly visible as a spheroidal or cylindric structure that may be either pedunculated (attached by a slender stalk) or sessile (relatively broad-based) (Fig 36–6).

Benign endometrial polyps are common in the endometrial cavity at all ages but particularly at age 29–59, with their greatest incidence after age 50. Risk factors include hypertension and obesity. A higher incidence of endometrial polyps is also noted in patients on tamoxifen therapy for breast cancer. Endometrial polyps must be differentiated from submucous

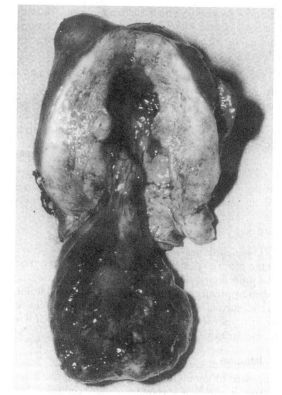

Figure 36–7. Large, partially infarcted endometrial polyp prolapsed through the cervical os.

myomas, malignant neoplasms (especially mixed sarcomas), and even retained fragments of placental tissue (which may grossly assume a polypoid architecture).

Polyps may be single or multiple and may range in size from 1–2 mm in diameter to masses that fill or even distend the uterine cavity. Most polyps arise in the fundal region and extend downward. Occasionally, an endometrial polyp may project through the external cervical os and may even extend to the vaginal introitus (Fig 36–7). Postmortem examinations have shown that about 10% of uteri contain presumably asymptomatic polyps.

Polyps may undergo malignant change, and isolated endometrial carcinomas and sarcomas have been identified in solitary polyps. When this occurs, the prognosis is more favorable than for uterine carcinoma or sarcoma in general, providing there is no evidence of spread beyond the polyp on analysis of the hysterectomy specimen.

The histogenesis of endometrial polyps is not clear. Unresponsive areas of endometrium often remain in

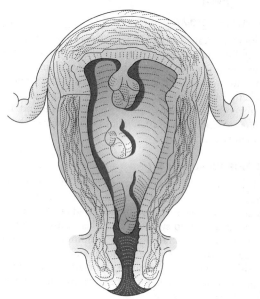

Figure 36–6. Endometrial polyps.

situ, along with the basalis, during menstrual shedding, and such an area may serve as the nidus of a polyp. However, not even the smallest polyps studied by histologic sectioning have given a wholly acceptable clue as to the precise mechanism of their formation. Polyps are considered to be estrogen-sensitive; their response to estrogen is similar to that of the surrounding endometrium, and their association with other proliferative endometrial lesions (such as hyperplasia and endometrial carcinoma) is well recognized.

Pathology

Grossly, an endometrial polyp is a smooth, red or brown, ovoid body with a velvety texture, ranging from a few millimeters to several centimeters in widest diameter. A large polyp usually tapers to an obvious pedicle; a small polyp, when cut longitudinally, often presents a rather cylindric silhouette, with rounding at the distal end. Uterine polyps are of the same color as the surrounding endometrium unless they are infarcted, in which case they are dark red. A sectioned polyp may have a spongy appearance if it contains many dilated glandular spaces.

The microscopic pattern of an endometrial polyp is a mixture of (1) generally dense fibrous tissue—the stroma; (2) impressively large and thick-walled vascular channels; and (3) glandlike spaces, of variable size and shape, lined with endometrial epithelium. The relative amounts of these 3 components vary considerably. The surface of an intact polyp in a functioning uterus usually is covered by a layer of endometrium resembling that of the remainder of the endometrial surface, but beneath this exterior there are glandular components that are seemingly much older, and these apparently do not participate in menstrual shedding.

Squamous metaplasia of the surface epithelium is not uncommon. The subsurface epithelial spaces are often compared with basal endometrial glands unresponsive to progesterone, but they tend to form bizarre shapes and become quite dilated. Hence, a fragment of polyp may be mistaken for the cystic variety of endometrial hyperplasia ("Swiss cheese" endometrium). The distal or dependent portion of a polyp may show marked engorgement of blood vessels, hemorrhage into the stroma, inflammatory cells, and perhaps ulceration at the surface.

Adenocarcinoma may develop within an otherwise benign polyp, usually at some distance from its base or pedicle. On the other hand, a benign polyp may exist in an area of endometrial carcinoma. Thus, when a harmless-appearing polyp is recovered from the bleeding uterus of a postmenopausal woman, there is no guarantee that a more serious lesion does not exist elsewhere in the cavity.

Polyps that contain interlacing bands of smooth muscle are called pedunculated adenomyomas. Generally, these have broad bases and are associated with adenomyosis of the uterus. In the same uterine cavity, endometrial polyps may coexist with pedunculated leiomyomas. In cases of hyperplasia of the endometrium, the abundant overgrowth of tissue may produce a gross pattern called multiple polyposis. Curettage of such lesions may suggest the presence of adenocarcinoma because of the unexpected volume of tissue obtained.

Clinical Findings

A. Symptoms and Signs

Patients with endometrial polyps can present with menorrhagia and intermenstrual and premenstrual bleeding. Presumably, a large polyp, with its central vascular component, may contribute to menstrual bleeding and add greatly to the total blood loss. Polyps may be the source of minor premenstrual and postmenstrual bleeding, allegedly because the polyp's dependent tip is the first endometrial area to degenerate and the last to obtain a new epithelial covering and cease bleeding after the menstrual slough.

The sudden occurrence of considerable bleeding in a postmenopausal woman, often accompanied by crampy uterine pain, may result from an infarcting large polyp. Such bleeding episodes usually are of limited duration and are not life-threatening.

These explanations are highly speculative, but it is true that duration and volume of menstruation often are lessened and the end points of the bleeding phase become more clear-cut by the removal of one or more endometrial polyps. In the postmenopausal woman, bleeding from polyps is usually light and is often described as "staining" or "spotting." A polyp should be suspected when bleeding continues following a D&C that has produced only benign normal tissue.

B. Imaging

Transvaginal ultrasound is a helpful tool in identifying endometrial polyps; a homogeneous hyperechoic intracavitary mass is characteristic of a benign polyp. Polyps may be evident on a hysterosalpingogram as irregularities in the outline of the uterine cavity or as filling defects. However, this technique has largely been replaced by office hysteroscopy and saline sonohysterography.

C. Special Examinations

Hysteroscopy and saline sonohysterography are excellent techniques for evaluating endometrial polyps. Treatment can also be accomplished using hysteroscopic resection

Treatment

A. SURGICAL EXCISION

Direct visualization of polyps by hysteroscopy has greatly aided in their identification and removal. The stalk may be identified, and, under direct visualization, hysteroscopic instruments used to remove the polyp. With larger polyps it may be necessary to section the tumor into portions that may be removed through the cervix. Many authorities recommend curettage of the point of insertion of the stalk into the endometrium-myometrium. Additionally, the direct visualization of the endometrium and selected biopsies can rule out endometrial atypias or dysplasias.

To avoid overlooking a polyp during curettage of the uterus (D&C), the endometrial cavity must be explored separately with a grasping forceps (such as an Overstreet polyp forceps [Fig 36–8] or a Randall stone clamp), preferably at the beginning of the curettage procedure.

Despite this precaution, all too frequently polyps are missed and remain in the uterus after curettage, only to be discovered later when menorrhagia persists and a hysterectomy is performed. At other times, only a portion of a polyp may be removed by curettage, and rather brisk bleeding will continue postoperatively from the residual basal portion of the lesion. A very large polyp may have to be severed at its base with a wire snare or scissors. In all cases, a fractional curettage should follow any nonvisualizing attempt at polyp removal, whether it was successful or not, in order to rule out endometrial carcinoma.

The imprecision of the nonvisualizing techniques has led to the emergence of hysteroscopy as the gold standard for both diagnosis and treatment of endometrial polyps.

A polyp should be labeled as such, preserved separately in fixative solution, and sent to the pathology laboratory as a separate specimen, because it may prove to be the most significant portion of the total tissue sample. If it is intermingled with other curettings or biopsies, there is no assurance that it will be part of the material chosen for histologic sectioning.

B. CHEMOTHERAPY

There is no specific hormonal therapy for endometrial polyps, although progestin therapy may cause them to regress somewhat.

C. HYSTERECTOMY

Simple excision is adequate for a benign polyp, but if areas of carcinoma or sarcoma are discovered, hysterectomy should be performed. In a premenopausal patient, persistence of abnormal uterine bleeding after removal of an apparently benign polyp (or some portion of it) may require further diagnostic steps and/or more invasive treatment (Fig 36–9). Uteri removed for this reason occasionally contain additional polyps, submucous leiomyomata, or (rarely) a small area of carcinoma in a relatively inaccessible location.

Prognosis

Removal is curative for that polyp, but recurrence is frequent. Hysterectomy is definitive but usually unnecessary if cancer has been ruled out.

REFERENCES

Uterine Leiomyomas

Agency for Healthcare Research: Management of Uterine Fibroids. Summary, Evidence Report/Technology Assessment: No. 34. AHRQ Pub. No. 01-E051, 2001.

Anderson J: Factors in fibroid growth. Bailliere's Clin Obstet Gynecol 1998;12:223.

Ang WC et al: Effect of hormone replacement therapies and selective estrogen receptor modulators in postmenopausal women with uterine leiomyomas: a literature review. Climacteric 2001;4:284.

Broder MS et al: Uterine artery embolization: a systematic review of the literature and proposal for research. RAND Report MR-1138. RAND, August 1999.

Carlson KJ et al: The Maine Women's Health Study. Obstet Gynecol 1994;83:556.

Lumsden MA, Wallace EM: Clinical presentation of uterine fibroids. Bailliere's Clin Obstet Gynecol 1998;12:177.

Parker W et al: Uterine sarcomas in patients operated on for presumed leiomyoma and rapidly growing leiomyoma. Obstet Gynecol 1994;83:414.

Reiter R et al: Routine hysterectomy for large asymptomatic uterine leiomyomata: a reappraisal. Obstet Gynecol 1992;79:481.

Schwartz SM: Epidemiology of uterine leiomyomata. Clin Obstet Gynecol 2001;44:316.

Verallaini P et. al: Abdominal myomectomy for infertility: a comprehensive review. Hum Reprod 1998;13:873.

West CP: Hysterectomy and myomectomy by laparotomy. Bailliere's Clin Obstet Gynecol 1998;12:317.

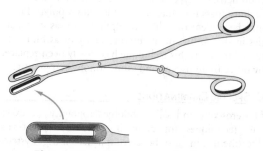

Figure 36–8. Overstreet polyp forceps.

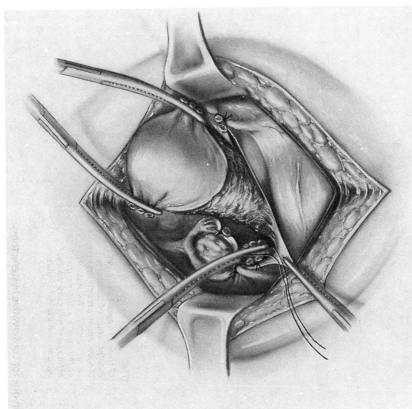

A. Uterine vessels are clamped, divided, and ligated.

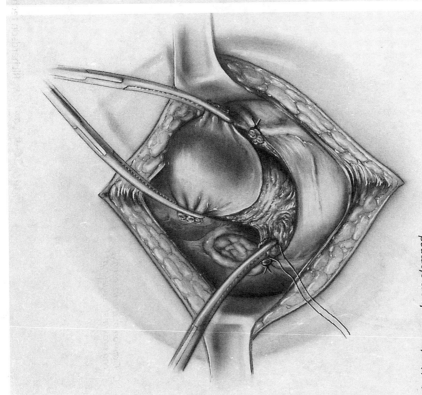

B. Base of broad ligament, including transverse cervical ligament and accompanying vasculature, clamped, divided, and ligated.

Figure 36–9. Richardson technique for conservative hysterectomy.

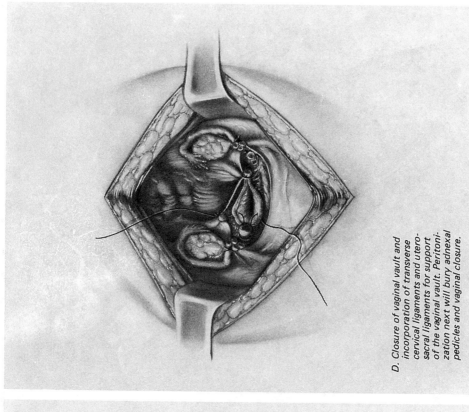

D. Closure of vaginal vault and incorporation of transverse cervical ligaments and uterosacral ligaments for support of the vaginal vault. Peritonization next will bury adnexal pedicles and vaginal closure.

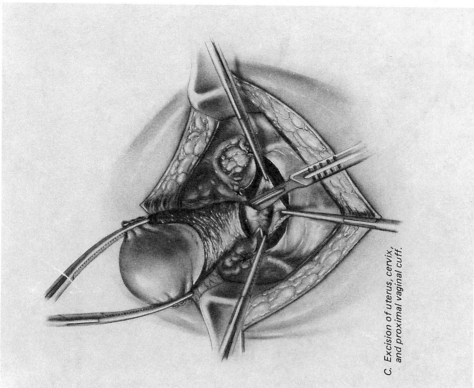

C. Excision of uterus, cervix, and proximal vaginal cuff.

Figure 36-9 (cont'd). Richardson technique for conservative hysterectomy.

Adenomyosis

Arnold LL, Ascher SM, Schrenfer J: The nonsurgical diagnosis of adenomyosis. Obstet Gynecol 1995;86:461.

Azziz R: Adenomyosis: Current perspectives. Obstet Gynecol Clin North Am 1989;16:221.

Falk RJ, Mullin BR: Exacerbation of adenomyosis symptomatology by estrogen progesterone therapy. A case report and histopathologic observation. Int J Fertil 1989;34:386.

Hernandez E, Woodruff DJ: Endometrial adenocarcinoma arising in adenomyosis. Am J Obstet Gynecol 1980;138:827.

Kilkku P, Erkkola R, Grauonroos M: Non-specificity of symptoms related to adenomyosis: A prospective comparative study. Acta Obstet Gynecol Scand 1984;63:229.

Luciano AA, Pitkin RM: Endometriosis: Approaches to diagnosis and treatment. Surg Annu 1984;16:297.

Siegler AM, Camilien L: Adenomyosis. J Reprod Med 1994;3 9:841.

Thomas JS Jr, Clark JF: Adenomyosis: a retrospective view. J Natl Med Assoc 1989;81:969.

Endometrial Polyps

Holst J, Koskela O, von Schoultz B: Endometrial findings following curettage in 2018 women according to age and indications. Ann Chir Gynaecol 1983;72:274.

Kupfer MC, Schiler VL, Hansen G: Transvaginal sonographic evaluation of endometrial polyps. J Ultrasound Med 1994; 13:757.

Reslova T, Toner J, Resl M: Endometrial polyps: A clinical study of 245 cases. Arch Obstet Gynecol 1999;26:133.

Siegler AM: Panoramic CO2 hysteroscopy. Clin Obstet Gynaecol 1983;26:242.

Benign Disorders of the Ovaries & Oviducts

Karen Purcell, MD, PhD, & James E. Wheeler, MD

37

Benign adnexal masses are common in the reproductive age group and are caused by physiologic cysts or benign neoplasms. The management of these benign masses is dictated by their presentation. If the patient is symptomatic with hemorrhage of a ruptured cyst or has acute pain indicative of ovarian torsion, then operative intervention is indicated. However, most benign adnexal masses are discovered as incidental findings. In this situation, the risk of malignancy must be excluded (see Chapter 49 for proper evaluation). Expectant management is then indicated because many of these cysts will be physiologic in nature and are therefore expected to regress over time. The patient should be reevaluated in 6 weeks, and any persistent mass should be considered a potentially benign or malignant neoplasm and operative evaluation pursued. For most benign ovarian cysts, laparoscopy is the preferred method due to its shorter recovery time, as well as less pain, blood loss, and overall cost when compared to laparotomy. For most patients, ovarian cystectomy is favored over oophorectomy in order to retain fertility.

■ PHYSIOLOGIC ENLARGEMENT

FUNCTIONAL CYSTS

Follicular Cysts

Follicular cysts (Fig 37–1) are common and vary in size from 3 to 8 cm in diameter. Histologically, they are lined by an inner layer of granulosa cells and an outer layer of theca interna cells which may or may not be luteinized. These cysts result from a failure in ovulation, most likely secondary to disturbances in the release of the pituitary gonadotropins. The fluid of the incompletely developed follicle is therefore not reabsorbed, producing an enlarged follicular cyst. Typically they are asymptomatic, although bleeding and torsion can occur. Large cysts may cause aching pelvic pain, dyspareunia, and occasionally abnormal uterine bleeding associated with a disturbance of the ovulatory pattern. Most follicular cysts disappear spontaneously within 60 days without treatment. Use of oral contra-

ceptive pills (OCPs) has often been recommended to help establish a normal rhythm; however, recent data show that this may not produce more rapid resolution than expectant management.

Corpus Luteum (Granulosa Lutein) Cysts

These are thin-walled unilocular cysts ranging from 3 to 11 cm in size. Following normal ovulation, the granulosa cells lining the follicle become luteinized. In the stage of vascularization, blood accumulates in the central cavity, producing the corpus hemorrhagicum. Resorption of the blood then results in a corpus luteum, which is defined as a cyst when it grows larger than 3 cm. A persistent corpus luteum cyst may cause local pain or tenderness. It can also be associated with either amenorrhea or delayed menstruation, thus simulating the clinical picture of an ectopic pregnancy. A corpus luteum cyst may be associated with torsion of the ovary, causing severe pain; or it may rupture and bleed, in which case laparoscopy or laparotomy is usually required to control hemorrhage into the peritoneal cavity. Unless acute complications develop, symptomatic therapy is indicated. As with follicular cysts, corpus luteum cysts usually regress after 1 or 2 months in menstruating patients and OCPs have been recommended but may be of questionable benefit.

Theca Lutein Cysts

Elevated levels of chorionic gonadotropin can produce theca lutein cysts, and thus are seen in patients with hydatidiform mole, choriocarcinoma, and chorionic gonadotropin or clomiphene therapy. Rarely, they may be seen in normal pregnancy. They are lined by theca cells which may or may not be luteinized, and they may or may not have granulosa cells. They are usually bilateral and are filled with clear, straw-colored fluid. Abdominal symptoms are minimal, although a sense of pelvic heaviness or aching may be described. Rupture of the cyst may result in intraperitoneal bleeding. Continued signs and symptoms of pregnancy, especially hyperemesis and breast paresthesias, are also reported. The cysts disappear spontaneously following termination of the molar pregnancy, treatment of the choriocarcinoma, or discontinuation of fertility therapy; however, such reso-

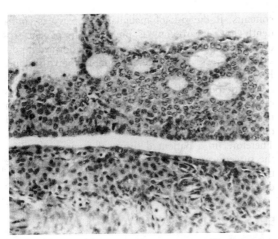

Figure 37–1. The wall of a follicular cyst showing the proliferating granulosa cells with tiny cystic Call-Exner bodies in the upper portion of the figure. They have artifactually pulled away from the underlying theca cells.

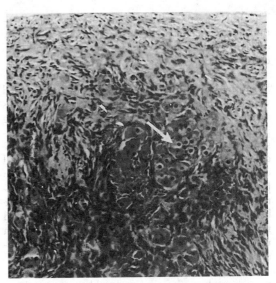

Figure 37–2. In hyperthecosis, nests of rounded eosinophilic luteinized stroma cells are found in the ovarian cortex.

lution may take months to occur. Surgery is reserved for complications such as torsion or hemorrhage.

HYPERTHECOSIS

Hyperthecosis, or thecomatosis, commonly produces no gross enlargement of the ovary (Fig 37–2). Thus, the lesions are demonstrable only by histologic examination of the excised gonad. They are characterized by nests of stromal cells demonstrating increased cytoplasm, simulating the changes seen in the normal theca after stimulation by pituitary gonadotropin. In the premenopausal woman, hyperthecosis is associated with virilization and clinical findings similar to those seen in polycystic ovarian disease (see following text). These alterations may also be associated with postmenopausal bleeding and endometrial hyperplasia.

POLYCYSTIC OVARIAN SYNDROME (PCOS) (Stein-Leventhal Syndrome)

Polycystic ovarian syndrome (PCOS) is characterized by bilaterally enlarged polycystic ovaries, secondary amenorrhea or oligomenorrhea, and infertility as a result of anovulation. About 50% of patients are hirsute, and many are obese. A presumptive diagnosis of polycystic ovarian syndrome often can be made from the history and initial examination. A normal puberty and early adolescence with menses are followed by episodes of amenorrhea that become progressively longer. The enlarged ovaries are identifiable on pelvic examination in about 50% of patients. Grossly they have been called "oyster ovaries" because they are enlarged and "sclero-

cystic" with smooth, pearl-white surfaces without indentations. Many small, fluid-filled follicle cysts lie beneath the thickened fibrous surface cortex (Fig 37–3). Luteinization of the theca interna is usually observed, and occasionally there is focal stromal luteinization. Laboratory testing often reveals mildly elevated serum androgen levels, an increased luteinizing hormone:follicle-stimulating hormone (LH:FSH) ratio, lipid abnormalities, and insulin resistance. Basal body temperature records and endometrial biopsies confirm anovulation.

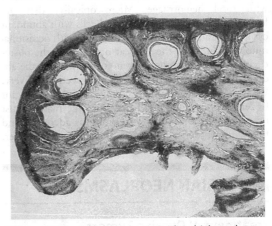

Figure 37–3. Polycystic ovary with a thickened capsule and prominent subcapsular cysts. Note lack of corpora lutea or corpora albicantia due to anovulation.

The disorder is presumably related to hypothalamic pituitary dysfunction and insulin resistance. A primary ovarian contribution to the problem has not been clearly defined.

Most patients with PCOS seek treatment either for hirsutism or infertility. The hirsutism can be treated with any agent that lowers androgen levels, and OCPs are typically the first choice in patients not desiring pregnancy. Infertility in PCOS patients is usually responsive to clomiphene citrate, 50–100 mg/d for 5–7 days cyclically. In the recalcitrant case, the experienced clinician may add human menopausal gonadotropin to produce the desired ovulation. Rarely is wedge resection necessary; however, the results of such surgery have been eminently successful in restoring ovulation and fertility. Recent studies also indicate that therapy with metformin may improve fertility rates although randomized controlled trials have yet to be performed.

Since patients with PCOS are chronically anovulatory, the endometrium is stimulated by estrogen alone. Thus endometrial hyperplasia, both typical and atypical, and endometrial carcinoma are more frequent in patients with PCOS and long-term anovulation. Many of these markedly atypical endometrial features can be reversed by large doses of progestational agents such as megestrol acetate, 40–60 mg/d for 3–4 months. Follow-up endometrial biopsy is mandatory to determine endometrial response and subsequent recurrence.

LUTEOMA OF PREGNANCY

Tumor-like nodules of lutein cells may form in the ovaries during pregnancy, and are often both multifocal and bilateral. The nodules range up to 20 cm in diameter, but most often are in the 5–10 cm range. On section they reveal well-delineated, soft, brown masses with focal hemorrhage. Microscopically, they are formed of sheets of large luteinized cells with abundant cytoplasm and relatively uniform nuclei with occasional mitoses. Clinically, they appear ominous to the obstetrician, who only becomes aware of them when the abdomen is open at the time of cesarean section delivery. Unilateral salpingo-oophorectomy may be done for frozen section in the belief that the large masses must be malignant. A confirmatory biopsy is adequate, and follow-up will reveal total regression a few months later.

■ OVARIAN NEOPLASMS

Treatment of Ovarian Tumors

The preferred treatment for all ovarian tumors is surgical excision with careful exploration of the abdominal contents. If the risk of malignant neoplasia is confidently low, laparoscopy is preferred. In patients requesting future fertility, cystectomy is performed if possible, otherwise a unilateral oophorectomy is done. Frozen section is helpful in identifying the type and neoplastic potential of the tumor. However, since it is often impossible to adequately sample a large ovarian neoplasm, final opinion and prognosis *must* be based on analysis of permanent, rather than frozen, sections. Therefore, in a patient desirous of retaining fertility, the surgeon must err on the side of retention of the uterus and contralateral ovary if there is the slightest doubt as to malignancy on the part of the pathologist.

EPITHELIAL TUMORS

Epithelial tumors account for approximately 60–80% of all true ovarian neoplasms and include the common serous, mucinous, endometrioid, clear cell, and transitional cell (Brenner) tumors, and the stromal tumors with an epithelial element. The epithelium of these tumors arises from a common anlage, ie, the mesothelium lining the coelomic cavity and ovarian surfaces (Fig 37–4). This basic thesis explains the similarity of the epithelia of the upper genital canal—endocervix, endometrium, and endosalpinx—to those found in the ovarian tumors. Most tumors presumably arise from invaginated surface epithelium (Fig 37–4) and proliferation or malignant degeneration in the epithelial lining of the resulting surface inclusion cyst (Fig 37–5). The epithelial tumors are classified on the basis of their histologic appearance.

Serous Tumors

Serous tumors have been reported in all age groups and are responsible for about 30% of all epithelial ovarian neoplasms. Low-grade neoplasms generally are found in patients in their 20s and 30s, whereas their anaplastic counterparts occur more commonly in peri- and postmenopausal women. Serous cystadenomas are benign lesions, commonly unilocular, with a smooth surface, and containing thin, clear yellow fluid. The cells lining the cyst are a mixed population of ciliated and secretory cells similar to those of the endosalpinx. They may grow large enough to fill the abdominal cavity, but they are usually smaller than their mucinous counterparts. About 10–15% are bilateral. Focal proliferation of the underlying stroma may produce firm papillary projections into the cyst, forming a serous cystadenofibroma (Fig 37–6). It is important to study these papillary projections thoroughly to rule out atypical proliferation. Some serous tumors consist of benign stromal proliferation interspersed with tiny serous cysts; these are known as serous adenofibromas.

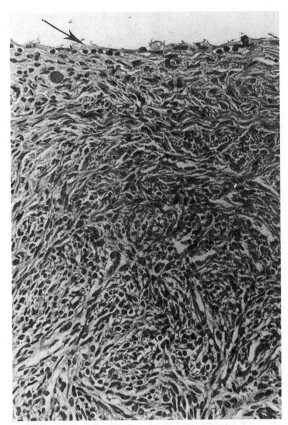

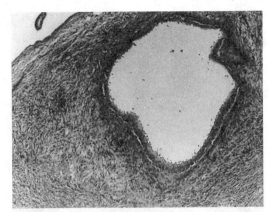

Figure 37–5. Most surface (germinal) inclusion cysts, such as the one shown here, undergo a serous (tubal) metaplasia. If larger than 1 cm in diameter, by definition they are termed cystadenomas.

Histologically, they are usually smooth-walled; true papillae are rare (compared with the serous variety). The tumors generally are multilocular, and the mucus-containing locules appear blue through the tense capsule (Fig 37–7). The internal surface is lined by tall columnar cells with dark, basally situated nuclei and mucinous cytoplasm as shown in Figure 37–8.

The epithelium of mucinous cysts resembles that of the endocervix in about 50% of cases; in the other 50%, mucin-containing goblet cells resembling intestinal epithelial cells are present. Careful study of mucinous neoplasms has shown that there may be great variation in histologic appearance from area to area, with some areas appearing benign while others are of low

Figure 37–4. The surface epithelium (mesothelium; indicated by the arrow) of the ovary forms an inconspicuous, usually flat, layer of cells over the underlying ovarian cortex.

Mucinous Tumors

Mucinous tumors account for approximately 10–20% of all epithelial ovarian neoplasms; about 75%–85% of them are benign. The benign tumors are typically found in women in the third through the fifth decades. Bilateral tumor development occurs in 8–10% of all cases, whether the tumors are benign or malignant. They are the largest tumors found in the human body; 15 reported tumors have weighed over 70 kg (154 lb). Consequently, the more massive the tumor, the greater the possibility that it may be mucinous. They generally are asymptomatic, and the patient is seen because of either an abdominal mass or nonspecific abdominal discomfort. In postmenopausal patients, luteinization of the stroma may rarely result in hormone production (usually estrogen) leading to associated endometrial hyperplasia with vaginal bleeding. During pregnancy, hormonal stimulation may result in virilization.

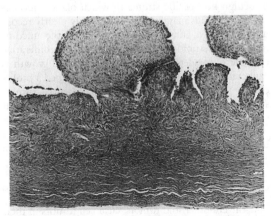

Figure 37–6. Serous cystadenofibromas usually form unilocular cysts with firm white papillations protruding into the cyst, seen here microscopically.

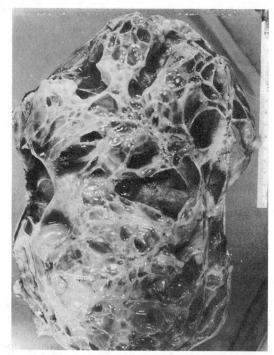

Figure 37–7. Multilocular mucinous cystadenoma of the ovary.

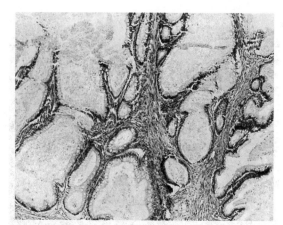

Figure 37–8. Mucinous cystadenoma. The lining cells are tall and columnar with basally situated nuclei. Generous sampling of these tumors is necessary to rule out a higher-grade lesion.

malignant potential or frankly malignant. Hence sampling must be more extensive than in the typical serous tumor. Metastases from appendiceal and other primary tumors may simulate closely a mucinous cystadenoma.

Endometrioid Lesions

Endometrioid tumors are characterized by proliferation of benign nonspecific stroma in which bland endometrial-type glands may be found. The only clearly recognizable benign endometrioid tumors are the uncommon endometrioid adenofibroma and the proliferative endometrioid adenofibroma. If the epithelial growth is exuberant but cytologically benign, it is termed a proliferative rather than a low malignant potential tumor, since the prognosis appears to be invariably excellent (Fig 37–9).

Endometriosis of the ovary (see Chapter 40) represents a benign "tumor-like" condition rather than a true neoplasm.

Clear Cell (Mesonephroid) Tumors

Like the endometrioid tumors, clear cell tumors in their benign form are rare, and are virtually limited to clear cell adenofibromas in which a solid proliferation of nonspecific stroma contains small cytologically bland

glands formed by columnar cells with clear cytoplasm. Clinically they appear like any other benign ovarian mass and are diagnosed only on histologic examination. The prognosis is excellent.

Transitional Cell (Brenner) Tumors

Transitional cell tumors are adenofibromas in which the proliferating epithelial element has a transitional

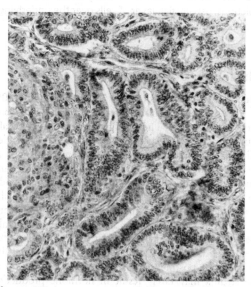

Figure 37–9. Endometrioid cystadenomas contain a proliferation of bland endometrial-like glands without the stroma of endometriosis.

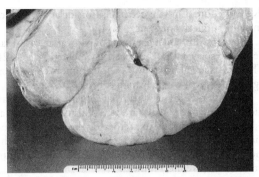

Figure 37–10. The cut surface of a Brenner tumor is firm, solid, and yellowish-white, and resembles a fibrothecoma.

cell appearance, which represents metaplasia. Brenner tumors account for 1–2% of primary ovarian tumors; over 98% are benign, and nearly 95% of cases are unilateral. They are frequently so small as to be incidental operative findings. However, the tumor may reach 5–8 cm in diameter and present as an adnexal mass at pelvic examination. On section they are firm and pale yellow or white (Fig 37–10). The epithelium is composed of nests of cells with ovoid nuclei with a prominent longitudinal groove ("coffee-bean nuclei"; Fig 37–11). Occasionally there is a mucinous metaplasia of the cells in the center of one or more of these nests, which may account for the 10% incidence of mucinous cystadenomas found associated with Brenner tumors.

SEX CORD-STROMAL TUMORS

Thecoma

This type of tumor can occur at any age, although they are most commonly found in postmenopausal women. They account for only 2% of all ovarian tumors and may not be a true neoplasm but instead a condition of hyperplasia of the cortical stroma. Histologically, the mass is filled with lipid-containing cells which are similar to theca cells, and the tumor is known to produce estrogen. As such, these tumors often present with dysfunctional uterine bleeding or postmenopausal bleeding; occasionally they have presented with adenocarcinoma of the endometrium given the unopposed estrogen production by the tumor. The tumors range from nonpalpable to more than 20 cm in size. They are rarely bilateral and rarely malignant.

Fibroma

Unlike thecomas, fibromas produce no hormones. They can occur at any age, but most often in the years prior to menopause. They range in size from incidental findings

to greater than 20 cm. They are multinodular, whorled, and formed from bundles of collagen-producing spindle cells. They can be found as part of Meig's syndrome, in which a patient is found to have a pelvic mass in concert with ascites and hydrothorax. Fibromas are also part of a hereditary basal cell nevus syndrome in which basal cell carcinoma is found with mesenteric cysts, calcification of the dura, and keratocysts of the jaw.

Hilus Cell Tumor

These tumors are a subset of Leydig cell tumors, which originate from the ovarian hilum or less frequently from the ovarian stroma. The typical presentation includes hirsutism, virilization, and menstrual irregularities. Hilus cell tumors rarely attain a palpable size. Histologically, groups of steroid cells containing eosinophilic cytoplasm and lipochrome pigment are found. For the tumor to be defined as a Leydig cell neoplasm, elongated eosinophilic crystalloids of Reinke must be found.

GERM CELL TUMORS

Mature Teratomas

Mature cystic teratomas, commonly referred to as dermoid cysts, comprise some 40–50% of all benign ovarian neoplasms. They contain well-differentiated tissue derived from any of the three germ cell layers, including hair and teeth as ectodermal derivatives. They account for the majority of benign ovarian neoplasms in reproductive-age women and are usually asymptomatic unless complications such as torsion or rupture occur. Transvaginal ultrasound is known to be very accurate in the diagnosis of dermoid cysts, with the hair and sebum, rather than calcium, creating highly reflective

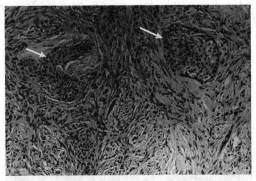

Figure 37–11. In a transitional cell (Brenner) tumor, islands of bland transitional cells (arrows) proliferate, accompanied by a prominent proliferation of benign spindly fibroblast-like cells.

irregular solid components within fluid-containing masses.

Studies have detailed several advantages to the laparoscopic approach to removal of dermoids, including less postoperative pain and blood loss, shorter hospital stay, and lower overall cost. Recent studies have shown that dermoid cysts can often be removed laparoscopically without intraperitoneal spillage. If intraoperative spillage does occur, the potential for chemical peritonitis or excess adhesion formation has led to the recommendation that copious saline irrigation be used until the lavage is clear. Current studies show the risk of peritonitis to be low (< .2%) with laparoscopic removal of dermoid cysts.

While most mature teratomas contain cells from all germ cell layers, a subset of monodermal teratomas exists. Those tumors composed mostly or entirely of thyroid tissue are called struma ovarii. These tumors account for only 3% of all teratomas, and only 5% of these will produce symptoms of thyrotoxicosis.

■ BENIGN TUMORS OF THE OVIDUCT

Since benign lesions of the uterine tube are routinely asymptomatic and rarely large enough to be palpable— with the exception of the paratubal or parovarian cyst—the diagnosis is made incidentally at the operating table or in the pathology laboratory.

CYSTIC TUMORS

Hydatid cysts of Morgagni are cystic tumors of the uterine tube located at or near the fimbriated end. They are lined by tubal-type epithelium, filled with clear fluid, and are usually about 1 cm in diameter. They are most often found inadvertently during a pelvic opera-

tive procedure. On rare occasions, torsion may produce an acute surgical emergency.

Occasionally, larger paratubal or parovarian cysts may develop, especially in the broad ligament (Fig 37–12). These cysts are almost always serous tumors of low malignant potential with a benign clinical outcome.

A third type of cyst associated with the fallopian tubes is known as a Walthard rest. This type is found as a 1-mm cyst beneath the serosa of the fallopian tube that appears to represent an inclusion cyst in which the mesothelium has undergone metaplasia similar to transitional cell (Brenner) tumors.

EPITHELIAL TUMORS

Benign epithelial tumors of the uterine tube are extremely rare. The polyps that occur in the cornual portion appear to be of endometrial rather than tubal origin.

ADENOMATOID TUMORS

The adenomatoid tumor is probably the most common benign tumor found in the uterine tube. It actually represents a benign mesothelioma, but the compact nature of the adenomatous pattern may be mistaken for malignancy (Fig 37–13). Adenomatoid lesions rarely measure

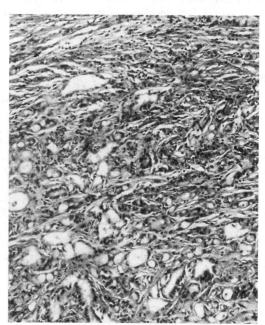

Figure 37–13. Adenomatoid tumor (benign mesothelioma) with tiny slit-like spaces and glands invading the muscular wall of the tube.

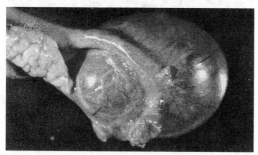

Figure 37–12. Parovarian cyst. Note the orientation of the cyst to the fimbriated end of the oviduct.

more than 1–1.5 cm. They are always incidental findings when the adnexa are removed for other purposes. Similar lesions, usually cystic, may involve the myometrium or ovary.

OTHER BENIGN TUBAL AND PARATUBAL TUMORS

Other benign tubal tumors, such as leiomyomas and teratomas are rare, as are benign adnexal tumors of probable wolffian origin. Adrenal cortical nests, however, are common incidental embryologic rests found in the broad ligament, seen as yellowish ovoid nodules 3–4 mm in diameter.

REFERENCES

Allias F et al: Value of ultrasound-guided fine-needle aspiration in the management of ovarian and paraovarian cysts. Diag Cytopathol 2000;22:70.

Canis M et al: Managemenet of adnexal masses: role and risk of laparascopy. Sem Surg Oncol 2000;19:28.

Ginsburg KA, McGinnis KT: Ovarian cystectomy: perioperative considerations and operative technique. Operative Tech Gynecol Surg 2000;5:224.

Jermy K, Luise C, Bourned T: The characterization of common ovarian cysts in premenopausal women. Ultrasound Obstet Gynecol 2001;17:140.

Lewis V: Polycystic ovary syndrome. A diagnostic challenge. Obstet Gynecol Clin N Amer 2001;28:1.

Mane S et al: Laparoscopic management of benign ovarian disease. Sem Laparascop Surg 1999;6:10.

Scully RE et al: Tumors of the ovary, maldeveloped gonads, fallopian tube, and broad ligament. AFIP Atlas of Tumor Pathology, 3rd Series, Washington, DC, 1998.

Strauss JF 3rd et al: Molecular mysteries of polycystic ovary syndrome. Mol Endocrinol 1999;13:800.

Templeman CL et al: Managing mature cystic teratomas of the ovary. Obstet Gynecol Surv 2000;55:738.

Yuen PM et al: A randomized prospective study of laparoscopy and laparotomy in the management of benign ovarian masses. Am J Obstet Gynecol 1997;177:109.

Zanetta G et al: Laparoscopic excision of ovarian dermoid cysts with controlled intraoperative spillage. Safety and effectiveness. J Reprod Med 1999;44:815.

Sexually Transmitted Diseases & Pelvic Infections

38

Steven W. Ainbinder, MD, & Susan M. Ramin, MD

■ SEXUALLY TRANSMITTED DISEASES

The term "sexually transmitted diseases" is used to denote disorders spread principally by intimate contact. Although this usually means sexual intercourse, it also includes close body contact, kissing, cunnilingus, anilingus, fellatio, mouth-breast contact, and anal intercourse. Many sexually transmitted diseases can be acquired by transplacental spread, by passage through the birth canal, and via lactation during the neonatal period. The organisms involved are peculiarly adapted to growth in the genital tract and are present in body secretions or blood.

Physicians have a critical role in preventing as well as treating sexually transmitted diseases (STDs). The clinician's role is fourfold. First, to understand the microbiology of STDs in order to appropriately diagnose and treat patients. Second, to alleviate the symptoms and prevent future sequelae. Third, to prevent the transmission to others including health care professionals. Finally, to do all of the above combined with patient education and counseling. As the future continues to bring advancement in therapy, the physician must be able to adapt to these changes. Today, preexposure vaccinations appear to be the trend in future therapy. For now, however, prevention through lifestyle and behavioral modification is the primary weapon against the spread of sexually transmitted diseases. Multiple cohort studies have demonstrated the protective effects of both male and female condoms.

The list of organisms traditionally thought of as causing sexually transmitted diseases has been extended to include cytomegalovirus, herpes simplex virus types I and II, *Chlamydia*, group B *Streptococcus*, molluscum contagiosum virus, *Sarcoptes scabiei*, hepatitis viruses, and human immunodeficiency virus (HIV). Some diseases spread by body contact but not necessarily by coitus—eg, pediculosis pubis and molluscum contagiosum—are discussed with the dermatitides rather than here; herpes genitalis is discussed in Chapter 34.

VULVAR LESIONS & GENITAL ULCERS

In the United States genital herpes, syphilis, and chancroid are the most prevalent ulcerative lesions. The diagnosis is difficult to make by physical examination alone. Thus, the work-up for all genital ulcers should include serologic screening for syphilis, culture/antigen testing for herpes simplex virus (1 and 2), and culture for *H ducreyi*. More than one infectious etiology may be present in a single lesion. In today's environment it is very important to recognize that human immunodeficiency virus (HIV) is a risk factor for genital ulcers.

1. Herpes Simplex

Vulvovaginal infections with herpes simplex virus have assumed a primary role in sexually transmitted diseases. HSV (1 and 2) is a highly prevalent (5 million cases in the U.S.), incurable, recurrent viral disease. Patient education and clinical skills are mandatory in obstetrics in order to prevent vertical transmission to the fetus or newborn. Systemic antiviral agents are commonly used during the first clinical episode to reduce symptoms, shorten duration of the lesion, and decrease the number of cesarean deliveries among infected mothers. These infections are discussed in Chapter 34.

2. Condylomata Acuminata (Venereal Warts)

See Chapter 34.

3. Chancroid (Soft Chancre)

 ESSENTIALS OF DIAGNOSIS

- *Painful, tender genital ulcer.*
- *Culture positive for* Haemophilus ducreyi.
- *Inguinal adenitis with erythema or fluctuance.*

General Considerations

Chancroid is a sexually transmitted disease characterized by a painful genital ulcer. However, there have been studies showing asymptomatic carriers among commercial sex workers. Although this can be a very difficult clinical diagnosis, suppurative inguinal adenopathy with painful ulcers is pathognomonic and may assist with a preculture diagnosis. It is endemic in many areas of the U.S., although it occurs more frequently in Africa, the West Indies, and Southeast Asia. The causative organism is the gram-negative rod *H ducreyi*. Exposure is usually through coitus, but accidentally acquired lesions of the hands have occurred. The incubation period is short: the lesion usually appears in 3–5 days or sooner. An increased rate of HIV infection has been reported among patients with this genital ulcer disease; chancroid is a cofactor for HIV transmission. Moreover, 10% of patients with genital chancroid may have coinfection with herpes or syphilis.

Clinical Findings

A. Symptoms and Signs

The early chancroid lesion is a vesicopustule on the pudendum, vagina, or cervix. Later, it degenerates into a saucer-shaped ragged ulcer circumscribed by an inflammatory wheal. Typically, the lesion is very tender and produces a heavy, foul discharge that is contagious. A cluster of ulcers may develop.

Painful inguinal adenitis is noted in over 50% of cases. The buboes may become necrotic and drain spontaneously.

B. Laboratory Findings

Syphilis must first be ruled out. Clinical diagnosis is more reliable than smears or cultures because of the difficulty of isolating this organism. Isolation of *H ducreyi* is diagnostic, but isolation occurs in less than one-third of cases. Aspirated pus from a bubo is the best material for culture. Serum adsorption enzyme immunoassays (EIAs) have been evaluated, and currently have a limited sensitivity. But polymerase chain reaction (PCR) testing of genital samples is becoming widely available.

Differential Diagnosis

Syphilis, granuloma inguinale, lymphogranuloma venereum, and herpes simplex may coexist with chancroid and need to be ruled out.

Prevention

Chancroid is a reportable disease. Routine antibiotic prophylaxis is not warranted. Condoms can give protection. Soap and water liberally used are relatively effective. Education is essential.

Treatment

A. Local Treatment

Good personal hygiene is important. The early lesions should be cleansed with mild soap solution. Sitz baths are beneficial.

B. Antibiotic Treatment

The susceptibility of *H ducreyi* to antimicrobial agents varies by locality. Consultation with the nearest STD clinic may reveal information about current susceptibilities and effective treatment regimens. Guidelines issued by the CDC for genital chancroid are as follows: (1) Recommended regimens are (a) azithromycin 1 g orally once; (b) ceftriaxone 250 mg intramuscularly as a single dose; (c) erythromycin base 500 mg orally 3 times daily for 7 days; and (d) ciprofloxacin 500 mg orally twice daily for 3 days in nonpregnant patients who are not lactating over 17. The course may have to be repeated. Fluctuant lymph nodes may need to be aspirated through normal adjacent skin. Incision and drainage of the nodes is not recommended, since it will delay healing.

Prognosis

Untreated or poorly managed cases of chancroid may persist, and secondary infection may develop. Frequently, the ulcers heal spontaneously. They should improve within 7–10 days. If no improvement is noted, coinfection, HIV, resistant strains, and non-compliance must be considered. If not treated, they may cause deep scarring with sequelae in men.

4. Granuloma Inguinale (Donovanosis)

 ESSENTIALS OF DIAGNOSIS

- Ulcerative vulvitis, chronic or recurrent.
- Donovan bodies revealed by Wright's or Giemsa's stain.

General Considerations

Granuloma inguinale is a chronic ulcerative granulomatous disease that usually develops in the vulva, perineum, and inguinal regions (Fig 38–1). The disease is almost nonexistent in the U.S. It is most common in India, Brazil, the West Indies, some South Pacific islands, and parts of Australia, China, and Africa. The causative organism is *Calymmatobacterium granulomatis* (Donovan body). Donovan bodies are bacteria encapsulated in mononuclear leukocytes. Transmission is via coitus, and the incubation period is 8–12 weeks.

Clinical Findings

A. Symptoms and Signs

Although granuloma inguinale most often involves the skin and subcutaneous tissues of the vulva and inguinal regions, cervical, uterine, orolabial, and ovarian sites have been reported. A malodorous discharge is characteristic. The disorder often begins as a papule, which then ulcerates, with the development of a beefy-red granular zone with clean, sharp edges. The ulcer shows little tendency to heal, and there are usually no local or systemic symptoms. Healing is very slow, and satellite ulcers may unite to form a large lesion. Lymphatic permeation is rare, but lymphadenitis may result when the cutaneous lesion becomes superimposed on lymphatic channels. Inguinal swelling is common, with late formation of abscesses (buboes). Rarely, granuloma inguinale may be manifested by chronic cervical lesions. These lesions usually take the form of redness

or ulceration, or they form granulation tissue. They produce a chronic inflammatory exudate characterized histologically by lymphocytes, giant cells, and histiocytes. They may mimic carcinoma of the cervix and must be distinguished from this as well as other neoplastic diseases.

The chronic ulcerative process may involve the urethra and the anal area, causing marked discomfort. Introital contraction may make coitus difficult or impossible; walking or sitting may become painful. The possibility of the coexistence of another venereal disease must be considered. Spread to other areas occurs in about 7% of patients.

B. Laboratory Findings

Direct smear from beneath the surface of an ulcer may reveal gram-negative bipolar rods within mononuclear leukocytes. These are seen best in Wright-stained smears. When smears are negative, a biopsy specimen should be taken. Biopsy of the lesion generally shows granulation tissue infiltrated by plasma cells and scattered large macrophages with rod-shaped cytoplasmic inclusion bodies (Mikulicz cells). Pseudoepitheliomatous hyperplasia often is seen at the margin of the ulcer.

The diagnosis of granuloma inguinale is made by demonstrating, in biopsy or smear material stained with Wright's, Giemsa's, or silver stain, large mononuclear cells having one or more cystic inclusions containing the so-called Donovan bodies—small round or rod-shaped particles that stain purple in traditional hematoxylin and eosin preparations.

Prevention

Personal hygiene is the best method of prevention. Therapy immediately after exposure may abort the infection.

Treatment

Trimethoprim-sulfamethoxazole, 1 double strength tablet orally twice daily for at least 3 weeks or doxycycline 100 mg twice daily for 3 weeks are the CDC-recommended agents. Ciprofloxacin 750 mg twice daily for 3 weeks, erythromycin base, 500 mg 4 times daily for 2–3 weeks, or Azithromycin 1 gm orally once per week for 3 weeks are alternate regimens. Penicillin is not effective.

Sex partners must be considered for treatment. If the partners have had sexual contact during the 60 days preceding the onset of symptoms or is clinically symptomatic, they should be treated by one of the above regimens. Also, special consideration for HIV and gravid women should be made. There are recommendations to add intravenous gentamycin to the oral protocol.

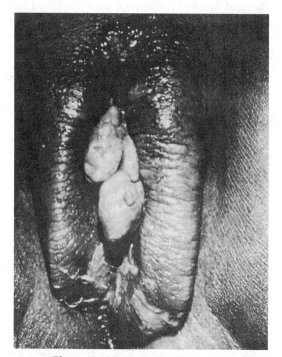

Figure 38–1. Granuloma inguinale.

5. Lymphogranuloma Venereum

ESSENTIALS OF DIAGNOSIS

- Rectal ulceration, inguinal lymphadenopathy, or rectal stricture.
- Positive complement fixation test.

General Considerations

The causative agent of lymphogranuloma venereum is one of the aggressive L serotypes (L1, L2, or L3) of *C trachomatis*. It is encountered more frequently in the tropical and subtropical nations of Africa and Asia but is also seen in the southeastern U.S. Transmission is sexual; men are affected more frequently than women (6:1). The incubation period is 7–21 days.

Clinical Findings

A. SYMPTOMS AND SIGNS (FIG 38–2)

Early in the course of the disease, a vesicopustular eruption may go undetected; with inguinal (and vulvar) ulceration, lymphedema, and secondary bilateral invasion, excruciating conditions arise. Sitting or walking may cause pain. During the inguinal bubo phase, the groin is exquisitely tender. A hard cutaneous induration (red to purplish-blue) is a notable feature. This usually occurs within 10–30 days after exposure and may be bilateral. Anorectal lymphedema occurs early; defecation is painful, and the stool may be blood-streaked.

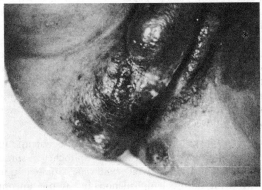

Figure 38–2. Lymphogranuloma venereum. Note involvement of perineum and spread over buttocks.

Later, as the lymphedema and ulceration undergo cicatrization, rectal stricture makes defecation difficult or impossible. Vaginal narrowing and distortion may end in severe dyspareunia. In the late phase, systemic symptoms—fever, headache, arthralgia, chills, and abdominal cramps—may develop.

B. LABORATORY FINDINGS

The diagnosis can be proved only by isolating *C trachomatis* from appropriate specimens and confirming the immunotype. These procedures are seldom available, so less-specific tests are used.

A complement fixation test using a heat-stable antigen that is group-specific for all *Chlamydia* species is available. This test is positive at a titer of ≥ 1:16 in more than 80% of cases of lymphogranuloma venereum. If acute or convalescent sera are available, a rise in titer is particularly helpful in making the diagnosis. Application of the microimmunofluorescent test may also be useful.

Differential Diagnosis

As with any disseminated disease, the systemic symptoms of lymphogranuloma venereum may resemble meningitis, arthritis, pleurisy, or peritonitis. The cutaneous lesions must be differentiated from those of granuloma inguinale, tuberculosis, early syphilis, and chancroid. In the case of colonic lesions, proctoscopic examination and mucosal biopsy are needed to rule out carcinoma, schistosomiasis, and granuloma inguinale.

Complications

Perianal scarring and rectal strictures—late complications—can involve the entire sigmoid, but the urogenital diaphragm is rarely involved. Vulvar elephantiasis (esthiomene) produces marked distortion of the external genitalia.

Prevention

Lymphogranuloma venereum is reportable. Avoiding infectious contact with a carrier is achieved by use of a condom or by refraining from coitus. Definite exposure can be treated with sulfonamides or tetracyclines.

Treatment

A. CHEMOTHERAPY

Doxycycline 100 mg twice daily orally should be given for 21 days according to tolerance. If disease persists, the course should be repeated. An alternative regimen is erythromycin 500 mg orally 4 times daily for 21 days.

B. LOCAL AND SURGICAL TREATMENT

Anal strictures should be dilated manually at weekly intervals. Severe stricture may require diversionary colostomy. If the disease is arrested, complete vulvectomy may be done for cosmetic reasons. Abscesses should be aspirated, not excised.

6. Syphilis

 ESSENTIALS OF DIAGNOSIS

Primary syphilis:

- *Painless genital sore (chancre) on labia, vulva, vagina, cervix, anus, lips, or nipples.*
- *Painless, rubbery, regional lymphadenopathy followed by generalized lymphadenopathy in the third to sixth weeks.*
- *Darkfield microscopic findings.*
- *Positive serologic test in 70% of cases.*

Secondary syphilis:

- *Bilaterally symmetric extragenital papulosquamous eruption.*
- *Condyloma latum, mucous patches.*
- *Darkfield findings positive in moist lesions.*
- *Positive serologic test for syphilis.*
- *Lymphadenopathy.*

Tertiary syphilis:

- *Cardiac, neurologic, ophthalmic, and auditory lesions.*
- *Gummas.*

Congenital syphilis:

- *History of maternal syphilis.*
- *Positive serologic test for syphilis.*
- *Stigmata of congenital syphilis (eg, x-ray changes of bone, hepatosplenomegaly, jaundice, anemia).*
- *Normal examination or signs of intrauterine infection.*
- *Often stillborn or premature.*
- *Enlarged, waxy placenta.*

Latent syphilis:

- *History or serologic evidence of previous infection.*
- *Absence of lesions.*
- *Serologic test usually reactive; titer may be low.*

General Considerations

The rates of syphilis in women during their reproductive years are the highest seen since the 1940s. Syphilis is caused by *Treponema pallidum,* transmitted by direct contact with an infectious moist lesion. Treponemes pass through intact mucous membranes or abraded skin. Ten to 90 days after the treponemes enter, a primary lesion (chancre) develops. The chancre persists for 1–5 weeks and then heals spontaneously, but may persist with signs of secondary disease. Serologic tests for syphilis are usually nonreactive when the chancre first appears, but become reactive 1–4 weeks later. Two weeks to 6 months (average, 6 weeks) after the primary lesion appears, the generalized cutaneous eruption of secondary syphilis may appear. The skin lesions heal spontaneously in 2–6 weeks. Serologic tests are almost always positive during the secondary phase. Latent syphilis may follow the secondary stage and may last a lifetime, or tertiary syphilis may develop. The latter usually becomes manifest 4–20 or more years after the disappearance of the primary lesion.

In one-third of untreated cases, the destructive lesions of late (tertiary) syphilis develop. These involve skin or bone (gummas), the cardiovascular system (aortic aneurysm or insufficiency), and the nervous system (meningitis, tabes dorsalis, paresis). The complications of tertiary syphilis are fatal in almost one-fourth of cases, but one-fourth never show any ill effects.

Clinical Findings

A. SYMPTOMS AND SIGNS

1. Primary syphilis—The chancre (Fig 38–3) is an indurated, firm, painless papule or ulcer with raised borders. Groin lymph nodes may be enlarged, firm, and painless. Genital lesions are not usually seen in women unless they occur on the external genitalia; however, careful examination may reveal a typical cervical or vaginal lesion. Primary lesions may occur on any mucous membrane or skin area of the body (nose, breast, perineum), and darkfield examination is required for all suspect lesions. Serologic tests should be done every week for 6 weeks or until positive.

2. Secondary syphilis—Signs of diffuse systemic infection become evident as the spirochetes spread hematogenously. A "viral syndrome" presentation, often with diffuse lymphadenopathy, is not uncommon. The characteristic dermatitis appears as diffuse,

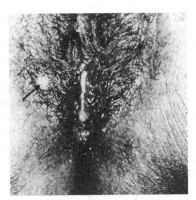

Figure 38–3. Chancre of primary syphilis (arrow).

bilateral, symmetric, papulosquamous lesions that often involve the palms and soles. Lesions may also cover the trunk and be macular, maculopapular, papular, or pustular. Other systemic manifestations include patchy alopecia, hepatitis, and nephritis. Moist papules can be seen in the perineal area (condyloma lata). Mucous patches may also be seen; like condyloma lata, they are darkfield-positive, infectious lesions. Serologic tests for syphilis are invariably reactive in this stage.

3. Latent syphilis—With resolution of the lesions of primary and secondary infection or the finding of a reactive serologic test without a history of therapy, a patient passes into latency. Persons are infectious in the first 1–2 years of latency, with clinical relapses resembling the secondary stage occurring in about 25% of cases in the first year. The United States Public Health Service defines early latent syphilis as disease of less than 1 year duration, and includes it in the category of "early or infectious syphilis, with primary and secondary lues." Late latent syphilis is an infection of indeterminate or greater than 1 year duration; consideration must be given to possible asymptomatic neurosyphilis in this setting, and CSF examination is recommended.

4. Neurosyphilis—Although the central nervous system is always vulnerable to *T pallidum,* it is most commonly infected during latent syphilis. Neurologic involvement of ophthalmic and auditory systems can be detected. Cranial nerve palsy and meningeal signs should be tested for on physical exam. All patients require cerebrospinal fluid (CSF) sampling with laboratory testing for cell count, protein, VDRL, and FTA-ABS. FTA-ABS is less specific but very sensitive when diagnosing neurosyphilis.

5. Syphilis during pregnancy—The course of syphilis is unaltered by pregnancy, but misdiagnoses are common. The chancre is often unnoticed or internal

and not brought to medical attention. Chancres, mucous patches, and condyloma lata are often thought to be herpes genitalis. The dermatoses can resolve prior to diagnosis, or they may be misdiagnosed.

The effect of syphilis on pregnancy outcome can be profound. The risk of fetal infection depends on the degree of maternal spirochetemia (greater in the secondary stage than in the primary or latent stages) and the gestational age of the fetus. Treponemes may cross the placenta at all stages of pregnancy, but fetal involvement is rare before 18 weeks because of fetal immunoincompetence. After 18 weeks, the fetus is able to mount an immunologic response, and tissue damage may result. The earlier in pregnancy the fetus is exposed, the more severe the fetal infection and the greater the risk of premature delivery or stillbirth. Antepartum infection in late pregnancy does not necessarily result in congenital infection, since only 40–50% of such infants will have definite congenital infection. Placental infection can occur with resultant endarteritis, stromal hyperplasia, and immature villi. Grossly, the placenta looks hydropic (pale yellow, waxy, and enlarged). Because hydramnios is frequently associated with symptomatic congenital infection, fetuses are ultrasonographically followed throughout pregnancy.

6. Congenital syphilis—Most infants with congenital syphilis are born to women of low socioeconomic status with inadequate or no prenatal care. Either these neonates may be affected at birth from intrauterine infection (hepatosplenomegaly, osteochondritis, jaundice, anemia, skin lesions, rhinitis, lymphadenopathy, nervous system involvement), or symptoms may develop weeks or months later. The clinical spectrum of congenital infection is analogous to adult secondary disease, since the disease is systemic from onset due to transplacental hematogenous inoculation.

Since the antibodies from the maternal compartment are of the IgG class, they freely cross the placenta, giving most neonates a reactive serologic test if the mother's test was reactive. With symptomatic neonatal infection, often the cord blood serologic test will be higher in titer than the maternal test. There is no clinically reliable neonatal IgM serologic test. Other diagnostic aids include long-bone survey and lumbar puncture, which may help diagnose asymptomatic systemic infection requiring more intense therapy.

The newborn may have lymphadenitis and an enlarged liver and spleen. The bones usually reveal signs of osteochondritis and an irregular epiphyseal juncture (Guaaerin's line) on x-ray. The eyes, central nervous system structures, and other organs may reveal abnormalities at birth, or defects may develop later in untreated cases.

Any infant with the stigmata of syphilis should be placed in isolation until a definite diagnosis can be made and treatment administered.

Newborns with congenital syphilis may appear healthy at birth but often develop symptoms weeks or months later. Examine the body for stigmata of syphilis at intervals of 3 weeks to 4 months. If the mother's serologic test is positive at delivery, the baby's test will also be positive. Obtain serial quantitative serologic tests of the infant's blood for 4 months. A rising titer indicates congenital syphilis, and treatment is indicated.

B. Laboratory Findings

1. Identification of the organism—*T pallidum* can usually be identified by darkfield examination of specimens from cutaneous lesions, but the recovery period of the treponeme is very brief; in most cases, diagnosis depends on the history and serologic tests. An immunofluorescent technique is now available for dried smears. Silver staining for *T pallidum* of biopsy specimens, placental sections, or autopsy material may confirm the diagnosis in difficult cases. Motile spirochetes can be identified in amniotic fluid obtained transabdominally in women with syphilis and fetal death. Polymerase chain reaction is extremely specific for detection of *T pallidum* in amniotic fluid and neonatal serum and spinal fluid.

2. Serologic tests—Diagnostic tests after the primary or secondary moist lesion has disappeared are confined largely to serologic testing. Serologic tests become positive several weeks after the primary lesion appears.

a. Nontreponemal tests—These measure reaginic antibody detected by highly purified cardiolipin-lecithin antigen. They can be performed rapidly, relatively easily, and inexpensively. Nontreponemal tests are used principally for syphilis screening, but they are relatively specific, so they are not absolute for syphilis and false-positive reactions may occur. Nontreponemal tests currently in use are flocculation procedures that include the VDRL slide test, rapid reagin test, and automated reagin test for screening procedures in the field. The latter tests are more sensitive but less specific than the VDRL. If they are positive, the activity should be verified, and the degree of reactivity should be checked by the VDRL test. Complement fixation tests (eg, Kolmer) are no longer used in the U.S.

The VDRL test (the nontreponemal test in widest use) generally becomes positive 3–6 weeks after infection, or 2–3 weeks after the appearance of the primary lesion; it is almost invariably positive in the secondary stage. The VDRL titer is usually high in secondary syphilis and tends to be lower or even nil in late forms of syphilis, although this is highly variable. A fourfold falling titer in treated early syphilis or a falling or stable titer in latent or late syphilis indicates satisfactory therapeutic progress. False-positive serologic reactions are frequently encountered in a wide variety of situations, including collagen diseases, infectious mononucleosis, malaria, many febrile diseases, leprosy, vaccination, drug addiction, old age, and possibly pregnancy. False-positive reactions are usually of low titer and transient and may be distinguished from true positives by specific treponemal antibody tests.

b. Treponemal antibody tests—The fluorescent treponemal antibody absorption (FTA-ABS) test and microhemagglutination assay for *T pallidum* (MHA-TP) detect antibody against *Treponema* spirochetes. Both tests are more sensitive and specific than nontreponemal tests (except the MHA-TP test with primary disease; Table 38–1). These tests remain positive despite therapy, and so are not given in titers or used to follow serologic response to treatment.

Differential Diagnosis

Primary syphilis must be differentiated from chancroid, granuloma inguinale, lymphogranuloma venereum, herpes genitalis, carcinoma, scabies, trauma, lichen planus, psoriasis, drug eruption, aphthosis, mycotic infections, Reiter's syndrome, and Bowen's disease.

Secondary syphilis must be differentiated from pityriasis rosea, psoriasis, lichen planus, tinea versicolor, drug eruption, "id" eruptions, perlèche, parasitic infections, iritis, neuroretinitis, condyloma acuminatum, acute exanthems, infectious mononucleosis, alopecia, and sarcoidosis.

Prevention

If the patient is known to have been exposed to syphilis, do not wait for the disease to develop to the clinical or reactive serologic stage before giving preventive treatment.

Table 38–1. Percent sensitivity of serologic tests in untreated syphilis.

Type of Test	Stage of Disease			
	Primary	Secondary	Latent	Late
VDRL	59–87	100	73–91	37–94
FTA-ABS	86–100	99–100	96–99	96–100
MHA-TP	64–87	96–100	96–100	94–100

Reproduced, with permission, from Holmes KK et al (editors): *Sexually Transmitted Diseases.* McGraw-Hill, 1984.

Even so, every effort should be made to reach a diagnosis, including a complete physical examination, before administering preventive treatment. It is recommended that if a patient is exposed and becomes symptomatic within 90 days of sexual contact and is seronegative they should still be treated. Also, if the exposure occurred > 90 days earlier and seroconversion takes place, the exposed person should be treated. Finally, if the duration since exposure is unknown and the nontreponemal antibody titer is > 1:32, treatment is indicated.

Prenatal care is often underutilized or unavailable in geographic areas where congenital syphilis occurs. Education concerning the preventive value of prenatal care in these high-risk, generally low socioeconomic groups is essential. All pregnant women should undergo a routine serologic test for syphilis at the first visit. The test should be repeated between 28 and 32 weeks of gestation in high-risk regions. If the test is positive, attention must be given to the patient's prior serologic test and therapy (if any) for syphilis. If doubt exists as to whether or not the patient has active syphilis, repeat therapy is far better than the risk of congenital syphilis.

Syphilis is still a serious public health problem. Teaching young people about the disease and its consequences is still the best method of control. Use of a condom, together with soap and water decontamination after coitus, would prevent most cases. If a lesion develops, a physician should be notified at once. All exposed persons must be sought and treated and the case reported to the communicable disease service in the city or state.

Treatment

A. Early Syphilis and Contacts

Primary, secondary, and early latent syphilis (less than 1 year duration).

(1) Benzathine penicillin G, 2.4 million units intramuscularly once.

(2) Tetracycline hydrochloride, 500 mg orally 4 times daily or 100 mg doxycycline twice daily for 14 days, for nonpregnant penicillin-allergic patients.

Erythromycin estolate should not be administered to pregnant women because of potential drug-related hepatotoxicity.

Ceftriaxone 1 gm daily IM or IV for 8–10 days may be effective but data with this regimen are limited.

B. Late Syphilis

Includes latent syphilis of indeterminate duration or more than 1 year duration, except neurosyphilis.

(1) Benzathine penicillin G, 2.4 million units intramuscularly weekly for 3 successive weeks (7.2 million units total).

(2) Tetracycline hydrochloride, 500 mg orally 4 times daily, or 100 mg doxycycline twice daily for 14 days, for penicillin-allergic patients.

C. Syphilis in Pregnancy

Treat as indicated above, except that tetracycline or erythromycin are not recommended. If serologic tests are equivocal (eg, possible biologic false-positive), it is better to err on the side of early treatment. Because of the increased risk of treatment failure, a second dose of 2.4 million units of penicillin intramuscularly is often recommended. Penicillin-allergic patients may be given oral desensitization therapy using gradually larger doses of phenoxymethyl penicillin suspension to achieve a temporary tolerant state that allows parenteral penicillin therapy. This is particularly useful in circumventing compliance problems due to hyperemesis or drug-induced gastric upset.

D. Congenital Syphilis

Adequate maternal treatment before 16–18 weeks' gestation prevents congenital syphilis. Treatment thereafter may arrest fetal syphilitic infection, but some stigmata may remain.

(1) Benzathine penicillin G, 50,000 U/kg intramuscularly as a single injection, for asymptomatic infants without neurosyphilis.

(2) Aqueous crystalline penicillin G, 50,000 U/kg intravenously every 8–12 hours, or procaine penicillin G, 50,000 U/kg intramuscularly once daily for 10–14 days, for symptomatic infants or those with neurosyphilis.

E. Jarisch-Herxheimer Reaction

A febrile reaction may occur in 50–75% of patients with early syphilis treated with penicillin. This occurs 4–12 hours after injection and is completed by 24 hours. Its cause is uncertain but may involve a release of treponemal toxic products upon organism lysis. The reaction is generally benign but may trigger labor or fetal distress. Prophylaxis with antipyretics or corticosteroids is of unknown value.

F. Coexisting Infection With HIV

No specific changes in treatment are currently necessary, but close follow-up is necessary to ensure adequate treatment. Recommendations include serology tests every 3 months for 1 year and twice during the second year.

VAGINITIS

Vaginitis is a clinical syndrome that is characterized by vaginal discharge, vulvar irritation, or malodorous discharge. This is often broken down into two entities: infectious vaginitis and atrophic vaginitis. This chapter will focus on infectious vaginitis. Infectious vaginitis is most frequently caused by one of three diseases: trichomoniasis, bacterial vaginosis, or candidiasis.

1. Bacterial Vaginosis (Corynebacterium vaginale Vaginitis; Gardnerella vaginalis Vaginitis)

Although bacterial vaginosis is the most prevalent vaginal infection, almost 50% of affected women are asymptomatic. The term bacterial vaginosis refers to the intricate changes of vaginal bacterial flora with a loss of lactobacilli, an increase in vaginal pH (pH > 4.5), and an increase in multiple anaerobic and aerobic bacteria. Clinical criteria for diagnoses include: (1) homogeneous white, noninflammatory discharge; (2) microscopic presence of > 20% clue cells; (3) vaginal discharge with pH > 4.5; and (4) fishy odor with or without addition of 10% KOH. *Gardnerella vaginalis* (formerly designated *C vaginale* and *Haemophilus vaginalis*) is a small, nonmotile, nonencapsulated, pleomorphic rod that stains variably with Gram's stain. It may be spread by sexual contact and, though of low virulence, causes vaginitis. The disorder may be atypical and even more troublesome when *G vaginalis* coexists with more virulent organisms. *G vaginalis* is not the only cause of bacterial vaginosis. The characteristic fishy odor of bacterial vaginosis is due to anaerobic bacteria, such as *Bacteroides, Prevotella, Peptostreptococcus,* and *Mobiluncus* spp., and genital mycoplasmas.

G vaginalis infection is often overlooked. It may be suspected on the basis of the microscopic appearance of unstained exfoliated vaginal cells in a wet preparation that appears to be dusted with many small dark particles, actually *G vaginalis* organisms. These "clue cells" are presumptive evidence of the presence of this organism. In case of mixed infection (eg, with *Candida albicans*), it may not be possible to make the diagnosis except by culture. Gram stain is another method useful in making the diagnosis of bacterial vaginosis.

Treatment

Specific therapy for vaginal infection caused by *G vaginalis* and *C vaginale* has been neglected, owing in part to the rather innocuous symptoms reported. Therapy should always be initiated for symptomatic relief. Pregnant women who are at high risk for preterm labor may benefit from treatment. Low-risk groups during pregnancy are also recommended to receive treatment if infected and symptomatic. A third cohort of patients who are thought to benefit from therapy are asymptomatic carriers before pelvic/abdominal surgery. Guidelines issued by the CDC for therapy are as follows: (1) recommended regimen—(a) oral metronidazole, 500 mg

twice daily for 7 days; (b) clindamycin cream 2%, one applicatorful (5 g) intravaginally at night for 7 days; and (c) metronidazole gel 0.75%, one applicatorful (5 g) intravaginally, once daily for 5 days. (2) alternative regimens—(a) oral metronidazole, 2 g in a single dose; (b) oral clindamycin, 300 mg twice daily for 7 days; (c) clindamycin ovules 100 g intravaginally once at bedtime for 3 days. Four randomized controlled trials have demonstrated overall cure rates of 95% for the 7-day metronidazole regimen and 84% for the single 2-g regimen. During pregnancy oral treatment is preferred to local agents to ensure adequate tissue levels of the bactericidal drug. The recommended regimen is metronidazole 250 mg orally three times daily for 7 days or clindamycin 300 mg orally twice daily for 7 days.

2. Trichomonas Vaginalis

See Chapter 34.

3. Candidiasis

See Chapter 34.

URETHRITIS AND CERVICITIS

Urethral mucopurulent or purulent discharge is commonly caused by *Neisseria gonorrhoeae, Chlamydia trachomatis,* or genital herpes. Although asymptomatic infections are common, some patients experience slow-onset dysuria with vaginal discharge and/or irregular bleeding. Urethritis and cervicitis are often coinfections. Both are reportable sexually transmitted diseases, and clinicians must mandate that partners of patients obtain diagnostic and therapeutic interventions.

Cervicitis is an inflammation of either the ectocervical cells or the glandular cells composing the cervical epithelium. The ectocervical squamous cells are contiguous with the vaginal epithelium and can be infected by the same organisms that cause inflammatory vaginitis. The glandular cells of the endocervix are more commonly inflamed by *Neisseria gonorrhoeae* and *Chlamydia trachomatis.*

1. Gonorrhea

ESSENTIALS OF DIAGNOSIS

- *Most affected women are asymptomatic carriers.*
- *Purulent vaginal discharge.*
- *Frequency and dysuria.*
- *Recovery of organism in selective media.*

· *May progress to pelvic infection or disseminated infection.*

General Considerations

Neisseria gonorrhoeae is a gram-negative diplococcus that forms oxidase-positive colonies and ferments glucose. The organism may be recovered from the urethra, cervix, anal canal, or pharynx. Optimal recovery of the organism is with use of Thayer-Martin or Martin-Lester (Transgrow) medium. *N gonorrhoeae* is rapidly killed by drying, sunlight, heat, and most disinfectants.

The columnar and transitional epithelium of the genitourinary tract is the principal site of invasion. The organism may enter the upper reproductive tract (Fig 38–1), causing salpingitis with its attendant complications. Approximately 600,000 new infections occur each year in both men and women. It has been estimated that after exposure to an infected partner, 20–50% of men and 60–90% of women become infected. Without therapy, 10–17% of women with gonorrhea develop pelvic infection. Depending on the geographic location and population involved, *N gonorrhoeae* is often present with other sexually transmitted diseases. Traditionally, women with gonorrhea are considered to be at risk for incubating syphilis. It has been shown that 20–40% also have *Chlamydia* infection.

Clinical Findings

A. Symptoms and Signs

1. Early symptoms—Most women with gonorrhea are asymptomatic. When symptoms occur, they are localized to the lower genitourinary tract and include vaginal discharge, urinary frequency or dysuria, and rectal discomfort. The incubation period is only 3–5 days.

2. Discharge—The vulva, vagina, cervix, and urethra may be inflamed and may itch or burn. Specimens of discharge from the cervix, urethra, and anus should be taken for culture in the symptomatic patient. A stain of purulent urethral exudate may demonstrate gram-negative diplococci in leukocytes. Similar findings in a purulent cervical discharge are less conclusively diagnostic of *N gonorrhoeae.*

3. Bartholinitis—Unilateral swelling in the inferior lateral portion of the introitus suggests involvement of Bartholin's duct and gland. In early gonococcal infections, the organism may be recovered by gently squeezing the gland and expressing pus from the duct. Enlargement, tenderness, and fluctuation may develop, signifying abscess formation. *N gonorrhoeae* is then less frequently recovered; however, the prevalence of infection with other bacteria merits a search for these pathogens. Spontaneous evacuation of pus often occurs if drainage by incision is not done. The infection may result in asymptomatic cyst formation.

4. Anorectal inflammation—Anal itching, pain, discharge, or bleeding occurs rarely. Most women are asymptomatic and acquire infection by perineal spread of vaginal secretions rather than by anal intercourse.

5. Pharyngitis—Acute pharyngitis and tonsillitis rarely occur; most infections are asymptomatic.

6. Disseminated infection—For unknown reasons, asymptomatic carriers can develop systemic infection. Commonly, a triad of polyarthralgia, tenosynovitis, and dermatitis is seen, or purulent arthritis without dermatitis. Septicemia is more common in the former clinical setting and *N gonorrhoeae* cultured from joint aspirates in the latter. Endocarditis and meningitis have been described.

7. Conjunctivitis—In adults, ophthalmic infection is usually due to autoinoculation. Ophthalmia neonatorum may result from delivery through an infected birth canal.

8. Vulvovaginitis in children—Gonococcal invasion of nonkeratinized membranes in prepubertal girls produces severe vulvovaginitis. The typical sign is a purulent vaginal discharge with dysuria. The genital mucous membranes are red and swollen. Infection is commonly introduced by adults, and in such cases the physician must consider the possibility of child abuse.

B. Laboratory Findings

A presumptive diagnosis of gonorrhea can be made based on examination of the stained smear; however, confirmation requires positive identification on selective media. Secretions are examined under oil immersion for presumptive identification. Gram-negative diplococci that are oxidase-positive and obtained from selective media (Thayer-Martin or Transgrow) usually signify *N gonorrhoeae.* Carbohydrate fermentation tests may be performed, but, in addition to being time-consuming and expensive, they occasionally yield other species of *Neisseria.* Cultures therefore are reported as "presumptive for *N gonorrhoeae.*" Chlamydial cultures or direct smear testing (ELISA or immunofluorescent staining) of the cervix and a serologic test for syphilis should also be obtained.

Complications

The major complication in the female is salpingitis and the complications that may arise from salpingitis (see section on acute salpingitis-peritonitis). *N gonorrhoeae* can be recovered from the cervix in about 50% of women with salpingitis. It is important to note that asymptomatic carriers can also develop tubal scarring, infertility, and increased risk of ectopic gestations. Resistant strains of *N gonorrhoeae* have emerged in some geographic areas owing to their capacity to produce penicillinase or owing to chromosome-mediated resistance. Some strains are also resistant to spectinomycin and tetracycline. Follow-up cultures are essential in these settings, at least by 7 days to 3 weeks after completion of therapy.

Differential Diagnosis

See Chapter 34.

Prevention

Gonorrhea is a reportable disease that can be controlled only by detecting the asymptomatic carrier and treating her and her sexual partners. It is crucial to instruct patients to abstain from sexual relations for the 7 days after therapy is initiated. All high-risk populations should be screened by routine cultures. Reexamination 3 weeks after treatment is mandatory to rule out reinfection or failure of therapy. The use of condoms will protect against gonorrhea.

Treatment

Any patient with gonorrhea must be suspected of also having other sexually transmitted diseases (eg, syphilis, HIV, and chlamydial infection) and managed accordingly. Treatment should cover *N gonorrhoeae, Chlamydia trachomatis,* and incubating syphilis. Dual therapy has contributed greatly to the declining prevalence of chlamydial infections. Therefore, if chlamydial infection is not ruled out, the regimens below should be given with doxycycline (for nonpregnant patients) or azithromycin.

Quinolone-resistant *N gonorrhoeae* (QRNG) is common in parts of Asia and the Pacific. It is becoming increasingly common in areas on the U.S. West coast, particularly California. Because of this, quinolones are no longer recommended for treatment of gonorrhea acquired in Asia and the Pacific (including Hawaii). Quinolones may not be advisable for treatment of gonorrhea acquired in California.

A. UNCOMPLICATED INFECTIONS

Guidelines issued by the Centers for Disease Control (CDC) for therapy of uncomplicated infection in adults are as follows: (1) Recommended regimens: (a) ceftriaxone, 125 mg intramuscularly once, plus doxycycline, 100 mg orally twice daily for 7 days (for nonpregnant patients), or azithromycin 1 g orally in a single dose if chlamydial infection is not ruled out; (b) cefixime 0.4 g orally once, plus doxycycline or azithromycin as

above; and (c) ofloxacin 0.4 g, levofloxacin .25 g, or ciprofloxacin 0.5 g, orally once in nonpregnant, nonlactating patients over 17 years of age, plus doxycycline or azithromycin as above. For patients residing in, or who may have acquired infection in Asia and the Pacific (including Hawaii), quinolones should not be used. The use of fluoroquinolones in California is probably inadvisable. According to one study, the advantage of oral cefixime over ceftriaxone is the reduced potential for needlesticks (HIV, hepatitis C) and increased patient comfort. (2) Alternative regimens: (a) spectinomycin, 2 g intramuscularly once, followed by doxycycline or azithromycin as above, for patients who cannot take cephalosporins or quinolones (not reliable for pharyngeal infection); (b) ceftizoxime, 0.5 g, cefotaxime 0.5 g, or cefoxitin 2 g, intramuscularly once with probenecid 1 g orally, plus doxycycline or azithromycin as above; and (c) gatifloxacin 0.4 g, norfloxacin 0.8 g, or lomefloxacin 400 mg orally once in nonpregnant, nonlactating patients over 17, plus doxycycline or azithromycin as above. Azithromycin 2 g orally is equally effective for *N gonorrhoeae,* but may be limited due to its higher cost and potential for gastrointestinal distress.

Pregnant women should not be treated with quinolones or tetracyclines. They should be treated with a recommended or alternate cephalosporin. If cephalosporins are not tolerated, spectinomycin 2 g IM should be given along with treatment for diagnosed or presumptive *C. trachomatis.*

The incidence of penicillanse-producing strains of *N gonorrhoeae* (PPNG) is increasing and is spreading from coastal areas to the center of the U.S. They are unresponsive to previously recommended conventional therapy such as penicillin, ampicillin, or amoxicillin. Currently recommended cephalosporins and quinolones and regimens with β-lactamase inhibitors are effective therapy against PPNG strains.

B. ACUTE SALPINGITIS

(See section on acute salpingitis-peritonitis.)

C. DISSEMINATED INFECTIONS

Disseminated gonococcal infection should be treated in the hospital initially. Evidence for endocarditis or meningitis should be sought. Recommended regimens include ceftriaxone, 1 g intramuscularly or intravenously every 24 hours, or cefotaxime or ceftizoxime, 1 g intravenously every 8 hours. For patients with β-lactamase allergy, spectinomycin, 2 g intramuscularly every 12 hours can be used. Testing for chlamydia should be performed or therapy given. Therapy should be given for a total of 1 week; oral medications include cefixime, 0.4 g every 12 hours, ciprofloxacin, 0.5 g every 12 hours, ofloxacin .4 g every 12 hours, or levofloxacin .5 g once daily if not pregnant or lactating.

D. NEONATES AND CHILDREN

Infants born to women with untreated gonorrhea should be treated with ceftriaxone, 25–50 mg/kg intravenously or intramuscularly, not to exceed 125 mg. It should be given cautiously to premature or hyperbilirubinemic infants.

Prognosis

The prognosis for patients with gonorrhea with prompt treatment is excellent. Infertility may result from even a single episode. Fewer cases have reported to the CDC in the recent years than previously.

2. Chlamydial Infections

ESSENTIALS OF DIAGNOSIS

- *Mucopurulent cervicitis.*
- *Salpingitis.*
- *Urethral syndrome.*
- *Nongonococcal urethritis in males.*
- *Neonatal infections.*
- *Lymphogranuloma venereum.*

General Considerations

The spectrum of genital infections caused by serotypes of *Chlamydia trachomatis* has only recently become appreciated. Over 4 million cases of chlamydial infection occur yearly. In 1994 the complications of untreated chlamydial infections cost approximately $2 billion in the United States. Genital infection with this organism is the most common sexually transmitted bacterial disease in women. Chlamydiae are obligate intracellular microorganisms that have a cell wall similar to that of gram-negative bacteria. They are classified as bacteria and contain both DNA and RNA; they divide by binary fission, but like viruses, they grow intracellularly. They can be grown only by tissue culture. With the exception of the L serotypes, chlamydiae attach only to columnar epithelial cells without deep tissue invasion. As a result of this characteristic, clinical infection may not be apparent. For example, infections of the eye, respiratory tract, or genital tract are accompanied by discharge, swelling, erythema, and pain localized to these areas only. *C trachomatis* infections are associated with many adverse sequelae due to chronic inflammatory changes as well as fibrosis (eg, tubal infertility and ectopic pregnancy). The proposed mechanism for the pathogenesis of chlamydial disease is an immune-mediated response. This has been supported by the observations of *C trachomatis* vaccine studies in humans and monkeys as well as other animal model studies. There is evidence that a 57-kDa chlamydial protein, which is a member of 60-kDa heat-shock proteins, plays a role in the immunopathogenesis of chlamydial disease.

Certain factors may be predictive of women with a greater likelihood of acquiring *C trachomatis*. Sexually active women younger than 20 years of age have chlamydial infection rates 2–3 times higher than those of older women. The number of sexual partners, and in some studies lower socioeconomic status, are associated with higher chlamydial infection rates. Persons who use barrier contraception are less frequently infected by *C trachomatis* than those who use no contraception, and women who use oral contraceptives may have a higher incidence of cervical infection than women not using oral contraceptives. Cervical infection in pregnant women varies from 2–24%, and is most prevalent in young, unmarried women of lower socioeconomic status in inner-city environments. The CDC recommends screening sexually active adolescent girls at their routine yearly gynecologic examination, as well as women aged 20–24 years, especially those who have new or multiple partners, and those who inconsistently use barrier contraceptives.

Clinical Findings

A. SYMPTOMS AND SIGNS

It is not uncommon for women with chlamydial infection to be asymptomatic. Women with cervical infection generally have a mucopurulent discharge with hypertrophic cervical inflammation. Salpingitis may be unassociated with symptoms.

B. LABORATORY FINDINGS

The diagnosis of chlamydial infection is based solely on laboratory tests. Diagnosis of *C trachomatis* using cell culture isolation has a sensitivity of 70–90%; however, this specialized modality is not yet widely available. Cell culture is the detection method of greatest specificity (almost 100%), but the cost can be prohibitive, and a 3- to 7-day delay in diagnosis is required. Despite its disadvantages, cell culture is presently the standard for quality assurance of nonculture chlamydia tests. The CDC recommends cell culture for specimens from the urethra, rectum, and vagina of prepubertal girls, and the nasopharynx of infants. In infants with inclusion conjunctivitis, Giemsa stain of purulent discharge from the eye is used to identify chlamydial inclusions, but similarly stained slides of exudates in adults with genital infections are only about 40% accurate in the diagnosis of these infections. Serologic methods, either the complement fixation or microimmunofluorescence test, are not totally accurate, because 20–40% of sexually active women have positive antibody titers. In fact, most women with microimmunofluorescent antibody do not have a current infection.

Moss and colleagues examined antibody responses to chlamydia species in patients who attended a genitourinary clinic and found that up to 50% of all chlamydia-IgG-positive cases were due to nongenital chlamydiae (*C pneumoniae* and *C psittaci*). The low specificity of the chlamydia serology tests is attributed to these antibodies as well as to the presence of group-specific antibodies. It is therefore of utmost importance to use serologic tests capable of distinguishing antibodies to *C trachomatis* from antibodies to *C pneumoniae* and *C psittaci* (nongenital chlamydial pathogens). Direct-smear fluorescent antibody testing requires a fluorescence microscope, and processing time is only 30–40 minutes. Sensitivity is 90% or higher, with a specificity of 98% or higher if an experienced microscopist and a satisfactory specimen are available. This appears to be the most promising test, and when tissue samples (endometrial or uterine tube) are being evaluated, it has been reported to be more accurate. Polymerase chain reaction (PCR), ligase chain reaction, and current DNA probes used in the detection of *C trachomatis* may be more rapid and less expensive. Nucleic acid hybridization methods (DNA probe) require only 2–3 hours for processing time. The DNA probe assay is specific for *C trachomatis;* cross-reactivity with *C pneumoniae* and *C psittaci* has not been reported. To ensure high specificity, a competitive probe assay has been produced and is currently undergoing evaluation in clinical trials. Recent reports indicate PCR positivity with negative culture. PCR may be the most sensitive and specific test method for chlamydia.

Differential Diagnosis

Mucopurulent cervicitis is frequently caused by *N gonorrhoeae,* and selective cultures for this organism should be performed. As discussed above, *C trachomatis* alone may be associated with as many as 20–35% of cases of acute salpingitis in the U.S. In both cervicitis and salpingitis, cultures may frequently be positive for both organisms.

Complications

Adverse sequelae of salpingitis, specifically infertility due to tubal obstruction and ectopic pregnancy, are the most dire complications of these infections. Pregnant women with cervical chlamydial infection can transmit infections to their newborns; there is evidence that up to 50% of infants born to such mothers will have inclusion conjunctivitis. In perhaps 10%, an indolent chlamydial pneumonitis develops at 2–3 months of age. This pathogen may also cause otitis media in the neonate. Whether or not maternal cervical infection with *Chlamydia* causes significantly increased fetal and perinatal wastage by abortion, premature delivery, or stillbirth remains uncertain.

Increasing evidence exists that chlamydial infection in pregnancy is a risk marker for premature delivery and postpartum infections. Women at greatest risk are those with recent chlamydial infection detected by antichlamydial IgM. Those with chronic or recurrent infection do not have increased risks of preterm delivery. It is hypothesized that asymptomatic cervicitis predisposes to mild amnionitis. This event activates phospholipase A_2 to release prostaglandins, which cause uterine contractions that may lead to premature labor. Chlamydial infection is associated with higher rates of early postpartum endometritis as well as a delayed infection from *Chlamydia* that often presents several weeks postpartum.

Treatment

In most cases, *Chlamydia* can be eradicated from the cervix by doxycycline, 100 mg orally twice daily for 7 days (for nonpregnant patients), or azithromycin, 1 g orally as a single dose. Compliance with treatment may play a major role in controlling chlamydial infections. One set of researchers evaluated the compliance with antichlamydial and antigonorrheal therapy and found that 63% of patients being treated with the standard 7-day regimen of tetracycline or erythromycin were compliant. Erythromycin base, 500 mg, or erythromycin ethylsuccinate, 800 mg, orally 4 times a day should be given for a minimum of 7 days as an alternate regimen. Patients who cannot tolerate erythromycin should consider ofloxacin, 300 mg twice daily or levofloxacin 500 mg orally once daily for 7 days. Giving high doses of ampicillin has resulted in the elimination of *C trachomatis* from the cervices of women with acute salpingitis. Addition of the irreversible β-lactamase enzyme inhibitor sulbactam increases in vitro antichlamydial activity.

Pregnant women are advised to take erythromycin base, 500 mg, 4 times per day for 7 days, or amoxicillin, 500 mg, 3 times a day for 7 days. Alternate regimens incude erythromycin base 250 mg orally 4 times daily for 14 days, erythromycin ethylsuccinate 800 mg orally 4 times daily for 7 days, erythromycin ethylsuccinate 400 mg orally 4 times daily for 14 days, or Azithromycin 1 g orally as a single dose.

Current studies indicate that 3–5% of pregnant women and as many as 15% of sexually active nonpregnant women have an asymptomatic chlamydial cervical colonization. It is not known whether attempts to eradicate asymptomatic colonization will prevent chlamydial cervicitis, salpingitis, or neonatal infections. Posttreatment cultures are not usually advised if doxycycline, azithromycin, or ofloxacin is taken as above and symptoms are not present; cure rates should be higher than 95%. Retesting may be considered 3 weeks after completing treatment with erythromycin. A positive posttreatment culture is more likely to represent noncompliance by the patient or sexual partner or reinfection rather than antibiotic resistance. It is important to ensure that the sexual partner is treated, since most post-treatment reinfections occur because the sexual partner was not treated. Clinicians should advise all women with chlamydial infection to be re-screened 3–4 months after treatment.

PELVIC INFECTIONS

Because of their common occurrence and often serious consequences, infections are among the most important problems encountered in the practice of gynecology. A wide variety of pelvic infections, ranging from uncomplicated gonococcal salpingo-oophoritis to septicemic shock following rupture of a pelvic abscess, confront the general physician as well as the gynecologist.

The following is a general classification of pelvic infections by frequency of occurrence:

(1) Pelvic inflammatory disease
   (a) Acute salpingitis
      (i) Gonococcal
      (ii) Nongonococcal
   (b) IUD-related pelvic cellulitis
   (c) Tubo-ovarian abscess
   (d) Pelvic abscess
(2) Puerperal infections
   (a) Cesarean section (common)
   (b) Vaginal delivery (uncommon)
(3) Postoperative gynecologic surgery
   (a) Cuff cellulitis and parametritis
   (b) Vaginal cuff abscess
   (c) Tubo-ovarian abscess
(4) Abortion-associated infections
   (a) Postabortal cellulitis
   (b) Incomplete septic abortion
(5) Secondary to other infections
   (a) Appendicitis
   (b) Diverticulitis
   (c) Tuberculosis

"Pelvic inflammatory disease" (PID) is a general term for acute, subacute, recurrent, or chronic infection

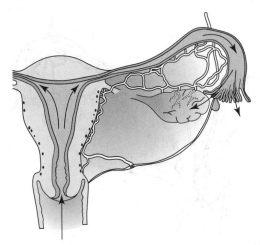

Figure 38–4. Intra-abdominal spread of gonorrhea and other pathogenic bacteria.

of the oviducts and ovaries, often with involvement of adjacent tissues. Most infections seen in clinical practice are bacterial, but viral, fungal, and parasitic infections may occur. The term PID is vague at best and should be discarded in favor of more specific terminology. This should include identification of the affected organs, the stage of the infection, and if possible, the causative agent. This specificity is especially important in light of the rising incidence of venereal disease and its complications.

The three proposed pathways of dissemination of microorganisms in pelvic infections are depicted in Figs 38–4, 38–5, and 38–6. Lymphatic dissemination (Fig 38–5), typified by postpartum, postabortal, and some IUD-related infections, results in extraperitoneal para-

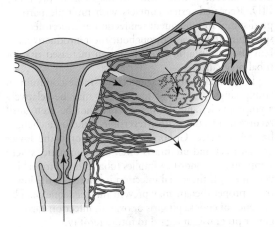

Figure 38–5. Lymphatic spread of bacterial infection.

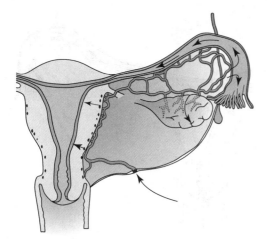

Figure 38–6. Hematogenous spread of bacterial infection (eg, tuberculosis).

metrial cellulitis. In Fig 38–4, the endometrial-endosalpingeal-peritoneal spread of microorganisms is depicted; this represents more common forms of nonpuerperal PID, in which pathogenic bacteria gain access to the lining of the uterine tubes, with resultant purulent inflammation and egress of pus through tubal ostia into the peritoneal cavity. These infections are represented by endometritis, adnexal infection, and peritonitis. In rare instances, certain diseases (eg, tuberculosis) may gain access to pelvic structures by hematogenous routes (Fig 38–6).

Early recognition and treatment of the various entities that make up PID are mandatory so that specific therapy can be instituted to prevent damage to the reproductive system. Laparoscopic studies have confirmed a 65–90% positive predictive value for tubal disease among patients with the diagnosis of presumed PID. Repeated sexual contacts with multiple partners predisposes to subsequent reinfection or superinfection, spreading the disease throughout the reproductive system and resulting in sterility and an increased risk for tubal pregnancy.

The initial gonococcal infection (more common in young single women of low parity) may be relatively asymptomatic, and the patient may not be seen until recurrent infection with irreversible pathologic changes has taken place. Gonorrhea involving only the lower genital tract and urethra is often asymptomatic; severe symptomatic gonorrhea implies tubal and peritoneal involvement. If the initial infection is limited to the lower tract, proper therapy may prevent further sequelae. The presence of endosalpingitis or ovarian infection carries a graver prognosis in regard to future fertility.

Originally, it was thought that the gonococcus was the only organism responsible for nonpuerperal acute

pelvic inflammation. More recent data indicate that *N gonorrhoeae* is isolated in only 40–60% of women with acute salpingitis. In Sweden, *C trachomatis* was estimated to cause 60% of cases of salpingitis. Although direct evidence of such infection, eg, recovery from tubal culture, is lacking in most studies done in the U.S., authorities believe that this pathogen may be responsible for 20–35% of such pelvic infections. It is unclear how frequently salpingitis is caused by chlamydiae alone or by chlamydia in association with other invasive microorganisms. Regardless of the initiating factors, nongonococcal pathogens that comprise the normal vaginal flora may become involved in many cases of acute salpingitis-peritonitis.

N gonorrhoeae was present alone or with other pathogens in 65% of the specimens. One set of researchers reported positive cul-de-sac fluid cultures in 18 (90%) of 20 patients with acute salpingitis compared with 8 normal patients with negative results.

If the infectious process continues, pelvic adhesions become more pronounced, and tissue planes are lost. It becomes difficult to identify the tubes and ovaries in the inflammatory mass, which may include omental and intestinal attachments. Further progression causes tissue necrosis with abscess formation. Containment of the purulent exudate under pressure becomes impossible at certain sites, and pus is released into the peritoneal cavity. This is usually at the site of an adhesion to a nearby organ, and the point of rupture can often be identified at operation. Abscess formation may be localized in either or both of the tubes and ovaries without leakage or rupture. Another possibility is accumulation of purulent material walled off in the cul-de-sac.

Recent observations have shown these pelvic infections to be polymicrobial with mixed anaerobic and aerobic bacteria. Anaerobes predominate and frequently coexist with aerobes. In some cases, aerobes alone are isolated. With further advanced disease, such as abscess formation, anaerobic organisms seem to predominate. All these bacteria are members of the normal vaginal and endocervical flora and include *Bacteroides, Escherichia coli,* aerobic streptococci, and anaerobic cocci (*Peptostreptococcus* and *Peptococcus*). Virtually any organism indigenous to the normal vaginal or gastrointestinal flora may be isolated if specific techniques are used. Direct immunofluorescent antibody testing of cervical smears of 500 asymptomatic women showed *C trachomatis* in 10%. Moreover, of women recently treated as outpatients for acute salpingitis, 16% had *C trachomatis* in endocervical specimens and 8% had the organism in the endometrial cavity (obtained with a double-lumen catheter-protected brush). These numbers should not be taken lightly when considering the cost of chlamydia-related PID. Also, many retrospective studies point to recurrent infections and delays in treatment as the major behavioral risk factors contributing to PID. From the same sites, *N gonorrhoeae* was identified in 68% and 65% of specimens, respectively. Great numbers of both aerobes and anaerobes were recovered from endometrial cultures; 10% had group B *Streptococcus*, 10% had *Bacteroides fragilis*, 55% had *Streptococcus faecalis*, 65% had *Staphylococcus epidermidis*, 75% had anaerobic *Streptococcus* spp., and 65% had *Prevotella bivius* in that location. Whether this is a result of infection or is flora from the lower tract and endometrium is under evaluation.

Many factors may account for adverse sequelae of these pelvic infections, eg, infertility and pain. Delay in initiation of treatment is associated with later symptomatology. Likewise, inadequate therapy due to improper antimicrobial selection, insufficient dosage, or inadequate duration of therapy may be responsible for subsequent problems. An inflammatory process that is allowed to continue—for whatever reason—results in anatomic derangements with adhesive attachments to nearby organs. An ovulation site in an ovary may serve as a portal of entry for extension of the infection into the ovarian stroma, and this sets the stage for formation of tubo-ovarian abscesses.

The most important factor in the diagnosis in women with pelvic infections is clinical awareness by the physician. For patients with high-risk factors (eg, postoperative pelvic surgery, postpartum, or postabortal) fever is usually the first clue. For women without these factors, a high index of suspicion is important. If gonorrhea is suspected, a Gram-stained smear of endocervical purulent material or fluid obtained by culdocentesis may be helpful. The Gram-stained smear may be life-saving, especially in the woman seen with a rare serious infection due to *Clostridium perfringens*. Except for isolation of *N gonorrhoeae* with specialized media, cultures taken from women with pelvic infections currently are not useful for clinical management. Since these infections are usually polymicrobial, sophisticated techniques are necessary for microbiologic identification. These are time-consuming, and by the time the results become available to the clinician, the woman has usually been cured with empiric antimicrobial drug therapy.

PELVIC INFLAMMATORY DISEASE

1. Acute Salpingitis-Peritonitis

 ESSENTIALS OF DIAGNOSIS

- Onset of lower abdominal and pelvic pain, usually following onset or cessation of menses and associated with vaginal discharge, abdominal,

uterine, adnexal, and cervical motion tenderness, plus one or more of the following:

 (a) Temperature above 38.3 °C (101 °F).

 (b) Leukocyte count greater than 10,000/μL or elevated C-reactive protein.

 (c) Inflammatory mass (examination or sonography).

 (d) Gram-negative intracellular diplococci in cervical secretions.

 (e) Purulent material (WBC) from peritoneal cavity (culdocentesis or laparoscopy).

 (f) Elevated erythrocyte sedimentation rate.

General Considerations

There is generally an acute onset of pelvic infection, often associated with invasion by *N gonorrhoeae* and involving the uterus, tubes, and ovaries, with varying degrees of pelvic peritonitis. In the acute stage, there is redness and edema of the tubes and ovaries with a purulent discharge oozing from the ostium of the tube.

Clinical Findings/Diagnosis

A. SYMPTOMS AND SIGNS

The insidious or acute onset of lower abdominal and pelvic pain usually is bilateral and only occasionally unilateral. There may be a sensation of pelvic pressure, with back pain radiating down one or both legs. In most cases, symptoms appear shortly after the onset or cessation of menses. There is often an associated purulent vaginal discharge.

Nausea may occur, with or without vomiting, but these symptoms may be indicative of a more serious problem (eg, acute appendicitis). Headache and general lassitude are common complaints.

Fever is not necessary for the diagnosis of acute salpingitis, although its absence may indicate other disorders, specifically ectopic pregnancy. In one study, only 30% of women with laparoscopically confirmed acute salpingitis had fever. Although standardization of criteria for diagnosis of acute salpingitis to include fever greater than 38.3 °C (101 °F) may greatly aid clinical research, such a distinction may result in many women with acute pelvic infection being erroneously diagnosed and inadequately treated.

Abdominal tenderness is often encountered, usually in both lower quadrants. The abdomen may be somewhat distended, and bowel sounds may be hypoactive or absent. Pelvic examination may demonstrate inflammation of the periurethral (Skene) or Bartholin glands as well as a purulent cervical discharge. Bimanual examination typically elicits extreme tenderness on movement of the cervix and uterus and palpation of the parametria.

B. LABORATORY FINDINGS

Leukocytosis with a shift to the left is usually present; however, the white count may be normal. A smear of purulent cervical material may demonstrate gram-negative kidney-shaped diplococci in polymorphonuclear leukocytes. These organisms may be gonococci, but definitive cultures on selective media are advised. Penicillinase production should also be confirmed.

Culdocentesis generally is productive of "reaction fluid" (cloudy peritoneal fluid) which, when stained, reveals leukocytes with or without gonococci or other organisms. Culture and sensitivity testing of organisms from culdocentesis samples may be done.

C. RADIOLOGIC FINDINGS

X-ray examination of the abdomen may show signs of ileus, but this finding is nonspecific. Air may be seen under the diaphragm with a ruptured tubo-ovarian or pelvic abscess and demands immediate laparotomy in addition to combination antimicrobial therapy.

D. ULTRASOUND

Due to the introduction of transvaginal sonography, the female reproductive tract can now be visualized at bedside. Markers for acute and chronic PID can be differentiated. Incomplete septation of the tubal wall ("cogwheel sign") is a marker for acute disease, and a thin wall ("beaded string") indicates chronic disease. Thickening is noted in the pelvic areas during the inflammatory process. When ultrasound diagnosis is compared with laparoscopic diagnosis, it is about 90% accurate. Ultrasonography is most valuable in following the progression or regression of an abscess after it has been diagnosed. The borders of an abscess conform to the surrounding pelvic structures and as such do not give a well-defined border as noted in an ovarian cyst.

E. CULDOCENTESIS

Culdocentesis (cul-de-sac tap) may be helpful in the diagnosis of suspected pelvic infection. Other conditions that may simulate infection can be ruled out by means of this simple procedure. The rectouterine pouch (of Douglas) is punctured with a long spinal needle to obtain a sample of the contents of the peritoneal cavity after vaginal membrane prep with povidone-iodine or similar agents. Culdocentesis is easy to perform and may be done with or without local anesthesia in the hospital or in the office. One milliliter of sterile saline anesthetizes the vaginal membrane and peritoneum. Culdocentesis is indicated whenever peritoneal material is needed for diagnosis. Cultures for aerobic and anaer-

Table 38–2. Differential evaluation of fluid contained by culdocentesis.

Finding	Implications for Diagnosis
Blood	Ruptured ectopic pregnancy. Hemorrhage from corpus luteum cyst. Retrograde menstruation. Rupture of spleen or liver. Gastrointestinal bleeding. Acute salpingitis.
Pus	Ruptured tubo-ovarian abscess. Ruptured appendix or viscus. Rupture of diverticular abscess. Uterine abscess with myoma.
Cloudy	Pelvic peritonitis (such as is seen with acute gonococcal salpingitis). Twisted adnexal cyst. Other causes of peritonitis: appendicitis, pancreatitis, cholecystitis, perforated ulcer, carcinomatosis, echinococcosis.

obic organisms may also be obtained. Contraindications include a cul-de-sac mass or a fixed retroflexed uterus. For differential evaluation of fluid obtained by culdocentesis, see Table 38–2.

Differential Diagnosis

Acute salpingitis must be differentiated from acute appendicitis, ectopic pregnancy, ruptured corpus luteum cyst with hemorrhage, diverticulitis, infected septic abortion, torsion of an adnexal mass, degeneration of a leiomyoma, endometriosis, acute urinary tract infection, regional enteritis, and ulcerative colitis.

Complications

Complications of acute salpingitis include pelvic peritonitis or generalized peritonitis, prolonged adynamic ileus, severe pelvic cellulitis with thrombophlebitis, abscess formation (pyosalpinx, tubo-ovarian abscess, cul-de-sac abscess) with adnexal destruction and subsequent infertility, and intestinal adhesions and obstruction. Rarely, dermatitis, gonococcal arthritis, or bacteremia with septic shock may occur.

Prevention

Approximately 15% of women with asymptomatic gonococcal cervical infection develop acute salpingitis. Detection and treatment of these women and their sexual partners should therefore prevent a substantial number of cases of gonococcal pelvic infection. Early diagnosis and eradication of minimally symptomatic disease (cervicitis, urethritis) also usually prevent salpingitis.

Treatment

As with most female pelvic infections, the microbial etiologic agents are not readily apparent when clinical infection is diagnosed, and because of the myriad of pathogens described above, empiric therapy is given as soon as a presumptive diagnosis is made. It is also important to note that negative cultures do not preclude upper reproductive tract disease. The majority of women who present with acute salpingitis-peritonitis have clinical disease of mild to moderate severity that usually responds well to outpatient antibiotic therapy. Hospitalization usually is warranted for women who are more severely ill as well as for women in whom the exact diagnosis is uncertain. Prepubertal children and pregnant women with this diagnosis should be hospitalized for therapy, as should women with a suspected abscess, women unable to tolerate outpatient oral therapy, and women who have not responded to outpatient therapy. Although it has not been clinically proved that inpatient therapy is associated with improved future fertility, those women who desire future fertility may benefit from inpatient therapy if only by reason of compliance. Some authors believe that all women with this infection should receive inpatient therapy.

A. OUTPATIENT THERAPY

Outpatient therapy for women with acute salpingitis may be undertaken if the temperature is less than 39 °C (102.2 °F), lower abdominal findings are minimal, and the patient is not "toxic" and can take oral medication. These women may be treated with antibiotics, IUD removal, analgesics, and bedrest. Regimens recommended by the CDC include (1) ofloxacin 400 mg, orally twice daily or levofloxacin 500 mg orally once daily for 14 days, plus clindamycin 450 mg, orally 4 times daily, or metronidazole 500 mg, orally twice daily for 14 days; (2) ceftriaxone 250 mg, intramuscularly, or equivalent cephalosporin (eg, ceftizoxime or cefotaxime) intramuscularly, with probenecid 1 g orally, followed by 14 days of doxycycline 100 mg, orally twice daily, with or without metronidazole 500 mg twice daily; or (3) cefoxitin 2 g, intramuscularly, plus probenecid 1 g, orally followed by 14 days of doxycycline 100 mg, orally twice daily, with or without metronidazole 500 mg twice daily. If after 72 hours a response to therapy has not been seen, the patient should be admitted for inpatient therapy. Refer the patient to the city or county health department or STD clinic for contact surveillance. All male sexual partners of women treated for this acute infection should be examined for sexually transmitted diseases and promptly treated with a regimen effective against uncomplicated gonococcal and chlamydial infections.

B. INPATIENT THERAPY

Inpatient therapy is prudent for patients with a temperature over 39 °C (102.2 °F), for those with guarding and rebound tenderness in lower quadrants, or for patients who look "toxic." Hospitalization of these patients is necessary for therapy and for watching for signs of complications or deterioration. Patients who fail outpatient therapy should be evaluated for a suspected tubo-ovarian abscess. The following measures should be taken:

(1) Maintain bedrest.

(2) Restrict oral feeding.

(3) Administer intravenous fluids to correct dehydration and acidosis.

(4) Use nasogastric suction in the presence of abdominal distention or ileus.

(5) No standardization of inpatient antimicrobial therapy for women with acute salpingitis has yet been established. Symptomatic response and adverse sequelae are related to the severity of tubal inflammatory disease and the development of adnexal abscesses. The CDC recommends one of the following regimens: (1) doxycycline, 100 mg intravenously or orally twice daily, plus cefoxitin, 2 g intravenously 4 times daily, or cefotetan, 2 g intravenously twice daily, for at least 24 hours after the patient shows clinical improvement, followed by doxycycline, 100 mg orally twice a day to complete 14 days of therapy; (2) clindamycin, 900 mg intravenously 3 times daily, plus gentamicin, 2 mg/kg intravenously and then 1.5 mg/kg intravenously every 8 hours (single daily dosing of gentamicin may be substituted), given as above in women with normal renal function, followed by doxycycline, 100 mg twice daily or clindamycin, 450 mg orally 4 times daily for 14 days. The incidence of infertility after the first episode of salpingitis is about 12%. Because infertility increases with the degree of inflammatory response, intensive broad-spectrum therapy should reduce complications. If there is an elevated suspicion for tubo-ovarian abscess, a regimen employing metronidazole or clindamycin should be utilized both inpatient, and for continued outpatient therapy for increased anaerobic coverage.

(6) Exploratory laparotomy should be performed if there is clinical suspicion of abscess rupture. More gynecologists are successfully performing just a linear salpingostomy, as might be done for ectopic pregnancy, when pyosalpinx is identified. Percutaneous drainage may avoid operation.

(7) Continual evaluation by the same experienced clinician is of paramount importance to maintain accuracy and continuity of clinical observation.

Prognosis

A favorable outcome is directly related to the promptness with which adequate therapy is begun. For example, the incidence of infertility is directly related to the severity of tubal inflammation judged by laparoscopic examination. A single episode of salpingitis has been shown to cause infertility in 12–18% of women. Tubal occlusion was demonstrated in only about 10% of these patients regardless of whether or not there had been a gonococcal or nongonococcal infection. Nongonococcal infection predisposed more commonly to ectopic pregnancy, and thus carried a worse prognosis for subsequent viable pregnancy. The ability and willingness of the patient to cooperate with her physician are important to the outcome of patients with the milder cases who are adequately treated on an outpatient basis. Follow-up care and education are necessary to prevent reinfection and complications.

2. Recurrent or Chronic Pelvic Infection

 ESSENTIALS OF DIAGNOSIS

- *History of acute salpingitis, pelvic infection, or postpartum or postabortal infection.*
- *Recurrent episodes of acute reinfection or recurrence of symptoms and physical findings less than 6 weeks after treatment for acute salpingitis.*
- *Chronic infection may be relatively asymptomatic or may provoke complaints of chronic pelvic pain and dyspareunia.*
- *Generalized pelvic tenderness on examination; usually less severe than with acute infection.*
- *Thickening of adnexal tissues, with or without hydrosalpinx (often).*
- *Infertility (commonly).*

General Considerations

Recurrent pelvic inflammatory disease begins as does primary disease, but preexisting tubal tissue damage may result in more severe infection. Chronic pelvic infection implies the presence of tissue changes in the parametria, tubes, and ovaries. Adhesions of the peritoneal surfaces to the adnexa as well as fibrotic changes in the tubal lumen are usually present. Hydrosalpinx or tubo-ovarian "complexes" may be present. Chronic inflammatory lesions usually are secondary to changes induced by previous acute salpingitis but may represent an acute reinfection.

The diagnosis of chronic pelvic infection generally is difficult to make clinically. It has been erroneously applied to almost any cause of chronic pelvic pain. However, it may be the cause of pain in less than 50% of such women.

Clinical Findings

A. Symptoms and Signs

Recurrent infection usually has the same manifestations as acute salpingitis (see previous text), and a history of pelvic infection can usually be obtained. Pain may be unilateral or bilateral, and dyspareunia and infertility are often reported. The patient may be febrile, with tachycardia; however, unless an acute reinfection is present, the fever is minimal. There is tenderness upon movement of the cervix, uterus, or adnexa. Adnexal masses may be present, as well as thickening of the parametria.

B. Laboratory Findings

Cultures from the cervix usually do not show gonococci unless reinfection is present. Leukocytosis may be demonstrated if active infection is superimposed on chronic changes.

Differential Diagnosis

Any patient with suspected chronic pelvic infection who presents with pelvic tenderness but without fever must be suspected of having an ectopic pregnancy. Other conditions to be considered include endometriosis, symptomatic uterine relaxation, appendicitis, diverticulitis, regional enteritis, ulcerative colitis, ovarian cyst or neoplasm, and acute or chronic cystourethritis.

Complications

The complications of chronic or recurrent pelvic infection include hydrosalpinx, pyosalpinx, and tubo-ovarian abscess; infertility or ectopic pregnancy; and chronic pelvic pain of varying degrees.

Prevention

Prompt and adequate treatment of acute pelvic infections is the essential preventive measure. Education about avoidance of sexually transmitted diseases is also important.

Treatment

A. Recurrent Cases

Treat for acute salpingitis (see previous text). If an IUD is in place, treatment may be started, and the IUD should be removed.

B. Chronic Cases

Long-term antimicrobial administration is of questionable benefit but is worthy of trial in young women of low parity. Therapy with a tetracycline, ampicillin, or a cephalosporin may occasionally be beneficial, but changes responsible for symptoms are usually not due to active infection. Symptomatic relief can be achieved by use of analgesics such as ibuprofen or acetaminophen with or without codeine. Careful follow-up, preferably by the same physician, may detect serious sequelae, eg, tubo-ovarian abscess.

If the patient remains symptomatic after 3 weeks of antibiotic therapy, other causes must be considered. Consider laparoscopy or exploratory laparotomy to rule out other causes, eg, endometriosis.

If infertility is a problem, verify tubal patency by means of hysterosalpingography or laparoscopy and retrograde injection of methylene blue solution. It is important to prescribe antibiotics prior to and following either procedure because acute retrograde reinfection is common.

Total abdominal hysterectomy with bilateral adnexectomy may be indicated if the disease is far advanced and the woman is symptomatic or if an adnexal mass is demonstrated. Consideration may be given to resection or drainage of the abscess if preservation of fertility is desired. In many instances, CT- or ultrasound-directed percutaneous drainage may avoid laparotomy.

Prognosis

With each succeeding episode of recurrent pelvic infection, the prognosis for fertility dramatically decreases. Likewise, the chances of an ectopic gestation increase with ensuing episodes of acute infection. These sequelae are undoubtedly due to chronic infection, which is the postinflammatory end result of one or multiple infections. Superimposition of acute infection on chronic disease is also associated with a higher incidence of tubo-ovarian and other pelvic abscesses.

3. Pelvic (Cul-De-Sac) Abscess

Pelvic abscess is an uncommon complication of chronic or recurrent pelvic inflammation. It may occur as a sequela to acute pelvic or postabortal infection. Abscess formation is frequently associated with organisms other than the gonococcus, commonly anaerobic species, especially *Bacteroides*. Occasionally, resistant gram-negative bacteria can be found such as *B bivias* and *B fragilis*.

Any of the symptoms of acute or chronic pelvic inflammation may be present together with a fluctuant mass filling the cul-de-sac and dissecting into the rectovaginal septum. These patients usually have more severe symptoms. They may complain of painful defecation and severe back pain, rectal pain, or both. The severity of symptoms is often directly proportionate to the size of the abscess, but occasionally even a large pelvic abscess may be totally asymptomatic. One woman who was admitted to the obstetric service with "fetal heart tones" was ultimately drained of 3000 mL of pus through a colpotomy incision.

Differential Diagnosis

The following conditions must be considered: tubo-ovarian abscess, periappendiceal abscess, ectopic pregnancy, adnexal torsion, ovarian neoplasm, uterine leiomyoma (especially those undergoing torsion or degeneration), retroflexed and incarcerated uterus, endometriosis, carcinomatosis, and diverticulitis with perforation.

Treatment

In addition to the measures outlined in the previous section, the following are required:

(1) Antibiotics to include anaerobic as well as aerobic microorganisms: (a) penicillin G, 20–30 million units or ampicillin, 2 g intravenously 4 times per day; clindamycin, 900 mg intravenously 3 times daily; and gentamicin, 5 mg/kg intravenously per 24 hours. Metronidazole may be substituted for clindamycin at a dose of 15 mg/kg loading dose, then 7.5 mg/kg 4 times daily; (b) cefoxitin, 8–12 g intravenously per 24 hours (2 g every 4–6 hours), and gentamicin or tobramycin, 5 mg/kg intravenously per 24 hours; (c) cefotaxime, 6–8 g intravenously per 24 hours in divided doses. With almost any effective therapeutic regimen, antibiotic-associated enterocolitis (diarrhea) is a complication that demands immediate evaluation, including testing for the presence of *Clostridium difficile* toxin. Pseudomembranous colitis is rare.

(2) Reevaluate abdominal findings frequently to detect peritoneal involvement.

(3) If the abscess is dissecting the rectovaginal septum and is fixed to the vaginal membrane, colpotomy drainage with dissection of sacculations is indicated. This space should be actively drained with a large catheter, such as a Cook catheter, and preferably irrigated with sterile saline solution every 4 hours until the space is obliterated.

(4) If fever persists in the face of altered antimicrobial therapy but there is no evidence of abscess rupture or dissection of the rectovaginal septum, percutaneous drainage and irrigation may obviate laparotomy (Figs 38–7, 38–8, and 38–9).

(5) If the patient's condition deteriorates despite aggressive management, perform exploratory laparotomy. In patients with recurrent infections and loss of repro-

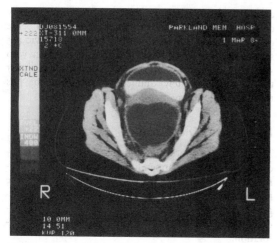

Figure 38–7. Pelvic CT scan, with bladder and contrast medium on top, uterus and thickened broad ligaments centrally, and the posterior pelvis filled with abscess.

ductive function, total abdominal hysterectomy with bilateral salpingo-oophorectomy and lysis of adhesions offers the only cure. The patient's age and parity and the degree of involvement of the tubes and ovaries determine the extent of surgery when there is some likelihood of preservation of reproductive function. Clinical judgment is difficult and tends to favor surgery. Conservative surgery for women desiring future fertility is appropriate in many cases.

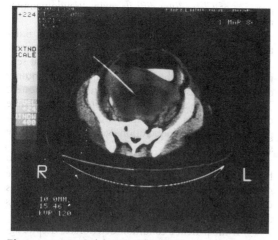

Figure 38–8. Pelvic CT scan with percutaneous drainage in process.

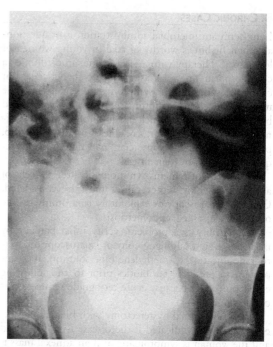

Figure 38–9. Cook catheter is in abscess cavity. Note the mild bilateral hydroureter caused by abscess compression at the pelvic brim.

Prognosis

With early treatment, the prognosis for the woman with a well-localized abscess is good. Antibiotic treatment is essential; drainage may be necessary. Rupture into the peritoneum is a serious complication and demands immediate abdominal exploration. The prognosis for fertility is very poor following this type of abscess.

4. Tubo-Ovarian Abscess

 ESSENTIALS OF DIAGNOSIS

- *History of pelvic infection. Tubo-ovarian abscess may present as a complication of acute salpingitis, including the initial episode.*
- *Lower abdominal and pelvic pain of varying degrees.*
- *Nausea and vomiting.*
- *Adnexal mass, usually extremely tender.*
- *Fever, tachycardia.*
- *Rebound tenderness in lower quadrants.*

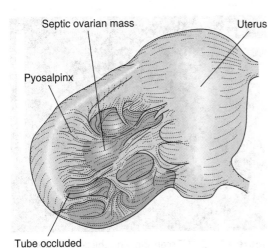

Figure 38–10. Tubo-ovarian abscess. (Reproduced, with permission, from Benson RC: *Handbook of Obstetrics & Gynecology*, 8th ed. Lange, 1983.)

- *Adynamic ileus.*
- *Culdocentesis productive of gross pus in case of rupture. (Contraindicated in cases of posterior pelvic abscess.)*

General Considerations

Tubo-ovarian abscess (TOA) formation may occur following an initial episode of acute salpingitis, but is usually seen with recurrent infection superimposed on chronically damaged adnexal tissue. It is strongly believed that fallopian tube necrosis and epithelial damage by bacterial pathogens create the environment necessary for anaerobic invasion and growth. Initially there is salpingitis with or without ovarian involvement. The inflammatory process may subside spontaneously or in response to therapy; however, the result may be anatomic derangement, with fibrinous attachments to nearby organs (Figs 38–10 and 38–11). Involvement of the adjacent ovary, usually at an ovulation site, may serve as the portal of entry for extension of infection and abscess formation. Pressure of the purulent exudate may cause rupture of the abscess with resultant fulminating peritonitis, necessitating emergency laparotomy.

Slow leakage of the abscess may cause formation of a cul-de-sac abscess (see previous text). Culdocentesis into an abscess of this type will yield exudate like that of a ruptured tubo-ovarian abscess. Clinical appraisal usually will differentiate the two conditions, but if any doubt exists, treatment should be as specified for ruptured tubo-ovarian abscess.

These abscesses may occur in association with use of an IUD or in the presence of granulomatous infection (eg, tuberculosis, actinomycosis). Disease can be bilateral, although unilateral disease is more common than previously observed and may account for up to 60% of such abscesses even in the absence of IUD usage. Abscesses are usually polymicrobial.

Actinomyces israelii, a normal anaerobic commensal of the gastrointestinal tract, has been identified in 8–20% of women who have an IUD. Most patients are asymptomatic, but up to 25% are reported to develop symptoms of pelvic infection. Controversy exists as to whether an IUD should be removed from an asymptomatic woman with evidence of *Actinomyces* on Papanicolaou smear or culture. If the IUD is removed, a new IUD should not be inserted until the organism is no longer present; this rarely takes longer than one menstrual cycle. Antimicrobial therapy with penicillin should be reserved for symptomatic patients. Surgical drainage is usually required for actinomycotic abscesses, which are almost always the result of intestinal infections such as appendicitis but may be associated with use of an IUD.

Clinical Findings

A. SYMPTOMS AND SIGNS

The clinical spectrum varies greatly and may range from total absence of symptoms in a woman who, on routine pelvic examination, is found to have an adnexal mass to a moribund patient presenting with acute abdomen and septicemic shock.

The typical patient with TOA is usually young and of low parity, with a history of previous pelvic infection. However, no age group is exempt. The duration of symptoms for these women is usually about 1 week, and the onset is usually about 2 weeks or more after a

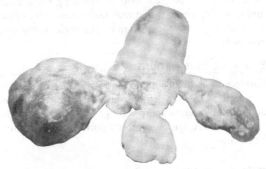

Figure 38–11. Uterus with myoma, unruptured right tubo-ovarian abscess, and chronic inflammatory left tubo-ovarian cyst.

menstrual period, in contrast to that which occurs in uncomplicated acute salpingitis, in which symptoms usually appear shortly after the onset or cessation of menses. The typical symptoms are pelvic and abdominal pain, fever, nausea and vomiting, and tachycardia. Four-quadrant abdominal tenderness and guarding may be present. Adequate pelvic examination is often impossible because of tenderness, but an adnexal mass may be palpated. Culdocentesis may lacerate (rupture) a pelvic abscess, so this procedure must be performed with extreme caution, if at all.

Signs and symptoms of ruptured TOA may resemble those of any acute surgical abdomen, and a careful history and an alert clinician are essential to ensure an accurate diagnosis. Signs of actual or impending septic shock frequently accompany a ruptured abscess and include fever (occasionally hypothermia), chills, tachycardia, disorientation, hypotension, tachypnea, and oliguria.

B. LABORATORY FINDINGS

Laboratory findings are generally of little value. The white count may vary from leukopenia to marked leukocytosis. Urinalysis may demonstrate pyuria without bacteriuria. Mean erythrocyte sedimentation rate (ESR) of at least 64 mm/h and mean acute C-reactive protein (CRP) of at least 20 mg/L may be used to assist in the diagnosis of TOA. Monitoring these levels has proven useful in following disease course.

C. X-RAY FINDINGS

Plain films of the abdomen (KUB) usually demonstrate findings of a dynamic ileus and may arouse suspicion of adnexal mass. Free air may be seen under the diaphragm with ruptured TOA.

D. ULTRASONOGRAPHY

Ultrasonography is the radiologic modality of choice and can be used with fewer complications to the patient. It can be of great help in following the patient and detecting changes that may take place such as progression, regression, formation of pus pockets, rupture, and so on.

E. SPECIAL EXAMINATIONS

Culdocentesis fluid obtained in a woman with an unruptured TOA may demonstrate the same cloudy "reaction fluid" seen in acute salpingitis. With a leaking or ruptured TOA, however, grossly purulent material may be obtained.

Differential Diagnosis

An unruptured TOA must be differentiated from an ovarian cyst or tumor with or without torsion, unrup-

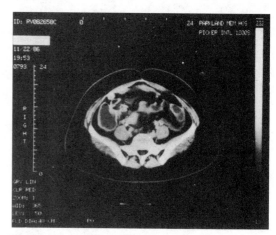

Figure 38–12. CT scan showing thickened appendix with intraluminal purulence. The source of this woman's pelvic abscess was a ruptured appendix.

tured ectopic pregnancy, periappendiceal abscess, uterine leiomyoma, hydrosalpinx, perforation of the appendix, perforation of a diverticulum or diverticular abscess, perforation of peptic ulcer, and any systemic disease that causes acute abdominal distress (eg, diabetic ketoacidosis, porphyria). If an abscess does not respond to medical therapy and colpotomy is not possible, CT or MRI scanning may disclose the cause (Fig 38–12).

Complications

Unruptured TOA may be complicated by rupture with sepsis, reinfection at a later date, bowel obstruction, infertility, and ectopic pregnancy.

Ruptured TOA is a surgical emergency and is frequently complicated by septic shock, intra-abdominal abscess (eg, subphrenic abscess), and septic emboli with renal, lung, or brain abscess.

Treatment

A. UNRUPTURED ASYMPTOMATIC TUBO-OVARIAN ABSCESS

Treatment is similar to that of chronic salpingitis: long-term antibacterial therapy and close follow-up. If the mass does not begin to subside within 15–21 days or becomes larger, drainage is indicated. At exploration, total hysterectomy and bilateral adnexectomy are usually performed; however, in selected cases, unilateral salpingo-oophorectomy or linear salpingostomy with copious irrigation and suction drainage may be considered (see recurrent or chronic pelvic infection, above).

B. Unruptured Symptomatic Tubo-Ovarian Abscess

Treatment consists of immediate hospitalization, bedrest in the semi-Fowler position, close monitoring of vital signs and urinary output, frequent gentle abdominal examination, nasogastric suction if necessary, and intravenous sodium-containing fluids. Intensive antimicrobial therapy should be instituted and should include either clindamycin or metronidazole because of their specific activity against anaerobes. The following combinations, given in appropriate intravenous doses, are recommended for these severely ill patients: (1) penicillin G or ampicillin, and gentamicin plus metronidazole or clindamycin. One set of researchers suggest a regimen of 48–72 hours of triple antibiotics. If the patient demonstrates clinical rupture (peritonitis), an increase in the size of the abscess, or persistent fever, she should be taken to the operating room.

Laparoscopy or laparotomy is mandatory in all cases of suspected leakage or rupture as well as in all cases that do not respond to medical management and percutaneous drainage.

If initial therapy is successful, the patient is kept on antibiotics (eg, oral tetracycline, 500 mg 4 times daily, or doxycycline, 100 mg twice daily) for a minimum of 10–14 days and must have frequent follow-up examinations. If the abscess persists—and many do—laparotomy may be necessary. The reported incidence of surgery for clinically diagnosed, unruptured TOA varies from 30–100%. On one service, approximately 57% of cases undergo surgery, and the remaining 43% seemingly respond to aggressive medical management. A recent prospective study found that aggressive antimicrobial treatment with cefotaxime was successful in 95% of 40 women with abscesses ranging in size from 4×4 to 13×15 cm. Only 12% of these patients underwent hysterectomy and bilateral adnexectomy 1–33 months following initial therapy because of a persistent adnexal mass. These patients did not wish to retain reproductive function. Of the remainder, 7 conceived and delivered 26 months (mean) following study entry; 6 of the 7 had bilateral abscesses at sonography. These data support the theory that conservative therapy can be successful.

C. Ruptured Tubo-Ovarian Abscess

This is an acute life-threatening catastrophe requiring immediate medical therapy associated with operation. In addition to the procedures described above, the following may be necessary:

(1) Monitoring of the hourly urinary output with an indwelling catheter in place.

(2) Monitoring of central venous pressure.

(3) Administration of oxygen by mask.

(4) Rapid replacement of fluid and perhaps blood to maintain blood pressure and ensure urine output of 30 mL/h.

(5) Rapid evaluation and preparation for immediate operation. The patient's systemic deficiencies should first be corrected by intravenous fluids and blood if needed.

(6) Surgical measures: The anesthesiologist must be well informed of the patient's condition. A low midline incision is made to allow for cephalad extension. When the abdomen is opened, pus is obtained for aerobic and anaerobic cultures. The bowel is inspected and all loculated abscesses identified and drained. The subphrenic and subhepatic spaces are explored and loculations lysed to allow drainage of pus. Careful irrigation and suction are performed to minimize spread of infection. Total hysterectomy and bilateral salpingo-oophorectomy were standard treatment; however, occasional supracervical hysterectomy may significantly shorten the operating time. The abscess wall is dissected from the adjacent structures. This is usually thick, indurated, and densely adherent to bowel, in which case it is best to dissect within the abscess wall, leaving a small portion of outer rim, rather than risk perforation of bowel wall. Careful surgical technique is necessary to avoid perforation of the bowel or ligation and transection of the ureters. The vaginal cuff is left open after a hemostatic interlocking continuous suture has been applied around the edge of the cuff.

Active drainage of the pelvis is done routinely. Active suction through the abdominal wall provides the best result with the least contamination. The drains are left in place as long as purulent material is recovered. The fascia is closed with wide monofilament synthetic or wire sutures. Retention sutures may be used. The subcutaneous space is left open. In some cases, only drainage may be possible.

Prognosis

A. Unruptured Abscess

Generally the patient with an unruptured abscess has an excellent prognosis. Medical therapy, followed by judicious surgical treatment, yields good results in the most cases. Unruptured localized abscesses that do not respond to aggressive medical management by improvement in signs and symptoms and decreasing size are best drained or removed surgically if inaccessible to percutaneous or transvaginal drainage. Many clinically diagnosed unruptured TOAs may represent only acute salpingitis with omental and intestinal adhesions, which respond promptly to adequate antibiotic therapy. Serial ultrasonography may help to identify the true unruptured TOAs. The outlook for fertility, however, is greatly reduced, ranging from 5–15% from retrospective analysis. There is also an increased risk for ectopic pregnancy. The risk of reinfection must be considered if definitive surgical treatment has not been performed, but the incidence of reinfection in our prospectively studied patient population is less than 10%.

B. RUPTURED ABSCESS

Before effective means of treating overwhelming septicemia became available and the need for immediate surgical intervention was recognized, the mortality rate from ruptured tubo-ovarian abscess was 80–90%. With modern therapeutic resources, both medical and surgical, the mortality rate should be less than 2%.

5. Postoperative Pelvic Infections

ESSENTIALS OF DIAGNOSIS

- Recent pelvic surgery.
- Pelvic or low abdominal pain or pressure.
- Fever and tachycardia.
- Purulent, foul discharge.
- Constitutional symptoms: malaise, chills, etc.
- Vaginal cuff tenderness with cellulitis or abscess.

General Considerations

Patients who have had gynecologic surgery, especially hysterectomy, may develop postoperative infections of the remaining pelvic structures. These infections include simple cuff induration (cellulitis), infected cuff hematoma (cuff abscess), salpingitis, pelvic cellulitis, suppurative pelvic thrombophlebitis, and tubo-ovarian abscess with or without rupture. The incidence of such infections has been significantly reduced, from 32% after abdominal hysterectomy and 57% after vaginal hysterectomy in women given placebo to about 5% in women given a single dose of antimicrobial prophylaxis. It is also important to note that severe pelvic abscess formation may occur following the relatively benign procedure of oocyte pickup used with in vitro fertilization.

The pathogenesis of posthysterectomy infection is simple and straightforward; the apex of the vaginal vault consists of crushed, devitalized tissue, and the loose areolar tissue in the parametrial areas usually oozes postoperatively. These conditions provide an ideal medium for the myriad of pathogens that normally inhabit the vagina and are inoculated into the operative site during surgery.

The term "pelvic cellulitis" implies that the soft tissue of the vaginal apex and adjacent parametrial tissues have been invaded by bacteria. In addition, the serum and blood at the cuff apex may become infected, resulting in an infected hematoma, which is in essence a cuff abscess. The infection is treated at this point by establishing adequate drainage combined with antibiotic therapy. Infection may extend via lymphatic channels to the adnexa, resulting in salpingitis. Pelvic veins may become involved in the infectious process, particularly if *Bacteroides* or anaerobic streptococci are predominant pathogens. Rarely, septic emboli to the lungs, brain, spleen, and elsewhere may occur.

Clinical Findings

The diagnosis of postoperative pelvic infection is made clinically; laboratory studies may be useful in establishing the specific etiologic diagnosis and determining the sensitivity of the recovered bacteria to various antibiotics.

A. SYMPTOMS AND SIGNS

Any postoperative gynecologic patient who develops fever may have atelectasis, phlebitis, upper urinary tract infection, or pelvic infection; these conditions may or may not require antimicrobial therapy. Although some investigators have stated that fever due to postoperative pelvic infection usually does not occur before the third or fourth postoperative day, up to 50% of patients develop temperatures of 38.3–39.4 °C (101–103 °F) by the 24th–36th postoperative hour. Recurrent temperature elevation without symptoms occurs a mean of 50 hours after hysterectomy in our patient population and disappears without therapy. Temperature elevations associated with symptoms and physical findings of infection occur later. The mean time of this diagnosis in our patients is about 80 hours. Those who ultimately require parenteral antimicrobial therapy do not experience early asymptomatic temperature elevation.

Within 2 days following hysterectomy, the surgical margin of the vagina (vaginal cuff) appears hyperemic and edematous, and there is almost always a purulent or seropurulent exudate, regardless of the clinical condition of the patient and whether or not fever is present. When palpated, this site is usually indurated and tender—findings common to most healing wounds and not indicative of a need for antimicrobial therapy. When natural defense mechanisms of the host are inadequate for the inoculum, lymphatic extension of the infection to adjacent tissues results in pelvic cellulitis, demonstrable on pelvic examination as tender induration in the parametrial areas. The infection may involve the tubes and ovaries, with resultant abscess formation in unresponsive patients. At this point, the patient will begin to complain of lower abdominal, pelvic, or back pressure or pain. Abdominal distention due to ileus may develop, as may urinary symptoms due to perivesical irritation.

The diagnosis of suppurative pelvic thrombophlebitis is rare and usually is not apparent until after the sixth postoperative day, at which time the patient continues to have hectic spiking fever of 39–40.5 °C (102.2–105 °F) with a diurnal variation. The pelvic findings are usually unrevealing except for mild pelvic tenderness. Surprisingly, the woman's general health often is good unless septic embolization has occurred. CT scan is the diagnostic tool of choice for these diagnoses.

An infected pelvic hematoma is impossible to palpate early, but it can be diagnosed by sonography. Recurring temperature elevation is the principal indicator of this type of infection. Rarely do these patients have symptoms, and their examination is usually unremarkable. This problem can be suspected when the hematocrit is lower than anticipated. Onset is frequently at the same time other pelvic infections begin.

B. Laboratory Findings

Unfortunately, as previously outlined, the polymicrobial nature of these infections prohibits accurate identification of the offending microorganisms in a reasonable time period. For this reason, broad-spectrum empirical antimicrobial administration is necessary.

Serial complete blood counts usually demonstrate leukocytosis but occasionally enable the physician to detect concealed hemorrhage, which may harbor a large pelvic abscess. Urinalysis is rarely helpful.

C. X-Ray Findings

Chest films are unrevealing in most cases but can be useful if pulmonary complications are suspected.

D. Ultrasonography

Pelvic sonograms may prove helpful in detecting hematomas or either retroperitoneal or tubo-ovarian abscesses that develop as a complication of cuff infection.

Differential Diagnosis

Pulmonary atelectasis may become manifest within 12–36 hours after operation. This can usually be detected by auscultation and confirmed by chest x-ray. Aspiration pneumonitis must always be considered if pulmonary problems develop.

Deep vein thrombophlebitis of the lower extremities is rarely detected clinically and, when present, is seldom accompanied by significant fever. Superficial phlebitis of the upper extremity due to an indwelling venous catheter may cause significant pyrexia. Long-term (48–72 hours) infusion of intravenous antimicrobials increases the likelihood of phlebitis. Although the routine of changing the intravenous site every 48 hours may prevent this complication, it will respond to warm soaks and anti-inflammatory agents such as aspirin if it does develop.

Upper urinary tract infection may also account for the fever. Because of the liberal use of indwelling catheters in gynecologic surgery, significant bacteriuria commonly develops; however, this rarely causes fever unless pyelonephritis develops.

Fever from abdominal wound infection usually becomes manifest on or after the fourth postoperative day. Examination of the abdominal wound is mandatory in all febrile patients. It may be necessary to probe the abdominal incision carefully, regardless of its appearance, especially if the pelvic examination is unrevealing.

Complications

Complications of postoperative pelvic infection include extensive pelvic or intra-abdominal abscesses, tubo-ovarian abscess with or without rupture, intestinal adhesions and obstruction, septic pelvic thrombophlebitis with metastatic abscesses, and septicemia.

Prevention

Many attempts have been made to decrease infectious morbidity following gynecologic surgical procedures. None have been uniformly successful, but the following measures may be of some help:

(1) Preoperative insertion of antibacterial vaginal creams or suppositories, especially if cervicitis, bacterial vaginosis, or vulvovaginitis is present.

(2) Preparation of the vagina with hexachlorophene or povidone-iodine solution just prior to surgery.

(3) Meticulous attention to hemostasis at operation and gentle handling of tissues. The use of large, strangulating hemostatic sutures should be avoided; nonreactive suture material should be used.

(4) If hemostasis is less than desirable but maximal under given circumstances, suction drainage of that area should be accomplished. This may be done with the vaginal surgical margin left open or closed at hysterectomy.

(5) Antimicrobial prophylaxis beginning preoperatively has been shown by many to significantly reduce pelvic infectious morbidity following vaginal and abdominal hysterectomy. Some controversy regarding this treatment still exists, however. Before using prophylaxis, one should consider these guidelines: (a) Morbidity on a specific service should be significant enough to warrant attempts to decrease it. (b) Antimicrobials of relatively insignificant toxicity but proved value should be used. (c) The first dose should be given preoperatively to ensure adequate tissue concentrations at the time of surgery. Increasingly, studies show that a single preoperative dose is as effective as multiple doses in preventing major infection. Use of many different antimicrobials has been associated with dramatic lowering of pelvic infection morbidity rates. Recent comparative

studies indicate that the newer, more expensive semi-synthetic cephalosporins and penicillins are more effective than the older agents. In otherwise uncomplicated cases, pelvic infections developing despite prophylaxis generally are mild in nature, although severe infections and resultant complications are not always prevented.

(6) Severe, more advanced infections may be prevented by early diagnosis, drainage (including an open vaginal cuff), and prompt treatment of mild infections.

Treatment

If a cuff hematoma or abscess is found, adequate drainage may be established by separating the apposed vaginal edges with ring forceps or some other suitable instrument. Care must be taken not to disrupt the intact peritoneum. The usual supportive measures are instituted, and antibiotic therapy is begun. Many of the newer semi-synthetic cephalosporins and expanded spectrum penicillins have proved valuable as single-agent therapy for these infections. Rarely, the addition of metronidazole to these regimens may be necessary to effect a cure.

In most cases, the patient with postoperative pelvic infection becomes afebrile within 48–72 hours. If a large, infected pelvic hematoma has developed, more prolonged treatment will be necessary. Large hematomas may be drained and irrigated from below by means of a Foley catheter or Penrose drain introduced into the abscess cavity. Suction drains should be used whenever possible.

A postoperative tubo-ovarian abscess is treated expectantly as outlined above in the section on unruptured tubo-ovarian abscess. If intra-abdominal rupture of a pelvic abscess or tubo-ovarian abscess is suspected, immediate laparotomy is indicated.

Persistent fever and clinical signs of unresponsiveness to therapy may indicate septic pelvic thrombophlebitis, which is generally a diagnosis of exclusion after a 7- to 10-day course of antibiotics. Intermittent intravenous heparin therapy, 5000 U every 4 hours, should be given. Persistence of fever in spite of heparin therapy suggests abscess formation. Abscesses—as well as septic thrombophlebitis—are usually associated with anaerobic bacteria, and antimicrobial therapy should include clindamycin or metronidazole in addition to other agents effective against aerobic microorganisms.

6. Pelvic Tuberculosis

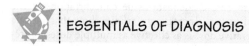

ESSENTIALS OF DIAGNOSIS

- Infertility.
- Active or healed pulmonary tuberculosis.

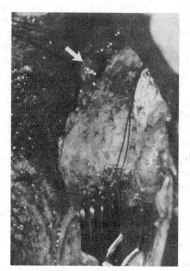

Figure 38–13. Miliary tuberculosis involving the uterus and peritoneum.

- Findings by hysterosalpingography or laparoscopy.
- Recovery of Mycobacterium tuberculosis from either menstrual fluid or biopsy specimen.

General Considerations

In the U.S., pelvic tuberculosis is becoming a rare entity. When it does occur, it usually represents secondary invasion from a primary lung infection via the lympho-hematogenous route (Fig 38–6). The overall incidence of pelvic tuberculosis in patients with pulmonary tuberculosis is approximately 5%. Prepubertal tuberculosis rarely results in genital tract infection.

After the pelvic organs become affected (Fig 38–13), direct extension to adjacent organs may occur. Older studies in the U.S. indicated that the oviducts were most frequently involved (90%) and the endometrium next most frequently (70%). More recent studies in Scotland, where the disease is still prevalent, showed endometrial involvement in more than 90% of cases and tubal involvement in only 5%.

Clinical Findings

A. SYMPTOMS AND SIGNS

The only complaint may be infertility, although dysmenorrhea, pelvic pain, and evidence of tuberculous peritonitis may also be present. Endometrial involvement may result in amenorrhea or some other disturbance of the cycle. Abdominal or pelvic pain from this infection is commonly associated with low-grade fever, asthenia, and weight loss. The diagnosis can usually be established on the basis of a complete history and physical examination, chest x-ray and lung scan, and appropriate tests such as a tuberculin (Mantoux) test, sputum smears, and sputum cultures. Tuberculosis of the female genital tract is usually secondary to hematogenous spread involving the endometrium, tubes, and ovaries. The manifestations are usually those of chronic pelvic disease and sterility. Gross ascites with fluid containing more than 3 g of protein per 100 mL of peritoneal fluid is characteristic of tuberculous peritonitis.

Pelvic tuberculosis is usually encountered in the course of a gynecologic operation done for other reasons. Although it may be mistaken for chronic pelvic inflammation, some distinguishing features usually can be found: extremely dense adhesions without planes of cleavage, segmental dilatation of the tubes, and lack of occlusion of the tubes at the ostia. If the internal genitalia are involved, with disseminated granulomatous disease of the serosal surfaces, ascites usually is present. Clinical diagnosis is difficult.

B. LABORATORY FINDINGS

The best direct method of diagnosis in suspected genital tuberculosis is detection of acid-fast bacteria by means of the Ziehl-Neelsen stain followed by culture on Lowenstein-Jensen medium. The specimen may be from menstrual discharge, from curettage or biopsy, or from peritoneal biopsy in cases where ascites is present. A rapid sedimentation rate, peripheral blood eosinophilia, and a strongly positive Mantoux test are additional evidence of tuberculous infection.

C. X-RAY FINDINGS

1. Chest x-ray—A chest x-ray should be taken in any patient with proved or suspected tuberculosis of other organs or tissues.

2. Hysterosalpingography—The tubal lining may be irregular, and areas of dilatation may be present. Saccular diverticula extending from the ampulla and giving the impression of a cluster of currants are characteristic of granulomatous salpingitis. Other findings that should arouse suspicion are calcifications of the periaortic or iliac lymph nodes.

D. SPECIAL EXAMINATIONS

Visual inspection (laparoscopy) as well as aspiration of fluid for culture and biopsy of affected areas is possible and often diagnostic.

Differential Diagnosis

Pelvic tuberculosis should be differentiated from schistosomiasis, enterobiasis, lipoid salpingitis, carcinoma, chronic pelvic inflammation, and mycotic infections.

Complications

Sterility and tuberculous peritonitis are possible sequelae of pelvic tuberculosis.

Treatment

A. MEDICAL MEASURES

To prevent the emergence of drug-resistant strains, the initial therapy of tuberculous infection should include four drugs. The drug regimen for the first 2 months of treatment should include isoniazid, rifampin, pyrazinamide, and streptomycin or ethambutol. Once drug susceptibility results are available, the drug regimen can be appropriately changed. Treatment should be continued for 24–36 months, since extrapulmonary tuberculosis is more difficult to eradicate.

B. SURGICAL MEASURES

The primary mode of treatment for pelvic tuberculosis is medical therapy; however, surgical intervention may be necessary. Medical therapy should be attempted for 12–18 months prior to evaluation for surgery. The ultimate indications for surgery include (1) masses not resolving with medical therapy, (2) resistant or reactivated disease, (3) persistent menstrual irregularities, and (4) fistula formation.

Prognosis

The prognosis for life and health is excellent if chemotherapy is instituted promptly, although the prognosis for fertility is poor.

7. Toxic Shock Syndrome

ESSENTIALS OF DIAGNOSIS

- *Fever of 38.9 °C (102 °F) or higher.*
- *Diffuse macular rash.*
- *Desquamation (1–2 weeks after onset of illness; particularly affects palms and soles).*
- *Hypotension (systolic < 90 mm Hg for adults or orthostatic syncope).*
- *Involvement of 3 or more of the following organ systems: gastrointestinal, muscular, mucous*

membrane, renal, hepatic, hematologic, central nervous system.

General Considerations

Toxic shock syndrome was first described in children in 1978, but was quickly identified as an illness occurring primarily in menstruating women 12–24 years of age. An association with use of superabsorbent tampons was made by the CDC. The majority of cases have occurred in California, Minnesota, Wisconsin, Utah, and Iowa. Peak incidence was reported in August, 1980. It is not known whether the abrupt decline in incidence has been due to changes in tampon use, improvements in manufacture, or reduction in disease severity due to early recognition. Of the approximately 30 million menstruating women in the U.S., it is estimated that 70% use tampons and over 50% of those use superabsorbent types. Almost 1,000,000 women are at theoretic risk. The incidence in menstruating women is now 6–7:100,000 annually. Toxic shock syndrome has also been reported in women after delivery and in those using a diaphragm, in men and women following surgical procedures, or associated with soft tissue abscesses or osteomyelitis. The incidence of nonmenstrual disease has shown only a slight increase in the past 10 years.

The cause of toxic shock syndrome is preformed toxins produced by *Staphylococcus aureus,* so that colonization or infection by this microorganism must occur. A pyrogenic toxin induces high fever and may enhance susceptibility to endotoxins that cause shock as well as liver, kidney, and myocardial damage. Other unrecognized toxins may play a role. How toxins gain access to the circulatory system is unknown. Tampon use has been associated with this syndrome, but evidence for the mechanism of toxin entry remains obscure. Insertion could cause mucosal damage. Vaginal ulcerations due to pressure changes usually are not observed, although vaginal erythema commonly is present. Superabsorbent tampons may obstruct the vagina, resulting in retrograde menstruation and peritoneal absorption of bacteria or toxin. Tampons may be associated with increased numbers of aerobic bacteria due to oxygen trapped in interfibrous spaces. The longer a tampon is left in place, the greater the risk for development of this syndrome.

Clinical Findings

A. Symptoms and Signs

Onset is usually sudden, with high fever, watery diarrhea, and vomiting—the triad often seen with viral gastroenteritis. Myalgia, headache, and sometimes sore throat may be present as well as erythroderma and con-

junctivitis, as frequently seen with viral infections. Unlike most viral infections, however, this disorder may progress to hypotensive shock within several hours (usually < 48 hours). Timely diagnosis is critical, and the key is the fact that the woman is menstruating or using tampons. The patient will appear obviously acutely ill, with a fever of 39 °C (102.2 °F) or higher. An erythematous, sunburn-like rash is seen over the face, proximal extremities, and trunk. Dehydration is evident, and the patient will have tachycardia and perhaps hypotension. The conjunctiva will be erythematous as will the pharynx, and there usually will be muscle and abdominal tenderness. A vaginal examination must be performed; if a tampon is present, it must be removed. Mucosal lesions should be sought, and a culture for *S aureus* performed. If nuchal rigidity, headache, or disorientation unexplained by hypotension or fever is present, a lumbar puncture must be performed to rule out meningitis. During convalescence, desquamation can be striking.

B. Laboratory Findings

Tests should include a complete blood count with differential, electrolyte measurements, urinalysis, urea nitrogen measurement, creatinine measurement, and hepatic function tests. Other tests are performed as indicated by clinical symptoms and signs. Cultures should be made of blood, throat secretions, and probably cerebrospinal fluid. A vaginal culture will yield penicillinase-producing *S aureus.*

Differential Diagnosis

Other systemic diseases characterized by rash, fever, and systemic complications should be considered. Most patients will not have an obvious source of infection such as a recent incision, soft tissue abscess, or osteomyelitis, but these should be sought. Kawasaki's disease of young children is similar but not as severe, since hypotension, renal failure, and thrombocytopenia do not occur and the incidence of myalgia, diarrhea, and hepatic damage is greatly decreased. Scarlet fever must be excluded. Rocky Mountain spotted fever, leptospirosis, and measles may be excluded by appropriate serologic tests. Gram-negative sepsis must be excluded by both blood and cerebrospinal fluid cultures.

Complications

Approximately 30% of women who develop toxic shock syndrome have recurrences. The greatest risk for recurrence is during the first 3 menstrual periods following treatment, and the recurrent episode may be less or more severe than the initial one. The incidence is reduced to less than 5% if antistaphylococcal antibiotic therapy is given during therapy of the initial occurrence. Half of the women who developed this disease in Wisconsin during the infancy of its recognition have had 3 recurrences. Cervicovaginal and nasal cultures for *S aureus* should be negative twice, 4 weeks apart, prior to resumption of tampon use. Women can almost entirely eliminate the risk of this illness by not using tampons and may substantially reduce the risk by intermittent use of tampons during menstruation.

Treatment

Aggressive supportive therapy is imperative for a successful outcome. Appropriate initial management begins with fluid and electrolyte resuscitation—up to 12 L/d. Packed red blood cells and coagulation factors may be necessary. Central venous or pulmonary wedge pressures and urine output must be monitored to guide therapy. Laboratory studies and appropriate cultures must be obtained early. Dopamine infusion at 2–5 µg/kg/min may be necessary if fluid volume alone does not correct hypotension. Mechanical ventilation may be necessary if acute respiratory syndrome develops, and hemodialysis may be necessary if renal failure develops. Corticosteroid therapy (methylprednisolone, 30 mg/kg, or dexamethasone, 3 mg/kg as a bolus and repeated every 4 hours as necessary), if instituted early, may reduce the severity of illness and duration of fever. Naloxone has resulted in reversal of hypotension in seriously compromised patients by antiendorphin activity. Although *S aureus* is not present in the blood, treatment with a β-lactamase-resistant antibiotic such as nafcillin, or oxacillin, (2 g intravenously every 4 hours) should be given. If penicillin allergy is present, vancomycin should be given. Dose reduction is necessary with renal impairment. Until gram-negative sepsis has been excluded, an aminoglycoside should be included with caution, since there will be altered renal function. The mortality rate associated with toxic shock syndrome is 3–6%. The 3 major causes of death are acute respiratory distress syndrome, intractable hypotension, and hemorrhage secondary to disseminated intravascular coagulopathy.

8. Human Immunodeficiency Virus (HIV) Infection

ESSENTIALS OF DIAGNOSIS

Asymptomatic Infection

- *HIV antibody, antigen, or ribonucleic acid or culture.*
- *High-risk group member.*

- *Mononucleosis-like syndrome with weight loss, fever, night sweats.*
- *Neurologic involvement.*
- *Lymphadenopathy.*
- *Pharyngitis.*
- *Erythematous maculopapular rash.*
- *Extragenital lymphadenopathy.*

Acquired Immunodeficiency Syndrome (AIDS)

- *HIV antibody, antigen, ribonucleic acid, or culture.*
- *Any of the above signs or symptoms.*
- *Opportunistic infections.*
- *Cognitive difficulties or depression.*
- *Kaposi's sarcoma.*
- *CD4+ counts below 200 CD4 lymphocytes/mm³.*
- *Cervical neoplasia.*

General Considerations

The World Health Organization estimates that the number of people living with HIV/AIDS is approaching 50 million, with women constituting 40–50% of the total. As of 1998, in North America there were approximately 890,000 cases of HIV infection with 20% of cases occurring in women. The best estimates of the incidence of HIV infection in the U.S. are likely to come from ongoing serologic surveillance studies in sentinel areas and hospitals. In the general population, HIV infection is most prevalent in gay or bisexual men, intravenous drug abusers, and hemophiliacs. The high-risk groups for women are intravenous drug abusers, those with heterosexual contacts with men in high-risk groups, recipients of unscreened transfusions, and prostitutes.

Over 80% of the cases of AIDS in women occur in women of reproductive age, making heterosexual and perinatal transmission important concerns. Minorities are disproportionately represented in the reported AIDS cases. Most HIV infections in the United States are due to HIV-1. The prevalence of HIV-2 in this country is very low. HIV-2 is endemic in parts of West Africa and has been reported increasingly in Angola, Mozambique, Portugal, and France.

Modes of Transmission

Although there has been much speculation about the modes of HIV transmission, HIV infection may be acquired in only 3 ways.

First, HIV infection may be acquired by sexual contact. Transmission has been reported from male to male, male to female, female to male, and recently, female to female. The risk appears to be greatest for the female sexual partners of men with AIDS, followed in decreasing order by intravenous drug abusers, bisexual men, transfusion recipients, and hemophiliacs. Other factors that increase the risk for heterosexual acquisition of HIV infection are the number of exposures to high-risk sexual partners; anal-receptive intercourse; and infection with other sexually transmitted diseases such as syphilis, genital herpes, chancroid, and condylomata acuminata.

The second means by which HIV transmission can occur is by parenteral exposure to blood or bodily fluids such as with intravenous drug use or occupational exposure.

The third means by which HIV infection can occur is by transmission from an infected woman to her fetus or infant.

Course of Infection

The chance of acquiring HIV infection through sexual contact is unknown. In American women, approximately 40% of the cases reported appear to be acquired through heterosexual contact; some of the cases without risk factors may be heterosexually acquired. The percentage of cases arising from heterosexual contact is significantly larger in women than in men, probably because transmission can occur more easily from male to female. This is due to 2 reasons: (1) the concentration of HIV in semen is high and (2) coitus causes more breaks in the introital mucosa than in the penile skin. It is hypothesized that these breaks in the mucosa, similar to those that occur with anal-receptive intercourse, increase the chances for acquiring HIV through sexual contact. The presence of a genital ulcerative disease also increases the risk of infection in a similar fashion.

The natural course of HIV infection is becoming better understood. HIV is a single-stranded RNA-enveloped retrovirus that attaches to the CD4 receptor of the target cell and integrates into the host genome. If they become infected, most patients develop anti-HIV antibody within 12 weeks and 95% within 6 months after exposure. As many as 45–90% of patients develop an acute HIV-induced retroviral infection in the first few months after infection. This is similar to mononucleosis, with symptoms of weight loss, fever, night sweats, pharyngitis, lymphadenopathy, erythematous maculopapular rash, and extragenital lymphadenopathy. Critical awareness of this acute syndrome is important because of improved prognoses associated with early antiretroviral treatment. This syndrome usually resolves within several weeks, and the patient becomes asymptomatic. HIV-infected individuals ultimately show evidence of progressive immune dysfunction and the condition progresses to AIDS as immunosuppression continues and systemic involvement becomes more severe and diffuse. AIDS develops in the majority of untreated HIV-infected individuals within 17 years after contracting the virus. All women diagnosed with HIV require counseling, an extensive STD work-up, Pap smear, CBC, chemistry panel, toxoplasma antibody, hepatitis panel, PPD, and chest radiograph. All patients should also be offered vaccinations for hepatitis B, influenza, and pneumococcus. The CDC case definition of AIDS is an HIV-infected person with a specific opportunistic infection (eg, *Pneumocystis carinii* pneumonia, central nervous system toxoplasmosis), neoplasia (eg, Kaposi's sarcoma), dementia, encephalopathy, wasting syndrome, rapid progression of cervical dysplasia to cancer, or a CD4 lymphocyte count less than $200/mm^3$. A patient without laboratory evidence of infection may also be diagnosed with AIDS if one of the indicator diseases is present and there is no explanation for the immune dysfunction.

Unfortunately, the mortality rate for patients with established AIDS is high, and at present does not appear to be altered by antiviral agents such as zidovudine. Further research in the development of antivirals and vaccines is in progress. Recent guidelines in this rapidly changing environment for antiviral agents are available by calling 800-HIV-0440.

Prevention of HIV Infection

To decrease the risk of acquiring HIV infection through sexual contact, "safer sex" guidelines have been established. These include a reduction in the number of sexual partners, especially those who are in high-risk groups, and use of condoms for all coital activity. Latex condoms are the most effective. Condoms lubricated with spermicides such as nonoxynol-9 (N-9) are no more effective than other lubricated condoms in protecting against transmission of HIV. In addition, recent data indicate that N-9 may increase the risk for HIV transmission during vaginal intercourse possibly via development of genital lesions that have been associated with N-9 use.

Education and counseling for detection of HIV-infected patients and prevention of HIV infection are difficult tasks. HIV infection in women appears to be a disease of drug users and sexual partners of high-risk men. Groups to whom information must be targeted are intravenous drug users and ethnic minorities, particularly blacks and Hispanics. Counseling must not only stress behavior modification, but also reinforce those behavioral changes through culturally significant and sensitive messages. In general, reduction of high-risk behavior and use of safer sex guidelines have been the 2 main areas of education and counseling.

The general preventive guidelines for seropositive women include the following:

(1) Refraining from donating blood, plasma, organs, or tissue.

(2) Being in a mutually monogamous sexual relationship.

(3) Using condoms with spermicide.

(4) Avoiding pregnancy.

HIV Infection During Pregnancy

Maternal transmission of HIV can occur transplacentally before birth, peripartum by exposure to blood and bodily fluids at delivery, or postpartum through breast-feeding. Hence, all pregnant women should be offered HIV testing. The range of the perinatal infection rate has been 15–30% without treatment. The risk appears to be higher in subsequent pregnancies if a patient has delivered one infected infant; in this setting the risk may be 37–65%. The mode of delivery may play a role in increasing or decreasing the risks of developing pediatric AIDS. It is recommended that membranes not be ruptured longer than 4 hours. Also, fetal scalp electrodes and scalp sampling are contraindicated.

Many of the concerns about the effect of pregnancy on HIV infection are unanswered. Does the altered immune status of pregnancy accelerate the progression of HIV infection? Clinically, progression from asymptomatic infection to AIDS is uncommon in pregnancy. However, 45–75% of women will develop symptomatic HIV infection within 2–3 years postpartum if their child was infected. Whether this represents an accelerated progression of HIV infection or demonstrates more effective perinatal transmission in women with longstanding infection is unknown. Delays in the diagnosis of acute HIV infection may occur, since some of the symptoms of early HIV infection may mimic those of the first trimester of pregnancy.

Prenatal care must be individualized, with referral to support systems ideally occurring during the pregnancy rather than postpartum. Screening for other sexually transmitted diseases (eg, syphilis, gonorrhea, and herpes simplex virus infection) is important. Other specific HIV-related infections must be sought, including *Pneumocystis carinii* pneumonia, *Mycobacterium* tuberculosis, cytomegaloviral infection, toxoplasmosis, and candidiasis. As a minimum, HIV-infected patients should receive a shielded chest x-ray, a tuberculin skin test with controls, and cytomegalovirus and toxoplasmosis baseline serologic tests. Susceptible patients

should receive hepatitis B virus, pneumococcal, and influenza vaccines. CD4+ lymphocyte cell counts should be monitored each trimester. A CD4+ count of less than 200/mm^3 is an indication for prophylaxis against *Pneumocystis carinii* pneumonia. Plasma viral load (HIV-1 RNA) is also monitored throughout pregnancy.

Zidovudine (ZDV) administered during the second and third trimester, during labor, and for 6 weeks to the newborn has been shown to decrease vertical transmission from 25–30% to 5–8%. Newer protocols that utilize a combination of drugs are now being used and comprise what is referred to as highly active antiretroviral therapy (HAART). The three main classes of drugs used in HAART are nucleoside analogue reverse transcriptase inhibitors, nonnucleoside reverse transcriptase inhibitors, and protease inhibitors. Perinatal transmission rates appear to have declined even further with the use of HAART. Pregnant women should be treated according to standard guidelines for antiretroviral therapy in adults with the goal being reduction of plasma viral load (plasma HIV-1 RNA). However, specific recommendations for antiretroviral treatment in pregnant patients continue to evolve so that all pregnant patients with HIV infection should be under the supervision of experts in the management of HIV in pregnancy.

There are data suggesting that cesarean section prior to the onset of labor and rupture of membranes further decreases the risk of vertical transmission. However, the bulk of these data were obtained prior to the routine use of viral load testing and combination antiretroviral therapy. More recent data suggest that the risk of vertical transmission is proportional to the viral load. In two separate analyses, when the viral load was less than 1000 copies per milliliter the perinatal transmission rate was zero (upper limits of the 95% confidence interval were 2.8% and 5.1%). Therefore, it is reasonable to offer scheduled cesarean section prior to the onset of labor and rupture of membranes to HIV-infected women with viral loads greater than 1000 copies per milliliter. The increased maternal morbidity associated with cesarean section must be taken into account, however, when making decisions regarding mode of delivery. It is unclear if cesarean section is beneficial when the mother has received HAART and/or has low to undetectable viral loads.

Peripartum care should include universal application of infection control guidelines to avoid exposure to blood and bodily fluids. These include water-repellant gowns, double gloves, hand-washing between patient contacts, goggles for significant splash exposures, and wall or bulb suction. Needles should not be recapped. A 1:10 sodium hypochlorite solution should be used to clean instruments. Fetal scalp sampling and scalp electrodes should be avoided because they could become portals of entry for infection.

Postpartum care should entail a continuance of blood and bodily fluids precautions with proscription of breastfeeding. Family planning and safer sex counseling can be continued in the postpartum period with consideration given to tubal ligation. Medical and support system referrals should be initiated prior to discharge from the hospital, if possible.

Pediatric HIV Infection

In the United States as of 1999, approximately 90% of pediatric AIDS cases were perinatally acquired, occurring in infants born to women in high-risk groups: intravenous drug users, partners of high-risk men, or women with AIDS. The progression to infection appears to be faster than in adults, and pediatric AIDS carries a mortality rate similar to that found in adults.

Identification of infected neonates is difficult, because maternal anti-HIV IgG crosses the placenta. Thus, most infants are born with HIV seropositivity, which may persist up to 15 months by the enzyme immunoassay (EIA) technique. Nucleic acid or antigen HIV studies are necessary to help identify fetal infection. An HIV embryopathy similar to the fetal alcohol syndrome has been described. Since many of the high-risk mothers have multifactorial perinatal problems, assigning the cause of the syndrome to HIV is uncertain.

Infant care involves many of the same guidelines as maternal peripartum care. Blood and bodily fluid precautions, as well as immunosuppression care guidelines, should be exercised. Consultation with a pediatric immunologist to plan neonatal and follow-up care should begin prior to discharge from the hospital. Circumcision should be discouraged. Prior to discharge, detailed home-care instruction should be given regarding avoidance of bodily secretions.

Guidelines for HIV Testing

HIV serologic testing should include pretest and posttest counseling about interpretation of the test results. After obtaining informed consent from the patient, confidentiality must be maintained concerning the test results. Situations in which HIV testing should be offered include the following:

(1) Women who have used intravenous drugs.

(2) Women who have engaged in prostitution.

(3) Women with sex partners who are HIV-infected or are at risk for HIV infection.

(4) Women who have sexually transmitted diseases.

(5) Women who have lived in communities or were born in countries where the prevalence of HIV infection (especially heterosexually acquired HIV infection) among women is high.

(6) Women who received blood transfusions between 1978 and 1985.

(7) Women undergoing medical evaluation or treatment for clinical signs and symptoms of HIV infection.

(8) Women who have been inmates in correctional systems.

(9) Women who consider themselves at risk.

(10) Pregnancy.

HIV Antibody Testing

The diagnosis of HIV infection is usually by HIV-1 antibody tests. Routine testing for HIV-2, other than at blood banks, is currently not recommended unless a patient is at risk for HIV-2 infection or has clinical findings of HIV disease and has had a negative HIV-1 antibody test. Refer to recent reviews cited in the references for details of the criteria for HIV antibody detection. In general, the enzyme-linked immunosorbent assay (ELISA) functions as a screening test for exposure to HIV. Most patients exposed to HIV develop detectable levels of antibody against the virus by 12 weeks after exposure. The presence of antibody indicates current infection, although the patient may be asymptomatic for years. The sensitivity and specificity of the ELISA test is 99% when it is repeatedly reactive. Thus, the test for HIV antibody is considered negative if the ELISA is nonreactive, and indicates a lack of HIV infection unless it is too early to detect antibody production.

The probability of a false-negative test in an uninfected woman is remote unless she is in the "window" before antibody is produced. A positive test result occurs when an ELISA is repeatedly reactive followed by a positive Western blot assay. The Western blot assay is reactive when a critical pattern of specific antibodies is detected against the 3 main gene products of HIV. The probability that an abnormal testing sequence will falsely identify a patient as HIV-infected is from < 1 to 5 in 100,000 persons. Individuals in high-risk groups should be retested in 3 months; they are likely to become positive. The status of those without associated risk factors is likely to remain indeterminate, but persistent indeterminate status is not diagnostic of HIV infection.

REFERENCES

General

Centers for Disease Control and Prevention: 2002 Sexually transmitted diseases, treatment guideliness. MMWR 2002; 51:RR06;1–80.

Fontanet AL et al: Protection against sexually transmitted diseases by granting sex workers in Thailand the choice of using the male or female condom: results from a randomized controlled trial. AIDS 1998;12:1851.

Levinson ME, Bush LM: Peritonitis and other intra-abdominal infections. In: Mandell GL, Douglas RG, Bennett JE (editors): *Principles and Practice of Infectious Diseases,* 3rd ed. Churchill Livingstone, 1990, p. 643.

McGregor JA et al: Assessment of office-based care of sexually transmitted diseases and vaginitis and antibiotic decision making by obstetrician-gynecologists. Infect Dis Obstet Gynecol 1988;6:247.

Miller HG et al: Correlates of sexually transmitted bacterial infections among U.S. women in 1995. Fam Plann Perspect 1999;31:4, 23.

Gonorrhea

Friedland LR et al: Cost-effectiveness decision analysis of intramuscular ceftriaxone versus oral cefixime in adolescents with gonococcal cervicitis. Ann Emerg Med 1996;27:299.

Chlamydial Infections

Chlamydia trachomatis infections—United States, 1995. MMWR 1997;46:193.

Faaunders A et al: The risk of inadvertent intrauterine device insertion in women carriers of endocervical *Chlamydia trachomatis.* Contraception 1998;58:105.

Lea AP, Lamb HM: Azithromycin: A pharmacoeconomic review of its use as a single-dose regimen in the treatment of uncomplicated urogenital *Chlamydia trachomatis* infections in women. Pharmacoeconomics 1997;12:596.

Chancroid

Chen CY et al: Comparison of enzyme immunoassays for antibodies to *Haemophilus ducreyi* in a community outbreak of chancroid in the United States. J Infect Dis 1997;175:1390.

Hawkes S et al: Asymptomatic carriage of *Haemophilus ducreyi* confirmed by the polymerase chain reaction. Genitourinary Med 1995;71:224.

Mertz KJ et al: An investigation of genital ulcers in Jackson, Mississippi, with the use of a multiplex polymerase chain reaction assay: high prevalence of chancroid and human immunodeficiency virus infection. J Infect Dis 1998;178:1060.

Genital Ulcers

Dillon SM et al: Prospective analysis of genital ulcer disease in Brooklyn, New York. Clin Infect Dis 1997;24:945.

Mertz KJ et al: Etiology of genital ulcers and prevalence of human immunodeficiency virus coinfection in 10 U.S. cities. The Genital Ulcer Disease Surveillance Group. J Infect Dis 1998;178:1795.

Human Immunodeficiency Virus

Anderson JR (editor): *A Guide to the Clinical Care of Women with HIV.* U.S. Department of Health and Human Services, HIV/AIDS Bureau, 2001, pp. 1, 77.

American College of Obstetricians and Gynecologists: Scheduled cesarean delivery and the prevention of vertical transmission of HIV infection. ACOG Committee Opinion No. 234, 2000.

Blattner W et al: Effectiveness of potent antiretroviral therapies on reducing perinatal transmission of HIV-1. XIII International AIDS Conference, Durban, South Africa (Abstr. LbOr4), July 9–14, 2000.

Garcia PM et al: Maternal levels of plasma human immunodeficiency virus type 1 RNA and the risk of perinatal transmission. Women and Infants Transmission Study Group. N Engl J Med 1999;341:394.

The European Mode of Delivery Collaboration: Elective caesarean section versus vaginal delivery in prevention of vertical HIV-1 transmission: a randomized clinical trial. Lancet 1999; 353:1035.

Mofenson LM et al: Risk factors for perinatal transmission of human immunodeficiency virus type 1 in women treated with zidovudine. Pediatric AIDS Clinical Trial Group Study 185 Team. N Engl J Med 1999;341:385.

Staszewski S et al: Safety and efficacy of lamivudine-zidovudine combination therapy in zidovudine-experienced patients: a randomized controlled comparison with zidovudine monotherapy. JAMA 1996;276:111.

U.S. Department of Health and Human Services—Centers for Disease Control and Prevention: Estimated incidence of AIDS and deaths of persons with AIDS, adjusted for delays in reporting, by quarter-year of diagnosis/death, United States, January 1985 through June 1997. HIV AIDS Surveil Rep 1997;9(2):1.

U.S. Department of Health and Human Services—Centers for Disease Control and Prevention: Guidelines for the use of antiretroviral agents in pediatric HIV infection. MMWR 1998;47:RR-4.

Pelvic Inflammatory Disease

Arredondo JL et al: Oral clindamycin and ciprofloxacin versus intramuscular ceftriaxone and oral doxycycline in the treatment of mild-to-moderate pelvic inflammatory disease in outpatients. Clin Infect Dis 1997;24:170.

Aral SO, Wasserheit JN: Social and behavioral correlates of pelvic inflammatory disease. Sex Transm Dis 1998;25:378.

McNeeley SG, Hendrix SL, Mazzoni MM: Medically sound, cost effective treatment for pelvic inflammatory disease and tubovarian abscesses. Am J Obstet Gynecol 1998;178:1272.

Reljic M, Gorisek B: C-reactive protein and the treatment of pelvic inflammatory disease. Int J Gynecol Obstet 1998;60:143.

Teisala K, Heinonen PK: C-reactive protein in assessing antimicrobial treatment of acute pelvic inflammatory disease. J Reprod Med 1990;35:955.

Timor-Tritsch IE et al: Transvaginal sonographic markers of tubal inflammatory disease. Ultrasound Obstet Gynecol 1998; 12:56.

Tubo-Ovarian Abscess

Golde SH, Israel R, Ledger WJ: Unilateral tubo-ovarian abscess: a distinct entity. Am J Obstet Gynecol 1977;127:807.

Henry-Suchet J, Soler A, Loffredo V: Laparoscopic treatment of tubovarian abscesses. J Reprod Med 1984;29:579.

Landers VD, Sweet LR: Current trends in the diagnosis and treatment of tubovarian abscess. Am J Obstet Gynecol 1985; 151:1098.

Lavy G, Hilsenrath RE: Management of tubo-ovarian abscess. Infertil Reprod Med Clin North Am 1992;3:821.

Reed SD, Landers DV, Sweet RL: Antibiotic treatment of tuboovarian abscess: comparison of broad-spectrum lactam agents versus clindamycin-containing regimens. Am J Obstet Gynecol 1991;164:1556.

Wilson JR, Black RJ: Ovarian abscess. Am J Obstet Gynecol 1964;90:34.

Younis JS et al: Late manifestation of pelvic abscess following oocyte retrieval for in vitro fertilization, in patients with severe endometriosis and ovarian endometriomata. J Assist Reprod Genet 1997;14:343.

Antimicrobial Chemotherapy

Ronald S. Gibbs, MD

■ ANTIMICROBIAL CHEMOTHERAPY

Although microbial infection has always been a threat to obstetric or gynecologic patients, gratifying developments in antimicrobial therapy have led to marked improvements in outcome and have contributed greatly to decreases in puerperal and postoperative mortality.

PRINCIPLES OF SELECTION OF ANTIMICROBIAL DRUGS

Several special conditions are pertinent to most infections encountered in obstetric and gynecologic practice. First, our patients (with the exception of some elderly and some oncology patients) are generally healthy and free of debilitating illness. Second, most infections, especially postpartum, postoperative infection and pelvic inflammatory disease, are polymicrobial in origin, involving an array of aerobes, anaerobes, genital mycoplasmas, and often *Chlamydia trachomatis*. Third, when a clinical diagnosis of infection is made, empiric antibiotic therapy is usually indicated before culture results are available. Fourth, because of limitations in laboratory technique, culture results may not be available in a timely fashion or tests may not even be performed at all. Thus, although general principles of good antimicrobial selection should generally be applied, knowledge of these special conditions is also essential.

To serve as a guide to antibiotic selection, 4 tables are provided. Table 39–1 provides the classification of β-lactam and related antibiotics. Table 39–2 provides a classification of antibiotics commonly used in obstetric and gynecologic practice and their main adverse effects, both in adults and in the fetus. Table 39–3 shows recommended drugs and alternatives for suspected or proved etiologic microorganisms, whereas Table 39–4 shows appropriate selections by clinical diagnosis.

The following steps merit consideration in each patient.

A. ETIOLOGIC DIAGNOSIS

Formulate an etiologic diagnosis based on clinical observations. The physician must attempt to decide on clinical grounds (1) whether the patient has a microbial infection that can probably be influenced by antimicrobial drugs and (2) the most probable infectious agent causing the disorder ("best guess") (Table 39–4).

B. "BEST GUESS"

Based on a best guess about the probable cause of the patient's infection, the physician should choose a drug (or drug combination) that is likely to be effective against the suspected microorganism.

C. LABORATORY CONTROL

Before beginning antimicrobial drug treatment, obtain meaningful specimens, if available, for laboratory examination to determine the causative infectious organism and, if appropriate, its susceptibility to antimicrobial drugs.

D. CLINICAL RESPONSE

Based on the clinical response of the patient, evaluate the laboratory reports and consider the desirability of changing the antimicrobial drug regimen. Laboratory results should not automatically overrule clinical judgment.

E. DRUG SUSCEPTIBILITY TESTS

Some microorganisms are uniformly susceptible to certain drugs; if such organisms are isolated from the patient, they need not be tested for drug susceptibility. For example, group A and B streptococci and clostridia respond predictably to penicillin. On the other hand, enteric gram-negative rods are sufficiently variable in their response to warrant drug susceptibility testing when they are isolated from a significant specimen.

Antimicrobial drug susceptibility tests may be done on solid media as "disk tests," in broth tubes, or in wells of microdilution plates. The latter method yields results usually expressed as MIC (minimal inhibitory concentration). In some infections, the MIC permits a better estimate of the amount of drug required for therapeutic effect in vivo. Disk tests usually indicate whether an isolate is susceptible or resistant to drug concentrations achieved in vivo with conventional dosage regimens, thus providing valuable guidance in selecting therapy.

When there appear to be marked discrepancies between in vitro test results and in vivo response, the following possibilities must be considered:

Table 39–1. Classification of beta-lactam and related antibiotics.

Group	Selected Members
Natural penicillins	Penicillin G, penicillin V
Antistaphylococcal penicillins	Methicillin, nafcillin, oxacillin, dicloxacillin
Aminopenicillins	Ampicillin, amoxicillin
Antipseudomonas penicillins	Carbenicillin, ticarcillin
Extended spectrum penicillins	Mezlocillin, piperacillin
Amidino penicillins	Mecillinam
Penicillin/ß-lactamase inhibitor combinations	Amoxicillin/clavulanic acid (Augmentin)
	Ticarcillin/clavulanic acid (Timentin)
	Ampicillin/sulbactam (Unasyn)
	Piperacillin/tazobactam (Zosyn)
First-generation cephalosporins	Cephalothin (Keflin)
	Cefazolin (Ancef, Kefzol)
	Cephalexin (Keflex)
	Cephradine (Velosef, Anspor)
	Cephapirin (Cefadyl)
	Cefadroxil (Duricef, Ultracef)
Second-generation cephalosporins	Cefamandole (Mandol)
	Cefoxitin (Mefoxin)
	Cefotetan (Cefotan)
	Cefuroxime (Zinacef)
	Cefaclor (Ceclor)
	Cefonacid (Monicid)
	Cefmetazole (Zefazone)
Third-generation cephalosporins	Cefotaxime (Claforan)
	Cefoperazone (Cefobid)
	Moxalactam (Moxam)
	Ceftizoxime (Ceftizox)
	Ceftriaxone (Rocephin)
	Ceftazadime (Fortaz)
	Cefixime (Suprax)
Carbapenems	Imipenem
Monobactam	Aztreonam

(1) Failure to drain a collection of pus or to remove a foreign body.

(2) Choice of inappropriate drug, dose, or route of administration.

(3) Failure of a poorly diffusing drug to reach the site of infection (eg, central nervous system) or to reach intracellular phagocytosed bacteria.

(4) Emergence of drug-resistant or tolerant organisms.

(5) Participation of two or more microorganisms in the infectious process, of which only one was originally detected and used for drug selection.

Table 39–2. Classification of antibiotics commonly used in obstetric-gynecologic practice and their adverse effects.

	Main Adverse Effect	
Antibiotic	Adult	Fetus
Penicillins	Allergic reaction	None known
Cephalosporins	Allergic reaction	None known
Monobactams Aztreonam	Rash, abnormal serum-transaminases	None known
Carbapenems Imipenem	Allergic reaction; seizures rarely	None known
Macrolides Erythromycins[1] Clarithromycin (Biaxin)	GI[2] Interaction with some antihistamines	None known
Azithromycin	GI	None known
Tetracyclines	GI, hepatotoxicity renal failure (rarely)	Discoloration of teeth; abnormal bone growth
Clindamycin	GI pseudomembranous colitis[3]	None known
Aminoglycoside Gentamicin	Oto- and nephrotoxicity, increased neuromuscular blockade	Ototoxicity reported with other aminoglycosides
Folate antagonists Trimethoprim-sulfamethoxazole	Rash, GI, allergic reaction	Possibly teratogenic due to inhibition of folate metabolism
Metronidazole	GI, alcohol intolerance, CNS at high doses	None known
Vancomycin	Allergic reaction; rare hearing loss; hypotension if given rapidly	None known
Quinolones	GI, headache, dizziness	Possible, due to inhibition of DNA gyrose

[1]Erythromycin esolate may be hepatotoxic.
[2]GI = gastrointestinal side effects.
[3]Pseudomembranous colitis may result from use of any antibiotic.

Table 39–3. Recommended and alternative drugs used to treat commonly encountered organisms in obstetric-gynecologic practice.

Suspected or Proved Etiologic Agent	Recommended Drug(s)	Alternative Drug(s)
Gram-negative cocci		
Gonococci	Cefixime, ceftriaxone, ciprofloxacin, oflox-acin	Spectinomycin, other single dose cephalosporins; other single dose quinolones (also treat *C trachomatis*)
Gram-positive cocci		
Pneumococci (*Streptococcus pneumoniae*)	Penicillin[1]	Vancomycin, clindamycin, clarithromycin
Streptococcus, hemolytic, groups A, C, G	Penicillin[1]	Erythromycin,[2] cephalosporin, clindamycin, vancomycin
Group B *Streptococcus*	Penicillin,[1] ampicillin	Erthromycin,[2] clindamycin, vancomycin, cephalosporins
Streptococcus viridans	Penicillin[1] ± aminoglycosides	Cephalosporin, vancomycin
Staphylococcus, penicillinase-producing	Penicillinase-resistant penicillin	Vancomycin, cephalosporin
Streptococcus faecalis	Ampicillin + aminoglycoside	Vancomycin
Gram-negative rods		
Acinetobacter (Mima-Herellea)	Aminoglycoside ± imipenem	TMP-SMX[3]
Bacteroides, oropharyngeal strains	Penicillin,[1] clindamycin	Metronidazole, cephalosporin
Bacteroides, gastrointestinal and pelvic strains	Metronidazole, clindamycin	Cefoxitin, chloramphenicol, cefotetan
Enterobacter	Newer cephalosporins	Aminoglycoside, TMP-SMX[3]
Escherichia coli (sepsis)	Aminoglycoside ± cephalosporin or extended spectrum penicillin	Some second- or third-generation cephalosporins, TMP-SMX[3]
Escherichia coli (first urinary tract infection)	TMP-SMX,[3] TMP	Cephalosporin, nitrofurantoin
Klebsiella	Newer cephalosporins, aminoglycoside	TMP-SMX[3]
Proteus mirabilis	Ampicillin, amoxicillin	Newer cephalosporins, aminoglycoside, TMP-SMX,[3] quinolones
Proteus vulgaris and other species	Newer cephalosporins	Aminoglycoside
Pseudomonas aeruginosa	Aminoglycoside + ticarcillin	Newer cephalosporins ± aminoglycoside
Serratia, Providencia	Newer cephalosporins, aminoglycoside	TMP-SMX[3]
Gram-positive rods		
Actinomyces	Penicillin[1]	Tetracycline[4]
Clostridium, (eg, gas gangrene, tetanus)	Penicillin,[1] clindamycin	Metronidazole
Listeria	Ampicillin ± aminoglycoside	TMP-SMX[3]
Mycoplasma	Tetracycline[4]	Erythromycin (for *U urealyticum*); Clindamycin (for *M hominis*)

± = alone or combined with.
[1]Penicillin G is preferred for parenteral injection; pencillin V for oral administration, to be used only in treating infections due to highly sensitive organisms.
[2]Erythromycin estolate is best absorbed orally but should be avoided in pregnancy because of risk of hepatotoxicity.
[3]TMP-SMX is a mixture of 1 part trimethoprim and 5 parts sulfamethoxazole.
[4]All tetracyclines have similar activity against microorganisms. Dosage is determined by rates of absorption and excretion of various preparations. Tetracyclines should not be used in pregnancy.

Table 39–4. Drugs used to treat suspected or proved infections.

Suspected or Proved Infection	Recommended Drug(s)	Alternative Drug(s)
Sexually Transmitted Infections		
Syphilis	Benzathine penicillin	A tetracycline
Genital herpes	Acyclovir, famciclovir, valacyclovir	
Gonorrhea	See Table 39–3	
C trachomatis	Azithromycin, tetracycline	Erythromycin, ofloxacin; amoxicillin or clindamycin in pregnancy
Pelvic inflammatory disease	Cefoxitin (or alternate) plus doxycycline OR clindamycin plus gentamicin for parenteral treatment; ofloxacin plus metronidazole OR ceftriaxone (or alternate) plus doxycylcline for oral treatment.	See CDC Guidelines for multiple alternatives.[1]
Vaginitis		
Trichomonas vaginalis	Metronidazole	
Candidiasis	Topical imidazoles; fluconazole	
Bacterial vaginosis	Metronidazole, clindamycin	
Obstetric Infection		
Puerperal endometritis	Clindamycin plus gentamicin	Several including cefoxitin or cefotetan; ampicillin plus sulbactam
Clinical chorioamnionitis	Ampicillin plus gentamcin, plus clindamycin if cesarean delivery	As for endometritis
Sepsis	Clindamycin plus gentamicin, plus ampicillin	Metronidazole plus gentamicin, plus ampicillin
Pyelonephritis, first episode	Ceftriaxone, TMS-SMX,[2] ofloxacin or ciprofloxicin	Third-generation cephalosporin
Urinary Tract Infection		
Recurrent	Ampicillin plus gentamicin	Same
Gynecologic Infection		
Posthysterectomy cuff infection	As for endometritis	As for endometritis
Abdominal wound infection	Drainage with or without antibiotics as for endometritis	

[1]Reproduced, with permission, from Centers for Disease Control and Prevention: 1998 Guidelines for Treatment of Sexually Transmitted Diseases. MMWR 1998;47:(RR-1).
[2]TMP-SMX is a mixture of 1 part trimethoprim and 5 parts sulfamethoxazole.

F. Adequate Dosage

To determine whether the proper drug is being used in adequate dosage, a serum assay may be performed. However, in obstetric-gynecologic practice, testing antibiotic levels is usually unnecessary except in selected cases of aminoglycoside use, such as in obese women, in women with renal insufficiency, in patients with longer courses (> 7 days), and in patients not responding to therapy.

G. Route of Administration

The absorption of oral penicillins, tetracyclines, erythromycin, etc, is impaired by food. Therefore, these oral drugs must be given between meals.

H. Duration of Antimicrobial Therapy

Generally speaking, effective antimicrobial treatment results in reversal of the clinical and laboratory parameters of active infection and marked clinical improvement within a few days. Treatment may, however, have to be continued for varying periods to effect cure. For instance, acute cystitis in women responds in just 1–3 days.

For most postoperative and postpartum infections, intravenous antibiotics may be discontinued after the patient has been afebrile for 48–72 hours. Furthermore, in most patients who respond promptly to such intravenous treatment, oral antibiotic therapy is unnecessary.

I. ADVERSE REACTIONS

The administration of antimicrobial drugs is occasionally associated with untoward reactions (see Table 39–2). These fall into several groups.

1. Hypersensitivity—The most common reactions are fever and skin rashes. Hematologic or hepatic disorders and anaphylaxis are rare.

2. Direct toxicity—Most common are nausea and vomiting and diarrhea. More serious toxic reactions are impairment of renal, hepatic, or hematopoietic functions or damage to the eighth nerve.

3. Suppression—Suppression of normal microbial flora and "superinfection" by drug-resistant microorganisms, or continued infection with the initial pathogen through the emergence of drug-resistant variants.

Oliguria, Impaired Renal Function, & Uremia

Oliguria, impaired renal function, and uremia have an important influence on antimicrobial drug dosage, since most of these drugs are excreted by the kidneys. Only minor adjustment in dosage or frequency of administration is necessary with renally excreted drugs when relatively nontoxic drugs (eg, penicillins) are used. On the other hand, aminoglycosides (gentamicin, tobramycin, amikacin, etc), tetracyclines, and vancomycin must be reduced in dosage or frequency of administration if toxicity is to be avoided in the presence of nitrogen retention. The administration of such drugs during renal failure should be guided by assay of drug concentration in serum.

Antimicrobial Drugs

PENICILLINS

The penicillins are a large group of antimicrobial substances, all of which share a common chemical nucleus (6-aminopenicillanic acid) that contains a β-lactam ring essential to their biologic activity (see Table 39–1). All β-lactam antibiotics inhibit formation of microbial cell walls. In particular, they block the final transpeptidation reaction in the synthesis of cell wall mucopeptide (peptidoglycan), and they activate autolytic enzymes in the cell wall. These reactions result in bacterial cell death.

One million units of penicillin G equal 0.6 g. Other penicillins are prescribed in grams. A blood level of 0.01–1 μg/mL of penicillin G or ampicillin is lethal for most susceptible gram-positive microorganisms. Most β-lactamase-resistant penicillins are 5–50 times less active against penicillin G-susceptible organisms.

Absorption, Distribution, & Excretion

After parenteral administration, absorption of most penicillins is complete and rapid. After oral administration, only a portion of the dose is absorbed (from {1/20} to {1/3}, depending on acid stability, binding to foods, and the presence of buffers). To minimize binding to foods, oral penicillins should not be preceded or followed by food for at least 1 hour.

After absorption, penicillins are widely distributed in body fluids and tissues. With parenteral doses of 3–6 g (5–10 million units) per 24 hours of any penicillin injected by continuous infusion or divided intramuscular injections, average serum levels of the drug reach 1–10 units (0.6–6 μg) per mL.

In many tissues, penicillin concentrations are equal to those in serum. Lower levels are found in the central nervous system. However, with active inflammation of the meninges, as in bacterial meningitis, penicillin levels in the cerebrospinal fluid exceed 0.2 μg/mL with a daily parenteral dose of 12 g.

Most of the absorbed penicillin is rapidly excreted by the kidneys into the urine—90% by tubular secretion. Tubular secretion can be partially blocked by probenecid, 0.5 g every 6 hours by mouth, to achieve higher systemic levels.

Renal excretion of penicillin results in very high levels in the urine. Thus, systemic daily doses of 6 g of penicillin may yield urine levels of 500–3000 μg/mL—enough to suppress not only gram-positive but also many gram-negative bacteria in the urine (provided they produce little β-lactamase).

Indications, Dosages, & Routes of Administration

The penicillins have been among the most effective and the most widely used antimicrobial drugs.

A. PENICILLIN G

In obstetric-gynecologic practice, this is the drug of choice for infections caused by group A and B streptococci, *Treponema pallidum,* aerobic gram-positive rods, clostridia, and *Actinomyces.*

Penicillin G is no longer used to treat gonococci because of widespread resistance. Enterococci are not susceptible to penicillin G alone, but are susceptible to a synergistic combination of penicillin G plus an aminoglycoside or, in milder infections (particularly in the urinary tract), to ampicillin alone.

1. Intramuscular or intravenous—Although most of the above-mentioned infections respond to aqueous penicillin G in daily doses of 0.6–5 million units administered by intermittent intramuscular injection, larger amounts (6–50 g daily) given by intermittent intravenous infusion are usually used. Sites for such intravenous administration are subject to thrombophlebitis and superinfection and must be rotated every 2–3 days. In enterococcal infections, an aminoglycoside is given simultaneously with large doses of a penicillin.

2. Oral—Penicillin V is indicated only in minor infections (eg, of the respiratory tract or its associated structures) in daily doses of 1–4 g (1.6–6.4 million units).

B. BENZATHINE PENICILLIN G

This penicillin is a salt of very low water solubility. It is injected intramuscularly to establish a depot that yields low but prolonged drug levels. An injection of 2.4 million units intramuscularly once a week for 1 or 3 weeks is the recommended treatment for early and late syphilis, respectively.

C. AMPICILLIN, AMOXICILLIN, CARBENICILLIN, TICARCILLIN, PIPERACILLIN, MEZLOCILLIN, AZLOCILLIN

These drugs have greater activity against gram-negative aerobes than penicillin G but are destroyed by penicillinases (β-lactamases).

Ampicillin can be given orally in divided doses, 2–3 g daily, to treat urinary tract infections with coliform bacteria, enterococci, or *Proteus mirabilis.* It is ineffective against *Enterobacter* and *Pseudomonas.* Amoxicillin, 500 mg every 8 hours, is similar to ampicillin but is better absorbed. Thus, it may be given at less frequent intervals.

Carbenicillin is more active against *Pseudomonas* and *Proteus,* but resistance emerges rapidly. Ticarcillin resembles carbenicillin but gives higher tissue levels. Because carbenicillin and ticarcillin also possess moderate activity against the wide array of bacteria involved in pelvic infections, they have been used with fairly good success as single-agent therapy. Carbenicillin indanyl sodium can be given orally for some urinary tract infections. Piperacillin resembles ticarcillin but is somewhat more active against some gram-negative aerobes, especially *Pseudomonas.* Mixtures of clavulanic acid with amoxicillin or ticarcillin are somewhat protected against destruction by β-lactamases and have been used for treatment of some lactamase producers, eg, *Haemophilus influenzae.*

D. β-LACTAMASE-RESISTANT PENICILLINS

Cloxacillin, nafcillin, and others are relatively resistant to destruction by β-lactamase. The main indication for the use of these drugs is infection by β-lactamase-producing staphylococci.

1. Oral—Oxacillin, cloxacillin, dicloxacillin, or nafcillin may be given in doses of 0.25–0.5 g every 4–6 hours in mild or localized staphylococcal infections. Food markedly interferes with absorption.

2. Intravenous—For serious systemic staphylococcal infections, nafcillin, 6–12 g, is given intravenously, by adding 1–2 g every 2 hours to a continuous infusion of 5% dextrose in water.

E. COMBINATIONS OF PENICILLINS PLUS β-LACTAMASE INHIBITORS

Because of their wide spectrum of activity against bacteria involved in pelvic infections, these combinations have been successful in many circumstances, particularly pelvic infections. For example, ampicillin plus sulbactam (Unasyn), 3 g every 6 hours, or carbenicillin plus clavulanic acid (Timentin), 3.1 g every 6 hours, may be the regimen given in such polymicrobial infections (Table 39–1).

Adverse Effects

Most of the serious side effects of the penicillins are due to hypersensitivity.

A. ALLERGY

All penicillins are cross-sensitizing and cross-reacting. In general, sensitization occurs in direct proportion to the duration and total dose of penicillin received in the past. Skin tests with penicilloylpolylysine, with alkaline hydrolysis products (minor antigen determinants), and with undegraded penicillin can identify many hypersensitive individuals. Among positive reactors to skin tests, the incidence of subsequent immediate (IgE-mediated) penicillin reactions is high. Although many persons develop IgG antibodies to antigenic determinants of penicillin, the presence of such antibodies is not correlated with allergic reactivity (except rare hemolytic anemia). A history of a penicillin reaction in the past is not reliable; however, in such cases the drug should be administered with caution; ie, have available an artificial airway, 1% epinephrine in a syringe, running intravenous fluids, and competent personnel standing by, or a substitute drug should be given.

Allergic reactions may occur as anaphylactic shock, serum sickness-type reactions (urticaria, fever, joint swelling, angioneurotic edema, intense pruritus, and respiratory embarrassment occurring 7–12 days after exposure), skin rashes, oral lesions, fever, nephritis, eosinophilia, hemolytic anemia and other hematologic disturbances, and vasculitis. The incidence of hypersensitivity to penicillin is estimated to be 3–5% among adults. Acute anaphylactic life-threatening reactions are fortunately very rare (0.05%). Ampicillin produces skin rashes (mononucleosis-like) 3–5 times more frequently than other penicillins, but some ampicillin rashes are not allergic. Methicillin and other penicillins can induce interstitial nephritis; nafcillin is less nephrotoxic than methicillin. In circumstances where penicillin is the clear drug of choice and where alternatives are likely to be less effective, an oral desensitization protocol may be employed safely. One such indication would be in the treatment of a patient with syphilis. One widely used protocol is to employ penicillin G suspensions starting at 100 units and giving incremental doses at 15-minute intervals.

B. TOXICITY

Since the action of penicillin is directed against a unique bacterial structure, the cell wall, it is virtually without effect on animal cells. The toxic effects of penicillin G are due to the direct irritation caused by intramuscular or intravenous injection of exceedingly high concentrations (eg, 1 g/mL). A patient receiving more than 50 g of penicillin G daily parenterally may exhibit signs of cerebrocortical irritation as a result of the passage of large amounts of penicillin into the central nervous system. With doses of this magnitude, direct cation toxicity (Na^+, K^+) can also occur. Potassium penicillin G contains 1.7 mEq of K^+ per million units (2.7 mEq/g), and potassium may accumulate in the presence of renal failure. Carbenicillin contains 4.7 mEq of Na^+ per gram—a risk in heart failure.

Large doses of penicillins given orally may lead to gastrointestinal upset, particularly nausea and diarrhea. These symptoms are most marked with oral ampicillin or amoxicillin. Oral therapy may also be accompanied by luxuriant overgrowth of staphylococci, *Pseudomonas, Proteus,* or yeasts, which may occasionally cause enteritis. Penicillins have caused pseudomembranous colitis. Superinfections in other organ systems may occur. Carbenicillin and ticarcillin may damage platelet function, cause bleeding, or result in hypokalemic alkalosis.

CEPHALOSPORINS

The cephalosporins are structurally related to the penicillins. They consist of a β-lactam ring attached to a dihydrothiazoline ring. Substitutions of chemical groups at various positions on the basic structure have resulted in a proliferation of drugs with varying pharmacologic properties and antimicrobial activities.

The mechanism of action of cephalosporins is analogous to that of the penicillins: (1) binding to specific penicillin-binding proteins that serve as drug receptors on bacteria, (2) inhibition of cell wall synthesis, and (3) activation of autolytic enzymes in the cell wall that result in bacterial death.

Cephalosporins have been divided into 3 major groups or "generations," based mainly on their antibacterial activity (see Table 39–1). First-generation cephalosporins have good activity against aerobic gram-positive organisms and many community-acquired

gram-negative organisms; second-generation drugs have a slightly extended spectrum against gram-negative bacteria, and some are active against anaerobes; and third-generation cephalosporins have less activity against gram-positives but are extremely active against most gram-negative bacteria. Not all cephalosporins fit neatly into this grouping, and there are exceptions to the general characterization of the drugs in the individual classes; however, the generational classification of cephalosporins is useful for discussion purposes.

1. First-Generation Cephalosporins

Antimicrobial Activity

These drugs are very active against gram-positive cocci, including pneumococci, viridans streptococci, group A and B streptococci, and *Staphylococcus aureus*. Like all cephalosporins, they are inactive against enterococci and methicillin-resistant staphylococci. Among gram-negative bacteria, *Escherichia coli*, *Klebsiella pneumoniae*, and *Proteus mirabilis* are usually sensitive except for some hospital-acquired strains. There is no activity against such gram-negatives as *Pseudomonas aeruginosa*, indole-positive *Proteus* spp., *Enterobacter* spp., *Serratia marcescens*, *Citrobacter* spp., and *Acinetobacter* spp. Anaerobic cocci are usually sensitive, but most *Bacteroides* species are not.

Pharmacokinetics & Administration

A. ORAL

Cephalexin, cephradine, and cefadroxil are absorbed from the gut to a variable extent. After a 500-mg oral dose, serum levels range from 15 to 20 μg/mL. Urine concentrations are usually very high, but in other tissues the levels are variable and usually lower than in the serum. Cephalexin and cephradine are given orally in doses of 0.25–0.5 g 4 times daily (15–30 mg/kg/d). Cefadroxil can be given in doses of 0.5–1 g twice daily.

Dosage should be reduced in renal insufficiency: for Cl_{cr} 20–50 mL/min, give half the normal dose; for Cl_{cr} < 20 mL/min, give one-fourth the normal dose.

B. INTRAVENOUS

Cefazolin has a longer half-life than cephalothin or cephapirin. After an intravenous infusion of 1 g, the peak serum level of cefazolin is 90–120 μg/mL, whereas cephalothin and cephapirin reach levels of 40–60 μg/mL. The usual doses of cefazolin for adults are 1–2 g intravenously every 8 hours (50–100 mg/kg/d) and for cephalothin and cephapirin 1–2 g every 4–6 hours (50–200 mg/kg/d). In patients with impaired renal function, dosage adjustment as for oral dosage is needed.

C. INTRAMUSCULAR

Both cephapirin and cefazolin can be given intramuscularly, and pain on injection is less with cefazolin.

Clinical Uses

Although the first-generation cephalosporins have a broad spectrum of activity and are relatively nontoxic, they are rarely the drugs of choice. Oral drugs are indicated for treatment of urinary infections in patients who are allergic to TMP-SMX or penicillins, and they can be used for minor staphylococcal infections in penicillin-allergic patients. Oral cephalosporins may also be preferred for minor polymicrobial infections (eg, cellulitis, soft tissue abscess).

Intravenous first-generation cephalosporins penetrate most tissues well and are among the drugs of choice for gynecologic and cesarean section prophylaxis. More expensive second- and third-generation cephalosporins offer no advantage over the first-generation drugs for surgical prophylaxis and should not be used for that purpose.

Other major uses of intravenous first-generation cephalosporins include infections for which they are the least toxic drugs (eg, *Klebsiella* infections) and infections in persons with a history of mild penicillin allergy (not anaphylaxis).

2. Second-Generation Cephalosporins

Second-generation cephalosporins are a heterogeneous group with marked individual differences in activity, pharmacokinetics, and toxicity. In general, all of them are active against organisms also covered by first-generation drugs, but they have an extended gram-negative coverage. Indole-positive *Proteus* and *Klebsiella* spp. (including cephalothin-resistant strains) are usually sensitive. In addition, cefoxitin and cefotetan are active against *Bacteroides fragilis,* other gram-negative anaerobes, and some strains of *Serratia* but have poor activity against *Enterobacter* and *H influenzae.* Against gram-positive organisms, these drugs are less active than the first-generation cephalosporins. Like the latter, second-generation drugs have no activity against *P aeruginosa* or enterococci.

Pharmacokinetics & Administration

After an intravenous infusion of 1 g, serum levels range from 75–125 μg/mL. Because of differences in drug half-life and protein binding, intervals between doses vary greatly. For cefoxitin (short half-life), the interval is 4–6 hours; cefoxitin, 50–200 mg/kg/d.

Drugs with longer half-lives can be injected less frequently: cefotetan, 1–2 mg every 8–12 hours; and cefonicid or ceforanide, 1–2 g (15–30 mg/kg/d) once or twice daily. In renal failure, dosage adjustments are required.

Clinical Uses

Because of their activity against anaerobes, cefoxitin and cefotetan are widely used to treat polymicrobial obstetric and gynecologic infections. They are not more effective than first-generation cephalosporins for perioperative prophylaxis, and they are more expensive.

3. Third-Generation Cephalosporins

Antimicrobial Activity

These drugs are active against staphylococci (not methicillin-resistant strains) but less so than first-generation cephalosporins. They have no activity against enterococci but inhibit nonenterococcal streptococci. Most of these drugs are active against *N gonorrhoeae.* A major advantage of the new cephalosporins is their expanded gram-negative coverage. In addition to organisms inhibited by other cephalosporins, they are consistently active against *Enterobacter* spp., *Citrobacter freundii, S marcescens, Providencia* spp., *Haemophilus* spp., and *Neisseria* spp., including β-lactamase-producing strains. Two drugs—ceftazidime and cefoperazone—have good activity against *P aeruginosa,* whereas the others inhibit only 40–60% of strains. *Listeria* spp., *Acinetobacter* spp., and non-*aeruginosa* strains of *Pseudomonas* are variably sensitive to third-generation cephalosporins. Only ceftizoxime and moxalactam have good activity against *B fragilis.* Several of these drugs have relatively long half-lives.

Pharmacokinetics & Administration

After an intravenous infusion of 1 g, serum levels of these drugs range from 60 to 140 μg/mL. They penetrate well into body fluids and tissues. The half-life of these drugs is variable: ceftriaxone, 7–8 hours; cefoperazone, 2 hours; the others, 1–1.7 hours. Consequently, ceftriaxone can be injected every 12–24 hours in a dose of 15–30 mg/kg/d (or 30–50 mg/kg every 12 hours in adult meningitis and 50 mg/kg every 12 hours in infants). Cefoperazone can be given every 8–12 hours in a dose of 25–100 mg/kg/d, and the other drugs of the group every 6–8 hours in doses ranging from 2 to 12 g/d depending on the severity of the infection. Cefoperazone and ceftriaxone are eliminated primarily by biliary excretion, and no dosage adjustment is required in renal insufficiency. The other drugs are eliminated by the kidney and thus require dosage adjustments in renal insufficiency.

Clinical Uses

Ceftriaxone 250 mg intramuscularly and cefixime 400 mg orally are two recommended regimens for treating uncomplicated gonorrhea. They are combined with doxycycline or azithromycin for cotreatment of chlamydia.

In obstetric-gynecologic practice, these agents have been used to treat urinary infection.

ADVERSE EFFECTS OF CEPHALOSPORINS

Allergy

Cephalosporins are sensitizing, and a variety of hypersensitivity reactions occur, including anaphylaxis, fever, skin rashes, nephritis, granulocytopenia, and hemolytic anemia. The incidence of cross-allergy between cephalosporins and penicillins is not certainly known but is estimated to be about 6–10%. Persons with a history of anaphylaxis to penicillins should not receive cephalosporins.

Toxicity

Local pain can occur after intramuscular injection, or thrombophlebitis after intravenous injection. Hypoprothrombinemia is a potential adverse effect of cephalosporins that have a methylthiotetrazole group (eg, cefamandole, moxalactam, cefoperazone), but these are infrequently used in ob/gyn practice.

Superinfection

Many newer cephalosporins have little activity against gram-positive organisms, particularly staphylococci and enterococci. Superinfection with these organisms—as well as with fungi—may occur. Pseudomembranous colitis has occurred with use of these antibiotics.

NEW BETA-LACTAM DRUGS

Monobactams

Monobactams are drugs with a monocyclic β-lactam ring, which are resistant to β-lactamases and are active against gram-negative organisms (including *Pseudomonas*) but not against gram-positive organisms or anaerobes. Aztreonam resembles aminoglycosides in activity. The usual dose is 1–2 g intravenously every 6–8 hours. Clinical uses of aztreonam alone are limited because of the availability of third-generation cephalosporins with a broader spectrum of activity and minimal toxicity. However, in combination with a drug such as clindamycin, aztreonam provides a regimen with a broad activity and appears equivalent to clindamycin-gentamicin in efficacy. Although aztreonam has potentially less toxicity than gentamicin, gentamicin is much less expensive, and the majority of obstetric-gynecologic patients are at low risk for gentamicin toxicity. The place of aztreonam remains limited.

Carbapenems

This class of drugs is structurally related to β-lactam antibiotics. Imipenem, the first drug of this type, has a wide spectrum with good activity against many gram-negative rods, gram-positive organisms, and anaerobes. It is resistant to β-lactamases but is inactivated by dipeptidases in renal tubules. Consequently, it must be combined with cilastatin, a dipeptidase inhibitor, for clinical use.

The half-life of imipenem is 1 hour. Penetration into body tissues and fluids, including the cerebrospinal fluid, is good. The usual dose is 0.5–1 g intravenously every 6 hours. Dosage adjustment is required in renal insufficiency. Because imipenem has an unusual spectrum, it should be reserved for special cases such as treatment of highly resistant organisms. It should not be used as a first-line treatment for pelvic infections.

The most common adverse effects of imipenem are nausea, vomiting, diarrhea, reactions at the infusion site, and skin rashes. Seizures can occur in patients with renal failure. Patients allergic to penicillins may be allergic to imipenem as well.

ERYTHROMYCIN GROUP

The erythromycins inhibit protein synthesis and are bacteriostatic or bactericidal against gram-positive organisms in concentrations of 0.02–2 µg/mL. *Chlamydia, Ureaplasma urealyticum, Legionella,* and *Campylobacter* are also susceptible. Activity is enhanced at alkaline pH.

Erythromycins are the drugs of choice in chlamydial infections or in pneumonia caused by mycoplasmas or *Legionella.* They are useful as substitutes for penicillin in persons who are allergic to penicillin and for tetracyclines in pregnancy in the treatment of *Chlamydia* and *Ureaplasma.* Erythromycin preparations may also be used parenterally for prophylaxis of group B streptococcal infection in patients with penicillin allergy. Even though these drugs are listed as alternatives, the likelihood of resistance to group B streptococci is recently being reported as up to 15%.

Dosages

A. ORAL

Erythromycin base, stearate, or estolate, 0.25–0.5 g every 6 hours (for children, 40 mg/kg/d), or erythromycin ethylsuccinate, 0.4–0.6 g every 6 hours. The estolate derivative should not be used during pregnancy since it causes hepatic enzyme elevations.

B. INTRAVENOUS

Erythromycin lactobionate, 0.5 g every 6 hours.

Adverse Effects

Nausea and vomiting and diarrhea may occur after oral intake. Erythromycin estolate probably more than the other salts can produce acute cholestatic hepatitis (fever, jaundice, impaired liver function) because of hypersensitivity. Most patients recover completely.

AZITHROMYCIN

Azithromycin is the first of the azalide antibiotics that are chemically similar to the macrolides such as erythromycin. With excellent in vitro activity against *C trachomatis* and with favorable kinetics including sustained high concentration in tissue (even though serum concentrations are low), azithromycin (1 g orally once) has been as effective as doxycycline (100 mg twice daily for 7 days), 97% versus 95%, respectively, in treating chlamydia urethritis and cervicitis. Side effects were similar, mainly gastrointestinal, and were mild to moderate. Accordingly, azithromycin has become one of the recommended regimens for treatment of chlamydial infection as a 1-g dose given orally. In pregnancy, the 1-g dose of azithromycin is an alternative regimen to the recommended regimens in pregnancy of erythromycin base or amoxicillin. Because this 1-g dose of azithromycin is not adequate for treating gonorrhea, cotreatment with single-dose ceftriaxone (250 mg intramuscularly) is necessary.

CLINDAMYCIN

Clindamycin resembles erythromycin and is active against gram-positive organisms (except enterococci). Clindamycin, 0.15–0.3 g orally every 6 hours yields serum concentrations of 2–5 µg/mL. The drug is widely distributed in tissues. Excretion is through the bile and urine. It is an alternative to erythromycin as a substitute for penicillin. Clindamycin is a recommended alternative to penicillin G for group B streptococcal prophylaxis. It is also effective against most strains of *Bacteroides* and is an excellent drug in polymicrobial aerobic-anaerobic infections, when used in combination with an aminoglycoside. Seriously ill patients are given clindamycin intravenously during a 1-hour period, 900 mg every 8 hours. Vaginal clindamycin cream, when used nightly (5–7 mL) is highly effective in treating bacterial vaginosis.

Common side effects are diarrhea, nausea, and skin rashes. Impaired liver function and neutropenia have been noted. If 3–4 g is given rapidly intravenously, cardiorespiratory arrest may occur. Pseudomembranous colitis has been associated with clindamycin administration. This is due to necrotizing toxin produced by *Clostridium difficile*, which is clindamycin-resistant and increases in the gut with the selection pressure exerted by administration of this drug. *C difficile* is sensitive to vancomycin and metronidazole, and the colitis rapidly regresses during oral treatment with metronidazole, which is preferred to vancomycin because of its lower cost.

TETRACYCLINE GROUP

The tetracyclines have common basic chemical structures, antimicrobial activity, and pharmacologic properties. Microorganisms resistant to one tetracycline show cross-resistance to all tetracyclines.

Antimicrobial Activity

Tetracyclines are inhibitors of protein synthesis and are bacteriostatic for many gram-positive and gram-negative bacteria. They are strongly inhibitory for the growth of mycoplasmas, rickettsiae, chlamydiae, and some protozoa (eg, amebas). Equal concentrations of all tetracyclines in blood or tissue have approximately equal antimicrobial activity. However, there are great differences in the susceptibility of different strains of a given species of microorganism, and laboratory tests are therefore important. Because of the emergence of resistant strains, tetracyclines have lost some of their former usefulness against gram-negative and gram-positive bacteria, but they have ongoing usefulness in treating sexually transmitted organisms. Tetracyclines alone are no longer considered adequate therapy for gonorrhea, but are recommended for chlamydia.

Absorption, Distribution, & Excretion

Tetracyclines are absorbed somewhat irregularly from the gut. Absorption is limited by the low solubility of the drugs and by chelation with divalent cations, eg, Ca^{2+} or Fe^{2+}. A large proportion (80%) of orally administered tetracycline remains in the gut lumen, modifies intestinal flora, and is excreted in feces. With full systemic doses (2 g/d), levels of active drug in serum reach 2–10 µg/mL. Tetracyclines are specifically deposited in growing bones and teeth, bound to calcium.

Absorbed tetracyclines are excreted mainly in bile and urine. Up to 20% of oral doses may appear in the urine after glomerular filtration. With renal failure, doses of tetracyclines must be reduced or intervals between doses increased.

Minocycline and doxycycline are well absorbed from the gut but are excreted more slowly than others, leading to accumulation and prolonged blood levels. Doxycycline does not accumulate greatly in renal failure.

Indications, Dosages, & Routes of Administration

Tetracyclines are the drugs of choice in chlamydial and genital mycoplasmal infections.

A. Oral

Tetracycline hydrochloride is dispensed in 250-mg capsules. Give 0.25–0.5 g orally every 6 hours. Doxycycline, 100 mg twice daily, is as effective as tetracycline hydrochloride, 2 g/d.

B. Intravenous

Several tetracyclines are formulated for parenteral administration in individuals unable to take oral medication. The dose is generally similar to the oral dose (see manufacturer's instructions).

Adverse Effects

A. Allergy

Hypersensitivity reactions with fever or skin rashes are uncommon.

B. Gastrointestinal Side Effects

Gastrointestinal side effects are common. These can be diminished by reducing the dose or by administering tetracyclines with food. After a few days of oral use, the gut flora is modified so that drug-resistant bacteria and yeasts become prominent. This may cause functional gut disturbances, anal pruritus, and even enterocolitis.

C. Bones and Teeth

Tetracyclines are bound to calcium deposited in growing bones and teeth, causing fluorescence, discoloration, enamel dysplasia, deformity, or growth inhibition. Tetracyclines are contraindicated in pregnant women.

D. Liver Damage

Tetracyclines can impair hepatic function or even cause liver necrosis, particularly during pregnancy, in the presence of preexisting liver damage, or with doses of more than 3 g intravenously.

E. Kidney Damage

Outdated tetracycline preparations have been implicated in renal tubular acidosis and other renal damage.

Tetracyclines may increase blood urea nitrogen when diuretics are administered.

F. Other

Tetracyclines, principally demeclocycline, may induce photosensitization, especially in fair-complected individuals. Intravenous injection may cause thrombophlebitis, and intramuscular injection may induce local inflammation with pain. Minocycline causes vestibular reactions (dizziness, vertigo, nausea) in 30–60% of cases after doses of 200 mg daily.

AMINOGLYCOSIDES

This group includes widely used drugs such as gentamicin and tobramycin. These agents inhibit protein synthesis in bacteria by attaching to and inhibiting the function of the 30S subunit of the bacterial ribosome. Anaerobic bacteria are resistant to aminoglycosides because transport across the cell membrane is an oxygen-dependent energy-requiring process.

All aminoglycosides are potentially ototoxic and nephrotoxic, although to different degrees. All can accumulate in renal failure; therefore, dosage adjustments must be made in uremia.

Aminoglycosides are used widely against presumed or established gram-negative enteric bacteria. In the treatment of bacteremia or endocarditis caused by fecal streptococci or by some gram-negative bacteria, the aminoglycoside is given together with a penicillin to enhance permeability and facilitate the entry of the aminoglycoside.

General Properties of Aminoglycosides

A. Physical Properties

Aminoglycosides are water soluble and stable in solution. If they are mixed in solution with β-lactam antibiotics, they may form complexes and lose some activity. Aminoglycosides may be mixed with clindamycin in IV solutions.

B. Absorption, Distribution, Metabolism, and Excretion

Aminoglycosides are well absorbed after intramuscular or intravenous injection but are not absorbed from the gut. They are distributed widely in tissues and penetrate pleural, peritoneal, or joint fluid in the presence of inflammation. They accumulate in amniotic fluid, but not for 6 hours after maternal injection. They enter the central nervous system to only a slight extent after parenteral administration. There is no significant metabolic breakdown of aminoglycosides. The serum half-life is 2–3 hours; excretion is mainly by glomerular filtration. Urine levels are 10–50 times higher than serum levels.

C. DOSE AND EFFECT IN CASES OF IMPAIRED RENAL FUNCTION

In the past, the dose of gentamicin for a person with normal renal function was 3–7 mg/kg per day divided in three equal injections every 8 hours. In the past several years, dosing every 24 hours has become the regimen that is usually recommended. The usual dose of gentamicin is 4.0–5.0 mg/kg intravenously once daily, in an infusion given over a 30-minute period. Reasons for the once daily administration of gentamicin are that there is potentially less toxicity, there is less cost, and there is equivalent efficacy clinically. In persons with impaired renal function, excretion is diminished and the dosing interval may be prolonged beyond 24 hours.

Because of the increased glomerular filtration rate in pregnancy and the subsequent rapid excretion of aminoglycosides in pregnancy, doses greater than 5 mg/kg every 24 hours may be necessary. When 24-hour dosing is used, especially in seriously ill patients, gentamicin levels are usually determined and plotted on a nomogram to ascertain appropriateness of the dose. Studies of gentamicin in postpartum individuals have been carried out, but there have been few studies of 24-hour dosing of gentamicin during pregnancy. Accordingly, many clinicians prefer to continue to use dosing at 8-hour intervals for gentamicin in the pregnant patient.

D. ADVERSE EFFECTS

All aminoglycosides can cause varying degrees of ototoxicity and nephrotoxicity. Ototoxicity can present either as hearing loss (cochlear damage) that is noted first as a deficiency in hearing high frequencies or as vestibular damage, as evidenced by vertigo, ataxia, and loss of balance.

In very high doses, aminoglycosides can be neurotoxic, producing a curare-like effect with neuromuscular blockage that results in respiratory paralysis. This has been most common in gynecologic surgery when solutions containing aminoglycosides have been used for peritoneal irrigation. Calcium gluconate or neostigmine can serve as antidote. Rarely, aminoglycosides cause hypersensitivity and local reactions.

1. Gentamicin

Gentamicin is the most widely used aminoglycoside antibiotic on obstetric-gynecologic services. In concentrations of 0.5–5 µg/mL, gentamicin is bactericidal not only for staphylococci and coliform organisms but also for many strains of *Pseudomonas, Proteus,* and *Serratia.* Enterococci are resistant to gentamicin alone, but are susceptible to gentamicin plus a penicillin. With doses of 3–7 mg/kg/d, serum levels reach 3–8 µg/mL. Gentamicin may be synergistic with ticarcillin against *Pseudomonas.* However, the two drugs should not be mixed in vitro.

Indications, Dosages, & Routes of Administration

Gentamicin is used in severe infections caused by gram-negative bacteria, including *Klebsiella-Enterobacter, Proteus, Pseudomonas,* and *Serratia.* The dosage is usually 4–5 mg/kg every 24 hours in a single IV infusion. It is necessary to monitor renal function by checking serum creatinine every few days and to reduce the dosage or lengthen the interval between doses if renal function declines. About 2–3% of patients develop vestibular dysfunction and loss of hearing when peak serum levels exceed 10 µg/mL. Serum concentrations should be monitored in selected circumstances.

2. Tobramycin

Tobramycin is an aminoglycoside that closely resembles gentamicin in antibacterial activity and pharmacologic properties and exhibits partial cross-resistance. Tobramycin may be effective against some gentamicin-resistant gram-negative bacteria, especially *Pseudomonas.* Tobramycin may be less nephrotoxic than gentamicin; their ototoxicity is similar.

SPECTINOMYCIN

Spectinomycin is an aminocyclitol antibiotic, related to the aminoglycosides. Its sole indication is for the treatment of β-lactamase–producing gonococci or gonorrhea in a penicillin-hypersensitive person. One injection of 2 g (40 mg/kg) is given. There usually is pain at the injection site, and there may be nausea and fever.

SULFONAMIDES-TRIMETHOPRIM

The combination of sulfonamides, particularly sulfamethoxazole with trimethoprim, offers a combination of two folic acid antagonists which is useful under a number of circumstances. These indications are as follows:

(1) Urinary tract infection: Many coliform organisms that are the most common causes of urinary tract infections are susceptible to the combination of trimethoprim-sulfamethoxazole (TMP-SMX). For lower urinary tract infection TMP-SMX, 160/800 mg, is often given every 12 hours for a 3-day regimen. For uncomplicated pyelonephritis in women who do not have evidence of sepsis, TMP-SMX, 160/800 mg, may be

given orally every 12 hours for 10–14 days. Women who have pyelonephritis requiring hospitalization may be treated with TMP-SMX, 160/800 mg intravenously every 12 hours until the patient is able to tolerate oral nourishment and oral therapy, which should be continued to complete a 10- to 14-day course.

(2) Parasitic diseases: The combination of trimethoprim with sulfamethoxazole is often effective for prophylaxis or treatment of *Pneumocystis carinii* pneumonia. The combination of pyrimethamine with sulfadiazine is used in the treatment of toxoplasmosis. It should be given in combination with folinic acid in pregnant women.

(3) Sexually transmitted diseases: Sulfonamides are no longer considered as drugs to treat *Chlamydia trachomatis.*

Because trimethoprim and sulfonamides are both folate antagonists, there is a hypothetical possibility of teratogenesis. Accordingly, this combination should be avoided in the first trimester of pregnancy. Sulfonamides may lead to hemolysis in persons with G6PD enzyme deficiency. Sulfonamides also compete with bilirubin for binding sites. Accordingly, long-acting sulfonamides should be avoided at term in order to avoid the unusual complication of low-level kernicterus in the newborn infant. These infants do not develop hyperbilirubinemia, but they do develop kernicterus at low levels of bilirubin because of displacement of bilirubin from its binding sites to free bilirubin.

Adverse Effects

Sulfonamides produce a wide variety of side effects—due partly to hypersensitivity, partly to direct toxicity—which must be considered whenever unexplained symptoms or signs occur in a patient who may have received these drugs. Except in the mildest reactions, fluids should be forced and, if symptoms and signs progressively increase, the drugs should be discontinued.

A. Systemic Side Effects

Side effects may include fever, skin rashes, urticaria; nausea and vomiting or diarrhea; stomatitis, conjunctivitis, arthritis, exfoliative dermatitis; hematopoietic disturbances, including thrombocytopenia, hemolytic (in G6PD deficiency) or aplastic anemia, granulocytopenia, leukemoid reactions; hepatitis, polyarteritis nodosa, vasculitis, Stevens-Johnson syndrome; psychosis; and many others.

B. Urinary Tract Disturbances

Sulfonamides may precipitate in urine, especially at neutral or acid pH, producing hematuria, crystalluria, or even obstruction. They have also been implicated in

various types of nephritis and nephrosis. Sulfonamides and methenamine salts should not be given together.

Precautions in the Use of Sulfonamides

(1) There is cross-allergenicity among all sulfonamides. Obtain a history of past administration or reaction. Observe for possible allergic responses.

(2) Keep the urine volume above 1500 mL/d by forcing fluids. Check urine pH—it should be 7.5 or higher. Give alkali by mouth (sodium bicarbonate or equivalent, 5–15 g/d). Examine fresh urine for crystals and red cells every 5–7 days.

(3) Check hemoglobin, white blood cell count, and differential count once weekly to detect possible disturbances early in high-risk patients.

METRONIDAZOLE

Metronidazole is an antiprotozoal drug that also is active against most anaerobes, including *Bacteroides* species. Metronidazole is well absorbed after oral administration and is widely distributed. The drug is metabolized in the liver, and dosage reduction is required in the presence of hepatic insufficiency. Metronidazole can also be given intravenously or by rectal suppository, with serum levels equivalent for both routes. It is used to treat amebiasis and also the following:

(1) *Trichomonas* vaginitis: The recommended dose is 2 g orally (single dose). The alternative is 500 mg twice a day for 7 days. Both sexual partners should be treated.

(2) Bacterial vaginosis: Recommended regimens for nonpregnant women are 500 mg orally 2 times daily for 7 days or vaginal gel 0.75%, 5 g vaginally twice a day for 5 days. Single-dose treatment is less effective, and treatment of sexual partners is not recommended since this does not decrease recurrences in the female.

(3) In anaerobic or mixed infections, metronidazole can be given intravenously, 500 mg 3 times daily.

(4) For pseudomembranous colitis, give 500 mg 3 times daily orally.

Adverse effects of metronidazole include stomatitis, nausea, diarrhea, and disulfiram-like reactions. With prolonged use, peripheral neuropathy may develop.

VANCOMYCIN

Vancomycin is bactericidal for most gram-positive organisms, particularly staphylococci. Resistant mutants had been rare, but since the late 1980s development of vancomycin-resistant enterococci has become a major cause for concern. In many institutions, policies for control of use of vancomycin have been developed. Vancomycin is an alternative to metronidazole in the treatment of pseudomembranous colitis. For this indication, it is given 2 g/d orally, but metronidazole is preferred because it is less expensive and because of the concern that oral vancomycin may lead to increased selection pressure for vancomycin-resistant enterococci in the gut. For systemic effect, the drug must be administered intravenously. After intravenous infusion of 0.5 g over a period of 20 minutes, blood levels of 10 μg/mL are maintained for 1–2 hours. Vancomycin is excreted mainly through the kidneys, but may accumulate in the kidneys in the event of liver failure. In renal insufficiency, the half-life may be up to 8 days. Thus, only 1 dose of 0.5–1 g may be given every 4–8 days to a uremic individual undergoing hemodialysis.

The only indications for parenteral vancomycin are serious staphylococcal infection or enterococcal endocarditis (in combination with an aminoglycoside). Vancomycin, 0.5 g, is infused intravenously over a 20-minute period every 6–8 hours (for children, 20–40 mg/kg/d).

Vancomycin is irritating to tissues; chills, fever, and thrombophlebitis sometimes follow intravenous injection. Rapid infusion may result in diffuse hyperemia (red man syndrome); this can be avoided by giving infusions over 1 hour. Vancomycin is sometimes ototoxic and (perhaps) nephrotoxic.

QUINOLONES

Quinolones are synthetic analogs of nalidixic acid and are active against many gram-positive and gram-negative bacteria. All quinolones inhibit bacterial DNA synthesis by blocking the enzyme DNA gyrase. The earlier quinolones (nalidixic acid, oxolinic acid, cinoxacin) did not achieve systemic antibacterial levels and thus were useful only as urinary antiseptics. The newer fluoroquinolones (eg, norfloxacin, ciprofloxacin, enoxacin, oxofloxacin, pefloxacin, levofloxacin, and trovafloxacin) have greater antibacterial activity, achieve clinically useful levels in blood and tissues, and have low toxicity. They are active against a wide variety of aerobic bacteria, and some members of this group are active against clinically important anaerobes. After oral administration, these newer fluoroquinolones are well absorbed and widely distributed, with a serum half-life of 3–8 hours. They are excreted mainly by tubular renal secretion or glomerular filtration. Up to 20% of the dose is metabolized by the liver.

Indications for fluoroquinolones have been developed over the last few years, and are as follows:

(1) Urinary tract infection: Use of quinolones should be reserved for infection due to organisms resistant to first-line treatment with nitrofurantoin, trimethoprim, and trimethoprim/sulfamethoxazole. Quinolones should be used when resistant organisms are suspected (eg, for treatment of documented resistant strains), treatment failures, recurrent infection, or infection in patients with allergy to preferred drugs of choice. For complicated pyelonephritis, an oral quinolone may be used. For women with evidence of sepsis requiring hospitalization, a regimen including a fluoroquinolone may be used. For example, ofloxacin or ciprofloxacin in a dose of 200–400 mg IV every 12 hours may be used until the patient's course improves. Thereafter, when the patient may take oral nourishment, oral therapy should be started and continued to complete a 10- to 14-day course.

(2) Fluoroquinolones are widely used in the treatment of sexually transmitted diseases. For example, in the treatment of pelvic inflammatory disease, quinolones fit among the alternative parenteral regimens such as ofloxacin 400 mg IV every 12 hours in combination with IV metronidazole. Another alternative regimen is ciprofloxacin 200 mg IV every 12 hours in combination with IV doxycycline and in combination with IV metronidazole. Intravenous fluoroquinolones are not recommended as single-agent therapy for pelvic inflammatory disease. Fluoroquinolones are also recommended in combination with other agents for the treatment of pelvic inflammatory disease on an ambulatory basis. One recommended regimen is ofloxacin 400 mg orally twice a day for 14 days plus metronidazole 50 mg orally twice a day for 14 days.

For the treatment of chlamydial infections in adolescents and adults, ofloxacin 300 mg twice a day for 7 days is an alternative regimen.

Several fluoroquinolones are listed as recommended regimens for the treatment of uncomplicated gonococcal infection of the cervix, urethra, and rectum. For example, one regimen is ciprofloxacin 500 mg orally in a single dose or ofloxacin 400 mg orally in a single dose. Either of these regimens should be combined with either azithromycin or doxycycline for the treatment of chlamydia.

Because they inhibit DNA gyrase, they should not be used in pregnancy.

The most pronounced adverse effects are nausea, vomiting, diarrhea, headache, dizziness, insomnia, occasional skin rashes, impairment of liver function, seizures, and anaphylaxis.

NITROFURANTOIN

Nitrofurantoin is bacteriostatic and bactericidal for both gram-positive and gram-negative bacteria in urine. The drug has no systemic antimicrobial activity. Its activity in urine is enhanced at pH 5.5 or below. Microbial resistance does not emerge rapidly.

The usual daily dose in urinary tract infections is 100 mg orally twice daily for 3 days, taken with food.

Nitrofurantoin is also useful for continuous or post-coital suppression of urinary infection.

Oral nitrofurantoin may cause nausea and vomiting. Hemolytic anemia occurs in G6PD deficiency. Hypersensitivity may produce skin rashes and pulmonary infiltration. In uremia, there is virtually no excretion of nitrofurantoin into the urine and no therapeutic effect.

ANTIFUNGAL DRUGS

Most antibacterial drugs have no effect on yeasts and fungi. Others (eg, amphotericin B) are relatively effective in some systemic mycotic infections but are difficult to administer because of toxicity. New imidazoles are fairly effective and relatively nontoxic. Topical preparations such as 2% miconazole, 1% clotrimazole, 2% butoconazole, or 0.4% terconazole have all been used effectively in vaginal candidiasis. Ketoconazole can be given orally, 200–600 mg once daily, preferably with food. It is well absorbed, reaches serum levels of 2–4 µg/mL, and is degraded in tissues, thus requiring no renal or biliary excretion. It has a dramatic therapeutic effect on chronic vaginal candidiasis. Ketoconazole blocks the synthesis of adrenal steroids and can cause gynecomastia. Adverse effects are mild, with nausea, headache, skin rashes, and occasional elevations in transaminase levels. If evidence of liver dysfunction persists, the drug should be discontinued.

Fluconazole is an effective single-dose treatment of uncomplicated yeast infection. The dose is 150–200 mg orally as a single dose. The drug is also effective in recurrent or refractory vulvovaginal candidiasis and is less hepatotoxic than ketoconazole. One regimen for recurrent or refractory yeast infection is fluconazole 150 or 200 mg taken on days 1, 4, and 8. Because of its unusually long half-life, it does not need to be given more frequently. One prophylactic regimen for patients with frequent recurrent yeast infections (ie, > 4–6/year) is fluconazole 150 mg taken once weekly for up to 6 months.

ANTIMICROBIAL CHEMOPROPHYLAXIS IN SURGERY

A major portion of all antimicrobial drugs used in hospitals are used on surgical services with the stated intent of "prophylaxis." Several general features of "surgical prophylaxis" are applicable.

(1) Prophylactic administration of antibiotics should generally be considered only if the expected rate of infectious complications is high or where a possible infection would have a catastrophic effect.

(2) If prophylactic antimicrobials are to be effective, a sufficient concentration of drug must be present at the operative site to inhibit or kill bacteria that might settle there. Thus, it is essential that drug administration begin immediately before (or in cesarean section just after) operation begins.

(3) Prolonged administration of antimicrobial drugs tends to alter the normal flora of organ systems, suppressing the susceptible microorganisms and favoring the implantation of drug-resistant ones. Thus, antimicrobial prophylaxis should last only 1–3 doses.

(4) Systemic antimicrobial levels usually do not prevent wound infection, pneumonia, or urinary tract infection if physiologic abnormalities or foreign bodies are present.

In hysterectomy and nonelective cesarean section, the administration of a broad-spectrum bactericidal drug from just before until 1 day after the procedure has been found effective. Thus, for example, cefazolin 1 g intravenously given before pelvic operations and again for 1–2 doses after the end of the operation results in a demonstrable lowering of the risk of deep infections at the operative site.

Other forms of surgical prophylaxis are used to reduce normal flora or existing bacterial contamination at the site. Thus, the colon is routinely prepared not only by mechanical cleansing through cathartics and enemas, but also by the oral administration of poorly absorbed drugs (eg, neomycin 1 g, plus erythromycin base 0.5 g, every 6 hours) for 1–2 days before operation.

In all situations in which antimicrobials are administered with the hope that they may have a prophylactic effect, the risk from these same drugs (eg, allergy, toxicity, selection of superinfecting microorganisms) must be evaluated daily, and the course of prophylaxis must be kept as brief as possible.

ANTIVIRAL CHEMOPROPHYLAXIS & THERAPY

Several compounds can suppress development of viral diseases. Of these, acyclovir is important in gynecologic practice.

Acyclovir (acycloguanosine [Zovirax]) inhibits replication of herpesviruses in infected cells. When given intravenously (15 mg/kg/d), acyclovir is effective in controlling disseminating herpesvirus infections in immunocompromised patients; it can also markedly reduce pain and extent of lesions in primary genital herpes infections of women. In herpetic encephalitis and in neonatal herpetic dissemination, acyclovir is more effective than vidarabine. There is no effect on cytomegalovirus or Epstein-Barr virus infections, but acyclovir can arrest the progression of varicella and herpes zoster, especially in immunocompromised patients.

Oral acyclovir, 200 mg 5 times daily for adults, has therapeutic effects similar to those of intravenous acyclovir, particularly in primary genital herpes simplex infections. When taken prophylactically in patients with frequent (> 6/y) episodes, it can reduce the frequency of recurrent lesions for up to 3 years. However, no regimen of acyclovir can block the establishment of latency or permanently eliminate recurrences.

Within the past few years, two new effective antiviral drugs have become available: famciclovir and valacyclovir. The advantage of these preparations is that they have longer half-lives and may be given at less frequent dosing intervals than acyclovir. However, they appear to be no more effective. Valacyclovir, famciclovir, and acyclovir are all recommended for first-episode genital herpes, for recurrent episodes of genital herpes, and for daily suppressive therapy of frequent recurrences. Although its use in pregnancy has not been extensive, data so far are reassuring in that there have been no side effects peculiar to the pregnant woman or the fetus.

REFERENCES

American College of Obstetricians and Gynecologists: Antibiotics and gynecologic infections. ACOG Technical Bulletin No. 237. Washington, DC: ACOG, 1997.

American College of Obstetricians and Gynecologists: Antimicrobial therapy for obstetric patients. ACOG Technical Bulletin No. 245. Washington, DC: ACOG, 1998.

Centers for Disease Control and Prevention: 1998 Guidelines for treatment of sexually transmitted diseases. MMWR 1998;47:RR-1.

Gorbach SL et al: *Infectious Diseases,* 2nd ed. WB Saunders Company, 1998.

Kucers A et al: *The Use of Antibiotics: A Clinical Review of Antibacterial, Antifungal and Antiviral Drugs,* 5th ed. Butterworth-Heinemann, 1997.

Sweet RL, Gibbs RS: *Infectious Diseases of the Female Genital Tract,* 4th ed. Lippincott Williams & Wilkins, 2001.

Wendel GD et al: Penicillin allergy and desensitization in serious infections during pregnancy. N Engl J Med 1985;312:1230.

Endometriosis

40

Sanaz Memarzadeh, MD, Kenneth N. Muse, Jr., MD, & Michael D. Fox, MD

Endometriosis is a disorder in which abnormal growths of tissue, histologically resembling the endometrium, are present in locations other than the uterine lining. Although endometriosis can occur very rarely in post-menopausal women, it is found almost exclusively in women of reproductive age. All other manifestations of endometriosis exhibit a wide spectrum of expression. The lesions are usually found on the peritoneal surfaces of the reproductive organs and adjacent structures of the pelvis, but they can occur anywhere in the body (Fig 40-1). The size of the individual lesions varies from microscopic to large invasive masses that erode into underlying organs and cause extensive adhesion formation. Similarly, women with endometriosis can be completely asymptomatic or may be crippled by pelvic pain and infertility.

Endometriosis is a common and important health problem of women. Its exact prevalence is unknown because surgery is required for its diagnosis, but it is estimated to be present in 3–10% of women in the reproductive age group and 25–35% of infertile women. It is seen in 1–2% of women undergoing sterilization or sterilization reversal, in 10% of hysterectomy surgeries, in 16–31% of laparoscopies, and in 53% of adolescents with pelvic pain severe enough to warrant surgical evaluation. Endometriosis is the commonest single gynecologic diagnosis responsible for hospitalization of women aged 15–44, being found in over 6% of patients.

Adenomyosis, also called endometriosis interna, is the presence of endometrial glands and stroma within the myometrium; it is generally thought to be unrelated to endometriosis. Adenomyosis is discussed in Chapter 36.

Pathogenesis

The cause of endometriosis is unknown. The leading theories include retrograde menstruation with transport of endometrial cells, metaplasia of coelomic epithelium, and hematogenous or lymphatic spread of endometrial cells. A combination of these theories is likely to be responsible.

A theory of retrograde menstruation was proposed during the 1920s. It was postulated that endometriosis occurred because viable fragments of endometrium were shed at the time of menstruation and passed through the uterine tubes. Once in the pelvic cavity, the tissue became implanted on peritoneal surfaces and grew into endometriotic lesions. Subsequent observations have confirmed that some degree of retrograde menstruation normally occurs in women with patent tubes, that outflow tract obstructions (cervical stenosis, transverse vaginal septa) increase the incidence of endometriosis, and that intentional deposition of endometrium onto peritoneum can initiate endometriosis. Also, the risk of developing the disease is higher in women with prolonged menstrual flow and in those with short menstrual cycle lengths (more menses per year). This theory is simple, attractive, and easily explains why endometriosis is most commonly found on the peritoneal surfaces of the ovaries, cul-de-sac, and bladder and why lesions may develop in episiotomies and other incisions. However, it does not explain why all women do not develop endometriosis nor does it explain the rare cases of endometriosis in the lung, brain, or other soft tissues or in nonmenstruating subjects (women with Turner's syndrome or with absent uteri).

Other workers proposed that endometrial tissue could be transported by lymphatic or hematogenous routes, and a theory of coelomic metaplasia was postulated. In the latter, peritoneum is induced to undergo metaplasia into endometrial tissue by some stimulus (menstrual fluid or other irritants, cyclic ovarian hormones, etc).

A role for the immune system in the origin of endometriosis was suggested by workers studying monkeys with spontaneous endometriosis that mounted a lesser immune response to endometrial antigens than control animals. The activity of peritoneal natural killer and T lymphocytes is suppressed in women with endometriosis, but whether these immunologic deviations are the cause or the result of endometriosis is still unclear. Endometriosis may occur when a deficiency in cellular immunity allows menstrual tissue to implant and grow on the peritoneum.

Genetic influences in the development of endometriosis have been described. Studies have found that 7–9% of endometriosis patients' first-degree female relatives are diagnosed with the disease—significantly greater than the control rate of 1–2%. Further investigation has revealed a possible role for the HLA-B7 allele. The expression of HLA-B7 has been shown

767

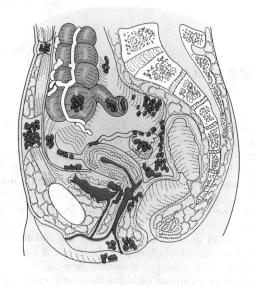

Figure 40–1. Common sites of endometrial implants (endometriosis). (Reproduced with permission from Way LW [editor]: *Current Surgical Diagnosis & Treatment*, 7th ed. Lange, 1985.)

to inhibit the cytotoxic activity of natural killerlike T lymphocytes, suggesting that the growth of ectopic endometrial cells might be under genetic control.

Pathology

The gross appearance of endometriosis at operation is usually quite characteristic and, to an experienced surgeon, is sufficient for diagnosis. The smallest (and presumably earliest) implants are red, petechial lesions on the peritoneal surface. With further growth, menstrual-like detritus accumulates within the lesion, giving it a cystic, dark brown, dark blue, or black appearance. The surrounding peritoneal surface becomes thickened and scarred. These "powder burn" implants typically attain a size of 5–10 mm in diameter. With progression of disease, the number and size of lesions increase, and extensive adhesions may develop. When present on the ovary, cysts may enlarge to several centimeters in size and are called "endometriomas" or "chocolate cysts." Severe disease can erode into underlying tissues and distort the remaining organs with extensive adhesions. In addition to these traditional presentations, endometriosis lesions can have a variety of nonclassical appearances: clear vesicles, white or yellow spots or nodules, circular folds of peritoneum ("pockets"), and visually normal peritoneum (lesions so small they can only be detected microscopically).

The distribution of lesions also exhibits a characteristic pattern. Solitary lesions are possible, but multiple implantations are the rule. The most common site of disease is the ovary (approximately half of all cases), followed by the uterine cul-de-sac, uterosacral ligaments, the posterior surfaces of the uterus and broad ligament, and the remaining pelvic peritoneum. Implants may occur over the bowel, bladder, and ureters; rarely, they may erode into underlying tissue and cause blood in the stool or urine, or their associated adhesions may result in stricture and obstruction of these organs. Implants can occur deep in tissue, especially on the cervix, posterior vaginal fornix, or within wounds contaminated by endometrial tissue. Very rarely, endometriosis is found distant from the pelvis, in such sites as the lung, brain, and kidney. Pleural implantations are associated with recurrent right pneumothoraces at the time of menses, termed "catamenial pneumothorax." Similarly, lesions in the central nervous system can cause catamenial seizures.

The microscopic finding that these lesions are composed of tissue histologically resembling endometrial glands and stroma gives endometriosis its name (Fig 40–2). The normal endometrial appearance is best seen in small, early lesions; with advanced disease, cyst formation, and fibrosis, the wall of the implant is lined by a monolayer of cells, if at all. Blood is present inside the cyst, and hemosiderin-laden macrophages are found in the cyst wall.

Although endometriosis resembles the uterine endometrium histologically, further assumptions about similarities between the tissues must be made with great caution. Simultaneous biopsies of implants and endometrium have found the implants often to be histologically out of phase with the uterine tissue. Also, the characteristic changes of estrogen and progesterone receptors present in endometrium across the menstrual cycle are absent in endometriosis implants. Endometriosis implants, unlike endometrium, do not respond to progesterone in vitro by the induction of 17β-hydroxysteroid dehydrogenase activity, the enzyme that in the luteal phase converts estradiol to the less potent estrone.

Pathologic Physiology

It is generally agreed that pelvic pain occurs premenstrually in endometriosis patients. Because of this, pain from endometriosis is thought to be due to stimulation from estrogen and progesterone during the menstrual cycle; the tissue of the implant is stimulated to grow in much the same way as is the endometrium. The implants enlarge and may undergo secretory change and bleeding; however, the fibrotic tissues surrounding the implants prevent the expansion and escape of hemorrhagic fluid that occurs in the uterus. With subsequent cycles, this process repeats itself. Pain is produced by

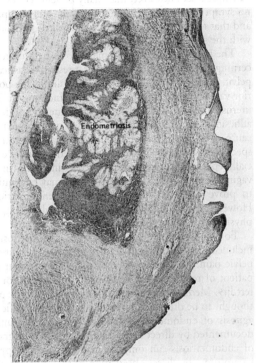 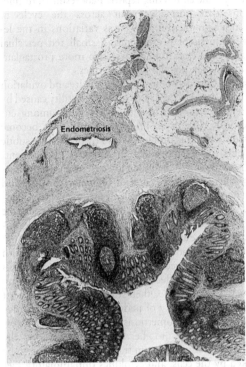

Figure 40–2. Histologic appearance of endometriosis. **Left:** Endometriosis of ovary. **Right:** Endometriosis of cervix. (Courtesy of Eugene H. Ruffolo, MD.)

pressure and inflammation within and around the lesion, by traction on adhesions associated with the lesions, by the number of implants and their proximity to nerves and other sensitive structures, and by the mass effect of large lesions. Although this sequence of events explains why premenstrual pelvic pain can occur in endometriosis, it is incomplete, because many patients with extensive endometriosis have no pain. It is a common observation that the occurrence and severity of pain from endometriosis bear little relationship to the amount and distribution of the disease. Severe pain in patients with endometriosis is associated with deeply infiltrating lesions, and it is thought that the degree of pain is perhaps determined by the depth of invasion.

The relationship between endometriosis and infertility has been more extensively investigated. Moderate and severe endometriosis is associated with pelvic adhesions that distort pelvic anatomy, prevent normal tuboovarian apposition, and encase the ovary. Implants can destroy ovarian and tubal tissue, although occlusion of uterine tubes is rare.

It is not difficult to understand how advanced disease can result in infertility, but minimal or mild endometriosis, in which pelvic anatomy is entirely normal

except for a few peritoneal surface lesions, can also cause infertility. The mechanism by which this occurs is unknown. Various theories have been proposed to explain this phenomenon.

Several investigators have examined peritoneal fluid abnormalities. The peritoneal fluid is an ultrafiltrate of plasma, with less than 5 mL normally present in the pelvis. After ovulation, a transient rise to approximately 20 mL occurs. The volume of peritoneal fluid and the concentrations of various hormones and other substances in it affect the processes of ovulation, ovum pickup, tubal function, and so on. The normal role of the peritoneal fluid and its constituents in these processes, and how it is altered by endometriosis, are largely unknown. Peritoneal fluid volume has been reported to be altered in endometriosis patients, but studies have led to inconsistent results.

Similarly, reports are contradictory as to whether endometriosis patients have elevations in peritoneal fluid prostaglandins F_2 and E_2. Prostaglandins are normally secreted by the endometrium and by endometriosis lesions; an increase in peritoneal fluid prostaglandin levels could theoretically decrease fertility by altering ovulation, tubal motility, nidation, and luteal phase adequacy. The conflicting reports may result from fluctuations that normally occur across the cycle in prostanoid production, as well as variations in the lesions' synthesis of prostaglandins; small red petechial implants have been found to secrete more prostaglandins than larger, powder burn-like ones.

Several disorders of menstrual cyclicity and ovulation have been suggested as a basis for the infertility caused by mild endometriosis. The rate of ovulation among endometriosis patients is 11–27%. Nearly half become pregnant when this problem is also treated. More subtle problems in folliculogenesis in endometriosis patients have been reported, including lower serum estradiol levels, smaller follicle size during follicular growth, and lower oocyte fertilization rates and pregnancy rates in assisted reproduction. Problems with ovum pickup by the fallopian tube and embryo implantation in the endometrium have also been suggested.

As noted previously, deficient cellular immunity to endometrium has been reported in endometriosis. This may also adversely affect normal nidation and other reproductive processes. Other studies have shown that the number or activity of peritoneal macrophages may be increased in endometriosis, possibly causing excessive prostaglandins to be released locally by the macrophages, causing sperm transport or function to be attacked by the cells, and cytokines (inflammatory mediators including interleukin-1) to be released from pelvic lymphocytes.

Clinical Findings

Endometriosis is common among women of reproductive age, and its prevalence increases to 30–40% among infertile women. Clinical findings vary greatly depending on the number, size, and extent of the lesions and on the patient population being examined.

The diagnosis of endometriosis is often strongly suspected from a patient's initial history. Infertility, dysmenorrhea and dyspareunia are the main presenting complaints. Most patients complain of constant pelvic pain or a low sacral backache that occurs premenstrually and subsides after menses begins. Dyspareunia is often present, particularly with deep penetration. Lesions involving the urinary tract or bowel may result in bloody urine or stool in the perimenstrual interval. Implantations on or near the external surfaces of the cervix, vagina, vulva, rectum, or urethra may cause pain or bleeding with defecation, urination, or intercourse at any time in the menstrual cycle. Adhesions from endometriosis may cause discomfort at any time during the cycle, and a sensation of pelvic pressure may result if large masses are present. Premenstrual spotting may occur and is more likely to be associated with endometriosis than with luteal phase inadequacy. It must

be emphasized, however, that many patients either have no symptoms or have infertility as their only symptom and that the extent of disease often has little correlation with the severity of symptoms.

The physical examination may also be helpful in discerning whether endometriosis is present. Classically, pelvic examination reveals tender nodules in the posterior vaginal fornix and pain upon uterine motion. The uterus may be fixed and retroverted due to cul-de-sac adhesions, and tender adnexal masses may be felt because of the presence of endometriomas. Careful inspection may reveal implants in healed wounds, especially episiotomy and cesarean section incisions, in the vaginal fornix, or on the cervix. Biopsy may be required to prove that the lesions are due to endometriosis. However, many patients have no abnormal findings on physical examination.

For the vast majority of patients, endometriosis is included in the differential diagnosis of infertility or pelvic pain. Endometriosis should be suspected in any patient of reproductive age complaining of pain or infertility. Medical treatment can be given for pelvic pain thought to be due to endometriosis, but the specific diagnosis of endometriosis should not be made unless documented by direct visualization. The final diagnosis of endometriosis can only be made at laparoscopy or laparotomy, by direct observation of the implants. Occasionally, an isolated endometrioma is removed, and the diagnosis must be made histologically by the demonstration of "endometrial" glands and stroma or of hemosiderin-laden macrophages in the cyst wall.

Except for special circumstances, such as urography or sigmoidoscopy for suspected bowel or urinary involvement, ancillary diagnostic studies (ultrasound, x-rays, CT scans) are of little help in diagnosis.

Complications

True complications of endometriosis are few. Implants over the bowel or ureters may cause obstruction and silent impairment of renal function. The erosive nature of the lesions in advanced aggressive disease can cause a myriad of symptoms, depending on the tissue damaged. Endometriomas can cause ovarian torsion or can rupture and spill their irritating contents into the peritoneal cavity, resulting in a chemical peritonitis. Excision of endometriosis causing catamenial seizures or pneumothorax may be necessary.

Differential Diagnosis

The varied presentations of endometriosis mandate that it be considered in the differential diagnosis of virtually all pelvic disease. In particular, the pain, infertility, and adhesions associated with endometriosis must be distinguished from similar symptoms accompanying pelvic inflammatory disease and pelvic tumors. Usually this will require operative evaluation. A patient with a persistent adnexal mass greater than 5 cm should never be presumed to have an endometrioma even if endometriosis has been diagnosed previously. Such masses require surgical diagnosis.

Prevention

Prevention of endometriosis is not currently possible. Traditionally, women with relatives affected by endometriosis—or in whom the diagnosis has recently been made—are advised not to postpone childbearing. The merits of this advice have not been proved. A more thorough understanding of the pathophysiology of endometriosis is required before preventative strategies can be devised.

Classification

Several classification schemes to assist in describing the anatomic location and severity of endometriosis at operation have been created. Although none is entirely satisfactory, the scoring systems are useful for reporting operative findings and for comparing the results of various treatment protocols. The revised American Fertility Society classification is given in Table 40–1 and Fig 40–3.

Treatment

Treatment options are dictated by the patient's desire for future fertility, her symptoms, the stage of her disease, and to some extent her age. It must be emphasized that therapy for endometriosis requires operative inspection of the lesions for correct diagnosis and staging and to be sure that the patient's symptoms are attributable to endometriosis only.

A. OBSERVATION

In asymptomatic patients, those with mild discomfort, or infertile women with minimal or mild endometriosis, expectant management may be appropriate. Although endometriosis is generally felt to be a progressive disease, there is no evidence that treating an asymptomatic patient will prevent or ameliorate the onset of symptoms later. Many reports have found expectant management of infertile women with minimal or mild endometriosis to be as successful as medical or surgical therapies.

B. ANALGESIC THERAPY

Analgesic treatments include nonsteroidal anti-inflammatory agents and prostaglandin synthetase-inhibiting drugs. These drugs are appropriate sole therapy for endometriosis when the patient has mild premenstrual pain

Table 40–1. American Society for Reproductive Medicine revised classification of endometriosis.

	Endometriosis	< 1 cm	1–3 cm	> 3 cm
Peritoneum	Superficial	1	2	4
	Deep	2	4	6
Ovary	R Superficial	1	2	4
	Deep	4	16	20
	L Superficial	1	2	4
	Deep	4	16	20
	Posterior Cul-de-sac Obliteration	Partial		Complete
		4		40
	Adhesions	< 1/3 Enclosure	1/3–2/3 Enclosure	> 2/3 Enclosure
Ovary	R Filmy	1	2	4
	Dense	4	8	16
	L Filmy	1	2	4
	Dense	4	8	16
Tube	R Filmy	1	2	4
	Dense	4[1]	8[1]	16
	L Filmy	1	2	4
	Dense	4[1]	8[1]	16

[1]If the fimbriated end of the fallopian tube is completely enclosed, change the point assignment to 16. Staging: Stage I (minimal): 1–5; stage II (mild): 6–15; stage III (moderate): 16–40; stage IV (severe): > 40. (Reproduced with permission from Revised ASRM classification. Fertil Steri 1997; 67:819.)

from minimal endometriosis, no abnormalities on pelvic examination, and no desire for immediate fertility.

C. HORMONAL THERAPY

The goal of treatment with hormonal therapy is to interrupt the cycles of stimulation and bleeding of endometriotic tissue. This can be achieved with various agents.

1. **Oral contraceptive pills (OCPs)**—Generally monophasic products are used and the patient is prescribed 1 pill a day continuously for 6–12 months. The continuous exposure to combination oral contraceptive pills results in decidual changes in the endometrial glands. In cases of breakthrough bleeding additional estrogen may be added. Use of oral contraceptive pills is considered suppressive and not curative in nature. Side effects are breast tenderness, bloating, headache, irri-

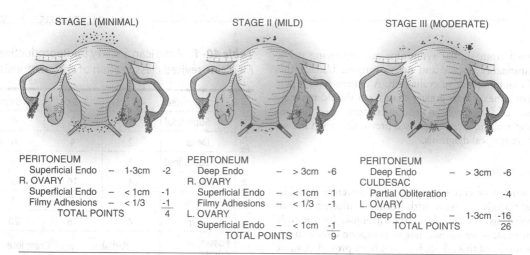

STAGE I (MINIMAL)		
PERITONEUM		
Superficial Endo	– 1-3cm	-2
R. OVARY		
Superficial Endo	– < 1cm	-1
Filmy Adhesions	– < 1/3	-1
TOTAL POINTS		4

STAGE II (MILD)		
PERITONEUM		
Deep Endo	– > 3cm	-6
R. OVARY		
Superficial Endo	– < 1cm	-1
Filmy Adhesions	– < 1/3	-1
L. OVARY		
Superficial Endo	– < 1cm	-1
TOTAL POINTS		9

STAGE III (MODERATE)		
PERITONEUM		
Deep Endo	– > 3cm	-6
CULDESAC		
Partial Obliteration		-4
L. OVARY		
Deep Endo	– 1-3cm	-16
TOTAL POINTS		26

STAGE III (MODERATE)		
PERITONEUM		
Superficial Endo	– > 3cm	-4
R. TUBE		
Filmy Adhesions	– < 1/3	-1
R. OVARY		
Filmy Adhesions	– < 1/3	-1
L. TUBE		
Dense Adhesions	– < 1/3	-16*
L. OVARY		
Deep Endo	– < 1cm	-4
Dense Adhesions	– < 1/3	-4
TOTAL POINTS		30

STAGE IV (SEVERE)		
PERITONEUM		
Superficial Endo	– > 3cm	-4
L. OVARY		
Deep Endo	– 1-3cm	-32**
Dense Adhesions	– < 1/3	-8**
L. Tube		
Dense Adhesions	– < 1/3	-8**
TOTAL POINTS		52

*Point assignment changed to 16
**Point assignment doubled

STAGE IV (SEVERE)		
PERITONEUM		
Deep Endo	– > 3cm	-6
CULDESAC		
Complete Obliteration		-40
R. OVARY		
Deep Endo	1-3cm	-16
Dense Adhesions	– < 1/3	-4
L. Tube		
Dense Adhesions	– > 2/3	-16
L. OVARY		
Deep Endo	– 1-3cm	-16
Dense Adhesions	– > 2/3	-16
TOTAL POINTS		114

Figure 40–3. Staging of endometriosis. Determination of the stage or degree of endometrial involvement is based on a weighted point system (see Table 40–1 for point values). Distribution of points has been arbitrarily determined and may require further revision or refinement as knowledge of the disease increases. To ensure complete evaluation, inspection of the pelvis in a clockwise or counterclockwise fashion is encouraged. Number, size, and location of endometrial implants, plaques, endometriomas, and/or adhesions are noted. For example, 5 separate 0.5-cm superficial implants on the peritoneum (2.5 cm total) would be assigned 2 points. (The surface of the uterus should be considered peritoneum.) The severity of the endometriosis or adhesions should be assigned the highest score only for peritoneum, ovary, tube, or cul-de-sac. For example, a 4-cm superficial and a 2-cm deep implant of the peritoneum should be given a score of 6 (not 8). A 4-cm deep endometrioma of the ovary associated with more than 3 cm of superficial disease should be scored 20 (not 24). In patients with only one set of adnexa, points applied to disease of the remaining tube and ovary should be multiplied by two. Points assigned may be circled and totaled. Aggregation of points indicates stage of disease (minimal, mild, moderate, or severe). The presence of endometriosis of the bowel, urinary tract, fallopian tube, vagina, cervix, skin, etc, should be documented under "additional endometriosis." Other pathology such as tubal occlusion, leiomyomata, uterine anomaly, etc, should be documented under "additional pathology." All pathology should be depicted as specifically as possible on the sketch of pelvic organs, and means of observation (laparoscopy or laparotomy) should be noted. (Copyright 1996, American Society for Reproductive Medicine. From: Revised ASRM classification for endometriosis: 1996. Fertil Steril 1997;67:820.)

tability, and the other side effects associated with oral contraceptive use. Rate of pregnancy following discontinuation of therapy can be as high as 50%.

2. Progestational agents—These agents work via a mechanism similar to that of the OCPs, causing decidualization in the endometriotic tissue. Oral medroxyprogesterone acetate can be prescribed as a 10–30 mg dosage daily. An alternative regimen is megestrol acetate prescribed as a 40-mg daily dose. Depot medroxyprogesterone acetate 150 mg IM can also be given as a single injection every 3 months. Side effects associated with these regimens include irritability, depression, breakthrough bleeding, and bloating. Treatment with progestational agents does not seem to affect pregnancy rates.

3. Danazol—Danazol is a weak androgen that is the isoxazole derivative of 17α-ethinyl testosterone (ethisterone). Danazol acts via several mechanisms to treat endometriosis. It acts at the hypothalamic level to inhibit gonadotropin release, inhibiting the midcycle surge of LH and FSH. Danazol inhibits steroidogenic enzymes in the ovary. As a result a hypoestrogenic environment is created. This, in addition to the androgenic effects of danazol, prevents the growth of endometriotic tissue.

The dosage of danazol is 800 mg/d in divided doses for 6 months. Because of its high cost, attempts have been made to reduce this daily dosage.

Side effects of danazol include acne, oily skin, deepening of the voice, weight gain, edema, and adverse plasma lipoprotein changes. Most changes are reversible upon cessation of therapy, but some (such as deepening of the voice) may not be.

Pain relief is achieved in up to 90% of patients taking danazol. However, upon discontinuation of therapy symptoms recur in 1 year.

4. Gestrinone—Gestrinone is a 19-nortestosterone derivative that suppresses the secretion of FSH and LH. It is not currently available in the U.S. Although use of gestrinone was effective, androgenic side effects were prominent, and ovulation was not inhibited.

5. GnRH agonists—Gonadotropin-releasing hormone (GnRH) agonists are analogues of the 10-amino-acid peptide hormone GnRH. With the continuous administration of GnRH analogues, suppression of gonadotropin secretion occurs, resulting in elimination of ovarian steroidogenesis and suppression of endometrial implants. Pain related to endometriosis is relieved in most cases by the second or third month of therapy. GnRH agonists can be administered intramuscularly as leuprolide acetate 3.75 mg once a month, intranasally as nafarelin 200 mg twice daily, or subcutaneously as goserelin 3.75 mg once a month.

The use of these agents is generally limited to 6 months because of the adverse effects associated with a hypoestrogenic state, particularly loss of bone mineral density. Other side effects include vasomotor symptoms, vaginal dryness, and mood changes.

Recent studies have examined the role of add-back therapy in addition to the GnRH agonists in the treatment of endometriosis. The addition of 2.5 mg of norethindrone or 0.625 mg of conjugated equine estrogen with 5 mg/d of medroxyprogesterone acetate seems to provide relief of vasomotor symptoms and decrease bone mineral density loss in a 6-month treatment period. The addition of 5 mg of norethindrone acetate alone or in conjunction with low-dose conjugated equine estrogen seems to eliminate the loss of bone mineral density effectively as well.

6. Surgical treatment—In women with complaints of infertility who have severe disease or adhesions or are older, conservative surgical therapy is the treatment of choice. This surgery attempts to excise or destroy all endometriotic tissue, remove all adhesions, and restore pelvic anatomy to the best possible condition. A recent randomized controlled trial evaluated the effects of laparoscopic surgery in infertile women with mild or minimal endometriosis. Results suggest that laparoscopic resection or ablation of minimal or mild endometriosis enhances fecundity in infertile women. Presacral neurectomy or uterosacral ligament ablation to relieve pain and a uterine suspension procedure may be performed as required, although the efficacy of these treatments is controversial. Conservative surgery has traditionally been performed at laparotomy, but a laparoscopic approach is associated with a shorter hospital stay and less morbidity, and it may be more cost effective. This is particularly true in contemporary practice, where this therapy is usually performed at the time of the initial diagnostic laparoscopy. Reported pregnancy rates following conservative surgery are inversely proportional to the severity of disease and vary greatly. In counseling patients, approximate pregnancy rates of 75% for mild disease, 50–60% for moderate disease, and 30–40% for severe disease should be quoted; however, individualization of therapy is stressed.

If the patient does not desire future childbearing and has severe disease or symptoms, definitive surgery is appropriate and often curative. This entails total abdominal hysterectomy, bilateral salpingo-oophorectomy, and excision of remaining adhesions or implants. If endometriosis remains after excision, postoperative medical therapy may be indicated. After this or after complete excision, hormone replacement therapy is indicated. Estrogen-progestin therapy may be used without reactivating the endometriosis, but individualization of therapy is required.

7. Assisted reproduction—Infertile women with endometriosis who are older, or who have failed other therapies for infertility, can undergo assisted reproduction (in vitro fertilization, gamete intrafallopian transfer, etc) with success rates similar to those seen in women with other diagnoses. The relatively short time required with this option may make it the most efficacious of all infertility therapies for endometriosis. Women with more severe disease have decreased success.

Prognosis

Proper counseling of patients with endometriosis requires attention to several aspects of the disorder. Of primary importance is the initial operative staging of the disease to obtain adequate information on which to base future decisions about therapy. The patient's symptoms and desire for childbearing dictate appropriate therapy. Most patients can be told that they will be able to obtain significant relief from pelvic pain and that treatment will assist them in achieving pregnancy.

Long-term concerns must be more guarded in that all current therapies offer relief but not cure. Even after definitive surgery, endometriosis may recur, but the risk is very low (about 3%). The risk of recurrence is not significantly increased by estrogen replacement therapy. After conservative surgery, reported recurrence rates vary greatly but usually exceed 10% in 3 years and 35% in 5 years. Pregnancy delays but does not preclude recurrence. Recurrence rates after medical treatment also vary and are similar to or higher than those reported following surgical treatment.

Although many patients are concerned that endometriosis will progress inexorably, experience has been that conservative surgery avoids the necessity for hysterectomy in the great majority of cases. The course of endometriosis in any individual is impossible to predict at present, and future treatment options should greatly improve what can now be offered.

REFERENCES

Epidemiology

Cramer DW: Epidemiology of endometriosis. In: Wilson EA (editor): *Endometriosis*, Alan R. Liss, Inc, 1987, p. 5.

Gruppos Italiano per lo Studio Dell'Endometriosi: Prevalence and anatomical distribution of endometriosis in women with selected gynaecological conditions: results from a multicentric Italian study. Hum Reprod 1994;9:1158.

Olive DL, Schwartz LB: Endometriosis. New Engl J Med 1993; 328:1759.

Wheeler JM: Epidemiology and prevalence of endometriosis. Infertil Reprod Med Clin North Am 1992;3:545.

Pathogenesis

American College of Obstetricians and Gynecologists: Endometriosis, ACOG Technical Bulletin No. 184, September 1993.

Coxhead D, Thomas EJ: Familial inheritance of endometriosis in a British population: A case control study. J Obstet Gynaecol 1993;13:42.

Ho HN et al: Peritoneal cellular immunity and endometriosis. Am J Reprod Immunol 1997;38:400.

Oosterlynck DJ et al: Immunosuppressive activity of peritoneal fluid in women with endometriosis. Obstet Gynecol 1993;82:206.

Ramey JW, Archer DF: Peritoneal fluid: Its relevance to the development of endometriosis. Fertil Steril 1993;60:1.

Semino C et al: Role of major histocompatibility complex class I expression and natural killer-like T cells in the genetic control of endometriosis. Fertil Steril 1995;64:909.

Pathology

Bergqvist A, Ferno M: Estrogen and progesterone receptors in endometriotic tissue and endometrium: Comparison according to localization and recurrence. Fertil Steril 1993;60:63.

Murphy AA et al: Unsuspected endometriosis documented by scanning electron microscopy in visually normal peritoneum. Fertil Steril 1986;46:52.

Pathologic Physiology

Koninckx PR et al: Suggestive evidence that pelvic endometriosis is a progressive disease, whereas deeply infiltrating endometriosis is associated with pelvic pain. Fertil Steril 1991;55:759.

Pittaway DE, Ellington CP, Klimek M: Preclinical abortions and endometriosis. Fertil Steril 1988;49:221.

Rodrigues-Escudero FJ et al: Does minimal endometriosis reduce fecundity? Fertil Steril 1988;50:522.

Steele RW, Dmowski WP, Marmer DJ: Deficient cellular immunity in endometriosis. Am J Reprod Immunol 1984;6:33.

Switchenko AC, Kauffman RS, Becker A: Are there endometrial antibodies in sera of women with endometriosis? Fertil Steril 1991;56:235.

Syrop CH, Halme J: Peritoneal fluid environment and infertility. Fertil Steril 1987;48:1.

Vercellini P et al: Endometriosis and pelvic pain: relation to disease stage and localization. Fertil Steril 1996;65:299.

Clinical Findings

Fedele L et al: Pain symptoms associated with endometriosis. Obstet Gynecol 1992;79:767.

Complications

Schorlemmer GR, Battaglini JW: Pneumothorax in menstruating females. Contemp Surg 1982;20:53.

Zwas FR, Lyon DT: Endometriosis: An important condition in clinical gastroenterology. Dig Dis Sci 1991;36:353.

Treatment

American College of Obstetricians and Gynecologists: Endometriosis. ACOG Technical Bulletin No. 184, September 1993.

Barbieri RL: Hormonal treatment of endometriosis: The estrogen threshold hypothesis. Am J Obstet Gynecol 1992;166:740.

Barbieri RL, Ryan KJ: Danazol: Endocrine pharmacology and therapeutic applications. Am J Obstet Gynecol 1981;141:453.

Cook AS, Rock JA: The role of laparoscopy in the treatment of endometriosis. Fertil Steril 1991;55:663.

Dlugi AM, Miller JD, Knittle J: Lupron depot (leuprolide acetate for depot suspension) in the treatment of endometriosis: A randomized placebo-controlled, double-blind study. Fertil Steril 1990;54:419.

Henzl MR et al: Administration of nasal nafarelin as compared with oral danazol for endometriosis: A multicenter double-blind comparative trial. N Engl J Med 1988;318:485.

Krasnow JS, Berga SL: Endometriosis and gamete intrafallopian transfer. Assisted Reprod Rev 1993;3:121.

Luciano AA, Turksoy RN, Carleo J: Evaluation of oral medroxyprogesterone acetate in the treatment of endometriosis. Obstet Gynecol 1988;72:323.

Maouris P: Asymptomatic mild endometriosis in infertile women: The case for expectant management. Obstet Gynecol Surv 1991;46:548.

Marcoux S et al: Laparoscopic surgery in infertile women with minimal or mild endometriosis. N Engl J Med 1997;337(4):217.

Speroff L et al: *Clinical Gynecologic Endocrinology and Infertility,* 6th ed. Lippincott Williams & Wilkins, 1999, 1063.

Surrey ES and the Add-Back Consensus Working Group: Add-back therapy and gonadotropin hormone agonists in the treatment of patients with endometriosis: can a consensus be reached? Fertil Steril 1999;71(3):1999.

Surrey ES et al: The effects of combining norethindrone with a gonadotropin-releasing hormone agonist in the treatment of symptomatic endometriosis. Fertil Steril 1990;53:620.

Relaxation of Pelvic Supports

41

Christopher M. Tarnay, MD, & Clyde H. Dorr, II, MD, FACOG

General Considerations

Defects in the pelvic supporting structures result in a variety of clinically evident pelvic relaxation abnormalities. Pelvic supportive defects may be classified according to their anatomic location.

Anterior Vaginal Wall Defects

- Cystocele—term to describe anterior vaginal wall defect where the bladder is associated with the prolapse
- Urethrocele—term to describe distal anterior vaginal wall defect where the urethra is associated with the prolapse
- Paravaginal/midline/transverse—indicates location of anterior vaginal wall defect
- Uterine prolapse
- Vaginal vault prolapse
- Enterocele—term to describe apical vaginal wall defect in which bowel is contained within the prolapsed segment. Can occur with or without the uterus in situ.

Posterior Vaginal Wall Defects

- Rectocele—term to describe posterior vaginal wall defect

Description and Staging of Pelvic Organ Prolapse

Two general classifications are used to describe and document the severity of pelvic organ prolapse.

The most commonly used system clinically is based on descent within the vaginal vault of the respective vaginal walls and uses terminology of cystocele, rectocele, enterocele, and uterine prolapse (Table 41–1). The most dependent position of the pelvic organs during maximum straining is used to rate the "degree" of prolapse.

Another system, introduced more recently, employs objective measurements from fixed anatomic points. The Pelvic Organ Prolapse Quantification (POP-Q) system standardizes terminology of female pelvic organ prolapse. This method for quantifying prolapse provides more precise description of the anatomy. This descriptive system contains series of site-specific measurements

of vaginal and perineal anatomy. Prolapse in each segment is evaluated and measured relative to the hymen, which is a fixed anatomic landmark that can be consistently identified. The anatomic position of the 6 defined points for measurement should be in centimeters above the hymen (negative number) or centimeters below the hymen (positive number). The plane at the level of the hymen is defined as zero (Table 41–2 and Fig 41–1). Stages are assigned according to the most severe portion of the prolapse when the full extent of the protrusion has been demonstrated. An ordinal system is utilized for measurements of different points along the vaginal canal which facilitates communication among clinicians and enables objective tracking of surgical results.

Better understanding of the pathophysiology of the pelvic supportive defects, their causes, and clinical presentations allows the individualization of the therapy most likely to successfully affect long-term therapy for each patient.

CYSTOCELE & URETHROCELE

 ESSENTIALS OF DIAGNOSIS

- *Sensation of vaginal fullness, pressure, "falling out."*
- *Feeling of incomplete emptying of the bladder, often stress incontinence, urinary frequency; perhaps a need to push the bladder up in order to void.*
- *Presence of a soft, reducible mass bulging into the vagina and distending through vaginal introitus.*
- *With straining or coughing, increased bulging and descent of the anterior vaginal wall and urethra.*

General Considerations

Cystocele, descent of a portion of the anterior bladder wall into the vagina, is usually associated with the trauma of parturition. The stretching, attenuation, or

Table 41–1. Classification of the severity of pelvic organ prolapse.

Cystocele

First degree: The anterior vaginal wall, from the urethral meatus to the anterior fornix, descends halfway to the hymen.

Second degree: The anterior vaginal wall and underlying bladder extend to the hymen.

Third degree: The anterior vaginal wall and underlying urethra and bladder are outside the hymen. This cystocele is often part of the third-degree uterine or posthysterectomy vaginal vault prolapse.

Uterine or Vaginal Vault Prolapse

First degree: The cervix or vaginal apex descends halfway to the hymen.

Second degree: The cervix or vaginal apex extends to the hymen or over the perineal body.

Third degree: The cervix and corpus uteri extend beyond the hymen or the vaginal vault is everted and protrudes beyond the hymen.

Rectocele

First degree: The saccular protrusion of the rectovaginal wall descends halfway to the hymen.

Second degree: The sacculation descends to the hymen.

Third degree: The sacculation protrudes or extends beyond the hymen.

Enterocele

The presence and depth of the enterocele sac, relative to the hymen, should be described anatomically, with the patient in the supine and standing positions during Valsalva maneuver.

Reproduced with permission from Bump RC et al: The standardization of terminology of female pelvic organ prolapse and pelvic floor dysfunction. Am J Obstet Gynecol 1996;175:10.

actual laceration of the so-called pubovesicocervical fascia produced by the birth of a large baby, multiple or operative deliveries, and prolonged labors increases the possibility and severity of cystocele (Figs 41–2 and 41–3). Urethrocele (sagging of the urethra) is commonly associated with cystocele. It is often seen in women who have urinary stress incontinence, and is a continuum of a cystocele involving the most distal aspect of the anterior vaginal wall.

Cystourethrocele (simultaneous occurrence of cystocele and urethrocele) may occur in nulliparous women, apparently as a result of congenital inadequacy of the endopelvic connective tissues or fascia and of the musculature of the pelvic floor. Contributing factors are likely inherent differences in collagen content and subtype.

Although a degree of cystourethrocele is demonstrable in virtually all parous women during childbearing years, the condition may not progress and may cause no

symptoms. However, progression of pelvic support defects may advance, particularly after the menopause. Hypoestrogenism may facilitate tissue and muscle atrophy and weakness. This then leads to more pronounced laxity. Treatment is unnecessary unless the woman becomes symptomatic or develops concomitant stress urinary incontinence.

Clinical Findings

A. Symptoms

A small cystocele causes no significant symptoms, and in many cases fairly large ones cause no noteworthy complaints. A cystocele may be large enough to bulge out of the vaginal introitus, and the patient may complain of vaginal pressure or a protruding mass that gives her the feeling that she is "sitting on a ball." Symptoms are aggravated by vigorous activity, prolonged standing, coughing, sneezing, or straining. Relief can be obtained by rest and by assuming a recumbent or prone position.

Although urinary incontinence is the most common and most important symptom associated with cystocele, this disorder as such does not cause incontinence,

Table 41–2. Staging of pelvic organ prolapse[1].

Stage 0   No prolapse is demonstrated. Points Aa, Ap, Ba, and Bp are all at –3 cm and either point C or D is between –TVL (total vaginal length) cm and –(TVL–2) cm (ie, the quantitation value for point C or D is ≤ –[TVL–2] cm).

Stage I   The criteria for stage 0 are not met, but the most distal portion of the prolapse is > 1 cm above the level of the hymen (ie, its quantitation value is < –1 cm).

Stage II   The most distal portion of the prolapse is ≤ 1 cm proximal to or distal to the plane of the hymen (ie, its quantitation value is ≥ –1 cm but ≤ + 1 cm).

Stage III   The most distal portion of the prolapse is > 1 cm below the plane of the hymen but protudes no further than 2 cm less than the total vaginal length in centimeters (ie, its quantitation value is > + 1 cm but < +[TVL–2] cm).

Stage IV   Essentially, complete eversion of the total length of the lower genital tract is demonstrated. The distal portion of the prolapse protrudes to at least (TVL–2) cm (ie, its quantitation value is ≥ +[TVL– 2] cm). In most instances, the leading edge of stage IV prolapse is the cervix or vaginal cuff scar.

---

[1]See Fig 41–2 for meaning of variables discussed here.
Reproduced with permission from Bump RC et al: The standardization of terminology of female pelvic organ prolapse and pelvic floor dysfunction, Am J Obstet Gynecol 1996;175:10.

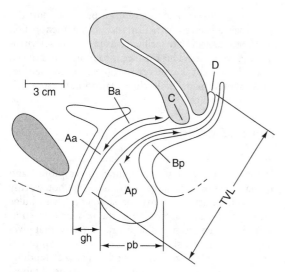

Figure 41–1. Six sites (points *Aa, Ba, C, D, Bp,* and *Ap*), genital hiatus *(gh)*, perineal body *(pb)*, and total vaginal length *(TVL)* used for pelvic organ quantitation. (Reproduced with permission from Bump RC et al: The standardization of terminology of female pelvic organ prolapse and pelvic floor dysfunction. Am J Obstet Gynecol 1996;175:10.)

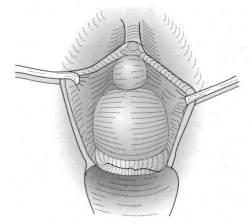

Figure 41–3. Cystocele.

and its repair does not correct stress incontinence. Stress incontinence is an anatomic condition, associated with relaxation of the musculofascial supporting tissues of the urethra. Unless special attention is directed to urethral support, operative correction of a large cystocele may cause rather than correct stress incontinence.

The vaginal pressure of a cystocele may be interpreted as incomplete bladder emptying and thus may lead to frequent efforts to empty the bladder. This has given rise to the popular misconception that cystocele is commonly responsible for large volumes of residual urine with accompanying problems of cystitis, trigonitis, urethritis, urinary urgency and frequency, and dysuria. It is true that a large cystocele projecting well outside the introitus is responsible for significant residual urine. This could lead to bladder infection and symptoms of inflammation. However, many patients in this category have learned through experience that complete bladder emptying can be achieved either by voiding again after several minutes ("double voiding") or by manually reducing the cystocele into the vagina prior to voiding. Unless the patient has significant volumes of residual urine as demonstrated by catheterization, cystocele operations performed primarily to relieve symptoms of chronic inflammation of the urinary tract (ie, urgency, frequency, dysuria, chronic cystitis) will be unsuccessful.

Sexual sensation is generally not impacted by vaginal wall prolapse unless the defect is so pronounced that it inhibits coital penetration or causes bladder or rectal discomfort.

B. Signs

Examination of the patient with cystocele reveals a relaxed vaginal outlet with a thin-walled, rather smooth, bulging mass involving the anterior vaginal wall below the cervix. Vaginal rugae are normally present. A loss of rugation denotes disruption of the connective tissue attachment below the epithelium. Utilization of the Sims speculum or the lower blade of a Graves speculum enables selective visualization of the vaginal walls. When the perineum is depressed and the patient is asked to strain, the mass descends and, depending on the degree of relaxation, distends or projects through the vaginal introitus. When there is an associated urethrocele, a downward and forward rotational "sliding" of the ure-

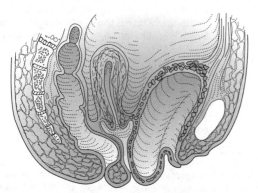

Figure 41–2. Cystocele.

thra and its external meatus is noted; asking the patient with a partially filled bladder to cough while straining may demonstrate stress incontinence of urine.

C. LABORATORY FINDINGS

Examination of a catheterized urine specimen may reveal evidence of infection. The volume of residual urine should be determined by catheterization after voiding. Unless the patient has a significant volume of residual urine, the cystocele is likely not responsible for urinary tract infection. Any urinary tract infection requires complete investigation prior to correction of the cystocele.

D. IMAGING STUDIES

In general a complete discriminative gynecologic examination is all that is necessary to accurately assess pelvic organ prolapse. In certain cases further diagnostic studies can be utililzed.

Traditional modalities to assist in the evaluation of all forms of pelvic relaxation include plain radiography and intravenous pyelography (IVP). More recently advances in radiologic medicine have allowed assessment of the pelvic floor with sonography, computed tomography (CT), and magnetic resonance imaging (MRI).

Despite newer techniques, IVP still holds great value, as it is a simple and safe method to visualize the urinary tract. It can be used to evaluate the bladder and ureters. The course of the ureters can be identified preoperatively if obstruction due to pelvic mass or scarring is suspected. IVP can be used to evaluate fistula, congenital anomalies, or suspected damage due to operative injury. However, it lacks sensitivity in imaging the pelvic floor and its associated defects, and does not yield much information regarding cystocele, rectocele, or enterocele.

Ultrasound techniques are an important tool to the urogynecologist. Compared to radiologic techniques, ultrasound is noninvasive and inexpensive, and does not require contrast media. Its main disadvantage is that the quality of the study depends heavily on the skill of the operator. When performed transabdominally, transvaginally, or transperineally and combined with Doppler or endoluminal transducers, the bladder, urethra, and surrounding structures can be visualized.

Videocystourethrography (VCUG)—VCUG combines a fluoroscopic voiding cystourethrogram with simultaneous recording of intravesical, intraurethral, and intra-abdominal pressure and urine flow rate. The contrast in the bladder allows dynamic evaluation of the bladder and bladder support.

Computed tomography (CT)—CT can be used in the evaluation of ureteral obstruction, urolithiasis, and the kidneys. It has poor resolution of soft tissues and has limited value in imaging the pelvic floor and associated defects.

Magnetic resonance imaging (MRI)—MRI has evolved into an important tool for the evaluation of the pelvic floor. It is an ideal modality as its resolution of soft tissues is superior to that of other radiologic techniques. The capability to image in multiple planes is also an advantage, particularly when visualizing the complex three-dimensional relationships of the pelvic floor. As this modality becomes less costly and techniques evolve to allow evaluation of patients in the upright position, the information provided by MRI will be invaluable in increasing our knowledge and understanding of functional pelvic support.

Differential Diagnosis

Tumors of the urethra and bladder are much more indurated and fixed than cystoceles.

A large urethral diverticulum may look and feel like a cystocele but usually is more lateral, sensitive, and painful; compression, as a rule, will express some purulent material from the urethral meatus.

A true bladder diverticulum is rare in the trigonal portion of the bladder. The diverticulum may appear somewhat asymmetric. Without cystoscopic or cinefluorographic study, it may go undetected.

Enterocele of the anterior vaginal wall (see discussion later in chapter), although rare, may occur in patients who have had a hysterectomy. These "anterior enteroceles" can be distinguished from a cystocele by identifying the loops of intestine contained in the hernial sac. Enterocele can be demonstrated by inserting a probe into the bladder; by vaginal palpation over the tip of the probe, one can detect the unusually thick anterior vaginal wall and perhaps note intestinal crepitation. This maneuver may also be helpful in differentiating the anterior vaginal mass produced by a previous interposition operation that interposed the uterine fundus (or just the uterine isthmus) between the bladder and the vaginal wall.

The terms urethrocele, distal cystocele, and cystourethrocele are also used and are similar to cystoceles in etiology as each results from a defect in the endopelvic fascia. The different terms distinguish where the breaks are along the anterior vaginal wall.

Complications

A large cystocele, perhaps in association with uterine prolapse, may lead to acute urinary retention. Recurrent urinary tract infection may occur in patients in whom bladder emptying is incomplete.

Prevention

Prevention of genital prolapse is becoming the focus of much debate. Antepartum and intrapartum and postpartum exercises, especially those designed to strengthen the levator and perineal muscle groups (Kegel), often help improve or maintain pelvic support. Obesity, chronic cough, straining, and traumatic deliveries must be corrected or avoided. Estrogen therapy following the menopause may help to maintain the tone and vitality of pelvic musculofascial tissues and thereby prevent or postpone the appearance of cystocele and other forms of relaxation.

Treatment

A. MEDICAL MEASURES

The patient with a small or moderate-sized cystocele requires reassurance that the pressure symptoms are not the result of a serious condition and that, even though the relaxation may progress slowly over several years, no serious illness will result. With this conservative approach, surgical correction of a cystocele is rarely indicated in a woman in her childbearing years who may still wish to have children. If the young woman does present with significant symptoms related to the cystocele—or with a disturbing degree of urinary incontinence—temporary medical measures may provide adequate relief until she has completed childbearing, whereupon a definitive operative procedure can be accomplished.

1. **Pessary**—Pessary use in selected patients may provide adequate relief of symptoms. For isolated cystocele, a ring pessary is usually sufficient. For the elderly patient with complicating medical factors who is therefore a poor operative risk, the temporary use of a vaginal pessary may provide relief of symptoms until her general condition has improved.

Prolonged use of pessaries, if not properly managed, may lead to pressure necrosis and vaginal ulceration.

2. **Exercises**—In younger patients, some improvement of pressure symptoms and of urinary control may be obtained by using Kegel isometric exercises for 6–12 months to tighten and strengthen the pubococcygeus muscles. Objective evidence of improved support of the pelvic floor may be noted. Kegel exercises can be of greatest benefit when used prophylactically, beginning in pregnancy and continuing during and after the puerperium. In older patients, Kegel exercises rarely provide more than partial relief.

3. **Estrogens**—In postmenopausal women, estrogen replacement therapy for a number of months may greatly improve the tone, quality, and vascularity of the musculofascial supports. Nevertheless, one cannot expect that severe anatomic injury (large cystocele with associated stress incontinence) will be corrected by estrogen or medical measures alone.

B. SURGICAL MEASURES

Cystocele alone (without concomitant uterine prolapse, rectocele, or enterocele) infrequently becomes large enough or causes symptoms that require operative correction. It is only when the cystocele is large, when it is responsible for urine retention and recurrent bladder infections, or when it is associated with bladder and urethral changes responsible for stress incontinence that operative repair is required.

Anterior vaginal colporrhaphy is the most common surgical treatment for cystocele (Fig 41–4). This may often be combined with vaginal hysterectomy and pos-

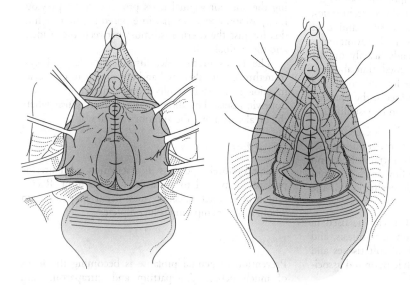

Figure 41–4. Repair of cystocele and plication of urethra for correction of anterior vaginal wall defect.

terior colpoperineorrhaphy because, ordinarily, the cystocele represents only one component of a generalized relaxation of pelvic supporting tissues.

Obliterative vaginal operations (vaginectomy, Le Fort's operation) are used primarily for severe uterovaginal prolapse in elderly patients and chronically ill patients who no longer desire coital function. It has the advantage of being done with regional or even local anesthesia (Fig 41–5). Unfortunately, operations of this type may not correct associated stress incontinence; in fact, traction produced by the obliterating scar tissue under the bladder neck and the urethra may actually cause or aggravate stress incontinence. Concomitant bladder neck suspension with a sling-type procedure can prevent stress incontinence.

Similarly, transabdominal repair of the cystocele (along with total abdominal hysterectomy) may be elected to correct the cystocele. When an abdominal approach is essential for other pelvic conditions, however, a retropubic urethrovesical suspension (Burch/Marshall-Marchetti-Krantz) can be combined with abdominal cystocele repair to correct or prevent the development of stress incontinence.

Prognosis

The prognosis after anterior colporrhaphy is excellent in the absence of a subsequent pregnancy or comparable factors (eg, constipation, obesity, large pelvic tumors, bronchitis, bronchiectasis, heavy manual labor) that increase intra-abdominal pressure. Recurrence of the cystocele after anterior colporrhaphy is rather common when a generalized relaxation of pelvic supports has been overlooked or ignored; in such cases, subse-

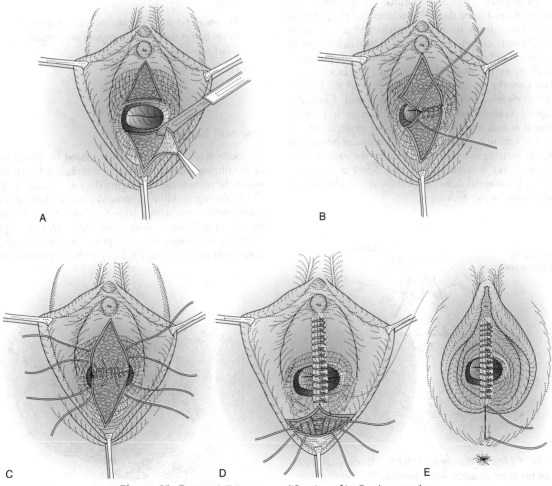

Figure 41–5. Goodall-Power modification of Le Fort's operation.

quent progression of uterine prolapse, enterocele, and rectocele may lead to disruption of the cystocele repair.

Vaginal Defects & Cystocele

PARAVAGINAL REPAIR

The etiology of the cystocele has been much debated over the last 80 years, beginning with White in 1912. The repair of defects in the anterior vaginal segment has been traditionally done by midline plication. An alternative method based on the anatomic observations by Richardson and colleagues advocates identification of the specific defect in the pubocervical fascia underlying the anterior vaginal epithelium and repairing the discrete breaks. These breaks are described as paravaginal, midline (central), distal, or transverse (superior) (Fig 41–6). This relationship may explain why no single operative repair should be applied to all patients with anterior vaginal wall defects.

Paravaginal repair is performed for cystoceles that are confirmed to be due to detachment of the pubocervical fascia from its lateral attachment at the arcus tendineus fascia pelvis (white line). These defects can be unilateral or bilateral. They can be confirmed preoperatively by noting loss of the lateral sulci and lack of rugation over the epithelium along the base of the bladder and elongation to the anterior vaginal wall. Clinically, vaginal examination using a speculum as it is withdrawn reveals a preponderance of the prolapse lateralized to one side. Further, a ring forceps can be used by gently exerting anterior traction along the vaginal sulci. If the defect is reduced, then the defect is consistent with a paravaginal defect and can be approached with a paravaginal repair technique.

The surgery can be performed either abdominally or vaginally. Both require identification of the white line and placement of serial sutures from the medial portion of the pubocervical fascia to the lateral sidewall at the level of the white line as it runs from the ischial spine over the obturator internus muscle to the posterior and inferior aspect of the pubic bone on the ipsilateral side. Reapproximation of the detached pubocervical fascia should reduce the anterior vaginal prolapse. This procedure can be done with other reconstructive procedures in the vagina as well as surgery to alleviate incontinence.

RECTOCELE

ESSENTIALS OF DIAGNOSIS

- *Sensation of vaginal fullness ("falling out" pressure).*
- *Presence of a soft, reducible mass bulging into the lower half of the posterior vaginal wall; frequently a flat, lacerated perineal body.*
- *Difficult evacuation of feces.*

General Considerations

Rectocele is a rectovaginal hernia caused by disruption of the fibrous connective tissue (rectovaginal fascia) between the rectum and the vagina (Figs 41–7 and 41–8). Often during childbirth, some degree of damage occurs—particularly with a large fetus or one presenting by the breech—and during multiple delivery. Episiotomy, once thought to be protective to the pelvic floor to minimize injury, is likely to be responsible for

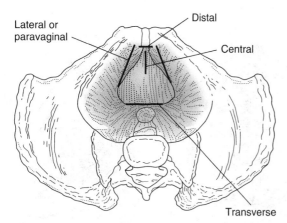

Figure 41–6. Four areas in which pubocervical fascia can break or separate—four defects. (Reproduced with permission from Contemp Ob-Gyn 1990;35:100.)

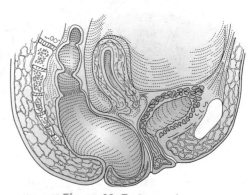

Figure 41–7. Rectocele.

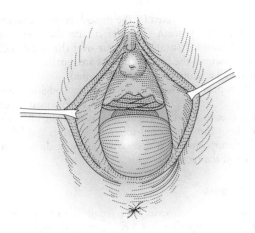

Figure 41–8. Rectocele.

compounding obstetrical trauma. Midline episiotomy is performed in over 50% of vaginal deliveries in the U.S. Midline episiotomy is associated with an increased rather than a decreased risk of severe lacerations. Additionally, after healing, the pelvic floor is scarred and the tissue strength is weakened and may predispose to pelvic organ prolapse in the future. Mediolateral episiotomy may protect against sphincter lacerations but does not appear to prevent the decreased pelvic floor strength seen with vaginal delivery. Episiotomy is not protective of the pelvic floor and should be used judiciously due to the potential long-term sequelae after obstetrical events.

Even though all multiparas have some degree of rectocele, the condition may not become manifest until the woman has passed the childbearing years and frequently not until several years after the menopause. This manifestation is due to the slowly progressive involutional changes in the pelvic musculofascial supporting tissues.

In addition to parturition and the inherent tone and quality of the patient's tissues, bowel habits are an important factor in the development of rectocele. Lifelong chronic constipation with straining may produce—or at least aggravate—a rectocele; conversely, a rectocele produced by the trauma of parturition, by pocketing of hard stool in the rectocele pouch, may aggravate mismanaged bowel function. Thus, the cause of rectocele may be difficult to distinguish from the effect of rectocele.

Clinical Findings

A. Symptoms

A small rectocele, demonstrable in virtually all multiparous patients, usually causes no symptoms. With more extensive relaxation (ie, with larger rectoceles), sensations of vaginal pressure, rectal fullness, and incomplete evacuation are typical complaints. The patient may report that it is necessary to manually reduce or "splint" the rectocele in order to defecate. Digital extraction of hard fecal material is sometimes required. The history may include prolonged, excessive use of laxatives or frequent enemas. Other nonspecific symptoms like low back pain, dyspareunia, or even fecal and gas incontinence may be reported.

B. Signs

Inspection of the area, with the patient straining and perhaps with slight depression of the perineum, discloses a soft mass bulging into the rectovaginal septum and distending the vaginal introitus. Examination (best accomplished rectovaginally, with the index finger in the vagina and the middle finger in the rectum) reveals a soft, thin-walled rectovaginal septum projecting well into the vagina. The septal defect may involve only the lower third of the posterior vaginal wall, but it often happens that the entire length of the rectovaginal septum is thinned out. The finger in the rectum confirms anterior sacculation into the vagina. Actually, a deep pocket into the perineal body may be noted, so that on apposition of the finger in the rectum and the thumb on the outside, the perineal body seems to consist of nothing but skin and rectal wall.

Previously unrecognized or unrepaired perineal lacerations may have almost destroyed the normally thick and strong musculature of the perineal body. Not infrequently, this traumatic attenuation involves some or all of the anal sphincter. Rarely, a small rectovaginal (or rectoperineal) fistula may also be present. Careful questioning about incontinence of feces or flatus and careful inspection of the area should disclose these associated defects.

C. Radiologic Findings

Although lateral x-ray views made after a barium enema will show the rectocele, this procedure is not essential for diagnosis. Dynamic cystoproctography can distinguish posterior vaginal wall defects from enteroceles, as can MRI. A rectocele frequently is associated with "hemorrhoidal bleeding"; when this occurs, proctoscopic study is necessary to exclude a concomitant colonic lesion.

Differential Diagnosis

What grossly appears to be a "high rectocele," ie, one involving the entire posterior vaginal wall, may consist partially or totally of an enterocele. With the patient standing, straining, and squatting slightly, rectovaginal examination will confirm the presence of abdominal contents sliding into the enterocele sac, and bowel crepitation may be noted. MRI is helpful in this setting.

Digital examination will also disclose tumors of the rectovaginal septum (lipomas, fibromas, sarcomas) that may produce a classic rectocele appearance.

Treatment

Treatment consists of avoidance of constipation by management of bowel function with daily stool softeners. Fecal impaction may require digital extraction or use of tap water enemas.

A. MEDICAL MEASURES

Medical management of a symptomatic rectocele is usually advisable until the patient has completed her childbearing. Increased fluid intake and stool softeners may be beneficial. Laxatives and rectal suppositories may be required. As a temporary measure, a large vaginal pessary of the Gehrung or doughnut type may provide relief if the perineum is adequate to retain the device in the vagina.

B. SURGICAL MEASURES

Rectocele alone (without associated enterocele, uterine prolapse, and cystocele) seldom requires surgical management. However, when the rectocele becomes so large that fecal evacuation is difficult, or the patient finds it necessary to manually reduce the rectocele into the vagina to expedite expulsion of feces, or the rectocele protrudes enough to cause discomfort or tissue breakdown, surgical repair is indicated (Fig 41–9).

There are two main surgical methods of a posterior vaginal defect (rectocele) repair. The traditional repair for colpoperineorrhaphy is the one described in most texts and involves posterior midline incision, often high, to the level of the posterior fornix. The vaginal epithelium is separated off the underlying fibromuscular layer and endopelvic fascia. Adequate repair includes plication of the levator ani muscles and bulk lateral plication of tissue oversewing the rectovaginal fascia. No attempt at identifying specific fascial defects is made.

The second method of posterior vaginal defect repair (rectocele) relies on the identification of discrete defects in the rectovaginal fascia. This anatomic description was first introduced by gynecologists advocating that rectoceles were caused by a variety of breaks in the rectovaginal fascia and that repairing these defects primarily was critical to anatomic restoration and lasting cure. This surgical technique included separating the vaginal epithelium off the underlying rectovaginal fascia as in a traditional colpoperineorrhaphy. Efforts are made to leave as much fascia on the rectum as possible. The surgeon inserts a finger of the nondominant hand into the rectum to inspect the rectovaginal fascia for defects. The rectal wall is brought forward to distinguish the uncovered muscularis (fascial defect) from the mus-

cularis that was covered by the smooth semitransparent rectal vaginal septum. The defects are then repaired with interrupted sutures to plicate over the rectal wall. In this manner the isolated defects are repaired and the functional anatomy is optimally restored.

Postoperative avoidance of straining, coughing, and strenuous activity is advisable. Careful instruction about diet to avoid constipation, about intake of fluids, and about the use of stool-softening laxatives and lubricating suppositories is necessary to ensure durable integrity of the rectocele repair.

Prognosis

Recurrence of rectocele after repair is uncommon if chronic constipation has been corrected, subsequent vaginal delivery is avoided, and a concomitant enterocele and uterine prolapse have not been overlooked.

ENTEROCELE

 ESSENTIALS OF DIAGNOSIS

- *Uncomfortable pressure and a falling-out sensation in the vagina.*
- *Associated with uterine prolapse or subsequent to hysterectomy in any age group; most common in postmenopausal women.*
- *Demonstration of a mass bulging into the posterior fornix and upper posterior vaginal wall.*

General Considerations

Enterocele is a herniation of the rectouterine pouch (pouch of Douglas) into the rectovaginal septum (Fig 41–10). This presents as a bulging mass in the posterior fornix and upper posterior vaginal wall. A similar hernial sac through the cul-de-sac, but extending posteriorly, may present through the anal canal as a rectal prolapse.

Enterocele may be congenital or acquired; the latter is much more common. The congenital form rarely causes symptoms. The acquired form of enterocele occurs in multiparous premenopausal or postmenopausal women and almost invariably is associated with other manifestations of musculofascial weakness such as uterine prolapse, cystocele, and rectocele. The trauma of many pregnancies and vaginal deliveries (perhaps breech extractions and forceps rotations), large pelvic tumors, marked obesity, ascites, chronic bronchitis, and

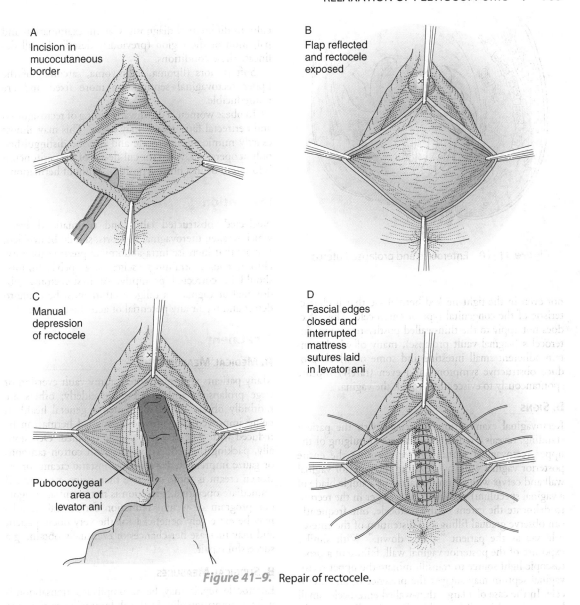

A
Incision in mucocutaneous border

B
Flap reflected and rectocele exposed

C
Manual depression of rectocele

Pubococcygeal area of levator ani

D
Fascial edges closed and interrupted mattress sutures laid in levator ani

Figure 41–9. Repair of rectocele.

other factors that increase intra-abdominal pressure are of etiologic importance.

Uterine prolapse is almost always accompanied by some degree of enterocele, and, as the degree of uterine descent progresses, the size of the hernial sac increases. Similarly, posthysterectomy prolapse of the vaginal vault usually is the result of an enterocele that was overlooked (not repaired) at the time of hysterectomy or develops as a result of poor repair and identification of cuff support structures. Rarely, after hysterectomy, the enterocele is located anterior to the vaginal vault, where it may be easily confused with ordinary cystocele.

Clinical Findings

A. SYMPTOMS

The pelvic and abdominal symptoms produced by an enterocele are nonspecific and perhaps are actually the result of downward traction of the lower abdominal viscera. Aching discomfort frequently is described, along with the sensation of vaginal pressure and fullness commonly noted with other forms of prolapse. Gastrointestinal symptoms can rarely, if ever, be attributed to an enterocele. Peculiarly, the small bowel almost never becomes adherent to or incarcerated in the enterocele—

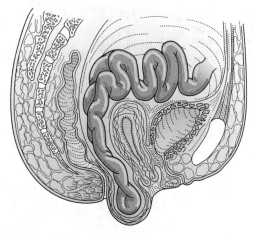

Figure 41–10. Enterocele and prolapsed uterus.

not even in the tight-necked hernial sac that is characteristic of the congenital type of enterocele. This effect does not apply to the thin-walled posthysterectomy enteroceles (vaginal vault prolapse), many of which contain adherent small intestine and some of which produce obstructive symptoms and even (rarely) rupture spontaneously to eviscerate through the vagina.

B. SIGNS

Rectovaginal examination, especially with the patient standing, reveals a reducible thickness or bulging of the upper rectovaginal septum. After exposing the entire posterior vaginal wall (by elevating the anterior vaginal wall and cervix with a Sims retractor or a single blade of a vaginal speculum) and inserting a finger in the rectum to delineate the extent of the rectocele, one frequently can observe gradual filling and distention of the enterocele sac as the patient "strains down." With similar exposure of the posterior vaginal wall, failure of a proctoscopic light source to transilluminate the upper rectovaginal septum may suggest the presence of an enterocele. In the case of a large, thin-walled enterocele, small bowel peristalsis will be visible. Occasionally, to obtain filling of the hernial sac, it is essential to examine the patient in a standing-straining position.

C. RADIOLOGIC FINDINGS

Lateral pelvic x-ray views obtained during barium studies of the small bowel may reveal prolapse of the ileum into the enterocele. MRI can facilitate distinction of high rectocele from an enterocele.

Differential Diagnosis

High rectocele and cystocele (when an anterior enterocele is suspected) are the most common causes of diffi-

culty in differential diagnosis. Careful examination and palpation of the region (previously described) will delineate these conditions.

Soft tumors (lipoma, leiomyoma, sarcoma) of the upper rectovaginal septum are more fixed and are nonreducible.

In obese women, a downward sliding of rectosigmoid and perirectal fatty tissues may occur. This may almost exactly mimic an enterocele and may be distinguished only at operation, when the cul-de-sac of the peritoneum is found to be in a normal position, without herniation.

Prevention

Neglected, obstructed labor and traumatic delivery, which weaken uterovaginal supports, should be avoided. Factors that increase intra-abdominal pressure (obesity, chronic cough, straining, ascites, large pelvic tumors) should be corrected promptly. At hysterectomy (abdominal or vaginal), a diligent effort must be made to detect and repair any potential or actual enterocele.

Treatment

A. MEDICAL MEASURES

Many patients with posthysterectomy vault eversion or large prolapsing apical defect are elderly; others are morbidly obese. While the patient's general health is being improved, the prolapsing vaginal hernia can be reduced with a pessary if it can be retained. Occasionally, packing the reduced vagina with cotton tampons or gauze impregnated with bacteriostatic creams or estrogen cream is more effective than using a pessary. If immediate operative correction is not essential, a rigorous program of weight reduction for several months may be extremely beneficial for the very obese patient and may increase her chances of eventually obtaining a successful repair.

B. SURGICAL MEASURES

Enterocele repair may be accomplished transabdominally or transvaginally. In the abdominal operation, the enterocele sac is obliterated and the uterosacral ligaments and endopelvic fascia are approximated with concentric purse-string sutures as described by Moschowitz. However, inasmuch as symptomatic enterocele almost invariably is associated with other forms of musculofascial weakness (uterine prolapse, cystocele, rectocele), a transvaginal operation may provide the best route of repair and offer the greatest likelihood of permanent correction of the enterocele. This procedure includes excision and high ligation of the enterocele sac (a cardinal principle of any hernia repair) and approximation of the uterosacral ligaments and endopelvic fascia anterior to the rectum (floor of the cul-de-sac).

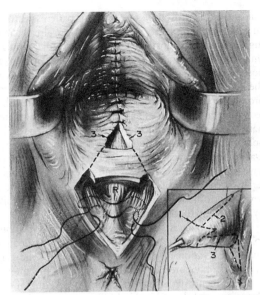
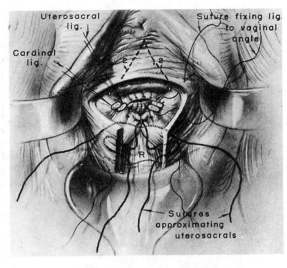

Figure 41–11. Correction of vaginal prolapse after hysterectomy. *R,* rectum.

Concomitant vaginal hysterectomy, anterior (cystocele) and posterior (rectocele) colporrhaphy, and perineorrhaphy may greatly augment the support.

Posthysterectomy enterocele with prolapse of the vaginal vault is also best managed by the transvaginal route. Numerous surgical techniques have been documented to correct posthysterectomy vault prolapse, including either a vaginal or an abdominal approach (Fig 41–11). A review of vaginal operations includes among others colpocleisis, sacrospinous ligament suspension

Table 41–3. Follow up and cure rate after sacrospinous ligament suspension.

Author (Year)	Duration of Follow-Up	No. Patients	No. Cured (%)
Nichols (1982)	>2 y	163	158 (97)
Morley and DeLancey (1988)	1 mo–11 y	92	75 (82)
Cruikshank and Cox (1990)	8 mo–3.2 y	48	40 (83)
Monk et al (1991)	1 mo–8.6 y	61	52 (85)
Shull et al (1992)	2–5 y	81	53 (65)
Peters and Christenson (1995)	Median 48 mo	30	22 (77)
Sze et al (1997)	7–72 m	75	53 (71)

Adapted from Sze EH, Karram MM: Transvaginal repair of vault prolapse: a review. Obstet Gynecol 1997;89:466.

(Table 41–3), endopelvic fascia vaginal vault fixation, iliococcygeal fixation, and high uterosacral ligament suspension (high McCall culdeplasty; see Fig 41–12).

Because the normal vaginal axis is directed some distance posteriorly (almost horizontally when the patient is in an erect position) over the levator plate, operative correction by any means, whether by the vaginal or the abdominal route, should restore a normal vaginal axis. This is accomplished by suspension of the vaginal apex far back on the uterosacral ligaments, the presacral fascia, or the sacrospinous ligaments. The suspension can be provided by use of nonabsorbable sutures, autogenous fascia, or prosthetic material (eg, Dacron, Teflon, or Marlex mesh). Techniques that suspend the vaginal vault from the anterior abdominal wall should be avoided because they bring the axis of the vagina too far forward and leave a hiatus posteriorly, which promotes recurrence of the enterocele.

A popular method of vaginal vault suspension is that of unilateral fixation to the sacrospinous ligament. In this technique the vaginal mucosa is separated from the rectovaginal tissues, and the associated enterocele is identified and repaired (as previously described). Perforation through the right or left rectal pillar is usually easily accomplished by directing blunt dissection toward the ischial spine through the loose areolar tissue. After an appropriate location on the sacrospinous ligament is identified (usually 2–3 cm medial to the ischial spine), one of several techniques may be used to safely pass 2 or more permanent (or delayed absorbable) ligatures through the ligament to the submucosal apex of

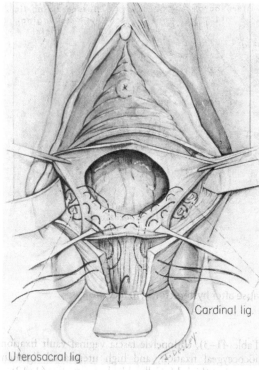

Figure 41–12. Symmonds' modification of the McCall enterocele repair (after vaginal hysterectomy and repair).

the vagina. Tying the sutures brings the vaginal apex to that sacrospinous ligament, and a posterior colporrhaphy is then performed (as noted previously). Closing the dead space by intermittently suturing the vaginal mucosa to the underlying reconstituted rectovaginal septum may be useful. Patients who have concomitant stress urinary incontinence should have a corrective procedure at this time. Needle urethropexies should be avoided due to high rates of recurrence.

The vaginal positioning to the right or left seemingly is minimal after healing occurs and has not constituted a problem. Indeed, vaginal connection to both sacrospinous ligaments is not recommended because it causes excessive lateral stretching of the vaginal apex. Vaginal vault suspension to one or both sacrospinous ligaments has the potential of injury to the pudendal nerve or pudendal vessels and is often technically difficult. Thus, it requires a skilled surgeon and should be undertaken only by those familiar with the technique.

Vaginal vault suspension can also be performed abdominally by attaching the vaginal cuff to the sacral promontory. Abdominal sacrocolopexy is an excellent primary procedure for vaginal vault prolapse and entero-

cele and is the procedure of choice for patients with recurrent vaginal prolapse or patients who are already having an abdominal approach for another indication. In this procedure a graft is used to bring the vaginal vault posteriorly along the hollow of the sacrum and affixed to the anterior longitudinal ligament overriding the sacral promontory. Numerous studies have demonstrated this technique to be curative (Table 41–4). A variety of materials have been used, including synthetic materials like polypropylene mesh, polytetrafluoroethylene mesh, and Dacron mesh; however, these types of materials appear to have higher erosion rates. Currently, biocompatible materials such as dermal allografts and biologic matrices have been utilized. Clinical results have shown durability, safety, and biocompatibility.

Vaginal obliterative procedures (Le Fort's operation, colpectomy) may be used in patients who do not require preservation of vaginal function. Unless the hernial sac is obliterated or removed, however, the enterocele may recur, perhaps in the form of a hernia of the perineum or of the ischiorectal fossa.

C. SUPPORTIVE MEASURES

As with hernias of other types, obesity, chronic cough, and constipation should be corrected. Strenuous lifting, straining, and vigorous activity (calisthenics, bowling, etc) should be avoided for at least 6 months postoperatively.

D. EMERGENCY MEASURES

With complete eversion of the vagina by the enterocele, trophic ulceration, edema, and fibrosis of the vaginal

Table 41–4. Follow–up and cure rate after abdominal sacral colpopexy.

Author (Year)	Duration of Follow-Up	No. Patients	No. Cured (%)
Cowan and Morgan (1980)	≤60 mo	39	38 (97)
Addision et al (1985)	6–126 mo	56	54 (96)
Baker et al (1990)	1–45 mo	51	51 (100)
Snyder and Krantz (1991)	≥6 mo	116	108 (93)
Timmons et al (1992)	9–216 mo	162	161 (99)
Iosif (1993)	12–120 mo	40	39 (96)
Grunberger et al (1994)	3–91 mo	48	45 (94)
Valatis and Stanton (1994)	3–91 mo	41	38 (96)

Adapted from Walters MD, Karram MM: *Urogynecology and Reconstructive Pelvic Surgery,* 2nd ed. Mosby, 1999.

walls may occur to such a degree that the prolapsing mass cannot be reduced. Rest in bed (with the foot of the bed elevated) and wet packs applied to the vagina will reduce edema and allow replacement of the vagina, and vaginal packing can be used to maintain reduction until local conditions permit operative correction.

Rupture of the enterocele, with evisceration of the small intestine, is rare and managed best by prompt reduction of the prolapsing loops of small intestine followed by simple closure of the tear in the vaginal wall.

Prognosis

The outlook after proper enterocele repair is excellent. Techniques that repair only the enterocele (neglecting the associated cystocele, rectocele, and uterine prolapse) and those that suspend the vaginal vault (or the intact uterus) without obliterating the hernial sac are associated with a high incidence of recurrence.

Failure to repair associated vaginal defects increases the risk of enterocele or recurrence (Table 41–4). Not only should these defects be repaired at the time of enterocele repair, prophylactic corrections should be carried out when an enterocele is not present, ie, shortening and plication of elongated, strong uterosacral ligaments; excision and high ligation of excessive posterior cul-de-sac peritoneum; wedging and closure of a wide vaginal cuff.

The surgical techniques used must be directed at the enterocele and all associated specific defects. A combination of procedures is most frequently necessary. There is no single surgical procedure that is always curative for this condition, and cure is effected by tailoring the operation to the patient. Possibly more than with any other pelvic support relaxation disorder, correct surgical treatment of complete vaginal prolapse requires a thorough understanding of all the vaginal defects present.

UTERINE PROLAPSE

 ### ESSENTIALS OF DIAGNOSIS

- *Firm mass in the lower vagina; cervix projecting through the vaginal introitus; vaginal eversion, with the cervix and uterus projecting between the legs.*
- *Sensation of vaginal fullness or pressure; lower abdominal pulling or aching; low backache.*

General Considerations

Uterine prolapse is descent of the uterus/cervix through the vaginal canal. It is due to defects in the support structures of the uterus and vagina, including the uterosacral ligaments, the cardinal ligament complex, and connective tissue of the urogenital membrane (Fig 41–13). Like cystocele, rectocele, and enterocele—conditions with which it is usually associated—uterine prolapse occurs most commonly in multiparous women as a gradually progressive result of childbirth injuries to the endopelvic fascia (and its condensations, the uterosacral and cardinal ligaments) and lacerations of muscle, especially the levator muscles and those of the perineal body. Additional factors promoting uterine prolapse are (1) systemic conditions, including obesity, asthma, chronic bronchitis, and bronchiectasis; and (2) local conditions such as ascites and large uterine and ovarian tumors. Uterine prolapse may also be the result of pelvic tumor; sacral nerve disorders, especially injury to S1–S4 (as in spina bifida); diabetic neuropathy; caudal anesthesia accidents; and presacral tumor.

A congenital weakness in the pelvic fascial supports may be causative of uterine prolapse as it is occasionally demonstrated in nulliparous, even virginal, females with intact, strong levator muscles and a narrow genital hiatus; apparently, prolapse in these cases is the result of an inherent weakness of the endopelvic fascial supports of the uterus and vagina. In uterine prolapse of the common type, symptoms may not occur until many years after the causative event (eg, traumatic delivery). This observation suggests that failure of the supporting

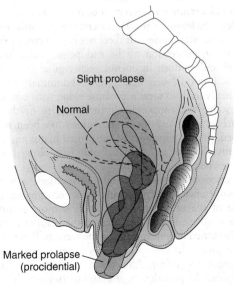

Figure 41–13. Prolapse of the uterus.

structures and attenuation of pelvic fascial support are potentially latent sequelae of neuronal injury that becomes clinically manifest with aging.

A uterus that is in a retroverted position is especially subject to prolapse; with the corpus aligned with the axis of the vagina, anything increasing intra-abdominal pressure exerts a piston-like action on the uterus, driving it down into the vagina.

Prolapse of a cervical stump (after subtotal abdominal hysterectomy) does not differ in any significant way from prolapse of an intact uterus. Admittedly, the oviducts and the utero-ovarian and round ligaments have been divided, but these structures do not normally contribute to the functional support of the uterus.

The degree of uterine prolapse parallels the extent of separation or attenuation of its supporting structures. In slight intravaginal or incomplete prolapse, the uterus descends only part of the way down the vagina; in moderate prolapse, it descends to the introitus, and the cervix protrudes slightly beyond; and in marked or complete prolapse (procidentia), the entire cervix and uterus protrude beyond the introitus and the vagina is inverted.

The principal components of the basin-like pelvic floor are the pelvic bones (including the coccyx), the endopelvic fascia, and the levator and perineal muscles. These structures normally support and maintain the position of the pelvic viscera despite great increments of intra-abdominal pressure that occur with straining, coughing, and heavy lifting when the patient is in the erect position. The urogenital hiatus ("anterior levator muscle gap"), which permits the urethra, vagina, and anus to emerge from the pelvis, is a site of potential weakness. Attenuation of the pubococcygeal and puborectal portions of the levator muscles, whether as the result of a traumatic delivery or of involutional changes, widens the levator gap and converts this potential weakness to an actual defect. If there has been a concomitant injury or attenuation of the endopelvic fascia (uterosacral and cardinal ligaments, rectovaginal and pubocervical fascia), heightened intra-abdominal pressure gradually leads to uterine prolapse along with cystocele, rectocele, and enterocele. If the integrity of the endopelvic fascia and its condensations has been maintained, the incompetency of the genital hiatus and levator muscles may be associated only with elongation of the cervix.

Anterior and posterior vaginal relaxation, as well as incompetence of the perineum, often accompanies prolapse of the uterus. Large cystocele is more common than rectocele in prolapse because the bladder is more easily carried downward than is the rectum. Prior to the menopause, the prolapsed uterus hypertrophies and is engorged and flabby. After the menopause, the uterus atrophies. In procidentia, the vaginal mucosa thickens and cornifies, coming to resemble skin.

Clinical Findings

A. SYMPTOMS AND SIGNS

With mild prolapse (first-degree; cervix palpable as a firm mass in the lower third of the vagina), few symptoms can be attributed to the relaxation. With moderate prolapse (second-degree; cervix visible and projecting into or through the vaginal introitus), the patient may experience a falling-out sensation or may report that she feels as if she is sitting on a ball; of less significance may be a sensation of heaviness in the pelvis, low backache, and lower abdominal and inguinal pulling discomfort. In cases of severe prolapse (procidentia; third-degree), the cervix and entire uterus project through the introitus and the vagina is totally inverted. Frequently, this large mass has one or more areas of easily bleeding atrophic ulceration.

In premenopausal women with prolapse, leukorrhea or menometrorrhagia frequently develops as a result of uterine engorgement. After the menopause, excessive vaginal mucus and bleeding may be due to atrophic ulceration and infection of the prolapse.

Compression, distortion, or herniation of the bladder by the displaced uterus and cervix may be responsible for accumulation of residual urine, which leads to urinary tract infection, frequency and urgency, and overflow voiding. Incontinence is rare, but does occur. Constipation and painful defecation occur with prolapse because of pressure and rectocele. Ease and completeness of voiding and defecation may follow manual reduction of the prolapse by the patient. Cramping and obstipation may follow intestinal constriction within a large enterocele.

B. PELVIC EXAMINATION

With the patient bearing down or straining (perhaps in a standing position), pelvic examination reveals descent of the cervix to the lower third of the vagina (mild prolapse), descent past the introitus (moderate prolapse), or descent of the entire uterus through the introitus (severe prolapse). As the uterus progressively descends, some degree of cystocele and enterocele must develop concomitantly as a result of anatomic fixation of the bladder base and of the cul-de-sac to anterior and posterior uterocervical surfaces. In fact, a supposed uterine prolapse unaccompanied by cystocele and enterocele is almost invariably the result of cervical elongation (see following section).

The uterine tubes, ovaries, bladder, and distal ureters are drawn downward by the prolapsing uterus. Uterine or adnexal neoplasms and ascites associated with uterine prolapse should be noted.

Rectovaginal examination may reveal a rectocele. An enterocele may be behind and perhaps below the cervix, but in front of a rectocele. Placement of a metal sound or firm catheter within the bladder may determine the extent of concomitant cystocele.

Differential Diagnosis

Cervical elongation presents the most troublesome problem in differential diagnosis. The distinction is important because vaginal hysterectomy (the customary operative treatment for uterine prolapse) may be difficult when performed for cervical elongation. With cervical elongation, vaginal examination discloses that the anterior, posterior, and lateral vaginal fornices are at their customary high level and descend minimally with straining; the anterior and upper posterior vaginal walls are well supported (little or no cystocele or enterocele); and the uterine corpus remains in a relatively high and posterior position.

Cervical tumors—as well as endometrial tumors (pedunculated myoma or endometrial polyps)—if prolapsed through a dilated cervix and presenting in the lower third of the vagina may be confused with mild or moderate uterine prolapse. Myomas or polyps may coexist with prolapse of the uterus and cause unusual symptoms.

Despite the variety of possibilities, the history and physical findings in uterine prolapse are so characteristic that diagnosis is usually not a problem.

Complications

Leukorrhea, abnormal uterine bleeding, and abortion may result from infection or from disordered uterine or ovarian circulation in prolapse. Chronic decubitus ulceration of the vaginal epithelium may develop in procidentia. Urinary tract infection may occur with prolapse because of cystocele; and partial ureteral obstruction with hydronephrosis may occur in procidentia. Hemorrhoids result from straining to overcome constipation. Small bowel obstruction from a deep enterocele is rare.

Prevention

Prenatal and postpartum Kegel exercises to strengthen the levator muscles may minimize prolapse. Prolonged estrogen therapy for menopausal and postmenopausal women tends to maintain the vascularity and vitality of the endopelvic fascia and pelvic floor musculature.

Treatment

A. MEDICAL MEASURES

A vaginal pessary (inflatable ball, doughnut, Menge, Gellhorn, bee cell) may be used either as palliative therapy if surgical treatment is contraindicated or as a tem-porary measure in mild to moderate prolapse. The use of a pessary may assist in determining whether or not the rather ambiguous symptoms reported by the patient are actually produced by the uterine prolapse. In procidentia, reduction of the uterus followed by packing of the vagina to maintain uterine position may be necessary in the preoperative management of an ulcerated, infected prolapse.

In postmenopausal patients, the administration of estrogen (systemically or vaginally) will improve the tissue tone and facilitate correction of an atrophic, perhaps ulcerative, vaginitis. Biopsies should be considered for ulcerated areas; D&C or biopsy may be necessary to investigate bleeding and to rule out cancer. Prescribe vaginal creams (eg, Aci-Jel), acetic acid douches, or topical estrogen for ulceration. Treat urinary tract infection, diabetes mellitus, or cardiovascular complications appropriately. Prescribe laxatives or enemas for constipation. Utilize a bowel preparation to evacuate distal sigmoid and rectum of feces to facilitate surgery of the vaginal compartment.

B. SURGICAL MEASURES

Uterine prolapse may remain constant for many years or may progress very slowly, depending somewhat on the patient's age and activity. Even though one can be certain that the condition will not regress and that operation may eventually be required, its correction is not urgent, and surgical treatment should be deferred until the prolapse gives rise to significant symptoms.

Selection of a surgical approach for uterine prolapse depends on a number of variables: the patient's age, her desire for pregnancy or preservation of vaginal function, the degree of prolapse, and the presence of associated conditions (cystocele, stress incontinence, enterocele, rectocele). In general, symptoms associated with mild to moderate uterine prolapse are not severe. Thus, in the younger patient whose subsequent pregnancy may well nullify any benefits derived from an operative repair, it is preferred to defer reparative surgery until childbearing is completed. Operations of the Manchester type were at one time recommended for the young patient with prolapse; but this procedure, which includes amputation of the cervix, has fallen into disfavor because it is associated with a high incidence of infertility and premature labor. The pelvic floor should be restored. Otherwise, vaginal hysterectomy with correction of hernial defects may be elected.

Most patients with uterovaginal prolapse have a composite lesion, ie, symptoms related to a moderate degree of uterine prolapse plus a moderate degree of cystocele, stress incontinence, enterocele, rectocele, and perineal relaxation. To provide good support for the vaginal vault and vaginal wall, the best surgical management consists of a composite operation. In addition to vaginal hysterectomy, the operation must include repair of actual or potential enterocele, careful anterior colporrhaphy to correct the cystocele and stress incontinence, and posterior colpoperineorrhaphy extending well up the posterior vaginal wall (Fig 41–14). If preservation of vaginal function is not important, narrowing and shortening the vagina by the removal of much of the anterior and posterior vaginal walls with the colporrhaphy, when combined with a high approximation of the levator muscles and with perineorrhaphy, will ensure the success of the operative repair. Vaginal obliterative operations (Le Fort's operation or vaginectomy) are rarely indicated in elderly women who are poor surgical candidates and who no longer desire coital function.

Uterine prolapse can be managed by an abdominal approach that includes total abdominal hysterectomy and the obliteration of any associated enterocele. However, this method can be more morbid and time-consuming; furthermore, it is optimal only when combined with transvaginal repair of cystocele and rectocele. Uterine suspensions—even ventrofixation of the corpus to the abdominal wall—are not effective in the treatment of prolapse and should be avoided.

In postmenopausal women who are sexually active, vaginal hysterectomy and repair of associated vaginal defects is preferred.

C. Supportive Measures

If the patient is obese, she should be encouraged to lose weight. Tight girdles and garments that increase intra-abdominal pressure and other factors (occupational or physical) that have a similar effect should be avoided or corrected.

D. Treatment of Complications

Infection of the operative area or of the urinary tract may require antibiotic therapy. Prescribe a pessary or reoperate for recurrence.

E. Emergency Measures

Infrequently, a patient with moderate to severe prolapse becomes pregnant. The rapidly enlarging uterus may become incarcerated within the true pelvis or, in procidentia, even outside the pelvis. It is imperative that the uterus be replaced and that the patient remain in bed until the uterus is large enough to prevent recurrence of the prolapse. An incarcerated, edematous procidentia may lead to urethral (or even ureteral) obstruction, anuria, and uremia; therefore, prompt reduction of the prolapse is essential.

Prognosis

Vaginal hysterectomy with an anterior repair and site-specific posterior repair provides excellent and lasting vaginal support and, if good healing occurs, preservation of vaginal function as well. Recurrent vaginal prolapse may result from generalized relaxation (unrepaired cystocele, rectocele, or enterocele) or from exertional factors such as heavy lifting or chronic straining.

Vaginal Defects & Uterine Prolapse

Uterine prolapse is the result of defects in the supravaginal supports, primarily the uterosacral and cardinal ligaments.

Depending on the exact defect or combination of defects present, abnormalities ranging from uterine retrodisplacement to procidentia associated with cystocele, rectocele, and enterocele may occur. Since these defects are usually progressive, failure to repair all defects present may lead to new difficulties or recurrence. For example, to perform a vaginal hysterectomy for early uterine descensus but not address the weaknesses in support at the vaginal cuff can lead to later development of an enterocele and/or vaginal vault prolapse. Additionally, failure to correct asymptomatic cystocele and rectocele at the time of hysterectomy not only increases the risk of vaginal vault prolapse, but also leaves the vagina with an abnormal depth and angle.

The importance of understanding the etiology of the various defects before attempting surgical correction of a prolapsed uterus cannot be overstated. Simply performing hysterectomy is insufficient.

MALPOSITIONS OF THE UTERUS ("TIPPED UTERUS")

Significant displacement of the uterus may cause signs or symptoms such as pelvic pain, backache, menstrual aberrations, and infertility. Virtually all women with symptoms that may be due to displacements are premenopausal. Almost all postpartum patients have a temporarily retroposed (tipped) uterus. Some retrodisplacements are secondary to defects in the supravaginal supports. It is unclear whether women with such defects may be at greater risk for developing other pelvic support problems, ie, uterine prolapse or vaginal wall defects.

The uterus is not a fixed organ, and the position may vary transiently as a result of pelvic inclination or prolonged sitting, standing, or lying. The body of the uterus is directed forward in 80% of women; in the remainder, it is directed backward, but fewer than 5% of these women have a bona fide complaint referable to posterior version of the uterus.

Retroversion implies that the axis of the body of the uterus is directed to the hollow of the sacrum, although the cervix remains in its normal axis. If angulation of

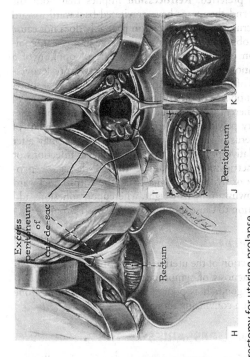

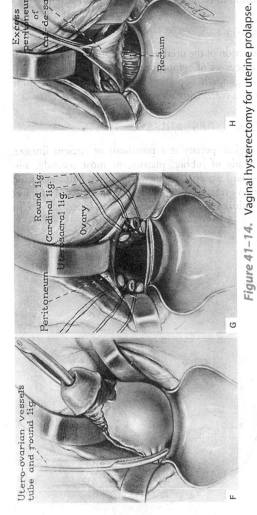

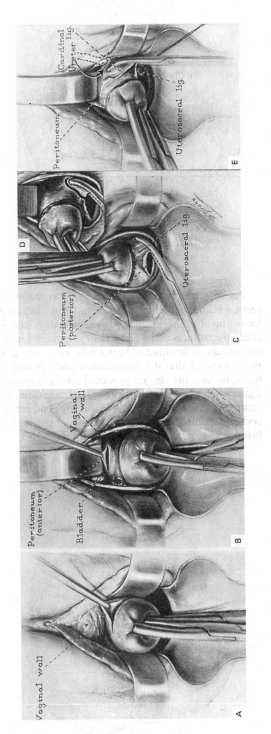

Figure 41-14. Vaginal hysterectomy for uterine prolapse.

the corpus on the cervix is extreme, the term **retroflexion** is preferred. **Retrocession** implies that both the cervix and the uterus have gravitated backward toward the sacrum. Acute **anteversion** probably does not cause either obstruction to uterine discharge or circulatory alteration or dysmenorrhea—a reversal of opinion of a generation or more ago. Free **dextroversion** or levoversion is of little clinical importance unless tumors, shortened supports, or other disorders are present.

Adherent lateral deviation of the uterus may indicate primary pelvic disease (eg, salpingitis). Enlargement of the uterus, whether by pregnancy or tumor, may alter the relative position of that organ. Pelvic infections or endometriosis may obliterate the cul-de-sac. A pyosalpinx or hydrosalpinx may drag the corpus backward and downward by its weight, whereupon adhesions add restriction to cause immobility (Figs 41–15 to 41–17).

Prognosis

If correction of the uterine malposition follows an accurate diagnosis of symptomatic displacement, the outlook is good. It is poor if uterine suspension is done without a convincing indication.

VAGINAL PESSARIES

The vaginal pessary is a prosthesis of ancient lineage, now made of rubber, plastics, or most recently, silicone-based material, often with a metal band or spring frame. A great many types have been devised, but fewer than a dozen are basically unique and specifically helpful.

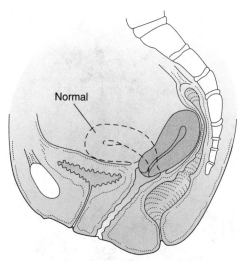

Figure 41–16. Retrocession of uterus.

Pessaries are principally used to support the uterus, cervical stump, or hernias of the pelvic floor. They are effective because they reduce vaginal relaxation and increase the tautness of the pelvic floor structures. Little or no leverage is involved. The retrodisplaced uterus remains forward after it is repositioned and a pessary inserted because the tension produced on the uterosacral ligaments draws the cervix backward. In most cases, adequate support anteriorly and a reasonably good perineal body are required; otherwise, the pessary may slip from behind the symphysis and extrude from the vagina.

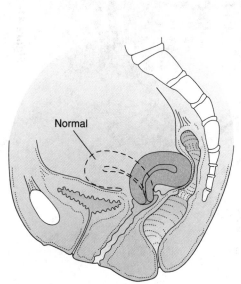

Figure 41–15. Retroflexion in an anteverted uterus.

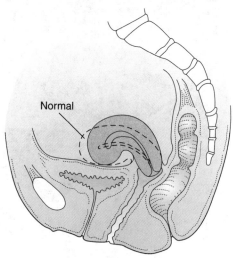

Figure 41–17. Acute anteflexion of uterus.

Indications & Uses

(1) To reduce cystocele or retrocele.

(2) To treat poor-risk patients or those who decline operation for uterine prolapse or other vaginal wall defects.

(3) To control urinary stress incontinence by exerting pressure beneath the urethra or by improving the posterior urethrovesical angle.

(4) To serve as a preoperative aid in the healing of vaginal or cervical stasis ulcerations associated with uterine prolapse.

Contraindications

Pessaries are contraindicated in acute genital tract infections and in adherent retroposition of the uterus.

Types of Pessaries (Fig 41–18)

A. Hodge Pessary (Smith-Hodge, or Smith and Other Variations)

This is an elongated, curved ovoid. One end is placed behind the symphysis and the other in the posterior vaginal fornix. The anterior bow is curved to avoid the urethra; the cervix rests within the larger, posterior bow. This type of pessary is used to hold the uterus in place after it has been repositioned.

B. Ring Pessary

A ring pessary with or without support provides relief of first and second degree uterine prolapse or cystocele.

C. Cube

This is a flexible rubber cube, with suction cups on each of its six sides that adhere to the vaginal walls. This is useful in elderly women with severe prolapse. Frequent monitoring initially to identify pressure ulcers is critical.

D. Doughnut

This doughnut is made of soft rubber or silicone, and this type of pessary provides support for severe uterine prolapse or vault prolapse.

E. Gellhorn and Menge Pessaries

Both of these types are uniquely shaped like a collar button and provide a ring-like platform for the cervix. The pessary is stabilized by a stem that rests on the perineum. These pessaries are used to correct marked prolapse when the perineal body is reasonably adequate.

F. Gehrung Pessary

The Gehrung pessary resembles 2 firm letter U's attached by crossbars. It rests in the vagina with the

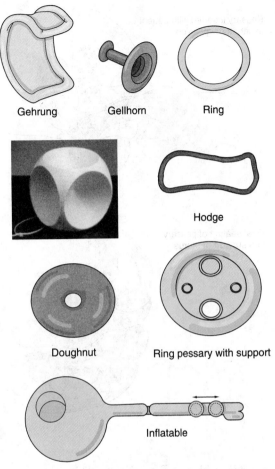

Figure 41–18. Types of pessaries.

cervix cradled between the long arms; this arches the anterior vaginal wall and helps reduce a cystocele.

G. Inflatable Pessary

The inflatable pessary (Milex) functions much like a doughnut pessary. The ball valve is moved up and down; when the ball is in the down position, air inflates the pessary; when in the up position, the air is sealed in and inflation is maintained.

FITTING OF PESSARIES

Pessaries that are too large cause irritation and ulceration. Those that are too small may not stay in place and may protrude.

In general, fitting a pessary is very much a trial and error endeavor. Once a type is selected based on the defects in the vaginal anatomy and on symptoms, sizing is

Pessary inserted with patient in lithotomy position

Patient in knee-chest position. Uterus anteverted and pessary seated

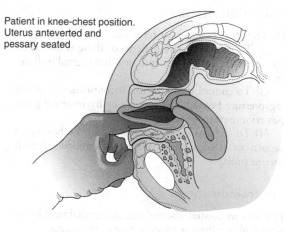

Final seating of pessary and support of uterus

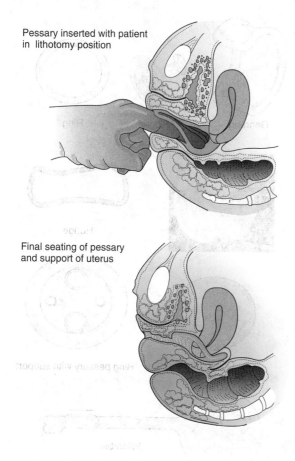

Figure 41–19. Insertion of Hodge type pessary.

best done with an office sizing set. This task is somewhat more complicated as each pessary has its own measurement system, but familiarity with each pessary over time with use simplifies this task. The pessary should be lubricated and inserted with its widest dimension in the oblique diameter of the vagina to avoid painful distention at the introitus. With a finger of the opposite hand, depress the perineum to widen the introitus.

The Hodge pessary should be rotated slightly after it is in the vagina; then, using the forefinger of one hand, slip the posterior bar behind the cervix. The anterior bar should then be brought upward so that the pessary will be wholly within the vagina (ie, no portion of it is visible; see Fig 41–19).

The forefinger should pass easily between the sides of the frame and the vaginal wall at any point; otherwise, the pessary is too large.

After the pessary has been fitted, the patient should be asked to stand, walk, and squat to determine whether pain occurs, whether the pessary becomes dis-

placed, and whether the uterus remains in position. She should be shown how to withdraw the pessary if it becomes displaced or is uncomfortable, and cautioned that a contraceptive vaginal diaphragm cannot be used while a vaginal pessary is in place.

During the initial period of pessary wear, any discomfort, bleeding, or disturbance in defecation or urinary function should be reported immediately. The patient should be examined 1 week after insertion to inspect for the presence of pressure and inflammatory or allergic reactions. A repeat exam in 4 weeks can be done, then visits should be done at 3- to 6-month intervals to assess for continued proper fit and to evaluate for vaginal erosion and inflammation as a result of pessary use. For women who are unable to remove and clean the pessary themselves, the pessary should be changed about every 2–3 months.

The pessary should be maintained with an acidic pH gel such as Trimo-san (Milex Products, Inc.). In postmenopausal patients topical estrogen can vitalize the vaginal mucosa and reduce ulceration. An estrogen-containing ring (Estring; Pharmacia-Upjohn) can also be used in conjunction by "piggy-backing" the ring with the pessary and then changing every 3 months.

Vaginal pessaries are not curative of prolapse, but they may be used for months or years for palliation with proper supervision.

A neglected pessary may cause fistulas or favor genital infections, but it is doubtful that cancer ever occurs as a result of wearing a modern pessary.

REFERENCES

General Pelvic Support

Goh V et al: Dynamic MR imaging of the pelvic floor in asymptomatic subjects. Am J Roentgenol 2000;174:661.

Shull BL: Pelvic organ prolapse: Anterior, superior, and posterior vaginal segment defects. Am J Obstet Gynecol 1999;181:6.

Cystocele

Walters MD, Karram MM: *Urogynecology and Reconstructive Pelvic Surgery,* 2nd ed. Mosby, 1999, p. 211.

Weber AM, Walters MD: Anterior vaginal prolapse: Review of anatomy and techniques of surgical repair. Obstet Gynecol 1997;89:311.

Rectocele

Cundiff GW et al: An anatomic and functional assessment of discrete defect rectocele repair. Am J Obstet Gynecol 1998; 179:1451.

Porter WE et al: The anatomic and functional outcomes of defect-specific rectocele repairs. Am J Obstet Gynecol 1999; 181:1353.

Enterocele

Lienemann A et al: Diagnosing enteroceles using dynamic magnetic resonance imaging. Dis Colon Rectum 2000;42:205.

Paraiso MF, Falcone T, Walters MD: Laparoscopic surgery for enterocele, vaginal apex prolapse and rectocele. Int Urogyn J 1999;10:223.

Walters MD, Karram MM: *Urogynecology and Reconstructive Pelvic Surgery,* 2nd ed. Mosby, 1999, p. 221.

Uterine Prolapse & Vaginal Vault Prolapse

Gemer O, Bergman M, Shmuel S: Prevalence of hydronephrosis in patients with genital prolapse. Eur J Obstet Gynecol 1999;86:11.

Sze EH, Karram MM: Transvaginal repair of vault prolapse: a review. Obstet Gynecol 1997;89:466.

Walters MD, Karram MM: *Urogynecology and Reconstructive Pelvic Surgery,* 2nd ed. Mosby, 1999, p. 235.

Webb MJ et al: Posthysterectomy vaginal vault prolapse: primary repair in 693 patients. Obstet Gynecol 1998;92:281.

Wheeless CR Jr: Total vaginal hysterectomy. In: *Atlas of Pelvic Surgery.* Lea & Febiger, 1981.

Urogynecology

Christopher M. Tarnay, MD, & Narender N. Bhatia, MD

Urinary incontinence affects well over 13 million people in the United States. Despite its prevalence and estimated costs in excess of $15 billion annually, most women do not seek help for incontinence, primarily because of social embarrassment or because they are unaware that help is available. The societal concept that incontinence is part of the "normal" aging process is no longer acceptable. The advances in modern medicine during the last 80 years have increased the life expectancy of women well into the eighth and ninth decades. We are caring for patients longer and better than ever, effectively managing chronic medical problems such as hypertension, cardiovascular disease, and diabetes, enabling women to enjoy longer and more productive lifetimes. This results in a large population of women living up to a third of their life after menopause, thereby introducing a whole host of medical issues and health concerns. The problems of urinary incontinence, voiding dysfunction, and fecal incontinence have become more prevalent as the population of aging women grows. The desire to improve quality of life by treating these potentially debilitating conditions has fostered the development of **urogynecology** as a specialized field within obstetrics and gynecology. The field continues to evolve, with continuing efforts to improve our understanding of the pathophysiology of urinary incontinence, to increase accuracy of the evaluation, and to develop new areas of research and management. The goal of urogynecology is to effectively deal with disorders of the lower urinary tract and pelvic floor dysfunction in women. In this chapter we will focus on the evaluation and treatment of women with urinary incontinence.

ANATOMY

The urinary and reproductive tracts are intimately associated during embryologic development. The lower urinary tract can be divided into three parts: the bladder, the vesical neck, and the urethra (Fig 42–1). The bladder is a hollow muscular organ lined with transitional epithelium designed for urine storage. The bladder musculature consists of three layers of smooth muscle, which are densely intertwined and constitute the detrusor muscle. The bladder stays relaxed to facilitate urine storage and contracts periodically to completely evacuate its contents when appropriate and acceptable. At the bladder base is the trigone, which is embryologically distinct from the bladder.

The two ureteral orifices and the internal urethral meatus form the boundaries of the trigone. The trigone has two distinct muscular layers: superficial and deep. The deep layer shares a similar cholinergic autonomic innervation as the detrusor muscle, while the superficial layer is densely innervated by noradrenergic nerves. The superficial detrusor layer extends muscular fibers that contribute to the distal urethra and posterior to the proximal urethra. The urethral "sphincter" itself is not a well-delineated structure, but rather a complex and intricate meshwork of intertwining smooth and striated muscle fibers that functionally responds neurophysiologically to variable degrees of vesicle pressures and facilitates urine storage and voiding.

The female urethra is about 3–4 cm long and the composition and support of the urethra and bladder neck play key roles in the function and maintenance of urinary continence. Together the striated urethral and periurethral muscles comprise the extrinsic urethral sphincter mechanism. The urethral sphincter, along with the contribution from the levator ani, function in the reflex contraction. The flow of urine may be voluntarily interrupted or the urethra occluded during stressful events such as coughing. The urethra is surrounded by dense vasculature that contributes to the urethral mucosal seal and urethral closure pressure. There is also an abundance of submucosal glands found along the dorsal surface. Most of the urethral diverticula arise from this area. The uroepithelium is stratified squamous (Fig 42–2).

Neuroanatomy

Neuronal innervation of the lower urinary tract is considered part of the autonomic and somatic nervous systems. The autonomic system (ie, the parasympathetic and sympathetic components) receives visceral sensation and regulates smooth muscle actively during conscious and involuntary lower urinary tract functions. The autonomic nervous system constitutes the bulk of neural control of the lower urinary tract. Sympathetic contributions from T1–L2 and parasympathetic contributions from S2–S4 comprise the neuronal control system (Fig 42–3). Voluntary control of micturition is

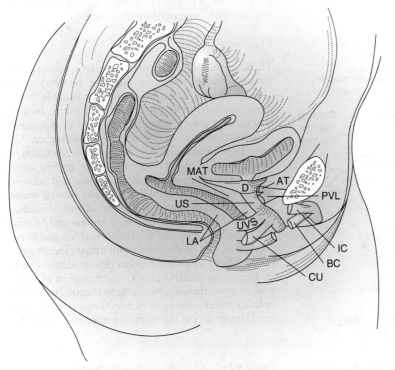

Figure 42–1. Interrelationships and approximate location of paraurethral structures. Levator ani muscles are shown as light lines running deep to the pelvic viscera. **AT,** arcus tendineus fasciae pelvis; **BC,** bulbocavernosus muscle; **CU,** compressor urethrae; D, detrusor loop; **IC,** ischiocavernosus muscle; **LA,** levator ani muscles; **MAT,** muscular attachment of the urethral supports; **PVL,** pubovesical ligament (muscle); **US,** urethral sphincter; **UVS,** urethrovaginal sphincter. (Reproduced, with permission, from DeLancey JOL: Correlative study of paraurethral anatomy. Obstet Gynecol 1986;68:91.)

controlled by the central nervous system. Cortical control of the detrusor muscle rests in the supramedial portion of the frontal lobes and in the genu of the corpus callosum. Receiving both sensory afferent and modulating motor efferent nerves, the net effect is that the brain provides tonic inhibition of detrusor contraction. Therefore lesions in the frontal lobe chiefly cause loss of voluntary control of micturition and thus loss of suppression of the detrusor reflex, resulting in uncontrolled voiding or urge urinary incontinence. The pons and mesencephalic reticular formation in the brainstem constitute the micturition center. A reflex activation in the central brainstem and peripheral spinal cord mediate a coordinated series of events, consisting of relaxation of the striated urethral musculature and detrusor contraction that result in opening of the bladder neck

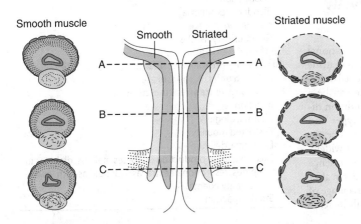

Figure 42–2. Urethral anatomy. The submucosal vascular plexus matures after puberty but undergoes great changes after menopause. The amount of smooth and especially striated muscles decreases with age, and the striated components become almost rudimentary. (Reproduced, with permission, from Rud T, Asmussen M: Neurophysiology of the lower urinary tract as measured by simultaneous urethral cystometry. In: Ostergard DR, Bent AE [editors]: *Urogynecology and Urodynamics: Theory and Practice,* 3rd ed. Williams & Wilkins, 1991, pp. 55–80.)

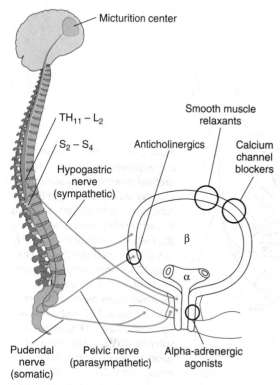

Figure 42–3. Schematic neuroanatomy of the lower urinary tract, with major sites of drug action. (Reproduced, with permission, from Sourander LB: Treatment of urinary incontinence. Gerontology 1990;36(Suppl 2):19–26. Copyright Karger S, with permission.)

and urethra. Lesions that interrupt these pathways have various effects depending on the level of interruption, essentially resulting in dyscoordination or dyssynergia of detrusor function.

URINARY INCONTINENCE—OVERVIEW

Definition

Urinary incontinence as defined by the International Continence Society (ICS) is the involuntary loss of urine that can be demonstrated objectively and is a social or hygienic problem for the patient. Incontinence can be a sign, a symptom (patient complaint), or a condition diagnosed by an examiner. There are many types and causes of urinary incontinence (Table 42–1). The reported incidence of urinary incontinence varies widely, ranging from 8–41% in women over 65. Incontinence becomes more common as one ages, particularly after menopause. In light of projections that the percentage of postmenopausal women in the population will increase

from 23% in 1995 to 33% in 2050, it is apparent that the problem of incontinence will be a major health and quality-of-life issue well into the future.

Etiology

There are numerous factors that play a role in maintaining urinary continence; therefore the development of incontinence is frequently not attributable to any single cause. Gender, age, hormonal status, birthing trauma, and genetic differences in connective tissue all contribute to the development of incontinence. Urinary incontinence is 2–3 times more common in women than in men because of shorter urethral length and the risk of connective tissue, muscle, and nerve injury associated with childbirth. Observational studies have consistently noted a high incidence of incontinence in the elderly population, with one study finding a 30% higher prevalence for each 5-year increase in age. The association of childbirth with urinary incontinence has long been suspected and has generated new interest in seeking to identify causes. Confirmation of higher rates of stress incontinence in parous compared to nulliparous women has been demonstrated in many studies. Damage to the pelvic floor neuromusculature dur-

Table 42–1. Classification and causes of urinary incontinence.

Genuine stress incontinence
    Bladder neck displacement
    Intrinsic sphincter dysfunction (ISD)
Detrusor instability/urge incontinence
    Idiopathic
    Neurologic detrusor hyperreflexia
Mixed incontinence (genuine stress and detrusor instability combined)
Overflow incontinence with urinary retention
    Obstruction
    Bladder hyporeflexia
Bypass incontinence
    Genitourinary fistulas
Urethral diverticulum
Congenital urethral abnormalities (eg, epispadias, bladder exstrophy, ectopic ureter)
Functional and transient incontinence
    Infection
    Pharmacologic
    Restricted mobility
    Dementia/delirium
    Excessive urine production (diabetes mellitus, diabetes insipidus, resorption of extravascular fluid as with lower extremity edema)
    Stool impaction

Table 42–2. Symptoms of urine storage problems.

Incontinence: involuntary loss of urine, which is a social or hygienic problem, and which is objectively demonstrable

Stress incontinence: loss of urine with increased intra-abdominal pressure as with sneezing, laughing, or coughing, or certain physical activities

Urge incontinence: loss of urine accompanied by a strong urge to void

Mixed incontinence: combined symptoms of both stress and urge incontinence

Increased frequency: high number of voids per day (generally more than 7 times per day is considered abnormal)

Nocturia: high number of times awakening with the urge to void (generally more than 2 times per night is considered abnormal)

Nocturnal enuresis: Urinary incontinence that occurs during sleep

ing vaginal delivery may lead to loss of pelvic muscle strength and nerve function, resulting in both stress urinary incontinence and pelvic floor support defects. Although muscle strength may be regained over time or with the help of pelvic floor muscle exercises, dysfunction may be permanent.

Aging and incontinence are closely associated. There is an increasing prevalence of incontinence as women age. However, it remains unclear if age alone is an independent risk factor. This theory has long been an argument in favor of the role of hypoestrogenism as a main factor in the development of incontinence. Although estrogen reduces urinary urgency, results from studies specifically examining menopausal status have been equivocal, with some studies showing a positive association and others no association.

Abnormalities in the muscular components and innervation of the pelvic floor and the connective tissue to this region also likely contribute to the multifactorial etiology of incontinence. Initial observations that the prevalence of abdominal hernias, lower leg varices, and uterine prolapse was higher in women with stress urinary incontinence suggested that connective tissue weakness may identify women at risk for developing incontinence. Subsequent studies have supported a connection between relative collagen deficiencies in the connective tissues of incontinent patients versus continent controls.

Incontinence affects a woman's quality of life, and it is an uncomfortable and embarrassing problem. The psychosocial impact is enormous on the patient as well as her family. Women with urinary incontinence are reported to be more depressed, have lower self-esteem, and are ashamed about their appearance and the odor.

Urinary incontinence impacts sexual desire and reduces sexual activity. This can curb social interactions to the point where individuals become isolated and even entirely homebound.

History

The first step in evaluating an incontinent patient is a thorough history. The nature and extent of the patient's symptoms should be elucidated. Knowledge of the duration, frequency, and severity of the urinary incontinence are essential to understanding the social implications and its impact on her life, and aids the clinician in determining the direction and extent of diagnostic and therapeutic measures (Table 42–2). There are a multitude of diagnostic and imaging studies available, but taking a thorough but focused urogynecologic history can isolate many of the easily reversible causes of incontinence.

By asking focused questions, the clinician can determine the character of the patient's symptoms, and the exact nature of the episodes can be better understood (Table 42–3). Knowledge of the use of protective items such as sanitary napkins, panty liners, absorbent pads, or adult diapers is very useful in quantitating urinary loss. Including questions about menopausal status and use of hormone treatment, history of urinary tract infections, previous surgery to remedy incontinence, and the patient's functional status are also essential.

Voiding Diary

A voiding diary, or urolog, that quantitates frequency and volume is a helpful tool. For a 24- to 48-hour period the patient records all fluid intake and measures

Table 42–3. Helpful questions when taking history of incontinence.

- Do you leak urine when you cough, sneeze, or laugh?
- Do you ever have such an uncomfortably strong need to urinate that if you don't reach the toilet you leak?
- How many times during the day do you urinate?
- How many times do you get up to void during the night after going to bed?
- Have you ever wet the bed?
- Do you leak during sexual intercourse?
- Do you wear a pad to protect your clothing?
- If yes, how often do you change the pad: when it has only a few drops, when it is damp, or when it is totally wet?
- After you urinate do you have dribbling or still feel the presence of urine in your bladder?
- Does it hurt when you urinate?
- Do you lose urine without the urge to go?

and records all urine output, including frequency and episodes of leakage (Fig 42–4). Numerous studies have validated the voiding diary as a reliable tool in the diagnosis and management of urinary urgency or urge incontinence. These data are beneficial to the physician because they clarify home voiding patterns, particularly in the elderly. They are often useful to patients as well, because they provide a focus on the problem and can serve as a baseline for treatment interventions such as behavioral training, bladder drill, and pharmacologic management.

Urinalysis

Examination of the urine is an essential part of the work-up of urinary incontinence or any patient with voiding complaints. Infection is an exceedingly common cause of urinary complaints, including frequency, urgency, and incontinence. A clean-catch voided specimen is suitable for routine urinalysis; however, a sterile "in and out" catheterized specimen is appropriate for patients unable to correctly perform collection or if urine culture has been previously equivocal due to skin flora contamination.

Urinary protein, glucose, ketones, hemoglobin, casts, and nitrates can indicate primary renal disease or injury. Microscopic evaluation of the urinary sediment may indicate renal tubular damage with the presence of casts or indicate infection with the presence of leukocytes and red blood cells. More than 6–8 white blood cells per high-power field along with the presence of bacteria are very suggestive of urinary tract infection.

Time	Amount Voided	Activity	Leak Volume	Urge Present	Amount/Type of Intake

Figure 42–4. Urinary diary (urolog).

Physical Examination

A general gynecologic and neurologic examination should be done on all patients, with a focus on the vaginal walls and pelvic floor. The patient should come to the clinic with a comfortably full bladder for spontaneous uroflowmetry and postvoid residual study. Then an examination should be performed with the patient in the lithotomy position. The examination should begin with an assessment of the vulvar area for atrophy and change in labial architecture due to estrogen deficiency. In elderly patients vulvar dystrophy may be coexistent with vulvar complaints ascribed to incontinence. The presence of inflammation or irritation from chronic moisture or pad usage should also be noted. The presence of discharge should be noted because this may mimic urinary incontinence. Examination of the urethra with palpation of the anterior vaginal wall under the urethra for fluctuance, masses, or discharge may reveal signs of urethral diverticulum, carcinoma, or an infection of the urethra. Tenderness may point to urethral syndrome.

Vaginal wall integrity needs to be assessed. Vaginal rugae, or the folds in the epithelium, are normal and tend to be absent if the underlying supportive endopelvic fascia is detached. The presence of anterior wall defects (cystoceles), posterior vaginal wall defects (rectoceles), and apical defects (enteroceles) can be quantified. The uterocervical position, or, if the woman has had a hysterectomy, the cuff position and its descent should be recorded. The position of the vaginal walls should be noted in the lithotomy position at rest and with Valsalva maneuver. A Sims speculum or the lower blade of a Graves' speculum allows easy visualization of either the anterior or posterior vaginal wall. The severity of vaginal laxity, which may be masked in the supine position, can often best be elicited by repeating the exam in the standing position while the patient places one foot on the step of the exam table or on a small portable step.

Mobility at the level of the bladder neck can be quantified with the use of a sterile cotton swab (Q-tip) test. The Q-tip test is one of the most commonly used tests to evaluate women with urinary problems because it effectively quantifies the degree of anatomic rotation of the support of the urethra and bladder neck. With the patient in the dorsolithotomy position, the labia are separated and urethral meatus is swabbed with antiseptic. A sterile Q-tip lubricated with 1–2% xylocaine jelly is inserted transurethrally into the bladder and then withdrawn slowly until definite resistance is felt. This places the tip of the Q-tip at the level of the bladder neck just distal to the internal urethral meatus. Using a standard protractor, resting angle is measured. The patient is then asked to Valsalva or cough and the maximum straining angle is noted. Net deflection is equal to the change from resting to maximum straining position (Fig 42–5). An angle of > 30 degrees is consid-

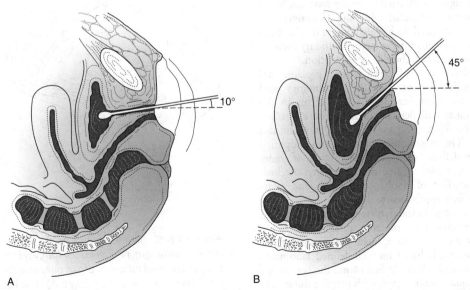

A **B**

Figure 42–5. The cotton-tipped swab (Q-tip) test for the assessment of urethral and bladder support. **A:** Angle of the Q-tip at rest. **B:** Angle of the Q-tip with Valsalva or cough (straining); the urethrovesical junction descends, causing upward deflection of the Q-tip.

ered abnormal. Urethral hypermobility must be interpreted with caution, as it may be present in women without incontinence. The utility of this simple test is that an angle of > 30 degrees is certainly present in the majority of women with genuine stress incontinence. In the absence of hypermobility, one has to question the diagnosis of anatomical stress incontinence and entertain the possibility of a damaged urethral sphincter (also called intrinsic sphincteric deficiency) to explain stress-related urinary loss.

Urinary Stress Test

Having the patient Valsalva or cough forcefully multiple times to reproduce urine loss at the beginning of the examination may reveal the presence of incontinence. If urine is lost immediately with a cough or Valsalva, this may obviate the need for more complex urodynamic testing if the complaint is minor. If no urine loss is exhibited, the patient is asked to stand with legs shoulder width apart and asked to cough. Immediate loss of urine suggests a diagnosis of stress urinary incontinence.

Other Studies

Bimanual examination to evaluate the uterine size, position, and descent within the vaginal canal and palpation of the ovaries should also be performed. A rectovaginal exam permits adequate examination of the posterior vaginal wall. Anal sphincter tone can be assessed at rest and with anal tightening. The presence of fecal impaction needs to be ruled out, as this has been shown to be a contributing factor to urinary incontinence, particularly in the elderly population.

The description of pelvic organ prolapse has lacked uniformity of standard terminology and methods for quantification. Existing terms to describe vaginal wall defects are imprecise and often refer to the adjacent organ, such as in cystocele and rectocele. The most commonly used and simplified system for defining such defects is a system of grades that allows a high degree of subjectivity. Accordingly, discussion of results of diagnosis and treatment is at best approximate.

In an attempt to standardize the terminology and grading of pelvic organ prolapse, a staging system has been proposed. In this system, description of the pelvic prolapse is based on well-defined landmarks using measured values. At first glance the system appears complicated; however, with practice the system becomes easier to use.

The examiner sees and describes the maximum protrusion, and the defects are confirmed by exami-

nation with the patient straining or standing. The examiner should be careful to describe the exact conditions present during the exam (eg, position, provocative maneuvers, type of speculum).

The system consists of a series of six site-specific points along the vaginal wall in profile, as well as three measured distances (Fig 42–6). Vaginal site-specific points are measured at maximal protrusion in centimeters and recorded. The measured distances of genital hiatus, perineal body, and total vaginal length are also recorded (Fig 42–7). The stage of pelvic organ prolapse is based on the most distal protrusion and specified. (See Description and Staging of Pelvic Organ Prolapse in Chapter 41 for more details; also see Table 42–4.)

Neurologic Exam

The control of micturition is complex and multitiered, with both autonomic and voluntary control. In addition to a complete history and screening for neurologic symptoms, a thorough physical examination is important because many neurologic diseases may present with voiding dysfunction in the absence of overt neurologic findings.

Mental status, cranial nerves, motor strength, sensory function, deep tendon reflexes, and sacral spinal cord integrity should all be assessed. Testing the patient's orientation to place and time and assessing

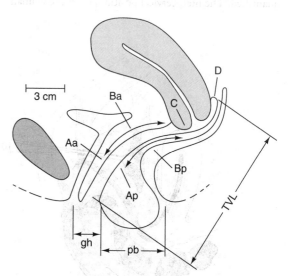

Figure 42–6. Six sites (points *Aa, Ba, C, D, Bp,* and *Ap*), genital hiatus (*gh*), perineal body (*pb*), and total vaginal length (*tvl*) used for pelvic organ quantitation. (Reproduced with permission from Bump RC et al: The standardization of terminology of female pelvic organ prolapse and pelvic floor dysfunction. Am J Obstet Gynecol 1996;175:10.)

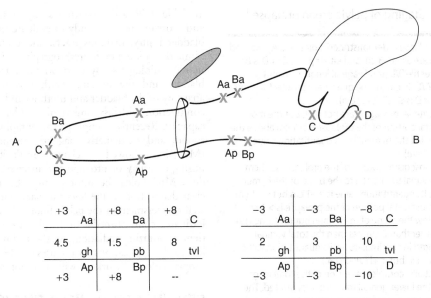

+3		+8		+8	
	Aa		Ba		C
4.5		1.5		8	
	gh		pb		tvl
	Ap		Bp		
+3		+8		--	

-3		-3		-8	
	Aa		Ba		C
2		3		10	
	gh		pb		tvl
	Ap		Bp		D
-3		-3		-10	

Figure 42–7. **A:** Grid and line diagram of complete eversion of vagina. Most distal point of anterior wall (point *Ba*), vaginal cuff scar (point *C*), and most distal point of the posterior wall (point *Bp*) are all at same position (+8), and points *Aa* and *Ap* are maximally distal (both at +3). Because total vaginal length equals maximum protrusion, this is stage IV prolapse. **B:** Normal support. Points *Aa* and *Ba* and points *Ap* and *Bp* are all –3 because there is no anterior or posterior wall descent. Lowest point of the cervix is 8 cm above hymen (–8), and posterior fornix is 2 cm above this (–10). Vaginal length is 10 cm, and genital hiatus and perineal body measure 2 and 3 cm, respectively. This represents stage 0 support. (Reproduced with permission from Bump RC et al: The standardization of terminology of female pelvic organ prolapse and pelvic floor dysfunction. Am J Obstet Gynecol 1996;175:10.)

speech and comprehension skills will help to ascertain her mental status. Motor control may be diminished in focal brain or cord lesions, most commonly Parkinson's, multiple sclerosis, and cerebrovascular accident. Motor strength is tested in the lower extremities by assessing hip, knee, and ankle flexion, as well as ankle eversion and inversion. Deep tendon reflexes are tested at the patella, ankle, and foot planus. Sensation can be tested at the dermatomes using light touch and pinprick over the perineum and thigh area. Deficits should be noted, but it should be kept in mind that there is considerable overlap in sensory innervation in the sensory nerve roots. The sacral spinal cord nerve roots 2–4 contain vital neurons controlling micturition. The anal wink reflex and the bulbocavernosus reflex can confirm integrity of neurovisceral and urethral reflex functions. These reflexes can be evoked by stroking the perianal area and looking for an external anal sphincter contraction, and by tapping or gently squeezing the clitoris and watching for contraction of the bulbocavernosus muscle, respectively. These reflexes are often easier to elicit at the beginning of the exam and it should be noted that their absence is not always indicative of neurologic

deficit. Clinically observed neurologic deficits should lead to a neurologic consult.

Urodynamics

A urodynamic study is any test that provides objective dynamic information about lower urinary tract function. There are many methods and tests available (Table 42–5). There are very simple methods, like diaries that track frequency and volume of urination, and more complex methods which require special equipment and training. A cystometrogram is necessary to rule out unstable bladder, overflow incontinence, reduced bladder capacity, or abnormalities of bladder sensation. A cystometrogram can be done utilizing water manometry or with more advanced methods. Complex urodynamic testing increases the diagnostic accuracy and may often identify why previous therapy has failed. Such testing is particularly helpful in difficult or complex cases.

The indications for more complex testing in the form of multichannel urodynamics are not standardized and each patient must be assessed individually (Table

Table 42–4. Staging of pelvic organ prolapse.[1]

Stage 0	No prolapse is demonstrated. Points Aa, Ap, Ba, and Bp are all at –3 cm and either point C or D is between –TVL (total vaginal length) cm and –[TVL–2] cm (ie, the quantitation value for point C or D is ≤ –[TVL–2] cm).
Stage I	The criteria for stage 0 are not met, but the most distal portion of the prolapse is > 1 cm above the level of the hymen (ie, its quantitation value is < –1 cm).
Stage II	The most distal portion of the prolapse is ≤ 1 cm proximal to or distal to the plane of the hymen (ie, its quantitation value is ≥ –1 cm but ≤ +1 cm
Stage III	The most distal portion of the prolapse is > 1 cm below the plane of the hymen but protrudes no further than 2 cm less than the total vaginal length in centimeters (ie, its quantitation value is > +1 cm but < +[TVL–2] cm).
Stage IV	Essentially, complete eversion of the total length of the lower genital tract is demonstrated. The distal portion of the prolapse protrudes to at least [TVL–2] cm (ie, its quantitation value is ≥ +[TVL–2] cm). In most instances, the leading edge of stage IV prolapse is the cervix or vaginal cuff scar.

[1]See Fig 42–6 for meaning of variables discussed here.
Reproduced with permission from Bump RC et al: The standardization of terminology of female pelvic organ prolapse and pelvic floor dysfuntion, Am J Obstet Gynecol 1996;175:10.

42–6). However, there are some basic criteria that, if met, indicate a need for urodynamic evaluation, which can aid in more accurate diagnosis, and thus appropriate medical or surgical management.

Cystourethroscopy

Endoscopic evaluation is an invaluable adjunct for the diagnosis and management of the urogynecologic patient. It is a simple office procedure that can yield important data when performed by experienced hands. Cystourethroscopy is indicated for hematuria, irritative voiding symptoms, obstructive voiding, suspicion of diverticula or fistula, persistent incontinence, and as a preoperative evaluation prior to reconstructive pelvic surgery.

Imaging Tests

Radiologic studies can be an integral component of the evaluation of lower urinary tract dysfunction and abnormalities. Traditionally, intravenous pyelography (IVP) and plain radiography were the main modalities available. IVP, a dye contrast study, is still the easiest and most inexpensive study to evaluate the presence of bladder injury, fistulous tracts, and ureteral integrity. Similarly, voiding cystourethrography (VCUG) is a dynamic radiologic study used primarily to evaluate the bladder and the urethra. With this technique, the anatomy of the bladder and urethra can be evaluated in conjunction with assessment of bladder function and capacity. Recently, computed tomography (CT), ultrasound, and particularly magnetic resonance imaging (MRI) have allowed clinicians more flexibility in diagnosing a variety of urologic and urogynecologic disorders. MRI holds the most promise because it allows clear delineation of the lower urinary tract anatomy as well as assessment of the pelvic floor, without the use of iodinated contrast media, and without exposing the patient to ionizing radiation. As the technique becomes less costly, applications for the uses of MRI to aid in the urogynecological work-up will no doubt expand.

GENUINE STRESS INCONTINENCE

The International Continence Society (ICS) defines genuine stress incontinence as the involuntary loss of urine that occurs when, in the absence of a detrusor contraction, the intravesical pressure exceeds the maximum urethral closure pressure.

Normally, while at rest the intraurethral pressure is greater than the intravesical pressure. The pressure difference between the bladder and the urethra is known as the urethral closure pressure. If intra-abdominal pressure increases as it does with a cough, sneeze, or strain, and if this pressure is not equally transmitted to the urethra, then continence is not maintained and leakage of urine occurs. What is thought to cause this inequity of pressure transmission is not universally accepted, but proposed mechanisms are listed below.

(1) Anatomic descent of the proximal urethra below its normal intra-abdominal position allows pressure to be unevenly transmitted to the urethra, and the subsequent rise in intraurethral pressure is not as great as the increase in intravesical pressure.

(2) Altered anatomic relationships between the urethra and bladder, so that increases in intra-abdominal pressure result in vector forces directed from the bladder along the axis of the urethra.

(3) Failure of neuromuscular and connective tissue components to preferentially increase intraurethral pressure in response to increase in intra-abdominal pressure in continent patients.

A subtype of genuine stress urinary incontinence known as intrinsic sphincteric deficiency is frequently an important cause of urinary incontinence. This entity involves inherent dysfunction of the urethral sphincter mechanism. It is commonly described as recurrent or

Table 42–5. Urodynamic testing methods.

Test	Purpose	Indications
Simple cystometry	Measures bladder pressure and volume	Useful in patients with clear-cut symptoms
Complex cystometry	Multiple parameters: bladder volume, filling rate, bladder pressure, abdominal pressure, and sub-tracted detrusor pressure	More accurate information on bladder function; most common type of urodynamics test
Uroflowmetry	Measures flow rate with special electronic flow-meters	Useful for general impression of voiding function
Pressure-flow	Combines complex cystometry and uroflowmetry. Measures bladder pressure, abdominal pressure, subtracted detrusor pressure, and uroflow	Provides accurate means of differentiating detrusor contraction, straining, and pelvic relaxation as mechanisms of urination
Leak point pressure	Using abdominal or bladder pressures, urethral resistance to abdominal strain is measured	Used in assessing urethral sphincter function
Urethral pressure profilometry	Using a dual transducer catheter, simultaneous bladder and urethral pressure can be recorded	
Electromyography	Surface or needle electrodes to determine striated muscle activity of the pelvic floor or the anal or urethral sphincters	

persistent high-grade urinary leakage after an incontinence procedure that may have repositioned the bladder neck, but nonetheless did not resolve the symptoms. This condition is also seen in patients after intensive pelvic radiation therapy or extensive or multiple operative procedures, resulting in the physical findings of a "drain pipe," "pipestem," or fixed urethra.

Treatment of Stress Urinary Incontinence

A. NONSURGICAL MEASURES

If the incontinence is mild or moderate, nonsurgical interventions should be tried first. Dietary measures are instituted, with identification of items that can be modified. Reduction in consumption of caffeinated beverages and alcoholic drinks should be encouraged. Fluid restriction in patients without chronic medical prob-

Table 42–6. Indications for multichannel urodynamic testing.

- Complicated symptoms and history
- Use when considering surgery for correction of incontinence or pelvic organ prolapse
- Underlying neurologic disease
- Urge incontinence refractive to initial conservative therapies
- Continuous leakage
- Previous anti-incontinence surgery
- Clinical findings do not correlate with symptoms
- Elderly patients > 65 years old

lems such as cardiovascular, renal, or endocrinologic disease can be attempted. Timed voiding to prevent filling the bladder to a capacity that causes urine loss should be undertaken with the use of a urine diary. The diary can also facilitate discussion between patient and clinician as therapy progresses.

Pelvic floor exercises or Kegel exercises have been found to be extremely helpful in patients with mild to moderate forms of incontinence. Focused repetitive voluntary contractions of the levator ani muscles (pubococcygeus, coccygeus, and iliococcygeus) by having the patient contract or "squeeze" the muscle as if to prevent the passage of rectal gas is an effective therapy. The contractions exert a closing force on the urethra and also increase muscle support to the pelvic organs. The patient should be provided written and verbal instructions on performing the exercises. Repetitions, with each contraction held for 3–5 seconds alternated with periods of relaxation, should be begun at 45–100 repetitions a day. In settings in which the patient is motivated and has individual instruction and thorough follow-up and support, results for cure or improvement of bladder control (reduction in urine loss) can be up to 75%.

1. Biofeedback—Biofeedback is an adjunct to pelvic floor exercises that is employed to facilitate the patient's comprehension of the proper muscles to contract. By using electronic pressure catheter and myographic monitoring, a visual or auditory signal of the physiologic response can be provided to the patient to help refine exercise skills. Utilizing surface electromyography (EMG) on the perineum to measure levator contraction and a pressure monitor in the vagina or rectum to indicate abdominal pressure, the patient can be instructed to preferentially contract the pelvic floor without concomitant abdominal contraction. Studies utilizing a variety of techniques demonstrate a 54–95% cure or improvement in incontinence. The efficacy of this modality is highly dependent on patient selection and proper clinical training.

2. Electrical stimulation—As an alternative to active patient contraction of the levator muscles, electrical stimulation of the muscles via small electrical currents can be used. Using intravaginal or transrectal electrodes with portable stimulators, the pelvic muscles automatically contract and artificially "train" the muscles for the patient. When used long term, weakened muscles are strengthened and innervation reestablished during activation. Experiences with the devices are variable, but they generally show a positive impact on incontinence and acceptable patient tolerance.

3. Pessaries—Intravaginal devices or pessaries to correct the anatomic deficits associated with stress incontinence have long been used to address this vexing problem. Many devices have been proffered, but long-term solutions to incontinence have yet to be proven in the general population. Pessaries, traditionally used for treatment of genital prolapse, have also been shown to have a potential role in supporting the bladder neck and urethra and preventing stress incontinence. Many pessary devices designed to fit within the vagina and elevate the bladder neck are available. Continence can often be achieved, because many devices adequately obstruct the bladder neck and urethra. As with all intravaginal devices, maintenance is essential to avoid urinary obstruction and vaginal erosion if the pessary is too compressive.

Other devices such as urethral plugs that are either placed over the external urethral meatus or transurethrally with an internal balloon are available and are often helpful in reducing wetting episodes.

B. SURGICAL MANAGEMENT

Surgical treatment should be offered for moderate to severe incontinence. Urinary incontinence is not a life-threatening condition and the decision to operate must be based on patient symptoms and their impact on daily life. Many patients are able to tolerate slight urine loss and what often provokes a desire for treatment is an increase in loss above a tolerable threshold. If medical management to improve bladder control is possible, and symptoms are reduced to below this threshold, this is most desirable. If not, surgery should be considered.

Since at least 130 operative procedures have been described for the treatment of female urinary stress incontinence, it is not surprising that many of these procedures have not had long-term success. Unfortunately,

Table 42–7. Surgical techniques to correct genuine stress urinary incontinence.

- Anterior colporraphy
- Needle urethropexy
- Retropubic colpocystourethropexy
- Suburethral slings
- Paravaginal repair
- Periurethral bulking agents
- Artificial sphincters

most of these procedures do not induce permanent urethrovesical elevation, and incontinence may recur with aging. For those patients who desire surgical correction, the options can be categorized by method of surgical approach (Table 42–7). Common to most surgical procedures is restoration of bladder neck support by elevation of the urethrovesical junction. Some procedures also reconstruct bladder neck supports and provide a stable suburethral layer.

Assessment of the cure rate of any surgical treatment for genuine stress incontinence must take into account the selection of patients, skill of the surgeon, accuracy of the preoperative diagnosis, length of postoperative follow-up, and criteria for cure. Reported cure rates for abdominal procedures range from 60–100%, with 85–90% being the generally accepted rate. Most failures appear to be due to incorrect preoperative diagnosis, poor surgical technique, and healing failures.

1. Anterior repair—Anterior colporraphy with Kelly plication is one of the oldest methods of surgical correction, and was introduced in 1914. Used for anterior vaginal defects (cystocele), the technique involves vaginal dissection of the epithelium below the bladder and bladder neck, identifying the perivesical fascia and pubocervical fascia, and plicating each side over the midline. The Kelly plication involves specific support at the bladder. Numerous studies have evaluated this approach, and long-term analysis does not support this method as an effective cure for stress incontinence, with > 60% failure rates over 5 years.

2. Needle urethropexy—Since the introduction of this procedure in 1957 by Armand Pereyra and its modifications with contributions by Thomas Lebherz, the needle urethropexy has become a fixture in anti-incontinence surgery. Numerous authors have published alterations of this technique (eg, Raz, Stamey, Gittes, and Musznai). All rely on a vaginal incision, dissection and mobilization of periurethral tissues, entry into the space of Retzius (retropubic space), and the passage of a needle ligature carrier from a small abdominal incision into the vaginal incision. The periurethral tissues and fascia are identified, secured with delayed absorbable suture, and brought through retropubically and secured above the abdominal rectus fascia. In this manner the bladder neck is elevated and continence restored. The heterogeneity of procedure and technique make generalized statements about this procedure difficult, but prospective long-term studies for individual procedures are available. The procedures appear to be effective initially with cure rates of approximately 80–85% with variable length of follow-up. When examining some studies, including one large prospective study, with at least 2 years of follow-up the cure rates drop dramatically to under 65%.

3. Abdominal retropubic colpopexy—The Marshall-Marchetti-Krantz (MMK) and Burch colposuspension are the two classic retropubic surgeries for incontinence. The two share the same mechanism of correction: First, both suspend the periurethral and paravaginal tissue at the level of the urethrovesical junction, and second, both utilize a firm point of attachment for fixation of these suspension sutures. In the case of the MMK, the sutures are fixed to the periosteum of the pubic bone, and in the Burch procedure the iliopectineal ligament (Cooper's ligament) (Fig 42–8). The Burch colposuspension has become the first choice for the treatment of patients with hypermobility

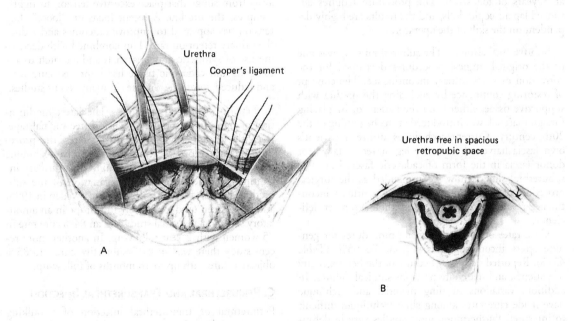

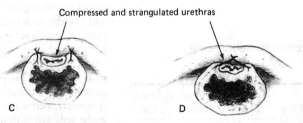

Figure 42–8. Abdominal surgical procedure to correct stress incontinence. **A:** Anterior vaginal wall has been mobilized. Two sutures have been placed on either side and far lateral from the midline. Distal sutures are opposite the mid urethra. Proximal sutures are at the end of the vesicourethral junction. Sutures are attached to Cooper's ligament. **B:** Cross-section shows urethra free in retropubic space with anterior vaginal wall lifting and supporting it. **C** and **D:** Urethra is compressed and strangulated against pubic bone when vaginal sutures are applied close to the urethra and then fixed to the pubic symphysis. (Reproduced, with permission, from Tanagho EA: Colpocystourethropexy. J Urol 1976;116:751. Copyright 1976 by The Williams & Wilkins Co.)

of the bladder neck and genuine stress urinary incontinence. In both longitudinal studies and randomized comparative trials against other procedures, the Burch procedure maintains the highest objective and subjective cure rates of 80% after 5 years, and 68% after 10 years of follow-up.

A laparoscopic approach to Burch colposuspension has been developed, which offers the benefit of minimally invasive surgery with the same level of efficacy. With the laparoscopic approach, hospital stay and postoperative recovery are minimized. Utilizing the transperitoneal or preperitoneal approach, this method has demonstrated cure rates comparable to the open procedure. Success rates with variable follow-up range between 87–97%, and in one prospective study, 85% at 5 years of follow-up. The procedure requires advanced laparoscopic skills, and the results are highly dependent on the skill of the operator.

4. Suburethral slings—The suburethral sling was one of the original surgical procedures developed for the correction of stress urinary incontinence. The concept of restoring continence by encircling the urethra with supportive tissue, either from the patient or by placing foreign material, was introduced at the beginning of the 20th century. Current techniques utilize a patient's own fascia harvested from the leg or rectus fascia, or donor fascia in the form of cadaveric fascia lata. The suburethral sling is now recommended as the surgical procedure of choice for the treatment of urinary incontinence resulting from intrinsic urethral sphincter deficiency.

Cure rates of suburethral sling procedures for genuine stress incontinence vary from 70–95% (Table 42–8). Reported rates vary because of the heterogeneity of patients, and many are previous surgical failures. In addition, variations in sling material and technique have made cure rates among sling techniques difficult to interpret. Furthermore, most studies vary in definition of cure and may not distinguish between cure and improvement.

In a large review study summarizing cure rates of surgical treatments for stress urinary incontinence, 16 studies comparing sling procedures to colposuspension were reviewed. Of the 4 that were randomized controlled trials comprising 150 patients, none reported a difference in cure. The remaining 12 were retrospective studies, with only one demonstrating a difference in outcome between procedures, 79% versus 95% cure for sling and colposuspension, respectively.

Finally, the sling procedure has undergone many modifications. Due to high postoperative urinary retention rates and renewed recognition of the importance of dynamic urethral function, there has been a movement away from slings that place excessive tension to tightly compress the urethra. A recent focus on "loose" sling tension has appeared to improve outcomes and reduce the urinary retention rate. This combined with decreasing use of synthetic graft materials and a switch to autologous and cadaveric tissue has improved cure rates and reduced complication rates in many recent studies.

5. Tension-free vaginal tape—The latest modification of the sling is the use of tension-free vaginal tape. Recently introduced in the United States, the procedure was developed as a minimally invasive technique for the surgical correction of genuine stress urinary incontinence. The technique is a variation of the suburethral sling and was first described in Sweden in 1995, and it has been used extensively in Europe in an ambulatory setting. The initial study had an 84% cure rate in 75 women with 2-year follow-up. In another more recent study there was an 87% subjective cure and 83% objective cure with up to 18 months of follow-up.

C. PERIURETHRAL AND TRANSURETHRAL INJECTION

Periurethral or transurethral injection of a bulking agent into the submucosal space of the bladder neck causes narrowing or coaptation of the proximal urethra and bladder neck opening. This increases urethral resistance to involuntary urine loss without changing resting urethral closure pressure. Currently glutaraldehyde cross-linked bovine collagen is the most commonly used material. This procedure is generally reserved for genuine stress urinary incontinence caused by intrinsic sphincteric deficiency. The injections can be performed under sedation with local anesthetic in an outpatient or office setting. The bovine collagen degrades over 9–19 months and repeat "booster" injections are often required. Improvement and cure rates are very high in the short term and complications are minimal. Nonabsorbable bulking agents like silicone and Teflon have also been employed with mixed results. Recently pyrolytic carbon beads (Durasphere) have been intro-

Table 42–8. Outcomes for suburethral sling procedures.

Author	Sling Type	No. of Pts. Cured	% Cured	Follow-up (m)
Parker et al	Fascia lata	42/51	84	12–24
Iosif	Mersilene	32/44	73	60–120
Beck et al	Fascia lata	56/61	92	
Blaivas and Jacobs	Rectus fascia	55/67	83	42
Stothers et al	Vaginal wall	129/134	96	11
Chaikin et al	Rectus fascia	231/251	92	12

duced as a permanent and hypoallergenic bulking agent that may obviate the need for repeat injections.

D. ARTIFICIAL SPHINCTERS

The artificial urethral sphincter is an effective option for patients with incontinence not amenable to standard surgical treatment because of urethral scarring or atony. The artificial urinary sphincter is best used in patients with incontinence due to poor urethral sphincter function. The sphincter obstructs the urethra by compressing the bladder neck via a pressure-regulated balloon and releases the compression when the patient desires to void. Reported success rates are up to 91%, but complications are high, with 21% of patients requiring surgical replacement of parts or the entire sphincter.

URGE INCONTINENCE (DETRUSOR INSTABILITY)

Definition

Urge incontinence is the involuntary loss of urine associated with a strong desire to void. Urge incontinence is usually associated with involuntary contractions of the bladder or detrusor contractions. Strictly speaking, detrusor instability (DI) is an urodynamic definition and term. Recent questions about the relevance and reproducibility about the role of involuntary contractions in the clinical presentation of incontinence have been raised. Additionally, the literature is at times confusing concerning the methodology (catheter type, bladder filling rate, provocative maneuvers, etc) for data acquisition. There are many different terms to describe DI, such as bladder dyssynergia, overactive bladder, uninhibited detrusor, and unstable bladder. In addition, when the cause of involuntary detrusor contractions is due to an underlying neurologic lesion, DI is called detrusor hyperreflexia. Detrusor instability will be the term applied in cases in which patients suffer from urinary symptoms due to involuntary bladder contractions.

Etiology

The incidence of DI varies depending on the population studied and the definition applied. Consequently, the reported prevalence varies widely from 8–50% in the general population and in women over 65 it is estimated to be at least 38%. An important concept is that involuntary detrusor contractions for bladder emptying are normally overridden by cortical inhibition of reflex bladder activity. In the majority of cases the cause of DI is unknown. Certainly patients with underlying neurologic disease may also manifest with urinary incontinence. Multiple sclerosis, cerebrovascular disease, Parkinson's disease, and Alzheimer's disease are most often associated with involuntary bladder contractions.

Diagnosis

Diagnosis of DI is suggested by urinary frequency often associated with a strong urge or a sense of impending urine loss. Incontinence often occurs prior to reaching the toilet. Loss of urine may occur seconds after stress, such as a cough or strain. Physical stimuli such as running water or hand washing also may elicit an urge. Patients also often describe "key in lock" syndrome. This is typically characterized by an uncontrollable urge to void when unlocking the door after returning from a trip out of the house. The first thing done upon return is to immediately rush to the toilet or risk losing urine. The diagnosis is confirmed with cystometry.

Treatment

Adequate therapy depends greatly on accuracy of diagnosis. History is most often suggestive, and the diagnosis of detrusor instability can be confirmed with office cystometry or more precisely with multichannel urodynamics. A more difficult challenge is differentiating between detrusor instability and sensory urge with irritative voiding symptoms.

Patients with detrusor instability should be offered simple treatments first. Behavioral modifications and medical therapy are the standard therapy for urinary incontinence due to detrusor instability. Surgical measures are methods of last resort for severe intractable DI. Recently, surgically implantable device like Interstim have been found very useful in patients with intractable urgency incontinence and voiding dysfunction.

Behavioral therapy includes bladder training, timed voiding, and pelvic floor muscle exercises.

Bladder training is an education program that combines written and verbal instruction to educate patients about mechanisms of normal bladder control with the teaching of relaxation and distraction skills to resist premature signals to urinate. Creating a voiding schedule for which the patient urinates at preset intervals while attempting to ignore the urge to urinate may progressively lead to the reestablishment of cortical voluntary control over the micturition reflex.

Timed voiding is a form of bladder retraining that again mandates regular scheduled voiding and attempts to match the person's natural voiding schedule. There is no effort made to motivate the patient to delay voiding by resisting the urge. This method is geared more for elderly patients with more challenging problems who have skilled help available.

Pelvic floor exercises may also aid in the treatment of DI. Evidence supports the utility of this modality in all types of incontinence. Particularly when augmented with biofeedback, pelvic floor exercises can greatly reduce symptoms of urinary frequency and urge incontinence, by up to 54–85%.

Pharmacologic Therapy

One of the most effective and popular treatments in urge urinary incontinence and detrusor instability is drug therapy. Numerous agents have been tried over the years in the management of these patients, but only a few have been demonstrated in controlled trials to have a substantial impact in reduction of symptoms. One of the main difficulties is that the cause of DI is not known. Therefore final results of treatment may vary considerably.

The drugs available can be broken into class by mechanism of action (Table 42–9).

Acetylcholine is the main neurotransmitter involved with bladder contraction, which occurs in response to parasympathetic nervous stimulation. It is the preganglionic and postganglionic neurotransmitter in the autonomic innervation of the bladder. The detrusor muscle of the bladder is heavily populated with cholinergic receptors. Anticholinergic activity, therefore, is a property of most drugs used to treat detrusor instability. The prototype medicine is propantheline. Used for many years, it has excellent results in uncontrolled case series, but only modest efficacy in controlled trials, providing benefit in up to 53% of patients.

Smooth muscle relaxants used to treat DI include oxybutynin chloride, tolterodine, and flavoxate hydrochloride. Oxybutynin chloride is the most commonly used drug, and has been shown to be effective. It has been demonstrated in randomized placebo-controlled trials to increase bladder capacity, decrease frequency of detrusor contractions, and improve symptoms of urinary urgency in approximately 70% of patients. It is both effective in idiopathic and neuropathic etiologies of DI.

Tolterodine is a relatively new medication designed specifically for overactive bladder. It too has anticholinergic activity with specificity for the bladder, and acts through muscarinic receptors as well as smooth muscle relaxation. In a multicenter randomized controlled trial, the medication compared favorably with oxybutynin in terms of reducing the number of micturitions in 24 hours and number of incontinent episodes. Because of its bladder specificity, tolterodine has a more favorable side effect profile than oxybutynin. It is also dosed less frequently and improves patient compliance.

Flavoxate is a tertiary amine that has smooth muscle relaxant properties in vitro that is sometimes used clinically. However, the only randomized controlled studies performed demonstrated no significant benefits.

Imipramine hydrochloride is a tricyclic antidepressant that acts through its anticholinergic properties to increase bladder storage. The drug improves bladder compliance rather than counteracting uninhibited detrusor contractions. It is given in doses greatly reduced from those recommended for use as an antidepressant. It also has pharmacologic activity in blockade of postsynaptic noradrenaline uptake and thereby increases bladder outlet resistance. With its dual action, imipramine may be effective in patients with both stress incontinence and detrusor instability (mixed incontinence). It has a low rate of discontinuation due to the main side effects of tremor and fatigue, but should be dosed in the evening as it may

Table 42–9. Pharmacologic agents used to treat for urge incontinence.

Drug Name	Trade Name	Drug Type	Dosage	Potential Side Effects
Oxybutynin chloride	Ditropan	Anticholinergic/smooth muscle relaxant	5–30 mg daily	Xerostomia, blurred vision, constipation, drowsiness, tachycardia
Oxybutynin chloride (OROS)	Ditropan XL	Same as above	5–30 mg daily	Same as above
Flavoxate hydrochloride	Urispas	Smooth muscle relaxant	200–800 mg daily	See above
Tolterodine	Detrol	Anticholinergic/smooth muscle relaxant	1–2 mg twice a day	See above
Imipramine hydrochloride	Tofranil	Tricyclic antidepressant: anticholinergic, alpha-adrenergic, antihistamine	25–100 mg daily	Drowsiness, orthostatic hypotension, hepatic dysfunction, xerostomia
Propantheline bromide	Probanthine	Anticholinergic	45–60 mg daily	Xerostomia, blurry vision, constipation, drowsiness, tachycardia

be sedating and used with caution in elderly patients due to potential orthostatic hypotension.

MIXED INCONTINENCE

Mixed incontinence occurs when both stress and detrusor instability occur simultaneously. Patients may present with symptoms of both types of incontinence. These patients present both a diagnostic and therapeutic dilemma. The prevalence of mixed incontinence is more common than most practitioners realize. A detailed history will reveal symptoms of stress urinary incontinence with urine loss associated with cough, sneeze, or other increase in Valsalva pressure, as well as urinary urgency, frequency, and concomitant incontinence. The coexistence of these two conditions may be brought about by many causes. Patients with stress incontinence often preemptively urinate to avoid a full bladder and subsequent urine loss, thereby conditioning the bladder to habituate to a low functional capacity. This may promote premature signaling of bladder fullness and result in frequent urge symptoms. Patients may have detrusor instability that is precipitated by coughing or laughing. Lastly, patients may have indolent involuntary bladder contractions that only manifest with the additional pressure of a cough, sneeze, or laugh. The cause is often difficult to ascertain, but the diagnosis should be confirmed with urodynamic studies that can assist in identifying the cause of urine loss.

Treatment

For mixed incontinence, treatment should be based on the patient's worst symptoms. Often patients can prioritize their symptoms, stating that one component impacts their life more than the other. By separating the symptoms for the patient a practical management plan with realistic expectations can be devised. A great disservice can be done by operating on a patient to restore bladder neck support and remove stress symptoms, when the patient's main concern is daily urge incontinence while she is at work. Conservative measures should be tried first, and if symptoms do not improve surgical measures can be entertained to alleviate the stress component. Occasionally the involuntary contractions are alleviated by restoration of bladder support and vaginal anatomy.

SENSORY URGE INCONTINENCE

Patients with irritative conditions of the lower urinary tract may lose urine either when they perform stressful activities or when bladder volume increases. A diagnosis of sensory urge incontinence is made when this leakage occurs in a stable bladder and is not due to excessive descent of the urethra and bladder. Infection, diverticula, neoplasia, and foreign bodies are common causes of sensory urge incontinence, as are psychological and neurologic factors.

Sensory urge incontinence is caused by either of two physiologic mechanisms: urethral relaxation or voluntary detrusor activity. As the bladder fills, reflex stimulation of the micturition reflex makes the patient aware of the initial urge to urinate: this urge is usually subconsciously inhibited in normal patients. Any condition that irritates the urethra or bladder (eg, infection, trauma) may overstimulate the afferent reflex arc. Urethral relaxation occurs intermittently, allowing small amounts of urine to dribble out and further stimulate the bladder. This urethral relaxation may be purely reflexive or may be voluntary, albeit subconscious, in order to relieve the discomfort the patient feels. During daily activities, when the patient is distracted and cannot concentrate on inhibiting the detrusor reflex, the bladder may contract after the urethra relaxes. However, the patient maintains this ability to inhibit detrusor contractions and does so when instructed during cystometry, demonstrating that her bladder is stable.

Sensory urge incontinence is usually associated with a small cystometric capacity, but a normal capacity may be present, and bladder capacity under anesthesia is almost always normal except when there is extensive scarring from radiation or trauma. Urethral relaxation or marked variation in urethral pressure may be found on urethral pressure profiles or simultaneous urethrocystometry. Repeated cystometrograms reveal absence of detrusor activity as long as the patient is encouraged to inhibit her desire to void.

Urethroscopy and cystoscopy are of utmost importance in the diagnosis of sensory urge incontinence, since most specific therapies are based on endoscopic findings.

Sensory urge incontinence is usually associated with multiple urinary complaints, including dysuria, which is not a common symptom of genuine stress incontinence or unstable bladder. When there is little or no anatomic defect present in a patient complaining of stress incontinence, sensory urge incontinence may be the correct diagnosis.

Treatment

Specific therapy is started if it is available. Acute infection responds rapidly to antibiotics, but chronic infection may be associated with residual inflammatory changes (eg, erythema, edema, exudate) that cause symptoms long after treatment has eliminated active infection. Mechanical treatments such as urethral dilation or instillation of anti-inflammatory agents in the bladder may be beneficial. Surgery is the treatment of choice for diverticula, calculi, and neoplasia. Estrogen deficiency and vaginal diseases (eg, infection, neoplasm, trauma) may cause sensory urge incontinence, and specific therapy for the underlying disorder usually relieves the urinary symptoms as well as the vaginal symptoms.

OVERFLOW INCONTINENCE

Definition

Overflow incontinence is defined as the involuntary loss of urine associated with bladder overdistention in the absence of a detrusor contraction. This classically occurs in men who have outlet obstruction secondary to prostatic enlargement that progresses to urinary retention. In women this is a relatively uncommon cause of urinary incontinence (Table 42–10).

Etiology

Overflow incontinence will most often occur due to postoperative obstruction if the bladder neck is overcorrected, or with a hyporeflexic bladder due to neurologic disease or spinal cord injury. The normal act of voiding is controlled centrally by sacral and pontine micturition centers. Impaired emptying can be due to a disruption of either central or peripheral neurons mediating detrusor function. Failure to identify the cause early may lead to permanent dysfunction and may lead to injury to the detrusor muscle or compromise in the parasympathetic ganglia in the bladder wall.

Diagnosis

Usually symptoms are loss of urine without awareness or intermittent dribbling and constant wetness. There may be associated suprapubic pressure or pain. Patients will often note a sensation of a full bladder, and having to strain to empty or apply suprapubic pressure to void. Patients are at risk for urinary tract infection secondary

Table 42–10. Causes of overflow incontinence.

Neurologic	Anatomic	Iatrogenic
Spinal cord trauma	Extrinsic compression	Surgery
Cerebral cortical lesions	Urethral mass	Obstetric
Diabetes mellitus		Anesthetic
Multiple sclerosis		
Infectious	Pharmacologic	
Cystitis		
Urethritis		

to persistent residual urine in the bladder which acts as a medium for bacterial growth. It is commonly seen after a bladder neck suspension. Complaints of poor urinary stream and sense of incomplete emptying combined with having to strain or apply hand pressure to void are likely.

Evaluation should always include a postvoid residual, and if the diagnosis is questionable, voiding pressure flow studies should be done. An imaging study of the upper urinary tract to evaluate the ureters and kidney should follow, as persistent high-volume retention can lead to reflux and hydroureter or hydronephrosis and renal damage if left unchecked.

Treatment

Bladder drainage to relieve retention is the first priority. Prolonged catheterization may be necessary, depending on resolution of the inciting cause. In cases of postoperative urinary retention, bladder function can be evaluated by serial postvoid residual urine determinations. Although no normal volume for residual urine is accepted, it is generally considered that less than 100 mL is within normal limits and greater than 150 mL is abnormal. More than one value is needed, as persistently high residual volumes will require prolonged catheterization.

When urinary retention occurs in the setting of neurologic disease, diabetes, or stroke, the correction of the underlying cause is often impossible; therefore, the goal is to prevent injury or damage to the upper urinary tract. Intermittent self-catheterization is preferable to an indwelling catheter, which may predispose to infection, bladder spasms, or erosion.

Medical therapy may assist in the care of these patients. Acetylcholine agonists can stimulate detrusor contractions in patients that have vesical areflexia. Alpha-adrenergic blockers can facilitate bladder emptying by relaxing tone at the bladder neck.

Behavior modification in the form of timed voiding on a preset schedule to empty regardless of urge will prevent accumulation of excess urine. Usually a voiding pattern of every 2–3 hours is preferable. In bladder areflexia, manual pressure or abdominal splinting may facilitate emptying.

BYPASS INCONTINENCE

Urinary loss due to abnormal anatomic variations is uncommon but extremely important to consider in the evaluation of the incontinent woman. Bypass incontinence may often mimic other forms of urinary incontinence, but usually presents as constant dribbling or dampness. Patients may also complain of positional loss of urine with urge or forewarning. Diagnosing this type of incontinence requires a high level of suspicion and an understanding of the underlying anatomic deviation in the lower urinary tract. Genitourinary fistulas (vesicovaginal or ureterovaginal) can be a debilitating cause of incontinence and are formed because of poor wound healing after a traumatic insult (eg, obstetric laceration, pelvic surgery, perineal trauma, or radiation exposure). Leakage due to fistulas is generally continuous although it may be elicited by position change or stress-inducing activities. Evaluation should include a careful examination of the vaginal walls for fistulas. This can be facilitated by filling the bladder with milk or dilute indigo carmine dye and looking for pooling in the vaginal canal. Pad testing can also be performed by having the patient ingest 200 mg of oral phenazopyridium hydrochloride (pyridium) several hours before a subsequent exam. By placing a tampon in the vagina and on the perineum the diagnosis may be confirmed by inspection of the pads after a period of time. Further imaging (intravenous urography) and cystoscopy can identify the exact location of the aberrant communication. Surgical correction is generally the only hope for cure. Prolonged catheterization after correction is necessary.

DIVERTICULUM

Another important but uncommon cause of involuntary urine loss is urethral diverticula. Diverticula are essentially weaknesses or "hernias" in the supportive fascial layer of the bladder or urethra. Urethral diverticulum is most likely to cause symptoms of urinary loss. It has an incidence of 0.3–3% in women and is thought to be largely an acquired condition due to obstruction and expansion of the paraurethral Skene's glands. The symptoms of constant small amounts of leakage or urethral discharge are often described. On physical exam a suburethral mass is visible and palpable. Urine or discharge may often be "milked" by palpation of the suburethral mass. Treatment is usually surgical excision of the diverticulum.

FUNCTIONAL AND TRANSIENT INCONTINENCE

Incontinence may be due to factors outside the lower urinary tract and are particularly significant in the geriatric population, because often there are a multitude of special circumstances that affect the health of the elderly. Physical impairment, cognitive function, medication, systemic illness, and bowel function are all factors that may contribute to incontinence. Many immobile patients are incontinent because of the inability to toilet. Cognitive disturbances will limit a patient's ability to respond normally to the sensation to void. Numerous medications have effects on the bladder that may reduce capacity, inhibit bladder function, increase diuresis and bladder load, or relax the urinary sphincter. Additionally, stool impaction and constipation have both been associated with increased prevalence of urinary incontinence. Treatments should first identify the etiologic factors of the incontinence, and then reduce or remove the cause.

REFERENCES

Anderson RU et al: Once daily controlled- versus immediate-release oxybutynin chloride for urge urinary incontinence. J Urol 1999;161:1809.

Bø K, Talseth AT: Long-term effect of pelvic floor muscle exercise 5 years after cessation of organized training. Obstet Gynecol 1996;87:261.

Comiter CV et al: Grading pelvic prolapse and pelvic relaxation using dynamic magnetic resonance imaging. Urology 1999; 54:454.

Danier M et al: The Burch procedure: a comprehensive review. Obstet Gynecol Surv 1998;54:49.

Elkins TE, Thompson JR: Lower urinary tract fistulas. In: Walters MD, Karram MM (editors): *Urogynecology and Reconstructive Pelvic Surgery*, 2nd ed. Mosby, 1999.

Leach GE et al: Female stress urinary incontinence clinical guidelines panel summary report on surgical management of female stress urinary incontinence. J Urol 1997;158:875.

Rosenman AR: Laparoscopic Burch colposuspension: an innovation whose time has come. J Gynecol Tech 1997;3:61.

Sarver R, Govier FE: Pubovaginal slings: past, present and future. Int Urogyn J 1997;8:358.

Sogor L: Suburethral diverticula. In: Walters MD, Karram MM (editors): *Urogynecology and Reconstructive Pelvic Surgery*, 2nd ed. Mosby, 1999.

Stanton SLR: What is the right operation for stress incontinence? A gynaecological view. Br J Urol 1997;80(supp 1):84.

Wang AC, Lo TS: Tension-free vaginal tape. A minimally invasive solution to stress urinary incontinence in women. J Reprod Med 1998;43:429.

Perioperative Considerations in Gynecology

43

Michael P. Aronson, MD, FACOG, FACS, Brendan P. Garry, MD & Mikio Nihara, MD, MPH

The central focus of the gynecologist is on the normal and pathologic anatomy and function of the female reproductive system. However, since no organ system functions independently, the gynecologist must also be familiar with many pathologic conditions not directly related to the reproductive system, but which might affect diagnosis and treatment. At no time is this more crucial than during the perioperative period, ie, just before, during, and immediately after gynecologic surgery.

The differential diagnosis of abdominopelvic pain and dysfunction not directly related to the reproductive system must be fully understood by the gynecologist because many of these entities can present with symptoms suggestive of uterine or adnexal origin. Conversely, the first evidence of nongynecologic disease may be an alteration in the function of the female reproductive system.

This chapter covers the perioperative period: the decision to operate (emergently or electively), and the pre- and postoperative management of these patients. Selected medical and surgical disorders of importance to the gynecologist are reviewed as they relate to management of the surgical patient.

■ ACUTE ABDOMEN

ESSENTIALS OF DIAGNOSIS

Essential Elements:

- *Acute onset of severe abdominal pain.*
- *Signs of peritoneal irritation with guarding and rebound tenderness.*

Frequently Seen:

- *Anemia or hypovolemic shock if intraperitoneal hemorrhage exists.*

- *Varying degrees of gastrointestinal irritation, nausea, and vomiting.*
- *Elevated white blood cell count (if cause is inflammatory or infectious).*
- *Fever (occasionally).*
- *Possible complication of pregnancy.*

General Considerations

The diagnosis of acute abdomen has traditionally been based on signs and symptoms of peritonitis, which can be caused by a diverse array of disease processes. Although the acute abdomen always requires an immediate surgical or medical decision, some patients suffer from a major intra-abdominal pathologic process not associated with peritonitis and should not be considered to have an acute abdomen. An example is the patient with acute gastrointestinal bleeding who requires emergency care but does not have an acute abdomen in the strictest sense. Although the acute abdomen is not precisely defined, a number of signs and symptoms generally accompany this diagnosis (Table 43–1).

It is important to note that although many perceive the acute abdomen as a problem always requiring surgical intervention, in many instances medical management is more appropriate. The presence of an acute abdomen does not dictate the type of management, only the need to come to a rapid decision and implement appropriate therapy as expeditiously as possible.

Finally, it should be stated that an abdomen with generalized peritonitis in all four quadrants is commonly termed a "surgical abdomen." If the patient has a rigid abdomen with guarding and rebound tenderness in all four quadrants, a clear diagnosis usually cannot be achieved except in the operating room. Ultrasonography, computed tomography (CT), culdocentesis, and other routine tests can often establish whether the process is hemorrhagic or inflammatory, but the specific diagnosis can typically be determined only during laparotomy or laparoscopy.

Table 43–1. Differential diagnosis of acute gynecologic intra-abdominal disease.

	Clinical and Laboratory Findings						
Disease	CBC	Urinalysis	Pregnancy Test	Ultrasound	Culdocentesis	Fever	Nausea and Vomiting
Ruptured ectopic pregnancy	Hematocrit low after treatment of hypovolemia.	Red blood cells rare.	Positive. ß-hCG low for gestational age.	Possible adnexal mass. Possible sac-like decidual reaction in uterus. Possible increased free fluid in cul-de-sac.	High hematocrit. Defibrinated, non-clotting sample with no platelets. Crenated red blood cells.	No.	Unusual.
Salpingitis	Rising white blood cell count.	White blood cells occasionally present.	Generally negative.	Negative unless pyosalpinx or tubo-ovarian abscess present.	Yellow, turbid fluid with many white blood cells and some bacteria.	Progressively worsening. Spiking.	Gradual onset with ileus.
Ruptured ovarian cyst (hemorrhagic)	Hematocrit may be low after treatment of hypovolemia.	Normal.	Usually negative.	No masses. Increase free fluid in cul-de-sac.	Hematocrit generally less than 10%.	No.	Rare.
Ruptured ovarian cyst (non-hemorrhagic)	Normal.	Normal.	Generally negative	No masses. Increased free fluid in cul-de-sac.	Increased clear fluid.	No.	Rare.
Torsion of adnexa	Normal or elevated white blood cell count with necrosis.	Normal.	Generally negative.	Adnexal mass common. Decreased flow on Doppler study.	Minimal clear fluid if obtained early.	Possibly with necrosis.	Possibly.
Degenerating leiomyoma	Normal or elevated white blood cell count.	Normal.	Generally negative.	Pedunculated or uterine mass often with central fluid areas.	Normal clear fluid.	Possibly.	Rare.

The patient with a surgical abdomen should never be delayed. The operating room should be notified, large-bore intravenous access obtained, and blood work including a complete blood count (CBC) and blood for cross-matching should be sent as the patient is being moved to the operating room. This is the exceptional case that demands the gynecologic surgeon's total attention and skills. For most patients with localized peritonitis, however, a diagnosis can be made outside the operating room, allowing more time for consideration of therapeutic options.

Etiology and Pathogenesis

The acute abdomen can be caused by a wide variety of problems. Their similar clinical presentation reflects the stimulation of pain receptors in the peritoneum by leakage of purulent matter into the peritoneal cavity, intraperitoneal bleeding, necrosis of an intra-abdominal structure, or inflammation due to infection. Stomach acid, bile, and pancreatic secretions cause intense peritoneal irritation when released into the peritoneal cavity, but urine and ascitic fluid generally do not.

Clinical Findings

A. Symptoms and Signs

The most common symptom of a patient with acute abdomen is pain. It can be generalized or have a maximum intensity in a specific area. The presence of guarding, rebound tenderness, or referred tenderness on abdominal examination can be helpful in localizing the area of greatest peritoneal irritation. On pelvic examination, the patient may exhibit uterine motion tenderness. Although commonly associated with pelvic inflammatory disease, this sign is nonspecific and is likely to be present with a number of irritative pelvic processes.

The irritated peritoneum is most sensitive to stretching and movement, so patients often minimize motion to reduce these stimuli. The patient's position may provide a useful clue to the site of greatest irritation. Patients with pelvic peritonitis are frequently most comfortable with one or both hips flexed, depending on the site and extent of the peritonitis.

The quality of the patient's pain is important. Patients with intermittent torsion of the adnexa or ruptured ovarian cyst may have had such pain before. The temporal relationship of the onset of pain to the patient's last menstrual period may give valuable clues, especially regarding possible complications of early pregnancy.

Gastrointestinal symptoms that often accompany the acute abdomen are anorexia, nausea, vomiting, or diarrhea. The extent of bowel involvement depends on the severity of the peritonitis. Patients with mild bowel irritation note decreased appetite. Nausea and vomiting may develop as the bowel becomes more directly involved in the inflammatory process. Further progression leads to inhibition of peristalsis with associated abdominal distention secondary to gas- and fluid-filled loops of bowel. As peristalsis decreases, bowel sounds may be decreased, and eventually may be absent. High-pitched bowel sounds and rushes may be heard if obstruction is present.

If the peritoneum covering the bladder or rectosigmoid is irritated first, the patient's initial complaint may be of painful bladder or bowel function. It can be a mistake to assume that a patient complaining of painful bladder filling and emptying merely has cystitis. For example, it is not unusual for a patient to note an episode of urinary or bowel urgency at the time of initial rupture of an ectopic pregnancy or an ovarian cyst.

While taking the history, keep in mind the progression and timing of the appearance of the patient's symptoms. While performing the physical examination, it is necessary to realize that the patient has an evolving process occurring, and a single examination only assesses one stage of that process. Several serial examinations may be necessary to guide clinical decision-making.

B. Laboratory Findings

Routine laboratory studies for all women with pelvic peritonitis should include CBC, urinalysis, and rapid pregnancy test. The CBC may demonstrate either acute blood loss or, if the white blood cell count is elevated, an infectious process.

A rapid, reliable pregnancy test should always be performed immediately in the female patient with pelvic pain. A patient whose history suggests salpingitis may actually have a ruptured ectopic pregnancy. In addition, a pregnancy may coexist with an independent pathologic process, in which case the pregnancy may influence management. For example, elective surgery for a degenerating leiomyoma in a pregnant patient would be deferred until the second trimester if possible.

Urinalysis may demonstrate urinary tract infection, but pyuria may also result from an abscess adjacent to the ureter, as occurs in ruptured retrocecal appendicitis. Gross or microscopic hematuria can reflect the passage of a stone or perhaps exacerbation of an underlying pathologic process such as interstitial cystitis.

Patients with diabetic ketoacidosis may present with severe acute abdominal pain; therefore, testing the blood and urine for glucose and ketones is essential. It is also possible for the stress of an acute abdomen from other causes to initiate or aggravate ketoacidosis in a normally well-controlled diabetic patient. Prior to operating on such patients every effort must be made to fully correct their fluid, glucose, electrolyte, and acidotic status.

Cervical cultures for *Neisseria gonorrhoeae* and *Chlamydia trachomatis* should also be obtained. Although not useful for immediate management decisions, they may aid in guiding antibiotic therapy if the patient is determined to have a pelvic infection. The erythrocyte sedimentation rate is a nonspecific test for the presence of inflammation and is not very useful in the initial evaluation of the acute abdomen.

A. SPECIAL EXAMINATIONS

1. Culdocentesis—Culdocentesis (discussed in Chapters 14 and 30) is an easily performed and important diagnostic procedure that is often overlooked in the modern era of high-resolution imaging studies, but it may be useful when those studies are not available. The contents of the peritoneal cavity can be evaluated by means of culdocentesis in any patient with pelvic peritonitis or pain during uterine and adnexal movement.

Clear, straw-colored peritoneal fluid represents a negative culdocentesis, indicating no intraperitoneal bleeding. An unruptured ectopic gestation could still be present. Large amounts of fluid of this type can indicate a ruptured, nonhemorrhagic ovarian cyst or ascites. Turbid peritoneal fluid containing white blood cells on Gram-stained smear suggests an intrapelvic inflammatory process.

A bloody, nonclotting peritoneal fluid sample with a hematocrit in the range of 15–40% reflects recent hemorrhage into the peritoneal cavity, possibly from ruptured ectopic pregnancy or a bleeding ovarian cyst. In this case, prior clotting of blood in the peritoneal cavity results in crenated red blood cells, defibrination, absence of platelets, and lack of clotting factors in the hemorrhagic fluid aspirated from the cul-de-sac. A bloody aspirate that forms a clot may represent blood inadvertently drawn from vaginal or uterine vessels. An attempted culdocentesis that returns no fluid at all is termed "nondiagnostic."

Given the increasing availability of transvaginal ultrasonography, the role of culdocentesis for the detection of hemoperitoneum is currently being reassessed. A review of 252 consecutive cases, in which patients underwent culdocentesis and subsequent surgery for presumed ectopic pregnancy revealed that 86% of the patients with a positive culdocentesis had a hemoperitoneum. However, 25 of the 42 patients with a negative result from culdocentesis were found to have a hemoperitoneum, a false-negative rate of 54%.

More recently, another study compared the sensitivity and specificity of culdocentesis and transvaginal ultrasound to identify hemoperitoneum. Among 46 patients who underwent surgery for the treatment of suspected ectopic pregnancy, the presence of "echogenic fluid" on transvaginal ultrasound had a sensitivity of 95% and a specificity of 100% for the detection of hemoperitoneum. A positive culdocentesis was found to have a sensitivity of 62% and a specificity of 89% for the detection of hemoperitoneum. Because culdocentesis is an invasive procedure whose sensitivity may be lower than previously thought, it should be primarily used when transvaginal ultrasound is not available.

2. Radiology—Transvaginal and transabdominal ultrasound studies have become extremely useful over the past decade for diagnosis of the acute abdomen. In the pelvis, ultrasonography is useful for characterizing the location and gestational age of early pregnancies, identifying adnexal or uterine masses, and determining the presence or absence of pelvic abscesses or excessive free fluid in the cul-de-sac. Outside the pelvis, ultrasonography is often the initial diagnostic modality used to investigate possible cholecystitis, choledocholithiasis, and appendicitis. In patients too uncomfortable to allow adequate abdominal or bimanual pelvic examination, ultrasound examination plays an even more important role. A number of CT techniques have also proved useful in the evaluation of the acute abdomen.

Plain x-ray films of the abdomen are less helpful in diagnosing gynecologic causes of acute abdomen, but may be helpful in detecting bowel obstruction or paralytic ileus if dilated loops of bowel with air-fluid levels are seen. Free air under the diaphragm on an upright film indicates perforation of a viscus organ and requires immediate intervention. An upright film that does not show the diaphragms should be considered inadequate in the work-up of the acute abdomen. Occasionally, loss of the psoas shadow on the right side is seen, supporting a diagnosis of appendicitis. In addition, renal calculi may be seen on plain films.

3. Microbiology—In the acute patient, Gram stains and cultures assume a role of lesser importance. Cervical cultures for *N gonorrhoeae* should be done; however, since this organism may be found on the cervix of asymptomatic as well as symptomatic patients, Gram-stained smears of cervical secretions to detect gram-negative diplococci may be unreliable. Finding *N gonorrhoeae* on the cervix does not prove that peritonitis is due to salpingitis. Conversely, many patients with laparoscopically proven pelvic infections have negative cervical cultures. In the patient who proves to have salpingitis, cervical cultures or cultures of washings done at laparoscopy may help to sharpen the focus of subsequent antibiotic therapy. Cervical material should be submitted for culture in all patients suspected of having gonococcal salpingitis, if only to determine the need for treatment of the sexual partner. Chlamydial culture or enzymatic assay is frequently done as well.

GYNECOLOGIC CAUSES OF ACUTE ABDOMEN

Ruptured ectopic pregnancy (Chapter 14), salpingitis (Chapter 38), and hemorrhagic ovarian cyst (Chapter 37) are the 3 most commonly diagnosed gynecologic conditions presenting as acute abdomen in the emergency room. Degenerating leiomyomas (Chapter 36) occur less frequently. Typical clinical and laboratory findings for these conditions are shown in Table 43–1. These gynecologic entities are discussed fully in their respective chapters.

Torsion, or twisting, of the ovary or both the ovary and tube is an unusual cause of acute abdomen. The most common etiology is ovarian enlargement by a benign mass. Patients present with acute, severe abdominal, pelvic pain which may be accompanied by nausea and vomiting. With progressive torsion venous and lymphatic obstruction occurs. Interruption of the arterial supply may follow, resulting in hypoxia, necrosis, fever and leukocytosis. Diagnosis is aided by ultrasound, where an adnexal mass is usually seen. Management is surgical. In a patient of reproductive age with a benign mass, it is acceptable to untwist the ovary and if the ovary is viable, remove the mass and stabilize the remaining ovary with sutures.

The challenge of the acute abdomen is expeditious arrival at an accurate diagnosis and the rapid implementation of a treatment plan. The gynecologist may be the only physician to evaluate the patient and must be capable of entertaining all possible diagnoses in the differential—both gynecologic and nongynecologic. The next section and Table 43–2 review the most common nongynecologic entities that need to be considered by the gynecologist evaluating the patient with an acute abdomen.

NONGYNECOLOGIC CAUSES OF ACUTE ABDOMEN

1. Appendicitis

More than 10% of the general population will develop appendicitis at some time in their lives. Appendicitis is widely recognized as a disease of childhood and is the most common reason for laparotomy in infants and children. In the older patient, however, appendicitis can manifest later and in a more subtle fashion. This

Table 43–2. Differential diagnosis of acute nongynecologic intra-abdominal disease.

Disease	CBC	Urinalysis	Pregnancy Test	Culdocentesis	Fever	Nausea and Vomiting
			Clinical and Laboratory Findings			
Appendicitis	Normal early; high white blood cell count later.	Normal.	If patient is pregnant, presentation of disease is atypical.	Yellow, turbid fluid with many white blood cells and no bacteria.	Not early in course.	Yes.
Retrocecal appendicitis	Normal early; high white blood cell count later.	Many white blood cells if abscess forms.	Not helpful.	May be normal.	Yes in advanced diseases.	Variable.
Regional enteritis (Crohn's disease)	High white blood cell count.	Normal.	Not helpful.	Yellow, turbid fluid with many white blood cells.	Yes if severe.	Yes if severe. Recent history of diarrhea.
Colonic diverticulitis	High white blood cell count.	Normal.	Not helpful.	Yellow, turbid fluid with many white blood cells and no bacteria.	Yes if severe.	Variable.
Bowel obstruction	High if ischemic bowel damage is present.	Normal.	Not helpful.	Increased amount of fluid with many white blood cells if bowel is ischemic.	Only if bowel is ischemic.	Yes.

can be of great clinical significance in these patients, who often have other significant underlying diseases. It is wise to consider the possibility of appendicitis in every patient—regardless of age—who presents in the emergency room with an acute abdomen.

In pregnancy the need to consider appendicitis is of paramount importance. One researcher found in a 10-year experience at a large teaching hospital a perinatal mortality rate of less than 3% for uncomplicated appendicitis as well as for negative laparotomy. When perforation occurred before surgery, the perinatal mortality rate rose to 20%. As the researcher put it, "the maxim regarding acute appendicitis—if in doubt, take it out—is never more true than in pregnancy."

Clinical Findings

A. SYMPTOMS AND SIGNS

It is prudent for the gynecologist to remember that the patient may not present with the "classic" symptoms of appendicitis, but may present with many variations that closely mimic other diagnostic entities.

The patient's first symptom may be nausea and loss of appetite. Pain typically begins in the periumbilical area and then gradually shifts to the right lower quadrant. Fever is usually not significant unless the appendix has ruptured. Bowel sounds are reduced, and often no bowel movement will have occurred since the onset of pain. After the patient's pain migrates to the right lower quadrant, tenderness to palpation is most severe at McBurney's point, approximately 5 centimeters medial to the right anterior superior iliac spine on a line between the anterior superior iliac spine and the umbilicus. As inflammation increases, guarding and rebound tenderness appear at this location. Palpation in the left lower quadrant may produce referred pain in the right lower quadrant.

Some patients note marked discomfort upon uterine motion as well as right adnexal tenderness on pelvic examination. These symptoms develop because the inflamed appendix irritates the peritoneum adjacent to the uterus and oviduct, and they may be improperly interpreted as signs of salpingitis. The patient is generally most comfortable in the supine position with the right hip flexed to minimize tension on the peritoneum adjacent to the appendix.

B. LABORATORY FINDINGS

The CBC may be normal, but an elevated white blood cell count may develop, especially after rupture of the appendix. Urinalysis results are usually normal unless the inflamed appendix rests adjacent to the ureter, or unless an abscess has formed near the ureter, producing pyuria. If the pregnancy test is positive, the presentation of appendicitis may be significantly altered (see Chapter 24).

C. RADIOLOGIC FINDINGS

High-resolution ultrasonography with graded compression has proven useful in the diagnosis of acute appendicitis. In one study, researchers claimed a diagnostic sensitivity varying from 80–95%, a specificity of 95–100%, and an accuracy rate of 91–95%. Ultrasonography also allows some differentiation between the acute appendix and the gangrenous and perforated appendix.

X-ray films of the abdomen may demonstrate an oval calcified fecalith up to 1–2 cm in diameter in the right lower quadrant. A dilated, gas-filled "sentinel loop" of the bowel may also be seen as a result of localized inflammation near the cecum on plain films.

D. SPECIAL EXAMINATIONS

Culdocentesis may demonstrate straw-colored, turbid peritoneal fluid containing numerous white blood cells. This finding is not diagnostic for appendicitis but merely reflects the existence of an intraperitoneal inflammatory process; similar findings may be seen in salpingitis and acute regional enteritis.

Laparoscopy may be appropriate in young, nulligravid patients in whom a missed diagnosis may have an adverse effect on future fertility. Considerable technical skill may be required to establish or rule out a diagnosis of appendicitis, depending on the location of the appendix and other intra-abdominal conditions. Removal of the appendix through the laparoscope may then also be possible as well.

Differential Diagnosis

On the basis of physical examination alone, it may be difficult to distinguish acute salpingitis from appendicitis. The irritation associated with pelvic inflammatory disease usually extends to both lower quadrants unless unilateral salpingitis (possibly associated with an intrauterine device) is suspected. In contrast to the patient with appendicitis, the patient with salpingitis is more likely to have a fever with an elevated white blood cell count at an earlier stage of her disease. The woman with salpingitis usually develops gastrointestinal symptoms later, since pelvic inflammation spreads from the oviducts to secondarily involve the bowel in the pelvic cavity.

A history of early gastrointestinal symptoms, decreased appetite, and nausea and vomiting is often the most reliable single factor in establishing a diagnosis of appendicitis rather than early pelvic inflammatory disease. The possibility of a ruptured right ovarian cyst must be entertained as well.

In the emergency setting, it is occasionally impossible to differentiate appendicitis from acute regional enteritis (Crohn's disease) with involvement of the terminal ileum. At laparotomy for suspected appendicitis in the patient with regional enteritis, the appendix is normal but the terminal ileum is inflamed. In contrast to the patient with appendicitis, a patient with regional enteritis usually has a history of recent diarrhea (Table 43–2).

Ruptured retrocecal appendicitis may be misdiagnosed as pyelonephritis. The fever, nausea, right-sided back pain, and pyuria from a retrocecal abscess may be mistakenly assumed to be of renal origin.

In the pregnant patient, the enlarging uterus displaces the appendix upward, thereby changing the site of the pain of appendicitis. Pregnant patients with appendicitis also demonstrate less dramatic gastrointestinal symptoms and may even continue to have an appetite. For these reasons, the diagnosis of appendicitis in the pregnant patient is much more likely to be made after appendiceal rupture and abscess formation have occurred than in the nonpregnant patient. This most often leads to premature labor. The risk of early surgical intervention in the gravid patient must be weighed against the considerable risk of premature delivery if appendicitis is indeed present and rupture occurs.

Treatment

The diagnosis of acute appendicitis requires immediate surgical removal of the appendix either by laparotomy or laparoscopy.

Complications

Early diagnosis and surgery are essential to prevent rupture of the appendix and the possible complications of recurrent pelvic abscess, wound infection, pelvic adhesions, and occasionally, infertility.

2. Acute Bowel Obstruction

Bowel obstruction may result from an intrinsic or extrinsic expanding neoplasm, compression of a segment of bowel by a hernia, constriction of the lumen by extrinsic bowel adhesions, or volvulus or intussusception of a segment of bowel. Because of the wide range of causes, all age groups or populations should be considered at risk for development of bowel obstruction. The cause is often not clear until laparotomy is performed. Obstruction due to adhesions is always a possibility if the patient has undergone previous abdominal surgery,

especially if the previous surgery was complicated by peritonitis.

Clinical Findings

A. SYMPTOMS AND SIGNS

Nausea and vomiting associated with abdominal distention and severe abdominal pain are the hallmarks of bowel obstruction. Bowel sounds may be absent if obstruction is total, or high-pitched if it is partial. The patient may complain of constipation and usually ceases to have bowel movements. A hernia or abdominal mass may be evident on physical examination. Abdominal palpation produces guarding and rebound tenderness.

B. LABORATORY FINDINGS

Loss of hydrochloric acid through protracted vomiting results in alkalosis with respiratory compensation. Serum bicarbonate levels may be high. Serum potassium levels may be low, indicating general depletion of electrolytes.

C. X-RAY FINDINGS

A supine x-ray view of the abdomen demonstrates one or more loops of gas-filled bowel. Air-fluid levels are evident in these loops in upright films (Fig 43–1).

Differential Diagnosis

Peritonitis with secondary inhibition of peristalsis, generally termed paralytic ileus, must be distinguished from bowel obstruction. The patient with paralytic ileus usually experiences constant abdominal pain rather than the cramping abdominal pain associated with bowel obstruction. Treatment of the condition causing peritonitis also results in gradual resolution of paralytic ileus.

Complications

Marked distention of a segment of bowel may result in vascular compromise, strangulation, and eventually, bowel perforation with spillage of toxic bowel contents into the abdominal cavity. Dehydration and loss of electrolytes are associated with accumulation of fluid within the bowel lumen. Hypokalemia may produce electrocardiographic abnormalities if the serum potassium level is lower than 3 mEq/L.

Treatment

Nasogastric suction may be effective in decompressing the distended bowel and may relieve the persistent vomiting and cramping pain associated with bowel obstruction. Surgical correction of the structural abnormality responsible for obstruction is the only definitive

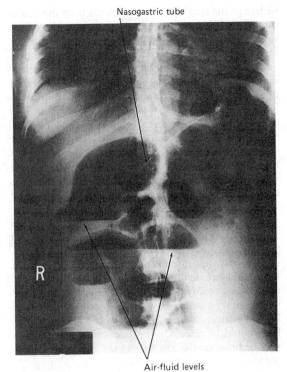

Nasogastric tube

R

Air-fluid levels

Figure 43–1. Upright abdominal film demonstrating air-fluid levels in a patient subsequently found to have small bowel obstruction.

treatment. Partial bowel obstruction due to adhesions occasionally subsides while the patient is undergoing nasogastric or long-tube suction. Fluid or electrolyte imbalance must also be corrected, and losses must be compensated for during prolonged suction drainage. Evidence of a perforated viscus organ requires immediate surgical intervention.

3. Inflammatory Bowel Disease (Ulcerative Colitis & Regional Enteritis [Crohn's Disease])

Ulcerative colitis and regional enteritis represent two distinct forms of inflammatory bowel disease. Inflammation restricted to the colon is termed ulcerative colitis. Regional enteritis (Crohn's disease, terminal ileitis) is characterized by multiple sites of small bowel or colonic inflammation, especially in the terminal ileum. Women are twice as likely to develop regional enteritis but carry the same risk as men for ulcerative colitis. Inflammatory bowel disease is most likely to develop during the reproductive years.

Clinical Findings

A. SYMPTOMS AND SIGNS

Patients suffering from inflammatory bowel disease generally complain of episodic bloody diarrhea and abdominal pain. Abdominal guarding and rebound tenderness are noted on palpation of the localized area of peritonitis associated with the inflamed segment of bowel. The severity of recurrent episodes of abdominal pain and diarrhea varies widely. Acute regional enteritis with terminal ileitis may mimic appendicitis, although the patient with acute regional enteritis is far more likely to give a history of recent diarrhea.

B. LABORATORY FINDINGS

The CBC generally shows an elevated white blood cell count with an increased number of polymorphonuclear leukocytes. Culdocentesis should be avoided if inflammatory bowel disease is suspected. If done, however, it would yield turbid fluid containing numerous white cells—largely a result of inflammatory transudate from the inflamed bowel.

C. X-RAY FINDINGS

Barium enema and an upper gastrointestinal study with small bowel follow-through may demonstrate either mucosal changes of the bowel consistent with acute inflammation, or induration and narrowing of bowel segments, suggesting chronic disease. Involvement of only one segment of colon suggests a diagnosis of ulcerative colitis; multiple sites of involvement, often including the terminal ileum, suggest regional enteritis. X-ray studies may be normal in patients with early or inactive inflammatory bowel disease.

D. SPECIAL EXAMINATIONS

Endoscopic evaluation with biopsy of areas of inflamed bowel mucosa is the most direct method of diagnosis.

Differential Diagnosis

Appendicitis, diverticulitis, torsion of the adnexa, and salpingitis may produce physical findings similar to those of acute terminal ileitis. Because of the great difference in appropriate therapy for each of these conditions and because of the serious results of inappropriate treatment, each disease must be ruled out whenever the diagnosis of acute inflammatory bowel disease is suspected.

Complications

Perforation of the colon and small bowel fistulas are serious inflammatory complications. Appendectomy in a patient with terminal ileitis carries an additional risk of poor healing, abscess formation, and fistula development, especially if the cecum and base of the appendix are involved in the inflammatory process.

Treatment

Acute inflammatory bowel disease generally responds to administration of corticosteroids. Intravenous metronidazole has been effective in some patients with acute illness. Recurrence may be prevented by long-term administration of sulfasalazine. Therapy is complex, however, and should be directed by a gastroenterologist. Surgical excision of segments of inflamed bowel may be appropriate in cases of stricture with obstruction, perforation, or massive hemorrhage, or in severe cases unresponsive to corticosteroids. Reanastomosis of bowel after resection for inflammatory bowel disease is often unsuccessful, and resection fails to prevent recurrence, which often occurs just proximal to the anastomotic site. Supportive care, including intravenous fluids, electrolytes, transfusion, antibiotics if sepsis is present, and nutritional replacement for patients with malabsorption, are essential general measures.

4. Colonic Diverticulitis

Diverticula of the distal colon are uncommon in women during the reproductive years, but as many as one-third of postmenopausal women have colonic diverticula demonstrable by barium enema or colonoscopy. Colonic diverticula appear to result from herniation of the bowel mucosa at a site of weakness of the colonic muscularis. The mucosa may be disrupted as the diverticulum enlarges, with resulting bleeding or localized infection. Bleeding may require partial colonic resection. Superficial infection may be self-limiting and associated with mild left lower quadrant pain, which spontaneously subsides as the bowel mucosa heals over a period of 2 or 3 days. Broad-spectrum antibiotics may be necessary if the patient with diverticulitis develops severe left lower quadrant pain, guarding, rebound tenderness, fever, and leukocytosis. Patients not responding to antibiotics or patients with associated pelvic abscess formation require surgical management, including drainage of the pelvic abscess, temporary colostomy, and possible resection of the segment of inflamed or obstructed colon. The surgeon must also rule out carcinoma of the colon, especially in the case of bowel obstruction.

5. Meckel's Diverticulitis

Meckel's diverticulum, a remnant of the vitelline duct, is found in 2–3% of the general population but is three times more common in men than in women. The diverticulum is generally found on the antimesenteric surface of the small bowel, about 8 cm from the ileocecal valve, although the exact distance from the cecum varies greatly. Ectopic secretory gastric mucosa may be found in 20% of patients with Meckel's diverticulum.

If secretory gastric mucosa is present in the diverticulum, ulceration of adjacent bowel mucosa may result in bleeding. Bleeding is an indication for laparotomy in 50% of patients subjected to surgery for complications arising from Meckel's diverticulum. Intestinal obstruction from intussusception of Meckel's diverticulum or obstruction due to volvulus around a vestigial band from the diverticulum to the umbilicus is the reason for an additional 25% of surgical procedures, and Meckel's diverticulitis is the reason for the remaining 25% of surgical cases.

Meckel's diverticulitis is associated with symptoms similar to those of appendicitis, except that abdominal pain is located more medially. Inflamed Meckel's diverticulum may rupture earlier than an inflamed appendix. If the cause of inflammatory peritonitis is unclear at the time of laparotomy, it is important to inspect the entire length of the small bowel for a possible inflamed Meckel's diverticulum. An inflamed Meckel's diverticulum should be resected. The base of the diverticulum may be broader than the base of the appendix, so simple ligation may not be possible.

6. Nephrolithiasis

Various metabolic factors, in combination with dehydration, may frequently produce supersaturated solutions of relatively insoluble substances that subsequently crystallize in the urine. Men are 2–3 times more likely than women to develop calcium renal stone disease. The less frequently detected struvite (magnesium-ammonium-phosphate), uric acid, and cystine stones are associated with chronic *Proteus* infection of the urinary tract, gout, and cystinuria, respectively.

Clinical Findings

A. SYMPTOMS AND SIGNS

Renal stones may be discovered in any portion of the urinary tract but are most likely to be symptomatic in the ureter. A renal stone passing from the ureteropelvic junction to the bladder usually causes severe ureteral spasm. Ureteral colic generally radiates from the flank on the affected side to the labia or bladder and may occur episodically over several hours or days until the stone passes into the bladder. Although the pain is usually prostrating, the patient experiences no peritonitis and may sometimes be able to remain mobile during the attack. A renal stone may remain lodged at the ureterovesical junction for a long time. In a patient with partial ureteral obstruction, symptoms caused by a renal stone at the ureterovesical junction may mimic the urinary frequency, urgency, bladder discomfort, and hematuria of hemorrhagic cystitis.

Abdominal and pelvic examinations remain normal during an acute attack of ureteral colic, but gentle flank percussion worsens ureteral pain.

B. LABORATORY FINDINGS

The most helpful initial laboratory test is evaluation for hematuria; blood is found in the urine sample of every patient with a renal stone unless total ureteral obstruction exists. Abdominal x-rays are helpful in locating calcium- and magnesium-containing stones. An intravenous pyelogram is useful in assessing ureteral obstruction and secondary renal structural damage. Intravenous pyelogram may also be necessary to locate stones not containing calcium or magnesium (< 10% of all stones), since these are not visible on x-rays. Renal ultrasonography will reveal hydronephrosis or hydroureter if distal obstruction is present.

C. SPECIAL EXAMINATIONS

After acute pain has subsided, efforts should be directed toward establishing the cause of renal stone disease. All urine should be filtered to collect stones for analysis of their mineral content. Appropriate metabolic studies to detect hyperuricosuria, hypercalciuria, hyperoxaluria, etc, are dictated by the composition of the stones.

Treatment

Treatment to prevent recurrent stone formation includes correction of any metabolic abnormalities in the minority of patients who demonstrate such disorders. The most helpful therapy for most patients appears to be conscientious efforts to maintain adequate hydration; consumption of more than 2 L of water daily is advised. Efforts to maintain hydration are especially important after meals and during the night. The pain caused by passage of a stone can be excruciating; adequate pain control is very important.

Obstructing stones lodged in the ureter must occasionally be removed surgically, either by laparotomy or through a cystoscope with the aid of a wire snare attached to a ureteral catheter. Large stones in the renal pelvis or proximal ureter may be pulverized by high-energy shock-wave therapy (extracorporeal shock-wave lithotripsy) to facilitate passage through the ureter.

7. Other Nongynecologic Causes

Other causes of acute onset of abdominopelvic pain in the female must also be entertained. Perforation of a peptic ulcer will allow entry of gastric secretions into the peritoneal cavity with resultant severe peritonitis. Acute cholecystitis is most often associated with right upper quadrant pain subsequent to a fatty ingestion. Always keep in mind the remote possibility of a nongynecologic intra-abdominal hemorrhage—either spontaneous or secondary to trauma. Trauma to the left upper quadrant can lead to intraperitoneal splenic hemorrhage that is delayed significantly from the event secondary to capsular containment. Sickle cell crisis can present with severe abdominal pain, as interstitial cystitis does occasionally.

THE DECISION TO OPERATE: SCHEDULED GYNECOLOGIC SURGERY

Emergent operations represent a small fraction of all the gynecologic surgical procedures performed. Most operations are planned in an elective fashion with varying degrees of urgency. The patient with a gynecologic malignancy does not have to be rushed to the operating room in the middle of the night, but will need to plan her procedure within a reasonable period of time. On the other hand, the patient who is having a uterovaginal prolapse repaired has much more leeway to fit her operation into her life rather than having to fit her life around her operation.

Scheduled surgery allows a patient time to get mentally prepared for the procedure. Patients should be encouraged to assemble support and assistance to help with their recovery, to help cover their responsibilities at work, and to help with child care during the postoperative period. The date for an elective gynecologic procedure should always be selected by the patient for the time that is most convenient in her life.

Patients should be encouraged to optimize their physical and emotional conditions prior to scheduled surgery. There is time to attempt to stop smoking, to donate autologous blood for surgery, to lose weight, to take preoperative estrogen or iron, and to take care of any concurrent medical problems before their surgery. In addition, the option exists to postpone a patient's surgery if a respiratory infection or other medical problem develops as the date for surgery approaches.

The indications, work-ups, and operations for benign and malignant gynecologic conditions are well documented elsewhere in this text. Hysterectomy, laparoscopy, hysteroscopy, and dilatation and curettage (Chapter 45); surgery for pelvic floor relaxation (Chapter 41); infertility surgery (Chapter 58); and surgery for urinary incontinence (Chapter 42) make up a large portion of procedures done for benign disease or dysfunction. Surgeries for gynecologic malignancies are well covered in Chapters 45 through 49.

■ PREOPERATIVE CARE

GENERAL CONSIDERATIONS IN PREOPERATIVE EVALUATION

Preoperative evaluation should include a general medical and surgical history, a complete physical examination, and laboratory tests. An anesthesiologist routinely sees patients preoperatively; however, a patient's medical status may warrant earlier consultation with an anesthesiologist and possibly with physicians in other specialties as well. The medical evaluation must be carried out in such a way as to identify all disorders that might complicate the operative procedure or convalescence. Although "diagnostic overkill" should be avoided, the responsibility of the operating gynecologist is to adequately assess—and take steps to minimize—a given patient's operative risk.

Records of prior hospitalizations should be obtained. Past records may be essential to the interpretation of present findings and may significantly influence the management plan. Patients' ability to recall illnesses and the details of previous surgeries is notoriously inaccurate.

Laboratory Studies

Although the efficacy of various preoperative testing regimens has not been established in a prospective, randomized fashion, most gynecologists would agree that preoperative laboratory studies should include at a minimum a CBC, a blood typing and antibody screen, and a urinalysis and culture. Further laboratory tests should be performed only when indicated by the patient's medical condition or by the type of surgery to be performed. A Papanicolaou smear should also be obtained.

A routine chest x-ray and electrocardiogram for all preoperative patients should be discouraged. One set of researchers found an overall positive yield for routine chest x-ray of 6%: 17% in patients than 60 years of age, and 2% in patients under 60. Routine electrocardiograms showed an overall positive yield of 7%: 7.4% in those over 40 and 4.5% in those under 40. Finally, they found that investigations prompted by history or physical findings yielded a high positive rate (34% for chest x-ray and 31% for electrocardiograms) and included most of the younger patients who would be missed by an age-only criterion for preoperative testing. It seems reasonable to obtain a preoperative chest x-ray and electrocardiogram on all patients over 45 years old, as well as all patients whose medical history or physical findings are matters of concern, regardless of their age.

Blood should be drawn for typing and cross-matching if a need for transfusion is anticipated, especially in patients with abnormal antibodies that would make intraoperative cross-matching time-consuming (see Chapter 30). If the patient's preoperative hematocrit and physical status permit, and if there is an appropriate interval before the anticipated surgery, the possibility of autologous blood donation should be discussed. Directed donor programs can be discussed as well.

Patients scheduled for surgery for menorrhagia with low hematocrit can often be allowed the time to build up their own blood supply through the use of a gonadotropin-releasing hormone (GnRH) agonist and iron supplementation. This can significantly lower the patient's risk for requiring transfusion by starting with a larger red blood cell mass. A GnRH agonist–induced reduction in the size of fibroids, if present, may also help reduce intraoperative blood loss.

More extensive testing tailored to the individual patient's needs can improve the safety of surgical procedures. Fasting and 2-hour postprandial plasma glucose determinations are helpful to exclude diabetes. Platelet count, bleeding time, prothrombin time, and partial thromboplastin time evaluate the adequacy of the clotting system. Liver, renal, and endocrine function testing should be obtained as indicated. A patient with poor pulmonary function might benefit from a baseline arterial blood gas determination. If prolonged parenteral dependency is anticipated, a preoperative laboratory assessment of the patient's nutritional status would be useful. Liver function tests and tumor markers are often obtained in the gynecologic cancer patient (see Chapters 45–49). Finally, testing for HIV antibodies and hepatitis B surface antigen and a serologic test for syphilis, although controversial, may also be appropriate.

Further imaging studies should be obtained only as indicated. Ultrasonography is useful for characterization of pelvic masses. CT also performs that function, as well as giving information regarding the course of the ureters and an assessment of retroperitoneal adenopathy. Intravenous pyelogram demonstrates renal function and architecture while providing information on the course of the ureters and ruling out a dual collecting system. Magnetic resonance imaging, with its superb soft tissue differentiation, can give much information regarding uterine, adnexal, and retroperitoneal architecture. Its clinical usefulness as a preoperative study has not been established. Double contrast barium enema can be useful in identifying bowel lesions or colonic involvement with pelvic masses.

Imaging studies as well as functional studies (eg, pulmonary function tests, stress electrocardiograms, multichannel urodynamics, or anal manometry) are informative but costly. They should be obtained on an individualized basis when the information they yield would decrease the patient's perioperative risk, influence the choice of the surgical procedure to be performed, or increase the chances for a successful surgical outcome for the patient. See the following section on Assessment and Minimization of Surgical Risk for further discussion of the extended preoperative evaluation.

Consultations

Patients should be seen well in advance of their surgical date by the anesthesiologist. This allows for the optimal selection of the type of anesthesia by considering the patient's physical status, prior anesthesia history, proposed surgery, and personal preferences. Consultation also gives the anesthesiologist an opportunity to allay the patient's anxieties.

Consultations with other physicians should be requested if the surgeon desires advice or assistance with a particularly high-risk surgical candidate or if the proposed procedure involves high risk. Medical preoperative consultation is of particular importance for the older surgery patient as well as the younger patient with known cardiovascular, pulmonary, renal, hematologic, or endocrinologic problems.

Preoperative urogynecologic consultation, individualized as noted in Chapter 42, can be considered in many cases requiring surgery for urinary incontinence. Consultation with a gynecologic oncologist should be considered preoperatively when the index of suspicion for malignancy is high.

Patient-Physician Communication

A. Informed Consent

It is imperative for every patient to have a complete understanding of exactly what her procedure will involve, why it is proposed, what alternatives are available, what the chances are for success, and what all the possible complications of the proposed procedure might mean to her in terms of further surgery, disability, or even death. It is important that this dialogue be carried out in layman's terms in the patient's native language and that the patient have ample opportunity to ask any questions that she may have.

To document that this important interaction took place to the satisfaction of the patient, she or her legal guardian should sign a consent form or note. All major points covered in the preoperative discussion should be written on the consent form or within the consent note before it is signed by the patient and the physician. If an interpreter was used, the interpreter should sign this document as well. Permission should be considered as being granted only for the procedures discussed in the preoperative conversation and designated in the consent form or note. This includes optional procedures such as appendectomy.

B. Patient Education

In view of the increasing complexity of operative procedures and the associated short- and long-term risks, audiovisual aids may be helpful in the patient counseling process. These aids can supplement, but should never replace, the actual communication between the gynecologic surgeon and the patient as outlined above.

A well-prepared video tape with simple diagrams can provide a consistent, in-depth presentation. Patient education pamphlets can serve a similar function. The patient should have an opportunity to ask questions about the video tape or pamphlet, and any modifications pertinent to her particular case should be explained. As documentation that this patient education was accomplished, it is appropriate to have the patient sign a form indicating that she has viewed the video tape, discussed it with the physician, and understands its content. If necessary, the video tape and signed form may serve as evidence that adequate preoperative counseling has been provided.

C. Documentation

All details of the history, physical examination, and diagnostic and therapeutic formulations and conclusions of all preoperative consultations must be entered in the patient's chart. This history and physical, or preoperative note, must include a problem-oriented assessment and a clearly delineated plan to address each problem. A note, or consent form as just described, documenting the scope of preoperative counseling must also be entered in the admission record. A carefully completed record is important for health care team communication and continuity of the patient's care as well as for hospital quality assurance.

ASSESSMENT AND MINIMIZATION OF SURGICAL RISK

1. Cardiovascular System

Cardiac Disease

The perioperative period is associated with significant cardiovascular stress. Any patient with heart disease should be considered a high-risk surgical candidate and must be fully evaluated preoperatively. Patients with symptoms of previously undiagnosed heart disease (eg, chest pain, dyspnea on exertion, pretibial edema or orthopnea), new electrocardiographic (ECG) changes, a recent history of congestive heart failure, recent myocardial infarction, or severe hypertension should be evaluated with the assistance of medical or cardiology consultation. Many factors may adversely affect cardiovascular function during and after surgery; for example, fluid shifts, hypotension, electrolyte imbalance, infection, severe pain, apprehension and tachycardia. Perioperative monitoring, anesthesia induction, maintenance techniques, and postoperative care can be tailored to the specific cardiovascular disease, thus improving the patient's chances for a good surgical outcome.

Special Studies

A. Electrocardiography

An ECG should be obtained on all patients over 45 years of age as well as on younger patients with a history of symptoms of cardiovascular disease. The ECG is of value in identifying the patient with coronary artery disease, ventricular hypertrophy, electrolyte disturbance, arrhythmia, and digitalis or other drug effect. Of prime interest are changes that might indicate coronary artery insufficiency such as ST- and T-wave changes; signs of infarct such as the appearance of Q waves or poor progression of R waves in the anterior chest leads; rhythm changes, particularly atrial fibrillation or flutter and atrioventricular or intraventricular block or ventricular ectopy; and others that might show the effect of systemic disease such as chronic hypertension, left ventricular hypertrophy, and electrolyte imbalance. The age when ECG changes are noted is important since patients with more recent infarcts have poorer postoperative outcomes than patients with older infarcts. Comparison with older ECGs is important when significant changes do exist. The preoperative ECG should serve as a baseline for subsequent studies if postoperative complications develop.

B. Echocardiography

If symptoms of cardiac disease are present, and particularly if an ECG demonstrates potential pathology, a consultation with a cardiologist should be obtained. Generally, an echocardiogram is performed, which will demonstrate any valvular or ventricular wall motion abnormalities resulting from coronary artery insufficiencies or cardiomyopathy. Left ventricular ejection fraction can also be estimated from an echocardiogram.

C. Dipyridamole/Thallium Stress Test

Patients with a significant cardiac history or an abnormal ECG should have a preoperative stress ECG under the direction of the patient's cardiologist. Dipyridamole or thallium stress tolerance scanning demonstrates older, fibrosed, fixed lesions or areas subject to ischemia and potential infarct. This test identifies ischemia under stress before the patient is subjected to the stress

of surgery. The result will guide the gynecologist and anesthesiologist in their invasive monitoring and surgical anesthesia maintenance decisions.

D. Intraoperative Central Monitoring

Invasive catheter measurements of intracardiac pressures can often provide useful information regarding cardiovascular dynamics. In most cases, the need for this intraoperative information can be evaluated simply by careful attention to aspects of the physical examination such as blood pressure, pulse, pulse pressure, heart rate, status of neck veins when supine, auscultation and percussion of the chest, presence or absence of edema, and size of the liver. If the preoperative evaluation raises a significant question, direct central venous pressure monitoring should be considered. A Swan-Ganz pulmonary artery catheter is particularly useful when surgery is likely to be prolonged, and the history, physical examination, and cardiology testing indicate depressed myocardial function or pulmonary artery hypertension. Specific references to the implementation of monitoring and management of these parameters are found in Chapter 59.

Varicose Veins and History of Deep Vein Thrombosis

Patients with large, extensive varicosities or a history of thrombophlebitis or thromboembolic events are at risk for developing lower-extremity thrombophlebitis or thromboembolic phenomena. This risk may be minimized by prevention of dehydration, early ambulation, and prompt and adequate treatment of cardiac disorders. Except in the patient in whom the risk of pregnancy is high, discontinuance of oral contraceptives 3–4 weeks preoperatively should be considered.

Before the operation, the patient should wear support stockings from toe to thigh. After surgery, these stockings should be worn continuously and discarded only after full ambulation is restored. Pressure on the calf or thigh should be avoided during a long operative procedure. Postoperative leg exercises should be initiated as soon as possible to prevent phlebitis. These may be begun even before ambulation by having the patient press against a footboard whenever supine. When discharged the patient should be advised to avoid prolonged sitting, eg, auto, train, or air travel, during the first month after surgery.

Prophylactic administration of heparin, 5000 U subcutaneously initiated just before surgery and every 8–12 hours thereafter until full ambulatory status is achieved, may be used to prevent thromboembolization in high-risk cases. No laboratory control is required. Similarly, the use of sequential compression boots intraoperatively and postoperatively until the patient is fully ambulatory helps to prevent thrombosis in high-risk patients. One researcher reviewed two meta-analyses of more than 70 published trials of deep venous thrombosis prophylaxis in general surgical patients. Both studies concluded that prophylaxis significantly reduced the rates of deep venous thrombosis and fatal pulmonary embolism and resulted in improved overall survival. Physical methods such as compression stockings and intermittent pneumatic compression were shown to be as effective as pharmacologic prophylaxis with heparin.

Valvular Heart Disease

Patients with a history of valvular heart disease or a heart murmur should have echocardiography done if they have not already been evaluated for this. Antibiotic prophylaxis should be administered according to the American Heart Association guidelines.

2. Pulmonary System

Elective surgery should be postponed if acute upper or lower respiratory tract infection is present. Even mild upper airway infection is associated with an irritable airway, which predisposes to laryngospasm or severe coughing on induction or emergence from anesthesia. Pulmonary infection causes poor ciliary motility, which predisposes to postoperative bronchitis and pneumonia. If emergency surgery is necessary in the presence of a respiratory tract infection, regional anesthesia should be used if possible and aggressive measures should be taken to avoid postoperative atelectasis or pneumonia. If the infection is severe, appropriate antibiotic therapy should be initiated promptly and modified as necessary when the results of cultures become available. The patient should be free from respiratory infection for 1–2 weeks before elective surgery.

Chronic obstructive pulmonary disease, which includes chronic bronchitis, emphysema, and asthma, puts the patient at increased risk in the perioperative period. Optimizing the patient's pulmonary status with chest physical therapy, breathing exercises, and appropriate antibiotics preoperatively decreases the potential for prolonged postoperative ventilation and suture line strain from coughing. Bronchiectasis, relatively uncommon at present, requires the patient to have rigorous chest physiotherapy and antibiotics before surgery. Preoperative pulmonary function tests should be performed to assess the severity and type of disease and to have as a baseline for reference in the postoperative period.

Asthmatic patients and those who smoke are at risk of developing pulmonary complications during or after surgery. Special care must be exercised in the management of such patients. Patients who smoke and for whom general anesthesia by endotracheal intubation is

planned should be encouraged to stop smoking for as long as possible before their surgery. Prolonged operations involving general anesthesia or hypoventilation increase the risk of postoperative hypoventilation and other pulmonary problems. Careful evaluation, including chest x-rays and pulmonary function tests, enable the surgeon and his or her consultant to decide when the operation may be safely undertaken and may influence the mode of anesthesia selected.

3. Renal System

Renal function should be appraised if there is a history of kidney disease, diabetes mellitus, or hypertension; if the patient is over 60 years of age; or if routine urinalysis reveals proteinuria, casts, or red cells.

It may be necessary to further evaluate renal function by measuring creatinine clearance, blood urea nitrogen, and plasma electrolyte determinations. An intravenous pyelogram or CT scan may sometimes be indicated for functional as well as anatomic reasons.

4. Hematologic System

Anemia

Anemia diagnosed in the preoperative obstetric or gynecologic patient usually is of the iron deficiency type caused by inadequate diet, chronic blood loss, or chronic disease. Care must be taken to differentiate iron deficiency anemia from other anemias, eg, sickle cell anemia. Iron deficiency anemia is the only type of anemia in which stained iron deposits cannot be identified in the bone marrow. Megaloblastic, hemolytic, and aplastic anemias usually are easily differentiated from iron deficiency anemia on the basis of the history and simple laboratory examinations. The diagnosis of obscure anemias may require the help of a hematologic consultation.

Patients with iron deficiency anemia respond to oral or parenteral iron therapy. Before elective surgery for menorrhagia, the patient's blood loss may be able to be stopped with a GnRH agonist long enough to allow reversal of the anemia. In emergencies or urgent cases, preoperative blood transfusions, preferably with packed red cells, may be given.

Von Willebrand's Disease

Von Willebrand's disease is a congenital bleeding disorder characterized by altered factor VIII activity and deficient platelet function. Inheritance is generally autosomal dominant, although a rare autosomal recessive form has been recognized. Clinical manifestations include epistaxis, easy bruisability, hypermenorrhea, and postpartum hemorrhage. Von Willebrand's disease is considered the most common congenital cause of hypermenorrhea. Vaginal bleeding between menses may also occur. Menstrual abnormalities are generally persistent and severe but may be intermittent or moderate, so that milder cases are less likely to be diagnosed. Hypermenorrhea may develop in affected persons at menarche and persist until the menopause or may not develop until after the second or third decade of life. Von Willebrand's disease is diagnosed in 10 persons per 100,000, but the true incidence is probably somewhat higher. It is possible that the true cause of menstrual abnormalities is undetected in some women with undiagnosed von Willebrand's disease who undergo hysterectomy for hypermenorrhea.

The diagnosis of von Willebrand's disease is confirmed by a prolonged bleeding time, decreased factor VIII activity, and abnormal platelet function. The platelet count is normal. All patients should avoid aspirin and nonsteroidal anti-inflammatory medications preoperatively, but this is especially true of the patient with von Willebrand's disease. Treatment with DDAVP 0.3 μg/kg intravenously immediately before surgery may help to improve platelet function. Patients should be given factor VIII and whole blood intraoperatively if needed.

Thrombocytopenia

The normal platelet count ranges from 150,000 to 350,000/μL. In the patient with thrombocytopenia but normal capillary function, platelet deficiency begins to manifest itself clinically as the count falls below 100,000/μL. Typical manifestations include petechiae on easily traumatized areas of the body, epistaxis, and menorrhagia. Epistaxis and hypermenorrhea may be severe enough to require transfusion. Bleeding into deep muscle and hemarthroses usually does not result spontaneously from thrombocytopenia, but intracranial hemorrhage is a serious risk if the platelet count is very low. The thrombocytopenic patient may require transfusion of platelets before surgery if the platelet count falls too low.

If thrombocytopenia is severe, the deficiency of platelet-produced factors involved in the coagulation cascade may result in some prolongation of clotting time. The most sensitive early clinical measure of platelet deficiency was thought to be the bleeding time. More recent literature suggests that bleeding time may not be a reliable indicator of platelet function and no study has established that bleeding time will predict the risk of hemorrhage in individual patients. Spontaneous hemostasis is not expected if the platelet count falls to 10,000/μL or less, and the patient may begin to bleed from all old puncture wounds as the platelet count approaches this threshold.

Bone marrow suppression, autoimmune disease, and platelet consumption are the chief causes of thrombocytopenia. Treatment revolves around treating the underlying cause and support with platelet transfusion and clotting factors as necessary. See also Chapter 22.

5. Endocrine System

Diabetes Mellitus

Diabetes is a common disease of disordered metabolism arising largely from altered pancreatic islet cell function. The incidence is higher with age, ranging from 0.1% in children to 2–3% in the general population. Diabetes in nonpregnant patients is defined by the American Diabetes Association as a fasting plasma glucose above 140 mg/dL on more than one occasion. Results of oral glucose tolerance testing are abnormal if fasting blood glucose is over 115 mg/dL, if the 2-hour value is over 140 mg/dL, and if the value in any sample exceeds 200 mg/dL.

Control of diabetes is made especially difficult by the stress of operation, acute infection, anesthesia, and electrolyte imbalance. The operative diabetic patient must be carefully observed and promptly treated before fluid and electrolyte abnormalities, ketosis, hyperglycemia, and infection develop. Diabetics whose disease is out of control are especially susceptible to postoperative sepsis. Preoperative consultation with an internist may be considered to ensure control of diabetes before, during, and after surgery.

Type II diabetes accounts for about 90% of cases and is seen in the older, usually more obese, patient population. Insulin production is close to or at normal values, but not appropriate for the blood sugar level. There is also peripheral insulin resistance. These patients develop neither ketoacidoses nor hyperosmolar states. The blood sugar is controlled by diet or oral medication. The oral medications most commonly used are the sulfonylurea derivatives, glyburide or glipizide. Their duration of action can be greater than 24 hours, and chlorpropamide may be effective for up to 50 hours. Therefore, it is important to avoid hypoglycemia by closely monitoring blood sugar on the day of surgery and possibly by not using the longer-acting agents for up to 2 days preoperatively.

Type I diabetics tend to be younger and nonobese and have little or no insulin production. They require insulin to avoid development of ketoacidoses, nonketotic hyperosmolar states, and hyperglycemia. Insulin-dependent diabetics with good control should be given half of their total morning insulin dose as regular insulin on the morning of surgery. This is preceded or immediately followed by the initiation of a 5% dextrose solution intravenously to prevent hypoglycemia in a fasting patient. Regular insulin should then be given every 6 hours in amounts dictated by plasma glucose or fingerstick determinations.

If the diabetes is severe, it may be necessary to admit the patient to the hospital before the operation for glycemic control. Regular insulin may be substituted for long-acting insulin to achieve tighter control. Serum electrolyte determinations should be recorded as points of reference for postoperative management. Fasting plasma glucose should be determined prior to surgery.

Some controversy exists regarding how tightly the blood sugar should be controlled perioperatively. It is generally accepted that keeping the blood sugar in the 100- to 250-mg/dL range in the perioperative period is adequate for most types of surgery. Cardiopulmonary bypass surgery, procedures in pregnancy or after a cerebral ischemic episode, and neurosurgical operations in which maintenance of cerebral autoregulation is important have better results if the blood sugar is more tightly controlled at about 80–130 mg/dL. Tight control is achieved by using an intravenous insulin infusion based on frequent blood sugar estimations.

Occasionally surgery is required emergently in a patient who presents in a hyperglycemic ketoacidotic state. It is important to first correct the fluid and electrolyte status, particularly the potassium levels, but it is not necessary to hold off surgery until complete resolution has occurred. The surgical condition may be the precipitating factor, and final correction may not be possible until surgery is completed. The hyperglycemic ketoacidotic state is treated by giving 10 U of regular insulin intravenously followed by an infusion of insulin based on the formula of the blood sugar level divided by 150 U/h. Normal saline solution is given to correct dehydration. Potassium must be supplemented because the insulin drives it into the cells. Total body potassium, despite its initial elevated serum level, may be very depleted. Because there are a fixed number of insulin receptors, there is nothing to gain by using higher doses of insulin. Blood glucose levels usually fall at a maximum rate of 100 mg/dL/h, except during the initial rehydration period when the fall is more precipitous.

Chronic medical conditions associated with diabetes may also complicate the perioperative period, eg, hypertension and coronary artery disease. Myocardial ischemia may often be silent in the diabetic with autonomic neuropathy. Autonomic neuropathy is also associated with gastric paresis and increased risk of aspiration. These patients should have an extended cardiac work-up and receive metoclopramide as well as a nonparticulate antacid before surgery. Intubation in some patients may be difficult because the atlanto-occipital joint may be involved with the diabetic process.

Thyroid Disease

Elective surgery should be postponed when thyroid function is suspected of being either excessive or inadequate. Hyperthyroidism is suspected clinically when the patient has a history of weight loss, muscle weakness, a persistently rapid pulse, agitation, tremor, heat intolerance, nervousness, or warm skin. The gland either may be diffusely enlarged, as in Graves' disease, or may have only an unobtrusive adenoma. Exophthalmos may be evident. Cardiac signs may be the only clue in the elderly patient (apathetic hyperthyroidism) and may include an unexplained atrial fibrillation or other tachyarrhythmia or dysrhythmia. A varying level of ventricular dysfunction is present in all patients with hyperthyroidism.

The patient should be rendered euthyroid before surgery if possible. This may take up to 2 months if antithyroid medications are used in combination with potassium iodide (Lugol's solution). The combination of a beta blocker, usually propranolol, and potassium iodide allows surgery in about 14 days. Propranolol blocks the peripheral effects of hyperthyroidism (ie, nervousness, sweating, tachycardia) and may slow the response to atrial fibrillation. It also impairs the conversion of T_4 to T_3 peripherally. Care must be exercised in the use of propranolol in patients with asthma or congestive heart failure. If surgery is immediately required, propranolol is titrated slowly intravenously in 0.5-mg aliquots until the peripheral signs of thyrotoxicosis have been brought under control. Regional or local anesthesia is preferable. If general anesthesia is required, the airway should be adequately assessed clinically and by x-ray or CT scan for severe tracheal compression or deviation that may interfere with placement of an intratracheal airway.

Severe stress such as that provided by surgery and anesthesia may precipitate a thyroid storm in a person with hyperthyroidism. Thyroid storm is a life-threatening event that manifests itself as hyperpyrexia, tachycardia, and cardiovascular instability, and it may be mistaken for malignant hyperthermia.

Hypothyroidism is relatively common in the elderly. It is usually of insidious onset; 95% of cases are due to primary failure of the thyroid to produce adequate T_4 and T_3. Goiter may be present, and a history of surgery or radioactive iodine treatment may be elicited. There is a slowing down of the metabolism affecting both mental and physical abilities, including a slowing of the heart rate and diminished ventricular contractility in response to catecholamines. Patients are very sensitive to respiratory depressant medications. There is blunting of the stress response, and corticosteroid supplementation may be needed.

In mild to moderate hypothyroidism, surgery and anesthesia need not be delayed before treatment is started. If the disease is severe, treatment should be started before surgery, if possible. In all cases, treatment must be started with a very low dose of thyroid replacement therapy to avoid sudden large demands on the myocardium, which may not yet be able to respond appropriately. The usual tests of thyroid function include total T_4 and T_3 levels, free T_4, T_3 resin uptake, and TSH levels. Preoperative consultation regarding the management of patients with thyroid dysfunction should be sought before major surgery.

Recent or Current Corticosteroid Use

Patients who are taking corticosteroids, or who have recently stopped them, are under the influence of the adrenal suppressive effects of their medication and are not able to respond to the stress of surgery appropriately. These patients must be provided with intravenous stress dose corticosteroids before, during, and after their surgery. While data do not exist to support one way of doing this over another, a representative regimen might be to provide hydrocortisone 100 mg three times a day on the day of surgery, 100 mg twice a day on postoperative day 1, and 100 mg on postoperative day 2.

6. Other Conditions Affecting Operative Risk

Pregnancy

The diagnosis of early pregnancy must be considered in the decision to do elective major surgery in the female. Elective surgery generally should be postponed until after delivery. Scheduled surgery that cannot be delayed, such as exploration for an adnexal mass, is best performed in the second trimester whenever possible.

Diagnostic or evaluative procedures necessary in the proper work-up for urgently needed surgery override theoretical fetal hazards in the pregnant patient. Appropriate protective measures should be taken to minimize these dangers, such as shielding the uterus from radiation during x-ray studies, using tocolytic agents to prevent premature labor, and considering possible fetal effects when pharmacologic and anesthetic agents are to be used. Hypotension and hypoxia must be meticulously avoided during anesthetic administration or surgical manipulation. Surgery should be performed in the left lateral decubitus position to optimize uterine perfusion. If the surgery is being performed after fetal viability, intraoperative fetal heart rate monitoring should be performed.

The new and more sensitive radioreceptor assay and radioimmunoassay for pregnancy are positive within 10 days of conception, ie, before the anticipated menstrual period. This capability may be important in scheduling elective surgery, especially in gynecologic procedures such as tubal ligation and hysterectomy.

Age

The 65-year-old and older segment of the population is currently undergoing the most rapid expansion of any demographic group in the U.S. This expansion is projected to continue and accelerate well into the new century. The majority of individuals in this age group are women. It has been estimated that over 50% of this older population will at some point undergo some surgical intervention. It is clear that the gynecologic surgeon will be caring increasingly for older patients requiring or desiring surgical procedures.

Care of the older patient can present a significant challenge. These persons often have multiple medical problems against a background of a general decline of their physiologic reserve. However, if care is taken with preoperative evaluation and perioperative management, these patients can do quite well. Age itself is not an independent predictor of surgical risk. The healthy elderly patient, or the carefully evaluated and managed elderly patient with medical problems, should not be discouraged from a beneficial elective procedure.

A careful history and review of systems must be taken and may require the assistance of family members or caretakers. A review of past medical records is crucial. A thorough physical examination must be performed. Appropriate preoperative consultation and extended preoperative evaluation as previously described should be obtained. The results should be reviewed with, and the patient seen by, the anesthesiologist well before the operative date so that an intraoperative management plan can be developed. Finally, meticulous and expeditious technique must be used during surgery to limit the patient's blood loss, operative time, and fluid shifts.

The principles and general considerations of good surgical practice become critically important when the elderly patient is being operated on. Serum electrolytes must be determined preoperatively and any imbalances corrected by appropriate parenteral solutions. Care should be taken not to overload the elderly patient's circulation when administering intravenous fluids, since cardiac, pulmonary, and renal reserves are often diminished. Nutritional deficiencies should be corrected before elective surgery is undertaken if possible. In older patients who are found to be significantly nutritionally deprived, total parenteral nutrition (TPN) may be required before and after surgery.

Fluid intake and urinary output should be monitored carefully and the patient's weight recorded daily. Early ambulation of the patient is very important. The older patient, or one who has been bedridden, requires frequent change of position to prevent the development of decubitus ulcers. Early ambulation, or aggressive active and passive physical therapy, may prevent many vascular and pulmonary complications.

The elderly patient often requires smaller dosages of medications such as narcotics and anesthetic agents. Barbiturates should especially be prescribed with caution, since mental confusion often results even from small doses.

Obesity

Obesity puts the patient and every member of the hospital team at a disadvantage in trying to avoid the increased perioperative morbidity associated with it. Every system in the body is affected by this disease.

The anesthesiologist is challenged by difficult intravenous access. These patients have markedly decreased functional residual capacity, making hypoxia a major concern, particularly in a supine or Trendelenburg position. Increased volume and acidity of gastric secretions, along with poor gastroesophageal sphincter tone, increases the risk of pulmonary aspiration. Poor neck extension makes intubation more difficult. The increased work of breathing and tendency for hypoxia occasionally necessitates later extubation and ambulation. In addition, obese patients have an increased potential for hypertension, coronary artery disease, and possibly diabetes.

The surgeon must struggle for exposure. Because of this, there is an increased risk of trauma to adjacent organs. Wound healing is inhibited, and there is an increased risk of postoperative wound seroma and infection. The gynecologic surgeon must plan ahead to make sure extra assistants are available as well as long instruments. The incision should be planned with the patient's body habitus in mind to provide maximal exposure. A mass closure technique with a delayed absorbable or permanent suture should be considered.

Postoperatively, nursing personnel are also at a serious disadvantage. Attempts to achieve ambulation and to prevent respiratory and thromboembolic complications are much more difficult because of the patient's size. These complications are far more likely to occur in patients with obesity than in patients of normal weight. Again, planning beforehand and extra personnel may be the key to a successful postoperative course.

Drug Allergies & Sensitivities

The obstetric or gynecologic patient who is being evaluated and prepared for a major operation may receive a variety of medications. Drug allergies, sensitivities, incompatibilities, and other adverse effects must be anticipated and prevented if possible. A history of serious reaction or sickness after injection, oral administration, or other use of any of the following substances should be noted and the medication avoided: (1) antibiotic medications, (2) narcotics, (3) anesthetics, (4) analgesics, (5) sedatives, (6) antitoxins or antisera, and (7) antiseptics. Untoward reactions to other medications, foods (eg, milk, chocolate), adhesive tape, and antiseptic solutions, especially iodine, should also be noted.

Immunologic Compromise

A patient may be considered an immunologically compromised or altered host if her capacity to respond normally to infection or trauma has been significantly impaired by disease or therapy. Obviously, preoperative recognition and special evaluation of these patients are important.

A. INCREASED SUSCEPTIBILITY TO INFECTION

Certain drugs may reduce a patient's resistance to infection by interfering with host defense mechanisms. Corticosteroids, immunosuppressive agents, cytotoxic drugs, and prolonged antibiotic therapy are associated with an increased incidence of superinfection by fungi or other resistant organisms. It is possible that the synergistic combination of radiation, corticosteroids, and serious underlying disease may set the stage for clinical fungal infection.

A high rate of wound, pulmonary, and other infections is seen in renal failure, presumably as a result of decreased host resistance. Granulocytopenia and diseases associated with immunologic deficiency (eg, lymphomas, leukemias, and hypogammaglobulinemia) are frequently complicated by sepsis. The uncontrolled diabetic is also observed clinically to be more susceptible to infection. The acquired immunodeficiency syndrome (AIDS) is associated with increased susceptibility to infection. For a full discussion of HIV infection and AIDS, see Chapter 38.

B. DELAYED WOUND HEALING

This problem can be anticipated in certain categories of patients whose tissue repair process may be compromised. Many systemic factors have been alleged to influence wound healing; however, only a few are of clinical significance: protein depletion, ascorbic acid deficiency, marked dehydration or edema, and severe anemia. It has been shown experimentally that hypovolemia, vasoconstriction, increased blood viscosity, and increased intravascular aggregation and erythrostasis due to remote trauma interfere with wound healing, probably by reducing oxygen tension and diffusion within the wound.

Large doses of corticosteroids depress wound healing. This effect apparently is increased by starvation and protein depletion. Wounds of patients who have received large doses of corticosteroids preoperatively should be closed with special care to prevent disruption that might delay healing.

Patients who have received anticancer chemotherapeutic agents are just as apt to require surgery as any other population group. Cytotoxic drugs may interfere with cell proliferation and may decrease the tensile strength of the surgical wound. It is wise to assume that healing may be delayed in patients receiving antitumor drugs.

Poor control of blood sugar in diabetic patients is associated with slow healing, poor scar formation, and an increased rate of wound infection. Slow healing sometimes is observed in debilitated patients, ie, those with advanced cancer, renal failure, gastrointestinal fistulas, or chronic infection. Protein and other nutritional deficiencies may be major causes of poor wound repair. Decreased vascularity and other local changes occur after a few weeks or months in tissues that have been heavily irradiated. These are potential deterrents to wound healing as well (see Chapter 51).

PREOPERATIVE ORDERS

Most patients are admitted to the hospital on the day of their surgery, or they have their surgery as outpatients. Much of the preoperative preparation of the patient that was formerly done in the hospital is now done at home by the patient and her family, since only a small percentage of gynecologic surgical patients are admitted before their surgical date. The following discussion reviews several areas of surgical concern that were formerly addressed in a patient's inpatient, night-before-surgery, preoperative orders.

A. Skin Preparation

Many gynecologic surgeons choose to have patients wash the skin over the operative site with povidone-iodine or hexachlorophene the night before the procedure is to be performed, and follow with a povidone-iodine preparation just before surgery. It has been shown that wound infection incidence is decreased by shaving the operative site in surgery rather than the night before the procedure. The wound infection rate is lower still with the use of clippers in the operating room or with no hair removal at all.

B. Diet

The patient should receive nothing by mouth for at least 8 hours before the operation so the stomach will be empty at the time of anesthesia.

C. Preparation of the Gastrointestinal Tract

Many gynecologic surgeons recommend that a patient use a cleansing enema the night before surgery to make certain that the examination under anesthesia will be accurate and to reduce the need for straining with a bowel movement during the early postoperative period. Mechanical (eg, enemas until clear or an oral osmotic and concentrated electrolyte agent such as GoLytely) and antibiotic bowel preparation (eg, a combination of oral neomycin and erythromycin) are necessary when the nature of the disease makes the possibility of bowel injury, resection, or purposeful entry likely. Some patients can comfortably complete a GoLytely, or a GoLytely and antibiotic, bowel preparation at home the night before surgery, while others may require admission the day before to accomplish this.

D. Sedation

A sedative-hypnotic may be prescribed to ensure restful sleep the night before the operation.

E. Preanesthetic Medication

Preanesthesia medication is not administered until after an intravenous line has been started on the day of surgery. It generally consists of a sedative such as midazolam, titrated to effect. See also Chapter 26.

F. Other Medications

The patient is generally advised to take all of her regular medications on the morning of surgery with sips of water sufficient to swallow them unless there are specific contraindications. Special preoperative orders sometimes must be given for modification of regularly required medications in diabetic patients and patients on anticoagulants or corticosteroids.

G. Antibiotics

Preoperative or prophylactic antibiotics are of value, especially in cases of expected bowel surgery, abdominal hysterectomy, all major vaginal surgery, and certain cesarean section deliveries. The first-generation cephalosporins have been particularly effective in decreasing postoperative febrile morbidity. Recent experience indicates that single-dose prophylaxis may be as effective as multiple doses.

H. Blood Transfusions

In circumstances in which transfusions are not usually required, a type and screen is satisfactory and cost-effective. If major blood loss is anticipated, a full crossmatch should be performed. Keep in mind that more blood can be prepared as you are transfusing the units you have already ordered.

Because of concerns about the risk of transmitting AIDS via transfusion, elective gynecologic surgery patients should be offered the option of autologous blood donation preoperatively. In addition, acute intraoperative autotransfusion should be considered if excessive intraperitoneal blood loss occurs either preoperatively, as in the case of ruptured ectopic pregnancy, or intraoperatively, as in the case of certain radical surgical procedures. Use of a cell-saver device, which processes blood aspirated from the surgical field and allows return of the patient's own red blood cells after washing in normal saline, is useful in these large blood loss situations and significantly cuts down on blood bank demand. The device is contraindicated in certain patients, such as those with infection near the operative site or those undergoing cesarean section or cesarean hysterectomy, because thromboplastins from decidual or amniotic fluid may become mixed with the blood.

I. BLADDER PREPARATIONS

For minor procedures, the patient voids prior to being moved to the operating room. If major pelvic surgery is planned, an indwelling Foley catheter should be placed when the vaginal preparation is done in the operating room. For prolonged bladder drainage, a suprapubic catheter provides a lower urinary tract infection rate along with the ability to allow voiding trials without multiple urethral catheterizations. Intermittent, clean self-catheterization is another bladder drainage modality that can be taught preoperatively and offers a low postoperative infection rate.

J. DOUCHES

An antiseptic douche, eg, povidone-iodine, is sometimes prescribed prior to gynecologic operations in an attempt to decrease the population of vaginal flora. Its value is not proved, and recent experience suggests that saline douches are as effective.

■ POSTOPERATIVE CARE

IMMEDIATE POSTOPERATIVE CARE

During the immediate postoperative period, maintenance of normal pulmonary and circulatory function should be emphasized. Vital signs and fluid balance should be monitored frequently to facilitate the early diagnosis of shock or pulmonary problems. Bleeding from the surgical site and persisting pulmonary or cardiovascular effects from anesthesia are risks that mandate careful surveillance of all patients in the immediate postoperative period.

Postoperative Orders

The postsurgical patient is taken to the recovery room, accompanied by the anesthesiologist and the surgeon or other qualified attendant, as soon as she responds. Patients with medical problems may require postoperative admission to an intensive care unit for prolonged ventilation or central monitoring. The nurse receiving the patient should be given a verbal report of her condition in addition to an operative summary and postoperative orders. These should include the following elements.

A. VITAL SIGNS

Record the blood pressure, pulse, and respiratory rate every 15–30 minutes until the patient is stable and hourly thereafter for at least 4–6 hours. Any significant change must be reported immediately. These measurements, including the oral temperature, should then be recorded 4 times a day for the remainder of the postoperative course.

B. WOUND CARE

Watch for excessive bleeding (inspect abdominal dressing or perineal pads). Determine the hematocrit the day after major surgery and, if there is a question of continued bleeding, repeat as indicated. An abdominal wound should be inspected daily. Skin sutures or clips generally are removed 3–5 days postoperatively and replaced with Steri-Strips.

C. MEDICATIONS

Following major surgery, give narcotic analgesics as needed (eg, meperidine, 75–100 mg intramuscularly every 4 hours, or morphine, 10 mg intramuscularly every 4 hours) to control pain. Injectable nonsteroidal anti-inflammatory drugs are available for postoperative pain control as well. Antiemetics such as promethazine or hydroxyzine may be helpful to suppress nausea as well as to potentiate analgesics.

Patient-controlled analgesia (PCA) is widely available. With PCA, patients are able to give themselves intravenous pain medication as they need it within the parameters set by the physician. Many patients prefer PCA because it allows them to avoid the "peak and valley" effect of scheduled pain injections.

Many centers are now using intrathecal or epidural opiate injection for relief of postoperative pain. This technique is particularly appropriate for patients who have been given regional anesthesia. A minimal dosage of less than 5 mg of morphine may allow several hours of complete pain relief without compromise of motor activity (ambulation, coughing). Respiratory depression is a hazard, however, and close monitoring of the patient is necessary. Following minor surgery, give mild analgesics as needed. Other medications required by the patient that were taken prior to surgery (insulin, digitalis, cortisone, or others) should be resumed as required.

D. POSITION IN BED

The patient is usually placed on her side to reduce the risk of inhalation of vomitus or mucus. Other positions desired by the surgeon should be clearly stated, eg, flat with foot of bed elevated.

E. DRAINAGE TUBES

Connect the bladder catheter to the gravity drainage system. Written orders for other postoperative drainage and suction catheters should be specific and clear, setting forth the degree of negative pressure desired and the intervals for measurement of drainage volume.

F. INTAKE AND OUTPUT

Record intake and output of all fluids as well as daily weight.

G. FLUID REPLACEMENT

Administer fluids orally or intravenously as needed. When deciding how to replace a particular patient's fluid needs, always take into account factors such as intraoperative blood loss and urine output, operating time, intraoperative fluid replacement, and the amount of fluid received in the recovery area. Although each patient and operation are different, an average healthy young patient who has been appropriately replaced intraoperatively will do well with 2400 mL to 3 L of a balanced crystalloid and glucose solution such as 5% dextrose in half normal saline over the first 24 hours. The rate of intravenous hydration must always be individualized, since many patients require less volume and may become fluid-overloaded at a faster rate. In the patient with normal renal function, adequate fluid replacement should result in a urine output of at least 30 mL/h.

H. DIET

Following minor surgery, offer food as desired and tolerated, when the patient is fully awake. Disagreement exists on how fast to advance a patient's diet after major surgery. This again must be individualized to the patient and depends on many factors.

One possible regimen is to allow the patient only sips of tap water on the day of surgery. Do not give ice water, because it may decrease bowel motility significantly. Give clear liquids on the first postoperative day if good bowel sounds are noted and until intestinal gas is passed. Change the diet thereafter to full regular. The time needed to progress to a full diet depends on the extent of the procedure, the duration of anesthesia, and individual variation among patients. Two randomized, controlled trials support the safety and efficacy of early oral feeding on postoperative day 1 following intra-abdominal gynecologic surgery in selected patients.

I. RESPIRATORY CARE

Encourage deep breathing every hour for the first 12 hours and every 2–3 hours for the next 12 hours. Incentive spirometry and the assistance of a respiratory therapist may be of great value, particularly in elderly, obese, or otherwise compromised or immobilized patients.

J. AMBULATION

Encourage early ambulation and bathroom privileges. If possible, require ambulation on the day of the operation after major surgery.

RECOVERY FROM MAJOR SURGERY

Even with the trend toward shorter hospital stays, the patient generally remains hospitalized until recovery of all bodily functions. Normal pulmonary function usually returns after resolution of inhalation anesthesia but may be influenced to some extent by surgical pain during the early postoperative period. Two or three days may pass before return of normal bowel function after laparotomy. The patient with febrile complications generally will not be discharged until she has remained asymptomatic and afebrile for 24 hours.

OUTPATIENT SURGERY

With the increasing number of outpatient procedures, the observation period following minor surgery becomes more critical. Following outpatient surgery, patients generally remain hospitalized until mental status and pulmonary and bladder functions return to normal. Occasionally, admission to the hospital becomes necessary for overnight observation or for further therapy. Although "ambulatory surgery" is designed for the healthy patient who is scheduled for less-extensive surgery, to become casual in preparation is to court disaster.

Because these patients play a more active role in the preparation and management of their surgery, the following additional elements must be considered: (1) Preoperative counseling should encompass the same information given the inpatient, but another responsible adult who will provide transportation and postoperative care for the patient should also be present at the session. (2) Emphasis should be placed on the importance of the "nothing by mouth" requirement and on the avoidance of any medications that the surgeon has not prescribed or approved. (3) A hospital must be available for backup if the facility is not hospital-based, and the patient must know where to report if problems arise;

this entails establishing 24-hour telephone service for access to medical advice and care. (4) A follow-up call from the physician within 24 hours is often beneficial for picking up early postoperative problems as well as for emotional support for the patient. (5) All postoperative instructions should be reviewed with the patient before her surgery.

POSTOPERATIVE COUNSELING & RELEASE FROM THE HOSPITAL

Following operation, the patient should receive a careful explanation (both oral and written) of the surgical procedure performed, the findings at surgery, and any postoperative procedures or findings. The postoperative course may be negatively influenced by the patient's anxiety regarding lack of information or unanswered questions. It may be helpful for the physician to refer to preoperative audiovisual aids during the postoperative counseling session.

Every postoperative patient should have a complete physical examination (including a pelvic assessment) before release from the hospital. Findings can be used as a baseline for subsequent follow-up examinations.

The patient should receive oral and written instructions regarding postoperative care at home, including which physical activities she may perform. Appointments should be made for outpatient or office follow-up examinations.

REFERENCES

Acute Abdomen

Ahmad TA et al: Experience of laparoscopic management in 100 patients with acute abdomen. Hepatogastroenterology 2001;48:733.

Mindelzun RE, Jeffrey RB: The acute abdomen: current CT imaging techniques. Semin Ultrasound CT MR 1999;20:63.

Tarraza HM, Moore RD: Gynecologic causes of the acute abdomen and the acute abdomen in pregnancy. Surg Clin North Am 1997;77:1371.

Appendicitis

Salky BA, Edye MB: The role of laparoscopy in the diagnosis and treatment of abdominal pain syndromes. Surg Endosc 1998;12:911.

Urbach DR, Cohen MM: Is perforation of the appendix a risk factor for tubal infertility and ectopic pregnancy? An appraisal of the evidence. Can J Surg 1999;42:101.

Viktrup L, Hee P: The diagnosis of appendicitis during pregnancy and maternal and fetal outcome after appendectomy. Int J Gynaecol Obstet 1999;65:129.

Diverticulitis and Inflammatory Bowel Disease

Farrell RJ, Farrell JJ, Morrin MM: Diverticular disease in the elderly. Gastroenterol Clin North Am 2001;30:475.

Iki K et al: Preoperative diagnosis of acute appendiceal diverticulitis by ultrasonography. Surgery 2001;130:87.

Lindner AE: Inflammatory bowel disease in the elderly. Clin Geriatr Med 1999;15:487.

Schoetz DJ Jr: Diverticular disease of the colon: a century-old problem. Dis Colon Rectum 1999;42:703.

Perioperative Evaluation and Care

Chen PC et al: Sonographic detection of echogenic fluid and correlation with culdocentesis in the evaluation of ectopic pregnancy. Am J Roentgenol 1998;170:1299.

Crapo RO: Pulmonary function testing. N Engl J Med 1994;331:25.

Graham GW, Unger BP, Coursin DB: Perioperative management of selected endocrine disorders. Int Anesthesiol Clin 2000;38:31.

Jacober SJ, Sowers JR: An update on perioperative management of diabetes. Arch Intern Med 1999;159:2405.

Muravchick S: Preoperative assessment of the elderly patient. Anesthesiol Clin North Am 2000;18:71.

Smetana GW: Preoperative pulmonary evaluation. N Engl J Med 1999;340:937.

Antibiotic Prophylaxis

American College of Obstetricians and Gynecologists: Antibiotics and gynecologic infections. ACOG Educational Bulletin No. 237. ACOG, June 1997.

Faro S: Can postoperative infection be prevented? Infect Dis Obstet Gynecol 1999;7:215.

Kamat AA, Brancazio L, Gibson M: Wound infection in gynecologic surgery. Infect Dis Obstet Gynecol 2000;8:230.

Smaill F, Hofmeyr GJ: Antibiotic prophylaxis for cesarean section. Cochrane Database Syst Rev 2000:CD000933.

Thromboprophylaxis

Green D: Current trends in the use of heparins in thromboprophylaxis. Semin Thromb Haemost 1999;25(Suppl 1):29.

Hull RD, Pineo GF: Prophylaxis of deep venous thrombosis and pulmonary embolism. Current recommendations. Med Clin North Am 1998;82:477.

Postoperative Care

Schilder JM et al: A prospective controlled trial of early postoperative oral intake following major abdominal gynecologic surgery. Gynecol Oncol 1997;67:235.

Intraoperative and Postoperative Complications of Gynecologic Surgery

44

Michael P. Aronson, MD, FACOG, FACS, David Chelmow, MD, & Sondra B. Lee, MD

■ INTRAOPERATIVE COMPLICATIONS

There are two commonly cited truisms concerning intraoperative complications of gynecologic surgery. The first is that if one performs enough gynecologic surgery, one will have complications. The second is that it is a venial sin to cause an intraoperative complication, but a mortal sin not to recognize that one has done so. In this chapter, we will review the keys to avoiding surgical misadventure and to recognizing it when it has occurred: understanding pelvic anatomy, using meticulous and methodical surgical technique, handling tissues gently, and maintaining a constant high index of suspicion. A detailed description of the management of each possible complication of gynecologic surgery is beyond the scope of this text. For this, the reader is referred to the many excellent references at the end of this chapter.

URINARY TRACT INJURY

Ureteral Damage

Ureteral injury has occurred in association with most major gynecologic surgical procedures, particularly pelvic cancer surgery, hysterectomy for benign indications, oophorectomy, and suspension of the bladder neck. The reported incidence of ureteral injury during gynecologic procedures ranges from about 0.5% in simple hysterectomies for benign disease up to 1.6% for laparoscopic cases, and to as high as 30% for some older series of Wertheim radical hysterectomies. Isolated statistics such as these, however, have little clinical significance; it is the knowledge, skill, and diligence of the surgeon as well as the difficulty of the surgical procedure that determine the incidence of ureteral injury.

The ureter may be accidentally ligated, kinked, transected, crushed, burned, or devascularized. In gynecologic surgery, injury to the ureter is most likely to occur

at the level of the infundibulopelvic ligament, the uterine artery, the uterosacral ligament, or the anterolateral fornix of the vagina as the ureter crosses it to enter the trigone of the bladder. Early recognition of ureteral injury can be crucial for preservation of function of the associated kidney. Repair is most likely to be successful if performed at the time of injury.

The best defense against injury to the ureter is knowledge of its anatomic relations and use of the avascular spaces of the pelvis to identify it intraoperatively (see Chapter 1). This can only be accomplished with good exposure through an adequate incision. On occasion, despite this careful attention, the question of ureteral integrity may arise.

A cystoscope or other endoscope can easily be used to prove bilateral ureteral patency at the end of a difficult operation. While the patient is being given 5 mL of indigo carmine intravenously, the bladder should be filled with 300 mL of normal saline. If vaginal surgery is being done, a 70-degree endoscope without its sheath can be gently introduced transurethrally. The ureteral orifices are visualized and a blue effluent can easily be seen emanating from the orifices if the ureters are patent. The rest of the bladder should also be examined for gross abnormality or evidence of operative trauma.

If an abdominal procedure is being performed and the entire course of the ureter cannot be visualized, patency can be demonstrated by introducing an endoscope through a purposeful cystotomy. The extraperitoneal dome of the bladder is dissected away from the symphysis pubis. Then a pursestring suture is placed and a small cystotomy made within it. A 0-degree or 30-degree endoscope is placed in the bladder and the pursestring suture cinched tightly. Again, the ureteral orifices can be identified along with the blue effluent of indigo carmine if there is ureteral patency. After the endoscope is removed, the pursestring suture is tied and imbricated. Postoperative catheter management is unchanged. If ureteral patency cannot be demonstrated by this technique, further steps can be initiated while the patient is still under anesthesia and the injury is fresh.

In the immediate postoperative period, a high index of suspicion should be maintained regarding the patient who develops flank pain. It should be noted that a patient with an obstructed ureter may not experience any flank pain at all. Urinary tract injury can be detected postoperatively by intravenous pyelogram (IVP) or retrograde x-ray studies. Renal ultrasonography may reveal hydronephrosis or hydroureter. A continuous postoperative watery vaginal discharge is suggestive of vesicovaginal or ureterovaginal fistula. A urinary fistula should also be suspected if laboratory analysis of the fluid draining from a surgical wound or drain demonstrates much higher levels of creatinine than found in the patient's blood sample.

As with all operative complications, the key to a good outcome is early recognition. Different types of ureteral injuries have different presenting symptoms and different management considerations.

A. Ureteral Ligation

Accidental ureteral ligation must be discovered within a few weeks if there is to be any hope of restoring renal function. Postoperative signs of ureteral ligation may include flank or pelvic pain, pyelonephritis and sepsis, abdominal swelling secondary to collection of urine (urinoma), and development of a ureterocutaneous fistula. In some patients, kidney failure occurs with no associated warning signs. One researcher reported on eight patients subjected to intentional ureteral ligation during colon cancer surgery. Two patients experienced asymptomatic loss of renal function on the ligated side, two developed pelvic urinomas, and three developed ureterocutaneous fistula; one patient died of pyelonephritis and septicemia.

B. Transection

Continuous leakage of urine into the operative site following ureteral transection increases the likelihood that the injury will be discovered during the operation. Hematuria may occur after transection but cannot be considered a reliable sign of ureteral damage. If unrepaired, ureteral transection can result in either a pelvic urinoma or ureterocutaneous fistula. A ureteroneocystotomy should be performed if the transection occurs within 5 centimeters of the bladder. Otherwise, the transected ureter above the pelvic brim may be repaired with an end-to-end anastomosis over a ureteral stent.

C. Crush Injury

There is a significant risk of segmental ureteral necrosis following a surgical clamp crush injury to the ureter. Resection of the crushed ureteral segment and reanastomosis, or performance of ureteroneocystostomy, depending on the site of injury, should be considered unless (1) the ureter was clamped for only a brief time as part of a larger pedicle, (2) there is no visible damage, and (3) peristalsis

persists at the site of injury. In such a case, a double-J ureteral stent should be placed and removed after 4–6 weeks with outpatient cystoscopy. An intravenous pyelogram should be obtained after removal to rule out extravasation and evaluate ureteral patency.

D. Devascularization

Extensive retroperitoneal dissection of the ureter may injure its adventitial vascular supply with subsequent necrosis of the devitalized segment. This risk is greatest in cancer surgery. In the 1950s, Dr. A. H. Palmrich of Vienna anatomically defined this complex of vessels and nerves that supply the ureter. Later series of radical hysterectomies that preserved this complex by avoiding skeletonization of the ureter resulted in a dramatic decline in ureteral complications.

Bladder Injury

Laceration of the bladder can be confirmed by filling the bladder with sterile milk or methylene blue through a urethral catheter and observing leakage of fluid. Use of milk has the advantage of not staining the operative field. All edges of the cystotomy must be visualized and mobilized if necessary. The bladder defect usually is then repaired with two layers of absorbable suture after which the bladder is again filled with milk to test for leakage. Uncomplicated recovery is generally the rule. Five to 10 days of catheter drainage, depending on the site and extent of injury, helps to promote healing by preventing bladder distention.

Very small bladder injuries caused by Verres needle insertion or small trocar insertion during laparoscopy can sometimes be managed conservatively with dependent drainage with a transurethral catheter. Small extraperitoneal defects will respond to 10–14 days of drainage. Intraperitoneal injuries require closure in two layers as described above.

GASTROINTESTINAL TRACT INJURY

Bowel is highly susceptible to injury during laparotomy, laparoscopy, and vaginal surgery. The moment of entry into the peritoneal cavity is a crucial step and should be approached cautiously. Patients with adhesions due to previous surgery, endometriosis, or salpingitis are at high risk for intraoperative bowel injury when adherent bowel is dissected away from the operative site. The risk of bowel laceration is even greater during the acute phase of pelvic infection because of the increased friability of the secondarily inflamed bowel. These factors should be taken into account when deciding on the operative approach: transvaginal versus laparotomy versus open or closed laparoscopy.

Tight abdominal packing, exposure of the bowel serosa with subsequent dehydration, indiscriminant use of unipolar electrocautery, and superficial abrasions from manipulation may be associated with apparently minimal trauma yet ultimately result in postoperative bowel adhesions. Bowel exposure and manipulation must therefore be kept to a minimum during laparotomy.

Complications associated with accidental penetration of bowel arise from bacterial and chemical peritonitis from spillage of bowel contents into the peritoneal cavity. Postoperative fever, abdominal distention, paralytic ileus, and diffuse peritonitis can develop within 24 hours after unrecognized bowel injury. Fecal contamination from colonic injury can prevent successful primary repair. Copious irrigation of the abdomen, followed by placement of a closed drainage system at the repair site, decreases the risk of generalized postoperative peritonitis. If unprepared colon is entered, or if the injury is extensive, a temporary diverting colostomy proximal to the site of injury may be necessary to allow healing. Abdominal abscess formation, wound infection, enterocutaneous fistula, and extensive bowel adhesions may follow fecal contamination of the abdominal cavity. The risk of bacterial peritonitis is clearly greater if the colon is the site of injury.

Small bowel injury may produce chemical peritonitis from leakage of secretions from the stomach, gallbladder, and pancreas. Injury to the small bowel or stomach can be successfully repaired with two layers of interrupted suture. It may be necessary to convert a longitudinal small bowel laceration into a transverse repair to avoid constriction of the bowel lumen. Larger injuries and thermal injuries may require segmental resection using suture techniques or stapling devices.

Perhaps even more dangerous is unrecognized, covert injury such as thermal bowel injury from electrocoagulation. A patient with such an injury may appear well in the immediate postoperative period. The delayed onset of symptoms of perforation may be misinterpreted or even overlooked. Such unrecognized injuries can prove lethal. Whether operating transvaginally, by laparotomy, or laparoscopically, keep in mind the possibility of unrecognized overt or covert intraoperative bowel injury as the patient moves through the postoperative period.

NEUROLOGIC INJURY

Damage From Patient's Position During Surgery

Unnatural positioning of the patient while under anesthesia may cause significant sensory and motor defects in the extremities. Hyperextension or hyperabduction of an extremity may stretch the corresponding major nerve trunk as it exits the thorax or pelvis. The upper roots of the brachial plexus are especially vulnerable to injury, and transient shoulder pain may occur postoperatively if the shoulder has remained hyperextended during surgery. Femoral neuropathy may occasionally follow procedures carried out in the lithotomy position when the hip has been hyperflexed and hyperabducted.

Nerves in the extremities are also vulnerable to injury where they cross over a skeletal prominence. External pressure on these sites during surgery may produce prolonged sensory and motor defects. The most common nerve injury during gynecologic surgery results from compression of the common peroneal nerve at the head of the fibula when the lateral aspect of the leg below the knee rests against a hard leg brace when the patient is in the lithotomy position. The result is loss of sensation in the dorsum of the ankle that is associated with footdrop due to loss of motor function of the peroneus longus and brevis muscles. Proper positioning and the use of sequential compression boots may help avoid this complication.

Prolonged pressure transmitted through the gluteal muscles may injure the sciatic nerves. Compression of the ulnar nerve against the medial epicondyle of the humerus occurs if the elbow is extended with the wrist pronated and results in nerve injury if the patient's arm remains in this position for prolonged periods.

Damage During Surgery

The tips of the blades of an improperly placed self-retaining retractor may rest on the psoas muscles. Prolonged pressure may be transmitted to the femoral, ilioinguinal, iliohypogastric, or genitofemoral nerve with resulting painful neuropathy, sensory loss, and muscle weakness. The risk is especially great in the thin patient. Often the external part of the retractor can be bolstered with folded sterile towels to relieve this pressure.

The sciatic or obturator nerves may be at significant risk during radical pelvic cancer surgery, and the long thoracic nerve can be easily damaged during surgery for breast cancer. Careful dissection and a strong anatomic background are the best defenses against these injuries.

VASCULAR INJURY

Major Vessel Injury

Incidental injury of major pelvic blood vessels is a rare but potentially catastrophic complication of pelvic surgery. The arteries, with their thick, muscular walls are less often damaged than the thin-walled veins. The inferior vena cava and iliac veins are delicate and are easily injured during lymphadenectomy and other procedures for invasive disease, whereas injury during procedures for benign disease is much less common.

Bleeding from even small injuries to these major vessels can be extremely heavy. If injury occurs, direct pressure should be applied to the injured vessel or the blood supply should be temporarily cut off by applying pressure proximal to the site of injury. This allows the surgeon time to obtain adequate exposure for repair, to carefully assess the nature and extent of the injury, to summon consultation if necessary, and to have blood products delivered to the operating room while limiting the patient's blood loss. Keeping up with replacement of blood volume with packed red blood cells and blood products is essential.

If the injury occurs during laparoscopy with penetration of a vessel by a Verres needle or trocar, the instrument should not be removed while the laparoscopy is being converted to a laparotomy. This allows the instrument to act as a tampon while identifying the site of penetration. A midline incision should be made to provide adequate exposure, and it can be easily extended as necessary.

Small injuries can often be repaired with carefully placed, very fine sutures after adequate exposure is obtained and the patient is stabilized. Larger injuries may require emergent consultation with a vascular surgeon about the need for vessel grafts. In the pregnant patient, many vessels are engorged, making them behave like major vessels. The uterine vessels carry 500 mL of blood per minute at term. Laceration of these vessels during cesarean delivery or cesarean hysterectomy can cause massive bleeding.

Hemorrhage

Even if major vessels are not injured, unexpected and hard-to-control bleeding from other sources can occur during any gynecologic surgery. The gynecologic surgeon should be comfortable with the technique of hypogastric artery ligation, which will frequently control such bleeding (see Fig 28–1). This technique involves dissection of the hypogastric artery distal to the bifurcation of the common iliac artery. Two silk ties are then passed under the internal iliac artery and tied approximately 1 cm apart. The artery itself should not be cut. Great care must be taken not to damage the delicate internal iliac vein located immediately posterior and lateral to the hypogastric artery. This ligation acts by decreasing the pulse pressure at the distal bleeding site sufficiently to allow clot formation. Rich collateral circulation exists distal to the ligation, especially from the lumbar and middle sacral circulations. Enough perfusion to the pelvis remains so that not only will the

pelvic organs remain viable, but the potential for future pregnancy is preserved.

Angiographically guided arterial embolization is another technique that has gained acceptance for control of massive pelvic hemorrhage. This technique can be used either intraoperatively or postoperatively in an attempt to avoid a subsequent return to the operating room. Arterial catheters are placed under fluoroscopic guidance, the bleeding sites identified, and embolization done by a variety of techniques. If hypogastric ligation has already been performed, angiographic catheters may not be able to reach the bleeding site, and angiographic embolization may not be possible.

Massive hemorrhage, defined as bleeding requiring transfusion of more than 10 units of blood, may occur in extensive pelvic and abdominal surgery such as tumor debulking, lymph node dissections, and pelvic exenterations. Any time the deep pelvic venous plexuses are encountered, this possibility exists. When other measures are unsuccessful, packing of the pelvis at the site of hemorrhage with long packs or with gauze rolls inside a bowel bag has been described. The abdomen is closed after it is packed, and the patient is brought back to the operating room 48–72 hours later for removal of the packing. In a case series of six patients with massive hemorrhage and abdominal packing, one patient died postoperatively.

ANESTHETIC COMPLICATIONS

Malignant Hyperthermia

One surgical patient in 14,000 has a congenital defect of calcium metabolism that presents as life-threatening hyperthermia during general anesthesia. The administration of succinylcholine or the volatile anesthetic agents can prevent the reuptake of calcium by the sarcoplasmic reticulum in skeletal muscle cells. Massive calcium levels stimulate a dramatic increase in cell metabolism, causing the characteristic symptoms of elevated body temperature, generalized skeletal muscle rigidity, and metabolic acidosis. Fatal cardiac arrhythmias may occur as hyperkalemia develops in association with acidosis.

If malignant hyperthermia develops, all anesthetic agents should be immediately discontinued and dantrolene given promptly intravenously. Dantrolene exerts its effects by interfering with the release of calcium from the sarcoplasmic reticulum. The dose should be repeated until symptoms subside or until a maximum of 10 mg/kg has been given. Dantrolene should be continued postoperatively. Treatment should also be directed toward stabilization of the patient through correction of cardiac arrhythmias, metabolic acidosis, hyperkalemia, and hyperthermia.

Bronchospasm

Bronchospasm is caused by increased airway reactivity and is detected by wheezing and increased difficulty in ventilating the patient. Patients with known asthma and cardiopulmonary disease are at increased risk for bronchospasm with general anesthesia. However, bronchospasm can also occur in patients without a known history of pulmonary disease. In patients with known disease, consideration is often given to performing procedures under regional anesthesia wherever possible. When bronchospasm does occur intraoperatively, pharmacologic measures such as inhaled beta-mimetics and intravenous corticosteroids should be instituted immediately.

Hypothermia

Prolonged exposure of the lightly clothed, anesthetized patient with an open abdomen to the relatively cool operating room environment can result in a drop of several degrees in the core body temperature. Severe hypothermia is unusual, but there are important implications for even minor hypothermia. The return to normal body temperature, which often involves shivering, can cause a large increase in oxygen requirements, which in turn can cause cardiovascular stress, particularly for patients with underlying cardiac or pulmonary disease. Careful attention to patient temperature, including covering the patient and using warmed intravenous fluids and warmed, humidified ventilation can reduce these problems.

Regional Anesthesia

Regional anesthetic techniques are being used more frequently for primary anesthesia as well as for relief of postoperative pain. Both epidural and spinal anesthetics are being used with increasing frequency in gynecologic surgery. The most common worrisome problem is respiratory depression. This occurs when the anesthetic level reaches to C3–C5, the level of innervation of the diaphragm. Whenever regional anesthesia is planned, equipment for intubation and mechanical ventilation must be readily available in the event of respiratory depression. These patients must be closely observed both during the procedure and afterward, until the anesthetic agents have been completely metabolized and the anesthetic block resolved, because delayed respiratory depression can occur.

The most common and aggravating postoperative problem with regional anesthesia is spinal headache, caused by persistent leakage of cerebrospinal fluid through the hole made by the spinal or epidural needle. In most instances, headache can be avoided by the use of very small-caliber needles and adequate hydration before, during, and after the procedure. Use of an epidural blood patch often gives immediate relief.

Other Complications

Teeth can be broken or chipped during intubation. Careful technique with the laryngoscope is always required. Some patients, particularly obese patients or patients with short necks, can be very difficult to intubate, resulting in laryngeal damage, laryngospasm, or abandonment of the procedure because of inability to intubate the patient. Esophageal intubation can be catastrophic if unrecognized, but can be avoided by careful attention to laryngeal visualization, CO_2 monitoring of exhalation, and careful auscultation. Pneumothorax and aspiration pneumonia, two other common complications, will be discussed at length in the section on pulmonary complications. It is thought that death due to anesthetic complication occurs in approximately 1 in 1500–2000 surgical procedures.

COMPLICATIONS OF ENDOSCOPIC PROCEDURES

In recent years, laparoscopy and hysteroscopy have become among the most frequently performed gynecologic procedures. These procedures are perceived as less invasive, with faster recovery times, and are frequently performed in an outpatient setting. It is becoming clear, however, that despite being considered "minimally invasive," major complications occur with endoscopic surgery. Recognized complications include bowel, bladder, and ureteral injuries, hernias at the trocar sites, catastrophic major vessel injury at the time of trocar insertion, and CO_2 embolism. In addition to complications specific to endoscopy, any of the complications associated with traditional gynecologic surgery may still occur.

Great care is necessary to minimize complications from endoscopic procedures. When inserting the Veress needle, careful attention should be paid to keeping the tip in the midline. The needle should be directed downward at approximately 45 degrees to avoid the bifurcations of the aorta and inferior vena cava, usually located 1–3 cm below the umbilicus. The umbilicus provides the shortest distance between skin and peritoneum because anatomic layers fuse there. Verres needle insertion at this site helps avoid the complication of extraperitoneal insufflation.

Many of the most serious complications occur at the time of trocar insertion. In patients with a high risk of bowel adhesions to the anterior abdominal wall, some surgeons advocate using an open trocar placement technique, although no objective evidence exists to support this. All other trocars should be placed under direct visualization, with careful attention paid to avoiding the inferior epigastric vessels. When performing operative procedures under laparoscopic guidance, the same attention must be paid to identification of the ureters and other anatomy as in open procedures. Bowel, bladder, and ureter, as well as major vessels, can be injured just as easily and seriously during endoscopic procedures as during laparotomy.

Hysteroscopy has some unique complications in addition to the risks of uterine perforation, visceral damage, and hemorrhage. The uterine distention media may cause life-threatening electrolyte imbalances as well as introduce air emboli into the uterine venous sinuses. Air emboli arise from bubbles in the distention media, room air introduced into the uterine cavity when the hysteroscope is placed, and from bubbles generated from vaporization or coagulation procedures within the distention media. Air emboli may cause pulmonary hypertension and hypoxic vasoconstriction, and result in pulmonary edema and respiratory distress. During the procedure, a drop in both oxygen saturation and end-tidal CO_2 should be recognized as a hallmark of air embolization.

Hyponatremia, hypokalemia, hypo-osmolality, and fluid overload develop when electrolyte-free distention media such as glycine and sorbitol enter into the venous circulation. The patient can present with headache, nausea, vomiting, arrhythmias, and altered mental status secondary to hyponatremic encephalopathy. The most effective means to avoid these complications is to closely record hysteroscopic fluid inputs and outputs. When a deficit of 1000 to 2000 ml of fluid is noted, the procedure should be abandoned. Serum sodium will decrease by 10 mmol/L per 1000 cc of hypotonic solution retained. Complications from fluid overload occur at a rate of 1–4% of all hysteroscopies.

■ POSTOPERATIVE COMPLICATIONS

CARDIOVASCULAR COMPLICATIONS

1. Shock

Shock is an acute emergency that takes precedence over all other problems except acute hemorrhage, cardiac arrest, and respiratory failure. Immediate correction of the underlying disorder is essential.

Shock, or failure of the circulation, may follow excessive blood loss, escape of vascular fluid into the extravas-

cular compartment ("third spacing"), marked peripheral vasodilatation, cardiac decompensation, sepsis, adrenocortical failure, and pain or emotional distress. A combination of causes may be responsible for shock. Ideally, correct diagnosis of the circulatory problem should be undertaken before proper treatment can be instituted. However, because this complication can be life-threatening, it may be necessary to institute treatment with a presumptive rather than a definitive diagnosis.

Treatment should be organized to stop hemorrhage, restore fluid and electrolyte balance, correct cardiac dysfunction, establish adequate ventilation, maintain vital organ perfusion, and avert adrenocortical failure.

Because multiple pathologic mechanisms may be involved, no simple and reliable pattern is seen in a patient going into shock or in her response to treatment. Survival depends on early diagnosis, correct appraisal of physiologic abnormalities, monitoring of essential parameters, and a flexible plan of therapy based on vital signs and laboratory data.

The primary cause of shock must be determined promptly. The history and gross physical findings often permit the differentiation of hemorrhagic, cardiogenic, septic, and allergic types of shock (Table 44–1). Pelvic examination, ultrasound examination, culdocentesis, or paracentesis may be of inestimable value in immediately establishing the presence or absence of postoperative hemoperitoneum. Except in neurogenic shock due to fainting, a self-limiting condition that is treated by placing the patient in the recumbent position and administering stimulants, antishock measures using additional therapy as required for specific problems should be instituted (Table 44–2).

Blood loss (hypovolemia) is the most common cause of postoperative shock. The rapid loss of up to 20% of blood volume is classified as mild shock. A healthy patient normally compensates well for a loss of less than 10–20% of their blood volume and is typically asymptomatic, with minimal changes in heart rate, blood pressure, or urine output. A loss of 20–40% usually yields moderate shock, with maximal use of the body's compensatory mechanisms including tachycardia, dropping of urine output, and vasoconstriction yielding cold, clammy, pallid skin. The affected patient's sensorium is usually altered. With unreplaced loss of more than 40% of the blood volume, the body's compensatory mechanisms are overwhelmed, and severe shock occurs. Large blood loss, unless promptly corrected, leads to a drop in cardiac output, a decrease in tissue perfusion, and eventual anoxia and permanent end-organ damage.

The accurate determination of parenteral fluid requirements depends on continuous clinical observation of blood pressure, temperature, pulse and respiratory rate, mental acuity, skin (color, temperature, and mois-

Table 44–1. Some characteristics of different types of shock.

Type of Shock	History	Physical Findings	Laboratory Findings
Hemorrhagic	Trauma, pregnancy complication.	Acute abdomen, trauma, obvious site of bleeding.	Low hemoglobin/hematocrit, possible clotting deficiency.
Cardiogenic	Heart disease.	Pulmonary edema, hepatospleno-megaly, anasarca.	Abnormal blood gases, cardio-megaly, or pulmonary edema on chest x-ray.
Septic	Infection, illness, abortion.	Febrile, evidence of infection.	High white blood cell count, urine white blood cell casts if pyelonephritis.
Anaphylactic (allergy)	Bee sting, acute medication administration.	Negative except for shock.	Negative.

ture), venous collapse, fluid intake, and urinary output. Frequent monitoring of central venous pressure and urine output with a transurethral catheter and serial determination of serum electrolytes, blood pH, PO_2, PCO_2, and lactate are essential. Pulmonary artery pressures, left ventricular function, and cardiac output can be assessed with a Swan-Ganz catheter. A peripheral arterial line is helpful for blood gas monitoring and blood drawing. Hemoglobin and hematocrit determinations are not dependable guides to blood replacement in the shock patient because they will not reflect the loss of whole blood until fluid replacement has been given.

Blood should be drawn promptly for cross-matching, hematocrit, coagulation studies, complete blood

Table 44–2. General antishock measures.

1. Place the patient in a recumbent position with foot of bed slightly elevated. Disturb the patient as little as possible. (The extreme Trendelenburg position is no longer recommended because it may interfere with breathing.)
2. Establish an adequate airway and make certain that pulmonary ventilation is unobstructed. Administer oxygen by nasal catheter, mask, or endotracheal tube as required, especially if dyspnea or cyanosis is present.
3. Keep the patient comfortably warm with blankets. Do not apply external heat, since this will cause peripheral vasodilatation.
4. Control pain and relieve apprehension. Shock patients often have very little discomfort, probably as a result of the physiologic endorphin response to trauma. When required, give a minimum effective parenteral dose of a sedative or, if absolutely necessary, morphine sulfate, 10–15 mg intravenously. Narcotics are contraindicated for patients in coma and those with head injuries or respiratory depression unless mechanical ventilation is immediately available. Avoid overdose of sedative and narcotic drugs.

count, and blood chemistry determinations prior to starting an infusion. If superficial veins have collapsed and peripheral venous access is not possible, a central line should be placed in the subclavian, internal jugular, or femoral vein for intravenous access and central monitoring.

Adequate blood volume must be restored as rapidly as possible. Replacement should be carried out with packed red blood cells (PRBCs) and blood components as necessary for coagulation factors. In general, 1 unit (U) of fresh frozen plasma should be administered with each 5 U of PRBCs to replace clotting factors. Acid-base deficits and electrolyte disturbances may require individual correction. In particular, if large blood volumes are being replaced, calcium should be monitored and replaced as necessary because the citrate in the replacement blood units decreases serum calcium.

Intravenous crystalloid solutions (normal saline or Ringer's lactate) should be infused while awaiting blood components from the blood bank. If the patient has not responded promptly to these measures or if her condition again deteriorates, further intensive monitoring and management will be necessary. (See Chapter 59 for further discussion of management of shock.)

2. Cardiac Arrest

Cardiac arrest occurs most frequently during the induction of anesthesia, but can also occur during surgery or in the postoperative period. Predisposing conditions include preexisting heart disease, previous myocardial infarction, shock, hypoventilation, airway obstruction, or drug reaction.

Clinical Findings

The signs of impending cardiac arrest are rapid fall in blood pressure and irregularity of pulse. The diagnosis should be verified by confirming the absence of pulse and heart sounds by auscultation, and cardiopulmonary resuscitation must be initiated immediately.

Prevention

Patients with cardiac risk factors require a multidisciplinary approach with preoperative consultation with anesthesiologists, cardiologists, and the surgeon. Frequently, a Swan-Ganz catheter and peripheral arterial line is placed before induction of anesthesia to allow intensive monitoring. All patients require careful attention to prevent hypotension and ensure adequate ventilation.

Treatment

Immediate resuscitation should be initiated per the American Red Cross Advanced Cardiac Life Support (ACLS) algorithms. The gynecologist should be trained in Red Cross Basic Life Support and is usually required to initiate emergency treatment only (Fig 44–1). The subsequent care of the patient should be the responsibility of an expert in critical care medicine. All patients at risk for major complications should be encouraged to complete a health care proxy prior to surgery.

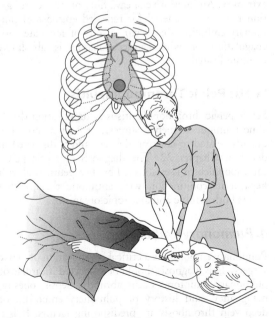

Figure 44–1. Technique of closed-chest cardiac massage. Heavy circle in heart drawing shows area of application of force. Circles on supine figure show points of application of electrodes for defibrillation. (Reproduced with permission, from Benson RC: *Handbook of Obstetrics & Gynecology*, 8th ed. Lange, 1983.)

3. Thrombophlebitis

Superficial Thrombophlebitis

Postoperative superficial thrombophlebitis is most common in the lower extremities of women with extensive varicosities or at intravenous access sites. The lithotomy position, with its localized pressure on the legs from supports, can also contribute. It usually occurs within the first few days after operation. The affected vein becomes inflamed, with erythema, localized heat, swelling, and tenderness. This disorder is generally limited to the superficial veins and pulmonary embolism is unusual. When superficial thrombophlebitis is diagnosed, treatment includes warm, moist packs, elevation of the extremity, and analgesics. Anticoagulants are rarely indicated when only the superficial vessels are involved. As soon as clinical improvement occurs, usually within 48 hours, the patient should be ambulated. Prolonged bedrest predisposes to thrombophlebitis of the deep veins.

Deep Vein Thrombosis

Thrombosis of the deep veins occurs most often in the calf but may also occur in the thigh or pelvis. It may be primary or an extension of more peripheral disease. Advanced age, obesity, cancer, pregnancy, oral contraceptive use, hyperlipidemia, diabetes, hemoconcentration following transfusion for severe anemia, and certain hypercoagulable states (protein C and S deficiencies, hyperhomocysteinemia) are predisposing factors, but the disease frequently occurs in otherwise healthy patients. Recently, the factor V Leiden mutation has been implicated as a potential important cause.

A. CLINICAL FINDINGS

Symptoms may be localized to the involved extremity, or the thrombus may be asymptomatic. Pulmonary embolism may be the first sign. The patient may complain of a dull ache or frank pain in the leg or calf. There may be tenderness or spasm in the calf muscle. Examination may reveal slight swelling of the calf. This swelling can be so slight that it may be evident only by precise measurement of the circumference of both calves at the same level. Dorsiflexion of the foot may elicit pain in the calf (Homans' sign). Although a positive Homans' sign is specific, the test is not very sensitive (about 25%). Slight elevation of the temperature and pulse is frequently noted. If the clot is in the femoral vein or in the pelvis, swelling of the extremity may be more severe.

The major complication of deep thrombophlebitis is pulmonary embolism. Chronic venous insufficiency may develop as a long-term consequence.

B. Diagnosis

Compression ultrasonography or impedance plethysmography usually provides a definite diagnosis. Both are noninvasive and are sensitive and specific. If these tests are not diagnostic, contrast venography is the gold standard and should be performed.

C. Treatment

1. Medical treatment—Once the diagnosis of a significant deep vein thrombosis extending into the veins proximal to the calf has been made, anticoagulants should be started immediately. Traditionally, intravenous unfractionated heparin has been the first-line therapy. Recently, subcutaneous low molecular weight heparin has gained acceptance. Coagulation studies, including international normalized ratio (INR) and partial thromboplastin time (PTT), should be done before anticoagulant therapy is started; these tests provide a basis for interpreting the degree of anticoagulation achieved with unfractionated heparin. When using unfractionated heparin, the PTT should be kept to 2–3 times the control value. The more predictable bioavailability, clearance, and activity of low molecular weight heparins obviates the need for laboratory monitoring except in unusual circumstances. Intravenous protamine sulfate can be used in emergencies to counteract the effects of heparin. Heparin should be continued at least 3–5 days after the disappearance of all signs and symptoms and effective long-term therapy has been established.

Oral anticoagulants such as dicumarol and warfarin are contraindicated in pregnant patients but are often started at the same time as heparin in other patients. The therapeutic effect of these agents is measured by the INR. Whereas heparin prolongs the clotting time almost immediately, the oral anticoagulants do not exert their full effect for 48–72 hours. Heparin is usually started for its immediate short-term effect, then replaced with oral anticoagulants for long-term treatment. Once-daily low molecular weight heparin can be used long-term in patients for whom bleeding is a particular risk or laboratory monitoring is problematic. If using warfarin, the INR should be determined daily until equilibrium levels of 2.0–3.0 are attained. Emergency reversal can be achieved with 2 units of fresh frozen plasma. Anticoagulation is usually continued empirically for 3 months.

Anticoagulation presents significant risks, and patients with deep vein thrombosis must be thoroughly counseled to recognize possible complications of therapy, including hematuria, hemoptysis, hematemesis, melena, and easy bruisability. These patients should be provided with a means of identification indicating that they are receiving anticoagulant therapy, in case of an accident in which they become unconscious. Patients should also be given a list of over-the-counter medications to avoid, including nonsteroidal anti-inflammatory drugs, aspirin, and antibiotics, which may affect their anticoagulation. Acetaminophen, previously thought not to affect coagulation, has been linked to a risk of over-anticoagulation in the outpatient setting.

Management of calf vein thromboses is somewhat controversial. They are often viewed as no problem unless they extend into the proximal veins. When suspected or confirmed, serial compression ultrasound can be performed with reservation of anticoagulation for the approximately 10% whose clots will extend into the proximal circulation.

2. Local measures—Local measures include elevation of the legs to provide good venous drainage and the application of full-leg gradient-pressure elastic hose. When inflammation has subsided, usually within 1–2 weeks of starting therapy, full activities may be permitted. The patient should be encouraged to continue to elevate her legs whenever she can. Prolonged sitting and the use of constrictive garments, especially knee-high support stockings or hosiery, is to be avoided.

3. Surgical treatment—Thrombectomy occasionally may be considered for persistent severe swelling of the extremity. An inferior vena cava filter or vena cava ligation may be considered for repeated episodes of pulmonary embolism that occur in spite of adequate anticoagulation or when anticoagulation is absolutely contraindicated.

Septic Pelvic Thrombophlebitis

Septic pelvic thrombophlebitis is a complication that is almost unique to pelvic surgery. It occurs most frequently related to cesarean delivery and is discussed in detail in Chapter 22. The diagnosis of septic pelvic thrombophlebitis is established by therapeutic trial with heparin in conjunction with antibiotic therapy that covers both aerobic and anaerobic organisms.

4. Pulmonary Embolism

Pulmonary embolism is a critical complication of pelvic surgery. This diagnosis should be suspected if cardiac or pulmonary symptoms occur abruptly. Sepsis, obesity, malignancy, and history of pulmonary embolism or deep vein thrombosis are predisposing factors. It is a complication of pelvic or proximal lower extremity deep vein thromboembolism; nonetheless, pulmonary embolism may precede the diagnosis of peripheral disease. Indeed, in some patients no evidence of thrombophlebitis can be found. Pulmonary embolism may occur at any time, but usually occurs around the seventh to tenth postoperative days. The differential diagnosis includes atelectasis, pneumonia, myocardial infarction, and pneumothorax.

Clinical Findings

A. Symptoms and Signs

Patients with large emboli have chest pain, severe dyspnea, cyanosis, tachycardia, hypotension or shock, restlessness, and anxiety. If the embolus is massive, sudden death may result from acute cor pulmonale. In patients with smaller emboli, the diagnosis is suggested by the sudden onset of pleuritic pain, sometimes in association with blood-streaked sputum. A dry cough may develop. Physical examination may reveal a pleural friction rub. In many cases, no classic diagnostic signs can be elicited.

B. Diagnosis

In the patient suspected of having a pulmonary embolus, an arterial blood gas, 12-lead ECG, and chest X-ray should be obtained. If the patient has a low PO_2 with no other explanation, a V/Q scan and angiography if necessary should be obtained. Lower extremity studies as discussed above can also be performed. Presence of thrombus in a proximal lower extremity vein in the presence of symptoms of a pulmonary embolus also confirms the diagnosis.

C. Laboratory Findings

A low arterial PO_2 is a key finding and should immediately raise suspicion of pulmonary embolus. Moderate leukocytosis (up to 15,000/μL) and elevated serum bilirubin, lactate dehydrogenase (LDH), or serum glutamate oxaloacetate transaminase (SGOT) can also occur. Rapid D-dimer assays are under development and receiving attention as a potential method of ruling out deep venous thrombosis and pulmonary embolism; insufficient data are available at present to recommend their routine use in the postoperative setting.

D. X-Ray Findings

Chest x-ray may show no abnormality, or changes may be delayed 24–48 hours. In about 15% of patients, a pulmonary density is present, which is in the periphery of the lung and roughly in the shape of a triangle with its base at the lung surface. Other possible findings are enlargement of the main pulmonary artery, small pleural effusion, and elevated diaphragm. Embolism involves the lower lobes in 75% of cases, more often on the right than the left.

E. Electrocardiography

The ECG may show characteristic changes of pulmonary embolism in one-third of cases. The ECG is principally of interest in differentiating pulmonary embolism from myocardial infarction, which can appear clinically similar.

F. Lung Scan

The ventilation-perfusion scan, or V/Q scan, is used to diagnose pulmonary embolism and differentiate it from atelectasis and pneumonia. A negative scan is reassuring but not totally reliable, because there is a 15% false-negative rate in patients in whom there is high clinical suspicion. In these patients, or in patients with inconclusive scans, pulmonary angiography should be performed.

If V/Q scan is unavailable or inconclusive, spiral computed tomography (CT) may be of some value. This technology, in which images are generated from continuous spiraling segments rather than the interval segment images of conventional CT, has up to 92% sensitivity and 96% specificity in detecting pulmonary emboli. This imaging modality, however, may not be as effective as pulmonary angiography in detecting smaller, peripheral emboli.

G. Angiography

Pulmonary angiography should be done if the clinical situation is suggestive and the V/Q scan is indeterminate. It is the most reliable procedure for confirming the diagnosis and determining the location and extent of large emboli. It should always be done before an embolectomy is undertaken. Embolectomy is performed only on selected patients, and a definitive diagnosis is essential. Pressures measured in the right heart and pulmonary artery in conjunction with catheterization for angiography aid in evaluating the degree of right heart failure secondary to pulmonary artery obstruction. Angiography should be preceded by a V/Q scan; if the scan is negative, massive pulmonary embolus can be virtually ruled out.

Treatment

Cardiopulmonary resuscitation measures should be instituted as necessary. Close monitoring is essential, as is treatment of acid-base abnormalities and shock. Immediate initiation of heparin is indicated. Because of the high mortality associated with pulmonary embolism, it is better to begin heparin therapy even in the absence of a definitive diagnosis if pulmonary embolism is likely. Management of anticoagulation follows the same procedure as for deep vein thrombosis.

Prevention

Deep vein thrombosis is a common complication of pelvic and abdominal surgery, and because death from pulmonary embolism often occurs before heparin anti-coagulation begins its effect, prevention is a critical strategy. International consensus recommendations exist for prevention of venous thromboembolism, and include specific recommendations for gynecologic surgery. Patients undergoing minor gynecologic surgery without risk factors may or may not receive prophylaxis. For patients at moderate and high risk (major surgery, age over 40, use of oral contraceptives), patients should receive prophylaxis with intermittent pneumatic compression stockings or heparin.

PULMONARY COMPLICATIONS

Pulmonary complications remain one of the major hazards of the postoperative period. About 30% of deaths that occur within 6 weeks after operation are due to pulmonary complications. Postoperative problems vary with the preoperative status of the patient. Chronic bronchitis, emphysema, and increased bronchial secretions, which are commonly present in smokers, make these patients particularly susceptible to postoperative respiratory problems. Atelectasis, pneumonia, pulmonary embolism, and acute respiratory distress syndrome (ARDS) from aspiration, left ventricular failure, fluid overload, or infection are the most common complications.

1. Atelectasis

Atelectasis is a complication of the very early postoperative period. It consists of areas of airway collapse and is more common in patients who already have chronic lung disease. Atelectasis is more common in the postoperative period because of diminished functional residual capacity in the supine position and "splinting" caused by pain from abdominal surgery. The blood that traverses the areas with atelectasis is not oxygenated, resulting in shunting and hypoxia. Massive atelectasis may occur when a mucus plug or aspirated vomitus occludes a large bronchus. Predisposing factors include chronic bronchitis, asthma, smoking, and respiratory infection.

Clinical Findings

The clinical findings vary with the extent of atelectasis. Mild atelectasis is the most common cause of fever in the immediate postoperative period. It is usually related to incomplete expansion of the lungs during and after the surgery. As the patient begins ambulating and mobilizing her secretions, it resolves.

The patient may complain of an excess of bronchial secretions, with rhonchi and cough. Patients frequently are febrile. On auscultation, the patient will have diminished breath sounds, particularly at the lung bases. They may also have areas of dullness to percussion, together with bronchial breathing and inspiratory rales. Chest x-ray findings include patchy opacities. If atelectasis is not treated, superimposed pneumonia can develop.

With massive atelectasis, the temperature, pulse, and respiratory rate increase sharply. Segments of lung, sometimes entire lobes, may be dull to percussion, with absent breath sounds. Cyanosis may be present and the patient will often exhibit shortness of breath. A lateral shift of the mediastinum (ie, displacement of the trachea and heart toward the atelectatic side) can occur. Multiple small areas of atelectasis and bronchopneumonia, which often have a similar clinical picture, may occur together.

Prevention

The prevention of atelectasis begins in the preoperative period. Patients should be encouraged to stop smoking preoperatively. Patients with chronic lung disease should be given antibiotics and chest physical therapy if an acute or chronic infection is suspected. If bronchospasm is present, bronchodilators may be advisable. If upper respiratory infection is present, elective surgery should be postponed.

Intraoperatively, the patient should be ventilated with adequate tidal volumes with the addition of positive end-expiratory pressure if signs of atelectasis such as decreasing oxygen saturation become apparent. Intraoperative atelectasis or small airway collapse is more commonly seen in patients with chronic lung disease or obesity and can be aggravated by the Trendelenburg position. Intraoperative humidification and suctioning of secretions are helpful.

Postoperatively, atelectasis is best avoided by minimizing pain, placing patients in the sitting position, and encouraging deep breathing and early ambulation. Incentive spirometry devices help patients to perform deep inspiration exercises. Patient-controlled analgesia or use of an epidural catheter for postoperative pain management can help by reducing respiratory depression.

Treatment

Treatment consists of intensive chest physical therapy and supplemental oxygen. Pain should be controlled, since it is an obstacle to deep breathing. If fever persists and pneumonia develops, antibiotics will be necessary. If there is inadequate tissue oxygenation, intubation and mechanical ventilation will be necessary.

2. Pneumonia

Pneumonia may follow atelectasis or aspiration of vomitus or another substance. Abundant tracheobronchial secretions from preexisting bronchitis also predispose to this complication. Fever in the first few postoperative days is usually from atelectasis. If this persists or is followed by higher temperatures, systemic toxicity, and respiratory difficulty, a presumptive diagnosis of pneumonia is justified.

If pneumonia develops, secretions become progressively more abundant and the cough becomes productive. Physical examination may reveal evidence of pulmonary consolidation, and numerous coarse rales often are present. Although the chest x-ray may show diffuse patchy infiltrates or lobar consolidation, this appearance may lag behind the clinical picture by as much as 24 hours.

The treatment of pneumonia includes deep breathing and coughing. The patient should be encouraged to change position frequently. Nasotracheal suction may be used to stimulate the cough reflex. Specific broad-spectrum antibiotic therapy should be instituted based on Gram's stain and knowledge of pathogens specific to the institution, and revised as indicated by subsequent sputum culture and sensitivity tests. Induced sputum is more reliable since oral contamination of expectorated specimens occurs frequently.

In desperately weak or debilitated patients with a poor cough reflex, tracheostomy may occasionally be necessary to permit adequate ventilation, suctioning, and bronchoscopy. Positive pressure ventilation may improve the depth of respiration and reduce the work of breathing in extremely ill patients.

3. Aspiration Pneumonitis

Aspiration of gastric contents into the trachea is associated with many factors such as neurologic disease affecting the gag reflex and vomiting in debilitated patients who do not have the strength to adequately cough. Aspiration of gastric contents into the trachea during induction of anesthesia is the best-known cause, although it is by no means the most common. Risk factors include difficult intubations, passive regurgitation in the patient with an incompletely empty stomach, poor gastroesophageal sphincter tone in patients with hiatal hernia, and inflation of the stomach with air. Pregnant patients are particularly at risk because of slow gastric emptying time and poor gastroesophageal sphincter tone.

The chance for pulmonary aspiration of acid gastric contents can be minimized by:

1. Doing an awake fiberoptic intubation on patients with predictably difficult airways.
2. Speeding the process of gastric emptying by administering metoclopramide, 10 mg intravenously.

3. Increasing the pH of gastric contents by means of a nonparticulate antacid and use of H_2 blockers (this helps minimize pulmonary damage if aspiration does occur).
4. Using a rapid sequence induction with pentothal and cricoid pressure. Cricoid pressure closes off the esophagus to prevent passively regurgitated material from reaching the larynx. This pressure is kept on until the positioning of the tube in the trachea is verified.

If aspiration of gastric contents occurs, an endotracheal tube should be placed immediately and the trachea and bronchi aggressively suctioned and lavaged with saline solution. Generally, a small amount of aspiration may be associated with mild atelectasis and cause temporary hypoxia. More severe aspiration may lead to serious hypoxia requiring ventilation. The role of corticosteroids in the management of aspiration remains controversial. Air bronchograms may appear on chest x-ray 12–24 hours after the event. The patient must be monitored for development of full-blown acute respiratory distress syndrome (ARDS). Treatment of ARDS is considered in Chapter 59.

4. Tension Pneumothorax

Tension pneumothorax is an uncommon complication and is most likely to occur during the first 24–48 hours after surgery. Pneumothorax can occur during positive pressure ventilation and may not be apparent until the ventilation is stopped. Pneumothorax presents as acute respiratory distress with distant breath sounds on the affected side and frequently a marked mediastinal shift away from the affected side. The diagnosis is made by chest x-ray. Immediate placement of a chest tube is essential; temporary improvement can be obtained by inserting one or more large-bore angiocatheters with the patient under local anesthesia through the intercostal space at approximately T6–T8 to allow escape of air until a chest tube can be inserted. Chest tube drainage is usually continued for several days, until the air leak has sealed.

5. Acute Respiratory Distress Syndrome (ARDS)

ARDS, a frequently catastrophic postoperative complication, is considered in Chapter 59.

GASTROINTESTINAL TRACT COMPLICATIONS

Gastrointestinal complications are most apt to occur after transabdominal operations, but they may complicate vaginal surgery as well. In fact, any serious illness or surgical procedure may cause malfunction of the gastrointestinal tract.

1. Ileus

Some degree of postoperative ileus must be expected whenever the peritoneal cavity is entered. The proper rate for advancement of diet remains a matter of style with few good studies to offer guidance. Many surgeons encourage their patients to sip tap water (not ice water) on the first day after uncomplicated gynecologic surgery. On the following day, clear fluids are often given if bowel sounds are normal, and solid food usually is withheld until the patient passes flatus. Some recent studies suggest that early oral intake (clear liquids on postoperative day 1), even among patients with major abdominal surgery, reduces length of hospitalization and is not associated with an increased incidence of ileus.

Clinical Findings

Nausea occurring in the immediate postoperative period may be troublesome and is usually anesthesia-related. It may be suppressed with prochlorperazine, 5–10 mg intramuscularly or in a 25-mg rectal suppository, promethazine, 25 mg intramuscularly, or trimethobenzamide, 200 mg intramuscularly. Nausea or vomiting later in the postoperative period demands diagnostic attention, because the symptom may be due either to ileus or to bowel obstruction.

Ileus is classically characterized by abdominal distention, absence of bowel sounds, and generalized abdominal tympany on percussion. The complication is noted usually within the first 48–72 hours after surgery. On KUB, there is generalized dilatation and gaseous distention of both small and large bowel, although the small bowel component may be more prominent. Obstipation is also characteristic of postoperative ileus. If ileus is persistent, especially if accompanied by a febrile course, a retained foreign body must be considered. Such an object usually can be ruled out by the same radiologic study. Urologic trauma with resultant extravasation of urine may be an unusual cause of persistent ileus. An intravenous urogram may aid in the diagnosis of urinary extravasation.

Treatment

If nausea, vomiting, or abdominal distention becomes severe, a nasogastric tube should be inserted into the stomach. Gastric aspiration usually reveals green to yellow fluids. The distention should lessen with this treatment; if no benefit is noted, bowel obstruction should

be suspected. Electrolytes should be monitored and corrected in patients undergoing prolonged nasogastric suctioning. Nasogastric or orogastric tube decompression has been implemented postoperatively as a prophylactic measure to prevent distention and ileus, but has not been shown to reduce the incidence of ileus or time to bowel function recovery. In fact, nasogastric tube decompression can cause pharyngeal irritation and eustachian tube discomfort and is associated with increased postoperative complaints.

Enemas and suppositories are frequently used, but can obscure the diagnosis of a small bowel obstruction by placing air and fluid in the rectum.

2. Postoperative Intestinal Obstruction

Bowel obstruction may occur as a complication of any intraperitoneal operation. It most frequently occurs as a consequence of peritonitis or generalized irritation of the peritoneal surface, resulting in varying degrees of adhesions between loops of bowel. Obstruction results when these adhesions trap or kink a segment of intestine.

The resultant partial or complete bowel obstruction is usually noted between the fifth and sixth postoperative days; however, obstruction can occur sooner. Dense, fibrous adhesions develop after 8–12 weeks and can entrap bowel and cause delayed obstruction with a high incidence of bowel strangulation.

Clinical Findings

Obstruction is associated with significant and even protracted vomiting, accompanied by cramping abdominal pain. On percussion, there may be a localized or focal tympanitic area noted. Bowel rushes heard on auscultation are noted to be synchronous with cramping pain.

Diagnosis

A flat film of the abdomen usually reveals distention of a portion of small bowel, with air-fluid levels apparent. In general, the colon is free of air. Enteroclysis, the observation of contrast medium infused through a tube under fluoroscopic guidance, is useful in delineating the location and determining the degree of obstruction. Computed tomography (CT) scan is also useful in recognizing small bowel obstruction, is less invasive than enteroclysis, and can differentiate obstruction due to extrinsic causes such as hematoma and tumor.

Treatment

Small bowel obstruction, with its high incidence of resultant bowel ischemia and infarction, is a life-threatening complication requiring immediate intervention. It is possible to treat postoperative bowel obstruction conservatively by bowel decompression with a nasogastric or long intestinal tube. Long intestinal tubes do not offer any advantage over nasogastric tubes unless properly placed, which generally requires fluoroscopic guidance. Tube decompression often results in realignment of the bowel and relief of the obstruction, or adhesions may relax or be released sufficiently to allow spontaneous decompression. When conservative management is elected, an arbitrary period of decompression should be decided on in advance; if the obstruction does not respond within that period—usually 48–72 hours—reoperation is necessary. Obstruction is associated with large fluid shifts into the bowel lumen, and vigorous hydration and careful electrolyte monitoring are required.

Incidence of delayed small bowel obstruction secondary to adhesions after hysterectomy has been quoted as high as 16.3 per 1000 cases. The median time to clinical presentation is 5.3 years postoperatively. It has been suggested that small bowel obstruction may be associated with peritoneal closure.

3. Acute Gastric Distention

Acute gastric distention is one of the most common postoperative complications. It is caused by accumulation of air, and to a lesser extent gastric juices, in the stomach. Most patients with nausea or paralytic ileus swallow air. If intestinal peristalsis is depressed, the swallowed gas accumulates in the stomach. In unusual cases, as gastric distention increases, the movement of the diaphragm may be inhibited. If the patient develops hyperpnea and appears to be splinting her diaphragm and acute gastric distention is the suspected cause, a nasogastric tube should be passed immediately and gastric aspiration continued as long as the ileus persists.

4. Constipation and Fecal Impaction

A reduction in the number of bowel movements is to be expected in the early postoperative period because of low food intake and ileus. In a postoperative patient with obstipation, where ileus and small bowel obstruction are not suspected, a mild laxative (milk of magnesia, 30 mL orally) may be prescribed. A clear water enema or rectal bisacodyl suppository can also be used.

Fecal impaction can also cause diarrhea in the postoperative patient. If suspected, a digital rectal examination should be performed. If hard stool is encountered in the ampulla, the diagnosis of fecal impaction is verified. The condition is caused by limitation of oral fluids and is especially common in elderly patients and others confined to bed. It may be aggravated by previous gastrointestinal series or barium enema with accumulation of barium in the colon. The treatment of fecal impaction is digital disimpaction of the firm fecal masses after an oil retention enema.

5. Diarrhea

Pseudomembranous enterocolitis may occur as a complication of any antibiotic administration, with penicillins and cephalosporins the most frequently implicated agents. The bacterial flora of the gastrointestinal tract is altered, resulting in overgrowth of *Clostridium difficile,* the etiologic organism. The patient typically develops severe diarrhea, and pseudomembranous changes are seen on colonoscopy. The diagnosis is made by detection of the *C difficile* toxin in stool specimens. This disease may be particularly devastating for the geriatric or debilitated patient.

Oral metronidazole, 250 mg 4 times a day for 10 days, is the first-line therapy. Oral vancomycin, 125 mg every 6 hours for 10 days, is equally effective, but considerably more expensive. Careful attention must be paid to replacing fluid and electrolytes in these patients. The infection is easily spread throughout hospitals, and once diagnosed, patients are usually isolated and infection precautions initiated.

6. Fistulas

While a full discussion of genital fistulas is beyond the scope of this chapter, this serious delayed postoperative complication bears mentioning. Fistulas in gynecologic surgery are associated with malignancy; prior radiation therapy; intraoperative bowel, bladder, or ureteral injury; and obstetric trauma (eg, fourth-degree lacerations, breakdown of episiotomy repairs). Vesicovaginal, rectovaginal, and enterocutaneous fistulas are the most commonly seen of this rare complication.

Vesicovaginal fistula should be suspected if the patient presents with a continuous watery discharge from the vagina. Diagnosis involves direct observation or instillation of methylene blue into the bladder and placement of cotton balls or a tampon in the vagina. Discoloration of the cotton or tampon indicates a communication between bladder and vagina. Approximately 20% of fresh postoperative vesicovaginal fistulas will close spontaneously with prolonged catheter drainage. The remainder are usually repaired with a transvaginal surgical approach, which has a good success rate.

Rectovaginal fistulas occur after obstetric trauma or vaginal surgery. Primary transvaginal repair has an approximately 90% success of closure. Larger, recurrent, or irradiated defects may require diverting colostomy while the repair heals.

Enterocutaneous fistulas may present initially with wound erythema, followed by feculent drainage from the incision site. Treatment of enterocutaneous fistulas consists of keeping the patient from oral intake over a period of 2–4 weeks, supplementation with total parenteral nutrition, and nasogastric decompression. If spontaneous closure does not occur, surgical repair will be necessary.

URINARY TRACT COMPLICATIONS

1. Urinary Retention

After a minor procedure, measurement of urinary output can await natural voiding. If fluid therapy has been adequate, the patient should void by 4–6 hours after surgery; if she has not voided by then, bladder distention should be suspected. The patient should be encouraged to get out of bed to void. If the normal capacity of the bladder is exceeded (500 mL), serious bladder dysfunction may result. Overdistention of the bladder can occur in the patient with a kinked or clotted suprapubic tube or transurethral catheter.

Inability of the patient to void or difficulty in voiding often is due to pain caused by using the voluntary muscles to start the urinary stream. With vaginal procedures or with suprapubic procedures like the Marshall-Marchetti-Krantz operation performed to treat urinary incontinence, sutures near the urethra or urethral edema may make voiding difficult or impossible.

Treatment

The treatment for urinary retention is immediate bladder drainage with sterile catheterization. If over 500 mL of urine is drained, the bladder muscle has likely lost tone, and 24–48 hours of continued drainage should be considered before another voiding trial. Decompression of the distended bladder can be complicated by hematuria, transient hypotension, and postobstructive diuresis. Patients with recurrent difficulties may have underlying urinary tract infections.

Prevention

After a major procedure in which postoperative bleeding or operative damage to the urinary tract is a possibility, bladder drainage by means of a urethral catheter or suprapubic cystotomy tube should be instituted despite the small risk of bladder infection. The catheter usually can be removed within 24–48 hours except after a vaginal plastic procedure, bladder neck suspension, or extended operation, which usually requires drainage for a longer period.

If prolonged drainage is required, suprapubic drainage is preferred by many operators over urethral catheter drainage because of increased patient comfort, ease of care, and a reduced incidence of infection. A suprapubic catheter is also useful in facilitating postoperative voiding trials after urogynecologic procedures. If a patient is facing a prolonged return to normal voiding function and has adequate visual acuity and manual dexterity, intermittent clean self-catheterization can also be a useful bladder drainage modality.

Anxiety can play a significant role in patients with difficulty voiding after surgery. Diazepam may be helpful in management for both its anxiolytic and skeletal muscle-relaxant effects.

2. Oliguria and Anuria

Oliguria is frequently defined as urinary output of less than 30 mL per hour. It usually results from volume depletion, which often can be demonstrated by diuresis following the rapid intravenous administration of 500 mL of 5% dextrose in normal saline. Disturbances of electrolyte balance (eg, "water intoxication syndrome") or diminished renal blood flow (cardiac failure, shock) may also cause oliguria as can volume overload causing congestive heart failure and pulmonary edema. After these possible causes of oliguria have been eliminated, an underlying serious disorder of the urinary tract should be considered.

Anuria must be identified promptly. It rarely may be due to bilateral ureteral obstruction, a complication that must be considered when there is no urinary output on the operating table or during the immediate postoperative period. If an IVP fails to reveal the cause of this serious postoperative complication, underlying kidney disease (acute tubular necrosis) should be suspected.

Treatment

Major surgery often will upset the patient's fluid and electrolyte balance. Prohibition of fluids for at least 12 hours before operation, large insensible water losses during the operation, and inability to tolerate food or fluids postoperatively require major adjustments.

The amount and type of fluid replacement should take into account the fact that preoperative dehydration may have occurred. In addition, loss of fluid into the bowel and insensible losses from the skin, peritoneal cavity, and lungs may have been substantial. Blood loss must be accurately estimated in the operating room, since excessive blood loss may deplete the vascular and extracellular fluids. These losses are generally increased as operating time is prolonged.

In gynecologic surgery, patients vary in their postoperative fluid replacement needs. The healthy 28-year-old myomectomy patient may require a volume of intravenous fluid that would prove fatal to the frail 68-year-old patient with cardiopulmonary disease who underwent reconstructive vaginal surgery. Postoperative fluid replacement must be individualized, but in general should maintain a urine output greater than 30 mL per hour.

The composition of these fluids should address electrolyte as well as glucose needs. Subsequent fluid requirements should be based on replacement of an average of 1000 mL of daily insensible water loss (higher in febrile patients) plus urinary output. A clinical estimate of the state of hydration can be made by noting the urinary output, moistness of the mucous membranes, and skin turgor. If the patient is unable to take fluids orally in adequate amounts after 48 hours, potassium may need to be added to the intravenous fluids after measurement of the serum electrolytes. If a complicated major procedure with substantial blood loss has been performed, albumin, plasma, or whole blood may be necessary.

3. Urinary Tract Infection

Urinary tract infection (UTI) may develop in the immediate postoperative period in any patient. This is due to the urinary retention that follows surgery, anesthesia, or immobilization. The bladder usually is sterile before surgery and remains so unless bacteria are introduced by instrumentation or catheterization. Catheter-associated urinary tract infection is the most common nosocomial infection.

While cystitis can cause frequency and dysuria, it should not cause fever. Pyelonephritis however, can cause extremely high fever. UTI should be considered in the evaluation of any patient with postoperative fever. Clinical signs such as high fever and flank tenderness may be present. Patients with urosepsis may appear quite toxic very rapidly. White blood cells and bacteria are seen on urinalysis. Postvoid residual urine, which is sometimes seen, tends to perpetuate the infection and predisposes to ascending infection and pyelonephritis.

Hydration should be increased and activity encouraged to facilitate complete emptying of the bladder. After urine specimens are obtained for culture, appropriate antibiotic therapy should be instituted. Antibiotic coverage may have to be adjusted based on culture and sensitivity results. Gram-negative organisms from the lower urogenital tract predominate. Reinstitution of catheter drainage may be necessary in patients with a postvoid residual urine of 100 mL or more, although in general discontinuing the catheter at the earliest possible time is useful for preventing and treating infection.

OTHER INFECTIOUS COMPLICATIONS

1. Hematoma and Pelvic Abscess

Small hematomas or seromas often resolve spontaneously, but some become infected. Closed-suction drainage is frequently used to prevent intra-abdominal hematoma. Gravity or Penrose drains have a limited role in gynecologic surgery.

Insidious accumulations may occur either in the pelvis or under the fascia of the rectus abdominis muscle. They may first be suspected because of a falling hematocrit in association with a low-grade fever. Ultrasonography is an excellent adjunct to physical examination for diagnosis. The subrectus collection, seen most frequently after a Pfannenstiel or Maylard incision or in conjunction with a retropubic urethropexy, may be difficult to outline clinically but can be clearly delineated by ultrasound.

Drainage of an infected hematoma should be accomplished extraperitoneally. This is simple if it is located in the anterior abdominal wall. Pelvic hematomas are usually not drained unless they are infected and antibiotic therapy has failed. If the pelvic hematoma is not easily accessible via the vaginal vault, an inguinal extraperitoneal approach would be necessary. Consideration should be given to percutaneous drainage. If the cavity is not readily accessible for operative drainage by either the abdominal or vaginal route, insertion of a large-caliber "pigtail" catheter under guidance of ultrasound or CT should be considered.

2. Wound Infection

The frequency and degree of postoperative wound infection depend on many factors, including the patient's age, health, nutritional status, and personal hygiene habits, as well as the presence of malignancy, history of smoking or diabetes, the use of corticosteroid medications, history of radiation therapy, and surgical technique. The method of skin preparation prior to surgery is also important. Shaving the operative site may cause folliculitis, resulting in a superficial wound infection. If a shave prep is to be done, it should be done in the operating room just before surgery. Using clippers or omitting shaving entirely yields a lower wound infection rate. Extensive guidelines have been drafted by the CDC for prevention of surgical site infection.

The use of antibiotic prophylaxis has long been known to reduce infection at the incision site of uncomplicated vaginal and radical abdominal procedures. Antibiotic prophylaxis has recently been shown by meta-analysis to be effective for routine abdominal hysterectomy as well. In obese patients a combination of subcutaneous drainage and prophylactic antibiotics has been shown to decrease wound morbidity. Active infection at the operative site (eg, pelvic abscess, ruptured appendix) or at a distant site will increase the risk of wound infection by direct contamination or hematogenous spread.

The diagnosis of wound infection usually is made during investigation of an unexplained postoperative fever, often on about the fourth or fifth day. This diagnosis is based on the physical findings of redness, induration at the operative site, or purulent drainage. Facultative and anaerobic gram-negative rods, beta-hemolytic streptococci, and staphylococci are the pathogens most commonly cultured from infected wounds. The wound should be explored and cultured. Ample drainage should be established and appropriate antibiotics ordered to treat adjacent cellulitis. If cellulitis is not present, wound opening and local care are adequate therapy. Damp to dry dressings should be changed three times a day and the wound debrided daily until definite improvement is noted. Hydrogen peroxide, iodine compounds, antibiotics, or other chemicals in the wound-irrigating solution are sometimes used but have not been proved beneficial and may even be toxic or impede healing. A drain or gauze packing may be required to keep the skin from prematurely sealing the wound.

Open wounds may be treated with irrigation, dressing changes, and periodic debridement until healing by secondary intention is complete. This often takes weeks or even months. One study supported a role for early secondary closure of these wounds after all infection is resolved and healing has begun. Healing times can thus be dramatically shortened. Delayed primary closure should be considered for cases with obvious contamination or infection.

3. Wound Dehiscence and Evisceration

The transverse lower abdominal incision used by many gynecologists rarely ruptures. Vertical incisions may carry a somewhat greater risk of breakdown. Risk factors for wound dehiscence and breakdown are similar to those for wound infections: age, nutritional status, diabetes, smoking, malignancy, and presence of a prior scar at the incision site.

Evisceration is disruption of all layers of the abdominal wall with protrusion of the intestines through the incision; it is a serious postoperative complication. The dreaded hallmark of this complication is a profuse serosanguineous discharge exuding from the abdominal incision. It must be emphasized that proper exploration and resolution of this problem should take place in the operating room and not on the ward or in the examining room. When the diagnosis of fascial dehiscence or evisceration is made, secondary closure must be performed immediately with the patient under general anesthesia. Interrupted nonabsorbable sutures through all layers of the abdominal wall are preferred. Broad-spectrum antibiotics should be initiated following wound culture. Consideration should be given to a mass closure technique when risk factors for dehiscence are present to help prevent this complication.

4. Necrotic Phenomena

Necrotizing fasciitis, a synergistic mixed facultative and anaerobic infection that involves the fascia and subcutaneous tissue, has been described in both abdominal and perineal sites and is extremely destructive and rapidly progressive. Despite early recognition, mortality is high. Group A streptococcus and anaerobes are important causes.

The skin near the incision site and surrounding area is cool, gray, and boggy. The patient usually appears floridly septic with fever and high white count. If necrotizing fasciitis is suspected, the patient should be brought to the operating room and fascial biopsy performed. If confirmed, radical debridement in the operating room is essential, followed by treatment with broad-spectrum antibiotics. Healing is usually by secondary intention with skin grafts often being necessary. This is a potentially lethal complication that requires timely intervention, and it should always be considered in the differential diagnosis when wound problems occur.

A second necrotic complication can result from a poorly planned incision. When a new incision is made near and parallel to an existing scar, sloughing of tissue secondary to ischemia can result. New incisions should either be made through the old incision, or at least several centimeters away to allow adequate blood supply for proper healing.

REFERENCES

Intraoperative Complications

American Heart Association: *Advanced Cardiac Life Support* (ACLS Guidelines). American Heart Association, 1997.

Bick RL, Haas SK: International consensus recommendations: summary statement and additional suggested guidelines. Med Clin North Am 1998;82:613.

Hemsell DL: Antibiotics and gynecologic infection. ACOG Educational Bulletin No. 237. American College of Obstetricians and Gynecologists, 1997.

Hoffman MS, Rozner MA: Hemorrhagic shock. ACOG Technical Bulletin No. 235. American College of Obstetricians and Gynecologists, 1997.

Mangram AJ et al: Guidelines for prevention of surgical site infection, 1999. Infect Control Hosp Epidemiol 1999;20:247.

Utri JW: Bladder and ureteral injury: prevention and management. Clin Obstet Gynecol 1998;41:755.

Postoperative Complications

Al-Took S, Platt R, Tulandi T: Adhesion-related small-bowel obstruction after gynecologic operations. Am J Obstet Gynecol 1999;180:313.

Cutillo G et al: Early feeding compared with nasogastric decompression after major oncologic gynecologic surgery: a randomized study. Obstet Gynecol 1999;93:41.

Ellozy S et al: Early postoperative small-bowel obstruction: a prospective evaluation of 242 consecutive abdominal operations. Dis Colon Rectum 2001;44:A5.

Hylek EM et al: Acetaminophen and other risk factors for excessive warfarin anticoagulation. JAMA 1998;279:657.

Janssen MCH et al: Rapid D-dimer assays to exclude deep venous thrombosis and pulmonary embolism: current status and new developments. Semin Thromb Hemosta 1998;24:393.

Kearson C et al: Noninvasive diagnosis of deep vein thrombosis. Ann Intern Med 1998;128:663.

Kim KI, Muller NL, Mayo JR: Clinically suspected pulmonary embolism: utility of spiral CT. Radiology 1999;210:693.

Schilder JM et al: A prospective controlled trial of early postoperative oral intake following major abdominal gynecologic surgery. Gynecol Oncol 1997;67:235.

Seal DV: Necrotizing fasciitis. Curr Opin Dis 2001;14:127.

Yassin SF et al: *Clostridium difficile*-associated diarrhea and colitis. Mayo Clin Proc 2001;76:725.

Laparoscopic and Hysteroscopic Complications

Isaacson KB: Complications of hysteroscopy. Obstet Gynecol Clin North Am 1999;26:39.

Lin P, Grow D: Complications of laparoscopy: strategies for prevention and cure. Obstet Gynecol North Am 1999;26:23.

Therapeutic Gynecologic Procedures

45

Dipika Dandade, MD, L. Russell Malinak, MD, & James M. Wheeler, MD, MPH

Four of the 10 most commonly performed operations in the U.S. are dilation and curettage (D&C), tubal sterilization, abdominal hysterectomy, and vaginal hysterectomy. This chapter will review these procedures, as well as other therapeutic operations. Indications, contraindications, technique, and complications will be discussed for each procedure.

DILATION AND CURETTAGE (D&C)

Indications

The procedure of cervical dilation and uterine curettage is usually performed for one of the following indications: diagnosis and treatment of abnormal uterine bleeding, management of abortion (incomplete, missed, or induced), stenosis, or cancer of the uterus. The diagnosis of abnormal bleeding is discussed in Chapters 32 and 36; D&C as a method of induced abortion is discussed in Chapter 33. This section will discuss the remaining therapeutic uses of D&C.

Technique

A. CERVICAL DILATION

Dilation of the cervix may be conducted under paracervical, epidural, spinal, or general anesthesia, depending largely on the indication for the procedure. Cervical dilation usually precedes uterine curettage but may be performed as a therapeutic maneuver for acquired or congenital cervical stenosis, dysmenorrhea, or insertion of an intrauterine contraceptive device (IUD) or radium device for treatment of cancer. Dilation may also precede hysterography or hysteroscopy.

The patient is placed in the dorsal lithotomy position, with the back and shoulders supported and the extremities padded. The inner thighs, perineum, and vagina are prepared as for any vaginal operation; the surgeon and assistant should adhere to surgical principles of asepsis. A thorough pelvic examination under anesthesia is mandatory prior to performing cervical dilation, in order to determine the size and position of the cervix, uterus, and adnexa and the presence of any abnormalities. The pa-

tient voids normally before the operation if possible; urinary catheterization is used only if significant residual urine is suspected.

A right-angle retractor is placed anteriorly to gently retract the bladder. A weighted speculum is placed posteriorly to reveal the cervix. Under direct vision, the anterior lip of the cervix is grasped with a tenaculum, avoiding the vascular supply at 3 and 9 o'clock. The cervix is grasped firmly but with care taken not to compromise, or especially perforate, the endocervical canal. With gentle traction, the cervix can be brought down toward the introitus. Before proceeding further, a complete visual examination should be made of the cervix and the four vaginal fornices, because the latter areas (especially posteriorly) are otherwise difficult to examine. Areas that appear abnormal (even benign inclusion cysts) should be noted and followed as appropriate. Areas that are clearly abnormal should be biopsied. After the cervix and vagina are evaluated, the uterine cavity is examined. A uterine sound is gently inserted into the endocervix and then advanced into the uterine cavity in the plane of least resistance and most compatible with the position of the uterus as revealed by pelvic examination. Perforation of the uterus during D&C is most likely to occur at the time of uterine sounding or cervical dilation. Perforation is more likely to occur if the woman has retroversion or anteversion of the uterus or cervical stenosis, is pregnant or has recently given birth, or is postmenopausal; or if the surgeon uses excessive force or faulty technique. If severe cervical stenosis is suspected from the preoperative office examination, cervical softening agents such as prostaglandin E$_2$ gel or *Laminaria* tents may be inserted the day before the planned D&C. The depth of the uterine cavity is recorded as well as any abnormalities such as leiomyomas or septa.

The two most common dilators used are the Hegar and Hank's dilators. Hegar dilators are relatively blunt, gently curved, and numbered sequentially according to width (ie, a No. 7 dilator is 7 mm wide). For most purposes, particularly preceding curettage, dilation to a No. 9 dilator suffices; if dilation is being performed for dysmenorrhea, infertility, or stenosis, dilation should proceed to a No. 11 dilator.

Hank's dilators differ from Hegar dilators in being more gradually tapered ("sharper"); they may have a solid core or a hollow center allowing egress of trapped blood and air. Hank's dilators are measured in French sizes (a No. 20F Hank's dilator is approximately the same diameter as a No. 9 Hegar dilator). The choice of dilator is largely based on surgical training; many prefer not to use the more pointed Hank's dilators in a small postmenopausal uterus.

B. ENDOCERVICAL CURETTAGE

Fractional curettage should be used for abnormal uterine bleeding or if genital tract neoplasia is suspected. The cervical canal should be curetted prior to dilation of the cervix and curettage of the endometrial cavity, in order to preserve the histologic characteristics of the endocervix and prevent contamination of the endometrial sample with endocervical cells. If cervical conization is planned for diagnosis or treatment of cervical intraepithelial neoplasia, uterine sounding precedes conization, but cervical dilation and fractional curettage follow in order to minimize denuding of the endocervical epithelium. The Gusberg curet is a small, slightly curved instrument particularly well suited for endocervical curettage. The curet is placed in the endocervical canal to the level of the internal os; with a firm touch, each of the four walls is curetted with a single stroke, with the specimen delivered onto a coated cellulose sponge with a twirling motion of the curet. (The coated cellulose sponge is preferred over ordinary surgical sponges because tissue is less likely to adhere to it.) The cervix is then dilated as described earlier and curettage of the endometrium performed. The endocervical and endometrial specimens are immersed in fixative in separate containers and submitted to the pathologist.

Complications from endocervical curettage are rare in nongravid patients. Because of obvious risks to the fetus and membranes, endocervical curettage is contraindicated in pregnant women. Healing of the curetted endocervix may take 3 weeks or more; the cervical epithelium commonly takes 2 weeks to heal following a routine Papanicolaou smear. Tissue should be allowed to heal before follow-up Papanicolaou smears are taken, because regenerating cells are often mistaken for dysplastic cells.

C. ENDOMETRIAL POLYPECTOMY

The uterine cavity is explored with polyp forceps prior to diagnostic or therapeutic endometrial curettage. It is easier to remove polyps prior to curettage, preserving the histologic integrity necessary to differentiate benign uterine polyps from neoplasia. In a large series advocating routine exploration of the endometrial cavity preceding curettage, 64% of 130 diagnosed endometrial polyps were removed by ureteral stone forceps. Pedunculated or submucous leiomyomas, intrauterine and in-

tracervical synechias, and uterine anomalies may be first suspected at passage of the polyp forceps.

The technique of polypectomy includes gentle insertion of the forceps in the plane most compatible with the position of the uterus (as for uterine sounding). The forceps are opened slightly, rotated 90 degrees, and removed. Many clinicians repeat this procedure through 360 degrees, completely exploring the uterine cavity.

Skillful use of hysteroscopy for diagnosis and treatment of synechias, septa, leiomyomas, and polyps is preferred to blind polypectomy and curettage. With the new, narrow hysteroscope, the procedure is easily done as an office procedure similar to colposcopy for biopsy or laser conization.

D. ENDOMETRIAL CURETTAGE

Endometrial curettage is indicated for treatment of complications of pregnancy, including incomplete or missed abortion, postpartum retention of products of conception, placental polyps, and perhaps, endomyometritis. The procedure is also used in treatment of abnormal uterine bleeding due to pedunculated leiomyomas or polyps or in the occasional case of dysfunctional uterine bleeding that is refractory to medical therapy or life-threatening. The D&C is often both diagnostic and therapeutic.

The technique of endometrial curettage is tailored to the individual patient. In determining the hormone responsiveness of the endometrium, a small but representative sample may be obtained from the anterior and posterior walls. When curettage is being performed therapeutically, a systematic, thorough approach is indicated. The largest sharp curet that can comfortably fit through the dilated cervix is chosen. A serrated curet may cause injury to the underlying basalis layer of the endometrium and myometrium. The anterior, lateral, and posterior walls are scraped with firm pressure in a clockwise or counterclockwise fashion from the top of the uterine fundus down to the internal os. The top of the cavity is curetted with a side-to-side motion. The curettings are retrieved onto the waiting gauze and immersed in fixative as soon as possible. If endometrial curettage is being used for diagnosis of infection (eg, tuberculous endometritis, salpingitis), a portion of the curettings should be placed in containers appropriate for culture (without fixative).

A single curettage will not remove the entire endometrium. Thorough curettage by an experienced gynecologist often removes 50–60% of the endometrium, as determined by immediate postcurettage hysterectomy. If risk factors for endometrial cancer are present and clinical suspicion for neoplasia persists despite a histologic diagnosis of benign endometrium, further evaluation with hysteroscopically guided biopsy or hysterectomy is indicated.

Perforation of the uterus occurred in 0.63% of a large series of D&Cs. Perforation is suspected when the sound or curet meets no resistance at the point expected by uterine size, consistency, and position determined by preoperative bimanual examination. Curettage may be continued if the area of suspected perforation is avoided. Should suction curettage be associated with perforation, laparoscopy must be used to continue the procedure to avoid aspiration of bowel into the uterine cavity. In the case of suspected perforation, the patient should be observed for at least 24 hours in the hospital for possible infection or hemorrhage. In a series of 70 uterine perforations, 55 were treated expectantly, and only one patient developed complications (pelvic abscess drained via colpotomy). In seven patients, hysterectomy was elected but not indicated by operative findings. Today, laparoscopy is the method of choice for evaluating perforations in the hemodynamically stable patient.

E. Endometrial Biopsy

Outpatient curettage, or endometrial biopsy, should always be a diagnostic and not a therapeutic technique. The many techniques available, all compared to D&C under adequate anesthesia, are discussed in Chapter 36.

HYSTEROSCOPY

This section will discuss therapeutic uses of hysteroscopy.

Indications & Contraindications

See Table 45–1.

Technique

The hysteroscope is a rigid endoscope similar in design to an operating laparoscope or a urologic resectoscope. Typically 6–10 mm in external diameter, the outer sleeve encloses a fiberoptic light source, a channel used to introduce a medium to distend the uterus, and a channel through which probes, forceps, and electrocautery or laser instruments may be visually directed in the uterine cavity. Viewing angles vary from 10 to 45 degrees.

The uterine cavity, which is normally collapsed, must be distended by a medium: dextran-70, CO_2, sodium chloride, lactated Ringer's, glycine, or sorbitol. Two disadvantages to the use of electrolyte solutions such as sodium chloride and lactated Ringer's are mix-

Table 45–1. Indications and contraindications for hysteroscopy.

Indications	Contraindications
Evaluation and treatment of abnormal uterine bleeding	**Absolute contraindications**
Premenopausal/postmenopausal bleeding with negative D&C.	Pelvic inflammatory disease, especially tubo-ovarian complex.
Directed biopsy in patient with atypical adenomatous hyperplasia but at high risk for hysterectomy.	Uterine perforation.
Evaluation of endocervix versus endometrium as origin of biopsy-proved adenocarcinoma.	Sensitivity to anesthetic or distention medium.
Suspicion (on history or hysterography) of uterine polyp or submucous leiomyoma amenable to hysteroscopic resection.	Lack of proper equipment, specifically, low-pressure insufflator for CO_2 distention.
Evaluation and treatment of infertility	Operator inexperience.
Habitual abortion.	**Relative contraindications**
Known uterine septum on previous hysterography or curettage.	Heavy bleeding limiting visual field.
Suspected foreign body (eg, broken or imbedded IUD).	Known gynecologic cancer, especially endometrial, cervical, tubal, and ovarian, because of theoretic risk of flushing cancer cells into the peritoneal cavity.
Suspected submucous leiomyoma on history, pelvic examination, or laparoscopy.	
Suspected cornual occlusion on hysterography.	
Suspected intracervical, intrauterine, or intracornual adhesions.	
Suspected congenital anomaly (eg, with known urologic anomaly).	
Possible intrauterine infection (eg, tuberculosis).	
Intrauterine insemination or embryo transfer in selected patients with known uterine fusion anomaly.	
Suspected endometrial polyp.	

ing of blood, which limits visualization, and the inability to use electrosurgery because these solutions are electroconductors. They should therefore only be used for diagnostic, rather than operative, hysteroscopy. Pressure no greater than 100 mm Hg is required to achieve adequate uterine distention. Instillation of high-viscosity dextran can be done via a 50 mL syringe attached to the hysteroscope. The disadvantage of using dextran is its sticky consistency. Anaphylactic reaction is a rare response to the use of dextran. Care must be taken to avoid intravascular volume expansion and possible pulmonary edema.

CO_2 gas insufflation is favored by some gynecologic surgeons for both office and outpatient hysteroscopy. The addition of a cervical suction cup to prevent leakage has lost favor. The flow rate must not exceed 40–60 mL/min to avoid uterine injury or gas embolism; thus laparoscopic insufflators must never be connected to a hysteroscope. The advantages of CO_2 gas over dextran are easier cleansing of instruments and improved comfort for the surgeon. A disadvantage is more difficult visualization due to mixing with blood or debris.

More and more instruments are available for use in hysteroscopic procedures, including blunt probes, microscissors, alligator clamps with electrocautery attachment, rollerball electrode, and a wire loop for excision and coagulation (resectoscope). The argon laser is useful for lysing septa, and the neodymium:YAG (yttrium, aluminum, garnet) laser is available for polyp and myoma removal and endometrial ablation (see Table 45–2).

Local or general anesthetics are chosen on the basis of expected hysteroscopic findings or procedures, concomitant operations planned, and the desires and cooperation of the patient. Most hysteroscopic examinations and virtually all therapeutic procedures are performed under general anesthesia. Following administration of anesthesia, the urinary bladder is drained, and the ante-

rior lip of the cervix is grasped with a tenaculum. The cervix should then be gradually dilated to the same diameter as the external sleeve of the hysteroscope in order to provide a snug fit. Concomitant laparoscopy is an option in any patient in whom a hysteroscopic therapeutic procedure is planned. Uterine perforation may be observed through the laparoscope, and excess distention media may be aspirated from the posterior cul-de-sac after a prolonged procedure.

An assistant must be constantly present during hysteroscopy to monitor uterine insufflation so that the pressure never exceeds 200 mm Hg, and the flow rate of the distending medium never exceeds 100 mL/min. The surgeon must be sitting comfortably, with all instruments available to perform the hysteroscopic procedure safely and expeditiously. Following the procedure, intrauterine instruments should be inspected for their integrity. The microscissors in particular are delicate and could break within the uterus. If dextran is used, it must be immediately flushed from the hysteroscope before it is allowed to dry.

Complications

Hysteroscopic surgery is generally safe in experienced hands. With laparoscopic observation, the serious complication of uterine perforation can almost always be prevented. If overt bleeding occurs during resection of a septum, polyp, or leiomyoma, the laparoscopic probe can be held against the uterine vessels to slow the blood flow. A Foley catheter may be inserted into the uterine cavity and inflated to provide a tamponade for heavy endometrial bleeding. Infection is an unusual complication following hysteroscopy, although there are surgeons who administer prophylactic antibiotics (doxycycline, 100 mg twice daily for 7 days). Complications of distending media include hyponatremia and pulmonary edema if an excessive amount results in vascular intervasation. These risks can be prevented with close monitoring of fluid use intraoperatively.

Prognosis

With proper selection of patients, hysteroscopic surgery has high success rates. Small pedunculated leiomyomas and polyps are usually retrieved by an experienced, patient surgeon. Submucous leiomyomas may be destroyed if they are not too vascular. In the treatment of intrauterine adhesions, the chance for success and restoration of a normal endometrial cavity depends on the density and extent of the adhesions and the area of normal endometrium remaining after dissection.

Following hysteroscopic surgery for infertility in which the endometrium is denuded, postoperative es-

Table 45–2. Comparison of lasers used in treatment of endometriosis.

	CO₂	Argon	Nd:YAG
Laser wavelength	10.6 µm	0.5 µm	1.06 µm
Depth of tissue destruction	0.1 mm	0.5 mm	4 mm
Beam scattering	None	Slight	Significant
Effect dependent on tissue color	None	Yes	Yes
Delivery by fiberoptic systems	Experimental	Yes	Yes

trogen therapy is prescribed by many physicians to promote rapid endometrial growth.

LAPAROSCOPY

Laparoscopy is a transperitoneal endoscopic technique that provides excellent visualization of the pelvic structures and often permits the diagnosis of gynecologic disorders and pelvic surgery without laparotomy.

Most basic laparoscopes are 4–12 mm in diameter and have a 180-degree viewing angle. The instrument has an effective length of over 25 cm and can be utilized with a fiberoptic light box. In order to facilitate visualization, CO_2 must be instilled into the peritoneal cavity to distend the abdominal wall.

Use of a pneumatic insufflator permits continuous monitoring of the rate, pressure, and volume of the gas used for inflation. In addition to the equipment used for observation, a variety of other instruments for resection, biopsy, coagulation, aspiration, and manipulation can be passed through separate cannulas or inserted through the same cannula as the laparoscope. A laser (CO_2 or Nd:YAG) may be used with the laparoscope.

The laparoscope has become an invaluable tool in both diagnostic and operative gynecologic procedures. However, its use requires considerable expertise, and it should always be used by a surgeon familiar with the management of complications. Laparoscopic procedures are *major* intra-abdominal operations performed through small incisions. This technique is rapidly performed and has a low morbidity rate and a short convalescence period. In many cases, laparoscopy may replace conventional laparotomy for diagnosis and treatment of gynecologic problems. It is a cost-effective outpatient procedure.

Indications

The indications will increase with the clinician's experience and as technical innovations permit even more complicated procedures.

A. DIAGNOSIS

1. Differentiation between ovarian, tubal, and uterine masses, eg, ectopic pregnancy, ovarian cyst, salpingitis, myomas, endometriosis, tuberculosis.
2. Pelvic pain, eg, possible adhesions, endometriosis, ectopic pregnancy, twisted or bleeding ovarian cyst, salpingitis, appendicitis, psychogenic pelvic pain.
3. Genital anomalies, eg, ovarian dysgenesis, uterine maldevelopment.
4. Ascites, eg, ovarian diseases versus cirrhosis.

5. Secondary amenorrhea of possible ovarian origin, eg, polycystic ovarian syndrome, arrhenoblastoma.
6. Pelvic injuries after penetrating or nonpenetrating abdominal trauma.
7. Staging of Hodgkin's disease and lymphomas.
8. Diagnosis of occult cancer.

B. EVALUATION

1. Infertility, eg, tubal patency, ovarian biopsy.
2. "Second look" after tubal surgery or treatment of endometriosis.
3. Assessment of pelvic and abdominal trauma.
4. Appraisal of bowel for viability after surgery, for mesenteric thrombosis.
5. Study of pelvic nodes after lymphography.
6. Peritoneal washings for cytology study.
7. Peritoneal culture.
8. Evaluation of uterine perforation.
9. Evaluation of pelvic viscera to determine the feasibility of vaginal hysterectomy.

C. THERAPY

1. Tubal sterilization:
   a. Electrical: Unipolar or bipolar technique.
   b. Mechanical: Silastic bands, Silastic rings, or metal clips.
2. Lysis of adhesions, with or without laser.
3. Fulguration of endometriosis by laser or thermal cautery.
4. Aspiration of small unilocular ovarian cyst or of fluid for culture.
5. Removal of extruded intrauterine device.
6. Uterosacral ligament division (denervation).
7. Treatment of ectopic pregnancy.
8. Myomectomy.
9. Salpingostomy for phimotic fimbriae.
10. Removal of tuboplastic hoods or splints.
11. Ova collection for in vitro fertilization.
12. GIFT (gamete intrafallopian transfer for fertilization).
13. Mini-wedge resection of ovary.
14. Biopsy of tumor, liver, ovary, spleen, omentum, etc.
15. Placement of intraperitoneal clips as markers for radiotherapy.
16. Oophorectomy.
17. Ovarian cystectomy.

18. Lysis of adhesions or adnexal surgery to allow vaginal hysterectomy ("laparoscopic assisted vaginal hysterectomy").

Contraindications

A. ABSOLUTE

Intestinal obstruction, generalized peritonitis, massive hemorrhage.

B. RELATIVE

Severe cardiac or pulmonary disease, previous periumbilical surgery, shock, cancer involving anterior abdominal wall.

Additional factors weighing against performing laparoscopic surgery include extremes of weight, intrauterine pregnancy after the first or early second trimester, presence of a large mass, inflammatory bowel disease, and known severe intraperitoneal adhesions.

Preparation for Laparoscopy

Careful explanation of the contemplated procedure must be given to each patient prior to surgery. Unless the individual is a poor operative risk, laparoscopy is usually an outpatient operation. Preparation includes no solid food for at least 8 hours prior to surgery, no liquids for more than 6 hours preoperatively, a history and physical examination, and routine blood studies. Abdominal or perineal shaving is usually unnecessary, but skin preparation with an antiseptic is routine.

Anesthesia

Local anesthesia, local anesthesia with systemic analgesia, spinal or epidural block techniques, or general anesthesia with or without endotracheal intubation may be used. Special hazards of anesthesia exist, eg, reduced diaphragmatic excursion because of the pneumoperitoneum and because the patient may be operated on in the Trendelenburg position. Because of these factors, most procedures in the U.S. are performed with the patient under general anesthesia with endotracheal intubation. With adequate understanding of the physiology involved, effective anesthesia and laparoscopy can be accomplished safely.

An alternative to general anesthesia is local anesthesia with intravenous sedation. The patient may experience transient discomfort during manipulation of the uterine tubes, but in selected patients this discomfort is easily tolerated.

Surgical Technique

The patient should be placed with her arms at her sides in the dorsal lithotomy position and draped after induction of anesthesia and preparation of the abdomen and pelvic area. The video monitor should be placed in a position that allows for easy viewing by the surgeon, usually at the patient's feet or side. The bladder must be emptied by catheterization to decrease the risk of injury during subsequent introduction and use of other instruments. After careful bimanual examination, a tenaculum is attached to the cervix, and a tubal insufflation cannula is inserted into the cervical canal and finally fixed to the tenaculum so that it can be used to manipulate the uterus. A 1-cm incision is made within or immediately below the umbilicus; a veress needle is inserted through this incision into the peritoneal cavity. Carbon dioxide should then be introduced and monitored by the pneumatic insufflator. The amount of gas insufflated will vary with the patient's size, the laxity of the abdominal wall, and the planned procedure. In most patients, 2–3 L of gas will be needed to obtain adequate visualization. The maximum insufflation pressure should not exceed 20 mm Hg. The needle is withdrawn and the laparoscopic trocar and cannula inserted. After proper abdominal entry, the trocar may be withdrawn and replaced with the fiberoptic laparoscope. The examiner manipulates the intrauterine cannula so that the pelvic organs can be observed. To test for tubal patency, methylene blue or indigo carmine solution can be injected through the intrauterine cannula. Direct observation of a lack of dye leakage attests to tubal patency. A second trocar with a cannula may be inserted under direct laparoscopic vision through a 5-mm transverse midline incision at the pubic hairline. Additional punctures are utilized as necessary for the placement of other instruments. A number of instruments are available including irrigators, the harmonic scalpel, forceps, scissors, and staple applicators. Surgical knots may be tied and sutures placed using specially made equipment.

The operation is terminated by evacuating the insufflated gas through the cannula, followed by removal of all instruments and placement of a 3-0 subcuticular suture for wound closure. Incisions greater than 10 mm require fascial closure to avoid incisional hernias. A small dressing is applied to the wound. In uncomplicated cases involving diagnosis only, operating time is about 10 minutes. In massively obese patients (> 250 lb) or in patients with previous periumbilical surgery, an open technique may be utilized. A small incision is dissected to the fascia, and the peritoneum is entered under direct visualization. The trocar sleeve is placed in the peritoneal cavity, and Allis forceps or a pursestring suture is used to create an airtight seal. Insufflation is then effected through the sleeve to create the pneumoperitoneum.

A. Sterilization

Electrical cautery, Silastic rings or bands, and metal spring clips achieve sterilization by occluding the uterine tubes. Following sterilization, about 20% of women younger than 30 years old and 5.9% older than 30 years old studied over a 14-year period regretted the procedure. For women under age 30 and of low parity, techniques resulting in lesser amounts of tissue destruction limited to the midportion of the tube are preferred. The advantages or disadvantages of the different techniques are of less significance than the skill with which a physician can perform any one technique; therefore, choice of method should depend on which technique is most comfortable for the physician. The failure rate of most sterilization methods is greater in women less than 28 years old.

1. Cautery—Laparoscopic sterilization with electrical cautery is associated with a very low pregnancy rate, especially when unipolar coagulation is used (7.5/1000 over 10 years). However, bipolar coagulation is less likely to cause injury to adjacent structures (eg, bowel). Excessive tubal destruction is associated with an unacceptably high incidence of ectopic pregnancy, since it may create a tiny fistula from the uterus into the peritoneal cavity through which sperm may travel. Therefore, when using either form (unipolar or bipolar) of electrical coagulation, one should destroy only a short section of the midportion of the uterine tube, avoiding the uterine cornu if possible. Generally, the tube is burned at two to three different locations, and division of the tube by cutting is not necessary.

2. Silastic bands—Tubal occlusion with Silastic bands or rings results in a slightly higher pregnancy rate (17.7/1000 over 10 years) but fewer ectopic pregnancies. Mechanical problems in placement of the bands and bleeding from the tubes during the procedure are more common.

3. Clips—Tubal occlusion with clips of several types is less frequently employed. Failure rates are higher (36.5/1000 over 10 years) than with other techniques and are probably related to poor clip placement.

4. Interval partial salpingectomy—Compared to postpartum tubal ligation, interval partial salpingectomy has a higher failure rate of 20.1/1000 over 10 years.

B. Infertility

In procedures of sterilization reversal, laparoscopic visualization may be needed prior to reanastamosis, particularly if the ligation procedure involved electrocautery.

Peritubal adhesions may be lysed with electric scissors, and salpingostomy may be accomplished. The minimal trauma of these procedures using laparoscopy and the saving of a major operative procedure are obvious benefits. Laparoscopy should be considered for women with complaints of abnormal bleeding and unexplained pelvic pain. More liberal use of the laparoscope has led to the diagnosis of many unsuspected cases of endometriosis.

Electrical fulguration of areas of endometriosis or laser destruction of these diseased areas by laparoscopy is a safe, effective, and rapid treatment. The use of laser obviously allows implants on structures such as bowel, bladder, and the fallopian tubes to be treated with a fairly wide margin of safety. Relief may be immediate and striking, whether the woman has complained of dysmenorrhea, dyspareunia, or generalized pelvic pain. Among infertile patients with lesser stages of endometriosis, pregnancy rates are similar to those in other published studies of treatment with danazol.

In infertility, the laparoscope has been important for ova collection for in vitro fertilization, GIFT, and other procedures. However, it is used less frequently now as most egg retrievals for in vitro fertilization are performed under ultrasound guidance.

C. Ectopic Pregnancy

In hemodynamically stable patients, laparoscopic linear salpingostomy is the preferred method for conservative management of tubal pregnancies. The laparoscopic approach has a similar rate of subsequent intrauterine pregnancy (61.0%) and recurrent ectopic pregnancy (15.5%) compared to abdominal salpingostomy. Advantages to laparoscopy include less blood loss, reduced length of hospital stay, lower cost, and decreased anesthesia requirements. An alternative conservative approach for those who meet the criteria is methotrexate administration.

D. Laparoscopic Hysterectomy

Laparoscopy can be used for total laparoscopic hysterectomy (LH), laparoscopic assisted vaginal hysterectomy (LAVH), and laparoscopic subtotal hysterectomy (LSH; see section on hysterectomy). Other procedures that can be done via the laparoscope include vault suspension and pelvic reconstruction such as retropubic Burch colposuspension.

E. Abdominal and Pelvic Pain

Laparoscopy has proved invaluable in differentiating various causes of acute and chronic pain. The technique may save the patient the necessity of a major exploratory operation. Fluid aspiration and tissue biopsy are possible through laparoscopy. Also, pelvic and intestinal disease can be differentiated. The appendix may be visualized and acute appendicitis may be diagnosed. Numerous cases of pain caused by intra-abdominal adhesions also have been diagnosed by laparoscopy, and relief has been obtained following laparoscopic adhesion resection.

F. Trauma

In cases of intra-abdominal trauma, laparoscopy can be utilized to exclude the need for a major abdominal operation.

G. Miscellaneous

"Missing" IUDs have been removed from the intra-abdominal cavity. Mulligan plastic hoods from tuboplasty procedures, "lost" drains, and other foreign material have been removed from the abdomen by operative laparoscopy.

Postsurgical Care

Patients may be sent home following full recovery from anesthesia, usually in 1–2 hours. Recovery from more extensive procedures such as LH may require a longer hospital stay of 1–2 days. Postoperative pain is usually minimal, and patients are discharged with a prescription for a simple oral analgesic. The most common complaint is shoulder pain secondary to subdiaphragmatic accumulation of gas. Patients are encouraged to resume full activity, except for sexual relations, the day following surgery. Sexual relations may be resumed several days postoperatively after a simple procedure, eg, tubal ligation. Following extensive operative laparoscopy or other gynecologic procedures, coitus should be delayed for an appropriate interval, ie, until it is unlikely to cause discomfort or damage to the operative site. Patients should routinely be seen in the office 1–2 weeks postoperatively.

Complications

A survey conducted by the American Association of Gynecologic Laparoscopists disclosed a complication rate (procedures requiring laparotomy) of 1.6:1000 with sterilization laparoscopy and 3.1:1000 with diagnostic laparoscopy. The higher incidence of complications when the instrument is used for investigation of disease is probably related to the fact that the patients often have had prior laparotomies. As laparoscopists become more experienced, the incidence of complications tends to fall. Complications are infrequent when meticulous care is exercised throughout the procedure.

A. Pain

Pain may be referred from the diaphragm to the shoulder or chest due to pressure from unabsorbed gas. Use of smaller volumes of gas will minimize pain. Gas is usually absorbed within hours. Mild analgesics and rest in the recumbent position should alleviate discomfort.

B. Bleeding

Insertion of a needle and trocar through the abdominal wall has inherent risks. Proper positioning of the penetrating instrument is essential.

(1) Small arterial or venous bleeding usually responds to electrocoagulation or pressure with biopsy forceps. Tubal damage resulting in significant bleeding requiring laparotomy is rare.

(2) Ecchymotic areas in the anterior abdominal wall or omentum need no treatment if no active bleeding is visualized.

(3) Laceration or puncture injuries of the iliac arteries or veins or of the aorta have been reported. If this is likely to have happened, immediate emergency blood replacement and laparotomy for vascular repair must be instituted.

C. Puncture Injury

Injury from a trocar requires laparotomy and repair. Puncture injury to the stomach or bowel by the needle during insufflation of gas usually requires no treatment. In selected cases, injuries to the bowel may be repaired via laparoscopy.

D. Misplacement of Gas

The risk of misplacement of gas into the anterior rectus sheath is minimized by the pneumatic insufflator monitoring equipment, but on occasion it is uncertain whether or not gas has been introduced into the abdominal cavity. Gas disperses rapidly and is absorbed through body tissues, and these qualities provide a safety factor.

E. Thermal Burns

Bipolar sterilization should reduce the number of thermal injuries occurring during laparoscopy, but some still occur. With increased operator experience, the number of serious injuries with unipolar cautery has been reduced drastically. Burn injuries are fewer with improved equipment and operator experience.

F. Vague Unexplained Lower Abdominal Discomfort

Abdominal discomfort in the days following the procedure must be assessed with the possibility of salpingitis in mind. This is uncommon in patients undergoing tubal ligation but is occasionally seen in patients with preexisting tubal disease and chronic pelvic inflammatory disease. Infections of the surgical wound are rare.

Mortality Rates Associated With Laparoscopic Sterilization

The Centers for Disease Control and Prevention studied deaths attributable to tubal sterilization in the U.S. from 1977–1981. Of the 17 deaths associated with laparoscopic sterilization, six followed complications of general anesthesia; five were due to sepsis (in three of these, sepsis was caused by thermal injury to the bowel during electrical sterilization); three were due to hemorrhage; and one each was due to myocardial infarction, pulmonary embolism, and complete heart block. Obesity was the most common preexisting condition in patients who died. Some deaths might have been prevented by the use of endotracheal intubation during general anesthesia. Local anesthesia is safe and effective but, regrettably, is not well accepted by patients or physicians in the U.S.

■ OPERATIONS FOR STERILIZATION OF WOMEN & MEN

Sterilization is a permanent method of contraception. By 1990, tubal sterilization became the most common method of contraception among women in the U.S. Sterilization is the most frequent indication for laparoscopy in the U.S. (> 1 million women per year). A similar number of men choose partial vasectomy for sterilization.

TUBAL STERILIZATION

Tubal sterilization was first performed in 1823 to prevent pregnancy in women who would need repeated cesarean sections. Since the first tubal sterilization was performed, over 200 different techniques have been described. Table 45–3 lists the most common methods of tubal sterilization and their failure rates.

Preoperative Counseling

Clear, comprehensive counseling is essential for women who are considering tubal sterilization. Possible medical and psychologic complications must be carefully outlined (see Complications, later); women are more likely to regret having had the operation if they do not know what to expect.

The physician should be alert to signs that the patient is undecided about having the operation or is being pressured by her husband or others. Regret or dissatisfaction is more common if the procedure is done postpartum than at another time, and these women are more than twice as likely to feel that preoperative counseling was inadequate. Temporary stress associated with

Table 45–3. Overall failure rates with tubal sterilization (over 10 years per 1000 procedures)

Postpartum partial salpingectomy	7.5
Unipolar coagulation	7.5
Bipolar coagulation	24.8
Spring clip	36.5
Silicone rubber band	17.7
Interval partial salpingectomy	20.1
All methods	18.5

Reproduced with permission from Peterson HB et al: The risk of pregnancy after tubal sterilization: findings from the U.S. Collaborative Review of Sterilization. Am J Obstet Gynecol 1996;174:1161.

the pregnancy may have influenced a premature decision for sterilization in these women.

Patients should be told that tubal sterilization is usually not reversible. Some methods are sometimes reversible (see Chapter 58). One article estimates that about 1% of women who undergo tubal sterilization request reversal. In general, success is directly related to the amount of normal tube preserved. Less destructive methods such as clips and bands have reversal rates of 84% and 72%, respectively. The reversal rate following the most commonly performed procedure (Pomeroy method) approaches 50%, and following electrocoagulation is 41%. Ectopic pregnancy rates vary from 1.7–6.5% following reversal; this incidence may increase to 15% when concomitant tubal disorders (eg, pelvic adhesions) exist at the time of anastomosis or develop subsequent to anastomosis.

It is also important for legal reasons that patients be fully informed of the risks, effectiveness, and chances of reversibility of this operation and of alternative procedures. According to the American College of Obstetricians and Gynecologists, there is no need for a hospital committee to approve or disapprove a request for sterilization if the patient is of legal age and sound mind, irrespective of parity. The United States Supreme Court has ruled that the husband's signature is not required for regulation of a woman's fertility. Guidelines have been established by the FDA Bureau of Medical Devices to ensure that safe, efficient endoscopes and other devices are used in sterilization procedures.

Complications

Pain and menstrual disturbances (postbilateral tubal ligation syndrome) have been reported following tubal sterilization. The theory holds that destruction of the mesosalpinx might alter the blood supply and subsequent gonadotropin delivery to the ovary. Ovarian function and hormone production may then be altered. However, prospective controlled studies show that these problems are no more common than in women who have not undergone sterilization. Menstrual changes seem to be related to use of contraceptives—before sterilization. Oral contraceptives are associated with decreased menstrual flow and relief of dysmenorrhea; once they are discontinued, heavier flow and pain may recur. Complaints of menstrual changes are much less frequent in the second half of the first postoperative year. Patients should be told that pelvic pain or menstrual disturbances may develop after tubal sterilization but are no more common than in other women of similar age and parity.

Patients who have undergone tubal sterilization require hysterectomy more frequently than patients who have not undergone this procedure. This is probably because most women who have tubal sterilizations have had children and are therefore more likely to have disorders typically treated with hysterectomy (eg, symptomatic pelvic relaxation, adenomyosis). Patients may have been sterilized secondary to medical reasons and gynecologic disorders that might eventually require further surgery. Some studies suggest that women are more likely to accept a surgical treatment if they have been sterilized.

Failure of sterilization is most often secondary to poor technique, for example, improper application of a clip or ring. Fistula formation may occur. A complication of failure is ectopic pregnancy.

Postoperative psychologic problems correlate well with preoperative problems. Even in patients sterilized in the postpartum period, adverse psychologic effects are rare, and psychiatric disturbance is no more common than in the general population.

An association between decreased risk of ovarian cancer and tubal sterilization has been shown in several studies.

Technique
(See Figures 45–1 through 45–4.)

Postpartum tubal ligation uses a small infraumbilical incision to access the tubes. Minilaparotomy involves a 2–3 cm incision made above the symphysis pubis. The incision is closed in two layers.

OTHER METHODS OF FEMALE STERILIZATION

Because of relatively high morbidity and mortality rates in comparison with tubal occlusion procedures, hysterectomy is justified for sterilization only if there is another unequivocal indication for hysterectomy. Transvaginal tubal ligation via culdotomy or culdoscopy is technically more difficult than transabdominal sterilization and has a higher infection rate. However, there may be less discomfort postoperatively. Experimental methods of transuterine tubal occlusion include electro-

coagulation, silicone plugs, clips, and sclerosing liquids. All are investigational at this time.

VASECTOMY

Vasectomy, or vas occlusion, accounts for 8% of sterilizations worldwide. Partial vasectomy is usually done under local anesthesia via a small incision in the upper outer aspect of the scrotum (Fig 45–5). Sutures or clips are placed tightly around the vas, demarcating a 1- to 1.5-cm segment, which is then excised. The ligated and fulgurated ends are tucked back into the scrotal sac, and the incision is closed. The same procedure is performed on the opposite side. The no-scalpel technique requires no incision because a sharpened dissection forceps is used to pierce the skin and dissect the vas. Studies are being done on the efficacy of intravasal plugs to confer sterility. Microscopic examination confirms excision of vasal tissue.

The failure rate with this technique is estimated to be less than 2 in 1000. Sterility is assumed only after ejaculates are completely free of sperm after 3 months and after periodic microscopic analysis.

Complications are infrequent, usually involving slight bleeding, hematoma formation, skin infection, and reactions to sutures or local anesthetics.

When vasal anastomosis is attempted (vasovasostomy), patency is achieved in 86–97% of patients depending on the interval between vasectomy and vasovasostomy. Pregnancy rates are lower (18–60%). Skillful microsurgery performed by an experienced urologist will optimize the chances of pregnancy.

■ HYSTERECTOMY

Hysterectomy is complete removal of the uterus. With over 575,000 procedures done per year, hysterectomy is the second most common major operation performed in the United States. With advancements in medical and conservative surgical therapy of gynecologic conditions, the need for hysterectomy has declined. More women now wish to avoid major surgery if equally efficacious alternatives exist. Regulatory boards of gynecologists now support the use of hysterectomy as treatment for conditions refractory to more conservative management.

Indications

The indications for hysterectomy can be practically divided into those for the treatment of gynecologic cancer, benign gynecologic conditions, and obstetric complications. Hysterectomy for cancer of the uterus, ovary, and cervix is discussed in Chapters 26 and

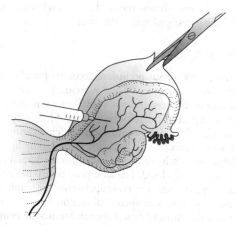

Saline with epinephrine injected below serosa, which becomes inflated locally. Muscular tube, and even blood vessels, can be separated from serosa, which is then cut open.

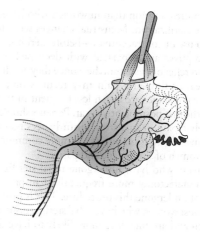

Muscular tube emerges through opening or is pulled out to form a U shape.

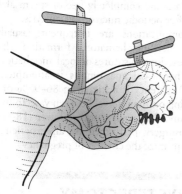

Fimbriated end is untouched, while the end leading to the uterus is stripped of serosa. This can usually be done without damaging blood vessels.

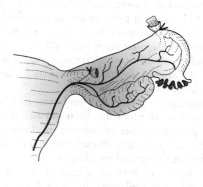

About 5 cm of muscular tube is cut away; the end is buried automatically in serosa. Fimbriated end and serosa opening are closed and tied together.

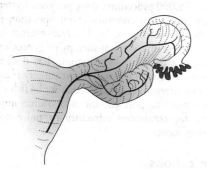

Blood supply continues normally between ovary and uterus. Hydrosalpinx or adhesion has not been noticed.

Figure 45–1. Uchida method of sterilization. (Reproduced, with permission, from Benson RC: *Handbook of Obstetrics & Gynecology*, 8th ed. Lange, 1983.)

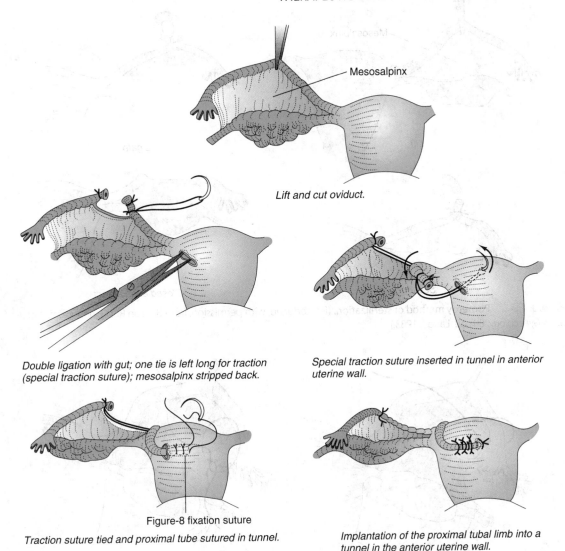

Mesosalpinx

Lift and cut oviduct.

Double ligation with gut; one tie is left long for traction (special traction suture); mesosalpinx stripped back.

Special traction suture inserted in tunnel in anterior uterine wall.

Figure-8 fixation suture

Traction suture tied and proximal tube sutured in tunnel.

Implantation of the proximal tubal limb into a tunnel in the anterior uterine wall.

Figure 45–2. **Irving** method of sterilization. (Reproduced, with permission, from Benson RC: *Handbook of Obstetrics & Gynecology,* 8th ed. Lange, 1983.)

47–49. Hysterectomy for obstetric complications, including excessive bleeding and molar pregnancy, is becoming less common (see Chapter 28).

The most common benign diseases and disorders that warrant hysterectomy are shown in Table 45–4.

Preoperative Evaluation

A. DIAGNOSTIC TESTS TO DETECT OCCULT CANCER

All patients anticipating hysterectomy should have a baseline evaluation to detect occult cancer. A Papani-

colaou smear should be performed within 3 months before operation, and abnormalities should be followed with colposcopic examination and biopsy before surgery. Cervical conization is indicated prior to hysterectomy if (1) colposcopy fails to demonstrate the entire squamocolumnar junction, where cervical cancers typically arise; (2) colposcopically guided biopsies reveal dysplasia that is more severe by two or more grades than that shown on the Papanicolaou smear (eg, carcinoma in situ on smear but mild dysplasia on biopsy); (3) endocervical curettage demonstrates atypical endocervical cells; and (4) biopsy reveals microinva-

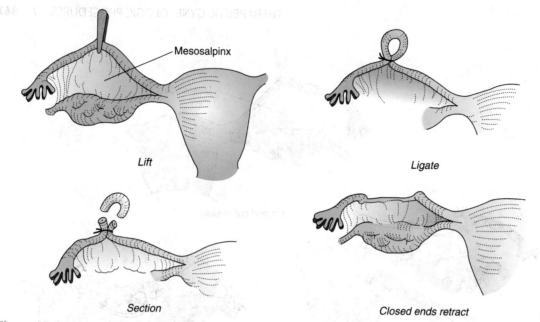

Mesosalpinx

Lift

Ligate

Section

Closed ends retract

Figure 45–3. Pomeroy method of sterilization. (Reproduced, with permission, from Benson RC: *Handbook of Obstetrics & Gynecology*, 8th ed. Lange, 1983.)

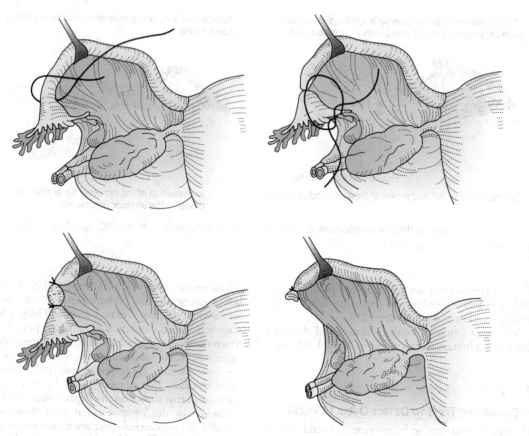

Figure 45–4. Sterilization by fimbriectomy.

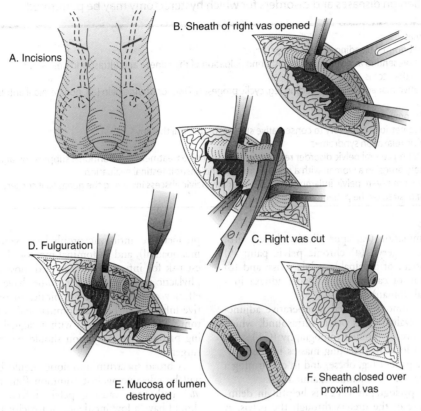

A. Incisions

B. Sheath of right vas opened

C. Right vas cut

D. Fulguration

E. Mucosa of lumen destroyed

F. Sheath closed over proximal vas

Figure 45–5. **Steps in vasectomy.** (Modified from a drawing by S. Taft. Reproduced, with permission, from Schmidt S: Vasectomy should not fail. Contemp Surg 1974;4:13.)

sive squamous cell carcinoma or squamous adenocarcinoma in situ.

Cervical conization for the previous indications is performed to ensure that occult invasive cancer is not present within the endocervical canal. Frozen-section analysis of cervical conization tissue correlates well enough with "permanent" (hematoxylin and eosin) slide analysis that if intraepithelial neoplasia with clear margins is found, the surgeon may, with reasonable certainty, perform a hysterectomy that will totally include the tumor.

Biopsy for endometrial neoplasia must also be considered. Generally any woman over age 35 who presents with abnormal uterine bleeding should have endometrial evaluation (D&C, directed biopsies) before hysterectomy. However, certain clinical situations that produce an unopposed estrogen effect on the endometrium warrant preoperative endometrial evaluation at any age: chronic anovulation and secondary oligomenorrhea, unopposed estrogen therapy for menopause, and known ovarian disorders associated

with endometrial neoplasia (eg, polycystic ovarian syndrome, granulosa cell tumors). Unfortunately, frozen-section analysis of endometrial curettings is neither practical nor accurate, so hysterectomy usually must wait for permanent section.

Occult cancer may also be present outside the genital tract. All patients should have their stool checked for occult blood preoperatively. In women 40 years of age or older, mammography is standard.

B. Preoperative Evaluation of the Pelvis

In the woman with a small, mobile uterus with mobile adnexa, little diagnostic evaluation beyond bimanual examination is indicated. However, pelvic disease may have caused disturbance of normal tissue planes that endanger the urologic and gastrointestinal tracts. The following conditions may indicate the need for more extensive evaluation of the pelvis prior to hysterectomy: (1) pelvic inflammatory disease, especially if repeated, chronic, or associated with a tubo-ovarian complex; (2) endometriosis; (3) pelvic adhesions due to other causes

Table 45–4. Benign diseases and disorders for which hysterectomy may be performed.

Uterine leiomyomas
    Symptomatic (abnormal bleeding or pelvic pressure)
    Asymptomatic (presenting as a large uterus obscuring palpation of the adnexa and ultrasound unavailable)
    Rapid growth of the uterus
    Failed conservative management of bleeding (eg, cyclic progestin, D&C) or uterine pain (eg, nonsteroidal anti-inflammatory
        medications)
Symptomatic adenomyosis
Symptomatic endometriosis refractory to conservative surgical or medical therapy
Symptomatic pelvic relaxation syndromes
Chronic incapacitating central pelvic disorder refractory to conservative treatment (eg, hormonal suppression and nonsteroidal
    antiinflammatory drugs) in a woman with a normal urologic and gastrointestinal evaluation
Definitive treatment of severe pelvic inflammatory disease or any pelvic abscess involving the genitalia if conservative therapy is
    not possible or desired by the patient

---

of pelvic inflammation (eg, appendicitis, cholecystitis, previous pelvic surgery); (4) chronic pelvic pain; (5) questionable origin of a palpable pelvic mass; and (6) clinical suspicion of cancer (eg, palpable adnexa in a postmenopausal woman).

The most commonly utilized preoperative adjunctive diagnostic evaluation is pelvic ultrasound, which has advantages over computed tomography (CT) scan. Ultrasound is helpful in detecting masses in the difficult-to-examine patient (eg, obese) and in confirming a pelvic mass detected on bimanual examination.

Intravenous pyelography (IVP) is helpful in delineating the course of the ureters through the pelvis. A preoperative intravenous pyelogram is especially useful for inflammatory conditions that could distort or obstruct the ureters. Also, patients with genital developmental anomalies should have a preoperative IVP to look for concomitant urologic anomalies.

Prehysterectomy evaluation of the colon (beyond screening for occult blood in the stool) is indicated in any patient with symptoms for rectal disease. In most cases, proctoscopy or flexible proctosigmoidoscopy is sufficient. In cases of severe pelvic inflammation, chronic pelvic pain, or suspected cancer, complete colonoscopy or barium enema is indicated. Preoperative diagnosis of bowel disease will aid in the selection of the incision. If necessary, a consultant gastrointestinal surgeon can be present during the operation.

C. Preoperative Bowel Preparation

See Chapter 43.

D. Prophylactic Antibiotics

Significant infection occurs in 6.6–25% of patients with abdominal hysterectomy versus 4–10% with vaginal hysterectomy. Certain risk factors are associated with a higher likelihood of operative site infection. These factors include long operation (> 2¾ hours), no

preoperative antibiotic prophylaxis, younger age (premenopausal), and abdominal incision. Patients at highest risk for infection were helped most by use of prophylactic antibiotics. Other studies have confirmed the efficacy of prophylactic antibiotics in reducing operative infection in both abdominal and vaginal hysterectomy. Patients diagnosed with a vaginal infection during preoperative evaluation should be treated prior to surgery.

A broad-spectrum antibiotic should be chosen that will be effective against common (but not necessarily *all*) pathogens causing pelvic infection. The agent should have a low incidence of toxicity and side effects and should be easily administered and cost-effective. The proper dosage should be administered 30 minutes prior to surgery. Therapeutic levels must be achieved in tissue at the surgical site. It should *not* be an antibiotic reserved for serious infection. Ampicillin, cefazolin, cefotetan, cefoxitin, cephaloradine, cephalothin, cephradine, doxycycline, metronidazole, clindamycin, and ticarcillin with clavulanic acid are all effective. Intravenous or intramuscular administration is usually used, but intraperitoneal irrigation with antibiotic solution is also effective in reducing cuff infections after abdominal hysterectomy. The ideal antibiotic for prophylaxis would be administered once at the time of surgery.

E. Thromboembolism Prophylaxis

The risk of calf vein thrombosis, proximal vein thrombosis, and pulmonary embolism can be minimized with the use of graduated compression stockings perioperatively and early ambulation postoperatively. Sequential compression devices will help prevent stasis as well. For patients at high risk for thromboembolic disease, a dose of 5000 U subcutaneous heparin is given preoperatively and then every 8–12 hours postoperatively. Risk factors include malignancy, obesity, previous radiation therapy, immobilization, estrogen use, prolonged anesthesia, radical surgery, history of thromboembolism, and personal or family history of hypercoagulability. Other less-often-used prophylactic modalities include low-dose dihydroergotamine-heparin, dextran-70, and low-molecular-weight heparin.

F. Blood Products

Cross-matching of blood is routine in hysterectomy patients. Two to four units of blood should be available. It may not be necessary to preoperatively cross-match all patients undergoing hysterectomy. Women who are not at particular risk of needing a transfusion during hysterectomy should at least have blood typing and antibody screening prior to surgery. Patients undergoing peripartum hysterectomy or hysterectomy for gynecologic cancer are more likely to need blood transfusion. Patients undergoing elective hysterectomy are more likely to need a transfusion if the hematocrit is low (30%), if they have pelvic inflammatory disease or pelvic abscess or adhesions, or if colporrhaphy is performed at the time of vaginal hysterectomy.

G. Informed Consent

Many women desire, and most insurance companies require, a second opinion prior to scheduling an elective hysterectomy. The patient must understand the diagnosis and be aware of alternative therapies and the risks and benefits of the operation. Common risks of surgery such as cuff cellulitis and blood loss are usually explained during preoperative counseling. The current medicolegal climate mandates the discussion of unusual complications, including the possibility of completing a vaginal operation via an abdominal route and the risks of viral illness following transfusion, severe postoperative infection (including adnexal abscess), ectopic pregnancy, and vaginal vault prolapse (see also Chapter 63).

TECHNIQUE

Vaginal Versus Abdominal Hysterectomy

The route of hysterectomy is chosen according to the following guidelines.

A. Pelvic Anatomy

The ideal candidate for vaginal hysterectomy has a gynecoid pelvis with a pubic arch radius greater than 100 degrees, divergent side walls with widely spread pubic rami, and flat sacrum. Some descent of the uterus is helpful but not mandatory; procidentia makes for a more complicated vaginal hysterectomy because of the greater vulnerability of the prolapsed ureters.

B. Uterine Size

Most gynecologists will perform vaginal hysterectomy on a uterus equivalent in size to a uterus at 12 weeks'

gestation or smaller. More experienced surgeons will perform what has been termed "heroic" removal of a uterus equivalent in size to that at 20 weeks' gestation.

C. Adnexa

In patients with symptoms or pelvic findings suggesting adnexal disease that may indicate adnexectomy, the abdominal route for hysterectomy is preferred. Such patients may be candidates for laparoscopic assisted vaginal hysterectomy (LAVH).

D. Gastrointestinal Tract

Especially in older patients or those with significant history of gastrointestinal complaints, the abdominal approach offers an opportunity for complete examination of the bowel. An exception to this rule is the patient planning concomitant cholecystectomy and hysterectomy; some surgeons feel a vaginal hysterectomy and subcostal incision are preferable to a single midline xiphoid-to-symphysis incision in terms of wound complications and recuperation time.

E. Urologic Disorders

If a retropubic urethropexy is planned, a laparoscopic or abdominal approach can be used. If anterior vaginal colporrhaphy only is planned, vaginal hysterectomy is preferred. Advanced degrees of cystocele, with marked prolapse of the urethrovesical angle, may be best treated with a combined vaginal and abdominal approach (see Chapter 41).

F. Pelvic Relaxation

In the case of isolated rectocele, a vaginal approach is preferred. Culdoplasty for enterocele may be performed by either route.

G. Plastic Procedures

As more women choose to undergo procedures such as abdominoplasty or suction-assisted lipectomy, an abdominal approach is indicated. Perineorrhaphy and vaginal repairs usually accompany vaginal hysterectomies but can also be done after abdominal hysterectomy.

H. Medical Disorders

In patients with significant heart or lung disease, the vaginal approach is preferable when possible because of a lower incidence of postoperative pulmonary complications and earlier ambulation.

I. Previous Surgery

Most surgeons are willing to perform a vaginal hysterectomy in patients with previous tubal ligation or cesarean section. The surgery would be more problematic in patients with a history of multiple cesarean births or complications (eg, postpartum endomyoparametritis) or with probable abdominal adhesions from previous laparotomy. LAVH may be used in these situations.

The preceding guidelines may certainly be adjusted to the individual patient based on the surgeon's experience and abilities. An examination performed under anesthesia when the physician first sees the patient may help to decide on the approach. Uterine size can be assessed with transvaginal ultrasound. Laparoscopic evaluation of the adnexa will further aid in the decision. All patients anticipating vaginal hysterectomy, LH, or LAVH should be told that the operation may have to be completed abdominally if difficulties arise.

Abdominal Hysterectomy

The technique of abdominal hysterectomy varies according to the indication for the operation, the size and placement of vital structures including the ureters (which may be distorted), and the pelvic anatomy. A standard, well-organized approach to abdominal hysterectomy is essential to avoid incidental injury. Modifications are made as necessary, always within an organized plan of operation.

The anesthetic of choice typically includes general endotracheal intubation, an inhalation agent, and an analgesic. Hysterectomies are of such duration and risk that using a mask alone is unwise. In patients with pulmonary compromise, spinal or epidural anesthesia may be used.

A sterile scrub of the abdomen and vagina is done, and a urinary catheter is placed so that the anesthesiologist can monitor urine output intraoperatively. The choice of incision is based on the suspected disease or disorder; in general, a midline incision extending from 2 fingerbreadths above the pubic symphysis to the umbilicus offers the greatest exposure. One modification of the low transverse incision to improve exposure is the Maylard muscle-splitting procedure or the Cherney detachment of the rectus muscles from their insertion on the pubic symphysis.

The surgeon and assistants should rinse excessive talcum powder from their gloves before making the incision to prevent granulomatous tissue reaction in the wound. Once the incision is complete, peritoneal fluid may be aspirated if the possibility of gynecologic cancer exists. The pelvic organs are then inspected and the upper abdomen palpated in a systematic fashion: right gutter, right hemidiaphragm, liver, gallbladder, pancreas, stomach (assessing the position of the indwelling gastric decompression tube), and spleen and right hemidiaphragm (gently, because of the risk of trauma to the spleen), left gutter, para-aortic lymph nodes, and omentum. Excessive bowel manipulation should be avoided to decrease the severity of postoperative ady-

namic ileus; at the least, the appendix and cecum should be inspected as well as the terminal meter of ileum. Older patients and those with gastrointestinal complaints would benefit from careful palpation and inspection of the bowel from rectum to ligament of Treitz. If desired, the wound may be protected with moist towels, a self-retaining retractor placed, and the bowel packed into the upper abdomen.

The classic extrafascial hysterectomy performed by Richardson remains the mainstay of surgical technique in abdominal hysterectomy (see Fig 36–9). Choice of suture and needle is made according to surgeon experience and preference; 2-0, 0, or 1 absorbable sutures on half-curved taper needles are standard choices. The uterus is grasped either by the fundus with a Massachusetts double-toothed clamp or at the cornu with Ochsner or Kocher clamps. The round ligament is clamped proximal to the uterus; at its midportion, it is ligated by suture, and the suture is tagged with a small hemostat. The round ligament is divided about 0.5 cm proximal to the suture, thus opening the broad ligament at its apex. The anterior uterine peritoneum may be incised at the vesicouterine junction in preparation for advancement of the bladder. The peritoneum only should be incised; the potentially vascular areolar tissue should be avoided. When this procedure is repeated on the contralateral side, the anterior leaves of the broad ligament are opened, the uterine vessels first become apparent, and attention is then directed to the posterior leaf of the broad ligament.

The posterior leaf of the broad ligament is incised beginning at the ligated round ligament. The extent of the incision is determined by the decision to preserve or remove the adnexa. If the adnexa are to be removed, the peritoneum is incised parallel to the infundibulopelvic ligament to the pelvic sidewall; the loose areolar tissue is dissected medial to the internal iliac (hypogastric) artery, which is typically 0.5 cm thick with a visually appreciable (and certainly palpable) pulse. The dissection will reveal a clear area of peritoneum under the infundibulopelvic ligament; below this area at a variable distance lies the ureter on this medial flap of peritoneum.

The intimate proximity of the ureters to the uterus makes ureteral dissection important. Whereas the ureter is usually 4–6 cm deep to the infundibulopelvic ligament at the lateral margin of the uterus, it is only 0.5–2 cm below this vascular bundle at the level of the pelvic brim. Observing the ureter through the peritoneum or palpating the characteristic "snap" of the ureter should serve only to guide dissection and should not be a substitute for identification of the entire ureter through its pelvic course. The ureter tolerates careful dissection well as long as its blood-carrying adventitia is not stripped away. The ureter can always be found and dissection begun at the pelvic brim, where the ureter passes over the bifurcation of the iliac artery. The most serious ureteral injury is the unrecognized insult. The most common ureteral injuries during hysterectomy occur during ligation of the infundibulopelvic ligament, clamping and suture ligation of the uterosacral-cardinal ligament complex, placement of vaginal angle sutures, ligation of the vesicouterine ligament, ligation of the hypogastric artery as an adjunctive measure to lessen operative blood loss, and reperitonealization of the pelvic floor.

Once the course of the ureters is well established, the adnexal component of the operation is completed. If the adnexa are to be removed, a ligating suture may be passed beneath the infundibulopelvic ligament and above the ureter; this step is repeated for a double ligature as a precaution. Traditionally, the infundibulopelvic ligament is clamped, divided, and ligated; the direct suture technique may avoid undue crushing of tissue. The ligament is ligated again adjacent to the uterus to avoid back bleeding; the infundibulopelvic ligament is divided and the peritoneum incised to the back of the uterine fundus, always cognizant of the proximity of the ureter. If the adnexa are to be preserved, a hole is made in the avascular portion of the posterior leaf of the broad ligament superior to the ureter. The utero-ovarian ligament and fallopian tube are doubly clamped, divided, and ligated, with care taken to avoid incorporation of ovarian tissue into the ligature.

The final step is extending the peritoneal incision posteriorly around the uterus between the medial portions of the uterosacral ligaments. If the incision of the posterior leaf of the broad ligament is extended over the uterosacral ligaments, there is typically significant bleeding just lateral to the insertion of the ligament at the uterus. The advantages of making an incision between the uterosacrals include clear identification of the rectum and its separation from the uterus, ease of suturing the vaginal cuff, and improved mobility of the peritoneum to allow reperitonealization under less tension.

The bladder is advanced down off of the lower uterine segment prior to clamping the uterine vessels. Surgeons-in-training have more difficulty with advancement of the bladder than with other aspects of abdominal hysterectomy. The principal difficulty in mobilization of the bladder is failure to identify the proper cleavage plane between the bladder and the uterus. At the attachment of the bladder to the lower uterine segment, a median raphe is variably present; it is typically a 1-cm long longitudinal band of thick connective tissue. The raphe is attenuated in pregnant or postmenopausal patients. The raphe is divided at midportion, and loose avascular fibroareolar tissue is seen immediately between the cervix and bladder. The

uterus is retracted posteriorly and superiorly, roughly at an angle of 30 degrees to the long axis of the vagina. The midpoint of the peritoneal incision of the bladder flap is gently lifted with forceps; the avascular plane of the vesicovaginal and vesicocervical areolar spaces is continuous once the median raphe is divided. Metzenbaum scissors are pointed to the uterus, and sharp dissection reveals the shiny white pubocervical fascia overlying the cervix. Properly done, the dissection is bloodless, and the plane is recognized by the ease with which the bladder falls away from the cervix. The vesicouterine space is developed 2 cm beyond the anterior vaginal fornix. Care must be exercised in any dissection laterally, because the vesicouterine ligaments ("bladder pillars") may bleed because of the paracervical and paravaginal veins present laterally.

The uterine vessels may be skeletonized by separating the loose avascular areolar connective tissue from the vessels. The intraligamentous course of the ureter is again checked; it is typically 2–3 cm inferolateral to the insertion of the uterine vessels into the uterus. The uterine vessels are clamped with a curved crushing clamp (eg, Heaney, Pfannen, or curved Ballantine clamp). Double-clamping is used for larger vessels. It is not necessary to place another clamp on the uterine side of the pedicle to prevent back bleeding if the uterine arteries on both sides of the uterus are clamped before either pedicle is incised. The clamp is applied at the level of the internal os, with the tip of the clamp at a right angle to the long axis of the cervix; the temptation to clamp the entire cervix and "slide off" dragging paracervical tissue into the pedicle should be avoided in order to minimize the risk of the pedicle slipping out of the clamp. The uterine vessels are then ligated by suture at the tip of the clamp. Occasionally, a second application of the curved clamp is necessary to complete ligation of the uterine vessels.

Next, the cardinal ligament is assessed. Ordinarily, a single application of a straight clamp (Ochsner, Kocher, or Ballantine clamp) will include the cardinal ligament to the level of its attachment at the lateral edge of the cervix and upper vagina. A deep knife is often useful in dividing the cardinal ligament adjacent to the uterus, leaving a larger pedicle, which is less likely to slip out of the suture than one remaining after cutting with scissors flush to the clamp. The suture ligature of the cardinal ligament is often tagged to aid in manipulation of the vaginal cuff.

The uterosacral ligaments are clamped at their insertion into the lower cervix, divided at their insertion, and ligated. Alternatively, they may be transected with large Mayo scissors while the vagina is entered posterolaterally. If division and suture ligation of either pedicle of the cardinal-uterosacral ligament complex fails to enter the vagina, the safest approach is to enter the vagina with the knife in the midline, either anteriorly or posteriorly, at the confluence of the vagina with cervix. Once entered, the cervix is circumferentially incised, with long Ochsner clamps used to control point bleeders and elevate the vaginal cuff. The cervix is inspected to ensure complete excision.

Sutures are placed at each lateral vaginal angle to ligate small paravaginal vessels coursing upward through the paravaginal tissues and to provide vaginal vault support. The suture is begun inside the vagina 1 cm from the upper border, then incorporates the cardinal and uterosacral ligaments, and finally transverses the vagina again to end up within the vagina. This suture is tagged, and the procedure is repeated on the contralateral side.

Surgical management of the cuff is individualized. In the case of marked pelvic inflammation and persistent oozing, the cuff may be left open to afford retroperitoneal drainage or allow egress of a closed drain system. In most cases, closing the cuff may reduce granulation tissue and possibly minimize ascension of bacteria from the vagina. The cuff may be closed with either interrupted figure-of-eight sutures or a double running suture; the key points with either closure are inversion of the cut edges into the vagina and hemostasis.

The pelvis is irrigated and hemostasis checked in a systematic fashion from one lateral pedicle to the ipsilateral round ligament pedicle to the cuff and on to the other side. Small bleeding vessels must be ligated to minimize the risk of retroperitoneal hematoma formation, which may expand or become infected. For diffuse oozing, hemostatic agents such as thrombin powder or thrombostatic absorbable sponges may be useful. There is no advantage to closing the parietal peritoneum.

Retained ovaries may be suspended to minimize the risk of torsion and adherence to the vaginal cuff. The utero-ovarian ligament can be conveniently attached to the round ligament stump to suspend the ovaries above the pelvis without placing the infundibulopelvic ligament under tension.

The abnormal appendix should be removed. In cases of hysterectomy for endometriosis, appendectomy will reveal microscopic endometriotic foci in some 3% of cases.

Supracervical Hysterectomy

Supracervical/subtotal hysterectomy, or removal of the uterine corpus without the cervix, made up 95% of hysterectomies prior to the 1940s. Despite Papanicolaou's introduction of his cervical smear, concern over neoplastic changes occurring in the retained cervix made total abdominal hysterectomy (TAH) the leading approach to surgery from the 1950s and on. Debate has been renewed about which approach leads to decreased morbidity. Proponents of supracervical hysterectomy believe that there is less damage to sympathetic and parasympathetic innervation that might occur with paracervical dissection. Thus, bladder function and orgasm are less likely to be affected with supracervical hysterectomy. Also, by leaving the cervix, vault prolapse and vaginal shortening might be avoided. Those in favor of TAH suggest that it decreases the risk of cervical cancer, especially in women who might not follow up for routine Pap smears. Current indications for supracervical hysterectomy include difficulty dissecting the cervix, distorted anatomy secondary to pelvic inflammatory disease or endometriosis, and compromised medical condition.

Following ligation of the uterine vessels, the uterine fundus may be amputated from the cervix; the level of amputation should be below the internal cervical os to avoid postoperative uterine bleeding from endometrial remnants. The cervical stump is closed with figure-of-eight sutures.

Vaginal Hysterectomy

Most vaginal hysterectomies are performed under general anesthesia. In the patient with medical complications, particularly pulmonary problems, spinal anesthesia may be elected. Following administration of the anesthetic, a bimanual examination is mandatory before beginning surgery. The perineum is shaved or trimmed as necessary and a sterile wash performed. The patient is placed in a modified dorsal lithotomy position and draped; the surgeon should participate in proper positioning of the patient, because excessive flexion of the hips can stretch the obturator nerves, and excessive extension of the knee can jeopardize the peroneal nerves. All bony prominences and soft tissues in contact with the leg stirrups should be carefully padded.

The urinary bladder may be drained by catheter, but this step is optional. The cervix is grasped with a tenaculum. Passage of a uterine sound will aid in determining the size and position of the uterus; some advocate performing a D&C at this point to rule out pyometra or endometrial neoplasia.

As the surgeon exerts gentle traction downward on the cervix, two assistants maintain exposure with lateral vaginal retractors and protect the bladder with an anterior Heaney retractor. If desired, the junction of the vagina and cervix can be injected with a 1% 1:1000 epinephrine solution to minimize blood loss during incision of the cervix. Beginning posteriorly to minimize obscuring the field with blood, the surgeon circumferentially incises the cervix down to the level of the pubovesicocervical fascia. Gentle traction with the bladder retractor and downward traction of the cervix will allow exposure of the fibers of fascia between bladder and cervix, which are incised. When the bladder has been advanced up off of the cervix, attention is given to the posterior attachment of the cervix. While the assistant pulls the uterus upward, the posterior vaginal mucosa is tented away from the cervix. With the patient in the Trendelenburg position to allow as much emptying of the posterior cul-de-sac as possible, the posterior cul-de-sac is incised with a single stroke of the scissors. A retractor is placed within the opening, exposing the uterosacral ligaments. The uterosacral ligaments are grasped with Heaney clamps, making certain that the peritoneum posterior to the ligament is within the clamp. The ligament is cut and ligated with 2-0 or 0 absorbable suture and tagged with a hemostat for later manipulation of the cuff.

The cardinal ligament may next be clamped if the bladder is safely advanced; likewise, the uterine vessels are included in the next application of the Heaney clamps. The anterior cul-de-sac is entered by blunt and sharp dissection to the anterior vesicouterine fold of peritoneum. The anterior retractor is placed within this opening and the bladder is gently lifted upward. The surgeon now clamps, incises, and ligates in pedicles the remaining portions of the broad ligaments bilaterally, incorporating the tissue between the anterior and posterior leaves of the broad ligament. The round ligament, utero-ovarian ligament, and fallopian tube are excised from the uterus and incorporated into these pedicles, and the uterus is removed from the field. A larger uterus may require special manipulation for delivery through the vaginal introitus (eg, bivalving the uterus in the midline, morcellation of the uterus into multiple extractable segments, or myomectomy).

The final suture on the utero-ovarian ligament is tagged to allow careful inspection of the tubes and ovaries. If ovarian disease is suspected or if prophylactic oophorectomy is planned, a clamp is placed above the ovary and uterine tube on the infundibulopelvic ligament for suture ligature, while traction is placed on the last stay suture. The entire ovary must be removed, because an ovarian remnant may become cystic and produce pain many years after the hysterectomy.

Once all pedicles are inspected and found to be hemostatic, the peritoneum is closed with a running 2-0 absorbable suture, incorporating the cardinal and uterosacral ligament pedicles for support of the vaginal vault. Lateral vaginal angle sutures are placed from the vaginal mucosa at 2 o'clock, inside the cuff and including the uterosacral pedicle, then out through the cuff to the 4 o'clock position. If anterior or posterior colporrhaphy is planned, that operation is completed prior to complete closure of the cuff. The cuff may be closed by an interrupted absorbable 0 suture, a running simple suture, or a running vertical mattress technique. The goals of closure are obliteration of the cuff's dead space back to the peritoneum and approximation of the cut edges of the vagina to afford healing and minimize postoperative granulation tissue. Modifications of the just-described technique are made by virtually every gynecologic surgeon based on operative findings and experience. Many surgeons will close the posterior cul-de-sac to prevent development of an enterocele or will shorten the uterosacral ligaments to suspend the vaginal vault. As in abdominal hysterectomy, the cuff can be left open to promote drainage with a running locked absorbable 0 suture. Another technique to drain the closure is insertion of a T-tube above the cuff, which is associated with a demonstrable reduction in postoperative febrile morbidity.

After the operation is completed, the vagina and perineum are gently cleansed. An indwelling bladder catheter is inserted and a vaginal pack may be placed. The patient is returned slowly to the dorsal supine position.

Laparascopic Hysterectomy

The laparoscope can be used to aid vaginal hysterectomy by freeing abdominal adhesions (laparoscopic assisted vaginal hysterectomy; LAVH) or to free the uterus in its entirety with removal via the vagina (total laparoscopic hysterectomy; LH). Supracervical hysterectomy can also be done laparoscopically with morcellation and removal by culdotomy or through extended trocar sites. Advantages to LH include decreased length of hospital stay, decreased postoperative analgesia, and decreased convalescence period. There may be a lower complication rate compared to TAH but there is no difference versus vaginal hysterectomy. However, the laparoscopic approach requires significantly more operating time and a well-trained, experienced surgeon. Because of the costs for the endoscopic equipment, LH has been found to be more expensive despite the shorter hospital stay. Complications with LH include hemorrhage and bowel or urinary tract damage. Conversion to abdominal hysterectomy may occur, especially in cases with large leiomyomas obstructing access to upper pedicles.

Postoperative Care of the Hysterectomy Patient

The details of postoperative care are dictated by the indications for surgery and the individual patient's overall medical condition. General guidelines include the following:

(1) A Foley catheter is left indwelling for 24 hours.

(2) Prophylactic antibiotics are given only within the first 24 hours postoperatively.

(3) Hydration, 2–3 L/d of balanced electrolyte solution, is given intravenously, depending on blood loss and intraoperative replacement.

(4) Sips of water are given the first night, followed by clear liquids on the next postoperative day or two. The diet is advanced based on return of bowel sounds and appetite, toleration of the diet, and the passage of flatus.

(5) Prophylactic heparin therapy, sequential compression device, or antiembolic stockings are used in patients according to risk for thromboembolic complications.

(6) Ambulation is begun on the first postoperative day.

(7) Adequate analgesia is given parenterally. Once the patient can tolerate a regular diet, she can be switched to oral analgesics.

Complications

Perioperative deaths may be due to cardiac arrest, coronary occlusion, or respiratory paralysis. Postoperative deaths are usually the result of hemorrhage, infection, pulmonary embolus, or intercurrent disease. A recent study of factors contributing to the risk of death found that abdominal hysterectomies performed for complications of pregnancy or cancer (8% of all hysterectomies) account for 61% of deaths due to hysterectomy. Overall mortality rates for abdominal or vaginal hysterectomy are 0.1–0.2%. Mortality rates increase with age and medical complications for both vaginal and abdominal hysterectomies.

The bladder may be injured in 1–2% of all hysterectomies. Consequences are slight if the injury is to the dome of the bladder—which is usually the case—away from the trigone. Ureteral injury occurs in 0.7–1.7% of abdominal hysterectomies and 0–0.1% of vaginal hysterectomies. The essential point is to recognize urologic injuries and correct them intraoperatively, avoiding the serious postoperative complications that occur from urinary extravasation.

Damage to the bowel is quite uncommon, particularly with vaginal hysterectomy. In preparation for abdominal hysterectomy for suspected extensive or inflammatory pathologic process (eg, ovarian cancer, endometriosis, pelvic inflammatory disease), preoperative bowel preparation will allow incidental colon surgery without the necessity of colostomy. Small bowel injuries, assuming no obstruction, are closed in layers perpendicular to the long axis of the bowel; a running layer of 3-0 sutures in the mucosa is supported by interrupted 2-0 silk sutures in the serosa. If a transmural large bowel injury occurs and no preoperative bowel preparation was given, a temporary diverting colostomy may be indicated to protect the suture line and lower the risk of peritonitis and sepsis.

The most serious postoperative complication is hemorrhage (0.2–2% of patients). Bleeding usually originates at the lateral vaginal angles and is amenable to vaginal resuturing in most cases. Blood products are replaced as needed.

Infection remains the most common complication following hysterectomy. Even with immaculate technique and careful patient selection, the gynecologic surgeon can still expect a 10% rate of postoperative febrile morbidity. A postoperative temperature of 38 °C (100.4 °F) or higher on two consecutive determinations 6 hours apart must be investigated by (1) careful interview of the patient for localizing symptoms (eg, productive cough, intravenous line pain), (2) thorough physical examination (including pelvic examination for inspection and palpation of the cuff), and (3) appropriate laboratory studies (eg, urinalysis, Gram-stained smear of sputum, or complete blood count).

Antibiotics are begun only if a focus of infection is identified or highly suspected. Broad-spectrum antibiotics covering anticipated pathogens are prescribed; single-agent semisynthetic penicillins (eg, piperacillin) and cephalosporins (eg, cefoxitin) offer sufficient coverage. In the presence of sepsis, multiagent comprehensive coverage (eg, a penicillin, an aminoglycoside, and an anaerobic agent such as clindamycin or metronidazole) must be prescribed.

Granulation of the vaginal vault is part of the normal healing process and is evident on speculum examination in over half of cases. The granulation is rarely troublesome; light cauterization with silver nitrate sticks or electrocautery eliminates the granulation tissue promptly in most cases. Many suggestions have been made on ways to minimize granulation, including management of the cuff (open versus closed), choice of suture (plain gut versus chromic versus newer synthetics), and drainage techniques. The most important common denominator is close apposition of the cut vaginal edges, which can be accomplished with any of the techniques.

REFERENCES

American College of Obstetricians and Gynecologists: Antibiotics and gynecologic infections. ACOG Technical Bulletin No. 237, 1997.

American College of Obstetricians and Gynecologists: Uterine leiomyomata. ACOG Educational Bulletin No. 192, 1994.

Bronz L: Hysteroscopy in the assessment of postmenopausal bleeding. Contrib Gynecol Obstet 2000;20:519.

Cha SH et al: Fertility outcome after tubal anastamosis by laparoscopy and laparotomy. J Am Assoc Gynecol Laparosc 2001;8:34852.

Cheong YC, Bajekal N, Li TC: Peritoneal closure—to close or not to close. Hum Reprod 2001;16:154852.

Christman GM, Uechi H: Female sterilization. Female Patient 2000;25:4856.

Cosson M et al: Vaginal, laparoscopic, or abdominal hysterectomies for benign disorders: immediate and early postoperative complications. Eur J Obstet Gynecol Reprod Biol 2001;98:2316.

Doucette RC, Scott JR: Comparison of laparoscopically assisted vaginal hysterectomy with abdominal and vaginal hysterectomy. J Reprod Med 1996;41:1.

Ewies AA, Olah KS: Subtotal abdominal hysterectomy: a surgical advance or a backward step. Br J Obstet Gynaecol 2000;107:13169.

Farquhar CM, Steiner CA: Hysterectomy rates in the United States 1990–1997. Obstet Gynecol 2002;99:22934.

Gentile GP, Kaufman SC, Helbig DW: Is there any evidence for a posttubal sterilization syndrome? Fertil Steril 1998;69:179.

Harris WJ. Early complications of abdominal hysterectomy and vaginal hysterectomy. Obstetrical and Gynecological Survey. 1995;50(1):795–805.

Hillis SD et al: Poststerilization regret: findings from the United States Collaborative Review of Sterilization. Obstet Gynecol 1999;93:889.

Holtz G: Laparoscopy in the massively obese female. Obstet Gynecol 1987;69:423.

Kim SH et al: Microsurgical reversal of tubal sterilization: a report on 1118 cases. Fertil Steril 1997;68:865.

Makinen J et al: Morbidity of 10,110 hysterectomies by type of approach. Hum Reprod 2001;16:14738.

Marlow JL: Media and delivery systems. Obstet Gynecol Clin North Am 1995;22:409.

Marana R et al: Current practical application of office endoscopy. Curr Opin Obstet Gynecol 2001;13:3837.

Mintz PD, Sullivan MF: Preoperative crossmatch ordering and blood use in elective hysterectomy. Obstet Gynecol 1985;65:389.

Munro MG, Deprest J: Laparoscopic hysterectomy: does it work?: A bicontinental review of the literature and clinical commentary. Clin Obstet Gynecol 1995;38:401.

Munro MG: Supracervical hysterectomy: . . . a time for reappraisal. Obstet Gynecol 1997;89:133.

Palmer RH et al: Cost and quality in the use of bloodbank services for normal deliveries, cesarean sections, and hysterectomies. JAMA 1986;256:219.

Peterson HB et al: The risk of pregnancy after tubal sterilization: findings from the U.S. Collaborative Review of Sterilization. Am J Obstet Gynecol 1996;174:1161.

Rhodes JC et al: Hysterectomy and sexual functioning. JAMA 1999;282:20.

Rowlands S: Counselling and consent in vasectomy. J Roy Soc Med 2002;95:567.

Sakellariou P et al: Management of ureteric injuries during gynecological operations: 10 years experience. Eur J Obstet Gynecol Reprod Biol 2002;101:17984.

Schafer M et al: Trocar and veress needle injuries during laparoscopy. Surg Endosc 2001;15:27580.

Smith GL, Taylor GP, Smith KF: Comparative risks and costs of male and female sterilization. Am J Public Health 1985; 75:370.

Summit RL et al: A multicenter randomized comparison of laparoscopically assisted vaginal hysterectomy and abdominal hysterectomy in abdominal hysterectomy candidates. Obstet Gynecol 1998;92:321.

Tadir Y et al: Actual effective CO_2 laser power on tissue in endoscopic surgery. Fertil Steril 1986;45:492.

Tittel A et al: New adhesion formation after laparoscopic and conventional adhesiolysis: a comparative study in the rabbit. Surg Endosc 2001;15:446.

Tulandi T, Saleh A: Surgical management of ectopic pregnancy. Clin Obstet Gynecol 1999;42:31.

Wadstrow J, Gerdin B: Closure of the abdominal wall: how and why? Acta Clin Scand 1990;156:75.

Wilson EW: Sterilization. Baillieres Clin Obstet Gynecol 1996; 10:103.

Wingo PA et al: The mortality risk associated with hysterectomy. Am J Obstet Gynecol 1985;152:803.

SECTION V
GYNECOLOGIC ONCOLOGY

Premalignant & Malignant Disorders of the Vulva & Vagina

46

Wendy A. Satmary, MD, Sanaz Memarzadeh, MD, Donna M. Smith, MD, & David L. Barclay, MD

PREINVASIVE DISEASE OF THE VULVA

General Considerations

The vulvar skin is one component of the anogenital epithelium, extending from the distal vagina to the perineum and perianal skin. The lower genital tract epithelium is of common cloacogenic origin. Neoplasia of the vulvar skin is often associated with multiple foci of dysplasia in the lower genital tract. A strong association exists between sexually transmitted diseases and vulvar intraepithelial neoplasia (VIN), primarily HPV, but also gonorrhea, syphilis, *Gardnerella vaginalis,* trichomonas, and HIV. Approximately 35–50% of VIN lesions are positive for high-risk HPV types, primarily HPV 16. Other risk factors include smoking and other genital precancers or cancers. VIN can also be classified into viral and nonviral etiologies. Younger women are more commonly affected by viral VIN than older women and are also more likely to exhibit multifocal disease. The incidence of VIN and HPV has been increasing over the past decade; however, the incidence of vulvar carcinoma has remained relatively constant. The long-term risk of malignant transformation of treated VIN III has been estimated at 3.4–7% and the risk for progression of untreated VIN is thought to be higher.

Premalignant lesions of the vulva occur in both premenopausal and postmenopausal women, with the median age being approximately 40. The average age is shifting towards younger women, with 75% of lesions occurring during the premenopausal period. There is no racial predisposition to VIN and the disease process is often asymptomatic. The most common presenting symptom is pruritus, which is seen in more than 60% of patients with VIN. The diagnosis is made by careful inspection of the vulvar area followed by biopsy of suspicious lesions.

Pathology

In 1989, the International Congress of the International Society for the Study of Vulvar Disease (ISSVD) adopted a standard of reporting vulvar dysplastic lesions as vulvar intraepithelial neoplasia (VIN) I, II, and III, depending on the degree of epithelial cellular maturation. This terminology has replaced the old and more confusing terms used to describe this disease process such as Bowen's disease, erythroplasia of Queyrat, and bowenoid papulosis. The degree of loss of epithelial cellular maturation in a given lesion defines the grade of VIN. In VIN I, immature cells occur in the lower one-third of the epithelium. Complete loss of cellular maturation in the full thickness of epithelium is defined as VIN III, which is also synonymous with carcinoma in situ of the vulva. VIN II is intermediate between VIN I and VIN III.

In contrast to intraepithelial carcinoma of the cervix, which seems to arise from a single point of origin, dysplasia of the vulva is often multicentric. These lesions may be discrete or diffuse, single or multiple, flat or raised. They even form papules and vary in color from the white appearance of hyperkeratotic tumors to a velvety red or black.

The microscopic appearance of dysplastic vulvar lesions is characterized by cellular disorganization and loss of stratification that involves essentially the full thickness of the epithelium. Cellular density is increased, and individual cells vary greatly in size, with giant and multinucleated cells, numerous mitotic figures, and hyperchromatism (Fig 46–1). HPV cyto-

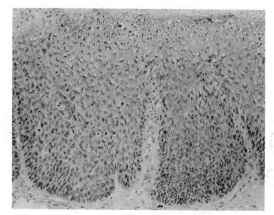

Figure 46–1. Carcinoma in situ demonstrating hyperkeratosis, acanthosis, and parakeratosis. The rete ridges are elongated and thickened, and individual cells are atypical.

pathic changes, such as perinuclear halos with displacement of nuclei, are also common.

Diagnosis

Possibly 1–2% of young women with cervical dysplasia will be found to have multifocal disease that tends to involve the upper third of the vagina and the vulva, perineum, and perianal areas—these surfaces arising from a common cloacogenic origin. A spectrum of disease may be found ranging from mild dysplasia to carcinoma in situ. Involvement may not be appreciated without careful inspection with and without the green colposcopy filter. Clinically, the appearance of VIN can be quite variable. Lesions are typically white and hyperkeratotic, but may also appear gray, pink, or brown. Colposcopy and biopsy of any suspicious lesion is the gold standard for diagnosis. In premenopausal women, lesions tend to be more multifocal, whereas in postmenopausal women, they are more often unifocal. An abnormal vascular pattern is most frequently associated with a severe degree of dysplasia, carcinoma in situ, or early invasive disease.

Treatment

Treatment options for VIN are wide local excision, laser ablation, or superficial vulvectomy with or without split-thickness skin grafting. Untreated VIN has the potential of progression to invasive carcinoma. This risk may be as high as 100% for women over age 40. In younger patients spontaneous regression may occur.

Treatment modality depends on the extent of involvement of the vulva, perineum, and perianal skin,

which is defined by colposcopy. Wide local excision of small foci of VIN is preferred. For unifocal lesions, a 1-cm margin of uninvolved skin is usually curative. Carbon dioxide laser may be used for multifocal disease. Disadvantages of the laser include painful recovery and lack of pathology specimens. The incidence of foci of microinvasion in VIN III has been reported to range from 10–22% in different series. Extensive disease may be best treated by superficial vulvectomy. The surgical goal is to preserve as much of the normal anatomy as possible. In the superficial "skinning" vulvectomy procedure, the excised vulvar skin can be closed with fine suture or may need to be replaced with a split-thickness skin graft (Figs 46–2 and 46–3) if the defect is too large.

Topical application of fluorouracil (5-FU), cryotherapy, and photodynamic therapy have historically been proven useful in the treatment of some lesions, but surgery remains the hallmark treatment modality for VIN. Promising future directions for treatment of VIN

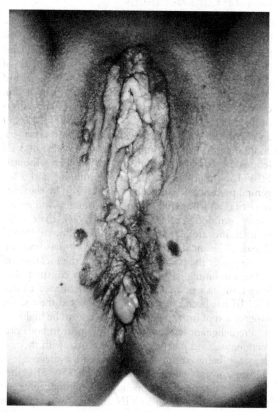

Figure 46–2. Diffuse, hypertrophic carcinoma in situ of the vulva and perianal skin. A skinning vulvectomy was performed.

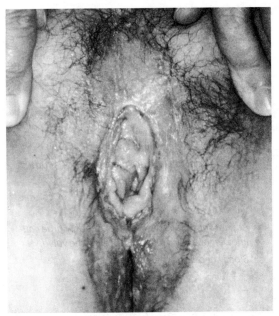

Figure 46–3. Appearance after skinning vulvectomy and split-thickness skin grafting of the lesion shown in Fig 46–2.

involve the development of a vaccine for HPV and use of immunomodulating agents, such as topical imiquimod.

Follow-up

Intraepithelial carcinoma of the vulva is often one manifestation of multifocal disease. For this reason, affected patients must be examined periodically for a number of years. Recommended follow-up includes thorough pelvic examinations with colposcopy every 3–4 months until the patient is disease-free for 2 years. If the patient is disease-free for a 2-year period, examinations can be done every 6 months.

EXTRAMAMMARY PAGET'S DISEASE

General Considerations

Paget's disease of the skin is an intraepithelial neoplasia or adenocarcinoma in situ. Reports of long-term survivals suggest that the in situ stage of the disease persists for a long time or that invasive disease is a different clinicopathologic entity. It appears that there are two separate lesions: intraepithelial extramammary Paget's disease and pagetoid changes in the skin associated with an underlying adenocarcinoma. Experts believe that an adenocarcinoma associated with Paget's disease arises as a primary adenocarcinoma of an underlying apocrine gland, Bartholin's gland, or anorectum, and represents two separate disease entities and not a spectrum. Unlike mammary Paget's disease, less than 20% of vulvar Paget's disease is associated with an underlying adenocarcinoma. Paget's disease with an underlying adenocarcinoma metastasizes frequently to regional lymph nodes and distally. Paget's disease without an underlying adenocarcinoma behaves like an intraepithelial neoplasia and can be treated as such.

Pathology

The initial lesion may be confused with a number of benign forms of chronic vulvar pruritus. It is a pruritic, slowly spreading, velvety-red discoloration of the skin that eventually becomes eczematoid in appearance with secondary maceration and development of white plaques; it may spread to involve the skin of the perineum, the perianal area, and the adjacent skin of the thigh. Grossly the lesion gives the impression of "cake icing." Because of the serpiginous growth pattern of Paget cells in the basal layer of the epidermis, the true extent of disease is difficult to assess.

Paget's disease of the vulvar skin is an intraepithelial disease. The typical Paget cell, pathognomonic of the disease process, apparently arises from abnormal differentiation of the cells of the basal layer of the epithelium (Fig 46–4). The appearance of malignant cells varies from that of the clear cell of the apocrine gland epithelium to a totally undifferentiated basal cell. It has been suggested that there may be both an intraepithelial and an invasive variety of the disease. The intraepithelial stage of the disease persists for years without evidence of an underlying adenocarcinoma.

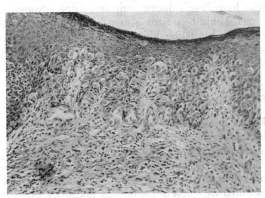

Figure 46–4. Paget's disease with typical cells in the basal layer of the epidermis.

Diagnosis

Paget's disease affects primarily postmenopausal Caucasian women in the seventh decade of life, but can be seen in younger patients. Pruritus and vulvar soreness are the most frequent symptoms. These symptoms may persist for years before the patient seeks medical attention. The lesion may be localized to one labium or involve the entire vulvar area. The lesion usually has an eczemoid appearance macroscopically and usually begins on the hair-bearing portions of the vulva. It is not unusual for the disease process to extend beyond the vulva to involve the perirectal area, buttocks, thighs, inguinal area, and mons. Intraepithelial extramammary Paget's disease presents as a lesion with hyperemic areas associated with a superficial white coating to give the impression of "cake icing." Although these lesions can be very extensive, most are confined to the epithelial layer. The diagnosis is made by vulvar biopsy. It is important to palpate the lesion in its entirety. A generous biopsy should be taken of any area that appears to be thickened to rule out an underlying adenocarcinoma.

Treatment

Since extramammary Paget's disease is an intraepithelial neoplasia it can be treated as such. Wide local excision is the primary treatment modality for this disease process. The lesion needs to be excised in its entirety; however, wide margins need to be removed around the primary lesion since disease often extends beyond the clinically visible erythematous area. The underlying dermis should be removed for adequate histologic evaluation. Often such a resection involves a complete vulvectomy. Careful histologic examination of the entire operative specimen is necessary to delineate the true extent of disease, ensure free surgical margins, and detect the remote possibility of underlying adenocarcinoma. For this reason, laser therapy is unsatisfactory. Patients who have Paget's disease with underlying adenocarcinoma should be treated with radical local excision of the vulva and bilateral inguinal lymph node dissection as they would for any other invasive tumor involving the vulvar area.

Prognosis

Paget's disease of the vulva has a great propensity for local recurrence, which may represent persistence of the disease or development of new disease in the remaining vulvar skin. Extramammary Paget's disease characteristically requires repeated local excisions of recurrent disease after treatment of the primary disease by total vulvectomy. Invasive disease without evidence of lymph node metastases has a favorable prognosis; however,

with nodal metastases, the disease is almost invariably fatal.

CANCER OF THE VULVA

ESSENTIALS OF DIAGNOSIS

- *Occurs in postmenopausal women.*
- *Long history of vulvar irritation with pruritus, local discomfort, and bloody discharge.*
- *Appearance of early lesions like that of chronic vulvar dermatitis.*
- *Appearance of late lesions like that of a large cauliflower, or a hard ulcerated area in the vulva.*
- *Biopsy necessary for diagnosis.*

General Considerations

Cancer of the vulva may arise from the skin, subcutaneous tissues, glandular elements of the vulva, or the mucosa of the lower third of the vagina. Approximately 90% of these tumors are squamous cell or epidermoid cancers. Less common tumors are extramammary Paget's disease with underlying adenocarcinoma, carcinoma of Bartholin's gland, basal cell carcinoma, melanoma, sarcoma, and metastatic cancers from other sites.

Cancer of the vulva is uncommon, accounting for approximately 5% of gynecologic cancers. Vulvar cancer is more common in the poor and elderly in most parts of the world, and no race or culture is spared. Vulvar cancer is primarily a disease of postmenopausal women, with a peak incidence in the 60s. The average age at the time of diagnosis is 65, and 75% of patients are over the age of 50. In general, the mean age of patients with carcinoma in situ is approximately 10 years less than that for patients with invasive cancer. Intraepithelial cancer of the vulva in women in their 20s and 30s has increased remarkably in recent years coincidentally with an increase in the incidence of diagnosis of dysplasia and carcinoma in situ of the cervix. HPV is strongly associated in younger women, whereas older women with vulvar cancer do not have tumors with HPV. Also, older women are more likely to have squamous hyperplasia in the tissue adjacent to the tumor.

Considering that cancer of the vulva is a disease of a body surface readily accessible to diagnostic procedures, early diagnosis should be the rule. This is not the case, however, and a 6- to 12-month delay in reporting symptoms of discovery of a tumor is common. Despite the advanced age of many of these patients and the frequent finding of a moderately large tumor, the disease is usually amenable to surgical therapy. In stage I and II disease, the corrected 5-year survival rate is greater than 90%. A 75% corrected 5-year survival rate for all stages of vulvar cancer is reported by most institutions.

Associated disorders found most frequently with carcinoma of the vulva are obesity, hypertension, and chronic vulvar irritation secondary to diabetes mellitus, granulomatous venereal disease, or vulvar dystrophy.

Pathology

The gross appearance of vulvar cancer depends on the origin and histologic type. These tumors progress by local extension and involvement of adjacent organs and, with few exceptions, by lymphatic permeation or embolism. The primary route of lymphatic spread is by way of the superficial inguinal, deep femoral, and external iliac lymph nodes (Fig 46–5). Contralateral spread may occur as a result of the rich intercommunicating lymphatic system of the vulvar skin. Direct extension to the deep pelvic lymph nodes, primarily the obturator nodes, occurs in about 3% of patients and seems to be related to midline involvement around the clitoris, urethra, or rectum, or to cancer of a vestibular (Bartholin's) gland. Extension of the tumor to the lower and

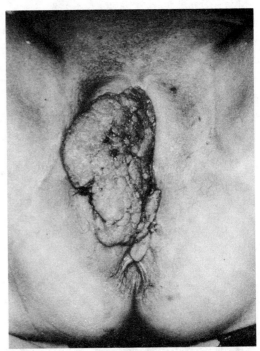

Figure 46–6. Large, exophytic epidermoid cancer of the vulva, which was treated by radical vulvectomy and regional lymphadenectomy.

middle thirds of the vagina may also allow access of tumor cells to lymph channels leading to the deep pelvic lymph nodes.

The gross and histologic appearance of the various types of vulvar cancers is as follows.

A. EPIDERMOID CANCER

Epidermoid cancer is by far the most common type of tumor and most frequently involves the anterior half of the vulva. In approximately 65% of patients, the tumor arises in the labia majora and minora, and in 25% the clitoris is involved. Over one-third of tumors involve the vulva bilaterally or are midline tumors. These tumors are most frequently associated with nodal spread and in particular bilateral nodal metastases. Midline tumors that involve the perineum do not worsen the outlook unless they extend into the vagina or to the anus and rectum.

Epidermoid cancer of the vulva varies in appearance from a large, exophytic cauliflower-like lesion to a small ulcer crater superimposed on a dystrophic lesion of the vulvar skin (Figs 46–6 and 46–7). Ulcerative lesions may begin as a raised, flat, white area of hypertrophic skin that subsequently undergoes ulceration. Exophytic lesions may become extremely large, undergo necrosis,

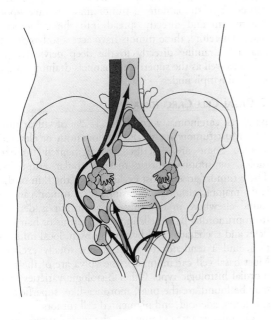

Figure 46–5. Lymphatic spread of cancer of the vulva.

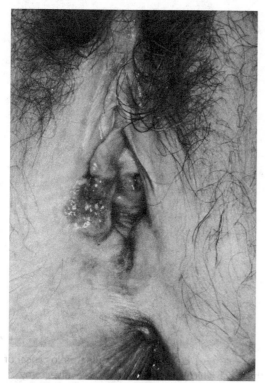

Figure 46–7. Ulcerative epidermoid cancer of the vulva.

and become secondarily infected and malodorous. A third variety arises as a slightly elevated, red velvety tumor that gradually spreads over the vulvar skin. There does not appear to be a positive correlation between the gross appearance of the tumor and either histologic grade or frequency of nodal metastases. The primary determinant of nodal metastases is tumor size.

Epidermoid cancers may be graded histologically from I to III. Grade I tumors are well differentiated, often forming keratin pearls; grade II tumors are moderately well differentiated; and grade III tumors are composed of poorly differentiated cells. The extent of underlying inflammatory cell infiltration into the stroma surrounding the invasive tumor is variable. The histologic grade of the tumor may be of some significance in small tumors less than 2 cm in diameter. However, the gross size of the tumor is the most significant factor in prognosis.

A variant of epidermoid cancer, **verrucous carcinoma,** is a locally invasive tumor that seldom metastasizes to regional lymph nodes. Grossly, the tumor looks like a mature condylomatous growth. Invading fronds of tumor tend to push the dermal tissue aside, causing diagnostic confusion. Local recurrence is common if a wide vulvectomy is not performed; lymphadenectomy is usually not recommended.

An attempt has been made to define a group of early vulvar cancers that might be described as microinvasive cancer and that exhibit little tendency for local recurrence or nodal metastases. Depth of stromal penetration has proved to be the key factor in determining invasive potential of the tumor. Early authors accepted 5 mm or less of dermal invasion as the definition of microinvasion, but this has not been universally accepted. A task force of the International Society for the Study of Vulvar Diseases suggested that the term "microinvasive cancer of the vulva" be discarded. They defined stage IA carcinoma of the vulva as a single lesion measuring 2 cm or less in diameter and exhibiting one focus of invasion to a depth of 1 mm or less. The depth of invasion was measured from the epidermal-stromal junction of the most superficial dermal papilla to the deepest point of tumor invasion.

B. CARCINOMA OF BARTHOLIN'S GLAND

Carcinoma of Bartholin's gland accounts for about 1% of vulvar cancers. Approximately 50% of the tumors are squamous cell. Other types of tumors arising in the Bartholin's glands are adenomatous, adenoid cystic (an adenocarcinoma with specific histologic and clinical characteristics), adenosquamous, and transitional cell.

It may be difficult to differentiate by clinical examination a tumor of Bartholin's gland or duct from a benign Bartholin's cyst. Because of its location deep in the substance of the labium, a tumor may impinge upon the rectum and directly spread into the ischiorectal fossa. Therefore, these tumors have access to lymphatic channels draining directly to the deep pelvic lymph nodes as well as the superficial channels draining to the inguinal lymph nodes.

C. BASAL CELL CARCINOMA

Basal cell carcinomas account for 1–2% of vulvar cancers. Most tumors are small papillomatous or elevated lesions. Some are described as pigmented tumors, moles, or simply pruritic maculopapular eruptions. These tumors arise almost exclusively in the skin of the labia majora, although occasionally a tumor can be found elsewhere in the vulva. The tumor is derived from primordial basal cells in the epidermis or hair follicles and is characterized by slow growth, local infiltration, and a tendency to recur if not totally excised. Most basal cell carcinomas of the vulva are of the primordial histologic type. Other histologic varieties that may be found are the pilar, morphea-like, superficially spreading, adenoid, and pigmented cell tumors.

On microscopic examination the typical tumor consists of nodular masses and lobules of closely packed, uniform-appearing basaloid cells with scant cytoplasm and spherical or oval dark nuclei. Peripheral margination by columnar cells is usually prominent. In larger tumor nodules, there may be areas of central degeneration and necrosis.

If a sufficiently wide local excision is not performed, there is a tendency for local recurrence, estimated to be about 20%. If a basal-squamous cell–type tumor is diagnosed, appropriate therapy for invasive epidermoid cancer of the vulva should be undertaken.

D. MALIGNANT MELANOMA

About 5% of vulvar cancers are malignant melanomas. Since only 0.1% of all nevi in women are on vulvar skin, the disproportionate frequency of occurrence of melanoma in this area may be due to the fact that nearly all vulvar nevi are of the junctional variety. Malignant melanoma most commonly arises in the region of the labia minora and clitoris, and there is a tendency for superficial spread toward the urethra and vagina. A nonpigmented melanoma may closely resemble squamous cell carcinoma on clinical examination. A darkly pigmented, raised lesion at the mucocutaneous junction is a characteristic finding; however, the degree of melanin pigmentation is variable, and amelanotic lesions do occur. The lesion spreads primarily through lymphatic channels and tends to metastasize early in the course of the disease; local or remote cutaneous satellite lesions may be found. All small pigmented lesions of the vulva are suspect and should be removed by excision biopsy with a 0.5- to 1-cm margin of normal skin. In the case of large tumors, the diagnosis should be confirmed by a generous biopsy.

E. UNUSUAL VULVAR MALIGNANCIES

Sarcomas of the vulva constitute a variety of malignant neoplasms that account for less than 2% of vulvar cancers. The most common is leiomyosarcoma, followed in frequency of occurrence by the fibrous histiocytoma group and an array of other sarcomas. Clinically, the tumor may be a subcutaneous nodule or may be exophytic and fleshy. Prognosis depends on histologic type, extent of local invasion, and treatment. In general, radical vulvectomy and regional lymphadenectomy are indicated, with the exception of tumors such as dermatofibrosarcoma protuberans, which is a locally aggressive tumor that tends to recur locally but does not metastasize.

Adenocarcinoma of the vulva is exceptionally rare unless it arises from Bartholin's gland or the urethra. Primary cancer of the breast from ectopic breast tissue has been reported. Rarely, a malignant tumor will arise from a vulvar sweat gland.

Metastatic cancers of the vulva have received scant attention in the medical literature. They usually originate from a genital tract tumor, and 18% arise from the kidney or urethra. Advanced cervical cancer is the most common primary tumor. Other primary tumors have been reported, including malignant melanoma, choriocarcinoma, and adenocarcinoma of the rectum or breast. Cloacogenic carcinoma is primarily an anorectal neoplasm occurring twice as often in women than in men; it may arise in anal ducts and present as a submucosal mass.

Metastatic epidermoid cancer tends to form nests of cells within the dermis. Adenocarcinoma, regardless of the primary site, invades the surface squamous epithelium. Because these tumors are a manifestation of advanced disease, the prognosis is uniformly grave.

Clinical Findings

The patient with vulvar cancer characteristically has had infrequent medical examinations. About 10% are diabetic, and 30–50% are obese or hypertensive or demonstrate other evidence of cardiovascular disease. The incidence of complicating medical illness exceeds that expected in the age group under consideration.

Invasive epidermoid cancer is a disease mainly of the seventh and eighth decades of life, though about 15% of patients are age 40 or younger. About 20% of patients have a second primary cancer that was diagnosed prior to, at the time of, or subsequent to the diagnosis of vulvar cancer; 75% of these second primaries are in the cervix.

A. SYMPTOMS AND SIGNS

Pruritus vulvae or a vulvar mass is the presenting complaint in over 50% of patients with vulvar cancer. Other patients complain of bleeding or vulvar pain, whereas approximately 20% of patients have no complaints, and the tumor is found incidentally during routine pelvic examination. A significant number of patients, about 25%, have seen a physician and received various medical treatments without benefit of a biopsy of the tumor or have undergone incomplete therapy consisting of a simple excision biopsy of an invasive tumor. The importance of performing a biopsy of any vulvar lesion cannot be overemphasized.

Differential Diagnosis

Differential diagnosis of vulvar disease and exclusion of cancer depend on an adequate biopsy. The tumor may be a diffuse white lesion, a discrete tumor, an ulcer, or diffuse papules, which may not be appreciated without thorough colposcopic examination of the skin of the vulva, perineum, and perianal area.

Benign ulcerative lesions may be due to a sexually transmitted disease (syphilis, herpes, or granuloma inguinale), pyogenic infections, or a benign tumor such as a granular cell myoblastoma.

Treatment

Staging and treatment for stage I and II vulvar cancer is surgical (Table 46–1). The primary treatment for invasive vulvar cancer is complete surgical removal of all tumor whenever possible. There has been a trend over recent years towards a more conservative surgical approach.

The number of preoperative studies ordered prior to surgery depends on the extent of disease and the general condition of the patient. A complete history and a thorough physical examination that includes cytologic study of the cervix and vulvoscopy should be per-

Table 46–1. International Federation of Gynecology and Obstetrics (FIGO) staging of invasive cancer.

Stage 0			
Cis			Carcinoma in situ, intraepithelial carcinoma
Stage I			
T1	N0	M0	Tumor confined to the vulva and/or perineum—2 cm or less in greatest dimension (no nodal metastasis)
Stage II			
T2	N0	M0	Tumor confined to the vulva and/or perineum—no more than 2 cm in greatest dimension (no nodal metastasis)
Stage III			
T3	N0	M0	Tumor of any size with
T3	N1	M0	(1) Adjacent spread to the lower urethra and/or the vagina, or the anus, and/or
T1	N1	M0	(2) Unilateral regional lymph node metastasis
T2	N1	M0	
Stage IVA			
T1	N2	M0	Tumor invades any of the following: Upper urethra, bladder mucosa, rectal mucosa, pelvic bone, and/or bilateral regional node metastasis
T2	N2	M0	
T3	N2	M0	
T4	Any N	M0	
Stage IVb	Any T	Any N	Any distant metastasis including pelvic lymph nodes
M1			

formed. A large tumor may interfere with adequate pelvic examination. Bleeding may be caused by a lesion higher in the genital tract rather than the obvious vulvar tumor. In that case, the pelvic examination may be performed under anesthesia, and endometrial biopsy or D&C considered.

Chest x-ray, complete blood count, and urinalysis are performed on all patients. Older patients require an electrocardiogram (ECG) and a biochemical profile. Other studies such as proctoscopy, pyelography, barium enema, and CT scans are ordered on an individual basis. Enlarged lymph nodes do not require biopsy; they will be excised by lymphadenectomy or thoroughly sampled at the time of operation. Mechanical bowel cleansing is recommended for most patients, particularly if the perineal skin is involved. An antibiotic bowel preparation is prescribed if extensive perianal dissection, skin grafting, or intestinal surgery (such as abdominoperineal resection) is anticipated. At least 2 units of packed red cells should be available for transfusion. Less than 50% of patients require a transfusion during or after the operation.

Historically the basic operation had been radical vulvectomy and regional lymphadenectomy. However, the trend has shifted away from standard en bloc radical vulvectomy and bilateral lymph node dissection towards wide radical local excision of the primary tumor with inguinal lymph node dissection. For a unifocal stage I lesion, wide radical local excision with surgical margins of at least 1 cm should be performed. Patients with unilateral lesions with depth of invasion more than 1 mm should undergo ipsilateral groin dissection in addition to the above to determine nodal status. For patients with bilateral lesions or lesions crossing the midline, bilateral inguinal femoral lymphadenectomy can be performed. However, when disease has spread to more than two lymph nodes, adjuvant radiation therapy is now preferred instead of pelvic lymphadenectomy. The role of sentinel node mapping is also being evaluated for patients with squamous vulvar carcinoma and melanomas. In general, lymphatic spread occurs in a sequential manner from the superficial to the deep inguinal lymph nodes. Therefore, if the superficial nodes harbor no metastatic disease, there is reasonable assurance that the deeper nodes are not involved.

When the disease involves the anus, rectum, rectovaginal septum, proximal urethra, or bladder, an adequate surgical resection is only possible with pelvic exenteration combined with radical vulvectomy. Operative mortality is high for these procedures and the postoperative psychologic impact is significant. In addition, with advanced stage disease where ulcerated or fixed lymph nodes are palpated, attempts at lymphadenectomy have yielded very poor results. Based on data from the Gynecologic Oncology Group, this group of patients may benefit from preoperative chemoradiation resulting in higher rates of successful resection and reduced need for more radical surgery. Chemotherapeutic agents such as cisplatin and 5-FU have been combined with radiation therapy. These chemotherapeutic agents are used as radiation sensitizers in large necrotic tumor beds, enhancing the radiation effects.

There is controversy concerning the extent of surgery required for treatment of malignant melanoma of the vulva. For some years, standard treatment consisted of vulvectomy with superficial and deep inguinal and pelvic lymphadenectomy. It is also generally treated with a more conservative surgical approach. If depth of the vulvar lesion is less than 0.76 mm, vulvar melanoma may be adequately treated with local incision. However, if the depth of invasion is greater, the excision requires a 2- to 3-cm margin in addition to a bilateral groin node dissection. Advanced or recurrent melanoma may be best treated with chemotherapy, radiation, or immunotherapy.

Locally invasive but nonmetastasizing sarcomas such as dermatofibrosarcoma protuberans can be removed by wide local resection. Most other sarcomas are treated by radical vulvectomy and regional lymphadenectomy. The primary determinant of cure appears to be adequate wide removal of the primary lesion.

Operative Morbidity & Mortality

The most frequently encountered complication is wound breakdown, which occurs in well over 50% of patients undergoing radical vulvectomy and bilateral inguinal dissection. This complication is related to the amount of skin removed during the procedure, particularly at the groin areas. Separate groin incisions and careful handling of skin flaps have reduced the incidence of wound breakdown. Vigorous wound care with debridement almost always results in adequate healing.

Lymphedema occurs in approximately 65% of patients who have had radical vulvectomy. Hemorrhage, lymphocyst formation, thromboembolic disease, urinary tract infections, and sexual dysfunction are other commonly associated morbidities.

Follow-up

After the immediate postoperative period, patients should be examined every 3 months for 2 years and every 6 months thereafter to detect recurrent disease or a second primary cancer. Nearly 80% of recurrent vulvar cancer occurs in the first 2 years. Treatment modalities depend on the location of recurrence. Malignant melanomas and sarcomas may recur locally or metastasize to the liver or lungs.

Prognosis

The principal prognostic factors in cancer of the vulva are the size and location of the lesion, the histologic type, and the presence or absence of regional lymph node metastases.

A 5-year survival rate of 75% and a 10-year survival rate of approximately 58% should be expected after complete surgical treatment of primary invasive squamous vulvar cancer. Lymph node status is the most important prognostic variable. Overall, the survival rate for patients with vulvar cancer and negative inguinal-femoral nodes is 90%, whereas rates drop to almost 40% with nodal metastasis. Several authors have reported no deaths from cancer among patients who were found to have negative lymph nodes. With tumors less than 2 cm in diameter, the incidence of nodal metastases is 10–15%. In general, about 30% of patients undergoing surgery will be found to have positive lymph nodes. With nodal metastases, the approximate 5-year cure rates are as follows: 1 node, 94%; 2 nodes, 80%; and 3 nodes or more, less than 15%. Patients who have 3 or more positive lymph nodes in the groin usually demonstrate palpably suspicious nodes preoperatively. These patients have a high incidence of metastases to the pelvic lymph nodes; however, pelvic lymphadenectomy apparently does not improve survival rates. Involvement of contiguous organs such as the bladder or rectum increases the incidence of nodal metastases and worsens the prognosis accordingly.

The cure rate for adequately treated cancer of Bartholin's gland has not been established. There is a propensity for unresectable local recurrences under the pubic ramus despite a thorough primary operation.

Wide local excision of basal cell carcinoma should be curative. Some authors have reported an approximately 20% recurrence rate after local excision that may represent cases of incomplete excision.

Results of treatment of malignant melanoma are related to the level of penetration of the tumor into the dermis of the vulvar skin or the lamina propria of the vaginal mucosa and to the presence or absence of nodal metastases. The 5-year survival rate ranges from 14–50%, but patients who have metastases to groin lymph nodes have a survival rate below 14%. Amelanotic cutaneous melanomas are particularly virulent tumors. The survival rate for patients with superficial spreading melanomas is much better than for those with the nodular variety, which tend to have a smaller diameter and exhibit aggressive vertical invasion, increased incidence of nodal metastases, treatment failures, and distant recurrences. The most common site of recurrence is at the site of resection or the groin lymph nodes (if not previously resected).

Sarcomas of the vulva tend to recur locally, particularly if the initial resection is not extensive, and metastasize to the liver and lungs.

PREINVASIVE DISEASE OF THE VAGINA

General Considerations

Vaginal intraepithelial neoplasia (VAIN) can occur as an isolated lesion, but multifocal disease is more common. Little is known regarding the natural history of VAIN; however, it is thought to be similar to that of CIN. Many patients may have similar intraepithelial neoplastic lesions involving the cervix or vulva. At least one-half to two-thirds of patients with VAIN have been treated for similar disease in either the cervix or the vulva. In addition, VAIN can reappear several years later, necessitating long-term follow-up in these patients. Several investigators have recognized a "field response" involving the squamous epithelium of the lower genital tract including the cervix, vagina, and vulva to be affected simultaneously by the same carcinogenic agent. The vagina lacks a transformation zone, where in the cervix immature epithelial cells are infected with HPV. Some theorize that the HPV entry mechanisms involve abrasions from coitus or tampon use. HPV may begin its growth in a healing abrasion in a similar fashion as in the transformation zone.

The upper third of the vagina is vulnerable to the development of dysplasia and carcinoma in situ whether or not hysterectomy has been performed previously for intraepithelial neoplasia. Each of these entities has a potential for progression to invasive cancer. For this reason, women who have had a hysterectomy with a history of HPV or intraepithelial neoplasia should continue to have periodic cytologic screening of the vaginal apex. A similar lesion may develop after prior irradiation for a pelvic malignancy; some authors report a 20% incidence of cervical or vaginal dysplasia. These tumors are usually asymptomatic and detected by routine vaginal cytologic studies. New invasive tumors in an irradiated field usually develop 15–30 years after therapeutic irradiation.

Condylomatous lesions of the lower genital tract often demonstrate associated dysplasias. For this reason a biopsy should be made of condylomatous growth of the vagina prior to treatment.

Pathology

As with other intraepithelial neoplasias occurring in the lower genital tract, VAIN is characterized by a loss of epithelial cell maturation. This is associated with nu-

clear hyperchromatosis and pleomorphism with cellular crowding. The thickness of the epithelial abnormality designates the various lesions as VAIN I, II, or III. VAIN III is a synonymous term for carcinoma in situ of the vagina.

Diagnosis

Almost all lesions of VAIN are asymptomatic. Lesions often accompany HPV infection, so patients may complain of vulvar warts. An abnormal Pap smear is usually the first sign of disease. The diagnosis is made by colposcopic examination of the vagina with a directed biopsy. Colposcopic examination of the vagina can be difficult to perform, particularly if a hysterectomy has already been done. Techniques similar to those used for colposcopic examination of the cervix are used for examination of the vagina. After application of 3–5% acetic acid to the vagina, a lesion under the colposcope may appear as white epithelium, and may have mosaicism or punctation. Lesions are often located along the vaginal ridges; they may appear to be raised or have spicules. Since the disease process tends to be multifocal, a thorough examination of the vagina from the introitus to the apex must be conducted.

Treatment

The primary treatment modality for VAIN is surgical excision or laser ablation. VAIN grade 1 lesions usually do not require treatment, as lesions typically regress, are multifocal, and often recur. VAIN grades 2–3 can be treated by laser ablation or excision. VAIN grade 3 lesions are more often associated with an early invasive lesion; therefore, adequate sampling should be performed before any ablative procedure is employed. If the lesion is focal, it is best removed in its entirety with local excision. When carcinoma in situ of the cervix extends to the upper vagina, the upper third of the vagina can be removed at the time of hysterectomy. If multifocal disease is present, a total vaginectomy may be performed with a split-thickness skin graft vaginal reconstruction. Topical 5-FU may also be used in treating multifocal VAIN. Approximately 80% of patients can expect to have evidence of dysplasia remit after one to two courses of treatment.

Follow-up

Intraepithelial neoplasia of the vagina tends to be multifocal, with involvement of the cervix and vulva in many cases. These lesions can be difficult to eradicate with only one treatment modality or treatment session. This group of patients must be monitored closely every 3–4 months with colposcopic examinations of not only the vagina but also the entire lower genital tract.

CANCER OF THE VAGINA

ESSENTIALS OF DIAGNOSIS

- Asymptomatic: abnormal vaginal cytology.
- Early: painless bleeding from ulcerated tumor.
- Late: bleeding, pain, weight loss, swelling.

General Considerations

Primary cancers of the vagina are rare, representing about 1–2% of gynecologic cancers. About 85% are epidermoid cancers, and the remainder, in decreasing order of frequency, are adenocarcinomas, sarcomas, and melanomas. A tumor should not be considered a primary vaginal cancer unless the cervix is uninvolved or only minimally involved by a tumor obviously arising in the vagina. By convention, any malignancy involving both cervix and vagina that is histologically compatible with the origin in either organ is classified as cervical cancer. Secondary carcinoma of the vagina is seen more frequently than primary vaginal cancers. Secondary, or metastatic, tumors may arise from cervical, endometrial, or ovarian cancer, gestational trophoblastic disease, colorectal cancer, or urogenital or vulvar cancer. Extension of cervical cancer to the vagina is probably the most common malignancy involving the vagina. HPV, early hysterectomy, and prior radiation are possible risk factors for vaginal cancer, but no specific etiologic agent has been identified.

Pathology

Squamous cell carcinoma may be ulcerative or exophytic. It usually involves the posterior wall of the upper third of the vagina, but may be multicentric. Direct invasion of the bladder or rectum may occur. The incidence of lymph node metastases is directly related to the size of the tumor. The route of nodal metastases depends on the location of the tumor in the vagina. Tumors in the lower third metastasize like cancer of the vulva, primarily to the inguinal lymph nodes (Fig 46–8). Cancers of the upper vagina, which is the most common site, metastasize in a manner similar to cancer of the cervix. The lymphatic drainage of the vagina consists of a fine capillary meshwork in the mucosa and submucosa with multiple anastomoses. As a consequence, lesions in the middle third of the vagina may metastasize to the inguinal lymph nodes or directly to the deep pelvic lymph nodes.

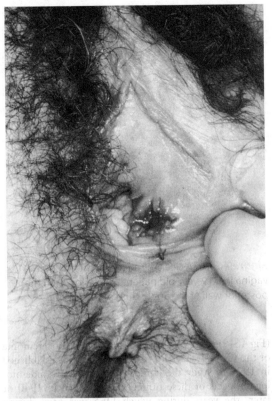

Figure 46–8. An ulcerated epidermoid cancer of the lower third of the vagina.

Melanomas and sarcomas of the vagina metastasize like epidermoid cancer, although liver and pulmonary metastases are more common. Nevi rarely occur in the vagina; therefore, any pigmented lesion of the vagina should be excised or biopsied. The anterior surface and lower half of the vagina are the most common sites. Grossly, the tumors are usually exophytic and described as polypoid or pedunculated with secondary necrosis.

Sarcomas of the vagina occur in children under 5 years of age and in women in the fifth to sixth decades. Embryonal rhabdomyosarcomas replace the vaginal mucosa of young girls and consist of polypoid, edematous, translucent masses that may protrude from the vaginal introitus. Leiomyosarcomas, reticulum cell sarcomas, and unclassified sarcomas occur in older women. The upper anterior vaginal wall is the most common site of origin. The appearance of these tumors depends on the size and the extent of disease at the time of diagnosis.

Clear cell adenocarcinomas arise in conjunction with vaginal adenosis, which in recent years has been detected most frequently in young women with a history of exposure to diethylstilbestrol (DES) in utero

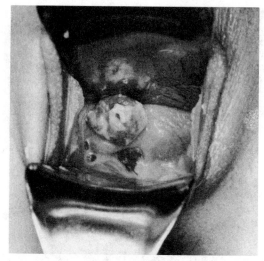

Figure 46–9. A clear cell adenocarcinoma of the vagina in a 19-year-old patient. The lesion is on the posterior wall of the upper third of the vagina.

(Fig 46–9). The Registry of Clear Cell Adenocarcinoma of the Genital Tract in Young Females was established in 1971 to study the clinicopathologic and epidemiologic aspects of these tumors in girls born in 1940 or later, the years during which DES was used during pregnancy. The risk of developing clear cell adenocarcinoma by age 24 has been calculated to be 0.14–1.4 per 1000 exposed female fetuses. Adenosis vaginae and adenocarcinoma do occur in sexually mature and postmenopausal women.

Metastatic adenocarcinoma to the vagina may arise from the urethra, Bartholin's gland, the rectum or bladder, the endometrial cavity, the endocervix, or an ovary; or it may be metastatic from a distant site. Hypernephroma of the kidney characteristically metastasizes to the anterior wall of the vagina in the lower third. These tumors would not be primary vaginal cancers.

Clinical Findings

Vaginal cancer is often asymptomatic, discovered by routine vaginal cytologic examination, and confirmed by biopsy after delineation of the location and extent of the tumor by colposcopy.

Postmenopausal vaginal bleeding and/or bloody discharge are the most common presenting symptoms. About 50% of patients with invasive vaginal cancer report for examination within 6 months after symptoms are noted. Less commonly, advanced tumors may impinge upon the rectum or bladder or extend to the pelvic wall, causing pain or leg edema.

A diagnosis of primary cancer of the vagina cannot be established unless metastasis from another source is eliminated. A complete history and physical examination should be performed, including a thorough pelvic examination, cervical cytologic examination, endometrial biopsy when indicated, complete inspection of the vagina, including colposcopy, and biopsy of the vaginal tumor. Careful bimanual examination with palpation of the entire length of the vagina can detect small submucosal nodules not visualized during the examination.

The staging system for cancer of the vagina is clinical and not surgical (Table 46–2).

Differential Diagnosis

Benign tumors of the vagina are uncommon, are usually cystic, arise from the mesonephric (wolffian) or paramesonephric ducts, and are usually an incidental finding on examination of the anterolateral wall of the vagina (Gartner's duct cyst).

An ulcerative lesion may occur at the site of direct trauma, following an inflammatory reaction due to prolonged retention of a pessary or other foreign body, or occasionally following a chemical burn. Granulomatous venereal diseases seldom affect the vagina but may be diagnosed with appropriate laboratory studies and a biopsy.

Endometriosis that penetrates the cul-de-sac of Douglas into the upper vagina cannot be differentiated from cancer except by biopsy.

Cancer of the urethra, bladder, rectum, or Bartholin's gland may penetrate or extend into the vagina. Cloaco-

Table 46–2. FIGO staging of carcinoma of the vagina.

Preinvasive carcinoma	
Stage 0	Carcinoma in situ, intraepithelial carcinoma.
Invasive carcinoma	
Stage I	The carcinoma is limited to the vaginal mucosa.
Stage II	The carcinoma has involved the subvaginal tissue but has not extended to the pelvic wall.
Stage III	The carcinoma has extended to the pelvic wall.
Stage IV	The carcinoma has extended beyond the true pelvis or has involved the mucosa of the bladder or rectum. A bullous edema as such does not permit allotment of a case to stage IV.
Stage IVA	Spread of the growth to adjacent organs.
Stage IVB	Spread to distant organs.

FIGO, Federation of Gynecology and Obstetrics.

genic carcinoma is a rare tumor of the anorectal region originating from a persistent remnant of the cloacal membrane of the embryo. The tumor accounts for 2–3% of anorectal carcinomas and occurs more than twice as often in women. Although these metastatic tumors often penetrate into the vagina as fungating or ulcerating lesions, they may present as a submucosal mass.

Biopsy should be performed to establish a histologic diagnosis.

Treatment

Following biopsy confirmation of disease, all patients should undergo a thorough physical examination and evaluation of the extent of local and metastatic disease. Pretreatment evaluation may include the following studies: chest x-ray, intravenous pyelogram, cystoscopy, proctosigmoidoscopy, and often CT scan of the abdomen and pelvis. The treatment of patients with invasive vaginal cancer primarily consists of combined external beam and internal radiation therapy. In patients in whom coitus is an important factor, surgery should be considered. Also in patients with stage I and IIA lesions, radical hysterectomy with an upper vaginectomy may be performed. Therapy is complicated by the anatomic proximity of the vagina to the rectum, bladder, and urethra. Most primary invasive epidermoid cancers of the vagina are treated by irradiation. Irradiation consists of whole-pelvis external therapy supplemented by internal radiation treatment. Interstitial therapy is commonly utilized unless there exists a small vault lesion, which may be adequately managed by a tandem and ovoid implant.

A selected group of patients with stage III or IV disease may benefit from preoperative whole pelvic radiation followed by radical surgery. However, most affected patients are treated by irradiation, which consists of whole-pelvis external irradiation followed by intracavitary or interstitial implants, or additional external therapy through a treatment field that has been reduced in size and localized to the affected parametrium. In some cases carcinoma at the introitus may be treated like cancer of the vulva, utilizing radical vulvectomy and bilateral superficial and deep inguinal lymphadenectomy. A very small and early lesion may be treated by total vaginectomy. However, the close proximity of the bladder and the rectum often precludes conservative surgery. Irradiation is essentially the same as that used for cancers of the upper vagina. When the lower third of the vagina is involved, the inguinal nodes must be treated with either irradiation or inguinal lymphadenectomy.

The principles of treatment of primary adenocarcinoma of the vagina are the same as those for epidermoid cancer. However, preferred therapy for clear cell carcinoma of the vagina and cervix in young women has not been established. Approximately 60% of tumors occur in the upper half of the vagina, and the remainder occur in the cervix. The incidence of nodal metastases is approximately 18% in stage I and 30% or more in stage II disease. If the disease is found sufficiently early and is confined to the upper vagina and cervix, radical abdominal hysterectomy, upper vaginectomy, and pelvic lymphadenectomy with ovarian preservation can be performed. More advanced lesions are treated with irradiation.

Sarcoma botryoides, a variety of rhabdomyosarcoma, is usually seen in patients less than 5 years of age. Radiation therapy or local excision has yielded poor results; thus historically pelvic exenteration was the standard of therapy. Primary chemotherapy with vincristine, actinomycin D, and cyclophosphamide plus radiation has led to excellent results in treating patients with this disease. Melanoma of the vagina may be treated with radiation, conservative excision, and/or radical surgery.

Epidermoid cancers that recur after primary radiation therapy are usually treated by pelvic exenteration. Chemotherapy for recurrent disease has been relatively ineffective, but multidrug regimens incorporating cisplatin may prove to be more useful.

Prognosis

The size and stage of the disease at the time of diagnosis are the most important prognostic indicators in squamous cell cancers. The 5-year survival rate is 77% in patients with stage I disease, 45% in patients with stage II disease, 31% in patients with stage III disease, and 18% in patients with stage IV disease.

Melanomas—even small ones—are very malignant, and few respond to therapy. The tumor recurs locally and metastasizes to the liver and lungs. Chemotherapy and immunotherapy have been used as adjunctive treatment.

Too few sarcomas of the vagina have been reported to generate survival data; these tumors have a propensity for local recurrence and distant metastases, and the prognosis is usually poor.

REFERENCES

General

Berek JS: *Novak's Gynecology.* Wilkins & Wilkins, 1996.

Preinvasive Disease of the Vulva & Vagina

Benedet JL, Wilson PS, Matisic JP: Epidermal thickness measurements in vaginal intraepithelial neoplasia: a basis for optimal CO_2 laser vaporization. J Reprod Med 1992;37:899.

Davis GD: Colposcopic examination of the vagina. Obstet Gynecol Clin North Am 1993;20:217.

Davis G, Wentworth J, Richard J: Self-administered topical imiquimod treatment of vulvar intraepithelial neoplasia. J Reprod Med 2000;45:619.

Hart WR: Vulvar intraepithelial neoplasia: historical aspects and current status. Int J Gynecol Pathol 2001;20:116.

Hatch K: Colposcopy of vaginal and vulvar human papilloma virus and adjacent sites. Obstet Gynecol Clin North Am 1993;20:203.

Jones RW et al: Human papilloma virus in women with vulvar intraepithelial neoplasia III. J Reprod Med 1990;35:1124.

Jones RW, Rowan DM: Spontaneous regression of vulvar intraepithelial neoplasia 2–3. Obstet Gynecol 2000;96:470.

Joura EA et al: Increasing incidence of vulvar intraepithelial neoplasia and squamous cell carcinoma of the vulva in young women. J Reprod Med 2000;45:613.

Krebs HB: Treatment of vaginal intraepithelial neoplasia with laser and topical 5-fluorouracil. Obstet Gynecol 1989;73:657.

Muderspach L et al: A phase I trial of a HPV peptide vaccine for women with high grade cervical and vulvar intraepithelial neoplasia who are HPV 16 positive. Clin Cancer Res 2000;6:3406.

Petrilli ES et al: Vaginal intraepithelial neoplasia: biologic aspects and treatment with topical 5-fluorouracil and the carbon dioxide laser. Am J Obstet Gynecol 1980;138:321.

Schneider A, de Villiers E-M, Schndeider V: Multifocal squamous neoplasia of the female genital tract: Significance of human papillomavirus infection of the vagina after hysterectomy. Obstet Gynecol 1987;70:294.

Sillman FH, Sedlis A, Boyce JG: A review of lower genital intraepithelial neoplasia and the use of topical 5-fluorouracil. Obstet Gynecol Surv 1985;40:190.

Sturgeon SR et al: In situ and invasive vulvar cancer incidence trends (1973 to 1987). Am J Obstet Gynecol 1992;166:1482.

Twiggs LB et al: A clinical, histopathologic and molecular biologic investigation of vulvar intraepithelial neoplasia. Int J Gynecol Pathol 1988;7:48.

Extramammary Paget's Disease

Bergen S et al: Conservative management of extramammary Paget's disease of the vulva. Gynecol Oncol 1989;33:151.

Curtin JP et al: Paget's disease of the vulva. Gynecol Oncol 1990;39:374.

Feuer GA, Shevchuk M, Calanog A: Vulvar Paget's disease: the need to exclude an invasive lesion. Gynecol Oncol 1990;38:81.

Gunn RA, Gallager HS: Vulvar Paget's disease: A topographic study. Cancer 1980;46:590.

James LP: Apocrine adenocarcinoma of the vulva with associated Paget's disease. Acta Cytol 1984;28:178.

Cancer of the Vulva

Ansink A, van der Velden J: Surgical interventions for early squamous cell carcinoma of the vulva. Cochrane Database Syst Rev 2000:CD002036.

Balat O, Edwards C, Delclos L: Complications following combined surgery (radical vulvectomy versus wide local excision) and radiotherapy for the treatment of carcinoma of the vulva: report of 73 patients. Eur J Gynaecol Oncol 2000;21:501.

Balch CM et al: Efficacy of 2-cm surgical margins for intermediate thickness melanomas (1–4 mm): results of a multi-institutional randomized surgical trial. Ann Surg 1993;218:262.

Benedet JL et al: FIGO staging classifications and clinical practice guidelines in the management of gynecologic cancers. FIGO Committee on Gynecologic Oncology. Int J Gynaecol Obstet 2000;70:209.

Berek JS et al: Concurrent cisplatin and 5-fluorouracil chemotherapy and radiation therapy for advanced stage squamous cell carcinoma of the vulva. Gynecol Oncol 1991;42:197.

Boice CR et al: Microinvasive squamous carcinoma of the vulva: Present status and reassessment. Gynecol Oncol 1984;18:71.

Bradgate MG et al: Malignant melanoma of the vulva: A clinicopathological study of 50 women. Br J Obstet Gynaecol 1990;97:124.

Buscema J, Woodruff JD: Progressive histologic alterations in the development of vulvar cancer. Am J Obstet Gynecol 1980;138:146.

Carlson JA et al: Vulvar lichen sclerosis and squamous cell carcinoma: a cohort, case control, and investigational study with historical perspective; implications for chronic inflammation and sclerosis in the development of neoplasia. Hum Pathol 1998;29:932.

Copeland LJ et al: Bartholin gland carcinoma. Obstet Gynecol 1986;67:794.

Crowther ME, Lowe DG, Shepherd JH: Verrucous carcinoma of the female genital tract: A review. Obstet Gynecol Surv 1988;43:263.

Fisher M, Marsch WC: Vulvodynia: an indicator or even an early symptom of vulvar cancer. Cutis 2001;67:235.

Groff DB: Pelvic neoplasms in children. J Surg Oncol 2001;77:65.

Hacker NF: Current management of early vulvar cancer. Ann Acad Med Singapore 1998;27:688.

Hacker NF et al: Individualization of treatment for stage I squamous cell vulvar carcinoma. Obstet Gynecol 1984;63:155.

Homesley HD et al: Assessment of current International Federation of Gynecology and Obstetrics staging of vulvar carcinoma relative to prognostic factors for survival (a Gynecologic Oncology Group study). Am J Obstet Gynecol 1991;164:997.

Homesley HD et al: Radiation therapy versus pelvic node resection for carcinoma of the vulva with positive groin nodes. Obstet Gynecol 1986;68:733.

Johnson TL et al: Prognostic features of vulvar melanoma: A clinicopathologic analysis. Int J Gynecol Pathol 1986;5:110.

Lea JS, Miller DS: Optimum screening interventions for gynecologic malignancies. Tex Med 2001;97:49.

Leminen A, Forss M, Paavonen J: Wound complications in patients with carcinoma of the vulva. Comparison between radical and modified vulvectomies. Eur J Obstet Gynecol Reprod Biol 2000;93:193.

Lin JY et al: Morbidity and recurrence with modifications of radical vulvectomy and groin dissection. Gynecol Oncol 1992;47:80.

Menczer J: A trend toward more conservative surgery in gynecologic oncology. Obstet Gynecol Surv 1996;51:628.

Mirhashemi R, Nieves-Neira W, Averette HE: Gynecologic malignancies in older women. Oncology 2001;15:580, discussion 592, 597.

Modesitt SC, Waters AB, Walton L: Vulvar intraepithelial neoplasia III: Occult cancer and the impact of margin status on recurrence obstetrics and gynecology. Obstet Gynecol 1998; 92:962.

Moore DH et al: Preoperative chemoradiation for advanced vulvar cancer: A phase II study of The Gynecologic Oncology Group. Int J Radiat Oncol Biol Phys 1998;42:79.

Montana GS et al: Preoperative chemo-radiation for carcinoma of the vulva with N2/N3 nodes: A Gynecologic Oncology Group Study. Int J Radiat Oncol Biol Phys 2000;48:1007.

Morgan MA, Mikuta JJ: Surgical management of vulvar cancer. Semin Surg Oncol 1999;17:168.

Moscarini M et al: Surgical treatment of invasive carcinoma of the vulva. Our experience. Eur J Gynaecol Oncol 2000; 1:393.

Nucci MR, Fletcher CDM: Vulvovaginal soft tissue tumors: update and review. Histopathology 2000;36:97.

Rodolakis A et al: Squamous vulvar cancer: a clinically based individualization of treatment. Gynecol Oncol 2000;78(3 Pt 1): 346.

Rouzier R et al: Prognostic significance of epithelial disorders adjacent to invasive vulvar carcinomas. Gynecol Oncol 2001; 81:414.

Scurry JP, Vanin K: Vulvar squamous cell carcinoma and lichen sclerosis. Australas J Dermatol 1997;38(Suppl 1):S20.

Senkus E et al: Second lower genital tract squamous cell carcinoma following cervical cancer. A clinical study of 46 patients. Acta Obstet Gynecol Scand 2000;79:765.

Cancer of the Vagina

Aho M et al: Natural history of vaginal intraepithelial neoplasia. Cancer 1991;68:195.

Andersen ES: Primary carcinoma of the vagina: A study of 29 cases. Gynecol Oncol 1989;33:317.

Borazjani G et al: Primary malignant melanoma of the vagina: A clinicopathological analysis of 10 cases. Gynecol Oncol 1990;37:264.

Copeland LJ et al: Sarcoma botryoides of the female genital tract. Gynecol Oncol 1985;66:262.

Davis KP et al: Invasive vaginal carcinoma: analysis of early stage disease. Gynecol Oncol 1991;42:131.

Friedman M et al: Modern treatment of vaginal embryonal rhabdomyosarcoma. Obstet Gynecol Surv 1986;41:614.

Gallup DG et al: Invasive squamous cell carcinoma of the vagina: A 14-year study. Obstet Gynecol 1987;69:782.

Hays DM et al: Clinical staging and treatment results in rhabdomyosarcoma of the female genital tract among children and adolescents. Cancer 1988;61:1893.

Herbst A, Anderson D: Clear cell adenocarcinoma of the vagina and cervix secondary to intrauterine exposure to diethylstilbestrol. Semin Surg Oncol 1990;6:343.

Herbst AL et al: Clear cell adenocarcinoma of the genital tract in young females: Registry report. N Engl J Med 1972; 287:1259.

Herbst AL et al: Risk factors of the development of diethylstilbestrol-associated clear cell adenocarcinoma. Am J Obstet Gynecol 1986;154:814.

Melnick S et al: Rates and risks of diethylstilbestrol-related clear-cell adenocarcinoma of the vagina and cervix. N Engl J Med 1987;316:514.

Peters WA et al: Primary sarcoma of the adult vagina: A clinicopathologic study. Obstet Gynecol 1985;65:699.

Perez CA, Camel HM: Long-term follow-up in radiation therapy of carcinoma of the vagina. Cancer 1982;49:1308.

Peters WA, Kumar NB, Morley GW: Carcinoma of the vagina: Factors influencing treatment outcome. Cancer 1985;55:892.

Reddy S et al: Radiation therapy in primary carcinoma of the vagina. Gynecol Oncol 1987;26:19.

Rubin SC, Young J, Mikuta JJ: Squamous carcinoma of the vagina: Treatment, complications, and long-term follow-up. Gynecol Oncol 1985;20:346.

Thigpen JT et al: A phase II trial of cisplatin in advanced recurrent cancer of the vagina: A GOG study. Gynecol Oncol 1986;23:101.

Tjalama WA et al: The role of surgery in invasive squamous carcinoma of the vagina. Gynecol Oncol 2001;81:360.

Wagner W et al: Vulvar carcinoma: a retrospective analysis of 80 patients. Arch Gynecol Obstet 1999;262:99.

Premalignant & Malignant Disorders of the Uterine Cervix

47

Christine H. Holschneider, MD

CERVICAL INTRAEPITHELIAL NEOPLASIA

ESSENTIALS OF DIAGNOSIS

- *The cervix often appears grossly normal.*
- *Dysplastic or carcinoma in situ cells are noted in a cytologic smear preparation (traditional Pap smear or liquid-based cytology).*
- *Colposcopic examination reveals an atypical transformation zone with thickened acetowhite epithelium and coarse punctate or mosaic patterns of surface capillaries.*
- *Iodine-nonstaining (Schiller-positive) area of squamous epithelium is typical.*
- *Biopsy diagnosis of cervical intraepithelial neoplasia (dysplasia or carcinoma in situ).*

General Considerations

Lower genital tract squamous intraepithelial neoplasia is often multicentric (ie, affecting multiple anatomic sites which embryologically are derived from the same anogenital epithelium): cervical intraepithelial neoplasia (CIN), vaginal intraepithelial neoplasia (VAIN, see Chapter 46), vulvar intraepithelial neoplasia (VIN, see Chapter 46), and perianal intraepithelial neoplasia (PAIN). Approximately 10% of women with CIN have concomitant preinvasive neoplasia of the vulva, vagina, or anus. Conversely, 40–60% of patients with VIN or VAIN have synchronous or metachronous CIN.

Cervical intraepithelial neoplasia (CIN), formerly called dysplasia, means disordered growth and development of the epithelial lining of the cervix. There are various degrees of CIN. Mild dysplasia or CIN I is defined as disordered growth of the lower third of the epithelial lining. Abnormal maturation of two-thirds of the lining is called moderate dysplasia or CIN II. Severe dysplasia, CIN III, encompasses more than two-thirds of the epithelial thickness with carcinoma in situ (CIS)

representing full-thickness dysmaturity (Fig 47–1). While histologically evaluated lesions are characterized using the CIN nomenclature, cytologic smears are classified according to the Bethesda system (Table 47–1). Briefly, in this recently revised system atypical squamous cells are divided into those of undetermined significance (ASC-US) and those in which a high grade lesion cannot be excluded (ASC-H). Low-grade squamous intraepithelial lesion (LGSIL or LSIL) encompasses cytologic changes consistent with koilocytic atypia or CIN I. High-grade squamous intraepithelial lesion (HGSIL or HSIL) denotes the cytologic findings corresponding to CIN II and CIN III (see also Chapter 30). CIN may be suspected because of an abnormal cytologic smear, but the diagnosis is established by cervical biopsy. Spontaneous regression, especially of CIN I, occurs in a significant number of patients, allowing for expectant management with serial cytologic smears in the reliable patient. A certain percentage of all dysplasias, especially high-grade lesions, will progress to an invasive cancer if left untreated. Because it is not presently possible to predict which lesions will progress, it is recommended that all patients with CIN II and III be treated when diagnosed.

Epidemiology & Etiology

Prevalence figures for CIN vary according to the socioeconomic characteristics and geographic area of the population studied, from as low as 1.05% in some family planning clinics to as high as 13.7% in women attending STD clinics. CIN is most commonly detected in women in their 20s, the peak incidence of carcinoma in situ is in women aged 25–35, while the incidence of cervical cancer rises after the age of 40.

The epidemiologic risk factors for CIN are similar to those for cervical cancer and include multiple sexual partners, early onset of sexual activity, a high-risk sexual partner (history of multiple sexual partners, HPV infection, lower genital tract neoplasia, or prior sexual exposure to someone with cervical neoplasia), a history of STDs, as well as cigarette smoking, immunodeficiency, multiparity, and long-term oral contraceptive pill use.

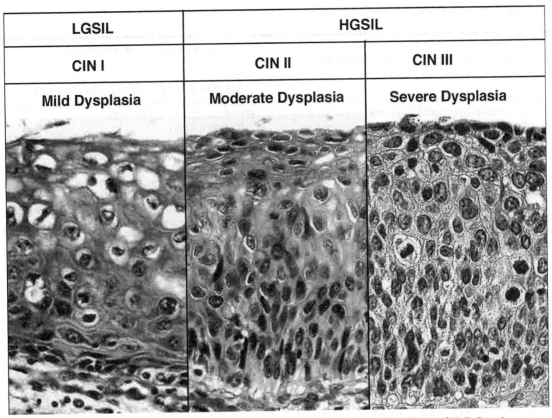

LGSIL	HGSIL	
CIN I	CIN II	CIN III
Mild Dysplasia	Moderate Dysplasia	Severe Dysplasia

Figure 47–1. Changes in the terminology for cervical intraepithelial neoplasia. (Courtesy of UpToDate in Oncology.)

Human papillomaviruses (HPVs) are a prime etiologic factor in the development of CIN and cervical cancer. In fact, most of the above behavioral and sexual risk factors for cervical neoplasia become statistically insignificant as independent variables after adjusting for HPV infection. Analyses of cervical neoplasia lesions show the presence of HPV in over 80% of all CIN lesions and over 90% of all invasive cervical cancers.

Infection with HPV is extremely common and varies with the patient's age. In the U.S., the prevalence of detectable HPV infection rises from 1% in newborns, to 20% in teenagers, to 40% in women 20–29 years of age, with a slow decline thereafter to a plateau of 5% in women age 50 and older. Condoms are not as protective against HPV as they are against other sexually transmitted diseases since transmission can occur from labial-scrotal contact.

Women who have persistent HPV infections, especially with high viral loads, have a higher likelihood of developing CIN and cervical cancer. However, over 90% of immunocompetent women will have a spontaneous resolution of their HPV infection over a 2-year period and only about 5% will have cytologically detectable CIN. Thus, the vast majority of women infected with HPV do not develop CIN or cervical cancer. This suggests that infection with HPV alone is not sufficient for the development of CIN or cervical cancer and underscores the importance of other cofactors, such as cigarette smoking or immunosuppression.

There are over 70 HPV subtypes, half of which infect the anogenital epithelium. Based on their malignant potential, HPV subtypes are categorized into low-risk, intermediate-risk, and high-risk types. Low-risk HPV types (6, 11, 42, 43, and 44) are associated with condylomata and low-grade lesions (CIN I). Intermediate-risk HPV types (33, 35, 51, and 52) are found in higher-grade lesions (CIN II and CIN III) that tend to persist but rarely progress, whereas high-risk HPV (16, 18, 31, 39, 45, 56, 58, 59, and 68) is, in addition to high-grade lesions (CIN II and CIN III), found in invasive cancer.

Cigarette smoking and HPV infection have synergistic effects on the development of CIN, and cigarette smoking is associated with a two- to fourfold increase

Table 47–1. The Bethesda System 2001.

Specimen Type	Glandular cells status posthysterectomy
Indicate conventional smear (Pap smear) vs liquid-based vs. other	Atrophy
Specimen Adequacy	**OTHER**
Satisfactory for evaluation (*describe presence or absence of endocervical transformation zone component and any other quality indicators, eg, partially obscuring blood, inflammation, etc*)	Endometrial cells (in a woman ≥ 40 years of age) (*Specify if negative for squamous intraepithelial lesion*)
	EPITHELIAL CELL ABNORMALITIES
	SQUAMOUS CELL

Specimen Type

Indicate conventional smear (Pap smear) vs liquid-based vs. other

Specimen Adequacy

  Satisfactory for evaluation (*describe presence or absence of endocervical transformation zone component and any other quality indicators, eg, partially obscuring blood, inflammation, etc*)

  Unsatisfactory for evaluation . . . (*specify reason*)

    Specimen rejected/not processed (*specify reason*)

    Specimen processed and examined, but unsatisfactory for evaluation of epithelial abnormality because of (*specify reason*)

General Categorization (optional)

Negative for intraepithelial lesion or malignancy

Epithelial cell abnormality: See Interpretation/Result (*specify squamous or glandular as appropriate*)

Other: See Interpretation/Result (*eg, endometrial cells in a woman ≥ 40 years of age*)

Automated Review

If case examined by automated device, specify device and result

Ancillary Testing

Provide a brief description of the test methods and report the result so that it is easily understood by the clinician

Interpretation/Result

  NEGATIVE FOR INTRAEPITHELIAL LESION OR MALIGNANCY (*when there is no cellular evidence of neoplasia, state this in the General Categorization above and/or in the Interpretation/Result section of the report, whether or not there are organisms or other non-neoplastic findings*)

    ORGANISMS:

      Trichomonas vaginalis

      Fungal organisms morphologically consistent with *Candida* spp.

      Shift in flora suggestive of bacterial vaginosis

      Bacteria morphologically consistent with *Actinomyces* spp.

      Cellular changes consistent with herpes simplex virus

    OTHER NON-NEOPLASTIC FINDINGS (*Optional to report; list not inclusive*):

    Reactive cellular changes associated with inflammation (includes typical repair)

    Radiation

    Intrauterine contraceptive device (IUD)

Glandular cells status posthysterectomy

Atrophy

OTHER

  Endometrial cells (in a woman ≥ 40 years of age) (*Specify if negative for squamous intraepithelial lesion*)

EPITHELIAL CELL ABNORMALITIES

  SQUAMOUS CELL

    Atypical squamous cells

      of undetermined significance (ASC-US)

      cannot exclude HSIL (ASC-H)

    Low-grade squamous intraepithelial lesion (LSIL) encompassing: HPV/mild dysplasia/CIN

    High-grade squamous intraepithelial lesion (HSIL) encompassing: moderate and severe dysplasia, CIN 2 and CIN 3/CIS

    Squamous cell carcinoma

  GLANDULAR CELL

    Atypical (AGC)

      endocervical cells

      endometrial cells

      glandular cells not otherwise specified (NOS)

    Ayptical, favor neoplastic

      endocervical cells

      glandular cells NOS

    Endocervical adenocarcinoma in situ (AIS)

    Adenocarcinoma

      endocervical

      endometrial

      extrauterine

      not otherwise specified (NOS)

  OTHER MALIGNANT NEOPLASMS: (*specify*)

Educational Notes and Suggestions (*optional*)

  Suggestions should be concise and consistent with clinical follow-up guidelines published by professional organizations (references to relevant publications may be included)

in the relative risk for developing cervical cancer. Cigarette smoke carcinogens have been found to accumulate locally in the cervical mucus, and the cumulative exposure as measured by pack-years smoked is related to the risk of developing CIN or carcinoma in situ. However, the mechanisms by which cigarette smoking contributes to cervical carcinogenesis are poorly understood.

The incidence of cervical neoplasia is increased in HIV-infected women who in some studies have a 20–30% incidence of colposcopically confirmed CIN. With increasing immunosuppression there is an increase in the risk of de novo HPV infection, persistent HPV infection, and progressive cervical neoplasia. Since 1993, invasive cervical cancer has been included as an AIDS-defining illness.

Pathology

On cytologic examination, the dysplastic cell is characterized by anaplasia, an increased nuclear:cytoplasmic ratio (ie, the nucleus is larger), hyperchromatism with changes in the nuclear chromatin, multinucleation, and abnormalities in differentiation.

Histologically, involvement of varying degrees of thickness of the stratified squamous epithelium is typical of dysplasia. The cells are anaplastic and hyperchromatic, and show a loss of polarity in the deeper layers as well as abnormal mitotic figures in increased numbers. Benign epithelial alterations, particularly those of an inflammatory nature, the cytopathic effects of HPV, and technical artifacts may be mistaken for CIN I and CIN II.

The columnar epithelium of the mucus-secreting endocervical glands can also undergo neoplastic transformation. Adenocarcinoma in situ (ACIS) is defined as the presence of endocervical glands lined by atypical columnar epithelium that cytologically resembles the cells of endocervical adenocarcinoma, but that occur in the absence of stromal invasion. The diagnosis of ACIS can be made only by cone biopsy.

Clinical Findings

A. SYMPTOMS AND SIGNS

There are usually no symptoms or signs of CIN, and the diagnosis is most often based on biopsy findings following an abnormal routine cervical cytology smear. Because high-grade dysplasia probably is a transitional phase in the pathogenesis of many cervical cancers, early detection is extremely important. As recommended by the American College of Obstetricians and Gynecologists, all women who have been sexually active or reached age 18 should have a pelvic and cytologic examination at least once a year. After three or more consecutive, satisfactory, normal annual examinations, the screening interval may be extended in selected low-risk patients. However, annual screening should be continued in women with any risk factors for CIN.

B. SPECIAL EXAMINATIONS

All abnormal Pap smears require further evaluation, such as visual inspection of the cervix, repeat cytology, HPV testing, staining with Lugol's solution (Schiller test) or toluidine blue, colposcopy, directed biopsy, endocervical curettage, or diagnostic conization (see treatment section) (Fig 47–2). The objective is to exclude the presence of invasive carcinoma and to determine the degree and extent of any CIN.

1. Repeat cervical cytology—There are three acceptable initial evaluation steps for patients with minimally abnormal cervical cytology smears (eg, atypical squa-

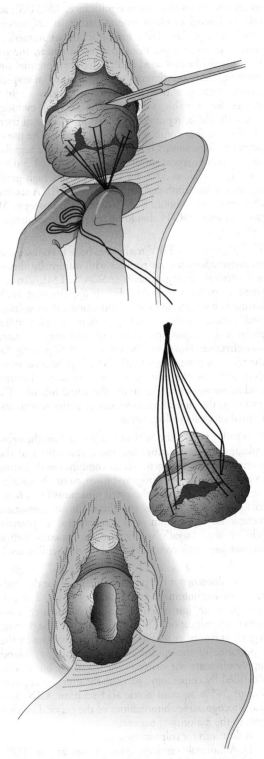

Figure 47–2. Conization of the cervix.

mous cells of undetermined significance; ASC-US): accelerated serial cytology smears, triage to colposcopy based on a positive HPV testing result, or immediate referral to colposcopy. Prior to a repeat smear, the patient should be evaluated and treated for potential underlying conditions that might contribute to an atypical smear, such as antimicrobials for infectious or hormones for atrophic vaginitis. The cervical cytology smear should be repeated every 4–6 months until there are three to four consecutive normal smears. The use of serial cytologic smears is important, as the false negative rate of a single repeat smear following an ASC-US diagnosis is as high as 33% for biopsy-proven high-grade squamous intraepithelial lesions (CIN II/III). A second abnormal smear should be evaluated by colposcopy. All patients with ASC-H should be referred for immediate colposcopy.

2. HPV testing—HPV testing has been investigated as an intermediary test for patients with minimally abnormal cervical cytology smears (ASC-US, LSIL). In the triage of patients with ASC-US, it appears that HPV testing is comparable to the performance of an accelerated repeat cervical cytology smear in identifying patients for colposcopic evaluation and may be more cost-effective. However, the value of HPV testing for the triage of patients with LSIL is limited because more than 80% of the lesions are HPV-positive. Further studies are needed to determine the actual role of HPV testing in the clinical management of patients with abnormal cervical cytology smears.

3. Schiller test—The Schiller test is based on the principle that normal mature squamous epithelium of the cervix contains glycogen, which combines with iodine to produce a deep mahogany-brown color. Nonstaining, therefore, indicates abnormal squamous (or columnar) epithelium, scarring, cyst formation, or immature metaplastic epithelium and constitutes a positive Schiller test. Lugol's solution is an aqueous iodine preparation and is commonly used for the Schiller test.

4. Colposcopic examination (see also Chapter 30)—Colposcopy is the primary technique for the evaluation of an abnormal cervical cytology smear. The colposcope is an instrument that uses illuminated low-power magnification (5–15×) to inspect the cervix, vagina, vulva, or anal epithelium. Abnormalities in the appearance of the epithelium and its capillary blood supply often are not visible to the naked eye but can be identified by colposcopy, particularly after the application of 3–5% aqueous acetic acid solution. CIN produces recognizable abnormalities of the cervical epithelium in the majority of patients.

Indications for colposcopy are:

1. Abnormal cervical cytology smear or HPV testing;

2. Clinically abnormal or suspicious-looking cervix;

3. Unexplained intermenstrual or postcoital bleeding;

4. Vulvar or vaginal neoplasia; or

5. History of in utero DES exposure.

Details of the colposcopy technique are described in Chapter 30.

Normal colposcopic findings are those of:

(a) The original squamous epithelium, which extends from the mucocutaneous vulvovaginal junction to the original squamocolumnar junction.

(b) The transformation zone, which is the metaplastic squamous epithelium between the original squamocolumnar junction and the active squamocolumnar junction. The original squamocolumnar junction is the junction between the stratified squamous epithelium of the vagina and ectocervix, and the columnar epithelium of the endocervical canal. In two-thirds of female infants, this original squamocolumnar junction is located on the ectocervix, in close to a third in the endocervical canal, and in a very small subset out in the vaginal fornices. During a woman's life cycle the squamocolumnar junction "migrates" due to various hormonal and environmental influences which alter the cervical volume and cause squamous metaplasia of everted endocervical columnar cells. Following menarche the squamocolumnar junction is generally found on the ectocervix, with further eversion during pregnancy. In the postmenopausal patient, the squamocolumnar junction is frequently within the endocervical canal. This squamous metaplasia is a dynamic process and cervical neoplasia almost invariably originates within the transformation zone. If the new squamocolumnar junction is visualized in its entirety, the colposcopic examination is called satisfactory; if it cannot be fully visualized, the examination is called unsatisfactory.

(c) The columnar epithelium of the endocervical canal.

Abnormal findings indicative of dysplasia and CIS are those of:

1. Leukoplakia or hyperkeratosis, which is an area of white, thickened epithelium which is appreciated prior to the application of acetic acid and may indicate underlying neoplasia.

2. Acetowhite epithelium, which is epithelium that stains white after the application of acetic acid.

3. Mosaicism or punctation reflecting abnormal vascular patterns of the surface capillaries. As a general rule, capillary thickness and intercapillary distances correlate with the severity of the lesion and thus tend to be larger and coarser in higher-grade lesions.

4. Atypical vessels with bizarre capillaries with so-called corkscrew, comma-shaped, or spaghetti-like configurations suggest early stromal invasion (Figs 47–3 through 47–5).

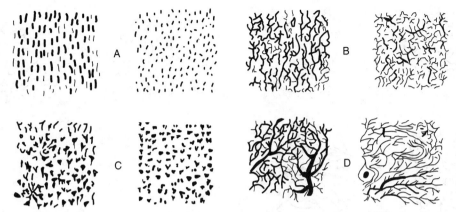

Figure 47–3. Schematic drawing of different types of terminal vessels as observed in the normal squamous epithelium: hairpin capillaries (**A**), network capillaries (**B**) both found in normal states, double capillaries (**C**) seen in *Trichomonas* inflammation, and branching vessels (**D**) seen in the transformation zone. (Reproduced, with permission, from Johannisson E, Kolstat P, Soderberg G: Cytologic, vascular, and histologic patterns of dysplasia, carcinoma in situ and early invasive carcinoma of the cervix. Acta Radiol Suppl [Stockh] 1966;258.)

A colposcopically directed punch biopsy of the most severely abnormal areas should be done. The transformation zone extends into the endocervical canal beyond the field of vision in 12–15% of premenopausal women and in a significantly higher percentage of postmenopausal women. Evaluation of the nonvisualized portion of the endocervical canal by endocervical curettage (ECC) should be performed in every case in which colposcopy is unsatisfactory, where the lesion is extending into the endocervical canal, or where the colposcopic impression does not explain the cervical cytology findings. In up to 20% of patients with CIN, the endocervical curettage is positive for dysplasia.

5. Diagnostic cone biopsy—Following expert colposcopic evaluation, diagnostic cone biopsy of the cervix (Fig 47–2) is indicated if colposcopy is unsatisfactory, for a high-grade cervical cytology smear, if the lesion extends into the cervical canal beyond the view afforded by the colposcope, if there is a significant discrepancy between the histologic diagnosis of the directed biopsy specimen and the cytologic examination, if adenocarci-

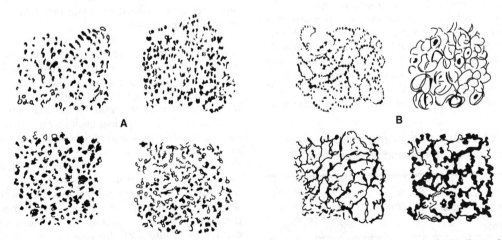

Figure 47–4. Schematic drawing of punctation terminal vessels (**A**) and mosaic terminal vessels (**B**). (Reproduced, with permission, from Johannisson E, Kolstat P, Soderberg G: Cytologic, vascular, and histologic patterns of dysplasia, carcinoma in situ and early invasive carcinoma of the cervix. Acta Radiol Suppl [Stockh] 1966;258.)

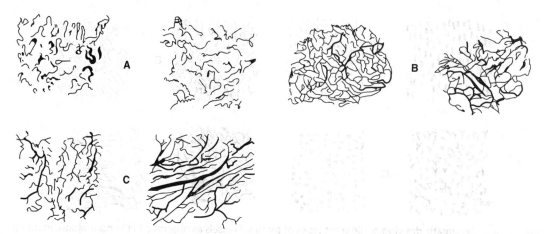

Figure 47–5. Schematic drawing of atypical vessels: hairpin-like (**A**); network-like (**B**); and branching type (**C**). (Reproduced, with permission, from Johannisson E, Kolstat P, Soderberg G: Cytologic, vascular, and histologic patterns of dysplasia, carcinoma in situ and early invasive carcinoma of the cervix. Acta Radiol Suppl [Stockh] 1966;258.)

noma in situ is suspected, or if microinvasive carcinoma is suspected.

Natural History

Understanding the natural history of the various degrees of CIN is central to the appropriate clinical management of these patients. In addition to the degree of dysplasia, it is likely that the course of a specific lesion is also influenced by a number of other factors, such as the inciting HPV type, the patient's immune competence, or smoking habits. As is summarized in Table 47–2, the majority of CIN I lesions will spontaneously regress without treatment. However, 2–21% of patients with CIN I are reported to have disease progression to CIN III or worse over a 2- to 5-year follow-up. Therefore, it is reasonable to expectantly follow the compliant patient with CIN I using surveillance with serial cervical cytology smears at 4- to 6-month intervals. Since we currently lack the means to identify individuals at risk for progressive disease, immediate treat-

Table 47–2. Approximate rates of spontaneous regression, persistence, and progression of CIN.

	CIN I	CIN II	CIN III
Regression to normal	60%	40%	30%
Persistence	30%	35%	48%
Progression to CIN III	10%	20%	—
Progression to cancer	< 1%	5%	22%

ment might be appropriate for high-risk patients likely to be lost to follow-up, because up to 40% of these women may have persistent or progressive disease that will require therapy. The majority of high-grade lesions will persist or progress (Table 47–2), so immediate treatment is generally warranted.

Treatment

Patient management is based on the correlation of the results of the cervical cytology smear; findings at colposcopy, biopsy, and ECC results, as well as individual patient characteristics, such as pregnancy, HIV infection, and the likelihood of compliance with management recommendations.

Treatment options fall into one of two main categories: procedures that ablate the abnormal tissue and do not produce a tissue specimen for additional histologic evaluation and procedures that excise the area of abnormality, allowing for further histologic study. Prior to any therapeutic intervention an assessment has to be made as to whether a patient qualifies for ablative therapy (eg, satisfactory diagnostic evaluation has excluded invasive disease) or if she requires an excisional procedure (conization) for further diagnostic work-up. In most cases conization is also the appropriate therapeutic intervention. If the intraepithelial lesion is confined to the ectocervix, treatment with cryotherapy, laser ablation, or a superficial excision by the loop electrosurgical excision procedure (LEEP) is appropriate. If the lesion extends into the endocervical canal, the endocervical curettage contains dysplastic epithelium, or the colposcopic examination is otherwise unsatisfactory, the en-

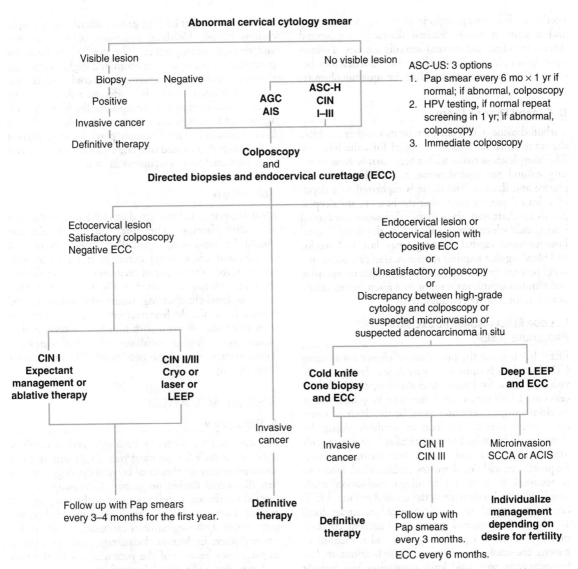

Abnormal cervical cytology smear

Visible lesion

Biopsy —— Negative

Positive

Invasive cancer

Definitive therapy

No visible lesion

ASC-US: 3 options
1. Pap smear every 6 mo × 1 yr if normal; if abnormal, colposcopy
2. HPV testing, if normal repeat screening in 1 yr; if abnormal, colposcopy
3. Immediate colposcopy

AGC
AIS

ASC-H
CIN
I–III

Colposcopy
and
Directed biopsies and endocervical curettage (ECC)

Ectocervical lesion
Satisfactory colposcopy
Negative ECC

Endocervical lesion or ectocervical lesion with positive ECC
or
Unsatisfactory colposcopy
or
Discrepancy between high-grade cytology and colposcopy or suspected microinvasion or suspected adenocarcinoma in situ

CIN I
Expectant management or ablative therapy

CIN II/III
Cryo or laser or LEEP

Cold knife
Cone biopsy
and ECC

Deep LEEP
and ECC

Invasive cancer

Invasive cancer

CIN II
CIN III

Microinvasion
SCCA or ACIS

Follow up with Pap smears every 3–4 months for the first year.

Definitive therapy

Definitive therapy

Follow up with Pap smears every 3 months.

ECC every 6 months.

Individualize management depending on desire for fertility

Figure 47–6. Plan for management of the abnormal cytologic smear with visible or no visible cervical lesion.

docervical canal must be included in the treatment by a deeper LEEP or cone biopsy (Fig 47–6).

The five most common techniques for the treatment of CIN include two ablative techniques, cryotherapy or laser ablation, and three excisional procedures, cold knife conization, laser cone excision, and LEEP. Evidence from controlled trials show that these techniques are of equal efficacy, averaging approximately 90% success rates in the treatment of CIN. Cure depends on the size of the lesion, endocervical gland involvement, margin status of any excisional specimen, and ECC results.

A. CRYOTHERAPY

In cryotherapy, an office procedure not requiring anesthesia, nitrous oxide or carbon dioxide is used as the refrigerant for a supercooled probe. The cryoprobe is positioned on the ectocervix where it must cover the entire lesion, which at times is not easily achieved. It is then activated until blanching of the cervix extends at least 7 mm beyond the probe. Introduction of a two-cycle freeze-thaw-freeze technique has improved efficacy. The advantages of cryotherapy include ease of use, low cost, widespread availability and a low complication rate. Side effects include mild uterine cramping and a copious watery vaginal discharge for several weeks. Infection and cervical stenosis are rare. Follow-up colposcopic examinations can be unsatisfactory because of the inability to visualize the squamocolumnar junction.

B. Carbon Dioxide Laser

Carbon dioxide (CO_2) laser can be used either to ablate the transformation zone or as a tool for cone biopsies. The laser destroys tissue with a very narrow zone of injury around the treated tissue, and is therefore both precise and flexible. The tissue is vaporized to a depth of at least 7 mm to assure that the bases of the deepest glands are destroyed, since dysplastic lesions can extend into glands which have a maximum depth of 7 mm. Posttreatment vaginal discharge may last 1–2 weeks, and bleeding that requires reexamination can occur in a small percentage of patients. The technique is expensive and requires significant training and attention to safety, as well as local or general anesthesia.

C. Loop Electrosurgical Excision Procedure (LEEP)

LEEP has become the procedure of choice for treating CIN II and III because of its ease of use, low cost, provision of tissue for histologic evaluation, and high success rate. LEEP uses a small, fine wire loop attached to an electrosurgical generator to excise the tissue of interest. Various sizes of wire loop are available. Again, lesions should be excised to a depth of at least 7 mm. Following LEEP excision of the transformation zone, frequently an additional narrow endocervical specimen is removed to allow for histologic evaluation while avoiding excessive damage to the cervical stroma. LEEP can be performed as an office procedure under local anesthesia. An insulated speculum to prevent conduction of electricity, a grounding pad, and a vacuum to remove the smoke are necessary. Complications are less frequent than with cold knife conization and include bleeding, infection, and cervical stenosis.

D. Cold Knife Conization

Cold knife conization of the cervix refers to the excision of a cone-shaped portion of the cervix using a scalpel. This technique can be individualized to accommodate the size and shape of the specimen. For example, a wide, shallow cone specimen can be obtained from a young patient whose squamocolumnar junction is on the ectocervix. In an older patient, in whom the squamocolumnar junction tends to move more cephalad into the endocervical canal, a narrower, deeper cone is preferable. An endocervical curettage is performed after the conization to assess the remaining endocervical canal. Cervical cone biopsy is generally done in the op-

erating room under local or general anesthesia. Complications include bleeding, infection, cervical stenosis, and cervical incompetence. The need to perform the procedure in the operating room and higher complication rate are distinct disadvantages of cold knife conization. However, it results in a specimen devoid of any thermal artifact that may complicate the histologic diagnosis and margin assessment seen with LEEP and laser conization. This becomes particularly important with lesions that extend into the endocervical canal and with suspected adenocarcinoma in situ.

Follow-up

Most treatment failures are diagnosed within the first year after therapy. Therefore, careful examination should be performed, with Pap smears every 3–4 months and endocervical curettage if the endocervix was involved. Treatment of recurrent dysplasia follows the same guidelines outlined in Fig 47–6. If a woman has completed childbearing, recurrent dysplasia can be treated by a simple hysterectomy after invasion has been ruled out. Women with a history of cervical dysplasia have a higher incidence of vaginal dysplasia. These women continue to need yearly Pap smears after hysterectomy.

SPECIAL SITUATIONS

A. Pregnancy

Pregnant women routinely undergo cervical cytology screening at their first prenatal visit. As a result, it is not uncommon that an abnormal cervical cytology smear is first discovered during pregnancy. Colposcopy is performed for the same indications as in the nonpregnant patient. However, biopsies are limited unless there are colposcopic signs suggestive of carcinoma in situ or invasive disease. Endocervical curettage is not performed in pregnancy because of the potential risk of abortion and infection. The physiologic changes of pregnancy render the transformation zone easily accessible for satisfactory colposcopy by 20 weeks' gestation in almost all women. Colposcopy during pregnancy can be challenging because pregnancy may produce changes in the cervical epithelium that mimic those of cervical dysplasia. Although the gravid cervix is more vascular, directed ectocervical biopsies can be performed safely with minimal increase in the risk of significant bleeding. After the diagnosis of dysplasia has been established, the patient can be carefully followed with serial colposcopic examinations and treated postpartum. Even high-grade lesions discovered during pregnancy have a high rate of regression in the postpartum period. Conization during pregnancy is indicated only if microinvasive disease is suspected. Complications of a cone biopsy in pregnancy include abortion, hemorrhage, infection, and incompetent cervix.

B. Atypical Glandular Cells (AGC) on Cervical Cytology Smear

Patients with atypical glandular cells of undetermined significance (prior Bethesda system) on a cervical cytology smear have a 30–50% risk of having high-grade cervical neoplasia. The underlying lesion is most commonly CIN II or III, which is diagnosed in up to 25% of cases. Cervical adenocarcinoma in situ, invasive cervical adenocarcinoma, and endometrial disease, including hyperplasia and cancer, comprise the remaining 20%. The 2001 Bethesda System divides glandular cell abnormalities into atypical glandular cells (AGC), AGC-favor neoplasia, endocervical adenocarcinoma in situ (AIS) and adenocarcinoma. Given the high risk for significant pathology, any patient with glandular cell abnormalities on a cervical cytology smear requires immediate evaluation, which includes at a minimum colposcopy with careful evaluation of the endocervical canal. Assessment of the endometrium is recommended in all patients with abnormal bleeding or age > 35 years. Diagnostic conization is indicated in all cases of AGC-favor neoplasia, AIS, or suspected adenocarcinoma as well as persistent AGC-NOS, unless a definitive diagnosis has been made on the colposcopy directed biopsy or endometrial sampling.

C. Adenocarcinoma In Situ (AIS)

The reported incidence of glandular neoplasia of the cervix is increasing, especially in young women, with up to 30% of cases occurring in women under 35 years of age. Adenocarcinoma of the cervix represents about 25% of all cervical cancers and there is convincing evidence that ACIS is a precursor lesion. Half of the women with ACIS have concomitant squamous CIN. Management is difficult. The lesion may be located high in the endocervical canal, involve the deeper portions of the endocervical clefts, or be multifocal with skip lesions. Conization is required to make the diagnosis. Follow-up surveillance after conization is difficult as cervical cytology, endocervical curettage, or endocervical cytobrush sampling each have a sensitivity of only about 50%. This is of particular concern because the incidence of residual ACIS or invasive adenocarcinoma following conization for ACIS may be higher than 50% with positive conization margins, and 35% even with negative conization margins. Therefore, conservative management should be undertaken only in the young patient with a negative conization margin who is fully counseled and desires to maintain her fertility. In all other patients, hysterectomy should be performed as a definitive therapeutic intervention because even with negative margins, as many as 8–16% may have invasive disease on the hysterectomy specimen. For the same reason, consideration should be given to the performance of a modified radical hysterectomy in this situation.

D. HIV Infection

Management of CIN in the HIV-infected patient presents a great challenge. Following treatment, the risk of recurrent CIN is high, especially in the immunocompromised patient with low CD4 counts and high viral loads. Recurrence rates may reach 80% within 3 years in markedly immunocompromised women. Use of highly active antiretroviral therapy (HAART) appears to reduce the risk of recurrent or progressive cervical neoplasia.

CANCER OF THE CERVIX

 ESSENTIALS OF DIAGNOSIS

- Early disease is frequently asymptomatic, underscoring the importance of cervical cytology screening.
- Abnormal uterine bleeding and vaginal discharge are the most common symptoms.
- A cervical lesion may be visible on inspection as a tumor or ulceration; cancer within the cervical canal may be occult.
- Diagnosis must be confirmed by biopsy.

General Considerations

Cancer of the cervix is the sixth most common solid cancer in American women. In the U.S. an estimated 12,900 new cases of invasive cervical cancer are diagnosed annually, and there are 4400 deaths from the disease. In contrast, with more than 370,000 new cases diagnosed annually and a 50% mortality rate, cervical cancer is the second most common cause of cancer-related morbidity and mortality among women in developing countries. This dichotomy is largely due to a 75% decrease in the incidence of cervical cancer in developed countries following the implementation of population-based screening programs and treatment of preinvasive disease. The average age at diagnosis of patients with cervical cancer is 51 years. However, the disease can occur in the second decade of life and during pregnancy. Over 95% of patients with early cancer of the cervix can be cured.

Etiology & Epidemiology

The major epidemiologic risk factors for cervical cancer are the same as those for CIN and have been discussed above. HPV is central to the development of cervical neoplasia. HPV DNA is found in 95% of all squamous cell carcinomas, and in over 90% of all adenocarcinomas and adenosquamous carcinomas. High-risk oncogenic HPV types account for approximately 80% of HPV types in cervical cancer, with HPV 16 being the most prevalent in squamous cell carcinoma, and HPV 18 most prevalent in adenocarcinoma. Other associated risk factors are immunosuppression, infection with HIV or a history of other sexually transmitted diseases, tobacco use, high parity, or oral contraceptive use.

Pathogenesis & Natural History

HPV is epitheliotropic. Once the epithelium is acutely infected with HPV, one of three clinical scenarios ensues:

(a) Asymptomatic latent infection;

(b) Active infection in which HPV undergoes vegetative replication, but not integration into the genome (eg, leading to condyloma or CIN I); or

(c) Neoplastic transformation following integration of oncogenic HPV DNA into the human genome.

Integration of HPV into the human genome is associated with cell immortalization allowing for malignant transformation. This involves an upregulation of the viral oncogenes E6 and E7. These oncoproteins interfere with cell cycle control in the human host cell. E6 and E7 have the ability to complex with the tumor suppressor genes p53 and Rb, respectively. The disabling of these two major tumor suppressor genes is thought to be central to host cell immortalization and transformation induced by HPV.

Incipient cancer of the cervix is generally a slowly developing process. Most cervical cancers probably begin as a high-grade dysplastic change (see previous section) or carcinoma in situ with gradual progression over a period of several years. At least 90% of squamous cell carcinomas of the cervix develop from the intraepithelial layers, almost always within 1 cm of the squamocolumnar junction of the cervix either on the portio vaginalis of the cervix or slightly higher in the endocervical canal.

Early stromal invasion (stage IA1) to a depth of 1–3 mm below the basement membrane is a localized process, provided there is no pathologic evidence of lymphovascular space involvement. Penetration of the stroma beyond this point carries an increased risk of lymphatic metastasis (Table 47–3). As the tumor grows, it also spreads by direct extension to the parametria. When the lymphatics are involved, tumor cells are carried to the regional pelvic lymph nodes (parametrial, hypogastric, obturator, external iliac, and sacral) (Fig 47–7). The more pleomorphic or extensive the local disease, the greater the likelihood of lymph node involvement. Squamous cell carcinoma clinically confined to the cervix involves the regional pelvic lymph nodes in 15–20% of cases. When the cancer involves the parametrium (stage IIB), tumor cells can be found in the pelvic lymph nodes in 30–40% and in the para-aortic nodes in about 15–30% of cases. The more advanced the local disease, the greater the likelihood of distant metastases. The para-aortic nodes are involved in about 45% of patients with stage IVA disease.

Ovarian involvement is rare, occurring in approximately 0.5% of squamous cell carcinomas and 1.7% of adenocarcinomas. The liver and lungs are the most common sites of blood-borne metastasis, but the tumor may involve the brain, bones, bowels, adrenal glands, spleen, or pancreas.

When cancer of the cervix is untreated or fails to respond to treatment, death occurs in 95% of patients within 2 years after the onset of symptoms. Death can occur from uremia, pulmonary embolism, or hemor-

Table 47–3. Risk of any lymph node metastasis for patients with microscopic squamous cell carcinoma of the cervix.

Depth of Tumor Invasion	Risk of Lymph Node Metastasis
FIGO stage IA1	
Early stromal invasion (< 1 mm)	3/1543 (0.2%)
Microinvasion (1–3 mm)	5/809 (0.6%)
FIGO stage IA2	
Microscopic 3–5 mm invasion	14/214 (6.5%)

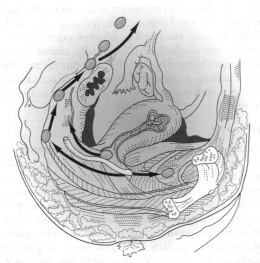

Figure 47–7. Lymphatic spread of carcinoma of the cervix.

rhage from direct extension of tumor into blood vessels. Life-threatening sepsis from complications of pyelonephritis or vesicovaginal and rectovaginal fistulas is possible. Large-bowel obstruction from direct extension of tumor into the rectosigmoid can be the terminal event. Pain from perineural extension is a significant management problem of advanced disease.

Pathology

About 70–75% of cervical carcinomas are squamous cell; the remainder are composed of various types of adenocarcinomas (20–25%), adenosquamous carcinomas (3–5%), and undifferentiated carcinomas.

A. Squamous Cell Carcinomas

Cervical squamous cell carcinomas have been classified according to the predominant cell type: large cell nonkeratinizing, large cell keratinizing, and small cell carcinomas. The large cell nonkeratinizing variety accounts for the majority of tumors. The small cell type of squamous carcinoma carries a notably worse prognosis than either the large cell keratinizing or large cell nonkeratinizing tumors.

B. Verrucous Carcinoma

Verrucous carcinoma, which has been associated with HPV 6, is a rare subtype of well-differentiated squamous carcinoma. It is a slow-growing, locally invasive neoplasm. Histologically, this tumor is composed of well-differentiated squamous cells with frondlike papil-

lae and little apparent stromal invasion, but it is potentially lethal. Radical resection is the mainstay of therapy.

C. Adenocarcinoma

Adenocarcinoma of the cervix is derived from the glandular elements of the cervix. The incidence of adenocarcinomas, including the mucinous, endometrioid, clear cell, and serous types, has been rising over the last several decades, especially in women younger than 35 years of age. Part of this increase may be due to an increasing prevalence of HPV infection and part to improvements in screening and prevention of squamous preinvasive disease, thus leading to a histologic shift toward adenocarcinoma. When the initial growth of adenocarcinoma of the cervix is within the endocervical canal and the ectocervix appears normal, this lesion may not be diagnosed until it is advanced and ulcerative. The so-called clear cell variety may be related to in utero exposure to DES. It has a prognosis comparable to that of other adenocarcinomas of the cervix. The villoglandular-papillary variety of adenocarcinoma of the cervix tends to occur in younger women and have a more favorable prognosis.

D. Adenoma Malignum

Adenoma malignum or minimal deviation adenocarcinoma is an extremely well-differentiated adenocarcinoma that may be difficult to recognize as a malignant process. It represents approximately 1% of adenocarcinomas of the cervix and has been associated with Peutz-Jeghers syndrome. It occurs mainly in the fifth and sixth decades of life. Diagnosis is often delayed due to frequently normal cervical cytology smears. Punch biopsies are often nondiagnostic, requiring conization for further evaluation.

E. Adenoid Cystic Carcinoma

Another uncommon variant of adenocarcinoma is adenoid cystic carcinoma. This lesion is considered more aggressive than most cervical adenocarcinomas and occurs more commonly in black women of high parity in their sixth and seventh decades of life. It should not be confused with adenoid basal carcinomas, which have an indolent growth pattern.

F. Adenosquamous Carcinoma

Adenosquamous carcinomas contain an admixture of malignant squamous and glandular cells. In most series, adenosquamous carcinomas are found to have a worse prognosis. Glassy cell carcinoma is a poorly differentiated form of adenosquamous carcinoma and is considered to have an extremely aggressive course. It accounts for about 1–2% of cervical cancers. Synchronous adenocarcinomas and squamous cell carcinomas that invade each other are called collision tumors.

G. Neuroendocrine Carcinomas

Approximately one-third of small cell carcinomas of the cervix stain positive for neuroendocrine markers. These tumors need to be distinguished from small cell type of squamous tumors. They have a high frequency of lymphovascular space invasion, lymph node metastases, recurrence, and poor survival. Carcinoid tumors, arising from the argyrophil cells of the endocervical epithelium, are malignant but have rarely been associated with the carcinoid syndrome. Because of their propensity for early systemic spread, systemic chemotherapy is an integral part of the treatment of neuroendocrine tumors of the cervix.

H. Other Malignant Tumors

Direct extension of metastatic tumors to the cervix include those originating from the endometrium, rectum, and bladder. Lymphatic or vascular metastases occur less often but are associated with endometrial, ovarian, gastric, breast, colon, kidney, and pancreas carcinomas. Sarcomas, lymphomas, choriocarcinomas, and melanomas are encountered rarely in the cervix.

Clinical Findings

A. Symptoms and Signs

Abnormal vaginal bleeding is the most common symptom of invasive cancer and may take the form of a blood-stained leukorrheal discharge, scant spotting, or frank bleeding. Leukorrhea, usually sanguineous or purulent, odorous, and nonpruritic, is frequently present. A history of postcoital bleeding may be elicited on specific questioning.

Pelvic pain, often unilateral and radiating to the hip or thigh, is a manifestation of advanced disease, as is the involuntary loss of urine or feces through the vagina, a sign of fistula formation. Weakness, weight loss, and anemia are characteristic of the late stages of the disease, although acute blood loss and anemia may occur in an ulcerating stage I lesion.

Physical examination findings include a grossly normal-appearing cervix with preclinical disease. As the local disease progresses, physical signs appear. Infiltrative cancer produces enlargement, irregularity, and a firm consistency of the cervix and eventually of the adjacent parametria. The growth pattern can be endophytic, leading to a barrel-shaped enlargement of the cervix, or exophytic, where the lesion generally appears as a friable, bleeding, cauliflower-like lesion of the portio vaginalis. Ulceration may be the primary manifestation of invasive carcinoma; in the early stages the change often is superficial, so that it may resemble an ectropion or chronic cer-

vicitis. With further progression of the disease, the ulcer becomes deeper and necrotic, with indurated edges and a friable, bleeding surface. The adjacent vaginal fornices may become involved next. Eventually, extensive parametrial involvement by the infiltrative process may produce a nodular thickening of the uterosacral and cardinal ligaments with resultant loss of mobility and fixation of the cervix.

B. Biopsy

Because of the failure of malignant cells to desquamate and the obscuring effect of inflammatory cells, it is not uncommon for an invasive carcinoma of the cervix to exist despite a negative cytologic smear. Any suspicious lesion of the cervix should be sampled by adequate biopsy, regardless of cytologic examination result. Biopsy of any Schiller-positive areas or of any ulcerative, granular, nodular, or papillary lesion provides the diagnosis in most cases. Colposcopically directed biopsies with endocervical curettage or conization of the cervix may be required when reports of suspicious or probable exfoliated carcinoma cells are made by the pathologist and a visible or palpable lesion of the cervix is not evident. Colposcopic warning signs of early invasive cancer in a field of CIN include capillaries which are markedly irregular, appearing as commas, corkscrews, and spaghetti-shaped vessels with great variation in caliber and abrupt changes in direction, often causing acute angles. Ulcerations or a markedly irregular appearance of the cervix with a waxy, yellowish surface and numerous bizarre, atypical blood vessels are common. Bleeding may occur also after slight irritation.

C. Conization

In the setting of a biopsy revealing carcinoma in situ, where invasion cannot be ruled out, or in the setting of a negative colposcopy in the face of a significantly abnormal cervical cytology smear, conization of the cervix should be performed to determine the presence or absence of invasion. If a cervical biopsy shows microinvasive cancer (less than 3 mm of invasion), a cone biopsy is necessary to rule out deeper invasion. The conization specimen should be properly marked for the pathologist (eg, with a pin or small suture), so that the area of involvement can be specifically localized in relation to the circumference and margins of the cervix. Conization for a lesion grossly suggestive of invasive cancer is not indicated, as it only delays the initiation of appropriate therapy and predisposes the patient to serious pelvic infections and bleeding. The diagnosis of such a lesion can almost always be confirmed by simple cervical biopsy.

D. Radiologic Findings

Chest x-rays are indicated in all patients with cervical cancer and an intravenous pyelogram (IVP) or computed tomography (CT) urogram should be performed to determine if there is any ureteral obstruction producing hydroureter and hydronephrosis. Magnetic resonance imaging (MRI), CT scan, lymphangiography, or positron emission tomography (PET) scanning may demonstrate involvement of the pelvic or periaortic lymph nodes or other sites of metastases. The sensitivity and specificity of each of these imaging modalities for metastases is limited.

Clinical Staging

It is important to estimate the extent of the disease not only for prognostic purposes but also for treatment planning. Clinical staging also affords a means of comparing methods of therapy for various stages of the disease worldwide. The classification adopted by the International Federation of Gynecology and Obstetrics (FIGO) is the most widely used staging system (Table 47–4). Cervical cancer is staged by clinical examination, and evaluation of the bladder, ureters, and rectum. If the lesion is clearly confined to the cervix by office examination, only chest x-ray and evaluation of the ureters by IVP or CT scan with intravenous contrast is necessary to assign the stage. If it is not possible to evaluate the parametria in the office, examination under anesthesia with cystoscopy and proctoscopy may be necessary. Although CT scan, MRI, lymphangiography, or PET scan may at times offer information helpful for treatment planning, these findings do not change the FIGO stage of disease. The FIGO stage of disease is also not changed by surgicopathologic findings of metastatic disease at the time of radical hysterectomy or lymphadenectomy.

Table 47–4. FIGO staging of cervical cancer (adopted from FIGO Annual Report on the Results of Treatment in Gynecologic Cancer 1998).

FIGO Stage	Definition
Stage 0	Carcinoma in situ
Stage I	Cervical carcinoma confined to the cervix (extension to the corpus would be disregarded)
Stage IA[1]	Invasive cervical cancer diagnosed by microscopy only
Stage IA1	Stromal invasion no deeper than 3 mm, no wider than 7 mm in horizontal spread
Stage IA2	Stromal invsion greater than 3, but less than 5 mm and no wider than 7 mm in horizontal spread
Stage IB	Clinically visible lesion confined to the cervix or microscopic disease greater than stage IA
Stage IB1	Lesion not greater than 4 cm
Stage IB2	Lesion greater than 4 cm
Stage II	Tumor extends beyond uterus but not to pelvic sidewall or lower third of vagina
Stage IIA	Vaginal involvement without parametrial involvement
Stage IIB	Parametrial involvement
Stage III	Tumor extends to pelvic sidewall and/or causes hydronephrosis and/or extends to lower third of vagina
Stage IIIA	Involvement of lower third of vagina with no extension to sidewall
Stage IIIB	Extension to pelvic sidewall and/or hydronephrosis
Stage IV	Extension beyond the true pelvis or into mucosa of rectum or bladder
Stage IVA[2]	Extension into adjacent organs
Stage IVB	Distant metastases

[1]The depth of invasion should be no more than 5 mm from the epithelial basement membrane of the adjacent most superficial epithelial papilla to the deepest point of invasion where the cancer originates. Vascular space invasion, venous or lymphatic, does not affect staging, but should be noted as it may affect future therapy. All macroscopically visible lesions (even with superficial invasion only) are allotted to stage IB.

[2]The presence of bullous edema is not sufficient to classify a tumor as stage IVA. The finding of malignant cells in cytologic bladder washings requires further histologic confirmation in order to be considered stage IVA.

Differential Diagnosis

A variety of lesions of the cervix may be confused with cancer. Entities that must sometimes be ruled out include cervical ectropion, acute or chronic cervicitis, condyloma acuminata, cervical tuberculosis, ulceration secondary to sexually transmitted disease (syphilis, granuloma inguinale, lymphogranuloma venereum, chancroid), abortion of a cervical pregnancy, metastatic choriocarcinoma or other cancers, and rare lesions such as those of actinomycosis or schistosomiasis. Histopathologic examination is usually definitive.

Complications

The complications of cervical cancer, for the most part, are those related to tumor size or invasion, necrosis of the tumor, infection, and metastatic disease. The natural history of the disease has been outlined above. There are also problems pertaining to treatment of the disease (eg, radical surgery or radiation therapy; see Treatment, below).

Prevention

While prophylactic HPV vaccines are under development and investigation, prevention of morbidity and death from cervical cancer largely involves recognition and treatment of preinvasive and early invasive disease. Currently, approximately 60% of women who develop cervical cancer in developed countries either never had been screened or have not been screened in the preceding 5 years.

Risk factors must be recognized, and screening, treatment intervention, and patient education must be modified respectively. Universal cytologic screening of all postpubertal women must be continued on a regular basis until better, more sensitive and specific means of screening are found, and outreach into underserved areas is improved. Women with preinvasive cervical neoplasia should be treated and followed up closely (Fig. 47–6). It is important to remember that cervical cytology smears are of limited value in detecting frankly invasive disease, with some studies finding false negative rates up to 50%. Sexual abstinence is an effective but impractical prophylactic measure. Education of young women and men about risk factors and the necessity for regular screening, as well as information about the association of HIV infection and smoking with the development of cervical cancers, is crucial.

Treatment

Invasive carcinoma of the cervix spreads primarily by direct extension and lymphatic dissemination. The therapy of patients with cervical cancer needs to address not only the primary tumor site, but also the adjacent tissues and lymph nodes. This is generally accomplished by either radical hysterectomy and pelvic lymphadenectomy, radiation with concomitant chemotherapy, or a combination thereof.

A. Treatment of Early Stage Disease (Stage IA2 to IIA)

Patients with early stage cervical cancer may be treated with either radical hysterectomy and pelvic lymphadenectomy or with primary radiation with concomitant chemotherapy. The overall 5-year cure rates for surgery and for radiation therapy in operable patients are approximately equal. The advantage of surgery is that the ovaries may be left intact and be transposed out of the radiation field if adjuvant postoperative therapy appears necessary, that the extent of disease can be determined surgicopathologically, and that grossly metastatic lymph nodes can be resected. Furthermore, surgery may be more appropriate in sexually active women with early stage disease since radiation causes vaginal stenosis and atrophy. Adjuvant radiation with concomitant chemotherapy is administered to selected patients at increased risk for recurrence following radical hysterectomy.

1. **Radical hysterectomy and therapeutic lymphadenectomy**—Radical hysterectomy (techniques initially described by Wertheim, Meigs, and Okabayashi) with pelvic lymphadenectomy is the surgical procedure for invasive cancer limited to the cervix (stages I and II). The operation is technically difficult and should be performed only by those experienced in radical pelvic surgery. Surgery involves dissection of the ureters from the paracervical structures so that the ligaments supporting the uterus and upper vagina can be removed. When the operation is done vaginally, a deep Schuchardt (paravaginal) incision is required for exposure. Five different types of hysterectomy have been described based upon the extent of parametrial dissection and vaginal tissue removed (Table 47–5). Typically a type I hysterectomy is indicated for patients with stage IA1 squamous cell carcinoma. An alternative treatment is cervical conization in the young patient wishing to preserve fertility. Stage IA2 is treated with a type II (modified radical) hysterectomy, while stage IB and IIA disease is classically treated with a type III hysterectomy. It is rarely necessary to remove as much vaginal tissue as was initially recommended. As long as complete tumor clearance can be provided, a modified radical hysterectomy appears to provide therapeutic outcomes comparable to a radical hysterectomy for stage IB and IIA disease, but with shorter operating time and lower urologic morbidity. Full pelvic lymphadenectomy is indicated at the time of radical hysterectomy,

Table 47–5. Types of hysterectomy based on radicality.

Type of Hysterectomy	Principles of Procedure
Type I	Extrafascial hysterectomy with removal of all cervical tissue without dissecting into the cervix itself.
Type II	The uterine artery is ligated where it crosses over the ureter. The uterosacral and cardinal ligaments are divided midway towards their attachment to sacrum and pelvic sidewall. The upper third of the vagina is resected.
Type III	The uterine artery is ligated at its origin from the superior vesical or internal iliac artery. Uterosacral and cardinal ligaments are resected at their attachments to the sacrum and pelvic sidwall. The upper half of the vagina is resected.
Type IV	The ureter is completely dissected from the vesicouterine ligament, the superior vesical artery is sacrificed, and three fourths of the vagina is resected.
Type V	Involves the additional resection of a portion of the bladder or the distal ureter with ureteral reimplantation into the bladder

followed by para-aortic lymphadenectomy. Resection of all grossly enlarged lymph nodes provides a distinct survival advantage. Microscopic evaluation of the lymph nodes allows for tailoring of the postoperative radiation field, if indicated.

2. Adjuvant postoperative radiation—Postoperative adjuvant radiation therapy with concomitant chemotherapy is indicated in women with localized cervical cancer at high risk for recurrent disease, such as positive lymph nodes, positive or close resection margins, or microscopic parametrial involvement. In this setting, adjuvant radiation with platinum-based chemotherapy is superior to adjuvant radiation alone, with an improvement in the 4-year progression-free interval from 63% to 80%. Women with intermediate risk factors for recurrent disease, such as large tumor size, deep cervical stromal invasion, and lymphovascular space invasion, also benefit from postoperative adjuvant radiation. These patients have an improved 2-year recurrence-free survival of 88% with adjuvant radiation versus 79% without adjuvant therapy.

3. Primary radiation with concomitant chemotherapy—For the treatment of early cervical cancer (stages IA to IIA), primary therapy with definitive radiation and radical surgery followed by tailored radiation if indicated by the surgical findings produce comparable outcomes. The choice of treatment depends on the tumor size, the general condition of the patient, and preferences of the oncologists at the treating institution. Surgery has often been preferred for young patients in the hope of preserving ovarian function. If it is likely that the patient will need postoperative radiation therapy, transposition of the ovaries to a location outside the radiation field can be performed. For primary radiation of cervical cancer, external beam radiation is generally used in combination with intracavitary irradiation (see Chapter 51). At least five controlled trials have demonstrated the superiority of radiation with concomitant platinum-based chemotherapy over radiation alone. This has led to the adoption of radiation plus concomitant chemotherapy as the standard of care whenever radiation therapy is given for the treatment of cervical cancer over a broad spectrum of disease stages.

Special Situations

A. Stage IA1 Disease

The definitive diagnosis of microinvasive squamous cell carcinoma of the cervix can be made by conization only. These patients may be treated by simple abdominal or vaginal hysterectomy. For a young woman desiring to maintain fertile, conization alone is an acceptable treatment modality for microinvasive squamous cell carcinoma with a depth of invasion of 3 mm or less, if the conization margins are negative, and if there is no evidence of lymphovascular space invasion. If margin and endocervical curettage are positive, the risk of residual disease is as high as 33%. FIGO staging is not influenced by the presence of lymphovascular space invasion, which occurs in close to 10% of patients with stage IA1 disease. These patients have a small but significant risk for lymph node metastases to parametrial and pelvic lymph nodes. This subgroup of patients should therefore be treated like patients with stage IA2 disease. There is considerable controversy regarding the existence of microinvasive adenocarcinoma and its pathologic diagnostic criteria, which is beyond the scope of this chapter.

B. Radical Trachelectomy

During the last decade, radical trachelectomy has evolved as an alternative to radical hysterectomy in carefully selected young women with early stage (IA2 or small IB1) cervical cancer who wish to preserve fertility. A therapeutic lymphadenectomy is performed and following radical resection of the cervix a cerclage is placed. Although experience with this technique is limited, the oncologic outcome appears comparable to radical hysterectomy in carefully selected patients. While successful near-term cesarean deliveries have been reported in close to half of the patients who attempted pregnancy following the procedure, infertility and an up to 25% second trimester miscarriage rate characterize some of the reproductive difficulties following the procedure.

C. Bulky Cervical Cancer

The management of patients with stage IB2 and bulky IIA disease is a matter of considerable debate. Proposed management strategies include the following.

1. Primary radiation therapy with concomitant chemotherapy and the option of a subsequent adjuvant extrafascial hysterectomy—Radiation therapy has usually been recommended for patients with bulky cervical cancers, recently with the addition of concomitant chemotherapy. Many of these tumors, however, contain hypoxic central areas which do not respond well to radiation, as is reflected in a 15–35% pelvic failure rate. This has provided the rationale for the performance of an adjuvant hysterectomy following radiation, which has been associated with a significant reduction in pelvic recurrences to 2–5%. However, the impact of adjuvant hysterectomy on extrapelvic recurrences and survival is less well established.

2. Primary radical hysterectomy and therapeutic lymphadenectomy, followed by tailored radiation with concomitant chemotherapy when indicated by pathological findings—Potential benefits of this approach include the removal of the large primary tumor, complete surgical staging with the opportunity to resect any grossly involved lymph nodes, and the preservation of ovarian function as ovarian transposition can be performed if adjuvant radiation therapy is likely. If postoperative radiation becomes necessary, the radiation field can be tailored to the surgicopathologic findings. The resection of macroscopically involved lymph nodes has a therapeutic benefit because it improves survival to that of patients with microscopic lymph node metastases only. A primary surgical approach should be taken in patients with acute or chronic pelvic inflammatory disease, an undiagnosed coexistent adnexal mass, or anatomic alterations that make radiation therapy difficult.

3. Neoadjuvant chemotherapy followed by radical hysterectomy and lymphadenectomy and subsequent chemoradiation when indicated by pathological findings—Neoadjuvant chemotherapy, frequently three cycles of platinum-based combination therapy followed by radical hysterectomy and lymphadenectomy, has recently been proposed as a novel treatment strategy for these patients. Neoadjuvant chemotherapy has been reported to improve the resectability of bulky lesions,

pelvic disease control, and possibly long-term survival. Although this is a provocative treatment strategy, in most studies patients ultimately received multimodality treatment with chemotherapy, radical surgery, and radiation. Further randomized studies are needed to determine the precise role of neoadjuvant chemotherapy in the treatment of these patients.

B. Treatment of Locally Advanced Disease (Stage IIB to IVA)

Patients with locally advanced cervical cancer are best treated with primary radiation (external beam plus brachytherapy; see Chapter 51) with concomitant chemotherapy. Extended field radiation should be considered in the presence of para-aortic lymph node metastases documented at surgical staging or empirically in patients at high risk for para-aortic lymph node metastases. The benefit of cisplatin-based combined modality therapy over radiation alone for advanced disease has been demonstrated in at least three randomized controlled trials, which have found a 30–50% reduction in the risk of death from cervical cancer for patients treated with chemoradiation compared to those treated with radiation alone. This difference is most significant for patients with stage II disease (and bulky IB disease) in whom in one study chemoradiation improved 5-year survival rates compared to radiation alone from 58% to 77%. For patients with more advanced disease, the benefits associated with chemoradiation versus radiation alone appear less pronounced, with the same study showing a small, statistically insignificant improvement in 5-year survival from 57% to 63%. The optimal drug regimen is not known, but combination therapy did not show superior results over weekly single-agent cisplatin, and the latter was associated with substantially less toxicity.

C. Treatment of Disseminated Primary (Stage IVB) and Persistent or Recurrent Disease

The use of chemotherapeutic agents in the treatment of cervical carcinoma has been discouraging. This is partly because most patients who may be candidates for this type of treatment either present with disseminated disease or have cancer that has already failed to respond to radical surgery or radiation therapy. Modest activity in recurrent or disseminated cervical cancer has been observed with single-agent cisplatin, ifosfamide, paclitaxel, and vinorelbine. There may be a small therapeutic advantage to multiagent chemotherapy with cisplatin and paclitaxel or cisplatin and ifosfamide with 31% and 36% response rates, respectively. These responses are short-lived, with progression-free intervals of 4.6 and 4.8 months, respectively. Palliative pelvic radiation therapy may be indicated. If a patient develops a palpable mass in the left supraclavicular region, it can be palliated with radiation therapy with concomitant chemotherapy, with or without resection.

D. TOTAL PELVIC EXENTERATION FOR ISOLATED CENTRAL PELVIC RECURRENCE OF DISEASE

Patients who develop a central recurrence of cervical cancer after primary therapy with radiation or after surgery followed by radiation may be candidates for this extensive, potentially curative surgical procedure if a complete evaluation fails to reveal evidence of metastatic disease. In a small proportion of patients with cancer of the cervix treated initially with radiation, a small recurrence of the cancer may be noted centrally within the cervix. A radical hysterectomy may be an alternative to total pelvic exenteration in this selected subgroup of patients. Surgery is the only potentially curative method of treating cancers that persist or recur centrally following adequate radiation therapy. In such instances, pelvic exenteration is often necessary to make certain that all of the cancer has been removed.

Pelvic exenteration is one of the most formidable of all gynecologic operations and requires removal of the bladder, rectum, and vagina, along with the uterus if hysterectomy has not yet been performed. This is followed by the reconstructive phase of the procedure. Urinary diversion needs to be provided, necessitating the creation of either a continent ileocolonic pouch or a noncontinent ileal conduit. In either case, a stoma is created in the anterior abdominal wall. If extensive rectal resection was required, a sigmoid colostomy serves for the passage of feces. If a low rectal anastomosis could be accomplished, a temporary diverting colostomy should be performed in all patients who had received prior radiation. The vagina can be reconstructed using various myocutaneous flaps, such as transverse rectus abdominis or gracilis myocutaneous flaps. Depending on the location of the lesion, an anterior (preservation of the rectosigmoid) or posterior (preservation of the bladder) exenteration is at times an alternative.

Because of the high surgical morbidity and mortality rates, stringent criteria are necessary to justify these procedures. Pelvic exenteration should be reserved primarily for problems that cannot be effectively managed in any other manner. In essence, this means (1) a biopsy-proven persistence or recurrence of cervical cancer following an adequate course of radiation therapy or radical surgery in which the recurrent or persistent tumor occupies the central portion of the pelvis (without metastases) and is completely removable; and (2) a patient who is able to cope with the urinary and fecal stomas in the abdomen created by the operation. Both psychological and physical preparation of the patient for this operation and its aftermath are of vital importance. Because of the extreme difficulties encountered in making an accurate assessment preoperatively, only about half of the patients explored for a total pelvic exenteration will intraoperatively be confirmed to have resectable, nonmetastatic disease. The 5-year survival rate following pelvic exenteration for recurrent cervical cancer averages 30–40%.

E. PALLIATIVE CARE

Comprehensive care of a patient with cancer involves in addition to antitumor therapy, good symptom relief, as well as personal and family support. The palliative care for patients with progressive cervical cancer poses many challenges. The emphasis should be to facilitate comfort, dignity, autonomy, and personal rehabilitation and development, especially in the face of an incurable disease.

Most patients with progressive cervical cancer eventually develop symptoms related principally to the site and extent of the malignant disease. Ulceration of the cervix and adjacent vagina produces a foul-smelling discharge. Tissue necrosis and slough may initiate life-threatening hemorrhage. If the bladder or rectum is involved in the tissue breakdown, fistulas result in incontinence of urine and feces. Pain due to involvement of the lumbosacral plexus, soft tissues of the pelvis, or bone is frequently encountered in advanced disease. Ureteral compression leading to hydronephrosis and, if bilateral, to renal failure and uremia is a common terminal event. The comfort and well-being of the patient can be considerably enhanced even though cure cannot be effected. A foul, purulent discharge may be ameliorated by astringent douches and antimicrobial vaginal creams or suppositories. Hemorrhage from the vagina often can be controlled by packing the area with gauze impregnated with a hemostatic agent; occasionally emergent radiation or hypogastric artery embolization is indicated.

Current management of severe pain combines the use of a long-acting narcotic such as morphine or a transdermal fentanyl patch with short-acting narcotics for breakthrough pain and nonsteroidal anti-inflammatory agents or selective cyclooxygenase inhibitors. Anxiolytics and antidepressants may be of considerable value. For patients with significant pain who are no longer responding to oral medications, a subcutaneous or intravenous morphine drip can be started. In patients with lower back or extremity pain, a peridural catheter can be placed and connected to a subcutaneous pump with a reservoir for continuous morphine instillation. This method gives pain relief without the sedating effects of oral and parenteral narcotics.

Radiation therapy may be very helpful in the relief of pain due to bony metastases or in the treatment of lesions that recur following primary surgical treatment of cervical cancer. In general, if initial therapy has been accomplished by adequate radiation therapy, re-treatment is contraindicated since it does little good and carries the potential of massive radiation necrosis.

Special Situations

A. CARCINOMA OF THE CERVIX DURING PREGNANCY

Invasive carcinoma of the cervix in pregnancy is found more frequently in areas where routine prenatal cytologic examination is done. Abnormal cervical cytology in pregnancy calls for immediate colposcopic evaluation and any other diagnostic modalities necessary to exclude invasive cancer (see section on preinvasive disease).

Invasive cervical cancer complicates approximately 0.05% of pregnancies. As is the case with nonpregnant patients also, the principal symptom is bleeding, but the diagnosis is frequently missed because the bleeding is assumed to be related to the pregnancy rather than to cancer. The possibility of cancer must be kept in mind. The diagnosis and management of invasive cervical cancer during pregnancy presents the patient and the physician with many challenges. Pregnancy does not appear to affect the prognosis for women with cervical cancer and the fetus is not affected by the maternal disease, but may suffer morbidity from its treatment (eg, preterm delivery).

If the pregnancy is early and the disease is stage I to IIA, radical hysterectomy and therapeutic lymphadenectomy can be performed with the fetus left in situ, unless the patient is unwilling to terminate the pregnancy. Women at a gestational age closer to fetal viability or who are unwilling to lose the baby may decide to continue the pregnancy after careful discussion regarding the maternal risks. Delivery in patients with cervical dysplasia and carcinoma in situ may be via the vaginal route. Patients with invasive cervical cancer should be delivered by cesarean section to avoid potential cervical hemorrhage and dissemination of tumor cells during vaginal delivery. A cesarean radical hysterectomy with therapeutic lymphadenectomy is the procedure of choice for patients with stage IA2–IIA disease as soon as adequate fetal maturity is established.

As in the nonpregnant patient, radiation with concomitant chemotherapy is used for the treatment of more advanced disease. In the first trimester, irradiation may be carried out with the expectation of spontaneous abortion. In the second trimester, interruption of the pregnancy by hysterotomy prior to radiation therapy is preferred, although some physicians advocate proceeding with immediate radiation treatment, again awaiting spontaneous evacuation of the uterus. In selected cases with locally advanced disease in which the patient declines pregnancy termination, consideration may be given to neoadjuvant chemotherapy in an effort to prevent disease progression during the time needed to achieve fetal maturity. Delivery should be by cesarean section. A lymphadenectomy can be performed at the same time. Postpartum the patient should receive chemoradiation following guidelines established for the nonpregnant patient.

B. CARCINOMA OF THE CERVICAL STUMP

Early stage cervical cancer noted on a cervical stump (left in situ following supracervical hysterectomy for an unrelated indication) should be treated with radical trachelectomy and therapeutic lymphadenectomy in the medically fit patient. Surgery is preferred over chemoradiation in this setting as the delivery of an adequate radiation dose may be difficult in a patient with a short cervical stump. However, radiation with concomitant chemotherapy is the preferred treatment modality for patients with more advanced disease.

C. CERVICAL CANCER INCIDENTALLY DIAGNOSED AFTER SIMPLE HYSTERECTOMY

Women who are found to have microinvasive disease after a simple hysterectomy do not require any additional therapy. Patients with microinvasive disease who do not have gross parametrial disease are candidates for a radical parametrectomy, upper vaginectomy, and lymphadenectomy. This approach may be particularly desirable for young women in whom ovarian function can be preserved or for any surgically fit women with enlarged lymph nodes which should be debulked prior to adjuvant chemoradiation. Indications for chemoradiation follow the same guidelines as outlined above.

Complications of Therapy

A. RADICAL SURGERY

The operative mortality rate in radical hysterectomy with lymphadenectomy has been reduced to less than 1%. The most common complication is prolonged bladder dysfunction. Approximately 75% of patients have adequate recovery of bladder function within 1–2 weeks after radical hysterectomy, and most patients will have satisfactory voiding function by 3 weeks. Serious complications include fistula formation; ureterovaginal fistula is the most common type (1–2%), followed by vesicovaginal and rectovaginal fistulas. Modified radical hysterectomy as compared to radical hysterectomy is associated with a shorter operating time, a more rapid return of bladder function, and fewer fistulas. Other complications are urinary tract infections, lymphocysts and lymphedema, wound sepsis, dehiscence, throm-

Table 47–6. Survival of patients with cervical cancer based on FIGO stage.

Stage	Number of Patients (%)	Survival		
		1 year	2 years	5 years
IA1	518 (4.3%)	99.2%	97.4%	95.1%
IA2	384 (3.2%)	98.9%	97.9%	94.9%
IB	4657 (39.0%)	95.5%	89.3%	80.1%
IIA	813 (6.8%)	91.8%	80.8%	66.3%
IIB	2551 (21.4%)	92.1%	78.9%	63.5%
IIIA	180 (1.5%)	79.4%	57.4%	33.3%
IIIB	2350 (19.7%)	76.7%	55.3%	38.7%
IVA	294 (2.5%)	52.2%	30.9%	17.1%
IVB	198 (1.7%)	35.1%	23.4%	9.4%

boembolic disease, ileus, postoperative hemorrhage, and intestinal obstruction.

The surgical mortality rate from pelvic exenteration has been reduced from about 25% to less than 5%, but as many as 50% of patients experience major morbidity. Complications include intraoperative and postoperative hemorrhage, infectious morbidity, urinary fistulas or obstruction, urinary pouch dysfunction, pyelonephritis, bowel obstruction or intestinal leaks and fistulas, stomal retraction, electrolyte disturbances, and other less common occurrences.

B. Radiation Therapy With Concomitant Chemotherapy

See Chapter 51.

Posttreatment Follow-up

Approximately 35% of patients with invasive cervical cancer will have recurrent or persistent disease following therapy. Death from recurrent or persistent cervical cancer occurs most frequently in the first year of observation following primary therapy. About half the deaths occur in the first year, another 25% in the second year, and 15% in the third year. This explains the generally accepted schedule of posttreatment surveillance in asymptomatic patients of every 3 months in the first year, every 4 months in the second year, and every 6 months in years 3–5. Symptomatic patients should be evaluated with appropriate examinations immediately when symptoms occur. The most common signs and symptoms of recurrent malignant disease are positive cytologic examination, palpable tumor in the pelvis or abdomen, ulceration of the cervix or vagina, pain in the pelvis, back, groin, and lower extremity, unilateral lower extremity edema, vaginal bleeding or discharge, supraclavicular lymphadenopathy, ascites, unexplained weight loss, progressive ureteral obstruction, and cough (especially with hemoptysis or chest pain).

Prognosis

The major prognostic factors affecting survival are stage, lymph node status, tumor volume, depth of cervical stromal invasion, lymphovascular space invasion and, to a lesser extent, histologic type and grade. After stage of disease, lymph node status is the most important prognostic factor. For example, following radical surgery, patients with stage IB or IIA disease have a 5-year survival of 88–96% with negative lymph nodes, compared to 64–73% in the presence of lymph node metastases.

Table 47–6 summarizes survival rates by stage of disease. These are based on the FIGO Annual Report on the Results of Treatment in Gynecological Cancer, in which results of treatment for each stage of cervical cancer are reported by more than 100 participating institutions worldwide. The results are equated in terms of 5-year cure rates, or those patients who are living and show no evidence of cervical cancer 5 years after beginning therapy.

Recurrences following radiation therapy are not often centrally located and thus amenable to exenteration procedures. Only about 25% of recurrences are localized to the central portion of the pelvis. The most common site of recurrence is the pelvic side wall.

REFERENCES

Cervical Intraepithelial Neoplasia

Ahdieh L et al: Cervical neoplasia and repeated positivity of human papillomavirus infection in human immunodeficiency virus-seropositive and -seronegative women. Am J Epidemiol 2000;151:1148.

Arends MJ, Buckley CH, Wells M: Etiology, pathogenesis, and pathology of cervical neoplasia. J Clin Pathol 1998;51:96.

Denehy TR, Gregori CA, Breen JL: Endocervical curettage, cone margins, and residual adenocarcinoma in situ of the cervix. Obstet Gynecol 1997;90:1.

Economos K et al: Abnormal cervical cytology in pregnancy: a 17-year experience. Obstet Gynecol 1993;81:915.

Follen Mitchell M et al: Cervical human papillomavirus infection and intraepithelial neoplasia: A review. J Natl Cancer Inst Monogr 1996;21.

Ho GY et al: Natural history of cervicovaginal papillomavirus infection in young women. N Engl J Med 1998;338:423.

Holowaty P et al: Natural history of dysplasia of the uterine cervix. J Natl Cancer Inst 1999;91:252.

Im DD, Duska LR, Rosenshein NB: Adequacy of conization margins in adenocarcinoma in situ of the cervix as a predictor of residual disease. Gynecol Oncol 1995;59:179.

Kennedy AW et al: Results of the clinical evaluation of atypical glandular cells of undetermined significance (AGUS) detected on cervical cytology screening. Gynecol Oncol 1996; 63:14.

Kim TJ et al: Clinical evaluation of follow-up methods and results of atypical glandular cells of undetermined significance (AGUS) detected on cervicovaginal Pap smears. Gynecol Oncol 1999;73:292.

Kinney WK et al: Where's the high-grade cervical neoplasia? The importance of minimally abnormal Papanicolaou diagnoses. Obstet Gynecol 1998;91:973.

Maiman M et al: Cervical cancer as an AIDS-defining illness. Obstet Gynecol 1997;89:76.

Manos MM et al: Identifying women with cervical neoplasia. Using human papillomavirus DNA testing for equivocal Papanicolaou results. JAMA 1999;281:1605.

Martin-Hirsch PL, Paraskevaidis E, Kitchener H: Surgery for cervical intraepithelial neoplasia. Cochrane Database Syst Rev 2000;CD001318.

McIndoe WA et al: The invasive potential of carcinoma in situ of the cervix. Obstet Gynecol 1984;64:451.

Melnikow J et al: Natural history of cervical squamous intraepithelial lesions: A meta-analysis. Obstet Gynecol 1998;92:727.

Moreno V et al: Risk factors for progression of cervical intraepithelial neoplasia grade III to invasive cervical cancer. Cancer Epidemiol Biomarkers Prev 1995;4:459.

Olsen AO et al: Combined effect of smoking and human papillomavirus type 16 infection in cervical carcinogenesis. Epidemiology 1998;9:346.

Poynor EA, Barakat RR, Hoskins WJ: Management and follow-up of patients with adenocarcinoma in situ of the uterine cervix. Gynecol Oncol 1995;57:158.

Prokopczyk B et al: Identification of tobacco-specific carcinogen in the cervical mucus of smokers and nonsmokers. J Natl Cancer Inst 1997;89:868.

Solomon D, Dowey D, Kurman R, et al: The 2001 Bethesda system terminology for reporting results of cervical cytology. JAMA 2002;287:2114–2119.

Solomon D, Schiffman M, Tarone R: Comparison of three management strategies for patients with atypical squamous cells of undetermined significance: baseline results from a randomized trial. J Natl Cancer Inst 2001;93:293.

Soutter WP et al: Invasive cervical cancer after conservative therapy for cervical intraepithelial neoplasia. Lancet 1997;349:978.

The Atypical Squamous Cell of Undetermined Significance/Low-Grade Squamous Intraepithelial Lesions Triage Study (ALTS) Group: Human papillomavirus testing for triage of women with cytologic evidence of low-grade squamous intraepithelial lesions: baseline data from a randomized trial. J Natl Cancer Inst 2000;92:397.

The 1988 Bethesda system for reporting cervical/vaginal cytological diagnoses. National Cancer Institute Workshop. JAMA 1989;262:931.

Wallin KL et al: Type-specific persistence of human papillomavirus DNA before the development of invasive cervical cancer. N Engl J Med 1999;341:1633.

Wolf JK et al: Adenocarcinoma in situ of the cervix: significance of cone biopsy margins. Obstet Gynecol 1996;88:82.

Ylitalo N et al: Consistent high viral load of human papillomavirus 16 and risk of cervical carcinoma in situ: a nested case-control study. Lancet 2000;355:2194.

Yost NP et al: Postpartum regression rates of antepartum cervical intraepithelial neoplasia II and III lesions. Obstet Gynecol 1999;93:359.

Cancer of the Cervix

Anderson B et al: Ovarian transposition in cervical cancer. Gynecol Oncol 1993;49:206.

Anttila T et al: Serotypes of *Chlamydia trachomatis* and risk for development of cervical squamous cell carcinoma. JAMA 2001;285:47.

Arends MJ, Buckley CH, Wells M: Aetiology, pathogenesis, and pathology of cervical neoplasia. J Clin Pathol 1998;51:96.

Averette HE et al: Radical hysterectomy for invasive cervical cancer: A 25-year prospective experience with the Miami technique. Cancer 1993;71:1422.

Benedet J et al: Carcinoma of the cervix. FIGO Annual Report on the Results of Treatment in Gynecological Cancer. J Epidemiol Biostat 1998;3:5.

Benedet JL et al: FIGO staging classifications and clinical practice guidelines in the management of gynecologic cancers. FIGO Committee on Gynecologic Oncology. Int J Gynaecol Obstet 2000;70:209.

Bosch FX et al: Prevalence of human papillomavirus in cervical cancer: A worldwide perspective. J Natl Cancer Inst 1995;87:796.

Cosin JA et al: Pretreatment surgical staging of patients with cervical carcinoma: the case for lymph node debulking. Cancer 1998;82:2241.

Covens A et al: Is radical trachelectomy a safe alternative to radical hysterectomy for patients with stage IA–B carcinoma of the cervix? Cancer 1999;86:2273.

Dargent D et al: Laparoscopic vaginal radical trachelectomy: a treatment to preserve the fertility of cervical carcinoma patients. Cancer 2000;88:1877.

Eifel PJ et al: The relationship between brachytherapy dose and outcome in patients with bulky endocervical tumors treated with radiation alone. Int J Radiat Oncol Biol Phys 1994;28:113.

Feeney DD et al: The fate of the ovaries after radical hysterectomy and ovarian transposition. Gynecol Oncol 1995;56:3.

Gallion HH et al: Combined radiation therapy and extrafascial hysterectomy in the treatment of stage IB barrel-shaped cervical cancer. Cancer 1985;56:262.

Greenlee RT et al: Cancer statistics, 2001. CA Cancer J Clin 2001;51:15.

Hacker NF, Wain GV, Nicklin JL: Resection of bulky positive lymph nodes in patients with cervical carcinoma. Int J Gynaecol Cancer 1995;5:250.

Hopkins MP, Lavin JP: Cervical cancer in pregnancy. Gynecol Oncol 1996;63:293.

Keys HM et al: Cisplatin, radiation, and adjuvant hysterectomy compared with radiation and adjuvant hysterectomy for bulky stage IB cervical carcinoma. N Engl J Med 1999;340:1154.

Klaes R et al: Detection of high-risk cervical intraepithelial neoplasia and cervical cancer by amplification of transcripts derived from integrated papillomavirus oncogenes. Cancer Res 1999;59:6132.

Landoni F et al: Randomised study of radical surgery versus radiotherapy for stage IB–IIA cervical cancer. Lancet 1997;350:535.

Landoni F et al: Class II versus class III radical hysterectomy in stage IB–IIA cervical cancer: A prospective randomized study. Gynecol Oncol 2001;80:3.

Lazo PA: The molecular genetics of cervical carcinoma. Br J Cancer 1999;80:2008.

Lee YN et al: Radical hysterectomy with pelvic lymph node dissection for treatment of cervical cancer: A clinical review of 954 cases. Gynecol Oncol 1989;32:135.

Metcalf KS et al: Site specific lymph node metastasis in carcinoma of the cervix: Is there a sentinel node? Int J Gynecol Cancer 2000;10:411.

Moore DH et al: A randomized phase III study of cisplatin versus cisplatin plus paclitaxel in stage IVB, recurrent or persistent squamous cell carcinoma of the cervix: a Gynecologic Oncology Group study (abstract). Proc Am Soc Clin Oncol 2001;20:201a.

Morris M et al: Pelvic radiation with concurrent chemotherapy compared with pelvic and para-aortic radiation for high-risk cervical cancer. N Engl J Med 1999;340:1137.

Omura GA: Chemotherapy for stage IVB or recurrent cancer of the uterine cervix. J Natl Cancer Inst Monogr 1996;123.

Omura GA et al: Randomized trial of cisplatin versus cisplatin plus mitolactol versus cisplatin plus ifosfamide in advanced squamous carcinoma of the cervix: a Gynecologic Oncology Group study. J Clin Oncol 1997;15:165.

Parkin DM, Pisani P, Ferlay J: Global cancer statistics. CA Cancer J Clin 1999;49:33.

Perez CA et al: Irradiation alone or combined with surgery in stage IB, IIA, and IIB carcinoma of uterine cervix: update of a nonrandomized comparison. Int J Radiat Oncol Biol Phys 1995;31:703.

Peters WA III et al: Concurrent chemotherapy and pelvic radiation therapy compared with pelvic radiation therapy alone as adjuvant therapy after radical surgery in high-risk early-stage cancer of the cervix. J Clin Oncol 2000;18:1606.

Piver MS, Rutledge F, Smith JP: Five classes of extended hysterectomy for women with cervical cancer. Obstet Gynecol 1974;44:265.

Roman LD et al: Risk of residual invasive disease in women with microinvasive squamous cancer in a conization specimen. Obstet Gynecol 1997;90:759.

Rose PG et al: Concurrent cisplatin-based radiotherapy and chemotherapy for locally advanced cervical cancer. N Engl J Med 1999;340:1144.

Sardi JE et al: Long-term follow-up of the first randomized trial using neoadjuvant chemotherapy in stage IB squamous carcinoma of the cervix: The final results. Gynecol Oncol 1997;67:61.

Sasieni PD, Cuzick J, Lynch-Farmery E: Estimating the efficacy of screening by auditing smear histories of women with and without cervical cancer. The National Co-ordinating Network for Cervical Screening Working Group. Br J Cancer 1996;73:1001.

Sedlis A et al: A randomized trial of pelvic radiation therapy versus no further therapy in selected patients with stage IB carcinoma of the cervix after radical hysterectomy and pelvic lymphadenectomy: A Gynecologic Oncology Group Study. Gynecol Oncol 1999;73:177.

Sevin BU et al: Microinvasive carcinoma of the cervix. Cancer 1992;70:2121.

Sood AK et al: Cervical cancer diagnosed shortly after pregnancy: Prognostic variables and delivery routes. Obstet Gynecol 2000;95:832.

Sutton GP et al: Ovarian metastases in stage IB carcinoma of the cervix: A Gynecologic Oncology Group study. Am J Obstet Gynecol 1992;166:50.

Tewari K et al: Neoadjuvant chemotherapy in the treatment of locally advanced cervical carcinoma in pregnancy: a report of two cases and review of issues specific to the management of cervical carcinoma in pregnancy including planned delay of therapy. Cancer 1998;82:1529.

Vizcaino AP et al: International trends in the incidence of cervical cancer: I. Adenocarcinoma and adenosquamous cell carcinomas. Int J Cancer 1998;75:536.

Whitney CW et al: Randomized comparison of fluorouracil plus cisplatin versus hydroxyurea as an adjunct to radiation therapy in stage IIB–IVA carcinoma of the cervix with negative para-aortic lymph nodes: a Gynecologic Oncology Group and Southwest Oncology Group study. J Clin Oncol 1999;17:1339.

Womack C, Warren AY: Achievable laboratory standards: a review of cytology of 99 women with cervical cancer. Cytopathology 1998;9:171.

Premalignant & Malignant Disorders of the Uterine Corpus

Oliver Dorigo, MD, & Annekathryn Goodman, MD

48

■ ENDOMETRIAL HYPERPLASIA & CARCINOMA

ESSENTIALS OF DIAGNOSIS

- Bleeding: hypermenorrhea, intermenstrual, or postmenopausal.
- Hyperestrogenism: conditions with possible alterations in estrogen metabolism, ie, ovarian granulosa cell tumor, polycystic ovarian syndrome, obesity, late menopause, and exogenous estrogens, and tamoxifen use.
- Susceptible persons: classic—obese, white, diabetic, hypertensive, anovulatory; other—thin, genetic predisposition, no hyperestrogenic state, unusual histologic subtypes.
- Diagnosis: endometrial sampling, ultrasonography.

General Considerations

In the U.S., white women have a lifetime risk of endometrial carcinoma of 2.4% compared with 1.3% for black women. The peak incidence of onset is in the sixth and seventh decades, but 2–5% occur before age 40 years, and the disease has been reported in women aged 20–30. Endometrial carcinoma is now the most common pelvic genital cancer in women. A doubling of the incidence of endometrial cancer in the 1970s correlated with unopposed estrogen use in hormone replacement and sequential oral contraceptives over the previous 10 years. The declining incidence in the 1980s paralleled progesterone use in hormone replacement regimens and low-dose estrogen combination birth control pills. The incidence of endometrial cancer has now remained stable over the past 10 years. The estimated incidence for the year 2000 is 36,100 new cases

with 6500 deaths occurring from the disease. The onset of endometrial bleeding facilitates detection in the earlier stages of disease. Consequently, the overall prognosis is considerably better than for the other major gynecologic cancers.

Estrogens have been implicated as a causative factor in endometrial carcinoma, because there is a high incidence of this disease in patients with presumed alterations in estrogen metabolism and in those who take exogenous estrogens. Furthermore, patients with anovulatory cycles are at higher risk of developing endometrial cancer because of prolonged periods of estrogenic stimulation of the endometrium without the counteracting effect of progesterone. Classically, it affects the obese, nulliparous, infertile, hypertensive, and diabetic white woman, but it can occur in the absence of all these factors. Unlike cervical cancer, it is not related to sexual history. Fortunately for the victim, there is a warning: abnormal bleeding usually occurs early in the course of the disease and alerts the patient or physician to an endometrial abnormality. In the elderly patient with an obliterated endocervical canal, severe cramps from hematometra or pyometra may be the presenting symptom. In the asymptomatic patient, a fortuitous diagnosis may occur from an abnormal Papanicolaou (Pap) smear, but cytologic discovery of endometrial cancer is not consistent and should not be relied on for early diagnosis. A total hysterectomy with bilateral salpingo-oophorectomy is usually the first step in treatment. Further postoperative therapy depends on the particular histologic characteristics and the extent of the tumor.

Etiology

Although the exact cause of endometrial cancer remains unknown, the argument that estrogens are somehow implicated is becoming increasingly more difficult to refute. It has been known for many years that the administration of estrogen to laboratory animals can produce endometrial hyperplasia and carcinoma. Furthermore, certain constitutional states such as diabetes mellitus, hypertension, polycystic ovary syndrome, and obesity, perhaps having in common elevated endogenous estrogen levels, are associated with a higher incidence of endometrial carcinoma. Patients receiving exogenous estrogen replacement therapy for Turner's syndrome or gonadal agenesis and patients with endogenous elevations from granulosa cell tumors of the ovary are also more susceptible to endometrial carcinoma. Recently tamoxifen, which has weak estrogenic effects on the endometrium, has been associated with both endometrial hyperplasia and carcinoma.

More than a dozen case-control studies indicate an association between estrogen administration and endometrial carcinoma. These studies report a 2- to 10-fold increase in the incidence of endometrial carcinoma in women receiving exogenous unopposed estrogens. The risk of cancer is related to both the dose and the duration of exposure and diminishes with cessation of estrogen use. The risk seems to be neutralized by the addition of cyclic progestin for 10 days at least every 3 months. Basic research also reveals increased conversion of androstenedione to estrone in women with recognized risk factors for endometrial cancer (advanced age, obesity, and polycystic ovary syndrome). This collective body of information has raised serious questions about the carcinogenic effects of unopposed estrogens on the endometrium. Women on replacement estrogens or women suspected of having elevated levels of endogenous estrogen require close clinical follow-up. Progestin should be added to the treatment program to counteract the effect of estrogen on the endometrium. Endometrial biopsies to rule out endometrial hyperplasia or pelvic ultrasonography to evaluate the thickness of the endometrial stripe should be obtained if abnormal bleeding occurs.

Evidence is accumulating that there is a genetic factor in the development of endometrial cancer. Those women with a personal history of ovarian, colon, or breast cancer as well as those with a family history of endometrial cancer may be at higher risk. Certain oncogenes such as Ha-, K-, and N-*ras*, *c-myc*, and Her-2/neu have been found in endometrial cancers. Furthermore, alterations in the p53 and even more frequently in the PTEN tumor suppressor gene have been identified recently. Certain vascular growth promoting factors like VEGF (vascular endothelial growth factor) have been found to be overexpressed in endometrial cancer. The biological role of these factors for the development and growth of endometrial cancer remains to be elucidated.

Surgical Staging
(Table 48–1)

Prior to 1988, a clinical staging system classified cancers of the endometrium. Presently the stage of an endometrial carcinoma is based on abdominal explora-

Table 48–1. FIGO surgical staging of carcinoma of the corpus uteri (1988).[1]

Stage I
  Stage Ia G123 Tumor limited to endometrium
  Stage Ib G123 Invasion to less than one-half the myometrium
  Stage Ic G123 Invasion to more than one-half the myometrium
Stage II
  Stage IIa G123 Endocervical glandular involvement only
  Stage IIb G123 Cervical stromal invasion
Stage III
  Stage IIIa G123 Tumor invades serosa and/or adnexa, and/or positive peritoneal cytology
  Stage IIIb G123 Vaginal metastases
  Stage IIIc G123 Metastases to pelvic and/or para-aortic lymph nodes
Stage IV
  Stage IVa G123 Tumor invades bladder and/or bowel mucosa
  Stage IVb Distant metastases including intra-abdominal and/or inguinal lymph nodes

[1]From Internatinal Federation of Gynecology and Obstetrics: Annual Report on the results of treatment in gynecologic cancer. Int J Gynecol Obstet 1991;36(Suppl):132.

tion, pelvic washings, total hysterectomy with salpingo-oophorectomy, and selective pelvic and periaortic lymph node biopsies. Grade of the tumor is included in the staging description. Grade 1 tumors have less than 5% of a nonsquamous solid growth pattern. Grade 2 tumors contain 6–50% of a nonsquamous solid growth pattern. Tumors with more than 50% of a solid pattern are classified as grade 3. Notable nuclear atypia that is not congruent with architectural grade raises the grade of a tumor by 1 point.

Surgical stage I tumors account for 75% of all endometrial carcinomas, which explains the relatively good overall prognosis. Eleven percent of cancers are surgical stage II, and the remaining 11% and 3% are surgical stage III and IV, respectively.

Classification

A. ENDOMETRIAL HYPERPLASIA

The glandular hyperplasias of the endometrium are benign conditions that may produce symptoms clinically indistinguishable from early endometrial carcinoma. Because of their association with hyperestrogenic states, some of the hyperplasias, even though reversible, are considered premalignant lesions. Since endometrial hyperplasia and endometrial carcinoma present clinically as abnormal bleeding, thorough endometrial sampling or fractional curettage is always necessary when hyperplasia is present to rule out coexisting carcinoma. Hyperplasia can be classified as simple or complex and with or without atypia.

1. Hyperplasia without atypia—Microscopically, this type of hyperplasia has crowding of glands in the stroma. There is no nuclear atypia. In simple hyperplasia (previously called "cystic hyperplasia"), the glands are cystically dilated and give a "Swiss cheese" appearance histologically. Frequently this type of hyperplasia is asymptomatic and is an incidental finding at hysterectomy. When followed without treatment over a 15-year period, 1% progressed to a cancer whereas 80% spontaneously regressed.

Complex hyperplasia without atypia (previously designated "adenomatous hyperplasia") describes a complex, crowded appearance to the glands with very little intervening stroma. There can be epithelial stratification and mitotic activity. Left untreated over 13 years, complex hyperplasia regresses in 83% of cases and progresses to cancer in 3% of cases. In general, the hyperplasias without atypia are not considered premalignant. Eighty-five percent of women have reversal of the lesions with progestin therapy.

2. Hyperplasia with atypia—Atypical hyperplasia may be simple or complex. It is characterized histologically by endometrial glands lined by enlarged cells with increased nuclear:cytoplasmic ratios. The nuclei may be irregular with coarse chromatin clumping and prominent nucleoli. These hyperplasias are generally considered premalignant. Progression to carcinoma occurs in 8% and 29% of simple atypical and complex atypical hyperplasias, respectively. Fifty to 94% of lesions regress with progestin therapy but have a higher rate of relapse when therapy is stopped compared with that of lesions without atypia. In peri- and postmenopausal patients with atypical hyperplasias who relapse after progestin therapy or who cannot tolerate its side effects, vaginal or abdominal hysterectomy is recommended.

3. Carcinoma in situ—The term carcinoma in situ has been used to denote an entity at the extreme end of the continuum from hyperplasia to carcinoma. It is distinguished from carcinoma by the presence of intervening stroma between abnormal glands. There is no evidence of invasion, but sometimes this is impossible to identify in regions of crowded glands. Many authorities do not feel this is a uniform and replicable diagnosis.

B. ENDOMETRIAL CARCINOMA

This cancer is characterized by obvious hyperplasia and anaplasia of the glandular elements, with invasion of underlying stroma, myometrium, or vascular spaces. As previously noted, it has been postulated that it may represent the end process of a spectrum beginning with hyperplasia, passing through atypical hyperplasia, and ending with frank cancer. Despite the attractiveness of this theory, only about 25% of patients with endometrial carcinoma have a history of hyperplasia. What really happens is not known, but it is likely that endometrial cancer, although it may follow atypical hyperplasia, can develop independently of it.

In recent years, careful reevaluation of the pathologic findings and spread pattern of endometrial cancer has clarified our understanding of this disease. Important prognostic factors include histologic grade and cell type, depth of myometrial invasion, presence of lymph vascular space involvement, lymph node metastases, and positive peritoneal cytology. There is some evidence that tumor aneuploidy and an increased proportion of cells in S phase as determined by DNA flow cytometry is predictive of a poorer outcome.

Endometrial cancers of any grade are almost never associated with lymph node metastases if there has been no myometrial invasion. After myometrial invasion occurs, the incidence of pelvic and aortic lymph node metastases is directly proportional to the depth of invasion and the degree of differentiation. Patients with poorly differentiated deeply invasive cancers have about a 35% incidence of involved pelvic nodes and a 10–20% incidence of aortic node metastases. Since patients with lymph node metastases are at very high risk for recurrence, these pathologic features have serious implications for treatment planning.

Endometrial cancer can spread by four possible routes: direct extension, lymphatic metastases, peritoneal implants after transtubal spread, and hematogenous spread. It is believed that the tumor remains confined to the body of the uterus for a relatively long time, but eventually it invades the myometrium and cervix. It may then spread to the parametria, the pelvic wall and aortic nodes, the serosa of the uterus, the ovaries, and ultimately the peritoneal surfaces. Undifferentiated lesions (grade 3) may spread to the pelvic and aortic nodes while still confined to the superficial myometrium. In serous and clear cell subtypes (see text that follows), the spread pattern is similar to that of ovarian cancer, and upper abdominal peritoneal relapses are common. Hematogenous metastases to the lungs are uncommon with primary tumors limited to the uterus but do occur with recurrent or disseminated disease. In contrast to the former belief that endometrial carcinoma spreads primarily to the aortic lymph nodes through infundibulopelvic and broad ligament lymphatics, recent studies indicate a dual pathway of spread to the pelvic and aortic lymph nodes (Fig 48–1). The aortic nodes are rarely involved when the pelvic nodes are free of metastases, but the pelvic nodes are sometimes involved when the aortic nodes are not.

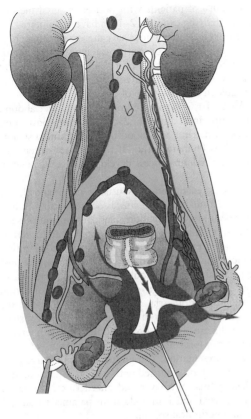

Figure 48-1. Dual lymphatic spread pattern of endometrial carcinoma.

Vaginal metastases occur by submucosal lymphatic or vascular metastases in approximately 3–8% of patients with clinical stage I disease. The concept that these metastases occur by spillage of tumor through the cervix at the time of surgery lacks convincing support. However, vaginal metastases are more common with higher histologic grade and with lower uterine segment or cervical involvement.

Malignant cells identified in the peritoneal washings obtained at the time of hysterectomy are usually associated with the finding of other risk factors such as deep myometrial invasion of lymph node metastases. When these cells are present in the absence of other risk factors, they convey a prognosis in proportion to their number and degree of differentiation. Vascular and lymphatic invasion in the hysterectomy specimen is also associated with a poorer outcome.

Pathologists recognize three major histologic types of endometrial carcinoma: adenocarcinoma, adenocarcinoma with squamous differentiation, and adenosquamous carcinoma. All three types have identical present-ing symptoms and signs, patterns of spread, and general clinical behavior. For this reason, they can be considered collectively for purposes of clinical work-up, differential diagnosis, and treatment. Papillary serous and clear cell carcinomas of the endometrium are other unusual histologic subtypes that appear to carry a poor prognosis even when apparently confined to the superficial myometrium.

1. Adenocarcinoma—The most common type of endometrial carcinoma is adenocarcinoma, composed of malignant glands that range from very well-differentiated (grade 1)—barely distinguishable from atypical complex hyperplasia—to anaplastic carcinoma (grade 3). To determine stage and prognosis, the tumor is usually graded by the most undifferentiated area visible under the microscope (Fig 48–2). In the U.S., adenocarcinoma comprises 70–80% of endometrial carcinomas, but this figure is higher in other countries.

2. Adenocarcinoma with squamous differentiation—This entity is composed of malignant glands and benign squamous metaplasia. It makes up approximately 5% of endometrial carcinomas. Although these cancers have a reputation for running a more benign course, this is probably due to the very well-differentiated pattern they usually display. Grade for grade, adenocarcinomas with squamous differentiation are probably no better or worse than other histologic types.

3. Adenosquamous carcinoma—Adenosquamous carcinoma of the endometrium is composed of malignant glands and malignant squamous epithelium and makes up approximately 10–20% of endometrial cancers in the U.S. The reason for its high incidence in this country is unknown; however, there seems to be some variability in incidence from institution to institution, and the difference may be explained in the basis of pathologic interpretation. The tumor is often poorly

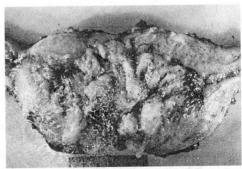

Figure 48-2. Adenocarcinoma of the endometrium. Note the sharp demarcation of the tumor at the isthmus.

differentiated (grade 3), which makes pathologic interpretation difficult. Because of the poor differentiation, prognosis is worse than that of endometrial carcinoma as a whole, since the overall statistics of endometrial carcinoma are heavily weighted in favor of better-differentiated lesions.

4. Serous carcinoma—Histologically, this cancer is identical to the complex papillary architecture seen in serous carcinomas of the ovary. Women with serous carcinoma are more likely to be older and less likely to have hyperestrogenic states. These tumors account for 50% of all relapses in stage I tumors. Serous tumors spread early and involve peritoneal surfaces of the pelvis and abdomen. The tumors also have a propensity for myometrial and lymphatic invasion. The prognosis is unfavorable, and patients with serous tumors should be treated in a manner similar to that of patients with ovarian tumors.

5. Clear cell carcinoma—This subtype is not associated with clear cell carcinomas of the cervix and vagina that are seen in young women with diethylstilbestrol exposure. Its microscopic appearance is significant for clear cells or hobnail cells. Solid, papillary, tubular, and cystic patterns are possible. Clear cell carcinoma is commonly high grade and aggressive with deep invasion and is seen at an advanced stage. It occurs in older women (average age, 67 years), and like the serous subtype is not associated with a hyperestrogenic state.

6. Miscellaneous subtypes—Mucinous carcinomas make up 9% of endometrial adenocarcinomas; they contain periodic acid-Schiff (PAS)-positive, diastase-resistant intracytoplasmic mucin. Secretory carcinoma, present in 1–2% of cases, exhibits subnuclear or supranuclear vacuoles resembling early secretory endometrium. These rare cancers behave in a manner similar to that of typical endometrial carcinomas. Pure squamous cell carcinomas are extremely rare and are associated with cervical stenosis, pyometra, and chronic inflammation.

Clinical Findings

A. SYMPTOMS AND SIGNS

Abnormal bleeding occurs in about 80% of patients and is the most important warning sign of endometrial carcinoma. An abnormal vaginal discharge especially after menopause is present in some patients. During the premenopausal years, the bleeding is usually described as excessive flow at the time of menstruation. However, bleeding may occur as intermenstrual spotting or premenstrual and postmenstrual bleeding. In the postmenopausal woman, intermittent spotting, described as lighter than a normal menstrual period, is more common. As a presenting symptom, hemorrhage is rare.

About 20% of patients with postmenopausal bleeding have underlying cancer; 12–15% have endometrial carcinoma; and the remainder have uterine sarcoma or cervical, vaginal, tubal, or ovarian carcinoma. Endometrial carcinoma as a cause of postmenopausal bleeding increases with age, so that after the age of 80, cancer is responsible in fully 50–60% of cases.

About 10% of patients complain of lower abdominal cramps and pain secondary to uterine contractions caused by detritus and blood trapped behind a stenotic cervical os (hematometra). If the uterine contents become infected, an abscess develops and sepsis may supervene.

Physical examination is usually unremarkable but may reveal medical problems associated with advanced age. Speculum examination may confirm the presence of bleeding, but since it may be minimal and intermittent, blood may not be present. Atrophic vaginitis is frequently identified in these elderly women, but postmenopausal bleeding should never be ascribed to atrophy without a histologic sampling of the endometrium to rule out endometrial carcinoma. Bimanual and rectovaginal examination of the uterus in the early stages of the disease will be normal unless hematometra or pyometra is present. If the cancer is extensive at the time of presentation, the uterus may be enlarged and soft and may be confused with benign conditions such as leiomyoma. With very advanced cases, the uterus may be fixed and immobile from parametrial adnexal and intraperitoneal spread.

Vaginal metastases are rarely identified in early disease but are not uncommon in advanced cases or with recurrence following treatment. Ovarian metastases may cause marked enlargement of these organs.

When feasible, endocervical curettage with a small Kevorkian curet followed by endometrial biopsy may obviate the need, risk, and expense of fractional curettage.

B. LABORATORY FINDINGS

Routine laboratory findings are normal in most patients with endometrial carcinoma. If bleeding has been prolonged or profuse, anemia may be present.

Cytologic study of specimens taken from the endocervix and posterior vaginal fornix reveals adenocarcinoma in about 60% of symptomatic patients. More important, endometrial carcinoma will be missed in 40% of symptomatic patients by routine cytologic examination. Accuracy has been greatly increased by aspiration cytologic study or biopsy (discussed under Special Examinations). The Pap smear is nevertheless an integral part of the examination of all patients, because it identifies a small but definite percentage of patients with asymptomatic disease. Furthermore, the presence of benign endometrial cells in the cervical or vaginal smear of a menopausal or postmenopausal woman is associated with occult endometrial carcinoma in 2–6% of cases. Thus, any postmenopausal woman who shows endometrial cells on a routine cervical Pap smear requires evaluation for endometrial cancer.

Routine blood counts, urinalysis, endocervical and vaginal pool cytology, chest x-ray, intravenous urography, stool guaiac, and sigmoidoscopy have proved to be useful ancillary diagnostic tests in patients with endometrial carcinoma. Liver function tests, blood urea nitrogen, serum creatinine, and a blood glucose test (because of the known relationship to diabetes) are considered routine. Serum Ca-125, a well-established tumor marker for epithelial ovarian cancer, can also be useful for endometrial cancer. About 20% of patients with clinical stage I (preoperatively, the tumor appears to be confined to the uterus) have an elevated Ca-125. Eighty percent of surgically upstaged patients have an elevated preoperative value.

C. X-RAY FINDINGS

Chest x-ray may reveal metastases in patients with advanced disease but is rarely positive in the early stages. Intravenous urography establishes the presence of a normal genitourinary system and rules out deviation or compression of the ureters by enlarged pelvic nodes or other unsuspected extrauterine spread. Barium enema is usually not necessary in a patient with a negative stool guaiac test and normal sigmoidoscopic examination but should always be performed in the patient with gross or occult gastrointestinal bleeding or symptoms.

Hysterosalpingography and hysteroscopy have been widely used in some foreign countries and in many institutions within the U.S. for the evaluation of endometrial carcinoma. Although investigators consistently report no adverse effects from these procedures, the possibility of transtubal spread of cancer is nevertheless real. However, the significance of positive peritoneal cytologic results is controversial. For example, in patients with stage I disease, an incidence of 10–20% positive peritoneal cytology has been reported without influence on survival. In a study conducted by the Gynecologic Oncology Group, a relative risk of 3 for death was found in patients with positive washings. For this reason, these procedures should not be used to evaluate this disease.

Magnetic resonance imaging (MRI) appears to improve the accuracy of clinical staging and is particularly helpful in identifying myometrial invasion and lower uterine segment or cervical involvement.

D. SPECIAL EXAMINATIONS

1. Fractional curettage—Dilatation and fractional curettage is the definitive procedure for diagnosis of endometrial carcinoma. It should be performed with the patient under anesthesia to afford an opportunity for thorough and more accurate pelvic examination. It is carried out by careful and complete curettage of the endocervical canal followed by dilatation of the canal and circumferential curettage of the endometrial cavity. When obvious cancer is present with the first passes of the curet, the procedure should be terminated as long as sufficient tissue for analysis has been obtained from the endocervix and endometrium. Perforation of the uterus followed by intraperitoneal contamination with malignant cells, blood, and bacteria is a common complication in patients with endometrial carcinoma and can usually be avoided by gentle surgical technique and limitation of the procedure to the extent necessary for accurate diagnosis and staging. D&C is never considered curative in these circumstances and should not be performed with the same vigor as therapeutic curettage.

2. Endometrial biopsy—This procedure is attractive because it can be performed in an outpatient setting, resulting in a substantial savings in cost. It can usually be done without anesthesia, although paracervical block is effective when necessary. Currently, some form of negative pressure attached to an aspiration curet is the most popular method, but gentle curettage with a Kevorkian nonaspirating curet is also successful.

All types of endometrial biopsy are notoriously inaccurate for diagnosing polyps and will miss a significant number of cases of endometrial hyperplasia as well. Therefore, it must be emphasized that when these tests cannot be completed for technical reasons or when the tissue obtained is insufficient for diagnosis or for accurate grading and staging of the lesion, complete fractional curettage must be performed.

a. Aspiration biopsy—This procedure is performed with a variety of aspirating or nonaspirating curets designed for easy entry into the endometrial cavity. The Novak curet is a good example (Fig 48–3). While slight negative pressure is maintained on the syringe, the endometrial cavity is sampled, preferably in all four quadrants. Overall, the procedure is 80–90% accurate for the diagnosis of endometrial carcinoma when the tissue sample is adequate and when it can be successfully accomplished. It does, however, have a wide range of accuracy (between 67% and 97%), and negative findings in the symptomatic (bleeding) patient should never be considered definitive. The pipelle, a thin plastic cannula, is another office instrument that can adequately sample the endometrium. Because of its small diameter, it usually causes less cramping than other curets.

b. Aspiration curettage—The Vabra aspirator is another form of endometrial biopsy technique that uses a 3- or 4-mm suction curet with approximately 300–600 mm of negative pressure (Fig 48–4). To date, aspiration curettage is the most accurate outpatient method for evaluating endometrial cancer, with an

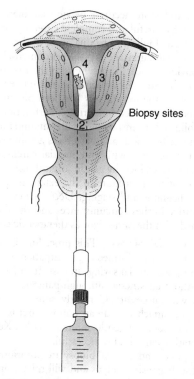

Biopsy sites

Figure 48–3. Technique of endometrial biopsy with Novak curet.

overall accuracy rate of 95–98%. However, the range of accuracy may be as low as 80%, and various technical problems preclude completion of the procedure in about 10% of cases. In another 6–7%, the sample is considered insufficient for histologic interpretation. Consequently, negative findings in a symptomatic patient cannot be considered definitive.

3. Pelvic ultrasonography—Ultrasonography can be helpful in deciding whether high-risk patients (such as those with a hyperestrogenic state, breast cancer pa-

tients on tamoxifen, and women with strong family histories of endometrial cancer) who do not have symptoms should undergo endometrial sampling. In postmenopausal women, 5 mm is the cutoff for a normal unilateral endometrial stripe. Color flow imaging may increase specificity.

4. Estrogen and progesterone receptor assays—Estrogen and progesterone receptor assays should be obtained from the neoplastic tissue. This information helps in planning adjuvant or subsequent hormone therapy. Estrogen and progesterone receptor content are inversely proportional to histologic grade. In general, patients with tumors positive for one or two receptors have longer survival than patients with receptor-negative tumors.

Differential Diagnosis

Clinically, the differential diagnosis of endometrial carcinoma generally includes all the various causes of abnormal uterine bleeding. In the premenopausal or menopausal patient, complications of early pregnancy such as threatened or incomplete abortion must be high on the list; a pregnancy test usually clarifies the issue. Other causes of bleeding in this group are leiomyoma, endometrial hyperplasia and polyps, cervical polyps, and various genital or metastatic cancers. Cervical, endometrial, tubal, and ovarian neoplasms all can cause abnormal uterine bleeding. Although rare, metastatic cancers from the bowel, bladder, and breast have also been reported to cause abnormal uterine bleeding.

In the postmenopausal age group, the emphasis will be shifted to atrophic vaginitis, exogenous estrogens, endometrial hyperplasia and polyps, and various genital neoplasms. The older the patient, the more likely that her bleeding will prove to be due to endometrial cancer. In any event, the diagnosis will be evident following adequate evaluation of the endocervical and endometrial cavities. In the patient with a normal pelvic examination and recurrent postmenopausal bleeding following

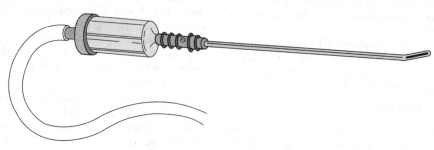

Figure 48–4. Vabra aspirator.

a recent negative D&C, tubal and ovarian cancer must be strongly considered. Patients with recurrent unexplained episodes of postmenopausal uterine bleeding may be considered for total hysterectomy and bilateral salpingo-oophorectomy.

Pathologically, the differential diagnosis of endometrial carcinoma is usually not difficult except in the well-differentiated forms, where the distinction from atypical hyperplasia can be perplexing. Whenever doubt or disagreement exists, consultation with a pathologist skilled in the diagnosis of gynecologic neoplasms usually resolves the problem.

Complications

If the patient has ignored her symptoms of bleeding over a long period of time and allowed the cancer to extensively invade the myometrium, she may present with severe anemia secondary to chronic blood loss or acute hemorrhage. If bleeding is significant and continuous, high-dose bolus radiation therapy is usually effective in slowing the hemorrhage.

The presence of a hematometra can be confirmed by sounding the uterus under anesthesia, followed by dilatation of the cervix to allow adequate drainage. When a pyometra is present, the patient may present with peritonitis or generalized sepsis, with all the consequent complications.

Perforation of the uterus at the time of dilatation and fractional curettage or endometrial biopsy is not an uncommon problem. If the perforating instrument is large, loops of small bowel may be inadvertently retrieved through the cervical canal. A large perforation warrants laparoscopy or laparotomy to evaluate and repair the damage. If significant contamination of the peritoneal cavity with blood or necrotic tumor has occurred, the patient should be treated with broad-spectrum antibiotics to prevent peritonitis. Perforation in the patient with endometrial cancer should be viewed as a serious complication, since spillage of tumor into the peritoneal cavity may drastically alter her prognosis.

Prevention

The constitutional and other risk factors for endometrial carcinoma are well known. Obese, diabetic, hypertensive, nulliparous women with a history of infertility or repeated D&C for abnormal bleeding certainly require close surveillance. Women with late menopause or previous pelvic radiation therapy and those taking estrogens should be under closer observation than women in the general population. Very little can be done for the constitutional risk factors other than gen-

eral health measures to control diabetes and hypertension and maintain ideal body weight.

If the patient desires hormone replacement therapy, estrogens should be administered cyclically, 25–31 days each month, using the lowest dose that controls symptoms. Progesterone (10 mg of medroxyprogesterone acetate or 200 mg of micronized progesterone) should be added for the last 10–14 days of the cycle to neutralize the risk of endometrial carcinoma. Alternatively, estrogen and progesterone can be administered continuously; 2.5 mg of medroxyprogesterone acetate is given daily.

Treatment

The treatment of cancer anywhere in the body depends on its natural history and pattern of spread. The clinician is confronted with familiar questions in each case: What is it? Where is it now or where is it most likely to be? What are its pathways of dissemination or invasion? Recent studies have done much to clarify the lymphatic spread pattern of endometrial carcinoma; nodal metastases, vaginal recurrence, and survival have been demonstrated to be directly proportionate to the depth of myometrial invasion, degree of anaplasia, and the presence of cervical involvement. Any one of these features implies a high risk of treatment failure and recurrence. It follows that any rational treatment plan for endometrial carcinoma must take these risk factors into consideration.

Surgery and radiation therapy are the only methods of treatment that have consistently shown a high degree of success in treating this disease. It has been repeatedly demonstrated that radiation therapy can cure endometrial carcinoma in some patients, but when irradiation is used alone the survival rates have been clearly inferior to those achieved with surgery alone. Radiation therapy averages about a 20% lower cure rate than surgery in stage I disease. Surgery is therefore the treatment of choice whenever feasible, but some form of adjuvant therapy is necessary in patients at high risk for metastasis. Because chemotherapy is not reliable for this purpose, radiation therapy is the clear choice for adjuvant treatment. Even though preoperative or postoperative radiation therapy in combination with surgery for stage I disease has not significantly improved 5-year survival rates over rates achieved by surgery alone, considerable evidence supports the use of adjuvant radiation therapy in this disease.

It is well known that radiation therapy alone can cure endometrial carcinoma in some patients, and when used preoperatively it completely eradicates the primary tumor in over 50% of stage I cases. Furthermore, adjuvant radiation therapy has reduced the incidence of vaginal vault recurrence following surgery for stage I patients from an average of 3–8% to 1–3%. Intracavitary vaginal irradiation can be performed by using colpostats to deliver a surface dose of 5500–6000 cGy. Also, regional radiation therapy has eliminated microscopic nodal metastases in other tumor systems, and some patients with surgically proved nodal metastases from endometrial carcinoma are now alive more than 5 years following adjuvant radiation therapy to pelvic and aortic nodes. Accordingly, in the presence of extrauterine extension, lower uterine segment or cervical involvement, poor histologic differentiation, papillary serous or clear cell histology, or myometrial penetration greater than one-third of the full thickness, adjuvant radiation therapy is recommended. In the absence of these findings, it is difficult to justify the risk and morbidity of any additional treatment beyond simple total abdominal hysterectomy and bilateral salpingo-oophorectomy.

A. Emergency Measures

Infrequently, the patient with endometrial adenocarcinoma may present in a critical state. When bleeding has been ignored for long periods of time, profound anemia may exist; or when blood loss is acute and massive, the patient may be in shock. After vital signs have been stabilized and adequate blood is in reserve, emergency dilatation and fractional curettage should be performed with the utmost caution and gentleness. If the uterus is obviously full of necrotic tumor, instrumentation only increases the bleeding. If bleeding persists following D&C, high-dosage bolus radiation therapy to the whole pelvis should be administered. Rarely, in the face of very advanced lesions, embolization of the hypogastric arteries via percutaneous selective angiography may be required to control hemorrhage before treatment can be initiated. Hysterectomy should always be considered if it can be accomplished safely without jeopardizing curative therapy.

Elderly patients may present with severe lower abdominal pain and cramping secondary to hematometra or pyometra; these complications result from endometrial carcinoma in over 50% of cases. When adequate blood levels of broad-spectrum antibiotics are established, the cervix should be dilated and the endometrial cavity adequately drained. In this setting, vigorous D&C is contraindicated because of the high risk of uterine perforation. If the cervix is well dilated, an indwelling drain is usually not necessary, but if sepsis is not controlled within 24–48 hours, the patient should be reexamined to ascertain cervical patency. Once the infection has completely subsided and the patient has been afebrile for 7–10 days, gentle fractional curettage should be performed if the diagnosis was not confirmed at the initial procedure.

B. Radiation Therapy

Radiation therapy is used as primary therapy in patients considered too medically unstable for laparotomy. Adjuvant preoperative radiation is no longer used unless the patient presents with gross cervical involvement. In this situation, after preoperative whole pelvic radiation and an intracavitary implant, an extrafascial hysterectomy is performed. Contraindications to preoperative radiation therapy include the presence of a pelvic mass, a pelvic kidney, pyometra, history of a pelvic abscess, prior pelvic radiation, and previous multiple laparotomies (see Chapter 51).

C. Surgical Treatment

Because bleeding is usually an early sign of endometrial carcinoma, most patients present with early disease and can be adequately and completely treated by simple hysterectomy. In this situation, the results are the same whether hysterectomy is accomplished vaginally or abdominally, but the abdominal approach is superior for removal of the ovaries and for assessment of the peritoneal cavity and retroperitoneal nodes. It also permits the surgeon to obtain peritoneal washings for cytologic identification of occult spread. For these reasons, the abdominal approach is preferred except in patients with very early disease and a small uterus, in whom the risk of occult cervical involvement or deep myometrial invasion is minimal and who also have other compelling reasons for vaginal surgery.

Pelvic and para-aortic lymphadenectomy plays an important role in the surgical staging of endometrial cancer. The uterus should be opened in the operating room to determine the need for surgical staging in patients with grade 1 or 2 tumors. Patients that require surgical staging in stage I are patients with grade 3 lesions; grade 2 tumors greater than 2 cm in diameter; histologic adenosquamous, clear cell, or papillary serous carcinomas; and tumors with greater than 50% myometrial invasion and/or cervical extension. The therapeutic role of lymphadenectomy is still unclear. However, a number of studies have suggested that if the lymph nodes are negative, external-beam therapy may be omitted and brachytherapy only performed to prevent vaginal vault recurrence. Furthermore, it might be therapeutically beneficial to remove bulky, positive nodes, which are unlikely to respond to external beam radiation.

Radical hysterectomy has been recommended by some, particularly for stage II tumors, but the results have been no better than with simple hysterectomy combined with radiation therapy. Furthermore, most patients are elderly or have concurrent diabetes, hypertension, or other medical problems that preclude radical surgery. However, radical hysterectomy can be effective treatment for patients with recurrence following treatment with radiation therapy alone or for those who have previously received therapeutic doses of pelvic radiation therapy for other pelvic cancers. The high risk of bowel or urinary tract injury in this setting must be understood and accepted by both patient and physician.

As with patients presenting with gross cervical involvement, those with vaginal and parametrial involvement should receive initial pelvic radiation. Exploratory laparotomy should then be considered in patients whose disease seems resectable. Hormonal therapy or chemotherapy is most appropriate for patients with clinical evidence of extrapelvic metastases. Palliative radiation to bone or brain metastases is beneficial for symptomatic relief. Pelvic radiation can be helpful for local tumor control and alleviation of bleeding.

D. Hormone Therapy

Progesterone has been the time-honored agent for the treatment of recurrent endometrial carcinoma not amenable to irradiation or surgery. This type of therapy can be administered orally or parenterally. Oral megestrol, parenteral medroxyprogesterone acetate suspension, and parenteral hydroxyprogesterone caproate appear to have similar effectiveness. In patients with recurrent endometrial cancer, progestins should be used initially, particularly for tumors with positive hormone receptors. The average duration of response is 20 months, and patients who respond survive more than four times longer than nonresponders. About 30% of responders survive 5 years; virtually all nonresponders die before this time. Patients who are young and have localized recurrence respond better than older patients and those with disseminated disease; those with well-differentiated tumors respond better than those with poorly differentiated ones; and patients with late recurrences respond better than those with early ones (indicating a more indolent, well-differentiated form of the disease). Because some patients do not achieve remission until after 10–12 weeks of therapy, the minimum duration of treatment should be over 3 months. Overall, about 13% of patients with recurrent disease appear to achieve long-term remissions with progesterone therapy.

Although progesterones have a somewhat encouraging record in the treatment of recurrent endometrial adenocarcinoma, they are disappointing as prophylactic agents. They have not improved survival or decreased recurrence when used following definitive treatment of early stage disease.

Tamoxifen has been used as another hormonal agent in advanced or recurrent endometrial cancer. It may be as effective as progesterone. As with progesterone, the patients who respond generally have well-differentiated tumors and long disease-free intervals. Tamoxifen is administered orally at 10–20 mg twice daily. For single-agent tamoxifen, the overall response rate is 22%. Studies using combination tamoxifen-progestin therapy have suggested a possibly better clinical response.

E. Antitumor Chemotherapy

Doxorubicin and cisplatin are the two most active agents in the treatment of advanced or recurrent endometrial cancer. Doxorubicin used as a single agent has shown an overall response rate of 38% with 26% of the patients achieving a complete response. Other agents with antitumor activity against endometrial cancer include carboplatin, cyclophosphamide, and 5-fluorouracil.

F. General and Supportive Measures

When the patient presents without acute symptoms of hemorrhage or sepsis, the work-up, although it should be efficient and thorough, can be less urgent. Patients with endometrial carcinoma are often elderly and medically feeble. They may be weak, anemic, diabetic, or hypertensive, and specific attention to these problems is necessary before the cancer can be treated.

Prognosis

Contemporary studies of the clinical, surgical, and pathologic findings in patients with endometrial carcinoma have identified subsets of patients at greater risk for recurrence. The prognosis is proportionately worse with increasing age, higher pathologic grade and clinical stage, and greater depth of myometrial invasion. Malignant cells in the peritoneal fluid or washings and adnexal metastases are ominous findings.

Survival of patients with cancer of the endometrium is dependent on stage and histological grade. The overall 5-year survival rates are 81–91% for surgical stage I, 67–77% for stage II, 31–60% for stage III, and 5–20% for stage IV.

These figures underline the increasing risk for treatment failure and recurrence with increasing bulk and extension of tumor. Consequently, identification of the known risk factors by thorough preoperative and intraoperative evaluation and careful examination of the histopathologic material is vital for treatment planning.

When no risk factors are identified, conservative surgery (simple total abdominal hysterectomy and bilateral salpingo-oophorectomy) should result in corrected survivals greater than 95% at 5 years. The presence of risk factors mandates an aggressive approach using adjuvant radiation therapy and, in some instances, chemotherapy as well. It is hoped that properly controlled prospective randomized studies will determine the success of such treatment.

SARCOMA OF THE UTERUS (LEIOMYOSARCOMA, ENDOMETRIAL SARCOMAS)

ESSENTIALS OF DIAGNOSIS

- Bleeding: intermenstrual, hypermenorrhea, post-menopausal, preadolescent.
- Mass: rapid enlargement of the uterus or of a leiomyoma.
- Pain: discomfort in the pelvis from pressure on surrounding organs.
- Malignant tissue: obtained by biopsy, D&C, or hysterectomy, confirming uterine sarcoma.

General Considerations

The uterine sarcomas, which are sometimes composed of a great variety of mesodermally derived elements, such as bone, cartilage, fat, and striated muscle, are the subject of great histogenetic speculation and innumerable pathologic classification systems. Consequently, they are surrounded by more confusion and controversy than most gynecologic tumors. In fact, for a group of cancers that make up only 2–3% of all malignant tumors of the corpus, they have received an inordinate amount of attention, and they occupy a disproportionate volume of controversial literature.

No common etiologic agent has been identified with uterine sarcomas, but in some reports prior pelvic radiation therapy has been associated with the mixed forms of uterine sarcoma in an unexpectedly high number of cases.

Sarcomas can occur at any age but are most prevalent after age 40. They are well known as a source of hematogenous metastases, but with the exception of leiomyosarcomas, lymphatic permeation and contiguous spread are probably the most common methods of extension. Endometrial sarcomas can usually be diagnosed by endometrial biopsy or dilatation and fractional curettage, but the sarcomas derived from the myometrium (leiomyosarcoma) frequently require hysterectomy to obtain adequate tissue for analysis.

There is no universal agreement on the histologic features that determine outcome, but most authorities agree that the number of mitotic figures per high-power field, vascular and lymphatic invasion, serosal extension, and in some cases degree of anaplasia are all helpful. Lack of discriminating histologic features and ana-

lytic sophistication often cause arbitrary assignment of a specific tumor to an improper category. This is regrettable, since treatment is largely predicated on correct histologic diagnosis. Historically, surgery has been the favored treatment for uterine sarcomas, but some evidence shows that a combination of radiation therapy and surgery is more beneficial for patients with endometrially derived uterine sarcomas. Chemotherapeutic agents reported to be active against sarcomas include doxorubicin, cisplatin, and ifosfamide. Clinical response rates have been reported to range between 8% and 31%. However, most responses are partial and only temporary.

Histogenesis, Classification, & Staging

From a clinical standpoint, the uterine sarcomas can be separated into four categories: leiomyosarcomas (LMSs), endometrial stromal sarcomas (ESSs), malignant mixed mesodermal tumors (MMMTs), and adenosarcomas. A brief review of the histogenesis of these tumors will help the reader to understand the conflicting literature on this subject.

LMSs are thought to arise from the myometrial smooth muscle cell or a similar cell lining blood vessels within the myometrium. A less plausible explanation proposes an origin from the endometrial stromal cell, but almost no data support this contention.

The ESS and MMMT arise from undifferentiated endometrial stromal cells, which retain the potential to differentiate into malignant cell lines that histologically appear native (homologous) or foreign (heterologous) to the human uterus. Because the undifferentiated stromal cells of the endometrium arise from specialized mesenchymal cells of the müllerian apparatus in the genital ridge and ultimately from the mesoderm during embryogenesis, endometrial sarcomas have been variously termed "mesodermal," "müllerian," or "mesenchymal" sarcomas. The prognoses of patients with homologous and heterologous tumors is similar stage for stage, and this terminology has limited clinical usefulness. ESSs have been categorized in the older literature as "pure" and homologous endometrial sarcomas because they are composed of a single cell line. MMMTs, previously designated as "mixed" because of containing two or more cell lines, arise from an undifferentiated malignant stem cell. MMMTs contain both a carcinomatous element and a sarcomatous element and have also been called "carcinosarcomas." The origin of this confusing terminology is better understood by study of Figure 48–5, which graphically represents the histogenesis of uterine sarcomas. Table 48–2 combines the prevailing histogenetic terminology for endometrial sarcomas and depicts the various possibilities in each category.

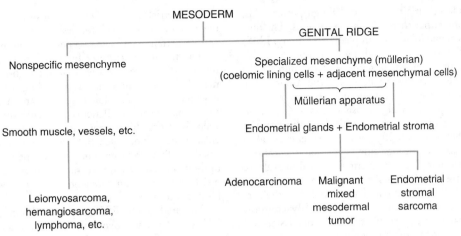

Figure 48–5. Histogenesis of uterine sarcomas.

Pure heterologous sarcomas such as rhabdomyosarcoma, chondrosarcoma, osteosarcoma, and liposarcoma are extremely rare. Finally, the other uterine sarcomas (hemangiosarcoma, fibrosarcoma, reticulum cell sarcoma, lymphosarcoma, and others) are exceedingly rare, and, being indistinguishable from identical sarcomas elsewhere in the body, are not considered specialized tumors of the uterus.

No staging system is designated for uterine sarcomas, but most authors use the FIGO system for endometrial carcinoma (Table 48–1).

Major Types of Sarcomas of the Uterus

A. LEIOMYOSARCOMAS

LMSs make up 35–40% of all uterine sarcomas and 1–2% of all uterine cancers. It usually occurs between ages 25 and 75, with a mean incidence at about age 50.

Table 48–2. Classification of uterine sarcomas.

Leiomyosarcoma (tumors of the uterine smooth muscle)
Endometrial stromal sarcoma (pure homologous endometrial sarcoma)
  High grade
  Low grade (endolymphatic stromal myosis)
Malignant mixed mesodermal tumor (mixed epithelial/stromal tumors)
  Homologous carcinosarcoma
  Heterologous carcinosarcoma
Adenosarcoma (mixed epithelial/stromal tumors)
  Homologous
  Heterologous

Younger patients with this disease seem to have a more favorable outcome than postmenopausal women. Like the benign leiomyomas, which are much more common in blacks, LMSs are 1.5 times more common among black women than among white women. Leiomyomas are commonly identified in uteri containing leiomyosarcomas, but the incidence of malignant transformation of leiomyoma is only 0.1–0.5%. Only about 5–10% of LMSs are reported to originate in a leiomyoma.

Abnormal uterine bleeding is the most common symptom of LMS, occurring in about 60% of patients; 50% describe some type of abdominal pain or discomfort; 30% complain of gastrointestinal or genitourinary symptoms; and only about 10% are aware of an abdominal mass. Occasionally a pedunculated tumor prolapses through the cervix, where it is accessible for biopsy. The deeply situated intramural position of most tumors impedes diagnosis by D&C, which is accurate in only 25% of cases. The Pap smear may be abnormal; more frequently, however, the true nature of the disease becomes evident after the fact, when pathologic analysis of a hysterectomy specimen reveals cancer.

LMSs spread by contiguous growth, invading the myometrium, cervix, and surrounding supporting tissues. Lymphatic dissemination is common in the late stages. Pelvic recurrence and peritoneal dissemination following resection are also common. In the more malignant types, hematogenous metastasis to the lungs, liver, kidney, brain, and bones probably occurs early but is clinically evident only in the lungs until the advanced stages.

The clinical behavior of the tumor can usually be predicted by the number of mitotic figures identified on microscopic examination. Low-grade LMSs are those with less than 5 mitoses per 10 high-power fields, with pushing rather than infiltrating margins. The outcome is favorable following simple hysterectomy. LMSs with 5–10 mitoses per 10 high-power fields are considered to be of intermediate grade, but the outcome is unpredictable—usually favorable if the tumors are completely removed, but with potential to recur or metastasize. Tumors with mitosis counts greater than 10 per 10 high-power fields are highly malignant and usually lethal; less than 20% of these patients are alive at 5 years. Some authors emphasize that the mitosis count should not be the only criterion used to evaluate the aggressiveness of LMS. An invasive pattern, particularly into the blood and lymphatic vessels and the surrounding smooth muscle, is important. By contrast, cellular characteristics such as atypia, anaplasia, and giant cells are not accurate prognosticators of aggressive behavior. Clinically, the most reliable prognostic feature of LMS is stage; that is, when the tumor has extended beyond the uterus, the outcome is uniformly fatal. However, most patients with LMS present at stage I.

Other unusual smooth muscle tumors of the uterus such as benign metastasizing leiomyoma and intravenous leiomyomatosis should be considered low-grade LMS. Although they are histologically benign, they are notorious for local recurrence and can cause death by compression of contiguous or distant vital structures. Intravenous leiomyomatosis has been known to grow up the vena cava into the right atrium, impeding venous return and precipitating congestive heart failure. Because of their slow growth, they can frequently be controlled by repeated local excision. The metastatic lung lesions of benign metastasizing leiomyoma have disappeared following resection of the primary lesion in some cases, perhaps indicating hormone dependency.

B. ENDOMETRIAL SARCOMAS

1. Endometrial stromal sarcomas (ESSs)—ESSs make up 8% of all sarcomas. They occur predominantly in postmenopausal women. Patients with these tumors most commonly present with bleeding or lower abdominal discomfort and pain. The diagnosis can be made accurately by D&C in approximately 75% of cases. Although no etiologic relationship to hormones has been established, a small number of metastatic lesions has responded to progesterone therapy.

ESSs can be divided into two distinct subtypes; low-grade and high-grade. The indolent low-grade ESSs—also called endolymphatic stromal myosis—have fewer than 10 mitoses per 10 high-power fields, with infiltrating margins and myometrial invasion. A benign form, the stromal nodule, has been described; it contains pushing rather than infiltrating margins and fewer than 15 mitoses per 10 high-power fields, with no vascular or myometrial invasion. The diagnosis of stromal nodule should be reserved for lesions with low mitotic counts, certainly fewer than 5 per 10 high-power fields.

The mean age at onset for endolymphatic stromal myosis is 5–10 years earlier than for high-grade sarcomas. This tumor infiltrates surrounding structures and is characterized by indolent growth and a propensity to vascular invasion. Patients frequently present with yellowish worm-like extensions into the periuterine vascular spaces. Under such circumstances, it may be confused grossly with intravenous leiomyomatosis, as previously described. It tends to recur late, sometimes after 5–10 years, and can often be controlled by repeated local excisions.

The high-grade ESSs display infiltrating margins and vascular and myometrial invasion and contain more than 10 mitoses per 10 high-power fields. These tumors are highly malignant and are associated with a poor prognosis, particularly when they extend beyond the uterus at the time of diagnosis. They spread by contiguous growth and lymphatic metastasis. After they move out to the serosal surface of the uterus, they spread to the adnexa and throughout the abdomen. Distant hematogenous metastases to the lungs and liver are usually a late event.

2. Malignant mixed mesodermal tumors (MMMTs)—MMMTs account for 50% of all uterine sarcomas and 3–6% of all uterine tumors. They characteristically occur in postmenopausal women, with the exception of embryonal rhabdomyosarcoma of the cervix or vagina (sarcoma botryoides), which occurs also in infants and children. Radiation therapy may be a predisposing cause. Many published series are available containing a significant number of patients with a history of pelvic radiation for benign or malignant conditions (Fig 48–6).

As with the other types, the presenting symptom of MMMT is usually bleeding. Abdominal discomfort

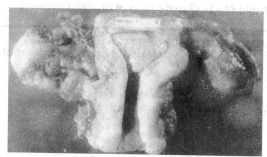

Figure 48–6. Mixed sarcoma of the uterine fundus. Prior full pelvic radiation therapy had little effect on the tumor.

and pain or a neoplastic mass prolapsed into the vagina also occur. Since the tumors are endometrial in origin, about 75% can be diagnosed accurately by D&C. In contrast to the other two major types—LMS and ESS—mitotic counts are not helpful in predicting the outcome of patients with these tumors. Histologically, they are usually highly anaplastic, with many bizarre nuclei and mitotic figures. They usually contain malignant glands and heterotopic elements such as bone, striated muscle, cartilage, or fat, and are then termed "carcinosarcoma." Like the high-grade ESSs, MMMTs spread by contiguous infiltration of the surrounding tissues and by early lymphatic dissemination. Hematogenous metastases are common.

The metastatic deposits are usually composed of malignant glands, but sarcomatous elements have been identified in some cases. The prognosis depends chiefly on the extent of the tumor at the time of primary surgery; there are virtually no long-term survivors among those whose tumor has extended beyond the confines of the uterus at the time of diagnosis.

C. ADENOSARCOMAS

Adenosarcoma is a distinctive mixed müllerian tumor that accounts for 1–2% of uterine sarcomas. It arises from the endometrium and is composed of a combination of benign-appearing glands and a stromal sarcoma or fibrosarcoma. Adenosarcomas usually occur in the postmenopausal age group but have been reported in adolescents and women of reproductive age. Bleeding is the most common symptom. Recurrence occurs in 25% of patients and is usually late. The primary treatment is removal of uterus, tubes, and ovaries. Postoperative radiation therapy is recommended for those tumors with deep myometrial invasion.

D. OTHER UTERINE SARCOMAS

Embryonal rhabdomyosarcoma of the cervix (sarcoma botryoides), which occurs in infants and children, was previously lethal. However, combination therapy using surgery, radiation, and chemotherapy has considerably improved the outlook for these patients.

Fibrosarcoma, hemangiosarcoma, reticulum cell sarcoma, hemangiopericytoma, and other esoteric and bizarre uterine sarcomas are rare. In general, these sarcomas behave like the other intermediate-grade uterine sarcomas, but treatment must be individualized according to age, histologic type, and the patient's state of health.

Clinical Findings

A. SYMPTOMS AND SIGNS

Abnormal uterine bleeding is the most common manifestation of uterine sarcoma. Other recurring complaints include pelvic discomfort or pain, constipation, urinary frequency and urgency, and the presence of a mass low in the abdomen. Uterine sarcoma should be suspected in any nonpregnant woman with a rapidly enlarging uterus. Severe uterine cramps may exist if the tumor has prolapsed into the endometrial cavity or through the cervix. Pelvic examination may reveal the characteristic grapelike structures of sarcoma botryoides protruding from the cervix or the presence of velvety fronds of ESS in the cervical canal. A necrotic fungating mass at the vaginal apex should suggest an infarcted myoma, LMS, or MMMT. The uterus is usually enlarged and often soft and globular. If the cancer has involved the cervix, cul-de-sac, or cardinal ligaments, fixation or asymmetry of the parametria may be found. In advanced cases, inguinal or supraclavicular node metastases may be evident. Patients with advanced uterine sarcomas may present with a large omental mass or ascites secondary to abdominal carcinomatosis.

B. LABORATORY FINDINGS

Standard laboratory evaluation of patients with uterine sarcoma should include a complete blood count and urinalysis, liver function studies (especially serum alkaline phosphatase, prothrombin time, and serum lactic dehydrogenase), blood urea nitrogen, and serum creatinine. Ca-125 may be elevated. Estrogen and progesterone receptor analysis may indicate which patients are likely to respond to hormone therapy. Cytologic study of tissue recovered from the endometrial cavity or endocervical canal is often positive in endometrial sarcomas but not in the more deeply situated LMSs. Office endometrial biopsy or punch biopsy of a prolapsed vaginal mass is helpful only if positive.

C. X-RAY FINDINGS

The chest x-ray may contain metastatic coin lesions characteristic of uterine sarcomas. Because uterine sarcomas commonly metastasize to the lung, a chest computed tomography (CT) scan should be considered when the routine films are negative, particularly before any radical extirpative surgery in the pelvis is performed. An intravenous urogram is indispensable in the work-up of any patient with a pelvic mass. It may reveal ureteral deviation, compression, obstruction, or anomaly, and will demonstrate clearly the number and location of the kidneys and ureters. The combination of the chest x-ray and the intravenous urogram (scout film) may be used as a survey of the axial skeleton, ribs, and pelvic bones, which are most frequently involved by metastases.

CT scan of the abdomen and pelvis is not warranted routinely but may delineate enlarged retroperitoneal nodes in advanced cases. MRI should provide an accurate preoperative assessment of uterine size and degree of involvement.

D. SPECIAL EXAMINATIONS

Pelvic ultrasonography, although not usually indicated in the evaluation of palpable pelvic masses, may occasionally confirm the presence of a pelvic mass or help to differentiate an adnexal from a uterine mass in the obese patient. Sigmoidoscopy should always be performed in older women, or in young women if gastrointestinal bleeding or masses suspected of being malignant are present. Cystoscopy is indicated in locally advanced disease or in the presence of gross or microscopic hematuria.

Differential Diagnosis

The clinical diagnosis of uterine sarcoma is frequently overlooked. Diagnostic accuracy can be increased if the physician keeps these tumors in mind while investigating any pelvic mass. The tumor frequently does not present the classic picture of abnormal bleeding accompanied by a symmetrically enlarged soft globular uterus. It can masquerade as any condition causing uterine enlargement or a pelvic mass; of these, pregnancy, leiomyoma, adenomyosis, and adherent ovarian neoplasms or pelvic inflammatory disease are most likely to cause misinterpretation. When cytologic studies, endometrial biopsy, or dilatation and fractional curettage fails to provide the diagnosis—a situation not uncommon with LMS—laparotomy is necessary. At laparotomy, thorough evaluation is critical to the future management of the patient with uterine sarcoma and must include inspection (where possible) and palpation of all abdominal viscera, peritoneal and mesenteric surfaces, liver, both diaphragms, and retroperitoneal structures, especially the pelvic and aortic lymph nodes. Cytologic examination of peritoneal exudate is indispensable for treatment planning; if no free fluid is present, samples may be obtained by instilling 50–100 mL of normal saline into the abdominal cavity. If a sarcoma is identified on frozen section of the hysterectomy specimen, suspicious lymph nodes should be removed. This information, gathered at the time of the initial exploration and carefully documented in the operative records, is critical for identification and staging of the neoplasm and for predicting outcome.

The pathologic diagnosis of uterine sarcoma is often extremely difficult and may require consultation with a gynecologic pathologist familiar with these tumors. As each cancer becomes more anaplastic, the parent cell or tissue becomes more difficult to identify histologically. Since proper treatment is predicated on accurate histologic diagnosis, every effort should be expended to identify the cell of origin.

Complications

Severe anemia from chronic blood loss or acute hemorrhage may be present. The severity and extent of other complications due to uterine sarcomas are directly related to the size and virulence of the primary tumor. A pedunculated mass may protrude into the uterine cavity or prolapse through the cervix, causing bleeding or uterine cramps as the uterus attempts to expel the tumor. Infarction with subsequent infection and sepsis may ensue. Rupture of the uterus and kidney due to rapidly growing uterine sarcomas has been reported. Obstructed labor and postpartum uterine inversion secondary to endometrial sarcomas have also been noted. Extensive pulmonary metastases can produce hemoptysis and respiratory failure. Ascites is common in advanced disease with peritoneal metastases.

A wide variety of complications has been reported secondary to pressure or compression of a neighboring viscus or resulting from extension or metastases to other vital structures. Urethral elongation due to stretching of the bladder over a rapidly growing mass can simultaneously produce obstruction and loss of sphincter control, with subsequent overflow incontinence. Colon compression may result in ribbon stools and, eventually, complete bowel obstruction. Ureteral obstruction is common, especially with recurrent pelvic sarcomas. Urinary diversion or colostomy may be required prior to treatment if life-threatening viscus obstruction is present in an untreated patient, but urinary diversion should not be performed unless there is some hope for cure or meaningful palliation, since it precludes a painless death from uremia.

Prevention

Indiscriminate use of radiation therapy for benign conditions in the pelvis should be avoided, since several clinical studies have suggested an etiologic role of pelvic radiation in the development of MMMT.

Treatment

A. EMERGENCY MEASURES

Hemorrhage from uterine sarcomas can be exsanguinating and requires prompt attention. When there has been acute hemorrhage, blood volume should be replaced with whole blood; patients with severe or profound anemia secondary to chronic intermittent bleeding should have blood volume replaced with packed red blood cells over a somewhat prolonged time course. Rapid replacement with whole blood in these patients can precipitate congestive heart failure.

Emergency D&C should be used only to obtain tissue for analysis. Vigorous curettage is likely to aggravate or provoke bleeding. High-dose bolus radiation is a more reliable and safe method of controlling bleeding. A dose of 400–500 cGy administered daily to the whole pelvis over 2–3 days usually controls acute hemorrhage; this does not appreciably interfere with future management. If these measures are not successful, emergency embolization or ligation of the hypogastric arteries sometimes controls hemorrhage when hysterectomy is not indicated or technically feasible.

B. SURGICAL MEASURES

Extirpative surgery provides the best chance for long-term palliation or cure for patients with uterine sarcomas. Surgery is the cornerstone of the treatment plan and should be the central focus of attack against these cancers.

Low-grade uterine sarcomas (some LMSs, endolymphatic stromal myosis, intravenous leiomyomatosis) have a propensity for isolated local spread and central pelvic recurrence; therefore, such patients should be considered for radical hysterectomy and bilateral salpingo-oophorectomy. The benefits of this type of therapy have not been conclusively shown, but theoretically the problem of local recurrence should be improved by more radical excision of the primary tumor. Lymph node metastases in these low-grade tumors are negligible; consequently, pelvic lymphadenectomy can be reserved for patients with enlarged or suspicious nodes. Pelvic recurrences of low-grade uterine sarcomas have been successfully treated by repeated excisions of all resectable tumor. Patients have been known to survive for many years following this type of conservative treatment. Partial or complete pelvic exenteration may occasionally be useful for recurrence of indolent tumors.

The high-grade uterine sarcomas (some LMSs, ESSs, all MMMTs) display early lymphatic, local, and hematogenous metastases even when apparently confined to the uterus. For this reason, radical surgery has been abandoned in favor of simple total abdominal hysterectomy and bilateral salpingo-oophorectomy preceded or followed by adjunctive radiation therapy. The addition of radiation therapy for LMS, although still controversial, is being discarded by many centers because it has not improved survival and because it substantially interferes with subsequent chemotherapy.

At the time of surgical exploration, a thorough examination and evaluation of the abdominal contents must be performed and documented. Cytologic specimens and omental tissue should be obtained, and suspicious papillations, excrescences, and adhesions should be excised for pathologic analysis. The more information obtained at the primary exploration, the less difficult will be the design of an appropriate postoperative treatment plan.

When uterine sarcomas recur in the lung and the metastatic survey is negative, unilateral isolated metastases should be excised after a chest CT scan has ruled out other lesions not apparent on the routine chest x-ray. Considering all sources, resection of isolated sarcoma metastases to the lung carries about a 25% 5-year cure rate.

C. CHEMOTHERAPY

Adjuvant doxorubicin has been shown to reduce the distant recurrence rate for LMS. Although the data are not statistically significant, some authorities recommend the use of doxorubicin-based chemotherapy in high-grade LMS.

Because of the high hormone receptor content in ESS, adjuvant progestin or tamoxifen therapy has been recommended. For receptor-negative tumors, doxorubicin-based chemotherapy is used.

Doxorubicin, cisplatin, and ifosfamide display significant activity against MMMTs. Cyclophosphamide and vincristine have also shown activity. Some data suggest that combination chemotherapy is more effective than single-agent therapy. In advanced or metastatic disease, adjuvant combination chemotherapy is recommended.

D. RADIATION THERAPY

When used as the only modality of treatment for uterine sarcomas, radiation has produced dismal results—very few survivors are reported in the literature following treatment with radiation therapy alone for any of the uterine sarcomas. Radiation therapy does seem to improve survival and reduce local recurrences when used in combination with surgery for the treatment of some endometrial sarcomas. Collected data indicate that adjuvant radiation therapy improves the 2-year survival rate in patients with ESS by approximately 20% and may also improve survival for those with MMMTs, although less convincingly. Although an occasional 5-year survivor with LMS has been reported following radiation therapy alone, analysis of large numbers of patients from different institutions does not support its use for these tumors. Nevertheless, in advanced forms of LMS, radiation may prove useful for palliation and control of pelvic symptoms such as massive bleeding or pain.

Prognosis

In determining the prognosis for patients with uterine sarcomas, a constellation of factors must be examined simultaneously. Such considerations as the patient's age, state of health, and ability to withstand major surgery or radiation therapy (or both) must be evaluated. The most important clinical characteristic—and probably the overriding prognostic feature affecting the prognosis of these patients—is the stage of the disease at the time of diagnosis. In the high-grade sarcomas (LMS and mixed endometrial sarcoma), the presence of tumor outside the uterus at the time of diagnosis is a clear prognostic omen: fewer than 10% of patients survive 2 years. Even when the disease is apparently limited to the uterus, the prognosis is poor: 10–50% survive 5 years. In the intermediate-grade LMS and high-grade ESS, the outcome is improved, with up to 80–90% of patients surviving 5 years if the disease is clinically limited to the uterus at the time of surgery. Low-grade ESS and low-grade LMS have a generally favorable outcome: 80–100% of patients survive 5 years following complete excision of the uterus. Low-grade stromal tumors have been known to recur locally after 10–20 years; this confuses the survival statistics. Undoubtedly, these patients must be followed closely for life.

REFERENCES

Endometrial Hyperplasia & Carcinoma

Abeler V, Kjorstad KE: Clear cell carcinoma of the endometrium: A histopathological and clinical study of 97 cases. Gynecol Oncol 1991;40:207.

American College of Obstetricians and Gynecologists: Estrogen replacement therapy and endometrial cancer. ACOG Committee Opinion No. 126. ACOG, August 1993.

Belloni C et al: Magnetic resonance imaging in endometrial carcinoma staging. Gynecol Oncol 1990;37:172.

Bloss JD et al: Use of vaginal hysterectomy for the management of stage I endometrial cancer in the medically compromised patient. Gynecol Oncol 1991;40:74.

Boring CC et al: Cancer statistics, 1992. Cancer 1992;42:19.

Borst MP et al: Oncogene alterations in endometrial carcinoma. Gynecol Oncol 1990;38:364.

Bourne TH et al: Detection of endometrial cancer by transvaginal ultrasonography with color flow imaging and blood flow analysis: A preliminary report. Gynecol Oncol 1991;40:253.

Britton LC et al: DNA ploidy in endometrial carcinoma: Major objective prognostic factor. Mayo Clin Proc 1990;65:543.

Burke TW et al: Treatment failure in endometrial carcinoma. Obstet Gynecol 1990;75:96.

Goff BA, Rice LW: Assessment of depth of myometrial invasion in endometrial adenocarcinoma. Gynecol Oncol 1990;38:46.

Granberg S et al: Endometrial thickness as measured by endovaginal ultrasonography for identifying endometrial abnormality. Am J Obstet Gynecol 1991;164:47.

Greenlee RT et al: Cancer statistics, 2000. CA Cancer J Clin 2000;50:7.

Hirsch M, Lilford RJ, Jarvis GJ: Adjuvant progestogen therapy for the treatment of endometrial cancer: review and metaanalysis of published, randomized controlled trials. Eur J Obstet Gynecol Reprod Biol 1996;65:201.

Koh WJ et al: Radiation therapy in endometrial cancer. Baillieres Best Pract Res Clin Obstet Gynaecol 2001;15:417.

Lalloo F, Evans G: Molecular genetics and endometrial cancer. Baillieres Best Pract Res Clin Obstet Gynaecol 2001;15:355.

Lehoczky O et al: Stage I endometrial adenocarcinoma: Treatment of nonoperable patients with intracavitary radiation alone. Gynecol Oncol 1991;43:211.

Morrow CP et al: Relationship between surgical-pathological risk factors and outcome in clinical stage I and II carcinoma of the endometrium: A gynecologic oncology group study. Gynecol Oncol 1991;40:55.

Pettersson F: Annual report on the results of treatment in gynecological cancer. Int J Gynecol Obstet 1991;36(Suppl):132.

Quinn MA, Campbell JJ: Tamoxifen therapy in advanced/recurrent endometrial carcinoma. Gynecol Oncol 1989;32:1.

Rubin GL et al: Estrogen replacement therapy and the risk of endometrial cancer: Remaining controversies. Am J Obstet Gynecol 1990;162:148.

Seouid MAF, Johnson J, Weed JC: Gynecologic tumors in tamoxifen-treated women with breast cancer. Obstet Gynecol 1993; 82:165.

Stringer CA, Gershenson DM, Burke TW: Adjuvant chemotherapy with cisplatin, doxorubicin, and cyclophosphamide (PAC) for early stage high-risk endometrial cancer: A preliminary analysis. Gynecol Oncol 1990;38:305.

Thigpen T et al: A randomized trial of medroxyprogesterone acetate (MPA) 200 mg versus 1000 mg daily in advanced or recurrent endometrial carcinoma: A gynecologic oncology group study. Proc Am Soc Clin Oncol 1991;10:185.

Sarcoma of the Uterus

Berchuk A et al: Treatment of endometrial stromal tumors. Gynecol Oncol 1990;36:60.

Clement PB, Scully RE: Mullerian adenosarcoma of the uterus: A clinicopathologic analysis of 100 cases with a review of the literature. Hum Pathol 1990;21:363.

Echt G et al: Treatment of uterine sarcomas. Cancer 1990;66:35.

Leibsohn S et al: Leiomyosarcoma in a series of hysterectomies performed for presumed uterine leiomyomas. Am J Obstet Gynecol 1990;162:968.

Silverberg SG et al: Carcinosarcoma (malignant mixed mesodermal tumor) of the uterus: A Gynecologic Oncology Group Pathologic Study of 203 cases. Int J Gynecol Pathol 1990;9:1.

Thigpen JT et al: Phase II trial of cisplatin as first line chemotherapy in patients with advanced or recurrent uterine sarcomas: A Gynecologic Oncology Group Study. J Clin Oncol 1991; 9:1962.

Premalignant and Malignant Disorders of the Ovaries and Oviducts

49

Oliver Dorigo, MD, & Vicki V. Baker, MD

General Introduction

Ovarian cancer is the fifth most common cancer in women and the fifth most frequent cause of cancer death. In the year 2000, 23,100 new ovarian cancer cases were diagnosed and 14,000 patients succumbed to the disease. About 23,000 cases were diagnosed in 1993, and 14,000 women died as a result of this disease. Approximately 1 in 70 newborn girls will develop ovarian cancer during her lifetime. In general, ovarian cancer is a disease of the postmenopausal woman and the prepubescent girl, although it is documented to occur in females of all ages.

ETIOLOGY OF OVARIAN CANCER

The cause of ovarian cancer is unknown, although a number of predisposing risk factors have been identified. It has been proposed that repeated ovulation is causally related to the development of this disease. Ovulation is accompanied by disruption of the germinal epithelium and the activation of cellular repair mechanisms. Repeated ovulation may provide ample opportunity for somatic gene deletions and mutations to occur, which in turn can contribute to tumor initiation and progression. Supporting this theory are the observations that chronic anovulation, multiparity, and a history of breastfeeding are protective. Pregnancy is associated with a risk reduction of 13–19% per pregnancy. Infertility treatment may be associated with a slightly increased risk of ovarian cancer as suggested by a meta-analysis. Furthermore, women with polycystic ovarian syndrome (PCOS) were found to have a 2.5-fold increased risk of developing epithelial ovarian cancer. Hormone replacement therapy has not been found to increase the overall risk of ovarian cancer. However, unopposed estrogen therapy may be associated with a significant increase in risk of endometroid, epithelial ovarian tumors. Use of oral contraceptives decreases the risk of epithelial ovarian cancer by 50% for users of 5 years and longer. This risk reduction is also evident in high-risk families with a genetic predisposition.

A number of different studies have suggested an association between dietary factors and ovarian cancer. Diets high in saturated animal fats seem to confer an increased risk by unknown mechanisms. Interestingly, Japanese women who move to the United States have been found to have an increased ovarian cancer risk. Other factors like alcohol and milk product consumption have been hypothesized as risk factors but never confirmed. Exposure to talc has also been proposed as a risk factor in women who place talcum powder on the external genitalia. The presence of talc granulomas in the ovaries of patients who have never been previously operated on has been well documented and can be explained by the continuity of the introitus and peritoneal cavity via the endocervical canal, the endometrial cavity, and the fallopian tubes (Fig 49–1). The ability of foreign materials, including talc and asbestos, to act as carcinogenic substances is established in several models, but their role in ovarian carcinogenesis remains speculative.

Over 90% of ovarian cancer develops sporadically. However, an estimated 10% of epithelial ovarian cancers are based on genetic predisposition. Chromosomal abnormalities are commonly associated with ovarian malignancies. Patients with Turner's syndrome (45,XO) are at increased risk of dysgerminoma and gonadoblastoma. Women with two first-degree relatives with ovarian cancer have a 50% likelihood of developing ovarian cancer until age 70. Hereditary ovarian cancer occurs in two forms, either as breast and ovarian cancer syndrome (BOC), or the less common Lynch II syndrome, also known as hereditary nonpolyposis colorectal cancer syndrome (HNPCC syndrome). BOC is most often associated with germline mutations in the *BRCA1* gene located on chromosome 17 and less commonly with *BRCA2* mutations on chromosome 13. The overall frequency of *BRCA1* mutation carriers in the United States is approximately 1 in 800 women. Greater mutation frequencies have been found in Ashkenazi Jews and Icelandic women. These mutations are inherited in an autosomal dominant fashion and

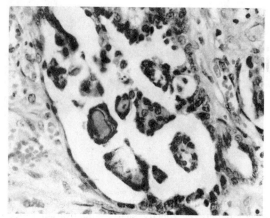

Figure 49–1. Papillary lesion with incorporated talc granules.

therefore require a careful pedigree analysis. Women with *BRCA1* mutations from high-risk families have a lifetime risk of ovarian cancer as high as 28–44%.

The HNPCC syndrome involves a combination of familial colon cancer and a high rate of ovarian, endometrial, and breast cancer as well as other gastrointestinal malignancies. Genes involved in this syndrome include mainly DNA mismatch repair genes like *hMSH2* or *hMLH1*.

A number of molecular mechanisms related to ovarian cancer pathogenesis have been described. Allelic loss and mutations of the p53 tumor suppressor gene are found in about 55% of all ovarian cancers. The c-erb-B2 (HER2/*neu*) proto-oncogene is activated in about 30% of ovarian cancers, providing the potential for increased proliferation and metastasis. Other molecular pathways include *bcl*-2, k-*ras*, Ki67 and interleukin-6. Several novel therapeutic approaches have been developed based on the identification of these different pathologic mechanisms, including replacing missing p53 tumor suppressor gene function and blocking the activation of HER2/*neu.*

HISTOPATHOLOGY OF OVARIAN CANCER

Ovarian cancer may be divided into three major categories, based on the cell type of origin (Table 49–1). The ovary may also be the site of metastatic disease by primary cancer from another organ site. Unlike carcinomas of the cervix and endometrium, precursor lesions of ovarian carcinoma have not been defined.

1. Epithelial Neoplasms

Epithelial neoplasms are derived from the ovarian surface mesothelial cells and include six cell types: **serous, mucinous, endometrioid, clear cell, transitional cell,** and **undifferentiated.** Epithelial tumors account for over 60% of all ovarian neoplasms and more than 90% of malignant ovarian tumors.

Ovarian **serous cystadenocarcinoma** is the most common malignant tumor of the ovary, accounting for 35–50% of all epithelial tumors. Grossly, these neoplasms are bilateral in 40–60% of cases, and 85% are associated with extraovarian spread at the time of diagnosis. Over 50% of serous tumors exceed 15 cm in diameter, and cut section reveals solid areas, areas of hemorrhage, necrosis, cyst wall invasion, and adhesions to adjacent structures. Unilocular or multilocular cysts often contain coarse papillae that project into the cystic lumen (Fig 49–2).

Histologically, serous carcinomas of the ovary exhibit mild to moderate nuclear atypia and occasional mitotic figures of the stratified squamous epithelium, which often forms budding tufts. Psammoma bodies, which are irregular calcifications, are characteristic of serous tumors. The grade of differentiation of these neoplasms is based on the degree of preservation of the papillary architecture. Most serous carcinomas are poorly differentiated with trabecular and solid growth patterns.

Serous ovarian neoplasms of low malignant potential exhibit histologic features suggestive of both carcinoma and benignity. Although marked cellular pleomorphism and mitotic figures are often present, there is no stromal invasion. Psammoma bodies are often present. As will be discussed in a later section, the prognosis and therapy of serous carcinoma of low malignant

Table 49–1. Major histopathologic categories of ovarian cancer.

Epithelial
Serous, mucinous, endometrioid, clear cell, transitional cell (Brenner), undifferentiated
Germ Cell
Dysgerminoma, endodermal sinus tumor, teratoma (immature, mature, specialized), embryonal carcinoma, choriocarcinoma, gonadoblastoma, mixed germ cell, polyembryona
Sex Cord and Stromal
Granulosa cell tumor, fibroma, thecoma Sertoli-Leydig cell, gynandroblastoma
Neoplasms Metastatic to the Ovary
Breast, colon, stomach, endometrium, lymphoma

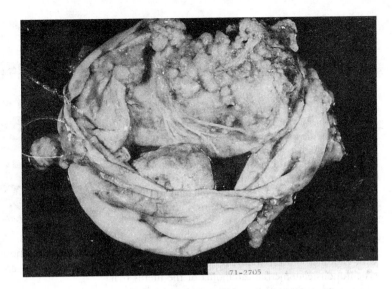

Figure 49–2. Internal papillae characteristic of the papillary serous cystadenocarcinoma.

potential are different from invasive serous carcinoma, and an accurate diagnosis is essential.

Mucinous neoplasms of the ovary account for 10–20% of all epithelial ovarian tumors and are the second most common type of epithelial ovarian cancer. In contrast to serous tumors, mucinous tumors are bilateral in less than 10% of cases.

Mucinous tumors are notable for the large size that they may attain; neoplasms over 150 pounds have been reported. However, the average size of these lesions is 16–17 cm. Cut sections of these tumors typically reveal multilocular cysts filled with viscous mucin (Fig 49–3). The lining of these tumors is composed of atypical cells with numerous mitotic figures.

Histologically, mucinous adenocarcinoma of the ovary is composed predominantly of intestinal-like cells that invade the surrounding stroma. The cells have large hyperchromatic nuclei and prominent nucleoli. Invasive mucinous ovarian carcinoma exhibits marked histologic variability from area to area within the tumor, and extensive sampling is required. It is recommended that at least one section per centimeter of tumor be examined. The differentiation of mucinous cystadenocarcinoma is related to the preservation of glandlike architecture of the tumor.

Analogous to serous ovarian neoplasms, both invasive carcinomas and tumors of low malignant potential of the mucinous variety are recognized. Mucinous tumors of low malignant potential are characterized histologically by several cell types, including endocervical-like columnar cells, intestinal-like columnar cells with eosinophilic cytoplasm, goblet cells, and basal endocrine cells. Although cellular atypia may be mild to moderate and a moderate number of mitotic figures

may be present, cellular stratification does not exceed 2–3 layers and stromal invasion is absent.

Pseudomyxoma peritonei is an unusual condition that may occur in association with mucinous neoplasms of the ovary resulting from the progressive accumula-

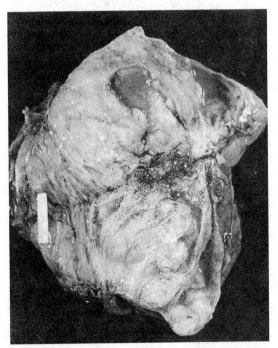

Figure 49–3. Mucinous cystadenocarcinoma. Note the obvious mucinous component and the solid, more malignant areas.

tion of mucin in the abdominal cavity following its slow leakage from a neoplasm. It most commonly occurs in association with lesions of low malignant potential, although it is also reported to occur in association with cystadenocarcinoma of the ovary and appendix as well as mucocele of the appendix. Although rare and histologically benign in appearance, pseudomyxoma peritonei has a protracted and potentially morbid course secondary to repeated bowel obstruction, with a mortality rate that approaches 50%.

An **endometrioid neoplasm** of the ovary exhibits an adenomatoid pattern that resembles endometrial adenocarcinoma (Fig 49–4). It is bilateral in 30–50% of cases. Rarely, this neoplasm arises in foci of endometriosis (less than 10% of cases). The degree of differentiation is based on the extent to which the glandular architecture is retained. As many as 30% of patients with endometrioid carcinoma of the ovary also have a synchronous endometrial carcinoma of the uterus that is a second primary rather than a metastatic focus of disease.

Clear cell carcinoma of the ovary, also referred to as **mesonephroid carcinoma** of the ovary, accounts for approximately 5% of epithelial ovarian cancers. It rarely

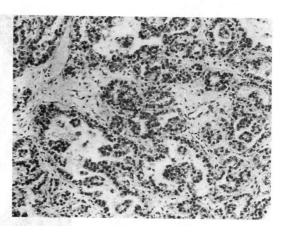

Figure 49–5. Adenomatous pattern with papillary infolding and "hobnail epithelium." In many areas, clear cells can be seen with transitions to the hobnail type.

attains the size of serous and mucinous neoplasms of the ovary. Clear cell carcinomas of the ovary are biologically aggressive and may be associated with hypercalcemia and hyperpyrexia. On cut section, both cystic and solid areas are present. The external surface is smooth but has a bosselated contour. Histologically, two cell types may be present: the clear cell and the "hobnail cell" (Fig 49–5). Occasionally, clear cell carcinomas may be difficult to differentiate from mucinous neoplasms. The periodic acid-Schiff reaction can be used to differentiate the two since it is only weakly positive in clear cell neoplasms but strikingly positive in mucinous tumors.

Transitional cell (Brenner) carcinoma of the ovary is a newly described entity composed of cells that resemble low-grade transitional cell carcinoma of the urinary bladder. Patients typically present with advanced stage disease and exhibit a poorer prognosis when compared with that of other histologic types of epithelial ovarian cancer.

Undifferentiated carcinoma of the ovary accounts for less than 10% of epithelial neoplasms. This neoplasm is characterized by the absence of any distinguishing microscopic features that permit its placement in one of the other histologic categories.

2. Germ Cell Neoplasms

Germ cell neoplasms arise from the germ cell elements of the ovary and include dysgerminoma, endodermal sinus tumor, embryonal cell carcinoma, choriocarcinoma, teratoma, polyembryona, and mixed germ cell tumors. Unlike the epithelial neoplasms, which tend to occur during the sixth decade of life, this group of tu-

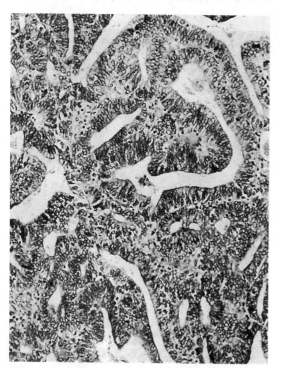

Figure 49–4. Endometrioid carcinoma as seen with high-power field. Note the tall epithelium—not a tubal type or the mucoid variety.

Table 49–2. Tumor markers that may be elevated in the presence of germ cell neoplasms.

Neoplasm	AFP	hCG
Dysgerminoma	–	+/–
Endodermal sinus tumor	+	–
Immature teratoma	+/–	–
Mixed germ cell tumor	+/–	+/–
Choriocarcinoma	–	+
Embryonal carcinoma	–	+

AFP, alpha-fetoprotein; hCG, human chorionic gonadotropin.
– = negative (not elevated);
+ = positive (elevated above normal level).

mors tends to occur during the second and third decades and as a group is associated with a better prognosis. Many of these neoplasms produce biologic markers, which can be monitored to assess response to therapy (Table 49–2).

Dysgerminoma of the ovary is the female counterpart of the seminoma in the male. It occurs primarily in young females and accounts for about 30–40% of germ cell tumors. Grossly, the tumor is rather rubbery in consistency, smooth, rounded, and thinly encapsulated, with a brown or grayish-brown color. This neoplasm is unilateral in 85–90% of cases. It is a solid neoplasm, which may contain areas of softening due to degeneration.

Histologically, dysgerminoma mimics the pattern seen in the primitive gonad, ie, it has nests of germ cells that appear as large, rounded cells with central nuclei that contain one or two prominent nucleoli surrounded by undifferentiated stroma (Fig 49–6). Lymphocytes may invade the stroma and occasionally giant cells are identified. A lymphocytic infiltrate is considered a favorable prognostic indicator.

Endodermal sinus tumor of the ovary, previously called a **yolk sac tumor,** is the second most common germ cell neoplasm, occurring in approximately 20% of cases. It is bilateral in less than 5% of cases. It holds the distinction of being the most rapidly growing neoplasm that occurs at any site. These lesions are friable, focally necrotic, and hemorrhagic. Patients commonly present with an acute abdomen.

Microscopically, endodermal sinus tumor is composed of primitive epithelial cells that form architectural patterns that recapitulate the primitive gut and the primitive liver. The pathognomonic finding is the Schiller-Duval body, which is a single papilla lined by tumor cells with a central blood vessel. This neoplasm commonly contains cells that produce alpha-fetoprotein (AFP).

Immature teratomas of the ovary are the malignant counterpart of the mature cystic teratoma or dermoid and also account for about 20% of germ cell neoplasms. This malignancy is bilateral in less than 5% of cases, although the contralateral ovary commonly contains a dermoid cyst. The serum AFP is usually elevated in patients with an immature teratoma.

Microscopic examination reveals a disordered collection of tissues derived from the three germ layers with at least some of the components having an immature, embryonic appearance. The immature elements are commonly neuroectodermal and consist of small round malignant cells that may be associated with glia formation. Hyaline bodies stain positive for AFP. Immature teratomas may be graded from 1 to 3 based on the amount of immature neural tissue that they contain. Tumor grade is correlated with prognosis and also guides recommendations regarding the need for chemotherapy. Metastatic implants may be composed entirely of mature neuroectodermal tissue. In this circumstance, the stage of the tumor is not increased nor is the prognosis diminished.

Mature teratomas or dermoids are common ovarian neoplasms, occurring primarily in women aged

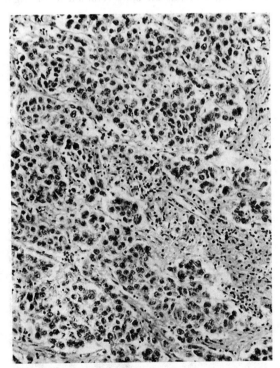

Figure 49–6. Classic histologic picture of dysgerminoma. Note nests of germ cells of various sizes separated by fibrous trabeculae.

20–30 years. They represent the most common neoplasm diagnosed during pregnancy. Rarely, the squamous component undergoes malignant transformation (less than 2%) in women over the age of 40.

Embryonal carcinoma of the ovary is a very rare germ cell tumor in pure form, although foci may occasionally be found admixed with other germ cell neoplasms. Histologically, this neoplasm consists of solid sheets of large polygonal cells with pale, eosinophilic cytoplasms that appear to merge together as a syncytium because the cell membranes are poorly defined. Serum human chorionic gonadotropin (hCG) and AFP values are usually elevated.

Choriocarcinoma of the ovary is another rare germ cell tumor that is unrelated to pregnancy. Unlike gestational choriocarcinoma, primary ovarian choriocarcinoma is associated with somewhat lower elevations of hCG. The endocrine activity of this neoplasm may cause precocious puberty, uterine bleeding, or amenorrhea. Microscopically, this neoplasm is composed of cytotrophoblasts, intermediate trophoblasts, and syncytiotrophoblasts.

Gonadoblastoma of the ovary is a rare neoplasm composed of nests of germ cells and sex cord derivatives that are surrounded by connective tissue stroma (Fig 49–7). These tumors are more common in the right ovary than in the left and usually occur during the second decade of life. Gonadoblastomas are found in patients with abnormal gonadal development in the presence of a Y chromosome.

Mixed germ cell tumors of the ovary account for approximately 10% of germ cell neoplasms. As implied by the name, these neoplasms contain two or more germ cell elements. A dysgerminoma and endodermal sinus tumor occur together most frequently. These neoplasms must be meticulously evaluated by the pathologist to identify all elements correctly, since different components may require treatment with different chemotherapeutic regimens.

SEX CORD-STROMAL TUMORS OF THE OVARY

Granulosa cell tumors represent 1–2% of all ovarian neoplasms and are the most common malignant tumors of the sex cord-stromal tumor category. They are associated with hyperestrogenism and may cause precocious puberty in young girls and adenomatous hyperplasia and vaginal bleeding in postmenopausal women. Microscopically, the granulosa cells, which exhibit characteristic grooved or coffee bean nuclei, may exhibit microfollicular, macrofollicular, trabecular, insular, or solid growth patterns. Call-Exner bodies are associated with the microfollicular growth pattern and represent multiple small cavities that contain eosinophilic fluid. Theca cells are present in varying amounts.

Like the granulosa cell tumors, an ovarian thecoma is often associated with hyperestrogenism. This benign ovarian tumor consists of lipid-laden stromal cells, which give the tumor a yellow color on cut section. An ovarian fibroma is another benign tumor that is noteworthy because of its association with Meigs' syndrome. Meigs' syndrome refers to the occurrence of an ovarian fibroma, ascites, and pleural effusion, which collectively mimic the presentation of ovarian cancer.

Sertoli-stromal cell tumors are rare and consist of testicular structures at different stages of development. They are usually virilizing and occur most commonly during the third decade of life. They are rarely bilateral. Microscopically, both Sertoli and Leydig cells are present. A variety of architectural patterns have been described.

NEOPLASMS METASTATIC TO THE OVARY

Cancer metastatic to the ovary accounts for as many as 25% of all ovarian malignancies. Clinically, these tumors often mimic primary ovarian cancer and usually present as bilateral adnexal masses, although a unilateral mass occurs in as many as 25% of patients. These

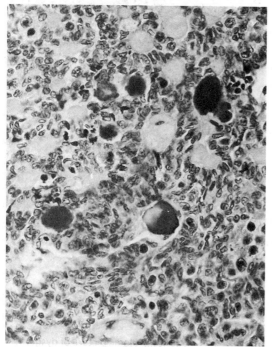

Figure 49–7. Gonadoblastoma with folliculoid pattern, focal calcifications, and concretions.

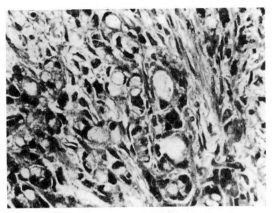

Figure 49–8. Metastatic ovarian cancer. Note the "signet cells," characteristic of the mucocellular nature of the tumor.

masses are usually smooth and bosselated, solid, and mobile. The most common primary cancers that metastasize to the ovary are those of the breast, stomach, colon, and endometrium. Ovarian metastases in patients with breast cancer are found in up to 40% of cases.

Microscopically, cancer metastatic to the ovary can present a variety of potentially confusing patterns. For example, when the primary lesion is a breast carcinoma, the histologic appearance of the ovary may vary from one that accurately reflects the primary pathology to a pattern of diffuse invasion of the stroma by undifferentiated cells. Gastrointestinal carcinoma metastatic to the ovary often simulates a primary mucin-secreting adenocarcinoma of the ovary with the presence of characteristic signet ring cells (Fig 49–8). Large locules lined by tall columnar mucin-secreting epithelial cells are separated by fibrous trabeculae. The epithelium may be well, moderately, or poorly differentiated.

Krukenberg tumors by definition represent carcinomas of the stomach metastatic to the ovary. However, the eponym is commonly used to denote any gastrointestinal carcinoma metastatic to the ovary.

■ DIAGNOSIS OF OVARIAN CANCER

Ovarian cancer typically develops as an insidious disease, with few warning signs or symptoms. Most neoplastic ovarian tumors produce few symptoms until the disease is widely disseminated throughout the abdominal cavity. A history of nonspecific gastrointestinal complaints, including nausea, dyspepsia, and altered bowel habits, is particularly common. Early satiety and abdominal distention as a result of ascites are generally signs of advanced disease. A change in bowel habits, such as constipation and decreased stool caliber, is occasionally noted. Large tumors may cause a sensation of pelvic weight or pressure. Rarely, an ovarian tumor may become incarcerated in the cul-de-sac and cause severe pain, urinary retention, rectal discomfort, and bowel obstruction.

Menstrual abnormalities may be noted in as many as 15% of reproductive age patients with an ovarian neoplasm. Abnormal vaginal bleeding may occur in patients with ovarian cancer in the presence of a synchronous endometrial carcinoma or as a consequence of metastatic disease to the lower genital tract. Rarely, excess androgens or estrogens may be present in women with ovarian neoplasms, presumably because of stimulation of normal theca, granulosa, or hilar cells that surround the neoplasm. Ovarian stromal hyperplasia or hyperthecosis may also be associated with excess androgen production, which alters the normal menstrual cycle. Granulosa theca cell tumors are classically estrogen-producing tumors that present with abnormal vaginal bleeding.

The prognosis of ovarian cancer is significantly improved when the disease is detected while still confined to the ovary. Several screening methods for the early detection of ovarian cancer are available. Routine pelvic examination has limited sensitivity and specificity and a significant percentage of tumors are missed. Ultrasonographic evaluation can detect the majority of ovarian neoplasms but has poor specificity. One of the best characterized tumor markers in epithelial ovarian cancer is CA-125. CA-125 is an antigen from fetal amniotic and coelomic epithelium and its level can be detected in serum using immunoassay. The accepted upper limit of normal is 35 IU/mL, but this is a rather arbitrary cutoff. Routine screening of low-risk, asymptomatic women with the CA-125 tumor marker cannot be recommended at this time. However, CA-125 might have a role in screening of high-risk patients with genetic predisposition. Other currently studied markers include TAG 72, M-CSF and OVX1. Ovarian cancer screening to detect early stage disease will remain difficult until more specific and sensitive markers are defined. Unfortunately, routine pelvic examination is a notoriously poor screening method with limited sensitivity and specificity. Ten percent of masses less than 10 cm in size are missed on routine examination, and the size of a mass is correctly predicted within 2 cm in only 68% of patients. Current strategies for screening focus on the detection of tumor-associated antigens, such as CA-125, and ultrasound examinations of the adnexa. However, the limited prevalence of ovarian cancer and the sensitivity and specificity of currently available tests such as ultrasound and CA-125 contraindicate the implementation of routine ovarian cancer screening in the general population.

EVALUATION OF THE PATIENT WITH A SUSPECTED OVARIAN NEOPLASM

A patient found to have a pelvic mass must be evaluated in a timely and cost-effective manner that is tailored to a realistic list of possible diagnoses. The differential diagnosis of a pelvic mass is influenced by the age of the patient, the characteristics of the mass on pelvic examination, and the radiographic appearance of the mass. In general, the prepubescent child and the postmenopausal woman are at greatest risk for developing a pelvic mass that subsequently proves to be a malignant ovarian neoplasm. The reproductive age woman is more likely to have a functional ovarian cyst or endometrioma.

Physical Examination

Although the natural focus of the physical examination of the patient with a suspected adnexal neoplasm is the pelvis, it is important to perform a comprehensive examination. Particular attention should be paid to the lymph-node–bearing areas, particularly the supraclavicular and inguinal areas. Metastatic disease to the skin rarely occurs in the presence of ovarian cancer. Sister Mary Joseph's nodule is the term that refers to a metastatic implant in the umbilicus.

Examination of the abdomen often provides important information. Abdominal distention is one of the more common findings. The presence of flank fullness and shifting dullness implies the presence of ascites or a large pelvic-abdominal mass. Together with these signs, a tympanitic percussion note over the lateral abdomen is consistent with a large mass that displaces the bowel to the periphery. In contrast, a central tympanitic percussion note is suggestive of ascites. Recent eversion of the umbilicus in a patient with abdominal distention may result from an increase in intra-abdominal pressure secondary to ascites.

A careful and thorough pelvic examination provides many helpful clues concerning the etiology of a pelvic mass and should never be replaced by a cursory examination or radiographic evaluation. The characteristics of the mass that should be noted on pelvic examination are listed in Table 49–3.

Unilateral, cystic masses in reproductive age women are benign in up to 95% of cases. These masses, particularly when less than 6–8 cm in size, are observed through a menstrual cycle since many represent functional cysts and spontaneously resolve. An enlarging

Table 49–3. Characteristics of a pelvic mass that should be noted on physical examination.

Benign	Malignant
Mobility	Fixed
Consistency	Solid or form
Bilateral or unilateral	Bilateral
Cul-de-sac	Nodular
Mobile	
Cystic	
Unilateral	
Smooth	

mass or one that is associated with pain merits prompt intervention. A cystic, somewhat immobile adnexal mass may represent a hydrosalpinx or tubo-ovarian abscess. Fixed, bilateral masses and firm masses with nodularity are suggestive of, but not diagnostic of, an ovarian malignancy. Because no features seen on physical examination consistently distinguish malignant from benign neoplasms, further characterization must be accomplished with select radiographic examinations.

Radiographic Evaluation

Ultrasonography is the most common radiographic test to evaluate adnexal masses. Transabdominal examinations require a full bladder as an acoustic window for optimal visualization of the adnexa. In contradistinction, a transvaginal examination does not have this requirement but may not be as useful for the assessment of large adnexal masses. Examples of ultrasonographic characteristics of benign compared to malignant ovarian masses are shown in Table 49–4. A number of different scoring systems are used, including ovarian volume, outline, presence of papillary projections, and cyst complexity. Persistence of ultrasonic findings on a re-

Table 49–4. Radiographic characteristics that help to differentiate benign and malignant adnexal masses.

Benign	Malignant
Simple cyst, < 10 cm in size	Solid or cystic and solid
Septations < mm in thickness	Multiple septations > 3 mm in size
Unilateral	Bilateral
Calcification, especially teeth	Ascites
Gravity-dependent layering of cyst contents	

peat scan after 4–6 weeks may help reduce the false-positive rate. However, there is no standardized system for evaluation of ovarian masses. The correlation between the ultrasonic appearance of an adnexal mass and the pathologic findings is imprecise. Color flow Doppler studies that evaluate the vascular patterns of adnexal masses show promise as a means to improve the sensitivity and specificity of the radiographic diagnosis of benign and malignant lesions. Angiogenesis accompanying malignancy results in vascular abnormalities and increased blood flow compared with the vascular architecture and patterns of blood flow in nonmalignant lesions.

Characterization of adnexal masses by computed tomography (CT) or magnetic resonance imaging (MRI) may provide clinically useful information in select instances. CT scanning provides information about the retroperitoneal structures in addition to the pelvic organs. MRI scans can add more information regarding the nature of the ovarian neoplasm. Because of the high cost and questionable benefit, this diagnostic procedure is infrequently used for ovarian tumors. However, it may be of particular benefit in the evaluation of pregnant patients because it avoids radiation exposure of the fetus.

When a patient has a suspected ovarian malignancy based on her clinical presentation, physical examination, and the ultrasonographic appearance of the mass, a radiograph of the chest is done to exclude metastatic parenchymal disease and to detect a pleural effusion.

If the patient notes a change in bowel habits or if guaiac-positive stools are detected, a barium enema should be obtained. Patients who appear to have advanced ovarian cancer, evidenced by a nodular pelvic mass with or without ascites may actually have colon cancer. Because of the genetic links among ovarian cancer, colon cancer, and breast cancer, a patient with a suspected ovarian malignancy should also undergo a screening mammogram study.

Laboratory Evaluation

When an ovarian malignancy is included in the list of diagnostic possibilities, a limited number of laboratory tests are indicated. A complete blood count (CBC) and serum electrolyte test should be obtained in all patients. Coagulation tests are not indicated in the absence of a suggestive history of bleeding after minor trauma or increased bruisability. Similarly, routine liver function tests are rarely helpful.

The serum hCG level should be measured in any female in whom pregnancy is a possibility. In addition, a serum AFP and lactate dehydrogenase (LDH) should be measured in young girls and adolescents who present with adnexal masses because the younger the patient, the greater the likelihood of a malignant germ cell tumor. The serum CA-125 level should also be determined whenever an ovarian malignancy is included in the differential diagnosis. An elevated CA-125 in the postmenopausal patient is particularly suggestive of the presence of an ovarian malignancy, although it is not specific for this diagnosis. Cancers of the colon, breast, pancreas, stomach, uterus, and fallopian tube are also associated with an elevated CA-125 value. Benign conditions commonly diagnosed in younger women, including pregnancy, endometriosis, leiomyomata, and adenomyosis, limit the usefulness of this test in premenopausal women. A normal CA-125 level does *not* exclude the diagnosis of cancer and does not represent a reason to delay surgery.

Paracentesis is not advocated as a routine procedure for the patient with ascites and a pelvic mass and in whom renal, cardiac, and hepatic failure has been excluded. False-negative results may occur in as many as 40% of patients with widespread intra-abdominal disease. The presence or absence of a malignant effusion does not diminish the need for surgery. Furthermore, insertion of a trocar may rupture an encapsulated neoplasm, spilling tumor cells into the peritoneal cavity, or it may result in implantation of neoplastic cells along the insertion site.

In contrast to the role of paracentesis, diagnostic thoracentesis to remove an aliquot of a pleural effusion for cytology is recommended prior to surgical intervention. In the presence of a malignant pleural effusion, the patient has stage IV disease. Many surgeons would not perform ultraradical surgical resections in patients with stage IV disease because of the very poor prognosis.

SURGICAL TREATMENT OF EPITHELIAL OVARIAN CANCER

Surgery is the cornerstone of therapy for ovarian cancer, regardless of cell type or stage of disease. Whenever ovarian cancer is considered a likely diagnosis, a gynecologic oncologist should be consulted and actively involved in the evaluation and subsequent management of the patient. A gynecologic oncologist is trained to address both the surgical and the medical needs of these patients.

Ultrasonically directed cyst aspiration and laparoscopic cyst decompression are not generally recommended. Simple cyst aspiration is associated with a high recurrence rate, and the cytology of the cyst fluid is unreliable to establish or confidently exclude a diagnosis of cancer. In addition, the laparoscopic resection of a mass that is suggestive of malignancy is not advocated because of concerns related to the intra-abdominal spillage of neoplastic cells and the adequacy of surgical staging. Simply because a procedure can be accomplished using the laparoscope does not mean that it is in the patient's best interest to do so.

Intraoperatively, several features have been described that assist in the differentiation of malignant from benign adnexal masses (Table 49–5). However, gross examination of a mass is never a substitute for histologic examination. Whenever the pathology of a pelvic or adnexal mass is in question, a frozen section pathologic study should be requested. In the hands of experienced pathologists, false-positive and false-negative diagnoses occur in less than 2% of cases. Patients diagnosed with ovarian cancer have to undergo surgical staging to reduce the amount of disease and evaluate the extent of spread. Removal of the primary tumor as well as the associated metastatic disease is referred to as debulking or cytoreductive surgery. In early stages and when fertility is desired, removal of the involved adnexa alone may be considered.

The full extent of disease must be carefully documented. At the time of diagnosis, over 70% of patients with epithelial ovarian cancer have metastases beyond the pelvis. The most common locations of metastases secondary to advanced stage ovarian cancer are the peritoneum (85%), omentum (70%), liver (35%), pleura (33%), lung (25%), and bone (15%). Lymphatic metastasis occurs frequently, with up to 80% involving pelvic lymph nodes and 67% involving para-aortic lymph nodes, depending on the stage of disease.

The information gained from accurate surgical staging guides discussion of prognosis and also influences treatment decisions. Surgical staging requires documentation of the primary neoplasm and determination of the extent of disease by inspection, biopsy of peritoneal and intra-abdominal lesions, and biopsy of the retroperitoneal lymph nodes. The procedures included in surgical staging of ovarian cancer are listed in Table 49–6. Any fluid in the peritoneal cavity should be aspirated. In the absence of free fluid, peritoneal washings should be obtained and submitted for cytologic study. It is recommended that 100 mL of saline be lavaged into the right paracolic gutter, the left paracolic gutter, the pelvic cul-de-sac, and the right subdiaphragmatic surface, and collected and submitted to the laboratory. Complete surgical staging of ovarian cancer requires biopsy of pelvic and para-aortic lymph nodes. It is emphasized that palpation of the retroperitoneal node-bearing areas is inaccurate and is not a substitute for biopsy and histologic examination. The current staging of ovarian cancer approved by the International Federation of Gynecology and Obstetrics (FIGO) is provided in Table 49–7.

In general, the contralateral adnexa should be removed even when they are grossly normal. They are often the site of occult metastatic disease, and there is a significant risk of subsequent cancer. Exceptions to this generalization are made for young women with an apparent stage I epithelial ovarian neoplasm. When future fertility is an issue and the patient fully understands the potential for recurrent disease, a more conservative approach may be followed when certain conditions are satisfied. Obviously, the conservative management of invasive ovarian cancer requires a thorough staging procedure. The histology and grade of the neoplasm, as well as the findings at the time of surgery, guide these decisions. Well-differentiated stage I lesions are associated with a much better 5-year survival rate than are moderately and poorly differentiated lesions. Mucinous and endometrioid neoplasms are associated with a better prognosis than serous and clear cell carcinomas of the ovary. The presence of adhesions, capsular rupture, ascites, or excrescences on the capsular surface constitute arguments against the performance of a conservative operation. When the decision to preserve or remove the contralateral adnexa is unclear, it is advisable to await the results of the permanent pathology before performing a bilateral adnexectomy.

Table 49–6. Procedures in the surgical staging of ovarian cancer.

Sample of ascites or peritoneal washings from the paracolic gutters and pelvic and subdiaphragmatic surface for cytology
Complete abdominal exploration
Intact removal of tumor
Hysterectomy
Infracolic omentectomy
Biopsies of abdominal peritoneal implants; if present, random biopsies from the paracolic gutter peritoneum, pelvic peritoneum, and right subdiaphragmatic peritoneal surface
Pelvic and para-aortic lymph node biopsies
Cytoreductive surgery to remove all visible disease

Table 49–5. Intraoperative differentiation of benign and malignant masses.

Benign	Malignant
Simple cyst	Adhesions
Unilateral	Rupture
No adhesions	Ascites
Smooth surfaces	Solid areas
Intact capsule	Areas of hemorrhage or necrosis
	Papillary excrescences
	Multioculated mass
	Bilateral

Table 49–7. International Federation of Gynecology and Obstetrics (FIGO) staging of ovarian neoplasms.

Stage I. Growth limited to the ovaries
 Ia—one ovary involved
 Ib—both ovaries involved
 Ic—Ia or Ib and ovarian surface tumor, ruptured capsule, malignant ascites, or peritoneal cytology positive for malignant cells
Stage II. Extension of the neoplasm from the ovary to the pelvis
 IIa—extension to the uterus or fallopian tube
 IIb—extension to other pelvic tissues
 IIc—IIa or b and ovarian surface tumor, ruptured capsule, malignant ascites, or peritoneal cytology positive for malignant cells
Stage III. Disease extension to the abdominal cavity
 IIIa—abdominal peritoneal surfaces with microscopic metastases
 IIIb—tumor metastases < 2 cm in size
 IIIc—tumor metastases > 2 cm in size or metastatic disease in the pelvic, para-aortic, or inguinal lymph nodes
Stage IV. Distant metastatic disease
 Malignant pleural effusion
 Pulmonary parenchymal metastases
 Liver or splenic parenchymal metastases (not surface implants)
 Metastases to the supraclavicular lymph nodes or skin

A hysterectomy is generally performed because the uterus is a common site for metastatic disease. There is also a risk of synchronous endometrial cancer in patients with endometrioid carcinoma of the ovary. In addition, removal of the uterus facilitates subsequent follow-up examinations and obviates potential problems secondary to uterine bleeding.

An infracolic omentectomy is recommended, even in the absence of gross tumor involvement, because it is a common site of microscopic metastatic disease. In addition, removal of the omentum facilitates the distribution of intraperitoneal agents, may decrease the rate of accumulation of ascites postoperatively, and provides palliation to those patients with omental metastases.

Cytoreductive surgery should always be attempted if possible. The rationale for aggressive reduction of tumor burden is based on three main considerations. First, the removal of tumor mass often relieves gastrointestinal symptoms and improves the overall nutritional status. Reduction of tumor cell mass also leads to a therapeutically favorable change in tumor cell kinetics since large bulky tumors are often poorly vascularized and oxygenated and thus are more resistant to chemo- and radiation therapy. Furthermore, large tumor masses consist of

a higher proportion of cells in the resting phase of the cell cycle. Finally, a number of tumors including ovarian cancer are known to produce immunosuppressive factors that block antitumor immune responses, eg, by inhibiting the generation of cytotoxic T-lymphocytes.

Peritoneal implants should always be sampled to confirm the clinical impression of metastatic disease. Potential "look-alikes" include endometriosis, tuberculous peritonitis, and talc or suture granulomas. Nodular, roughened, or otherwise suspicious areas should be biopsied.

After completion of initial therapy for ovarian cancer, patients without clinical evidence of disease may undergo a second-look operation to determine the therapeutic response and assess the persistence of tumor disease. This is usually done in the setting of an investigational protocol. A laparotomy is performed to obtain multiple specimens from peritoneal surfaces and suspicious areas. About 30% of patients without evidence of macroscopic disease are found to have microscopic metastasis. Patients with negative second-look laparotomy have significantly longer survival than those with residual disease. The likelihood of negative findings at second-look laparotomy is higher in patients that were initially diagnosed with early stage disease, low-grade tumors, residual tumor disease < 5 mm, and chemotherapy containing paclitaxel. However, even patients with negative biopsies have a recurrence rate of 30–50% after 5 years.

The indications for and realistic benefits of surgery in the patient with recurrent or persistent ovarian cancer require individualization and considerable surgical judgment. Removal of tumor disease after primary surgery is referred to as secondary cytoreductive surgery. These procedures are performed in selected patients for whom resection may prolong life expectancy by reducing tumor burden to less than 5 mm metastatic disease or for whom resection of tumor will relieve symptoms like gastrointestinal obstruction. Patients in whom complete resection of residual tumor burden is possible have a significantly longer survival compared to patients without complete resection.

■ SURGICAL TREATMENT OF GERM CELL NEOPLASMS

In contrast to epithelial ovarian neoplasms, most germ cell neoplasms are early stage at the time of diagnosis. This observation, in conjunction with the low incidence of bilaterality and the young age of most patients, for whom future fertility is an issue, influences the surgical management of this group of neoplasms. For young women with a germ cell neoplasm of the ovary, removal of the involved adnexa with preservation of the normal-appearing contralateral adnexa and uterus is generally advocated. In view of the low incidence of bilaterality, biopsy or bivalving the contralateral ovary is not recommended because of the risk of peritubal and periovarian adhesions. Complete surgical staging of germ cell neoplasms is the same as for epithelial ovarian neoplasms and should be performed in all cases.

Certain characteristics unique to germ cell neoplasms make an impact on their surgical management. Dysgerminoma of the ovary has a propensity to metastasize to the pelvic and para-aortic lymph nodes in the absence of other evidence of metastatic disease; biopsies of these structures is particularly important. Endodermal sinus tumor of the ovary is the most rapidly growing neoplasm known to occur at any site. When a young woman presents with a rapidly enlarging mass and abdominal pain, this diagnosis must be considered and surgery undertaken as soon as possible. Immature teratoma of the ovary may present with numerous peritoneal implants consistent with metastatic disease. It is important to adequately sample these lesions to determine whether or not they contain malignant elements.

CHEMOTHERAPY OF EPITHELIAL OVARIAN CANCER

In patients with stage Ia disease and grade 1 tumors, chemotherapy following initial surgical treatment has no influence on survival. Therefore, this group of patients, if selected carefully, does not require chemotherapeutic treatment. However, all other patients should undergo systemic chemotherapy. Agents shown to be active against epithelial ovarian cancer include cisplatin, carboplatin, cyclophosphamide, and paclitaxel. Combination therapies have been demonstrated to be superior to single-agent treatment.

Currently the most effective regimen uses a combination of paclitaxel and cisplatin or carboplatin. This combination has replaced the former treatment with cyclophosphamide and cisplatin since it was shown to more efficacious in a number of clinical trials. A typical regimen includes systemic administration of cisplatin at 75 mg/m^2 and paclitaxel at 175 mg/m^2 for 6 cycles at 3-week intervals. Potential toxicities of this treatment include nausea, vomiting, diarrhea, alopecia, nephro- and ototoxicity, and myelosuppression.

Carboplatin is a second-generation platinum analog that shows clinical efficacies and survival rates similar to cisplatin when used in combination with paclitaxel. However, the frequency of gastrointestinal side effects and neurotoxicity associated with carboplatin were found to be lower compared to cisplatin. Therefore carboplatin is currently widely used instead of cisplatin in combination with paclitaxel.

Assessment of response to combination chemotherapy is based on physical examination, changes in size of palpable or radiographically measurable lesions, and changes in the CA-125 level. Although the preoperative CA-125 level does not correlate with tumor burden, changes in response to chemotherapy appear to be of some prognostic benefit. An elevated CA-125 (> 35 IU/mL) predicts persistent disease at second look in > 97% of patients. However, a normal CA-125 level does not completely exclude the possibility of residual, subclinical disease.

Most if not all patients develop resistance to platin-based regimens during the course of treatment. Salvage therapy for ovarian cancer is rarely curative, although significant prolongation of survival may be achieved in some instances. The response to re-treatment with cisplatin is influenced by the time interval between completion of the initial regimen and subsequent disease recurrence—the greater the interval, the greater the likelihood of a beneficial response.

Patients with platinum- or paclitaxel-sensitive tumors as evidenced by the clinical response to initial chemotherapy will likely benefit from re-treatment with a platinum- or paclitaxel-based regimen.

Chemotherapy of Germ Cell Neoplasms

Significant advances have been made in the treatment of germ cell neoplasms of the ovary. Once associated with 5-year survival rates of less than 20–30%, these neoplasms are now considered curable in a majority of cases following the introduction and refinement of combination chemotherapy.

Dysgerminoma is the most radiation-sensitive neoplasm identified. Historically, it has been treated with whole abdominal radiation therapy with excellent results. More recently, chemotherapy with cisplatin-containing regimens has been administered with excellent results. A significant advantage of chemotherapy is the potential to preserve future reproductive potential compared with radiation therapy.

The other germ cell neoplasms are rare, and the optimal chemotherapy and duration of therapy have not been established. Regimens including vinblastine-bleomycin-cisplatin, vincristine-actinomycin D-cyclophosphamide, and bleomycin-etoposide-cisplatin have been used with encouraging results. Response to chemotherapy is based on physical examination and the decrease in serum tumor markers, if initially elevated.

Complications of Chemotherapy

Combination chemotherapy invariably makes an impact on the patient's day-to-day activities and may be associated with a variety of potentially life-threatening

Table 49–8. Chemotherapy-associated toxicities.

Agent	Toxicity
Cisplatin	Nephrotoxicity, neurotoxicity, ototoxicity
Carboplatin	Thrombocytopenia, neutropenia
Cyclophosphamide	Hemorrhagic cystitis, pulmonary fibrosis
Paclitaxel	Myelosuppression
Altretamine	Peripheral neuropathy
Etoposide	Myelosuppression
Bleomycin	Pulmonary fibrosis
Doxorubicin	Cardiac toxicity
Vincristine	Neuropathy
Ifosfamide	Hemorrhagic cystitis, central neurotoxicity

side effects. The most common toxicities of some of the more commonly used drugs in the treatment of ovarian cancer are listed in Table 49–8.

Nausea, vomiting, and alopecia are side effects anticipated and feared by many patients. The development of new, more effective antiemetics permits improved control of nausea and a reduction in the number of emesis episodes. Unfortunately, suggested strategies to prevent alopecia, such as scalp tourniquets and local hypothermia, are generally ineffective. Patients should be counseled that all chemotherapy regimens do not invariably result in hair loss.

Myelosuppression is another common side effect of chemotherapy. CBCs with differential and platelet counts are typically monitored between cycles of therapy. Most regimens cause granulocytopenia and thrombocytopenia between days 10 and 18. Synthetic erythropoietin and colony-stimulating factor can be administered to lessen the severity and duration of anemia and granulocytopenia. In the future, agents to decrease chemotherapy-induced thrombocytopenia will be commercially available.

RADIATION THERAPY

Currently, radiation therapy plays a very limited role in the treatment of patients with epithelial ovarian cancer. It is difficult to subject the entire abdominal cavity to therapeutic doses without causing life-threatening side effects because of damage to the small bowel, liver, and kidneys. Radioisotopes such as intraperitoneal P^{32} may be of benefit in patients with stage Ic disease and those with microscopically positive second-look operations.

With respect to germ cell neoplasms, radiation therapy has been used successfully in the treatment of patients with dysgerminoma.

ALTERNATIVE THERAPIES

In the last decade, a number of alternative therapies have been applied for the treatment of epithelial ovarian cancer. Immunotherapeutic approaches include the systemic or intraperitoneal administration of recombinant cytokines like interleukin-2 or interferons, and the use of ex vivo stimulated tumor-infiltrating lymphocytes. In general, these approaches have shown up to 30% response rates in otherwise chemotherapy-resistant patients. However, immunotherapy is still experimental and the approach that may yield the most promising results for secondary or even primary treatment still has to be defined.

Similarly, several gene therapeutic approaches have been developed. These strategies include the replacement of missing tumor-suppressor gene functions like p53 or BRCA1, stimulation of the immune system by expression of immunostimulatory gene products, or the targeting of oncogenes commonly overexpressed in ovarian cancer. A number of preclinical studies have shown promising results with these approaches. Clinical trials are underway to evaluate clinical responses.

PROGNOSIS

The prognosis for patients with ovarian cancer is primarily related to the stage of disease. The 5-year survival rate for patients with stage I epithelial ovarian cancer is, depending on tumor grade, between 76% and 93%. The 5-year survival rate for those with stage II disease is 60–74%. Stage III ovarian cancer is associated with a 5-year survival rate of approximately 23–41%. The survival rate for a patient with stage IV disease is about 11%. Within each stage of disease, other factors are related to response to chemotherapy, disease-free survival, and overall survival. In general, patients with well-differentiated, diploid neoplasms with an S-phase fraction of less than 8–10% do better than patients who have poorly differentiated, aneuploid, rapidly proliferating (eg, high S-phase fraction) neoplasms.

In general, germ cell tumors are associated with better 5-year survival rates than epithelial ovarian neoplasms. Patients with dysgerminoma have a 5-year survival rate of 95%. Immature teratomas are associated with 5-year survival rates of 70–80%. An endodermal sinus tumor is associated with a 5-year survival rate of 60–70%. Embryonal carcinoma, choriocarcinoma, and polyembryona are very rare lesions, and it is difficult to assess 5-year survival estimates. Epithelial ovarian neoplasms of low malignant potential are characterized by 5-year survival rates of 95%, reflecting their protracted and indolent biologic behavior.

DIAGNOSIS AND MANAGEMENT OF CANCER METASTATIC TO THE OVARY

Typically, patients with cancer metastatic to the ovary present as if they have primary ovarian cancer. Several clinical scenarios may be encountered. Primary colon cancer or gastric carcinoma may present as a pelvic mass, ascites, and a change in bowel habits or early satiety. Recurrent metastatic breast cancer may present as an asymptomatic pelvic mass.

The role of surgery in patients with cancer metastatic to the ovary must be individualized. When the diagnosis is unclear, exploratory laparotomy to establish the diagnosis is appropriate in most cases. However, the role of tumor-reductive surgery in patients with known metastatic disease is less clear. No long-term survivors of gastric cancer metastatic to the ovary are known, regardless of treatment. Survival following surgery and combination chemotherapy for breast and colon cancer metastatic to the ovary is poor, ranging from 4–12 months.

■ MALIGNANT NEOPLASMS OF THE FALLOPIAN TUBE

Etiology

Primary carcinoma of the fallopian tube is the least common cancer arising in the female genital tract, accounting for approximately 0.3% of all such cancers. Fallopian tube cancers are similar to epithelial ovarian cancer regarding clinical presentation and biological behavior.

Clinical Presentation

The patient with carcinoma of the fallopian tube is usually in the sixth decade of life. The signs and symptoms are often similar to those noted in patients with ovarian cancer. In fact, it is difficult to differentiate tubal from ovarian carcinomas preoperatively.

Rarely, patients with carcinoma of the fallopian tube present with the symptom complex referred to as **hydrops tubae profluens,** or **Latzko's sign,** which is a watery vaginal discharge and a palpable adnexal mass.

Positive vaginal cytology in the absence of endometrial or cervical neoplasia suggests the possibility of a tubal cancer, but this is rarely diagnostic.

Histopathology

At least 95% of all primary carcinomas of the fallopian tube are papillary carcinomas. Bilaterality is found in 40–50% of cases, and this is believed to represent synchronous neoplasms rather than metastatic disease from one tube to the other. Grossly, the affected tube is fusiform or sausage-shaped. On initial inspection, these neoplasms resemble pyosalpinx or tubo-ovarian inflammatory disease. However, there is usually little associated serosal reaction with adhesion formation, as is noted with an inflammatory process.

Classically, the neoplastic fallopian tube contains solid or necrotic cancer tissue and a dark-brown or serosanguineous fluid. The fimbriated end of the fallopian tube is patent in as many as 50% of cases, and often tumor extrudes from the ostium to adhere to adjacent structures. Histologically, papillary carcinomas may exhibit papillary, papillary-alveolar, and alveolar growth patterns. There is no prognostic significance attached to these differences.

Treatment

The surgical therapy of fallopian tube carcinoma is the same as that recommended for epithelial ovarian cancer. In addition, the same type of surgical staging should be performed if for no other reason than it is often not clear at the time of surgery whether the primary cancer is of ovarian or fallopian tube origin. The staging system for ovarian cancer is often applied to neoplasms of the fallopian tube, although this is by custom rather than FIGO recommendations.

Chemotherapy for fallopian tube cancer has evolved along the same lines as that for epithelial ovarian cancer. The currently used chemotherapeutic regimen is similar to that of epithelial ovarian cancer and includes carboplatin and paclitaxel.

Prognosis

The prognosis for patients with fallopian tube carcinoma is based on the stage of disease. The overall 5-year survival rate is about 50%.

REFERENCES

Christian J, Thomas H: Ovarian cancer chemotherapy. Cancer Treat Rev 2001;27:99.

Runnebaum IB, Stickeler E: Epidemiological and molecular aspects of ovarian cancer risk. J Cancer Res Clin Oncol 2001;127:73.

Gestational Trophoblastic Diseases

Tricia E. Markusen, MD, & April Gale O'Quinn, MD

ESSENTIALS OF DIAGNOSIS

- *Uterine bleeding in first trimester.*
- *Absence of fetal heart tones and fetal structures.*
- *Rapid enlargement of the uterus; uterine size greater than anticipated by dates.*
- *β-hCG titers greater than expected for gestational age.*
- *Expulsion of vesicles.*
- *Hyperemesis.*
- *Theca lutein cysts.*
- *Onset of preeclampsia in the first trimester.*

General Considerations

Gestational trophoblastic neoplasms include the tumor spectrum of hydatidiform mole (complete and partial), invasive mole (chorioadenoma destruens), placental-site trophoblastic tumor (PSTT), and choriocarcinoma. They arise from fetal tissue within the maternal host and are composed of both syncytiotrophoblastic and cytotrophoblastic cells, except PSTT, which is derived from intermediate trophoblastic cells. In addition to being the first and only disseminated solid tumors that have proved to be highly curable by chemotherapy, they elaborate a unique and characteristic tumor marker, human chorionic gonadotropin (hCG).

Hydatidiform mole is the most common gestational trophoblastic neoplasm. Its incidence varies worldwide from 1 in 125 deliveries in Mexico and Taiwan to 1 in 1500 deliveries in the U.S. The incidence is higher in women under 20 and over 40 years of age, in patients of low economic status, and in those whose diets are deficient in protein, folic acid, and carotene. Molar pregnancy occurs in fewer than 2% of subsequent gestations in women with a history of mole.

Hydatidiform mole should be suspected in any woman with bleeding in the first half of pregnancy, passage of vesicles, hyperemesis gravidarum, or preeclampsia-eclampsia with onset before 24 weeks. Absent fetal heart tones and a uterus too large for the estimated duration of gestation on physical examination support the diagnosis. Ultrasonography and serial β-hCG determinations are necessary to establish a firm diagnosis of hydatidiform mole.

Invasive mole is reported in 10–15% of patients who have had primary molar pregnancy. Although considered a benign neoplasm, invasive mole is locally invasive and may produce distant metastases.

PSTT is a rare variant of gestational trophoblastic tumor. It may arise from a hydatidiform mole or less commonly from a normal term pregnancy. The tumor is generally confined to the uterus and metastasizes late in its course. Syncytiotrophoblastic cells are generally absent from this tumor, resulting in minimal secretion of β-hCG in relation to tumor burden. However, human placental lactogen (hPL) is secreted and these levels can be monitored to follow response.

Choriocarcinoma is rare, reported in 2–5% of all cases of gestational trophoblastic neoplasia. The incidence in the U.S. is 1 in 40,000 pregnancies, but it is higher in Asia. In about half of all cases of choriocarcinoma, the antecedent gestational event is hydatidiform mole. One-fourth follow term pregnancy, and the remainder occur following abortion.

A generalization worth repeating is that any woman presenting with bleeding or a tumor in any organ who has a recent history of molar pregnancy, abortion, or term pregnancy should have at least one β-hCG assay to be sure that metastatic gestational trophoblastic neoplasia is not the cause. This is important, for the cure rate of properly treated metastatic gestational trophoblastic neoplasia is approximately 90%.

Etiology & Pathogenesis

Gestational trophoblastic tumors arise in fetal rather than maternal tissue. Cytogenetic studies have demonstrated that true moles are usually (perhaps always) euploid, paternal in origin, and sex chromatin-positive 46,XX or 46,XY; transitional moles are usually trisomic; and partial moles are triploid. The development of an ovum under the influence of a sperm nucleus requires the absence or inactivation of the ovum nucleus and the presence of a dispermic fertilization or the duplication of its chromosomes. This provides important insight into the pathogenesis of gestational trophoblastic neoplasms, because this process results in a homozygous conceptus with a propensity for altered growth.

To date, hydatidiform mole has been considered to be derived from extraembryonic trophoblasts. Histologic similarities between molar vesicles and chorionic villi support the view that one is derived from the other. However, detailed morphologic study of a hysterectomy specimen containing an intact molar pregnancy presents a new concept regarding genesis of hydatidiform mole as a transformation of the embryonic inner cell mass at a stage just prior to the laying down of endoderm. At this stage in embryogenesis, the inner cell mass has the capability of developing into trophoblasts, ectoderm, and endoderm. If normal development is interrupted, such that the inner cell mass loses its capacity to differentiate into embryonic ectoderm and endoderm, a divergent development pathway is created. This pathway may then result in formation of trophoblasts (from the inner cell mass) that develop into cytotrophoblasts and syncytiotrophoblasts with sufficient differentiation to produce extraembryonic mesoderm, giving rise to molar vesicles with loose primitive mesoderm in their villous core. In contrast, choriocarcinoma is less well differentiated and, lacking this capability, is composed of only cytotrophoblasts and syncytiotrophoblasts.

Thus, the ultimate cause of gestational trophoblastic disease may be genetic. Nonetheless, there are interesting clinical correlates, some of which were mentioned earlier. Additionally, evidence indicates that the distribution of ABO blood groups in women with gestational trophoblastic neoplasms and their sexual partners differs from that of the general population. The most remarkable findings are that group A women impregnated by group O men have an almost 10-fold greater risk of developing choriocarcinoma than group A women with group A partners and that women with group AB have a relatively poor prognosis. A study of the ABO blood groups of children resulting from pregnancies prior or subsequent to choriocarcinoma revealed fewer instances than expected in which the child was ABO-incompatible with its mother. The leukocytes of these children frequently showed antigenic differences from the mothers' cells. Although these antigens are regarded as strong transplantation antigens, they seem notably weaker than the ABO factors—evidence that choriocarcinoma is able to grow and to kill in spite of the immune response it evokes. Further, gestational trophoblastic tissue may suppress the maternal immune response via such factors as interleukins and tumor necrosis factor (TNF).

Pathology

Four distinct forms of gestational trophoblastic neoplasia are recognized: hydatidiform mole, invasive mole (chorioadenoma destruens), placental-site trophoblastic tumor (PSTT), and choriocarcinoma.

A. HYDATIDIFORM MOLE

Hydatidiform mole is an abnormal pregnancy characterized grossly by multiple grapelike vesicles filling and distending the uterus, usually in the absence of an intact fetus (Fig 50–1). Most hydatidiform moles are recognizable on gross examination, but some are small and may seem to be ordinary abortuses.

Microscopically, moles may be identified by three classic findings: edema of the villous stroma, avascular villi, and nests of proliferating syncytiotrophoblastic or cytotrophoblastic elements surrounding villi (Fig 50–2). Today with earlier clinical diagnosis, the classic pathologic presentation of molar pregnancies is less common. Therefore, it can be more difficult to differentiate histologically between a molar pregnancy and a nonmolar hydropic abortion. The likelihood of malignant sequelae is increased in patients whose trophoblastic cells show increased proliferation and anaplasia. Although histologic study of the trophoblast provides some basis for predicting a benign or malignant course for the mole, the correlation is not absolute, and it is

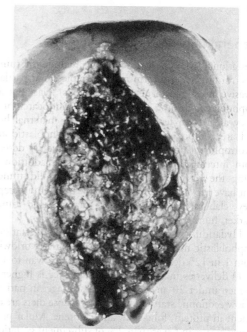

Figure 50–1. Hysterectomy specimen with anterior wall incised, displaying typical miliary, clear, "grapelike" vesicles filling the uterine cavity. Hysterectomy was performed for primary treatment for molar gestation.

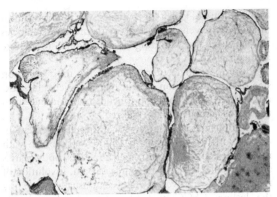

Figure 50–2. Photomicrograph of hydatidiform mole characterized by well-developed but avascular villi with stromal edema and minimal trophoblastic proliferation.

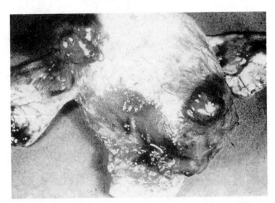

Figure 50–3. Hysterectomy specimen showing invasive mole penetrating the myometrium and serosal surface of the uterus that resulted in life-threatening intraperitoneal hemorrhage.

essential to obtain accurate, sensitive gonadotropin assays in all patients who have had hydatidiform moles.

Two forms of hydatidiform moles exist—complete (true) and partial moles. The clinical, pathologic, and genetic characteristics of both are outlined in Table 50–1.

B. INVASIVE MOLE (CHORIOADENOMA DESTRUENS)

Invasive mole is a hydatidiform mole that invades the myometrium or adjacent structures. It may totally penetrate the myometrium and be associated with uterine rupture and hemoperitoneum (Fig 50–3). The microscopic findings are the same as in hydatidiform mole (Fig 50–4). Since adequate myometrium is rarely obtained at curettage, the diagnosis is made by histologic study less frequently now than formerly, because fewer hysterectomies are performed in patients with tro-

phoblastic disease. Metastatic lesions may contain invasive mole, but most will be choriocarcinoma regardless of the morphologic features of the uterine tumor.

C. PLACENTAL-SITE TROPHOBLASTIC TUMOR

PSTT is derived from the intermediate trophoblasts of the placental bed, with minimal or absent syncytiotrophoblastic tissue. Histologically, local invasion occurs into the myometrium and lymphatics. Vascular invasion is less common. It may occur with any type of pregnancy.

D. CHORIOCARCINOMA

Choriocarcinoma is a pure epithelial tumor composed of syncytiotrophoblastic and cytotrophoblastic cells. It may accompany or follow any type of pregnancy. Histologic examination discloses no villi, but instead sheets

Table 50–1. Comparison of complete and partial hydatidiform moles.

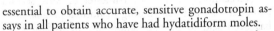

	Complete	Partial
Karyotype	Diploid (46,XX or 46,XY)	Triploid (69,XXX or 69,XXY)
Embryo	Absent	Present
Villi	Hydropic	Few hydropic
Trophoblasts	Diffuse hyperplasia	Mild focal hyperplasia
Implantation-site trophoblast	Diffuse atypia	Focal atypia
Fetal RBCs	Absent	Present
β-hCG	High (> 50,000)	Slight elevation (<50,000)
Frequency of classic clinical symptoms[1]	Common	Rare
Risk for persistent GTT	20–30%	< 5%

[1]Hyperemesis, hyperthyroidism, excessive uterine enlargement, anemia, and preeclampsia. The frequency of these symptoms has decreased due to earlier diagnosis of molar pregnancies through evaluating β-hCG levels and ultrasound.
GTT = gestational trophoblastic tumor.

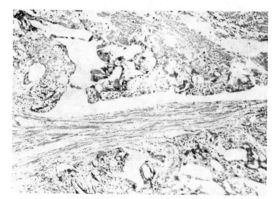

Figure 50–4. Photomicrograph of invasive mole. The pattern of hydatidiform mole is maintained with avascular villi and stromal edema, but they are deep within the uterine wall, interspersed among smooth-muscle bundles.

or foci of trophoblasts on a background of hemorrhage and necrosis. A histopathologic diagnosis of choriocarcinoma in any site is an indication for prompt treatment after confirmation by gonadotropin excretion measurements. Assessment of trophoblastic tissue following or accompanying pregnancy may be difficult because of the histologic similarity of the trophoblastic pattern in very early human pregnancy and in choriocarcinoma. The entire specimen must be processed for histologic study when curettage is done, because specimens may reveal only small, isolated areas of choriocarcinoma. Careful search usually discloses the villous pattern in the tissue of early normal pregnancy.

Choriocarcinoma may also arise from ectopic pregnancy. In confusing situations, β-hCG testing may clarify the diagnosis and document the need for therapy.

Malignant gestational trophoblastic neoplasia is diagnosed in the setting of invasive mole, placental-site trophoblastic tumors, choriocarcinomas, and postmolar rising or plateauing (decline of < 10% for at least 3 values over more than 14 days) β-hCG values.

Clinical Findings

A. SYMPTOMS AND SIGNS

Abnormal uterine bleeding, usually during the first trimester, is the most common symptom, occurring in over 90% of patients with molar pregnancies. Three-fourths of patients with bleeding have this symptom before the end of the third month of pregnancy. Only one-third of patients have profuse vaginal bleeding.

Nausea and vomiting, frequently excessive but at times difficult to distinguish from similar complaints normally occurring in pregnancy, have been reported

to occur in 14–32% of patients with hydatidiform mole. Ten percent of patients with molar pregnancies have nausea and vomiting severe enough to require hospitalization.

Disproportionate uterine size is the most common sign of molar gestation. About half of patients have excessive uterine size for gestational date, but in one-third the uterus is smaller than expected.

Multiple theca lutein cysts causing enlargement of one or both ovaries occur in 15–30% of women with molar pregnancies. In about half the cases, both ovaries are enlarged and may be a source of pain. Involution of the cysts proceeds over several weeks, usually paralleling the decline of hCG level. Operation is indicated only if rupture and hemorrhage occur or if the enlarged ovaries become infected. Patients with associated theca lutein cysts appear to have a greater likelihood of developing malignant sequelae of gestational trophoblastic neoplasia.

Preeclampsia in the first trimester or early second trimester—an unusual finding in normal pregnancy—has been said to be pathognomonic of hydatidiform mole, although it occurs in only 10–12% of those patients.

Hyperthyroidism from production of thyrotropin by molar tissue occurs in up to 10% of patients with hydatidiform mole. The manifestations disappear following evacuation of the mole. An occasional patient may require brief antithyroid therapy. These classic symptoms and signs are becoming less prevalent today due to the earlier diagnosis of molar pregnancies. For instance, at the New England Trophoblastic Disease Center, the incidence of excessive uterine enlargement, hyperemesis, and preeclampsia is 28%, 8%, and 1%, respectively. Hyperthyroidism and respiratory insufficiency have become negligible. Although these classic signs and symptoms have decreased, the incidence of persistent postmolar gestational trophoblastic disease has remained static, stressing the continued importance of postmolar β-hCG surveillance.

B. LABORATORY FINDINGS

The most important characteristic of gestational trophoblastic neoplasms is their capacity to produce hCG. This hormone may be detected in serum or urine in virtually all patients with hydatidiform mole or malignant trophoblastic disease. Careful monitoring of β-hCG levels is necessary for diagnosis, treatment, and follow-up in all cases of trophoblastic disease.

The amount of hCG found in the serum or excreted in the urine correlates closely with the number of viable tumor cells present. Studies indicate that one tumor cell produces from about 5×10^{-5} to 5×10^{-4} IU of hCG in 24 hours. Thus, a patient excreting 10^6

IU of hCG in 24 hours has about 10^{11} viable tumor cells.

The usefulness of a gonadotropin assay depends on the level of the patient's β-hCG titer and the sensitivity of the test. Today, sensitive and specific immunoassays are available to differentiate hCG from LH by measuring the beta chain of hCG. Serial fl-hCG levels are best monitored in the same laboratory using the same immunoassay technique.

The rate and constancy of the decline in hCG titer are important. Using the serum β-hCG radioimmunoassay, a normal postmolar pregnancy hCG regression curve based on weekly determinations in patients undergoing spontaneous remission has been constructed (Fig 50–5). This provides a reference with which random or serial values can be compared. In most instances, the β-hCG values exhibit a progressive decline to normal within 14 weeks following evacuation of a molar pregnancy. If metastases are detected or if the hCG titer rises or plateaus, it must be concluded that viable tumor persists.

C. X-RAY FINDINGS

Transabdominal amniocentesis combined with amniography may be used to confirm the presence of hydatidiform mole, although this is rarely utilized today given the extensive use of transvaginal and transabdominal ultrasound and β-hCG levels.

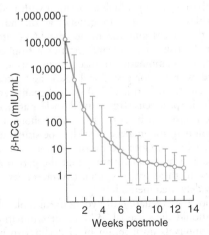

Figure 50–5. Normal postmolar pregnancy regression curve of serum β-hCG measured by radioimmunoassay. Vertical bars indicate 95% confidence limits. (Reproduced, with permission of the American College of Obstetricians and Gynecologists, from Schlaerth JB et al: Prognostic characteristics of serum human chorionic gonadotropin titer regression following molar pregnancy. Obstet Gynecol 1981;58:478.)

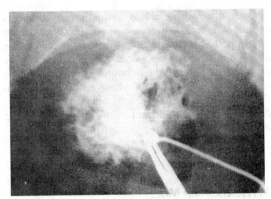

Figure 50–6. A gray-scale ultrasonogram depicting the typical intrauterine multiple-echo pattern of hydatidiform mole.

D. SPECIAL EXAMINATIONS

The simplicity, safety, and reliability of ultrasonography make it the diagnostic method of choice for patients with suspected molar pregnancy. In a molar pregnancy, the characteristic ultrasound pattern includes multiple echoes formed by the interface between the molar villi and the surrounding tissue without the presence of a normal gestational sac or fetus (Fig 50–6). This study should be done in any patient who experiences bleeding in the first half of pregnancy and has a uterus greater than 12 weeks' gestational size. Even when the uterus is smaller, ultrasonography may be very specific in differentiating between a normal pregnancy and hydatidiform mole.

Differential Diagnosis

Gestational trophoblastic disease must be distinguished from normal pregnancy. Ultrasonography is useful, and quantitative hCG levels afford another means of differentiation. In general, β-hCG assays with values greater than 100,000 mIU/mL are usual with molar pregnancies, in contrast to normal pregnancy values below 60,000 mIU/mL.

Complications

The maternal/fetal barrier contains leaks large enough to permit passage of cellular and tissue elements. Trophoblastic deportations to the lungs are frequent and have totally unpredictable manifestations, including spontaneous regression. A dramatic but now less common life-threatening complication of molar pregnancy in patients with uterine enlargement beyond 16 weeks' gestational size is a syndrome of acute pulmonary insufficiency characterized by sudden onset of dyspnea, often with cyanosis. Symptoms usually begin within 4–6 hours after evacuation. Historically, the syndrome has been attributed to massive deportation of trophoblasts to the pulmonary vasculature, but the most likely cause may be pulmonary edema secondary to cardiac dysfunction and excessive fluid administration. Nevertheless, massive fatal pulmonary embolization by gross deportation of villous tissue masses may occur, as documented by postmortem examination.

Treatment

A. Hydatidiform Mole

1. Evacuation—When the diagnosis has been confirmed, molar pregnancy should be terminated.

Suction curettage is the method of choice. It is safe, rapid, and effective in nearly all cases. Intravenous oxytocin should be started after a moderate amount of tissue has been removed and may be continued for 24 hours postevacuation if necessary. Suction curettage with the largest curette possible should be followed by gentle sharp curettage, and tissue from the decidua basalis should be submitted for pathologic study separately. Suction curettage can be safely accomplished even when the uterus is as large as in a 28-week pregnancy. Blood loss usually is moderate, but precautions should be taken for massive transfusion. When a large hydatidiform mole (> 12 weeks in size) is evacuated by suction curettage, a laparotomy setup should be readily available, since hysterotomy, hysterectomy, or bilateral hypogastric artery ligation may be necessary if perforation or hemorrhage occurs.

Before the use of suction curettage, hysterectomy was frequently used for patients with uteri beyond 12–14 weeks in size. Hysterectomy remains an option for good surgical candidates not desirous of future pregnancy and for older women (who are more likely to develop malignant sequelae). If theca lutein cysts are encountered at hysterectomy, the ovaries should remain intact, because regression to normal size will occur as the hCG titer diminishes. Hysterectomy does not eliminate the need for careful follow-up and β-hCG testing, although the likelihood of metastatic disease following hysterectomy for gestational trophoblastic disease is low (decreases from 20% to 3.5%).

Hysterotomy is no longer a method of choice in typical cases. The higher incidence of malignant disease following hysterotomy is probably attributable to greater uterine enlargement in patients selected for this therapy. Current recommendations restrict hysterotomy to cases complicated by hemorrhage.

Prostaglandin induction, oxytocin induction, and intra-amniotic instillation of prostaglandin or hypertonic solutions (saline, glucose, urea, etc) are no longer acceptable methods for evacuation of a molar pregnancy.

2. Prophylactic chemotherapy—It is controversial whether prophylactic chemotherapy (with methotrexate or dactinomycin) following a complete hydatidiform molar pregnancy should be offered to patients considered at high risk for persistent gestational trophoblastic disease (age > 35 years, history of prior molar pregnancy, trophoblastic hyperplasia) or in whom poor follow-up is anticipated. Several studies indicate that the incidence of postmolar gestational trophoblastic disease may be decreased with prophylactic chemotherapy. However, further studies are required to determine if the potential side effects warrant such treatment.

3. Surveillance following molar pregnancy—Regardless of method of termination, close follow-up with serial β-hCG titers is essential for every patient because of the incidence of malignant disease. The incidence is commonly thought to be 20–30%. Despite earlier diagnosis of molar pregnancies, the incidence of persistent gestational trophoblastic disease has not decreased. Three-fourths of patients with malignant nonmetastatic trophoblastic disease and half of patients with malignant metastatic disease develop these tumors as sequelae to hydatidiform mole. In the remainder, disease arises following term pregnancy, abortion, or ectopic pregnancy.

Several clinical features of hydatidiform mole are recognized as having a high association with malignant trophoblastic neoplasia. In general, at diagnosis, the larger the uterus and the higher the hCG titer, the greater the risk for malignant gestational trophoblastic disease. The combination of theca lutein cysts and uterine size excessive for gestational age is associated with an extremely high risk (57%) of malignant sequelae. Pathologic specimens with marked nuclear atypia, presence of necrosis or hemorrhage, and trophoblastic proliferation may also increase the risk of persistent disease.

Effective contraceptive measures should be implemented and maintained throughout the period of surveillance in these patients. Oral contraceptives are the most widely used method.

Following evacuation of hydatidiform mole, the patient should have serial β-hCG determinations at weekly intervals until serum hCG declines to nondetectable levels (β-hCG radioimmunoassay) on three successive assays. If titer remission occurs spontaneously within 14 weeks and without a titer plateau, the β-hCG titer than should be repeated monthly for at least 1 year before the patient is released from close medical supervision (in cases of partial moles, β-hCG may be followed for 6–12 months). Thereafter, the patient may enter into a regular gynecologic care program.

Gynecologic examination should be done 1 week after evacuation, at which time blood may be taken for the first postevacuation hCG titer. Estimates of uterine size and presence of adnexal masses (theca lutein cysts) and a careful search of the vulva, vagina, urethra, and cervix should be made for evidence of genital tract metastases. Unless symptoms develop, the examination should be repeated at 4-week intervals throughout the observation period.

Chest x-ray should be obtained prior to evacuation, and if pulmonary metastases are noted, at 4-week intervals thereafter until spontaneous remission is confirmed, then at 3-month intervals during the remainder of the surveillance period.

A patient who has entered into spontaneous remission with negative titers, examinations, and chest x-rays for 1 year and who is desirous of becoming pregnant may terminate contraceptive practices. Successful pregnancy is usual, and complications are similar to those of patients in the general population. The risk of repeat molar pregnancy is 1–2%, but increases to approximately 25% following the second molar pregnancy.

Therapy for progressive gestational trophoblastic neoplasia after delivery of a hydatidiform mole is usually instituted because of an abnormal hCG regression curve. While the hCG titer usually returns to normal within 1–2 weeks after evacuation of a hydatidiform mole, it should be normal by 8 weeks. The most critical period of observation is the first 4–6 weeks postevacuation. Few patients whose hCG titers are normal during this interval will require treatment. Approximately 70% of patients achieve a normal hCG level within 60 days postevacuation.

In the past, therapy was recommended if the hCG titer remained elevated at or beyond 60 days after termination of molar pregnancy. However, current data suggest that an additional 15% of patients demonstrate a continuous decline in titers and ultimately achieve normal titers without treatment. About 15% of patients who have elevated titers at 60 days postevacuation demonstrate a rising or plateauing titer. Nearly half of these patients have histologic evidence of choriocarcinoma, and the rest have invasive mole.

Delayed postevacuation bleeding is uncommon after molar pregnancy, but it signifies the presence of invasive mole or choriocarcinoma and is invariably attended by an enlarging uterus and abnormal hCG regression pattern. On pelvic examination, the enlarged uterus may have the characteristics of an intrauterine pregnancy. Curettage is effective in stopping the bleeding, although little intracavitary tissue will be present in most of these cases.

In summary, the indications for initiating chemotherapy during the postmolar surveillance period are (1) β-hCG levels rising for 2 successive weeks or constant for 3 successive weeks; (2) β-hCG levels elevated at 15 weeks' postevacuation; (3) rising β-hCG titer after reaching normal levels; and (4) postevacuation hemorrhage. Treatment should also be instituted whenever there is a tissue diagnosis of choriocarcinoma. However, histologic confirmation is unnecessary, because the development of metastasis is a sufficient justification for chemotherapy.

B. MALIGNANT GESTATIONAL TROPHOBLASTIC NEOPLASIA

Once the diagnosis of malignant trophoblastic disease has been established, obtain an accurate history and perform a physical examination, including pelvic examination. Most patients have an enlarged uterus, and ovarian enlargement due to theca lutein cysts is common. Sites of metastasis must be sought, especially in the lower genital tract. Obtain a chest x-ray and scans of the liver and brain. CT scan is now the diagnostic procedure of choice for brain, lung (40% of patients with negative chest x-rays may show evidence of pulmonary micrometastases on chest CT), liver, and renal metastases. In brain metastasis, evaluation of the ratio of serum hCG to the concentration of hCG in cerebrospinal fluid (normal > 60:1) may be helpful. Carefully consider the baseline hematologic counts as well as hepatic and renal function, which may be critical in the risk and monitoring of drug toxicity.

After sites of metastases or of abnormal function have been identified, the patient's desires for preservation of reproductive function are known, and the disease has been categorized as nonmetastatic or metastatic, specific therapy should be started.

1. Nonmetastatic gestational trophoblastic disease—Trophoblastic disease confined to the uterus is the most common malignant lesion seen in gestational trophoblastic neoplasia. The diagnosis is usually made during follow-up after evacuation of molar pregnancy. If there is no evidence of spread outside the uterus, histologic examination may be important, for nonmetastatic choriocarcinoma is a more serious condition than nonmetastatic hydatidiform mole. Therapy for patients with nonmetastatic malignant trophoblastic disease includes (1) single-agent chemotherapy; and (2) combined chemotherapy and hysterectomy, with surgery done on the third day of drug therapy if the patient does not wish to preserve reproductive function and her disease is known to be confined to the uterus.

Table 50–2 summarizes the recommended chemotherapy regimens available for nonmetastatic gestational trophoblastic disease (and low-risk gestational trophoblastic disease). Single-agent chemotherapy using methotrexate or dactinomycin has demonstrated clear-cut superiority over other protocols. The therapeutic ef-

Table 50–2. Chemotherapy regimens for nonmetastatic or low-risk gestational trophoblastic disease.

Drug/dosage:

Methotrexate 30–60 mg/m^2 IM once a week.[1]

Methotrexate 0.4 mg/kg/d IV or IM for 5 days, repeat every 14 days

Methotrexate 1 mg/kg IM on days 1, 3, 5, and 7 and folinic acid 0.1 mg/kg IM on days 2, 4, 6, and 8, repeat every 15–18 days

Dactinomycin 1.25 mg/m^2 IV every 14 days

Dactinomycin 10–12 μg/kg/d IV for 5 days, repeat every 14 days

Follow-up:

Follow β-hCG titer weekly. Switch to alternative drug if β-hCG titer rises 10-fold or more, titer plateaus at an elevated level, or new metastasis appears.

Obtain labs daily during treatment cycle or weekly as indicated. Hold chemotherapy for WBC count < 3000 (absolute neutrophil count < 1500); platelets < 100,000; significantly elevated BUN, Cr, AST, ALT, or bilirubin; or for significant side effects (severe stomatitis, gastrointestinal ulceration, or febrile course).

Oral contraceptive agents or other form of birth control should be taken concurrently, and continued for at least 1 year following remission.

Chemotherapy continued for one course after negative β-hCG titer.

Follow-up program: β-hCG titer weekly until 3 consecutive normal titers; monthly β-hCG titer for 12 months thereafter; β-hCG titer every 2 months for 1 additional year or every titer for 6 months indefinitely.

Physical examination including pelvic examination and chest x-ray monthly until remission is induced; at 3-month intervals for 1 year thereafter; then at 6-month intervals indefinitely.

---

[1]For nonmetastatic disease only.

ficacy of the two drugs is apparently equivalent; however, no randomized controlled study has compared the response rate and side effect profile of single-agent chemotherapy with methotrexate to that of dactinomycin. The regimen of choice has therefore not been standardized. However, weekly intramuscular methotrexate injections provide a convenient and cost-effective alternative to the more intense 5-day regimens with methotrexate or dactinomycin, and with minimal side effects. Treatment failure (indicated by rising β-hCG or presence of new metastasis) or intolerable side effects with one regimen should result in administration of the other agent. Overall, the complete response rate ranges from 60–98% with salvage rates approaching 100%. Methotrexate is contraindicated in the presence of hepatocellular disease or when renal function is impaired. Each treatment cycle should be repeated as soon as normal tissues (bone marrow and gastrointestinal mucosa) have recovered, with a minimum 7-day window between the last day of one course and the first day of the next.

During treatment, weekly quantitative β-hCG titers and complete blood counts should be obtained. Before each course of therapy, liver and renal function assessments should be done. At least one course of drug therapy should be given after the first normal β-hCG determination. The number of treatment cycles necessary to induce remission is proportionate to the magnitude of the β-hCG concentration at the start of therapy. An average of 3 or 4 courses of single-agent therapy is required. After remission has been induced and treatment is completed, β-hCG assays should be obtained monthly for 12 months.

2. Metastatic gestational trophoblastic disease—Treatment in metastatic disease utilizes either single-agent chemotherapy (Table 50–2) or multiple-agent chemotherapy. Multiple-agent chemotherapy is used in cases where resistance to a single agent is anticipated. Several systems have been developed to help determine which patients will require at onset more aggressive therapy:

3. Clinical Classification of Malignant Gestational Trophoblastic Disease

National Cancer Institute—This system is utilized in the United States to determine if the patient has a good or poor prognosis to respond well to single-agent chemotherapy (Table 50–3).

Table 50–3. Categorization of gestational trophoblastic neoplasia.

A. **Nonmetastatic disease:** No evidence of disease outside uterus.

B. **Metastatic diease:** Any disease outside uterus.

   1. **Good-prognosis metastatic disease—**

     a. Short duration (< 4 months).

     b. Serum β-hCG < 40,000 mIU/mL.

     c. No metastasis to brain or liver.

     d. No significant prior chemotherapy.

   2. **Poor-prognosis metastatic disease—**

     a. Long duration (> 4 months).

     b. Serum β-hCG > 40,000 mIU/mL.

     c. Metastasis to brain or liver.

     d. Unsuccessful prior chemotherapy.

     e. Gestational trophoblastic neoplasia following term pregnancy.

Table 50–4. WHO prognostic scoring system for gestational trophoblastic disease.

Parameter	Score			
	0	1	2	3
Age (y)	< 39	> 39		
Antecedent pregnancy	Mole	Abortion	Term	
Interval (mo)[1]	< 4	4–6	7–12	> 12
Pretreatment β-hCG level	10^3	10^3–10^4	10^4–10^5	> 10^5
ABO group (female × male)		O × A, A × O	B, AB	
Largest tumor (cm)		3–5	> 5	
Site of metastases		Spleen, kidney	Gastrointestinal, liver	Brain
Number of metastases		1–4	4–8	> 8
Prior chemotherapy failed			Single	> 2

[1]Interval = time between end of antecedent pregnancy and the initiation of chemotherapy. Obatin total score by adding the individual score from each parameter. Total score: > 5 = low risk, 5–7 = medium risk, > 7 = high risk.

World Health Organization—This scoring system is based on an individual's risk factors, including age, type of antecedent pregnancy, interval from antecedent pregnancy to initiation of chemotherapy, pretreatment β-hCG level, blood type (but this criterion not consistently used), size of largest tumor, site of metastases, number of metastases, and prior chemotherapy. Patients are categorized into low-, medium-, and high-risk based on their total score (Table 50–4).

Revised FIGO (International Federation on Gynecology and Obstetrics)—This staging system is based on site of disease extension with presence or absence of 2 risk factors: β-hCG level and interval since antecedent pregnancy (Table 50–5).

Table 50–5. 1992 Revised FIGO staging system for gestational trophoblastic disease.

Stage
I Disease confined to uterus
II Disease extending outside of the uterus but limited to the genital structures (adnexa, vagina, broad ligaments)
III Disease extending to the lungs, with or without known genital tract involvement
IV Disease at other metastatic sites
Substage
A. No risk factors
B. One risk factor
C. Two risk factors
Risk Factors
1. β-hCG > 100,000 mIU/mL
2. Duration from termination of the antecedent pregnancy to diagnosis > 6 months

No single system is consistently being used internationally, thereby making comparisons in treatment success difficult.

a. Good-prognosis patients—Based on the clinical classification of malignant disease, patients can be expected to respond satisfactorily to single-agent chemotherapy if (1) metastases are confined to the lungs or pelvis; (2) serum β-hCG levels are below 40,000 mIU/mL at the onset of treatment; and (3) therapy is started within 4 months of apparent onset of disease.

The most common site of metastasis is the lung. When a patient develops pulmonary metastases and elevation of hCG titer, choriocarcinoma is a more likely cause than metastatic mole. Invasive mole may also metastasize to the lungs, and hydatidiform mole has occasionally been reported to metastasize to the chest. Probably any form of metastasis (even benign deportation) should suggest metastatic trophoblastic disease.

In these patients, single-agent chemotherapy (Table 50–2) is generally successful. Methotrexate is considered the drug of choice. Ideally, the 5-day treatment cycle is given every other week, because tumor regrowth becomes significant after treatment gaps of 2 weeks or longer. Once negative titers have been achieved, an additional course is administered. If resistance to methotrexate occurs, manifested either by rising or plateauing titers or by the development of new metastases, or if negative titers are not achieved by the fifth course of methotrexate, the patient should be given dactinomycin. Dactinomycin should be initiated as well for patients who experience severe side effects with methotrexate.

The advantage of single-agent chemotherapy is that it is less toxic and its toxicity is less apt to be irreversible than is the case with multiple-agent chemotherapy.

There is a tendency to approach the treatment of these patients too lightly, probably because of the "good-prognosis" (low-risk) designation. But failure of drug therapy does occur in about 10% of cases, and meticulous care by physicians familiar with these problems is necessary for good results.

b. Poor-prognosis patients—Poor-prognosis patients, based on the Clinical Classification of Malignant Disease, are those with any of these risk factors: (1) serum β-hCG titers greater than 40,000 mIU/mL; (2) disease diagnosed more than 4 months after molar pregnancy; (3) brain or liver metastases; (4) prior unsuccessful chemotherapy; or (5) onset following term gestation. These patients respond poorly (< 40% response rate) to single-agent therapy. A poor response is also seen in patients with revised FIGO stage IIIC and all stages of IV and with WHO scores > 7. These patients present a serious challenge. Many have been previously treated with chemotherapy and have become resistant to that treatment while accumulating considerable toxicity and depleting bone marrow reserves. Prior unsuccessful chemotherapy is one of the worst prognostic factors.

Generally, these patients require prolonged hospitalization and many courses of chemotherapy. They often need specialized care and other life-support measures, including hyperalimentation, antibiotics, and transfusions to correct the effects of marrow depression.

Central nervous system involvement, particularly brain metastasis with focal neurologic signs suggestive of intracranial hemorrhage, is common in choriocarcinoma. Since patients with brain or liver metastases are at great risk of sudden death from hemorrhage from these lesions, it has been standard practice when treating them to include immediate institution of whole-brain or whole-liver irradiation concomitantly with combination chemotherapy. It is uncertain whether radiation therapy exerts its beneficial effect by destroying tumor in combination with drug therapy or by preventing fatal hemorrhage and thus keeping the patient alive until remission with chemotherapy can be achieved. For acute bleeding episodes, surgical intervention or angiographic embolization can be considered.

Cerebral metastasis should be treated over a 2-week period with radiation given in a dosage of 300 rads daily, 5 days a week, to a total organ dose of 3000 rads. Whole-liver irradiation is usually accomplished over 10 days to attain a 2000-rad whole-organ dose given at a rate of 200 rads daily, 5 days a week. Other treatment options include selective hepatic artery chemotherapy infusion.

Prior treatments for poor prognosis/high-risk gestational trophoblastic disease have included MAC (methotrexate, dactinomycin, and chlorambucil or cyclophosphamide) and the modified Bagshawe protocol (CHAMOCA: cyclophosphamide, hydroxyurea, methotrexate, vincristine, cyclophosphamide, and dactinomycin). Currently, EMA/CO (etoposide, methotrexate, dactinomycin, cyclophosphamide, and vincristine) chemotherapy (Table 50–6) provides the best response rate (approximately 80%) with the lowest side effect profile. The cycle is repeated every 2 weeks. The same tests must be employed to detect toxicity as are used when single-agent chemotherapy is given, but monitoring must be even more vigilant because of the possibility of combined toxicity.

Treatment of malignant trophoblastic disease must be continued with repeated courses of combination chemotherapy until β-hCG titers return to nondetectable levels. Complete remission is documented only after three consecutive weekly normal β-hCG titers have been achieved. It is recommended that all high-risk patients receive at least three courses of triple-agent chemotherapy after β-hCG titers have returned to normal. After remission is achieved, follow-up is the same as for hydatidiform mole and nonmetastatic or good-prognosis disease.

Salvage therapy for disease not responsive to EMA/CO substitutes cisplatin and etoposide (EP-EMA) for cyclophosphamide and vincristine (CO) (Table 50–6). Close monitoring of renal function is required because of nephrotoxicity secondary to cisplatin and as methotrexate is renally excreted. Other treatment options include such agents as paclitaxel, topotecan, and high-dose chemotherapy with autologous bone marrow transplantation.

In resistant cases, adjunctive measures along with chemotherapy may include hysterectomy, resection of metastatic tumors, or irradiation of unresectable lesions.

4. Placental-Site Trophoblastic Tumor (PSTT)—Treatment of PSTT generally is resistant to chemotherapy. Therefore hysterectomy is the recommended route of treatment. Partial uterine resection involving the tumor is possible if the patient desires to retain fertility. Chemotherapy is indicated in cases of metastatic disease. EP-EMA is the preferred regimen over EMA/CO, with paclitaxel and topotecan used when resistance develops. The greatest adverse outcomes are associated with an interval > 2 years from antecedent pregnancy to diagnosis.

Prognosis

The prognosis for hydatidiform mole following evacuation is uniformly excellent, though surveillance is needed as outlined in the text. The prognosis for malignant nonmetastatic disease with appropriate therapy is also quite good, since almost all patients are cured. Over 90% of patients have been able to preserve reproductive function, but first-line therapy failed in 6.5% of

Table 50–6. Current treatment regimens for high-risk gestational trophoblastic disease.

EMA/CO[1]

Day

1	Etoposide	100 mg/m^2 IV (infused over 30 minutes)
	Actinomycin D	0.5 mg IV bolus
	Methotrexate[2]	100 mg/m^2 IV bolus
		200 mg/m^2 IV (infused over 12 hours)
2	Etoposide	100 mg/m^2 IV (infused over 30 minutes)
	Actinomycin D	0.5 mg IV bolus
	Folinic acid	15 mg IM infusion or orally every 12 hours for four doses beginning 24 hours after start of methotrexate
8	Cyclophosphamide	600 mg/m^2 IV infusion
	Vincristine	1 mg/m^2 IV bolus

Other options:

Salvage therapy: Substituting etoposide (100 mg/m^2 IV) and cisplatin (80 mg/m^2 IV) (EMA-EP) for cyclophosphamide and vincristine. Adjuvant surgery (hysterectomy and thoracotomy) for chemotherapy-resistant disease.

With failure of EMA-EP, treatment with: BEP (cisplatin 20 mg/m^2 IV, etoposide 100 mg/m^2 IV on days 1–4 every 21 days, with bleomycin 30 units IV on day 1 then every week), G-CSF (granulocyte colony-stimulating factor) 300 μg SC on days 6–14.

VIP (etoposide 75 mg/m^2 IV, ifosfamide 1.2 g/m^2 IV, cisplatin 20 mg/m^2 IV each day for 4 days every 21 days). Mesna 120 mg/m^2 IV bolus prior to first ifosfamide dose, followed by 1.2 mg/m^2 12-hour IV infusion daily after each ifosfamide dose, G-CSF 300 μg SC on days 6–14.

High-dose chemotherapy with autologous bone marrow transplantation.

Taxanes (paclitaxel and docetaxel) and camptothecins (topotecan and irinotecan).

[1]Mild toxicity with 5-year survival 80%. Repeat cycles on days 15, 16, and 22 (every 2 weeks).

[2]Increase to 1 g/m^2 as 24-h infusion with CNS metastases, with folinic acid increased to 15 mg every 8 h for nine doses beginning 12 h following completion of methotrexate infusion. Also may receive methotrexate 12.5 mg by intrathecal injection on day 8. Another option is whole-brain irradiation 3000 cGY in 200-cGY fractions given over 10–14 days during chemotherapy.

Chemotherapy should be continued for at least 3 cycles after negative β-hCG.

As with nonmetastatic and low-risk disease, oral contraceptive pills or other form of birth control should be utilized if not contraindicated.

patients with nonmetastatic disease. In one large reported series, no death from toxicity occurred, and only one patient died of the disease.

In poor-prognosis metastatic disease, the best results are with EMA/CO chemotherapy and concurrent radiation as indicated. Seventy-five to 85% of patients achieve remission with a 69% salvage rate. This is a similar response to agents used previously (MAC) but with fewer side effects. Brain and liver metastases have the worst prognosis with reports of survival ranging from 0–60% for hepatic involvement and 50–80% for CNS involvement at diagnosis. Survival decreases to < 20% when prior chemotherapy agents have been utilized or if CNS metastases develop while undergoing treatment. Deaths from toxicity have decreased considerably. Recurrence, when it happens, is usually in the first several months after termination of therapy but may be as late as 3 years.

Secondary Tumors

Multiple-agent chemotherapy (specifically utilizing etoposide) but not single-agent chemotherapy has been

associated with a 50% increased risk for secondary tumors. One retrospective study found that the relative risk for developing myeloid leukemia and colon cancer was 16.6 and 4.6, respectively. When survival exceeded 25 years, the relative risk for developing breast cancer was 5.8.

Subsequent Pregnancy Outcome

Subsequent pregnancies are not at increased risk for complications such as preterm labor, anomalies, or stillbirth. These pregnancies should, however, be monitored early with ultrasound and β-hCG levels because there is a small risk of recurrent gestational trophoblastic disease (1–2%). Following delivery, the placenta should be sent to pathology and a β-hCG level should be checked at the 6-week postpartum visit.

In cases where pregnancy occurs prior to the completion of standard postmolar surveillance (less than 1 year), the pregnancy may be continued with close observation, and the risks discussed with the patient. Most pregnancies end with a good outcome, but there is a small risk for delayed diagnosis of recurrence.

REFERENCES

Berkowitz RS, Goldstein DP: Recent advances in gestational trophoblastic disease. Curr Opin Obstet Gynecol 1998;10:61.

Berkowitz RS et al: Management of gestational trophoblastic diseases: Subsequent pregnancy experience. Semin Oncol 2000;27:678.

Cohn DE, Herzog TJ: Gestational trophoblastic diseases: New standards for therapy. Curr Opin Oncol 2000;12:492.

Goldstein DP et al: Revised FIGO staging system for gestational trophoblastic tumors. J Reprod Med 1998;43:37.

Homesley HD: Single-agent therapy for nonmetastatic and low-risk gestational trophoblastic disease. J Reprod Med 1998;43:69.

Newlands ES et al: Management of placental site trophoblastic tumors. J Reprod Med 1998;43:53.

Tham KF, Tatnam SS: The classification of gestational trophoblastic disease: a critical review. Int J Gynaecol Obstet 1998;60 (Suppl 1):S39.

Truncer ZS et al: Outcome of pregnancies occurring before completion of human chorionic gonadotropin follow-up in patients with persistent gestational trophoblastic tumor. Gynecol Oncol 1999;73:345.

Radiation Therapy for Gynecologic Cancers

Julie Jolin, MD, & Harrison G. Ball, MD

Two European discoveries in the late 1800s led to future radiation treatment of human malignancies. While studying the penetrating power of cathode ray emission in Germany, Wilhelm Roentgen discovered x-rays on November 8, 1895. The Curies in France isolated radium from uranium ore in 1898. Soon thereafter, Robert Abbe of New York City introduced radium for medical therapy, and Howard Kelly of Baltimore pioneered radium treatment of cervical cancer. Since then radiation therapy has evolved to become a major modality in the treatment of many cancers, particularly those of the female reproductive tract.

Definitions

Radiation oncology may be defined as the therapeutic manipulation of **ionizing radiation,** high-energy radiation capable of separating one or more orbital electrons from their affiliated atoms or molecules. Such radiation may be electromagnetic or particulate, both of which transfer energy to the electrons or nuclei of cellular components. Conventional radiation comprises **electromagnetic radiation,** in which photons produced interact with cellular water in the cell, resulting in the formation of free radicals that then lead to cellular damage.

The most familiar forms of electromagnetic radiation, x-rays and gamma rays, are generated from different sources but possess the same physical characteristics in that they both lack mass and charge. When accelerated electrons strike the atoms of a positioned target, x-rays result from the energy liberated, whereas the decay of radioactive isotopes results in gamma rays.

Particulate radiation includes electrons and nuclear forms such as protons, neutrons, and pions (negative π mesons), which are negatively charged particles that have a mass 273 times that of an electron. New radiation modalities attempt to harness the ability of such high linear energy transfer (LET) radiations since they are more effective against hypoxic cells than conventional, low LET radiation.

Conventional x-rays and gamma rays may be considered as discrete units of radiant energy called **photons.** The energy of each unit is proportional to the frequency of the wave associated with the photon. Radiation with a shorter wavelength has greater frequency and consequently carries greater energy per photon to allow deeper tissue penetration. It is the amount of energy imparted to the individual photons rather than the total invested energy that distinguishes ionizing radiation, which possesses more energy per photon packet, from nonionizing radiation.

The transfer of radiant energy in the form of photons to another material occurs through the photoelectric effect, the Compton effect, or pair production. With the **photoelectric effect,** absorption is influenced by atomic number; the tissues bearing elements of higher atomic number (eg, calcium in bone) will absorb proportionately greater and possibly detrimental levels of radiation. The photoelectric effect involves electron ejection from matter when a photon strikes it. The **Compton effect** involves the interaction of incident photons with the outer-shell electrons of bombarded atoms, with resulting change in the wavelength of x-ray or gamma radiation due to production of a recoil electron and a scattered photon of reduced energy (Fig 51–1). The atomic number of the tissue elements does not determine the amount of absorbed radiation. **Pair production** refers to the complex interaction of an incident photon with the nucleus of a target atom, resulting in a positron electron pair.

In the lower range of energy transfer, the photoelectric effect predominates, while in the transfer of higher levels of energy, the Compton effect and pair production are more prevalent.

Dosage Theory

Radiant energy produces biologic change by damaging the DNA molecule of target tissues and thus hampering further effective replication. Such damage is incurred initially by the production of the hydroxyl radical, which is formed by the collision of radiant energy and water, and is irreversible only in the presence of molecular oxygen. Normal tissue as well as malignant cells are susceptible to toxicity induced by radiation therapy, the extent of which depends on total dose, fractionization, and tumor volume.

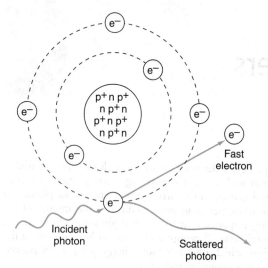

Figure 51–1. Absorption of an x-ray photon by the Compton process. The photon interacts with a loosely bound planetary electron of an atom of the absorbing material. Part of the photon energy is given to the electron as kinetic energy. The photon, deflected from its original direction, proceeds with reduced energy. e^- = electron; p^+ = proton; n = neutron. (Reproduced, with permission, from Hall EJ: *Radiobiology for the Radiologist*, 4th ed. JB Lippincott, 1994, p. 7.)

After exposure to radiation, tissue survival follows a predictable curve that essentially constitutes the number of viable clone cells (Fig 51–2). The shoulder represents the cell's enzymatic ability to reverse damage due to radiant energy. As radiation increases, cells become incapable of self-repair and a logarithmic pattern of cell destruction occurs. Importantly, for every increase in dosage that occurs beyond the shoulder, a constant fraction of cells is eliminated (**log-kill hypothesis**).

The implications of these observations provide some of the rationale for dividing (fractionating) the total dose of radiation therapy administered in the clinical setting. It is helpful to consider the so-called "4 R's" of radiobiology to understand the effects of fractionated doses at the cellular level.

A. REPAIR OF SUBLETHAL INJURY

When a specified radiation dose is divided into two doses given at separate times, the number of cells surviving is higher than that seen when the same total dose is given at one time. Fractionation allows the administration of amounts of radiation that would not be tolerated if the specified dose were given in only one treatment.

B. REPOPULATION

The reactivation of stem cells that occurs when radiation is stopped is necessary for further tissue growth; therefore those tissues with increased numbers of progenitor cells have a greater ability to regenerate.

C. REOXYGENATION (OXYGEN EFFECT)

Hypoxic cells are known to be relatively resistant to radiation. Experimental and clinical evidence has con-

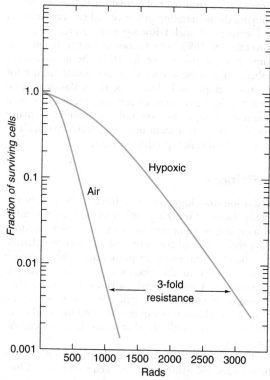

Figure 51–2. Typical radiation survival curve for mammalian cells. These cells have been irradiated and then plated out in culture, and the number of survivors has been determined by measuring the colonies (clones) of cells that survive. The curve is characterized by an initial shoulder followed by a log-linear region. Cells irradiated in air are considerably more sensitive than those irradiated in nitrogen (hypoxic), and the difference between the levels of killing is frequently about threefold. It is believed that most clinically demonstrable tumors have areas of hypoxia that lead to radioresistance. (Reproduced, with permission, from Morrow CP, Curtin JP, Townsend DE [editors]: *Synopsis of Gynecologic Oncology*, 4th ed. Churchill Livingstone, 1993, p. 449.)

firmed that molecular oxygen must be present before radiation damage can occur. Cells located farther than 100 mm from capillary flow are at risk for hypoxia and may not be killed by radiation therapy. If these hypoxic cells are malignant, they may not be killed by radiation therapy. For this reason, it is important to correct anemia in patients undergoing radiation treatment so that tissue oxygen perfusion will be enhanced and tissues will become more radiosensitive. As tumor regresses with radiation treatment, previously anoxic areas may be brought into contact with capillary flow and increased oxygenation. However, malignant cells in these sites may then be exposed to now sublethal amounts of radiation, since cells undergoing reoxygenation are only affected after surrounding tissues have received significant radiation doses. Thus, the reoxygenated tumor will be able to receive only a portion of the optimum tumoricidal dose.

D. RADIATION-INDUCED SYNCHRONY

Malignant cells are most sensitive to radiation while in the mitotic phase of the cell cycle. If a segment of the malignant cell population can be destroyed in this phase of the cell cycle, the remaining malignant cells may be synchronized for selective destruction at a later time.

Clinical experience has shown that prolonged interruption of radiation therapy has a deleterious effect on cure, since malignant cells have a greater chance to regenerate.

Dosimetry

Dosimetry is the measurement of the amount of radiation absorbed by target tissue. Units are expressed in rads or in gray (1 cGy = 1 rad). External pelvic irradiation is expressed in those terms, whereas internal irradiation is also described in milligram hours. This latter unit is obtained by multiplying the number of milligrams of radioactive substance (usually radium or cesium) used in the internal applicators by the number of hours the applicators have been in place.

The exact conversion factor between milligram hours and gray is difficult to determine, but computer-directed dosimetry permits the calculation of isodose curves, points of equal dose surrounding a radioactive source, that permit critical considerations in avoiding overdose to the bladder and rectum. Unfortunately, the radiation tolerance of the bladder and rectum is close to the dosage levels required for curative radiation therapy of common pelvic cancers.

TREATMENT METHODS

External Irradiation (Teletherapy)

Early radiation therapists used electric x-ray sources that were basically modifications of Roentgen's experi-

mental apparatus. Electrons were accelerated across a vacuum tube to strike a tungsten target with the subsequent liberation of photons. These orthovoltage (140–400 keV) units were limited in their power to penetrate tissue effectively because of their relatively low energy output. Consequently, pronounced fibrotic skin changes and high absorbed bone radiation levels limited their usefulness in some patients.

As units generating higher levels of energy were developed, the penetrating power of the x-rays produced was enhanced, and less scattering of radiation was seen at the margins of the treatment area. The surface skin dose was also diminished, of particular importance in the treatment of obese patients, and less-toxic bone radiation was achieved (Fig 51–3).

Cobalt 60 teletherapy units are in the supervoltage range (500 keV–1 MeV) and use the radiant energy released by the nuclear decay of cobalt 60. Megavoltage (> 1 MeV) radiation sources, such as linear accelerators, allow even more precise delineation of the area receiving radiation therapy.

Local Irradiation (Brachytherapy)

Brachytherapy is radiation therapy in which the source of therapeutic ionizing radiation is placed close to the treatment area. The appliances most commonly used in gynecologic cancer patients are intracavitary devices and interstitial implants.

The chief advantage of local irradiation is that a relatively high dose of radiation can be applied to a limited anatomic region. The **inverse square law** has critical implications in clinical applications. The principle of the inverse square law states that the intensity of radiation is inversely proportional to the square of the distance from the source. An important implication is that the rapid falloff of radiant energy supplied by a central source precludes the achievement of cancerocidal doses at the margins of the pelvis. Therefore, external therapy must be used to provide adequate radiation to eliminate tumor at the periphery of large lesions and at the pelvic side walls, where metastatic disease may be present.

An additional therapeutic possibility is the use of spacers in the vagina that increase the distance between vaginal epithelium and the source of radiation. The surface dose, and thus radiation damage, is diminished, but the effective radiation dose applied to the parametrial tissue is essentially unchanged.

Though not widely used now, a few institutions have begun to perform operative procedures in which areas of disease are carefully defined, and 1500 cGy–2500 cGy radiation fractions are delivered to the areas intraoperatively. Some gynecologic oncologists have used intraoperative radiation in treating biopsy-

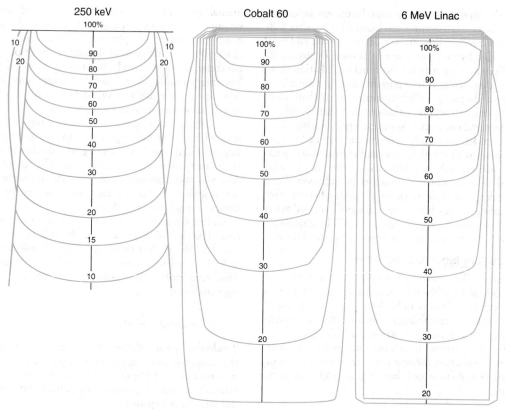

250 keV · Cobalt 60 · 6 MeV Linac

Figure 51–3. Typical isodose curves for orthovoltage (250 keV), cobalt 60, and a 6-MeV linear accelerator. The most important difference between the megavoltage (cobalt 60 and Linac) beams in comparison with the 250-keV unit is the movement of the 100% isodose line several millimeters beneath the surface. This results in elimination of the severe skin reactions characteristic of earlier radiation sources. In addition, it can be seen that the higher energy leads to deeper penetration as the energy of the beam increases. The lateral spreading of the beam (penumbra or shadow) is less with cobalt 60 than with the 250-keV unit and is further reduced in the accelerator beam. The reduction of the penumbra with the accelerator beam is due to its possessing a source with smaller physical dimensions. (Reproduced, with permission, from Morrow CP, Curtin JP, Townsend DE [editors]: *Synopsis of Gynecologic Oncology*, 4th ed. Churchill Livingstone, 1993, p. 443.)

proven positive periaortic nodes at time of staging laparotomy for cervical carcinoma.

TREATMENT OF GYNECOLOGIC CANCER

Cervical Cancer

Treatment of cervical cancer is considered a prime example of the successful application of radiation therapy. The relative accessibility of the central lesion, a metastatic pattern of cervical squamous cell carcinoma that can be predicted with reasonable accuracy, and the radiation tolerance of the cervix and surrounding tissues often permit curative radiation therapy.

Radiation therapy with curative intent uses both external-beam and intracavitary radiation. Palliative radiation for advanced cervical cancer may utilize either modality for control of bleeding, management of disease in the pelvis, and relief of pain.

The goal of external irradiation is to sterilize metastatic disease to pelvic lymph nodes and the parametria and to decrease the size of the cervix to allow optimal placement of intracavitary radioactive sources.

The size of the portal used to treat a patient with carcinoma of the cervix must be carefully designed to encompass those structures at risk for regional spread of the cancer. To spare normal structures within the pelvis, particularly bowel and bladder, a 4-field technique with both anterior-posterior and lateral portals can be used. The superior border of the anterior-posterior field is usually the L4–L5 interspace, but may need to extend more cephalad if the common iliac lymph nodes are to be included in the treatment field. The inferior border is the obturator foramen, but if the vagina is involved by the cancer, the field may be extended to the introitus. Laterally, the field should extend 1–2 cm lateral to the bony pelvis. The lateral field includes the pubic symphysis anteriorly and the sacral hollow posteriorly. For patients with stage IB cervical cancer, a typical field would approximate 15 × 15 cm, whereas stage IIA to IVA cancer would require larger field sizes. Patients with known or suspected metastatic disease to periaortic lymph nodes may be considered for extended field irradiation. External irradiation is administered using a cobalt 60 machine or a linear accelerator.

Various techniques are used to maximize the effect of therapy while decreasing the chances of damage to surrounding organs. With the aid of computerized dosimetry, radiation can be increased to compensate for asymmetric parametrial disease. In large lesions, the size of the field can be progressively restricted to concentrate on a defined tumor burden.

In the U.S., most intracavitary therapy is delivered via the Fletcher-Suit afterloading applicator. This method permits optimal placement of the tandem and colpostats within the cervical canal and vagina in the operating room. Since the radioactive sources are placed in the devices later, this minimizes exposure to radiation in personnel involved in intracavitary placement. It is crucial that the devices be placed so as to maximize the dose to the target region and at the same time minimize the possibility of radiation damage to the bladder and rectum.

Combining pelvic radiation with concomitant chemotherapy (cisplatin and fluorouracil were administered in recent trials) for locally advanced cervical cancer (stages bulky IB to IVA) was shown to provide survival advantage over pelvic and para-aortic radiation alone. The success of combined treatment decreased the risk of death from cervical cancer by 30–50%. Advantages of combined treatment theoretically include no delay time in starting definitive irradiation; decreased treatment time overall; and possible interaction of chemotherapy with radiotherapy by mechanisms such as repair of sublethal and lethal damage, cell phase distribution changes, effect on vascularity of tumor, effects on repopulation, effects on hypoxic cells, alteration of cell survival curve, and modification of apoptosis.

Endometrial Cancer

Adenocarcinoma of the endometrium tends to present with disease confined to the uterus. Although a variety of combinations of surgery and radiation therapy have been employed in treatment, there has been a trend in the U.S. toward surgical staging followed by individualized postoperative irradiation. Total abdominal hysterectomy with bilateral salpingo-oophorectomy and aspiration of peritoneal fluid for cytologic evaluation is performed for all patients. Patients chosen on the basis of poor prognostic factors undergo pelvic and periaortic lymph node biopsies.

After the pathologist examines the uterus, tubes, ovaries, and lymph nodes, a decision to use postoperative radiation therapy is based on the presence or absence of poor prognostic factors. Patients with deep myometrial invasion (greater than one-third) or with metastatic disease to fallopian tubes, ovaries, or pelvic lymph nodes receive 4500–5000 cGy of whole-pelvis irradiation. If there is involvement of the cervix, additional treatment is given to the vaginal apex utilizing a vaginal cylinder delivering an additional 2500–3000 cGy to the vaginal mucosa. Metastatic disease to periaortic lymph nodes can be managed with extended-field radiation. Patients with stage III and stage IV disease may be considered for whole abdominal radiation of 2500–3000 cGy with a pelvic boost of 4500–5000 cGy.

Patients with gross involvement of the cervix are ideally treated with preoperative whole-pelvic and intracavitary radiation followed by extrafascial hysterectomy.

Endometrial cancer can be managed with radiation therapy alone for the high-risk patient with medical problems who is not a candidate for abdominal surgery. Patients with well-differentiated adenocarcinoma may be managed with tandem and ovoids or intrauterine Simon capsules. Patients with moderately or poorly differentiated cancers or those with involvement of the cervix are at risk for parametrial and pelvic lymph node spread and should receive whole-pelvic irradiation prior to brachytherapy.

Ovarian Cancer

Since the introduction of combination chemotherapy, the use of radiation therapy in the treatment of epithelial ovarian cancer has become increasingly uncommon in the U.S. Irradiation is used as adjuvant therapy in patients with early-stage epithelial ovarian cancer, as definitive therapy for minimal residual advanced ovarian cancer, and in the management of recurrent and persistent ovarian cancer. However, despite its proven benefit in patients with microscopic or minimal residual disease, radiation therapy's overall role in treating ovarian cancer remains controversial.

Patients who have been adequately staged and have stage IA1 and IB1 adenocarcinoma have not been shown to benefit from adjuvant therapy. All other patients with stage I disease and those with stage II disease currently receive adjuvant therapy. In these patients, a randomized trial has shown no difference in survival between those receiving intraperitoneal colloidal chromic phosphate (^{32}P) and single-agent melphalan. If ^{32}P is considered for therapy, it is imperative that adequate staging has been performed, including sampling of pelvic and periaortic nodes, since ^{32}P has limited penetration and the dosage to pelvic and periaortic nodes is considered subtherapeutic. ^{32}P has the advantages of convenience of a single treatment, minimal toxicity, and low cost.

Generally, whole abdominal irradiation is considered as second-line treatment in selected patients who fail initial chemotherapy, particularly in those debulked to small amounts of residual disease. Since the tolerance of the kidneys, liver, and bone marrow limits the dose of radiation that can be delivered to the whole abdomen, the size of residual disease in the upper abdomen should be microscopic and no greater than 2 cm in the pelvis. Current treatment regimens use 2000–3000 cGy to the abdomen with appropriate shielding of the kidneys and liver, and 4500–5500 cGy to the pelvis. The treatment can be delivered by either the moving-strip or the open-field technique; randomized studies have shown no differences in patient survival or in complications between the two methods.

European and American studies suggest that patients with stage I, II, III, or IV ovarian cancer with residual disease following aggressive cytoreductive therapy and multiple-drug, platinum-based chemotherapy benefit from whole abdominopelvic irradiation. One such study revealed that survival rates of optimally debulked patients who received adjuvant chemotherapy were significantly higher than those of patients who received adjuvant chemotherapy alone. Radiation therapy may play an important role in palliation for patients with advanced disease not responsive to chemotherapy. For example, recurrence in the pelvis impinging on the rectum may lead to large bowel obstruction. The judicious use of external-beam irradiation may control disease in the pelvis and prevent the need for a diverting colostomy.

Vaginal Cancer

Radiotherapy remains the primary treatment for vaginal cancer, which is one of the rarest human malignancies, and historically one of the gravest. A 1954 review of a published series of 992 patients reported an overall 5-year survival rate of 18%. More recent studies, however, have shown overall 5-year cure rates of 40–50%. Such improvement in survival rates has been attributed to megavoltage external therapy along with physical and technical advances in local irradiation. With squamous cell carcinoma comprising the most common form of vaginal cancer, these patients undergo whole-pelvic radiation therapy followed by a vaginal cylinder

and interstitial needle irradiation. Patients with lesions involving the lower third of the vagina should have the inguinal and femoral lymph nodes included in the external-beam treatment field.

Vulvar Cancer

Slightly more common than vaginal cancer (5% versus 2% of female malignancies), vulvar cancer also is usually squamous cell in origin. However, the mainstay of treatment of vulvar cancer is surgical, often consisting of radical vulvectomy plus inguinal and pelvic lymphadenectomy. Combined radiation therapy with surgical treatment has been studied recently, based on earlier reports that vulvar cancer is sensitive to radiation therapy. Thus, the Gynecologic Oncology Group reported in 1998 that preoperative chemoradiation therapy in advanced squamous cell vulvar cancer may reduce the need for more radical surgery, including primary pelvic exenteration. And previously it was reported by the GOG that there is a survival advantage in patients with more than one positive groin node when treated postoperatively with pelvic lymph node irradiation therapy versus lymph node dissection.

Complications of Radiation Therapy

Radiation therapy regimens are formulated to maximize the chances for cure while incurring the smallest amount of damage to normal tissues. In gynecologic cancers, the most serious complications are those involving the gastrointestinal or genitourinary systems.

Complications of radiation therapy are classified as early or delayed. Early problems that occur, especially with whole-pelvis teletherapy, include enteritis, proctosigmoiditis, cystitis, vulvitis, and, occasionally, depression of bone marrow elements. Bowel side effects usually comprise cramping and diarrhea that require dietary adjustments and the judicious use of antidiarrheal agents. Such problems usually respond to appropriate medication, but occasionally radiation therapy must be interrupted or curtailed because of fulminant acute reactions.

Delayed radiation injury may be manifested by chronic proctosigmoiditis, hemorrhagic cystitis, small and large bowel strictures, and the formation of rectovaginal and vesicovaginal fistulas. Pelvic fibrosis and loss of ovarian function may affect sexual activity in younger patients.

New Directions in Radiation Therapy

In addition to radiation sensitizers, other treatment methods including hyperbaric oxygen administration, fast neutrons, hyperthermia, negative pions, and altered fractionation schemes are being evaluated for effectiveness against the tumor-protective effects of hypoxia, which is a common problem with gynecologic cancers. With the current emphasis on cost containment in medical care, continuing study of high-dose-rate brachytherapy is likely to shorten the time course of intracavitary treatment. As newer computer technologies are wedded to imaging techniques, further advances in anatomic contouring for planning and treatment are expected to translate into better local control rates as well as improved survival with a wider margin of safety.

REFERENCES

Cardenes H, Randall ME: Integrating radiation therapy in the curative management of ovarian cancer: Current issues and future directions. Semin Radiat Oncol 2000;10:61.

Cmelak AJ, Kapp DS: Long-term survival with whole abdominopelvic irradiation in platinum-refractory persistent or recurrent ovarian cancer. Gynecol Oncol 1997;65:453.

Greven KM, Corn BW: Endometrial cancer. Curr Prob Cancer 1997;21:94.

Keys H et al: Cisplatin, radiation, and adjuvant hysterectomy compared with radiation and adjuvant hysterectomy for bulky stage IB cervical carcinoma. N Engl J Med 1999;340:1154.

Moore DH et al: Preoperative chemoradiation for advanced vulvar cancer: A phase II study of the Gynecologic Oncology Group. Int J Radiat Oncol Biol Phys 1998;42:79.

Morris M et al: Pelvic radiation with concurrent chemotherapy compared with pelvic and para-aortic radiation for high-risk cervical cancer. N Engl J Med 1999;340:1137.

National Institutes of Health Consensus Development Conference Statement on Cervical Cancer. Gynecol Oncol 1997;66:351.

Okada M et al: Indication and efficacy of radiation therapy following radical surgery in patients with stage IB to IIB cervical cancer. Gynecol Oncol 1998;70:61.

Pickel H et al: Consolidation radiotherapy after carboplatin-based chemotherapy in radically operated advanced ovarian cancer. Gynecol Oncol 1999;72:215.

Pinilla J: Cost minimization analysis of high-dose-rate versus low-dose-rate brachytherapy in endometrial cancer. Int J Radiat Oncol Biol Phys 1998;42:87.

Rose P et al: Concurrent cisplatin-based radiotherapy and chemotherapy for locally advanced cervical cancer. N Engl J Med 1999;340:1144.

Thomas G et al: A randomized trial of standard versus partially hyperfractionated radiation with or without concurrent 5-fluorouracil in locally advanced cervical cancer. Gynecol Oncol 1998;69:137.

U.S. Dept of Health and Human Services: Concurrent chemoradiation for cervical cancer. National Cancer Institute Clinical Announcement, Feb 1999.

Chemotherapy for Gynecologic Cancers

52

Oliver Dorigo, MD, April Gale O'Quinn, MD, & Simie Degefu, MD

General Considerations

Effective chemotherapy for gynecologic cancers exploits characteristic differences between tumor cells and normal cells to selectively kill malignant cells without producing serious, irreversible harm to vital organs and tissues. Knowledge of the scientific basis of cancer chemotherapy is derived from research in molecular biology and cell kinetics and is indispensable to the development of better drugs, establishment of a more rational basis for the design of protocols, and the optimal use of presently available antineoplastic drugs.

Long-lasting remissions and occasional cures for several types of cancer have been achieved with antitumor drugs. For example, up to 90% of patients with metastatic choriocarcinoma achieve a normal life expectancy, and almost 100% of those without metastases are cured now that the effect of drugs may be monitored by the level of β-hCG (human chorionic gonadotropin), which provides a reliable index of tumor growth. For most tumors, however, no such specific and sensitive assay or tumor marker exists. Now that multiple-drug regimens are being used for primary chemotherapy of carcinoma of the ovary, objective response rates of 60–80% are achieved. The objective response rate of 20–40% achieved by chemotherapy in patients with primary carcinoma of the breast and endometrium warrants the use of chemotherapy as an integral part of an initial treatment program.

In spite of extensive experience, the use of cytotoxic agents for carcinomas of the cervix, vagina, and vulva is still on a clinical trial basis, since these tumors usually grow more slowly, and cytotoxic drug treatment has been palliative but not curative; these types of cancer are better controlled by surgery and radiation therapy, and chemotherapy should be considered only when these standard methods have proved ineffective.

Among the uncommon gynecologic cancers that may require chemotherapy are germ cell tumors of the ovary and primary ovarian, uterine, vaginal, or vulvar sarcomas. Because these tumors are rare, little is known about their sensitivity to antitumor drugs.

The Normal Cell Cycle

Figure 52–1 represents the cell cycle in a clockwise progression. The phases and their durations are depicted, and the phases during which some specific chemotherapeutic agents exert their effects are included for reference.

Cell Kinetics

Knowledge of tumor cells has been derived from clinical and laboratory methods of tumor growth measurement, including direct measurement of cell cycle parameters, clinical measurement of doubling times, and use of biologic markers such as hormone production or polyamines and other abnormal proteins. A knowledge of the terminology of cell kinetics is helpful in understanding the dynamics of tumor cells, in which some cells divide more slowly than others, some cells enter or leave a nondividing state, and some are lost from the tumor population entirely.

The **mitotic index (MI)** is the fraction of cells in mitosis in a steady-state condition. The MI may be calculated by giving a drug such as a *Vinca* alkaloid that halts further cellular progression through mitosis and then counting the number of cells in mitosis. Another method uses tritiated thymidine, which is incorporated only into the DNA of cells in the S phase; the tritiated thymidine emits β rays that can then expose the silver in a photographic emulsion during cell mitosis to produce **percent-labeled mitosis (PLM)** curves. Radioactive tagging of DNA during synthesis provides the **labeling index (LI)**, which is the percentage of cells in the S phase at a particular time.

Growth fraction (GF) is the overall proportion of proliferating tumor cells in a given tumor. The growth fraction is important because most antitumor drugs inhibit only proliferating cells. Therefore, a major difference between tumor and normal cell populations may be the relative percentage of each in the growth fraction. The selective effect of antitumor drugs on tumor cells may be explained by the characteristic higher growth fraction of tumor cells. Toxicity results from the effects of antitumor drugs on normal cells in the mitotic cycle or

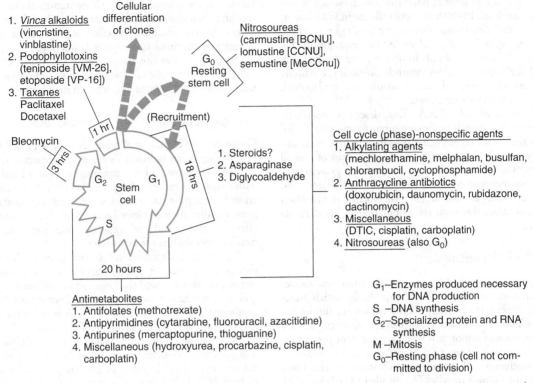

Figure 52–1. Model of the cell cycle, with progression proceeding clockwise. Phases and their durations are depicted, along with points in the cell cycle at which some chemotherapeutic agents exert their effects.

growth fraction; consequently, the toxicity of most antitumor drugs occurs in those normal cell populations with rapid turnover, eg, the hematopoietic and gastrointestinal systems. Therefore, alopecia, bone marrow suppression and diarrhea are common side effects.

Cell cycle time denotes the amount of time needed by a proliferating cell to progress through the cell cycle and produce a new daughter cell. Cell cycle times vary widely according to histologic type (18–217 hours in solid tumors) but are relatively constant for a specific tumor type.

Doubling time is the time required for the tumor cell population to double. Human tumors often have doubling times greater than those of comparable normal tissues and, in advanced stages of disease, may exhibit a range of doubling times, but 30–60 days is typical. In the model ascites system, cell doubling time remains constant at nearly 100% throughout almost the entire life cycle of the tumor, whereas in solid tumor systems, a gradual slowing of the tumor doubling time and reduction of the proliferation rate of

cells occur with tumor enlargement as a result of decreased accessibility to nutrients.

Cell loss may be a major determinant of the tumor growth rate. Cells are lost from a tumor mass in various ways, including death, migration, or metastases. Cell loss is frequently high in advanced tumors.

Stem Cell Theory

The stem cell theory states that only certain relatively undifferentiated cells, or stem cells, of a particular tissue type are able to divide and reproduce the entire tissue. Examples include rapidly proliferating tissues such as bone marrow, the lining of the gastrointestinal tract, and the basal cell layer of the skin. In other words, most cells making up a particular tissue have matured or have become highly differentiated after clonal division from the reproducing cell or a specific stem cell.

Not all cells of a particular stem cell population are committed to division at a given time. A significant proportion of stem cells are in the G_0 or resting phase, as is the case in normal bone marrow, in which at any one time from 15–50% of stem cells are in G_0. Numerous stimuli may recruit this reserve (resting) population of stem cells into the cell cycle. The equilibrium between the number of cells in division and those at rest, and the requirement for controls on such growth, are important. Some of the controls are understood, whereas others are unknown.

The stem cell theory also describes neoplastic growth. The clonality of many tumors such as epithelial ovarian cancer suggests that tumors originate from single stem cells. Therefore, tumors may consist of a small percentage of stem cells that due to failed growth control mechanisms continuously provide malignant cells. Based on this assumption, any therapeutic intervention should target this stem cell population to avoid recurrences.

Cell-Kill Hypothesis

The fundamental kinetic consideration in cancer chemotherapy is the cell-kill hypothesis, which states that the effects of cancer chemotherapy on tumor cell populations demonstrate first-order kinetics; ie, the proportion of tumor cells killed is a constant percentage of the total number of cells present. In other words, chemotherapy kills a constant proportion of cells, not a constant number of cells. The number of cells killed by a particular agent or combination of drugs is proportional to one variable: the dose used. The relative sensitivity of cells is not considered, and the growth rate is assumed to be constant.

Since chemotherapy follows an exponential (log-kill) model, treatment may be said to have a specific exponential, or log-kill, potential. For example, a log kill of 2 reduces a theoretical human tumor burden of 10^9 cells to 10^7 cells. Although this represents a reduction of 99%, at least 10 million (10^7) viable cells remain. A log kill of 3 achieves a reduction of 99.9%, but 1 million (10^6) cells remain. Theoretically, therefore, such fractional reductions by antineoplastic agents can never reduce a tumor cell population to zero. This traditional cell-kill model is based mainly on exponentially growing tumors in laboratory models, eg, L-1210 murine leukemia.

Although the cell-kill hypothesis probably explains some aspects of drug selectivity, other mechanisms are involved. The more responsive tumors are those with large growth fractions. Normal tissue can withstand greater cell loss due to chemotherapy than can tumors, although the proportion killed in both systems may be identical.

Another theory states that clinical tumor regression as a result of chemotherapy is best explained by the relative growth fraction in the tumor at the time of treatment. Thus very small and very large tumors are less responsive than those of intermediate size, which have the biggest growth fraction. Therefore, log kills occur only at times of maximal tumor growth fraction. Although this hypothesis has not been directly confirmed clinically, it explains some clinical observations of responses to chemotherapy in large and small human tumors.

Gompertzian Model of Tumor Growth

Gompertz, a German insurance actuary, depicted the relationship of an individual's age to the expected time of death by means of an asymmetric sigmoid curve. This mathematical model approximates tumor proliferation in experimental systems wherein tumors initially grow rapidly. As the tumor increases in size, a plateau effect develops, and the apparent doubling time is much longer than at the beginning.

Figure 52–2 demonstrates several current chemotherapeutic principles plotted against a Gompertzian tumor growth curve and the large tumor cell burden required to produce clinical expression of symptoms. The minimum palpable subcutaneous lesion is about 60 mg and contains 6×10^7 cells. In superficial tumors, 1 cm^3 or 1 g of tumor is not an uncommon size at the time of diagnosis and contains about 10^9 cells, whereas most patients with visceral tumors of 10–100 g are estimated to have 10^{10}–10^{11} tumor cells at the time of diagnosis. Since death occurs with a tumor burden of 10^{12} cells, which is only 1–2 orders of magnitude less than the total number of cells in the human adult, a significant proportion of the life cycle of a clinically recognizable tumor has already transpired when it is finally detected. The importance of early diagnosis of malignant disease therefore becomes even more essential.

The outcome of the two chemotherapeutic treatment regimens, A and B; the influence of the fractional kill achieved by drug therapy; and the effect of volume of tumor at the onset of therapy are illustrated in Figure 52–2. Chemotherapy treatment A in a patient with a visceral solid tumor composed of 10^{11} cells achieves a good response when the tumor cell population is reduced by the characteristic percentage of first-order kill, regardless of the actual number of tumor cells present. Thus, an agent with a one-log cell kill reduces the cell concentration by 90% from a palpable 10-g mass to a nonpalpable 1-g mass and induces an apparently tumor-free state, yet a residual tumor burden remains that may contain more than 1 billion cells. After a brief delay, the remaining 10% of tumor cells resume their former rate of proliferation. After tumor cell repopulation has occurred, treatment again results in reduction of tumor volume, but resistance develops that results in death of the host at a predictable time.

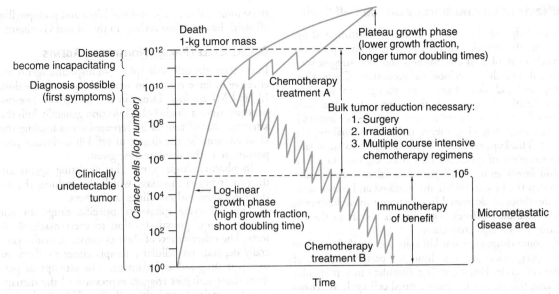

Figure 52–2. Gompertzian tumor growth curve. The model depicts the relationship between tumor growth and diagnosis, appearance of symptoms, and various treatment regimens.

Although normal tissues do not develop resistance to antitumor drugs, the larger the initial tumor volume and the smaller the fractional kill, the more likely is the development of resistance in tumor cells. The effect of successive drug doses in sensitive tumors depends on the number of existing cells when treatment is begun, the fractional kill, the number of cells surviving the preceding treatment, and the tumor cell production between treatment cycles. Obviously, cell destruction must exceed cell production for chemotherapy to be successful.

Nonlethal damage to cells can occur due to chemotherapy and is well known after radiation therapy. A key principle of theory, therefore, is to schedule chemotherapy, radiation therapy, or both at appropriate intervals to allow normal cells to recover from nonlethal damage but to preclude the recovery of tumor cells, which is slower. It is important that the interval between treatments be reduced to the bare minimum required for restoration and recovery of normal tissues.

In chemotherapy treatment B, repeated doses of a chemotherapeutic agent are used to destroy a large tumor cell population. Such consecutive log-kill reductions cannot be consistently achieved because the cell-kill potential of a drug is limited in comparison with the size of the tumor cell population in most clinical situations; however, in Figure 52–2, a reduction of a 10^{10} (10 billion) cell population by 90% as a result of a single course of drug therapy produces complete clinical remission. Repeated treatment at shorter intervals may result in enhanced destruction of tumor cells as long as toxic effects remain tolerable and resistant cell lines are not selected out by the drug. A drug becomes curative once the tumor cell kill exceeds the order of magnitude of repopulation and (statistically) less than one tumor cell remains. Additional courses of drug therapy are required to eradicate the last surviving cell of the so-called exponential iceberg if each course kills the same fraction of cells and not the same number.

On the other hand, fewer cycles of chemotherapy may produce a tumor-free host if subclinical tumor containing only 10^4 cells is present at diagnosis. Unfortunately, the usual inability to detect tumors so early in clinical situations makes this model less realistic.

Alternatively, the tumor population may be reduced by surgery or radiation so that subsequent adjuvant chemotherapy has a rational basis. Initial theapy for many solid tumors involves surgery or irradiation to reduce tumor bulk. Adjuvant chemotherapy, immunotherapy, or both are added as appropriate to eradicate micrometastatic or subclinical tumor masses. The same general principle guides therapy of hematologic cancer, in which intensive induction chemotherapy is used to achieve reduction of tumor bulk and induce remission; less intensive consolidation and remission maintenance doses of chemotherapy are then used to control subclinical tumor burdens.

Effects of Chemotherapy on the Cell Cycle

Knowledge of the site of action of antitumor drugs within the mitotic cell cycle may help to explain the mechanism of their effectiveness and may suggest ways to enhance their carcinostatic properties. Chemotherapy and radiation therapy are thought to alter the proliferation kinetics of both tumor and normal cells. Initially, individual sensitive cells are killed or incapacitated, thereby leaving a more resistant residual population. This large reduction in tumor cell mass stimulates recruitment of quiescent cells from G_0 into G_1. This shift favors an increased growth fraction in the tumor, so that the LI and the MI are increased and tumor doubling times are decreased (ie, the tumor mass doubles in less time than before). The effect is a shift to the left along the Gompertzian curve.

Some drugs may not kill cells but can halt or slow the progression of a cell through a particular phase of the cell cycle. Because cells accumulate in a particular phase, this process has been termed **cell cycle synchronization.** Generally, these effects occur at lower doses than those necessary for cell killing. Blockage may be either temporary or permanent and does not occur predictably in all cell populations treated.

The effects of various classes of anticancer agents on tumors depend on the basic events occurring in the 4 main phases of the cell cycle and the pharmacologic mechanisms of drug action, and these cytotoxic effects influence the design of rational drug regimens. Two basic classes of antineoplastic drugs are recognized: cell cycle (phase)-specific agents and cell cycle (phase)-nonspecific agents.

A. CELL CYCLE (PHASE)-SPECIFIC DRUGS

Cell cycle (phase)-specific drugs are much more effective in tumors in which a large proportion of cells are actively dividing, as occurs when the cell mass is low. The major cytotoxic activities of anticancer drugs in this class are manifested during a particular phase of the cell cycle, and these drugs are technically **phase-specific** rather than **cycle-specific** agents. These drugs have been termed **schedule-dependent** agents because they produce a greater cell kill if the drug is given in multiple, repeated fractions rather than as a large single dose.

In pharmacologic terms, these cell cycle (phase)-specific agents are most often described as antimetabolites, because each drug causes some type of unique biochemical blockade of a particular reaction that occurs in a single phase of the cell cycle.

Most cell cycle (phase)-specific agents, such as methotrexate and fluorouracil, exert their most significant effects in the S phase. Corticosteroids and asparaginase appear to be most active in G_1, bleomycin appears to be most active in G_2, and the *Vinca* and podophyllin alkaloids have marked activity in the M and G_2 phases.

B. CELL CYCLE (PHASE)-NONSPECIFIC AGENTS

In contrast, the cell cycle (phase)-nonspecific agents are effective in large tumors in which the growth fraction, LI, and MI are low. Drugs in this group are dose-dependent, since a single bolus injection generally kills the same number of cells as do repeated doses totaling the same amount; ie, the degree of cell kill is directly proportionate to the absolute dose given.

In pharmacologic terms, the alkylating agents are the prototypes of this class, which also includes the nitrosoureas, the anthracyclines, and others.

The cell cycle (phase)-nonspecific drugs do not require a large growth fraction to exert maximal effects. The effectiveness of their cytotoxic activities generally depends on cellular attempts either to divide or to repair drug-induced damage. The attempt to perform these activities triggers expression of the damage already sustained, and the cell dies. This mechanism of cell death is important, since cancer cells in G_0 (resting phase) are not generally susceptible to cytotoxic agents, with the possible exception of the cell cycle (phase)-nonspecific mustard-type alkylators and the nitrosoureas.

Selectivity of Anticancer Drugs

There is a common belief that cancer chemotherapy is generally nonselective and kills normal as well as cancerous tissues. However, most anticancer drugs are more active against tumor than normal tissues. The cell-kill hypothesis probably explains some drug selectivity, but other mechanisms are involved as well. The selectivity of cytotoxic agents appears to correlate inversely with cell cycle specificity, since cell cycle (phase)-nonspecific agents such as the nitrosoureas and mechlorethamine (an alkylator) tend to be more toxic in normal bone marrow than in tumor cells. The selectivity of most antitumor drugs must still be based largely on differences in the cell kinetics of normal and neoplastic cell lines. Normal systems can withstand greater cellular losses due to chemotherapy than can tumors, even though the proportion of cells killed in both might be identical. Recovery from damage produced by a tumor-inhibiting drug may be more protracted in tumor cells than in normal host cells. Increased antitumor selectivity can be provided by the judicious use of a second dose of drug following return of normal tissue function but before recovery of tumor cell function. This approach to selective recovery from chemotherapeutic damage may provide enormous benefit by enhancing the antitumor activity of presently available drugs.

Most agents are equally effective at key enzymatic sites in either normal or neoplastic cells, but some anticancer drugs kill cancer cells by taking advantage of unique biochemical differences in the cancer cells; eg, the enzyme asparaginase takes advantage of a relative deficiency of aspartic acid synthetase in some leukemic cells to cause cell death. Cancer cells demonstrate a selective uptake of high concentrations of methotrexate, and this selectivity can be experimentally enhanced by vincristine or asparaginase and inhibited by aminoglycosides and cephalosporins.

Sensitivity to drugs based on the type of tissue is recognized in some anticancer agents; eg, the antimetabolite fluorouracil is more active in neoplasms arising from endodermal tissues such as the gastrointestinal tract and the breast. Dacarbazine has some selective action for melanoma cells, and bleomycin is active against epithelial tumors such as squamous cell cancers of the lung and cervix. When a tumor is derived from an organ characterized by a distinct biochemical feature (eg, the thyroid gland's ability to accumulate iodine, the sensitivity of the adrenal cortex to mitotane, or the selective destruction of the pancreatic islet cells by streptozocin), chemotherapy can be devised that attacks that tumor preferentially.

Although individual differences between the cells of a particular tumor and normal cells have been discovered, no single biochemical feature has been detected that pertains exclusively to one or the other. Studies suggest numerous possibilities for exploiting small quantitative differences between tumor and normal tissue. These include selective uptake of drugs into tumors, enhanced anabolism in tumors of "pro-drugs" requiring activation, diminished catabolism of drugs by tumors, diminished repair of tumor cell damage, and reduced availability of a protecting metabolite in tumor tissue.

Chemotherapy Resistance of Cancer Cells

One of the major problems in the treatment of cancers with chemotherapeutic agents is the development of drug resistance. According to the Goldie-Coldman hypothesis, most mammalian cells start with intrinsic sensitivity to antineoplastic agents but subsequently develop resistance at variable rates. This model has important clinical implications; tumors are only curable if no resistant cell lines are present or develop during the course of chemotherapy. To minimize the development of drug resistance, multiple drug regimens are preferred to single drug therapies.

Development of resistance is mainly based on the occurrence of spontaneous mutations which occur at a frequency of 1 in 10,000 to 1 in 1,000,000 cells. Mechanisms of drug resistance involve decreased cellular uptake or increased efflux of the chemotherapeutic agents

via cellular pumps, decrease in drug activation, increase in drug degradation, inactivation of active metabolites by binding to sulfhydryl compounds, increase in DNA repair mechanisms, or increase in level of target enzyme (dihydrofolate reductase). Several genes have been implicated in drug resistance, eg, the multiple drug resistance (MDR) gene. Gene therapy approaches are currently being studied to reverse drug resistance in tumor cells. Alternatively, the transfer of drug resistance genes into normal cells like bone marrow cells might confer increased protection to chemotherapeutic agents and possibly allow a dose increase.

Poor Host Defenses

The normal individual's immunologic defenses against an invading tumor cell population are unreliable and still poorly understood. They operate only if the tumor mass is relatively small, and they become less effective as the person ages. As tumor growth progresses, the body's diminishing immunocompetence compounds the difficulties of therapy. A complicating factor is the immunosuppressant properties of most antitumor drugs. Treatment schedules to minimize immunosuppression while permitting adequate therapeutic effectiveness should be more intensive but actually must be practiced sparingly because of the lack of antitumor selectivity. Current studies are attempting to enhance immunologic host defenses by immunostimulation with reagents such as bacille Calmette-Guérin (BCG) or *Corynebacterium parvum* and by restoration of immunocompetence with agents such as levamisole, thymosin, or interferon, as well as with combinations of two or more kinds of immunotherapy. Cyclophosphamide at low doses can stimulate CD4$^+$ helper cells and has been used in clinical immunotherapy trials in conjunction with immunostimulatory cytokines.

Protected Tumor Sanctuaries

Antitumor drugs frequently fail to reach all sites of tumor cells, and so-called "sanctuaries" may exist that permit the establishment and unimpeded proliferation of a tumor once it has been successfully eradicated from the remainder of the body. Sanctuaries may develop because of the metastatic spread of tumors to distant sites, and the problem may be accentuated by a lack of knowledge regarding the mechanism of drug access to such secondary neoplasms and their susceptibility to various drugs.

The central nervous system is impermeable to many drugs and often represents such a protected site. Attempts to reach sequestered cells have included intrathecal administration of drugs or use of more highly lipid-soluble drugs capable of rapidly penetrating the blood–brain barrier. The success of peripheral chemotherapy in the leukemias is due in part to the ease with which high levels of drug can be achieved in tumor cells; on the other hand, leukemic cells that have penetrated the central nervous system are no longer affected by most drugs, and disease progresses.

A more common problem, however, is the diminished blood supply in many solid tumors that blocks delivery of antitumor drugs to the tumor core, which, although necrotic, may still contain active cells sensitive to antitumor drugs. It should be remembered that high doses of radiation (as used in the primary treatment of many gynecologic cancers) produce vascular damage leading to the formation of ischemic sanctuaries for cells that might otherwise be sensitive to drug treatment.

Secondary Malignancies

Antineoplastic agents have the potential to induce secondary malignancies. The alkylating agent melphalan is associated with a cumulative 7-year risk of acute non-lymphocytic leukemia in 9.6% of patients treated for more than 1 year. The development of acute leukemia is also associated with combined chemotherapy and radiation. Secondary malignancies usually occur between 4 and 7 years after successful therapy.

Route of Administration

Chemotherapeutic drugs can be administered orally, intravenously, intramuscularly, or intra-arterially. The particular localization of gynecologic tumors has led to the development of intraperitoneal and intrapleural chemotherapy regimens. Pleural and intraperitoneal clearance of the agent is usually slower than plasma clearance, leading to prolonged and increased concentrations of the drug. Clinical trials in ovarian cancer have used intraperitoneal cisplatin and paclitaxel with significantly improved survival compared to systemic chemotherapy. The treatment is usually well tolerated. Frequent local side effects include peritoneal irritation with abdominal discomfort and complications related to the intraperitoneal administration, such as infection at the catheter site. Systemic side effects were unexpectedly reported to be worse with intraperitoneal treatment. An ongoing study by the Gynecologic Oncology Group is currently evaluating the effect of systemic paclitaxel combined with intraperitoneal cisplatin and paclitaxel therapy.

Principles of Clinical Chemotherapy

The chief aim of therapy is to achieve maximum cell kill with minimum toxicity. To this end, the dose and schedule of drugs critically influence the therapeutic index. The steep dose–response curve for most drugs indicates that the highest tolerable dose producing an acceptable degree of reversible toxicity should be used in the treatment of sensitive tumors, in which a twofold increase in dose may produce a tenfold increase in the fractional kill.

Therapy must also take into account the length of time a therapeutic concentration of drug is maintained. The maximal effectiveness of some oncolytic drugs depends mainly on peak tissue concentration, whereas that of others depends on the duration of exposure.

In principle, a therapeutic concentration of the cell cycle (phase)-specific drugs is best maintained by 5-day courses of treatment (about 2 average cell generation times). Such prolonged exposure permits a higher fraction of proliferating cells to pass through vulnerable phases of the cell cycle, since proliferating cells do not progress through the cell cycle in a synchronized fashion. In contrast, the cell cycle (phase)-nonspecific drugs are best administered as an intravenous bolus of the highest tolerable dose, and the dose repeated when normal target tissues have recovered.

High-dose, intermittent therapy has been the most successful schedule against tumors with a large growth fraction. Slow-growing tumors have a large component of permanently nondividing cells and a small growth fraction. Theoretically, drugs active against cells in G_0 and given on a continuous basis should produce the best results in these tumors.

Chronic therapy is feasible only if toxicity is negligible. Some myelosuppression is acceptable, since recovery occurs between treatment cycles. Immunosuppression is a side effect of most cytotoxic drugs and is more pronounced when drugs are given continuously.

Antitumor drugs have been combined concurrently or sequentially in an effort to increase their effectiveness. It is logical to assume that drugs with different dose-limiting toxicities and different modes of action may increase the fractional cell kill without a parallel rise in damage to normal tissues and immunocompetent cells. Since tumors are composed of numerous cell clones that vary in their sensitivity to drugs, the use of multiple agents should lessen the chance of development of resistance and repopulation of the tumor by a resistant cell clone. Sequential, concomitant, or complementary blockade of metabolic pathways should avoid the problem of drug resistance secondary either to the utilization of alternative pathways or the emergence of a protective random mutation.

As a rule, drugs selected for multidrug therapy must be effective as single agents if improved results are to be expected. Unfortunately, the toxicities of most antitumor drugs are similar, and selecting drugs that have no overlapping side effects is usually not possible. Nevertheless, combination chemotherapy has proved superior to single-agent therapy in leukemia, lymphoma, and some rapidly proliferating solid tumors including ovarian cancer.

In summary, successful drug therapy requires the administration of an effective agent using the best possible dose and schedule. The tumor must have a high growth fraction and must be accessible to drugs so that they can exert their antitumor effects (ie, cells must not be in tumor sanctuaries). The tumor volume must be small or the fractional cell kill large to avoid the emergence of a resistant cell clone or the development of tolerance in previously sensitive cell clones. Normal tissue must recover from drug injury faster than tumor can regenerate to pretreatment levels.

CANCER CHEMOTHERAPEUTIC AGENTS

Cancer chemotherapeutic agents are commonly classified into six general categories on the basis of their mechanism of action: alkylating agents, antimetabolites, plant alkaloids, miscellaneous agents, hormonal agents, and immunotherapeutic agents. This section presents a broad overview of the mechanism of action and general toxicities of the four major groups of cytotoxic cancer chemotherapy drugs.

Alkylating Agents

A. CLASSIC ALKYLATING AGENTS

The alkylating agents evolved from products developed for chemical warfare. The parent chemical, dichloroethyl sulfide (sulfur mustard), was first synthesized during the mid-19th century and used during World War I because of its blistering properties on skin and mucous membranes. These agents also produced atrophy of lymphoid and myeloid tissues, a finding that led workers to explore their use in treating lymphomas and leukemias.

The 3 chemical subgroups of classic alkylating agents in use today are (1) the bis(chloroethyl)amines, which include chlorambucil, cyclophosphamide, ifosfamide, mechlorethamine, melphalan, and uracil mustard; (2) the ethylenimines, which include triethylenethiophosphoramide (thiotepa); and (3) the alkylsulfonates, which include busulfan and improsulfan hydrochloride.

Alkylating agents induce cytotoxic effects on cells by binding to DNA, particularly at the N-7 position of guanine. This binding interferes with correct base pairing and produces single- and double-stranded DNA breaks. DNA replication in S phase is consequently inhibited. In addition to these cytotoxic and mutagenic effects, alkylating agents also inhibit cellular glycolysis, respiration, and synthesis of various enzymes, protein, and nucleic acids.

Most alkylating agents are cell cycle (phase)-nonspecific drugs that are active against both resting and dividing cells; they may therefore be used effectively in tumors with a small growth fraction. Cyclophosphamide is unique in that it appears to inhibit DNA synthesis in certain tumors and may therefore have some cell cycle (phase) specificity in the S phase not possessed by the other alkylating agents.

The major toxicities associated with the classic alkylating agents are related to their cytotoxic effects, although each drug has its own unique side effects. Normal tissues most affected are those with a rapid growth rate, eg, the hematopoietic system, the gastrointestinal tract, and gonadal tissue. Nausea and vomiting occur with use of most of these agents, particularly with the intravenous route, and may result from a direct effect on the chemoreceptor trigger zone in the medulla. If extravasation of mechlorethamine occurs during administration or if skin or mucous membranes are exposed to this agent, tissue necrosis develops, and sloughing will occur later, producing a slow-healing ulcer. The myelosuppression associated with classic alkylating agents is mainly a leukopenia, with the lowest cell counts occurring in 10–14 days and recovery occurring in 21–28 days. Busulfan and chlorambucil have slightly more prolonged myelosuppressive effects. Bone marrow depression causes the most serious complications of therapy associated with the alkylating agents; patients are at increased risk for bleeding episodes due to thrombocytopenia and infection due to leukopenia. Anemia from depressed levels of erythrocyte production occurs less frequently.

B. NITROSOUREAS

The nitrosoureas include carmustine (BCNU), lomustine (CCNU), semustine (methyl CCNU), estramustine, streptozocin, and chlorozotocin. Although nitrosoureas probably act mainly as alkylating agents, they may also cause the inhibition of several key enzymatic steps necessary for the formation of DNA. The cytotoxic activity of these drugs is thought to be mediated through the action of metabolites that can alkylate DNA. Like other alkylating agents, the nitrosoureas are cell cycle (phase)-nonspecific. The nitrosoureas are lipid-soluble and cross the blood–brain barrier. These agents may undergo some enterohepatic circulation, but they are rapidly metabolized. The largest fraction of these drugs is excreted in the urine as metabolites, with only a small fraction excreted in the active form. Streptozocin is a naturally-occurring nitrosourea that is particularly useful in the treatment of insulinomas because of its marked specificity for pancreatic B and exocrine cells.

The major adverse reaction associated with the nitrosoureas is a notable delayed and dose-dependent depression of the hematopoietic system occurring with commonly used dosage levels. In contrast to the classic alkylating agents, maximal depression of the white cell count occurs in 3–5 weeks with use of the nitrosoureas; it may persist for several weeks or longer. Severe nausea and vomiting may limit the dosage that can be given. Pain at the injection site is associated with the use of carmustine.

C. ANTITUMOR ANTIBIOTICS

The antitumor antibiotics are products of microbial fermentation and include the anthracyclines and the chromomycins. Although most antitumor antibiotics exert some antimicrobial properties, the cytotoxic effects of these agents generally preclude their use as such.

1. Anthracyclines—The anthracyclines include daunorubicin, doxorubicin, and rubidazone. These drugs effectively interfere with nucleic acid synthesis and block DNA-directed RNA and DNA transcription. The anthracyclines are probably effective in all phases of the cell cycle and are therefore cell cycle (phase)-nonspecific.

Disposition kinetics of the anthracyclines are complex. Their half-life is relatively long, ranging from 15 hours to several days for doxorubicin. These drugs are extensively metabolized in the liver, and some of the metabolites retain antitumor activity. Biliary excretion appears to be the major means of elimination, but a small portion of drug is excreted in the urine.

Many of the adverse effects of the anthracyclines are similar to those of the alkylating agents. Acute toxicity is manifested as bone marrow depression that may be severe enough to require limiting of dosage; the nadir usually occurs in 10–14 days, with recovery by 21 days in most patients. The anthracyclines also produce tissue necrosis and sloughing if extravasation occurs during intravenous injection. A unique cardiomyopathy has been observed when high cumulative doses of the anthracyclines have been administered.

2. Chromomycins—Another group of antitumor antibiotics is the chromomycins, which include chromomycin A_3, mithramycin (plicamycin), and dactinomycin. All act similarly to block DNA-directed RNA synthesis by intercalating and anchoring in DNA, as do the anthracyclines. Bone marrow depression due to use of chromomycins is a significant but usually not dose-limiting toxicity characterized by thrombocytopenia with some leukopenia.

Chromomycin A_3 (Toyomycin) is rapidly cleared from plasma, is excreted via the urinary and biliary tracts, and causes nausea and vomiting, renal toxicity, and severe local reactions at the injection site.

Mithramycin crosses the blood–brain barrier and is well distributed in the cerebrospinal fluid. It is excreted mainly in the urine. Gastrointestinal effects include nausea and vomiting, anorexia, and diarrhea. Liver and kidney toxicity is common. A toxicity unique to this agent is a hemorrhagic syndrome heralded by facial flushing. Mithramycin has been used to lower serum calcium levels in patients with hypercalcemia.

Dactinomycin is rapidly cleared from serum and is excreted mainly in the bile with minimal biotransformation. Gastrointestinal effects include mucositis characterized by oral ulceration. Nausea and vomiting may be severe enough to limit the dosage. Other toxicities include bone marrow depression and alopecia.

3. Other antitumor antibiotics—Other antitumor antibiotics include mitomycin, piperazinedione, and bleomycin. Mitomycin probably functions as an alkylating agent by causing cross-linking of DNA. Mitomycin is rapidly cleared from the vascular compartment and is found in most body tissues except the brain; it is excreted via the kidneys and in bile. Delayed bone marrow depression may occur, with the nadir occurring 3–5 weeks after administration. Myelosuppression may be more severe with repeated doses and is the major dose-limiting toxicity. Renal toxicity may be observed, whereas gastrointestinal effects and alopecia occur less frequently.

Piperazinedione appears to function as an alkylating agent by inhibiting the incorporation of several DNA nucleotides into DNA synthesis. Although cell progression through G_2 is delayed, piperazinedione is probably not cell cycle (phase)-specific. Myelosuppression is the major dose-limiting toxic effect and is manifested as granulocytopenia followed by thrombocytopenia, with the nadir and recovery from myelosuppression varying by patient. The level of activity against neoplasms resistant to alternative alkylating agents and antimetabolites has not been high enough to warrant expanded clinical trials.

Bleomycins are antineoplastic antibiotics produced by fermentation of *Streptomyces verticillus*. More than a dozen fractions have been isolated, but the major constituent of commercially available preparations is bleomycin A_2. Inasmuch as the exact composition of the drug may vary, the drug is rated in units of activity. Bleomycin contains DNA- and ion-binding moieties. The mechanism of action most likely involves the production of single- and double-stranded breaks leading to inhibition of DNA synthesis, and to a lesser extent inhibition of RNA and protein synthesis. Bleomycin is cell cycle (phase)-specific for mitosis and G_2. This cycle specificity has been useful experimentally to achieve cell cycle synchronization in combination chemotherapy. Bleomycin appears to exert much less myelosuppressive activity than most other antineoplastic drugs and is therefore useful in patients who already have depressed bone marrow counts. Cutaneous reactions are dose-related and include hyperpigmentation, edema, erythema, and thickening of the nail beds. They are the most common side effects because the drug is concentrated in the skin. The most serious toxicity is pneumonitis related to the total dose received; the disease is characterized by dyspnea, rales, and infiltrates that progress to fibrosis. A high incidence of hypersensitivity reactions ranging from fever and chills to anaphylaxis is also associated with bleomycin.

Antimetabolites

The antimetabolites exert their major activity during the S phase and therefore are most effective against tumors that have a high growth fraction. The antimetabolites are structural analogs of naturally-occurring metabolites and interfere with normal synthesis of nucleic acids by substituting different compounds for the normal purines or pyrimidines in metabolic pathways. The antimetabolites are subdivided into the folate antagonists, the purine antagonists, and the pyrimidine antagonists.

A. FOLATE ANTAGONISTS

Methotrexate is a 4-amino-4-deoxy-N-methyl analog of folic acid and is the classic antimetabolite prototype. Methotrexate is a cell cycle (phase)-specific agent that exerts its cytotoxic effect in the S phase by binding to dihydrofolate reductase and thereby blocking the reduction of folic acid. Thymidine and purine synthesis are halted, thus arresting DNA, RNA, and protein synthesis. For maximal effect, intracellular levels of methotrexate must be sufficiently high to bind almost all of the dihydrofolate reductase, of which only small quantities are required to maintain adequate levels of the reduced folate pool. Resistance is thought to develop as a consequence either of increased levels of dihydrofolate reductase or of decreased cell uptake.

Methotrexate enters the cell through an active carrier-mediated cell membrane transport system that it shares with leucovorin calcium (folinic acid, citrovorum factor) and its metabolite, 5-methyltetrahydrofolate. When this transport system is functional in tumor cells, adequate intracellular levels of methotrexate are easily achieved. Because some tumors lack or have reduced transport capabilities, high levels of methotrexate are required to facilitate transport by a passive method instead. To limit toxicity, treatment requiring high doses of methotrexate is followed by "rescue" of normal cells with leucovorin calcium.

Another antifolate is ethane sulfonic acid compound, or Baker's antifol (triazinate). It is actively transported into the cell by a different transport carrier than is methotrexate, but the target enzyme is the same. Thus, these two antifolates may have different tumor specificity, even though their general mechanism of action is the same.

Both compounds produce bone marrow depression, with the lowest cell counts occurring in 7–14 days. Stomatitis and gastrointestinal distress are frequent. Skin rashes are common side effects of ethane sulfonic acid compound, but occur in fewer patients treated with methotrexate. Central nervous system abnormalities may also occur with either agent.

B. PURINE ANTAGONISTS

Mercaptopurine and thioguanine are analogs of the natural purines hypoxanthine and guanine. The purine antagonists have specific antitumor effects on the S phase.

Mercaptopurine acts as a false metabolite because of its close chemical similarity to hypoxanthine. It competes for the enzymes responsible for the conversion of inosinic acid to adenine and xanthine ribotides, and thus interferes with normal DNA and RNA synthesis. Simultaneous administration of allopurinol may block the metabolism of mercaptopurine and azathioprine by xanthine oxidase and require reduction of the dose to one-fourth or one-third the normal amount. This drug interaction does not occur with thioguanine, because its detoxification occurs by methylation.

Thioguanine also acts as a false metabolite; its substitution for the corresponding guanine nucleotide blocks purine synthesis.

The indications for use and efficacy of thioguanine and mercaptopurine are the same. Their toxicities are identical, and the two drugs are mutually cross-resistant.

Azathioprine is an imidazolyl derivative. It is used as an immunosuppressant but has cytotoxic properties similar to those of mercaptopurine and thioguanine because it is extensively metabolized to mercaptopurine.

The major dose-limiting toxicity of the purine antagonists is myelosuppression consisting mainly of leukopenia, with lesser effects on platelets and red blood cells. Gastrointestinal distress is common, and hepatotoxicity may occur with use of any of the purine antagonists.

C. PYRIMIDINE ANTAGONISTS

Fluorouracil (5-fluorouracil, 5-FU) is the classic antimetabolite. It is cell cycle (phase)-specific and inhibits the enzyme thymidylate synthetase to block DNA synthesis. It is catabolized in the liver by dihydrouracil dehydrogenase.

Two other closely related fluoropyrimidines, ftorafur and floxuridine (FUDR, 5-fluorodeoxyuridine), have recently been used in clinical trials.

Ftorafur is hydrolyzed to 5-FU in the liver and stomach and therefore may act as a depot form of 5-FU.

Fluorouracil and ftorafur cause myelosuppression that reaches a nadir in 1–14 days, but ftorafur appears to cause less myelosuppression, which may be due to its slower release of 5-FU. Both agents commonly produce gastrointestinal toxicities, including occasional glossitis and stomatitis. Neurotoxicities may also occur because these drugs cross the blood–brain barrier.

The cytidine and deoxycytidine analogs include cytarabine, cyclocytidine (ancitabine), and azacitidine. The active form of these nucleoside analogs stops DNA synthesis by competitively inhibiting DNA polymerase and production of deoxycytidine. Cytarabine is metabolized by cytidine deaminase in the liver, granulocytes, and gastrointestinal tract. Small amounts of cytarabine cross the blood–brain barrier. Because cyclocytidine is not inactivated by cytidine deaminase, it slowly releases the more active cytarabine, which prolongs plasma levels; cyclocytidine can therefore be regarded as a depot form of cytarabine that has a biphasic half-life occurring at 3–15 minutes and at 2 hours.

Cytarabine and cyclocytidine are active only in the S phase. Although azacitidine is most active during the S phase, it appears to exert activity in all phases of the cell cycle by inhibiting DNA, RNA, and protein synthesis. Although it has some cross-resistance with the other cytidine analogs, this is not complete. These facts suggest that azacitidine has an additional mechanism of action not found in cytarabine and cyclocytidine.

The toxicities of cytarabine, cyclocytidine, and azacitidine are similar to those of other pyrimidine antagonists and include myelosuppression and gastrointestinal abnormalities, which may be severe. Cytarabine produces a flu-like syndrome, and cyclocytidine commonly produces unusual jaw pain and hypotension.

Plant Alkaloids

A. VINCA ALKALOIDS

Although the periwinkle plant has a long history in folklore medicine, clinical research to evaluate its possible therapeutic effects was not begun until 1945; by 1958, several active alkaloids had been isolated, but to date, only vinblastine and vincristine have had extensive clinical use. Although they are quite similar chemically and structurally, vincristine and vinblastine have markedly different clinical activities and toxicities. The precise mechanism of action of these compounds is not clearly understood, but they appear to cause arrest of metaphase by crystallization of the microtubular spindle proteins. Vinca alkaloids may also inhibit nucleic acid and protein synthesis, but these effects become apparent only after high concentrations are reached. There appears to be no cross-resistance between the

Vinca alkaloids and radiation therapy, alkylating agents, or each other. The differences in their therapeutic spectrum, toxicity, and potency may be related to each drug's ability to enter different types of cells.

The dose-limiting toxicity of vinblastine and vindesine is bone marrow depression, manifested chiefly by leukopenia 4–10 days after administration, with recovery occurring within 10–21 days. Vincristine does not usually cause leukopenia and can be given with relative safety to leukopenic patients.

Neurotoxicity is a major dose-limiting effect of vincristine and vindesine but occurs infrequently with vinblastine. Vincristine neurotoxicity consists of peripheral neuropathy with loss of deep tendon reflexes, numbness, and eventually severe weakness. Cranial nerve palsies, vocal cord paralysis, and autonomic nervous system dysfunction, manifested as urinary retention, tachycardia, or gastrointestinal symptoms of constipation or paralytic ileus may occur. All of the Vinca alkaloids cause severe local necrosis if extravasation occurs, and vindesine may produce pain and phlebitis even without evidence of infiltration.

B. PODOPHYLLOTOXINS

The 2 podophyllotoxins presently used are semisynthetic compounds derived from the root of the mayapple plant. The mechanism of action of etoposide (VP-16) and teniposide (VM-26) is similar to that of Vinca alkaloids in that they cause a mitotic spindle toxicity resulting in arrest of metaphase. Podophyllotoxins prevent cells from entering mitosis, thereby causing an increase in the MI; at high concentrations, the drugs cause lysis of cells entering mitosis. They also suppress DNA synthesis and, to a lesser degree, RNA and protein synthesis. Thus both the Vinca alkaloids and podophyllotoxins are cell cycle (phase)-specific and exert their major activity in the M phase; they also demonstrate some activity in the G2 and S phases.

Etoposide and teniposide are extensively protein-bound and are mainly eliminated by biliary excretion, with some enterohepatic recirculation. Both drugs may cause severe hypotension if infused too rapidly. Other adverse effects include nausea and vomiting, diarrhea, alopecia, and phlebitis at the injection site. The podophyllotoxins produce mild bone marrow depression and leukopenia, with the nadir occurring from 3–14 days following therapy.

C. TAXANES

The taxanes, paclitaxel and docetaxel, are relatively novel antimitotic agents. Taxanes arrest cells at the G2/M phase of the cell cycle by preventing depolymerization of the microtubuli structure. The cells therefore are unable to divide and will eventually undergo apoptosis. Both taxanes have demonstrated significant activity against many solid tumors as single agents and in combination with other chemotherapeutic agents. In addition, taxanes have been used in combination with chemotherapy in a variety of cancers including non-small-cell lung cancer (NSCLC), cancers of the head and neck, and cancers of the gastrointestinal tract.

Paclitaxel has been used extensively in patients with gynecologic malignancies, particularly ovarian and endometrial cancer. Major side effects include bone marrow toxicity, hypersensitivity reactions, arthralgias, peripheral neuropathy, and alopecia.

Miscellaneous Agents

Cisplatin was the first inorganic compound to be used to treat human cancers. Crosslinking of DNA may be somewhat different from that of other alkylators, in that the interatomic distance is much smaller than with the traditional alkylating agents; this characteristic may account for some of the toxicity associated with cisplatin. Cisplatin is cell cycle (phase)-nonspecific and is excreted mainly unchanged in the urine. Adverse reactions include anaphylaxis, nausea and vomiting, nephrotoxicity, ototoxicity, and myelosuppression that is usually mild.

Carboplatin is a derivative of cisplatin with equal clinical efficacy. Compared to cisplatin, it causes more hematopoietic toxicity but less ototoxicity, neuropathy, and nephrotoxicity.

Dacarbazine was originally thought to be an antimetabolite but is now recognized as an alkylating agent that is activated in the liver and excreted in the urine. It has somewhat less bone marrow toxicity than standard alkylating agents but typically causes severe nausea and vomiting similar to that due to cisplatin.

Hexamethylmelamine does not act as an alkylating agent in vitro, although it is structurally similar to triethylenemelamine, which is an alkylator. Although the precise mechanism is unknown, it is possible that hexamethylmelamine is activated to an alkylating agent in vivo. Hexamethylmelamine is rapidly metabolized in the liver and excreted in the urine. Gastrointestinal, neurologic, and hematologic toxicities occur.

Hydroxyurea is cell cycle (phase)-specific for the S phase. In addition to holding cells in G_1, the drug exerts a lethal effect on cells in the S phase by inhibiting ribonucleotide reductase and DNA synthesis without interfering with RNA or protein synthesis. Hydroxyurea may also act as an antimetabolite in that incorporation of thymidine into DNA appears to be inhibited. The major adverse reactions are bone marrow depression, gastrointestinal disturbances, and rarely, dermatologic reactions and renal impairment.

Procarbazine appears to be cell cycle (phase)-specific for the S phase; it apparently interferes with DNA synthesis, but its exact mechanism of action is unclear. Oxidative breakdown products, hydrogen peroxide, formaldehyde, azoprocarbazine, and free hydroxyl radicals may be responsible for the characteristic chromosomal breakage observed after use of procarbazine. Procarbazine may demonstrate dangerous interactions with a number of other drugs. Adverse reactions include myelosuppression, a flu-like syndrome, and dermatologic and various central nervous system reactions.

Most normal cells possess the ability to synthesize the amino acid asparagine. Some tumor cells, such as those in acute lymphoblastic leukemia, do not possess this ability and require exogenous asparagine. Asparaginase converts asparagine to nonfunctional aspartic acid and thereby deprives the tumor cell of this crucial amino acid to block protein synthesis. Side effects include protein depletion and pancreatic and hepatic damage. Allergic reactions are frequent, since asparaginase is a biologic product obtained from bacteria.

Chemotherapy in Gynecologic Cancers

A. OVARIAN CANCER

Chemotherapy is standard in most ovarian cancers after initial surgery. Of all gynecologic malignancies, ovarian cancer responds best to chemotherapeutic regimens. A wide variety of antineoplastic drug regimens has been studied in the last two decades to determine the optimal choice of drugs, route, and timing of administration.

Before the introduction of the taxanes, chemotherapeutic regimens included a combination of cisplatin, cyclophosphamide, and doxorubicin. In 1989, the first drug in the taxane group, paclitaxel, showed response rates of 24% in platinum-resistant cancers. Further trials comparing cisplatin and cyclophosphamide with cisplatin and paclitaxel showed an improvement in survival with the latter regimen. Currently, systemic chemotherapy with a platinum-based drug (cisplatin or its derivative, carboplatin) and paclitaxel is the most commonly used drug regimen in ovarian cancer. In patients with hypersensitivity to paclitaxel, an alternative drug like cyclophosphamide or topotecan is substituted.

The treatment of refractory or recurrent ovarian cancer is less standardized. Patients that are resistant to platin-based regimens are likely to be resistant to other drugs. Agents that have shown effects in these clinical situations include the topoisomerase I inhibitor topotecan, etoposide, the semisynthetic taxane docetaxel, liposome-encapsulated doxorubicin, and gemcitabine. In general, these drugs show a 13–26% clinical response rate in cisplatin-refractory and recurrent ovarian cancer.

B. Endometrial Cancer

Chemotherapy in endometrial cancer is mainly confined to patients with advanced or recurrent metastatic disease. The most active single agents are doxorubicin, platinum-based regimens, and paclitaxel.

C. Cervical Cancer

Similarly to endometrial cancer, chemotherapy for cervical cancer plays a role mainly in the treatment of advanced or recurrent disease. Antineoplastic agents found to be effective in cervical cancer include platinum compounds, ifosfamide, and paclitaxel. Combinations of cisplatin with ifosfamide have shown response rates of up to 31%. In a series of recent clinical trials, the combination of platinum-based chemotherapy with radiation has shown increased survival rates in cervical cancer in early-stage disease. Patients with bulky stage IB cervical cancer showed significantly prolonged survival and disease-free intervals when preoperative radiation was combined with cisplatin chemotherapy.

REFERENCES

Christian J, Thomas H: Ovarian cancer chemotherapy. Cancer Treat Rev 2001;27:99.

Keys HM et al: Cisplatin, radiation, and adjuvant hysterectomy compared with radiation and adjuvant hysterectomy for bulky stage IB cervical carcinoma. N Engl J Med 1999; 15:1154.

Lehne G: P-glycoprotein as a drug target in the treatment of multidrug resistant cancer. Curr Drug Targets 2000;1:85.

SECTION VI
Reproductive Endocrinology & Infertility

Infertility

53

Niloofar Eskandari, MD, & Mary Cadieux, MD

Definitions & Statistics

Infertility is generally defined as the inability of a couple to conceive within a certain period of time, usually 1 year. Infertility defies categorization as a single disease entity; there are few symptoms and few definitive tests. The goal of treatment is absolute—a successful delivery—so a sense of progress is seldom felt. Time is seen as the enemy and often the couple feels a sense of personal loss and frustration.

Sterility implies an intrinsic inability to achieve pregnancy, whereas infertility implies a decrease in the ability to conceive; infertility is synonymous with **subfertility. Primary infertility** applies to those who have never conceived, whereas **secondary infertility** designates those who have conceived at some time in the past. Approximately 90% of couples with unprotected intercourse will conceive within 1 year. **Fecundity** is the probability of achieving a live birth in 1 menstrual cycle. **Fecundability** is expressed as the likelihood of conception per month of exposure. In normal fertile couples having frequent intercourse, the chances of pregnancy are estimated to be approximately 20% per month.

The prevalence of infertility ranges from 7–28%, depending on the age of the woman. Sterility affects 1–2% of couples. An inverse relationship exists between fecundability and the age of the woman. The decline in fecundability begins in the early thirties and progresses rapidly in the late thirties and early forties. The number of infertility visits has increased in the last few decades. The reasons for the increase in attention given infertility are multiple.

Couples in some cases have voluntarily delayed childbearing in favor of establishing careers and may experience an age-related decline in fertility. In some cases the choice of prior contraceptive method may have contributed to infertility, as with the use of some intrauterine devices (IUDs); having an increased number of sexual partners leads to a greater potential for exposure to sexually transmitted diseases, which may contribute to infertility; and couples are less willing to simply accept childlessness and are increasingly aware of the available services and options for resolving infertility.

Both partners in a relationship contribute to potential fertility, and both may be subfertile. A primary diagnosis of a male factor (see section on Evaluation of Male Factors) is made in about 30% of infertile couples, and the man may be contributory in another 20–30%. An abnormality in the woman is responsible for the remaining 40–50% of cases.

A conscientious evaluation of the factors contributing to fertility usually indicates a probable cause in 85–90% of couples. It is important to remember that about 15% of normal fertile couples require more than 1 year to conceive and some of the "unexplained" causes of infertility may simply be a part of this normal 15%. The success rates of treatment for infertility depends on a variety of factors, including cause of infertility, woman's age, duration of infertility, and many times cost of treatment. Health insurance plans vary a great deal in the amount and type of infertility treatments that are covered. For those couples without infertility coverage, treatment choices are frequently dictated by financial rather than medical considerations. Many times infertility treatment does not actually make the difference between conceiving and not conceiving, but in sooner rather than later conception.

PSYCHOLOGIC ASPECTS OF INFERTILITY

Along with the increasing level of sophistication in evaluation and treatment of infertility has come a growing awareness of the psychologic consequences of this problem. When an anticipated conception fails to occur in a timely fashion, and a couple begins to consider infertility as a diagnosis that may pertain to them, their reactions can be intense and overwhelming. Self-images are threatened, sexuality can be affected, and feelings of adequacy may be destroyed; feelings of loss of control, anger, guilt, shame, and resentment can alter behavior and become contributing factors as relationships are threatened. As an individual or couple actually confronts infertility, they may progress through stages, including denial, anger, grief, and resolution. A recognition of these stages may assist the practitioner in providing appropriate support and counseling. Particularly when denial gives way to anger, the practitioner may be the recipient of the frustration, rage, or resentment expressed by couples in response to the results of tests or the failure of a proposed therapy. Insight into these profound reactions may assist partners in maintaining and strengthening their relationship, reaffirming the desirability of their mates, and preventing depression from becoming despair.

The advent of new therapies, while expanding the options for some, may open old wounds for others. Couples who had resolved their feelings about their infertility may feel obligated to explore new options when they hear of yet another treatment or technique. Infertility, even when secondary, remains a chronic reality, and honest advice about probabilities for success should be offered at frequent intervals to assist couples in maintaining an appropriate perspective.

It is known that participation in infertility evaluation and treatment can be one of the most stressful and devastating experiences in a couple's life. Often, feelings of grief and depression are present prior to the initiation of treatment. Treatment cycles often begin with high hopes and expectations and end with disappointment. Professional counseling should be offered and encouraged for all infertility patients, both to treat and prevent feelings of depression, and to address marital stability, financial security, psychological stability, social support, and coping strategies.

The feelings of grief experienced by many infertile couples may be exacerbated by well-meaning but hurtful advice from friends, relatives, and even strangers.

DIAGNOSIS OF INFERTILITY

The goals of the infertility evaluation are to determine the probable cause of infertility; to provide accurate information regarding prognosis; to provide counseling, support, and education throughout the process of evaluation; and to provide guidance regarding options for treatment. It is hoped that in the process of their infertility evaluation and treatment a couple may achieve their goal of a desired child; it is also hoped that they may benefit from a strengthened relationship, gain information about the causes of their difficulty, and achieve the certainty that all that could reasonably be done was done in an expeditious and conscientious manner.

The organization of the infertility evaluation is based on a consideration of the various individual factors required for successful reproduction. These factors are discussed in terms of whether they are male or female (ovulatory, pelvic, and cervical); a detailed list of male and female factors is contained in Table 53–1. The efficiency in completing the evaluation is determined in large part at the initial assessment visit, when the expenses, invasiveness, risks, and probabilities of significant findings of various procedures and tests are discussed. Reassessment will occur at intervals determined by the completion of various evaluations or the discovery of a contributing factor.

The Initial Assessment

The initial visit should be the opportunity to begin to accomplish several of the stated goals of the infertility evaluation. Participation of both partners is ideal and can assist the practitioner in assessing the dynamics of the relationship. Some determination of the couple's level of understanding of the problem and of their individual acceptance of the concept of infertility can be made.

The initial clinical assessment, while focusing on the history and physical status of the female partner, should also include the historical factors of importance that pertain to the male partner and to the couple. Important historical information beyond that obtained in a general medical history is outlined in Table 53–2 for the female and in Table 53–3 for the male.

General information regarding reproduction and the timing of events may assist in correcting any misunderstandings about coital frequency, and some myths regarding infertility may be dispelled. The timing of various investigative studies, which should be conducted within the framework of the work and life situation of the couple, can be discussed. In most cases, an initial basic investigation can be completed in 6–8 weeks. The aggressiveness of the approach taken should be agreed on and is determined by the age of the couple, any historical factors suggesting a cause of infertility, the affordability of various tests, and the availability of each partner for testing.

A realistic schedule of tests should be planned, and then an estimate of costs determined, with a discussion of their potential financial obligation and the variability

Table 53–1. Causes of infertility.

Male Factor	**Peripheral defects**
Endocrine disorders	Gonadal dysgenesis
Hypothalamic dysfunction (Kallmann's syndrome)	Premature ovarian failure
Pituitary failure (tumor, radiation, surgery)	Ovarian tumor
Hyperprolactinemia (drug, tumor)	Ovarian resistance
Exogenous androgens	Metabolic disease
Thyroid disorders	Thyroid disease
Adrenal hyperplasia	Liver disease
Anatomic disorders	Renal disease
Congenital absence of vas deferens	Obesity
Obstruction of vas deferens	Androgen excess, adrenal or neoplastic
Congenital abnormalities of ejaculatory system	**Pelvic Factor**
Abnormal spermatogenesis	Infection
Chromosomal abnormalities	Appendicitis
Mumps orchitis	Pelvic inflammatory disease
Cryptorchidism	Uterine adhesions (Asherman's syndrome)
Chemical or radiation exposure	Endometriosis
Abnormal motility	Structural abnormalities
Absent cilia (Kartagener's syndrome)	DES exposure
Varicocele	Failure of normal fusion of the reproductive tract
Antibody formation	Myoma
Sexual dysfunction	**Cervical Factor**
Retrograde ejaculation	Congenital
Impotence	DES exposure
Decreased libido	Müllerian duct abnormality
Ovulatory Factor	Acquired
Central defects	Surgical treatment
Chronic hyperandrogenemic anovulation	Infection
Hyperprolactinemia (drug, tumor, empty selia)	
Hypothalamic insufficiency	
Pituitary insufficiency (trauma, tumor, congenital)	

of insurance policies. After the anticipated time investment and expenses have been discussed, a planned consultation for evaluation of test results should be offered, so that a discussion of diagnoses and appropriate therapies can then be held. When a team approach to the infertility evaluation is utilized, the members of the team and their roles should be identified and the strategies for providing emotional support and counseling discussed. In many cases, the couple will be attempting to absorb significant amounts of information, some of which may be highly technical, at a time of heightened emotion. It is therefore helpful to offer literature or a written summary of the discussion and to plan a subsequent review of the information; this written summary and plan can form the basis for the chart note, which assists in maintaining a consistent approach.

Frequently, the initial history will indicate a probable diagnosis or a contributing cause of infertility, but it is important to complete a basic evaluation of all of the major factors so a secondary diagnosis is not ignored.

Evaluation of Male Factors

The initial evaluation of the male should include a general health history and a specific assessment of factors contributing to infertility, as listed in Table 53–3.

A. SEMEN ANALYSIS

A normal semen analysis will usually exclude a significant male factor. The male partner should abstain from coitus for 2–3 days before collecting the sample and the specimen should be received in the lab within 1 hour of collection. Normal values are given in Table 53–4. If fundamental parameters of count and motility are normal, the assessment of the morphology of the sperm becomes more critical. Specialized expertise in determining sperm morphology and strict application of criteria should be used before declaring the semen normal.

The semen parameters in normal fertile males may vary significantly over time, and the first response to any abnormal result should be to wait an interval of several

Table 53–2. Medical history for female factor infertility.

In utero DES exposure
History of pubertal development
Present menstrual cycle characteristics (length, duration, molimina)
Contraceptive history
Prior pregnancies, outcomes
Previous surgeries, especially pelvic
Prior infection
History of abnormal Pap smear, treatment
Drugs and medications
General health (diet, weight stability, exercise patterns, review of systems)

Table 53–4. Normal semen parameters.

Liquification	30 minutes
Count	20 million/mL or more
Motility	> 50%
Volume	2 mL or more
Morphology	≥ 30% normal
Strict criteria	> 14% normal
pH	7.2–7.8
WBC	< 1 million/mL

days to weeks and repeat the test. Although low counts, decreased motility, and increased numbers of abnormal forms are most frequently associated with infertility, unfavorable semen parameters may still be found in 20% of males undergoing vasectomy after having completed their families. If the semen analysis reveals abnormal or borderline parameters, the history should be reviewed for any proximate cause of an abnormality, keeping in mind that the cycle of spermatogenesis takes about 74 days. Abnormal parameters warrant further investigation and possible referral to a urologist with a special interest and expertise in infertility.

B. MUCUS STUDIES

The functional sperm must interact normally with the egg and surrounding cells in the uterine tube. The normal migration of sperm is affected by attrition and filtering, and it is estimated that less than 1000 sperm will be found in the environment of the oocyte. The initial interaction of sperm and female genital tract can be determined by postcoital examination of the cervical mucus (Sims-Huhner test).

Table 53–3. Medical history for male factor infertility.

In utero DES exposure
Congenital abnormalities
Prior paternity
Frequency of intercourse
Exposure to toxins
Previous surgery
Previous infections, treatment
Drugs and medications
General health (diet, exercise, review of systems)

The purpose of the postcoital test is to determine the number of active spermatozoa in the cervical mucus and the length of sperm survival (in hours) after coitus. The test should be performed in the late follicular phase, as close to ovulation as possible, the couple should abstain from intercourse for 2 days prior, and the lab should evaluate the mucus from 9–24 hours after coitus. The actual test involves aspirating cervical mucus with a syringe after coitus and checking under a microscope for the number and the motility of the sperm; less than 10 motile sperm per high-power field is considered abnormal. The postcoital test is a fairly common but controversial test in the infertility workup. Its value in assessing cervical hostility to sperm has never been proven and some argue that it leads to more tests and treatments, but has no effect on pregnancy rate.

Cervical mucus is a heterogeneous secretion containing over 90% water. It has intrinsic properties including consistency, spinnbarkeit (stretchability), and ferning. When mucus is obtained from the cervical canal in the preovulatory phase, it normally exhibits a response to the high estrogen environment. The mucus is thin, watery, and acellular; it dries in a crystalline pattern (ferning), and acts as a facilitative reservoir for the sperm. A satisfactory test results in large numbers of forwardly progressive sperm seen in thin, acellular mucus and indicates a healthy sperm-mucus interaction. Findings of few to rare sperm have been observed in cycles of conception and in many fertile couples serving as controls for studies of sperm-mucus interaction.

In cases of sufficient numbers of sperm seen with poor motility, an assessment of the quality of the mucus and timing of the test is critical to interpretation. When the mucus and timing appear favorable, but the sperm appear immobile, tests for autoantibodies in the male or serum antibodies in the female are appropriate. When the mucus is unfavorable in appearance or amount, the timing of the test should be investigated. Evaluation of a contributing female factor may also be necessary. Immediate feedback regarding the timing of the test can be obtained during an office visit by use of vaginal ultrasound to determine the presence or absence of a dominant follicle.

C. OTHER TESTS

When the initial evaluation of both partners does not reveal a probable cause of infertility or when repeated semen analyses are abnormal, the male factor can be investigated further. More detailed assessment of sperm function may include antibody studies, a sperm penetration assay (hamster egg penetration assay), or more sophisticated assessment of the sperm parameters previously described. Such assessments are designed to investigate more subtle problems or abnormalities of function not revealed by the assessment of sperm number and motility. Although helpful in some cases, the sensitivity of these assays in detecting fertility is still uncertain and varies with the particular laboratory where the test is performed. No universal methodology has yet been accepted, and consequently the interpretation of these tests requires close communication with the laboratory selected.

A test developed to predict the fertilizing ability of sperm is the zona-free hamster egg penetration test, also called the sperm penetration assay. This assay tests the ability of sperm to penetrate the zona-free hamster egg (a hamster egg in which the zona pellucida has been enzymatically digested) and compares it to sperm from a known fertile donor. The value of this test remains controversial and it is not generally used as part of the infertility evaluation. The hemizona test is yet another way to assess sperm functional capacity. Human zonae are exposed to the man's sperm, and the ability of the sperm to bind or penetrate the zona is measured and compared with that of a known fertile man. Clinical application has been limited, but hemizona assay results often correlate with in vitro fertilization (IVF) rates.

Sperm possess antigens and semen may contain antibodies including sperm-agglutinating, sperm-immobilizing, or cytotoxic antibodies. The antibodies can be measured in semen or in serum. The immunobead test is the antibody assay used in most labs, and is considered positive when only 20% or more of motile spermatozoa have immunobead binding. However, the test is considered to be clinically significant when 50% of sperm are coated with immunobeads.

In some cases, more detailed analysis of the sperm morphology, of the type of flagellar movement, or of the capacity for sperm to undergo the acrosome reaction can be assessed in special centers. Subtle abnormalities in these parameters may explain a previously undiagnosed cause of infertility.

The ultimate test of sperm function may occur with IVF, and this may be the last recourse for both diagnosis and attempted therapy for cases of poor sperm parameters or unexplained infertility. Failure to achieve fertilization in a cycle of IVF when an adequate number of apparently healthy mature fertilizable eggs are exposed to sperm may lead to an acceptance of the diagnosis of male factor infertility. The diagnosis is strengthened if a negative sperm penetration assay is obtained, and it is further substantiated if donor sperm are able to penetrate eggs when partner sperm has failed to do so.

Evaluation of Female Factors

A. OVULATORY FACTORS

An ovulatory dysfunction is responsible for approximately 20–25% of infertility cases. The problem should be investigated first by review of historical factors, including the onset of menarche; present cycle length (intermenstrual interval); and presence or absence of premenstrual symptoms (molimina), such as breast tenderness, bloating, or dysmenorrhea. Signs and symptoms of systemic disease, particularly of hyperthyroidism or hypothyroidism, and physical signs of endocrine disease (eg, hirsutism, galactorrhea, and obesity) should be noted. The degree and intensity of exercise, a history of weight loss, and complaints of hot flushes all are clinical clues to possible endocrine or ovulatory dysfunction.

If regular menses with molimina and mild dysmenorrhea occur at intervals of 28–32 days, and particularly if the patient notes reliable mittelschmerz, then the initial evaluation can focus on confirming ovulation with a serum progesterone assay performed in the mid-luteal phase, or the third week of the cycle. The value accepted as confirming ovulation must be determined in each endocrine laboratory. Using very specific assay reagents, the follicular-phase progesterone will be less than 1 ng/mL, and values from 3–10 ng/mL are consistent with ovulation having occurred, depending on the lab. In the case of oligomenorrhea, amenorrhea, or short or very irregular menstrual cycles, evaluation of the hypothalamic-pituitary-ovarian axis is warranted, beginning with determination of the serum concentrations of luteinizing hormone (LH), follicle-stimulating hormone (FSH), and prolactin.

In some women with delayed childbearing who are seeking evaluation in their fifth decade, an evaluation of the level of FSH and estradiol in the early follicular phase may provide helpful guidance in terms of the likelihood of achieving success, as mild elevations in either FSH or estradiol may precede overt ovulatory dysfunction but still indicate a poor prognosis for successful pregnancy. The specific cause of oligo-ovulation or anovulation is determined by the history, physical examination, and appropriate laboratory studies.

1. Follicular phase—If menstrual cycles are normal by history, but no cause for infertility is determined after completing the initial testing, a more detailed assessment of the normalcy of the cycle is indicated. The follicular phase can be examined with the assistance of vaginal ultrasound monitoring, so the development of a normal dominant follicle of adequate size can be detected. The dominant follicle usually is selected early in the follicular phase and can be detected by ultrasound around or before the 10th day of the cycle, with subsequent linear growth of about 1–2 mm per day, ultimately achieving a preovulatory size of 18–26 mm prior to rupture. The occurrence of ovulation can be suggested by the disappearance of, or change in, the preovulatory follicle and free fluid in the cul de sac. This change can be predicted by using either serum testing or home monitoring with commercially available urinary LH kits to detect the LH surge, which predicts the occurrence of ovulation within 24 hours. Ovulation occurs 24–36 hours after the onset of the LH surge and 10–12 hours after the peak of the LH surge. The LH surge affects the final maturation of the egg within the follicle, induces the preovulatory changes in the follicle that lead to rupture and extrusion of the egg in the cumulus mass, and initiates the luteinization of the granulosa cells.

2. Luteal phase—The luteal phase is characterized by the production of progesterone, and the clinical assessment of the luteal phase relies on determination of the adequacy of progesterone's effects. Indirect evidence of progesterone production can be determined by assessing the following biologic effects of progesterone.

a. Basal body temperature—The basal body temperature (BBT) is the temperature obtained in the resting state, and should be taken shortly after awakening in the morning after at least 6 hours of sleep and prior to ambulating. It is most easily obtained by use of a basal body thermometer that shows a wide range of a few degrees, usually 96–100 °F. Progesterone has a central thermogenic effect; when it is produced in sufficient concentrations, it causes the basal body temperature to become elevated. Usually, the rise represents a change of 0.5 °F during the luteal phase. The luteal phase is thus characterized by a temperature elevation lasting about 10 days. Some women exhibit a greater sensitivity to the thermogenic effect than others. When a biphasic monthly temperature pattern is recorded, it is confirmatory evidence of luteinization, but the absence of a biphasic pattern may be seen in ovulatory cycles. In some cases, use of an electric blanket or a heated waterbed may reduce the observed fluctuations. The BBT is not useful for predicting ovulation; instead it only confirms ovulation retrospectively. The exact day of ovulation is difficult to predict, but is likely 1 day before the temperature elevation, and no prediction of the adequacy of ovulation can be made based on the BBT

chart. For some couples, the daily ritual of taking morning temperatures can be a symbol of frustration since the information gained from BBT charts is usually more readily available by other means.

b. Endometrial sampling—The finding of secretory endometrium confirms ovulation. The use of an endometrial biopsy (EMB) near the end of the luteal phase can provide reassurance of an adequate maturational effect on the endometrial lining. Generally, the EMB is performed 2–3 days before the expected onset of menses. It can also be timed from the LH surge and the cycle day should be within 1–2 days of the pathologically diagnosed cycle day. The pathologist determines this by examination of the morphology of glands and stroma.

c. Premenstrual molimina—Premenstrual molimina are largely due to the cyclic hormonal influences of estrogen followed by progesterone with estrogen. The particular constellation of symptoms that affect each woman is usually fairly constant, so headaches, bloating, cramping, and emotional lability may be experienced differently, but often repetitively, by different women. When questioned, over 95% of ovulatory women can identify molimina associated with the premenstrual interval.

d. Mucus changes—Within 48 hours of ovulation, the cervical mucus changes under the influence of progesterone to become thick, tacky, and cellular, with loss of the crystalline fernlike pattern on drying.

The only absolute documentation of release of a fertilizable egg is the establishment of pregnancy. The production of progesterone, whether determined by clinical signs or by assay of serum concentration, is usually accepted as evidence of the luteinization of the follicle that normally follows the LH surge. The value of serum progesterone adequate to prepare and maintain the secretory endometrium, however, is difficult to determine by measurement.

The subject of the inadequate luteal phase remains an area of controversy. There is disagreement on how to make the diagnosis, when the diagnosis is significant, and how best to treat the problem if diagnosed. The diagnosis of luteal phase deficiency or defect requires a histologic diagnosis that lags 3 days or more behind the expected pattern at the time of EMB. Dating should be established using ultrasound for this purpose. Luteal phase defects have never been established as a cause of infertility and subjective interpretation of histology by pathologists further complicates this test. Treatment of luteal phase defect is also controversial; the use of progestogens, clomiphene citrate, and human chorionic gonadotropin (hCG) have been described but are not established. Women with repetitive short cycles, galactorrhea, persistent low levels of progesterone, or repeated out-of-phase endometrial biopsies should also have their serum prolactin level determined. Elevated prolactin secretion has been shown to be associated with luteal phase defects.

B. THE PELVIC FACTOR

1. **History and pelvic examination**—The pelvic factor includes abnormalities of the uterus, fallopian tubes, ovaries, and adjacent pelvic structures. Factors in the history that are suggestive of a pelvic factor include any history of pelvic infection, such as salpingitis or appendicitis, use of intrauterine devices, endometritis, and septic abortion. Endometriosis is included as a pelvic factor in infertility and may be suggested by worsening dysmenorrhea, dyspareunia, or previous surgical reports. Any history of ectopic pregnancy, adnexal surgery, leiomyomas, or exposure to diethylstilbestrol (DES) in utero should be noted as possibly contributory to the diagnosis of a pelvic factor. A transvaginal office ultrasound examination can be an efficient means of supplementing information gained from the standard bimanual examination. Hydrosalpinges, leiomyoma, and ovarian cysts and tumors can be often be observed, and the appropriate focused evaluations initiated sooner.

2. **Hysterosalpingogram**—After the pelvic examination, the evaluation of the pelvic factor usually begins with the hysterosalpingogram. Radiographic liquid dye is instilled into the uterine cavity using either a pediatric Foley catheter or a suction catheter passed through the cervical canal. After 3–5 mL of dye is instilled an image is obtained, and additional dye is added to fill the uterine tubes. The procedure is witnessed by the practitioner under image intensification—or key films are obtained by a radiologist skilled in the procedure—in order to determine the uterine contour, the patency of the tubes, and the ability of the dye to freely spill into the pelvis. Abnormal findings include congenital malformations of the uterus, submucous leiomyomas, intrauterine synechiae (Asherman's syndrome) intrauterine polyps, salpingitis isthmica nodosa, and proximal or distal tubal occlusion. The hysterosalpingogram can be obtained in an outpatient setting, with minimal analgesia consisting of premedication with an antiprostaglandin synthetase medication. The test is usually scheduled for the interval after menstrual bleeding and prior to ovulation. Either water-based dye or oil-based dye may be selected; the advantages and disadvantages of each are summarized in Table 53–5. Several studies have suggested a fertility-enhancing effect of the procedure that is more pronounced with the oil-based dye. On this basis, many practitioners inject oil-based dye, but only after confirmation of tubal patency with water-based dye.

Table 53–5. Comparison of oil-based versus water-based dye used in the hysterosalpingogram.

Fertility enhancement	Oil: higher pregnancy rates
Patient discomfort	Water: less cramping
Image quality	Water: rugae seen / Oil: better image
Embolization	Minimal risk with either dye
Granuloma	Greater risk for retained oil

If tubal patency is verified on the hysterosalpingogram and no infertility factor is identified, it is sometimes appropriate to allow an interval of several months without further therapy in order to capitalize on the benefit of the procedure. In studies of high-risk populations, an exacerbation of apparent preexisting salpingitis has been observed in 1–3% of women. For women with a history suggestive of salpingitis, a sedimentation rate may be obtained prior to the procedure—to decrease the likelihood of testing in the face of active disease—and a short course of broad-spectrum antibiotics is frequently advocated when tubal occlusion is demonstrated. The issue of universal antibiotic prophylaxis for hysterosalpingogram is controversial, but many practitioners routinely give doxycycline, 100 mg twice daily for 3 days, beginning the day before the study. A lack of correlation between the interpretation of the hysterosalpingogram and subsequent findings at laparoscopy has been reported in up to 35% of cases. A hysterosalpingogram is contraindicated in the presence of an adnexal mass or an allergy to iodine or radiocontrast dye. Dye embolization is rare and is usually preceded by dye intravasation, which can be seen during the procedure. If dye intravasation occurs, infusion of dye should be terminated.

Some studies investigating the use of ultrasonography instead of fluoroscopy to monitor the passage of injected fluid suggest that in some cases a diagnosis of tubal patency may be established without exposure to diagnostic radiation.

3. **Laparoscopy**—The information regarding the pelvic factor obtained with a hysterosalpingogram is complemented by a laparoscopy with dye instillation. When hysteroscopy is also done, supplementary information about the uterine contour can be obtained at the same time as the laparoscopy. Tubal abnormalities such as agglutinated fimbria or filmy adhesions (which restrict motion of the tubes) or peritubal cysts may suggest tubal disease that would not necessarily be detected

on hysterosalpingogram. The diagnosis of endometriosis is usually based on laparoscopic findings. Endometriosis may be suggested by the history but can be diagnosed only by laparoscopy or laparotomy. The association between endometriosis and infertility is strong, although the understanding of the mechanism by which the disease contributes to infertility is as yet poor. In some cases, significant anatomic distortion can result from the irritative foci of endometriosis leading to dense adhesions, but in other cases extensive disease may be present without significant compromise of pelvic structures, and the disease is an unexpected finding at laparoscopy.

The timing of the laparoscopy is one of the key aspects of the discussion of the pace at which the couple and the practitioner feel the investigation should proceed. In a young couple with a negative history, it is usually offered after all other tests are completed and discussed; in an older couple, or if the history suggests a pelvic factor, it is often indicated as one of the primary evaluations. In some patients with longstanding infertility, laparoscopy might be offered in conjunction with stimulation of the ovaries and ovum retrieval in order to combine the diagnostic potential with an attempt to achieve pregnancy. This may be done either by IVF, to confirm the ability of the eggs and sperm to interact, or by placing sperm and egg in the normal uterine tube to attempt normal transport to the uterus (see Chapter 56).

Documentation of the laparoscopic procedure, by either video or still photography, can be a valuable aid for the couple and may assist in determining subsequent therapy, particularly if referral to a consultant is indicated. With thoughtful preparation and discussion prior to the procedure, it is frequently possible to accomplish treatment of pathologic findings at the time of laparoscopy. Particularly if significant endometriosis is encountered, it may be possible to eliminate much of the disease at the time of diagnosis. If uterine abnormalities are encountered during hysteroscopy, they can be resected through the hysteroscope in some cases. The skill and training of the surgeon will determine the extent of intervention that can be offered, and this should be considered in discussion with the couple.

Laparoscopy is usually done in an outpatient surgery center with the patient under general anesthesia, although in some settings it is offered under local anesthesia with good results. The expense of the procedure, as well as the fact that it is the most invasive of the diagnostic strategies, are factors that may influence a couple's decision whether or not to progress to this step.

C. THE CERVICAL FACTOR

A cervical factor may be indicated by a history of abnormal Pap smears, postcoital bleeding, cryotherapy, conization, or DES exposure in utero. The major evaluation of the cervical factor is by physical examination and properly timed postcoital test. In some cases of apparently normal cervical mucus that repeatedly fails to yield reassuring numbers of sperm, a cross-check of donor sperm and donor mucus can be performed to determine the possible contribution of the cervical mucus as opposed to that of the sperm. The value of routine cervical cultures is controversial, and the role of infectious agents, such as *Chlamydia* and *Ureaplasma*, is not universally accepted, particularly when the organisms are identified in cervical or vaginal cultures.

Combined Factors & Unexplained Infertility

After completion of the basic evaluation, it is frequently necessary to repeat some of the initial tests in order to confirm abnormalities or accurately time some assessments. This can be frustrating for the couple and the investigator and requires careful communication regarding anticipation of progress. After all test results are available and interpretable, an opportunity exists for review and discussion of the factors contributing to infertility. A review of what has been found to be normal as well as any probable cause of subfertility should be presented. This will then permit a discussion of treatment options available (see text that follows), with an attempt to convey prognosis for success with each approach. Because infertility statistics are the result of population studies and are seldom derived from controlled comparisons, it is very difficult to give unbiased recommendations.

Often, certain treatments will have been popularized in the mass media without substantiation of benefit, and the practitioner may be pressured to participate in unproved therapies. The individual circumstances, including attitudes toward surgery, financial status, previous experiences, and reports from friends, may determine the choice of therapy. The costs of each possible option, in terms of time and energy, required visits, side effects, loss of intimacy, and expense, should be presented. In some cases seeking a second opinion might be suggested, so that the couple may feel comfortable with the therapeutic choices they have made and ready for whatever degree of commitment is required.

In about 20% of couples, combinations of factors will have been found to be suboptimal, and multiple therapies need to be arranged, either sequentially or simultaneously. Perhaps the most disheartening situation confronting a couple may be when the initial evaluation has been completed and no diagnosis made. When this occurs, a review of more subtle causes of infertility is appropriate, and additional testing should be described and offered. For the couple with unexplained infertility, the options for testing may seem endless, and a discussion regarding the statistics that apply to unexplained infertility may lead them to choose to delay additional intervention, since 30–80% may ultimately achieve pregnancy within 3 years. If age and length of time of infertility limit this option, superovulation, intrauterine insemination, and advanced reproductive technologies should be discussed.

THERAPY FOR INFERTILITY

Male Factor Infertility

Many causes of male factor infertility require therapy in consultation with a urologist. Conditions that may respond to specific medical therapy include hypothyroidism, hypogonadotropic hypogonadism, congenital adrenal hyperplasia, hyperprolactinemia, abnormal sperm parameters, and retrograde ejaculation. Treatment with thyroxine replacement, hCG and human menopausal gonadotropin (hMG), glucocorticoid therapy, and bromocriptine can help those with endocrine abnormalities. For those with high or low semen volumes, treatment with sperm washing, concentration, and extraction of the best swimming sperm from the ejaculate followed by intrauterine insemination is often successful. Patients with asthenospermia, or a decrease in general sperm motility, should be evaluated for antisperm antibodies, and treated with sperm washing and intrauterine insemination. For those with antibodies present, steroid therapy is one option but it carries with it significant side effects, including aseptic necrosis of the hip. The other treatment options include artificial insemination, IVF, and intracytoplasmic sperm injection. Retrograde ejaculation can be treated with alpha sympathomimetics to encourage antegrade ejaculation. Also, urine specimens can be centrifuged and insemination can be attempted with sperm from the urine sample.

Intracytoplasmic sperm injection (ICSI) offers a new and powerful option for couples with severe male factor infertility associated with a variety of sperm abnormalities. It involves the mechanical insertion of a single spermatozoon into the oocyte cytoplasm. Indications for ICSI include fertilization failure with standard IVF and those whose semen analysis is such that they could not benefit from IVF, such as those with severe oligospermia or asthenospermia. ICSI can be performed with spermatozoa collected from the epididymis and testis as well. There exists a concern about chromosomally abnormal embryos from ICSI due to the high risk of fertilization with genetically abnormal gametes. Also, the oocytes are exposed to intense light, temperature fluctuations, hyaluronidase, and an artificial opening in the zona pellucida and the oolemma. A few reports have indicated that sperm microinjection does not increase the incidence of chromosomally abnormal embryos. Once sexing of spermatozoa becomes available, prefertilization diagnosis may help prevent sex-linked diseases.

A varicocele is a dilatation of scrotal veins in the pampiniform plexus. A clinical varicocele is one that is detected by examination and is present in 15% of men. Subclinical varicoceles can be detected by ultrasound or venography. There is evidence that varicoceles can cause a decline in semen quality and that a minority of men are subfertile due to varicoceles. There also exists evidence to suggest that correction of varicocele improves fertility rates, but some experts do not agree. Subclinical varicoceles, those not evident on exam, have not been proven to have an effect on fertility, and treating these is controversial. Studies have shown that for treatment of varicocele-associated infertility, surgery is more cost-effective than primary treatment with assisted reproduction.

When semen parameters are normal but results from postcoital examinations are repeatedly poor, treatment with intrauterine insemination of washed concentrated sperm has been effective in overcoming an apparent barrier to fertility.

When male infertility is not amenable to therapy, donor insemination offers an opportunity for pregnancy. The use of a donor raises medical, emotional, ethical, and legal issues for the potential parents and the practitioner. The husband may experience grief, confusion regarding the concepts of fertility versus masculinity, concern over acceptance of the child, and guilt. Decisions about what to tell the child are often difficult to face. Because of the potential for infection with use of fresh sperm, and the concern for risk of AIDS in particular, it is the recommendation of the American Fertility Society to rely on frozen semen. The freezing process results in semen with slightly lower fecundability and consequently a longer interval to pregnancy for most couples. Most pregnancies will result within 6–9 cycles; if this method is not successful, a reappraisal of female fertility factors is in order.

Female Factor Infertility

There are data to suggest that women with infertility, whether treated or untreated, are at high risk of having a perinatal death. Much of this increased risk is due to the increase in multiple gestations from infertility drugs. However, even women who conceive spontaneously may be at increased risk of delivering premature infants, and thus at increased risk of perinatal death.

A. THE OVULATORY FACTOR

The treatment of specific ovulatory disorders is determined by the diagnosis. The chances for conception are good; in each cycle of treatment, the range of conception is 15–25%, depending on the degree of stimulation. If there is inexplicable failure to conceive after several ovulatory cycles, assisted reproduction techniques such as IVF or gamete intrafallopian transfer (GIFT) may be considered. With IVF, one can control the number of oocytes or embryos transferred, which is especially beneficial in women who are difficult to control in regard to multiple ovulation.

If an elevated FSH is detected, ovarian failure or resistance is present and fertility cannot be restored; no biopsy information is necessary or helpful. The options that may then be considered include adoption, surrogate pregnancy, embryo donation, or egg donation. Success rates for embryo and egg donation are in the range of 40% pregnancies achieved per transfer with fresh embryos, and they are lower if cryopreservation has been used. The ethical, psychologic, and legal issues are similar to those involved in donor sperm options.

Induction of ovulation can be accomplished in 90–95% of patients with chronic anovulation and normal FSH and prolactin. Usually, a progression of therapy will be planned, with the use of clomiphene citrate as the first approach. Clomiphene citrate is the agent of choice for women with oligomenorrhea or amenorrhea but who have sufficient ovarian estradiol production to have an estradiol level of 40 pg/mL. Clomiphene citrate is given by mouth, and acts by competing with endogenous estrogen for estrogen binding sites on the hypothalamus and thus blocks the negative feedback of endogenous estrogen. GnRH is then released in a pulsatile manner, stimulating LH and FSH. It is usually given for 5 days, starting on day 5 of menses. Success with clomiphene may require adjustment of dosage and timing and combining it with other supplementary medications, such as corticosteroids, estrogen, or midcycle hCG. The risk of ectopic pregnancy is not increased. The amount of monitoring required depends on the response. Until a normal follicle with apparent ovulation has been consistently achieved, ultrasound and hormonal testing may be required for interpretation of response. After a regimen has been shown to achieve ovulation, 3–6 cycles with timed intercourse should be attempted. Clomiphene will be successful in inducing ovulation in about 70% of women with ovaries that are producing estrogen but not ovulating regularly. In more than 50% of the stimulated cycles, more than one follicle can be shown to be stimulated and will progress to dominance, correlating with an incidence of twins of 8%. Side effects with clomiphene are common, including hot flushes, emotional lability or depression, bloating, and visual changes; most are mild and all disappear with discontinuation of the drug. If ovulation occurs but no pregnancy results (50% of cases), reevaluation of the regimen and possible progression to more aggressive therapy may be considered.

Patients in whom there is no response to clomiphene, or those in whom there is ovulatory response to clomiphene but no pregnancy, patients with pituitary insufficiency, those with hypothalamic insufficiency, and patients with unexplained infertility usually respond to stimulation with human gonadotropins. Human menopausal gonadotropin (hMG) is a formulation of equal amounts of FSH and LH, obtained from urine of postmenopausal women, and it is given by intramuscular injection. Removal of most of the LH from the urine led to development of a more purified preparation of FSH, also administered intramuscularly. Recombinant FSH is now available and is free of contamination by proteins and thus can be given subcutaneously. There is no evidence that any of these gonadotropins yields better results when used for ovulation induction. The use of gonadotropins is more time consuming and expensive than clomiphene, and there is an increased risk of side effects such as multiple gestation and ovarian hyperstimulation syndrome. Usually hCG is required as an ovulatory trigger, and monitoring is required to determine the intensity of the ovarian response. A combination of frequent ultrasonic scanning and estrogen determinations will indicate the number of follicles stimulated and their degree of maturity, so that hCG can be appropriately administered or withheld. With perseverance and appropriate adjustment of therapy, 85–90% of patients can be stimulated to ovulate with gonadotropin treatment, but even with careful monitoring there is a 20% risk of multiple births. The cost of treatment is high due to the expense of the drug and requisite monitoring. Used judiciously, the major complication of hyperstimulation from gonadotropin will occur in 1–3% of cycles. The expense, risk, and side effects of these therapies will determine their feasibility.

When modification of lifestyle or body habitus does not successfully restore ovulation in the patient diagnosed with hypothalamic insufficiency, pulsatile GnRH is successful in restoring normal ovulation in nearly 100% of correctly diagnosed patients. Normal fertility is then restored during cycles of treatment, and most pregnancies occur within 3–6 cycles.

Elevated prolactin levels can cause abnormalities of ovulation, including inadequate luteal phase or amenorrhea. An elevated prolactin level should lead to a verification of normal thyroid-stimulating hormone (TSH) secretion, because primary hypothyroidism can cause increased prolactin. Prolactin elevations are attributable to many different medications and drugs, including phenothiazines, tricyclic antidepressants, opiates, oral contraceptives, alpha-methyldopa, and metoclopramide, and the history should be reviewed. The elevated prolactin can often be treated with bromocriptine, leading to normalization of the endocrinology of the cycle. The woman can be advised to discontinue the drug once pregnancy is verified, but she can be reassured by a growing body of information confirming the safety of the medication when it is taken during early pregnancy.

There exists some concern about a possible association between ovulation induction agents and ovarian cancer. The possibility that ovulation induction increases the risk of ovarian cancer remains unproven. Both infertility and endometriosis themselves may be independent risk factors. The fact that ovarian cancer is relatively rare makes it difficult to prove an association with infertility drugs. Future studies in this area are needed.

B. THE PELVIC FACTOR

Endometriosis and the effects of salpingitis are two of the most common problems confronting infertile couples. When definitive treatment cannot be accomplished during diagnosis at laparoscopy, referral to experienced surgical specialists is advised, as the best opportunity for pregnancy will usually occur following the primary conservative procedure. However, much controversy exists surrounding the use of tubal surgery for tubal disease such as tubal occlusion or peritubal adhesions. Comparing results of IVF and tubal surgery reveals success rates in the range of 3–5% monthly fecundability for tubal surgery. The success rates after IVF are much closer to that of the normal fertile population, 15–20%. Also, the rate of ectopic pregnancy with tubal surgery is much higher than with IVF. As for endometriosis, it is generally accepted that laparoscopic resection or ablation of moderate or advanced endometriosis enhances fecundity in infertile women. It is more controversial in those with mild disease because these patients exhibit only a slightly lower than normal rate of conceiving naturally. There are, however, some data to suggest that laparoscopic ablation of endometriosis is beneficial even in those with mild or minimal disease.

The role of fibroids in infertility is unclear, and most surgeons reserve myomectomy for treatment of recurrent abortion, to relieve symptoms of discomfort or excessive blood loss, or when a submucosal fibroid has been demonstrated. The fibroids considered significant will usually distort the endometrial cavity and may be diagnosed by hysterosalpingogram, ultrasonography, hysteroscopy, or magnetic resonance imaging.

When to abandon conservative surgical therapy in favor of IVF is a matter of assessing multiple factors that will influence the probabilities of conceiving. The nature and extent of pelvic adhesions, the presence of hydrosalpinges, the age of the patient, and associated fertility factors will influence the degree of enthusiasm for recommendation of surgical treatment.

C. THE CERVICAL FACTOR

The absence of adequate nurturing mucus at midcycle can be treated either by attempts to improve the mucus or by bypassing the mucus with intrauterine insemination. To improve the amount of mucus, estrogen can be administered during the mid- to late follicular phase of the cycle. The potential for interfering with the normal follicular dynamics exists, and if low doses of estrogen are ineffective, an attempt to increase endogenous follicular estrogen using hMG may result in improved cervical mucus. In most cases, this will be a direct result of the recruitment of additional follicles and must be carefully monitored for the intensity of the response in order to reduce the risk of multiple gestation and prevent hyperstimulation syndrome. When the cervical mucus appears to be affected by cervicitis and inflammatory changes, empiric treatment of patient and partner with doxycycline is advocated by some authors. When the cervix is altered by congenital malformation or past surgical treatment that has rendered endocervical glands absent or nonfunctional, intrauterine insemination with washed sperm can be anticipated to result in pregnancy in 20–30% of patients who complete at least 3 cycles of treatment. Cervical factor patients who do not respond to these therapies can be offered IVF, GIFT, or zygote intrafallopian transfer (ZIFT) (see Chapter 56), although GIFT and ZIFT are now rarely utilized.

Unexplained Infertility

A diagnosis of unexplained infertility is assigned to couples with normal results of a standard infertility work-up. The likelihood of this is about 15%. The main treatment options include expectant observation with timed intercourse, ovarian stimulation, intrauterine insemination, GIFT, and IVF. Expectant management is an option that leads to conception rates of 30–80% over 3 years, depending on the woman's age and the duration of infertility. Studies support the use of clomiphene with intrauterine insemination for up to 4 cycles. The next step is usually hMG with intrauterine insemination for 3 cycles, and if unsuccessful, assisted reproductive techniques should be considered. The rationale for treatment with superovulation in women with documented ovulation is that it may overcome a subtle defect in ovulatory function not detected by standard tests or that by increasing the number of eggs available, the likelihood of pregnancy is increased. GIFT, or gamete intrafallopian transfer, involves the aspiration of eggs, mixing eggs and sperm in culture media, and transferring the mixture to the tube. IVF is useful because fertilization is inherent whereas in GIFT it is simply assumed. In instances in which unexplained infertility may be due to a fundamental defect in fertilization or in embryo transfer to the uterus, IVF may play a role in treatment. Regardless, IVF is now considered the treatment of choice, rather than GIFT (or ZIFT), when other infertility treatments have failed.

For many, the hardest course to contemplate is no therapy at all. A time limit with expectation of resolution of infertility should be presented, and in some cases guidance toward acceptance of childless living, adoption, use of surrogate pregnancy, or donor insemination should be offered before extensive time and resources are expended on procedures or regimens that offer little potential.

REFERENCES

Burmeister L, Healy DL: Ovarian cancer in infertility patients. Ann Med 1998;30:525.

Chuang AT, Howards SS: Male infertility, evaluation and nonsurgical therapy. Urol Clin North Am 1998;25:703.

Draper ES et al: Assessment of separate contributions to perinatal mortality of infertility history and treatment: a case-control analysis. Lancet 1999;353:1746.

Guzick DS et al: Efficacy of treatment for unexplained infertility. Fertil Steril 1998;70:207.

Hull MGR, Cahill DJ: Female infertility. Endocrinol Metabol Clin North Am 1998;27:851.

Luske MP, Vacc NA: Grief, depression, and coping in women undergoing infertility treatment. Obstet Gynecol 1999;93:245.

Marcoux S et al: Laparascopic surgery in infertile women with minimal or mild endometriosis. N Engl J Med 1997;337:217.

Oei SG et al: Effectiveness of the postcoital test: randomised controlled trial. BMJ 1998; 317: 502.

Van Voorhis BJ et al: Cost-effectiveness of infertility treatments: a cohort study. Fertil Steril 1997;67:830.

Van Voorhis BJ et al: Cost-effective treatment of the infertile couple. Fertil Steril 1998;70:995.

World Health Organization: *WHO Laboratory Manual for the Examination of Human Semen and Sperm-Cervical Mucus Interaction*, 3rd ed. Cambridge University Press, 1992.

Zayed F, Abu-Heija A: The management of unexplained infertility. Obstet Gynecol Survey 1999;54:121.

Amenorrhea

Donelle Laughlin, MD, & Ian H. Thorneycroft, MD, PhD

DEFINITION & INCIDENCE

Approximately 97.5% of females begin normal menstruation by age 16 in the U.S. When a female fails to have her first menstrual cycle by age 16 in the face of normal secondary sexual characteristics or by age 14 in the absence of secondary sexual characteristics this condition is considered **primary amenorrhea.** The incidence of primary amenorrhea is 2.5%.

Secondary amenorrhea is the absence of menses for 6 months in a woman in whom normal menstruation has been established or for the equivalent of 3 cycles in a woman with oligomenorrhea. The incidence of secondary amenorrhea is quite variable from, 3% in the general population to 100% under conditions of extreme physical or emotional stress (eg, in prisoners awaiting execution). A list of the most common causes of secondary amenorrhea is seen in Table 54–1. **Oligomenorrhea** is menses occurring at an interval exceeding 35 days.

Amenorrhea is important for several reasons. It can be associated with infertility, osteoporosis, genital atrophy, and major social and psychosexual dysfunction. Unopposed estrogen, which may occur in some women with amenorrhea, may lead to the development of endometrial hyperplasia and carcinoma.

ETIOLOGY & PATHOGENESIS

Pregnancy is the most common cause of amenorrhea and must be considered in every patient presenting for evaluation of amenorrhea. Amenorrhea caused by aberrations of the normal menstrual cycle is discussed in Chapter 6. Chapter 31 and Chapter 55 discuss developmental anomalies of the reproductive organs and masculinization respectively. This chapter will discuss amenorrhea associated with 46,XX and 46,XY karyotypes, anatomic defects, and defects in the hypothalamic-pituitary-ovarian axis, as well as systemic disorders that affect menstruation.

Amenorrhea in Women With 46,XY Karyotype

The details of embryonic sexual differentiation are discussed in Chapter 4. Briefly, the sexually undifferentiated male fetal testis secretes müllerian inhibiting factor (MIF) and testosterone. MIF promotes regression of all müllerian structures: the uterine tubes, the uterus, and the upper two-thirds of the vagina. Testosterone and its active metabolite dihydrotestosterone (DHT) are responsible for embryonic differentiation of the male internal and external genitalia.

A. TESTICULAR FEMINIZATION

In testicular feminization, all müllerian-derived structures are absent. The external genital anlagen and mesonephric ducts cannot respond to androgens, because androgen receptors are either absent or defective. Affected individuals are therefore phenotypic females lacking a uterus and a complete vagina. They produce some estrogen, develop breasts, and are reared as girls and therefore present with primary amenorrhea.

B. PURE GONADAL DYSGENESIS

If the primitive germ cells do not migrate to the genital ridge, a testis will not develop, and a streak gonad will be present. Affected individuals have normal female internal and external genitalia, since neither MIF nor androgens are secreted by the streaks. Because these individuals produce no estrogen, they will not develop breasts. They are reared as girls and present clinically with either delayed puberty or primary amenorrhea.

C. ANORCHIA

If the fetal testes regress before 7 weeks' gestation, neither MIF nor testosterone is secreted, and affected individuals will present with a clinical picture identical to that of pure gonadal dysgenesis. Individuals whose testes regress between 7 and 13 weeks' gestation present with ambiguous genitalia.

D. TESTICULAR STEROID ENZYME DEFECTS

A testis with defective enzymes 1–4 will produce MIF but not testosterone (Fig 54–1). Affected individuals have female external genitalia and no müllerian structures. They will be reared as girls and present clinically with either delayed puberty or primary amenorrhea.

A defect in enzyme 6 (17-hydroxysteroid dehydrogenase) results in ambiguous genitalia and virilization at puberty.

Table 54–1. Causes of secondary amenorrhea.

Common
  Pregnancy
  Hypothalamic amenorrhea
  Androgen disorders: polycystic ovarian syndrome, congenital adrenal hypreplasia
  Galactorrhea-amenorrhea syndrome
Less Common
  Premature ovarian failure
  Asherman's syndrome
  Sheehan's syndrome
Rare
  Diabetes
  Hyperthyroidism or hypothyroidism
  Cushing's syndrome or Addison's disease
  Cirrhosis
  Tuberculosis
  Malnutrition
  Irradiation or chemotherapy
  Surgery

Anatomic Abnormalities Associated With Amenorrhea (see Chapter 31)

A. MÜLLERIAN DYSGENESIS

Müllerian dysgenesis is characterized by congenital absence of the uterus and the upper two-thirds of the vagina. Affected individuals have a 46,XX karyotype.

B. VAGINAL AGENESIS

Vaginal agenesis is characterized by failure of the vagina to develop.

C. TRANSVERSE VAGINAL SEPTUM

This anomaly results from failure of fusion of the müllerian and urogenital sinus-derived portions of the vagina.

D. IMPERFORATE HYMEN

If the hymen is complete, menstrual efflux cannot occur.

E. ASHERMAN'S SYNDROME

In Asherman's syndrome, amenorrhea is due to intrauterine synechiae. The usual cause is a complicated D&C (eg, infected products of conception, vigorous elimination of the endometrium), but the syndrome can occur after myomectomy, cesarean section, and tuberculous endometritis.

Hypothalamic Defects

Under normal physiologic circumstances, the arcuate nucleus releases pulses of gonadotropin-releasing hormone (GnRH) into the hypophyseal portal system approximately every hour. Discharge of GnRH releases luteinizing hormone (LH) and follicle-stimulating hormone (FSH) from the pituitary; LH and FSH in turn stimulate ovarian follicular growth and ovulation. Anovulation and amenorrhea will occur as a result of interference with GnRH transport, GnRH pulse discharge, or congenital absence of GnRH (Kallmann's syndrome). Any of these situations will lead to hypogonadotropic hypogonadism.

A. DEFECTS OF GnRH TRANSPORT

Interference with the transport of GnRH from the hypothalamus to the pituitary may occur with pituitary stalk compression or destruction of the arcuate nucleus. Pituitary stalk section from trauma, craniopharyngioma, germinoma, glioma, Hand-Schuller-Christian disease, midline teratomas, endodermal sinus tumor, tuberculosis, sarcoidosis, and irradiation will all either destroy parts of the hypothalamus or prevent transport of hypothalamic hormones to the pituitary.

B. DEFECTS OF GnRH PULSE PRODUCTION

The metabolic consequence of any significant reduction in the normal GnRH pulse frequency or amplitude is that little or no LH or FSH can be released, with the result that no ovarian follicles develop, virtually no estradiol is secreted, and the patient is amenorrheic. This is the biochemical status in normal prepubertal girls and those with constitutional delayed puberty, such as in anorexia nervosa, severe stress, extreme weight loss, or prolonged vigorous athletic exertion, and in hyperprolactinemia. Amenorrhea on this basis may also be an idiopathic phenomenon.

Less severe reductions in GnRH pulse amplitude and frequency result in diminished LH and FSH secretion with some follicular stimulation. The stimulation is insufficient to result in full follicular development and ovulation, but estradiol is secreted. This may occur with stress, hyperprolactinemia, as a result of vigorous athletic activity, or in the early stages of eating disorders. It may also be idiopathic.

C. KALLMANN'S SYNDROME

These patients have a congenital absence of GnRH and, consequently, do not release LH or FSH from the pituitary. Ovulation does not occur. Anosmia is an associated phenomenon.

Pituitary Defects

Pituitary causes of amenorrhea are rare; most are secondary to hypothalamic dysfunction.

A. CONGENITAL PITUITARY DYSFUNCTION

Congenital absence of the entire pituitary is a rare and lethal condition. Isolated defects of LH or FSH pro-

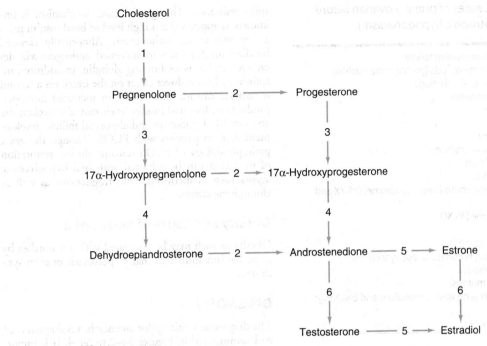

Cholesterol

1

Pregnenolone — 2 → Progesterone

3   3

17α-Hydroxypregnenolone — 2 → 17α-Hydroxyprogesterone

4   4

Dehydroepiandrosterone — 2 → Androstenedione — 5 → Estrone

6   6

Testosterone — 5 → Estradiol

Key to enzymes
1 = Cholesterol 20- and 22-desmolase and 20-hydroxylase
2 = 3β-Hydroxysteroid dehydrogenase
3 = 17α-Hydroxylase
4 = 17- and 20-Desmolase
5 = Aromatase
6 = 17-Hydroxysteroid dehydrogenase

Figure 54–1. Steroidogenesis in the ovary.

duction do occur (rarely), resulting in anovulation and amenorrhea.

B. ACQUIRED PITUITARY DYSFUNCTION

Sheehan's syndrome, characterized by postpartum amenorrhea, results from postpartum pituitary necrosis secondary to severe hemorrhage and hypotension and is a rare cause of amenorrhea. Surgical ablation and irradiation of the pituitary as management of pituitary tumors also cause amenorrhea.

Iron deposition in the pituitary may result in destruction of the cells that produce LH and FSH. This occurs only in patients with markedly elevated serum iron levels (ie, hemosiderosis) usually resulting from extensive red cell destruction. Thalassemia major is an example of a disease that causes hemosiderosis.

Pituitary microadenomas and macroadenomas also lead to amenorrhea due to elevated prolactin levels, but the mechanism(s) underlying this cause of amenorrhea are unclear. Hypothyroidism may also lead to elevated prolactin levels and thereby lead to amenorrhea.

Ovarian Failure

Primary ovarian failure is characterized by elevated gonadotropins and low estradiol (**hypergonadotropic hypogonadism**). Secondary ovarian failure is almost always due to hypothalamic dysfunction and is characterized by normal or low gonadotropins and low estradiol (**hypogonadotropic hypogonadism**).

Causes of primary ovarian failure are listed in Table 54–2.

A. STEROID ENZYME DEFECTS

Figure 54–1 depicts normal steroidogenesis in the ovary. Genetic females with defects in enzymes 1–4 have normal internal female genitalia and 46,XX karyotype. However, they cannot produce estradiol and thus they fail to menstruate or have breast development.

B. OVARIAN RESISTANCE (SAVAGE'S) SYNDROME

Patients with this syndrome have elevated LH and FSH levels, and the ovaries contain primordial germ cells. A

Table 54–2. Causes of primary ovarian failure (hypergonadotrophic hypogonadism).

Idiopathic premature ovarian failure
Steroidogenic enzyme defects (primary amenorrhea)
   Cholesterol side-chain cleavage
   3β-ol-deghydrogenase
   17-hydroxylase
   17-desmolase
   17-ketoreductase
Testicular regression syndrome
True hermaphroditism
Gonadal dysgenesis
   Pure gonadal dysgenesis (Swyer syndrome) (46,XX and 46,XY)
   Turner's syndrome (45,XO)
   Turner variants
Mixed gonadal dysgenesis
Ovarian resistance syndrome (Savage syndrome)
Autoimmune oophoritis
Postinfection (eg, mumps)
Postoophorectomy (also wedge resections and bivalving)
Postirradiation
Postchemotherapy

defect in the cell receptor mechanism is the presumed cause.

C. Ovarian Dysgenesis

If the primitive oogonia do not migrate to the genital ridge, the ovaries fail to develop. Streak gonads, which do not secrete hormones, develop instead, and the result is primary amenorrhea (pure gonadal dysgenesis; **Swyer's syndrome**).

In patients with **Turner's syndrome** (45,XO) or mosaicism (45,XO/XX), the oogonia migrate normally to the ovary but undergo rapid atresia, so that by puberty no oogonia remain. These patients usually have primary amenorrhea, but some—particularly those with the mosaic abnormality—may menstruate briefly, and a few have conceived (see Chapter 5).

D. Premature Ovarian Failure

Menopause occurs when the ovaries fail secondary to depletion of ova. If this occurs before age 40, it is considered premature. It is marked by amenorrhea, increased gonadotropin levels and estrogen deficiency.

Ovarian Dysfunction

One of the most common causes of amenorrhea is **polycystic ovarian syndrome** (**PCOS**) or Stein-Leventhal syndrome. PCOS is the constellation of hyperandrogenemia, hirsutism, anovulation, obesity, and in-

sulin resistance. Though the exact mechanism is unknown, it appears that a high level of basal insulin plays a key role in its pathogenesis. Abnormally elevated baseline insulin leads to increased androgens via decreased sex-hormone binding globulin. In addition, insulin may have a direct effect on the ovary via a second messenger cascade that results in increased androgen production. Elevated insulin levels may also explain the abnormal LH pulsation and abnormal follicle development seen in patients with PCOS. Though the exact pathophysiology of PCOS remains elusive, restoration of ovulation can be achieved with oral hypoglycemic agents such as metformin and troglitazone as well as clomiphene citrate.

Obesity as a Cause of Amenorrhea

Obesity as such may be associated with amenorrhea by a mechanism similar to that of polycystic ovarian syndrome.

DIAGNOSIS

The diagnostic work-up for amenorrhea is diagrammed and summarized in Figures 54–2 to 54–4. It is important at the outset to determine which organ is dysfunctional and then to identify the exact cause. Once this has been done, specific therapy can be planned.

Any patient with amenorrhea who has a uterus should be tested for pregnancy and for serum levels of thyroid-stimulating hormone (TSH) and prolactin. Galactorrhea should be identified or ruled out by physical examination.

Diagnosis of Primary Amenorrhea

The diagnostic scheme for primary amenorrhea is outlined in Figure 54–2. Pelvic examination should be done to establish the presence of a vagina and uterus and no vaginal septum or imperforate hymen that might account for the failure of appearance of menses. Because pelvic examination of an adolescent girl may be difficult, pelvic ultrasound or examination under anesthesia may be required to establish the presence of a uterus.

If no uterus is present, serum testosterone levels should be measured and karyotyping done to differentiate between müllerian agenesis and testicular feminization.

Diagnosis of Amenorrhea Associated With Galactorrhea-Hyperprolactinemia

The diagnostic work-up of patients with galactorrhea or hyperprolactinemia is outlined in Figure 54–3. The differential diagnosis of galactorrhea-amenorrhea is summarized in Table 54–3.

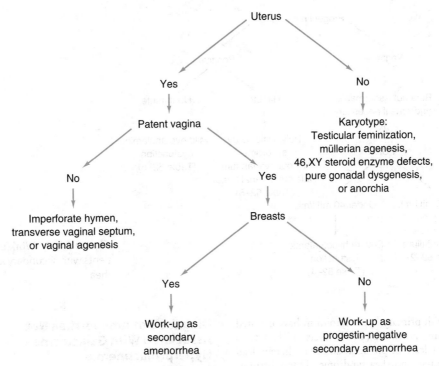

Figure 54–2. Work-up for patients with primary amenorrhea.

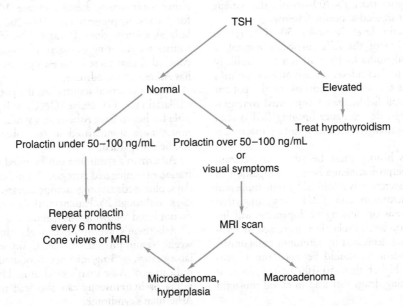

Figure 54–3. Work-up for patients with amenorrhea-galactorrhea-hyperprolactinemia.

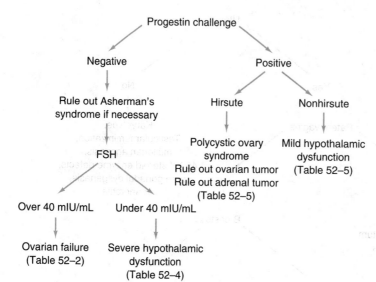

Progestin challenge

Negative — Positive

Negative → Rule out Asherman's syndrome if necessary

Positive → Hirsute / Nonhirsute

Rule out Asherman's syndrome if necessary → FSH

Hirsute → Polycystic ovary syndrome
Rule out ovarian tumor
Rule out adrenal tumor
(Table 52–5)

Nonhirsute → Mild hypothalamic dysfunction
(Table 52–5)

FSH → Over 40 mIU/mL / Under 40 mIU/mL

Over 40 mIU/mL → Ovarian failure
(Table 52–2)

Under 40 mIU/mL → Severe hypothalamic dysfunction
(Table 52–4)

Figure 54–4. Work-up for patients with secondary amenorrhea.

Patients with primary hypothyroidism have elevated thyroid-releasing hormone (TRH) levels. TRH acts to stimulate the release of prolactin and may thereby lead to galactorrhea-amenorrhea syndrome. Thyroid-stimulating hormone (TSH) is also elevated and easier to measure and thus is the screening test for hypothyroidism.

Once hypothyroidism is adequately treated serum prolactin must be measured again after thyroid function has become normal. If prolactin remains elevated or is initially higher than 50–200 ng/mL, the patient should be further studied as outlined below.

If the prolactin level is under 50–100 ng/mL and the cone view of the sella turcica is normal, a pituitary macroadenoma (> 10 mm) is a very unlikely diagnosis. If the prolactin level exceeds 50–100 ng/mL, the cone view of the sella is abnormal, or the patient has restricted visual fields, then a computed tomography (CT) or magnetic resonance imaging (MRI) scan of the sella is required to rule out pituitary macroadenoma.

A meticulous history must be taken to ascertain whether the hyperprolactinemia is due to ingestion of drugs. Prolactin secretion is inhibited by dopamine and stimulated by serotonin and TRH. Any drug that blocks the synthesis or binding of dopamine will increase the prolactin level. Prolactin is increased by serotonin agonists and decreased by serotonin antagonists. Pituitary macroadenoma should be ruled out if prolactin levels are higher than 50–100 ng/mL, even if the patient is taking drugs that lead to raised prolactin levels.

Diagnosis of Amenorrhea Not Associated With Galactorrhea-Hyperprolactinemia

These patients are studied according to the scheme outlined in Figure 54–4.

The first step is the progestin challenge, which indirectly determines whether the ovary is producing estrogen. If the endometrium has been primed with estrogen, exogenous progestin will produce menses. Give either medroxyprogesterone acetate, 10 mg orally daily for 5 days, or progesterone, 100–200 mg intramuscularly as a single dose. If vaginal bleeding follows, the ovaries are secreting estrogen. If it does not, it can be concluded that there is no estrogen or that the patient has Asherman's syndrome.

From a practical standpoint, if a patient has not had a dilatation and curettage (D&C), it is virtually impossible for her to have Asherman's syndrome, so the diagnostic steps summarized in the following paragraphs can be disregarded.

Asherman's syndrome can be ruled out by administration of conjugated estrogen, 2.5 mg orally daily for 25 days, plus medroxyprogesterone acetate, 10 mg orally on days 16 through 25. Patients with Asherman's syndrome do not bleed following this regimen.

Asherman's syndrome can also be diagnosed by weekly serum progesterone tests. Any value in the ovulatory range (> 3 ng/mL) not associated with menses is indicative of Asherman's syndrome. Hysterosalpingography or hysteroscopy can also lead to a diagnosis of Asherman's syndrome.

Table 54–3. Differential diagnosis of galactorrhea-hyperprolactinemia.

Pituitary tumors secreting prolactin
  Macroadenomas (> 10 mm)
  Microadenomas (< 10 mm)
Hypothyroidism
Idiopathic hyperprolactinemia
Drug-induced hyperprolactinemia
  Dopamine antagonists
    Phenothiazines
    Thioxanthenes
    Butyrophenone
    Diphenylbutylpiperidine
    Dibenzoxazepine
    Dihydroindolone
    Procainamide derivatives
  Catecholamine-depleting agents
  False transmitters (α-methyldopa)
Interruption of normal hypothalamic-pituitary relationship
  Pituitary stalk section
Peripheral neural stimulation
  Chest wall stimulation
    Thoracotomy
    Mastectomy
    Thoracoplasty
    Burns
    Herpes zoster
    Bronchogenic tumors
    Bronchiectasis
    Chronic bronchitis
  Nipple stimulation
    Stimulation of nipples
    Chronic nipple irritation
  Spinal cord lesion
    Tabes dorsalis
    Syringomyelia
Central nervous system disease
  Encephalitis
  Craniopharyngioma
  Pineal tumors
  Hypothalamic tumors
  Pseudotumor cerebri

In a patient who does not have Asherman's syndrome and does not respond to the progestin challenge, ovarian dysfunction may be of hypothalamic or ovarian origin. The distinction is based on the FSH level. Primary ovarian dysfunction resulting in low estradiol secretion is associated with high serum FSH. Values vary in different laboratories, but in general an FSH level higher than 40 mIU/mL indicates primary ovarian failure. A patient whose FSH level is less than 40 mIU/mL

has hypothalamic-pituitary dysfunction and secondary ovarian failure.

Diagnosis of Amenorrhea Due to Primary Ovarian Failure

The causes of primary ovarian failure are set forth in Table 54–2.

Karyotyping is indicated for all women who present with premature menopause, particularly if their amenorrhea is primary. Patients with primary amenorrhea may have a steroid enzyme defect. Autoimmune oophoritis is a reversible cause of ovarian failure that must be investigated.

Diagnosis of Amenorrhea Associated With Hypothalamic-Pituitary Dysfunction

The differential diagnosis of hypoestrogenic amenorrhea is presented in Table 54–4. The category includes amenorrhea associated with athletic activity, weight loss, or stress. Differentiation of hypothalamic from pituitary dysfunction can be achieved by giving GnRH, but is generally not a worthwhile effort, since pituitary causes are rare and can often be diagnosed on the basis of the history. Moreover, in Kallmann's syndrome, a single bolus dose of GnRH may not elicit a normal response. Up to 40 doses of GnRH have been required to prime the pituitary so that it will respond normally. A GnRH pump has also been utilized.

If there is a significant history consistent with Sheehan's syndrome, pituitary function testing is indicated

Table 54–4. Differential diagnosis of hypoestrogenic amenorrhea (hypogonadotropic hypogonadism).

Hypothalamic dysfunction
  Kallmann's syndrome
  Tumors of hypothalamus (craniopharyngioma)
  Constitutional delay of puberty
  Severe hypothalamic dysfunction
  Anorexia nervosa
  Severe weight loss
  Severe stress
  Exercise
Pituitary disorder
  Sheehan's syndrome
  Panhypopituitarism
  Isolated gonadotropin deficiency
  Hemosiderosis (primarily from thalassemia major)

in order to determine the functional capacity of the gland—particularly the integrity of the pituitary-adrenal axis.

In girls with primary amenorrhea, observing the pattern of LH and FSH release after administration of GnRH will help to determine whether the patient is undergoing late pubertal changes.

Patients who bleed in response to the progestin challenge (ie, whose ovaries are secreting estrogen) fit into one of 4 categories: (1) virilized, with or without ambiguous genitalia; (2) hirsute, with polycystic ovaries, hyperthecosis, or mild maturity-onset adrenal hyperplasia; (3) nonhirsute, with hypothalamic dysfunction; or (4) amenorrheic secondary to systemic disease. The differential diagnosis is set forth in Table 54–5. The LH:FSH ratio is a helpful clue to etiologic diagnosis. If the ratio exceeds 2:1 or if the LH level is persistently above 26–30 mIU/mL, a diagnosis of polycystic ovaries is a strong possibility. A vaginal ultrasound may be helpful in making the diagnosis of PCOS. However, 25% of normal patients have polycystic ovaries. Ultrasound cannot therefore be the sole criterion for diagnosis.

TREATMENT

1. Management of Patients Desiring Pregnancy—Ovulation Induction

Ovulation Induction in Patients With Amenorrhea-Galactorrhea With Pituitary Macroadenoma

Bromocriptine remains the mainstay for medical therapy. If the lesion is large and causing symptoms such as visual changes or headaches, surgical therapy may be needed. Surgical therapy involves transsphenoidal or frontal removal of the pituitary adenoma or the entire gland. About half of surgically treated patients will menstruate normally after this procedure.

Ovulation Induction in Patients With Amenorrhea-Galactorrhea Without Macroadenoma (Including Patients With Microadenomas)

These patients ovulate readily in response to bromocriptine therapy. The usual dose is 2.5 mg orally twice daily, but it is generally titrated until serum prolactin is normal—often possible with as little as 1.25 mg daily. Once pregnancy has been achieved bromocriptine may be discontinued. Patients with macroadenomas may need to continue therapy throughout pregnancy to avoid further growth of the lesion.

Table 54–5. Differential diagnosis of eugonadotropic eugonadism (progestin-challenge positive).

Mild hypothalamic dysfunction
  Emotional stress
  Psychologic disorder
  Weight loss
  Obesity
  Exercise-induced
  Idiopathic
Hirsutism-virilism
  Polycystic ovarian syndrome (Stein-Leventhal syndrome)
  Ovarian tumor
  Adrenal tumor
  Cushing's syndrome
  Congenital and maturity-onset adrenal hyperplasia
Systemic disease
  Hypothyroidism
  Hyperthyroidism
  Addison's disease
  Cushing's syndrome
  Chronic renal failure
  Many others

Patients taking drugs that raise the prolactin level should discontinue them if possible, but continued use of such drugs is not a contraindication to bromocriptine therapy.

Ovulation Induction in Patients With Hypothyroidism

Amenorrheic patients with hypothyroidism frequently respond to thyroid replacement therapy.

Ovulation Induction in Patients With Primary Ovarian Failure

According to Rebar and associates, patients with primary ovarian failure can be made to ovulate only under very rare circumstances. Patients with reversible ovarian failure include those with autoimmune oophoritis, who can be successfully treated with corticosteroids. Otherwise, almost all patients with primary ovarian failure fall into the category of idiopathic premature ovarian failure and cannot be made to ovulate. In vitro fertilization (IVF) with donor oocytes is the only way they can have children.

Any patient with a Y chromosome should undergo oophorectomy to prevent tumor development.

Ovulation Induction in Patients With Hypoestrogenic Hypothalamic Amenorrhea (Progestin-Challenge Negative)

In these patients with low estrogen levels, the pituitary does not release high quantities of LH and FSH (as would be expected with an intact, normally-functioning negative feedback mechanism). Therefore, even though clomiphene citrate (an antiestrogen) is not likely to stimulate gonadotropin release, many reproductive endocrinologists treat such patients successfully with a single course of clomiphene citrate, 150 or 250 mg daily for 5 days, on the chance that ovulation will occur.

Human menopausal gonadotropin (hMG or other synthetic gonadotropin) is usually first line therapy. Patients showing some ovarian stimulation by clomiphene can be treated with a combination of clomiphene and hMG—the advantage being a reduction in the amount of hMG required and thus a substantial cost savings. Ovulation induction with gonadotropins must be carefully monitored with serial ultrasound and estradiol determinations to avoid hyperstimulation. Hyperstimulation is the stimulation of too many follicles, with associated ovarian enlargement and ascites as well as other systemic abnormalities.

If a specific and potentially reversible cause of amenorrhea can be identified (eg, marked weight loss), it should be corrected.

Ovulation Induction in Patients Who Bleed in Response to Progestin Challenge

Virtually all of these patients respond to clomiphene citrate. The starting dose is 50 mg orally daily for 5 days. This can be increased to a maximum of 250 mg orally daily in 50-mg increments until ovulation is induced. Efficacy of clomiphene, however, plateaus at 100 mg per day. Ovulation occurs 5–10 days after the last dose. Patients with elevated androgens who do not respond to clomiphene citrate may respond to combined treatment with an oral hypoglycemic agent and clomiphene.

If clomiphene therapy with or without oral hypoglycemic agents is not effective, gonadotropin therapy may be attempted. Care must be taken in using hMG in these patients, as they are likely to become hyperstimulated.

Surgical wedge resection of the ovary in patients with polycystic ovary disease will frequently lead to ovulation. Unfortunately, wedge resection may cause postoperative pelvic adhesions, resulting in mechanical infertility. There is no place for a wedge resection today. The placement of multiple holes in the ovary with either cautery or the CO_2 laser appears to give similar results to wedge resection. Adhesions have also been noted with this technique.

Again, if a specific reversible cause of amenorrhea can be identified as outlined in Table 54–5, it should be corrected before drug therapy is attempted.

2. Management of Patients Not Desiring Pregnancy

Patients who are hypoestrogenic must be treated with a combination of estrogen and progesterone to maintain bone density and prevent genital atrophy. The dose of estrogen varies with the age of the patient. Oral contraceptives are good replacement therapy for most women. Combinations of 0.625–1.25 mg of conjugated estrogens orally daily on days 1 through 25 of the cycle with 5–10 mg of medroxyprogesterone acetate on days 16 through 25 are a suitable alternative. Calcium intake should be adjusted to 1–1.5 g of elemental calcium daily.

Patients who respond to the progestin challenge require occasional progestin administration to prevent the development of endometrial hyperplasia and carcinoma. Oral contraceptive pills may be used to regulate the menstrual cycle. Oral contraceptives also help with management of hirsutism. Alternatively, medroxyprogesterone acetate, 10 mg orally daily for 10–13 days every month or every other month, is sufficient to induce withdrawal bleeding and to prevent the development of endometrial hyperplasia.

Patients with hyperprolactinemia need periodic prolactin measurements and radiographic cone views of the sella turcica to rule out the development of macroadenoma.

COMPLICATIONS

The complications of amenorrhea can be numerous, including infertility and psychosocial developmental delays with lack of normal physical sexual development. Hypoestrogenic patients can develop severe osteoporosis and fractures, the most hazardous to life being femoral neck fracture (see Chapter 57). The complications associated with amenorrhea in patients who respond to progestin challenge are endometrial hyperplasia and carcinoma (see Chapter 48) resulting from unopposed estrogen stimulation.

PROGNOSIS

The prognosis for amenorrhea is good. It is not usually a life-threatening clinical event, since with proper work-up, tumors can be recognized and treated. Many patients with hypothalamic amenorrhea will spontaneously recover normal menstrual cycles.

Virtually all amenorrheic women who do not have premature ovarian failure can be made to ovulate with bromocriptine, clomiphene citrate, hypoglycemic agents, and gonadotropins.

REFERENCE

Nestler JE: Role of hyperinsulinemia in the pathogenesis of polycystic ovarian syndrome and its clinical implications. Semin Reprod Endocrinol 1997;15:111.

Hirsutism

M.K. Guess, MD, D. Ellene Andrew, MD, Carol L. Gagliardi, MD, & Adelina M. Emmi, MD

Definition

Hirsutism is defined as excessive growth of androgen-dependent sexual hair. This is most often manifested as increased "midline hair" on the upper lip, chin, ears, cheeks, lower abdomen, back, chest, and proximal limbs. The interpretation of what constitutes excessive growth is subjective and may range from an occasional hair on the upper lip to a full male-pattern beard. The psychological implications of hirsutism must not be underestimated. In Western society, excessive facial or body hair in women is unacceptable. Women who do not conform to a prevailing feminine ideal of physical appearance because of hirsutism may feel unattractive and suffer from low self-esteem, and such women may find social interactions difficult. Hirsutism is more than a cosmetic problem, however, because it usually represents a hormonal imbalance, resulting from a subtle excess of androgens that may be of ovarian origin, adrenal origin, or both.

Etiology

Excessive growth of sexual hair may be due to excessive production of androgens, increased sensitivity of the hair follicle to androgens, or increased conversion of weak androgens to potent androgens. Potential sources of increased androgens include the ovaries, the adrenal glands, exogenous hormones and other medications (Table 55–1).

A. Ovarian Disorders Causing Hirsutism

1. Nonneoplastic disorders—The most common cause of hirsutism is **polycystic ovarian syndrome.** Polycystic ovarian syndrome is typically associated with menstrual irregularities, infertility, obesity, and hirsutism. The histologic changes seen in polycystic ovary disease include a thickened ovarian capsule and numerous follicular cysts surrounded by a hyperplastic, luteinized theca interna. The pathophysiology of this disease is not fully understood; proposed causes include ovarian dysregulation, a disturbance of the hypothalamic-pituitary axis, adrenal androgen excess, and increased insulin resistance. Regardless of the underlying defect, the degree of hyperandrogenism and the individual's sensitivity to androgens may result in the complaint of hirsutism in 80% of these patients.

Other nonneoplastic ovarian disorders associated with hirsutism include stromal hyperplasia and stromal hyperthecosis. **Stromal hyperplasia** results in the hypersecretion of androgens from hypertrophic ovaries. It has a peak incidence between 60 and 70 years of age and is usually associated with uniform enlargement of both ovaries. **Stromal hyperthecosis** is a proliferation of stroma with foci of luteinized thecal cells, and also results in bilateral ovarian involvement. It frequently results in the clinical manifestations of virilism, obesity, hypertension, and disturbances of glucose metabolism, with most patients showing histologic evidence of concurrent stromal hyperplasia. A syndrome known as **Hy-perAndrogenism, Insulin Resistance, Acanthosis Nigricans** (HAIR-AN) has also been described; however, this is thought to most likely represent a variation of one of the nonneoplastic disorders, rather than denoting a separate disease entity.

2. Neoplastic disorders—Androgen-secreting ovarian neoplasms usually present with rapidly developing hirsutism, amenorrhea, and virilization, and are rare causes of hirsutism. The most common androgen secreted by these tumors is testosterone, with serum testosterone levels usually in excess of 200 ng/dL. Most hormone-secreting neoplasms are palpable on pelvic examination and are unilateral.

Sertoli-Leydig cell tumors and **hilar (Leydig) cell tumors** are ovarian neoplasms typically associated with hirsutism and virilization. Sertoli-Leydig cell tumors constitute less than 0.5% of all ovarian tumors and occur mainly in young, menstruating females. Hilar cell tumors are rare neoplasms and are usually encountered in older women. Their presentation is often more indolent and less dramatic than that of Sertoli-Leydig cell tumors. Other ovarian neoplasms that may be associated with hirsutism are the gynandroblastomas, germ cell tumors, granulosa cell tumors, and gonadoblastomas. The latter occur mainly in male patients, with gonadal dysgenesis and resultant female phenotypes.

Ovarian tumors with functional stroma are categorized as germ cell tumors containing syncytiotrophoblast cells and idiopathic and pregnancy-related tumors (see below). In these tumors, the neoplastic cells do not secrete steroid hormones directly, but stimulate secretion by the ovarian stroma either within or immediately adjacent to the tumor. These tumors have been

Table 55–1. Differential diagnosis of hirsutism.

Ovarian nonneoplastic causes
  Polycystic ovarian syndrome
  Stromal hyperplasia
  Stromal hyperthecosis
  Hyperandrogenism, insulin resistance, acanthosis nigricans
  (HAIR-AN)
Ovarian neoplastic causes
  Sertoli-Leydig cell tumors
  Hilar cell tumors
  Germ cell tumors
  Gynandroblastomas
  Granulosa cell tumors
  Gonadoblastomas
  Ovarian tumors with functional stroma
Pregnancy-related causes
  Theca lutein cysts
  Luteoma of pregnancy
Adrenal causes
  Congenital adrenal hyperplasia (CAH)
  Adrenal tumors
  Cushing's syndrome
  Hyperprolactenemia
Iatrogenic causes
  Methyltestosterone
  Danazol
  Anabolic steroids
  19-Nortestosterones
Idiopathic hirsutism

described in essentially all tumors that occur in the ovary, whether benign or malignant, metastatic or primary.

3. Pregnancy-related disorders—During pregnancy, elevated androgen levels that lead to severe hirsutism and virilization may be due to any of the above-mentioned conditions; however, pregnancy-specific disorders also exist. **Theca lutein cysts** (hyperreactio luteinalis) are benign neoplasms that can cause bilateral ovarian enlargement, hirsutism, and infrequently, virilization. These cysts occur almost exclusively in pregnancy and have an increased incidence in pregnancies complicated by gestational trophoblastic disease. Ovarian biopsy reveals cysts lined mostly with luteinized theca cells, but luteinized granulosa cells may also be present. Typically, resolution of the cysts occurs after pregnancy.

Luteoma of pregnancy is a benign human chorionic gonadotropin (hCG)–dependent ovarian tumor that may develop during pregnancy. High levels of testosterone and androstenedione are present, and virilization may occur in up to 25% of affected mothers

and 65% of female fetuses. In most patients, spontaneous regression of the neoplasm and return of androgen levels to normal occur in the postpartum period.

B. ADRENAL DISORDERS CAUSING HIRSUTISM

1. Enzyme deficiencies—Enzyme deficiencies affecting adrenal and ovarian steroidogenesis represent the second most common cause of hyperandrogenism in postmenarchal females and **congenital adrenal hyperplasia (CAH)** represents the most common disorder in this group. CAH is inherited as an autosomal recessive trait, and is present in 1–5% of women who complain of hirsutism. It results from mutations in enzymes required for adrenal steroidogenesis. The most common form of CAH is characterized by a deficiency of 21-hydroxylase with case reports of similar occurrences in patients with 3β-hydroxysteroid dehydrogenase and 11β-hydroxylase deficiencies. These defects prohibit cortisol synthesis from its precursor 17β-hydroxyprogesterone. The expectant decrease in serum cortisol stimulates pituitary secretion of adrenocorticotropic hormone (ACTH) in an effort to normalize cortisol levels. Higher levels of ACTH stimulate adrenal production of intermediates in the biosynthetic pathway of cortisol. Consequently, these intermediates cannot be used for cortisol production because of enzyme defects, and are instead shunted into the biosynthetic pathways for androgens, with resultant increases in testosterone and androstenedione.

Classical CAH is usually diagnosed in females during the neonatal period because of androgen-induced ambiguous genitalia (pseudohermaphroditism); however, a minor enzyme deficiency may go unrecognized until puberty or later when hirsutism, amenorrhea, and virilization may occur. Such disease is termed acquired, late-onset, or adult-onset CAH.

2. Neoplastic disorders—Adrenal tumors are a rare cause of hirsutism, although when present, symptoms may be acute and quite severe. The main androgen produced by adrenal neoplasms is dehydroepiandrosterone sulfate (DHEAS), with serum levels usually greater than 700–800 μg/dL. Rarely, adrenal neoplasms may secrete testosterone; when this occurs, testosterone values are usually higher than 200 ng/dL.

3. Cushing's syndrome—Cushing's syndrome and the associated overproduction of cortisol may increase androgen levels and cause hirsutism. The syndrome has three known etiologies: (1) adrenal tumor, (2) ectopic production of ACTH by a nonpituitary tumor, or (3) excess production of ACTH by the pituitary (**Cushing's disease**). Since androgens are formed from intermediates in the synthesis of cortisol, increased serum and tissue levels of cortisol and its intermediates may result in hyperandrogenism and clinically present as hirsutism, regardless of the underlying cause of this syndrome.

4. Other causes—**Hyperprolactinemia** has been shown to produce mild hirsutism. Several investigators have reported increased DHEAS levels with hyperprolactinemia. This likely results from adrenal stimulation after prolactin binds to its numerous receptors on the adrenal gland. Despite increased androgen secretion, clinical manifestations are mild or absent, due to the inhibitory effects of prolactin on the conversion of testosterone to dihydrotestosterone (DHT) and its metabolites.

The adrenal gland may be the source of excess androgen production in the absence of an identifiable cause. The cause of this adrenal hyperactivity is not clear, but mild enzyme deficiencies, stress and hyperfunctioning of the entire adrenal gland, have been postulated as probable causes.

C. IATROGENIC MECHANISMS CAUSING HIRSUTISM

Exogenous sources of androgens should also be considered as possible causes of hirsutism. Methyltestosterone, danazol, and anabolic steroids such as oxandrolone may lead to excessive hair growth. The 19-nortestosterones in low-dose oral contraceptives rarely cause hirsutism or acne.

D. IDIOPATHIC HIRSUTISM

Hirsutism that occurs without adrenal or ovarian dysfunction, in patients with normal menstrual cycles and in the absence of any exogenous source of steroid hormones is termed **idiopathic hirsutism.** The term idiopathic hirsutism is thought to be a misnomer, since a likely cause has been elucidated. When normal levels of testosterone, unbound testosterone, DHEAS, dihydrotestosterone, and androstenedione are present, increased 5α-reductase enzyme activity appears to be the major mechanism of action. This enzyme converts testosterone to the more potent dihydrotestosterone in the hair follicle. Many patients with idiopathic hirsutism have an elevated level of plasma 3α-androstanediol glucuronide, a metabolite of dihydrotestosterone, thought to reflect the increased peripheral androgen metabolism, which is responsible for the clinical manifestation of hirsutism.

In summary, hirsutism may result from an ovarian disorder, an adrenal disease, an iatrogenic cause, or an increase in peripheral androgen metabolism. Rarely, other endocrinologic disturbances such as hypothyroidism or acromegaly may be associated with excessive hair growth. An important clinical correlation is that hirsutism may be accompanied by infertility as a result of the underlying abnormality. Since infertility may be the inciting factor triggering a patient to seek medical care, questions regarding a history of hirsutism should be a part of any infertility work-up.

Physiology of Androgens

Androgens are steroids that stimulate the development of male secondary sex characteristics and consequently promote the growth of sexual hair. The major androgens are testosterone, dihydrotestosterone, androstenedione, dehydroepiandrosterone (DHEA), and DHEAS. In order to comprehend the role played by elevated levels of androgens in the development of hirsutism, one must understand the sources of androgens, their metabolic pathways and sites of action, and their interrelationship with other steroid hormones such as estrogens and corticosteroids.

A. PRODUCTION

All steroid hormone production begins with the two-stage rate-limiting step of cholesterol conversion to pregnenolone, which is regulated by trophic hormones. In the nonpregnant woman, androgens are produced by both the ovaries and the adrenals, as well as by peripheral conversion. The rate-limiting step in androgen formation is the regulation of P450c17 gene expression, which is dependent on the concentrations of luteinizing hormone (LH) in the ovary and ACTH in the adrenal cortex.

1. Ovarian production of androgens—Androgens are produced by the normal ovary as precursors in the synthesis of estrogens. When gonadotropin-releasing hormone (GnRH) is secreted in a pulsatile fashion, thecal cells are stimulated to secrete and bind LH. In response to ligand binding, the theca cells of the preantral follicle produce androstenedione, DHEA, and testosterone. In the normal female, follicle-stimulating hormone (FSH) secreted from granulosa cells stimulates the granulosa cells to aromatize these androgens to the estrogens, estrone and estradiol. This relationship produces a system of androgen anabolism and catabolism balanced and coordinated to meet the needs of the follicular cycle.

2. Adrenal production of androgens—Stimulation of the adrenal gland by ACTH results in androgen production in the zona reticularis and zona fasciculata of the adrenal cortex. The main androgen manufactured is DHEAS, with smaller amounts of DHEA and androstenedione. A phenomena called adrenarche occurs and is usually chronologically timed before menarche in females. During this period, the adrenal cortex has a significant increase in adrenal hormone production, as a result of increased responsiveness of androgens and their precursors to the circulating levels of ACTH. This results in adrenocortical secretion of DHEAS at a level

similar to that of cortisol secretion. Controversy remains regarding the causative factors.

B. CIRCULATION

1. Testosterone—Testosterone, by virtue of its plasma concentration and its potency, is one of the major androgens. It is the second most potent androgen after dihydrotestosterone, and circulating levels are 20–80 ng/dL in adult women. The ovary and the adrenals contribute equally to testosterone production, with each supplying about 25% of the total circulating level. The other 50% of circulating testosterone is derived from peripheral conversion of androstenedione, although the ovarian contribution to testosterone levels may increase during the periovulatory portion of the menstrual cycle. Peripheral levels of testosterone display a slight diurnal variation that parallels that of cortisol. In normal women, 99% of testosterone is protein-bound, of which 80% is bound to sex hormone-binding globulin (SHBG) and 19% is loosely bound to albumin. The remaining 1% is free and unbound. The free and albumin-bound testosterone are the biologically active forms of circulating testosterone.

2. Dihydrotestosterone—Circulating levels of dihydrotestosterone, the most potent androgen, are 2–8 ng/dL or one-tenth those of testosterone. Although both the ovary and the adrenal gland secrete it, most dihydrotestosterone is produced by peripheral conversion of testosterone by 5(-reductase.

3. Androstenedione—Androstenedione, one of the 17-ketosteroids, is not very potent, with only 20% of the effectiveness of testosterone. Synthesis and secretion occur mostly in the ovaries and adrenals in equal amounts, with the remaining 10% being produced peripherally. Androstenedione levels display a diurnal variation paralleling that of cortisol and may simultaneously increase by as much as 50% when cortisol levels rise. Moreover, periovulatory increases in androstenedione levels can also be observed. In contrast to testosterone, androstenedione is bound mainly to albumin and secondarily to SHBG.

4. DHEA and DHEAS—DHEA and DHEAS, both weak androgens, have approximately 3% of the effectiveness of testosterone, and are the other major precursors of 17-ketosteroids. DHEA is primarily produced by the adrenals (60–70%), with ovarian production and hydrolysis of DHEAS accounting for the remainder. DHEA has a large diurnal variation similar to that of cortisol. Conversely, DHEAS is derived almost entirely from the adrenal, has only slight diurnal variation, and circulates in high concentrations. The DHEAS level may provide a good clinical assessment of adrenal function.

C. ACTION

The skin and hair follicles are androgen-responsive and thus have the capacity to metabolize androgens. DHEA, androstenedione, and testosterone enter the target cell and are reduced to dihydrotestosterone by 5α-reductase. Dihydrotestosterone is then bound to a cytoplasmic receptor protein that transports the androgen into the cell nucleus, where it is bound to chromatin and initiates transcription of stored genetic information. In the hair follicle, this promotes hair growth, leading to increased hair growth and initiating the conversion of vellus to terminal hair.

In females a certain amount of androgenic stimulation is expected, with the greatest levels noted at puberty, when these increased levels result in the clinical appearance of pubic hair and axillary hair. Similarly, androgens stimulate the facial pilosebaceous glands resulting in the pubertal development of acne.

Metabolic conversion of androgens to dihydrotestosterone may be accelerated. This results in irreversible conversion of vellus hair to terminal hair in areas of androgen-sensitive skin. Thus, in excess androgens are pathologic, and the clinical signs and symptoms of hirsutism and virilization result.

Physiology of Hair Growth

The hair follicle and its sebaceous gland together make up the pilosebaceous unit. The hair follicle begins to develop within the first 2 months of gestation, and by birth, a child possesses all of the hair follicles he or she will ever have. Hair first appears as vellus hair, which is fine, short, and lightly pigmented. During puberty, adrenal and ovarian androgen levels rise, converting vellus hair to terminal hair, which is coarse, long, and more heavily pigmented.

Hair growth is cyclic. The three phases of the cycle are (1) anagen (growth), (2) catagen (rapid involution), and (3) telogen (inactivity). The length of each hair is determined by the relative duration of anagen and telogen and varies with different locations on the body, although each hair follicle has its own growth cycle independent of adjacent hair follicles. Scalp hair has a long anagen, from 2 to 6 years, with a short telogen.

The growth and development of the hair follicle may be influenced by several factors. First, the pilosebaceous unit is sensitive to the effects of sex hormones, especially androgens. During puberty, adrenal and ovarian androgen levels rise, converting testosterone to dihydrotestosterone, which can initiate growth and increase both the diameter and pigmentation of hair. Although conversion of vellus hair to terminal hair is essentially irreversible, removal of the androgenic stimulus will slow hair growth and stop the conversion of vellus to terminal hair. Conversely, estrogens can retard the growth rate and result in finer hair with less pigmentation.

Genetic factors may also influence the pilosebaceous unit. Although males and females are born with equal numbers of hair follicles, racial and ethnic differences are noted in the concentration of hair follicles; Caucasians have a greater number of hair follicles than African-Americans, who in turn have a greater number than Asians. Different ethnic groups within each race may also exhibit differences in hair follicle concentrations (eg, Caucasians of Mediterranean ancestry have a greater concentration of hair follicles than those of Nordic ancestry).

Understanding the role of exogenous factors on the pilosebaceous unit allows one to better understand how pathologic hirsutism develops, and what factors may affect the severity of the disease process.

Diagnosis & Clinical Findings

Appropriate questioning allows one to rule out any history of drug ingestion that might cause excessive hair growth, to determine the speed of onset of symptoms, and to correlate the timing of symptoms with age and puberty. Specific inquiry into the patient's menstrual history allows the classification of patients who are amenorrheic or oligomenorrheic, and to distinguish those whose pathology began with puberty from those with a later onset of hirsutism. Knowledge of a family history of hirsutism or of abnormal menstrual cycles may also be informative.

Finally, a physical examination should be performed to differentiate hypertrichosis from hirsutism and to evaluate for acanthosis nigricans or additional signs of virilization such as clitorimegaly, male pattern balding, deepening voice, or decreased breast contour. Particular attention should be paid to body habitus, hair distribution, and the pelvic examination. Employing the Ferriman-Gallwey grading system provides a subjective determination of the severity of hirsutism and may also be followed to determine treatment effectiveness.

A. SIGNS AND SYMPTOMS

Many of the disorders involving hirsutism have characteristic presentations that may aid in diagnosis. For example, in classical congenital adrenal hyperplasia, the stigmata are identified at birth and include clitorimegaly, labial fusion, and an abnormal urethral course. Hirsutism presenting in childhood may be due to androgen-producing tumors and usually presents with other pronounced signs of virilization and the presence of a pelvic mass. However, an androgen-producing tumor should also be suspected when a woman with a normal menstrual history presents with sudden

onset of irregular menses followed by amenorrhea, hirsutism, and virilization. Genetic anomalies such as mosaic cells containing Y chromosomes or incomplete androgen insensitivity syndrome may produce signs of androgen stimulation associated with primary amenorrhea at puberty. Moreover, if a patient presents with a long history of irregular menses with slow onset of hirsutism beginning at puberty or in the early 20s, polycystic ovary syndrome or late-onset congenital adrenal hyperplasia are suggested. A higher index of suspicion for CAH should be considered in individuals with a genetic predisposition (Ashkenazi Jews and Eskimos), short stature, or a strong family history of hirsutism. Similarly, menstrual irregularities, in the presence of galactorrhea or visual changes, should cause suspicion of hyperprolactinemia. Hirsutism or virilization during pregnancy raises the suspicion of a luteoma of pregnancy or bilateral theca-lutein cysts. The physical signs of Cushing's syndrome, including centripetal obesity, wasting of the extremities, fat deposition in supraclavicular areas and in the neck and face, facial plethora, and wide cutaneous striae are usually apparent if this syndrome exists. When acromegaly is present, overgrowth of the viscera and soft body tissues, as well as enlargement of the bones of the hands, feet, and face can be seen. Finally, if hypothyroidism is present, thickening of the skin of the lips, fingers, lower legs, or lower eyelids may be present, along with complaints of lethargy, cold intolerance, constipation, and voice changes.

While the medical history, the menstrual history, and the physical examination are directive and informative, significant overlap exists and laboratory studies and sometimes imaging studies are needed before a diagnosis can be confirmed.

B. LABORATORY FINDINGS

Investigators disagree about which androgens should be measured in the evaluation of hirsutism. Laboratory evaluation should seek to identify life-threatening conditions associated with hyperandrogenism, such as Cushing's syndrome, congenital adrenal hyperplasia, and ovarian or adrenal tumors. Serum testosterone, DHEAS, and 17β-hydroxyprogesterone levels can be obtained for screening purposes.

1. Screening tests

a. Testosterone—A serum testosterone level of less than 200 ng/dL will rule out almost all of the testosterone-secreting neoplasms. A total testosterone level higher than 200 ng/dL should be considered evidence of an ovarian tumor until proven otherwise; few adrenal tumors produce testosterone.

The presence of hirsutism in a patient with a normal testosterone level indicates increased androgen effects. In hirsute women, increased androgen levels may decrease production of SHBG by the liver, and the free, biologically active fraction of testosterone may increase 2–3%. Therefore, normal total serum levels of testosterone in a hirsute woman can reflect a decreased level of SHBG, with an increase in the free testosterone fraction. However, the determination of the serum free testosterone level is expensive and does not add any useful clinical information.

b. DHEAS—A normal or slightly elevated DHEAS level excludes significant adrenal pathology. Adrenal tumors usually produce DHEAS with plasma levels markedly elevated to greater than 700–800 μg/dL. The plasma DHEAS level is reliable and convenient and has replaced 24-hour urine collection for measurement of 17-ketosteroids in most laboratories.

c. 17α-Hydroxyprogesterone—17α-Hydroxyprogesterone is the single most accurate diagnostic test for congenital adrenal hyperplasia due to 21-hydroxylase deficiency. It is a cost-effective screen for women whose history suggests CAH. 17α-Hydroxyprogesterone should be measured immediately upon awakening, in the morning, and only during the follicular phase of the menstrual cycle. Normal levels are less than 200 ng/dL. Levels ranging between 200 and 400 ng/dL warrant further evaluation. Levels greater than 400 ng/dL are virtually diagnostic of 21-hydroxylase deficiency.

2. Directed tests—Further testing should be ordered based on history and physical examination. If a woman is oligo-ovulatory or anovulatory, determination of FSH, LH, thyroid-stimulating hormone (TSH), and prolactin levels is helpful. In patients with a mild enzyme deficiency or a partial block at the 21-hydroxylation step in the biosynthesis of cortisol, 17α-hydroxyprogesterone levels may not be elevated and ACTH stimulation may be required for diagnosis. If the DHEAS level is elevated or if Cushing's syndrome is suspected, then either an overnight dexamethasone suppression test or a 24-hour urinary free cortisol level should be obtained. If the above laboratory tests are normal in a hirsute female, the diagnosis of idiopathic hirsutism must be considered and an androstanediol glucuronide level may be evaluated.

a. FSH and LH—An elevated level of LH, particularly when the LH:FSH ratio is 3 or higher, suggests polycystic ovary syndrome; however, this value is neither sensitive nor specific and is not required for the diagnosis. Newer diagnostic tests being employed include the evaluation of the glusose:insulin ratio and SHBG. Low levels of these values indicate insulin resistance, which is often a contributing factor in the development of polycystic ovarian syndrome.

b. Prolactin—A mildly elevated prolactin level may be seen in patients with polycystic ovarian syndrome or those with increased adrenal stimulation. However, prolactin elevation above 200 μg/dL usually suggests a prolactinoma.

c. TSH—An increased TSH level is strongly suggestive of hypothyroidism. A free T_4 and T_4 index should be obtained to confirm the diagnosis in these individuals.

d. ACTH stimulation test—The ACTH-induced increase in 17α-hydroxyprogesterone is a sensitive diagnostic test for congenital adrenal hyperplasia. Generally, this test is reserved for individuals in high-risk populations, given the low prevalence of disease among hirsute women. For diagnosis, 17α-hydroxyprogesterone is measured 30 minutes after an intravenous injection of 250 μg of synthetic ACTH. Values rarely exceed 400 ng/dL in normal women and values above 1000 ng/dL are indicative of disease. Once the diagnosis is made, the nomogram by Marie New can be used to differentiate nonclassical and classical disease.

e. Tests used to diagnose Cushing's syndrome

(1) Overnight dexamethasone suppression test—An overnight dexamethasone suppression test may be used as a simple outpatient screening test. A baseline morning plasma cortisol level is drawn, then dexamethasone, 1 mg orally, is given at 11:00 PM. A second plasma cortisol level is obtained at 8:00 AM the next morning. In normal patients, cortisol levels are suppressed to 5 μg/dL, whereas in patients with Cushing's syndrome, cortisol levels fall but do not go below 5 μg/dL. This test is easily performed on an outpatient basis, but may result in false-negative results, particularly in patients with mild disease. The false-positive rate is much higher in obese patients, chronically ill or depressed patients, and patients taking carbamazepine.

(2) 24-hour urinary free cortisol—The most accurate screening test for documentation of hypercortisolism is measurement of urinary free cortisol over a 24-hour period. Values greater than 100 ng/24 h are considered abnormal and further evaluation is warranted. Values greater than 250 ng/24 h are virtually diagnostic of Cushing's syndrome. The 24-hour urinary free cortisol determination is an excellent screening test because it has a low incidence of false-negative results; however, false-positive values may occur in the presence of depression, polycystic ovarian syndrome, carbamazepine therapy, or increased fluid intake.

(3) Low-dose dexamethasone suppression test—If the above screening tests yield equivocal results, the low-dose dexamethasone suppression test may be employed. Low-dose suppression of urinary free cortisol to less than 25 mg/24 h or 17-hydroxycorticosteroids to less than 3 mg/24 h after the administration of 0.5 mg of dexam-

ethasone every 6 hours for 2 consecutive days rules out Cushing's syndrome. Unfortunately, this test also has remarkably low sensitivity and specificity, and some investigators questions its benefit in patient evaluation.

(4) Additional tests—Alternatively, newer tests may be employed. These include (1) evaluation of late night plasma or salivary cortisol levels; (2) assessment of plasma cortisol after dexamethasone and corticotropin-releasing hormone are given; and (3) evaluation of ACTH after administration of intravenous and oral hydrocortisone. While all of the above tests may assist when verification of disease is required, the ideal test for evaluation has yet to be identified.

f. Tests used to differentiate Cushing's disease from Cushing's syndrome

(1) High-dose dexamethasone test—Once the diagnosis of Cushing's syndrome has been made, the etiology should be further elucidated. The high-dose dexamethasone test is usually used for this purpose, although it is currently being reevaluated. It requires 6 days of urine collection and the sensitivity and specificity are poor. Despite efforts by many investigators to improve this test, limitations continue to exist. When this test is used diagnostically, Cushing's disease is diagnosed when urinary free cortisol and 17-hydroxycorticosteroid are suppressed by 90%.

(2) Corticotropin-releasing hormone (CRH) stimulation test—Measuring plasma ACTH levels before and after the administration of CRH yields better results than the high-dose dexamethasone test; however, the diagnostic accuracy is no better than 85–90%. Therefore, the addition of imaging studies or inferior petrosal sinus sampling may be justified (see below).

g. Androstanediol glucuronide levels

The measurement of serum androstanediol glucuronide has been proposed as a good marker of peripheral androgen production and activity in hirsutism. Serum androstanediol glucuronide may be elevated in idiopathic hirsutism as a result of altered metabolism or increased utilization of androgen in the skin and hair follicles. Although this test is useful for research, its clinical applicability remains limited. Because of high cost and limited usefulness, the test for androstanediol glucuronide levels is not currently recommended in the routine evaluation of hirsutism.

C. IMAGING STUDIES

Ultrasonography is usually reserved for patients suspected of having a pelvic mass contributing to their disease process. In general, pelvic examination reveals a palpable ovarian mass; however, if the examination is limited by the individual's body habitus, pelvic ultrasonography may help delineate an abnormal structure. Although patients with polycystic ovarian syndrome have characteristic small, peripheral ovarian follicles, the specificity of ultrasonography is extremely limited, since many individuals without this syndrome have been found to have polycystic ovaries. Hence, routine ultrasonography in the diagnosis of this syndrome is not a universal practice.

If the testosterone level is higher than 200 ng/dL and no ovarian mass is identified, computed tomography (CT) or magnetic resonance imaging (MRI) of the adrenal glands should be performed before laparotomy to rule out the rare testosterone-producing adrenal tumor. CT scan and MRI of the adrenal glands have proven to be sensitive diagnostic techniques that have generally replaced selective venous sampling and selective angiography. Selective bilateral venous catheterization of adrenal and ovarian veins has limited clinical usefulness, since it is technically difficult and hazardous to perform, and its diagnostic sensitivity is poor.

Primary adrenal disease is most often confirmed with adrenal CT scan. CT scan or MRI of the lung is indicated with ectopic ACTH secretion, since this is the most common site of ectopic ACTH production. Similarly, a CT scan or MRI of the sella turcica may be used to localize an ACTH-secreting tumor. Currently, MRI is the preferred study due to its increased sensitivity when enhancement and dynamic imaging are judiciously used. Still, detection of the more centrally located ACTH-secreting microadenomas is only about 45–71%, and only 40–50% of these lesions are visualized before surgical correction of the problem. Due to limitations in biochemical testing and conservative imaging studies for Cushing's disease, simultaneous bilateral inferior petrosal sinus sampling is usually necessary to confirm the disease and to localize the lesion. A petrosal sinus:peripheral venous ACTH ratio greater than 2 in the absence of CRH, or greater than 3 when CRH is administered, is diagnostic of Cushing's disease.

Differential Diagnosis

Hirsutism should be differentiated from both virilization and hypertrichosis, since the cause and treatment of these disorders may be different. **Virilization** is characterized by more extensive androgen-induced changes than hirsutism alone. These changes include acne, increased oiliness of the skin, temporal balding, clitoromegaly, deepening of the voice, development of male muscular pattern and body habitus (in extreme cases), and atrophy of the breasts.

Hypertrichosis is also characterized by excessive growth of hair, but the term denotes increased growth of nonsexual hair (eg, hair on the forehead, lower leg, or forearm). The hair is usually fine-textured and is not caused by androgen excess or abnormal androgen metabolism. Heredity, certain drugs, physical irritation (trauma to the skin), or even starvation may be responsible. However, drug ingestion is the most common cause. Phenytoin, diazoxide, and minoxidil are known to cause a generalized increase in hair growth. Penicillamine and streptomycin have been associated with increased hair growth in infants and children. In addition, inadvertent ingestion of the fungicide hexachlorobenzene has also caused hypertrichosis. Disorders such as porphyria, hypothyroidism, dermatomyositis, acromegaly, Hurler's syndrome, trisomy E, and Cornelia de Lange's syndrome may be associated with hypertrichosis.

Treatment

The selection of therapy for hirsutism depends on the physical and laboratory findings, as well as on the patient's desire for childbearing. After evaluation has ruled out neoplasm or a serious disease process, a mildly hirsute woman with normal menstrual cycles may require only reassurance. A moderately or severely hirsute woman with menstrual irregularities requires treatment. For women not desiring childbearing in the near future, medical therapy consisting of adrenal or ovarian suppression or the blocking of peripheral androgen effects is advised. If infertility is a major concern, ovulation induction with the appropriate drug (eg, clomiphene, bromocriptine, human menopausal gonadotropin [hMG], or gonadotropin-releasing hormone [GnRH]) is started after appropriate evaluation. In many patients, simultaneous use of mechanical depilators and rarely surgery may be necessary.

A. MEDICAL MANAGEMENT

The medical treatment of hirsutism is not completely successful. The response rate has been reported to be between 23% and 95%, depending on the drug and dosage used. The drugs most commonly used to treat hirsutism include oral contraceptives, GnRH analogs, androgen receptor antagonists, and corticosteroids.

All drug therapy should seek to alter at least one of the 5 major aspects of androgen metabolism: (1) decrease production; (2) increase the metabolic clearance rate; (3) inhibit androgen receptors; (4) inhibit the enzymes involved in the peripheral production of testosterone or dihydrotestosterone; or (5) increase SHBG.

1. Combination oral contraceptives—Oral contraceptives have been extensively used to treat hirsutism. Their effect is exerted through a wide range of actions. The combination pill contains both estrogen and progestins and prevents ovulation by inhibiting gonadotropin secretion. Inhibition of LH secretion is mainly accomplished by the addition of the progestational component. When adequate suppression of LH is achieved, ovarian steroidogenesis is suppressed, lead-

ing to decreased testosterone production by the ovary. A decline in plasma testosterone can be seen as early as 1 week after treatment has been started; levels may decrease to normal by 3 months. Hair growth is reportedly decreased 50–60% in patients taking combination birth control pills. This effect is seen with the administration of all combination oral contraceptives, regardless of the individual steroid concentrations. Use of a low-dose pill (less than or equal to 35 ng of estrogen) allows for suppression of testosterone production while minimizing estrogen-related side effects.

The estrogen component decreases the androgenic effects of plasma testosterone by increasing hepatic SHBG synthesis. Since only the unbound form of testosterone is available to initiate a biologic response, increasing the bound fraction of testosterone by increasing SHBG levels leads to a decrease in testosterone-mediated effects. However, this increase has not been shown to have a direct effect on hirsutism.

Several studies suggest that combination birth control pills may exert a significant suppressive effect on adrenal androgen synthesis. Although the mechanism of action is presently unclear, this effect is probably due (at least in part) to suppression of ACTH release. The ability of combination birth control pills to lower the serum levels of DHEAS has several therapeutic implications. First, although DHEAS is low in biologic potency, it can serve as a precursor for peripheral conversion to more biologically potent androgens, and elevated levels of DHEAS can therefore be clinically manifested as hirsutism. Second, the ability of combination birth control pills to suppress both adrenal and ovarian androgen production, resulting in a significant reduction of androstenedione, DHEAS, and testosterone, may make these pills an even more attractive therapeutic option.

Older combination pills contain progestins, which are derivatives of testosterone. These 19-nortestosterones have some androgenic properties, which may result in hirsutism, acne, or oily skin. However, newer generation oral contraceptives contain desogestrel, gestodene, norgestimate or drospirenone. These drugs have fewer androgenic side effects, but have not consistently been shown to be more beneficial in the treatment of hirsutism.

2. Gonadotropin-releasing hormone (GnRH) agonists—GnRH analogs inhibit the secretion of gonadotropins from the pituitary gland, thereby inhibiting the secretion of androgens and estrogens from the ovary. Although GnRH agonists acutely stimulate ovarian production of androgens and estrogens, continued therapy causes a sustained decrease in ovarian steroid production compared with pretreatment levels. This suppression continues for the duration of GnRH agonist therapy. Significant decreases in serum levels of estradiol, testosterone, and androstenedione occur during treatment, although adrenal androgens are usually unaffected.

As a result of the hypoestrogenism associated with ongoing GnRH therapy, a potential risk of osteoporosis and menopausal symptoms exists with long-term therapy. However, concomitant use of estrogen and progesterone replacement therapy may counteract the adverse effects. Newer studies suggest that spironolactone may also simulate this effect.

Most studies have shown greater improvement of hirsutism with the use of GnRH agonists alone or in combination with oral contraceptives as compared with combination oral contraceptives alone; however, some studies show comparable efficacy.

3. Androgen receptor antagonists—There are four androgen receptor antagonists currently being used for the treatment of hirsutism. Despite proven efficacy in numerous clinical trials, none of these drugs has been approved by the U.S. Food and Drug Administration for this indication. Additionally, similar reported efficacy has been reported with all of these medications. Hence the agent of choice should be dictated by the individual's response, reported side effects, and known contraindications.

a. Cyproterone acetate—This potent agent was the first androgen receptor antagonist used to treat hirsutism and is widely prescribed in Europe to treat hirsutism. Antiandrogenic effects result from competitive displacement of dihydrotestosterone from its receptor and reduction of 5α-reductase activity in the skin. Progestational activity results in gonadotropin suppression with subsequent suppression of ovarian testosterone secretion. Cyclical administration of 50–100 mg on days 1–10 of the menstrual cycle combined with oral estrogen on days 1–21 produces therapeutic levels. Additionally, this method counters hypoestrogenism and irregular bleeding and prevents pregnancy and the potential teratogenic complications that may result. Although effective in 50–75% of hirsute women, significant side effects include decreased libido, mental depression, and hepatotoxicity, which is rarely seen when cyclic administration is performed. Clinical studies have shown efficacy equivalent to that of spironolactone, with the latter showing fewer side effects (see below). Currently, cyproterone acetate is not available in the U.S.

b. Spironolactone—Spironolactone, an aldosterone antagonist traditionally used as a diuretic in the treatment of hypertension, is also used to treat hirsutism. It possesses antiandrogenic properties and exerts its peripheral antiandrogenic effects in the hair follicle by competing for androgenic receptors and displacing dihydrotestosterone at both nuclear and cytosol recep-

tors. It also lowers testosterone levels by inhibiting the cytochrome P450 monooxygenases that are required for biosynthesis of androgens in gonadal and adrenal steroid-producing cells. Serum levels of SHBG, DHEAS, and DHEA are unaltered by treatment with spironolactone. The dosage used for treatment of hirsutism has varied between 50 and 200 mg/d. Serum androgen levels will drop within a few days of the start of treatment, and a clinical response can usually be seen within 2–5 months. Side effects are mild—transient diuresis and polydipsia have been noted in the first few days of treatment, and disturbances in the menstrual cycle, breast tenderness, and fatigue have also been reported, but no long-term problems have been encountered. Because spironolactone is a potent antiandrogen, all women using it should use effective contraception.

c. Flutamide—Flutamide is a potent, highly specific, nonsteroidal antiandrogen with no intrinsic hormonal or antigonadotropin activity. Although the exact mechanism of action is unknown, it competitively inhibits target tissue androgen receptor sites. Recent studies suggest that 250 mg 1–3 times daily is a highly effective treatment for moderate to severe hirsutism. Side effects include decreased appetite, amenorrhea, decreased libido, or dry skin. A rare but serious reported side effect is hepatotoxicity. Consequently, flutamide is usually reserved for resistant cases of hirsutism, and liver enzymes should be checked regularly in patients on the drug. Additionally, because of possible teratogenic effects, contraception must be used with this therapy.

d. Finasteride—Finasteride is the newest antiandrogenic agent used for hirsutism. It is a selective type 2 5α-reductase inhibitor that blocks the conversion of testosterone to dihydrotestosterone. It has proven efficacy in up to 86% of patients with a subjective improvement rate of 21–45% when 5 mg is administered orally over 3 months to 1 year. Side effects at this dosage are usually mild or absent and include headaches, transient gastrointestinal upset, and an unexplained increase in total testosterone.

4. Glucocorticoids—Dexamethasone is used mainly to treat hirsutism in patients with hyperandrogenism of adrenal origin. Chronic low-dose dexamethasone, 0.5–1 mg orally taken at bedtime, will provide adequate adrenal androgen suppression. Diminution of hair growth is reported in 16–70% of patients. Glucocorticoid therapy has fallen out of favor due to frequent side effects, potential for adrenal suppression, and evidence that these agents are less effective than antiandrogens, even when there is a clear adrenal cause of hyperandrogenism. However, their use may be justified in some patients, since recent data suggest that concomitant use of glucocorticoids with GnRH agonists may prolong the disease-free interval when therapy is discontinued. Moreover, glucocorticoids are the treatment of choice to decrease ACTH levels and thereby decrease formation of androgenic precursors of cortisol for patients with congenital adrenal hyperplasia.

5. Other

a. Dopamine—Dopamine is a centrally acting inhibitor of prolactin secretion and is frequently used in the treatment of hyperprolactinemia. Recently, hirsutism scores were shown to decrease significantly during dopamine treatment of hyperandrogenic women with hyperprolactinemia.

b. Troglitazone—Troglitazone is an insulin-sensitizing agent of the thiazolidinedione class, which results in a dose-related decrease in androgen level in patients with polycystic ovarian syndrome. Additionally, it has been shown that the administration of 600 mg/d results in significant improvement of hirsutism in this population.

c. Cimetidine—Cimetidine, an H_2-receptor antagonist, has weak antiandrogenic properties. Recent studies show minimal or no beneficial effect in hirsutism.

d. Ketoconazole—Ketoconazole is a synthetic imidazole derivative that blocks adrenal and gonadal steroidogenesis; it has been advocated by some as a treatment for hirsutism. However, serious side effects result in poor compliance and preclude long-term use. Its use should be avoided since safer therapeutic regimens exist.

B. MECHANICAL THERAPY

The goal of mechanical therapy is to limit new hair growth without affecting existing hair. For this reason, mechanical depilators such as lasers, electrolysis devices, creams, and waxes are often used as supplemental therapy. Recent technology has made this procedure faster, easier, less painful, and generally free of any serious adverse effects.

C. SURGICAL TREATMENT

In the minority of hirsute patients in whom a specific cause can be identified, therapy should be directed toward the underlying disorder. For example, ovarian and adrenal tumors should be surgically excised. Additionally, women with Cushing's disease are treated with transsphenoidal pituitary microsurgery. Alternatively, when Cushing's syndrome is caused by an adrenal tumor, simple adrenalectomy is sufficient. Finally, acromegaly can be treated by transsphenoidal hypophysectomy. For persistent disease, bilateral adrenalectomy or pituitary irradiation is appropriate.

Similarly, a minority of older women may fail to respond to medical management for hyperthecosis despite good compliance. For these women, bilateral oophorectomy may be justified as definitive therapy.

Although wedge resection of the ovary has been successfully used to induce ovulation, it is not recommended for the treatment of hirsutism. This surgical procedure exposes patients to the risks of both anesthesia and possible formation of adhesions. More importantly, this procedure results in only a transient decrease in androgen levels and has successfully reduced the rate of hair growth in only 16% of patients. Wedge resection should not be used as a treatment for hirsutism.

Complications & Prognosis

The treatment for hirsutism can be frustrating for both patient and physician because of the physiologic properties of hair itself. The growth cycle of hair is long, varying between 6 and 24 months, and the conversion of vellus hair to terminal hair is essentially irreversible. Also, once hair growth has been stimulated by excessive androgen levels, maintenance of that same growth rate requires much less androgen. Patients must be advised that a response to therapy may not be seen for 6–12 months and that although it is possible to prevent further conversion of vellus hair to terminal hair, little change will be seen in the total number of terminal hairs. Some patients may note lightening of hair color and a decrease in the diameter of the hair shaft with therapy. Cosmetic treatment of excess hair consists of shaving, plucking, bleaching, waxing, or use of depilatories; however, shaving and plucking may cause infection and scarring and are not recommended. Permanent hair removal may be accomplished only by electrolysis (electrocoagulation of the hair root, or papilla), which is costly and uncomfortable, or by depilation. Unless there is excessive hirsutism, electrolysis should be delayed until after 6–12 months of medical therapy have been completed.

Patients who exhibit progressive hirsutism while receiving hormonal therapy or patients whose circulating androgen levels fail to decrease as expected should undergo further evaluation. If androgen levels are not suppressed with appropriate therapy, the possibility of a slow-growing neoplasm should be considered. Levels of testosterone and DHEAS should be monitored and the adrenal glands and ovaries reevaluated.

When adequate suppression of DHEAS and testosterone has been maintained for 6–12 months but a satisfactory reduction in new hair growth has not occurred, several options are available. The dose of the current medication can be increased, a new medication can be substituted, or a new medication can be added. It is frequently impossible to increase the dose of the initial medication, since the incidence of side effects may increase as the drug dosage increases. Likewise, it is not always easy to switch medications, since choice of the initial drug may have been guided by specific therapeutic considerations (eg, hirsute women who desire contraception may be treated with combination contraceptive pills, whereas hirsutism associated with hypertension may be treated with spironolactone). Some authors have recommended adding a second medication to the treatment regimen for hirsutism unresponsive to therapy. Newer evidence suggests that combination drug treatment for hirsutism with concomitant use of drugs that act at different sites may produce the best results (eg, combination birth control pills that act chiefly through decreased production of ovarian steroids may be combined with spironolactone, which acts mainly at the peripheral androgen receptors).

Treatment for hirsutism must be individualized and based on the results of a thorough history, physical examination, and laboratory studies. After therapy has begun, the patient's progress can be monitored on the basis of both clinical appearance and laboratory values. The patient should be educated about her disorder in order to prevent unrealistic expectations of therapy and to make her aware of any side effects that might manifest during therapy. Adjunctive therapy is almost always necessary with any medical treatment for hirsutism. Depilatories and electrolysis are frequently needed to remove the terminal hair already present; these methods, when combined with medical therapy, offer the best cosmetic result.

REFERENCES

Azziz R et al: Troglitazone improves ovulation and hirsutism in the polycystic ovary syndrome: a multicenter double blind, placebo-controlled trial. J Clin Endocrinol Metab 2001; 86:1626.

Barnes R: Diagnosis and therapy of hyperandrogenism. Balliere's Clin Obstet Gynaecol 1997;11:369.

Bencini PL et al: Long-term epilation with long-pulsed neodymium:YAG laser. Dermatol Surg 1999;25:175.

Carmina E, Lobo R: The addition of dexamethasone to antiandrogen therapy for hirsutism prolongs the duration of remission. Fertil Steril 1998;69:1075.

Castelo-Branco C et al: Gonadotropin-releasing hormone analog plus an oral contraceptive containing desogestrel in women with severe hirsutism: effects on hair, bone, and hormone profile after 1-year use. Metabolism 1997;46:437.

DeLeo V et al: Hormonal and clinical effects of GnRH agonist alone, or in combination with a combined oral contraceptive or flutamide in women with severe hirsutism. Gynecol Endocrinol 2000;14:411.

Deplewski D et al: Role of hormones in pilosebaceous unit development. Endocr Rev 2000;21:363.

Escobar-Morreale HF et al: Treatment of hirsutism with ethinyl estradiol-desogestrel contraceptive pills has beneficial effects on the lipid profile and improves insulin sensitivity. Fertil Steril 2000;74:816.

Falsetti L et al: Comparison of finasteride versus flutamide in the treatment of hirsutism. Eur J Endocrinol 1999;141:361.

Findling JW, Raff J: Newer diagnostic techniques and problems in Cushing's disease. Endocrinol Metab Clin North Am 1999;28:191.

Fox R: Transvaginal ultrasound appearances of the ovary in normal women and hirsute women with oligomenorrhoea. Aust N Z J Obstet Gynaecol 1999;39:63.

Fruzzetti F et al: Treatment of hirsutism: comparisons between different antiandrogens with central and peripheral effects. Fertil Steril 1999;71:445.

Gregoriou O et al: The effect of combined oral contraception with or without spironolactone on bone mineral density of hyperandrogenic women. Gynecol Endocrinol 2000;14:369.

Hagag P et al: Androgen suppression and clinical improvement with dopamine agonists in hyperandrogenic-hyperprolactinemic women. J Reprod Med 2001;46:678.

Hock DL et al: New treatments of hyperandrogenism and hirsutism. Obstet Gynecol Clin North Am 2000;27:567.

Judd HL et al: The effects of ovarian wedge resection on circulating gonadotropin and ovarian steroid levels in patients with polycystic ovary syndrome. J Clin Endocrinol Metab 1976; 43:347.

Lunde O et al: Polycystic ovarian syndrome: a follow-up study on fertility and menstrual pattern in 149 patients 15–25 years after ovarian wedge resection. Hum Reprod 2001;16:1479.

Moghetti P et al: Comparison of spironolactone, flutamide, and finasteride efficacy in the treatment of hirsutism: a randomized, double blind, placebo-controlled trial. J Clin Endocrinol Metab 2000;85:89.

Moran C et al: 21-Hydroxylase-deficient nonclassic adrenal hyperplasia is a progressive disorder: a multicenter study. Am J Obstet Gynecol 2000;183:1468.

Naidich MJ, Russell EJ: Current approaches to imaging of the sellar region and pituitary. Endocrinol Metab Clin North Am 1999;28:45.

Pazos F et al: Prospective randomized study comparing the long-acting gonadotropin-releasing hormone agonist triptorelin, flutamide, and cyproterone acetate, used in combination with an oral contraceptive in the treatment of hirsutism. Fertil Steril 1999;71:122.

Shin Y et al: Comparison of Diane 35 and Diane 35 plus finasteride in the treatment of hirsutism. Fertil Steril 2001; 75:496.

Simberg N et al: High bone density in hyperandrogenic women: effect of gonadotropin-releasing hormone agonist alone or in conjunction with estrogen-progestin replacement. J Clin Endocrinol Metab 1996;81:646.

Sonino N, Boscaro M: Medical therapy for Cushing's disease. Endocrinol Metab Clin North Am 1999;28:211.

Spritzer PM et al: Spironolactone as a single agent for long-term therapy of hirsute patients. Clin Endocrinol (Oxf) 2000; 52:587.

Tulandi T, Took SA: Surgical management of ovarian syndrome. Baillere's Clin Obstet Gynaecol 1998;12:541.

Venturoli S et al: A prospective randomized trial comparing low dose flutamide, finasteride, ketoconazole, and cyproterone acetate-estrogen regimens in the treatment of hirsutism. J Clin Endocrinol Metab 1999;84:1304.

In Vitro Fertilization & Related Techniques

56

Catherine M. Marin, MD, Alan H. DeCherney, MD, Alan S. Penzias, MD,
& Ian H. Thorneycroft, MD, PhD

IN VITRO FERTILIZATION

In vitro fertilization and embryo transfer (IVF-ET) is only one method of assisted reproduction that enables couples to turn their dream of having a child into a reality. It involves removing eggs from the ovary, fertilizing them in the laboratory, and replacing them into the patient's uterus. The first live birth resulting from this technique occurred in June 1978. Since then, thousands of children have been born throughout the world after IVF-ET was used to help women who otherwise could not conceive.

The IVF-ET techniques outlined here are not experimental; they are part of the armamentarium of every fully equipped infertility service. As the success rate of IVF-ET improves with new developments, many conventional infertility therapies may become second-line treatments, while in vitro fertilization could become the primary therapy. Such is the case today for severe tubal disease, when pregnancy following tuboplasty is much less likely than pregnancy following in vitro fertilization.

The data in Table 56–1 were drawn from the United States In Vitro Fertilization and Embryo Transfer registry for 1990. The table depicts the percentage of patients entering an IVF program who progress to oocyte retrieval and embryo transfer along with cycle outcome. The table also shows that not all patients who begin an IVF cycle reach the egg retrieval stage. Some patients may respond poorly to stimulatory medications or ovulate prior to oocyte aspiration. An additional group of patients may undergo oocyte retrieval but not have an embryo transfer. These cases generally involve a severe male factor in which oocyte fertilization fails to occur. Assisted reproductive techniques (ARTs) have come a long way with more programs reporting (increasing from 30 in 1985, to 267 in 1993, and 335 in 1997), increased number of cycles treated, an increase in pregnancy rate, and an increase in the delivery rate (increasing from 6.6% in 1985, to 16% in 1993, and 27.9% in 1997) for IVF. In 1997 there were 73,069 ART cycles, including 51,344 IVF cycles, 1943 gamete intrafallopian transfer (GIFT) cycles (delivery rate 30%), 1104 zygote intrafallopian transfer (ZIFT) cycles

(delivery rate 28%), 4616 donor oocyte cycles (delivery rate 40%), and 10,181 frozen embryo transfers (delivery rate 18.8%). From all these cycles 17,311 deliveries resulted in 25,059 babies.

Approximately 20% of patients who undergo egg retrieval will become pregnant with sonographic documentation of an intrauterine pregnancy (clinical pregnancy); 80% of these patients will carry to term. Many "biochemical pregnancies" occur, but these should not be included in pregnancy statistics. (A biochemical pregnancy is one in which serum levels of human chorionic gonadotropin (hCG) rise and then fall before sonographic detection of pregnancy is possible.) Eggs are almost always obtained by aspiration, and under ordinary circumstances, approximately 85% of eggs will fertilize and cleave. The clinical pregnancy rate of approximately 20% per embryo transfer per IVF cycle is close to the 20–25% pregnancy rate per cycle observed in spontaneous conceptions in the general population.

The success rate in IVF has been improved by replacing more than 1 embryo, but doing so increases the likelihood of multiple gestation. The ethical questions and medical problems associated with multiple gestation as IVF-ET becomes more successful are discussed at the end of this chapter.

Indications

IVF-ET bypasses the mechanical transport functions of the female reproductive tract. It was first developed for patients with severe tubal disease, and it clearly offers the only hope of conception to patients who have had a bilateral salpingectomy or whose tubes are so badly damaged that they cannot function. Subsequently, in vitro fertilization has been applied to a variety of other infertility problems such as antisperm antibodies, endometriosis, oligospermia, and unexplained infertility. When the probability of conception by IVF-ET exceeds that of conception by conventional therapy, IVF-ET appears to be the procedure of choice. Due to an increased incidence of infertility in our modern society where women work earlier and conceive later and where there is an increased awareness and availability of ART, IVF demand has grown.

Table 56–1. Success of IVF-ET at various stages.

Percentage of patients starting IVF	100%
Percentage undergoing oocyte retrieval	82%
Percentage having an embryo transfer (ET)	69%
Percentage of clinical pregnancies/ET	20%
Percentage of ectopic pregnancies/ET	1%
Percentage of deliveries/ET	16%
Percentage of multiple deliveries/ET	4%

Although IVF is successful in treating many infertility problems, its success hinges upon entry of sperm into the egg. It was initially hoped that routine IVF-ET could be used to compensate for severe oligospermia (< 5 million sperm per mL). However, early results were highly variable. Recent advances in this area are now being applied in clinical practice. Modern microsurgical techniques permit placement of sperm under the protective egg shell (zona pellucida) or even directly into the cytoplasm of the oocyte. This is discussed in detail below. In addition to male factor issues, another barrier to success with IVF is hydrosalpinx. This condition may interfere with implantation and additional surgery may be needed so that implantation and pregnancy rates improve.

Technique

A. SUPEROVULATION

All IVF-ET programs use superovulation to stimulate production of several eggs and to improve timing of egg aspiration. The type of ovulation induction therapy varies from group to group and is constantly changing. The following methods are used alone or in combination (Table 56–2):

(1) Clomiphene citrate.
(2) Human menopausal gonadotropins.
(3) FSH agonists.
(4) GnRH agonists.

Superovulation is carefully monitored with ultrasound scanning and serum estradiol and luteinizing hormone (LH) determinations. Ultrasound scanning monitors the number and growth of ovarian follicles. At least 2 or 3 follicles should be developing before proceeding with egg aspiration. Otherwise, the cycle is abandoned and an alternative stimulation regimen is selected for a subsequent cycle. Serum estradiol levels are complementary to ultrasonography in evaluating the maturation and growth of the developing follicles. There is evidence that the pattern of serum estradiol may predict the cycles most likely to result in pregnancy. A declining estradiol level prior to hCG administration is associated with a lower pregnancy rate. hCG

Table 56–2. Types of ovulation induction therapy.

Medication	Mechanism	Contraindications	Complications	Other
Clomiphene citrate	Estrogen agonisit/ antagonist	Liver disease, abnormal uterine bleeding, pregnancy	Multiple pregnancies, ovarian enlargement, hot flushes, visual disturbances, changes in coordination	Use with caution in polycystic ovarian syndrome, increased sensitivity
Human menopausal gonadotropins				
Menotropins	FSH/LH combination	High FSH levels, thyroid or adrenal dysfunction, pituitary tumor, abnormal uterine bleeding, ovarian enlargement	Multiple pregnancies, spontaneous abortion, ovarian, hyperstimulation syndrome, hypercoagulability	10% of all patients treated for IVF are poor responders to stimulation with exogenous gonadotropins
Urofollitrophins	FSH/some LH	Same as above	Same as above	Easy administration
Highly purified FSH	FSH/minimal LH			
Recombinant human	No LH; pure FSH			Greater purity, no human contaminants
Genetically engineered FSH				Increased half life

or a GnRH agonist are given to mature the oocytes when ultrasonography has determined the presence of an adequate number of preovulatory follicles (17–20 mm). Ovulation ordinarily begins 36 hours after hCG injection. Serum LH measurement is extremely important, since spontaneous LH peaks, which result in ovulation prior to egg aspiration, can occur. Detection of a premature LH peak permits either immediate egg aspiration or abandonment of the cycle. The introduction of GnRH-a to superovulation regimens has drastically reduced the likelihood of a premature LH surge; therefore it is used in the majority of IVF patients in the U.S. Treatment with superovulation induction and intrauterine insemination of sperm is also used to treat certain types of infertility and is much more likely to result in pregnancy than is the treatment with either superovulation or intrauterine insemination alone.

B. Aspiration of Eggs

Aspiration of the preovulatory follicles is performed approximately 34 hours after the hCG injection or 24 hours after the beginning of the natural LH surge.

Egg aspiration is performed using one of two methods. Laparoscopy was the first method to be used and is rarely used today. The second method uses ultrasonography to direct transvaginal aspiration. In transvaginal aspiration, a needle is passed through the posterior vaginal fornix using a vaginal ultrasound probe and directed into the ovary. The advantage of ultrasound aspiration is that it can be performed on an outpatient basis with the patient awake.

C. Fertilization With Capacitated Sperm and Intracytoplasmic Sperm Injection (ICSI)

Freshly ejaculated sperm cannot fertilize an egg; the sperm must be capacitated. Fortunately, capacitation is a very simple process in humans and involves only a short incubation period in a culture medium.

Due to the nature of the superovulatory process, eggs will be in different stages of maturation. Therefore, once the eggs have been identified, they are classified by the embryologist as either mature (preovulatory) or immature. Mature eggs have an expanded cumulus oophorus, whereas immature eggs have a very compact cumulus. Mature eggs have undergone the first meiotic division; immature eggs have not. Mature eggs are usually fertilized 5 hours after aspiration. Immature eggs are incubated in the laboratory for up to 36 hours prior to fertilization. If sperm and eggs are mixed too early, fertilization and cleavage will not take place. Between 10,000 and 50,000 motile sperm are placed with each egg.

For male factor infertility, intracytoplasmic sperm injection has emerged as an effective solution, resulting in higher fertilization rates and expanded possibilities for cryopreservation.

D. Culture of Fertilized Eggs in the Laboratory

Eggs are incubated in an atmosphere of 5% carbon dioxide. Some physicians advocate an oxygen content of 5%; others use atmospheric oxygen (20%). Various culture media are used and are often supplemented with either the patient's serum or bovine serum albumin. At various intervals after the attempted fertilization, the eggs are examined in order to identify pronuclei, which confirm fertilization, as well as blastomeres, which confirm cleavage.

Fertilization and culture of the eggs are probably the most crucial stages of IVF-ET. All media must be carefully prepared. As a means of quality control, mouse pronuclear or 2-cell embryos or human sperm are incubated in all media made for IVF-ET and in all Petri dishes and test tubes used. Nontoxicity is established if virtually all embryos develop to the blastocyst stage or if sperm maintain complete motility for 24 hours. If nontoxicity cannot be established, new media are prepared or that particular batch of plastic ware is discarded.

E. Replacement of Fertilized Egg into the Uterus

After 48–72 hours of laboratory culture, the fertilized eggs are replaced into the patient's uterus, usually at the 2-cell to 8-cell stage. A cumulative embryo score can first be obtained and used as a reference to determine an optimal number of embryos to transfer and to predict pregnancy outcome. Recently blastocyst transfers have also been done and they may offer better success rates in selected patients. The embryos are aspirated into a small catheter, the catheter is passed transcervically into the uterus, and the eggs are injected into the uterine cavity. The probability of pregnancy after embryo transfer can be affected by the patient's age, the cause of infertility, the endometrial thickness, and the average embryo morphology score.

Scientific Study of Human Embryos & Embryo Biopsy

Scientific study of human embryos is a very controversial subject and is generally restricted to abnormally fertilized embryos that are not compatible with life. Embryo research is not only discussed in medical centers but also in the White House. Karyotyping of apparently normal embryos in some European centers has revealed interesting findings (eg, haploid and aneuploid embryos have appeared morphologically normal at the 8-cell stage). No one advocates discarding healthy-appearing embryos.

Certain genetically heritable diseases can be identified using a variety of molecular biologic techniques. These techniques include but are not limited to polymerase chain reaction (PCR) and fluorescent in situ hybridization (FISH). Recent advances in embryo manipulation have made possible the removal of 1 or 2 cells from a developing 8-cell human embryo without harm to the embryo. In patients at risk of passing along a heritable genetic disease, application of PCR and FISH have made possible the identification of normal embryos (those with no risk of passing on the lethal heritable disease). These normal embryos without risk are then transferred back to the patient. Several live births have been reported following application of these techniques. The number of centers performing these techniques are few but growing.

Complications

Few risks are associated with IVF-ET. Congenital anomalies occur no more frequently than in normally conceived embryos. Some of the complications and drawbacks of IVF-ET include:

(1) Multiple gestations—Transferring more embryos does not necessarily lead to a greater IVF success rate (Table 56–3). IVF-ET clinics with the highest success rates transfer only 3–4 embryos, though they have many fertilized embryos from a single cycle. The remaining embryos can either be donated to another woman or frozen for later use. A frozen embryo is thought to have one-half the potential for successful implantation of a fresh embryo. Recently the methods for oocyte freezing have been improved as well.

(2) Ectopic and heterotopic pregnancies—A significant risk to mothers.

(3) Cost—Currently only 12 states allow health insurance to cover infertility treatment, which leaves many couples with tremendous expenses (the estimated cost per delivery is $66,667).

Table 56–3. Number and PE of embryos typically transferred by age group.

Age of Patient	Embryos Transferred
< 35	4 poor quality vs 2 fair quality vs 2 good quality
36–39	4 poor quality vs 3 fair quality vs 2 good quality vs
> 40	5 poor quality vs 4 good quality

(4) Pulmonary embolus—A result of superovulation that increases coagulability.

(5) Preterm birth and low birthweight infants.

(6) Ovarian hyperstimulation syndrome.

OTHER TECHNIQUES RELATED TO IVF-ET

Ovum Donation

Embryos have been donated from one woman to another with resultant live births. Women who receive donated embryos may be those who are not candidates for IVF-ET because of ovarian failure or absence, or gonadal dysgenesis. In these women, the endometrium must be primed with estrogen and progesterone prior to transfer of the donated embryo, and progesterone supplementation must be maintained for at least 10 weeks.

Ovum donation can occur under one of two circumstances. One is the infertile patient who produces a large number of oocytes during her own IVF or GIFT cycle and elects to donate some of them to another woman who is otherwise incapable of producing eggs. The other circumstance involves the recruitment of a woman who undergoes superovulation and oocyte retrieval purely for the purpose of donating her oocytes. The donor may be known to the patient (a family member or friend) or may be anonymous. Although the genetics of the resulting pregnancy is derived from the husband and the donor, the infertile woman incapable of producing her own eggs goes through the pregnancy. In these women the endometrium must be primed with estrogen and progesterone prior to transfer of the donated embryo and progesterone supplementation should be maintained for at least 6 weeks. This technique has resulted in live births, with remarkable success.

GIFT (Gamete Intrafallopian Tube Transfer)

GIFT is similar to IVF-ET. It was first used in 1984 and the number of cycles in North America increased 75-fold from 75 in 1985 to 5767 in 1992, and the pregnancy rate rose from 4% to 29.5%. Superovulation is induced as in IVF-ET; an hCG injection is given and the follicles are aspirated via laparoscopy. Prior to laparoscopy, semen is collected and capacitated. The eggs are identified in the laboratory. Sperm are then mixed with the eggs and drawn up into a catheter. The sperm and eggs can also be separated by an air bubble in the catheter. The eggs and sperm are then transferred to the uterine tubes, permitting natural fertilization and cleavage. A 20–30% pregnancy rate per cycle has been reported for this technique.

Obviously, GIFT is useful only in patients who have normal tube function and are not of advanced age. It has been argued that the requirement of normal tubal function renders the direct comparison of IVF-ET and GIFT results impossible. Among proponents of each technique, there is vigorous ongoing debate as to the advantages of GIFT over IVF-ET .

In unexplained infertility, IVF-ET will differentiate the etiology of fertilization problems between egg and sperm; GIFT will not. Additionally, GIFT exposes patients to the risks of general anesthesia and laparoscopy. GIFT is now rarely utilized.

ZIFT (Zygote Intrafallopian Transfer)

ZIFT is a procedure that combines IVF and GIFT. Ovulation is induced and the oocytes are removed and fertilized in vitro. Soon thereafter they are placed into the fallopian tubes by laparoscopy and the embryo travels to the uterine cavity. ZIFT is now rarely utilized.

REFERENCES

In Vitro Fertilization and ART

Assisted reproductive technology in the United States: 1997 results generated from the American Society for Reproductive Medicine/Society for Assisted Reproductive Technology Registry. Fertil Steril 2000;74:641.

Aboulghar M, Mansour R, Serour G: Controlled ovarian hyperstimulation and intrauterine insemination for treatment of unexplained infertility should be limited to a maximum of three trials. Fertil Steril 2001;75:88.

Abusheikha N, Salha O, Brinsden P: Extra-uterine pregnancy following assisted conception treatment. Hum Reprod Update 2000;6:80.

Aubard Y et al: Ovarian tissue cryopreservation and gynecologic oncology: a review. Eur J Obstet Gynecol Reprod Biol 2001;97:5.

Balasch J, Barri PN: Reflections on the cost-effectiveness of recombinant FSH in assisted reproduction. The clinician's perspective. J Assist Reprod Genet 2001;18:45.

Baird DT: Is there a place for different isoforms of FSH in clinical medicine? IV. The clinician's point of view. Hum Reprod 2001;16:1316.

Bergh T: Deliveries and children born after in-vitro fertilization in Sweden 1982–1995: a retrospective cohort study. Lancet 1999;354:1579.

Blazar A et al: The impact of hydrosalpinx on successful pregnancy in tubal factor infertility treated IVF. Fertil Steril 1997; 67:517.

Boulot P et al: Multifetal reduction of triplets to twins: a prospective comparison of pregnancy outcome. Hum Reprod 2000; 15:1619.

Desai NN et al: Morphological evaluation of human embryos and derivation of an embryo quality scoring system specific for day 3 embryos: a preliminary study. Hum Reprod 2000; 15:2190.

The ESHRE Capri Workshop Group: Multiple gestation pregnancy. Hum Reprod 2000;15:1856.

Forti G, Krausz C: Evaluation and treatment of the infertile couple. J Clin Endocrinol Metab 1998;83:4177.

Garcia-Velasco JA, Isaza V, Requena A: High doses of gonadotrophins combined with stop versus non-stop protocol of GnRH analogue administration in low responder IVF patients: a prospective, randomized, controlled trial. Hum Reprod 2000;15:2292.

Gleicher N et al: Reducing the risk of high-order multiple pregnancy after ovarian stimulation with gonadotropins. N Engl J Med 2000;343:2.

Graham J, Han T, Porter R: Day 3 morphology is a poor predictor of blastocyst quality in extended culture. Fertil Steril 2000;74:495.

Guzick DS, Sullivan MW, Adamson GD: Efficacy of treatment for unexplained infertility. Fertil Steril 1998;70:207.

Hugues JN, Bry-Gauillard H, Bstandig B: Comparison of recombinant and urinary follicle-stimulating hormone preparations in short-term gonadotropin releasing hormone agonist protocol for in vitro fertilization-embryo transfer. J Assist Reprod Genet 2001;18:191.

Kodama H, Takeda S, Fukuda J: Activation of plasma kinin system correlates with severe coagulation disorders in patients with ovarian hyperstimulation syndrome. Hum Reprod 1997; 12:891.

Lass A, Gerrard A, Abusheika N: IVF performance of women who have fluctuating early follicular FSH levels. J Assist Reprod Genet 2000;17:566.

Ludwig M, Rietmuller-Winzen H, Felberbaum RE: Health of 227 children born after controlled ovarian stimulation for in vitro fertilization using the luteinizing hormone-releasing hormone antagonist cetrorelix. Fertil Steril 2001;75:18.

Murray D et al: The adverse affect of hydrosalpinges on in vitro fertilization pregnancy rates and the benefit of surgical correction. Fertil Steril 1998;69:41.

Nargund G, Waterstone J, Bland J: Cumulative conception and live birth rates in natural (unstimulated) IVF cycles. Hum Reprod 2001;16:259.

Nikolettos N et al: Gonadotropin-releasing hormone antagonist protocol: a novel method of ovarian stimulation in poor responders. Eur J Obstet Gynecol Reprod Biol 2001; 97:202.

Racowsky C et al: Recombinant FSH preparations for controlled ovarian stimulation in assisted reproduction: A comparison of Gonal F and Follistim. Fertil Steril 2001;75(4 suppl 1):S15.

Senn A: Prospective randomized study of two cryopreservation policies avoiding embryo selection: the pronuclear stage leads to a higher cumulative delivery rate than the early cleavage stage. Fertil Steril 2000;74:946.

Shenfield F, Pennings G, Sureau C: The cryopreservation of human embryos. Hum Reprod 2001;16:1049.

Simon A et al: Comparison of cryopreservation outcome following ICSI and conventional IVF. J Assist Reprod Genet 1998;15:431.

Stone J, Eddleman K: Multifetal pregnancy reduction. Curr Opin Obstet Gynecol 2000;12:491.

Strandell A, Thorburn J, Hamberger L: Risk factors for ectopic pregnancy in assisted reproduction. Fertil Steril 1998;71:282.

Strehler E, Abt M, El-Danasouri I: Impact of recombinant follicle-stimulating hormone and human menopausal gonadotropins on in vitro fertilization outcome. Fertil Steril 2001;75:332.

Templeton A, Morris J: Reducing the risk of multiple births by transfer of two embryos after IVF. N Engl J Med 1998; 339:573.

Terriou P et al: Embryo scoring is a better predictor of pregnancy than the number of transferred embryos or female age. Fertil Steril 2001;75:525.

Tesarik J, Mendoza C: In vitro fertilization by intracytoplasmic sperm injection. Bioessays 1999;21:791.

Tesarik J, Mendoza C, Greco E: Treatment of severe male factor infertility by micromanipulation-assisted fertilization: news and views. Front Biosci 1998;15:E238.

Van Voorhis BJ, Barnett M, Sparks AE: Effect of the total motile sperm count on the efficacy and cost-effectiveness of intrauterine insemination and in vitro fertilization. Fertil Steril 2001;75:661.

Van Voorhis BJ, Stovall D, Allen B: Cost effective treatment of the infertile couple. Fertil Steril 1998;70:995.

Venn A, Jones P, Quinn M: Characteristics of ovarian and uterine cancers in a cohort of in vitro fertilization patients. Gynecol Oncol 2001;82:64.

Wakeley KE, Grendys EC: Reproductive technologies and risk of ovarian cancer. Curr Opin Obstet Gynecol 2000;12:43.

Yim SF, Lok IH, Cheung LP: Dose-finding study for the use of long-acting gonadotrophin-releasing hormone analogues prior to ovarian stimulation for IVF. Hum Reprod 2001;16:492.

Yunxiahu BS: Maximizing pregnancy rates and limiting higher order multiple conceptions by determining the optimal number of embryos to transfer based on quality. Fertil Steril 1998;69:650.

Zayed F, Abu-Heija A: The management of unexplained infertility. Obstet Gynecol Surv 1999;54:121.

Zayed F, Ghazawi I, Francis L: Predictive value of human chorionic gonadotropin in early pregnancy after assisted conception. Arch Gynecol Obstet 2001;265:7.

Zeynelogue HB, Arici A, Olive DL: Comparison of intrauterine insemination with timed intercourse in superovulated cycles with gonadotropins: a meta-analysis. Fertil Steril 1998; 69:486.

Ziebe S, Petersen K, Lindenberg S: Embryo morphology or cleavage stage: how to select the best embryos for transfer after in-vitro fertilization. Human Reprod 1997;12:1545.

Zuppa AA, Maragliano G, Scapillati ME: Neonatal outcome of spontaneous and assisted twin pregnancies. Eur J Obstet Gynecol Reprod Biol 2001;95:68.

Ovum Donation

Koopersmith TB et al: Outcomes of high-order multiple implantations in women undergoing ovum donation. J Matern Fetal Med 1997;6:268.

Licciardi F et al: a two versus three embryo transfer: the oocyte donation model. Fertil Steril 2001;75:510.

Schoolcraft WB, Gardner DK: Blastocyst culture and transfer increases the efficiency of oocyte donation. Fertil Steril 2000; 74:482.

Soderstrom-Antilla V: Oocyte donation in infertility treatment—a review. Acta Obstet Gynecol Scand 2001;80:191.

Soderstrom-Antilla V: Pregnancy and child outcome after oocyte donation. Hum Reprod Update 2001;7:28.

Tarlatzis BC, Pados G: Oocyte donation: clinical and practical aspects. Mol Cell Endocrinol 2000;161:99.

Wolff KM, McMahon MJ, Kuller JA: Advanced maternal age and perinatal outcome. Obstet Gynecol 1997; 89:519.

Yaron Y, Amit A, Kogosowski A: The optimal number of embryos to be transferred in shared oocyte donation: walking the thin line between low pregnancy rates and multiple pregnancies. Hum Reprod 1997;12:699.

GIFT/ZIFT

Chung PH: Gamete intrafallopian transfer: Comparison of epidural vs. general anesthesia. J Reprod Med 1998;43:681.

Eldar-Geva T et al: Different influence of incongruent follicular development on in vitro fertilization-embryo transfer and gamete intrafallopian transfer pregnancy rates. Fertil Steril 1998;70:1039.

Farhi J, Weissman A, Nahum H: Zygote intrafallopian transfer in patients with tubal factor infertility after repeated failure of implantation with in vitro fertilization-embryo transfer. Fertil Steril 2000;74:390.

Klonoff-Cohen H et al: Effects of female and male smoking on IVF and gamete intrafallopian transfer. Hum Reprod 2001; 16:1382.

Levran D, Mashiach S, Dor J: Zygote intrafallopian transfer may improve pregnancy rate in patients with repeated failure of implantation. Fertil Steril 1998;69:26.

Milki AA, Tazuke SI: Office laparoscopy under local anesthesia for gamete intrafallopian transfer: technique and tolerance. Fertil Steril 1997;68:128.

Silva PD, Olson KL, Meisch JK: Gamete intrafallopian transfer. A cost-effective alternative to donor oocyte in vitro fertilization in women aged 40–42 years. J Reprod Med 1998;43:1019.

Swisher ED, Wobster R, Armstrong A: Age-related pregnancy rates in GIFT patients. Mil Med 1998;163:449.

Menopause & Postmenopause 57

Norma L. Jones, MD, & Howard L. Judd, MD

General Considerations

According to the 1990 U.S. census, of the 139 million women in this country, 40 million were 50 years of age or older. Most of these women had or shortly would have their last menstrual period, thus becoming postmenopausal. Since a woman at age 50 can expect to live another 35 years, a large portion of the female population is without ovarian function and live about one-third of their lives after this function ceases. Consequently, physicians caring for women must understand the hormonal and metabolic changes associated with the menopause, or "change of life," and the potential benefits and risks of hormone replacement therapy (HRT).

According to the Comite des Nomenclatures de la Federation Internationale de Gynecologie et d'Obstetrique, the **climacteric** is the phase of the aging process during which a woman passes from the reproductive to the nonreproductive stage. The signals that this period of life has been reached are referred to as "climacteric symptoms" or, if more serious, as "climacteric complaints." **Premenopause** refers to the part of the climacteric before the menopause occurs, the time during which the menstrual cycle is likely to be irregular and when other climacteric symptoms or complaints may be experienced. The **menopause** is the final menstruation, which occurs during the climacteric. **Postmenopause** refers to the phase of life that comes after the menopause.

Etiology & Pathogenesis

A. MENOPAUSE

There are two types of menopause, classified according to cause.

1. Physiologic menopause—In the human embryo, oogenesis begins in the ovary around the third week of gestation. Primordial germ cells appear in the yolk sac, migrate to the germinal ridge, and undergo cellular divisions. It has been estimated that the fetal ovaries contain approximately 7 million oogonia at 20 weeks' gestation. After 7 months' gestation, no new oocytes are formed. At birth, there are approximately 1–2 million oocytes, and by puberty this number has been reduced to 300,000–500,000. Continued reduction of oocyte

number occurs during the reproductive years through ovulation and atresia. Nearly all oocytes vanish by atresia, with only 400–500 actually being ovulated. Very little is known about oocyte atresia. Animal studies have shown that estrogens prevent the atretic process while androgens enhance it.

Menopause apparently occurs in the human female because of two processes. First, oocytes responsive to gonadotropins disappear from the ovary, and second, the few remaining oocytes do not respond to gonadotropins. Isolated oocytes can be found in postmenopausal ovaries on very careful histologic inspection. Some of them show a limited degree of development, but most reveal no sign of development in the presence of excess endogenous gonadotropins.

The average age at menopause in the U.S. is 50–51 years. There does not appear to be any consistent relationship between age at menarche and age at menopause. Marriage, childbearing, height, weight, and prolonged use of oral contraceptives do not appear to influence the age of menopause. Smoking, however, is associated with early menopause.

Spontaneous cessation of menses before age 40 is called **premature menopause** or **premature ovarian failure.** It appears that approximately 0.9% of women in the U.S. may experience this early cessation of function. Cessation of menstruation and the development of climacteric symptoms and complaints can occur as early as a few years after menarche. The reasons for premature ovarian failure are unknown.

Disease processes, especially severe infections or tumors of the reproductive tract, can occasionally damage the ovarian follicular structures so severely as to precipitate the menopause. The menopause can also be hastened by excessive exposure to ionizing radiation; chemotherapeutic drugs, particularly alkylating agents; and surgical procedures that impair ovarian blood supply. The possibility of associated endocrine abnormalities should also be considered.

2. Artificial menopause—The permanent cessation of ovarian function brought about by surgical removal of the ovaries or by radiation therapy is called an artificial menopause. Irradiation to ablate ovarian function is rarely used today. Artificial menopause is employed as a treatment for endometriosis and estrogen-sensitive neoplasms of the breast and endometrium. More frequently, artificial menopause is a side effect of treatment of intra-abdominal disease; eg, ovaries are removed in premenopausal women because the gonads have been damaged by infection or neoplasia. When laparotomy affords the opportunity, elective bilateral oophorectomy is also employed to prevent ovarian cancer. For premenopausal women, this practice is controversial. For postmenopausal women, it is now generally accepted as good medical practice.

B. PREMENOPAUSAL STATE

The decades of mature reproductive life are characterized by generally regular menses and a slow, steady decrease in cycle length. Mean cycle length at age 15 is 35 days, at age 25 it is 30 days, and at age 35 it is 28 days. This decrease is due to shortening of the follicular phase of the cycle, with the luteal phase length remaining constant. After age 45, altered function of the aging ovary is detectable in regularly menstruating women (Fig 57–1). The mean cycle length is significantly

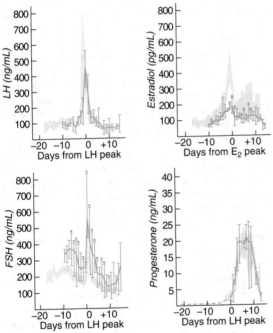

Figure 57–1. Mean and range of LH, FSH, estradiol (E₂), and progesterone levels in women over age 45 with regular menstrual cycles. Shaded area represents the mean (2 SEM in cycles found in young women. (Reproduced, with permission, from Sherman BM, Korenman SG: Hormonal characteristics of the human menstrual cycle throughout reproductive life. J Clin Invest 1975;55:699.)

shorter than in younger women and is attributable to a shortened follicular phase. The luteal phase is of similar length, and progesterone levels are no different from those observed in younger women. Estradiol levels are lower during portions of the cycle, including active follicular maturation, the midcycle peak, and the luteal phase. Concentrations of follicle-stimulating hormone (FSH) are strikingly elevated during the early follicular phase and fall as estradiol increases during follicular maturation. FSH levels at the midcycle peak and late in the luteal phase are also consistently higher than those found in younger women and decrease during the midluteal phase. Luteinizing hormone (LH) concentrations are indistinguishable from those observed in younger women. The mechanism responsible for this early rise of FSH is probably related to inhibin. **Inhibin** is a polypeptide hormone that is synthesized and secreted by granulosa cells. It causes negative feedback on FSH release by the pituitary. As the oocyte number decreases, inhibin levels fall, resulting in a rise in FSH levels.

The transition from regular cycle intervals to the permanent amenorrhea of menopause is characterized by a phase of marked menstrual irregularity. The duration of this transition varies greatly among women. Those experiencing the menopause at an early age have a relatively short duration of cycle variability before amenorrhea ensues. Those experiencing it at a later age usually have a phase of menstrual irregularity characterized by unusually long and short intermenstrual intervals and an overall increase of mean cycle length and variance.

The hormonal characteristics of this transitional phase are of special interest and importance. The irregular episodes of vaginal bleeding in premenopausal women represent the irregular maturation of ovarian follicles with or without hormonal evidence of ovulation. The potential for hormone secretion by these remaining follicles is diminished and variable. Menses are sometimes preceded by maturation of a follicle with limited secretion of both estradiol and progesterone. Vaginal bleeding also happens after a rise and fall of estradiol without a measurable increase in progesterone, such as is seen during anovulatory menses.

From these findings, it is clear that the transitional phase of menstrual irregularity is not one of marked estrogen deficiency. During the menopausal transition, high levels of FSH appear to stimulate residual follicles to secrete bursts of estradiol. Occasionally, estradiol levels will rise to concentrations 2 or 3 times higher than is normally seen, probably reflecting the recruitment of more than 1 follicle for ovulation. This may be followed by corpus luteum formation, often with limited secretion of progesterone. Because the episodes of follicular maturation and vaginal bleeding are widely spaced, premenopausal women may be exposed to persistent estrogen stimulation of the endometrium in the absence of regular cyclic progesterone secretion.

C. CHANGES IN HORMONE METABOLISM ASSOCIATED WITH THE MENOPAUSE

Following the menopause, there are major changes in androgen, estrogen, progesterone, and gonadotropin secretion, much of which occurs because of cessation of ovarian follicular activity (Fig 57–2).

1. Androgens—During reproductive life, the primary ovarian androgen is androstenedione, the major secretory product of developing follicles. In postmenopausal women, there is a reduction of circulating androstenedione to approximately 50% of the concentration found in young women, reflecting the absence of follicular activity. In the year following the last menstrual period, the levels of this hormone are steady. In older women, there is a circadian variation of androstenedione, with peak concentration between 8:00 AM and noon, and the nadir occurring between 3:00 PM and 4:00 AM. This rhythm reflects adrenal activity. The clearance rate of androstenedione is similar in pre- and postmenopausal women; therefore, the level of circulating hormone reflects production. Thus, the average production rate of androstenedione is approximately 1.5 mg/24 h in older women, a rate that is 50% of the rate found in premenopausal women. The source of most of this circulating androstenedione appears to be the adrenal glands, but continued secretion by the postmenopausal ovary accounts for approximately 20%.

For testosterone, the level found in postmenopausal women is minimally lower than that found in premenopausal women before oophorectomy and is distinctly higher than the level observed in ovariectomized young women. There is also a prominent circadian variation of this androgen, with the highest levels occurring at 8:00 AM and the nadir at 4:00 PM. There is no difference in the clearance rate of testosterone before and after the menopause. Thus, the production rate in older women is approximately 150 µg/24 h, a rate that is only one-third lower than the rate seen in young women.

The source of circulating testosterone is more complex than that of androstenedione. After the menopause, oophorectomy is associated with a nearly 60% decrease in testosterone. There is no change in the metabolic clearance rate of the androgen with oophorectomy; therefore, the fall in the circulating level reflects alterations of its production rate. About 15% of circulating androstenedione is converted to testosterone. The small simultaneous fall of androstenedione after oophorectomy can only account for a small portion of the total decrease of testosterone. The remainder presumably represents direct ovarian secretion and is larger than the amount secreted directly by the premenopausal ovary. Large increments in testosterone have been found in the ovarian compared with the peripheral veins of postmenopausal women. These increments are greater than those observed in premenopausal women, supporting the hypothesis that the postmenopausal ovary secretes more testosterone directly than the premenopausal ovary. Hilar cells and luteinized stromal cells (hyperthecosis) are present in most postmenopausal ovaries and have been shown to produce testosterone in premenopausal women. Presumably, these cells could do the same in postmenopausal subjects.

A proposed mechanism for increased ovarian testosterone production by postmenopausal ovaries is the stimulation of gonadal cells still capable of androgen production by excess endogenous gonadotropins, which in turn are increased because of reduced estrogen production by the ovaries. This increased ovarian testosterone secretion, coupled with a reduction of estrogen production, may in part explain the development of symptoms of defeminization, hirsutism, and even virilism occasionally seen in older women.

Levels of the adrenal androgens dehydroepiandrosterone (DHEA) and dehydroepiandrosterone sulfate (DHEAS) are reduced by 60% and 80%, respectively, with age. Whether these reductions are related to the

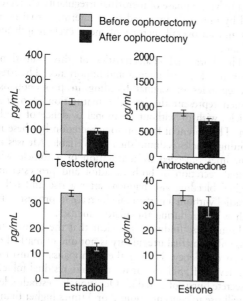

Figure 57–2. Serum androgen and estrogen levels in 16 postmenopausal women with endometrial cancer before and after oophorectomy. (Reproduced, with permission, from Judd HL: Hormonal dynamics associated with the menopause. Clin Obstet Gynecol 1976;1:775.)

menopause or to aging has not been determined. Again, a marked circadian variation of DHEA has been observed. Whether a similar rhythm is present for DHEAS is not known. As with younger subjects, the primary source of these two androgens is thought to be the adrenal glands, with the ovary contributing less than 15%. Thus, the marked decreases of DHEA and DHEAS reflect altered adrenal androgen secretion, and this phenomenon has been called the "adrenopause." The mechanism responsible for it is not known.

2. Estrogens—After a woman has passed the menopause, there is good clinical evidence of reduced endogenous estrogen production in most subjects. When circulating levels have been assessed, the greatest decrease is in estradiol. Its concentration is distinctly lower than that found in young women during any phase of their menstrual cycle and is similar to the level seen in premenopausal women following oophorectomy. A decrease of this estrogen occurs up to 1 year following the last menstrual period. There does not appear to be a circadian variation of the circulating concentration of estradiol following the menopause. The metabolic clearance rate of estradiol is reduced by 30%. The average production rate is 12 μg/24 h.

The source of the small amount of estradiol found in older women has been established. Direct ovarian secretion contributes minimally, but the adrenal glands are the major source. Investigators who have examined the concentrations of estradiol in adrenal veins have reported minimal increments, arguing against direct adrenal secretion being a major contributor. Although both estrone and testosterone are converted in peripheral tissues to estradiol, it is conversion from estrone that accounts for most estradiol in older women.

After the menopause, the circulating level of estrone decreases—not as much as that of estradiol—and overlaps with values seen in premenopausal women during the early follicular phase in menstrual cycles. There is a circadian variation of circulating estrone, with the peak in the morning and the nadir in late afternoon or early evening. This variation is not as prominent as that observed for the androgens. In postmenopausal women, there is a 20% reduction of estrone clearance, and the average production rate is approximately 55 μg/24 h.

The adrenal gland is the major source of estrone. Direct adrenal or ovarian secretion is minimal. Most estrone results from the peripheral aromatization of androstenedione. The average percent conversion is double that found in ovulatory women and can account for the total daily production of this estrogen. Aromatization of androstenedione has been shown to occur in fat, muscle, liver, bone marrow, brain, fibroblasts, and hair roots. Other tissues may also contribute but have not been evaluated. To what extent each cell type contributes to total conversion has not been determined, but fat cells and muscle may be responsible for only 30–40%. This conversion has been shown to correlate with body size, with heavy women having higher conversion rates and circulating estrogen levels than slender women.

3. Progesterone—In young women, the major source of progesterone is the ovarian corpus luteum following ovulation. During the follicular phase of the cycle, progesterone levels are low. With ovulation the levels rise greatly, reflecting the secretory activity of the corpus luteum. In postmenopausal women, the levels of progesterone are only 30% of the concentrations seen in young women during the follicular phase. Since postmenopausal ovaries do not contain functional follicles, ovulation does not occur and progesterone levels remain low. The source of the small amount of progesterone present in older women is felt to be due to adrenal secretion, since dexamethasone suppresses its level, adrenocorticotropic hormone (ACTH) stimulates its concentration, and human chorionic gonadotropin (hCG) administration has no effect.

4. Gonadotropins—With the menopause, both LH and FSH levels rise substantially, with FSH usually higher than LH. This is thought to reflect the slower clearance of FSH from the circulation. The reason for the marked increase in circulating gonadotropins is the absence of the negative feedback of ovarian steroids and inhibin on gonadotropin release. As in young women, the levels of both gonadotropins are not steady, but instead show random oscillations. These oscillations are thought to represent pulsatile secretion by the pituitary. In older women, these pulsatile bursts occur every 1–2 hours, a frequency similar to that seen during the follicular phase of premenopausal subjects. Although the frequency is similar, the amplitude is much greater. This increased amplitude is secondary to increased release by the hypothalamic hormone gonadotropin-releasing hormone (GnRH) and enhanced responsiveness of the pituitary to GnRH due to low estrogen levels. Studies with rhesus monkeys suggest that the site governing pulsatile LH release is in the arcuate nucleus of the hypothalamus. The large pulses of gonadotropin in the peripheral circulation are believed to maintain the high levels of the hormones found in postmenopausal women.

Clinical Findings

A. SYMPTOMS AND SIGNS

1. Reduced endogenous estrogens—

a. Reproductive tract—Alteration of menstrual function is the first clinical symptom of the climacteric, although a gradual reduction of fertility starts by age 25 and is prominent after age 40. Some premenopausal women also complain of hot flushes. Changes in menstrual function may conform to one or more of the following patterns:

(1) Abrupt cessation of menstruation is fairly rare, because the decline of ovarian function usually proceeds slowly.

(2) The most common pattern is a gradual decrease in both amount and duration of menstrual flow, tapering to spotting, and eventually to cessation. Irregularity of the cycle appears sooner or later, with skips and delays of menses occurring.

(3) A minority of patients have more frequent or heavier vaginal bleeding. Bleeding between periods may also occur. As mentioned earlier, the occurrence of this type of bleeding usually reflects continued follicular estrogen production with or without ovulation. However, it may also reflect organic disease, eg, atypical endometrial hyperplasia or endometrial carcinoma.

The diagnosis of permanent cessation of menses is of necessity retrospective. Amenorrhea lasting 6 months to 1 year is commonly accepted as establishing the diagnosis. Only rarely will vaginal bleeding reflecting ovarian follicular activity recur after 1 year of amenorrhea. In older women, when uterine bleeding does happen after prolonged amenorrhea, it is more suggestive of organic disease. As menstrual function declines, associated symptoms such as mastodynia, abdominal bloating, edema, headache, and cyclic emotional disturbances also subside, reflecting the decrease in ovarian hormone secretion.

Because estrogen functions as the major growth factor of the female reproductive tract, there are substantial changes in the appearance of all the reproductive organs. Most postmenopausal women experience varying degrees of atrophic changes of the vaginal epithelium. The vaginal rugae progressively flatten. As the epithelium thins, the capillary bed shines through as a diffuse or patchy reddening. Rupture of surface capillaries produces irregularly scattered petechiae, and a brownish discharge may be noted. Minimal trauma with douching or coitus may result in slight vaginal bleeding. Early in the process, local bacterial invasion is likely to initiate vaginal pruritus and leukorrhea. Further atrophy of the vaginal epithelium renders its capillary bed increasingly sparse, so that the hyperemic appearance gives way to a smooth, shiny, pale epithelial surface.

There are also atrophic changes of the cervix. It usually decreases in size, and there is a reduction of secretion of cervical mucus. This may contribute to excessive vaginal dryness, which may cause dyspareunia.

Atrophy of the uterus is also seen, with shrinkage of both the endometrium and myometrium. This shrinkage is actually beneficial to women who enter the climacteric with small to moderate-sized uterine myomas. Reduction in size and elimination of symptoms frequently prevent the necessity for surgical treatment. The same applies to adenomyosis and endometriosis, both of which usually become asymptomatic. With cessation of follicular activity, hormonal stimulation of the endometrium comes to an end. This tissue usually is atrophic and inactive, not only inside the uterus but also at ectopic sites. Hence, palpable and symptomatic areas of endometriosis generally become progressively smaller and less troublesome.

The oviducts and ovaries also decrease in size postmenopausally. Although this produces no symptoms, the smallness of the ovaries makes them difficult to palpate during pelvic examination. A palpable ovary in a postmenopausal woman must be viewed with suspicion, and the presence of an ovarian neoplasm must be considered.

The supporting structures of the reproductive organs suffer loss of tone as estrogen levels decline. Postmenopausal estrogen deficiency may lead to symptomatic progressive pelvic relaxation.

b. Urinary tract—Estrogen plays an important role in maintaining the epithelium of the bladder and urethra. Marked estrogen deficiency may produce atrophic changes in these organs similar to those that occur in the vaginal epithelium. This may give rise to atrophic cystitis, characterized by urinary urgency, incontinence, and frequency without pyuria or dysuria. Loss of urethral tone, with pouting of the meatus and thinning of the epithelium, favors the formation of a urethral caruncle with resultant dysuria, meatal tenderness, and occasionally hematuria.

c. Mammary glands—Regression of breast size during and after menopause is psychologically distressing to some women. To those who have been bothered by cyclic symptoms of breast pain and cystic formation, the disappearance of these symptoms postmenopausally is a great relief.

d. Hot flushes—The most common and characteristic symptom of the climacteric is an episodic disturbance consisting of sudden flushing and perspiration, referred to as a **hot flash** or **flush.** It has been observed in about 75% of women who go through the physiologic menopause or have a bilateral ovariectomy. Of those having flushes, 82% experience the disturbance for more than 1 year and 25–50% complain of the symptom for more than 5 years. Most women indicate that hot flushes begin with a sensation of pressure in the head, much like a headache. This increases in intensity until the physiologic flush occurs. Palpitations may also be experienced. The actual flush is characterized as a feeling of heat or burning in the face, neck, and chest, followed immediately by an outbreak of sweating that affects the entire body but is particularly prominent over the head, neck, upper chest, and back. Less common symptoms include weakness, fatigue, faintness, and vertigo. The duration of the whole episode varies from momentary to as long as 10 minutes; the average length is 4 minutes. The frequency varies from 1–2 an hour to 1–2 a week. In women with severe flushes, the mean frequency is 54 minutes.

Investigators have now characterized the physiologic changes associated with hot flushes and have shown that the symptoms result from true alterations in cutaneous vasodilation, perspiration, reductions of core temperature, and elevations of pulse rate. Fluctuations in electrocardiographic data probably reflect changes in skin conductance. Changes in heart rhythm and blood pressure have not been observed.

The patient's awareness of symptoms does not correspond exactly with physiologic changes. Women become conscious of symptoms approximately 1 minute after the onset of measurable cutaneous vasodilatation, and discomfort persists for an average of 4 minutes, whereas physical changes persist for several minutes longer.

The exact mechanism responsible for hot flushes is not known, but physiologic and behavioral data indicate that symptoms result from a defect in central thermoregulatory function. Several observations support this conclusion: (1) The 2 major physiologic changes associated with hot flushes—perspiration and cutaneous vasodilatation—are the result of different peripheral sympathetic functions. Excitation of sweat glands results from sympathetic cholinergic fibers, and cutaneous vasodilatation is under the control of tonic alpha-adrenergic fibers. It seems unlikely that any peripheral event could cause both cholinergic excitation of sweat glands and alpha-adrenergic blockade of cutaneous vessels, and it is well recognized that these are the two basic functions triggered by central thermoregulatory mechanisms that lower the central temperature. (2) During a hot flush, the central temperature decreases because of cutaneous vasodilatation and perspiration. If hot flushes were the result of some peripheral event, the body's regulatory mechanisms would be expected to prevent such a decrease. (3) There is also a change in behavior associated with hot flushes. Women feel warm and have a conscious desire to cool themselves by throwing off the bedcovers, standing by open windows or doors, fanning themselves, or by other means. This behavior is observed even in the presence of a steady or decreasing central temperature.

Most investigators believe the core temperature of the body is maintained near a central set point that is controlled by central thermoregulatory centers, particularly those in the rostral hypothalamus. This central set point temperature is analogous to a thermostat setting.

Hot flushes appear to be triggered by a sudden lowering of the central hypothalamic "thermostat." As a consequence, heat loss mechanisms, both physiologic and behavioral, are activated so that the core temperature will be brought in line with the new set point; this results in a fall of central temperature.

Because hot flushes occur after the spontaneous cessation of ovarian function or following oophorectomy, it has been presumed that the underlying mechanism is endocrinologic, related either to reduction of ovarian estrogen secretion or to enhancement of pituitary gonadotropin secretion. Low estrogen levels alone do not appear to trigger hot flushes; prepubertal children and patients with gonadal dysgenesis have low estrogen levels but not flushing. Patients with gonadal dysgenesis do experience symptoms if they are given estrogens that are later withdrawn. Thus, it appears that estrogen must be present and then withdrawn in order for hot flushes to be experienced.

Hot flushes appear to be related to gonadotropins. A close temporal association between the occurrence of flushes and the pulsatile release of LH has been demonstrated. The observation that flushes occur after hypophysectomy suggests that they are not due directly to LH release (Fig 57–3). The appearance of hot flushes in women with defects in GnRH release or synthesis (Kallman's syndrome) also suggests GnRH itself is not involved in the flushing mechanism. The absence of

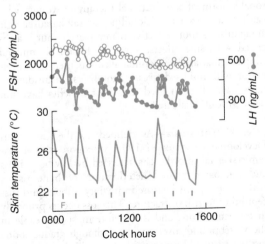

Figure 57–3. Skin temperature and LH and FSH levels in a woman with hot flushes. Note the close temporal relationship between the rises in skin temperature and the occurrence of pulsatile LH release. (Reproduced, with permission, from Tataryn IV et al: LH, FSH, and skin temperature during the menopausal hot flash. J Clin Endocrinol Metab 1979;49:152.)

hot flushes in women with hypothalamic amenorrhea and hypoestrogenemia is intriguing. These women have been shown to have defects in neurotransmitter or neurochemical input to their GnRH neurons. In particular, excessive endogenous opioid and dopamine input to GnRH neurons may account for chronic suppression of GnRH release, leading to hypothalamic amenorrhea. The absence of hot flushes in these women suggests that altered afferent input of neurotransmitters or neurochemicals to the GnRH neuron that is secondary to hypogonadism leads to hot flushes. Two likely candidates are norepinephrine and endogenous opioids.

Hot flushes are a greater annoyance than most physicians have recognized. Patients frequently complain of night sweats and insomnia. A close temporal relationship has been shown between the occurrence of hot flushes and nighttime awakening. Women with frequent flushes may experience flushes and awakening episodes hourly; this may cause a profound sleep disturbance that may in turn cause cognitive (memory) and affective (anxiety) disorders in some women.

Estrogens are the principal medications used to relieve hot flushes. Estrogens block both the perceived symptoms and the physiologic changes. Their use also relieves some aspects of the sleeping disorder. Estrogen administration has been shown to enhance hypothalamic opioid activity in postmenopausal women. This increase of hypothalamic opiates may be involved in the relief of hot flushes with estrogen administration.

Progestins also block hot flushes and represent a reasonable form of substitutional therapy in women who can't take estrogens. Clonidine, an alpha-adrenergic antagonist, is more effective than a placebo but is associated with side effects. Vitamins E and K, mineral supplements, and belladonna alkaloids used in combination with mild sedatives, tranquilizers, or antidepressants have all been tried, but their benefits have not been critically evaluated.

e. Osteoporosis—As defined by the Consensus Development Center in 1993, osteoporosis is a systemic skeletal disorder characterized by low bone mass and microarchitectural deterioration of bone tissue, with a consequent increase in fragility of bone and susceptibility to risk of fracture. This loss occurs primarily in trabecular bone and is therefore most noticeable in the vertebra and distal radius. Although gradual bone loss occurs in all humans with aging, this loss is accelerated in women after cessation of ovarian function. Following attainment of peak bone mass by age 25–30, bone loss begins, accelerates in women at menopause, and then slows again but continues into advanced years at a rate of 1–2% per year. Postmenopausal osteoporosis is responsible for fractures in 1 of every 2 postmenopausal women and is sometimes called type I os-

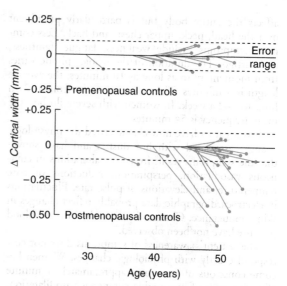

Figure 57–4. Changes in metacarpal cortical width, as determined by sequential measurements in pre- and postmenopausal women, age range 30–50. Note bone loss in postmenopausal women. (Reproduced, with permission, from Nordin BEC et al: Postmenopausal osteopenia and osteoporosis. Front Horm Res 1975;3:131.)

teoporosis (Fig 57–4). It is most severe in women who have had early oophorectomy, premature ovarian failure, and those with gonadal dysgenesis. Type II osteoporosis is age-related, is seen in both men and women, and affects both cortical and trabecular bone. The arguments for categorizing osteoporosis this way are reasonable, but are not supported by all experts. Symptomatic osteoporosis occurs most often in whites, followed by Asians, Hispanics and African-Americans. Estrogen loss, smoking, family history, corticosteroid use, excessive exercise, eating disorders, hyperthyroidism, excessive alcohol consumption, and slender body size are also risk factors. Bone loss produces minimal symptoms, but leads to reduced skeletal strength. Thus, osteoporotic bones are more susceptible to fractures. The most common site of fracture is in the vertebral body; however, fractures also occur in the humerus, upper femur, distal forearm, and ribs. Recent figures from the National Osteoporosis Foundation show that osteoporosis is responsible for 1.66 million fractures per year and that more than 20 million women are affected. Forty percent of all women will have one or more spinal fractures by the age of 80 (Fig 57–5). More than 275,000 hip fractures occur annually in the U.S. at a cost of more than $10 billion per year. The incidence of hip fractures in women is 2–3 times that in men.

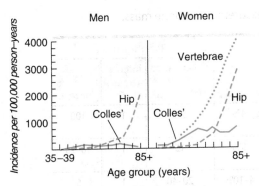

Figure 57–5. Incidences of the 3 common osteoporotic fractures (Colles', hip, and vertebral) in men and women, plotted as a function of age at time of fracture in the community population of Rochester, Minnesota. (Reproduced, with permission, from Riggs BL, Melton LJ III: Involutional osteoporosis. N Engl J Med 1986;314:1677.)

The mortality rate associated with hip fractures is between 5% and 20% within 12 months following the injury. Of survivors, 15–25% are permanently disabled.

The bone remodeling cycle involves a complex series of sequential steps that are closely regulated. The "activation" phase of remodeling is dependent on the effects of local and systemic factors on mesenchymal cells of the osteoblast lineage. With the adherence of monocytes to the collagen receptors on bone, interleukin-1 (IL-1) is released, which is a potent stimulator of osteoclast activity. These cells interact with hematopoietic precursors to form osteoclasts in the "resorption" phase. The "reversal" phase consists of mononuclear cells, which are present on the bone surface, completing the resorption process and producing signals that initiate formation. In the "formation" phase, mesenchymal cells differentiate into functional osteoblasts which lay down the matrix.

There are numerous substances involved in the bone remodeling process. In addition to IL-1, parathyroid hormone (PTH) is also involved in the genesis of osteoporosis. PTH stimulates bone resorption and absence of this hormone inhibits development of osteoporosis in animal and human studies. PTH receptors have been demonstrated on rat osteoblasts and PTH stimulates release of insulin-like growth factor 1 (IGF-1) in vitro. IGF-1 has several actions on bone: it stimulates differentiation of osteoclast precursors into mature osteoclasts, it is produced by osteoblasts and stimulates osteoblast proliferation, and it increases local density of trabecular bone. Thus far it does not appear that PTH is elevated in most women with osteoporosis or that the sensitivity of bone to PTH is enhanced. It is interesting

that the amino-terminus of PTH (1-34) has been shown to inhibit bone resorption in experimental settings. Growth hormone has been shown to stimulate bone remodeling; however, studies evaluating the effect of exogenous growth hormone administration on established osteoporosis are inconclusive. Recently, new factors have been discovered that are involved with the regulation of bone remodeling: osteoprotegerin, a naturally-occurring protein with potent osteoclastogenesis inhibitory activity; and RANKL (receptor activator of nuclear factor kappa beta ligand), a transmembrane ligand expressed on osteoblasts.

Ovarian estrogen production and hormone replacement after the menopause are protective against osteoporosis. It is likely that estrogens have direct effects on bone, since estrogen receptors exist in osteoblasts, osteoclasts, macrophages, and T cells. IL-1 activity in bone has been shown to increase immediately after the menopause or oophorectomy, but remains increased in osteoporotic women, whereas IL-1 levels return to the premenopausal range after 2 or 3 years in those who do not develop the disease. Estrogen inhibits release of IL-1 by monocytes and may also have a direct effect on osteoclasts. Estrogen also seems to enhance bone formation by a direct local action on osteoblasts. A possible mediator for this action is transforming growth factor B.

Although much has been done to study urinary and serum factors as predictors of osteoporosis, the most predictive test remains bone densitometry. Several different types of densitometry are available (Table 57–1). Single-photon absorptiometry can be used to measure appendicular bone mineral density (BMD). However, in order to measure axial bone, dual-energy x-ray absorptiometry is required for an accurate assessment. The variability of soft-tissue density around the spine and pelvis decreases the accuracy of single-photon testing. Results are given in grams or g/cm^2. In 1994, the World Health Organization created a clinically useful definition of osteoporosis. Bone mineral density results are reported using T and Z scores. The T score is the number of standard deviations (SD) above or below the mean bone mineral density for gender- and race-matched young controls. The Z score compares the patient with a population adjusted for age, gender, and race. Normal bone density is defined as a T score greater than −1.0 SD. Osteopenic patients have T scores between −1.0 and −2.5, whereas osteoporotic patients have T scores below −2.5. In most studies, a decrease by 1 SD in mass was associated with an increase of 50–100% in fracture risk. The assessment of specific bones for fracture has increased the predictive value. A decrease in hip density of 1 SD increases the risk of future hip fracture by 250–300%.

Assessment of risk factors has not been nearly as predictive of fracture risk as density measurement. Assess-

Table 57–1. Selected techniques for the measurement of bone mass.

Technique	Site	Precision	Accuracy	Radiation Dose Examination Time (Minutes)	Radiation Dose Internal Organs (μSV)	Radiation Dose Skin (mrem)
Radiographic absorptiometry (RA)	Hand	1–2%	4%	3–5	1	100
Single-photon absorptiometry (SPA)	Wrist, heel	1–3%	5%	15	1	10–20
Dual-photon absorptiometry (DPA)	Spine, hip, total body	2–4%	4–10%	20–40	1	5
Dual-energy x-ray absorptiometry (DXA)	Spine, hip, total body	0.5–2%	3–9%	3–7	1	1–3
Quantitative computed tomography (QCT)	Spine	2–5%	5–20%	10–15	60	150–250

At least 1 of the 5 specific methods of bone mass measurement should be available to any clinician.

ment of serum osteocalcin and bone-specific alkaline phosphatase, markers of bone formation, or of urinary pyridinium cross-links and serum/urinary type I collagen telopeptides, markers of bone resorption, have not been shown to be predictive of fracture risk.

In 1998 the National Osteoporosis Foundation created a set of guidelines for the use and interpretation of measurement of bone mineral density. Measurements of bone mineral density are recommended for the following groups: (1) all postmenopausal patients younger than age 65 who have one or more additional risk factors for osteoporosis (besides menopause); (2) all women aged 65 and older regardless of additional risk factors; (3) postmenopausal women who present with fractures; (4) women considering therapy for osteoporosis if testing would facilitate the decision; and (5) women who have been on hormone replacement therapy for prolonged periods.

Until recently estrogen was the mainstay of prevention and treatment of postmenopausal osteoporosis. In observational studies, estrogen seems to decrease the risk of hip fractures by 25–50%, of vertebral fractures by approximately 50%, and reduces the risk of other fractures. It is recommended that all postmenopausal women, including those with established osteoporosis and the elderly, be treated with estrogen unless contraindications exist or the therapy is not tolerated. Daily dosages of 0.625 mg of conjugated estrogens, 1.25 mg piperazine estrone sulfate, 0.5–1 mg micronized estradiol, and 0.05 mg of transdermal estradiol all have been approved for the prevention of osteoporosis. For best results, therapy should begin soon after the menopause.

Alternatives to estrogen are being used increasingly in the prevention and treatment of postmenopausal osteoporosis. Bisphosphonates are potent antiresorptive agents that bind to hydroxyapatite crystals on the surface of bones, enter osteoclasts, and decrease resorptive actions by reducing the production of hydrogen ions and lysosomal enzymes. In addition, they have indirect effects, causing osteoblasts to produce substances that inhibit osteoclasts. Bisphosphonates are useful for prevention and treatment of osteoporosis. They increase bone mineral density at the spine, wrist, and hip in a dose-dependent manner and decrease the risk of vertebral fractures by 30–50%. In addition, they reduce the risk of subsequent nonvertebral fractures in women with osteoporosis. There are two bisphosphonates currently available. Alendronate is approved by the Food and Drug Administration for the prevention of osteoporosis (5 mg daily) and for the treatment of established osteoporosis (10 mg daily). The FDA has also approved a 35-mg weekly dose for prevention and a 70-mg weekly dose for treatment of osteoporosis. Risedronate was approved by the FDA in April 2000. The recommended daily dose is 5 mg. Intestinal absorption is poor and therefore these medications should be taken in the morning with 8 ounces of water, prior to consumption of any food or beverage. Nothing else should be taken by mouth for at least 30 minutes after oral dosing. The patient should also remain upright for 30 minutes after administration. The most common side effects of bisphosphonates are gastrointestinal. Risks include gastric and esophageal ulceration.

Selective estrogen receptor modulators (SERMs) are nonhormonal agents that bind to estrogen receptors and may exhibit either estrogen agonist or antagonist activity. Currently, there are three SERMs approved for use in humans (tamoxifen, toremifene, and raloxifene); however, raloxifene is the only SERM approved for the prevention and treatment of osteoporosis. It exhibits estrogen agonist properties in the bone (inhibits osteoclast function) and the liver (decreases low-density lipoprotein cholesterol), and acts as an antagonist in the breast and uterus. Raloxifene 60 mg daily for 24 months is associated with a 1–2% increase in lumbar spine and hip bone density.

Calcitonin is a peptide hormone that inhibits osteoclast activity and therefore inhibits bone resorption. It demonstrates positive effects on bone mineral density at the lumbar spine, although less effectively than estrogen or bisphosphonates. Salmon calcitonin is the most potent form and is available for intranasal administration or as a subcutaneous injection. Calcitonin 100 IU is given subcutaneously daily or every other day. The intranasal calcitonin dose is 200 IU daily. The most frequent side effect with the intranasal route is rhinitis.

Progestins decrease biochemical markers of bone resorption and preserve bone density. When used as monotherapy for osteoporosis, they may be more effective at preserving bone in the wrist than in the spine. Fluoride has been used in Europe and the U.S. and was associated with a marked increase in trabecular bone, but did not improve fracture rates, and in some studies fracture rates were increased. This may be due to a lack of increase in cortical bone. There is insufficient evidence to support the safety and efficacy of sodium fluoride therapy for the treatment of osteoporosis. In experimental trials parathyroid hormone appears to stimulate bone growth if given intermittently or at low doses. It is not currently approved by the FDA for the treatment of osteoporosis. Phytoestrogens are plant-derived compounds which have weak estrogen-like effects. Although some animal studies are promising, no effects on the incidence of fractures in humans have been shown.

Finally, all postmenopausal women should receive calcium supplementation to achieve a total daily dose of calcium of 1000–1500 mg/d. Vitamin D supplements of 400–800 U daily are also recommended. Postmenopausal women should be encouraged to exercise regularly to improve grace and agility, which will decrease their risk of falls. Diet should be modified to decrease consumption of salt, animal protein, alcohol, and caffeine, all of which may increase the risk of osteoporotic fractures.

f. Cardiovascular system—The incidence of death from cardiovascular disease increases with age in all populations and both sexes. Substantially more heart disease is seen in younger men, with the onset of cardiovascular problems occurring an average of 10 years later in women. Before the age of menopause, very few women die of a heart attack. After the menopause, a woman's risk increases progressively until age 70 when it becomes equal to that of men. Heart disease affects nearly 3 million women in the U.S. Deaths due to heart disease number more than 478,000 per year, which is greater than the death rate in men. The rate in women has nearly doubled since 1984.

Until recently two types of studies attempted to ascertain whether cessation of ovarian function is associated with increased incidence of heart disease. The first has examined the relationship between the menopause and carefully-defined cardiovascular disease in an entire population. For example, the Framingham study, in which nearly 3000 women are examined biennially, revealed that following the menopause, there is indeed an increased incidence of heart disease that is not just age-related. In this study, the impact of the menopause was abrupt, and further (age-related) increases in incidence occurred only slowly, if at all. In the Nurses' Health Study cohort of 121,700 women, after controlling for age and cigarette smoking, women who had a natural menopause had no appreciable increase in risk compared to that of premenopausal women. However, women who underwent a bilateral oophorectomy and no estrogen replacement had an increased risk (RR 2.2) compared with that seen in premenopausal women.

In the second type of investigation, case-control studies have been performed comparing the degree of coronary heart disease or the incidence of myocardial infarction in women who had undergone early oophorectomy with age-matched premenopausal controls. Most of these studies revealed an increased risk of cardiovascular disease after ovarian excision. All these reports have been criticized because of patient selection bias, particularly the controls.

Numerous case-control and large cohort studies have been published with most showing a beneficial impact of estrogens. A meta-analysis found that estrogen use provided a 50% decrease in risk of mortality from heart disease. Although the magnitude of change and the consistency of results appear compelling, it must be recognized that all these studies are observational, and the choice of controls has been questioned. In particular, women who take estrogens are more health-conscious and must see a doctor regularly to receive their medication, whereas women who don't take estrogens may or may not receive regular medical checkups. Thus, some or all of the apparent benefits of estrogens on heart disease may have been due to these other considerations.

There are several mechanisms by which estrogen could protect against coronary artery disease. Evidence for both an indirect effect on circulating lipids and a direct action on the vascular system now exists. For years, the greatest emphasis of research has been to study the impact of estrogens on lipoproteins. Orally administered estrogens influence hepatic lipid metabolism and raise high-density lipoprotein (HDL) cholesterol and triglycerides and lower low-density lipoprotein (LDL) cholesterol. The impact of nonorally administered estrogens is of lesser magnitude and takes longer to become apparent. The Lipid Research Clinic study suggests that approximately 50% of the benefit of estrogen on heart disease is elicited through the action of estrogens on lipoproteins, whereas the remainder is through other mechanisms.

The PEPI (Postmenopausal Estrogen Progestin Intervention) Trial showed that there is a significant lowering of LDL cholesterol with oral conjugated equine estrogens (CEE), even with the addition of medroxyprogesterone acetate (MPA) or micronized natural progesterone. Of the four regimens studied, continuous CEE 0.625 mg without the addition of progestin had the most favorable effect on lipid profiles. All active HRT regimens lowered LDL cholesterol and fibrinogen levels.

Numerous studies have shown that estrogen and progesterone receptors are present in the heart and aorta. Thus, the subcellular components necessary for hormonal action exist in these tissues. Studies in castrated cynomolgus monkeys given atherogenic diets have shown estradiol administered by subcutaneous pellets prevents coronary atherogenesis in the absence of any measurable change in circulating lipoproteins. Endothelial cells of the arteries produce factors in response to estrogen. The most potent of these is believed to be nitric oxide (NO). NO exerts several effects on the arterial wall. It increases intracellular cyclic guanosine monophosphate in the arterial smooth muscle, which results in vasodilatation. It also inhibits platelet and macrophage adherence to the arterial endothelium. Both are important first steps to atheromatous plaque formation. Estrogen appears to increase NO production. Basal release of NO is greater in intact female rabbits than in either male rabbits or castrated females. Acetylcholine is known to stimulate vasodilatation of the coronary arteries of humans and monkeys. This effect is dependent on an intact vascular endothelium. Because superoxide radicals inhibit both NO and this acetylcholine-induced vasodilatation, NO is felt to be the endothelial factor responsible for this acetylcholine-induced vasodilatation. It has been theorized that estrogens may increase muscarinic receptors on endothelial cells, leading to acetylcholine-induced endothelial-dependent vasodilatation. Estrogen has also been shown in an animal model to prevent two of the earliest steps in the atherogenic process—adhesion and migraton of monocytes. Although these mechanisms are only partially understood, they emphasize the importance of studying the direct effects of estrogen on the vascular system.

Observational studies have suggested that the protective effect of estrogens on the heart is greatest in women with known risk factors for heart disease. These include obesity, smoking, and hypertension, among others. However, the HERS (Heart and Estrogen/Progestin Replacement Study) showed that treatment with oral conjugated CEE plus MPA did not reduce the overall rate of coronary heart disease events in postmenopausal women with established heart disease. In addition, there was an early increased risk of coronary heart disease (CHD) events within the first year of starting HRT. In addition, the ERA (Estrogen Replacement and Atherosclerosis) Trial, which is the first randomized angiographic endpoint trial to test the effect of ERT (estrogen replacement therapy) and HRT on the progression of atherosclerosis in postmenopausal women with documented coronary stenosis, showed no benefit of CEE combined with MPA on angiographic progression of disease. In addition, an estrogen-only arm showed no angiographic benefit compared with placebo. It is therefore suggested that physicians not prescribe ERT/HRT for the sole purpose of *secondary* cardiovascular protection.

Until recently, the primary prevention of CHD by HRT had not been evaluated in a prospective, randomized fashion. The Women's Health Initiative (WHI), a large, multi-center, prospective, randomized placebo-controlled trial of primarily healthy postmenopausal women, was initiated to assess the effects of a specifc regimen of HRT (conjugated equine estrogens alone in combination with medroxyprogesterone acetate) on several health-related outcomes, including CHD. The combined estrogen/progestin portion of the study was stopped after 5.2 years as overall health risks exceeded benefits. The increased risks included a greater number of cardiovascular events. While the absolute risk of harm was small, the authors concluded that this regimen of HRT should not be initiated or continued for the primary prevention of CHD. The estrogen-only arm of the study is continuing as the balance of overall risks and benefits remains uncertain.

There were several limitations of the study. The trial only tested one regimen of HRT. It did not assess different dosages, types of estrogens and progestogens, nor different routes of administration (i.e. transdermal vs. oral). Without the results of the estrogen-only arm it is difficult to determine whether the effects were mediated by the estrogen, progestin, or a combination of the two. Finally, it was also not possible to precisely ascertain from the study whether starting HRT with the onset of menopause, when initiation or more rapid acceleration of atherosclerosis may take place, is beneficial. Since estrogen has been shown in experimental models to prevent the very earliest steps in atherogenesis, but to raise cardiovascular risk in the setting of established atherosclerosis, it is possible that the adverse cardiovascular effects seen in this study may have been due to the possibility that many women started HRT following the onset of menopause when subclinical atherosclerotic changes may have already set in.

The decision to use HRT should be based primarily on the proven benefits of ERT/HRT on other systems, the potential risks of therapy, and patient preference. Short term use of HRT for relief of postmenopausal symptoms is still considered an option by many.

g. Skin and hair—With aging, noticeable changes occur in the skin. There is generalized thinning and an accompanying loss of elasticity, resulting in wrinkling. These changes are particularly prominent in the areas exposed to light (ie, the face, neck, and hands). "Purse-string" wrinkling around the mouth and "crow's feet" around the eyes are characteristic. Skin changes on the dorsum of the hands are particularly noticeable. In this area, the skin may be so thin as to become almost transparent, with details of the underlying veins easily visible.

Histologically, the epidermis is thinned, and the basal layers become inactive with age. Dehydration is typical. Reduction in the number of blood vessels to the skin is also seen. Degeneration of elastic and collagenous fibers in the dermis also appears to be part of the process of aging.

These skin changes are of cosmetic importance and have been related to the onset of the climacteric by women. It is commonly stated that women undergoing estrogen replacement look younger, and the cosmetic industry has been putting estrogens in skin creams for years for precisely this reason.

The possibility that estrogens may have effects on skin was suggested by the demonstration of estrogen receptors in skin. The number of receptors is highest in facial skin, followed by skin of the breasts and thighs. This gives credence to the hypothesis that estrogens affect the skin.

Skin circulation has been found to be decreased in women after oophorectomy. Radiolabeled thymidine incorporation (an index of new DNA metabolism) has been reported to decrease during the several months following oophorectomy. In animals, estrogens have been shown to increase the mitotic rate (a reflection of growth) of skin in some studies. Estrogens may alter the vascularization of skin. They also change the collagen content of the dermis, as reflected by mucopolysaccharide incorporation, hydroxyproline turnover, and alterations of the ground substance. In addition, dermal synthesis of hyaluronic acid and dermal water content are enhanced.

Skin collagen content and thickness have been studied in postmenopausal women. Decreases of both have been observed at a rate of 1–2% per year. The losses correlated with the number of years since the menopause, but not with chronological age. Estrogen replacement has been shown to prevent these losses or restore both parameters to premenopausal values. The greatest recovery is observed in women who began with low values. These data were interpreted to indicate that estrogen can prevent loss in women with high skin collagen levels, whereas it can restore content as well as prevent further loss in women with low collagen levels. Although these results are promising, it remains unclear whether they are clinically relevant.

After the menopause, most women note some change in patterns of body hair. Usually there is a variable loss of pubic and axillary hair. Often there is loss of lanugo hair on the upper lip, chin, and cheeks, together with increased growth of coarse terminal hairs; a slight moustache may become noticeable. Hair on the body and extremities may either increase or decrease. Slight balding is seen occasionally. All of these changes may be due in part to reduced levels of estrogen in the face of fairly well maintained levels of testosterone.

h. Psychologic changes—Early cross-sectional surveys of community or large general medical practice–based populations attempted to measure the temporal association of depression and irritability to the cessation of menses. Some reports indicated an increased incidence of minor symptoms such as irritability, dysphoria, and nervousness early in the menopausal transition.

Reports from community-based cohort studies have refined knowledge in the area of mood, mentation, and menopause. The initial longitudinal report of the U.S. cohort found an increase in overall nonspecific symptom reporting at the menopause. Depression for more than two interviews was noted in 26%. Perceived health, rather than menopause or coincident life stresses, was most related to depression in this study. These findings are consistent with the concept of variability in a woman's response to the menopause; individual characteristics and self-perceptions appear to be important determinants of each woman's experience of the climacteric.

Hypotheses as to the etiology of the affective complaints at the menopause also include a primary biologic cause (eg, an alteration in brain amines). Studies using the opioid antagonist naloxone have demonstrated that estrogen deficiency is associated with low levels of endogenous opioid activity and that estrogen supplementation increases opioid activity. These findings suggest that central neurotransmitters may contribute to the etiology of affective and cognitive complaints. Sociologic factors postulated to cause psychologic symptoms, such as negative cultural values attached to aging, may also promote a negative climacteric experience.

Double-blind studies have found improvements in self-reported irritability, mild anxiety, and dysphoria in women treated with estrogen alone or combined with progestin. Improvement of the Beck depression score in women without hot flushes indicates that estrogens likely have direct effects on brain function.

The determinants of sexual behavior are complex and interrelated. Sexual function is believed to be regulated by three general components: the individual's motivation (also called desire or libido), endocrine competence, and social-cultural beliefs. Decreased libido is reported with increasing age. However, the relative contributions of the primary decrease in desire, anatomic limitations to sexual function, or beliefs that sexual behavior is inappropriate in older women to this decreased libido are unknown.

The hypoestrogenemic state leads to atrophy of the internal genitalia. Although dyspareunia is the most obvious symptom of vaginal atrophy, suboptimal sexual functioning can occur without frank dyspareunia. Diminished genital sensation (and therefore decreased sensory output in the arousal phase), lessened glandular secretions, less vasocongestion, and decreased vaginal expansion may not be perceived as discrete symptoms by the postmenopausal female, but may influence her perception that she is less responsive.

Genital atrophy, one cause of postmenopausal sexual dysfunction, responds to estrogen therapy. The specific impact of estrogen on libido has been difficult to determine. Improved anatomy may also have a positive psychologic impact and may indirectly encourage sexual motivation.

i. Alzheimer's Disease—As life expectancy in women has risen, there has been more research regarding the effects of estrogen on cognitive functioning in postmenopausal women. Research indicates that estrogen influences areas of the brain known to be important for memory. Studies are ongoing to assess whether estrogens have a protective role in the prevention of dementia or Alzheimer's disease.

2. Excess endogenous estrogens—Not all women experiencing the climacteric have symptoms of estrogen deprivation. Some have no symptoms, whereas others actually experience symptoms and signs of estrogen excess, usually uterine bleeding but in some cases mastodynia, abdominal bloating, edema, growth of uterine myomas, and exacerbation of endometriosis as well. The problems of postmenopausal uterine bleeding are of particular concern, because this bleeding may reflect the presence of endometrial hyperplasia or adenocarcinoma.

Based on a variety of evidence, it has been suggested that continuous estrogen stimulation of the endometrium, unopposed by progesterone, can lead to a progression of changes from benign proliferation to simple hyperplasia, complex hyperplasia, and varying degrees of anaplasia, including invasive adenocarcinoma. When postmenopausal patients with hyperplasia or adenocarcinoma are studied, many have higher than usual levels of circulatory estrogens.

As mentioned earlier, the principal source of estrogens in older women is the peripheral aromatization of circulating androgens. Thus, there are three mechanisms that could conceivably result in increased endogenous estrogen production: (1) increased production of precursor androgens, (2) enhanced aromatization of precursor androgens, and (3) increased production of estrogens directly. The occurrence of each has been reported and has been associated with signs of estrogen excess.

Of particular importance is enhanced aromatization of androgens. A variety of conditions are associated with this phenomenon, including obesity, liver disease, and hyperthyroidism. The association of obesity with endometrial cancer has been known for years.

Comparisons have been made between postmenopausal women with and without endometrial cancer. When these comparisons have been conducted using control subjects matched to the cancer patients by age, there have been no differences in androgen and estrogen levels or in the conversion rate of androstenedione to estrone between the 2 groups. However, increasing body size has always shown a positive correlation with endogenous estrogen levels and with conversion rates of androstenedione to estrone, and it is well recognized that obese women are at greater risk of developing endometrial hyperplasia and adenocarcinoma than slender women. The high concentrations of endogenous estrogens found in obese subjects presumably play a role in the increased incidence of this tumor in obese older women.

3. Miscellaneous postmenopausal symptoms—Many other symptoms have been attributed to the endocrine changes of the postmenopausal state, but a direct cause-and-effect relationship has not been established for them. Some of these so-called climacteric symptoms are so common that they deserve brief mention.

Symptoms possibly related to specific autonomic nervous system instability—but equally attributable to anxiety or other emotional disturbances—are paresthesias (pricking, itching, formication), dizziness, tinnitus, fainting, scotomas, and dyspnea. Symptoms clearly not of endocrine origin are weakness, fatigue, nausea, vomiting, flatulence, anorexia, constipation, diarrhea, arthralgia, and myalgia.

Many women erroneously believe that the endocrine changes accompanying menopause will produce a steady weight gain. Women and men do tend to gain weight at this time of life, but the cause is a combination of decreased exercise and possibly increased caloric intake. There may be some redistribution of body weight occasioned by the deposition of fat over the hips and abdomen. Perhaps this is partly an endocrine effect, but more likely it is the result of decreased physical activity, reduced muscle tone, and other effects of aging.

Many of the previously mentioned symptoms occasionally respond promptly to administration of estrogen. This should not mislead physicians into assuming a specific endocrine action for what is actually a placebo effect.

B. Laboratory Findings

1. Vaginal cytologic smears—In certain laboratory animals, the degree of maturation of exfoliated vaginal epithelial cells, as revealed by stained vaginal smears, is an accurate index of estrogenic activity. When this method is applied to women, several staining techniques are available. Among the various methods of assessing the smears, the following are most commonly used: the **maturation index** consists of a differential count of three types of squamous cells—parabasal cells, intermediate cells, and superficial cells, in that order—expressed as percentages (eg, 10/85/5); and the **cornification count** is the percentage of precornified and cornified cells among total squamous cells counted. This is actually a simplified maturation index, because this percentage is essentially the same as that of the superficial cells.

The assessment of exfoliated vaginal epithelial cells is influenced not only by the level of estrogenic activity, but also by other hormones (particularly progesterone and testosterone), local vaginal inflammation, local medication ("hygiene"), vaginal bleeding, the presence of genital cancer, the location of the vaginal area sampled, and variations in end-organ (epithelial) responses to estrogenic influence. Thus, women with identical levels of circulating estrogens may have quite different cytograms. Moreover, even with extraneous factors eliminated, the vaginal smear does not indicate absolute levels of estrogenic function; rather, it reflects the net balance of the influence on vaginal epithelium of endogenous and exogenous estrogens, androgens, and progestogens. This is well demonstrated in women taking oral contraceptives. Despite the intake of relatively large doses of estrogen, the cornification counts are usually lower because of the concomitant effect of the progestin.

The great variation in cytologic findings leads to the following conclusions regarding the use of smears in the clinical management of postmenopausal women: (1) The smear is only a rough measure of estrogenic status, and it may sometimes be grossly misleading. (2) The vaginal cytogram cannot predict whether or not an individual woman is experiencing climacteric signs and symptoms. (3) The smear cannot be used as the sole guide to steroid supplementation therapy; clinical signs and symptoms are more dependable for this purpose. (4) The smear can be helpful in determining the dosage of estrogen needed to reverse vaginal atrophy.

2. Hormone production—Techniques of radioisotopic protein binding or radioimmunoassay are available for the determination of hormone levels in blood and other body fluids (Table 57–2).

a. Androgens—In premenopausal women, plasma androstenedione is approximately 1.5 ng/mL. Plasma testosterone is about 0.3 ng/mL. Mean DHEA and DHEAS levels are approximately 4 ng/mL and 1600 ng/mL, respectively, in samples drawn at 8:00 AM.

In postmenopausal women, the mean plasma androstenedione concentration is reduced by at least 50%, to approximately 0.6 ng/mL. Plasma testosterone levels are only slightly reduced (about 0.25 ng/mL). Plasma DHEA and DHEAS levels are decreased to mean levels of 1.8 ng/mL and 300 ng/mL in women in their 60s and 70s.

Table 57–2. Serum concentrations (mean ± SE) of steroids in premenopausal and postmenopausal women.

Steroid	Premenopausal (ng/mL)	Postmenopausal (ng/mL)
Progesterone	0.47 ± 0.03	0.17 ± 0.02
Dehydroepiandrosterone	4.2 ± 0.5	1.8 ± 0.2
Dehydroepiandrosterone sulfate	1600 ± 350	300 ± 70
Androstenedione	1.5 ± 0.1	0.6 ± 0.01
Testosterone	0.32 ± 0.02	0.25 ± 0.03
Estrone	0.08 ± 0.01	0.029 ± 0.002
Estradiol	0.05 ± 0.005	0.013 ± 0.001

b. Estrogens—During normal menstrual life, the mean plasma estradiol fluctuates from 50 to 350 pg/mL and estrone from 30 to 110 pg/mL. These fluctuations reflect the development and involution of the follicle and corpus luteum. In postmenopausal women, cyclic fluctuations disappear. The mean estradiol level is approximately 12 pg/mL, with a range of 5–25 pg/mL. The mean estrone level is approximately 30 pg/mL, with a range of 20–70 pg/mL. Estradiol levels in normal young women do not overlap with those observed in postmenopausal subjects. The finding of estradiol levels below 20 pg/mL can be helpful in establishing the diagnosis of menopause, since the fall of this estrogen is the last hormonal change associated with loss of ovarian function. There is substantial overlap of estrone levels in younger and older women. Measurement of this estrogen is not helpful in determining the ovarian status of a patient.

c. Progesterone—In young menstruating women, the mean progesterone level is approximately 0.4 ng/mL during the follicular phase of the cycle, with a range of 0.2–0.7 ng/mL. During the luteal phase, progesterone levels rise and fall, reflecting corpus luteum function; the mean level is approximately 11 ng/mL with a range of 3–21 ng/mL. In postmenopausal women, the mean progesterone level is 0.17 ng/mL. To date, no clinical use has been established for the measurement of progesterone in postmenopausal women.

d. Pituitary gonadotropins—One of the striking hormonal changes associated with the menopause is the increase in secretion of pituitary gonadotropins. During reproductive life, the levels of both FSH and LH range from 4–30 mU/mL except during the preovulatory surge, when they may exceed 50 mU/mL and 100 mU/mL, respectively. After the menopause, both rise to levels above 100 mU/mL, with FSH rising earlier and to higher levels than LH.

When contradictory or uncertain clinical findings make the diagnosis of the postmenopausal state questionable, measurement of plasma FSH, LH, and estradiol levels may be helpful. This situation occurs frequently in women following hysterectomy without oophorectomy. The findings of plasma estradiol below 20 pg/mL and elevated FSH and LH levels are consistent with cessation of ovarian function. In practical terms, it is not necessary to measure LH.

e. Thyroid function—There are changes in thyroid function with aging. Thyroxine (T_4) and free T_4 concentrations are similar in young and older women, but triiodothyronine (T_3) levels fall by approximately 25–40% during aging. This decrease of T_3 does not seem to reflect hypothyroidism, since the thyroid-stimulating hormone (TSH) concentration, a sensitive indicator of primary hypothyroidism, is not elevated. In addition, there is an age-related decrease in the responsiveness of TSH to thyrotropin-releasing hormone (TRH) rather than the increase seen in patients with hypothyroidism. T_4-binding globulin levels rise slightly and T_4-binding prealbumin falls, but the latter is a minor carrier of T_4. All these changes in thyroid function appear to be related to aging, not the climacteric, since they also occur in men.

There is an increased incidence of hypothyroidism (Hashimoto's thyroiditis) in older people, and this should be kept in mind when caring for the elderly.

3. Endometrial histology—As long as menses and occasional ovulation persist, all phases of endometrial growth may be found on histologic examination. After ovulation ceases, no further secretory changes are seen. After menopause, endometrial biopsy may reveal anything from a very scanty, atrophic endometrium to one that is moderately proliferative. Spontaneous postmenopausal bleeding may occur in the presence of any of these patterns. Endometrial tissue revealing glandular hyperplasia (with or without uterine bleeding) is an indication of enhanced estrogenic stimulation from either endogenous estrogen production (eg, increased conversion of androgen), or from exogenous intake of estrogen.

C. ULTRASONOGRAPHY

Increasingly, physicians are using vaginal ultrasonography to evaluate the pelvis in postmenopausal women. Besides the evaluation of pelvic masses, two other indications for pelvic ultrasound examination have been proposed. The first is evaluation of the endometrium or "endometrial stripe" to determine whether a woman has endometrial hyperplasia or cancer. This has been controversial, with investigators reporting the demarcation between normal and abnormal endometrium ranging from 4–10 mm. Others have recommended setting the criterion at a low thickness to exclude most people with a potential endometrial lesion. If the criterion is set low, such as at 4 mm, then published results indicate that the rare patient (1 in 128) will have endometrial hyperplasia or cancer with a stripe ≤ 4 mm. Conversely, approximately 20% will have normal endometrium with a stripe > 4 mm.

Differential Diagnosis

Signs and symptoms similar to those of the climacteric can be caused by a variety of other diseases. In general, seeing the entire clinical picture is helpful in establishing the proper diagnosis. The absence of evidence of other disease will point to cessation of ovarian function, whereas the presence of prominent features of other conditions, in the absence of other climacteric symptoms, will suggest a nonclimacteric origin.

A. AMENORRHEA

By definition, the primary symptom of the menopause is the absence of menstruation. Amenorrhea can occur for many reasons, of which physiologic menopause is only one. Cessation of ovarian function is by far the most common reason for amenorrhea to occur in women in their 40s or early 50s. Persistent amenorrhea in younger women may be due to premature cessation of ovarian function, but must be differentiated from other causes. Obvious features of specific disease often suggest the proper diagnosis (eg, extreme weight loss in anorexia nervosa, galactorrhea in hyperprolactinemia, hirsutism and obesity in polycystic ovarian disease). Although the reproductive tract commonly shows evidence of lowered estrogenic activity in these and other diseases associated with amenorrhea, true vasomotor symptoms are rare.

B. VASOMOTOR FLUSHES

Several diseases can produce sensations of flushing that may be misinterpreted as hot flushes. Notable are hyperthyroidism, pheochromocytoma, carcinoid syndrome, diabetes mellitus, tuberculosis, and other chronic infections. None of these disorders produces the specific symptoms associated with the climacteric (ie, short duration and specific body distribution). Moreover, the absence of other signs or symptoms of the climacteric suggest some other cause of the flushes should be sought.

C. ABNORMAL VAGINAL BLEEDING

Prior to the menopause, irregular vaginal bleeding is expected and does not necessitate a diagnostic work-up in most cases. However, organic disease can occur at this time, and some patients require evaluation. If a woman is in her 40s or 50s and experiences an increase in cycle length and a decrease in the quantity of bleeding, menopausal involution can be presumed and endometrial sampling is not necessary. However, if menses become more frequent and heavier, or spotting between menses occurs, assessment of the endometrium should be done. The usual procedure is an endometrial biopsy or D&C. The disadvantage of the former is that entry into the endometrial cavity may not be accomplished in the setting of a stenotic os, and the drawbacks of the latter are greater expense and risk. If normal endometrium is found, no further investigation is required. If hyperplastic or cancerous endometrium is obtained, treatment should be instituted.

It is most unusual for a woman to experience vaginal bleeding because of ovarian activity by 6 months after the menopause. Thus, postmenopausal bleeding is much more ominous and necessitates evaluation each time it occurs. The only exception to this rule is the uterine bleeding associated with estrogen replacement therapy. Other guidelines are recommended for this type of bleeding (see Treatment).

Organic disease is commonly associated with postmenopausal bleeding. Endometrial polyps may be found, which can be resected via the hysteroscope. Endometrial hyperplasia may be discovered, frequently in obese women. This can be treated by the periodic administration of progestin or by hysterectomy. If hyperplasia develops in a woman taking estrogens, the addition of progestins should be considered. If hyperplasia develops unrelated to hormone replacement, surgery should be considered if the patient is a good surgical risk or is not reliable in taking progestins. The finding of endometrial cancer necessitates appropriate therapy depending on the stage and grade of the tumor.

D. VULVOVAGINITIS

Many specific vulvar and vaginal diseases (eg, trichomoniasis and candidiasis) may mimic the atrophic vulvovaginitis of estrogen deficiency. Their special clinical characteristics usually suggest more specific diagnostic testing. When pruritus and thinning of the vaginal epithelium or the vulvar skin are the only manifestations, therapeutic testing with local applications of estrogen may help to establish the diagnosis of vulvovaginitis. When any whitening, thickening, or cracking of vulvar tissues is present, biopsy to rule out carcinoma is mandatory. Biopsy to rule out carcinoma is also necessary for a suspicious-looking localized vaginal or cervical lesion.

E. OSTEOPOROSIS

Occasionally, the pain of vertebral compression may mimic that of gastric ulcer, renal colic, pyelonephritis, pancreatitis, spondylolisthesis, acute back strain, or herniated intervertebral disk.

Prevention

Nothing can prevent the physiologic menopause (ie, ovarian function cannot be prolonged indefinitely), and nothing can be done to postpone its onset or slow its progress. However, artificial menopause can often be prevented. When ionizing radiation is used for the treatment of intra-abdominal disease, incidental ablation of ovarian function often cannot be avoided. In such cases, if an operation will serve equally well, it should be used in preference to radiation therapy in order to preserve the ovaries.

Elective removal of the ovaries to prevent ovarian cancer is frequently performed at laparotomy in premenopausal women, with deliberate acceptance of artificial menopause. This form of therapy, however, remains controversial.

Treatment

As long as ovarian function is sufficient to maintain some uterine bleeding, no treatment is usually required. Occasionally, women complain of hot flushes while menstrual function is still present. Treatment with low-dose oral contraceptive pills, if no contraindications exist, will relieve these symptoms and help to regulate menstrual cycles during the premenopause.

A. COUNSELING

Every woman with climacteric symptoms deserves an adequate explanation of the physiologic event she is experiencing, in order to dispel her fears and minimize symptoms such as anxiety, depression, and sleep disturbance. Reassurance should be emphasized. Specific reassurance about continued sexual activity is important.

B. ESTROGEN REPLACEMENT

1. Complications—Before discussing the management of estrogen replacement, it is necessary to review the complications and contraindications of this type of therapy. These play an important role in the ultimate decision regarding treatment for all patients.

a. Endometrial cancer—The role of estrogen therapy in the development of endometrial cancer has been one of the most highly charged issues related to the climacteric. Current concerns are based on several lines of investigation. Although none has been conclusive, the scope of investigative efforts and the consistent incrimination of estrogen lead to the conclusion that estrogen stimulation of the endometrium, unopposed by progesterone, causes endometrial proliferation, hyperplasia, and finally neoplasia. It is therefore recommended that a progestin be added to ERT to reduce the risk of endometrial hyperplasia or carcinoma.

The reports of estrogen replacement and endometrial carcinoma have received the greatest attention. In most studies, a strong association has been found, with two- to eightfold overall risk ratios. High dosage and prolonged treatment increased the risk. Disease is local in most cases, although invasive tumors have been reported. Concerns have been raised about these studies, particularly regarding the selection of controls. In most studies, controls had not undergone sampling of the endometrium to rule out asymptomatic endometrial cancer. Studies using controls who have undergone endometrial sampling have shown no greater incidence of estrogen use in women with cancer than in women without cancer. Based on autopsy studies, approximately 50% of the endometrial cancers found at postmortem examination were not apparent in the women while they were alive. Thus debates persist, and prudent physicians should discuss the risks with their patients and employ preventive measures.

b. Breast cancer—Early age at menarche and older age at menopause are known risk factors for breast cancer, and early oophorectomy is known to give protection against this disease. Ovarian activity is thus shown to be an important determinant of risk, and estrogen may play a role in the development of breast cancer. Studies in rodents support that view. More than 30 epidemiologic studies have been published since 1974 to determine the possible link between postmenopausal estrogen use and breast cancer. In general, the later studies have had better design, quality, and analytic strategies. The number of subjects in more recent studies has also been larger. At least six meta-analyses of this topic also have been conducted. These results have not always agreed. The recent prospective randomized Women's Health Initiative Trial also addressed this issue. In this study there was a trend toward an increased risk of invasive breast cancer in the estrogen/ progestin arm which did not reach statistical significance.

Despite this inconsistency in studies, some trends have been observed: (1) The overall risk of breast cancer with estrogen use has not uniformly been shown to be increased. (2) Long-term use (ie, 4–10 years) has been associated with mild increased risk (RR 1.2–1.5) in some of the meta-analyses and the Women's Health Initiative. (3) Increased estrogen dosage does not appear to increase risk. (4) The addition of a progestin does not appear to decrease risk. (5) Finally, risk does not vary in strata of family history of breast cancer or with benign breast disease.

Although these findings are somewhat reassuring, it must be remembered that all women are at risk for breast cancer. Thus, instructions for breast self-examination, a careful breast assessment, and routine screening mammography should be a part of the medical care of all older women.

c. Hypertension—Hypertension may develop during or may be exacerbated by use of oral contraceptives and usually disappears when the medications are discontinued. Hypertension has not been shown to be a risk of hormone replacement in women who are either normotensive or hypertensive at the beginning of replacement.

d. Thromboembolic disease—Use of oral contraceptives increases the risk of overt venous thromboembolic disease and subclinical disease extensive enough to be detected by laboratory procedures such as ^{125}I fibrinogen uptake and plasma fibrinogen chromatography. The risk of venous thromboembolic disease was also increased among users of combined estrogen/progestin in the WHI as well as the HERS trial.

The effects of estrogen on the clotting mechanism may contribute to or be responsible for a generalized hypercoagulable state. Estrogen increases vascular endothelial proliferation, decreases venous blood flow, and enhances coagulability of blood, involving changes in the platelet, coagulation, and fibrinolytic systems. Reports have found decreased platelet counts. Evaluation of clotting factors has shown increases in factors VII, IX, X, and X complex; these factors are hepatic in origin. Estrogen replacement therapy can also cause decreases in anticoagulant factors such as antithrombin III and antithrombin Xa. Antithrombin III is of particular interest. It is also hepatic in origin and inactivates thrombin, activated factor X, and other enzymes involved with the generation of thrombin. Ingestion of conjugated estrogens, 1.25 mg/d, has been reported to have no effect on this anticlotting factor. Studies have reported increases of plasminogen and α_1-antitrypsin with 1.25 mg of conjugated equine estrogens. The same has not been observed with nonoral (ie, transdermal) estrogen administration.

e. Lipid metabolism—An increased incidence of gallbladder disease has been reported following estrogen replacement therapy. Estrogens cause increased amounts of cholesterol to collect in bile. Two primary bile salts, cholate and chenodeoxycholate, are produced by liver cells. In women taking estrogen, decreased levels of chenodeoxycholate and increased levels of cholate are found in bile. Chenodeoxycholate inhibits activity of the enzyme β-hydroxy-β-methylglutaryl-CoA reductase, which regulates cholesterol synthesis, and a decrease in chenodeoxycholate may therefore cause increased activity of β-hydroxy-β-methylglutaryl-CoA reductase, leading to increased synthesis of cholesterol. Bile normally has a 75–90% saturation in cholesterol, and even small increases of this substance can initiate cholesterol precipitation and stone formation. Three-fourths of gallstones are composed predominantly of cholesterol.

Estrogen replacement also has an impact on circulating lipids. Most lipids are bound to proteins in the blood, and the concentrations of the various types of lipoproteins are associated with varying risks of heart disease. Lower levels of HDL cholesterol and higher concentrations of total cholesterol, LDL cholesterol, very low-density lipoprotein (VLDL) cholesterol, and triglycerides are associated with increased risk of atherosclerosis and coronary artery disease. Estrogen replacement decreases LDL cholesterol and increases HDL cholesterol and triglycerides. Use of conjugated estrogens, 0.625 mg/d or less, causes approximately a 10% increase in HDL cholesterol. Much attention has been focused on the impact of estrogens on lipoproteins to explain its apparent beneficial effect on heart disease.

In patients with familial defects of lipoprotein metabolism, estrogen replacement therapy has been associated with massive elevations of plasma triglycerides, leading to pancreatitis and other complications. However, this is a very unusual complication of estrogen replacement.

f. Miscellaneous—Other side effects of estrogen therapy include uterine bleeding, generalized edema, mastodynia and breast enlargement, abdominal bloating, signs and symptoms resembling those of premenstrual tension, headaches (particularly of a "menstrual migraine" type), and excessive cervical mucus. These side effects may be dose-related or idiosyncratic and are managed by lowering the dosage, by use of another agent, or by discontinuation of the medication.

2. Contraindications to estrogen replacement therapy—Undiagnosed vaginal bleeding, acute liver disease, chronic impaired liver function, acute vascular thrombosis (with or without emboli), neuro-ophthalmologic vascular disease, and endometrial or breast carcinoma are contraindications to estrogen replacement. Estrogen therapy may stimulate growth of malignant cells remaining after treatment of breast or endometrial carcinoma and may thus hasten the recurrence of cancer. Therefore, it is prudent to avoid estrogen therapy until arrest is likely. Recently, it has been suggested that women with early (stage 1) and well-differentiated (grade 1) endometrial cancer can be administered estrogens following primary treatment of the cancer. Care must be exercised in following this recommendation until it has been properly studied. Patients who have had estrogen receptor–positive malignant tumors of the breast probably should not receive estrogen supplements. Recently, this concept has also been questioned. Again, until it is properly studied, physicians should avoid administering estrogens to such patients. A history of treated carcinoma of the cervix or ovary is not a contraindication to estrogen therapy. Estrogens may have undesirable effects on some patients with preexisting seizures, hypertension, fibrocystic disease of the breast, uterine leiomyoma, collagen disease, familial hyperlipidemia, diabetes mellitus, migraine headaches, chronic thrombophlebitis, and gallbladder disease. At the low dosages recommended for replacement therapy, increased growth of uterine myomas, endometriosis, or chronic cystic mastitis is rarely a concern.

3. Management guidelines for estrogen replacement therapy—Only general guidelines can be offered, because risks and benefits must be evaluated for each patient. Current indications for estrogen therapy are relief of menopausal symptoms (including hot flushes and vaginal atrophy) and prevention of osteoporosis. Caution should be exercised in providing therapy for other reasons until more definitive studies have been performed. If symptoms of hot flushes and vaginal atrophy are severe, therapy should be recommended; minimal or no symptoms may not require hormones.

Table 57–3. Preparations of estrogens and progestins available in the U.S. for hormone replacement.

Agent	How Supplied	Special Features
Oral estrogens		
Conjugated equine estrogens	0.3 mg, 0.625 mg,[1] 0.9 mg, 1.25 mg, 2.5 mg	Well studied, well tolerated, long use.
Micronized estradiol	1 mg[1] scored tablet, 2 mg scored tablet	Well tolerated.
Piperazine estrone (estropipate)	0.625mg, 1.25 mg, 2.5 mg, 5.0 mg	The 1.25-mg dosage prevents bone loss from spine and hip.
Ethinyl estradiol	0.02 mg, 0.05 mg, 0.5 mg	Not approved for prevention of osteoporosis.
Quinestrol	100 µg	Not approved for prevention of osteoporosis.
Chlorotrianisene	12 to 25 mg capsules	Not approved for prevention of osteoporosis.
Diethylstilbestrol	1 mg, 5 mg enseals (enteric release), 1 mg, 5 mg tablets	Not approved for treatment of estrogen deficiency.
Systemic estrogens		
Transdermal estradiol	0.05 mg,[1] 0.1 mg patch	Well tolerated, 10% skin rash.
Injectable estrogens		
Estradiol valerate	20 mg/10 mL, 40 mg/10 mL, 4 mg/10 mL with 90 mg testosterone enanthate	Certainty of administration; peak blood levels. Not approved for prevention of osteoporosis.
Polyestradiol phosphate	40 ampules	Approved for use in prostate cancer only: not approved for treatment of estrogen deficiency.
Vaginal estrogens		
Conjugated equine estrogens	0.625 mg/g creme	Not approved for prevention of osteoporosis.
Micronized estradiol	0.1 mg/g creme	Not approved for prevention of osteoporosis.
Piperazine estrone sulfate	1.5 mg/g creme	Not approved for prevention of osteoporosis.
Oral progestogens		
Medroxyprogesterone acetate	2.5 mg, 5 mg, 10 mg tablets	Well tolerated.
Megestrol acetate	20 mg, 40 mg scored tablets	Well tolerated; dosage probably too large for routine use in hormone replacement.
Micronized progesterone	100 mg, 200 mg capsules	Well tolerated, possible somnolence
Norethindrone	0.35 µg	Available only as minipill.
Norethindrone acetate	5 mg scored tablets	Dosage probably too large for routine use in hormone replacement
Injectable progestins		
Depoprovera	100 mg/mL, 400 mg/mL	Approved for inoperable cancer and contraception.

[1]Indicates lowest dosage of estrogen approved by FDA for prevention of osteoporosis.

Prevention of osteoporosis depends on the bone density of a woman as measured by the newer techniques.

In women with menopausal symptoms, a standard dosage of estrogen, such as 0.625 mg of conjugated equine estrogens, should be given daily (Table 57–3). Higher doses may be necessary to relieve hot flushes. Progressive reduction of dosage should be attempted as soon as feasible. Either systemic estrogen or vaginal creams can be used for vaginal symptoms.

For prevention of osteoporosis, several guidelines are important. The 0.625-mg dosage of conjugated equine estrogens, the 1.25-mg dosage of piperazine estrone sulfate, and the 0.05-mg dosage of transdermal estradiol all have been shown to prevent bone loss from both the spine and the hip. The 0.5-mg dosage of micronized estradiol has been shown to prevent bone loss

from the spine, but the FDA has approved only the 1- and 2-mg dosages. Lower doses of estrogens, i.e. 0.3 mg conjugated equine estrogens, also prevent bone loss, but not as well as higher doses. Early commencement of prophylaxis following cessation of ovarian function will maintain the highest bone density. Delay in administration will stop bone loss when estrogen is begun, but will not return bone density to that which was present at the time of the menopause. Long-term prophylaxis is essential to prevent fractures. At least 5 years appears necessary to reduce the occurrence of fracture and increase bone density in older women. Treatment for 1 or 2 years will have little impact on the occurrence of fractures.

All preparations—synthetic, naturally-occurring, and nonsteroidal estrogens—probably yield equally good results, but only a few have been studied. We usually restrict the use of specific preparations to those that have been approved by the FDA for the prevention of osteoporosis. Many U.S. physicians are now using continuous instead of interrupted estrogen administration.

a. Progestogen-estrogen therapy—The most serious concern about estrogen replacement is the occurrence of endometrial hyperplasia or cancer. Progestins oppose the action of estrogen on the endometrium. Progestins reduce the number of estrogen receptors in glandular and stromal cells of the endometrium. These agents also block estrogen-induced synthesis of DNA, and they induce the intracellular enzymes estradiol dehydrogenase and estrogen sulfotransferase. The former reduces estradiol to the much less potent estrone, while the latter converts estrogen to estrogen sulfates for rapid elimination from endometrial cells. In addition, full secretory transformation occurs if the progestin is given at a large enough dosage for a sufficient length of time.

Progestins have been shown to reduce the occurrence of endometrial cancer. Epidemiologic studies have shown significant reduction of the occurrence of endometrial cancer with estrogen plus progestin compared with estrogen alone. One study indicated use of the progestin for greater than 10 days a month reduced the occurrence more than a shorter interval. In treating women with hormones, a more practical concern is the prevention of endometrial hyperplasia. Initially, British investigators showed that high-dose estrogens (1.25 mg or greater of conjugated equine estrogens) resulted in 32% hyperplasia, whereas low doses (0.625 mg or less) stimulated 16% hyperplasias in women followed for 15 months. In women given estrogen plus progestins, the occurrence of hyperplasia was 6% and 3%, respectively. In comparison of length of therapy, 7 days of progestin reduced the occurrence of hyperplasia to 4%, 10 days reduced it to 2%, and 12 days eliminated hyperplasia. Direct comparisons in drug trials have also shown reductions of hyperplasia in women given estrogens and progestins compared with those given estrogen alone. It should be pointed out that the majority of endometrial lesions observed in women in these trials were either cystic or simple hyperplasias, which could be reversed by giving a progestin or discontinuing the estrogen.

One option is to administer a progestin such as medroxyprogesterone acetate at a dosage of 5–10 mg/d for 12–14 days each month (see Table 57–3). If this is accomplished, 80–90% of women will experience some vaginal bleeding monthly toward the end of or after the progestin is administered. An alternative is to prescribe a lower dosage, 2.5 mg, continuously. The combined, continuous administration of estrogen plus progestin promotes endometrial atrophy and results in amenorrhea in 70–90% of women who use continuous therapy for more than 1 year. The remainder will bleed occasionally, with the bleeding usually being less frequent, shorter, and lighter than with sequential therapy.

Administration of progestins can be associated with other uncomfortable side effects including fatigue, depression, breast tenderness, bloating, menstrual cramps, and headaches. It is also important to keep in mind that it was a progestin-containing regimen that was utilized in the WHI trial which was discontinued largely due to a trend toward an increased risk of breast cancer. This raises concerns about the potential role of progestogens in increasing breast cancer risk. Until the estrogen-only arm of the WHI becomes available, patients and physicians may be reluctant to incorporate progestogens into HRT regimens. This concern combined with potential progestogen side effects may lead to elimination of or nonstandard progestogen administration. If lower dosages or shorter duration of progestogens are utilized, endometrial sampling to diagnose the development of hyperplasia should be performed.

Special Treatment Problems

A. ALTERNATIVES TO ESTROGEN THERAPY

Estrogen replacement is contraindicated in some patients, and others may want to avoid the risks of this type of therapy. Alternative medications are available for control of some of the symptoms and complaints associated with the climacteric.

For hot flushes, depo-medroxyprogesterone acetate, 150 mg/mo intramuscularly, oral administration of the same agent, 10–40 mg/d, or megestrol acetate 20–80 mg/d, have all been shown to be more effective than placebo but less efficacious than estrogen in reducing hot flashes. Clonidine and methyldopa have also been shown to reduce flushes, but cause their own side effects and usually have not been satisfactory medications. Plant-derived compounds, such as soy, may help alleviate some vasomotor symptoms.

For prevention of osteoporosis, calcium supplements have been shown to significantly reduce the loss of calcium from bone, particularly several years after menopause. Elemental calcium, 1000–1500 mg, should be given. Administration of bisphosphonates and SERMs have also been effective in preventing bone loss. Calcitonin also prevents bone loss. Vitamin D at 400–800 IU/d should be given to enhance calcium absorption. For vaginal atrophy, no good substitution therapy has been devised.

B. UTERINE BLEEDING

If patients are given sequential estrogen and progestins, the majority will experience some uterine bleeding.

This bleeding can occur during the treatment-free interval (scheduled bleeding) or while the medications are being administered (unscheduled bleeding). Hyperplastic endometrium can develop with this type of therapy. If the bleeding is heavy or prolonged, a biopsy should be performed. If endometrial hyperplasia is present, the medications can be discontinued, or a progestin can be given each day of estrogen administration. Whichever approach is adopted, a repeat biopsy should be performed to make certain that the hyperplastic endometrium has resolved. The cost effectiveness ratio for periodic biopsy in women who do not bleed or bleed only during the medication-free interval is poor and indicates that such biopsy is probably not necessary.

In women taking estrogen only, the incidence of endometrial hyperplasia can be as high as 25% after only 12 months of therapy. Hyperplasia occurs in women who do not experience vaginal bleeding, bleed only during the medication-free interval, or bleed during drug administration. Thus, a pretreatment biopsy and yearly endometrial biopsies are necessary in all women receiving estrogens alone to determine the presence of hyperplasia. Again, estrogen withdrawal or combined estrogen-progesterone therapy may be employed to treat the hyperplasia. It is presumed, but not established, that the incidence of endometrial cancer will be reduced if the programs discussed above are instituted.

Prognosis

The prognosis for the postmenopausal woman who does not develop clinically manifest estrogen deficiency includes only the ordinary hazards of disease and aging. For the woman who does develop signs of estrogen deficiency, steroid therapy can correct physical symptoms and signs, ameliorate associated emotional disturbances, and prevent the development of major metabolic estrogen deficiency disorders. Correction of minor distressing symptoms and signs can improve the general well-being of the postmenopausal woman and help her to pursue a vigorous life. On the other hand, steroid therapy for the postmenopausal woman who does not need it serves no purpose and can cause unpleasant side effects and impose unnecessary risks on her health.

REFERENCES

Abraham GE, Maroulis GB: Effect of exogenous estrogen on serum pregnenolone, cortisol, and androgens in postmenopausal women. Obstet Gynecol 1975;45:271.

Adams MR et al: Inhibition of coronary artery atherosclerosis by 17-beta estradiol in ovariectomized monkeys: Lack of an effect of added progesterone. Arteriosclerosis 1990;10:1051.

American College of Obstetricians and Gynecologists: Hormone replacement therapy. ACOG Educational Bulletin No. 247, 1998.

Antunes CM et al: Endometrial cancer and estrogen use. N Engl J Med 1979;300:9.

Aubin JE: Osteoprotegerin and its ligand: A new paradigm for regulation of osteoclastogenesis and bone resorption. Medscape Women's Health 2000;5:5.

Avioli LV: The role of calcitonin in the prevention of osteoporosis. Endocrinol Metab Clin North Am 1998;27:411.

Barrett-Connor E, Bush TL: Estrogen replacement and coronary heart disease. Cardiovasc Clin 1989;19:159.

Barrett-Connor E, Miller V: Estrogens, lipids, and heart disease. Clin Geriatr Med 1993;9:57.

Bergkvist L et al: The risk of breast cancer after estrogen and estrogen-progestin replacement. N Engl J Med 1989;321:293.

Bolognia J: Aging skin, epidermal and dermal changes. Prog Clin Biol Res 1989;320:121.

Bone HG et al: Alendronate and estrogen effects in postmenopausal women with low bone mineral density. Alendronate/Estrogen Study Group. J Clin Endocrinol Metab 2000;85:720.

Boston Collaborative Drug Surveillance Program, Boston University Medical Center: Surgically confirmed gallbladder disease, venous thromboembolism, and breast tumors in relation to postmenopausal estrogen therapy. N Engl J Med 1974;290:15.

Brincat M et al: Long-term effects of the menopause and sex hormones on skin thickness. Br J Obstet Gynecol 1985;92:256.

Brincat M et al: A study of the decrease of skin collagen content, skin thickness, and bone mass in the postmenopausal woman. Obstet Gynecol 1987;70:840.

Campbell S, Whitehead M: Estrogen therapy and the postmenopausal syndrome. Clin Obstet Gynecol 1977;4:31.

Cauley JA et al: Estrogen replacement therapy and mortality among older women: the study of osteoporotic fractures. Arch Intern Med 1997;157:2181.

Chetkowski RJ et al: Biologic effects of transdermal estradiol. N Engl J Med 1986;314:1615.

Collaborative group on hormonal factors in breast cancer: breast cancer and hormone replacement therapy. Lancet 1997;350:1047.

Creasman WT: Estrogen replacement therapy: is previously treated cancer a contraindication? Obstet Gynecol 1991;77:308.

Cummings SR et al: Bone density at various sites for prediction of hip fractures. Lancet 1993;341:962.

Dawson-Hughes B: Calcium supplementation and bone loss: A review of controlled clinical trials (1–3). Am J Clin Nutr 1991;54:274S.

Delmas PD: Biochemical markers of bone turnover: Methodology and clinical use in osteoporosis. Am J Med 1991;91:59S.

Delmas PD et al: Effects of raloxifene on bone mineral density, serum cholesterol concentrations, and uterine endometrium in postmenopausal women. N Engl J Med 1997;337:1641.

Erickson GE: Normal ovarian function. Clin Obstet Gynecol 1978;21:31.

Ettinger B et al: Low-dosage micronized 17β-estradiol prevents bone loss in postmenopausal women. Am J Obstet Gynecol 1992;166:479.

Ettinger B et al: Reduction of vertebral fracture risk in postmenopausal women with osteoporosis treated with raloxifene: results from a 3-year randomized clinical trial. Multiple Outcomes of Raloxifene Evaluation (MORE) Investigators. JAMA 1999;282:637.

Falkeborn M et al: The risk of acute myocardial infarction after estrogen and estrogen-progesterone replacement. Br J Obstet Gynaecol 1992;99:821.

Field CS et al: Preventive effects of transdermal 17β-estradiol on osteoporotic changes after surgical menopause: A two-year placebo-controlled trial. Am J Obstet Gynecol 1993;168:114.

Fogelman I et al: Risedronate reverses bone loss in postmenopausal women with low bone mass: results from a multinational, double-blind, placebo-controlled trial. BMD-MN Study Group. J Clin Endocrinol Metab 2000;85:1895.

Furchgott RF, Vanhoutte PM: Endothelium-derived relaxing and contracting factors. FASEB J 1989;3:2007.

Gambone J et al: Further delineation of hypothalamic dysfunction responsible for menopausal hot flashes. J Clin Endocrinol Metab 1985;59:1097.

Gibbons WE et al: Biochemical and biological effects of sequential estrogen/progestin therapy on the endometrium of postmenopausal women. Am J Obstet Gynecol 1986;154:456.

Grodstein F et al: Postmenopausal hormone therapy and mortality. N Engl J Med 1997;336:1769.

Hammond MG, Hatley L, Talbert LM: A double blind study to evaluate the effect of methyldopa on menopausal vasomotor flushes. J Clin Endocrinol Metab 1984;58:1158.

Harris ST et al: Effect of combined risedronate and hormone replacement therapies on bone mineral density in postmenopausal women. J Clin Endocrinol Metab 2001;86:1890.

Harris ST: Effects of risedronate treatment on vertebral and nonvertebral fractures in women with postmenopausal osteoporosis: a randomized controlled trial. Vertebral Efficacy with Risedronate (VERT) Study Group. JAMA 1999; 282:1344.

Hasselquist MB et al: Isolation and characterization of the estrogen receptor in human skin. J Clin Endocrinol Metab 1980; 50:76.

Hayashi T et al: Basal release of nitric oxide from aortic rings is greater in female rabbits than in male rabbits: Implications for atherosclerosis. Proc Natl Acad Sci U S A 1992;89:11259.

Hemminki E et al: Impact of postmenopausal hormone therapy on cardiovascular events and cancer: pooled data from clinical trials. Br Med J 1997;315:149.

Henderson BE et al: Re-evaluating the role of progestogen therapy after the menopause. Fertil Steril 1988;49(Suppl):9S.

Herrington DM, Reboussin DM, Brosnihan KB et al: The effects of estrogen replacement on the progression of coronary-artery atherosclerosis. N Engl J Med 2000;343:522.

Holloway L: Skeletal effects of cyclic recombinant human growth hormone and salmon calcitonin in osteopenic postmenopausal women. J Clin Endocrinol Metab 1997;82:1111.

Horwitz RI et al: Necropsy diagnosis of endometrial cancer and detection-bias in case/control studies. Lancet 1981;2:66.

Hulley S et al: Randomized trial of estrogen plus progestin for secondary prevention of coronary heart disease in postmenopausal women. Heart and estrogen/progestin replacement study research group. JAMA 1998;280:605.

Jensen J et al: Long-term effects of percutaneous estrogens and oral progesterone on serum lipoproteins in postmenopausal women. Am J Obstet Gynecol 1987;156:66.

Johnston CC Jr, Slemenda CW, Melton LJ III: Clinical use of bone densitometry. N Engl J Med 1991;324:1105.

Judd HL: Hormonal dynamics associated with the menopause. Clin Obstet Gynecol 1976;19:775.

Judd HL et al: Endocrine function of the postmenopausal ovary: Concentrations of androgens and estrogens in ovarian and peripheral vein blood. J Clin Endocrinol Metab 1974; 39:1020.

Judd HL et al: Origin of serum estradiol in postmenopausal women. Obstet Gynecol 1982;59:680.

Judd HL et al: Serum androgens and estrogens in postmenopausal women with and without endometrial cancer. Am J Obstet Gynecol 1980;136:859.

Kado DM et al: Vertebral fractures and mortality in older women: a prospective study. Study of Osteoporotic Fractures Research Group. Arch Intern Med 1999;159:1215.

Kimble RB: Alcohol, cytokines, and estrogen in the control of bone remodeling. Alcohol Clin Exp Res 1997;21:385.

Laufer LR et al: Effect of clonidine on hot flashes in postmenopausal women. Obstet Gynecol 1982;60:583.

Lindsay R et al: Bone response to termination of estrogen treatment. Lancet 1978;1:1325.

Meldrum DR et al: Elevations in skin temperature of the finger as an objective index of postmenopausal hot flashes: Standardization of the technique. Am J Obstet Gynecol 1979; 135:713.

Mendelsohn ME et al: The protective effects of estrogen on the cardiovascular system. N Engl J Med 1999;340:1801.

Meunier PJ: Fluoride salts are no better at preventing new vertebral fractures than calcium-vitamin D in postmenopausal osteoporosis: the FAVO study. Osteoporos Int 1998;8:4.

Mosca L et al: Hormone replacement therapy and cardiovascular disease: a statement for healthcare professionals from the American Heart Association. Circulation 2001;104:499.

Mosca L: The role of hormone replacement therapy in the prevention of postmenopausal heart disease. Arch Intern Med 2000;160:2263.

Nabulsi AA et al: Association of hormone-replacement therapy with various cardiovascular risk factors in postmenopausal women. N Engl J Med 1993;328:1069.

National Osteoporosis Foundation: *Physician's Guide To Prevention And Treatment Of Osteoporosis.* National Osteoporosis Foundation, 1998.

Nathan L, Pervin S, Singh R, Rosenfeld M, Chandhuri G: Estradiol inhibits leukocyte adhesion and transendothelial migration in vivo: possible mechanisms for gender differences in atherosclerosis. Circ Res 1999;85:377–385.

Osteoporosis Prevention, Diagnosis, and Therapy. National Institutes of Health Consensus Development Conference Statement 2001;17:1.

Phillips SM, Sherwin BB: Effects of estrogen on memory function in surgically menopausal women. Psychoneuroendocrinology 1992;17:485.

Reid IR et al: Effect of calcium supplementation on bone loss in postmenopausal women. N Engl J Med 1993;328:460.

Rickard DJ, Gowen M, MacDonald BR: Proliferative responses to estradiol IL-1 alpha and TGF beta by cells expressing alkaline phosphatase in human osteoblast-like cell cultures. Calcif Tissue Int 1993;52:227.

Rigg LA et al: Absorption of estrogens from vaginal creams. N Engl J Med 1978;298:195.

Roberts WC, Giraldo AA: Bilateral oophorectomy in menstruating women and accelerated coronary atherosclerosis: An unproved connection. Am J Med 1979;67:363.

Rosen CJ: Emerging anabolic treatments for osteoporosis. Rheum Dis Clin North Am 2001;27:215.

Rosen CJ: The pathophysiology and treatment of postmenopausal osteoporosis. An evidence-based approach to estrogen replacement therapy. Endocrinol Metab Clin North Am 1997;26:295.

Ross RK, Paganini-Hill A, Wan PC et al: Effect of hormone replacement therapy on breast cancer risk: estrogen versus estrogen plus progestin. J Natl Cancer Inst 2000;92:328.

Roux S: Bone loss. Factors that regulate osteoclast differentiation: an update. Arthritis Res 2000;2:6.

Rubin SM, Cummings SR: Results of bone densitometry affect women's decisions about taking measures to prevent fractures. Ann Intern Med 1992;116:990.

Shahrad P, Marks R: A pharmacologic effect of estrogen on human epidermis. Br J Dermatol 1977;97:383.

Sherman BM, Korenman SG: Hormonal characteristics of the human menstrual cycle throughout reproductive life. J Clin Invest 1975;55:669.

Shermin BB: Estrogen effects on cognition in menopausal women. Neurology 1997;48(5 Suppl 7):S21.

Stock JL et al: Calcitonin-salmon nasal spray reduces the incidence of new vertebral fractures in postmenopausal women: three year interim results of the "PROOF" study group. J Bone Miner Res 1997;12(Suppl 1):S187.

Storm T et al: Effect of intermittent cyclical etidronate therapy on bone mass and fracture rate in women with postmenopausal osteoporosis. N Engl J Med 1990;322:1265.

Stumpf WE et al: Estrogen target cells in the skin. Experientia 1974;30:196.

Sunyer T: Estrogen's bone-protective effects may involve differential IL-1 receptor regulation in human osteoclast-like cells. J Clin Invest 1999;103:1409.

Tataryn IV et al: LH, FSH, and skin temperature during the menopausal hot flash. J Clin Endocrinol Metab 1979;49:152.

Tsai KS, Ebeling PR, Riggs BL: Bone responsiveness to parathyroid hormone in normal and osteoporotic postmenopausal women. J Clin Endocrinol Metab 1989;69:1024.

Vermeulen A: The hormonal activity of the postmenopausal ovary. J Clin Endocrinol Metab 1976;42:247.

Vollman RF: *The Menstrual Cycle,* Vol. 7. WB Saunders, 1977, p. 193.

Weiss NS et al: Decreased risk of fractures of the hip and lower forearm with postmenopausal use of estrogen. N Engl J Med 1980;302:551.

Whitehead MI et al: Effects of estrogens and progestins on the biochemistry and morphology of the postmenopausal endometrium. N Engl J Med 1981;305:1599.

Williams JK, Adams MR, Klopfenstein HS: Estrogen modulates responses of atherosclerotic coronary arteries. Circulation 1990;81:1680.

Williams JK et al: Short-term administration of estrogen and vascular responses of atherosclerotic coronary arteries. J Am Coll Cardiol 1992;20:452.

Woitge HW et al: Biochemical markers to survey bone turnover. Rheum Dis Clin North Am 2001;27:49.

The Women's Health Initiative Study Group: Design of the Women's Health Initiative clinical trial and observational study. Control Clin Trials 1998;19:61.

World Health Organization: Assessment of fracture risk and its application to screening for postmenopausal osteoporosis. Report of a WHO Study Group. World Health Organ Tech Rep Ser 1994;843:1.

Writing Group for the Women's Health Initiative: Risks and benefits of estrogen plus progestin in healthy postmenopausal women: Principal results from the Women's Health Initiative randomized controlled trial. JAMA 2002:288:321–333.

SECTION VII.
Contemporary Issues

Critical Care Obstetrics

58

Johanna Weiss, MD, & Ramada S. Smith, MD

Critical care medicine has increasingly become an area of interest to the obstetrician-gynecologist. Pregnancy complications such as shock, thromboembolism, acute respiratory distress syndrome (ARDS), and coagulation disorders can lead to significant morbidity. Furthermore, the approach to these patients can be influenced by a variety of physiologic changes that are unique to pregnancy. This chapter provides a basic approach to some of the common clinical problems that often require complex multidisciplinary care and a knowledge of invasive hemodynamic monitoring.

PULMONARY ARTERY CATHETERIZATION

The flow-directed pulmonary artery catheter has been a major addition to the clinician's armamentarium because of its applicability to a wide range of cardiorespiratory disorders. The catheter allows simultaneous measurement of central venous pressure (CVP), pulmonary artery pressure (PAP), pulmonary capillary wedge pressure (PCWP), cardiac output, and mixed venous oxygen saturation. The pulmonary artery catheter is a 7F triple-lumen polyvinyl chloride catheter with a balloon and thermodilution cardiac output sensor at the tip. The distal port is used to measure PAP when the balloon is deflated and PCWP when inflated. A proximal lumen is present 30 cm from the balloon tip; this can be used to monitor the CVP and to administer fluids and drugs. Both ports can be used to withdraw blood. Oximetric catheters also have 2 optical fibers that permit continuous measurement of mixed venous oxygen saturation by reflection spectrophotometry.

Insertion Technique

A 16-gauge catheter is used to gain access to the internal jugular or subclavian vein (Fig 58–1). Pertinent

anatomic landmarks for the internal jugular vein approach are shown in Figure 58–2. A guidewire is then introduced into the vein through the catheter, and the 16-gauge catheter sheath is removed. A pulmonary artery catheter is inserted over the guidewire, and the guidewire is removed. The central venous and pulmonary artery ports are connected to a pressure transducer, so that the characteristic waveforms of the various heart chambers can be identified as the catheter is advanced (Fig 58–3). When the catheter is in the superior vena cava, the balloon is inflated with 1–1.5 mL of air, and the catheter is advanced forward into the main pulmonary artery. Table 58–1 shows the average distance in centimeters the catheter must be advanced from various insertion sites. From the main pulmonary artery, the flow of blood moves the catheter into a branch of the pulmonary artery, where it wedges and records the PCWP.

Criteria for verification of the true PCWP include (1) x-ray confirmation of catheter placement, (2) characteristic left atrial waveform configuration, (3) mean PCWP lower than mean PAP, (4) respiratory variation demonstrated by fluctuation of the PCWP waveform baseline with inspiration and expiration, and (5) blood samples showing higher oxygen tension and lower CO_2 tension than in arterial blood.

After deflation of the balloon, the pulmonary artery waveform should again be visualized. Fiberoptic catheters allow verification of PCWP by showing a sudden increase in mixed venous saturation to 95% or greater.

Indications for Invasive Monitoring

According to the American College of Obstetricians and Gynecologists, invasive hemodynamic monitoring may provide useful information for critical conditions during pregnancy such as:

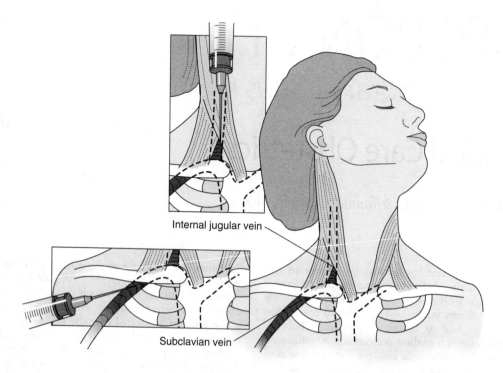

Figure 58–1. Comparison of right internal jugular vein and subclavian vein vascular access sites for right heart catheterization.

- Shock (septic, hemorrhagic, cardiogenic, unexplained).
- Pulmonary edema (eg, severe pregnancy-induced hypertension [PIH], congestive heart failure [CHF], unexplained or refractory).
- Severe PIH with persistent oliguria unresponsive to fluid challenge.
- Acute respiratory distress syndrome (ARDS).
- Severe cardiac disease.

Hemodynamic Parameters Available With Pulmonary Artery Catheterization

During the diastolic period of the cardiac cycle, the left ventricle, left atrium, and pulmonary vascular bed essentially become a common chamber (Fig 58–4). In a normal cardiovascular system, the left ventricular end-diastolic pressure (LVEDP), left atrial pressure, and PCWP are essentially interchangeable. A disparity may develop between PCWP and LVEDP when LVEDP is greater than 15 mm Hg; however, for clinical purposes, the PCWP provides a fairly accurate index of LVEDP, especially if the "a" wave (caused by retrograde transmission of the left atrial contraction) can be identified

in the wedge tracing. The relationships described earlier can be substantially altered by mitral or aortic valvular disease.

A. Cardiac Output

The thermal sensing device in the tip of a pulmonary artery catheter allows for rapid determination of cardiac output by the thermodilution method. Five milliliters of 5% dextrose in water is injected through the central venous port at a constant distance from the thermistor tip. The use of this solution at room temperature can minimize sources of potential error associated with inaccurate temperature measurements and catheter warming. The change in pulmonary artery temperature is detected by the thermistor. The cardiac output is inversely proportional to the fall in temperature and is computed by planimetric or computerized methods. The average of 3 values within 10% of each other is typically utilized to calculate cardiac output.

B. Systemic Vascular Resistance

Systemic vascular resistance (SVR) represents the total resistance to forward flow of blood through the body's vascular tree. SVR is calculated as follows:

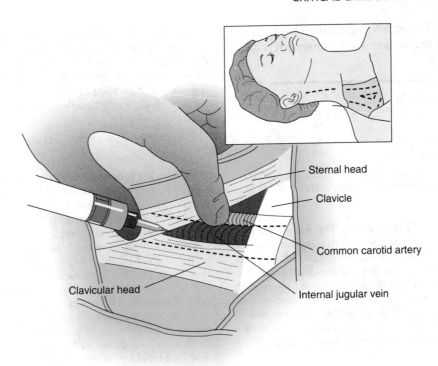

Figure 58–2. Important anatomic landmarks associated with the internal jugular vein approach for right heart catheterization.

$$SVR = \frac{[(MAP - CVP)] \times 80}{CO}$$

(MAP = mean arterial pressure; CVP = central venous pressure; CO = cardiac output)

During pregnancy, this parameter is usually in the range of 800–1200 dynes · s · cm^{-5}. Depending on the clinical condition, a reduction or increase in SVR may be desirable in the presence of normal blood pressure (eg, septic shock), in which a very low SVR may be seen despite normal or low blood pressure. In order to maintain vital organ perfusion, vasopressor therapy may be indicated to increase SVR.

C. PULMONARY CAPILLARY WEDGE PRESSURE

The PCWP provides important information on 2 basic parameters of cardiopulmonary function: (1) pulmonary venous pressure, which is a major determinant of pulmonary congestion; and (2) the left atrial and left ventricular filling pressures, from which ventricular function curves can be constructed.

Pulmonary capillary wedge pressure can be reliably assessed by CVP monitoring only in the absence of sig-

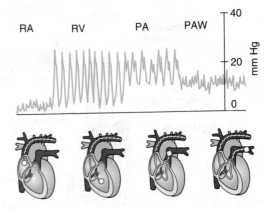

Figure 58–3. Changes in waveforms observed during placement of a pulmonary artery catheter. RA, right atrium; RV, right ventricle; PA pulmonary artery; PAW, pulmonary artery wedge. (Reproduced, with permission, from Rosenthal MH: Intrapartum intensive care management of the cardiac patient. Clin Obstet Gynecol 1981;24:796.)

Table 58–1. Distance to right atrium from various sites of insertion in pulmonary artery catheterizaton.

Vein	Distance to Right Atrium[1] (cm)
Internal jugular	15
Subclavian	15
Right antecubital	40
Left antecubital	50
Femoral	30

[1]Distance from right atrium to pulmonary artery is 8–15 cm.

nificant myocardial dysfunction. The measurement of PCWP has certain advantages over measurement of CVP alone. A disparity between right and left ventricular function may be seen in conditions such as myocardial infarction, valvular disease, sepsis, and severe PIH. Under these circumstances, the management of fluid therapy based on CVP alone could have adverse results. Additionally, cardiac output and mixed venous oxygen tension cannot be determined with a simple CVP catheter.

D. Ventricular Function Curves

Myocardial performance is best interpreted in terms of left ventricular function curves (ie, the Frank-Starling relationship). The cardiac output and PCWP are used to construct the ventricular function curve by plotting the ventricular stroke work index against the mean atrial pressure or ventricular end-diastolic pressure (usually the PCWP). The left ventricular stroke work index is calculated by the following formula:

$$LVSWI = SVI \times (MAP - PCWP) \times 0.0136$$

(LVSWI = left ventricular stroke work index [g-m/m²]; SVI = stroke volume index [mL/beat/m²]; MAP = mean arterial pressure [mm Hg]; PCWP = pulmonary capillary wedge pressure [mm Hg]).

Ventricular function curves provide a useful index of cardiovascular status to guide inotropic and vasoactive drug therapy. Evaluation of myocardial contractility by ventricular function curves allows one to obtain optimal filling pressures and stroke volume index in critically ill patients. The effects of therapy (eg, diuretics, antihypertensive agents, or volume expanders) can be evaluated on the basis of performance. Under normal conditions, a small rise in filling pressure is accompanied by a rapid rise in stroke work. Unfavorable conditions such as hypoxia or myocardial depression produce a shift in the curve to the right and downward such that lower stroke work indices are seen at higher filling pressures.

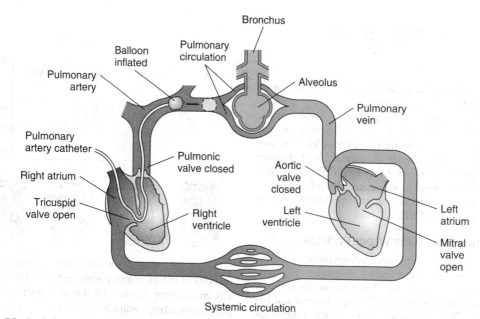

Figure 58–4. Pulmonary capillary wedge pressure in diastole (ventricles relaxed). (Reproduced, with permission, from *Understanding Hemodynamic Measurements Made With the Swan-Ganz Catheter.* American Edward Laboratories, 1982.)

E. Mixed Venous Oxygen Saturation

The mixed venous oxygen saturation (SvO_2) reflects the body's capacity to provide adequate tissue oxygenation. This parameter is affected by cardiac output, hemoglobin concentration, arterial oxygen saturation, and tissue oxygen consumption. An SvO_2 of 60–80% usually indicates normal oxygen delivery and demand with adequate tissue perfusion. An SvO_2 greater than 80% reflects increased oxygen delivery and decreased oxygen utilization. This situation may be seen in patients with hypothermia or sepsis who are receiving supplemental oxygen. A high SvO_2 may also provide confirmatory evidence that the pulmonary artery catheter is in the wedge position. Finally, a low SvO_2 (< 60%) indicates increased oxygen demands with decreased oxygen delivery due to anemia, low cardiac output, or decreased arterial oxygen saturation.

Measurement of SvO_2 allows for continuous monitoring of cardiorespiratory reserve by providing an index of tissue oxygen delivery and utilization. Changes in SvO_2 will be apparent with infusion of vasoactive drugs, volume loading, or afterload reduction. While many intensive care units rely on direct measurement of cardiac output alone, this parameter does not always accurately reflect tissue oxygenation. For instance, normal cardiac output might not be adequate to meet increased oxygen requirements in malignant hyperthermia or thyroid storm.

F. Maternal Oxygen Consumption

Mixed venous oxygen saturation results can be used with arterial blood gas analysis to provide useful information about the metabolic status of the critically ill obstetric patient. Resting maternal oxygen consumption progressively increases during pregnancy. Occasionally, one needs to pay particular attention to the metabolic status of critically ill women or those with ARDS. Factors such as tachycardia or fever that are associated with increased oxygen consumption should be minimized under these circumstances.

The Fick relationship:

$$CO = \frac{Vo_2}{AVo_2 \text{ diff.}} \times 100$$

provides a method for calculating oxygen consumption (VO_2), if the cardiac output (CO) and systemic arteriovenous oxygen (AvO_2) concentration difference is known. The AvO_2 difference can be calculated by subtracting the oxygen content of desaturated mixed venous blood from that of arterial blood that passes through the pulmonary artery catheter. For example, a patient with a cardiac output minus AvO_2 difference of

5 mL would have an oxygen consumption (VO_2) of 300 mL.

$$6000 \text{ mL min}^{-1} \times 5 \text{ mL per 100 mL blood}$$
$$Vo_2 \ 100 = 300 \text{ mL min}^{-1}$$

An understanding of these relationships will allow the clinician to better understand how to use physiologic variables for interpreting the hemodynamic and pulmonary condition of critically ill patients.

G. Colloid Osmotic Pressure

The plasma colloid oncotic pressure (COP) is another measurement that can be useful in critical care (Table 58–2). Plasma COP is the pressure exerted by certain plasma proteins that hold fluid in the intravascular space. Albumin accounts for 75% of the oncotic pressure of plasma, with the rest coming from globulin and fibrinogen. It has been demonstrated in dogs that iatrogenic reduction in plasma proteins resulted in pulmonary edema with only minimal increases in left atrial pressure. Subsequent studies in humans identified cases of pulmonary edema in which normal or slightly elevated PCWP was present. From these studies, the important concept of a COP-PCWP gradient evolved. It appears that when the COP-PCWP gradient is less than 4 mm Hg, the likelihood of pulmonary edema is increased, although not all patients with a decreased gradient will develop pulmonary edema. The determination of COP and its relationship to the PCWP can play a crucial role in the detection of patients likely to develop pulmonary edema in the face of normal left-sided filling pressures.

Studies of pregnant women have demonstrated that patients with certain conditions in which the risk of pulmonary edema is markedly increased tend to have lowered COP (eg, hypovolemic shock, severe PIH, prolonged tocolytic therapy, and frank pulmonary edema).

Complications

The most common complication associated with pulmonary artery catheter placement is dysrhythmia. More

Table 58–2. Serum colloid oncotic pressure during pregnancy.

	Normotensive (mm Hg)	Hypertensive (mm Hg)
Antepartum (term)	22.4 ± 0.5	17.9 ± 0.7
Postpartum (first 24 hours)	15.4 ± 2.1	13.7 ± 0.5

serious complications also include pulmonary infarction, thromboembolism, balloon rupture with air embolism, pulmonary artery or valve rupture, catheter knotting, infection, arterial puncture, thromboembolism, pneumothorax, and pulmonary hemorrhage. Table 58–3 summarizes the complication rates for pulmonary artery catheterization.

A. DYSRHYTHMIA

Premature ventricular contractions may transiently occur as the catheter tip enters the right ventricle. However, they usually resolve following advancement of the catheter into the pulmonary artery. If the dysrhythmia is refractory to lidocaine, 50–100 mg given intravenously, the catheter should be withdrawn from the cardiac chambers.

B. PULMONARY INFARCTION

Pulmonary infarction may occur when the catheter migrates distally and wedges spontaneously for a prolonged period. This complication, as well as thromboembolism, may be avoided by monitoring the PCWP at regular intervals and by using a continuous heparinized flow system.

C. BALLOON RUPTURE

Balloon rupture can be avoided by limiting the number of balloon inflations and by inflating only to the smallest necessary volume. Inflation of the balloon beyond 2 mL of air is unnecessary and may be harmful. To avoid rupture of a pulmonary artery branch, inflation of the balloon should be stopped immediately when the wedge tracing is seen.

Table 58–3. Complications of pulmonary artery catheterization.[1]

Complication	Incidence (%)
Premature ventricular contractions	15–27
Arterial puncture	8
Superficial cellulitis	3
Thromboembolism	?
Pneumothorax	1–2
Balloon rupture	< 1
Pulmonary infarction/ischemia	1–7
Pulmonary artery rupture	< 1
Catheter knotting	< 1
Catheter-related sepsis	1

[1]Reproduced, with permission, from Hankins GDV, Cunningham FG: Severe preeclampsia and eclampsia: Controversies in management. Williams Obstetrics 1991;18(suppl):11. Appleton & Lange.

D. CATHETER KNOTTING

Catheter knotting is usually the result of advancing the catheter 10–15 cm farther than is necessary to reach the right ventricle or pulmonary artery. Withdrawing the catheter while the balloon is still inflated may cause tricuspid rupture or chordae tendineae tears.

E. INFECTION AND PHLEBITIS

Infection and phlebitis can be minimized by using aseptic technique. The risk of associated sepsis is related to excessive catheter manipulation and the duration of catheterization.

NONINVASIVE MONITORING FOR CRITICALLY ILL PATIENTS

Pulse oximetry is a simple tool that can be used with invasive monitoring for patients with cardiovascular or respiratory compromise. The correlation between pulse oximetry and direct blood oxygen saturation is excellent when oxygen saturation is greater than 60%. Factors adversely affecting the accuracy of pulse oximetry include movement, peripheral vasoconstriction, hypotension, anemia, hypothermia, intravascular dye, and possibly nail polish.

■ OBSTETRIC DISORDERS REQUIRING CRITICAL CARE

OBSTETRIC SHOCK

Shock may be defined as an imbalance between oxygen supply and demand. The basic underlying defect is a significant reduction in the supply of oxygenated blood to various tissues due to inadequate perfusion. In obstetrics, this reduction often results from hemorrhage, sepsis, or pump failure. The physiologic compensation common to all shock states involves tachycardia and peripheral vasoconstriction to maximize cerebral and cardiac perfusion by way of the sympathetic nervous system. Failure of these compensatory mechanisms will lead to a predominance of anaerobic metabolism and lactic acidosis, which can be potentially devastating to the patient and fetus. Cardiogenic shock may be seen in pregnant women with cardiac dysrhythmias, congenital heart disease, peripartum cardiomyopathy, and congestive heart failure. The following discussion will focus on 2 of the more common shock syndromes complicating pregnancy—those related to hemorrhage and sepsis.

1. Hypovolemic Shock

 ESSENTIALS OF DIAGNOSIS

- Recent history of acute blood loss or excessive diuresis.
- Hypotension, tachycardia, tachypnea, and oliguria with progression to altered mental status.
- Precipitous drop in hematocrit.

General Considerations

Hypovolemic shock is a leading cause of maternal morality in the U.S. and is most commonly associated with obstetric hemorrhage. Bleeding severe enough to cause hemorrhagic shock may result from a wide variety of conditions, including ruptured ectopic pregnancy; abruptio placentae; placenta previa; placenta accreta; rupture, atony, or inversion of the uterus; surgical procedures; obstetric lacerations; or retained products of conception.

Pathophysiology

During normal pregnancy, the blood volume expands by approximately 1500 mL. This hypervolemia results from hormonal alterations and may be considered protective against peripartum bleeding. During acute hemorrhage, the body responds to volume loss by hemodynamic, volume-altering, and hormonal mechanisms.

Hemodynamic adjustments result from activation of the sympathetic nervous system. These changes include vasoconstriction of arteriolar resistance vessels, constriction of venous capacitance vessels, and redistribution of blood flow away from peripheral organs to preserve adequate cerebral and cardiac blood flow.

Volume adjustments occur from extravascular fluid shifts into the intravascular compartment. The rate of plasma refill depends on the magnitude of volume depletion.

If these mechanisms are insufficient to restore circulatory function, other compensatory effects, such as secretion of antidiuretic hormone (ADH), cortisol, aldosterone, and catecholamines will occur. Epinephrine, in addition to causing peripheral vasoconstriction, will have inotropic and chronotropic effects on the heart. ADH, cortisol, and aldosterone will help conserve water and salt, which may then result in reduced blood flow to the kidneys and decreased urine output.

These homeostatic mechanisms serve to maintain adequate tissue perfusion until approximately 25–30% of the circulating blood volume is lost. Inadequate tissue perfusion and oxygenation will then lead to anaerobic metabolism and lactic acidosis. Over a prolonged period of vasoconstriction, there may be decompensation of the peripheral vasculature leading to damaged or leaky capillaries. Observations of blood flow regulation during pregnancy suggest that uterine arteries have limited capacity to autoregulate fetoplacental perfusion. Thus uteroplacental blood flow is critically dependent upon systemic maternal cardiac output.

Clinical Findings

The clinical manifestations of hemorrhagic shock depend on the quantity and rate of volume depletion. Orthostatic signs and symptoms may be masked by the hypervolemia of pregnancy, especially if a source of bleeding is not evident. Obvious hypotension and tachycardia in the presence of external bleeding should alert the clinician to the possibility of shock. A careful physical examination will identify decreased tissue perfusion in several different organ systems, including the heart, brain, kidneys, lungs, and skin. Altered mental status, dizziness, diaphoresis, and cold, clammy extremities, as well as a fast, "thready" pulse are common findings in significant hemorrhagic shock. Oliguria (< 30 mL/h), CVP of less than 5 cm H_2O, and PCWP of less than 5 mm Hg are all consistent with significant volume depletion. The identification of intra-abdominal bleeding may require culdocentesis or peritoneal lavage. Fetal heart monitoring may reveal bradycardia or late decelerations.

Differential Diagnosis

Hypovolemic shock should be differentiated from other shock syndromes resulting from sepsis or heart failure. Usually, there is a history of profound bleeding. Since shock may affect several organ systems, it is essential that its underlying cause be identified. Patients with septic shock will tend to be febrile, with associated abnormal white blood cell counts and clinical evidence of infection. Cardiogenic shock may be associated with clinical and radiographic evidence of pulmonary congestion or a previous history of heart disease.

Complications

Electrolyte imbalance, acidosis, acute tubular necrosis, stress-induced gastric ulceration, pulmonary edema, and ARDS are common complications associated with hemorrhagic shock. Myocardial infarction is a rare complication in the obstetric population.

Treatment

The treatment of hemorrhagic shock should be directed toward replacing blood volume and optimizing cardiac performance. The source of bleeding should be controlled. Uterine atony that is unresponsive to massage and oxytocin may benefit from methylergonovine (0.2 mg intramuscularly), or 15-methyl prostaglandin $F_{2\alpha}$ (0.25 mg intramuscularly). Persistent bleeding may require uterine artery ligation, hypogastric artery ligation, or even cesarean hysterectomy (see Fig 28–1). Decisions regarding blood and fluid replacement should be guided by central pressures and urine output, although pulmonary artery catheterization is rarely necessary. Military antishock trousers (MAST suit) will mobilize blood pooled in the lower body and return it to the central circulation, improving systemic cardiac output and organ perfusion. Supplemental oxygen will minimize tissue hypoxia and fetal acidosis.

Initial rapid volume replacement with crystalloid solution given through a large-bore intravenous site is a temporizing measure until blood replacement is possible. Typically, 1–2 L of lactated Ringer's solution can be administered as rapidly as possible. Compared with normal saline, the electrolyte composition of lactated Ringer's solution more closely approximates plasma, and the metabolism of lactate to bicarbonate provides some buffering capacity for acidosis.

Guidelines for perioperative transfusion of red blood cells have been defined by the National Institutes of Health. Initial treatment of hemorrhagic shock should involve volume replacement by crystalloid or colloid solutions that do not carry risks for disease transmission or transfusion reaction. The use of perioperative red blood cell transfusion should not rely solely upon the dogma of "transfusing to a hematocrit above 30%" as the sole criterion since there is poor evidence supporting its usefulness. The decision whether or not to transfuse red cells should also take into account other factors such as patient age, hemodynamic status, anticipated bleeding, and medical or obstetrical complications. If it is necessary to transfuse large amounts of blood, it is important to note and correct the presence of electrolyte imbalances, acid-base abnormalities, hypothermia, and the dilution of platelets and coagulation factors, which may require the transfusion of other blood products.

The risk of posttransfusion hepatitis has been dramatically decreased by testing blood products with a commercially available hepatitis C assay. The test is a qualitative, enzyme-linked imunosorbent assay (ELISA) for the detection of antibody to hepatitis C virus (anti-HCV) in human serum or plasma. The ELISA test has a specificity of 99.84% in a low prevalence population. A supplemental assay, the recombinant immunoblot assay (RIBA), can be performed on blood that has a repeat reactive anti-HCV.

Fluid balance from intravenous infusions or urine output should be meticulously recorded with daily weights. Oliguria refractory to volume loading may be improved by the addition of intravenous dopamine in low doses (2–5 µg/kg/min) to improve renal perfusion. A diuretic such as bumetanide 0.5–1 mg IV, not to exceed 10 mg/day, should be considered for patients with prolonged oliguria despite normal elevated pulmonary capillary wedge pressures.

Blood tests should include complete blood count, serum electrolytes, creatinine, arterial blood gas analysis, and coagulation profile. Urinalysis is also important. A baseline chest radiograph and electrocardiogram are desirable. Typed and cross-matched transfusion products should be available from the blood bank. One to two ampules of sodium bicarbonate (50–100 mEq) can be administered intravenously to correct acidosis (pH < 7.20). Frequent serial hematocrits may provide an index of acute blood loss. A baseline hematologic profile (PT, PTT, fibrinogen, platelets) is necessary to evaluate the possibility of coagulopathy.

Prognosis

Maternal and fetal survival rates are directly related to the magnitude of volume depletion and length of time the patient remains in shock. If the hemorrhage is controlled and intravascular volume is restored within a reasonable interval, the prognosis is generally good in the absence of associated complications. However, the return of fetal blood flow may lag behind correction of maternal flow.

2. Septic Shock

ESSENTIALS OF DIAGNOSIS

- History of recent hospitalization or surgery.
- Pelvic or abdominal infection with positive confirmatory cultures.
- Temperature instability, confusion, hypotension, oliguria, cardiopulmonary failure.

General Considerations

Septic shock is a life-threatening disorder secondary to bacteremia. The American College of Obstetricians and Gynecologists defines septic shock as sepsis with hypotension despite adequate fluid resuscitation, with the presence of perfusion abnormalities including (but not limited to) lactic acidosis and oliguria. The incidence of bacteremia in obstetric patients has been estimated to be between 0.7% and 10%. Although gram-negative bacteria are usually responsible for most of these infections, septic shock may also result from infection with other bacteria, fungi, protozoa, or viruses. The most common cause of obstetric septic shock is postoperative endometritis (85%). Other commonly associated conditions include antepartum pyelonephritis, septic abortion, and chorioamnionitis.

Pathophysiology

Sepsis may lead to a systemic inflammatory response that can be triggered not only by infections but also by noninfectious disorders, such as trauma and pancreatitis. However, there is strong evidence to support the concept that endotoxin is responsible for the pathogenesis of gram-negative septic shock. *Escherichia coli* has been implicated in 25–50% of cases of septic hypotension, but a variety of other organisms may be causative, including *Klebsiella, Enterobacter, Serratia, Proteus, Pseudomonas, Streptococcus, Peptostreptococcus, Staphylococcus, Fusobacterium, Clostridium,* and *Bacteroides.* The gram-negative endotoxin theory does not explain gram-positive shock, although an understanding of the proposed mechanisms will serve to exemplify the multisystemic effects of this disorder.

Endotoxin is a complex lipopolysaccharide present in the cell walls of gram-negative bacteria. The active component of endotoxin, lipid A, is responsible for initiating activation of the coagulation, fibrinolysis, complement, prostaglandin, and kinin systems. Activation of the coagulation and fibrinolysis systems may lead to consumptive coagulopathy. Complement activation leads to the release by leukocytes of mediators that are responsible for damage to vascular endothelium, platelet aggregation, intensification of the coagulation cascade, and degranulation of mast cells with histamine release. Histamine will cause increased capillary permeability, decreased plasma volume, vasodilatation, and hypotension. Release of bradykinin and β-endorphins also contributes to systemic hypotension. Early stages of septic shock involve low SVR and high cardiac output with a relative decrease in intravascular volume. Late or cold shock subsequently involves an endogenous myocardial depressant factor that has not been isolated. This factor is associated with decreased cardiac output and continued low SVR in the absence of pressor agents. Recent studies suggest that tumor necrosis factor (TNF) may lead to depressed myocardial function during septic shock. Monocytes and macrophages incubated with endotoxin produce this 17-kDa polypeptide within 40 minutes. Direct injection of TNF into animals leads to many of the changes seen in endotoxic shock. Other possible factors include IL-1, IL-6, IL-8, interferon gamma, and granulocyte stimulating factor.

Clinical Findings

A. Symptoms and Signs

Septic shock can be divided into 3 stages: preshock, early shock (warm shock), and late (or cold) shock. In preshock, patients present with tachypnea and respiratory alkalosis. Their condition is best described as a moderate hyperdynamic state, with elevated cardiac output, decreasing SVR, and normal blood pressures. Response to therapy will be greatest at this stage. Early shock is a more hyperdynamic state. Blood pressure drops (SBP < 60 mm Hg), and SVR decreases dramatically (< 400 dynes · s · cm^{-5}). Altered mental status, temperature instability, and sinusoidal fluctuations in arterial blood pressure may be seen at this stage. As this condition progresses into late shock, activation of the sympathetic nervous system with release of catecholamines will lead to intense vasoconstriction, which serves to shunt blood from the peripheral tissues to the heart and brain (cold shock). The compensatory vasoconstriction results in increased cardiac work. Lactic acidosis, poor coronary perfusion, and the influence of myocardial depressant factor may also contribute to poor cardiac performance (Fig 58–5). The fetus is more resistant to the effects of endotoxin than the mother; however, alterations in uteroplacental flow can lead to hypoxia, acidosis, placental abruption, intracranial hemorrhage, and fetal demise.

The clinical manifestations of septic shock depend on the target organs affected (Table 58–4). The most common cause of death in patients with this condition is respiratory insufficiency secondary to ARDS.

B. Laboratory Findings

Complete blood cell count, serum electrolytes, urinalysis, baseline arterial blood gases, chest radiograph, and a coagulation profile are laboratory studies important in the management of these patients. Hematologic findings may include significant anemia, thrombocytopenia, and leukocytosis. Serum electrolytes are often abnormal because of acidosis, fluid shifts, or decreased renal perfusion. Urinalysis permits evaluation of renal involvement. In addition to urine cultures, aerobic and anaerobic blood cultures may be helpful to confirm the diagnosis and guide antibiotic therapy.

Arterial blood gas measurements and a chest radiograph will facilitate clinical assessment of the ventilatory and oxygenation status. Early stages of septic shock

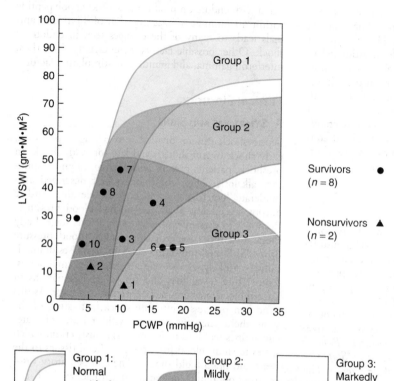

Figure 58–5. Presenting left ventricular function of 10 pregnant women with septic hypotension. LVSWI, left ventricular stroke work index; PCWP, pulmonary capillary wedge pressure. (Reproduced, with permission, from Lee W et al: Septic shock during pregnancy. Am J Obstet Gynecol 1988;159:410.)

Survivors ● (n = 8)

Nonsurvivors ▲ (n = 2)

Group 1: Normal ventricular function

Group 2: Mildly depressed ventricular function

Group 3: Markedly depressed ventricular function

Table 58–4. Effects on target organs in septic shock.[1]

Organ System	Clinical and Laboratory Findings
Brain	Confusion, obtundation
Hypothalamus	Hypothermia, hyperthermia
Cardiovascular	Myocardial depression, arrhythmias, tachycardia, hypotension
Pulmonary	Tachypnea, arteriovenous shunting, hypoxemia
Gastrointestinal	Vomiting, diarrhea
Hepatic	Increased AST (SGOT) and bilirubin
Kidneys	Oliguria, renal failure
Hematologic	Hemoconcentration, thrombocytopenia, leukocytosis, coagulopathy

[1]Adapted and reproduced, with permission, from American College of Obstetricians and Gynecologists: Septic shock. ACOG Technical Bulletin No. 75, March 1984.

will be associated with respiratory alkalosis, which later progresses to metabolic acidosis.

A baseline electrocardiogram (ECG) should be performed to rule out myocardial infarction or cardiac dysrhythmia. Abdominal radiographic studies may be useful to rule out other intrapelvic or intra-abdominal sources of obstetric sepsis (eg, bowel perforation, uterine perforation, tubo-ovarian abscess). Significant disseminated intravascular coagulation (DIC) will be identified by abnormal PT, PTT, or fibrinogen levels.

Differential Diagnosis

The differential diagnosis should include other hypovolemic and cardiogenic shock syndromes. Additional causes of acute cardiopulmonary compromise include amniotic fluid embolism, pulmonary thromboembolism, cardiac tamponade, aortic dissection, and diabetic ketoacidosis. The history, physical examination, and laboratory studies will usually be sufficient to distinguish between these diagnoses.

Complications

Numerous complications may occur with septic shock, depending on the target organs involved. Aside from ARDS, some of the more serious complications include congestive heart failure and cardiac dysrhythmias. Systemic hypotension and ischemic end-organ damage can lead to hepatic failure or renal insufficiency. Fetal or maternal demise are the most dire outcomes.

Treatment

Successful management of obstetric septic shock depends on early identification and aggressive treatment focused on stabilization of the patient, removal of underlying causes of sepsis, broad-spectrum antibiotic coverage, and treatment of associated complications. Febrile patients with mild hypotension who respond rapidly to volume infusion alone do not require invasive monitoring. In other cases, the pulmonary artery catheter should be used to guide specific therapeutic maneuvers for optimizing myocardial performance and maintaining systemic cardiac output and blood pressure. A hemodynamic approach for stabilizing pregnant

women with septic shock should include (1) volume repletion and hemostasis; (2) inotropic therapy with dopamine on the basis of left ventricular function curves; and (3) addition of peripheral vasoconstrictors (phenylephrine first, then norepinephrine) to maintain afterload (Fig 58–6).

A. GENERAL MEASURES

Septic shock during pregnancy should be treated with a broad-spectrum antibiotic regimen such as ampicillin, gentamicin, and clindamycin. Aminoglycoside maintenance doses should be titrated in relation to serum peak and trough levels or a 24-hour dosing regimen may be used. Newer antibiotics such as imipenem, cilastatin, vancomycin, and the extended spectrum penicillins (eg, ticarcillin) are also proving to be effective therapies. There must be a careful search for infected or necrotic foci that can result in persistent bacteremia, and surgical intervention may be necessary. In one study, 40% of septic obstetric patients required surgical removal of infected products of conception, and all survived. If chorioamnionitis is present in the septic obstetric patient, prompt delivery is necessary. However, if the pregnancy is not the cause of infection, immediate de-

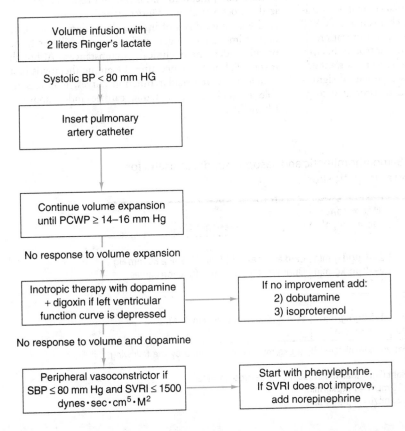

Figure 58–6. Hemodynamic algorithm for treatment of obstetric septic shock. SVRI, systemic vascular resistance index. (Reproduced, with permission, from Lee W et al: Septic shock during pregnancy. Am J Obstet Gynecol 1988;159:410.)

livery is usually not required. Supportive care should also include control of fever with antipyretics, hypothermic cooling blankets, or both. Correction of maternal acidosis, hypoxemia, and systemic hypotension will usually improve any abnormalities in the fetal heart tracing.

B. CARDIOVASCULAR SUPPORT

Aggressive treatment of obstetric septic shock must rapidly and effectively reverse organ hypoperfusion, improve oxygen delivery, and correct acidosis. Priority should be given to cardiopulmonary support with the additional understanding that other major organ systems can also be severely affected.

A sequential hemodynamic approach for stabilizing obstetric septic shock with volume repletion, inotropic therapy, and peripheral vasoconstrictors is recommended. Volume therapy initially begins with 1–2 L of lactated Ringer's solution infused over approximately 15 minutes. However, it is important that volume infusion not be withheld in a hypotensive patient pending placement of a pulmonary artery catheter. The total amount of crystalloid administered should be guided by the presence or absence of maternal hypoxemia secondary to pulmonary edema and left ventricular filling pressures, as estimated by PCWP.

In general, myocardial performance will be optimized according to the Starling mechanism at a PCWP of 14–16 mm Hg. Such preload optimization is mandatory prior to the initiation of inotropic therapy. Blood component therapy can also be an important adjunctive measure if the patient has experienced significant hemorrhage and has developed an associated coagulopathy.

If the shock state persists despite volume replacement and adequate hemostasis, efforts should be directed toward improving myocardial performance and vascular tone. Inotropic agents such as dopamine, dobutamine, or isoproterenol are excellent choices for improving myocardial contractility in an obstetric patient with a failing heart (Table 58–5). We recommend dopamine as the first-line drug of choice for treating septic hypotension when inotropic therapy is indicated. This substance is a chemical precursor of norepinephrine that has alpha-adrenergic, beta-adrenergic, and dopaminergic receptor stimulating actions. The dopamine infusion is initiated at 2–5 µg/kg/min and titrated against its effect on improving cardiac output and blood pressure in patients with obstetric septic shock. At low doses (0.5–5.0 µg/kg/min), this sympathomimetic amine acts primarily on the dopaminergic receptors, leading to vasodilation and improved perfusion of the renal and mesenteric vascular beds. Higher dopamine doses (5.0–15.0 µg/kg/min) are associated with predominant effects on the β receptors of the heart. The beta-adrenergic effects are responsible for improved myocardial contractility, stroke volume, and cardiac output. Much higher dopamine dosages (15–20 µg/kg/min) will elicit an alpha-adrenergic effect, similar to a norepinephrine infusion, and result in generalized vasoconstriction. Vasoconstrictive action associated with high doses of infused dopamine can actually be detrimental to organ perfusion and will rarely be useful under these clinical circumstances. Although myocardial performance after dopamine therapy is best evaluated by ventricular function curves, it is reasonable to maintain a systemic cardiac index above 3 $L/min/M^2$.

Table 58–5. Sympathomimetic and vasopressor drugs useful for therapy of obstetric spetic shock.

Agent	Maintenance Dose Range[1]	Therapeutic Goals
Inotropic		
Dopamine	2–10 µg/kg/min	Cardiac index ≥ 3 L/min/M² SBP ≥ 80 mm Hg
Dobutamine	2–10 µg/kg/min	Optimize left ventricular function curves
Isoproterenol	1–20 µg/min	
Vasopressors		
Phenylephrine	1–5 µg/kg/min	SVRI ≥ 1500 dynes · 5 · cm⁻⁵ · M²
Norepinephrine	1–4 µg/min	

[1]Drug dosages that are administered by µg/kg/min can be prepared by the following method:

1.5 mg × body weight (kg) = total mg in 250 mL 5% dextrose in water

10 mL/h = 1 µg/kg/min

20 mL/h = 2 µg/kg/min

If satisfactory ventricular function is not achieved with dopamine, a second inotropic agent such as dobutamine (2–20 µg/kg) should be added to the dopamine regimen. Dobutamine is a direct myocardial β_1 stimulant that increases cardiac output with only minimal tachycardia. Isoproterenol should be considered a third-line agent, which can be titrated at 1–20 µg/min. This drug acts primarily on beta-adrenergic receptors to increase contractility and heart rate. However, potential side effects may include ventricular ectopy, excessive tachycardia, and undesired vasodilatation. Digoxin is commonly added to the previously described regimen to improve the force and velocity of myocardial contraction. This agent is given in a loading dose of 0.5 mg IV, followed by 0.25 mg every 4 hours for a total dose of 1.0 mg. Intravenous digoxin should be given under continuous ECG monitoring with special attention to serum potassium levels. The usual maintenance dosage during pregnancy is 0.25–0.37 mg/dL depending on plasma drug levels.

A peripheral vasoconstrictor may be initiated if there is a reduced systemic vascular resistance index (SVRI; less than 1500 dynes $\cdot$ s $\cdot$ cm^{-5}) accompanied by a systolic blood pressure of less than 80 mm Hg despite inotropic therapy. It should be emphasized that maintenance of afterload appears to be a major hemodynamic determinant associated with maternal survival. Because of its pure alpha-adrenergic activity (which increases SVR), phenylephrine (1–5 µg/kg/min) is the initial drug of choice. Norepinephrine is only indicated for septic shock patients with decreased afterload who do not respond to volume loading, inotropic therapy, and phenylephrine. This drug is a mixed adrenergic agonist with a primary effect on the alpha receptors, which leads to generalized vasoconstriction and increased SVR. Although the therapy of septic shock should focus primarily on stabilization of maternal factors, vasopressor agents should be administered cautiously during pregnancy since they have been reported to decrease uterine blood flow in animals with experimentally-induced spinal hypotension.

Some investigators have advocated large doses of corticosteroids for the acute management of septic shock, but human clinical trials have failed to demonstrate any conclusive benefit.

Newer investigational agents include corticosteroids and antiendotoxin therapy. Multicenter trials of endotoxin antibodies have suggested a possible improvement in mortality rate and organ failure in some subgroups of nonpregnant septic patients.

Prognosis

Despite all medical and surgical therapeutic options, the overall maternal mortality rate in septic shock is approximately 50%. The prognosis is worsened by the presence of ARDS or preexisting medical problems.

AMNIOTIC FLUID EMBOLISM

 ### ESSENTIALS OF DIAGNOSIS

- Sudden, unexplained peripartum respiratory distress, cardiovascular collapse, and coagulopathy.
- Bleeding secondary to coagulopathy or uterine atony (common).
- Amniotic fluid debris in right side of the heart on autopsy.

General Considerations

Amniotic fluid embolism is a rare but potentially devastating complication of pregnancy that often results in poor obstetric outcome. Most of the information about amniotic fluid embolism has been derived from clinical reports, because the rarity of the disorder does not allow for clinical trials, and no suitable animal model exists. The first major review of the literature regarding this condition was by Morgan in 1979. This evaluated 272 cases. Since that time, a national registry was initiated by Clark. The incidence of amniotic fluid embolism is difficult to estimate, and may be anywhere from 1:8000 to 1:30,000.

Pathophysiology

The basic mechanism of disease is related to the effects of amniotic fluid on the respiratory, cardiovascular, and coagulation systems. One of the classic theories hypothesized that the following 3 primary acute events occur: (1) pulmonary vascular obstruction, leading to sudden decreases in left ventricular filling pressures and cardiac output; (2) pulmonary hypertension with acute cor pulmonale; and (3) ventilation-perfusion inequality of lung tissue, leading to arterial hypoxemia and its metabolic consequences.

Only a small volume of amniotic fluid (1–2 mL) is transferred to the maternal circulation during normal labor. Thus, enhanced communication between the amniotic fluid sac and the maternal venous system is necessary for amniotic fluid embolism to occur. Sites of entry may include endocervical veins lacerated during normal labor, a disrupted placental implantation site, and traumatized uterine veins. Squamous cells and trophoblastic tissue are often found in the maternal pulmonary vasculature of patients who underwent pulmonary artery catheterization. However, one must see more specific material like mucin, fetal debris, vernix, lanugo, and squamous cells coated with white blood cells and granular debris to confirm the diagnosis. If meconium is present, a more dramatic response is seen. Fetal demise has also been shown to worsen this condition. Once amniotic debris enters the venous system, it travels rapidly to the cardiopulmonary circulation, leading to shock and arterial hypoxemia. Myocardial dysfunction may result from ischemic injury or right ventricular dilatation. Some experimental evidence suggests that amniotic fluid may have a direct myocardial depressant effect. Endothelin, a vasoconstrictive peptide found in vascular endothelial cells, has been implicated. Other factors that may play a role include proteolytic enzymes, histamine, prostaglandins, complement, and biogenic amines (eg, serotonin). These mediators are seen in other shock states like sepsis and anaphylaxis, leading Clark to suggest that amniotic fluid embolism be termed "anaphylactoid syndrome of pregnancy." The effects of systemic hypotension and hypoxemia may lead to cardiopulmonary collapse, renal insufficiency, hepatic failure, seizures, and coma.

Amniotic fluid embolism is almost always associated with some form of DIC. The etiology of coagulopathy associated with amniotic fluid embolism is incompletely understood, but it is known that amniotic fluid has potent total thromboplastin and antifibrinolytic activity, both of which increase with advancing gestational age. Once clotting is triggered in the pulmonary vasculature, local thrombin generation can cause vasoconstriction and microvascular thrombosis.

Limited hemodynamic observations with pulmonary artery catheterization suggest that in humans with amniotic fluid embolism, left ventricular dysfunction is the only significant hemodynamic alteration that is consistently documented. The response to amniotic fluid embolus in humans may be biphasic, initially resulting in intense vasospasm, severe pulmonary hypertension, and hypoxia. The transient period of right heart failure with hypoxia is later followed by a secondary phase of left heart failure, as reflected by elevated pulmonary artery pressure with subsequent return of right heart function. This biphasic theory may account for the extremely high maternal mortality rate within the first hour (25–34%) and explains why pulmonary hypertension can be difficult to document in patients with this disorder.

Clinical Findings

A. SYMPTOMS AND SIGNS

In his classic review of 272 patients with amniotic fluid embolus, Morgan characterized the main presenting clinical features: 51% presented with respiratory distress and cyanosis, 27% with hypotension, and only 10% with seizures. The Clark national registry noted 30% of patients presented with seizures or seizure-like activity, 27% with dyspnea, 17% with fetal bradycardia, and 13% with hypotension. Between 37% and 54% of patients exhibited an associated bleeding diathesis. Risk factors identified in the Morgan study included multiparity, tumultuous labor, or tetanic uterine contractions. Other studies have noted risk factors including advanced maternal age, use of uterine stimulants, cesarean section, uterine rupture, high cervical lacerations, premature separation of the placenta, and intrauterine fetal demise. Clark, however, was unable to identify any notable risk factors. Other presenting signs that have been described include tachypnea, peripheral cyanosis, bronchospasm, and chest pain.

B. LABORATORY FINDINGS

Arterial blood oxygen tension typically indicates severe maternal hypoxemia. This hypoxemia may result from ventilation-perfusion inequality with atelectasis and associated pulmonary edema. The diagnosis of significant coagulopathy is manifested by the presence of microangiopathic hemolysis, hypofibrinogenemia, prolonged clotting times, prolonged bleeding time, and elevated fibrin split products. The chest radiograph is nonspecific, although pulmonary edema is often noted. The ECG typically reveals unexplained tachycardia, nonspecific ST- and T-wave changes, and a right ventricular strain pattern. Lung scans occasionally identify perfusion defects resulting from amniotic fluid embolism even though chest radiographic findings are normal.

Differential Diagnosis

Many conditions may mimic the effects of amniotic fluid embolism on the respiratory, cardiovascular, and coagulation systems. Pulmonary thromboembolism can result in severe hypoxemia with pulmonary edema. In contrast to amniotic fluid embolism, chest pain is a relatively common finding. Congestive heart failure due to fluid overload or preexisting heart disease may mimic the cardiorespiratory compromise observed during amniotic fluid embolism. Hypotension may result from several disorders, including septic chorioamnionitis or postpartum hemorrhage. Pulmonary aspiration (Mendelson's syndrome) is associated with tachycardia, shock, respiratory distress, and production of a frothy pink sputum, but is usually also associated with bronchospasm and wheezing. Other conditions in the differential diagnosis include air embolism, myocardial infarction, anaphylaxis, placental abruption, eclampsia, uterine rupture, transfusion reaction, and local anesthesia toxicity.

Treatment

Amniotic fluid embolism remains one of the most devastating and unpreventable conditions complicating pregnancy. Therapeutic measures are supportive and should be directed toward minimizing hypoxemia with supplemental oxygen, maintaining blood pressure, and managing associated coagulopathies. Patients with poor oxygenation often require intubation and positive end-expiratory pressure. Adequate oxygenation will minimize related cerebral and myocardial ischemia and acidosis-induced pulmonary artery vasospasm. Pulmonary artery catheterization should be considered in the absence of coagulopathy to guide inotropic therapy with dopamine. If invasive hemodynamic monitoring is not available, rapid digitalization should be considered. Finally, the development of consumptive coagulopathy may require replacement of depleted hemostatic components in cases with significant uncontrollable bleeding or abnormal clotting parameters.

Prognosis

Maternal mortality rates range from 60–80%; however, a recent study quoted a 26.4% mortality rate. Of those patients who do not survive, 25% die within the first hour, and 80% within the first 9 hours. Correspondingly high perinatal morbidity and mortality rates would be expected.

PULMONARY THROMBOEMBOLISM

ESSENTIALS OF DIAGNOSIS

- *Unexplained chest pain and dyspnea (most frequent presenting symptoms).*
- *History of pulmonary embolism, deep venous thrombosis, prolonged immobilization, or recent surgery.*
- *Physical examination: usually nonspecific, depending on extent of cardiopulmonary involvement, but may include tachycardia, wheezing, pleural friction rub, and pulmonary rales.*
- *Laboratory evaluation: decreased arterial blood oxygen tension to less than 90 mm Hg in the sitting position.*
- *Diagnostic studies: pulmonary radionuclide ventilation-perfusion scanning, spiral CT, and angiography.*

General Considerations

Pulmonary thromboembolism is a rare complication of pregnancy (0.09%) but is a significant cause of maternal morbidity and mortality. Mortality has been documented as 12.8% if untreated, and 0.7% if therapy is instituted. The diagnosis of deep venous thrombosis (DVT) occurs in the antepartum period approximately half the time, and is evenly distributed throughout each trimester. Pulmonary embolism has a higher incidence in the postpartum period. Predisposing factors commonly include advanced maternal age, obesity, traumatic delivery, abdominal delivery, thrombophlebitis, and endometritis. Patients with underlying thrombophilias or previous thrombotic events are at greater risk for this condition.

Pathophysiology

More than 100 years ago, Virchow postulated that the basic mechanism of thrombus formation is related to a combination of vessel injury, vascular stasis, and alterations in blood coagulability. Venous thrombi consist of fibrin deposits and red blood cells with varying amounts of platelet and white blood cell components. In most cases, lower extremity and pelvic thrombi are responsible for the pathologic sequelae.

Ordinarily, the vascular endothelium does not react with either platelets or the blood coagulation system unless it is disrupted by vessel injury. Such injury exposes subendothelial cells to blood elements responsible for activation of the extrinsic coagulation cascade. Disruption of the vascular endothelium may occur during traumatic vaginal delivery or cesarean section.

Pregnancy is also associated with venous stasis, especially in the lower extremities, because the enlarging uterus reduces blood return to the inferior vena cava by direct mechanical effects. Hormonal factors may contribute to venodilatation and stasis during pregnancy. Stasis prevents the hepatic clearance of activated coagulation factors and minimizes mixing of these factors with their serum inhibitors. In this manner, venous stasis becomes another predisposing factor for the formation of thrombi. Stasis secondary to prolonged bedrest for medical or obstetric complications will predispose a pregnant woman to increased venous stasis and formation of vascular thrombi. The period of greatest risk for thrombosis and embolism appears to be the immediate postpartum, especially after cesarean delivery.

The maternal circulation becomes hypercoagulable from alterations in the coagulation and fibrinolytic systems. Serum concentrations of most coagulation proteins, such as fibrinogen and factors II, VII, VIII, IX, and X, increase during pregnancy. These changes are also associated with decreased fibrinolytic activity, which is responsible for the conversion of plasminogen to the active proteolytic enzyme plasmin.

Women with congenital or acquired thrombophilias are at increased risk for thrombosis; in fact, up to half of women who have these events in pregnancy may have an underlying disorder. The most commonly recognized thrombophilia in the Caucasian population is factor V Leiden mutation (5%). Other less common but significant disorders include: prothrombin gene mutation G20210A (2–4%), antithrombin III deficiency (0.02–0.2%), protein C deficiency (0.2–0.5%), protein S deficiency (0.08%), and hyperhomocysteinemia (1%). The antiphospholipid antibody syndrome also significantly increases maternal risk.

Once a venous thrombus is formed, it may dislodge from its peripheral vascular origin and enter the central maternal circulation. Propagation of the original venous clot or recurrent pulmonary emboli are possible. DVTs limited to the calf rarely embolize, but approximately 20% extend to the proximal lower extremity.

Clinical Findings

A. Symptoms and Signs

The subsequent cardiopulmonary effects of pulmonary embolus will depend on the location and size of thrombi in the lung. A patient with a large embolus affecting the central pulmonary circulation may present with acute syncope, respiratory embarrassment, and shock. Smaller emboli may not have significant clinical sequelae.

No single symptom or combination of symptoms is specific for the diagnosis of pulmonary embolus. Classic triads (hemoptysis, chest pain, and dyspnea; or dyspnea, chest pain, and apprehension) are rarely seen (Table 58–6). Chest pain and dyspnea were the most common symptoms in patients with angiographically documented pulmonary emboli (over 80%). Physical findings include tachycardia, tachypnea (rate > 16/min), pulmonary rales, wheezing, and pleural friction rub.

B. Laboratory Findings

There are no specific routine laboratory findings associated with the diagnosis of pulmonary embolus, although arterial blood gas measurements will often reveal significant hypoxemia. In the upright position, almost all healthy young pregnant women will have an arterial blood oxygen tension greater than 90 mm Hg. An alveolar-atrial (A-a) gradient of greater than 20 is suspicious for pulmonary embolus. The ECG may reveal unexplained tachycardia associated with cor pulmonale (right axis deviation, S wave in lead I, Q wave plus T wave inversion in lead III). A chest roentgenogram may be normal or may show infiltrates, atelecta-

Table 58–6. Symptoms and signs in 327 patients with pulmonary embolus confirmed by angiography.[1]

Symptom or Sign	Frequency (%)
Chest pain	88
Pleuritic	74
Nonpleuritic	14
Dyspnea	84
Apprehension	59
Cough	53
Hemoptysis	30
Sweating	27
Syncope	13
Respiration more than 16/min	92
Pulmonary rales	58
Pulse more than 100/min	44
Fever (> 37.8 °C [99.7 °F])	43
Phlebitis	32
Heart gallop	34
Diaphoresis	36
Edema	24
Heart murmur	23
Cyanosis	19

[1]Adapted and reproduced, with permission, from Bell WR, Simon TL, DeMets DL: The clinical features of submassive and massive pulmonary emboli. *Am J Med* 1977;62:355.

sis, or effusions. Thirty percent of patients with a pulmonary embolus will have a normal chest x-ray.

It is generally accepted that a normal radionuclide perfusion study can effectively rule out pulmonary embolus. Perfusion studies are occasionally equivocal, and ventilation scanning may be required to clarify the diagnosis. Ventilation scanning will improve the specificity of the perfusion study, since this will rule out airway disorders that may be responsible for reduced pulmonary perfusion. The radiation exposure is minimal (< 0.1 rad). Unfortunately, a V/Q scan can only confirm a diagnosis if it is normal or indicates high probability of embolus. Therefore, 40–60% of patients will require further testing.

Spiral computed tomography is a newer form of imaging that has a sensitivity and specificity of 94% in the nonpregnant patient. Spiral CT may also be helpful in detecting other abnormalities causing pulmonary symptoms (eg, pleural effusions, consolidation, emphysema, pulmonary masses). However, this study may miss emboli below the segmental level. Magnetic resonance imaging has limited value in pregnancy because it has not been well studied.

If the above studies are equivocal, pulmonary angiography should be considered. Subsequent exposure of the fetus to the relatively low levels of ionizing radiation from angiography can be minimized with appropriate pelvic shielding and selective angiography on the basis of prior radionuclide scanning.

Noninvasive Doppler should be considered as an initial diagnostic test for suspected DVT involving the lower extremities. Compression ultrasound uses firm compression with the transducer probe to detect intraluminal filling defects. Imaging is most useful for the distal iliac, femoral, and popliteal veins. Doppler is also useful for the proximal iliac veins. Sensitivity is 95%, with a 96% specificity. Impedance plethysmography measures impedance flow with pneumatic cuff inflation. Sensitivity and specificity are 83% and 92%, respectively. Compression of the inferior vena cava by the gravid second- or third-trimester uterus may cause false-positive results.

If the above noninvasive tests are inconclusive, it may be helpful to confirm the extent of the original thrombotic event by venography with pelvic shielding. The soleal calf sinuses and the valves involving the popliteal and femoral veins are the sources of most deep venous thrombi. Venography is associated with induced phlebitis in approximately 3–5% of procedures performed. Radiofibrinogen methods to detect thrombus formation will result in placental transfer of radioactive iodine and are contraindicated in pregnant or nursing women.

Differential Diagnosis

Any condition potentially related to cardiopulmonary compromise during pregnancy should be included in the differential diagnosis. This includes amniotic fluid and air emboli, spontaneous pneumothorax, septic shock, and preexisting heart disease.

Treatment

A. PREVENTIVE TREATMENT

Once predisposing risk factors to pulmonary embolus are identified, it is important to minimize the possibility of further complications. In patients at higher risk for DVT, prophylactic measures should be directed toward preventing venous stasis that leads to clot formation. Mechanical maneuvers such as raising the lower extremities 15 degrees above the horizontal, keeping the legs straight rather than bent at the knees when sitting, or performing calf flexion exercises may be useful, as may external pneumatic compression. One method used to prevent perioperative thrombophlebitis includes minidose heparin prophylaxis, 5000 U subcutaneously 2 hours before surgery and every 12 hours until routine ambulation is achieved. Minidose heparin prophylaxis significantly decreases not only the incidence

of DVT but also the incidence of fatal pulmonary emboli. Subcutaneous minidose heparin may be reinstituted approximately 6 hours after delivery. Postpartum or postoperative ambulation is important in minimizing thromboembolic complications during this high-risk period. Some women may require therapeutic anticoagulation during pregnancy to prevent a thromboembolic event. Included in this category are women with artificial heart valves, antithrombin III deficiency, antiphospholipid antibody syndrome, history of rheumatic heart disease and atrial fibrillation, homozygosity for factor V Leiden or prothrombin gene mutation, and recurrent thromboembolic disease. Therapeutic anticoagulation can be achieved by using subcutaneous heparin 2–3 times a day, adjusting for a partial thromboplastin time (PTT) of 2.0–3.0 times normal. Low molecular weight heparin (LMWH) can also be used. LMWH does not cross the placenta, and it has been shown to be relatively safe in pregnancy. In addition, complications of heparin therapy (osteoporosis, thrombocytopenia) are not seen with this medication, and dosing in pregnancy usually does not require many adjustments. The PTT does not need to be followed; instead, peak antifactor Xa levels can be checked every 4–6 weeks. It is controversial whether other disorders, like protein C or S deficiency, or a family history of thrombophilias, require anticoagulation therapy. These patients may benefit from minidose heparin prophylaxis.

B. TREATMENT OF DOCUMENTED PULMONARY EMBOLISM

Once pulmonary embolism is documented, therapeutic intervention should be directed to correction of arterial hypoxemia and any associated hypotension. Other measures should prevent clot propagation or recurrent emboli. Supplemental oxygen should be given to achieve an arterial oxygen tension of at least 70 mm Hg. A loading dose of 5000–10,000 U of heparin should be given intravenously by continuous infusion, followed by a maintenance dose of approximately 1000 U/h. The PTT should be maintained at 1.5–2.5 times control values. Other investigators recommend the use of heparin levels for monitoring anticoagulation therapy. Heparin levels may be measured on the third or fourth day and should be about 0.2 µg/mL, not to exceed 0.4 µg/mL. Leg elevation, bedrest, and local heat will be beneficial to patients who have associated DVT. Intravenous morphine may be helpful in alleviating anxiety and ameliorating chest pain.

Intrapartum care of pulmonary embolus is complicated, and individual treatment approaches may vary. Selected patients with recent pulmonary thromboembolism, ileofemoral DVT, or heart valve prosthesis should probably continue full anticoagulation with high-dose heparin during labor or surgical procedures. Under these circumstances, the risk for potential bleeding complications from anticoagulant needs to be balanced against the risk of thromboembolism. Although there is a higher incidence of wound hematomas associated with peripartum anticoagulation, there is no clear evidence that this regimen is associated with excessive postpartum hemorrhage after normal vaginal delivery.

Postpartum patients receiving heparin may be switched over to warfarin once oral intake is tolerated. Heparin should be continued for the first 5–7 days of warfarin therapy. By the time heparin is discontinued, the international normalized ratio (INR) should be 2.0–3.0 times the normal value. Alternatively, it may be desirable to continue moderate doses of subcutaneous heparin (10,000 U twice daily), especially in nursing mothers. Postpartum anticoagulation should be continued for at least 3 months if the patient developed pulmonary embolus in the third trimester.

C. COMPLICATIONS OF TREATMENT

The major complication of anticoagulant therapy is maternal or fetal hemorrhage. Heparin does not cross the placenta due to its large molecular weight, but it has been associated with maternal thrombocytopenia and osteoporosis. These effects can be avoided with low molecular weight heparin. Warfarin is known to cross the placental barrier, and its use in the first trimester has been associated with embryopathy (nasal hypoplasia and stippled epiphyses). Fetal nervous system abnormalities (eg, hydrocephalus) have also been noted with the use of warfarin during pregnancy.

A small percentage of patients will experience recurrent pulmonary emboli despite full anticoagulation. These patients may be candidates for vena caval ligation by a transabdominal approach under general or regional anesthesia. If the pelvis is suspected as the source of embolus, the right ovarian vein should also be ligated. It has been estimated that approximately 95% of patients with pulmonary embolism massive enough to cause hypotension eventually die. In this context, pulmonary artery embolectomy may be life-saving.

Placement of a vena caval umbrella via the internal jugular vein is an option for unstable patients with recurrent emboli who would not be prime surgical candidates. Although abdominal radiography is required for this procedure, placement of the umbrella filter does not require general anesthesia. This strategy will prevent larger emboli from reaching the pulmonary circulation.

Prognosis

Pulmonary embolus, with a mortality rate of 12–15% if left untreated, will develop in approximately one-fourth of untreated patients with antenatal DVT. In a review of pregnancies complicated by DVT treated with anticoagulant therapy, the incidence of pulmonary embolus was 4.5% of patients, with a maternal mortality rate of less than 1%.

DISSEMINATED INTRAVASCULAR COAGULATION (DIC)

ESSENTIALS OF DIAGNOSIS

- *History of recent bleeding diathesis, especially concurrent with placental abruption, amniotic fluid embolism, fetal demise, sepsis, preeclampsia-eclampsia, or saline abortion.*

- *Clinical evidence of multiple bleeding points associated with purpura and petechiae on physical examination.*

- *Laboratory findings classically include thrombocytopenia, hypofibrinogenemia, and elevated PT, elevated D-dimer, and fibrin split products.*

General Considerations

Disseminated intravascular coagulation (DIC) is a pathologic condition associated with inappropriate activation of coagulation and fibrinolytic systems. It should be considered a secondary phenomenon resulting from an underlying disease state. The most common obstetric conditions associated with DIC are intrauterine fetal death, amniotic fluid embolism, preeclampsia-eclampsia, HELLP syndrome (hemolysis, elevated liver enzymes, and low platelet count), placenta previa, and placental abruption. Saline-induced abortion is also a cause.

Pathophysiology

The most widely accepted theory of blood coagulation entails a "cascade theory" (Fig 58–7). Basically, the coagulation system is divided into intrinsic and extrinsic systems. The intrinsic system contains all the intravascular components required to activate thrombin by sequential activation of factors XII, XI, IX, X, V, and II (prothrombin). The extrinsic system is initially activated by tissue thromboplastin, leading to sequential activation of factors VII, X, V, and prothrombin. Both the intrinsic and extrinsic pathways converge to activate factor X, which subsequently reacts with activated fac-

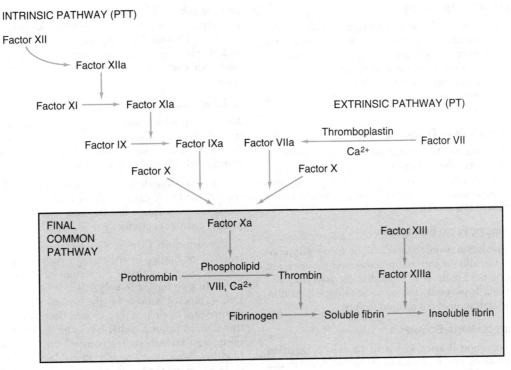

Figure 58–7. Coagulation cascade mechanism.

tor V in the presence of calcium and phospholipid to convert prothrombin to thrombin.

Thrombin is a proteolytic enzyme responsible for splitting fibrinogen chains into fibrinopeptides, leading to the formation of fibrin monomer. This central enzyme is capable of activating factor XIII to stabilize the newly formed fibrin clot and will enhance the activity of factors V and VIII.

Activation of the coagulation system also stimulates the conversion of plasminogen to plasmin as a protective mechanism against intravascular thrombosis. Plasmin is an enzyme that inactivates factors V and VIII and is capable of lysing fibrin and fibrinogen to form degradation products. Thus, the normal physiologic hemostatic mechanism represents a delicate and complex balance between the coagulation and fibrinolytic systems.

Pregnancy is considered to represent a hypercoagulable state. With the exception of factors XI and XIII, there is an overall increase in the activity of coagulation factors. Fibrinogen rises as early as 12 weeks' gestation and reaches a peak level of 400–650 mg/dL in late pregnancy. The fibrinolytic system is depressed during pregnancy and labor but returns to normal levels within 1 hour of placental delivery. The early puerperium is accompanied by a secondary rise in fibrinogen, factors VIII, IX, X, and antithrombin III; a return to nonpregnant levels occurs by 3–4 weeks postpartum.

The complex pathophysiology of DIC is characterized by (1) procoagulant system activation; (2) fibrinolytic system activation; (3) inhibitor consumption; (4) cytokine release; (5) cellular activation; and (6) resultant end-organ damage. DIC occurs as a secondary event in a wide variety of illnesses associated with excess production of circulating thrombin. The pathophysiologic factors responsible for inappropriate activation of the clotting mechanism include endothelial cell injury, liberation of thromboplastin from injured tissue, and release of phospholipid from red cell or platelet injury. All these mechanisms may contribute to development of a bleeding diathesis resulting from increased thrombin activity. Additionally, widespread DIC will cause increased platelet aggregation, consumption of coagulation factors, secondary activation of the fibrinolytic system, and deposition of fibrin into multiple organ sites, which can result in ischemic tissue damage. The associated thrombocytopenia and presence of fibrin split products will impair hemostasis.

Specific obstetric conditions associated with DIC include the following.

A. Placental Abruption

DIC may occur in placental abruption involving liberation of tissue thromboplastin or possible intrauterine consumption of fibrinogen and coagulation factors during the formation of retroplacental clot. This leads to activation of the extrinsic coagulation mechanism. Placental abruption is one of the most common obstetric causes of DIC.

B. Retained Dead Fetus Syndrome

Another cause of DIC is retained dead fetus syndrome involving liberation of tissue thromboplastin from nonviable tissue. This cause is less common in recent years due to advanced ultrasound technology and the earlier detection of this condition.

C. Amniotic Fluid Embolism

This involves not only the release of tissue thromboplastin but also the intrinsic procoagulant properties of amniotic fluid itself. It is likely that the associated hypotension, hypoxemia, and tissue acidosis will encourage the activation of coagulation factors.

D. Preeclampsia-Eclampsia

This condition is associated with chronic coagulation abnormalities that may lead to thrombocytopenia and elevation of fibrin degradation products. It is uncertain whether endothelial damage activates procoagulant proteins and platelets or the reverse, although the former is more likely. Eclampsia is associated with DIC 11% of the time; with HELLP syndrome this increases to 15%. Preeclampsia together with placental abruption also significantly increases this association.

E. Saline or Septic Abortion

Saline-induced abortion has been associated with subclinical DIC. Severe cases of DIC have occurred in 1:400–1:1000 cases. Disease may be related to the release of tissue thromboplastin from the placenta. Septic abortion may also cause release of tissue thromboplastin or release of bacterial endotoxin (phospholipids).

F. Other

Other triggers of DIC include septicemia, viremias (eg, HIV, varicella, CMV, hepatitis), drugs, and acidosis.

Clinical Findings

A. Symptoms and Signs

Acute clinical manifestations of DIC are variable and include generalized bleeding, localized hemorrhage, purpura, petechiae, and thromboembolic phenomena. Also, fever, hypotension, proteinuria, hypoxia, hemorrhagic bullae, acral cyanosis, and frank gangrene have been described. Widespread fibrin deposits may affect any organ system, including the lungs, kidneys, brain, and liver. Chronic DIC (eg, fetal demise) is associated with slower production of thrombin and may be associated with minimal or absent clinical signs and symptoms.

B. Laboratory Findings

Although histologic diagnosis of fibrin deposits is the only definitive manner by which DIC may be confirmed, there are a host of indirect tests suitable for the clinical evaluation of coagulopathy.

1. Platelets—Platelets are decreased ($< 100,000/\mu L$) in more than 90% of cases. In the absence of other causes, spontaneous purpura usually does not occur when platelet counts are greater than $30,000/\mu L$.

2. Prothrombin time (PT)—PT measures the time required for clotting by the extrinsic pathway and is dependent on the ultimate conversion of fibrinogen to fibrin. It is prolonged in only 50–75% of patients with DIC. The explanations for the normal PTs are, first, the presence of circulating activated clotting factors like thrombin or factor Xa, that accelerate the formation of fibrin; and second, the presence of early degradation products, which are rapidly clottable by thrombin; these may cause the test to register a normal or fast PT.

3. Partial thromboplastin time (PTT)—PTT is frequently normal in DIC (40–50% of the time) and is not as helpful for establishing the diagnosis. This test measures the function of the intrinsic and final common pathways of the coagulation cascade.

4. Thrombin time (TT)—TT is elevated in 80% of patients with DIC. It is affected only by the amount of circulating fibrinogen or the presence of thrombin inhibitors such as fibrin degradation products and heparin. This test specifically measures the time necessary for conversion of fibrinogen to fibrin.

5. Fibrinogen—Fibrinogen is often decreased, with approximately 70% of patients with DIC having a serum level less than 150 mg/dL. The normal physiologic increase of serum fibrinogen levels during pregnancy may mask a pathologic decrease in this parameter.

6. Fibrin split products—Values greater than 40 $\mu g/mL$ are suggestive of DIC. These are elevated in 85–100% of patients with DIC. These degradation products are diagnostic of the plasmin biodegradation of fibrinogen or fibrin, so indicate only the presence of plasmin.

7. Clotting time and clot retraction—Observation of clotting time and ability of the clot to retract can be performed by using 2 mL of blood in a 5-mL glass test

tube. These are relatively simple bedside tests that can provide qualitative evidence of hypofibrinogenemia. When the clot forms, it is usually soft but not reduced in volume (adding celite will hasten this reaction). Over the next half hour, the clot should retract, with the volume of serum exceeding that of the formed clot. If this phenomenon does not occur, low serum fibrinogen levels can be suspected.

8. Peripheral blood smear—A peripheral blood smear reveals schistocytes in approximately 40% of patients with DIC.

9. Bleeding time—The time required for hemostasis after skin puncture will become progressively prolonged as the platelet count falls below 100,000/μL. Spontaneous continuous bleeding from puncture sites may develop if the platelet count falls below 30,000/μL.

10. Newer tests—Several of these laboratory findings are more reliable than the classic studies.

a. D-dimer—This is a neoantigen formed as a result of plasmin digestion of cross-linked fibrin when thrombin initiates the transition of fibrinogen to fibrin, and activates factor XIII to cross-link the fibrin formed. The test is specific for fibrin (not fibrinogen) degradation products, and is abnormal in 90% of cases.

b. Antithrombin III level—This is abnormal in 89% of cases.

c. Fibrinopeptide A—This is abnormal 75% of the time.

Differential Diagnosis

Most acute episodes of generalized bleeding in obstetric patients will be related to pregnancy, but other rare causes of congenital or acquired coagulopathies need to be considered. These include idiopathic thrombocytopenic purpura, hemophilia, and von Willebrand's disease. Placental abruption is often associated with uterine tenderness, fetal bradycardia, and uterine bleeding. DIC associated with fetal demise usually does not become apparent until at least 5 weeks after the absence of heart tones has been documented. Amniotic fluid embolus is typically associated with acute onset of respiratory distress and shock. Preeclampsia is characterized by hypertension and proteinuria, which may lead to eclamptic seizures.

Complications

In addition to the potential complications of uncontrolled hemorrhage previously discussed, widespread fibrin deposition may affect any major organ system. This may include the liver (hepatic failure), kidneys (tubular necrosis), and lungs (hypoxemia).

Treatment

Although individual measures will be dictated by the specific obstetric condition, the primary, most important treatment of pregnancy-related DIC is correction of the underlying cause. In most cases, prompt termination of the pregnancy is required. Moderate or low-grade DIC may not be associated with clinical evidence of excessive bleeding and often will require close observation but no further therapy.

Supportive therapy should be directed to the correction of shock, acidosis, and tissue ischemia. Cardiopulmonary support, including inotropic therapy, blood replacement, and assisted ventilation, should be implemented with the patient in close proximity to a delivery suite. Fetal monitoring, careful recording of maternal fluid balance, and serial evaluation of coagulation parameters are extremely important. If sepsis is suspected, antibiotics should be employed. Central monitoring with a pulmonary artery catheter is relatively contraindicated due to potential bleeding complications. Vaginal delivery, without episiotomy if possible, is preferable to cesarean section. Failure of improvement in the coagulopathy within several hours after delivery suggests sepsis, liver disease, retained products of conception, or a congenital coagulation defect.

Blood component therapy should be initiated on the basis of transfusion guidelines reported by the National Institutes of Health. Criteria for red cell transfusions were discussed earlier (see Hypovolemic Shock). Fresh-frozen plasma has only limited and specific indications, which include massive hemorrhage, isolated factor deficiencies, reversal of warfarin, antithrombin II deficiency, immunodeficiencies, and thrombocytopenic purpura. Although most cases of severe obstetric hemorrhage will lead to laboratory evidence of coagulation abnormalities, transfusion of fresh-frozen plasma may not always benefit these patients; the amount transfused is usually insufficient for replacing coagulation factors lost by dilution or clot formation. Even with massive obstetric hemorrhage, most procoagulant levels are above 30% of normal values, which is sufficient for maintaining clinical hemostasis in most patients. Specific replacement of fibrinogen should be accomplished by cryoprecipitate. Each unit of cryoprecipitate carries approximately 250 mg of fibrinogen. Platelets should only be administered in the face of active bleeding with a platelet count < 50,000/μL or prophylactically with platelet count 20–30,000/μL or less or following massive transfusion (> 2 times blood volume). Platelets should be transfused on the basis of 1 U/10 kg body weight to raise the cell count above 50,000/μL. However, it should be noted that clotting factors containing fibrinogen may be associated with enhanced hemorrhage and also with thrombosis when given to patients with DIC. For this reason, they should be administered with extreme caution. Obstetricians should remember that Rh immune globulin should be given to Rh-negative recipients of platelets from Rh-positive donors.

Subcutaneous low-dose heparin or low molecular weight heparin may be effective in treating the intravascular clotting process of DIC. Heparin acts as an anticoagulant by activating antithrombin III but has little effect on activated coagulation factors. Anticoagulation is contraindicated in patients with fulminant DIC and central nervous system insults, fulminant liver failure, or obstetric accidents. The one instance, however, in which heparin has been demonstrated to benefit pregnancy-related DIC is in the case of the retained dead fetus with an intact vascular system, where heparin may be administered to interrupt the coagulation process and thrombocytopenia for several days until safe delivery may be implemented.

Prognosis

Most cases of obstetric DIC will improve with delivery of the fetus or evacuation of the uterus. The maternal and fetal prognosis will be more closely related to the associated obstetric condition than to the coagulopathy.

ACUTE RESPIRATORY DISTRESS SYNDROME (ARDS)

 ## ESSENTIALS OF DIAGNOSIS

- *History of gastric aspiration, infection/sepsis, preeclampsia-eclampsia, seizures, hemorrhage, coagulopathy, or amniotic fluid embolism.*
- *Progressive respiratory distress with decreased lung compliance.*
- *Severe hypoxemia refractory to oxygen therapy.*
- *Diffuse infiltrates on chest roentgenogram.*
- *Normal PCWP, with absence of radiographic evidence of congestive heart failure.*

General Considerations

Acute respiratory distress syndrome (ARDS) is a severe form of lung disease with acute onset, characterized by bilateral infiltrates on chest X-ray, no evidence of intravascular volume overload (PCWP no greater than 18 mm Hg), and severely impaired oxygenation, demonstrated by a ratio of arterial oxygen tension (PaO_2) to

the fraction of inspired oxygen (FIO_2) of less than 200 mm Hg. ARDS appears to occur more commonly in obstetric patients than in the general population. Its incidence in the nonpregnant population is 1.5 per 100,000, but it has been estimated to occur in between 1:3000 and 1:10,000 pregnant patients. ARDS has many causes, including gastric aspiration, amniotic fluid embolism, sepsis, coagulopathy, massive blood transfusion, and shock. It can be easily confused with cardiogenic pulmonary edema secondary to alterations in preload, myocardial contractility, or afterload. A basic understanding of the differences between cardiogenic and noncardiogenic pulmonary edema is essential before rational therapeutic intervention may be implemented.

Pathophysiology

The basic underlying pathologic change responsible for ARDS is lung injury that results in damage to the pulmonary epithelium and endothelial tissue. This, in turn, leads to enhanced vascular permeability. Factors determining the net flux of lung fluid between the capillary lumen and interstitial space are quantitatively related by the Starling equation:

$$Net\ fluid\ flux = k[(Pcap - Pis) - (\pi cap - \pi is)]$$

(k = filtration coefficient, Pcap = pulmonary capillary hydrostatic pressure, Pis = interstitial space hydrostatic pressure, πcap = pulmonary capillary serum colloid osmotic pressure, πis = interstitial space fluid colloid osmotic pressure)

Normally, fluid flows from the capillary system to the interstitial space and is returned to the systemic circulation by the pulmonary lymphatic system. An increase in left atrial pressure is observed when the left ventricle is unable to pump all the returning blood into the left atrium. Accordingly, the pulmonary capillary hydrostatic pressure increases, facilitating net movement of lung fluid into the interstitial space. When capillary fluid efflux into the interstitial space exceeds lymphatic resorption, the clinical presentation of pulmonary edema will occur. Although colloid osmotic pressure in the interstitial space and serum also plays a role in pulmonary edema, the most common factor is increased capillary hydrostatic pressure secondary to increased preload (fluid overload), afterload (severe hypertension), and decreased myocardial contractility (postpartum cardiomyopathy).

Capillary membrane permeability plays a much larger role in the genesis of noncardiogenic pulmonary edema (ARDS). Such injury due to hypoxic ischemia, vasoactive substances, chemical irritation, or microthrombi facilitates further efflux of capillary fluid and plasma proteins into the interstitium. This increase in permeability acutely produces atelectasis and diminished compliance of the lung, and damage is usually non-uniform. As the functional capability of atelectatic bronchioles diminishes, shunting and hypoxemia develop.

Maternal physiologic changes can contribute to the severity of ARDS. It has been suggested that decreased extrathoracic compliance, decreased functional residual capacity, higher oxygen deficit, limited cardiac output increases, and anemia may adversely affect the clinical presentation and course of ARDS during pregnancy.

Clinical Findings

A. SYMPTOMS AND SIGNS

Classic signs of respiratory distress are tachypnea, intercostal retractions, and even cyanosis, depending on the degree of hypoxemia. Fetal tachycardia or late decelerations may reflect maternal hypoxemia and uteroplacental insufficiency. Pulmonary rales in noncardiogenic pulmonary edema will be indistinguishable from those of cardiogenic pulmonary edema, but physical findings consistent with the cardiogenic disorder (ventricular gallop, jugular venous distention, and peripheral edema) are not typical features of ARDS. Unfortunately, the physiologic changes of pregnancy may mask the significance of these physical findings during the more subtle stages of respiratory distress.

B. LABORATORY FINDINGS

Arterial blood gas determinations will reveal a progressive moderate to severe hypoxemia despite oxygen therapy. Depending on the obstetric cause of ARDS, other laboratory findings will be variable or nonspecific. The initial chest roentgenogram will often be normal, even in the presence of clinically significant respiratory distress. Within the next 24–48 hours, patchy or diffuse infiltrates will progress to prominent alveolar infiltrates (Fig 58–8). Unlike in cardiogenic pulmonary edema, the heart will most likely be of normal size in a patient with ARDS. PCWP measured by right heart catheterization is the procedure most helpful in differentiating ARDS and pulmonary edema. The PCWP is elevated (> 20 mm Hg) in cardiogenic pulmonary edema but is often normal in ARDS.

Measurement of endobronchial fluid COP has also been utilized to differentiate capillary permeability-induced pulmonary edema from hydrostatic or cardiogenic pulmonary edema. In pulmonary edema secondary to capillary permeability, the COP of endobronchial fluid obtained from endotracheal tube suctioning is usually greater than 75% of the simultaneously obtained plasma COP. In cardiogenic pulmonary

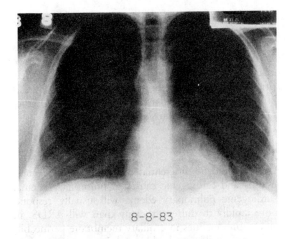

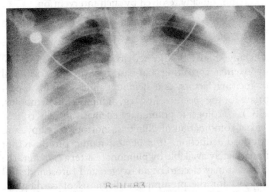

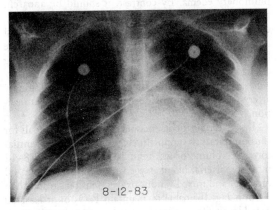

Figure 58–8. Sequence of chest radiographs from a 21-year-old woman during her first pregnancy with antepartum pyelonephritis and ARDS. **A:** Normal chest film. **B:** Bilateral patchy pulmonary densities have developed consistent with the diagnosis of ARDS. Much of the apparent increase in heart size is related to shallow inspiration and supine technique. **C:** ARDS has improved dramatically with only minimal residual pulmonary densities.

edema, the COP of the endobronchial fluid is usually less than 60% that of plasma.

Histopathologically, idiopathic pulmonary fibrosis and ARDS are remarkably similar. Both show evidence of acute alveolar injury, which is characterized by interstitial inflammation, hemorrhage, and edema. This is followed by a hypercellular phase, loss of alveolar structure, and pulmonary fibrosis.

Differential Diagnosis

ARDS should be differentiated from infectious pneumonitis and cardiogenic causes of pulmonary edema. Cardiogenic pulmonary edema will usually respond more rapidly to diuretic therapy than will ARDS, in which abnormalities in capillary membrane permeability are not quickly resolved by such intervention.

Treatment

Therapy should be directed toward the prevention of hypoxemia, correcting acid-base abnormalities, removal of inciting factors, and hemodynamic support appropriate for the specific cause (eg, amniotic fluid embolus, DIC). Cardiogenic pulmonary edema is usually treated with a combination of diuretics, inotropic therapy, and afterload reduction. If a hemodynamic profile is not immediately available by pulmonary artery catheter, the clinician may elect to begin oxygen and furosemide (20 mg IV) for the presumptive diagnosis of cardiogenic pulmonary edema. By contrast, it should be apparent that the basic therapy for ARDS is supportive. Endotracheal intubation with mechanical ventilation is almost always required. The pulmonary artery catheter will be helpful in guiding fluid management and optimizing cardiac performance. Additionally, mixed venous oxygen saturation from the distal port of the pulmonary artery catheter will provide an index of oxygen utilization.

In obstetric patients, reasonable therapeutic goals for cardiorespiratory support include a mechanical ventilator tidal volume of less than 10 mL/kg, PCWP 8–12 mm Hg, arterial blood oxygen tension greater than 60 mm Hg, and mixed venous oxygen tension greater than 30 mm Hg. If unable to maintain PaO_2 of at least 60 mm Hg on 50% or less inspired oxygen, positive endexpiratory pressure (PEEP) in amounts of up to 15 cm H_2O may be helpful. However, it is important to avoid barotrauma to the remaining functional alveolar units, so high tidal volumes and pressures should be avoided. If the mixed venous tension is low, transfusion of red blood cells or inotropic therapy may improve oxygen transport and delivery.

Since the presence of capillary membrane abnormalities in ARDS is associated with rapid equilibration of proteinaceous material between the capillaries and interstitial spaces, intravenous colloid replacement should be discouraged in lieu of crystalloid resuscitation. A policy of relative fluid restriction should be followed, but only if the following criteria are met: stable fetus, no evidence of metabolic acidosis, normal renal function, and no need for vasopressor therapy or PEEP. Sedation and pain relief should be used liberally, and may help to decrease oxygen consumption. Nutritional support for patients on prolonged mechanical ventilation must be considered; enteral feeding is preferred as it may reduce the translocation of gut bacteria into the body. Prospective controlled studies have not demonstrated the benefit of steroid therapy for ARDS. Once therapy for cardiopulmonary support has been implemented, a thorough search for predisposing factors to ARDS must be identified for specific intervention.

Potential future therapies for ARDS include high frequency ventilation, extracorporeal membrane oxygenation (ECMO), intravenous oxygen, inhaled nitric oxide, surfactant replacement, oxygen-free radical scavengers, arachidonic acid metabolite inhibitors, antiprotease agents, antiendotoxin antibodies, anti-tumor necrosis factor antibodies, and other immunologic therapies for sepsis.

The timing of delivery in these patients is unclear from the literature. Based on the high rates of fetal death, preterm labor, fetal heart rate abnormalities, and perinatal asphyxia, most authorities recommend delivery after a gestational age of 28 weeks. In one review, only 10 of 39 patients with antepartum ARDS were discharged undelivered, and all had pylelonephritis or *Varicella*. Cesarean section should be reserved for standard obstetrical indications.

Prognosis

Older series suggested a mortality rate as high as 50–60% for patients with ARDS. More recent reviews show rates of 39–44%. One study of 41 patients demonstrated a 24.4% mortality rate; this has been attributed to possible differences in patient population as well as improvements in critical care. Many affected patients developed pulmonary complications that included barotrauma and pneumothorax. Fortunately, survivors of ARDS usually do not demonstrate permanent long-term pulmonary dysfunction.

CARDIOPULMONARY RESUSCITATION DURING PREGNANCY

Many of the critical conditions discussed in this chapter can lead to cardiopulmonary arrest. Cardiopulmonary resuscitation should follow standard protocols, with some modifications for the pregnancy. It may be difficult to perform cardiac compressions due to a large uterus and engorged breasts. Compressions should not be performed in the supine position, as the gravid uterus may cause aortocaval compression, diminished venous return, and subsequent decreased cardiac output. Patients should be positioned with a left lateral tilt before compressions are applied. This can be accomplished using a moving table, a wedge, or with manual displacement of the uterus. Defibrillation and cardioversion been successfully used during pregnancy without disturbance of the fetal cardiac conduction system. It is important, however, to remove fetal monitors to prevent arcing. Finally, the decision to perform a perimortem cesarean section should be made rapidly, within 4–5 minutes of cardiac arrest. This extreme measure can maximize maternal survival by relieving aortocaval compression and increasing blood flow return back to the heart.

REFERENCES

Hypovolemic Shock

American College of Obstetricians and Gynecologists: Hemorrhagic shock. ACOG Educational Bulletin No. 235. ACOG, April 1997.

Amniotic Fluid Embolism

Clark LD et al: Amniotic fluid embolism: analysis of the national registry. Am J Obstet Gynecol 1995;172;1158.

Davies SD: Amniotic fluid embolus: a review of the literature. Canadian J Anesth 2001;48:88.

Locksmith GJ: Amniotic fluid embolism. Obstet Gynecol Clin North Am 1999;26:435.

Morgan M: Amniotic fluid embolism. Anaesthesia 1979;34:20.

Pulmonary Thromboembolism

American College of Obstetricians and Gynecologists: Thromboembolism in pregnancy. ACOG Practice Bulletin No. 19. ACOG, August 2000.

Ginsberg JS, Greer I, Hirsh J: Use of antithrombotic agents during pregnancy. Chest 2001;119:122S.

Ray JG, Chan WS: Deep vein thrombosis during pregnancy and the puerperium: a meta-analysis of the period of risk and the leg of presentation. Obstet Gynecol Surv 1999;54:265.

Disseminated Intravascular Coagulation

Bick RL: Syndromes of disseminated intravascular coagulation in obstetrics, pregnancy, and gynecology. Hematol Oncol Clin North Am 2000;13:5.

Acute Respiratory Distress Syndrome

Catanzarite V et al: Acute respiratory distress syndrome in pregnancy and the puerperium: causes, courses, and outcome. Obstet Gynecol 2001;97:760.

Perry KG: Maternal mortality associated with adult respiratory distress syndrome. South Med J 1998;91:441.

Van Hook JW: Acute respiratory distress syndrome in pregnancy. Semin Perinatol 1997;21:320.

Psychological Aspects of Obstetrics & Gynecology

59

Alexandra Haessler, MD, & Miriam B. Rosenthal, MD

■ PSYCHOLOGIC ASPECTS OF GYNECOLOGY

Gynecologic practice has always been influenced by folklore and taboos, as well as religious and civil sanctions to control and regulate sexual activity and reproduction. Recent changes in gynecologic practice and the growing number of female practitioners have greatly influenced women's perceptions of what gynecologic care should be.

Gynecologists care for women throughout their life cycle—from menarche through adolescence, young adulthood, pregnancy, menopause, and old age. To perform this function, gynecologists need to know about the psychosexual and physical development of women. The gynecologist needs to be prepared to be a pelvic surgeon, a reproductive endocrinologist, a sex counselor, an educator, and a confidant. Gynecologists need to be sensitive to their own attitudes, values, prejudices, and personality while understanding that these tendencies will influence their practice and their patients' willingness to work collaboratively with them.

THE DOCTOR-PATIENT RELATIONSHIP IN GYNECOLOGY

In the past, doctors and patients generally related to each other in accordance with a model in which a compliant, obedient patient viewed the doctor as omnipotent. Today, many women reject this model and demand a more active role in making decisions relating to their health care. Health and disease-related information are much more widely available. Thus, patients are generally better informed than in the past and have access to specific material relating to the concern that brings them to the physician. For better or worse, the lay media has a profound influence on a patient's understanding of her condition. A patient may arrive at a first visit with a physician having preconceived ideas about what her diagnosis is and how it should be treated. An open doctor-patient relationship is an es-

sential part of the therapeutic process and can lead to a healthy compliance with medical and surgical regimens. To achieve this relationship, it is essential to have some understanding of the personality style of each patient and her approach to thinking about her body and medical interventions.

There are still many women who do not want to participate in decisions about health care and who view their physicians as omnipotent and protective. They believe they will be protected and that nothing will go wrong. While these beliefs may be flattering to the physician, unrealistic expectations often lead to anger and disappointment on the part of the patient. The collaborative model of doctor-patient interaction is usually most effective for both doctor and patient. The patient interview is the place to begin this collaboration and to evaluate the woman's personality.

The Patient Interview

Gathering historical data is a necessary skill the practitioner must maintain. Failure to obtain an essential bit of information can be disastrous. The clinician must use both direct and indirect methods in history taking. It is important to actively listen, noting not only the words, but also the affect and the nonverbal cues accompanying them such as facial expressions, body posture, gestures, voice quality, or tears. The physician needs to learn why these complaints are being brought to his or her attention at the time of presentation. Did the patient recently undergo a hardship or trauma, or lose her ability to cope with a preexisting problem? Open-ended questions, followed by more specific ones, allow information to be gathered effectively. For example, in interviewing a woman with pelvic pain, it is better to ask the open-ended question, "What is the pain like and what is it associated with?" rather than the closed-ended, "Does the pain hurt badly, and does it happen in the morning or at night?" Psychologic symptoms such as problems with sleep or eating, fatigue, libido, and anxiety may relate to physical disorders. If one asks open-ended questions, the interviewer will glean a better understanding of all the factors that play a role in the patient's complaint.

1066

Understanding a patient's social context can also shed light on the medical issues at hand. It may be difficult for the patient to bring up these topics. In these circumstances, it is often best to ask personal questions in a direct way that demonstrates that the interviewer is comfortable discussing the topic. For example, instead of assuming a patient is in a monogamous, married relationship, ask her if she sleeps with men, women, or both. You will likely get to the core of the issues by using this technique when discussing personal topics.

Personality Style

The following personality styles are commonly seen in practice, and an understanding of how each type of patient views illness can assist with planning a patient's care.

(1) The dependent, demanding personality has insatiable needs. This patient becomes increasingly dependent on the physician, calls frequently and often creates frustration. The physician needs to set limits, but with some concessions such as telling the patient she can call at specific times. Interviews can be limited in frequency and duration. The dependent patient can make the physician angry by venting hostility in an indirect way. Illness is seen as a threat of abandonment. Assuring her of continued care that has definite limits is helpful.

(2) The orderly, obsessive, controlled, anxious personality has needs for control and uses the defense mechanisms of isolation and intellectualization. This patient needs much information and participation in decisions regarding care. Illness is seen as a punishment for letting things get out of control. Helping her feel in control of her care will likely help.

(3) The histrionic, dramatic, vivid, anxious personality is often seductive and flirtatious. This patient needs a physician with a caring but firm professional manner. Illness is seen as punishment or an attack on her femininity. This patient needs support but not overly detailed explanations.

(4) The long-suffering personality needs somatic symptoms to function. Illness may be considered as justly deserved and a punishment for worthlessness. The patient may need the physician to acknowledge her courage and not give too much reassurance.

(5) The paranoid personality is suspicious, blaming, and hypersensitive and is threatened by intimacy. A respectful distance is necessary to help this individual. Illness is viewed as an annihilating assault coming from outside the self. Helpful techniques include honest, simple explanations and assuring her that the medical team is there to help her.

(6) The schizoid personality is remote, unsociable, and uninvolved. Illness is viewed as a force that threatens to invade her privacy. A respect for privacy and distance is helpful.

PSYCHOLOGIC ASPECTS OF SPECIFIC GYNECOLOGIC PROBLEMS

Acute Gynecologic Emergency

When urgent medical or surgical care is needed, the relationship with the patient changes to one that requires submission (of a now passive and vulnerable patient) to the skills of a physician that the patient has likely never met. This role may be one the physician is comfortable with, but that terrifies the patient. Once the emergency has passed, it is essential to help the patient gradually resume a role in determining the nature of her care. Prolongation of the dominant role by the physician may easily lead to continued dependency after its justification has ceased. The patient recovering from surgery or a serious illness must not be suddenly abandoned to her own devices as long as she needs her doctor's help and support. Every effort should be made to hasten her return to full health without dependency on her doctor.

Emergent care for the sexual assault survivor deserves special mention. In this circumstance the care provider needs not only to be concerned with patient care, but also with obtaining important legal evidence. Many states require that at least the physician, a police representative, and a patient advocate be present during the interview and examination. It is essential to be familiar with your local government's guidelines and to take appropriate steps to ensure proper data collection. Obviously, sedatives and narcotic medications should only be used once the patient has given a full, recorded statement.

Chronic Pelvic Pain

Pain is one of the most common symptoms that prompt women to visit their gynecologists. It is also one of the most frustrating. Ten to 60% do not have evidence of pathology when examined at laparoscopy. These women are often labeled as having psychiatric problems, and the pain is seen as a result of emotional conflicts when this may not be the case. There are at least 4 reasons why women may complain of pain in the apparent absence of organic pelvic disease: (1) Disease processes are present but have not been detected; (2) pain may be associated with disorders that are not accompanied by objective evidence (migraine variant); (3) pain may be due to nongynecologic causes such as gastrointestinal, genitourinary, or skeletal system problems; and (4) complaints may be psychogenic.

The perception of pain can be influenced by several psychosocial variables. Examples include the anxiety that accompanies pain, childhood experiences with pain and punishment, the ability of an individual to control pain by cognitive and behavioral means, experiences with physical and sexual abuse, previous painful illnesses, the patient's current psychic state, and the patient's cultural expression of pain.

Chronic pain is pain of at least 6 months' duration. It may become more difficult to distinguish organic from psychogenic pain in patients who have had pain for 6 months or longer. It is essential to perform a thorough medical work-up before diagnosing a patient with chronic pelvic pain. Chronic pain may cause or exacerbate psychologic disorders. Patients with chronic pelvic pain are more often found to be depressed, and to suffer from substance abuse, sexual dysfunction, and somatization disorders. These patients often have histories of childhood and adult sexual abuse. One should determine which organic and psychiatric disorders are present and treat distinct symptoms. Over time the primary diagnosis may become clear. No one personality type is more susceptible to chronic pain.

Somatization disorders are psychiatric diagnoses that characterize patients with multiple, recurrent somatic complaints presenting over months and years despite the lack of an identifiable etiology. These disorders more commonly present in women and occur in 0.2–2% of patients. It is not uncommon for depression to present as physical manifestations.

The management of chronic pain and somatization requires careful history taking, physical examination, laboratory studies, psychologic assessment, and possibly laparoscopy. Unnecessary surgery should be avoided, and psychologic treatments along with suitable medications are helpful. Narcotics should be avoided except for extreme pain episodes. Biofeedback with pelvic vaginal blood flow has been used, as has relaxation training, hypnosis, and psychotherapy. Antidepressants have been used with good results. Advances in this field will come from research that integrates the biologic, psychologic, and cultural approaches, not from the labeling of the unknown as psychologic. A multidisciplinary approach appears to be the most effective in managing intractable pelvic pain syndromes.

Eating Disorders

The incidence of eating disorders has markedly increased in recent years and these disorders are often managed in gynecologic practice. Cultural pressure for females to maintain thinness contributes to this problem. The diagnostic criteria for the major entities of obesity, anorexia nervosa, and bulimia are still imprecise and the relationship among these 3 disorders is often nebulous. Anorexia, bulimia, and obesity are heterogeneous conditions with biologic, psychologic, and social dimensions. For each patient being evaluated, particular attention should be paid to history of the eating problem, weight and eating history, physical examination, and family dynamics, including affective mental disturbances in the family, personality style, substance abuse, and cultural background. Patients with anorexia nervosa or bulimia should have a psychologic assessment. Eating disorders may also reappear during pregnancy and interfere with appropriate nutrition.

A. Anorexia Nervosa

Anorexia nervosa is a disorder characterized by refusal to maintain a body weight within 85% of ideal body weight for age and height. Generally anorexia is seen in the cultural context of a society where food is abundant and thinness is desirable. It is characterized by markedly decreasing food intake, a preoccupation with a fear of becoming obese, a distorted body image, and often by amenorrhea for at least 3 consecutive menstrual cycles. People with this condition generally have body dysmorphic syndrome such that they view themselves as overweight, though they appear thin. Though the weight loss is generally dramatic, the patient does not consider it concerning. She often comes to the attention of the gynecologist because of her amenorrhea, infertility, or other endocrinologic disorders. Associated physiologic signs may include hypothermia, bradycardia, hypotension, edema, lanugo, and other metabolic changes.

Typically anorexia nervosa presents in early adolescence or the early twenties. Ninety-five percent of patients are female, and occurrence is rare in heterosexual males. Its prevalence is 0.13–1% in females 12–18 years old. The course may be episodic or chronic: 40% of patients recover, 30% significantly improve, 20% remain ill, and death occurs in more than 5%. Family patterns demonstrate that these disorders are more prevalent in sisters and mothers of affected individuals. Other family members may have a history of major depression or bipolar affective disorder. The onset may or may not coincide with a stressful life event. These patients often were model children and are perfectionists.

Management consists of referral to specialists trained in the treatment of this disorder, usually as a team with behavioral medicine specialists and nutritionists. Hospital treatment is indicated for severe cases. The primary physician should remain involved throughout each phase of treatment to provide continuity of care. Better prognosis is associated with earlier age of onset and poor prognosis with premorbid obesity, bulimia, vomiting, and laxative abuse.

B. Bulimia

Bulimia is an eating disorder characterized by recurrent bouts of rapid consumption of large amounts of food in a short time alternating with little or no food intake.

There is accompanying depression, anxiety, a lack of control over the eating, low self-esteem, and often social isolation. Other features include self-induced vomiting, use of laxatives and diuretics, dieting, fasting, and vigorous exercise, all designed to keep weight down. There is preoccupation with food, weight, and body shape. The diagnosis is made when there are at least 2 large binge-eating episodes per week for at least 3 months. The food eaten is usually high in calories, easily ingested, and eaten secretly. The binge may be followed by abdominal pain, distention, and vomiting. The individual may be obese, thin, or of normal weight. Stress or eating itself may precipitate binges, which usually occur in the late afternoon or evening after school or work.

Many bulimics are depressed or are afflicted with other affective disorders. Alcohol or drug abuse is often associated with bulimia, especially involving sedatives, amphetamines, and cocaine. A variety of personality types, including those with borderline personality disorders, develop this condition. Some physical complications include lethargy, impaired concentration, and abdominal pain. Dehydration and electrolyte disturbances (ie, hypokalemia, metabolic alkalosis, hypochloremia, and rarely metabolic acidosis) may result from fasting, diuretic use, and acute diarrhea. Arrhythmias may result from significant electrolyte disturbances. Other complications are gastric rupture, salivary gland swelling (usually the parotid), and dental problems including decalcification of teeth that result from frequent vomiting.

The neuroendocrine abnormalities include blunted thyroid-stimulating hormone response to thyroid-releasing hormone administration, increase in growth hormone following TRH or glucose administration, and elevated basal serum prolactin. Menstrual dysfunction may be due to disturbed gonadotropin production.

An exact etiology is unknown, but associated factors include a history of traumatic events, especially separation or loss and a history of being overweight. The mild form of bulimia is fairly common among women in college (4.5% of women and 0.4% of men reported in one study of college freshmen). Severe bulimia occurs in approximately 1% of the population. The course is chronic and intermittent over many years. The differential diagnosis must include schizophrenia, certain neurologic diseases such as central nervous system tumors, and epileptic equivalent seizures. A history of sexual assault is common. A recent survey of girls demonstrated that sexual assault survivors were three times more likely to binge and purge than girls who did not report a history of sexual abuse.

Management and treatment begin with a very careful history of eating patterns and psychologic function. This may be difficult to obtain since the patients are often secretive. Behaviors to inquire about include binge eating and use of diuretics, laxatives, diet pills, and enemas. The next step is careful physical examination including a neurologic work-up, noting the state of hydration, teeth, salivary glands, and cardiac function. Minimal laboratory work should include plasma glucose, complete blood count, liver function tests, thyroid function, and, if indicated, skull films with visual fields or CT scan. Hospitalization may be necessary. Psychologic approaches are usually behavioral or cognitive-behavioral, group therapy, and patient education (especially about nutrition). Drug treatment consists of anticonvulsants or antidepressants.

Obesity

Obesity is the excessive accumulation of fat; it is usually defined as a 20% increase over standard weight and a 20% increase in skinfold thickness. It affects approximately 25% of the adult population, is more common in women, increases with age, and is more prevalent in the U.S. in lower socioeconomic classes. There is no correlation with psychologic disturbance except for overeating behaviors, diet complications, and body image problems. Many treatment modalities are popular; nutritional-behavioral methods and self-help groups are useful for moderate obesity.

Sleep Disorders

A national survey indicates that one-third of the U.S. population has some degree of sleep disturbance. Complaints are frequently presented to gynecologists in the context of other disorders and may be minor or be part of a more serious physical or psychiatric disorder. Considerable diagnostic and treatment options are available.

Recent advances in the study of sleep have related sleep physiology and the stages of the sleep cycle. Stage 0 is wakefulness with closed eyes, high muscle tone, and some eye movement. Stages 1–4 are non-REM (rapid eye movement) sleep in humans and are characterized by specific encephalographic changes. REM or "desynchronized" sleep is characterized by extreme hypotonia, rapid eye movements, blood pressure and heart rate variability, muscle twitches, and nocturnal penile tumescence. There is high dream recall if one awakens during REM sleep. Sleep cycles vary with age, sex, and numerous other influences. In an ordinary 8-hour period of sleep, an adult 25 years old will go through 4–6 cycles, with the average cycle taking 90 minutes and REM periods 15 minutes.

Sleep and arousal problems have been classified into 4 groups. (1) The insomnias are disorders of initiating and maintaining sleep. They are a heterogeneous group associated with organic and psychiatric conditions. A history of the sleep-wakefulness pattern helps with diagnosis. A disturbance in falling asleep may be due to anxiety or worry. Staying asleep or early-morning awakening is often seen in depressive illness. Myoclonus or central apnea can disturb sleep. (2) Disorders of excessive somnolence can be due to narcolepsy, obstructive airway syndrome, depression, substance abuse, or other conditions. (3) Disorders of the sleep-wake schedule are those in which there is a misalignment between the individual's usual sleep-wake cycle and the internal circadian rhythms, eg, jet lag. (4) Parasomnias are a group of clinical conditions that happen during sleep, sleep stages, and partial arousals. Examples include somnambulism (sleep walking) and asthma (which may get worse during sleep). They are manifestations of atypical central nervous system activation during sleep with discharge into skeletal muscle or into channels of autonomic activity.

Treatment of sleep problems requires an accurate diagnosis. Insomnias that do not respond to treatment with relaxation, sleep hygiene methods, and benzodiazepines should be referred to a sleep laboratory for diagnosis and treatment. Sleep hygiene suggestions generally include curtail excess sleep; maintain regular awakening times; exercise regularly; avoid loud noises during sleep; keep sleeping room temperature comfortable; avoid hunger; limit caffeine and do not smoke; avoid alcohol; try to stop worrying; keep busy after a sleepless night; be flexible, but limit daytime naps. Hypnotic drugs are among the most widely used drugs in the U.S. The 3 most commonly used groups are the barbiturates, the benzodiazepines, and nonbarbiturate nonbenzodiazepines (eg, chloral hydrate, methaqualone). It is essential to be familiar with their pharmacology, action, potential for addiction or use for suicide, and teratogenicity before prescribing these drugs.

Premenstrual Syndrome

Premenstrual syndrome is a psychoneuroendocrine disorder related to menses with biologic, psychologic, and social parameters. A complete discussion of premenstrual syndrome can be found in Chapter 32.

PSYCHOLOGIC ASPECTS OF GYNECOLOGIC SURGERY

Most people are afraid of the prospect of surgery. There are several sources of fear: death and injury, physiologic stress, separation from family, and the forced dependency of being a patient. It is not abnormal to have a recurrence of childhood fears, especially related to punishment and abandonment, and feelings of aggression and control. The person who tends to handle the perioperative period well is one who has a clear understand-

ing of why they are having surgery, copes well with stress, has some anxiety, understands the risks of surgery, expects a reasonable outcome, is motivated to be healthy, and is free of psychiatric conditions.

Preoperative Preparation

Compared with unprepared patients, patients who are well prepared for surgery show less postoperative pain, use fewer pain medications, and have shorter hospital stays. Preparation means more than reassurance. It includes a careful description of the indications for surgery and an explanation of the preferred surgical approach. In addition, informed consent must be obtained, delineating the risks, benefits, and alternatives to the procedure. Obtaining informed consent is a process that allows the patient to make an informed decision about whether she understands and accepts the medical implications of the surgery. When the physician and patient sign the document, it serves as a legal statement of the patient's permission to proceed. Answering all of the patient's questions is a necessary component of informed consent. Patients often have strong feelings about their preferred surgical approach; for example, where the incision should be made. A clear preoperative discussion about patient preferences and concerns may prevent a great deal of anxiety, miscommunication, and dissatisfaction after the procedure.

It has been shown that patients who are anxious do not assimilate information well. For this reason the person obtaining consent must take the necessary time to communicate effectively with the patient. Consideration of a patient's social context and personality type may help the physician navigate this communication successfully. It can be helpful to have a family member or friend assist the patient in asking questions and assimilating information. A friend or family member may be the ideal person to facilitate communication between a nervous patient and the physician, but a representative of the professional staff should be used for translation whenever possible, since the physician cannot be sure that his or her words are being properly communicated.

Postoperative Preparation

Patients need a clear explanation of their procedure and potential postoperative outcomes. It is helpful to give anticipatory guidance regarding what to expect during the postoperative course. This includes a brief orientation to hospital procedures, rehabilitation, medication instructions, and follow-up arrangements. They should also understand how their body will change, for example, after oophorectomy. The possibility of hormone replacement should be discussed preoperatively, so that postoperative stressors are minimized.

Sexual function is a common concern for patients undergoing gynecologic surgery. It is important to address concerns directly and reassure patients that sexual function is minimally altered by hysterectomy. There is no indication that women with a history of depression have more depressive episodes or changes in sexual functioning or dyspareunia after surgery than other women. Interestingly, hysterectomy has not been shown to be related to decreased sexual functioning after surgery. Actually, the best predictor of sexual functioning postoperatively is a patient's level of sexual functioning preoperatively.

Hysterectomy: A Special Case

A woman tends to place special importance on her reproductive organs. Often, they represent how she views herself sexually, physically, and culturally. Many women are afraid that removing their reproductive organs will divest them of their womanhood. For some this may be because they consider menstruation an important confirmation of their feminine identity. The prospect of having a hysterectomy may bring sadness to one patient, while relieving another who considers her reproductive organs from a medical perspective. A woman's adaptation to hysterectomy is related to her age, stage of development, personality, style of coping, ideas regarding fertility, sexual relationships, experiences with close relatives or friends who had the surgery, and the rapport she establishes with medical personnel, especially her physician.

Preoperatively, it is helpful to inquire about attitudes toward femininity, prior losses, attitudes and expectations about surgery, baseline sexual functioning, and past history of anxiety or depression. Those with positive attitudes about femininity, an ability to adapt to loss, and some anxiety do best. Patients at high risk for psychologic difficulties after hysterectomy are those who seek surgery without a clear indication, those with chronic pelvic pain without any apparent pelvic disease, those who are depressed or who have past psychiatric history, those who have conflicts over sexuality and childbearing, those who have inappropriate levels of preoperative anxiety, and those with premonitions of death during surgery. Patients with somatization disorders should be identified prior to surgery. The patients who approach surgery with indifference or very high degrees of anxiety may have more trouble understanding the process and may have emotional reactions after they leave the hospital.

Postoperatively, the surgeon may note that a previously high functioning patient has developed delirium. This is a transient form of encephalopathy that is characterized by an alteration in consciousness, disorientation, perceptual abnormalities, and agitation or withdrawal. Other postoperative syndromes include tremors, postoperative depression or psychosis, or excessive pain. Interestingly, patients may recall comments made in the operating room during anesthesia if anesthesia is light. Care should be taken when conversing in the operating room when the patient is thought to be unconscious.

Gynecologic Oncology

The improved prognosis for many cancers makes the quality of life an increasingly important issue in the management of malignancy. The physician who cares for patients with gynecologic cancer needs to be familiar not only with the most current technical data, but also must be able to respond to the patient with empathy and understanding at all stages of the illness. For some patients, gynecologic cancers often have symbolic meanings related to sexuality and reproduction and are therefore highly emotionally charged.

With the diagnosis there is often a grief response characterized by shock, disbelief, anger, and fears of death, pain, losing a body part, and abandonment. This can occur even when the malignancy is treatable. A discussion of the treatment plan should cover expected functional losses, side effects of treatment, and effects on sexual functioning. Psychiatric disorders that may occur in the course of malignant disease (eg, organic brain syndromes, depressive syndromes, and anxiety syndromes) need recognition and treatment.

SEXUAL PROBLEMS IN GYNECOLOGIC PRACTICE

The most available resource for the woman with sexual difficulties is their gynecologist or family physician. Thus, a minimal sexual history is part of every gynecologic history. The gynecologist should be familiar with the sexual response cycle, with taking a sexual history, with the ability to make diagnoses of the most common sexual disorders, with the effects on sexuality of organic problems and drugs, and with the kind of sexual therapies that are available. Most sexual problems are managed by education, corrections of organic problems, and reassurance. More serious psychologic problems should be managed by gynecologists with added training in sexual therapy. Certain common dimensions of sexual identity warrant discussion for those providing primary sexual counseling. Sexuality and reproduction are central to one's identity as a male or female, whether or not one wants children. The sexual identity of any adult can be described along 3 major dimensions: gender identity, sexual orientation, and sexual intention.

Gender identity is the earliest aspect of sexual identity to form. Core gender identity is the sense one has of being male or female. It develops in the second year of life and is the result of: (1) biologic factors originating in fetal life and with the organization of the fetal brain; (2) sex assignment at birth by parents and medical staff; (3) parental attitudes; (4) conditioning and imprinting; and (5) development of body ego and body image, which comes in part from sensations from the genitals and other body parts. Masculinity and femininity are those behaviors that a person, parents, society, or the culture define as male or female. These may change from time to time. While many children show some evidence of gender confusion, 90% develop a core gender identity consistent with their biologic sex. **Gender role** is the sum of what one does that indicates to others the degree of maleness or femaleness. Gender identity continues to be influenced by identification with important adults as the child grows to adulthood.

Sexual orientation refers to the sex of the person in fantasy or reality that causes sexual arousal. Heterosexual individuals are sexually aroused by persons of the opposite sex, homosexual individuals by persons of the same sex, and bisexual individuals by persons of both sexes. There is increasing evidence of biologic contributions to sexual orientation, but further research is needed.

Sexual intention refers to what a person wants to do with his or her sexual partner, eg, kissing, caressing, or intercourse. There are two dimensions: fantasy and real-life behavior. The usual intention is giving and receiving pleasure. Some examples of abnormal sexual intention related to aggression are sadism, exhibitionism, rape, and pedophilia.

The ability to function sexually in adulthood is formed at birth with the earliest parent-infant bonds. The loving care a person receives in infancy and childhood prepares him or her for intimate relationships in adult life.

Phases of the Sexual Response Cycle*

Stages in the sexual response cycle are described below. A more detailed description can be found in the classic work of Masters and Johnson, *Human Sexual Response.*

A. Excitement Phase

Early sexual arousal in the male, whether initiated by tactile, visual, or psychic stimuli, results in engorgement and erection of the penis, with an increase in penile size and in the angle of protrusion from the body. In the woman, arousal in the excitement phase, also initiated by tactile, visual, or psychic stimuli, involves

vaginal lubrication. This lubrication, previously thought to be of uterine or cervical origin, has been demonstrated by Masters and Johnson to be a "sweating reaction" of the vagina; it is probably a true transudation that continues throughout sexual excitement. Coalescence of droplets provides a lubricating film; later in the response cycle, Bartholin's glands make a small contribution. The glans clitoridis swells, often to almost double its size, as a result of engorgement, but the degree of enlargement is apparently unrelated either to the woman's capacity for sexual response or to her ability to achieve orgasm. The shaft of the clitoris also increases in diameter. Engorgement of the glans clitoridis and shaft occur most rapidly with direct manual stimulation of the glans clitoridis and the mons veneris, by means of fantasy, or by stroking the breasts.

Breast changes in the sexually aroused woman consist of nipple erection and, later in the excitement phase, an increase in total size of the breasts. The labia majora, which in a resting state meet in the midline of the vagina, gape slightly and may be displaced toward the clitoris. In nulliparous women, the outer labia may also thin out and flatten against the surrounding tissue. In multiparous women, they may extend and be engorged to an exaggerated degree. The labia minora also swell. The vagina, which is in a collapsed state normally, now begins to expand in the inner two-thirds of the vaginal canal, alternating with a tendency to relax. As excitement increases, progressive distention of the vagina occurs. The vaginal walls also "tent" in response to upward and backward posterior movement of the cervix and uterus, so that the inner portion of the vagina swells dramatically. Engorgement changes the color of the vaginal wall to dark purple and causes the vaginal rugae to become smooth.

In both men and women, erotic tension causes increased muscle tone accompanied by tachycardia and blood pressure elevation. A "sex flush" begins over the upper abdomen and later spreads over the breasts as a morbilliform rash; this occurs in about 75% of women and 25% of men before orgasm. In the late phase, the man experiences shortening of the spermatic cords and retraction of the testes. The scrotum thickens and is flattened against the body.

B. The Plateau Phase

The delineation between the excitement and the plateau phases is imprecise. Ordinarily, the penis is completely erect in the first phase. In the plateau phase, there is usually a slight increase in the diameter of the coronal ridge and, in some men, a deepening of color of the glans to reddish-purple. Progressive excitement may increase testicular size by about 50%; at this point, the man is very close to orgasm and approaches an inevitable stage. In the late plateau phase, respiratory rate,

---

*This section contributed by Ralph Benson.

muscle tone, pulse rate, and blood pressure changes intensify, and muscle tension increases in the buttocks and anal sphincter. A few drops of fluid may appear in the male urethra from the bulbourethral (Cowper's) gland. Although this is not semen, it can contain large numbers of active sperm, which means that impregnation is possible before ejaculation.

In the woman, the "orgasmic platform" is formed by increased engorgement and swelling of the tissues of the outer third of the vagina, which reduces its interior diameter by 30–50%, tightening the grip on the penis and indicating that she is rapidly approaching orgasm. Elevation and ballooning of the inner two-thirds of the vagina increase, as does the size of the uterus (especially in multiparous women). The clitoris, now erect, rises from its position over the pubic bone, and retracts into its hood, shortening by about 50%. In this position the clitoris continues to respond, either to manual stimulation or to penile thrusts. Engorgement of the labia continues until they take on a deep wine color, indicating that climax is imminent.

C. ORGASMIC PHASE

In the woman, a series of rhythmic muscular contractions of the orgasmic platform signals the onset of climax. These contractions vary in number from 3–5 per minute to as many as 8–12 per minute in some women. They are intense at first but subside quickly. A series of uterine contractions quickly follows, beginning in the superior portion and moving downward toward the cervix. Occasionally, rhythmic contractions in the anal sphincter occur. In the man, the rhythmic contractions stimulate a discharge in the perineal floor, particularly in the bulbocavernosus muscle. Just before orgasm, increasing tension in the seminal vesicles causes the semen to empty into the bulbous urethra. Simultaneously, the prostate begins to contract, expelling fluid and distending the bulbous portion of the urethra as semen and prostatic fluid mingle. A series of rhythmic contractions at the bulb now eject the semen with great pressure. A series of minor contractions persists in the urethra for several seconds, continuing even after complete expulsion of the semen.

Changes in pulse rate, blood pressure, and respiratory rate reach a peak and quickly dissipate, but for both the man and the woman the height of orgasm is marked by generalized muscle tension. The facial muscles tighten, and the muscles of the neck, extremities, abdomen, and buttocks are strongly contracted. There may be grasping movements by both partners, followed by clutching and even carpopedal spasm. A fleeting period occurs in which each individual withdraws physiologically but not physically, concentrating almost solely on genital sensation, unaware perhaps of cries and uncontrollable behavior.

D. RESOLUTION PHASE

Muscle tension is released and engorgement subsides in the genitals and skin. The sex flush slowly fades. In the woman the nipples appear slightly prominent, but only because the swelling around them is subsiding. As the sex flush fades, some perspiration occurs. In some women, perspiration appears uniformly over the entire body, while men frequently perspire on the soles and palms. In either case, the amount of perspiration is unrelated to the degree of muscular effort expended before or during orgasm.

In the woman, the clitoris promptly returns to its unstimulated state but will not reach normal size for 5–10 minutes. Relaxation of the orgasmic platform then occurs, and the diameter of the outer third of the vagina increases. Vaginal ballooning diminishes, the uterus shrinks, and the cervix descends into its normal position. The slight enlargement of the cervical canal is maintained. Total resolution time varies; as much as 30 minutes may elapse before the woman is in a truly unstimulated state.

In men, loss of erection occurs in two stages: in the first, most of the erectile volume is lost; the second is a refractory stage during which he is unable to be aroused again, and the remainder of the shrinkage occurs. In young men, the refractory period may be very short, but it lengthens with age. In most men it will last for several minutes; in others it may last for hours or even days. Women are capable of multiple orgasms.

Sexual History Taking

A sexual history should be part of every gynecologic examination, although the amount of detail may vary.

Sexual dysfunction is very common, and patients usually appreciate suitable inquiry. Physicians need a knowledge base to respond to concerns, although their own anxiety may get in the way of adequate questioning. Time is usually not a major deterrent if one is skilled enough. The sexual history belongs in the review of systems. Language should begin with biologic terms and then move to simpler terms. General questions precede more specific ones. The physician should maintain a positive, empathetic, and professional manner with a patient and ask questions in a logical sequence. The sexual history can cover (1) areas of the sexual response cycle: sexual desire, sexual arousal (erection in males, lubrication in females), orgasm, and satisfaction; (2) concerns about gender identity and sexual orientation; (3) classification of problems: onset, course, best and worst functioning, frequency of sexual behaviors, and relationship of sexual behaviors to other life circumstances, ie, relationships, losses, financial problems, illness, medication, surgery, family difficulties, infertility, and contraception.

Sexual history taking should include the following information:

1. Identifying data
   a. Patient: age, sex, number of pregnancies and marriages
   b. Parents and family
   c. Partner
   d. Children
2. Childhood sexuality
   a. Family and religious attitudes toward sex
   b. Sexual learning
   c. Childhood sexual activity
   d. Childhood sexual abuse or incest
3. Adolescence
   a. Preparation for menses
   b. Menarche
   c. Masturbation
   d. Partner petting
   e. Intercourse
   f. Gender issues
4. Adolescence and adulthood
   a. Sexual fantasies
   b. Sexual orientation (heterosexual, homosexual)
   c. Partner choice
   d. Sexual activity
   e. Sexual deviations
   f. Sexual orientation
   g. Sexual function and dysfunction
   h. Contraception
5. Life changes in past year
   a. Losses
   b. Moves
   c. Pregnancy
   d. Other

Female Sexual Dysfunction

Considerable advances in the knowledge of female sexuality have occurred in the past decade. The major contributions of gynecologist William Masters and his colleague Virginia Johnson to the physiology and psychology of sexuality are well recognized. Women had been so inhibited by their culture that some had lived through courtship, marriage, childbearing, and menopause without ever experiencing their bodies in sexual arousal, orgasm, or a sense of sexual freedom. Though more women are comfortable exploring their sexual side, sexual dysfunction does persist. Sexual dysfunction includes psychogenic and organic causes of decreased sexual desire, arousal, orgasm, and pain causing personal distress. The most common types of female sexual dysfunction are noted in Table 59–1.

Inhibited sexual desire may be lifelong (primary) or occur after a period of normal functioning (secondary). Its presence does not necessarily imply a lack of ability to respond physiologically. Many women with primary inhibited sexual desire come from very sexually repressive backgrounds, have been sexually traumatized in childhood or adolescence, or have a poor partner relationship. They may avoid relationships in order to avoid sex. Treatment consists of behavioral and psychologic methods.

Secondary inhibited sexual desire often develops after problems with a partner, physical or emotional traumas, physical illnesses, drug or alcohol abuse, surgery, or psychologic depression. A careful history will usually reveal recent life changes, losses, and medical or drug problems. Other contributions to difficulties in sexual desire come from concern about pregnancy, partners with very different sexual appetites, and changes in body image.

Sexual phobias occur in many women who then develop patterns of avoidance and are thought to have low desire. The thought of sex arouses panic and anxiety. There may be avoidance of any mention of sex and social isolation. Treatment consists of education, support, psychotherapy, and behavioral desensitization. In severe cases, anxiolytics such as imipramine have been used with success.

A. ORGASMIC PROBLEMS

Orgasm is a genital reflex caused by sensory stimuli from the brain and periphery (clitoris, nipples, and

Table 59–1. Classification of female sexual dysfunctions.

Component	Symptom	Term
Desire	Decreased interest in sex	Inhibited sexual desire (ISD)
Excitement or arousal	Decreased lubrication	Excitement-phase dysfunction
Orgasm	No orgasm	Orgasmic dysfunction
Satisfaction	Decreased satisfaction	—
Other	Pain with intercourse	Dyspareunia
	Spasm of circumvaginal musculature	Vaginismus
	Fear of sex; fear of penetration	Sexual phobias Sexual panic

All: Primary or seondary, situational or absolute.

other body parts) that enter the spinal cord in the pudendal nerve at the sacral level. The efferent outflow is from T11 to L2 and involves the contraction of the perivaginal musculature. The reflex centers are close to those for bowel and bladder control, so that injuries to the lower cord may affect all 3 functions.

Orgasmic problems are very common. About 8–10% of adult women in the U.S. have never been orgasmic; another 10% may achieve orgasm with fantasy alone. Most women fall somewhere in between these two extremes, demonstrating a variety of responses. Women with primary orgasmic problems have never experienced orgasm in any situation, even after prolonged and effective sexual stimulation. Those with secondary orgasmic problems have had periods of normal functioning. In both primary and secondary cases, the women may lubricate easily, enjoy lovemaking, and feel satisfaction. Somehow, they get "stuck" in the plateau phase of the sexual response cycle. Some women are not sure if they have reached orgasm; others regularly "fake" orgasm in order to please their partner or live out their own fantasies. A number of women are orgasmic with clitoral stimulation but not during intercourse; this is a normal variant. For others, the presence of the penis or other erotic stimulus is necessary for orgasm.

In the female with adequate sensory stimulation, orgasm will bring about rhythmic contractions of pelvic musculature around the vagina at a rate of 8 per minute, plus pleasurable feelings. The uterus may also contract. Because of the connection between brain and spinal cord centers for orgasm, learned inhibition can occur as with other reflexes. Orgasm is under voluntary control so there may be neural connections between the orgasm center and the voluntary motor perception areas of the brain.

The woman with primary orgasmic dysfunction is likely to have some very basic fears about sexuality and relationships. She may fear losing control, urinating, getting pregnant, or giving herself pleasure. She may experience performance anxiety and may or may not be sexually inhibited in general. Not having a trusted partner is sometimes a factor.

There are innumerable orgasmic variations. Theories that labeled vaginal orgasms mature and clitoral orgasms immature have been laid to rest. The goal of any treatment is to help the individual achieve her first orgasm, if she has never had one, or to reestablish orgasmic achievement if it has ceased. Although every woman is physiologically capable of having an orgasm, the focus that our culture places on the achievement of orgasm may actually inhibit a woman's ability to reach orgasm. Pressure may also come from partners who insist that a woman's lack of orgasm is due to her partner's failure.

Treatment is aimed at enhancing sensory stimulation and extinguishing the woman's involuntary inhibitions. The therapist's first task is to make certain that the woman understands that sufficient clitoral stimulation is required and is able to communicate her needs to her partner. She needs to know that it is normal to be sexual. Sometimes these educational techniques alone are enough to overcome the problem. Barbach's book *For Yourself* has been very helpful to many women.

A woman with primary orgasmic dysfunction needs to learn what it feels like to have an orgasm. She may have to disregard her obsessive thoughts and distractions and focus on the erotic thoughts and premonitory feelings that directly precede orgasm. The use of fantasy can be very helpful. Women with very religious backgrounds may find the idea of erotic fantasy (ie, thinking of other partners and being overcome by a loving partner) more guilt-provoking than sex itself. Self-stimulation is often recommended as a means of learning what feels good and helps the woman become sexually aroused. The longstanding prohibition against masturbation in her value system may be difficult to overcome. She may prefer to masturbate in private, rather than with a partner. Some women have marked success with a vibrator, at first alone and then possibly with the partner. In addition to mastering the physical aspects of achieving orgasm, women need to address their fears. Many patients find it helpful to join a women's discussion group. Besides discussing educational issues, members are assigned specific sexual tasks to do at home alone. Tasks are performed in privacy and responses are later shared with the group members. They may also be able to share fantasies and give one another support.

Transferring orgasmic achievement to a partner situation is the final step in most treatment situations. Heterosexual women are encouraged to heighten arousal before penetration. They learn the clitoris may be stimulated by indirect friction of the hood being pulled back and forth over this organ, eg, during penile thrusting. Each woman needs to learn the most effective means of increasing her own pleasure, eg, active thrusting and use of pelvic and thigh musculature, avoidance of distracting thoughts, and free use of erotic and exciting fantasies. When there is a beloved, trusted partner, the prognosis is good.

Women who take selective serotonin reuptake inhibitors (SSRIs) often suffer from sexual dysfunction. In one study, approximately 50% complained of decreased libido, dyspareunia, decreased lubrication, anorgasmy and other problems. Patients often discontinue or change antidepressants as a result of these side effects. It is important to ask about these side effects when prescribing these medications.

Acquired sexual dysfunction is often due to vasomotor phenomena. Though conclusive studies have not been done regarding the use of sildenafil in female patients, patients using it have reported enhanced clitoral responsiveness, increased vaginal blood flow, and increased vaginal lubrication.

B. DYSPAREUNIA

Pain during sexual intercourse can be especially distressing. Even when the actual pain is gone, memory of the pain may persist and interfere with pleasure. Some women with no background of trauma or major inhibitions may assume that sex will be painful because they associate menstruation and childbirth with pain. A careful history and physical examination are essential. Table 59–2 lists the physical reasons for dyspareunia. It is also important to look for psychologic contributions. Management consists of treating the specific problem.

Vaginismus is the painful reflex spasm of the perivaginal and thigh adductor muscles that occurs in anticipation of any vaginal penetration. It occurs most often in young, inexperienced women from strict homes. Some patients may have been subjected to rape or incest as children or adults. Severe pain secondary to trauma or medical procedures in the vaginal area may sometimes cause the problem. Insufficient lubrication from lack of arousal or sexual phobias may also cause pain with intercourse and vaginismus.

Vaginismus must be diagnosed by history and physical examination. Gynecologists often institute a program of gradual vaginal dilation, using dilators, the woman's finger, or the partner's finger; not all women will respond to this prescription. Some may have more

Table 59–2. Some physical reasons for dyspareunia.

Vaginal opening
Hymen—rare
Tender episiotomy scar
Aging—with decreased elasticity
Labia—Bartholin gland abscess
Other lesions
Clitoris
Irritations
Infections
Vagina
Infections
Sensitivity reactions
Atrophic reactions
Decreased lubrication
Uterus, uterine tubes, ovaries
Endometriosis
Pelvic inflammatory disease
Ectopic pregnancy
Numerous others

Table 59–3. Classification of male sexual dysfunctions.

Component	Symptom	Term
Desire	Decreased interest in sex	Inhibited sexual desire (ISD)
Arousal of excitement	Difficulty with erection	"Impotence," erectile difficulty
Orgasm	No ejaculation No emission	Premature ejaculation, inhibited orgasm, retrograde ejaculation
Satisfaction	Decreased satisfaction	—

All: primary or secondary, situational or absolute.

serious problems that require psychotherapy. It is not unusual for a woman who has overcome her difficulty to find that her partner has developed erectile problems. This finding supports the belief that sexual problems are rarely limited to one partner.

Male Sexual Dysfunction

The term **impotence** used to refer to most male performance problems. Today, the word has an imprecise meaning since there has been a great increase in knowledge about sexual dysfunction and classification based on the physiology of the sexual response cycle (Table 59–3). The term impotence usually refers to erectile problems or the inability to sustain an erection for the time necessary for a desired sexual act. Erectile problems are common and increase with age.

Male sexual dysfunctions have been classified on the basis of an understanding of the sexual response cycle. The classification includes (1) problems of desire—diminished or excessive; (2) problems with arousal, ie, erectile difficulties (or impotence); and (3) problems with orgasm—premature ejaculation, inhibited orgasm, or retrograde ejaculation. These conditions may be caused by psychogenic, organic, or mixed psychogenic and organic factors. Performance anxiety leads to "spectatoring" in which a person becomes preoccupied in watching his or her own sexual responses. They may be primary (present all of one's life) or secondary (having developed after a period of normal functioning). The history should focus on the stage of life of the man, the quality of his sexual desire, the role of his partner, and significance of early and past life experiences. Organic contributions are more common than was previously thought and are related to illness, surgery, medication, drugs, alcohol, vascular disorders, and neuropathies.

Psychologic causes include performance anxiety, fear of women and intimacy, relationship problems, and depression or other mental illnesses. The purely psychogenic dysfunctions show more variability in erectile responses and are associated with normal nocturnal tumescence studies. An evaluation by a urologist knowledgeable about sexual function is often indicated.

Treatment is based on etiology. Organic causes need treatment if possible. The psychogenic forms of dysfunction are best managed by behavioral treatment approaches. Partners are seen together and their relationship helped with improved communication as well as special techniques for specific problems.

Drugs that cause sexual dysfunction commonly include antihypertensives, cimetidine, antipsychotic drugs, tricyclic antidepressants, and central nervous system depressants, such as sedatives, anxiolytics, cannabis, alcohol, and heroin.

Sexual Activity with Aging

Sexual changes occur in men and women as they grow older. Perimenopausal and postmenopausal women may have less sexual desire, with fewer sexual fantasies and a slower and lessened lubrication response to arousal with more vaginal dryness and discomfort with intercourse. Their breasts may have less nipple erection and enlargement. Sex flush diminishes, and the clitoris and labia enlarge to a lesser degree. The vaginal walls are thinner and less able to expand. Orgasm may be less intense, with weaker muscle contractions, and uterine contractions may be uncomfortable. Atrophic skin changes and altered peripheral nerve endings may diminish sensory perceptions.

Men show decreased sexual activity with aging. By age 60 men have about one erection a week. Sexual desire may diminish and erections take longer, require more stimulation, and are less firm. Ejaculation takes longer, with the feeling of ejaculatory inevitability less pronounced. There is less ejaculate, and the refractory period is longer. The sex flush is diminished.

Despite these normal changes with aging, the capacity for sexual activity and enjoyment persists. Many couples, freed from the worries of pregnancy, feel more able than ever to have the pleasure of an active sex life. A stenotic vagina after surgical procedures may make penetration difficult. Noncoital sexual activity may be a very satisfying form of intimacy and pleasure for some couples. The gynecologist can help the aging couple by educating them about normal changes, using estrogen and progesterone replacement when indicated, and accepting sexual activity as healthy behavior of older people.

■ PSYCHOLOGIC ASPECTS OF OBSTETRICS

A woman's psychology cannot be understood without considering the stage she is at in the course of her reproductive life and how her values and identity relate to the issues that arise at each stage. In recent decades, there have been many changes in women's lifestyles and attitudes that have an effect on the psychologic aspects of pregnancy. Family structure is changing. Many women now work outside the home, are single or divorced, or are having first babies in the teenage years or after age 35. Sexual values and practices have changed and they will continue to change. Women have more knowledge about their bodies, and most want to participate in important decisions regarding fertility, pregnancy, delivery, and infant care. Many men want a greater part in sharing their partner's pregnancy. Finally, the legal climate has greatly affected medical practice. These alterations significantly influence the practice of obstetrics and gynecology. Indeed, the clinician is faced with new challenges and stresses in caring for women from diverse ethnic, economic, and social backgrounds in a sensitive, caring, and highly skilled way.

Good obstetric and gynecologic care requires the consideration of each woman as an individual. To establish an effective working alliance with women who seek treatment, the clinician must not only be knowledgeable in medicine but also be a good observer and an able communicator. With a biopsychosocial approach, the clinician sees a person and not a disease. Objectivity, compassion, and a nonbiased approach are essential principles that foster appropriate care. Often a multidisciplinary approach is useful in evaluating and managing patients when psychological issues are intertwined with their medical problems. This involves employing physicians along with nurses, social workers, and psychiatrists or psychologists in the process of evaluation and treatment.

This section presents an overview of the important normal and abnormal psychologic aspects of pregnancy and the puerperium, and describes some of the syndromes and clinical situations that tend to affect female patients. Clinicians should bear in mind that individual psychosocial overtones come to bear on each woman's underlying physiologic or pathologic processes.

MOTIVATIONS FOR PREGNANCY

Pregnancy may be a welcomed and fulfilling experience for many women, but not for all. Motivations for pregnancy are varied and complex, and only some of them are conscious. The desire for a pregnancy is not always the same as the wish for a child. For example, a pregnancy may be wanted to confirm one's sexual identity or to give proof of one's reproductive integrity and capability. Desire for a pregnancy may also be a response to loss or feelings of loneliness. A woman may have a child so that she will always have someone to love who will love her in return. She may wish to preserve a relationship with a partner or she may be responding to family or cultural pressures to have a baby. In adolescents, peer pressure, rebellion against family, and feelings of depression are frequent motivations for pregnancy. Toward the end of their reproductive years, women may feel pressured to conceive before their personal and professional lives are ready to incorporate a child. Many of these feelings also exist in men. In some cultures, children represent immortality for parents, and it is natural as they grow older for many people to hope that some part of them will live on in future generations. Regardless of the multifactorial forces that play a role in women's reproductive choices, many women face similar stresses as the stages of pregnancy unfold.

Pregnancy as a Developmental Transition

Pregnancy is a major developmental step in the lives of women, often providing fulfillment of deep and powerful wishes that allow creativity, self-realization, and an opportunity for new growth. While pregnancy may bring a sense of joy and well-being, it is also a stressful experience. Conflicts may arise. How a woman responds to pregnancy is related to her early childhood experiences, coping mechanisms, personality style, life situation, emotional supports, and physical problems.

The father-to-be is also presented with challenges and conflicts. Men may have unusual symptoms during their partner's pregnancy and visit physicians more often with complaints reflecting their own anxieties and concerns about their new role. Infidelity often manifests when the female partner is pregnant. Men may envy their partner's new condition, have conflicts with sexuality and pregnancy, or may feel threatened by the baby's potential to replace them as the mother's focus of attention.

Though prenatal classes, friendships, and office visits are useful ways for patients to learn about the process of pregnancy and alleviate fears, professional consultation may be necessary. With a full understanding of the psychologic aspects of pregnancy, an insightful physician will be able to identify these issues and help a patient navigate though this developmental stage.

Normal Psychologic Processes During Pregnancy and the Puerperium

The basic developmental and psychologic tasks of pregnancy vary with the stage of pregnancy. During the first trimester, the woman's main task is to incorporate the fetus—part of the woman and part of her partner—as an integral part of her body and self. Ultrasound has led to earlier maternal and paternal bonding. In the second trimester, with recognition of fetal movement, it is necessary to perceive the fetus as a separate entity and to begin to visualize the fetus as a baby with needs of its own. In the third trimester and postpartum, the patient comes to see herself as a mother and begins to establish a nurturing relationship with the infant. She may have to resolve some lingering conflicts with her own parents. Her relationship with her partner may also change for better or worse.

A. First Trimester

The diagnosis of a wanted pregnancy is usually accompanied by a sense of excitement and anxiety. Even the most wanted pregnancy may cause ambivalence on the part of both parents because of the recognized major life transition. An unplanned pregnancy is not necessarily unwanted and may be readily accepted. However, the woman and her partner need time to process their feelings and thoughts. If a termination is being considered, counseling should begin as soon as possible and without ambivalence on the part of the professional staff. Such counseling should allow the woman, and her partner if possible, to understand the implications of each of their possible choices and to weigh the risks, benefits, and alternatives before making a decision. If a physician is unable to provide an unbiased approach to counseling, the patient should be referred for appropriate counseling.

The first trimester, with its attendant fatigue, breast tenderness, nausea, and urinary frequency, is often accompanied by an increased preoccupation with self and with the growth of the fetus. There may be a sense of fulfillment and well-being, but emotions may be labile. Sexual interest may decline, while a desire for affection may increase. Concern about weight gain may manifest. Apprehension concerning miscarriage, the baby's health, and changing roles is common. Interestingly, even the most educated individuals may harbor superstitious beliefs that serve to help patients understand or feel control over the process of pregnancy.

B. Second Trimester

During the second trimester, there is an increased sense of well-being and the resumption of outside interests. Fetal movement, commencing at approximately 16–18 weeks, often results in a greater sense of reality about the pregnancy. The fetus is perceived as a separate entity, and the parents fantasize about how the baby will look. The mother may experience increased feelings of dependency; sexual desire varies greatly, and changes in body image may be distressing.

C. THIRD TRIMESTER

During the latter part of pregnancy, fear or anxiety about labor and delivery may increase. Concerns arise about pain, injury, and the baby's health; about being a responsive mother; and about how relationships may be changed. Sleep is often disturbed, and somatic preoccupations may increase.

Childbirth education is invaluable. Ideally the woman will be in a setting where she and her partner feel free to ask questions, regardless of how inconsequential she may think they are. Questions to the mother-to-be should be open-ended, not "yes" or "no" questions. For example, "What worries or concerns are you having?" is far more likely to evoke a meaningful response than "Do you have any concerns?"

Some difficulties arise when a woman does not fulfill her own expectations concerning birth options and delivery methods. For example, she may feel like a failure if she requires anesthesia or surgical intervention during labor and delivery. Prospective discussion of these issues may prevent the patient from placing value judgements on treatment options. It is essential to remind patients that the ultimate goal is having a healthy baby and a healthy mother. In high-risk pregnancies, a patient should have realistic expectations about her options and their implications before entering the labor and delivery floor.

There is an increasingly high parental expectation that modern obstetric technology will prevent anything untoward from disrupting their expectation of a positive birth experience. Because patients think of childbirth as a natural process, patients often have a limited understanding of the inherent dangers involved. For these reasons it is essential to obtain informed consent before performing procedures. Obtaining informed consent not only offers an opportunity for physicians to explain all of the risks, benefits, and alternatives to procedures, but it also allows patients to discuss their concerns and make their preferences clear. It is important to respect a patient's wishes and incorporate her desired approach whenever possible. Good communication is essential for an informed exchange. Patience in listening is an invaluable aid to lessening patient anxiety and fear and improving the chance of successful communication.

D. LABOR AND DELIVERY

Labor and delivery are unique experiences for each woman. The professional support team's goals are to enhance the health and safety of mother and infant, to free the mother from excessive pain or complications without complete loss of fulfillment, and to establish a strong and loving relationship among mother, infant, and family.

The emphasis today is on active mastery of the birth experience with as much patient participation as possible. However, women vary tremendously in their ability to meet this goal. Fear and unfamiliarity can increase tension and pain. Some of the fear can be reduced by childbirth education classes, relaxation techniques, knowledge of both usual and unusual obstetric procedures, and familiarity with hospital facilities and delivery rooms. The presence during the labor of the partner, a close friend, or a family member offers invaluable support to the mother. Even having a doula (female labor coach unknown to the patient) has been shown to improve a woman's birth experience and is associated with decreased epidural use. Pain is related not only to biologic factors, length of labor, and complications, but also to fear, past experiences with pain, personality, style of expression, and cultural factors. The reassuring presence of a labor companion and childbirth preparation classes can help the mother handle the pain of labor and delivery.

The patient's attitude during pregnancy may *not* be a good predictor of her psychologic status in labor. Giving up the unity, the oneness with the child, is reported by some women as a stressor. Fears exist about death, bodily injury, loss of adequacy or control, and especially about exposing bodily functions. While women should be encouraged to take an active part in both labor and delivery, some women don't want to.

The number of home births in the U.S. remains low. The major concern is that there may be complications that can be handled only in a hospital. One-third of infants requiring immediate intensive care after home deliveries have been products of normal pregnancies. While the safety of mother and infant must be the first concern, hospitals should strive to provide a more homelike and less institutional atmosphere for the birthing experience.

Electronic fetal monitoring during labor is now commonly employed. Some patients find this practice intrusive, while others find it reassuring. Women who have experienced prior fetal loss are more accepting of its presence and find it reduces their anxiety. However, highly technical equipment does not eliminate the possibility of complications, nor is it a replacement for human skill. More studies are needed to relate psychologic factors to obstetric progress and complications. Women who freely express their concerns may do better than passive patients who suppress them. Communication between physician and patient remains crucial.

E. PUERPERIUM

Mothering is a learned skill, but the attachment of mother and infant begins long before birth. The term **bonding** refers to a sensitive period after birth, during which interactions between mother and infant facilitate a powerful connection. The attachment direction is from mother to infant, making her a more effective parent. Early visual and physical contact between mother and baby facilitates the attachment. Attachment behaviors include fondling, kissing, cuddling, and gazing—practices that maintain contact between mother and infant. Factors that may interfere with early bonding include lack of instinctual response, psychologic problems, inadequate preparation, physical illness in mother or baby, and hospital practices that separate mother and infant. To facilitate early bonding, sedation and separation should be minimal. Separation may have physical, biologic, and emotional consequences. However, a mother should not believe she will be a failure because something has interfered with her earliest contact with her infant. There is evidence that later bonding is also successful.

Bonding is especially important for women and infants who may have attachment problems. Some of these high-risk individuals are mothers who are very young, ill, or ambivalent about pregnancy, or who have suffered child abuse, have relational difficulties with their partner, or have a psychiatric disorder. Intervention includes recognition of the problem and referral to an appropriately trained mental health professional.

The father's presence in the labor and delivery room has contributed to earlier father-infant bonding, but fathers must be prepared for attending the delivery and should have a role in it (eg, coaching the mother's efforts). Whether the father will be present when complications occur or when operative delivery is required should be discussed in advance.

F. TRANSITION TO MOTHERHOOD

As noted earlier, although mothering has instinctual roots, it is largely a learned behavior. A mother's early experiences with a loving caregiver in her own infancy strengthen her capacity for mothering. Mothers of young infants in our culture are often isolated from family and friends, which makes the early days even more difficult. During this stressful time, the new mother needs supportive individuals in her environment. It is helpful if the professional staff knows about unusual home circumstances. Indeed, an evaluation of this environment should be part of discharge planning. Will this new mother be alone or with numerous relatives? Are there religious or cultural practices that will interfere with sexuality, reproduction, nursing, or motherhood? Will this woman be returning to work? If

so, when? Finally, if she was known to the staff during the pregnancy, have her personality and coping ability undergone abrupt changes?

Breastfeeding may have advantages, but women who bottle feed their babies must not be made to feel guilty or inadequate.

It is helpful for a woman to review her labor and delivery with her physician if she feels she has performed inadequately—whatever the setting and procedures may have been. Such communication may be encouraged by asking the woman, "How do you feel about your labor and delivery?"

Sources of Stress in Pregnancy and the Puerperium

Endocrine, somatic, and psychologic changes contribute to making pregnancy and the puerperium times of stress. The confirmation of pregnancy may be thrilling for some but devastating for others. Indeed, some degree of ambivalence is probably the usual response.

Women with preexisting health problems may be concerned about withstanding the physical demands. Most healthy women have some physical distress from the discomforts of abdominal enlargement, nausea, heartburn, or urinary frequency. Most women also experience psychologic distress from worries about body image, genetic problems, and role changes as well as the effect of the pregnancy on her partner, career, education plans, finances, or her ability to be a mother. A worry often not voiced, especially by a primigravida, is "Can I do this?"

Interpersonal relationships with the patient's partner, mother, coworkers, and friends change during and after the pregnancy. Her partner's sexual satisfaction may decline during pregnancy. Women who are sexually responsive are more likely to enjoy sex during pregnancy. Pregnancy is a public statement of a woman's sexual activity, which may be a source of pride or embarrassment.

While anxiety, emotional lability, and worries are normal during this time, the ability to cope depends on each woman's life experiences, personality style, social supports, and the care and technical expertise of the obstetric staff.

A. DENIAL OF PREGNANCY

Good prenatal care improves pregnancy outcome. Early recognition of pregnancy by a woman and her family leads her to seek prenatal health care, take extra care of herself, eat well, and get sufficient rest. Denial of pregnancy may interfere with the patient obtaining proper care. The woman most prone to denial of pregnancy may be psychotic, have borderline personality, or be from an extremely rigid background. The denial is usually an unconscious process in which the individual keeps the unpleasant reality of an unwanted pregnancy out of her awareness. She is often joined in this negativity by family and, on rare occasions, by physicians. She may go through an entire pregnancy forgetting missed periods, and unaware of breast changes, abdominal enlargement, or fetal movements. She may present in the emergency room in labor or deliver the infant at home. With the birth, a psychotic reaction may occur. These neonates are at high risk for injury or death. Obviously, these women need extra support in the postnatal period and, if identified during the course of pregnancy, may benefit from psychologic assistance.

B. SEXUALITY

There are many variations in sexual functioning during pregnancy and the puerperium. In general, women note a decrease of sexual interest during the first trimester, which is related to fatigue, nausea, and a feeling of turning inward. Women without a history of miscarriage, genital bleeding, or dyspareunia need not fear that intercourse will harm the fetus. In the second trimester there is often an increased interest and desire for sexual experience. Many women have an increased wish to be held or to masturbate. Some become orgasmic for the first time, possibly because of increased pelvic vasocongestion.

In the third trimester, sexual interest and performance are even more variable. The woman may feel awkward and have increased fears of harming the fetus. If there are no obstetric complications or physical discomfort, intercourse is not contraindicated; there is no evidence that intercourse precipitates premature labor, although orgasm does cause uterine contractions. Some men lose their sexual interest during their partner's pregnancy, or they fear harming the fetus. Noncoital techniques can be satisfying to the couple. Couples should be told that oral-genital sex must not include air blown into the vagina as this practice may cause an air embolism, which is potentially fatal to mother and fetus.

Sexual desire postpartum may not return for many weeks or months. This may be due to new interest in the baby, fatigue, depression, hormonal status, or concerns about body image. Breastfeeding may alter sexual feelings in the new mother or her partner. Fathers may feel excluded. The obstetrician can be helpful to a couple by discussing changes in sexuality with them.

C. VOMITING IN PREGNANCY

Vomiting in pregnancy can have several causes: the same as those seen in the nonpregnant state (eg, influenza, viral disorders, drug reactions); hormonal changes in the first trimester, which affect approximately 50% of pregnant women and are not associated with any particular psychologic syndrome; preeclampsia, liver disease, or other obstetric complication; or hyperemesis gravidarum (pernicious vomiting of pregnancy). The latter is a severe form of nausea that may occur at any time during pregnancy. The woman may become severely dehydrated, lose weight, and have metabolic disturbances and electrolyte imbalances. The incidence in the U.S. is 1 in 1000 pregnancies.

Biologic, psychologic, and social etiologies have been suggested for hyperemesis gravidarum. Biologic causes, still unconfirmed, relate to endocrine, metabolic, or immune system disorders. There is some support for an association with multiple birth and past pregnancy loss. Psychologically, this condition is considered to be a somatization disorder in which dysphoric feelings or psychic conflicts are expressed via physical symptoms, which are much more acceptable in our culture. There is often a history of early life experience colored by abdominal pain and nausea. The condition is not related to any one psychiatric diagnosis, although more severe psychiatric illness may be present. Social stress may contribute to its severity.

Treatment may require rehydration, antiemetics, or antihistamines; hospitalization may be necessary. Many practitioners believe that the most effective aspect of hospitalization is actually isolating the patient from the stressors of her life at home. A good response has been noted with hypnosis and relaxation techniques. Identification of stress in the individual's life and help with stress reduction are often useful.

D. SLEEP IN PREGNANCY AND THE PUERPERIUM

Sleep disturbances during pregnancy and the puerperium are common. There is often increased sleepiness in the early prepartum period associated with high levels of estrogen and progesterone. In the postpartum period, a demanding infant together with decreased ovarian hormone levels may lead to sleep deficiency. During pregnancy and the puerperium, sleep latency, the frequency of awakening, and stage 0 sleep are increased; REM sleep is decreased. Hormonal fluctuations are related to sleep pattern changes. Medication should be used cautiously.

ADOLESCENT PREGNANCY: PSYCHOLOGIC ISSUES

Approximately 1 million adolescents 15–19 years old (one-tenth of all women in this age range in the U.S.) become pregnant each year, and 500,000 give birth. This high teenage pregnancy rate is due to many factors, including a subculture in which there is glorification of sexual activity without education of young people regarding its consequences. Other motivations for pregnancy in adolescence may be related to peer pressure, rebellion, keeping a relationship, and desiring more emotional intimacy. Adolescent girls rarely enjoy their early sexual experiences as boys do, and a large number of teenage mothers have been sexually abused. First intercourse often takes place within a relationship the girl wants to keep. Psychologic traits associated with contraceptive use in adolescents are high self-esteem, an orientation toward the future, feelings of control over life, and acceptance of the sexual self.

Three psychologic subsets of adolescent mothers have been described. The problem-prone use alcohol, drugs, or both, are truant from school, and get poor grades in school. They act on impulse and are often part of a peer counterculture that rejects conventional society. The adequate copers are competent and open to alternative lifestyles but characteristically go through life transitions at an earlier age than their peers. The depressed idealize pregnancy as a way of dealing with their feelings of loss, sadness, and emptiness. It is useful to distinguish among these 3 groups and to offer assistance in response to their various needs.

Adolescents often strain the patience of health care personnel because they may be difficult to talk with, have values very different from those of the staff, arrive late for prenatal care, or be noncompliant. If the physician understands preadult development and sexuality well, adolescent care can be extremely gratifying. The importance of taking a responsible approach to prenatal care should be stressed. Counseling adolescents requires an ability to educate and communicate with them while offering privacy and confidentiality.

PSYCHIATRIC DISORDERS OF PREGNANCY AND THE PUERPERIUM

Pregnancy and the puerperium are emotionally stressful periods for many women. Mood swings are commonly manifested by emotional lability, weepiness, irritability, and feeling blue or high. Prenatal assessment for psychological difficulties should include the following:

(1) Prior personal or family history of psychiatric illness.

(2) Psychiatric disorder.

(3) Psychologic problems that accompanied maturational periods, eg, puberty.

(4) History of early maternal deprivation or mother's death.

(5) Difficulty separating from parents.

(6) Conflicts about mothering.

(7) Marital or family difficulties, including separation.

(8) Past difficulty with pregnancy, delivery, or postpartum depression.

(9) Recent death of family member or close friend.

(10) Familial or congenital disorders.

(11) History of infertility.

(12) History of repeat abortion.

(13) History of pseudocyesis or hyperemesis.

(14) Prior fetal death, miscarriage, or congenital abnormality.

(15) History of sexual, physical, or emotional abuse, current or past.

(16) History of premenstrual syndrome.

Psychiatric disorders during pregnancy and in the puerperium have been described throughout history, though there is disagreement as to whether these disorders are the same or different from those occurring at other times. Since untreated maternal mental illness is associated with deleterious effects on maternal-infant attachment and synchrony and child development, it is essential to diagnose and appropriately treat psychologic disorders that afflict pregnant patients. Though some psychotropic medications appear to be safe when used in breast-feeding mothers, few randomized controlled trials have been performed. For this reason, it is important to involve a pediatrician in the infant's care when treating a breastfeeding mother with psychotropic medications.

Depressive Disorders

The term **depression** refers to a mood, symptom, or group of syndromes. The mood—feeling "blue"—is part of human experience related to sadness, frustration, discouragement, and of feeling "down." Many women experience such moods, to greater or lesser degrees, in the weeks following delivery. The **symptom** can be part of another physical or psychologic illness such as alcoholism, schizophrenia, or viral illness. The **syndrome,** known as a major depressive or affective disorder, is characterized by a specific set of symptoms associated with a change in mood. This lasts for a period of at least 2 weeks and is severe enough to interfere with activities of daily living. The severity can vary considerably, from a very mild transient period of feeling blue, such as in the postpartum period (blues); to major clinical depression with vegetative signs and symptoms but normal reality testing; to severe psychotic depressions with hallucinations, delusions, and a possibility of suicide or infanticide. In the first 2 weeks to few months postpartum, most new mothers report feeling tired, weepy, moody, anxious about caring for a new baby, trapped, afraid, angry at the baby's father and at the baby, and guilty at having hostile thoughts. This has been called the "new mother syndrome." Treatment consists of support from family, health care providers, and other mothers. Generally the depressive reactions may be divided into 2 types.

A. POSTPARTUM BLUES

This condition (also called 3-day blues or baby blues) is a transitory mood disturbance following delivery (within 2 weeks) and usually occurs at the height of hormonal changes. It is frequent, occurring in about 50–85% of women. It is characterized by irritability, sensitivity to criticism, despondence, anxiety, sadness, or elation. It is unrelated to the health of mother or baby, obstetric complications, hospitalization, social class, or breast- or formula-feeding, although any of these factors can affect the patient's mood. It occurs cross-culturally but is less noticeable in cultures where emotions are expressed freely and when relatives and friends surround the new mother offering care and support. It may last a few days to 2–3 weeks. Though it is generally self-limited and does not require treatment, 20% of women who suffer from this disorder will go on to develop depression in the first postpartum year.

B. MAJOR DEPRESSION

This condition is a nonpsychotic depressive syndrome during pregnancy but most commonly occurs in the weeks and months after delivery. The incidence of moderate depression is 10–15%. Its symptoms include change in mood, sleep patterns, eating, mental concentration, or libido, and may involve somatic preoccupations, phobias, and fear of harming self or infant.

Discussion of her feelings may offer relief. To facilitate such discussion, a woman with symptoms of moderate depression should be asked about her symptoms. To elicit suicidal or homicidal ideas, the physician might ask "Have you felt so overwhelmed or that you might hurt yourself or your baby?" There seem to be few predictive factors, but there is a higher occurrence in women with past psychiatric disorders, family history of such disorders, life event and partner problems, and possibly the premenstrual syndrome. Depressions during pregnancy may differ from those occurring postpartum, but the exact nature of the differences is unclear.

Postpartum depression has a high rate of recurrence in subsequent pregnancies. Mental health consultation is advisable. Treatment may include providing the mother with environmental support, psychotherapy (with the partner included when possible), and antidepressant medication (carefully weighed against adverse effects in a pregnant or lactating woman). Suicidal or homicidal patients should be assessed immediately and should not be left alone. Hospitalization may be necessary.

Postpartum Psychoses

Postpartum psychoses occur in 1–2 per 1000 births. These are severe mental illnesses, usually requiring admission to mental hospitals because of delusions and the concern that the woman may harm herself or the infant. They are most frequently depressive illnesses (70–80%) but must be differentiated from schizophrenia or organic brain disease. Contributing factors include a family history of mental illness, past psychiatric disorders, marital and family problems, recent stressful life situations, and a lack of social supports, although none of these risk factors may be present. No single obstetric complication imposes a higher risk for these disorders. These individuals appear to be biologically vulnerable to mental disease. The discovery of neurotransmitter disorders, predominantly involving dopamine, in these patients has led to the development of useful medications. Risk of recurrence in subsequent pregnancies may be as high as 20–30%.

Symptoms develop most commonly from a few days to 4–6 weeks postpartum, although a careful history often reveals that the illness began in the third trimester of pregnancy. The woman may become restless, unable to sleep, irritable, have pressured speech, or become very withdrawn. Drug dependency, endocrinopathies such as thyroid disease, and other neurologic disorders must be ruled out.

Most postpartum psychoses are similar to those seen in nonpregnant women, although atypical disorders may not fit traditional classifications. Women at high risk for psychotic states are those with a past history of psychosis. Other symptomatologies to be followed closely after delivery are confusion, sleep disorders, increased emotional lability, unusual behavior, and obsessional or delusional thinking. Infant injury or infanticide by the mother is rare but does occur. Treatment of affective disorders is with antidepressant drugs or lithium and care in a psychiatric care facility.

Schizophrenia is a psychiatric disorder of at least 6 months' duration characterized in its acute phase by delusions, hallucinations, incoherent speech, catatonia, or flat affect. Generally, the level of the individual's function declines, with withdrawal and social isolation. The onset is usually during adolescence or young adulthood. Genetic as well as environmental and psychologic factors are involved. Schizophrenic women may have exacerbations during pregnancy and the puerperium and should be carefully monitored. Delusions in pregnancy often relate to bodily changes and fetal movements. The disease is considered to have an organic basis with biochemical abnormalities, and drug treatment is usually with neuroleptic antipsychotics such as phenothiazones, butyrophenones, and thioxanthenes. A psychiatric referral is indicated. Suicidal risk should be assessed.

Organic brain disease (delirium, organic brain syndrome) is often confused with acute psychosis. Toxic states, drugs, metabolic disorders, infection, and hemorrhage can cause neurodysfunction. There may be impairment of orientation, memory, intellectual function, and judgment as well as emotional lability. The individual is usually conscious and symptoms fluctuate. A neuropsychiatric consultation is indicated. It is best to avoid sedative drugs until an evaluation and diagnosis are made and treatment of the underlying disorder is begun.

In-hospital management includes keeping the surroundings familiar, the room well lit, and the woman oriented by using her name. The clinician must be alert to changes in mood, behavior, and thinking.

Psychoses require specialized psychiatric care, but a patient who becomes acutely disturbed or confused requires emergency management until the psychiatric consultation can be performed. Such patients can be divided into 5 categories according to the following features:

(1) Acute psychoses with disordered thought, hallucinations, and fear, possibly due to psychotic illness or drug reaction.

(2) Delirium due to an underlying medical problem with fluctuating disorientation to time, place, and person.

(3) Severe anxiety with somatic symptoms.

(4) Anger and belligerence with or without alcohol or drug abuse.

(5) Depression with suicidal ideas.

A medical and drug history should be obtained from relatives or friends. Accuracy diagnosis is essential (eg, insulin shock in a diabetic may be confused with psychogenic seizures). If possible, a blood sample should be drawn for drug and toxicity screening. The patient is calmed, and a relative or friend may remain with her unless she becomes violent. In such instances, security personnel should be alerted and the patient transferred to a psychiatric care facility as quickly as possible. Haloperidol may be given orally or parenterally to facilitate immediate management.

Anxiety Disorders in Pregnancy

Anxiety during pregnancy and the puerperium is normal; its total absence is as pathologic as is its excess. When anxiety increases enough to be considered a disorder, there are 2 major classifications: phobic disorders and anxiety state disorders. Phobic disorders include persistent and irrational fear of a specific object, activity, or situation that may lead to avoidance. In pregnancy, women with these disorders have irrational fears (eg, nonsubstantiated worries about food that might harm the fetus). Treatment ranges from simple reassurance to behavior modification.

Anxiety states are divided into 3 categories. Panic disorders include recurrent attacks of anxiety with sudden onset of intense fear and apprehension. There may be physical symptoms such as dyspnea, chest pains, palpitations, choking, and dizziness. Attacks may last minutes to hours with anxiety between attacks. They are thought to have a biochemical basis, but there is often a precipitating event. Their occurrence in pregnancy is not uncommon. Panic disorders may be part of the syndrome of depression. Treatment, if necessary, is with anxiolytics such as alprazolam.

Generalized anxiety disorders last a month or more with signs of motor tension, vigilance, scanning, autonomic hyperactivity, and apprehension. Other conditions causing anxiety must be ruled out.

Patients with obsessive compulsive disorder have ideas or thoughts that make them do or over-do certain things. In pregnancy, these may relate to harming the fetus or the infant after birth. This disorder may interfere with function and compliance. Diagnosis and therapy by a mental health professional are usually necessary.

Posttraumatic Stress Disorder (PTSD)

After an emotionally traumatic experience some patients develop a constellation of symptoms typical of posttraumatic stress disorder (PTSD). These symptoms include a sense of recurrently experiencing the event (flashbacks, dreams), avoiding stimuli associated with the trauma (activities, people, places), and heightened arousal (anxiety, irritability, trouble concentrating). Treatments include cognitive behavioral therapy and medical therapy with SSRIs. The traumatic event may have been a traumatic medical experience, fetal loss, infertility, sexual assault, or the death of a close relative or friend that the patient associates with pregnancy or labor.

When counseling a woman with any of the above disorders, the clinician needs to address several questions: Is there a medical condition causing the disorder? Is there a basic psychiatric disorder such as depression or schizophrenia present? Does substance abuse complicate the clinical presentation? Is this patient abusing alcohol or other drugs? Consultation with a mental health professional is recommended.

Psychotropic Medications During Pregnancy and Lactation

When SSRIs were first developed and their effects on pregnant women and the fetus were unknown, it was generally advised to avoid antidepressants in pregnancy. Only severely depressed patients were offered medical treatment for their depression in while pregnant. Retrospective reviews of this care and a few prospective studies have revealed that neither tricyclic antidepressants nor SSRIs are teratogens or are associated with adverse pregnancy outcomes.

Of note, TCAs occasionally cause a withdrawal syndrome in the fetus. As for breastfeeding while taking SSRIs, detectable levels are noted in breast milk. However, large studies have not been performed and long-term sequelae of SSRI exposure from breast milk is unknown. Breast feeding should be discontinued if lithuim is utilized. As a general rule, a patient and her physician should carefully discuss the risks and benefits on a case-by-case basis before prescribing psychotropic drugs in pregnancy and during lactation. Psychiatric consultation may be an important component of your evaluation, assessment, and planning.

Substance and Alcohol Abuse

Substance abuse can cause major problems in pregnancy and the puerperium. These problems may be mild or may be severe enough to lead to fetal abnormalities, morbidity, and death of infant and mother. Therefore, inquiry concerning drug use should be made during prenatal visits and documented in the record.

Management of Psychiatric Illness in Pregnancy and Lactation

Psychotropic drugs should be avoided if at all possible during pregnancy and lactation. However, there are many instances when this is not possible because there are psychiatric illnesses present that require medication. Nonpharmacologic methods such as psychotherapy, cognitive behavioral therapies, family and marital treatment, and even psychiatric hospitalization may be indicated before medications are used. A major problem is that there are few good data on the effects of these drugs on the fetus.

An antipsychotic drug of choice might be haloperidol in the lowest effective dosage and avoided in the first trimester. It may be used for the treatment of psychosis. SSRIs may be utilized when a depressive disorder is of significant enough magnitude to require medication. Lithium and carbamazepine should be avoided because of their teratogenic effects. If they must be used, patients should be warned of their possible harm, and these patients should be carefully monitored.

GRIEF & GRIEVING: PERINATAL LOSS

Despite modern medical technology, there is still significant pregnancy loss due to spontaneous abortion, stillbirth, or neonatal death. Relinquishment of a baby for adoption may have the same psychologic effects as loss due to death. While the fetus is in utero it becomes perceived by the mother as part of herself. Death of a fetus or baby is often felt to be a loss of part of the mother's self. Grief is the process of adapting to such a loss by detaching little by little through anger, pain, and sadness. The mother and father may feel an emptiness. Thoughtless comments such as "You can always have another," "You didn't know the baby anyway," or "Plan another pregnancy right away" may only serve to increase the couple's emotional pain.

Parents grieve for the lost fetus or infant in their own way and in their own time. One difficulty in grieving for a lost pregnancy is the lack of identification that is useful in detaching from a known person. Parents should be encouraged to make their own decisions concerning seeing or holding the baby, disposition of the remains (burial or cremation), religious observances, and naming the baby. They should not be discouraged from seeing a malformed infant; they often recall the positive aspects. Photos may be obtained if desired. Autopsies often give parents more information about the normal as well as the abnormal features. Mothers, perhaps more than fathers, suffer from guilt and helplessness. Participation in decision making can help them achieve more control in dealing with their loss.

Physicians may also feel helpless and sad. They must talk with patients, give them as much information as possible and assure them (if possible) that nothing the mother did caused the fetal or infant demise. Often, the anger that is part of the grieving process is displaced to hospital staff, especially physicians. It is important to deal with each set of parents individually, to meet with them, and encourage them to grieve in their own way. If severe grief persists beyond several months, psychiatric consultation should be obtained.

PSEUDOCYESIS

Pseudocyesis is a syndrome in which a nonpregnant woman believes she is pregnant and develops signs and symptoms suggestive of pregnancy. Pseudocyesis is a conversion reaction in which a psychic conflict is expressed in physical terms. It is an example of how a false belief may affect physiologic processes. It has been known since ancient times, and many cases have been described in women aged 7–79 years. The most common symptoms include menstrual abnormalities (oligomenorrhea, amenorrhea), abdominal enlargement, and breast changes. There may be nausea and vomiting. On examination, the uterus is not enlarged; the abdomen is firm to palpation and often tympanic to percussion. "Fetal movement" has been reported; it is usually intestinal activity or unconscious contractions of abdominal muscles. A supposed fetal heart rate may be maternal tachycardia. Galactorrhea may be present because of increased prolactin levels from other causes (ie, pituitary adenomas), long-term breast stimulation, or use of drugs such as phenothiazines. There are usually neuroendocrine abnormalities (eg, hypothalamic amenorrhea). Duration varies from 9 months to several years. Diagnosis of true pregnancy can be obtained with pregnancy tests and ultrasonography. However, negative test results may not convince a woman with this syndrome that she is not pregnant.

The clinical variants of pseudocyesis include "true" pseudocyesis, which should be distinguished from psychosis in women in whom the false belief in pregnancy is a delusion; factitious illness in which the woman knows she is not pregnant but simulates pregnancy for some secondary gain (eg, to keep a straying partner); organic diseases such as a pelvic tumor; and iatrogenic pseudopregnancy caused by administration of human chorionic gonadotropin to produce positive pregnancy tests in infertile women.

Management consists of a careful history, physical examination, and laboratory tests to rule out pregnancy and organic disease. Psychologic assessment and treatment are also indicated.

THE REFERRAL PROCESS

Referral to mental health professionals may be indicated for any psychologic processes the gynecologist believes to be beyond his or her ability, training, or willingness to treat. The gynecologist may prefer to work closely with a psychiatrist, psychologist, social worker, or psychiatric nurse. The attitude taken should be comfort in the feeling that counseling would be helpful, not that the patient is bothersome and therefore should be labeled or stigmatized by such referrals. Consultation-liaison psychiatrists have expertise in the psychologic aspects of medical and surgical problems as well as in the use of psychopharmacologic drugs. Most hospital staffs include social workers and psychiatric nurses who specialize in psychosocial issues. Marriage counselors offer much to those with relationship problems. As with obstetrics, the biopsychosocial approach is extremely useful.

REFERENCES

Psychologic Aspects of Obstetrics

Bryant RA, Friedman M: Mediation and non-medication treatment of post-traumatic stress disorder. Curr Opin Psychiatry 1999;14:119.

Ling FW: Randomized controlled trial of depot leuprolide in patients with chronic pelvic pain and clinically suspected endometriosis. Pelvic Pain Study Group. Obstet Gynecol 1999;93:51.

Schoen C et al: The Commonwealth Fund Survey of the Health of Adolescent Girls. The Commonwealth Fund, 1997.

Wisner KL et al: Pharmacologic treatment of depression during pregnancy. JAMA 1999;282:1264.

Psychologic Aspects of Gynecology

Barbach L: *For Yourself: The Fulfillment of Female Sexuality*. Doubleday, 1975.

Basson R et al: Report of the International Consensus Development Conference on Female Sexual Dysfunction: Definitions and classifications. J Urol 2000;163:888.

Gordon N et al: Effects of providing hospital-based doulas in HMOs. Obstet Gynecol 1999;93:422.

Grimes D: Role of the cervix in sexual response: Evidence for and against. Clin Obstet Gynecol 1999;42:972.

Kylstra W: Sexual outcomes following treatment for early stage gynecologic cancer: A prospective multicenter study. Int J Gynecologic Cancer 1999;9:387.

Masters W, Johnson V: *Human Sexual Inadequacy*. Little, Brown, 1970.

Montejo-Gonzalez AL et al: SSRI-induced sexual dysfunction: fluoxetine, paroxetine, sertraline and fluvoxamine in a prospective, multi-center and descriptive clinical study of 344 patients. J Sexual Ther 1997;23:176.

Rhodes J, Kjerulff K: Hysterectomy and sexual functioning. JAMA 1999;282:1934.

Singer ID: Patients are talking about Viagra. Strategic Med 1998;2:42.

Stewart DE et al: Psychosocial aspects of chronic clinically unconfirmed vulvovaginitis. Obstet Gynecol 1990;76:852.

Vivien K et al: The use of psychotropics during breast-feeding. Am J Psychiatry 2001;158:1001.

Walsh JM, Wheat ME, Freund K: Detection, evaluation, and treatment of eating disorders: the role of the primary care physician. J Gen Intern Med 2000;15:577.

Domestic Violence And Sexual Assault

60

Michael C. Lu, MD, MPH, Jessica S. Lu, MPH, & Vivian P. Halfin, MD

For many victims of domestic violence and sexual assault, the first contact with the health care system is with the obstetrician-gynecologist or primary care doctor. Therefore, it is critical that these physicians be knowledgeable in the identification, evaluation, and treatment of such patients.

DOMESTIC VIOLENCE

While the home is often thought of as a safe haven, it is the site of the most common manifestations of violence in our society today. Domestic or intimate partner violence typically refers to violence perpetrated against adolescent and adult females within the context of family or intimate relationships. Although victims of domestic violence may be male or female, 90–95% of the victims are women. It is a behavior pattern that is manifested in physical and sexual attacks, as well as psychological and economic coercion. The abuser utilizes the behavior in order to establish and maintain domination and control over the victim. Because abuse is usually accompanied by shame and guilt, the victim often does not report the abuse.

As a result of significant underreporting, it is difficult to compile exact data on the incidence of domestic violence. Every year, approximately 4–5 million women are believed to be battered by their intimate partners. Violence by an intimate partner accounts for about 21% of all the violent crime experienced by women. More than 40% of all female murder victims are murdered by their husbands, boyfriends or ex-partners. It is estimated that at least one-fifth of all American women will be physically assaulted by a partner or ex-partner during their lifetime.

Violent acts may include threats, throwing objects, pushing, kicking, hitting, beating, sexual assault, and threatening with or using a weapon. Domestic violence frequently includes verbal abuse, intimidation, progressive social isolation, and deprivation of things such as food, money, transportation, or access to health care. The violence typically occurs in a predictable, progressive cycle. The tension-building phase is characterized by arguing and blaming as anger intensifies. This leads to the battering phase that may involve verbal threats,

sexual abuse, physical battering, and use of weapons. The battering phase is followed by a honeymoon phase during which the abuser may deny the violence, make excuses for battering, apologize, buy gifts, and promise never to do it again, until the next cycle begins. While unemployment, poverty, and alcohol and substance abuse increase the likelihood of abuse, domestic violence cuts across all racial, ethnic, religious, educational, and socioeconomic lines. Domestic violence often occurs within a framework of family violence that can include child abuse, elder abuse, or abuse of adults who are disabled. It is estimated that child abuse occurs in 33–77% of families where adults are abused.

Clinical Presentation

Survivors of domestic violence or sexual abuse may present to health care professionals in a variety of clinical settings. The prevalence of domestic violence among patients in ambulatory care settings has been estimated to be between 20% and 30%.

Such patients commonly report chronic pelvic pain to their gynecologists. A history of sexual abuse has been found in significantly more women with chronic pelvic pain as compared with other gynecologic conditions. Others may complain of sexual dysfunctions such as decreased interest or arousal, dyspareunia, or anorgasmia. Incest victims have a very high rate of sexual dysfunction and may avoid sex or seek it out compulsively. Still others may present with chronic or recurrent vaginitis. Some women may present for a routine gynecologic appointment but become anxious and tearful before or during the pelvic examination.

Some women present to their primary care physicians with persistent multiple bodily complaints, such as chronic headaches, palpitations, abdominal complaints, or sleep and appetite disturbances. Eating disorders may be more common among abuse victims. Others may have a somatoform disorder. This condition is characterized by physical symptoms suggesting a physical condition for which there are no demonstrable organic findings or physiologic mechanisms. In the face of a negative work-up, there may be evidence or presumption that the symptoms are linked to psychologi-

1087

cal factors or conflicts. Women who meet the criteria for somatoform disorder often have a history of abuse.

In a mental health setting, victims of domestic violence or sexual assault may note feeling depressed or suicidal. They may have anxiety or sleep disorders that they may self-medicate with alcohol or other substances. Most commonly, these women may have post-traumatic stress disorder (PTSD), which occurs in individuals who have experienced a psychologically distressing event that is outside the range of usual human experience. Symptoms of PTSD include re-experiencing the traumatic event through intrusive memories, dreams, flashbacks, or exposure to events symbolic of the trauma. Patients with PTSD also exhibit a "psychic numbing," ie, they are detached from other people and have difficulty feeling emotions, especially those associated with intimacy or sexuality. Other clinical syndromes include personality disorders characterized by maladaptive character traits. In very extreme cases, patients may have multiple personality disorder (MPD), characterized by having two or more distinct personalities existing within them. This disorder is marked by a disturbance in the normally integrated functions of identity, memory, and consciousness as the result of dissociation from traumatic experiences.

The problem of domestic violence in pregnancy merits special mention because it is a threat to both the mother and her developing fetus. Estimates of prevalence of domestic violence in pregnancy are in the range of 1–20%, with most studies identifying rates between 4% and 8%. These estimates suggest that violence is a more common problem for pregnant women than preeclampsia, gestational diabetes, and placenta previa, conditions for which pregnant women are routinely screened and evaluated. Some evidence suggests that violence may escalate during pregnancy, especially in the postpartum period. Abuse is associated with increased physical and psychological stress, inadequate prenatal care utilization, poor nutrition and weight gain, and increased maternal behavioral risks (cigarette, alcohol, and substance abuse). These may lead to problems with fetal growth and development. Physical trauma can cause abruptio placentae, preterm labor, preterm premature rupture of membranes, and maternal and fetal injuries and demise.

Diagnosis & Treatment

Although battered women seek medical care frequently, as few as one in 20 are correctly identified by the practitioner to whom they turn for help. Barriers to diagnosis include practitioners' lack of knowledge or training, lack of recognition of the widespread prevalence of the problem, time constraints, fear of offending the patient, and a feeling of powerlessness in the area of treatment.

Research suggests that the use of abuse assessment questions on standard medical records may increase screening and documentation. In addition, since many women will not voluntarily disclose abuse, asking each patient directly about prior or ongoing victimization increases the likelihood of disclosure.

The screening assessment should be prefaced with a statement to establish that screening is universal, such as, "I would like to ask you a few questions about physical, sexual, and emotional trauma because we know that these are common and affect women's health." Direct questioning using behaviorally-specific phrasing should follow:

- Has anyone close to you ever threatened to hurt you?
- Has anyone ever hit, kicked, choked, or hurt you physically?
- Has anyone, including your partner, ever forced you to have sex?
- Are you ever afraid of your partner?

Disclosure rates will be higher when the questions are asked face to face by the health care provider rather than through a questionnaire, and when behaviorally-specific descriptions rather than the terms "abuse," "domestic violence," or "rape" are used. Abuse victims are often accompanied to health care appointments by the perpetrator, who may appear overprotective or overbearing, and may answer questions directed toward the woman. It is important to ask the patient questions in private, apart from the male partner. It is also important to ask the patient questions apart from children, family, or friends, and to avoid using them as interpreters when asking questions about violence.

In the office setting, the most effective and efficient strategy for providing assistance to a woman who has disclosed abuse involves acknowledging and documenting the trauma, assessing immediate safety and establishing a safety plan, and providing patient education and referrals to community support services. An essential first step is to acknowledge the trauma. It is important to reinforce to the victim that she is not to blame because many victims have trouble believing that they are not responsible for the abuse.

Documenting domestic violence is no different from documenting other patient interactions, but such documentation may provide important supportive evidence in the courtroom to put an end to the violence. Direct quotations of the patient's explanation of her injuries should be recorded. Photographs may be taken after consent is granted. Every effort should be made to maintain confidentiality to avoid retaliation by the perpetrators when they suspect disclosure of abuse. The physician or health care professional may be required by state law to report actual or suspected domestic violence.

Once domestic violence is acknowledged and documented, the next step is to assess immediate safety and to establish a safety plan. Lethality of the violence should be assessed by asking questions such as:

- Has your partner ever threatened to kill you or your children?
- Are there weapons in the house?
- Does your partner abuse alcohol or use drugs?
- Is it safe for you to go home?
- Are the children (or other dependents) safe?

If the violence has escalated to the point where she is afraid for her safety or that of her children, she should be offered shelter.

An important step in addressing ongoing violence is to help the victim establish a safety plan. The American College of Obstetricians and Gynecologists (www.acog. org) distributes pocket cards with suggested steps for making an exit plan. These cards can be handed to the patient or left in patient restrooms where a woman can pick it up without concern of being seen by an accompanying partner.

Providing educational materials about domestic violence and its consequences can sometimes help victims take action toward ending the violence. These materials demonstrate to women that their physicians' offices are both a resource and a safe place should they decide to take action. A list of referral resources should be readily available in medical offices. The list should include telephone numbers for police departments, emergency departments, shelters for battered women, rape crisis centers, counseling services, self-help programs, and advocacy agencies that can provide legal, financial, and emotional support.

Given the high rate of psychiatric symptomatology in this population, referral for psychiatric screening and counseling can be useful. Patients who are experiencing posttraumatic stress disorder can benefit from psychotherapy and possibly medication as well. Those with depression, substance abuse, or anxiety, personality, or dissociative disorders will also require ongoing treatment. Psychiatrists or other mental health professionals can serve to coordinate a variety of treatment modalities for the victims: individual, couples, and family therapy, detoxification and substance abuse treatment, and advocacy groups.

Despite the best efforts of physicians and other health care professionals, some women may initially be unable to extirpate themselves from victimization. For such women, an encounter with a health care system that they experience as nonblaming, accessible, and supportive will help maximize the chances of their making a positive life change at some future point.

SEXUAL ASSAULT

Sexual assault is any sexual act performed by one person on another without the person's consent. Sexual assault includes genital, oral, or anal penetration by a part of the accused's body or by an object. It may result from force, the threat of force either on the victim or another person, or the victim's inability to give appropriate consent. Many states have now adopted the gender-neutral legal term *sexual assault* in favor of *rape,* which has traditionally referred to forced vaginal penetration of a woman by a male assailant.

An estimated 700,000 to 1,000,000 American women are sexually assaulted every year. These estimates are higher than official crime reports because the majority of cases go unreported. According to one estimate, only 30% of rapes are reported to the police, and 50% of rape victims tell no one. At least 20% of adult women, 15% of college-age women, and 12% of adolescent girls have experienced sexual abuse and assault during their lifetime. Sexual assault occurs in all age, racial-ethnic, and socioeconomic groups, but its incidence may be higher for African American women and for adolescent females. In several studies, about one-fourth to one-half of the victims of sexual assault were under the age of 18. The very young, the elderly, and the physically or developmentally disabled may be particularly vulnerable to sexual assault.

Several variants of sexual assault deserve special mentioning. **Marital rape** is defined as forced coitus or related sexual acts within a marital relationship without the consent of a partner. **Acquaintance rape** refers to those sexual assaults committed by someone known to the victim. More than 75% of adolescent rapes are committed by an acquaintance of the victim. When the acquaintance is a family member, including step-relatives and parental figures living in the home, the sexual assault is referred to as **incest.** When the forced or unwanted sexual activity occurs in the context of a dating relationship, it is referred to as **date rape.** In this situation, the woman may voluntarily participate in sexual play but coitus occurs, often forcibly, without her consent. Alcohol use is frequently associated with date rape. "Date rape drugs" such as flunitrazepam (Rohypnol) and gamma hydroxybutyrate (GHB) have also been used to diminish a woman's ability to consent or to remember the assault.

Statutory rape refers to sexual intercourse with a female under an age specified by state law (ranging from 14–18 years of age); the consent of an adolescent younger than this age is legally irrelevant because she is defined as being incapable of consenting. **Child sexual**

abuse is defined as contact or interaction between a child and an adult when the child is being used for the sexual stimulation of that adult or another person. All 50 states and the District of Columbia mandate reporting of child abuse, including child sexual abuse. Nearly half of the states also require physicians to report statutory rape. Physicians should be familiar with the laws in their states; failure to report sexual assault against children may subject the physicians to fines and incarceration for up to 1 year.

Our society has many misperceptions about sexual assault. The victims are often blamed for having encouraged the assault by their behavior or dress, not sufficiently resisting the assault, being promiscuous, or having ulterior motives for pressing charges. This misplaced culpability is often internalized by the victims, which (in addition to fear of retribution) may explain their reluctance to report the violent crime to the authorities. Another common misperception is that rape is an impulsive or aggressive extension of normal sex drive on the part of the rapist. The motivation for most sexual assault, however, seems not to be sexual gratification but rather degradation, terrorization, and humiliation of the victim. The assault is often a demonstration of power (power rape), anger (anger rape), or sadism manifested in ritualized torture or mutilation of the victim (sadistic rape) on the part of the rapist.

Clinical Presentation

The majority of rape victims who come to emergency rooms do not openly admit to having been sexually assaulted. Instead, they may complain of having been mugged or may voice concerns about AIDS or other sexually transmitted diseases. Others may present with psychiatric symptoms including depression, anxiety, or a suicide attempt. Unless the primary care physician, obstetrician-gynecologist, or psychiatrist obtains a sexual history, assault victims will remain unidentified as such, and will therefore be inadequately treated.

A "rape-trauma" syndrome often occurs after a sexual assault. The initial response (acute phase) may last for hours or days and is characterized by a distortion or paralysis of the individual's coping mechanisms. The initial outward responses vary from complete loss of emotional control (crying, angry) to an unnatural calm and detachment (although some physical signs such as shaking or lowered skin temperature are usually present). The latter behavior represents the victim's need to reestablish control over herself and her environment while simultaneously abandoning the defense mechanism of denial and allowing the renewed invasion of privacy represented by the questioning and examination. The initial reactions of shock, numbness, withdrawal and denial typically abate after the first 2 weeks.

However, studies suggest there is a period, occurring from 2 weeks to several months postassault, in which symptomatology returns and may intensify. It is at this time that the victim may begin to seek help for her symptoms, often without telling the health care provider of the sexual assault that precipitated these symptoms.

The next phase (delayed phase) may occur months or years after the sexual assault and is characterized by chronic anxiety, feelings of vulnerability, loss of control, and self-blame. Long-term reactions include anxiety, nightmares, flashbacks, catastrophic fantasies, feelings of alienation and isolation, sexual dysfunction, psychological distress, mistrust of others, phobias, depression, hostility, and somatic symptoms. More than half of rape victims experience substantial difficulty in reestablishing sexual and emotional relationships with spouses or boyfriends. Thirty-three to fifty percent of victims report suicidal ideation; suicide attempts have been reported in nearly one in five rape victims not seeking treatment.

PTSD is a common long-term sequela of sexual assault, characterized by psychic numbing, intrusive reexperiencing of the trauma, avoidance of stimuli associated with the trauma, and intense psychological distress. Women with prior victimization histories often have more severe sequela. Women assaulted sexually by family members or dates experience as severe levels of distress as women assaulted by acquaintances or strangers.

Up to 40% of victims who are sexually assaulted sustain injuries. While most injuries are minor, about 1% of the injuries require hospitalization and major operative repair, and 0.1% are fatal. Somatic symptoms are common during the acute phase and include disturbed sleeping and eating patterns, gastrointestinal irritability (with nausea predominating), musculoskeletal soreness, fatigue, tension headaches, and intense startle reactions. Symptoms of vaginal irritation occur in more than 50% of victims, and rectal pain and bleeding are frequent in patients subjected to anal penetration. Ongoing health concerns include gynecological trauma, risk of pregnancy, and the potential for contracting infections or sexually transmitted diseases, including HIV. Victims may also seek to escape the pain of rape's effects through the use of alcohol and drugs.

Rape victims appear to be frequent users of medical services in the months and years following the assault. In one study, visits to physicians increased 18% in the year of the assault, 56% in the following year, and 31% in the year after, compared to previctimization levels. Reintegration of the self following sexual assault is a slow process that may take months to years as the victim works through the trauma and the loss of the event and replaces it with other life experiences. The prognosis for complete recovery is improved if health care professionals responsible for the victim's care have a supportive, nonjudgmental approach and a well-developed understanding and competent treatment of the emotional, as well as physical, consequences of sexual assault.

Diagnosis & Treatment

The physician evaluating the victim has both medical and legal responsibilities, and should be aware of state statutory requirements. Such requirements may involve the use of sexual assault assessment kits, which lists the steps necessary and the items to be obtained for forensic purposes. If personnel trained in collecting samples and information are available, it is appropriate to request their assistance.

Informed consent must be obtained prior to examining a sexual assault victim. A careful history and physical examination should be performed in the presence of a chaperon or victim advocate. The patient should be asked to state in her own words what happened, and to identify or describe her attacker if possible. The history should include inquiry about last menstrual period, contraceptive use, preexisting pregnancy and infection, and last consensual intercourse before the assault. The patient's activities in the interval between the assault and the examination—whether the patient has eaten, drunk, bathed, douched, voided, or defecated—might affect findings on physical examination; such activities must be recorded.

A careful physical examination of the entire body should be performed. The physician should search for bruises, abrasions, or lacerations about the neck, back, buttocks, and extremities. Bite marks should be noted, particularly about the genitalia and breasts. Injuries to the mouth and pharynx may result from oral penetration. Injuries should be documented with photographs or drawings in the medical record. *Rape* and *physical assault* are legal terms that should not be used in medical records. Instead, the physician should report findings as "consistent with the use of force."

A pelvic examination should be performed. Injuries to the vulva, hymen, vagina, urethra, and rectum should be noted. Occasionally, foreign objects may be found in the orifices. The speculum must be moistened only with saline. Two milliliters of normal saline are injected into the vaginal vault. Nonabsorbent cotton swabs should be used to sample fluid from this vaginal pool and should then be placed in sterile glass tubes and refrigerated. Air-dried, nonfixed smears of this same fluid should be placed on glass slides. A Pap test may also be obtained. Evidence of coitus will be present in the vagina for as long as 48 hours after the attack. Motile sperms may be noted in the vagina for up to 8 hours after intercourse, but may be present in the cervi-

cal mucus for as long as 2–3 days. Nonmotile sperm may be noted in the vagina for up to 24 hours and in the cervix for up to 17 days. Acid phosphatase is an enzyme found in high concentrations in the seminal fluid. Evidence of acid phosphatase should be sought by swabbing the vaginal secretions, even in the absence of sperm because the attacker may have had a vasectomy. DNA evaluation may also be performed from the vaginal swab. Nonmotile sperm may be found in the rectum for up to 24 hours after the assault, and acid phosphatase can also be detected in the rectum.

A wet mount or vaginal swab should be obtained to detect *Trichomonas vaginalis*. Testing for *Neisseria gonorrhoeae* and *Chlamydia trachomatis* should be performed from specimens from any sites of penetration or attempted penetration. A serum sample should be collected for subsequent serologic analysis if test results are positive. The risk of acquiring gonorrhea from sexual assault is estimated between 6% and 12%. Baseline serologic tests for hepatitis B virus, HIV, and syphilis should also be offered. The risk of acquiring syphilis from sexual assault is estimated to be 3%; that of acquiring HIV is undetermined.

An important part of the physician's legal responsibilities is to collect samples for forensic purposes. Pubic hair combings should be collected to look for pubic hair from the assailant. Fingernail scrapings should be obtained to look for skin or blood of the attacker. Skin washings and clothing should be investigated for the presence of blood or semen. A Wood light may be helpful because dried semen will fluoresce under its light. Saliva should be collected from the victim. Because seminal fluid is rapidly destroyed by salivary enzymes, identification of seminal fluid in the mouth after a few hours is difficult. Therefore, victims should be encouraged to come to a medical facility immediately following an assault, where they can be evaluated before they bathe, urinate, defecate, wash out their mouths, or clean their fingernails.

Proper processing and labeling of collected specimens is crucial. All collected specimens are placed in a larger sealed container and processed in a "chain of evidence" fashion. The person who collects the specimens verifies their completeness by signature on the sealed master container. The individual to whom they are transferred must verify by signature that all specimens were received in an untampered state. Thus, each individual who has "custody" of the specimens during processing must verify that they were transmitted without alteration until they are turned over to the responsible law enforcement agency. The name of the law enforcement agent who receives the specimens should be noted in the medical record.

Treatment of physical injuries sustained at the time of assault should be initiated immediately; prophylactic medical treatment may be indicated for prevention of sexually transmitted infections and pregnancy. For prophylaxis against sexually transmitted infections, empiric recommended antimicrobial therapy for chlamydial, gonococcal, and trichomonal infections may be given. One such regimen consists of

- Ceftriaxone 125 mg intramuscularly in a single dose, plus
- Metronidazole 2 g orally in a single dose, plus
- Doxycycline 100 mg orally two times a day for 7 days.

Alternative treatment may be given as recommended by the Centers for Disease Control and Prevention. In addition, it is recommended that hepatitis B immune globulin be administered intramuscularly as soon as possible, but certainly within 14 days of exposure. It should be followed by the standard three-dose active immunization series with hepatitis B vaccine at 0, 1 and 6 months, beginning at the time of passive immunization. Prophylaxis against HIV is controversial.

Emergency contraception can be offered as prophylaxis against pregnancy. The risk of pregnancy after sexual assault has been estimated to be 2–4% in victims who were not using some form of contraception at the time of the assault. A serum pregnancy test should be obtained prior to administration of emergency contraception to evaluate for preexisting pregnancy. Emergency contraception should be given within 72 hours of the assault, though it can still be effective up to 120 hours later. There are several different methods of emergency contraception; the most common method (Yuzpe method) involves the use of high-dose combined oral contraceptives within 72 hours of unprotected coitus, repeated 12 hours following the first dose. One randomized study showed that the use of levonorgestrel 0.75 mg, in two doses 12 hours apart, within 72 hours of unprotected coitus, is more effective and better tolerated than the Yuzpe method. Levonorgestrel prevented 85% of pregnancies that would have occurred without treatment.

As most patients suffer significant psychological trauma as a consequence of sexual assault, the physician must be prepared to provide access to counseling. It is preferable that follow-up psychological counseling be provided by individuals who have extensive experience in the management of crisis-response to rape. Even if the victim appears to be in control emotionally, she will probably experience aspects of rape-trauma syndrome at some time in the future. She should be made aware of the symptoms that she may experience, and advised to seek help if and when these symptoms occur. No patient should be released from the facility until specific follow-up plans are made and agreed upon by the patient, physician, and counselor.

A follow-up visit should be scheduled approximately 2 weeks after the assault for repeat physical examination and collection of additional specimens. Testing for *N gonorrhoeae, C trachomatis,* and *T vaginalis* should be repeated unless prophylactic antimicrobials have been provided. Follow-up counseling should be discussed again at the second visit. Additional visits may be scheduled according to the victim's needs; an additional follow-up visit approximately 12 weeks following the sexual assault is advisable to collect sera for detection of antibodies against *T pallidum,* hepatitis B virus (unless vaccine was given), and HIV (repeat test at 6 months). During each of these visits, assessment of the patient's psychological symptoms should be performed, and referrals for further counseling are made as indicated.

Much of this chapter addresses the role and responsibilities of the health care professional in caring for victims of domestic violence and sexual assault after they have occurred. One of the greatest challenges for health care and public health professionals working to improve women's health continues to be the epidemic of violence against women in our society, and around the world. A great deal remains to be learned and done about the primary prevention of violence.

REFERENCES

American College of Obstetricians and Gynecologists: Adolescent victims of sexual assault. ACOG Educational Bulletin No. 252, 1998.

American College of Obstetricians and Gynecologists: Domestic violence. ACOG Educational Bulletin No. 257, 1999.

American College of Obstetricians and Gynecologists: Sexual assault. ACOG Educational Bulletin No. 242, 1997.

American Medical Association, Council on Scientific Affairs: Violence against women: Relevance for medical practitioners. JAMA 1992;267:3184.

American Medical Association: Strategies for the treatment and prevention of sexual assault. AMA, 1995.

Bachman R, Saltzman LE: Violence against women: Estimates from the redesigned survey. Bureau of Justice Statistics Special Report. U.S. Department of Justice, 1995;NCJ-154348.

Bechtel K: Evaluation of the adolescent rape victim. Pediatr Clin North Am 1999;46:809.

Burgess AW, Holmstrom LL: Rape trauma syndrome. Am J Psychiatry 1974;131:981.

Centers for Disease Control and Prevention: 2002 sexually transmitted disease treatment guidelines. MMWR 2002; 51 (RR06): 1–80.

Commonwealth Fund Commission on Women's Health: Addressing domestic violence and its consequences. The Commonwealth Fund, 1998.

Gazmararian JA et al: Prevalence of violence against pregnant women. JAMA 1996;275:1915.

Haywood YC, Haile-Mariam T: Violence against women. Emerg Med Clin North Am 1999;17:603.

Kaplan DW: Care of the adolescent sexual assault victim. Pediatrics 2001;107:1476.

Linden JA: Sexual assault. Emerg Med Clin North Am 1999;17:685.

National Institute of Justice: The extent and costs of crime victimization: A new look. U.S. Department of Justice, 1996.

Newberger EH et al: Abuse of pregnant women and adverse birth outcome: Current knowledge and implications for practice. JAMA 1992;267:2370.

Patel M: Management of sexual assault. Emerg Med Clin North Am 1999;17:817.

Riggs N et al: Analysis of 1076 cases of sexual assault. Ann Emerg Med 2000;35:358.

Task Force on Postovulatory Methods of Fertility Regulation: Randomised, controlled trial of levonorgestrel versus the Yuzpe regimen of combined oral contraceptives for emergency contraception. Lancet 1998;352:428.

The Breast

Matthew M. Poggi, MD, & Kathleen F. Harney, MD

■ ANATOMY OF THE FEMALE BREAST

The breasts are secondary reproductive glands of ectodermal modified sweat gland origin. Each breast lies on the superior midsurface of the chest wall. In women, the breasts are the organs of lactation; in men, the breasts are normally functionless and undeveloped.

HISTOLOGY

The adult female breast contains glandular and ductal tissue, a stroma of fibrous tissue that binds the individual lobes together, and fatty tissue within and between the lobes.

Each breast consists of 12–20 conical lobes. The base of each lobe is close to the ribs; the apex, which contains the major excretory duct of the lobe, is situated close to the areola and nipple. Each lobe consists of a group of lobules, and the many lactiferous ducts in each lobule unite to form a major duct that drains a lobe as it converges toward the areola. Each of the major ducts widens to form an ampulla as it reaches the areola and then narrows for its individual opening on the nipple. The lobules are held in place by a meshwork of fatty areolar tissue. The fatty tissue increases toward the periphery of the lobule and gives the breast its bulk and its hemispheric shape.

About 80–85% of the normal breast is fat. The breast tissues are joined to the overlying skin and subcutaneous tissue by fibrous strands.

In the nonpregnant, nonlactating breast, the alveoli are small and tightly packed. During pregnancy, the alveoli enlarge and their lining cells increase in number. During lactation, the alveolar cells secrete milk proteins and lipids.

The deep surface of the breast lies on the fascia that covers the chest muscles. The fascial stroma, derived from the superficial fascia of the chest wall, is condensed into multiple fascial bands that run from the breast into the subcutaneous tissues and the corium of the skin overlying the breast. These fascial bands—Cooper's ligaments—support the breast in its upright position on the chest wall. These bands may be distorted by a tumor, resulting in skin dimpling.

HISTOLOGIC CHANGES IN THE FEMALE BREAST DURING THE LIFE SPAN

During puberty, in response to multiglandular stimulation, the female breast begins to enlarge and eventually assumes its conical or spherical shape. Growth is due to increase in acinar tissue, ductal size and branching, and deposits of fat (the main factor in breast enlargement). Also during puberty, the nipple and areola enlarge. Smooth muscle fibers surround the base of the nipple, and the nipple becomes more sensitive to touch.

Once menses are established, the breast undergoes a periodic **premenstrual phase** during which the acinar cells increase in number and size, the ductal lumens widen, and breast size and turgor increase slightly. Many women have breast tenderness during this phase of the cycle. Menstrual bleeding is followed by a **postmenstrual phase,** characterized by decrease in size and turgor, reduction in the number and size of the breast acini, and decrease in diameter of the lactiferous ducts. Individual response of the breast to cyclic hormonal influences is variable. This is true not only of breast size and turgor but also of the degree of hypertrophic and regressive histologic changes that may occur.

During pregnancy, in response to progesterone, breast size and turgidity increase markedly. These changes are accompanied by deepening nipple and areolar pigmentation, nipple enlargement, areolar widening, and an increase in the number and size of the lubricating glands in the areola. The breast ductal system branches markedly, and the individual ducts widen. The acini increase in number and size. In late pregnancy, the fatty tissues of the breasts are almost completely replaced by cellular breast parenchyma. After delivery, the breasts, now fully mature, start to secrete milk. With cessation of nursing or administration of estrogens to inhibit lactation, the gland rapidly returns to its prepregnancy state, with marked diminution of cellular elements and an increase in fat deposits.

Between the fifth and sixth decades of life, when menses cease, the breast undergoes a gradual process of involution. There is a decrease in the number and size of acinar and ductal elements, so that the breast tissue regresses to an almost infantile state. Adipose tissue may or may not atrophy, with disappearance of the parenchymal elements.

GROSS ANATOMY
(Fig 61–1)

The adult female breast usually forms an almost hemispheric protrusion on each side of the chest wall, usually extending from just below the level of the second rib inferiorly to the sixth or seventh rib. The gland is usually situated between the lateral sternal border and the anterior axillary fold. The superior surface of the breast emerges gradually from the chest wall, whereas the lateral and inferior borders are quite well defined. The major portion of the breast, lying atop the pectoralis major muscle, projects ventrally; smaller portions extend laterally and inferiorly to lie atop the serratus anterior and external oblique muscles and as far caudad as the rectus abdominis. A triangular tongue-shaped tail of breast tissue (the axillary tail of Spence) extends superiorly and laterally toward the axilla, perforates the deep axillary fascia, and enters the axilla, where it terminates in close apposition to the axillary lymph vessels and nodes and the axillary blood vessels and nerves.

The Nipple & Areola

The areola is a circular pigmented zone 2–6 cm in diameter at the tip of the breast. Its color varies from pale pink to deep brown depending on age, parity, and skin pigmentation. The skin of the areola contains multiple small elevated nodules beneath which lie the sebaceous glands (glands of Montgomery). The glands are responsible for lubrication of the nipple and help prevent nipple and areolar cracks and fissures. During the third trimester of pregnancy, the sebaceous glands hypertrophy markedly.

A circular smooth muscle band surrounds the base of the nipple. Longitudinal smooth muscle fibers branch out from the ring of circular smooth muscle to encircle the lactiferous ducts as they converge toward the nipple. The many small punctate openings situated at the top of the nipple are the terminals of the major lactiferous ducts. The ampullae of the lactiferous ducts lie just deep to the nipple and the areola.

Blood Vessels, Lymphatics, & Nerves

A. ARTERIES
(FIG 61–2)

The breast has a multiple arterial supply. Perforating branches from the internal thoracic artery that appear in interspaces 2, 3, and 4 supply blood to the medial quadrants of the breast. These arteries perforate the intercostal muscles and the anterior intercostal membrane to supply both the breast and the pectoralis major and minor muscles. During pregnancy and in advanced breast disease, the intercostal perforators generally enlarge. The breast is also supplied medially by small branches from the anterior intercostal arteries. It is nourished laterally by the pectoral branch of the thoracoacromial branch of the axillary artery and by the external mammary branch of the lateral thoracic artery, which also is a branch of the second segment of the axillary artery. The external mammary artery passes along the lateral free border of the pectoralis major muscle to reach the lateral half of the breast, the artery usually lying medial to the long thoracic nerve.

The medial and lateral arteries, as they reach the breast, tend to arborize mainly in the supra-areolar area; consequently, the arterial supply to the upper half of the breast is almost twice that of the lower half.

B. VEINS

Venous return from the breast closely follows the routes of arterial supply. Blood returns to the superior vena cava via the axillary and internal thoracic veins. It also returns via the vertebral venous plexuses, which are fed by the intercostal and azygos veins. There is some minor flow into the portal system via the azygos system. There is a rich subareolar anastomotic plexus of superficial breast veins. In thin-skinned, fair individuals, these veins are normally visible. They almost always become visible during pregnancy. Their presence makes for marked vascularity of sub- and para-areolar incisions. Venous flow in the superior quadrants is greater than in the inferior quadrants of the breast.

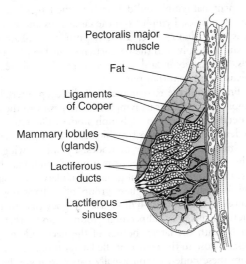

Pectoralis major muscle

Fat

Ligaments of Cooper

Mammary lobules (glands)

Lactiferous ducts

Lactiferous sinuses

Figure 61–1. Sagittal section of mammary gland.

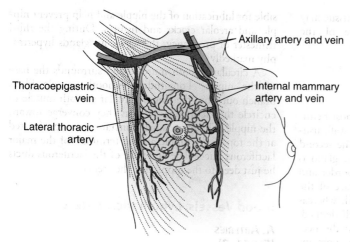

Axillary artery and vein

Thoracoepigastric vein

Internal mammary artery and vein

Lateral thoracic artery

Figure 61–2. Arteries and veins of the breast.

C. LYMPHATICS (FIG 61–3)

Study of the lymphatic drainage from the breast is of great importance for its implications in breast cancer. Modern surgical concepts of management of breast cancer are based to a large extent on an understanding of the pattern of lymphatic drainage from the breast.

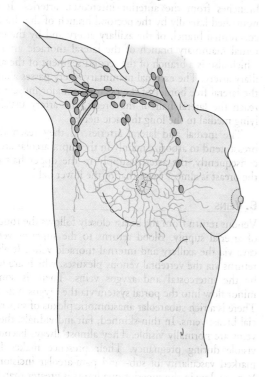

Figure 61–3. Lymphatics of the breast and axilla.

Lymphatic drainage from the breast may be divided into 2 main categories: superficial (including cutaneous) drainage and deep parenchymatous drainage.

1. **Superficial drainage**—A large lymphatic plexus lies in the subcutaneous tissues of the breast just beneath the areola and nipple. This plexus drains the areola and nipple areas and the cutaneous and subcutaneous tissues adjacent to the areola. It also drains the deep central parenchymatous region of the breast; the lymph rising from these areas pools in the superficial plexus.

2. **Deep parenchymatous drainage**—The deep parenchymatous lymph channels drain most of the breast as well as some lymph from the skin and subcutaneous tissues of the areolar and nipple areas. Small periductal and periacinal lymph channels collect parenchymal lymph and deliver it to the larger interlobar lymphatics. Lymph from the cutaneous and areolar areas may drain either directly into the subareolar plexus or deeply into the parenchymatous lymph channels and is secondarily delivered to the subareolar plexus for efferent transport.

From both the retroareolar and the deep interlobar lymphatics, most breast lymph usually passes to the ipsilateral axillary group of lymph nodes. There are no predetermined pathways by which breast lymph reaches the highest axillary node or nodes. Lymph flowing in either the superior or inferior mammary trunk may bypass the inferior or central group of axillary nodes and flow directly to the highest group of axillary nodes. However, most breast lymph usually goes first to the anterior axillary or subpectoral group of nodes that lie just beneath the lateral border of the pectoralis major muscle, close to the course of the lateral thoracic artery. From these nodes, lymph usually passes to nodes lying close to the lateral portion of the axillary vein. The lymph then passes superiorly, via the axillary chain of lymph vessels and nodes. The lymph eventually reaches the highest nodes of the axilla. Although this is the so-called normal pattern of lateral and superior breast lymphatic drainage, other paths of drainage are fairly common, particularly when the lateral and superiorly directed channels are obstructed by tumor masses. When plugging occurs, the following pathways are available for lymphatic flow from the breast:

a. From the breast directly to the highest axillary node, completely bypassing all other axillary nodal tissue. This may occur with superior quadrant breast tumors.

b. From the breast directly to the subscapular group of axillary nodes, subsequently progressing ventrally and superiorly through channels lying close to the axillary vein.

c. From the breast directly to the most inferior group of supraclavicular cervical nodes. Supraclavicular nodes are more commonly involved via direct extension from the apical axillary nodes.

d. From the breast across the sternal midline to the lymphatics of the contralateral breast.

e. From the breast directly to the contralateral axilla.

f. From the breast to the internal mammary group of nodes when the primary breast tumor is in the medial quadrant.

g. Rarely, from the breast to lymphatics that run to lymphatics closely related to the sheaths of the superior segments of the rectus abdominis and external oblique muscles and thence inferiorly toward the upper abdominal wall, the diaphragm, and the intra-abdominal viscera (especially the liver).

D. Nerves Encountered During Axillary Dissection

The lateral and anterior cutaneous branches of T4–6 supply the cutaneous tissues covering the breasts. Two major nerves and 2 smaller groups of nerves lie close to the breast area and thus assume importance in breast surgery:

(1) The **thoracodorsal nerve,** a branch of the posterior cord of the brachial plexus (C5–7), runs inferiorly along with the subscapular artery lying close to the posterior axillary wall and the ventral surface of the subscapular muscle. The nerve innervates the superior half of the latissimus dorsi muscle and is usually surrounded by a large venous plexus that drains into the subscapular veins.

(2) The **long thoracic nerve** (nerve of Bell) arises from the anterior primary divisions of C5–7 at the level of the lower half of the anterior scalene muscle. In the neck, the nerve descends dorsal to the trunks of the brachial plexus on the inferior segment of the middle scalene muscle. Further descent places it dorsal to the clavicle and the axillary vessels. On the lateral thoracic

wall, it descends on the external surface of the serratus anterior muscle along the anterior axillary line. The long thoracic nerve supplies filaments to each of the digitations of the serratus anterior muscle. Injury to this nerve results in a "winged" scapula.

(3) The **intercostal brachial nerves** are 3 relatively minor cutaneous nerves that supply the skin of the medial surface of the upper arm. They cross transversely from the lateral chest wall to the upper inner surface of the arm, passing across the base of the axilla.

(4) The **medial and lateral pectoral nerves** that supply the 2 pectoral muscles pass from the axilla to the lateral chest wall, reaching it by piercing the costocoracoid membrane. The medial pectoral nerve arises from the medial cord of the brachial plexus; the lateral pectoral nerve arises from the lateral cord of the plexus.

■ DISEASES OF THE BREAST

FIBROCYSTIC CHANGE

ESSENTIALS OF DIAGNOSIS

- *Painful, often multiple, usually bilateral masses in the breast.*
- *Rapid fluctuation in the size of the masses is common.*
- *Frequently, pain occurs or increases and size increases during the premenstrual phase of the cycle.*
- *Most common age is 30–50 years; occurrence is rare in postmenopausal women.*

General Considerations

This disorder, formerly known as mammary dysplasia, fibrocystic disease, or chronic cystic mastitis, is the most frequent benign condition of the breast. It is common in women 30–50 years of age but rare in postmenopausal women; this suggests that it is related to ovarian activity. The term **mammary dysplasia,** or **fibrocystic disease,** is imprecise and encompasses a wide variety of pathologic entities. These lesions are always associated with benign changes in the breast epithelium, some of which are found so commonly in normal breasts that they are probably variants of normal breast histology but have unfortunately been termed a "disease."

The microscopic findings of fibrocystic change include cysts (gross and microscopic), papillomatosis, adenosis, fibrosis, and ductal epithelial hyperplasia.

Clinical Findings

Fibrocystic change may produce an asymptomatic lump in the breast that is discovered by palpation, but pain or tenderness often calls attention to the mass. There may be discharge from the nipple. In many cases, discomfort occurs or is increased during the premenstrual phase of the cycle, at which time the cysts tend to enlarge. Some women seem to have more severe pain that is constant and not related to the menstrual cycle (**mastodynia**). Fluctuation in size and rapid appearance or disappearance of a breast tumor are common in cystic changes. Multiple or bilateral masses are common, and many patients give a history of a transient lump in the breast or cyclic breast pain. Pain, fluctuation in size, and multiplicity of lesions are the features most helpful in differentiation from carcinoma. However, if a dominant mass is present, it should be evaluated by biopsy.

Differential Diagnosis

Pain, fluctuation in size, and multiplicity of lesions help to differentiate these lesions from carcinoma and fibroadenoma. Final diagnosis often depends on biopsy. Mammography may be helpful, but the breast tissue in these young women may be too radiodense to permit a worthwhile study. Aspiration and/or sonography may be useful in differentiating a cystic from a solid mass.

Treatment

Because the condition of fibrocystic change is frequently indistinguishable from carcinoma on the basis of clinical findings, it is advisable to perform biopsy examination of suspicious lesions, which is usually done under local anesthesia. Surgery should be conservative, since the primary objective is to exclude cancer. Simple mastectomy or extensive removal of breast tissue is rarely, if ever, indicated for fibrocystic change.

When the diagnosis of fibrocystic change has been established by previous biopsy or is practically certain, because the history is classic, aspiration of a discrete mass suggestive of a cyst is indicated. The patient is reexamined at intervals thereafter. If no fluid is obtained or if the fluid is bloody, if a mass persists after aspiration, or if anytime during follow-up a persistent lump is noted, biopsy should be performed (Fig 61–4).

Breast pain associated with generalized fibrocystic change is best treated by avoiding trauma and by wearing a bra with good support.

The role of caffeine consumption in the development and treatment of fibrocystic change is controversial. Many patients report relief of symptoms after giving up coffee, tea, and chocolate.

Prognosis

Exacerbations of pain, tenderness, and cyst formation may occur at any time until menopause, when symptoms subside. The patient should be advised to examine her own breasts each month just after menstruation and to inform her physician if a mass appears. The risk of breast cancer in women with fibrocystic change showing proliferative or atypical changes in the epithelium is higher than that of women in general. Follow-up examinations at regular intervals should therefore be arranged.

FIBROADENOMA OF THE BREAST

This common benign neoplasm occurs most frequently in young women, usually within 20 years after puberty.

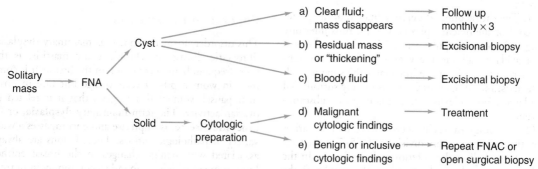

Figure 61–4. Algorithm for the use of fine needle aspiration (FNA) and fine needle aspiration cytology (FNAC) for office triage of breast lumps. (Reproduced, with permission, from Hindle WH: *Breast Disease for Gynecologists.* Appleton & Lange, 1990.)

It is somewhat more frequent and tends to occur at an earlier age in black than in white women. Multiple tumors in one or both breasts are found in 10–15% of patients.

The typical fibroadenoma is a round, firm, discrete, relatively movable, nontender mass 1–5 cm in diameter. The tumor is usually discovered accidentally. Clinical diagnosis in young patients is generally not difficult. In women over 30, cystic disease of the breast and carcinoma of the breast must be considered. Cysts can be identified by aspiration. Fibroadenoma does not normally occur after menopause, but postmenopausal women may occasionally develop fibroadenoma after administration of estrogenic hormone.

Treatment is either excision under local anesthesia or careful clinical observation.

Cystosarcoma phyllodes is a type of fibroadenoma with cellular stroma that tends to grow rapidly. This tumor may reach a large size and if inadequately excised will recur locally. The lesion is rarely malignant. Treatment is by local excision of the mass with a margin of surrounding breast tissue. The treatment of malignant cystosarcoma phyllodes is more controversial. In general, complete removal of the tumor and a rim of normal tissue should prevent recurrence. Since these tumors tend to be large, simple mastectomy is often necessary to achieve complete control.

NIPPLE DISCHARGE

General Considerations

The most common causes of nipple discharge in the nonlactating breast are carcinoma, intraductal papilloma, and fibrocystic change with ectasia of the ducts. The important characteristics of the discharge and some other factors to be evaluated by history and physical examination are as follows:

(1) Nature of discharge (serous, bloody, or other)
(2) Association with a mass or not
(3) Unilateral or bilateral
(4) Single duct or multiple duct discharge
(5) Discharge that is spontaneous (persistent or intermittent) or must be expressed
(6) Discharge produced by pressure at a single site or by general pressure on the breast
(7) Relation to menses
(8) Premenopausal or postmenopausal
(9) Patient taking contraceptive pills or estrogen for postmenopausal symptoms

Differential Diagnosis

Unilateral, spontaneous serous or serosanguineous discharge from a single duct is usually caused by an intra-

ductal papilloma or, rarely, by an intraductal cancer. In either case, a mass may not be present. The involved duct may be identified by pressure at different sites around the nipple at the margin of the areola. Bloody discharge is more suggestive of cancer but is usually caused by a benign papilloma in the duct. Cytologic examination of the discharge should be accomplished and may identify malignant cells, but negative findings do not rule out cancer, which is more likely in women over age 50. In any case, the involved duct, and a mass if present, should be excised.

In premenopausal women, spontaneous multiple duct discharge, unilateral or bilateral, most marked just before menstruation, is often due to fibrocystic change. Discharge may be green or brownish. Papillomatosis and ductal ectasia are also diagnostic possibilities. Biopsy may be necessary to establish the diagnosis of a diffuse nonmalignant process. If a mass is present, it should be removed.

Milky discharge (galactorrhea) from multiple ducts in the nonlactating breast may occur in certain syndromes (Chiari-Frommel syndrome, Argonz-Del Castillo [Forbes-Albright] syndrome), presumably as a result of increased secretion of pituitary prolactin. An endocrine workup may be indicated. Drugs of the chlorpromazine type and contraceptive pills may also cause milky discharge that ceases on discontinuance of the medication. Other medical illnesses may rarely cause galactorrhea (Table 61–1).

Oral contraceptive agents may cause clear, serous, or milky discharge from a single duct, but multiple duct discharge is more common. The discharge is more evident just before menstruation and disappears on stop-

Table 61–1. Causes of galactorrhea.

Idiopathic

Drug induced
  Phenothiazines, butyrophenones, reserpine, methyldopa, imipramine, amphetamine, metoclopramide, sulpride, pimozide, oral contraceptive agents

CNS Lesions
  Pituitary adenoma, empty sella, hypothalamic tumor, head trauma

Medical conditions
  Chronic renal failure, sarcoidosis, Schuller-Christian disease Cushing's disease, hepatic cirrhosis, hypothyroidism

Chest wall lesions
  Thoracotomy, herpes zoster

Reproduced, with permission, from Hindle WH: Breast Disease for Gynecologists. Appleton & Lange, 1990.

ping the medication. If it does not and is from a single duct, exploration should be considered.

Purulent discharge may originate in a subareolar abscess and require excision of the abscess and related lactiferous sinus.

When localization is not possible and no mass is palpable, the patient should be reexamined every week for 1 month. When unilateral discharge persists, even without definite localization or tumor, exploration must be considered. The alternative is careful follow-up at intervals of 1–3 months. Mammography should be done. Cytologic examination of nipple discharge for exfoliated cancer cells may be helpful in diagnosis.

Chronic unilateral nipple discharge, especially if bloody, is an indication for resection of the involved ducts.

FAT NECROSIS

Fat necrosis is a rare lesion of the breast but is of clinical importance because it produces a mass, often accompanied by skin or nipple retraction, that is indistinguishable from carcinoma. Trauma is presumed to be the cause, although only about half of patients give a history of injury to the breast. Ecchymosis is occasionally seen near the tumor. Tenderness may or may not be present. If untreated, the mass associated with fat necrosis gradually disappears. Should the mass not resolve in several weeks, a biopsy should be considered. The entire mass should be excised, primarily to rule out carcinoma.

BREAST ABSCESS

During nursing, an area of redness, tenderness, and induration may develop in the breast. In the early stages, the infection can often be reversed while continuing nursing with that breast and administering an antibiotic. If the lesion progresses to form a localized mass with local and systemic signs of infection, an abscess is present and should be drained. Nursing should be discontinued.

A subareolar abscess may develop (rarely) in young or middle-aged women who are not lactating. These infections tend to recur after incision and drainage unless the area is explored in a quiescent interval with excision of the involved lactiferous duct or ducts at the base of the nipple. Except for the subareolar type of abscess, infection in the breast is very rare unless the patient is lactating. Therefore, findings suggestive of abscess in the nonlactating breast require incision and biopsy of indurated tissue.

MALFORMATION OF THE BREAST

Many women consult their physicians for abnormalities in either the size or the symmetry of their breasts. It is common for there to be some difference in size between the two breasts, which, if extreme, may be corrected by plastic surgery. However, the breast tissue in these individuals is otherwise normal.

Similarly, woman may complain of overly large breasts (macromastia). Studies have failed to show any endocrinologic or pathologic abnormalities, and these patients may also be considered candidates for plastic surgery (breast reduction mammoplasty).

Less common malformations of the breast include amastia (complete absence of one or both breasts) or the presence of accessory nipples/breast tissue along the embryologic milk line (occurring in 1–2% of Caucasians).

PUERPERAL MASTITIS

See Chapter 28.

CARCINOMA OF THE FEMALE BREAST

 ESSENTIALS OF DIAGNOSIS

- *Early findings: Single, nontender, firm to hard mass with ill-defined margins; mammographic abnormalities and no palpable mass.*
- *Later findings: Skin or nipple retraction; axillary lymphadenopathy; breast enlargement, redness, edema, pain, fixation of mass to skin or chest wall.*
- *Late findings: Ulceration; supraclavicular lymphadenopathy; edema of arm; bone, lung, liver, brain, or other distant metastases.*

General Considerations

Cancer of the breast is the most common cancer in women, excluding skin cancers. After lung cancer, it is the second most common cause of cancer death for women. The American Cancer Society estimates 192,200 new cases of cancer of the breast and 40,200 deaths for 2001. Despite a slight increase in yearly incidence, the cancer death rate for malignancies of the breast decreased an average of 2.2% per year from 1990 to 1997. The probability of developing the disease increases throughout life. The mean and the median age of women with breast cancer is 60–61 years.

At the present rate of incidence, a woman's risk of developing invasive breast cancer in her lifetime from *birth* to *death* is 1 in 8. This figure from the Surveillance, Epidemiology, and End Results Program (SEER) of the National Cancer Institute (NCI) is often cited but needs clarification. The data include all age groups in 5-year intervals with an open-ended interval at 85 years and above. When calculating risk, each age interval is weighted to account for the increasing risk of breast cancer with increasing age. A woman's risk of being diagnosed with breast cancer is:

- By age 30: 1 out of 2000
- By age 40: 1 out of 233
- By age 50: 1 out of 53
- By age 60: 1 out of 22
- By age 70: 1 out of 13
- By age 80: 1 out of 9
- In a lifetime: 1 out of 8

While a woman's lifetime risk of developing breast cancer is 1 in 8, it must be emphasized that she still has a 7 out of 8 chance of never developing breast cancer. Women whose mothers or sisters had breast cancer are more likely to develop the disease than controls. Risk is increased when breast cancer has occurred before menopause, was bilateral, or was present in 2 or more first-degree relatives. However, there is no history of breast cancer among female relatives in over 90% of patients with breast cancer. Nulliparous women and women whose first full-term pregnancy was under age 35 have a slightly higher incidence of breast cancer than multiparous women. Late menarche and artificial menopause are associated with a lower incidence of breast cancer, whereas early menarche (under age 12) and late natural menopause (after age 50) are associated with a slight increase in risk of developing breast cancer. Fibrocystic change of the breast, when accompanied by proliferative changes, papillomatosis, or atypical epithelial hyperplasia, is associated with an increased incidence of cancer. A woman who has had cancer in one breast is at increased risk of developing cancer in the other breast. Women with cancer of the uterine corpus have a breast cancer risk significantly higher than that of the general population, and women with breast cancer have a comparably increased risk of endometrial cancer. In the United States, breast cancer is more common in whites than in nonwhites. The incidence of the disease among nonwhites (mostly blacks), however, is increasing, especially in younger women. In general, rates reported from developing countries are low, whereas rates are high in developed countries, with the notable exception of Japan. Some of the variability may be due to underreporting in the developing countries, but a real difference probably exists.

Women who are at greater than normal risk of developing breast cancer should be identified by their physicians and followed carefully. Screening programs involving periodic physical examination and mammography of asymptomatic high-risk women increase the detection rate of breast cancer and may improve the survival rate. Unfortunately, more than 50% of women who develop breast cancer do not have significant identifiable risk factors.

Growth potential of tumor and resistance of host vary over a wide range from patient to patient and may be altered during the course of the disease. The doubling time of breast cancer cells ranges from several weeks in a rapidly growing lesion to nearly a year in a slowly growing one. If one assumes that the rate of doubling is constant and that the neoplasm originates in one cell, a carcinoma with a doubling time of 100 days may not reach clinically detectable size (1 cm) for about 8 years. On the other hand, rapidly growing cancers have a much shorter preclinical course and a greater tendency to metastasize to regional nodes or more distant sites before a breast mass is discovered.

The relatively long preclinical growth phase and the tendency of breast cancers to metastasize have led many clinicians to believe that breast cancer is a systemic disease at the time of diagnosis. Although it may be true that breast cancer cells are released from the tumor prior to diagnosis, variations in the host-tumor relationship may prohibit the growth of disseminated disease in many patients. For this reason, a pessimistic attitude concerning the management of localized breast cancer is not warranted, and many patients can be cured with proper treatment.

Staging

The physical examination of the breast and additional preoperative studies are used to determine the clinical stage of a breast cancer. Clinical staging is based on the TNM system (of the International Union Against Cancer). This classification considers tumor size, clinical assessment of axillary nodes, and the presence or absence of metastases. The assessment of the clinical stage is important in planning therapy. Histologic (or pathologic) staging is determined following surgery and along with clinical staging helps determine prognosis (Table 61–2).

Clinical Findings

The patient with breast cancer usually presents with a lump in the breast or an abnormal screening mammogram. Clinical evaluation should include assessment of the local lesion, including a bilateral mammogram if not previously performed, and a search for evidence of metastases in regional nodes or distant sites. After the diagnosis of breast cancer has been confirmed by

Table 61–2. Staging of breast carcinoma.

				Stage			
Tis carcinoma in situ				**Stage 0**			
				Tis	N0	M0	
T1				**Stage I**			
T1mic microinvastion ≤ 0.1 cm				T1	N0	M0	
T1a > 0.1 but ≤ 0.5 cm							
T1b > 0.5 but ≤ 1.0 cm				**Stage IIa**			
T1c > 1.0 but ≤ 2.0 cm				T0	N1	M0	
				T1	N1	M0	
T2 > 2 but ≤ 5 cm				T2	N0	M0	
T3 > 5 cm				**Stage IIb**			
				T2	N1	M0	
T4				T3	N0	M0	
T4a extension to chest wall							
T4b edema or ulceration of skin				**Stage IIIa**			
T4c both T4a & T4b				T0	N2	M0	
T4d inflammatory carcinoma				T1	N2	M0	
				T2	N2	M0	
N1 movable ipsilateral axillary lymph nodes				T3	N1	M0	
				T3	N2	M0	
N2 fixed ipsilateral axillary lymph nodes							
N3 ipsilateral internal mammary lymph nodes				**Stae IIIb**			
				T2	any N	M0	
M1 distant metastasis (including ipsilateral supraclavicular lymph node)				Any T	N3	M0	
				Stage IV			
				Any T	any N	M1	

(Reproduced with permission, from Fleming ID et al (editors): AJCC Cancer Staging Manual, 5th ed. Lippincott, 1997, p. 174.)

biopsy, additional studies are often needed to complete the search for distant metastases or an occult primary lesion in the other breast. Then, before any decision is made about treatment, all the available clinical data are used to determine the extent or "stage" of the patient's disease.

A. SYMPTOMS

When the history is taken, special note should be made of menarche, pregnancies, parity, artificial or natural menopause, date of last menstrual period, previous breast lesions, hormonal supplementation, radiation exposure, and a family history of breast cancer. Back or other bone pain may be the result of osseous metastases. Systemic complaints or weight loss should raise the question of metastases, which may involve any organ but most frequently the bones, liver, and lungs. The more advanced the cancer in terms of size of primary lesion, local invasion, and extent of regional node involvement, the higher is the incidence of metastatic spread to distant sites. Lymph node involvement is the most significant prognostic feature and also increases with increasing tumor size.

The presenting complaint in about 70% of patients with breast cancer is a lump (usually painless) in the breast. About 90% of breast masses are discovered by the patient herself. Less frequent symptoms are breast pain; nipple discharge; erosion, retraction, enlargement, or itching of the nipple; and redness, generalized hardness, enlargement, or shrinking of the breast. Rarely, an axillary mass, swelling of the arm, or bone pain (from metastases) may be the first symptoms. About 35–50% of women involved in organized screening programs have cancers detected by mammography only.

B. SIGNS

The relative frequency of carcinoma in various anatomic sites in the breast is shown in Figure 61–5.

Inspection of the breast is the first step in physical examination and should be carried out with the patient sitting, arms at sides and then overhead. Abnormal variations in breast size and contour, minimal nipple retraction, and slight edema, redness, or retraction of the skin can be identified. Asymmetry of the breasts and retraction or dimpling of the skin can often be accentuated by having the patient raise her arms overhead or

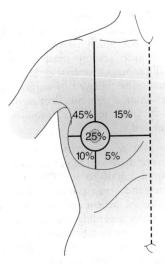

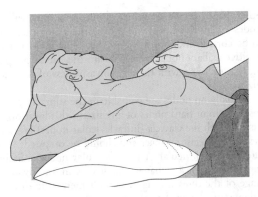

Figure 61–7. Palpation of breasts. Palpation is performed with the patient supine and the arm abducted.

Figure 61–5. Frequency of breast carcinoma at various anatomic sites.

press her hands on her hips in order to contract the pectoralis muscles. Axillary and supraclavicular areas should be thoroughly palpated for enlarged nodes with the patient sitting (Fig 61–6). Palpation of the breast for masses or other changes should be performed with the patient both seated and supine with the arm abducted (Fig 61–7).

Breast cancer usually consists of a nontender, firm, or hard lump with poorly delineated margins (caused

by local infiltration). Slight skin or nipple retraction is an important sign since it may affect staging. Minimal asymmetry of the breast may be noted. Very small (1–2 mm) erosions of the nipple epithelium may be the only manifestation of Paget's carcinoma. Watery, serous, or bloody discharge from the nipple is an occasional early sign but is more often associated with benign disease.

A lesion smaller than 1 cm in diameter may be difficult or impossible for the examiner to feel and yet may be discovered by the patient. She should always be asked to demonstrate the location of the mass; if the physician fails to confirm the patient's suspicions, radiographic evaluation should be attempted and the examination should be repeated in 1 month. During the premenstrual phase of the cycle, increased innocuous nodularity may suggest neoplasm or may obscure an underlying lesion. If there is any question regarding the nature of an abnormality under these circumstances, the patient should be asked to return after her period.

The following are characteristic of advanced carcinoma: edema, redness, nodularity, or ulceration of the skin; the presence of a large primary tumor (> 5 cm); fixation to the chest wall; enlargement, shrinkage, or retraction of the breast; marked axillary lymphadenopathy; edema of the ipsilateral arm; supraclavicular lymphadenopathy; and distant metastases.

Metastases tend to involve regional lymph nodes, which may be clinically palpable. With regard to the axilla, 1 or 2 movable, nontender, not particularly firm lymph nodes 5 mm or less in diameter are frequently present and are generally of no significance. Any firm or hard nodes larger than 5 mm in diameter are highly suspicious for metastases. Axillary nodes that are matted or fixed to skin or deep structures indicate locally advanced disease (at least stage III). Histologic studies show that microscopic metastases are present in about 40% of patients with clinically negative nodes. On the

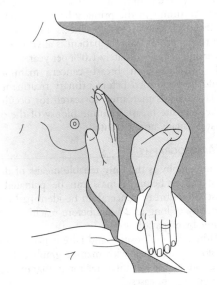

Figure 61–6. Palpation of axillary region for enlarged lymph nodes.

other hand, if the examiner thinks that the axillary nodes are involved, this will prove on histologic section to be correct in about 85% of cases. The incidence of positive axillary nodes increases with the size of the primary tumor and with the local invasiveness of the neoplasm.

Usually no nodes are palpable in the supraclavicular fossa. Firm or hard nodes of any size in this location or just beneath the clavicle (infraclavicular nodes) are suggestive of metastic cancer and should be biopsied. Ipsilateral supraclavicular or infraclavicular nodes containing cancer indicate that the patient is in an advanced stage of the disease (stage IV) with metastatic disease. Edema of the ipsilateral arm, commonly caused by metastatic infiltration of regional lymphatics, is also a sign of advanced (stage IV) cancer.

C. Special Clinical Forms of Breast Carcinoma

1. Paget's disease—This refers to eczematous changes about the nipple and is associated with cancer in 99% of cases. An underlying mass is palpable in 60% of patients with Paget's disease. Of these masses, 95% are found to be an invasive cancer, mostly infiltrating ductal. For patients with Paget's disease and no palpable mass, 75% of breast biopsies are found to harbor ductal carcinoma in situ, a noninvasive breast malignancy. The nipple epithelium is infiltrated, but gross nipple changes are often minimal, and a tumor mass may not be palpable. The first symptom is often itching or burning of the nipple, with a superficial erosion or ulceration. The diagnosis is established by biopsy of the erosion.

Paget's disease is not common (about 1% of all breast cancers), but it is important because it appears innocuous. It is frequently diagnosed and treated as dermatitis or bacterial infection, leading to an unfortunate delay in detection. If detected early, Paget's disease rarely involves the axillary lymph nodes. Treatment can be modified radical mastectomy or breast conservation therapy, which includes post-lumpectomy radiation, with an expected 8-year disease free survival of 90% or greater.

2. Inflammatory carcinoma—This is a clinical, pathologic entity defined as diffuse, brawny induration of the skin of the breast with an erysipeloid border, usually without an underlying palpable mass. Generally this is a clinical diagnosis with pathologic confirmation of tumor embolization in the dermal lymphatics by biopsy of the overlying skin. Inflammatory breast cancer is the most aggressive form of breast cancer. It represents less than 5% of cases. At presentation, nearly 35% of patients with inflammatory breast cancer have evidence of metastases. The inflammatory component, often mistaken for an infectious process, is caused by

the blockage of dermal lymphatics by tumor emboli, which results in edema and hyperemia. If a suspected skin infection does not rapidly respond (1–2 weeks) to a course of antibiotics, biopsy must be performed. Treatment usually consists of several cycles of neoadjuvant polychemotherapy followed by surgery or radiation depending on tumor response. Because of its severity and relatively small incidence, protocol therapy should be encouraged.

3. Occurrence during pregnancy or lactation—Cancer of the breast diagnosed in pregnancy has a ratio of occurrence from 1:3000 to 1:10,000. The association of pregnancy and breast cancer presents a therapeutic dilemma for the patient and the physician. Numerous studies differ regarding the prognosis; some show poorer outcome, while others demonstrate no difference. Termination of the pregnancy, formerly performed routinely in the first two trimesters, has not been demonstrated to improve outcome. In addition, the use of radiotherapy is contraindicated because of the potential for fetal damage. The use of chemotherapy, for similar reasons, is debatable.

In most instances, modified radical mastectomy in pregnancy is the minimal treatment of choice, with the possible exception of the latter part of the third trimester, wherein lumpectomy and radiotherapy in the puerperium may be considered.

4. Bilateral breast cancer—Clinically evident simultaneous bilateral breast cancer occurs in less than 1% of cases, but there is a 5–8% incidence of later occurrence of cancer in the second breast. Bilaterality occurs more often in women under age 50 and is more frequent when the tumor in the primary breast is lobular. The incidence of second breast cancers increases directly with the length of time the patient is alive after her first cancer and is approximately 1.0% per year.

In patients with breast cancer, mammography should be performed before primary treatment and at regular intervals thereafter, to search for occult cancer in the opposite breast. Routine biopsy of the opposite breast is usually not warranted.

D. Mammography

Mammography is the only reliable means of detecting breast cancer before a mass can be palpated in the breast. Some breast cancers can be identified by mammography as long as 2 years before reaching a size detectable by palpation.

Although false-positive and false-negative results are occasionally obtained with mammography, the experienced radiologist can interpret mammograms correctly in about 90% of cases.

Other than for screening, indications for mammography are as follows: (1) to evaluate each breast when a diagnosis of potentially curable breast cancer has been made, and at yearly intervals thereafter; (2) to evaluate a questionable or ill-defined breast mass or other suspicious change in the breast; (3) to search for an occult breast cancer in a woman with metastatic disease in axillary nodes or elsewhere from an unknown primary; (4) to screen at regular intervals a selected group of women who are at high risk for developing breast cancer (see below), (5) to screen women prior to cosmetic operations or prior to biopsy; and (6) to follow women who have been treated with breast-conserving surgery and radiation.

Patients with a dominant or suspicious mass must undergo biopsy regardless of mammographic findings. The mammogram should be obtained prior to biopsy so that other suspicious areas can be noted and the contralateral breast can be checked. Mammography is never a substitute for biopsy because it may not reveal clinical cancer in a very dense breast, as may be seen in young women with fibrocystic change, and it often does not reveal medullary-type cancer.

E. CYTOLOGY

Cytologic examination of nipple discharge or cyst fluid may be helpful on rare occasions. As a rule, mammography and breast biopsy are required when nipple discharge or cyst fluid is bloody or cytologically equivocal.

F. BIOPSY

The diagnosis of breast cancer depends ultimately on examination of tissue removed by biopsy. Treatment should never be undertaken without an unequivocal histologic diagnosis of cancer. The safest course is biopsy examination of all suspicious masses found on physical examination and, in the absence of a mass, of suspicious lesions demonstrated by mammography. About 30% of lesions thought to be definitely cancer prove on biopsy to be benign, and about 15% of lesions believed to be benign are found to be malignant. These findings demonstrate the fallibility of clinical judgment and the necessity for biopsy.

The simplest method is needle biopsy, either by fine needle aspiration (FNA) of tumor cells or by obtaining a small core of tissue with a stereotactic core needle biopsy. A negative FNA should be followed by open biopsy because false-negative needle biopsies may occur in 10% of cancers.

The definitive diagnostic method is open biopsy under local anesthesia as a separate procedure prior to deciding on treatment. Palpable masses are readily evaluated by a general surgeon. With the aid of diagnostic radiology, a nonpalpable, radiographically detected mass may be biopsied with the use of needle localization. The patient need not be admitted to the hospital. Decisions on additional workup for metastatic disease and on definitive therapy can be made and discussed

with the patient after the histologic diagnosis of cancer has been established. This approach has the advantage of avoiding unnecessary hospitalization and diagnostic procedures in many patients since cancer is found in the minority of patients who require biopsy for diagnosis of a breast lump.

In general, outpatient biopsy followed by definitive surgery at a later date gives patients time to adjust to the diagnosis of cancer, meet with members of the multidisciplinary team involved with managing breast cancer, and consider a second opinion as well as alternative forms of treatment. Studies have shown no adverse effects from the short (1–2 weeks) delay of the 2-step procedure, and this is the current recommendation of the National Cancer Institute.

At the time of the initial biopsy of breast cancer, it is important for the physician to preserve a portion of the specimen for immunohistochemical staining for hormone and growth factor (HER-2-Neu) receptors. At the time of pathological confirmation of a breast cancer diagnosis, patients on hormone replacement therapy (HRT) should be instructed to stop hormone use until counseled by an oncologist.

G. LABORATORY FINDINGS

A complete blood cell count (CBC), chemistry panel including liver function tests (LFTs), and a β-HCG in premenopausal patients to diagnose pregnancy should be obtained as part of the initial evaluation. An elevation in alkaline phosphatase or liver function may be an indication of metastatic disease and warrants further investigation. Hypercalcemia may be seen in advanced cases of metastatic cancer.

H. RADIOGRAPHIC FINDINGS

A baseline posteroanterior and lateral chest radiograph may reveal pulmonary disease involvement, which could include parenchymal metastases, plural thickening or studding, and effusions. A chest x-ray also provides for a radiographic evaluation of the cardiac silhouette prior to interventions, which could tax the cardiovascular system. Computed tomography (CT) scans of the brain and liver should be obtained sparingly and are generally reserved for locally advanced cases (stage IIIa or greater) as well as early stage cases in which there is a strong clinical suspicion of metastatic disease. Magnetic resonance (MR) scans of the previously surgically altered breast in which there is a question of malignancy or in the T0 N1 patient may be helpful in better characterizing the soft tissue of the breast but are otherwise not routinely used.

I. RADIONUCLIDE SCANNING

Bone scans using technetium 99m–labeled phosphonates are an important tool for the evaluation of metastatic breast cancer. There is no role for this imaging in screening or in the routine workup of a patient. The incidence of a positive bone scan increases with advancing disease stage. Stage I and II patients have a 7% and 8% possibility, respectively, of having a positive bone scan, while a stage III patient has roughly a 25% risk. Therefore bone scans are reserved for the locally advanced patient (stage IIIa or greater) or for the patient in whom there is clinical suspicion for metastatic disease.

Early Detection

A. Screening Programs

Mammography remains the single best screening procedure for the early detection of breast cancer. Both physical examination and mammography are necessary for maximum yield in detecting early breast cancer, since about 40% of early malignancies can be discovered only by mammography and another 40% can be detected by palpation. In general, depending on a woman's age and the density of her breasts, the sensitivity of mammography is 70–90% and specificity is greater than 90%. Yearly mammogram screening among women continues to increase so that in 1997 roughly 85% of women had had a mammogram at least once previously. This was an increase of 15% from 1990 and 47% from 1987. Women of color, however, have been shown to have more advanced stages of disease at the time of diagnosis and are less likely to engage in screening practices than white women. It has been postulated that socioeconomic status, education, and medical access may account for these differences.

Despite a consensus on the importance of mammographic screening, mammography has still not been demonstrated unequivocally to decrease breast cancer mortality across all age groups. In women between 50 and 69 years of age, there is reasonable evidence based largely on 8 randomized controlled trials that screening mammography is beneficial. For younger women, however, the evidence is not as clear. In the age group 40–49, there may be a small benefit, but this benefit emerges only after meta-analyses with varying levels of statistical significance and confidence intervals. Nevertheless, in the Health Insurance Plan screening study from the United States with the longest follow-up of any randomized mammography screening study of 18 years, there was a 30% reduction in mortality in women over 50 years of age.

Current screening recommendations from the American College of Radiology, the American Cancer Society, and the American Medical Women's Association call for annual mammograms starting at age 40. There is no recommendation for a "baseline" examination prior to age 40, nor is there any evidence to support this practice in women below this age. Women with a first-degree relative who had breast cancer typically are requested to obtain a first mammogram 5 years prior to the age at which the relative was diagnosed with breast cancer. Mammographic patterns are not a reliable predictor of the risk of developing breast cancer.

Breast ultrasonography is very useful in distinguishing cystic from solid lesions but should be used only as a supplement to physical examination and mammography in screening for breast cancer.

B. Self-Examination

Once women have reached puberty and start to develop breasts, breast self-examination should be encouraged. Initially, this allows the woman to become acquainted with her body and foster good self-examination habits for the future. All women over age 20 should be advised to examine their breasts monthly. Premenopausal women should perform the examination 5–7 days after the completion of the menstrual cycle when breast tissue is less dense. High-risk patients may wish to perform another self-examination in midcycle. Postmenopausal women should pick a particular date each month, perhaps the anniversary of a special occasion, to perform breast self-examination.

Breast self-examination consists of two parts: (1) inspection and (2) palpation. Using a mirror, the breasts should be inspected while standing with arms at sides, with arms overhead and palms pressed together, and with hands on hips pressing firmly to contract the pectoralis muscles. Gross asymmetry of the breasts, masses, and skin dimpling and/or retraction may be more apparent through the use of these maneuvers. In the supine position, each breast should be palpated with the fingertips of the opposite hand. Numerous techniques are advocated but methodical palpation is the goal.

The American Cancer Society publishes instructive guides, which can be viewed online at www.cancer.org. Their recommendations along with breast self-examination starting at age 20 are for a clinical breast examination to be performed by a health professional at least once every 3 years between 20–39. After age 40, a clinical breast examination should be performed annually. Physicians should instruct women in the technique of self-examination and advise them to report at once for medical evaluation if a mass or other abnormality is discovered. Many women report easier detection of breast abnormalities when the skin is moist while bathing or showering.

C. Genetic Testing

A positive family history of breast cancer is recognized as a risk factor for the subsequent development of breast cancer. With the discovery of 2 major breast cancer predisposition genes, *BRCA1* (17q21) and *BRCA2* (13q12-13), there has been increasing interest in genetic testing. Mutations in these 2 genes are associated with an elevated risk for breast cancer as well as ovarian, colon, prostate, and pancreatic cancers. Of all women with breast cancer, approximately 5–10% may have mutations in *BRCA1* or *BRCA2*. The estimated risk of a patient developing cancer with a *BRCA1* or *BRCA2* mutation is believed to be between 40% and 85%. Particular mutations may be more common in specific ethnic groups like the Ashkenazi Jewish population. Genetic testing is available and may be considered for members of high-risk families. Currently, there are no established guidelines or recommendations for genetic testing. Because of the complexities of genetic testing, genetic counseling before and after testing is necessary.

Differential Diagnosis

The lesions most often to be considered in the differential diagnosis of breast cancer include, in order of frequency, fibrocystic change, fibroadenoma, intraductal papilloma, and fat necrosis. The differential diagnosis of a breast lump should be established without delay by biopsy, either open or with localization guidance, or aspiration. Observation—even for a short, defined period—should be entertained with considerable caution.

Pathologic Types

Numerous pathologic subtypes of breast cancer can be identified histologically (Table 61–3). These pathologic types are distinguished by the histologic appearance and growth pattern of the tumor. In general, breast cancer arises either from the epithelial lining of the large or intermediate-sized ducts (ductal) or from the epithelium of the terminal ducts of the lobules (lobular). The cancer may be invasive or in situ. Most breast cancers arise

Table 61–3. Histologic types of breast cancer.

Type	Percent Occurrence
Invasive ductal (not otherwise specified)	80–85
Medullary	3–6
Colloid (mucinous)	3–6
Tubular	3–6
Papillary	3–6
Invasive lobular	4–10
Noninvasive	15–20
Intraductal	80
Lobular in situ	20

from the intermediate ducts and are invasive (invasive ductal, infiltrating ductal), and most histologic types are merely subtypes of invasive ductal cancer with unusual growth patterns (colloid, medullary, scirrhous, etc). Ductal carcinoma that has not invaded the extraductal tissue is intraductal or in situ ductal. Lobular carcinoma may be either invasive or in situ.

The histologic subtypes have only a little bearing on prognosis when outcomes are compared after accurate staging. Colloid (mucinous), medullary, papillary, adenoid cystic, and tubular histologies are generally believed to have a more favorable prognosis. Other histological criteria have been studied in an attempt to substratify patients based on features such as tumor differentiation, lymph vascular space invasion, and tumor necrosis. While these characteristics are important, stage is predominant and paramount in predicting outcome.

The noninvasive cancers by definition lack the ability to spread. However, in patients whose biopsies show noninvasive intraductal cancer, associated invasive ductal cancers are present in 1–3% of cases. Lobular carcinoma in situ is considered by some to be a premalignant lesion that by itself is not a true cancer. It lacks the ability to spread but is associated with the subsequent development of invasive ductal cancer in 25–30% of cases within 15 years.

Hormone Receptor Sites

The presence or absence of estrogen receptors in the cytoplasm of tumor cells is of paramount importance in managing patients with recurrent or metastatic disease. Up to 60% of patients with metastatic breast cancer will respond to hormonal manipulation if their tumors contain estrogen receptors. However, fewer than 10% of patients with metastatic, estrogen receptor–negative tumors can be successfully treated with hormonal manipulation.

Progesterone receptors may be an even more sensitive indicator than estrogen receptors of patients who may respond to hormonal manipulation. Up to 80% of patients with metastatic progesterone receptor–positive tumors seem to respond to hormonal manipulation. Receptors probably have no relationship to response to chemotherapy.

Estrogen receptors may be of prognostic significance, especially in the node-negative patient, but current evidence is still unclear. If there is a survival benefit, it is of a small magnitude, less than 10%. The defined role of establishing a tumor's hormone status is to help guide hormonal and systemic therapies. Two randomized trials (NSABP B-14, B-20) have shown a disease-free survival and an overall survival advantage for women with node-negative, estrogen-positive tumors who received tamoxifen.

It is advisable to obtain an estrogen-receptor assay for every breast cancer at the time of initial diagnosis. Receptor status may change after hormonal therapy, radiotherapy, or chemotherapy. The specimen requires special handling, and the laboratory should be prepared to process the specimen correctly.

Curative Treatment

Treatment may be curative or palliative. Curative treatment is advised for clinical stage I and II disease (see Table 61–2). Treatment is palliative for patients in stage IV and for previously treated patients who develop distant metastases or unresectable local recurrence.

A. THERAPEUTIC OPTIONS

1. **Radical mastectomy**—Historically, Halsted is credited with performing the first modern **radical mastectomy** as early as 1882 in the United States. This surgical procedure was the en bloc removal of the breast, pectoral muscles, and axillary lymph nodes. It was the standard surgical procedure performed for breast cancer in the United States from the turn of the century until the 1950s. During the 1950s, emerging information about lymph node drainage patterns prompted surgeons to undertake the **extended radical mastectomy,** which was a radical mastectomy and the removal of the internal mammary lymph nodes. It was postulated that a more extensive dissection of the draining lymphatics would improve control rates and translate into improved survival. A randomized trial, however, proved no benefit to the extended radical mastectomy versus the radical mastectomy, and the former was abandoned. Moreover, the failure of the extended radical mastectomy underscored the complications and morbidity of breast cancer surgery. This morbidity coupled with inadequate disease control led surgeons to explore less invasive and disfiguring techniques. Currently, radical mastectomy is rarely indicated or performed. Even in settings where radical resection may be entertained such as invasion of the pectoralis muscles or large tumors, less invasive surgery coupled with neo- or adjuvant treatments like radiation and chemotherapy are preferred.

2. **Modified radical mastectomy**—Replacing radical mastectomy, the **modified radical mastectomy** (MRM) is the removal of the breast, underlying pectoralis major fascia but not the muscle, and some of the axillary lymph nodes. Variations of this procedure include sacrificing the pectoralis minor muscle or not and retracting, splitting, or transecting the pectoralis major to access the apex of the axilla for dissection. Since it is less invasive and less disfiguring, MRM provides a better cosmetic and functional result than radical mastec-

tomy. Two prospective randomized trials, single institution data, and several retrospective studies have all demonstrated no difference in disease-free or overall survival between radical mastectomy and MRM for early-stage breast cancer. Until the early 1980s and the emergence of breast conservation therapy (BCT), MRM was the standard treatment available to women for early-stage cancer. For locally advanced breast cancer and when the patient is not a candidate for BCT or if she is not motivated for breast conservation, MRM remains a valid treatment option. A **total mastectomy** (simple mastectomy) is the removal of the whole breast, like a MRM, without the axillary dissection. Because an axillary evaluation is critical for staging purposes, total mastectomy is not performed for invasive cancers and is generally reserved for in-situ lesions with their low metastatic potential.

3. **Breast conservation therapy**—BCT involves a surgical procedure such as a **lumpectomy**—an excision of the tumor mass with a negative surgical margin—an axillary evaluation, and postoperative irradiation. Several other operations more limited in the scope of surgical dissection than MRM such as **segmental mastectomy, partial mastectomy,** and **quadrantectomy** are also used in conjunction with radiation and are part of the surgical component of BCT. As a result of 6 prospective randomized trials that showed no significant difference in local relapse, distant metastases, or overall survival between conservative surgery with radiation and mastectomy, BCT has gained increasing acceptance as a treatment option for stage I and II breast cancers.

B. CHOICE OF LOCAL THERAPY

Breast cancer is a multidisciplinary disease in which surgeons, radiation and medical oncologists, radiologists, pathologists, nurses, and psychosocial support staff all play fundamental roles. Working with the patient, this team recommends the most appropriate treatment strategy. Clinical and pathological stage (see Table 61–2) as well as biological aggressiveness are the principal determinants guiding local therapy, treatment strategy, and outcome. For early-stage breast cancer, including node-positive cases, much of the decision for initial local therapy rests with the patient. MRM is always a valid choice for addressing the local treatment of breast cancer. A patient's decision to undergo MRM does not necessarily obviate the role of radiation in the further management of breast cancer, and postmastectomy irradiation may still be recommended. To be a candidate for BCT, the patient must not be pregnant and cannot have multicentric breast cancer (evidence of cancer in more than 1 quadrant of the breast), locally advanced disease, diffuse microcalcifications on mammogram, or a prior history of ipsilateral breast irradiation. Relative contraindications are collagen-vascular disorders that could lead to a poor cosmetic outcome with irradiation and breast implants or psychiatric issues that would make close follow-up and surveillance difficult. These restrictions are only a portion of the decision-making process that must be completed before embarking on BCT.

Perhaps most importantly, the patient must be motivated and desire to maintain her breast in the face of a cancer diagnosis. This may entail some degree of physical, emotional, and psychological distress. For example, a patient may have to endure multiple reexcisions to obtain a negative surgical margin on the lumpectomy specimen. A patient may also experience resistance to BCT in areas where it is not commonly offered and where a multidisciplinary approach to breast cancer is not practiced. It has been shown that the surgical management of breast cancer differs considerably based on geographic location in the United States, independent of patient and tumor characteristics. Nevertheless, both physicians and patients pursue BCT because it allows the patient to keep her breast without any decrement to survival, and the vast majority of women are pleased with the cosmetic result.

Since the treatment options for locally advanced and inflammatory breast cancers are in some ways less flexible than those for early-stage breast cancer, it is even more critical to engage the patient in the decision-making process for the choice of initial therapy. Many different strategies, which include mastectomy and less invasive surgeries, with or without neoadjuvant chemotherapy and adjuvant chemotherapy, radiation, and further maintenance interventions, are commonly used. In many settings, protocol therapy may be the most desirable treatment option.

Mastectomy

For about three-quarters of a century, radical mastectomy was considered standard therapy for breast cancer. The procedure was designed to remove the primary lesion, the breast in which it arose, the underlying muscle, and, by dissection in continuity, the axillary lymph nodes that were thought to be the first site of spread beyond the breast. When radical mastectomy was introduced by Halsted, the average patient presented for treatment with advanced local disease (stage III), and a relatively extensive procedure was often necessary just to remove all gross cancer. This is no longer the case. Patients present now with much smaller, less locally advanced lesions. Most of the patients in Halsted's original series would now be considered incurable by surgery alone, since they had extensive involvement of the chest wall, skin, and supraclavicular regions.

Although radical mastectomy is rarely performed today, MRM is a valid initial local treatment for breast cancer. Radical mastectomy is seldom, if ever, indicated given advances in surgical technique and other more modern treatment modalities. Radical mastectomy has the disadvantage of being one of the most deforming of any of the available treatments for the management of primary breast cancer. Since the 1960s, MRM has supplanted the radical mastectomy because of its comparable disease control and a substantial decrease in morbidity and disfiguration.

In many cases, adjuvant therapy following MRM, eg, radiation, can even further reduce the incidence of local recurrence in certain patients with unfavorable tumor characteristics. In addition, 3 recent randomized trials of postmastectomy radiation, which confirmed a local control advantage, demonstrated an overall survival benefit in certain subsets of both pre- and postmenopausal women. For patients with ≥ 4 positive lymph nodes or an advanced primary tumor, postmastectomy radiation is strongly recommended. The role of postmastectomy radiation in patients with 1–3 positive nodes is not as clear. When deciding on initial local therapy, therefore, a patient must keep in mind that choosing MRM does not necessarily exclude a recommendation for adjuvant radiation.

Breast Conservation Therapy

Since studies comparing radical mastectomy and MRM demonstrated no decrement in local control or survival, radical mastectomy has given way to MRM. With less invasive surgery, there are fewer side effects, less morbidity, and ultimately an improvement in quality of life. Simple mastectomy performed alone, however, has an unacceptably high failure rate. (In part, this is because the lymph nodes are not removed. As many as 40% of patients with clinically negative nodes will have evidence of metastatic spread within these nodes at dissection, and roughly half of these patients subsequently develop regional recurrences.)

In the 1980s, 6 prospective randomized trials were conducted worldwide that showed no significant difference in local-regional relapse or overall survival between breast-conserving surgery and radiation versus MRM for early-stage invasive breast cancer. Two of these studies included patients with node-positive breast cancer. With the addition of radiation to breast-conserving surgery techniques such as lumpectomy with an axillary evaluation, local failure is reduced to rates comparable to MRM with no compromise to overall survival.

The next step has been to perform breast-conserving surgery without the addition of adjuvant radiation. Several trials including a seminal study by the National Surgical Adjuvant Breast Project (NSABP) established the efficacy of BCT for noninvasive breast cancer. For in situ disease, a group from Van Nuys, California, has proposed a prognostic index to determine which patients might not benefit from or need radiation after excision. With the exception of a small number of highly selected cases, the work of this group has not yet produced results to justify omitting radiation as standard practice.

Axillary Evaluation

It is important to recognize that axillary evaluation is valuable both in planning therapy and in staging of the cancer. Surgery is extremely effective in preventing axillary recurrences. While the removal of even occult cancer in axillary lymph nodes generally does not translate into an improvement in overall survival rates, regional failures will be lower. In addition, lymph nodes removed during the procedure can be pathologically assessed. This assessment is essential for the planning of adjuvant therapy, which is often recommended for patients with gross or occult involvement of axillary nodes.

An emerging alternative to formal axillary dissection for the pathological assessment of the clinically negative axilla is sentinel lymph node biopsy (SLNB). This procedure uses a tracer material, which is injected into the tumor bed to map the tumor drainage to the primary or "sentinel" axillary lymph node(s). The sentinel lymph node is excised and pathologically examined. If the sentinel lymph node is found to harbor metastatic disease, a subsequent formal dissection is done. Conversely, if the sentinel lymph node is negative, no further surgical evaluation need be performed. Although this procedure relies heavily on the surgeon's expertise with a new technique and has some inherent limitations, SLNB is another step toward less invasive breast cancer management. Potential side effects and complications are minimized, and recovery is quick without sacrificing diagnostic or therapeutic results. A practical example of the benefits of SLNB is that, when used in conjunction with BCT, reported rates of lymphedema are lower than with axillary dissection.

Current Recommendations

We believe that BCT, which includes radiation, with an axillary evaluation or MRM is the best initial local treatment for most patients with potentially curable carcinoma of the breast. It cannot be overemphasized, however, that a diagnosis of breast cancer should be managed with a multidisciplinary approach and treatment should be individualized. Treatment of the axillary nodes is not indicated for noninfiltrating cancers, because by definition in situ lesions do not have metastatic potential. Nevertheless, axillary nodal metastases are detected in a small minority of cases, most of which are subsequently found to harbor microinvasive disease.

Preoperatively, full discussion with the patient regarding the rationale for BCT and mastectomy as well as the manner of coping with the cosmetic and psychological effects of the operation is essential. Patients often have numerous questions about BCT and MRM and wish detailed explanations of the risks and benefits of the various procedures. If a patient decides on MRM, breast reconstruction should be discussed. Time spent preoperatively in educating the patient and her family is time well spent.

Adjuvant Systemic Therapy

A. Chemotherapy

Cytotoxic chemotherapy is commonly offered to women as adjuvant treatment for early-stage as well as locally advanced breast cancer. The goal of adjuvant chemotherapy is to eliminate occult microscopic metastases that are often responsible for late recurrences. It is systemic treatment and should not be confused with efforts to address known local disease. In the past, only premenopausal women with lymph node–positive cancers were routinely candidates for cytotoxic chemotherapy. For a host of reasons, recent guidelines recommend the use of chemotherapy on a more individualized basis and thus broaden the scope of who may be a candidate for therapy. Node-negative patients are now stratified into risk categories to help guide the decisions for adjuvant systemic therapy (see Table 61–4).

The NIH Consensus Statement on Adjuvant Therapy for Breast Cancer recommends that chemotherapy be offered to most women with localized breast cancer > 1 cm regardless of nodal, menopausal, or hormone receptor status. Polychemotherapy ($\geq$ 2 agents) has been found to be superior to single-agent chemotherapy. Duration for 3–6 months or 4–6 cycles appears to offer optimal benefit without subjecting the patient to undue toxicity associated with more prolonged treatment, which adds little benefit in terms of overall outcome. Cytotoxic chemotherapy with an anthracycline-based (doxorubicin [A] or epirubicin [E]) regimen is favored since a small but statistically significant improvement in survival has been demonstrated compared with nonanthracycline-containing regimens. Traditional regimens using 6 cycles of cyclophosphamide, methotrexate, and 5-fluorouracil (CMF), which do not cause alopecia, are not necessarily inferior to regimens now commonly used, such as 4 cycles of doxorubicin and cyclophosphamide (AC), but if an anthracycline-containing regimen is being considered, cyclophosphamide, doxorubicin, and 5-fluorouracil (CAF) or cyclophosphamide, epirubicin, and 5-fluorouracil (CEF) should be chosen. The cardiac toxicity caused by anthracyclines is not

Table 61–4. NIH Consensus Conference on adjuvant treatment for women with breast cancer risk categories for node-negative patients.

	Low Risk (All listed factors)	Intermediate Risk	High Risk (≥ 1 factor)
Tumor size	< 1.0 cm	1–2 cm	> 2 cm
ER or PR	+	+	–
Tumor grade	Grade I	Grade I–II	Grade II–III

Abbreviations: ER, estrogen receptor; PR, progesterone receptor.

considered detrimental in women without significant cardiac disease but does occur in 1% of cases or less.

Several areas concerning chemotherapy have generated considerable interest but suffer from a lack of data or inconclusive evidence. For instance, the current data are inconclusive with regard to the administration of taxanes (paclitaxel or docetaxel) to node-positive patients. For node-negative patients, there is no evidence to justify their use, and it is considered nonstandard. High-dose chemotherapy with bone marrow or stem cell rescue is also not recommended. There is no evidence that high-dose regimens are superior to standard-dose polychemotherapy. Stem cell support or bone marrow transplant should be offered only on protocol.

Further investigations need to be performed to clarify the role of high-dose regimens and new chemotherapy as well as biological agents and dosing schedules. Trials need to enroll more patients older than 70 years to assess the benefits and toxicities of adjuvant chemotherapy in this population. Finally, studies designed to measure quality of life need to be done to place the benefits versus toxicity question of adjuvant therapies into context.

B. HORMONAL THERAPY

Adjuvant hormonal therapy or manipulation is recommended for all women whose breast cancer expresses hormone receptors. Even if the tumor does not express estrogen hormone receptor protein but only progesterone, hormonal therapy may be beneficial. This recommendation is made regardless of age, menopausal status, involvement or number of positive lymph nodes, or tumor size. The benefit of adjuvant hormonal therapy is seen across all subgroups of breast cancer patients, with both invasive and in situ lesions. While the absolute decrease in recurrence, second primary breast cancer, and death may vary from group to group, there is a firmly established role for adjuvant hormonal intervention. Two possible exceptions, according to the NIH Consensus Conference, are the premenopausal

patient with a tumor < 1 cm who wants to avoid estrogen loss and the elderly patient with a similar size tumor and a history of thromboembolic events. Because of the overwhelming benefit of hormonal therapy, however, this determination should be made by an experienced medical oncologist (see Tables 61–5 and 61–6).

Five years of tamoxifen is currently the most common regimen of hormonal therapy, although other forms of manipulation such as ovarian ablation exist. Randomized trials support the 5-year duration, which is superior to shorter courses and does not expose the patient to the increased risk of adverse effects associated with longer use. Furthermore, use longer than 5 years doesn't appear to enhance the long-term benefit seen with just 5 years of use. Although tamoxifen carries a slight increased risk of endometrial cancer and venous thromboembolism (5–6 events per 1000 patient-years of treatment), the benefits outweigh the risks for the vast number of patients. Surveillance screening procedures such as transvaginal ultrasound and endometrial biopsy are not necessary in asymptomatic patients on tamoxifen. Raloxifene and aromatase inhibitors are currently being investigated as alternate adjuvant hormonal therapies.

Follow-Up Care

After primary treatment, breast cancer patients should be followed for life because of the long, insidious natural history of breast cancer. The goals of close breast cancer follow-up are to detect recurrences after treatment in the ipsilateral breast and to detect new second primary cancers in the contralateral breast. The risk of a second primary in the contralateral breast of a patient with a history of breast cancer is believed to be roughly 0.5–1% per year. Although there are no universally accepted guidelines, several consensus conferences have met to establish recommendations. After the completion of treatment, it is recommended that the patient

Table 61–5. Summary of NIH Conference on adjuvant treatment for women with axillary node-negative breast cancer.

Patient Group	Low Risk	Intermediate Risk	High Risk
Premenopausal ER/PR–	None or TAM	TAM + CT TAM Ablation GnRH	CT + TAM CT + Ablation/GnRH CT + TAM + Ablation/GNRH
Premenopausal ET/PR–	N/A	N/A	CT
Postmenopausal ER/PR +	None or TAM	TAM + CT TAM	TAM + CT TAM
Postmenopausal ER/PR–	N/A	N/A	CT
> 70 years	None or TAM	TAM TAM ± CT	TAM ± CT if receptor–

Abbreviations: Ablation, ovarian ablation; CT, chemotherapy; ER, estrogen receptor; GnRH, GnRH analogue; PR, progesterone receptor; TAM, tamoxifen.

undergo a physical examination every 4 months for the first 2 years, then every 6 months until year 5 and annually thereafter. A mammogram should be obtained annually for all patients. For patients who received irradiation, a chest radiograph is also obtained yearly. Routine laboratory tests including CBC, chemistry profile, and liver function tests can be ordered annually, especially if the patient received chemotherapy, or else as needed otherwise. There is no role for routine bone scans or additional imaging unless the patient is symptomatic or there is clinical suspicion of an abnormality. Patients taking tamoxifen should have annual pelvic examinations and be counseled to report any irregular vaginal bleeding.

Table 61–6. Summary of NIH Consensus Conference on adjuvant treatment for women with axillary node-positive breast cancer.

Patient Group	Treatment
Premenopausal ER/PR +	CT + TAM CT + Ablation/GnRH CT + TAM + Ablation/GnRH
Premenopausal	CT
Postmenopausal ER/PR +	TAM + CT
Postmenopausal ER/PR–	CT
> 70 years	TAM + CT if ER/PR–

Abbreviations: See Table 61–5.

A. LOCAL RECURRENCE

The development of local recurrence correlates with stage and thus tumor size as well as the presence and number of positive axillary lymph nodes, margin status, nuclear grade, and histologic type. The median time to recurrence is roughly 4 years with a 1–2% risk per year for the first 5 years and a 1% risk per year thereafter. Late failures occurring 15 years or more after treatment, however, do occur. The risk of local recurrence following BCT or MRM is generally < 15% 10 years after treatment. Positive axillary lymph nodes are prognostic for local failure at the chest wall following MRM, but they are not prognostic for a local failure following BCT.

The treatment of local recurrences depends on the initial local therapy. In the breast, failures after BCT can be treated with salvage mastectomy with salvage rates of approximately 50%. In general, there is no difference in overall survival for an isolated breast recurrence successfully treated with salvage mastectomy. Node failures are more ominous. Axillary failures have roughly a 50% 3–5 year disease-free survival and supraclavicular failures 0–20% 3-year disease-free survival. All chest wall abnormalities should be biopsied to rule out recurrence and resected with a wide local excision if possible. Adjuvant salvage therapies such as radiation, cytotoxic chemotherapy, and hormonal therapy may also be instituted.

Local recurrence may signal the presence of widespread disease and is an indication for bone and liver scans, posteroanterior and lateral chest x-rays, and other examinations as needed to search for evidence of metastases. When there is no evidence of metastases beyond the chest wall and regional nodes, radical irradiation for cure and complete local excision should be attempted. Most patients with locally recurrent tumors will develop distant metastases within 2 years. For this reason, many physicians use systemic therapy for treatment of patients with local recurrence. Although this seems reasonable, it should be pointed out that patients with local recurrence may be cured with local resection or radiation. Systemic chemotherapy or hormonal treatment should be used for patients who develop disseminated disease or those in whom local recurrence occurs following adequate local therapy.

B. Edema of the Arm

Lymphedema of the arm is a significant and often dreaded complication of breast cancer treatment. Lymphedema occurs as a result of lymphatic disruption and insult caused primarily by local treatment modalities like surgery and radiation. While each of these modalities carries its own a risk with respect to arm edema, a combined modality approach further increases this risk. With a typical level I/II axillary lymph node dissection and radiation, the risk of lymph edema is roughly < 10%. This risk approached 30% when a more aggressive level III dissection was more commonly performed in the past. The rates of clinically significant lymphedema—that is edema, that affects function and is not merely detectable with sophisticated measurement tools—are generally considered to be much lower. With the advent of SLNB, lymphedema rates are expected to continue to improve.

Late or secondary edema of the arm may develop years after MRM, as a result of axillary recurrence or of infection in the hand or arm, with obliteration of lymphatic channels. There is usually no obvious cause of late arm swelling.

C. Breast Reconstruction

Breast reconstruction, with the implantation of a prosthesis or transverse rectus abdominis myocutaneous flap (TRAM), is usually feasible after MRM. Reconstruction should be discussed with patients prior to mastectomy because it offers an important psychological focal point for recovery. Reconstruction is not an obstacle to the diagnosis of recurrent cancer.

Prognosis

The stage of breast cancer is the single most reliable indicator of prognosis. Patients with disease localized to the breast and no evidence of regional spread after microscopic examination of the lymph nodes have by far the most favorable prognosis. Estrogen and progesterone receptors appear to be an important prognostic variable because patients with hormone receptor–nega-

tive tumors and no evidence of metastases to the axillary lymph nodes have a much higher recurrence rate than do patients with hormone receptor–positive tumors and no regional metastases. The histologic subtype of breast cancer (eg, medullary, lobular, comedo) seems to have little, if any, significance in prognosis once these tumors are truly invasive.

As mentioned above, several different treatment regimens achieve approximately the same results when given to the appropriate patient. Localized disease can be controlled with local therapy—either MRM or BCT, which includes radiation. However, the criteria for selection of patients to be treated with conservative resection and radiation therapy require further clarification.

Many patients who develop breast cancer will ultimately die of breast cancer. The mortality rate of breast cancer patients exceeds that of age-matched normal controls for nearly 20 years. Thereafter, the mortality rates are equal, although deaths that occur among the breast cancer patients are often directly the result of tumor. Five-year statistics do not accurately reflect the final outcome of therapy.

When cancer is localized to the breast, with no evidence of regional spread after pathologic examination, the clinical cure rate with most accepted methods of therapy is 75–80%. Exceptions to this may be related to the hormonal receptor content of the tumor, tumor size, host resistance, or associated illness. Patients with small estrogen and progesterone receptor–positive tumors and no evidence of axillary spread probably have a 5-year survival rate of nearly 90%. When the axillary lymph nodes are involved with the tumor, the survival rate drops to 50–60% at 5 years and probably less than 25% at 10 years. In general, breast cancer appears to be somewhat more malignant in younger than older women, and this may be related to the fact that relatively fewer younger women have estrogen receptor–positive tumors.

TREATMENT OF ADVANCED BREAST CANCER

This section covers palliative therapy of disseminated disease incurable by surgery (stage IV).

Radiotherapy

Palliative radiotherapy may be advised for locally advanced cancers with distant metastases in order to control ulceration, pain, and other manifestations in the breast and regional nodes. As part of multimodality treatment, radical irradiation of the chest wall and the axillary, internal mammary, and supraclavicular nodes should be undertaken in an attempt to cure locally advanced and inoperable lesions when there is no evidence of distant metastases. A small number of patients in this group are cured in spite of extensive breast and regional node involvement. Adjuvant chemotherapy also plays a valuable role in the treatment of such patients.

Palliative irradiation is also of value in the treatment of certain bone or soft tissue metastases to control pain or avoid fracture. Radiotherapy is especially useful in the treatment of the isolated bony metastasis and chest wall recurrences.

Hormonal Therapy

Disseminated disease may respond to prolonged endocrine therapy such as ovarian ablation or administration of drugs that block hormone receptor sites or that block hormone synthesis or production. Hormonal manipulation is usually more successful in postmenopausal women. If treatment is based on the presence of estrogen receptor protein in the primary tumor or metastases, however, the rate of response is nearly equal in premenopausal and postmenopausal women. A favorable response to hormonal manipulation occurs in about one-third of patients with metastatic breast cancer. Of those whose tumors contain estrogen receptors, the response is about 60% and perhaps as high as 80% for patients whose tumors contain progesterone receptors as well. Tumors negative for both estrogen and progesterone receptors have response rates to hormonal therapy that are 10% or less.

Since the quality of life during a remission induced by endocrine manipulation is usually superior to a remission following cytotoxic chemotherapy, it may be best to try endocrine manipulation as a first-line systemic treatment.

In general, only one type of systemic therapy should be given at a time, unless it is necessary to irradiate a destructive lesion of weight-bearing bone while the patient is on another regimen. The regimen should be changed only if the disease is clearly progressing but not if it appears to be stable. This is especially important for patients with destructive bone metastases, since minor changes in the status of these lesions are difficult to determine radiographically. A plan of therapy that would simultaneously minimize toxicity and maximize benefits is often best achieved by hormonal manipulation.

The choice of endocrine therapy depends on the menopausal status of the patient. Women within 1 year of their last menstrual period are considered to be premenopausal, while women whose menstruation ceased more than 1 year ago are postmenopausal. The initial choice of therapy is referred to as primary hormonal manipulation; subsequent endocrine treatment is called secondary or tertiary hormonal manipulation.

A. PRIMARY HORMONAL THERAPY

In the past, bilateral oophorectomy was the standard method of hormone manipulation employed in premenopausal women with advanced breast cancer. However, it has subsequently become clear that tamoxifen is equally effective and has none of the attendant risks of surgical ablation of the ovaries. Tamoxifen is recommended as the treatment of choice for hormonal therapy in the premenopausal woman with advanced breast cancer. Tamoxifen, 10 mg twice daily, is also the initial therapy of choice for postmenopausal women with metastatic breast cancer amenable to endocrine manipulation.

B. SECONDARY OR TERTIARY HORMONAL THERAPY

A favorable response to initial hormonal therapy with tamoxifen is predictive of future responses to hormonal maneuvers.

Other hormonal agents have been found effective in premenopausal patients. GnRH agonists that act on the pituitary to eventually suppress FSH and LH and the pituitary ovarian axis, thereby decreasing estrogen production, have been used since the 1980s. They are an alternative to oophorectomy if used alone or can be combined with tamoxifen to provide a slight improvement in progression-free survival and overall survival.

The use of aromatase inhibitors, which work by blocking the conversion of testosterone to estradiol and androstenedione to estrogen both in the adrenal cortex and in peripheral tissue including breast cancers themselves, has been shown to be effective in postmenopausal patients.

Progestins, megestrol acetate, and medroxyprogesterone acetate are alternative agents reserved mainly for cases resistant to tamoxifen.

Chemotherapy

Cytotoxic drugs should be considered for the treatment of metastatic breast cancer in the following instances: (1) if visceral metastases are present (especially brain or lymphangitic pulmonary), (2) if hormonal treatment is unsuccessful or the disease has progressed after an initial response to hormonal manipulation, or (3) if the tumor is estrogen and progesterone receptor–negative. With response rates of 35–55% in many series, the taxanes are quickly eclipsing the anthracyclines in the single-agent treatment of hormone-refractory metastatic breast cancer. Where once doxorubicin could achieve response rates of 40–50%, in some trials the taxanes seem to offer a small overall survival advantage. In addition, they are generally well tolerated with an acceptable side-effect profile. Questions about dosing, schedule of administration, and use with other agents, however, still have to be thoroughly answered.

Combination chemotherapy using multiple agents is appealing because theoretically the risk of drug resistance and cumulative toxicity is decreased. When compared to single agent doxorubicin, combination chemotherapy provides higher response rates and longer intervals until first progression. Nevertheless, the use of combination chemotherapy has never been shown to decrease drug resistance or toxicity in breast cancer. When combination chemotherapy has been compared to a single-agent taxane, while response rates were slightly lower, quality of life measurements were higher for the single agent. Thus either a single-agent taxane or an anthracycline-containing combination regimen is frequently used as a first-line treatment. The use of cytotoxic chemotherapy or any other treatment modality should always be highly individualized in the palliative setting.

Bisphosphonate Therapy

After the treatment of primary breast cancer, bone is the most common site of breast cancer recurrence. It is also the most common site of metastatic disease. Metastases are often detected with a bone scan obtained in the staging of locally advanced cases or obtained because of clinical suspicion in the previously treated patient. Confirmation with plain radiographs, MR, and/or CT is frequently needed since 100% of lytic lesions may not be detected with a nuclear medicine scan. These other radiographic studies also help delineate the extent of the metastatic disease. After bone metastases are confirmed, bisphosphonate therapy should be started. Although no survival advantage has been demonstrated, bisphosphonates have been shown to reduce bony as well as visceral metastases. Bisphosphonate therapy should be administered with other palliative systemic treatments such as hormonal manipulation or chemotherapy. It is typically given intravenously every 3–4 weeks for 2 years or for the duration of other systemic treatment.

REFERENCES

Andersson M et al: Tamoxifen in high-risk premenopausal women with primary breast cancer receiving adjuvant chemotherapy. Report from the Danish Breast Cancer Co-operative Group DBCG 82B Trial. Eur J Cancer 1999;35:1659.

Bishop JF et al: Initial paclitaxel improves outcome compared with CMFP combination chemotherapy as front-line therapy in untreated metastatic breast cancer. J Clin Oncol 1999; 17:2355.

Diel IJ et al: Reduction in new metastases in breast cancer with adjuvant clodronate treatment. N Engl J Med 1998;339:357.

Erickson VS et al: Arm edema in breast cancer patients. J Natl Cancer Inst 2001;93:96.

Fisher B et al: Five versus more than five years of tamoxifen for lymph node–negative breast cancer: Updated findings from the National Surgical Adjuvant Breast and Bowel Project B-14 randomized trial. J Natl Cancer Inst 2001;93: 684.

Fisher B et al: Tamoxifen and chemotherapy for lymph node–negative, estrogen receptor–positive breast cancer. J Natl Cancer Inst 1997;89:1673.

Fisher B et al: Tamoxifen in treatment of intraductal breast cancer: National Surgical Adjuvant Breast and Bowel Project B-24 randomized controlled trial. Lancet 1999;353:1993.

Fisher ER et al: Fifteen-year prognostic discriminates for invasive breast carcinoma. Cancer 2001;91:1679.

Fisher ER et al: Pathologic findings from the National Surgical Adjuvant Breast Project (NSABP) eight-year update of Protocol B-17: Intraductal carcinoma. Cancer 1999;86:429.

Fleming ID et al (editors): AJCC Cancer Staging Manual, 5th ed. Lippincott, 1997, p. 174.

Freedman GM, Fowble BL: Local recurrence after mastectomy or breast-conserving surgery and radiation. Oncology (Huntingt) 2000;14:1561.

Greenlee RT et al: Cancer statistics, 2001. CA Cancer J Clin 2001;51:15.

Haagensen CD: Diseases of the Breast, 2nd ed. Saunders, 1971.

Harris JR et al: Consensus statement on postmastectomy radiation therapy. Int J Radiat Oncol Biol Phys 1999;44:989.

Hayes DF: Evaluation of patients after primary therapy. In: Harris JR et al (editors): Diseases of the Breast, 2nd ed. Lippincott, 2000.

Kerlikowske K: Efficacy of screening mammography among women aged 40 to 49 years and 50 to 69 years: Comparison of relative and absolute benefit. J Natl Cancer Inst Monogr 1997;22:79.

Klauber-DeMore N et al: Sentinel lymph node biopsy: Is it indicated in patients with high-risk ductal carcinoma-in-situ and ductal carcinoma-in-situ with microinvasion? Ann Surg Oncol 2000;7:636.

Krag D et al: The sentinel node in breast cancer. N Engl J Med 1998;339:941.

McCarthy EP et al: Local management of invasive breast cancer. In: Harris JR et al (editors): Diseases of the Breast, 2nd ed. Lippincott, 2000.

McMasters KM et al: Sentinel-lymph-node biopsy for breast cancer—not yet the standard of care. N Engl J Med 1998; 3 39:990.

Miner TJ et al: Sentinel lymph node biopsy for breast cancer: The role of previous biopsy on patient eligibility. Am Surg 1999;65:493.

Moskowitz MA: Mammography use helps to explain differences in breast cancer stage at diagnosis between older black and white women. Ann Intern Med 1998;128:729.

Myers RE et al: Baseline staging tests in primary breast cancer: A practice guideline. Can Med Assoc J 2001;164:1439.

National Institutes of Health Consensus Development Conference: Adjuvant Therapy for Breast Cancer, November 1–3, 2000.

Overgaard M et al: Postoperative radiotherapy in high-risk postmenopausal breast-cancer patients given adjuvant tamoxifen: Danish Breast Cancer Cooperative Group DBCG 82c randomised trial. Lancet 1999;353:1641.

Pendas S et al: Sentinel node biopsy in ductal carcinoma in situ patients. Ann Surg Oncol 2000;7:15.

Petrek JA, Pressman PI, Smith RA: Lymphedema: Current issues in research and management. CA Cancer J Clin 2000;50:292.

Ragaz J et al: Adjuvant radiotherapy and chemotherapy in node-positive premenopausal women with breast cancer. N Engl J Med 1997;337:956.

Recht A et al: Locoregional failure 10 years after mastectomy and adjuvant chemotherapy with or without tamoxifen without irradiation: Experience of the Eastern Cooperative Oncology Group. J Clin Oncol 1999;17:1689.

Ries LAG et al (editors): SEER Cancer Statistics Review, 1973–1998, National Cancer Institute. http://seer.cancer.gov/Publications/CSR1973_1998/ accessed October 2001.

Roetzheim RG et al: Effects of health insurance and race on early detection of cancer. J Natl Cancer Inst 1999;9:1409.

Sakorafas GH, Tsiotou AG: Selection criteria for breast conservation in breast cancer. Eur J Surg 2000;166:835.

Schrenk P et al: Morbidity following sentinel lymph node biopsy versus axillary lymph node dissection for patients with breast carcinoma. Cancer 2000;88:608.

Self-reported use of mammography and insurance status among women aged > or = 40 years—United States, 1991–1992 and 1996–1997. MMWR 1998;47:825.

Shapiro S: Periodic screening for breast cancer: The HIP randomized controlled trial. J Natl Cancer Inst Monogr 1997;22:27.

Silverstein MJ et al: A prognostic index for ductal carcinoma in situ of the breast. Cancer 1999;77:2267.

Swenson KK et al: Prognostic factors after conservative surgery and radiation therapy for early stage breast cancer. Am J Clin Oncol 1998;21:111.

Theriault RL: Medical treatment of bone metastases. In: Harris JR et al (editors): *Diseases of the Breast,* 2nd ed. Lippincott, 2000.

The Borderland Between Law & Medicine

62

John Patrick O'Grady, MD, Dennis R. Anti, JD, & Despina E. Hoffman, BA

> *The web of life*
> *is a mingled yarn*
> *good and ill together*
>
> *All's Well That Ends Well (IV, iii, 74)*
> *William Shakespeare (1564–1616)*

Introduction

Obstetric and gynecologic medicine is involved with the processes of human conception, pregnancy, parturition, and sexual and urologic function, so inevitable problems in practice occur, including maternal or fetal birth injuries or surgical complications. Such imperfect outcomes distress both patients and their families, prompting critical review of management. Not surprisingly, legal entanglements are a frequent consequence. Defense against malpractice allegations requires an understanding of basic American legal processes and an appreciation of the principles of law and medicine that establish prevailing standards of medical care.

Both the practice of medicine and the accepted standards of practice have changed rapidly in recent years. This is due in part to scientific advances, the increasing influence of third party payers, the introduction of new government regulations concerning the organization and financing of medical care, and changes in societal expectations for medicine. Unfortunately, even minor deviations from accepted standards of care have the potential to result in adverse legal judgments. Thus, physicians must continually incorporate medical advances into current practice while remaining cognizant of new legal concepts of potential liability.

This chapter explores several aspects of the interdependent and contentious relationship between law and medicine. Selected concepts of legal theory are examined and a number of medicolegal issues pertinent to specific clinical problems in modern obstetric and gynecologic practice are discussed. A bibliography is provided for readers interested in additional study.

Anatomy of the Legal System

Most malpractice claims proceed under rules of **common law,** the body of legal judicial opinion derived from precedent cases rather than statutory or legislative rules. The strength of common law is its ability to adapt its rulings and interpretations to the changes in society, including advances in medical science. However, less happily for clinicians, as standards of care and legal interpretations change, so do the potential grounds for litigation.

Elements of Tort

Alleged acts of medical malpractice are almost always tried as torts, governed by the rules of common law. A **tort** is a civil wrong committed against persons or property. Torts can be intentional, unintentional (or negligent), strict liability, or concomitant torts. In these proceedings, monetary compensation is awarded by the court as a remedy for a perceived harm or injury (damages). As is briefly discussed in the following sections, the majority of medical malpractice claims are filed as negligence torts.

A. Intentional Torts

Intentional torts include battery, assault, and false imprisonment. Most intentional torts in the context of medical practice are claims of battery. However, even these are rare in the physician-patient context. Battery is broadly defined as unwanted, harmful, or offensive bodily contact that occurs without consent. Claims of battery against obstetrician/gynecologists usually arise from an alleged improper extension of a previously consented to—but originally contemplated as less extensive—surgical procedure or from alleged improper events during examinations. In the case of surgery, the legal burden falls to the practitioner to prove that a proper informed consent was obtained **or** that the clinical circumstances were such that consent was implied. When an individual consents to a surgical procedure or to an examination and there is proof of informed consent and proper professional behavior, an intentional tort claim of battery is usually defeated. The prevention of potential claims of battery in surgery hinges on the content of the consent process. This requires appropriate communication between the clinician, patient, and family.

1117

B. Unintentional Torts

Most malpractice claims are filed as unintentional or negligence torts. These claims are based on allegations that damages resulted from the violation of one or more standards of care. In such negligence torts, liability is established by proving 4 elements: duty, breach of duty, causation, and damages.

Burden of Proof: The burden of proof, or the proof necessary to establish liability, is normally the requirement of the plaintiff. The plaintiff must demonstrate that the 4 elements—**duty, breach, causation,** and **damages**—are present by a fair preponderance of the evidence. This is not a requirement for scientific proof or proof beyond a reasonable doubt, but the simple demand that one side in the case is stronger than the other. This is an area in which physicians often have substantial difficulty, because the burden of proof accepted in science or medicine is not the "51% certainty" employed in torts. The testimony of expert medical witnesses concerning breaches of care standards and causation is central in establishing liability.

Duty and the Breach of Duty: The duty of the physician is the legal sanction to cause no harm and to act in accordance with established standards of care. Accepting an individual for care usually establishes the physician-patient relationship and duty. A breach of duty occurs when the physician does not adhere to established methods of diagnosis and treatment or to applicable standards of care. The existence of a breach in duty is supported by the testimony of expert witnesses who practice in the same medical specialty.

Causation: Causation is the link or proximate cause between a breach of duty and the injury sustained by the patient. Unless there is proof of causation, no liability exists. As an example, despite proof that a physician failed to diagnose an inoperable tumor in a timely manner, he or she will likely not be held liable to the plaintiff if the injury allegedly suffered was inevitable given the patient's condition and not *caused* by an act of the practitioner or by the practitioner's negligence in tardy diagnosis.

Proving causation in obstetric cases is often problematic and almost invariably complex. The etiology of many birth injuries is not established and honest disagreement among well-meaning experts is common. Here again, the testimony of expert witnesses is essential to either prosecute or to defend these cases. Important aspects of birth injury evaluation and expert testimony are discussed later.

Damages: The final component in a negligence suit is damages, or the harm(s) suffered by the patient. A damage must be a discernible injury in order for the plaintiff to recover compensation. Damages can either be economic (medical expenses, lost wages, etc) or noneconomic (emotional distress, loss of consortium, pain and suffering, etc). Amounts assigned for noneconomic injuries are subjective and depend largely upon the response of the judge or jury to the plaintiff's presentation. In some jurisdictions there are statutory limits to these noneconomic damages.

New Legal Theories and Issues

In response to advances in medical practice, especially those in prenatal diagnosis and the reproductive technologies, new legal theories of physician liability have developed. A brief discussion of the nature and complexity of these claims exemplifies the type of novel legal problems now developing in obstetric and gynecologic practice as a result of technologic advances.

A. Wrongful Birth

A wrongful birth is an alleged claim against a clinician for the *fact of birth as opposed to a specific birth injury.* Wrongful birth claims are usually brought by patients following the birth of an infant with serious or disfiguring disabilities such as central nervous system defects (eg, hydrocephalus, meningomyelocele, encephalocele) or various chromosomal abnormalities (eg, trisomy 18 or trisomy 21). The plaintiff usually alleges that the genetic or hereditary basis for a potentially serious condition was not recognized by the clinician, or that appropriate diagnostic testing was not offered early enough for pregnancy prevention or termination. In these proceedings the parents must prove that if they had been informed of the potential for a defective fetus prior to pregnancy or of the existence of an abnormal infant during pregnancy, they would have sought to either avoid pregnancy altogether or to terminate the affected pregnancy. Thus, the personal convictions of the parents concerning both prenatal testing and pregnancy termination become legitimate areas of examination.

If a wrongful birth claim is successful, potential damages depend upon both the condition of the infant as well as precedents in the jurisdiction where the action is brought. As an example, some state courts have allowed recovery for the extraordinary expenses in raising the impaired child as compared to the expenses of raising a nonimpaired child. Wrongful birth claims are uncommon proceedings and are not permitted in all jurisdictions.

Allegations of wrongful birth emphasize the importance of obtaining a complete family or genetic history and informing pregnant women of the available methods of genetic testing. Currently, at-risk families are often referred to prenatal centers for genetic testing and evaluation by perinatal geneticists. Perinatal genetics has rapidly become a highly complex field combining various antepartum tests, prenatal ultrasound examinations, and in-depth family histories in the effort to establish fetal condition and evaluate risk. Routine referral to a genetics counselor for evaluation is not yet considered the standard of care. However, practitioners should be aware that in event of a legal claim, the *content* of their genetic counseling will likely be evaluated against the standard of a trained geneticist as opposed to that of an obstetric generalist. Given the increasing complexity and sophistication of genetic evaluation, the trend toward referral to specially trained geneticists can only accelerate.

B. WRONGFUL LIFE

Wrongful life is an action claiming that negligent prenatal testing on the part of the health care provider resulted in the birth of a "damaged" child. Wrongful life differs from wrongful birth in that the claim is brought *in the name of the physically or mentally disabled child and not of the parents.* Such claims usually involve devastated infants with serious genetic disorders or those born with major injuries as a result of undiagnosed maternal disease or early pregnancy drug exposure. The legal theory for these claims is that the duty of the clinician owed to the unborn child is similar to that owed to the parents.

Due to the unique and controversial assertion that the child would have preferred nonexistence rather than life with impairments, and that because of the specified abnormalities compensation can be claimed for the child's continued life, only a minority of state courts will accept this type of claim.

C. WRONGFUL CONCEPTION

Wrongful conception claims are brought by the parents of a healthy, normal infant. In this instance, the alleged negligence is in the improper performance of a sterilization operation or the improper provision of contraceptive techniques leading to the birth of an otherwise normal but unwanted child. A common problem is women who become pregnant following a postpartum tubal ligation procedure. Another possible scenario involves a woman who undergoes tubal ligation only to discover that an early, undiagnosed pregnancy was already present at the time the surgery was performed. In such cases, potentially all costs relating to prenatal treatment and labor and delivery are recoverable as damages, as well as the expenses related to the failed sterilization. However, the courts remain divided on whether parents may recover for the economic expenses of rearing a normal infant. The unique facts of each case, the jurisdiction in which the case is brought, and the amount of "credit" the court assigns as a benefit for a normal pregnancy versus the "deduction" for this unwanted but normal child determines the final judgment.

Governmental Regulations

A. EMTALA

In 1986, Congress required all hospitals with Medicare participation to comply with the Emergency Medical Treatment and Active Labor Act, or EMTALA. The regulations established by this legislation are intended to protect individuals treated in hospital emergency services. The most important EMTALA requirements are that institutions offering emergency care facilities provide "appropriate medical screening" and "stabilization" of individuals with urgent medical problems prior to their transfer to another institution.

For purposes of EMTALA, "stabilized" for pregnant women *in labor* is interpreted to mean the delivery of the newborn and placenta. Uterine contractions are considered an emergency medical condition under the Act when there is either: (1) inadequate time to effect a safe transfer to another hospital before delivery; or (2) if transfer poses a threat to the health or safety of the woman or to the fetus.

The EMTALA legislation was intended to preclude the arbitrary exclusion of certain patients from hospital admission, especially when transfer would potentially endanger either mother or infant. It interdicts the practice of "dumping" these often indigent or otherwise undesirable individuals on other institutions. The most frequent problems for clinicians under the Act include the failure to see patients at risk, failure to take a proper history, and the failure to conduct basic examinations before deciding upon a transfer.

For the purposes of an EMTALA claim, the clinical outcome of the emergency visit is irrelevant. The issue simply becomes, were the established rules violated? Emergency physicians, obstetricians, or midwives—all practitioners involved in patient transfers—need to closely follow the proper procedures and complete the necessary institutional forms. The potential penalties are draconian—up to $50,000 for each violation! In addition, individuals who suffer personal harm as a result of an EMTALA violation are permitted to bring to a separate civil action for damages. Such cases would prove difficult to defend. The imposition of an EMTALA fine would be excellent evidence of the violation of a care standard.

Issues in Medical Malpractice

A. STANDARD OF CARE

The term **standard of care** defines a management prescription for a specified medical condition that is nationally accepted as best practice by a medical specialty. Note that obstetric and gynecologic clinicians are held to national standards, not simply a standard specific to their state or local area. Determining the standard of care when innovation and rapid change occur is not always easy. In fact, standards of practice for many common conditions during pregnancy remain both controversial and poorly defined. While experienced clinicians can usually identify the broad outlines of acceptable or standard practices, there is often disagreement concerning details. An example would be management of an individual with gestational diabetes and elevated blood sugar. In general, clinicians would concur that treatment is indicated. However, there would be vigorous disagreement concerning the best methods for treatment. Potential therapies might include dietary manipulation, a specific insulin regimen by pump or periodic injection, the administration of an oral hypoglycemic drug, or some combination of these methods.

In practical terms, the review and critique of a specific case by an expert witness are the principal means by which the applicable care standards for a given situation are identified. There are a number of sources for information about standards, including those derived from data in governmental regulations, the opinion of learned bodies of the profession, textbook chapters, articles in scientific literature, institution protocols and practice guidelines, the acts of legislature, and other sources. Often the practice guidelines, protocols, or opinion papers published by specialty groups such as the American College of Obstetricians and Gynecologists (ACOG) or individual institutions are highly influential in establishing the standard of care.

A care standard may seem a nebulous concept; however, these management prescriptions are of great importance. Legally, they are the benchmarks against which the practitioner's actions are measured. Standards also immediately affect clinical practice because they are major influences on the content of institutional protocols and practice guidelines. Such guidelines and protocols also represent an effort to improve patient care and encourage compliance with scientifically sound medicine, while regularizing practice and reducing the costs associated with defensive medicine. Despite these good intentions, these institutional documents can also increase a practitioner's legal risk if there is noncompliance. Overly rigid, inappropriate, or dated guidelines not reflective of best practice can actually *increase* legal risk rather than reduce it. Therefore, clinicians are well advised to be aware of the content of these institutional documents and challenge the care prescriptions if they are inappropriate, incomplete, or overly restrictive.

B. THE EXPERT WITNESS

The testimony of expert witnesses concerning applicable standards of care and causation is crucial to the fair litigation of a medical malpractice case. The expert is charged with reviewing the various medical records, considering best practice, identifying the clinical issues, and outlining the standards of care. Experts also provide learned opinions concerning how an individual physician deviated—or did not deviate—from the identified standards of care and how the alleged deviations either caused or could not have caused the injury in question. The problem is that not all experts deserve the title. Most individuals acting as experts are conscientious. However, there are also compliant "others" who selectively interpret standards of care or develop unique theories of causation to the advantage of their benefactor (either the plaintiff or the defense). Expert testimony is virtually unregulated by the specialties and is often highly rewarding financially. Perhaps not surprisingly, large numbers of willing experts and unique interpretations of practice standards are not rare. Caveat emptor.

Daubert Ruling: An important response to concerns about dubious experts is the Daubert rule, a Supreme Court decision bearing on the criterion used by courts in evaluating expert opinions. In *Daubert*, the Supreme Court abandoned the previously utilized "general acceptance in the field" standard for scientific testimony. Under the new rule, courts can and must assess whether the reasoning and methodology upon which an expert opinion is based have scientific merit and relevance to the facts at issue. In *Daubert*, the Court held that "scientific knowledge" connotes more than an expert's subjective belief or unsupported speculation concerning an issue in the case in question. This means that the inferences or assertions presented as expert evidence must be based upon the scientific method and supported by appropriate data. Who wins here? This ruling potentially benefits the defense if the medical opinion testimony offered by the plaintiff is based on "junk-science." However, it can also work to the detriment of the defense when the technique or methodology upon which the defense expert bases his or her opinion involves a novel or innovative concept that is an extrapolation from an established or accepted idea.

Since *Daubert* was decided in 1993, the Courts have taken very seriously their role as gatekeeper by allowing or denying the introduction of scientific evidence at trial. The Supreme Court in *Daubert* directed trial judges to consider at least 4 factors when determining the admissibility of scientific evidence: (1) whether the theory or technique can be tested; (2) whether the proffered work has been subject to peer review; (3) whether the rate of error is acceptable; and (4) whether the method at issue has widespread acceptance. Since the decision in *Daubert*, the trial courts have been inundated with claims from attorneys asking courts to deny the admission of opinions considered to be "junk science." These claims have met with varying success as courts struggle with implementation of these new requirements.

C. RISK MANAGEMENT:

The improvement in quality and organization of care and the prevention of legal entanglements are both important issues to clinicians. Obstetricians and gynecologists are at heightened risk for claims of medical negligence. The American College of Obstetricians and Gynecologists reports that 80% of obstetrician/gynecologists can anticipate being sued one or more times in their careers. According to the Physician Insurers Association of America, nearly 30% of doctors are now first sued during their residencies! Also, there is the strong suspicion in the specialty that concerns about possible malpractice claims are the cause of many unnecessary tests and procedures. Such "defensive medicine" inflates the cost of medical care while providing no demonstrable benefit. Risk management is a partial answer to these problems.

Risk management is a prospective process which identifies factors prompting legal action and attempts to improve the medical system to prevent future losses. Risk management involves the participation of health care providers of all types, attorneys, various technicians, health insurance providers, hospital administrators and many others. When a potential risk is identified, there are several possible resolutions. These might include the development of education programs, a review of the performance of clinicians, the purchase of new equipment, or changes in existing protocols and practice guidelines. A full discussion of this interesting and important topic is beyond the scope of this chapter.

D. PHYSICIAN-PATIENT RELATIONSHIP

The physician-patient relationship describes the unique interaction between a medical practitioner and an individual. This relationship is the foundation of a number of basic medicolegal principles. Society vests the physician with important powers over people's lives including conducting examinations, providing advice concerning matters of intimate sexual conduct and other intensely personal matters, the prescribing of drugs, and performing surgery—all of which potentially affect the individual's lifestyle and well being. Further, practitioners enjoy an elevated social status due to their special knowledge and access to highly personal information. Major concepts emerging from this position of trust and obligation are that of assured confidentiality and informed consent. **Informed consent** requires that the physician accept the duty to disclose all significant medical information to an individual that is material in medical decision making. The physician risks liability if there is a failure to disclose a risk or potential complica-

tion of a procedure for which the patient later claims would have led to consent being withheld.

Other concepts emerging from the duty of a physician in a patient-physician relationship are those of abandonment or lack of diligence. Throughout the duration of the patient-physician relationship, the physician is obliged to provide his or her patients with the required medical services. Abandonment, the abrupt termination of the physician-patient relationship without appropriate referral, and the lack of diligence, or the omission of proper treatment, are potential breaches of this basic duty.

E. MANAGED CARE

Health Care Reform: Many different schemes for health care reform have been proposed, focusing on disease prevention and cost containment. It is not clear if this restructuring of American medicine will improve the nation's health care, assuring that illusive characteristic of "quality care," while better serving a larger percentage of the populace. What is certain is that these reorganizations have altered the practice of both law and medicine and emphasized the need for additional reforms. Further, the changes wrought have become a hot political issue.

The Physician/Patient Relationship in A Managed Care Environment: The traditional role of the physician as patient advocate takes on greater significance in a managed care environment. The rules and regulations of a specific health care plan do not take precedence over the accepted medical standards for patient treatment. The physician has the legal duty to fully disclose to the patient the potential risks of not undertaking "ideal" management. If the physician believes that the practice standards promulgated by the managed care entity do not meet appropriate standards of care, he or she has the ethical obligation to challenge these standards and not simply acquiesce in accepting the recommended treatment.

Technology, Medicine & Law: New Legal Theories & Issues

A. PERINATAL DATA SYSTEMS

The need for data organization and demands for case quality improvement and quality assurance review and cost-benefit evaluations have sparked the increasing involvement of computers in medical practice. Beyond standard office applications for basic billing and record-keeping, new programs used by hospitals to manage clinical data have been developed.

The stated aim of hospital obstetric computer systems is to replace most or all of the traditional paper records with an immediately available, legible electronic patient record. The best of these systems combines maternal and fetal monitoring capabilities with programs for clinical data management. Such systems record important clinical information that in the past were entered into the paper medical record, such as nursing assessments, laboratory findings, and procedural or operative notes. For obstetrics, these programs also archive labor and delivery monitoring data. Computers do reduce or eliminate errors caused by missing or incomplete information or the vagaries of poor penmanship. Systems that organize data and generate statistical reports are also potentially useful in obtaining important birth and delivery statistics, monitoring physician conduct, and supporting quality improvement programs.

Obstetric services are now installing the next generation of perinatal programs, the so-called "smart" electronic record systems. These systems continuously monitor the course of labor and the actions of clinicians. The clinician's management is judged against the prescriptions in institutional protocols and practice guidelines. As the labor progresses, the program periodically suggests laboratory tests or prompts the clinician to perform physical evaluations, to consider alternative diagnoses, or to request specific consultations. With smart systems, clinicians are warned by electronic reminders when actions that deviate from institutional practice norms or contraindicated treatments have been chosen. These systems are highly complex and not easily developed. Their success in improving standardization of care, controlling costs, and helping to avoid errors remains to be proven, but early experience is encouraging. The greatest barriers to more widespread use of the systems remain cost, complexity, and provider resistance.

A few of the potential legal issues arising from computerization of patient records include system errors, inaccurate input of information resulting in either improper analyses or inappropriate guidelines for patient management, and maintenance of the confidentiality of clinical data and the related issues of privacy rights and informed consent. Perinatal data management systems offer much promise, but the potential of the creation of whole new areas of litigation is great.

B. OUTCOMES EVALUATIONS

A common impasse in the litigation of many cases involving imperfect obstetric outcomes is the assignment of responsibility, especially when the etiology of a birth defect is in dispute among the experts. Any clinician who attempts to analyze the causes of birth defects will soon discover the immense difficulty in identifying the reasons for adverse outcomes in many cases and in linking the presumed etiology to defects in the provision of care.

Among the most vexing cases for review are those involving neurologically impaired neonates with or without seizures where the extant data are inconclusive. Many of these cases involve initially depressed babies for whom their subsequent clinical condition was either poorly described in the medical record or the recorded data is contradictory. The data in these cases are invariably incomplete and inconsistencies and errors in recordkeeping are common. Such instances provide ample ground for acrimonious debate among well meaning experts. There are other problems as well. The retrospective report by the responsible clinician of his or her management intentions during a case, rendered in deposition years after the events in question, is often suspect. Also, the standards of management and scientific knowledge have changed over the years, in some instances dramatically. These problems and others demonstrate the difficulties in the fair but necessarily retrospective analysis of complex clinical events and emphasize the importance of thorough and accurate recording of clinical data at the time of delivery.

Such complexities in the analysis of clinical events have led to the use of various objective tests to better evaluate causation. It is safe to conclude that the utility of the various techniques briefly presented in the following sections will remain controversial in medicolegal proceedings. Nonetheless, the potential contribution of these studies to the problem of the pathophysiology of an observed neurologic injury cannot be ignored.

Genetic Studies and Placental Examination: Both genetic studies and forensic placental examination can help establish the etiology of an infant's disability or death. Certain histologic findings on placental examination, such as large numbers of nucleated red blood cells, intimal thickening, intervillous fibrin, acute and chronic meconium staining, and funisitis or villitis, can help to determine whether acute or chronic neonatal asphyxia or an occult infection was a factor in the etiology of a child's observed deficits. In the placental examination the plaintiff will seek data indicating that the fetus was normal or that a dysfunction occurred intrapartum that was potentially subject to amelioration by clinical management. The defendant will try to prove that an occult process existed that either injured the unborn child prior to the onset of labor or was otherwise beyond the ability of the attending physician to control.

If a case can be made that an occult but chronic process was present, the defendant's expert witness may claim that the intrapartum abnormalities noted (abnormal electronic fetal monitor tracing, meconium passage, etc) were not directly related to acute prenatal hypoxia or asphyxia, but reflect a prior injury that led to a limited reserve and the inability of the fetus to withstand the normal stresses of parturition. Alternatively, the plaintiff's expert may claim that failure to employ aggressive intervention at the first suggestion of difficulty—when the defendant knew or should have known of the pregnancy's enhanced susceptibility—increased the extent of the damage.

Due to the possible value of placental analysis, formal examination of the placenta by the pathologist is appropriate when a gross structural abnormality of the infant is identified, when the baby's condition is compromised, when the infant is stillborn, or in other settings of diagnostic uncertainty. Examination of the placenta is usually also advised for infants with low Apgar scores (ie, 5- or 10-minute scores ≤ 3) or when neurobehavioral abnormalities are identified in the neonatal period.

Many institutions have implemented programs for placental storage for a number of days to permit delayed study or for the routine examination of selected specimens. The costs associated with even a single "bad baby" judgment can far exceed the expenses of placental block storage and gross examination programs.

Genetic studies are also frequently used to investigate the cause of a neonate's dysfunction, the reasons for structural abnormalities, or to explain a stillbirth. Also, parental and fetal chromosomal analysis and selected biochemical tests may diagnose inborn errors of metabolism or unmask maternal disease causing or contributing to observed neurological deficits. A caveat of genetic testing is that many of these studies are invasive. A judge may be required to order that a child undergo these examinations and their performance is likely to be resisted by the family.

Forensic Radiology: Various imaging techniques (eg, ultrasound [US], magnetic resonance imaging [MRI], computed tomography [CT] scanning, positron emission tomography [PET] scanning) are used to evaluate neonates with neurologic abnormalities. These tests help to distinguish cases of congenital cranial malformations from brain damage resulting from hypoxia, anoxia, or other intrapartum insult. Such tests are most useful when performed soon after birth.

Each test has specific advantages and limitations. An ultrasound examination is an inexpensive bedside study that can identify many sources of CNS pathology. However, ultrasound is less useful than CT scanning or MRI in evaluating cerebral edema, intraparenchymal lesions, and structural malformations of the brain. CT scanning is rapid but requires patient transport to the scanner and is limited in its ability to study certain areas of the brain such as the brainstem and posterior fossa. MRI is often the most useful study for brain evaluation, but is the most difficult in terms of patient transfer, time required for study, and high expense. MRI is best for visualization of such disorders as cerebral edema, intraparenchymal lesions, or malformations.

Adverse effects suffered by the fetal or neonatal brain depend on the nature and timing of the insult and the maturity of the CNS at the time of injury. Important variables include blood oxygenation, perfusion pressure, temperature, and glucose level. Because of this, imaging techniques may not reveal abnormalities until 20 hours (for CT and routine MRI) to 2 days (for US) following delivery. The full extent of an injury is often not revealed until the 60th–90th days of life. Repeat studies are therefore indicated. Using selected techniques, some neuroradiologists claim the ability to determine precisely the time a CNS injury occurred, establishing whether or not the observed injury occurred before, during, or after the time of delivery.

Evaluation of a Stillborn: In cases of fetal death, the most useful studies include a gross and microscopic examination of the placenta and a necropsy. In general, the necropsy alone can provide a diagnosis in 30% or more of unexplained stillbirths, and can occasionally approximate the time of death. The gross and microscopic information from the necropsy requires correlation with other data including the history (maternal exposure to drugs, gestational age, etc), data on intrauterine growth, and the results of antepartum ultrasound exams. Potential barriers to complete evaluation of stillbirths include the availability of skilled pathologists, high cost, and parental consent.

Clinical Scenarios

A. NEUROLOGIC INJURIES

Serious injuries to a newborn that result in permanent neurological dysfunction or physical disfigurement are almost invariably followed by legal review. New concepts are developing concerning the etiology of certain neurologic injuries.

Prematurity: Preterm infants suffer a higher frequency of defects than term infants. Problems with the diagnosis and management of preterm infants provide fertile ground for lawsuits because of this high incidence of complications. While the causes of many cases of preterm labor cannot be established, recent data reveals the important role of bacterial infection of the cervix and membranes as a major risk factor. New tests (eg, fetal fibronectin) can help identify a population at high risk for preterm labor and delivery. In recent years the importance of tocolysis has been deemphasized, while the use of corticosteroid administration to enhance fetal pulmonary maturity have been encouraged.

Determination of best practices in preterm labor management has become much less certain than it was even 5 years ago. Even as modern medicine struggles to implement new tests and management protocols, the high incidence of complications from prematurity will assure an ample supply of legal claims.

Role of Infection: Epidemiologic data supports a causal relationship between infection of the fetal membranes (chorioamnionitis) and the development of premature labor and permanent neurological dysfunction in neonates. This is a previously unrecognized etiology for fetal injury. A number of inflammatory substances including interferon, cytokines, interleukin-6, and tumor necrosis factor have been implicated. Intrauterine exposure to these or related vasoactive substances that are either released by the infecting organism or elaborated by the body's inflammatory mechanisms in response to the infection predispose to both premature labor and brain injury in utero. Recent data link these perinatal infections to cerebral palsy and other permanent neurological deficits in term pregnancies and perhaps in premature infants as well.

It should be pointed out that the pathophysiology of this process is not yet fully elucidated. While additional study is needed, most observers believe that some relationship between inflammation and neurologic injury will be proven. Establishing pre- or intrapartum infection as one of the causes for permanent neurologic injury has the potential to substantially alter current clinical practice and is likely to increase opportunities for litigation.

B. Ectopic Pregnancy

Ectopic pregnancy is a common obstetric complication, with approximately 110,000 cases diagnosed each year. Over 95% of ectopic pregnancies occur in the fallopian tube, with 80% in the ampullary region. Potential causes for ectopic pregnancy include prior treatment for pelvic inflammatory disease, tubal surgery, and prior use of modern reproductive technologies. The growth of an undiagnosed ectopic pregnancy can result in rupture of the fallopian tube, cardiovascular collapse, and, in rare instances, maternal death. The small number of nontubal ectopic pregnancies or interstitial and cornual pregnancies is especially problematic. The diagnosis of these pregnancies is difficult and the risk of serious complications associated with catastrophic rupture remains high.

Litigation surrounding ectopic pregnancies usually results from claims of delayed diagnosis that leads to an increase in morbidity and unnecessary surgery. Due to recent biochemical advances and improvements in ultrasound, both the presence and the status of a normal early pregnancy is now easily determined. The firm diagnosis of ectopic pregnancy remains more of a challenge. If an ectopic is diagnosed early, either medical management (methotrexate or other drug administration) or surgery (laparoscopy or laparotomy with salpingostomy or salpingectomy) can be undertaken. In general, it is the failure of a clinician to suspect an ectopic in a given setting that leads to grief, and not a lack of familiarity with the appropriate and available diagnostic and therapeutic techniques.

Conclusions

The technological advances of the last 2 decades have profoundly altered the practice of obstetrics and the legal demands on the specialty. This chapter has briefly discussed a selected number of these technological advancements and their impact on both medicine and law.

The problem clinicians face is partially of their own making. The recent, dramatic improvements in reproductive capability, prenatal screening, and prenatal therapy, and the enthusiastic promotion of these capabilities through the media have led to increased public expectations and the unfortunate impression that these new technologies involve no risk. However, as practitioners are well aware, our scientific knowledge is still incomplete and the inherent imperfections in the reproductive process remain unchanged. Biologic limitations, the inevitable problems caused by human error, and the uncertainties inherent in all clinical diagnoses and in therapy are not going to disappear. Thus the continuation of the complex, interdependent, and contentious relationship between the law and obstetric and gynecologic medicine is assured.

REFERENCES

Andersen HF: Use of fetal fibronectin in women at risk for preterm delivery. Clin Obstet Gynecol 2000;43:746.

Badawi N et al: Intrapartum risk factors for newborn encephalopathy: the Western Australian case-control study. Br Med J 1998;317:1554.

Goldenberg RL, Hauth JC, Andrews WW: Intrauterine infection and preterm delivery. N Engl J Med 2000;342:1500.

Grether JK, Nelson K, Dambrosia J: Interferons and cerebral palsy. J Pediatr 1999;134:324.

Joffee G et al: Impact of fetal fibronectin assay on admissions of preterm labor. Am J Obstet Gynecol 1999;180:581.

Lawson EE: Antenatal corticosteroids: Too much of a good thing? JAMA 2001;286:1628.

Mercer BM et al: The preterm prediction study: Prediction of preterm premature rupture of membranes through clinical findings and ancillary testing. The National Institute of Child Health and Human Development Maternal-Fetal Medicine Units Network. Am J Obstet Gynecol 2000;183:738.

Niswander KR, Gordon M: The collaborative perinatal study of the national institute of neurological diseases and stroke: The women and their pregnancies. U.S. Department of Health, Education and Welfare, 1972.

Wing KR: Health care reform in the year 2000: The view from the front of the classroom. Am J Law Med 2000;26:277.

Yetter JF: Examination of the placenta. Am Fam Phys 1998;57:1045.

Zimmerman R, Winkler P: Perinatal brain injuries. In: Zimmerman R, Carmody Gibby W (editors): *Neuroimaging: Clinical and Physical Principles.* Springer-Velag, 1999, p. 531.

Index

NOTE: Page numbers in **boldface** type indicate a major discussion. A *t* following a page number indicates tabular material, an *f* following a page number indicates a figure.

CASE FILES: OBSTETRICS & GYNECOLOGY

a LANGE medical book

**Eugene C. Toy, MD, Benton Baker III, MD, Patti Jayne Ross, MD, and
Larry C. Gilstrap III, MD, all of University of Texas-Houston Medical School, Houston, Texas.**

0-07-140284-5 ◆ Softcover ◆ 500 pp. ◆ illus. ◆ Available October 2002

An invaluable bridge from the conventional textbook to the clinical setting, *Case Files: Obstetrics & Gynecology* presents clinical cases to equip medical students with a solid approach to obstetrics and gynecology. These in-depth case studies provide a wealth of medical information in the context of the patient and reinforce learning by emphasizing the mechanisms of disease.

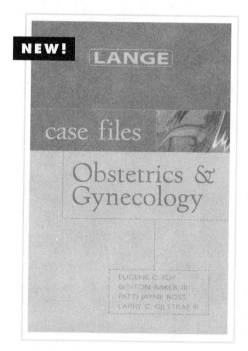

BASED ON THE AUTHORS' MANY YEARS OF WORKING EXPERIENCE WITH MEDICAL STUDENTS, *CASE FILES: OBSTETRICS & GYNECOLOGY* FEATURES:

◆ **60 clinical cases in ob/gyn that teach diagnosis and treatment in the context of the patient**

◆ **Clinical pearls and concise discussions that deepen knowledge of the medical approach used for each case**

◆ **USMLE-style questions & answers that reinforce key terms and concepts in each case and serve as a guide to studying for the shelf exam and USMLE Step 2**

◆ **An up-to-date list of suggested readings for each case**